a LANGE medical book

CURRENT
Diagnosis & Treatment Pediatrics

TWENTY-FIRST EDITION

Edited by

William W. Hay, Jr., MD
Professor, Department of Pediatrics
Section of Neonatology and the Division of Perinatal Medicine
University of Colorado School of Medicine and Children's Hospital Colorado

Myron J. Levin, MD
Professor, Departments of Pediatrics and Medicine
Section of Pediatric Infectious Diseases
University of Colorado School of Medicine and Children's Hospital Colorado

Robin R. Deterding, MD
Professor, Department of Pediatrics
Section of Pediatric Pulmonary Medicine
University of Colorado School of Medicine and Children's Hospital Colorado

Mark J. Abzug, MD
Professor, Department of Pediatrics
Section of Pediatric Infectious Diseases
University of Colorado School of Medicine and Children's Hospital Colorado

Judith M. Sondheimer, MD
Professor Emerita, Department of Pediatrics
Section of Pediatric Gastroenterology, Hepatology and Nutrition
University of Colorado School of Medicine and Children's Hospital Colorado
Professor of Pediatrics and Chief of Pediatric Gastroenterology, Georgetown University School of Medicine
Clinical Professor of Pediatrics, George Washington University School of Medicine

and Associate Authors

The Department of Pediatrics at the University of Colorado School of Medicine is affiliated with Children's Hospital Colorado.

Mc Graw Hill **Medical**

New York Chicago San Francisco Lisbon London Madrid Mexico City
Milan New Delhi San Juan Seoul Singapore Sydney Toronto

The McGraw-Hill Companies

CURRENT Diagnosis & Treatment: Pediatrics, Twenty-First Edition

1 2 3 4 5 6 7 8 9 0 DOC/DOC 17 16 15 14 13 12

ISBN 978-0-07-177970-8
MHID 0-07-177970-1
ISSN 0093-8556

Notice

Medicine is an ever-changing science. As new research and clinical experience broaden our knowledge, changes in treatment and drug therapy are required. The authors and the publisher of this work have checked with sources believed to be reliable in their efforts to provide information that is complete and generally in accord with the standards accepted at the time of publication. However, in view of the possibility of human error or changes in medical sciences, neither the authors nor the publisher nor any other party who has been involved in the preparation or publication of this work warrants that the information contained herein is in every respect accurate or complete, and they disclaim all responsibility for any errors or omissions or for the results obtained from use of the information contained in this work. Readers are encouraged to confirm the information contained herein with other sources. For example and in particular, readers are advised to check the product information sheet included in the package of each drug they plan to administer to be certain that the information contained in this work is accurate and that changes have not been made in the recommended dose or in the contraindications for administration. This recommendation is of particular importance in connection with new or infrequently used drugs.

This book was set by Cenveo Publisher Services.
The editors were Alyssa K. Fried and Peter J. Boyle.
The production supervisor was Sherri Souffrance.
Project management was provided by Vastavikta Sharma, Cenveo Publisher Services.
The interior designer was Alan Barnett.
RR Donnelley was printer and binder.

This book is printed on acid-free paper.

International Edition ISBN 978-0-07-179289-9; MHID 0-07-179289-9.

Contents

Authors

Frank J. Accurso, MD
Professor, Department of Pediatrics, Head, Section of Pediatric Pulmonary Medicine, University of Colorado School of Medicine and Children's Hospital Colorado
frank.accurso@childrenscolorado.org
Chapter 46: Chemistry & Hematology Reference Intervals

Joseph A. Albietz III, MD
Assistant Professor, Department of Pediatrics, Section of Pediatric Critical Care, University of Colorado School of Medicine and Children's Hospital Colorado
joseph.albietz@childrenscolorado.org
Chapter 14: Critical Care

Daniel R. Ambruso, MD
Professor, Department of Pediatrics, University of Colorado School of Medicine, Associate Medical Director, Belle Bonfils Blood Center
daniel_ambruso@bonfils.org
Chapter 30: Hematologic Disorders

Marsha S. Anderson, MD
Associate Professor, Department of Pediatrics, Section of Pediatric Infectious Diseases, University of Colorado School of Medicine and Children's Hospital Colorado
marsha.anderson@childrenscolorado.org
Chapter 42: Infections: Bacterial & Spirochetal

Christopher D. Baker, MD
Assistant Professor, Department of Pediatrics, Section of Pediatric Pulmonary Medicine, University of Colorado School of Medicine and Children's Hospital Colorado
christopher.baker@ucdenver.edu
Chapter 19: Respiratory Tract & Mediastinum

Vivek Balasubramaniam, MD
Assistant Professor, Department of Pediatrics, Section of Pediatric Pulmonary Medicine, Director, Pediatric Heart Lung Center Laboratory, University of Colorado School of Medicine and Children's Hospital Colorado
vivek.balasubramaniam@ucdenver.edu
Chapter 19: Respiratory Tract & Mediastinum

Jennifer M. Barker, MD
Assistant Professor, Department of Pediatrics, Section of Pediatric Endocrinology, University of Colorado School of Medicine and Children's Hospital Colorado
jennifer.barker@ucdenver.edu
Chapter 34: Endocrine Disorders

Timothy J. Bernard, MD
Assistant Professor, Departments of Pediatrics and Neurology, Section of Pediatric Neurology, University of Colorado School of Medicine and Children's Hospital Colorado
timothy.bernard@ucdenver.edu
Chapter 25: Neurologic & Muscular Disorders

Mark Boguniewicz, MD
Professor, Department of Pediatrics, Section of Pediatric Allergy, University of Colorado School of Medicine, Department of Clinical Immunology, National Jewish Health
boguniewiczm@njhealth.org
Chapter 38: Allergic Disorders

Rebecca Sands Braverman, MD
Assistant Professor, Department of Ophthalmology, University of Colorado School of Medicine and Children's Hospital Colorado
rebecca.sandsbraverman@ucdenver.edu
Chapter 16: Eye

Maya Bunik, MD, MSPH
Associate Professor, Department of Pediatrics, Section of General Academic Pediatrics, Medical Director, Child Health Clinic, University of Colorado School of Medicine and Children's Hospital Colorado
maya.bunik@childrenscolorado.org
Chapter 9: Ambulatory & Office Pediatrics

Casey J. Burg, MD
Pediatric Pulmonary Fellow, Pediatric Sleep Specialist, Department of Pediatrics, Section of Pediatric Pulmonary Medicine, University of Colorado School of Medicine and Children's Hospital Colorado
casey.burg@childrenscolorado.org
Chapter 19: Respiratory Tract & Mediastinum

Adam Burstein, DO
House Staff, Department of Psychiatry, Psychiatry Residency Training Program, University of Colorado School of Medicine and Children's Hospital Colorado
adam.burstein@ucdenver.edu
Chapter 7: Child & Adolescent Psychiatric Disorders & Psychosocial Aspects of Pediatrics

Todd C. Carpenter, MD
Associate Professor, Department of Pediatrics, Section of Pediatric Critical Care Medicine, University of Colorado School of Medicine and Children's Hospital Colorado
todd.carpenter@ucdenver.edu
Chapter 14: Critical Care

H. Peter Chase, MD
Professor, Department of Pediatrics, Clinical Director Emeritus, Barbara Davis Center for Childhood Diabetes
University of Colorado School of Medicine and Children's Hospital Colorado
peter.chase@ucdenver.edu
Chapter 35: Diabetes Mellitus

Antonia Chiesa, MD
Senior Instructor, Department of Pediatrics, University of Colorado School of Medicine, Kempe Child Protection Team, Kempe Center for the Prevention and Treatment of Child Abuse and Neglect and Children's Hospital Colorado
antonia.chiesa@childrenscolorado.org
Chapter 8: Child Abuse & Neglect

Gerald H. Clayton, PhD
Instructor, Department of Physical Medicine and Rehabilitation Administration, University of Colorado School of Medicine and Children's Hospital Colorado
jerry.clayton@ucdenver.edu
Chapter 28: Rehabilitation Medicine

Rachel A. Cole, MD, PhD, FAAP, CAQSM
Assistant Professor, Department of Orthopedics, Co-Medical Director, Sports Medicine Program, University of Colorado School of Medicine and Children's Hospital Colorado
rachel.coel@childrenscolorado.org
Chapter 27: Sports Medicine

Kathryn K. Collins, MD
Associate Professor, Department of Pediatrics, Section of Pediatric Cardiology, University of Colorado School of Medicine and Children's Hospital Colorado
kathryn.collins@childrenscolorado.org
Chapter 20: Cardiovascular Diseases

Ronina A. Covar, MD
Associate Professor, Department of Pediatrics, Section of Pediatric Allergy and Clinical Immunology, University of Colorado School of Medicine, National Jewish Health, and Children's Hospital Colorado
covarr@njhealth.org
Chapter 38: Allergic Disorders

Angela S. Czaja, MD, MSc
Assistant Professor, Department of Pediatrics, Section of Pediatric Critical Care Medicine, University of Colorado School of Medicine and Children's Hospital Colorado
angela.czaja@childrenscolorado.org
Chapter 14: Critical Care

Matthew F. Daley, MD
Associate Professor, Department of Pediatrics, Section of General Academic Pediatrics, University of Colorado School of Medicine and Children's Hospital Colorado, Senior Investigator, Institute for Health Research, Kaiser Permanente, Colorado
matthew.f.daley@kp.org
Chapter 10: Immunization

Jeffrey R. Darst, MD
Assistant Professor, Department of Pediatrics, University of Colorado School of Medicine
jeffrey.darst@ucdenver.edu
Chapter 20: Cardiovascular Diseases

Richard C. Dart, MD, PhD
Associate Professor, Director, Rocky Mountain Poison and Drug Center, Denver Health and Hospital Authority, University of Colorado School of Medicine
rdart@rmpdc.org
Chapter 13: Poisoning

Robin R. Deterding, MD
Professor, Department of Pediatrics, Section of Pediatric Pulmonary Medicine, University of Colorado School of Medicine and Children's Hospital Colorado
robin.deterding@childrenscolorado.org
Chapter 19: Respiratory Tract & Mediastinum

Emily L. Dobyns, MD, FCCM
Associate Professor, Department of Pediatrics, Section of Pediatric Critical Care Medicine, University of Colorado School of Medicine and Children's Hospital Colorado
emily.dobyns@childrenscolorado.org
Chapter 14: Critical Care

Samuel R. Dominguez, MD, PhD
Assistant Professor, Department of Pediatrics, Section of Pediatric Infectious Diseases, University of Colorado School of Medicine and Children's Hospital Colorado
samuel.dominguez@ucdenver.edu
Chapter 43: Infections: Parasitic & Mycotic

George S. Eisenbarth, MD, PhD
Professor, Department of Pediatrics, Executive Director, Barbara Davis Center for Childhood Diabetes, University of Colorado School of Medicine and Children's Hospital Colorado
george.eisenbarth@ucdenver.edu
Chapter 35: Diabetes Mellitus

Ellen R. Elias, MD
Associate Professor, Departments of Pediatrics and Genetics, Section of Clinical Genetics and Metabolism, University of Colorado School of Medicine, Director, Special Care Clinic, Children's Hospital Colorado
ellen.elias@childrenscolorado.org
Chapter 37: Genetics & Dysmorphology

Mark A. Erickson, MD
Associate Professor, Department of Orthopedic Surgery, University of Colorado School of Medicine, Chairman, Department of Pediatric Orthopedics, Orthopedic Institute, Children's Hospital Colorado
mark.erickson@childrenscolorado.org
Chapter 26: Orthopedics

Jennifer Exo, DO
Assistant Professor, Department of Pediatrics, Section of Critical Care Medicine, University of Colorado School of Medicine and Children's Hospital Colorado
jennifer.exo@ucdenver.edu
Chapter 14: Critical Care

Monica J. Federico, MD
Assistant Professor, Department of Pediatrics, Section of Pediatric Pulmonology Medicine, University of Colorado School of Medicine and Children's Hospital Colorado
monica.federico@childrenscolorado.org
Chapter 19: Respiratory Tract & Mediastinum

David M. Fleischer, MD
Assistant Professor, Department of Pediatrics, Section of Pediatric Allergy and Clinical Immunology, University of Colorado School of Medicine and National Jewish Health
fleischerd@njhealth.org
Chapter 38: Allergic Disorders

Douglas M. Ford, MD
Professor, Department of Pediatrics, Section of Pediatric Nephrology, Director, Home Dialysis & Renal Transplantation, University of Colorado School of Medicine and Children's Hospital Colorado
douglas.ford@childrenscolorado.org
Chapter 23: Fluid, Electrolyte, & Acid-Base Disorders & Therapy

Nicholas K. Foreman, MD
Professor, Department of Pediatrics, Section of Pediatric Hematology/Oncology/Bone Marrow Transplant, University of Colorado School of Medicine and Children's Hospital Colorado
nicholas.foreman@childrenscolorado.org
Chapter 31: Neoplastic Disease

David Fox, MD
Assistant Professor, Department of Pediatrics, Section of General Academic Pediatrics, University of Colorado School of Medicine and Children's Hospital Colorado
david.fox@childrenscolorado.org
Chapter 9: Ambulatory & Office Pediatrics

Norman R. Friedman, MD
Associate Professor, Department of Otolaryngology, University of Colorado School of Medicine and Children's Hospital Colorado
norman.friedman@childrenscolorado.org
Chapter 18: Ear, Nose, & Throat

Glenn T. Furuta, MD
Associate Professor, Department of Pediatrics, Section of Pediatric Gastroenterology, Director, Gastrointestinal Eosinophil Disease Program National Jewish Hospital, University of Colorado School of Medicine and Children's Hospital Colorado
glenn.furuta@childrenscolorado.org
Chapter 21: Gastrointestinal Tract

Jeffrey L. Galinkin, MD
Associate Professor, Department of Anesthesiology, University of Colorado School of Medicine and Children's Hospital Colorado
jeffrey.galinkin@ucdenver.edu
Chapter 32: Pain Management & Pediatric Palliative & End-of-Life Care

Roger H. Giller, MD
Professor, Department of Pediatrics, Director, Pediatric Bone Marrow Transplant Program, University of Colorado School of Medicine and Children's Hospital Colorado
roger.giller@childrenscolorado.org
Chapter 31: Neoplastic Disease

Neil A. Goldenberg, MD, PhD
Assistant Professor, Departments of Pediatrics and Medicine, Co-Director, Hemophilia & Thrombosis Center and Stroke Programs, Section of Pediatric Hematology/Oncology/Bone Marrow Transplant, University of Colorado School of Medicine and Children's Hospital Colorado
neil.goldenberg@ucdenver.edu
Chapter 30: Hematologic Disorders

Edward Goldson, MD
Professor, Department of Pediatrics, Section of Child Developmental and Behavioral Pediatrics, University of Colorado School of Medicine and Children's Hospital Colorado
edward.goldson@childrenscolorado.org
Chapter 3: Child Development & Behavior

Douglas K. Graham, MD, PhD
Associate Professor, Department of Pediatrics, Section of Pediatric Hematology/Oncology/Bone Marrow Transplant, University of Colorado School of Medicine and Children's Hospital Colorado
doug.graham@ucdenver.edu
Chapter 31: Neoplastic Disease

Eva Nozik Grayck, MD
Associate Professor, Department of Pediatrics, Section of Pediatric Critical Care Medicine, University of Colorado School of Medicine and Children's Hospital Colorado
eva.grayck@ucdenver.edu
Chapter 14: Critical Care

Brian S. Greffe, MD
Professor, Department of Pediatrics, Section of Pediatric Hematology/Oncology/Bone Marrow Transplant, University of Colorado School of Medicine and Children's Hospital Colorado
brian.greffe@childrenscolorado.org
Chapter 31: Neoplastic Disease
Chapter 32: Pain Management & Pediatric Palliative & End-of-Life Care

Joseph A. Grubenhoff, MD
Assistant Professor, Department of Pediatrics, Section of Emergency Medicine, University of Colorado School of Medicine and Children's Hospital Colorado
joe.grubenhoff@childrenscolorado.org
Chapter 12: Emergencies & Injuries

Matthew Haemer, MD
Assistant Professor, Department of Pediatrics, Section of Nutrition, University of Colorado School of Medicine and Children's Hospital Colorado
matthew.haemer@childrenscolorado.org
Chapter 11: Normal Childhood Nutrition & Its Disorders

Ann Halbower, MD
Associate Professor, Department of Pediatrics, Section of Pediatric Pulmonary Medicine, University of Colorado School of Medicine and Children's Hospital Colorado
ann.halbower@childrenshospital.org
Chapter 19: Respiratory Tract & Mediastinum

Pia J. Hauk, MD
Assistant Professor, Department of Pediatrics, Section of Pediatric Allergy and Clinical Immunology, University of Colorado School of Medicine and National Jewish Health
haukp@njhealth.org
Chapter 33: Immunodeficiency

Taru Hays, MD
Professor, Department of Pediatrics, Section of Pediatric Hematology/Oncology/Bone Marrow Transplant, University of Colorado School of Medicine and Children's Hospital Colorado
taru.hays@childrenscolorado.org
Chapter 30: Hematologic Disorders

Quynh B. Hoang, MD
Assistant Professor Department of Orthopedics, Sports Medicine Program, University of Colorado School of Medicine and Children's Hospital Colorado
quynh.hoang@childrenscolorado.org
Chapter 27: Sports Medicine

Edward J. Hoffenberg, MD
Professor, Department of Pediatrics, Section of Pediatric Gastroenterology, Hepatology and Nutrition, University of Colorado School of Medicine and Children's Hospital Colorado
edward.hoffenberg@childrenscolorado.org
Chapter 21: Gastrointestinal Tract

Daniel Hyman, MD, MMM
Chief Quality Officer, Department of Pediatrics, University of Colorado School of Medicine and Children's Hospital Colorado
daniel.hyman@childrenscolorado.org
Chapter 1: Advancing the Quality and Safety of Care

Richard B. Johnston Jr., MD
Professor, Department of Pediatrics, Section of Allergy and Clinical Immunology, Associate Dean for Research Development, University of Colorado School of Medicine and National Jewish Health
richard.johnston@ucdenver.edu
Chapter 33: Immunodeficiency

David W. Kaplan, MD, MPH
Professor, Department of Pediatrics, Head, Section of Adolescent Medicine, University of Colorado School of Medicine and Children's Hospital Colorado
david.kaplan@childrenscolorado.org
Chapter 4: Adolescence

Michael S. Kappy, MD, PhD
Professor, Department of Pediatrics, Section of Pediatric Endocrinology, University of Colorado School of Medicine and Children's Hospital Colorado
michael.kappy@childrenscolorado.org
Chapter 34: Endocrine Disorders

Paritosh Kaul, MD
Associate Professor, Department of Pediatrics, Section of Adolescent Medicine, University of Colorado School of Medicine, Denver Health, and Children's Hospital Colorado
paritosh.kaul@childrenscolorado.org
Chapter 5: Adolescent Substance Abuse

Amy K. Keating, MD
Assistant Professor, Department of Pediatrics, Section of Pediatric Hematology/Oncology/Bone Marrow Transplant, University of Colorado School of Medicine and Children's Hospital Colorado
amy.keating@ucdenver.edu
Chapter 31: Neoplastic Disease

Sita Kedia, MD
Clinical Instructor, Departments of Pediatrics and Neurology, Section of Pediatric Neurology, University of Colorado School of Medicine and Children's Hospital Colorado
sita.kedia@ucdenver.edu
Chapter 25: Neurologic & Muscular Disorders

Peggy E. Kelley, MD
Associate Professor, Department of Otolaryngology, University of Colorado School of Medicine and Children's Hospital Colorado
peggy.kelley@childrenscolorado.org
Chapter 18: Ear, Nose, & Throat

Megan Moriarty Kelsey, MD
Instructor, Department of Pediatrics, Section of Pediatric Endocrinology, University of Colorado School of Medicine and Children's Hospital Colorado
megan.kelsey@childrenscolorado.org
Chapter 34: Endocrine Disorders

Gwendolyn S. Kerby, MD
Associate Professor, Department of Pediatrics, Section of Pediatric Pulmonary Medicine, University of Colorado School of Medicine and Children's Hospital Colorado
gwendolyn.kerby@childrenscolorado.org
Chapter 19: Respiratory Tract & Mediastinum

Nancy A. King, MSN, RN, CPNP
Senior Instructor, Department of Pediatrics, Section of Pediatric Hematology/Oncology/Bone Marrow Transplant, University of Colorado School of Medicine and Children's Hospital Colorado
nancy.king@childrenscolorado.org
Chapter 32: Pain Management & Pediatric Palliative & End-of-Life Care

Ulrich Klein, DMD, DDS, MS
Associate Professor, Chair, Department of Pediatric Dentistry, University of Colorado School of Dental Medicine and Children's Hospital Colorado
ulric.klein@childrenscolorado.org
Chapter 17: Oral Medicine & Dentistry

Kelly Knupp, MD
Assistant Professor, Departments of Pediatrics and Neurology, Section of Pediatric Neurology, University of Colorado School of Medicine and Children's Hospital Colorado
kelly.knupp@childrenscolorado.org
Chapter 25: Neurologic & Muscular Disorders

Robert E. Kramer, MD
Assistant Professor, Department of Pediatrics, Section of Pediatric Gastroenterology, University of Colorado School of Medicine and Children's Hospital Colorado
robert.kramer@childrenscolorado.org
Chapter 21: Gastrointestinal Tract

Nancy F. Krebs, MD, MS
Professor, Department of Pediatrics, Head, Section of Nutrition, University of Colorado School of Medicine and Children's Hospital Colorado
nancy.krebs@ucdenver.edu
Chapter 11: Normal Childhood Nutrition & Its Disorders

Myron J. Levin, MD
Professor, Departments of Pediatrics and Medicine, Section of Pediatric Infectious Diseases, University of Colorado School of Medicine and Children's Hospital Colorado
myron.levin@ucdenver.edu
Chapter 40: Infections: Viral & Rickettsial
Chapter 43: Infections: Parasitic & Myotic

Paul M. Levisohn, MD
Associate Professor, Departments of Pediatrics and Neurology, University of Colorado School of Medicine and Children's Hospital Colorado
paul.levisohn@childrenscolorado.org
Chapter 25: Neurologic & Muscular Disorders

Andrew H. Liu, MD
Associate Professor, Department of Pediatrics, Section of Allergy and Immunology, University of Colorado School of Medicine, National Jewish Health and Children's Hospital Colorado
liua@njhealth.org
Chapter 33: Immunodeficiency

Gary M. Lum, MD
Professor, Department of Pediatrics, Head, Section of Pediatric Nephrology, University of Colorado School of Medicine and Children's Hospital Colorado
gary.lum@childrenscolorado.org
Chapter 24: Kidney & Urinary Tract

Kelly Maloney, MD
Associate Professor, Department of Pediatrics, Section of Pediatric Hematology/Oncology/Bone Marrow Transplant, University of Colorado School of Medicine and Children's Hospital Colorado
kelly.maloney@childrenscolorado.org
Chapter 31: Neoplastic Disease

David K. Manchester, MD
Professor, Department of Pediatrics, Section of Clinical Genetics and Metabolism, University of Colorado School of Medicine and Children's Hospital Colorado
david.manchester@childrenscolorado.org
Chapter 37: Genetics & Dysmorphology

Maria J. Mandt, MD
Assistant Professor, Department of Pediatrics, Section of Emergency Medicine, University of Colorado School of Medicine and Children's Hospital Colorado
maria.mandt@childrenscolorado.org
Chapter 12: Emergencies & Injuries

Elizabeth J. McFarland, MD
Professor, Department of Pediatrics, Section of Pediatric Infectious Diseases, University of Colorado School of Medicine and Children's Hospital Colorado
betsy.mcfarland@ucdenver.edu
Chapter 41: Human Immunodeficiency Virus Infection

Conor Merritt, BS
Research Assistant II, Department of Orthopedics, University of Colorado School of Medicine and Children's Hospital Colorado
conor.merritt@childrenscolorado.org
Chapter 26: Orthopedics

Shelley D. Miyamoto, MD
Assistant Professor, Department of Pediatrics, Section of Pediatric Cardiology, University of Colorado School of Medicine and Children's Hospital Colorado
shelley.miyamoto@childrenscolorado.org
Chapter 20: Cardiovascular Diseases

Paul G. Moe, MD
Professor, Departments of Pediatrics and Neurology, University of Colorado School of Medicine and Children's Hospital Colorado
paul.moe@childrenscolorado.org
Chapter 25: Neurologic & Muscular Disorders

Joseph G. Morelli, MD
Professor, Departments of Dermatology and Pediatrics, University of Colorado School of Medicine and Children's Hospital Colorado
joseph.morelli@ucdenver.edu
Chapter 15: Skin

Peter M. Mourani, MD
Assistant Professor, Department of Pediatrics, Section of Pediatric Critical Care Medicine, University of Colorado School of Medicine and Children's Hospital Colorado
peter.mourani@ucdenver.edu
Chapter 14: Critical Care

Kristen Nadeau, MD
Assistant Professor, Department of Pediatrics, Section of Pediatric Endocrinology, University of Colorado School of Medicine and Children's Hospital Colorado
kristen.nadeau@ucdenver.edu
Chapter 34: Endocrine Disorders

Michael R. Narkewicz, MD
Professor, Department of Pediatrics, Hewitt-Andrews Chair in Pediatric Liver Disease, Medical Director, The Pediatric Liver Center and Liver Transplantation Program, Section of Pediatric Gastroenterology, Hepatology and Nutrition, University of Colorado School of Medicine and Children's Hospital Colorado
michael.narkewicz@childrenscolorado.org
Chapter 22: Liver & Pancreas

Rachelle Nuss, MD
Professor, Department of Pediatrics, Section of Pediatric Hematology/Oncology/Bone Marrow Transplant and the Sickle Cell Center, University of Colorado School of Medicine and Children's Hospital Colorado
rachelle.nuss@childrenscolorado.org
Chapter 30: Hematologic Disorders

Ann-Christine Nyquist, MD, MSPH
Associate Professor, Department of Pediatrics, Section of Pediatric Infectious Diseases, University of Colorado School of Medicine and Children's Hospital Colorado
ann-christine.nyquist@childrenscolorado.org
Chapter 10: Immunization
Chapter 44: Sexually Transmitted Infections

John W. Ogle, MD
Professor and Vice Chairman, Director, Department of Pediatrics, Denver Health, and University of Colorado School of Medicine
jogle@dhha.org
Chapter 39: Antimicrobial Therapy
Chapter 42: Infections: Bacterial & Spirochetal

Sean T. O'Leary, MD, MPH
Assistant Professor, Department of Pediatrics, Section of Pediatric Infectious Diseases, University of Colorado School of Medicine and Children's Hospital Colorado
olearysea@gmail.com
Chapter 10: Immunization

Sarah K. Parker, MD
Assistant Professor, Department of Pediatrics, Section of Pediatric Infectious Diseases, University of Colorado School of Medicine and Children's Hospital Colorado
sarah.parker@ucdenver.edu
Chapter 45: Travel Medicine

K. Brooke Pengel, MD, FAAP, CAQSM
Assistant Professor, Department of Orthopedics, University of Colorado School of Medicine and Children's Hospital Colorado
brooke.pengel@healthonecares.com
Chapter 27: Sports Medicine

John D. Polousky, MD
Assistant Professor, Department of Orthopedics, University of Colorado School of Medicine and Children's Hospital Colorado
john.polousky@childrenscolorado.org
Chapter 26: Orthopedics

Laura E. Primak, RD, CNSD, CSP
Coordinator/Professional Research Assistant/Dietitian, Department of Pediatrics, Section of Nutrition, University of Colorado School of Medicine
laura.primak@ucdenver.edu
Chapter 11: Normal Childhood Nutrition & Its Disorders

Lori D. Prok, MD
Assistant Professor, Department of Pediatric Dermatology and Dermatopathology, University of Colorado School of Medicine and Children's Hospital Colorado
lori.prok@ucdenver.edu
Chapter 15: Skin

Ralph R. Quinones, MD
Associate Professor, Department of Pediatrics, Section of Pediatric Hematology/Oncology/Bone Marrow Transplant, University of Colorado School of Medicine and Children's Hospital Colorado
ralph.quinones@childrenscolorado.org
Chapter 31: Neoplastic Disease

Suchitra Rao, MBBS
Instructor, Department of Pediatrics, Section of Pediatric Infectious Diseases, University of Colorado School of Medicine and Children's Hospital Colorado
suchitra.rao@childrenscolorado.org
Chapter 45: Travel Medicine

Daniel H. Reirden, MD
Assistant Professor, Department of Pediatrics, Section of Pediatric Infectious Diseases, University of Colorado School of Medicine and Children's Hospital Colorado
daniel.reirden@childrenscolorado.org
Chapter 44: Sexually Transmitted Infections

Marian Rewers, MD, PhD
Professor & Clinical Director, Barbara Davis Center for Childhood Diabetes, University of Colorado School of Medicine and Children's Hospital Colorado
marian.rewers@ucdenver.edu
Chapter 35: Diabetes Mellitus

Ann Reynolds, MD
Assistant Professor, Department of Pediatrics, Section of Child Developmental and Behavioral Pediatrics, Director, The Child Development Unit, University of Colorado School of Medicine and Children's Hospital Colorado
ann.reynolds@childrenscolorado.org
Chapter 3: Child Development & Behavior

Adam A. Rosenberg, MD
Professor, Department of Pediatrics, Section of Neonatology, University of Colorado School of Medicine and Children's Hospital Colorado
adam.rosenberg@childrenscolorado.org
Chapter 2: The Newborn Infant

Barry H. Rumack, MD
Clinical Professor, Department of Pediatrics, University of Colorado School of Medicine, Director Emeritus, Rocky Mountain Poison and Drug Center, Denver Health Authority
barry@rumack.com
Chapter 13: Poisoning

Scott D. Sagel, MD
Associate Professor, Department of Pediatrics, University of Colorado School of Medicine and Children's Hospital Colorado
scott.sagel@childrenscolorado.org
Chapter 19: Respiratory Tract & Mediastinum

Amy E. Sass, MD, MPH
Assistant Professor, Department Pediatrics, Section of Adolescent Medicine, University of Colorado School of Medicine and Children's Hospital, Colorado
amy.sass@childrenscolorado.org
Chapter 4: Adolescence

Eric J. Sigel, MD
Associate Professor, Department of Pediatrics, Section of Adolescent Medicine, University of Colorado School of Medicine and Children's Hospital Colorado
eric.sigel@childrenscolorado.org
Chapter 6: Eating Disorders

Georgette Siparsky, PhD
Supervisor, Clinical Chemistry Laboratory, Department of Pathology, University of Colorado School of Medicine and Children's Hospital Colorado
georgette.siparsky@childrenscolorado.org
Chapter 46: Chemistry & Hematology Reference Intervals

Andrew P. Sirotnak, MD
Associate Professor, Department of Pediatrics, University of Colorado School of Medicine, Director, Kempe Child Protection Team, Kempe Center for the Prevention and Treatment of Child Abuse and Neglect, and Children's Hospital Colorado
andrew.sirotnak@childrenscolorado.org
Chapter 8: Child Abuse & Neglect

Jennifer B. Soep, MD
Assistant Professor, Department of Pediatrics, Section of Pediatric Rheumatology, University of Colorado School of Medicine and Children's Hospital Colorado
jennifer.soep@childrenscolorado.org
Chapter 29: Rheumatic Diseases

Ronald J. Sokol, MD
Professor and Vice Chair, Department of Pediatrics, Head, Section of Pediatric Gastroenterology, Hepatology and Nutrition; Director, Colorado Clinical and Translational Sciences Institute; University of Colorado School of Medicine and Children's Hospital Colorado
ronald.sokol@childrenscolorado.org
Chapter 22: Liver & Pancreas

Judith M. Sondheimer, MD
Professor Emerita, Department of Pediatrics, University of Colorado School of Medicine; Professor of Pediatrics and Chief of Pediatric Gastroenterology, Georgetown University School of Medicine; Clinical Professor of Pediatrics, George Washington University School of Medicine
judith.sondheimer@gmail.com
Chapter 21: Gastrointestinal Tract

Brian Stafford, MD, MPH
Assistant Professor, Departments of Psychiatry and Pediatrics, University of Colorado School of Medicine and Children's Hospital Colorado
brian.stafford@childrenscolorado.org
Chapter 7: Child & Adolescent Psychiatric Disorders & Psychosocial Aspects of Pediatrics

Paul Stillwell, MD
Senior Instructor, Department of Pediatrics, Section of Pediatric Pulmonary Medicine, University of Colorado School of Medicine and Children's Hospital Colorado
paul.stillwell@childrenscolorado.org
Chapter 19: Respiratory Tract & Mediastinum

Shikha S. Sundaram, MD, MSCI
Assistant Professor, Department of Pediatrics, Section of Pediatric Gastroenterology, Hepatology and Nutrition, University of Colorado School of Medicine and Children's Hospital Colorado
shikha.sundaram@childrenscolorado.org
Chapter 21: Gastrointestinal Tract

Ayelet Talmi, PhD
Assistant Professor, Departments of Psychiatry and Pediatrics, Associate Director, Irving Harris Program in Child Development and Infant Mental Health, University of Colorado School of Medicine and Children's Hospital Colorado
talmi.ayelet@ucdenver.edu
Chapter 7: Child & Adolescent Psychiatric Disorders & Psychosocial Aspects of Pediatrics

Elizabeth H. Thilo, MD
Associate Professor, Department of Pediatrics, Section of Neonatology, University of Colorado School of Medicine and Children's Hospital Colorado
elizabeth.thilo@childrenscolorado.org
Chapter 2: The Newborn Infant

Janet A. Thomas, MD
Associate Professor, Department of Pediatrics, Section of Clinical Genetics and Metabolism, University of Colorado School of Medicine and Children's Hospital Colorado
janet.thomas@childrenscolorado.org
Chapter 36: Inborn Errors of Metabolism

Sharon H. Travers, MD
Associate Professor, Department of Pediatrics, Section of Pediatric Endocrinology, University of Colorado School of Medicine and Children's Hospital Colorado
sharon.travers@childrenscolorado.org
Chapter 34: Endocrine Disorders

Meghan Treitz, MD
Assistant Professor, Department of Pediatrics, Section of General Academic Pediatrics, University of Colorado School of Medicine and Children's Hospital Colorado
meghan.treitz@childrenscolorado.org
Chapter 9: Ambulatory & Office Pediatrics

Anne Chun-Hui Tsai, MD, MSc
Associate Professor, Departments of Pediatrics and Genetics, Section of Clinical Genetics and Metabolism, University of Colorado School of Medicine and Children's Hospital Colorado
chun-hui.tsai@childrenscolorado.org
Chapter 37: Genetics & Dysmorphology

Johan L.K. Van Hove, MD, PhD, MBA
Associate Professor, Department of Pediatrics, Head, Section of Clinical Genetics and Metabolism, University of Colorado School of Medicine and Children's Hospital Colorado
johan.vanhove@childrenscolorado.org
Chapter 36: Inborn Errors of Metabolism

Kathleen Ventre, MD
Assistant Professor, Department of Pediatrics, Section of Pediatric Critical Care Medicine, University of Colorado School of Medicine and Children's Hospital Colorado
kathleen.ventre@childrenshospital.org
Chapter 14: Critical Care

Armando Vidal, MD
Assistant Professor, Department of Orthopedics, Sports Medicine Program, University of Colorado School of Medicine and Children's Hospital Colorado
armando.vidal@ucdenver.edu
Chapter 27: Sports Medicine

Adriana Weinberg, MD
Professor, Department of Pediatrics, Director, Clinical Virology Laboratory, Section of Pediatric Infectious Diseases, University of Colorado School of Medicine and Children's Hospital Colorado
adriana.weinberg@udenver.edu
Chapter 40: Infections: Viral & Rickettsial

Pamela E. Wilson, MD
Assistant Professor, Department of Rehabilitation Medicine, Rehabilitation Center, University of Colorado School of Medicine and Children's Hospital Colorado
pamela.wilson@childrenscolorado.org
Chapter 27: Sports Medicine
Chapter 28: Rehabilitation Medicine

Michele L. Yang, MD
Assistant Professor, Departments of Pediatrics and Neurology, Section of Pediatric Neurology, University of Colorado School of Medicine and Children's Hospital Colorado
michele.yang@childrenscolorado.org
Chapter 25: Neurologic & Muscular Disorders

Patricia J. Yoon, MD, FACS
Assistant Professor, Department of Pediatrics, Section of Pediatric Otolaryngology, University of Colorado School of Medicine and Children's Hospital Colorado
patricia.yoon@childrenscolorado.org
Chapter 18: Ear, Nose, & Throat

Philip S. Zeitler, MD, PhD
Professor, Department of Pediatrics, Head, Section of Pediatric Endocrinology, University of Colorado School of Medicine and Children's Hospital Colorado
phil.zeitler@ucdenver.edu
Chapter 34: Endocrine Disorders

Edith T. Zemanick, MD
Associate Professor, Department of Pediatrics, Section of Pediatric Pulmonary Medicine, University of Colorado School of Medicine and Children's Hospital Colorado
edith.zemanick@childrenscolorado.org
Chapter 19: Respiratory Tract & Mediastinum

Preface

The 21st edition of *Current Diagnosis & Treatment: Pediatrics (CDTP)* features practical, up-to-date, well-referenced information on the care of children from birth through infancy and adolescence. *CDTP* emphasizes the clinical aspects of pediatric care while also covering important underlying principles. *CDTP* provides a guide to diagnosis, understanding, and treatment of the medical problems of all pediatric patients in an easy-to-use and readable format.

INTENDED AUDIENCE

Like all Lange medical books, *CDTP* provides a concise yet comprehensive source of current information. Students will find *CDTP* an authoritative introduction to pediatrics and an excellent source for reference and review. *CDTP* provides excellent coverage of The Council on Medical Student Education in Pediatrics (COMSEP) curriculum used in pediatric clerkships. Residents in pediatrics (and other specialties) will appreciate the detailed descriptions of diseases as well as diagnostic and therapeutic procedures. Pediatricians, family practitioners, nurses and nurse practitioners, and other health-care providers who work with infants and children will find *CDTP* a useful reference on management aspects of pediatric medicine.

COVERAGE

Forty-six chapters cover a wide range of topics, including neonatal medicine, child development and behavior, emergency and critical care medicine, and diagnosis and treatment of specific disorders according to major problems, etiologies, and organ systems. A wealth of tables and figures provides quick access to important information, such as acute and critical care procedures in the delivery room, the office, the emergency room, and the critical care unit; anti-infective agents; drug dosages; immunization schedules; differential diagnosis; and developmental screening tests. The final chapter is a handy guide to normal laboratory values.

NEW TO THIS EDITION

The Editors of *CDTP* would like to welcome Dr. Mark Abzug as our new Editor. Mark brings to *CDTP* a wealth of knowledge and experience in pediatric infectious diseases, editing, and clinical research. Mark is replacing Judy Sondheimer, who has retired from the University of Colorado, but continues active work at Georgetown University. The 21st edition of *CDTP* has been revised comprehensively by the editors and contributing authors. New references as well as up-to-date and useful Web sites have been added, permitting the reader to consult original material and to go beyond the confines of the textbook. As editors and practicing pediatricians, we have tried to ensure that each chapter reflects the needs and realities of day-to-day practice.

CHAPTERS WITH MAJOR REVISIONS INCLUDE:

3 Child Development & Behavior
9 Ambulatory & Office Pediatrics
10 Immunization
14 Critical Care
15 Skin
19 Respiratory Tract & Mediastinum
21 Gastrointestinal Tract
25 Neurologic & Muscular Disorders
31 Neoplastic Disease
32 Pain Management & Pediatric Palliative & End-of-Life Care
33 Immunodeficiency
37 Genetics & Dysmorphology
40 Infections: Viral & Rickettsial
41 Human Immunodeficiency Virus Infection
42 Infections: Bacterial & Spirochetal
43 Infections: Parasitic & Mycotic

NEW CHAPTERS INCLUDE:

1 Advancing the Quality and Safety of Care

CHAPTER REVISIONS

The 16 chapters that have been extensively revised, with new authors added in several cases, reflect the substantially updated material in each of their areas of pediatric medicine. Chapters on Skin, Immunodeficiency, and Neoplastic Disease are markedly updated with the latest information. Especially important are updates to the chapters on Infectious Diseases, including information on methicillin-resistant staphylococcus, tropical diseases such as dengue and malaria, and respiratory viral infections, including influenza. All laboratory tables in Chapter 46 Chemistry & Hematology Reference Intervals have been updated. All other chapters are substantially revised and references have been updated. Eighteen new authors have contributed to these revisions.

ACKNOWLEDGMENTS

The editors would like to thank Bonnie Savone for her expert assistance in managing the flow of manuscripts and materials among the chapter authors, editors, and publishers. Her attention to detail was enormously helpful. The editors also would like to thank Tia Brayman at Children's Hospital Colorado who produced the cover photographs.

William W. Hay, Jr., MD
Myron J. Levin, MD
Robin R. Deterding, MD
Mark J. Abzug, MD
Judith M. Sondheimer, MD

Denver, Colorado
June 2012

Advancing the Quality and Safety of Care

1

Daniel Hyman, MD

While the history of the patient safety movement can be traced back to Hippocrates' famous dictum *primum non nocere* some 2500 years ago, the more modern safety effort was galvanized by the Institute of Medicine's (IOM) 1999 landmark report *To Err Is Human*. The most quoted statistic from this report, that between 44,000 and 98,000 Americans die each year as a result of medical error, was based upon studies of hospital mortality in Colorado, Utah, and New York and extrapolated to an annual estimate for the country. The IOM followed up this report with a second publication, *Crossing the Quality Chasm*, in which they said, "*Health care today harms too frequently, and routinely fails to deliver its potential benefits.... Between the health care we have and the care we could have lies not just a gap, but a chasm.*" These two reports have served as central elements in an advocacy movement that has engaged stakeholders across the continuum of our health care delivery system and changed the nature of how we think about the quality of care we provide, and receive.

In *Crossing the Quality Chasm,* the IOM included a simple but elegant definition of the word "Quality" as it applies to health care. They defined six domains of health care quality: SAFE—free from preventable harm, EFFECTIVE—optimal clinical outcomes; doing what we should do, not what we should not do according to the evidence, EFFICIENT—without waste of resources—human, financial, supplies/equipment, TIMELY-without unnecessary delay, PATIENT/FAMILY CENTERED—according to the wishes, values of patients and their families, EQUITABLE—eliminating disparities in outcomes between patients of different race, gender, and socioeconomic status.

In the years since these two reports were published, the multiple stakeholders concerned about the effectiveness, safety and cost of health care in the United States, and indeed throughout the world, have accelerated their individual and collective involvement in analyzing and improving care. In the United States, numerous governmental agencies, large employer groups, health insurance plans, consumers/patients, health care providers, and delivery systems are among the key constituencies calling for and working toward better and safer care at lower cost. Similar efforts are occurring internationally. Indeed, the concept of the Triple Aim is now being promoted as an organizing framework for considering the country's overall health care improvement goals.

Kohn L, Corrigan JM: *To err is human: building a safer health system*. Washington, DC: National Academy Press; 2000.

Committee on Quality Health Care in America, Institute of Medicine: *Crossing the quality chasm: a new health system for the 21st century*. Washington, DC: National Academy Press; 2001.

CURRENT CONTEXT

The health care industry is in a period of transformation being driven by at least four converging factors: the recognition of serious gaps in the safety and quality of care we provide (and receive), the unsustainable increases in the cost of care as a percent of the national economy, the aging of the population, and the emerging role of health care information technology as a potential tool to improve care. These are impacting health care organizations, as well as individual practitioners, in numerous ways that can also be traced to expectations regarding transparency and increasing accountability for results. As depicted in Figure 1–1, the Triple Aim includes the simultaneous goals of better care (outcomes/experience) for individual patients, better health for the population, and lower cost overall. Practitioners and trainees must adapt to a new set of priorities that focus attention on new goals to extend our historic focus on the doctor/patient relationship and autonomous physician decision making. Instead, new imperatives are evidence-based medicine, advancing safety, and reducing unnecessary expense.

The impact of health care quality improvement will increasingly influence clinical practice and the delivery of pediatric care in the future. This chapter provides a summary

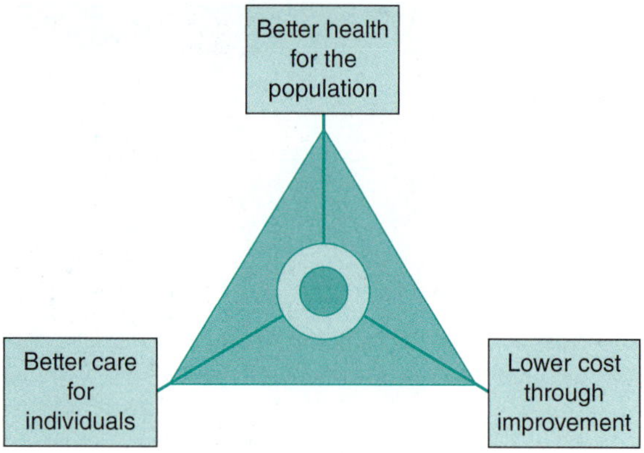

▲ **Figure 1–1.** Triple Aim. (Adapted from the Center for Medicare and Medicaid Services.)

of some of the central elements of health care quality improvement and patient safety, and offers resources for the reader to obtain additional information and understanding about these topics.

To understand the external influences driving many of these changes, there are at least six key national organizations central to the transitions occurring.

1. Center for Medicare and Medicaid Services (Department of Health and Human Services)—www.cms.gov
   Center for Medicare and Medicaid Services (CMS) oversees the United States' federally funded health care programs including Medicare, Medicaid, and other related programs. CMS and the Veterans Affairs Divisions together provide funding for more than 35% of the United States national healthcare spending at an annual cost of 925 billion dollars.
   CMS is increasingly promoting payment mechanisms that withhold payment for the costs of preventable complications of care and giving incentives to providers for achieving better outcomes for their patients, primarily in its Medicare population. The agency has also enabled and advocated for greater transparency of results and makes available on its website comparative measures of performance for its Medicare population. CMS is also increasingly utilizing its standards under which hospitals and other health care provider organizations are licensed to provide care as tools to assure greater compliance with these regulations. It has adopted a list of Hospital Acquired Conditions (HACs) in 10 categories for which hospitals are no longer reimbursed. This list of HACs includes: foreign object retained after surgery, air embolism, blood incompatibility, stage III and IV pressure ulcers, falls and trauma, manifestations of poor glycemic control, catheter-associated urinary tract infection (not in children), vascular catheter-associated infection, and surgical site infection or deep vein thrombosis/pulmonary embolism after selected procedures. It is worth noting that CMS is able to generate comparative national data only for its Medicare population because it, unlike Medicaid, is a single federal program with a single financial database. Because the Medicaid program functions as 51 state/federal partnership arrangements, patient experience and costs are captured in 51 separate state-based program databases. This segmentation has limited the development of national measures for pediatric care in both inpatient and ambulatory settings. Similarly, while the reporting of HACs is uniform across the United States for Medicare patients, in the Medicaid population it varies by individual state.
2. National Quality Forum—www.qualityforum.org/Home
   National Quality Forum (NQF) is a private, not-for-profit organization whose members include consumer advocacy groups, health care providers, accrediting bodies, employers and other purchasers of care, and research organizations. The NQF's mission is to promote improvement in the quality of American health care primarily through defining priorities for improvement, approving consensus standards and metrics for performance reporting, and through educational efforts. The NQF, for example, has endorsed a list of 29 "serious reportable events" in health care that include events related to surgical or invasive procedures, products or device failures, patient protection, care management, environmental issues, radiologic events, and potential criminal events. This list and the CMS list of HACs are both being used by insurers to reduce payment to hospitals/providers as well as to require reporting to state agencies for public review. In 2011, NQF released a set of 41 measures for the quality of pediatric care, largely representing outpatient preventive services and management of chronic conditions, and population-based measures applicable to health plans, for example immunization rates and frequency of well childcare.
3. Leapfrog—www.leapfroggroup.org
   Leapfrog is a group of large employers who seek to use their purchasing power to influence the health care community to achieve big "leaps" in health care safety and quality. Leapfrog promotes transparency and issues public reports of how well individual hospitals meet their recommended standards, including computerized physician order entry, ICU staffing models, and rates of hospital acquired infections. There is some evidence that meeting these standards is associated with improved hospital quality and/or mortality outcomes.
4. Agency for Health care Research and Quality—www.ahrq.gov
   Agency for Health care Research and Quality (AHRQ) is one of 12 agencies within the US Department of

Health and Human Services. AHRQ's primary mission has been to support health services research initiatives that seek to improve the quality of health care in the United States. Its activities extend well beyond the support of research and now include the development of measurements of quality and patient safety, reports on disparities in performance, measures of patient safety culture in organizations, and promotion of tools to improve care among others. AHRQ also convenes expert panels to assess national efforts to advance quality and patient safety and to recommend strategies to accelerate progress.

5. Specialty Society Boards
   Specialty Society Boards, eg, American Board of Pediatrics (ABP). The ABP, along with other specialty certification organizations, has responded to the call for greater accountability to consumers by enhancing its maintenance of certification programs (MOC). All trainees, and an increasing proportion of active practitioners, are now subject to the requirements of the MOC program, including participation in quality improvement activities in the diplomate's clinical practice. The Board's mission is focused on assuring the public that certificate holders have been trained according to their standards and also meet continuous evaluation requirements in six areas of core competency: patient care, medical knowledge, practice-based learning and improvement, interpersonal and communication skills, professionalism, and systems-based practice. These are the same competencies as required of residents in training programs as certified by the Accreditation Council on Graduate Medical Education. Providers need not only to be familiar with the principles of quality improvement and patient safety, but also must demonstrate having implemented quality improvement efforts within their practice settings.
6. The Joint Commission—www.jointcommission.org
   The Joint Commission (JC) is a private, nonprofit agency that is licensed to accredit health care provider organizations, including hospitals, nursing homes, and other health care provider entities in the United States as well as internationally. Its mission is to continuously improve the quality of care through evaluation, education, and enforcement of regulatory standards. Since 2003, JC has annually adopted a set of National Patient Safety Goals designed to help advance the safety of care provided in all health care settings. Examples include the use of two patient identifiers to reduce the risk of care being provided to an unintended patient; the use of time-outs and a universal protocol to improve surgical safety and reduce the risk of wrong site procedures; adherence to hand hygiene recommendations to reduce the risk of spreading hospital acquired infections, to name just a few. These goals often become regulatory standards with time and widespread adoption. Failure to meet these standards can result in actions against the licensure of the health care provider, or more commonly, requires corrective action plans, measurement to demonstrate improvement, and resurveying depending upon the severity of findings. The JC publishes a monthly journal on quality and safety, available at http://www.jcrinc.com/Periodicals/THE-JOINT-COMMISSION-JOURNAL-ON-QUALITY-AND-PATIENT-SAFETY/903/.

Finally, advances in quality and safety will be impacted by the provisions of the American Recovery and Reinvestment Act (ARRA) and Patient Protection and Affordable Care Act (PPACA) enacted by the United States government in the past 2 years. These laws and their implications are only beginning to be understood in the United States. The landmark 2010 federal health care legislation will provide for near universal access to health care, but it is still being debated in the courts and the legislatures, and its future status and structure remain unknown. It is likely that changes in payment mechanisms for health care will continue irrespective of ARRA/PPACA, and current and future providers' practices will be economically, structurally, and functionally impacted by these emerging trends. Furthermore, changes in the funding and structure of the US health care system may ultimately also result in changes in other countries. Many countries have single payer systems for providing health care to their citizens and often are leaders in defining new strategies for health care improvement.

Center for Medicare and Medicaid Services: Triple Aim.

Berwick D, Nolan T, Whittington J: The triple aim: Care, health, and cost, doi 10.1377/hlthaff.27.3.759 Health Affairs 2008: 27(3); 759-769.

https://www.cms.gov/nationalhealthexpenddata/02_national-healthaccountshistorical.asp

Accessed 9/21/11 (reference on federal health care spending)

Center for Medicare and Medicaid Services: www.cms.gov

Rosenthal M, Engi N: Beyond Pay for Performance — Emerging Models of Provider-Payment. Reform Med 2008;359:1197-1200.

http://www.nejm.org/doi/full/10.1056/NEJMp0804658 accessed 10/4/11

Straube B, Blum JD: The Policy On Paying For Treating Hospital-Acquired Conditions: CMS Officials Respond. Health Affairs 2009;28(5):1494-1497.

CMS list of Hospital Acquired Conditions

Miller T, Leatherman S: The National Quality Forum: a 'me-too' or a breakthrough in quality measurement and reporting? Health Affairs 1999;18(6):233-237.

http://www.qualityforum.org/News_And_Resources/Press_Releases/2011/NQF_Releases_Updated_Child_Quality_Health_Measures.aspx3 Accessed 9/21/11 (reference on 41 NQF pediatric measures)

Leapfrog: www.leapfroggroup.org

Jha A, Oray J, Ridgway A, Zheng J, Eptein A: Does the Leapfrog Program Help Identify High-Quality Hospitals? *The Joint Commission Journal on Quality and Patient Safety* 2008;34(6).

Agency for Healthcare Research and Quality: www.ahrq.gov

Shekelle P, Pronovost P, Wachter R et al: Advancing the Science of Patient Safety. 2011;154(10):693-696.

American Board of Pediatrics, https://www.abp.org/ABPWebStatic/?anticache=0.6997913528065516

Hawkins RE, Weiss KB: Commentary: *Building the Evidence Base in Support of the American Board of Medical Specialties Maintenance of Certification Program*, doi: 10.1097/ACM.0b013e318201801b. Academic Medicine 2011;86(1):6-7.

The Joint Commission: www.jointcommission.org, http://www.jcrinc.com/Periodicals/THE-JOINT-COMMISSION-JOURNAL-ON-QUALITY-AND-PATIENT-SAFETY/903/

Connors E, Gostin L: Health Care Reform—A Historic Moment in US Social Policy, doi: 10.1001/jama.2010.856. JAMA 2010;303(24):2521-2522.

STRATEGIES AND MODELS FOR QUALITY IMPROVEMENT (QI)

There are a number of commonly employed approaches to improving the quality of care in health care settings. This section highlights three representative approaches to conducting clinical improvement work, but they are by no means the only potential strategies that physicians and staff may see or utilize. The Model for Improvement is primarily emphasized because of its ease of adoption, and because it is the foundation for most improvement efforts included in the Maintenance of Certification program of the American Board of Pediatrics. Briefer summaries of Lean and Six-Sigma methods are also included, with listings of resources where the reader can find additional information.

"MODEL FOR IMPROVEMENT"

Widely taught and promoted by the Boston-based educational and advocacy organization the Institute for Healthcare Improvement (IHI), the Model for Improvement (MFI) is grounded in three simple questions that guide the work of the improvement leader and team. The model's framework includes an Aim statement, a measurement strategy and then the use of "rapid cycle" changes to achieve the aim. The IHI web site, www.ihi.org, has an extensive resource library, and hosts an "Open School" that includes a QI/Patient safety modular curriculum for health professional students and their faculty at www.ihi.org/openschool.

AIM STATEMENT

The Aim statement answers the question, "What do we want to accomplish?" The measure question is "How will we know that a change is an improvement?" and the Change component is focused on "What changes can we make that will result in improvement?" This model is represented in Figure 1–2.

Aim statements are a *written* description of what the team's improvement goal is, and also include information on who comprises the patient population, and a time frame within which the improvement will be achieved. They identify a "stretch" but achievable improvement target goal, and, often, some general statement regarding how the improvement will be achieved. Aim statements are sometimes characterized using the pneumonic SMAART: specific, measurable, achievable, actionable, relevant, and timely. Aim statements should be unambiguous and understandable to the stakeholders, and are most likely to be achieved if they are aligned with the strategic goals of the team or organization.

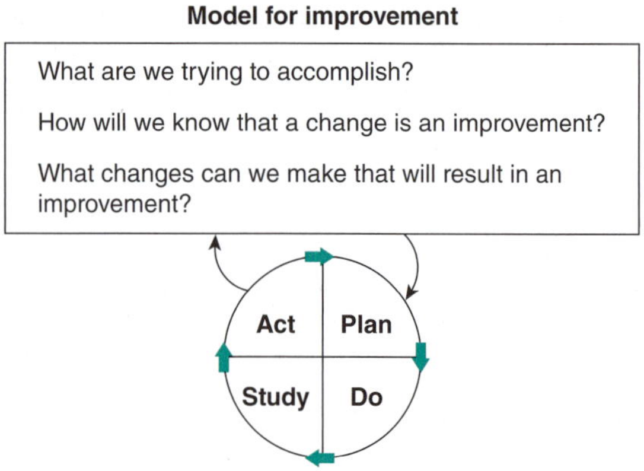

▲ **Figure 1–2.** Model for Improvement. (Adapted, with permission, from The Improvement Guide: AIM Model for Improvement. San Francisco, CA: Jossey-Bass; 2009:24.)

For example, the following statement meets the criteria for a SMAART Aim statement, "*We will reduce the frequency of emergency department visits and hospitalizations for patients with asthma seen at E Street Pediatrics by 25% by December 31, 2012.*" Whereas, this next statement does not,

"*We will improve the care for patients with asthma by appropriately prescribing indicated medications and better educating families in their use.*"

The first example provides a specific measurable goal, a time frame, and clarity with respect to who the patients are. A 25% reduction in ED/inpatient asthma visits will require a change in the system for asthma care delivery for the entire population of children with asthma; that extent of level of improvement is a stretch, but it is much more achievable than a goal would be if it was set to "eliminate" such encounters. The second example is unclear in terms of the measure for improvement, the time frame for the goal to be met, and even the population in question. The statement provides some sense of processes that could be utilized to improve asthma care but is missing needed specificity.

MEASURES

Specific measures provide a means to assess whether or not the improvement effort is on track. Three types of measures are useful. *Outcome measures* answer questions concerning the health care impact for the patients, such as how has their health status changed? *Process measures* are related to the health care delivery system itself. They answer questions like how is the system performing? *Balancing measures* seek to identify potential unintended consequences that are related to the improvement effort being undertaken. Examples are helpful to contextualize these conceptual definitions.

Continuing with asthma as an example of the improvement effort, and utilizing the first aim statement example, here are some examples of measures that might be employed, and the type of measure each is.

Examples of measures for an asthma improvement project:

1. Proportion of children with an asthma severity assessment in their medical record in the past year (process).
2. Percent of children with asthma in the practice seen in the ED or hospitalized for asthma in the past 6 months (outcome).
3. Average difference in the time between the last office patient's scheduled appointment time and the actual office close time (balancing).
4. Staff satisfaction with their job (balancing).
5. Percent of children with persistent asthma, of any severity, prescribed a controller medication at their most recent visit (process).
6. Percent of children prescribed a controller medication who report taking their medicine (process—this one might seem surprising, but an outcome measures the health status of the patient, not the taking of a medication. One might argue that adherence to a treatment plan is an outcome of the work of the practice/practitioner prescribing the medication. It is more consistent, however, to consider the translation of the treatment plan into action as a part of the process of care, and that the health status or outcome measure will be improved by fully improving the measured processes of care, including patient adherence to the treatment plan.)
7. Percent of children in a practice asthma registry provided with a complete asthma action plan in the past twelve months (process).
8. Percent of children who missed any school days due to asthma in the past 6 months (outcome).

Measures are essential elements of any improvement work. It is a good idea to choose a manageable (4-6) number of measures, all of which can be obtained with limited or no extra effort, and with a mix of outcome, process and balancing measures. Ideally, the best process measures are those that are directly linked to the outcome goal. The hypothesis in this specific example would be that assessing asthma severity and appropriately using controller medications and action plans would all contribute to reducing the number or frequency of missed school days and the need for ED/hospital utilization.

It is important to note that measurement in the setting of an improvement project is different from measurement in a research study. Improvement projects require "just enough" data to guide the team's continuing efforts. Often the results seen in a sequence of 10 patients is enough to tell you whether a particular system is functioning consistently or not. For example, considering measure example number 1, if in the last 10 patients seen with asthma, only two had their asthma severity documented, how many more charts need be checked to conclude that the system is not functioning as intended and that changes are needed? Other measures may require larger sample sizes, especially when assessing the impact of care changes on a population of patients with a particular condition. See Randolph's excellent summary for a fuller description of measurement for improvement.

CHANGES AND IDEAS

Once the team's aim is established and the measures are selected, the third component of the Model for Improvement focuses on what changes in the system must be made that will result in the targeted improvements. Here, the model draws from the field of industrial engineering and the work of improvement pioneers W. Edwards Deming and Walter Shewhart. To answer the question "What changes will result in improvement?", the improvement team should incorporate "Plan-Do-Study (or check)-Act" cycles, typically referred to as PDSA cycles. The cycles include the following steps:

Plan: what will we do that will likely improve the process measures linked to the outcome target goal? Who will do it? Where? When? How? How will the data be collected?

Do: implementation of the planned change(s). *TIP!* It is good to make the change cycles as small as possible, for example, trying a new process on the next five patients being seen by one provider as opposed to wide scale implementation of a new chart documentation form across an entire clinic.

Study (or check): Once the small test of change is tried, its results are assessed. How many times did the process work as planned for the five patients included in the cycle?

Act: Based upon the results of the study of the cycle, recommendations are made as to what the next steps ought to be to achieve the goal. At this point, the cycle then resumes and planning begins for the next cycle.

Over the course of an improvement effort, multiple tests of change might be implemented for any or all of the process measures felt to be likely to impact the outcome measures relevant to the project.

The Model for Improvement has been used by improvement teams across numerous health care settings around the world. Further information about the model and examples can be found at www.ihi.org/openschool, or in *The Improvement Guide* (Langley, Moen, Nolan, et al).

The IHI Open School modules are an excellent online resource for clinicians interested in learning more about the fundamentals of quality improvement and patient safety. These educational lessons are free of charge to health professional students, residents, and university faculty members, and for a modest subscription fee to other clinicians. They are also free to health care practitioners in the developing world. An excellent original resource on implementing this model in clinical practice is in Berwick's summary article from 1998.

G. Langley, R. Moen, K. Nolan, T. Nolan, C. Norman, L. Provost: The Improvement Guide: AIM model for Improvement. San Francisco, CA: Jossey-Bass; 2009:24.

Randolph G, Esporas M, Provost L, Massie S, Bundy D: Model for Improvement Part Two: *Measurement and Feedback for Quality Improvement Efforts.* Ped Clin N Am 2009;56(4):779-798; Developing and Testing Changes in Delivery of Care Berwick, Donald M. MD, MPP. This paper is also available at http://www.acponline.org.Ann Intern Med. 1998;128:651-656.

Berwick D: The Science of Improvement. JAMA; 2008: 299(10): 1182-1184.

"LEAN"

Also grounded in industrial engineering, an increasingly popular method for driving improvement efforts in health care settings is "Lean" or "Lean processing". Early thinking about lean processes is credited to the Toyota Manufacturing Company in Japan. The crossover to health care from manufacturing is a relatively recent phenomenon, but numerous hospitals and health care delivery settings, including individual clinics, have benefited from the application of these principles to their clinical operations. Lean improvement methods focus on reducing errors and variability in repetitive steps that are part of any process. In health care, examples of repeated processes would include how patients are registered and their information obtained; how medications are ordered, compounded, distributed, and administered; how consent forms are accurately completed in a timely manner prior to surgical procedures; how antibiotics are reliably and efficiently delivered prior to surgical procedures.

"Lean" is a philosophy of continuous improvement. It is grounded in recognizing that the way we do things today is merely "current state". With time, effort, focus, and long-term thinking, we can create a "future state" that is better than the status quo. It does so by focusing on identifying the value of all steps in any process and eliminating those steps that do not contribute to the value sought by the customer, or in health care, the patient/family. In doing so, improvements in outcomes, including cost and productivity, and in clinical measures of effectiveness can be realized. See Young for an early critical assessment of the incorporation of Lean into healthcare settings.

There are four categories that describe the essential elements of Toyota's adoption of "Lean" as a management strategy. These four categories are: *Philosophy* (emphasize long-term thinking over short-term gain); *Process* (eliminate waste through very defined approaches including an emphasis on process flow and the use of pull systems to reduce overproduction, for example); *People/Partners* (respect, challenge, and grow staff); and *Problem Solving* (create a culture of continuous learning and improvement).

There are a number of hospitals that have fully integrated Lean management as a primary basis for its organizational approach to improvement. Several were featured in a "White Paper" published by the Institute for Healthcare Improvement in 2005.

Young TP, McClean SI: A critical look at Lean Thinking in health care. BMJ Quality and Safety Health Care 2008; 17:382-386.

Liker: *The Toyota Way*. Madison, WI: McGraw-Hill; 2004

Going Lean in Health Care, Innovation Series White Paper, Institute for Healthcare Improvement: 2005: http://www.ihi.org/knowledge/Pages/IHIWhitePapers/GoingLeaninHealthCare.aspx

"SIX-SIGMA"

A third quality improvement methodology also arose in the manufacturing industry. Motorola is generally credited with promoting Six-sigma as a management strategy designed to reduce the variability in its processes and thereby reducing the number of defects in its outputs. Organizations adopting Six-sigma as an improvement strategy utilize measurement-based strategies that focus on process improvement and variation reduction to eliminate defects in their work and to reduce cycle times, thereby increasing profitability and enhancing customer satisfaction. Sigma is the statistical measure of standard deviation and Motorola adopted "Six-sigma" as a performance indicator, promoting consistency of processes in order to have fewer than 3.4 defects per million opportunities. This performance goal has since become the common descriptor for this approach to improvement both in manufacturing and in service industries, including health care. Similar to "Lean", the translation of business manufacturing strategies into health care has various challenges, but there are many processes that repeatedly occur in health care that can be routinized and made more consistent. Many health care processes fail far more frequently than 3.4 times per million opportunities. Consider pharmacy dispensing errors, medication ordering or administration errors, and patient scheduling errors, just to name a few. These are a few of many examples of processes that could potentially benefit from the kind of rigorous analysis that is integral to the Six-sigma approach.

In a typical Six-sigma structured improvement project, there are five phases generally referred to as DMAIC—Define (what is the problem, what is the goal?), Measure (quantify the problem and improvement opportunity), Analyze (use of observations and data to identify causes), Improve (implementation of solutions based on data analysis), and finally, Control (sustainable change).

One of the central aspects of Six-sigma as an improvement strategy is its defined focus on understanding the reasons for defects in any process. By understanding these drivers, it is then possible to revise the approach to either the manufacturing process or the service functions, in order to reduce these errors and failures.

"Lean-Six Sigma" is a newer entity that draws from both methodologies in order to simplify the improvement work where possible, but retain the rigorous statistical method that is a hallmark of Six-sigma projects. "Lean" focuses on where time is lost in any process and can identify opportunities to eliminate steps or reduce time. Six-Sigma aims to reduce or eliminate defects in the process, thereby resulting in a higher quality product through a more efficient and lower cost process.

Regardless of the method used, improvement happens because an organization, team, or individual sets a goal to improve a current process through systematic analysis of the way things are done now, and then implementing planned changes to see how they impact the outputs or outcomes.

For additional information on "Lean" and Six-sigma, see www.isixsigma.com or www.asq.org/sixsigma.

Pande P, Holpp L: *What is Six Sigma?* New York, NY: McGraw-Hill; 2002.

PRINCIPLES OF PATIENT SAFETY (INCIDENT REPORTING, JUST CULTURE, DISCLOSURE, FMEA, RCA, RELIABILITY, CHECKLISTS)

Safe patient care avoids preventable harm; it is care that does not cause harm as it seeks to cure. The list of adverse events that are considered to be preventable is evolving. As mentioned earlier, both CMS and NQF have endorsed lists of various complications of care as being "never events" or "serious reportable events" for which providers are often now not reimbursed, and which are increasingly reportable to the public through various state transparency programs.

Irrespective of one's views about whether various complications are entirely preventable at the current state of science or not, these approaches reflect a changing paradigm that is impacting many aspects of health care delivery. Transparency of results is increasingly expected. Perspectives and data on how these kinds of efforts are impacting actual improvement in outcomes are mixed.

Given these trends, health care providers need to have robust systems for measuring and improving the safety of care provided to patients. The methods for improving quality reviewed above are frequently used to reduce harm, just as they can be used to improve effectiveness or efficiency. For example, hospitals attempting to reduce infections have successfully used these types of process improvement approaches to improve antibiotic use prior to surgical procedures or to improve hand hygiene practices.

Common patient safety tools are summarized here.

Incident Reporting Systems—Efforts to advance safety in any organization require a clear understanding of the kinds of harm occurring within that organization, as well as the kinds of "near-misses" that are occurring. These reporting systems can range from a simple paper reporting form to a "telephone hot-line" to a computerized database that is available to staff (and potentially patients) within the organization. Events are traditionally graded according to the severity of harm that resulted from the incident. One example is the NCC MERP Index, which grades events from A (potential to cause harm) to I (resulting in patient death). Errors that are recognized represent only a fraction of the actual errors and near-misses that are present in the system. Incident reporting systems depend upon people recognizing the error or near-miss, being comfortable reporting it, knowing how and when to report, and then actually doing so. It is no surprise therefore, that estimates for how frequently incidents that could or should be reported into incident reporting systems range from 1.5% to 30% depending on the type of adverse or near-miss event. "Trigger tools" (either manual chart reviews for indications of adverse events, or automated reports from electronic medical records) are increasingly being used to increase the recognition of episodes of harm in health care settings.

"Just culture"—The effectiveness of incident reporting systems is highly dependent upon the culture of the organization within which the reporting is occurring. Aviation industry safety reporting systems are often highlighted for their successes over the past few decades in promoting reporting of aviation events that might have led to accidents. The Aviation Safety Reporting System (ASRS) prioritizes confidentiality in order to encourage reporting and protects reporters from punishment, with certain limitations when they report incidents, even if related to non adherence to aviation regulations. Although the system is voluntary, more than 880,000 reports have been submitted and used by the Federal Aviation Administration to improve air travel safety.

In health care, the variable recognition of adverse events as well as any fear about reprisal for reporting events both work to reduce the consistent reporting of events. The concept of "just culture" has been promoted as a strategy to increase the comfort of staff members to report the occurrence of errors or near-misses, even if they may have done something incorrectly. See the work of David Marx and the "Just Culture Community" for more information on how to evaluate error so as to support reporting and safer practices in organizations. A great deal more information about "just culture" principles is available at http://www.justculture.org.

Failure Modes and Effects Analyses (FMEA)—An FMEA is a systematic methodology used to proactively identify ways in which any process might fail, and then to prioritize among strategies for reducing the risk or impact of identified potential failures. In conducting an FMEA, which all hospitals are required to do annually, a team will carefully describe and analyze each step in a particular process, consider what and how anything might go wrong, why it would happen and what the impact would be of such failures. Like "Lean" and Six-sigma, the FMEA has been adopted into health care from its origins in military and industrial settings. The FMEA is an effective method for identifying strategies to reduce risks in health care settings, thereby protecting patients if interventions are put into place as a result of the analysis. A tool to use in conducting an FMEA is available from the IHI (http://www.ihi.org/knowledge/Pages/Tools/FailureModesandEffectsAnalysisTool.aspx). Their site includes additional information and resources about the FMEA process.

Root Cause Analyses (RCA) (Post Event reviews)—As contrasted with the proactive FMEA process, an RCA is a retrospective analysis of an adverse occurrence (or near-miss) that has already happened. It too is a systematic process that in this case allows a team to reach an understanding of why certain things occurred, what systems factors and human factors contributed to the occurrence, and what defects in the system might be changed in order to reduce the likelihood of recurrence. Key to an effective RCA process, and similar to the principles discussed above related to "just culture", RCAs are designed not to ask who was at fault, but rather what system reasons contributed to the event. "Why", not "who" is the essential question to be asked. The answer to the question "why did this occur" almost invariably results in a combination of factors, often illustrated by a series of pieces of Swiss cheese where the holes all line up. Taken from the writings of James Reason, the "Swiss Cheese Model" illustrates the many possible system failures that can contribute to an error, and contributes to identifying potential system changes that reduce the risk of error recurrence. Strategies for approaching retrospective RCA are available at http://www.ncbi.nlm.nih.gov/pmc/articles/pmc1117770.

Communication and Team Training—Because failures of communication are the most common identified factors in the analysis of reported serious health care events, many health care organizations have incorporated tools from other industries, particularly aviation, in order to enhance patient safety. As a result of the knowledge gained through analysis of tragic aviation accidents, the airline industry implemented methods like crew resource management training to assure that communication among cockpit team members is effective and clear, thereby reducing risk of air accidents. Similar methods have been used to train teams in operating rooms, delivery rooms, and other team-based settings. Most of these curricula include a few common elements: introductions to be sure all team members know one another's name, promoting the likelihood of speaking up; leader clarity with team members about the expectation that all will speak up if anyone has a concern; and structured language and other tools like verbal read-back of critical information to assure clarity in interpersonal or interdisciplinary communications. Such training also seeks to flatten the hierarchy, making it more likely that potential risks or problems will be identified and effectively addressed. Common tools used in promoting effective team communication include structured language like SBAR (situation, background, assessment, and recommendation), taken from the navy, to promote clarity of communication.

A number of resources exist in the public domain to support better teamwork and communication. One good place to start is the TeamSTEPPS program from the Agency for Healthcare Research and Quality. It can be found at http://teamstepps.ahrq.gov/.

Shekelle P, Pronovost P, Wachter R et al: Advancing the Science of Patient Safety. 2011;154(10):693-696.

Incident Reporting Systems: http://www.nccmerp.org/.

http://www.qualityforum.org/News_And_Resources/Press_Releases/2011/NQF_Releases_Updated_Serious_Reportable_Events.aspx (Accessed 9/21/11-reference on 29 serious reportable events NQF).

Mills R: *COLLABORATING WITH INDUSTRY TO ENSURE REGULATORY OVERSIGHT: THE USE OF VOLUNTARY SAFETY REPORTING PROGRAMS BY THE FEDERAL AVIATION ADMINISTRATION*, http://etd.ohiolink.edu/send-pdf.cgi/Mills%20Russell%20William.pdf?kent1302102713; 2011:46.

Marx D: A Primer for Health Care Executives: *Patient Safety and the "Just Culture"*. New York, NY: Columbia University

http://www.mers-tm.org/support/Marx_Primer.pdf : 2001.

Ashley L, Armitage G, Neary M, Hoolingsworth G: "A Practical Guide to Failure Mode and Effects Analysis in Health Care: *Making the Most of the team and its meetings*". Joint Commission Journal on Quality and Patient Safety, 2010;36(8):351-358.

http://www.ihi.org/knowledge/Pages/Tools/FailureModesandEffectsAnalysisTool.aspx

Reason J: "Human Error: Models and Management". BMJ 320:768, doi: 10.1136/bmj.320.7237.768:2000.

The Newborn Infant

2

Elizabeth H. Thilo, MD
Adam A. Rosenberg, MD

The newborn period is defined as the first 28 days of life. In practice, however, sick or very immature infants may require neonatal care for many months. There are three levels of newborn care. Level 1 refers to basic care of well newborns, neonatal resuscitation, and stabilization prior to transport. Level 2 refers to specialty neonatal care of premature infants greater than 1500 g or more than 32 weeks' gestation. Level 3 is subspecialty care of higher complexity ranging from 3A to 3D based on newborn size and gestational age, availability of general surgery, cardiac surgery, and extracorporeal membrane oxygenation. Level 3 care is often part of a perinatal center offering critical care and transport to the high-risk mother and fetus as well as the newborn infant.

THE NEONATAL HISTORY

The newborn medical history has three key components:

1. maternal and paternal medical and genetic history,
2. maternal past obstetric history, and
3. current antepartum and intrapartum obstetric history.

The mother's medical history includes chronic medical conditions, medications taken during pregnancy, unusual dietary habits, smoking history, occupational exposure to chemicals or infections of potential risk to the fetus, and any social history that might increase the risk for parenting problems and child abuse. Family illnesses and a history of congenital anomalies with genetic implications should be sought. The past obstetric history includes maternal age, gravidity, parity, blood type, and pregnancy outcomes. The current obstetric history includes the results of procedures during the current pregnancy such as ultrasound, amniocentesis, screening tests (rubella antibody, hepatitis B surface antigen, serum quadruple screen for genetic disorders, HIV [human immunodeficiency virus]), and antepartum tests of fetal well-being (eg, biophysical profiles, nonstress tests, or Doppler assessment of fetal blood flow patterns). Pregnancy-related maternal complications such as urinary tract infection, pregnancy-induced hypertension, eclampsia, gestational diabetes, vaginal bleeding, and preterm labor should be documented. Significant peripartum events include duration of ruptured membranes, maternal fever, fetal distress, meconium-stained amniotic fluid, type of delivery (vaginal or cesarean section), anesthesia and analgesia used, reason for operative or forceps delivery, infant status at birth, resuscitative measures, and Apgar scores.

ASSESSMENT OF GROWTH & GESTATIONAL AGE

It is important to know the infant's gestational age because normal behavior and possible medical problems can be predicted on this basis. The date of the last menstrual period is the best indicator of gestational age, if known, and if menses were regular. Fetal ultrasound provides supporting information. Postnatal physical characteristics and neurologic development are also clues to gestational age. Table 2–1 lists the physical and neurologic criteria of maturity used to estimate gestational age by the Ballard method. Adding the scores assigned to each neonatal physical and neuromuscular sign yields a score corresponding to gestational age.

Disappearance of the anterior vascular capsule of the lens is also helpful in determining gestational age. Until 27–28 weeks' gestation, the lens capsule is covered by vessels; by 34 weeks, this vascular plexus is completely atrophied. Foot length, from the heel to the tip of the longest toe, also correlates with gestational age in appropriately grown infants. The foot measures 4.5 cm at 25 weeks' gestation and increases 0.25 cm/wk until term.

If the physical examination indicates a gestational age within 2 weeks of that predicted by the obstetric dates, the gestational age is as assigned by the obstetric date. Birth weight and gestational age are plotted on standard grids (Figure 2–1) to determine whether the birth weight is appropriate for gestational age (AGA), small for gestational age (SGA, also known as intrauterine growth restriction or IUGR), or large for gestational age (LGA). Birth weight for gestational age in

Table 2–1. New Ballard score for assessment of fetal maturation of newly born infants.[a]

Neuromuscular Maturity								
Neuromuscular Maturity Sign	**Score** −1	0	1	2	3	4	5	**Record Score Here**
Posture 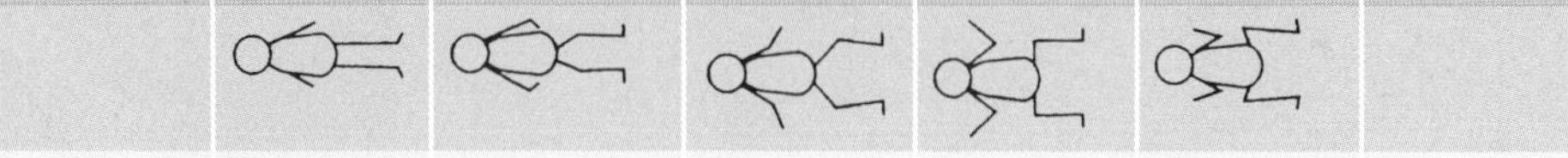								
Square window (wrist) 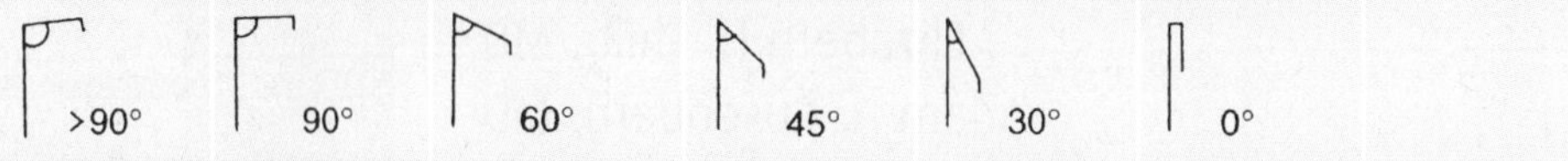	>90°	90°	60°	45°	30°	0°		
Arm recoil 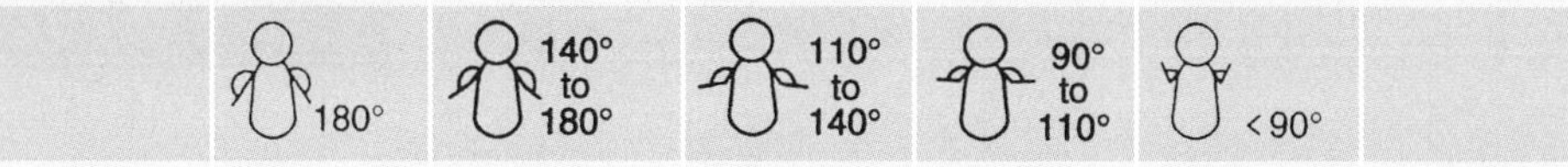		180°	140° to 180°	110° to 140°	90° to 110°	< 90°		
Popliteal angle 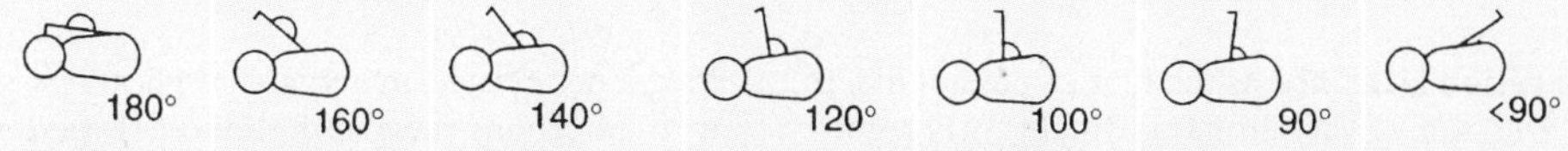	180°	160°	140°	120°	100°	90°	<90°	
Scarf sign 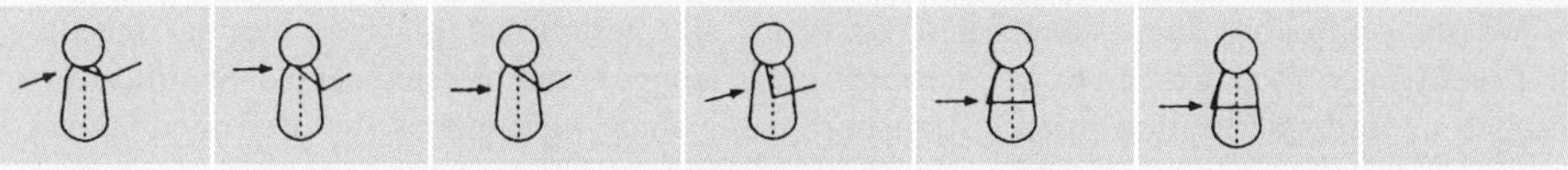								
Heel to ear 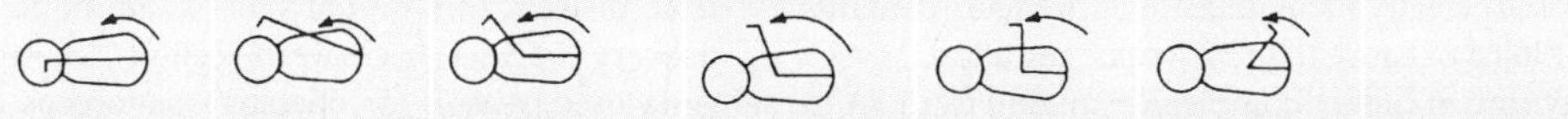								
					Total Neuromuscular Maturity Score			

Physical Maturity								
Physical Maturity Sign	**Score** −1	0	1	2	3	4	5	**Record Score Here**
Skin	Sticky, friable, transparent	Gelatinous, red, translucent	Smooth, pink, visible veins	Superficial peeling &/or rash; few veins	Cracking, pale areas; rare veins	Parchment, deep cracking; no vessels	Leathery, cracked, wrinkled	
Lanugo	None	Sparse	Abundant	Thinning	Bald areas	Mostly bald		
Plantar surface	Heel toe 40–50 mm: -1 < 40 mm: -2	> 50 mm: no crease	Faint red marks	Anterior transverse crease only	Creases anterior 2/3	Creases over entire sole		
Breast	Imperceptible	Barely perceptible	Flat areola; no bud	Stippled areola; 1- to 2-mm bud	Raised areola; 3- to 4-mm bud	Full areola; 5- to 10-mm bud		
Eye/Ear	Lids fused loosely: −1 tightly: −2	Lids open; pinna flat; stays folded	Slightly curved pinna; soft; slow recoil	Well-curved pinna; soft but ready recoil	Formed & firm instant recoil	Thick cartilage; ear stiff		
Genitals (male)	Scrotum flat, smooth	Scrotum empty; faint rugae	Testes in upper canal; rare rugae	Testes descending; few rugae	Testes down; good rugae	Testes pendulous; deep rugae		
Genitals (female)	Clitoris prominent & labia flat	Prominent clitoris & small labia minora	Prominent clitoris & enlarging minora	Majora & minora equally prominent	Majora large; minora small	Majora cover clitoris & minora		
						Total Physical Maturity Score		

Maturity Rating														
Maturity	Score	−10	-5	0	5	10	15	20	25	30	35	40	45	50
Rating	Weeks	20	22	24	26	28	30	32	34	36	38	40	42	44

[a]See text for a description of the clinical gestational age examination.

Reproduced, with permission, from Ballard JL et al: New Ballard Score, expanded to include extremely premature infants. J Pediatr 1991;119:417.

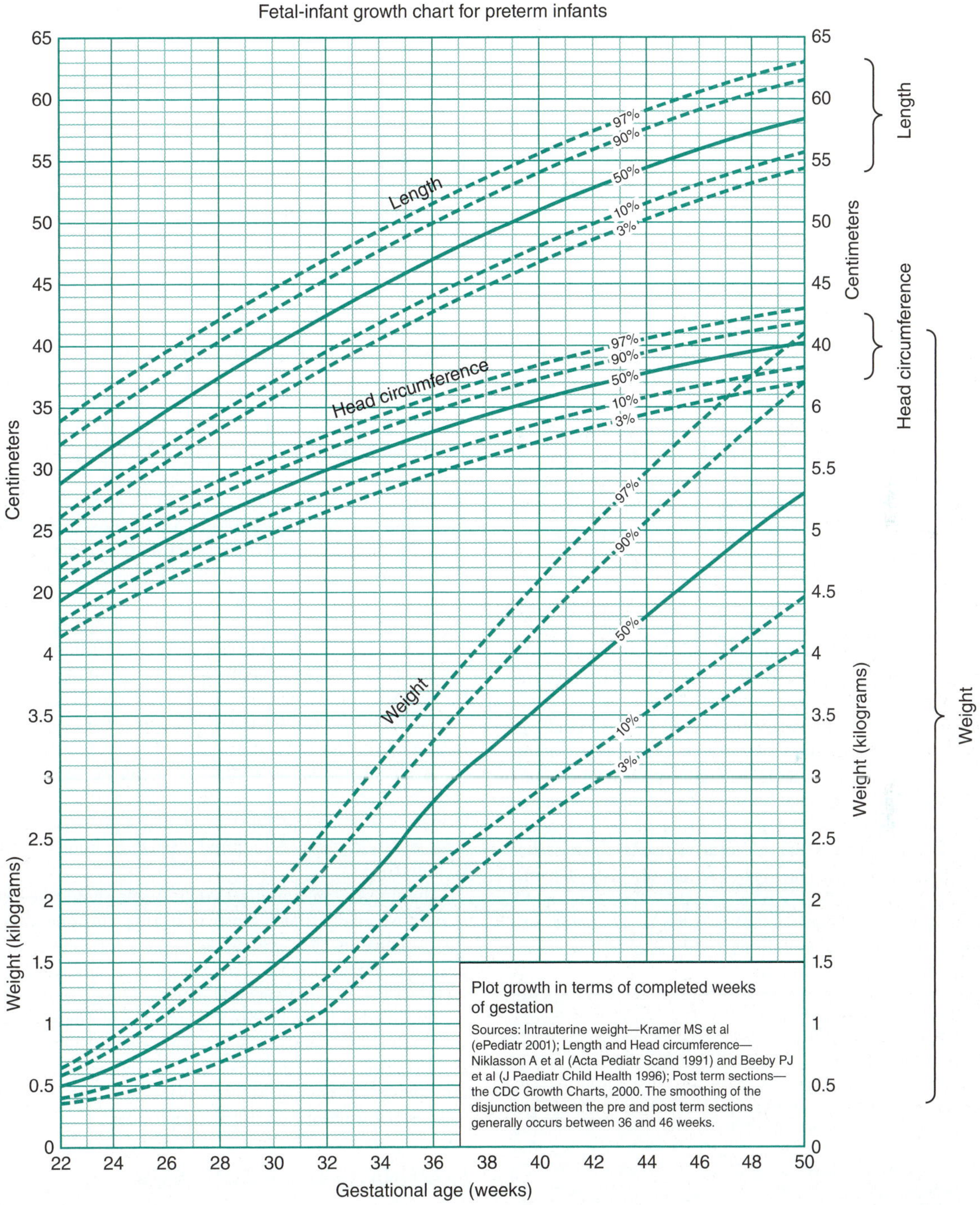

▲ **Figure 2–1.** Fetal-infant growth chart for weight, length, and head circumference. Sources: intrauterine weight (Kramer MS et al: ePediatr 2001), length and head circumference (Niklasson A et al: Acta Pediatr Scand 1991 and Beeby PJ et al: J Pediatr Child Health 1996), post term sections – CDC growth charts 2000. URL. http://www.biomedcentral.com/1471-2431/3/13.

normal neonates varies with race, maternal nutrition, access to obstetric care, and environmental factors such as altitude, smoking, and drug and alcohol use. Whenever possible, standards for newborn weight and gestational age based on local or regional data should be used. Birth weight related to gestational age is a screening tool that should be supplemented by clinical data when entertaining a diagnosis of IUGR or excessive fetal growth. These data include the infant's physical examination and other factors such as parental size and the birth weight–gestational age of siblings.

An important distinction, particularly in SGA infants, is whether a growth disorder is symmetrical (weight, length, and occipitofrontal circumference [OFC] all ≤ 10%) or asymmetrical (only weight ≤ 10%). Asymmetrical growth restriction implies a problem late in pregnancy, such as pregnancy-induced hypertension or placental insufficiency. Symmetrical growth restriction implies an event of early pregnancy: chromosomal abnormality, drug or alcohol use, or congenital viral infections (Table 2–2). In general, the outlook for normal growth and development is better in asymmetrically growth-restricted infants whose intrauterine brain growth has been spared.

The fact that SGA infants have fewer problems (such as respiratory distress syndrome) than AGA infants of the same birth weight but a lower gestational age has led to the misconception that SGA infants have accelerated maturation. SGA infants, when compared with AGA infants of the same gestational age, actually have increased morbidity and mortality rates.

Knowledge of birth weight in relation to gestational age allows anticipation of some neonatal problems. LGA infants are at risk for birth trauma; LGA infants of diabetic mothers are also at risk for hypoglycemia, polycythemia, congenital anomalies, cardiomyopathy, hyperbilirubinemia, and hypocalcemia. SGA infants are at risk for fetal distress during labor and delivery, polycythemia, hypoglycemia, and hypocalcemia.

Table 2–2. Causes of variations in neonatal size in relation to gestational age.

Infants large for gestational age
Infant of a diabetic mother
Infants small for gestational age
Asymmetrical
Placental insufficiency secondary to pregnancy-induced hypertension or other maternal vascular disease
Maternal age > 35 y
Poor weight gain during pregnancy
Multiple gestation
Symmetrical
Maternal drug abuse
Narcotics
Cocaine
Alcohol
Chromosomal abnormalities
Intrauterine viral infection (eg, cytomegalovirus)

American Academy of Pediatrics Committee on Fetus and Newborn: Levels of neonatal care. Pediatrics 2004;114:1341 [PMID: 15520119].

Leviton A et al: The wealth of information conveyed by gestational age. J Pediatr 2005;146:123 [PMID: 15644836].

Rosenberg A: The IUGR newborn. Semin Perinatol 2008;32:219 [PMID: 18482625].

EXAMINATION AT BIRTH

The extent of the newborn physical examination depends on the condition of the infant and the setting. Examination in the delivery room consists largely of observation plus auscultation of the chest and inspection for congenital anomalies and birth trauma. Major congenital anomalies occur in 1.5% of live births and account for 20%–25% of perinatal and neonatal deaths. Because infants are physically stressed during parturition, the delivery room examination should not be extensive. The Apgar score (Table 2–3) should be recorded at 1 and 5 minutes of age. In severely depressed infants, scores can be recorded out to 20 minutes. Although the 1- and 5-minute Apgar scores have almost no predictive value for long-term outcome, serial scores provide a useful description of the severity of perinatal depression and the response to resuscitative efforts.

Skin color is an indicator of cardiac output because of the normal high blood flow to the skin. Stress that triggers a catecholamine response redirects cardiac output away from the skin to preserve oxygen delivery to more critical organs. Cyanosis and pallor are thus two useful signs suggestive of inadequate cardiac output.

Skeletal examination at delivery serves to detect obvious congenital anomalies and to identify birth trauma, particularly in LGA infants or those born after a protracted second stage of labor where a fractured clavicle or humerus might be found.

The number of umbilical cord vessels should be determined. Normally, there are two arteries and one vein. In 1% of deliveries (5%–6% of twin deliveries), the cord has only one artery and one vein. This minor anomaly slightly increases the risk of associated defects. The placenta should be examined at delivery. Small placentas are always associated with small infants. The placental examination includes identification of membranes and vessels (particularly in multiple gestations) as well as placental infarcts or clots (placental abruption) on the maternal side.

EXAMINATION IN THE NURSERY

The purpose of the newborn examination is to identify abnormalities or anomalies that might impact the infant's well-being, and to evaluate for any acute illness or difficulty in the transition from intrauterine to extrauterine life. The examiner should have warm hands and a gentle approach. Start with observation, then auscultation of the chest, and then palpation of the abdomen. Examination of the eyes,

Table 2–3. Infant evaluation at birth—Apgar score.[a]

	Score		
	0	1	2
Heart rate	Absent	Slow (< 100)	> 100
Respiratory effort	Absent	Slow, irregular	Good, crying
Muscle tone	Limp	Some flexion	Active motion
Response to catheter in nostril[b]	No response	Grimace	Cough or sneeze
Color	Blue or pale	Body pink; extremities blue	Completely pink

[a]One minute and 5 minutes after complete birth of the infant (disregarding the cord and the placenta), the following objective signs should be observed and recorded.
[b]Tested after the oropharynx is clear.
Data from Apgar V et al: Evaluation of the newborn infant—Second report. JAMA 1958;168:1985.

ears, throat, and hips should be performed last, as these maneuvers are most disturbing to the infant. The heart rate should range from 120 to 160 beats/min and the respiratory rate from 30 to 60 breaths/min. Systolic blood pressure on day 1 ranges from 50 to 70 mm Hg and increases steadily during the first week of life. Blood pressure is influenced more significantly by perinatal asphyxia and mechanical ventilation than it is by gestational age. An irregularly irregular heart rate, usually caused by premature atrial contractions, is common, benign, and usually resolves in the first days of life.

Approximately 15%–20% of healthy newborns have one minor anomaly (a common variant that would not impact the infant's well-being; eg, a unilateral transverse palmar (simian) crease, or a single umbilical artery). Those with a minor anomaly have a 3% risk of an associated major anomaly. Approximately 0.8% of newborns have two minor anomalies, and 0.5% have three or more, with a risk of 10% and 20%, respectively, of also having a major malformation. Other common minor anomalies requiring no special investigation in healthy infants include preauricular pits, a shallow sacral dimple without other cutaneous abnormality within 2.5 cm of the anus, and three or fewer café au lait spots in a white infant or five or fewer in an African-American infant.

Skin

Observe for bruising, petechiae (common over the presenting part), meconium staining, and jaundice. Visible jaundice in the first 24 hours is never normal, and generally indicates either a hemolytic process, or a congenital hepatitis, either of which requires further evaluation. Peripheral cyanosis is commonly present when the extremities are cool or the infant is polycythemic. Generalized cyanosis merits immediate evaluation. Pallor may be caused by acute or chronic blood loss or by acidosis. In dark-skinned infants, pallor and cyanosis should be assessed in the lips, mouth, and nail beds. Plethora suggests polycythemia. Note the presence of vernix caseosa (a whitish, greasy material covering the body that decreases as term approaches) and lanugo (the fine hair covering the preterm infant's skin). Dry skin with cracking and peeling of the superficial layers is common in postterm infants. Edema may be generalized (hydrops) or localized (eg, on the dorsum of the feet in Turner syndrome). Check for birthmarks such as capillary hemangiomas (lower occiput, eyelids, and forehead) and mongolian spots (bluish-black pigmentation over the back and buttocks). There are many benign skin eruptions such as milia, miliaria, erythema toxicum, and pustular melanosis that are present in the newborn period. See Chapter 15 for a more in-depth description of these conditions.

Head

Check for cephalohematoma (a swelling over one or both parietal bones that is contained within suture lines) and caput succedaneum (edema of the scalp over the presenting part that crosses suture lines). Subgaleal hemorrhages (beneath the scalp) are uncommon but can cause extensive blood loss into this large potential space, resulting in hypovolemic shock. Skull fractures may be linear or depressed and may be associated with cephalohematoma. Check for the presence and size of the fontanelles. The anterior fontanelle varies from 1 to 4 cm in any direction; the posterior fontanelle should be less than 1 cm. A third fontanelle is a bony defect along the sagittal suture in the parietal bones and may be seen in syndromes, such as trisomy 21. Sutures should be freely mobile, but are often overriding just after birth. Craniosynostosis, a prematurely fused suture causing an abnormal cranial shape, is more easily diagnosed a few days or more after birth.

Face

Unusual facies may be associated with a specific syndrome. Bruising from birth trauma (especially with face presentation) and forceps application should be identified. Face presentation may cause soft tissue swelling around the nose and mouth and significant facial distortion. Facial nerve palsy is most obvious during crying; the unaffected side of the mouth moves normally, giving an asymmetric grimace.

Eyes

Subconjunctival hemorrhages are a frequent result of birth trauma. Less commonly, a corneal tear (presenting as a clouded cornea), or a hyphema (a layering of blood in the anterior chamber of the eye) may occur. Ophthalmologic consultation is indicated in such cases. Extraocular movements should be assessed. Occasional uncoordinated eye movements are common, but persistent irregular movements are abnormal. The iris should be inspected for abnormalities such as speckling (Brushfield spots seen in trisomy 21) and colobomas. Retinal red reflexes should be present and symmetrical. Dark spots, unilateral blunted red reflex, absent reflex, or a white reflex all require ophthalmologic evaluation. Leukokoria can be caused by glaucoma (cloudy cornea), cataract, or tumor (retinoblastoma). Infants with suspected or known congenital viral infection should have a retinoscopic examination with pupils dilated to look for chorioretinitis.

Nose

Examine the nose for size and shape. In-utero compression can cause deformities. Because infants younger than 1 month of age are obligate nose breathers, any nasal obstruction (eg, bilateral choanal atresia or stenosis) can cause respiratory distress. Unilateral choanal atresia can be diagnosed by occluding each naris, although patency is best checked by holding a cold metal surface (eg, a chilled scissor) under the nose, and observing the fog from both nares on the metal. Purulent nasal discharge at birth suggests congenital syphilis ("snuffles").

Ears

Malformed or malpositioned (low-set or posteriorly rotated) ears are often associated with other congenital anomalies. The tympanic membranes should be visualized. Preauricular pits and tags are common minor variants, and may be familial. Any external ear abnormality may be associated with hearing loss.

Mouth

Epithelial (Epstein) pearls are benign retention cysts along the gum margins and at the junction of the hard and soft palates. Natal teeth may be present and sometimes must be removed to prevent their aspiration. Check the integrity and shape of the palate for clefts and other abnormalities. A small mandible and tongue with cleft palate is seen with Pierre-Robin syndrome and can present as respiratory difficulty, as the tongue occludes the airway; prone positioning can be beneficial. A prominent tongue can be seen in trisomy 21 and Beckwith-Wiedemann syndrome. Excessive oral secretions suggest esophageal atresia or a swallowing disorder.

Neck

Redundant neck skin or webbing, with a low posterior hairline, is seen in Turner syndrome. Cervical sinus tracts may be seen as remnants of branchial clefts. Check for masses: mid-line (thyroglossal duct cysts), anterior to the sternocleidomastoid (branchial cleft cysts), within the sternocleidomastoid (hematoma and torticollis), and posterior to the sternocleidomastoid (cystic hygroma).

Chest & Lungs

Check for fractured clavicles (crepitus, bruising, and tenderness). Increased anteroposterior diameter (barrel chest) can be seen with aspiration syndromes. Check air entry bilaterally and the position of the mediastinum by locating the point of maximum cardiac impulse and assessment of heart tones. Decreased breath sounds with respiratory distress and a shift in the heart tones suggests pneumothorax (tension) or a space-occupying lesion (eg, diaphragmatic hernia). Pneumomediastinum causes muffled heart sounds. Expiratory grunting and decreased air entry are observed in hyaline membrane disease. Rales are not of clinical significance at this age.

Heart

Cardiac murmurs are common in the first hours and are most often benign; conversely, severe congenital heart disease in the newborn infant may be present with no murmur at all. The two most common presentations of heart disease in the newborn infant are (1) cyanosis and (2) congestive heart failure with abnormalities of pulses and perfusion. In hypoplastic left heart and critical aortic stenosis, pulses are diminished at all sites. In aortic coarctation and interrupted aortic arch, pulses are diminished in the lower extremities.

Abdomen

Check for tenderness, distention, and bowel sounds. If polyhydramnios was present or excessive oral secretions are noted, pass a soft catheter into the stomach to rule out esophageal atresia. Most abdominal masses in the newborn infant are associated with kidney disorders (eg, multicystic or dysplastic, and hydronephrosis). When the abdomen is relaxed, normal kidneys may be felt but are not prominent. A markedly scaphoid abdomen plus respiratory distress suggests diaphragmatic hernia. Absence of abdominal musculature (prune belly syndrome) may occur in association with renal abnormalities. The liver and spleen are superficial in the neonate and can be felt with light palpation. A distended bladder may be seen as well as palpated above the pubic symphysis.

Genitalia & Anus

Male and female genitals show characteristics according to gestational age (see Table 2–1). In the female infant during the first few days, a whitish vaginal discharge with or without blood is normal. Check the patency and location of the anus.

Skeleton

Check for obvious anomalies such as absence of a bone, club-foot, fusion or webbing of digits, and extra digits. Examine for hip dislocation by attempting to dislocate the femur posteriorly and then abducting the legs to relocate the femur noting a clunk as the femoral head relocates. Look for extremity fractures and for palsies (especially brachial plexus injuries) and evidence of spinal deformities (eg, scoliosis, cysts, sinuses, myelomeningocele). Arthrogryposis (multiple joint contractures) results from chronic limitation of movement in utero that may result from lack of amniotic fluid or from congenital neuromuscular disease.

Neurologic Examination

Normal newborns have reflexes that facilitate survival (eg, rooting and sucking reflexes), and sensory abilities (eg, hearing and smell) that allow them to recognize their mother soon after birth. Although the retina is well developed at birth, visual acuity is poor (20/400) because of a relatively immobile lens. Acuity improves rapidly over the first 6 months, with fixation and tracking becoming well developed by 2 months.

Observe the newborn's resting tone. Normal term newborns should exhibit flexion of the upper and lower extremities and symmetrical spontaneous movements. Extension of the extremities should result in spontaneous recoil to the flexed position. Assess the character of the cry; a high-pitched cry with or without hypotonia may indicate disease of the central nervous system (CNS) such as hemorrhage or infection, a congenital neuromuscular disorder, or systemic disease. Check the following newborn reflexes:

1. Sucking reflex: The newborn sucks in response to a nipple in the mouth; observed by 14 weeks' gestation.
2. Rooting reflex: Head turns to the side of a facial stimulus, present by 28 weeks' gestation.
3. Traction response: The infant is pulled by the arms to a sitting position. Initially, the head lags, then with active flexion, comes to the midline briefly before falling forward.
4. Palmar grasp: Evident with the placement of the examiner's finger in the newborn's palm; develops by 28 weeks' gestation and disappears by age 4 months.
5. Deep tendon reflexes: A few beats of ankle clonus and an upgoing Babinski reflex may be normal.
6. Moro (startle) reflex: Hold the infant supine while supporting the head. Allow the head to drop 1–2 cm suddenly. The arms will abduct at the shoulder and extend at the elbow with spreading of the fingers. Adduction with flexion will follow. This reflex develops by 28 weeks' gestation (incomplete) and disappears by age 3 months.
7. Tonic neck reflex: Turn the infant's head to one side; the arm and leg on that side will extend while the opposite arm and leg flex ("fencing position"). This reflex disappears by age 8 months.

Ben-Sira L et al: Low-risk lumbar skin stigmata in infants: the role of ultrasound screening. J Pediatr 2009;155:864 [PMID: 19643444].

Bishara N, Clericuzio CL: Common dysmorphic syndromes in the NICU. NeoReviews 2008;9:e29.

Drolet BA et al: Prospective study of spinal anomalies in children with infantile hemangiomas of the lumbosacral skin. J Pediatr 2010;157:789 [PMID: 20828712].

CARE OF THE WELL NEONATE

The primary responsibility of the Level 1 nursery is care of the well neonate—promoting mother-infant bonding, establishing feeding, and teaching the basics of newborn care. Staff must monitor infants for signs and symptoms of illness, including temperature instability, change in activity, refusal to feed, pallor, cyanosis, early or excessive jaundice, tachypnea, respiratory distress, delayed (beyond 24 hours) first stool or first void, and bilious vomiting. Several preventive measures are routine in the normal newborn nursery.

Prophylactic erythromycin ointment is applied to the eyes within 1 hour of birth to prevent gonococcal ophthalmia. Vitamin K (1 mg) is given intramuscularly or subcutaneously within 4 hours of birth to prevent hemorrhagic disease of the newborn.

All infants should receive hepatitis B vaccine. Both hepatitis B vaccine and hepatitis B immune globulin (HBIG) are administered if the mother is positive for hepatitis B surface antigen (HBsAg). If maternal HBsAg status is unknown, vaccine should be given before 12 hours of age, maternal blood should be tested for HBsAg, and HBIG should be given to the neonate before 7 days of age if the test is positive.

Cord blood is collected from all infants at birth and can be used for blood typing and Coombs testing if the mother is type O or Rh-negative to help assess the risk for development of jaundice.

Bedside glucose testing should be performed in infants at risk for hypoglycemia (infants of diabetic mothers, preterm, SGA, LGA, or stressed infants). Values below 45 mg/dL should be confirmed by laboratory blood glucose testing and treated. Hematocrit should be measured at age 3–6 hours in infants at risk for or those who have symptoms of polycythemia or anemia (see section on Hematologic Disorders).

State-sponsored newborn genetic screens (for inborn errors of metabolism such as phenylketonuria [PKU], galactosemia, sickle cell disease, hypothyroidism, congenital adrenal hyperplasia, and cystic fibrosis) are performed prior to discharge, after 24–48 hours of age if possible. In many states, a repeat test is required at 8–14 days of age because the PKU test may be falsely negative when obtained before 48 hours of age. Not all state-mandated screens include the same panel of diseases. The most recent addition in many states is an expanded screen that tests for other inborn errors of metabolism such as fatty acid oxidation defects and amino or organic acid disorders. Some states are also now beginning to screen for severe combined immunodeficiency syndrome.

Infants should routinely be positioned supine to minimize the risk of sudden infant death syndrome (SIDS). Prone positioning is contraindicated unless there are compelling clinical reasons for that position. Bed sharing with adults and prone positioning are associated with increased risk of SIDS.

FEEDING THE WELL NEONATE

A neonate is ready for feeding if he or she is (1) alert and vigorous, (2) has no abdominal distention, (3) has good bowel sounds, and (4) has a normal hunger cry. These signs usually occur within 6 hours after birth, but fetal distress or traumatic delivery may prolong this period. The healthy full-term infant should be allowed to feed every 2–5 hours on demand. The first breast feeding may occur in the delivery room. For formula-fed infants, the first feeding usually occurs by 3 hours of life. The feeding volume generally increases from 0.5 to 1 oz per feeding initially to 1.5–2 oz per feeding on day 3. By day 3, the average full-term newborn takes about 100 mL/kg/d of milk.

A wide range of infant formulas satisfy the nutritional needs of most neonates. Breast milk is the standard on which formulas are based (see Chapter 11). Despite low concentrations of several vitamins and minerals in breast milk, bio-availability is high. All the necessary nutrients, vitamins, minerals, and water are provided by human milk for the first 6 months of life except vitamin K (1 mg IM is administered at birth), vitamin D (400 IU/d for all infants beginning shortly after birth), and vitamin B_{12} and zinc (if the mother is a strict vegetarian and takes no supplements). Other advantages of breast milk include (1) immunologic, antimicrobial, and anti-inflammatory factors such as immunoglobulin A (IgA) and cellular, protein, and enzymatic components that decrease the incidence of upper respiratory and gastrointestinal (GI) infections; (2) possible decreased frequency and severity of childhood eczema and asthma; (3) improved mother-infant bonding; and (4) improved neurodevelopmental outcome.

Although about 70% of mothers in the United States start by breast feeding, only 33% continue to do so at 6 months. Hospital practices that facilitate successful initiation of breast feeding include rooming-in, nursing on demand, and avoiding unnecessary supplemental formula. Nursery staff must be trained to recognize problems associated with breast feeding and provide help and support for mothers in the hospital. An experienced professional should observe and assist with several feedings to document good latch-on. Good latch-on is important in preventing the common problems of sore nipples, unsatisfied infants, breast engorgement, poor milk supply, and hyperbilirubinemia.

Table 2–4 presents guidelines the nursing mother and health care provider can use to assess successful breast feeding.

Abrams SA: Dietary guidelines for calcium and vitamin D: a new era. Pediatrics 2011;127:566 [PMID: 21339264].

Kinney HC, Thach BT: The sudden infant death syndrome. N Engl J Med 2009;361:795 [PMID: 19692691].

Martinez JA, Ballew MP: Infant formulas. Pediatr Rev 2011;32:179 [PMID: 21536776]

Wagner CL, Greer FR: Section on Breastfeeding and Committee on Nutrition: Prevention of rickets and vitamin D deficiency in infants, children, and adolescents. Pediatrics 2008;122:1142 [PMID: 18977996].

EARLY DISCHARGE OF THE NEWBORN INFANT

Discharge at 24–36 hours of age is safe and appropriate for some newborns if there are no contraindications (Table 2–5) and if a follow-up visit within 48 hours is ensured. Most infants with cardiac, respiratory, or infectious disorders are identified in the first 12–24 hours of life. The exception may be the infant treated intrapartum with antibiotic prophylaxis for maternal group B streptococcal (GBS) colonization or infection. The Centers for Disease Control and Prevention (CDC) and the American Academy of Pediatrics (AAP) recommend that such infants be observed in hospital for 48 hours if they received no or inadequate intrapartum antibiotic prophylaxis (< 4 hours prior to delivery, or drug other than ampicillin, penicillin, or cefazolin). Hospital observation beyond 24 hours may not be necessary for well appearing full-term infants who received adequate intrapartum chemoprophylaxis (penicillin, ampicillin, or cefazolin ≥ 4 hours prior to delivery), and for whom ready access to medical care can be ensured if needed. Other problems, such as jaundice and breast-feeding problems, typically occur after 48 hours and can usually be dealt with on an out-patient basis.

The AAP recommends a follow-up visit within 48 hours for all newborns discharged before 72 hours of age. Infants who are small or late preterm—especially if breast feeding—are at particular risk for inadequate intake; the early visit is especially important for these infants. Suggested guidelines for the follow-up interview and physical examination are presented in Table 2–6. The optimal timing of discharge must be determined in each case based on medical, social, and financial factors.

Table 2–4. Guidelines for successful breast feeding.

	First 8 Hours	First 8–24 Hours	Day 2	Day 3	Day 4	Day 5	Day 6 Onward
Milk supply	You may be able to express a few drops of milk.		Milk should come in between the second and fourth days.			Milk should be in. Breasts may be firm or leak milk.	Breasts should feel softer after feedings.
Baby's activity	Baby is usually wide-awake in the first hour of life. Put baby to breast within 30 min after birth.	Wake up your baby. Babies may not wake up on their own to feed.	Baby should be more cooperative and less sleepy.	Look for early feeding cues such as rooting, lip smacking, and hands to face.			Baby should appear satisfied after feedings.
Feeding routine	Baby may go into a deep sleep 2–4 h after birth.	Use chart to write down time of each feeding. Feed your baby every 1–4 h or as often as wanted—at least 8–12 times a day.				May go one longer interval (up to 5 h between feeds) in a 24-h period.	
Breast feeding	Baby will wake up and be alert and responsive for several more hours after initial deep sleep.	As long as the mother is comfortable, nurse at both breasts as long as baby is actively sucking.	Try to nurse both sides each feeding, aiming at 10 min per side. Expect some nipple tenderness.	Consider hand expressing or pumping a few drops of milk to soften the nipple if the breast is too firm for the baby to latch on.	Nurse a minimum of 10–30 min per side every feeding for the first few weeks of life. Once milk supply is well established, allow baby to finish the first breast before offering the second.		Mother's nipple tenderness is improving or is gone.
Baby's urine output		Baby must have a minimum of one wet diaper in the first 24 h.	Baby must have at least one wet diaper every 8–11 h.	You should see an increase in wet diapers (up to four to six) in 24 h.	Baby's urine should be light yellow.	Baby should have six to eight wet diapers per day of colorless or light yellow urine.	
Baby's stool		Baby may have a very dark (meconium) stool.	Baby may have a second very dark (meconium) stool.	Baby's stools should be in transition from black-green to yellow.		Baby should have three or four yellow, seedy stools a day.	The number of stools may decrease gradually after 4–6 wk.

Modified, with permission, from Gabrielski L: Lactation support services. Childrens Hospital Colorado, 1999.

Table 2–5. Contraindications to early newborn discharge.

Contraindications to early newborn discharge
1. Jaundice ≤ 24 h
2. High risk for infection (eg, maternal chorioamnionitis); discharge allowed after 24 h with a normal transition
3. Known or suspected narcotic addiction or withdrawal
4. Physical defects requiring evaluation
5. Oral defects (clefts, micrognathia)

Relative contraindications to early newborn discharge (infants at high risk for feeding failure, excessive jaundice)
1. Prematurity or early term infant (< 38 weeks' gestation)
2. Birth weight < 2700 g (6 lb)
3. Infant difficult to arouse for feeding; not demanding regularly in nursery
4. Medical or neurologic problems that interfere with feeding (Down syndrome, hypotonia, cardiac problems)
5. Twins or higher multiples
6. ABO blood group incompatibility or severe jaundice in previous child
7. Mother whose previous breast-fed infant gained weight poorly
8. Mother with breast surgery involving periareolar areas (if attempting to nurse)

Table 2–6. Guidelines for early outpatient follow-up evaluation.

History

Rhythmic sucking and audible swallowing for at least 10 min total per feeding?

Infant wakes and demands to feed every 2-3 h (at least 8-10 feedings per 24 h)?

Do breasts feel full before feedings, and softer after?

Are there at least 6 noticeably wet diapers per 24 h?

Are there yellow bowel movements (no longer meconium)—at least 4 per 24 h?

Is infant still acting hungry after nursing (frequently sucks hands, rooting)?

Physical assessment

Weight, unclothed: should not be more than 8%-10% below birth weight

Extent and severity of jaundice

Assessment of hydration, alertness, general well-being

Cardiovascular examination: murmurs, brachial and femoral pulses, respirations

CIRCUMCISION

Circumcision is an elective procedure to be performed only in healthy, stable infants. The procedure has medical benefits, including prevention of phimosis, paraphimosis, balanoposthitis, and urinary tract infection. Important later benefits of circumcision include decreased incidence of penile cancer, decreased incidence of sexually transmitted diseases (including HIV), and decreased incidence of cervical cancer in female sexual partners. Most parental decisions regarding circumcision are religious and social, not medical. The risks of circumcision include local infection, bleeding, removal of too much skin, and urethral injury. The combined incidence of complications is less than 1%. Local anesthesia by dorsal penile nerve block or circumferential ring block using 1% lidocaine without epinephrine, or topical anesthetic cream are safe and effective methods that should always be used. Techniques allowing visualization of the glans throughout the procedure (Plastibell and Gomco clamp) are preferred to blind techniques (Mogen clamp) as occasional amputation of the glans occurs with the latter technique. Circumcision is contraindicated in infants with genital abnormalities (eg, hypospadias). A coagulation screen should be performed prior to the procedure in infants with a family history of serious bleeding disorders.

HEARING SCREENING

Normal hearing is critical to normal language development. Significant bilateral hearing loss is present in 1–3 infants per 1000 well neonates and in 2–4 per 100 neonates in the intensive care unit population. Infants should be screened for hearing loss by auditory brainstem evoked responses or evoked otoacoustic emissions as early as possible because up to 40% of hearing loss will be missed by risk analysis alone. Primary care providers and parents should be advised of the possibility of hearing loss and offered immediate referral in suspect cases. With the use of universal screening, the average age at which hearing loss is confirmed has dropped from 24–30 months to 2–3 months. If remediation is begun by 6 months, language and social development are commensurate with physical development.

American Academy of Pediatrics: Committee on the Fetus and Newborn: Policy statement-Hospital stay for healthy term newborns. Pediatrics 2010;125:405 [PMID: 20100744].

Berg AL et al: Hearing screening in a well infant nursery: profile of automated ABR-fail/OAE-pass. Pediatrics 2011;127:269 [PMID: 21262886].

Flynn P et al: Male circumcision for prevention of HIV and other sexually transmitted diseases. Pediatrics 2007;119:821 [PMID: 17403855].

Prevention of perinatal Group B Streptococcal disease revised guidelines from CDC, 2010. MMWR 2010;59:1-32 [PMID: 21088663].

US Preventive Services Task Force: Universal screening for hearing loss in newborns: US Preventive Services Task Force recommendation statement. Pediatrics 2008;122:143 [PMID: 18595997].

COMMON PROBLEMS IN THE TERM NEWBORN

NEONATAL JAUNDICE

General Considerations

Sixty-five percent of newborns develop visible jaundice with a total serum bilirubin (TSB) level higher than 6 mg/dL during the first week of life. Bilirubin, a potent antioxidant and peroxyl scavenger, may protect the normal newborn, who is deficient in antioxidants such as vitamin E, catalase, and super-oxide dismutase, from oxygen toxicity in the first days of life. Approximately 8%–10% of newborns develop excessive hyper-bilirubinemia (TSB > 17 mg/dL), and 1%–2% have TSB above 20 mg/dL. Extremely high and potentially dangerous TSB levels are rare. Approximately 1 in 700 infants have TSB higher than 25 mg/dL, and 1 in 10,000 have TSB above 30 mg/dL. Such high levels can cause kernicterus, characterized by injury to the basal ganglia and brainstem.

Kernicterus caused by hyperbilirubinemia was common in neonates with Rh-isoimmunization until the institution of exchange transfusion for affected infants and postpartum high-titer Rho (D) immune globulin treatment to prevent sensitization of Rh-negative mothers. For several decades after the introduction of exchange transfusion and phototherapy aimed at keeping the neonate's TSB below 20 mg/dL, there were no reported cases of kernicterus in the United States. Since the early 1990s, however, there has been a reappearance of kernicterus, with more than 120 cases reported. Common factors in the recent cases are newborn discharge before 48 hours (all but one), breast feeding (100%), delayed measurement of TSB, unrecognized hemolysis, lack of early post discharge follow-up, and failure to recognize the early symptoms of bilirubin encephalopathy.

Bilirubin is produced by the breakdown of heme (iron protoporphyrin) in the reticuloendothelial system and bone marrow. Heme is cleaved by heme oxygenase to iron, which is conserved; carbon monoxide, which is exhaled; and biliverdin, which is converted to bilirubin by bilirubin reductase. Each gram of hemoglobin yields 34 mg of bilirubin (1 mg/dL = 17.2 mmol/L of bilirubin). This unconjugated bilirubin is bound to albumin and carried to the liver, where it is taken up by hepatocytes. In the presence of the enzyme uridyldiphosphoglucuronyl transferase (UDPGT; glucuronyl transferase), bilirubin is conjugated to one or two glucuronide molecules. Conjugated bilirubin is then excreted through the bile to the intestine. In the presence of normal gut flora, conjugated bilirubin is metabolized to stercobilins and excreted in the stool. Absence of gut flora and slow GI motility, both characteristics of the newborn, cause stasis of conjugated bilirubin in the intestinal lumen, where mucosal β-glucuronidase removes the glucuronide molecules and leaves unconjugated bilirubin to be reabsorbed (enterohepatic circulation).

Excess accumulation of bilirubin in blood depends on both the rate of bilirubin production and the rate of excretion. It is best determined by reference to an hour-specific TSB level above the 95th percentile for age in hours (Figure 2–2).

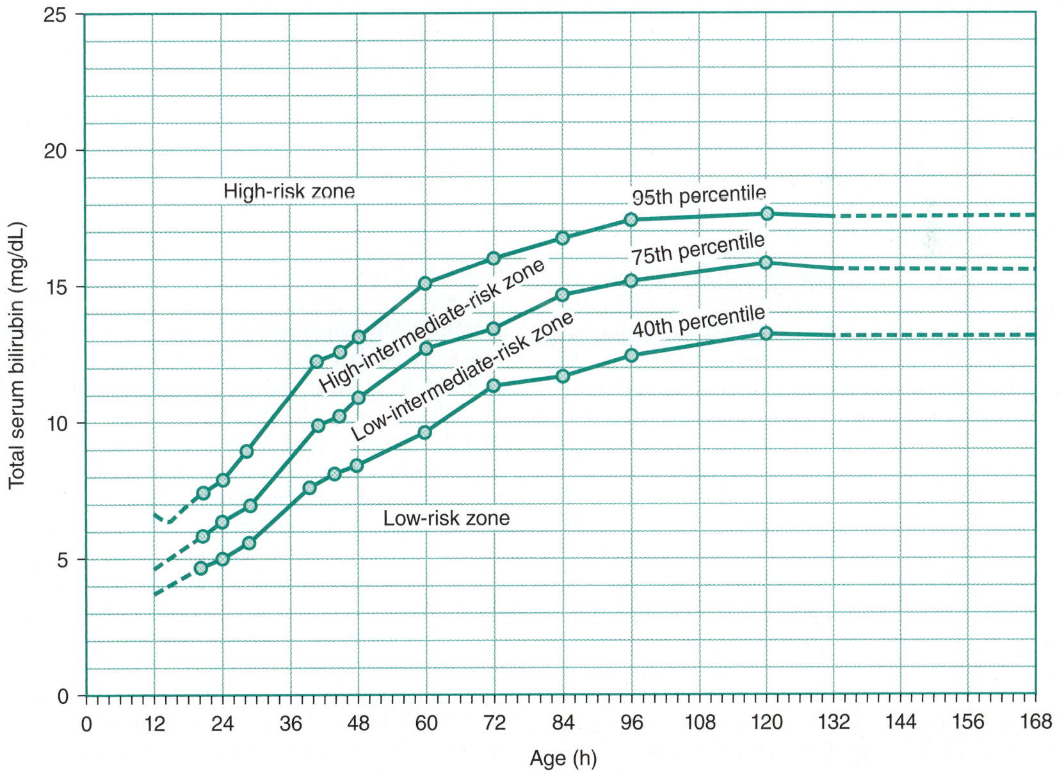

▲ **Figure 2–2.** Risk designation of full-term and near-term newborns based on their hour-specific bilirubin values. (Reproduced, with permission, from Bhutani VK et al: Predictive ability of a predischarge hour-specific serum bilirubin test for subsequent significant hyperbilirubinemia in healthy term and near-term newborns. Pediatrics 1999;103:6.)

1. Physiologic Jaundice

ESSENTIALS OF DIAGNOSIS & TYPICAL FEATURES

- Visible jaundice appearing after 24 hours of age.
- Total bilirubin rises by < 5 mg/dL (86 mmol/L) per day.
- Peak bilirubin occurs at 3–5 days of age, with a total bilirubin of no more than 15 mg/dL (258 mmol/L).
- Visible jaundice resolves by 1 week in the full-term infant and by 2 weeks in the preterm infant.

Factors contributing to physiologic jaundice in neonates include low UDPGT activity, relatively high red cell mass, absence of intestinal flora, slow intestinal motility, and increased enterohepatic circulation of bilirubin in the first days of life. Hyperbilirubinemia outside of the ranges noted in Figure 2–2 is not physiologic and requires further evaluation.

2. Pathologic Unconjugated Hyperbilirubinemia

Pathologic unconjugated hyperbilirubinemia can be grouped into two main categories: overproduction of bilirubin or decreased conjugation of bilirubin (Table 2–7). The TSB is a reflection of the balance between these processes. Visible jaundice with a TSB greater than 5 mg/dL before 24 hours of age is most commonly a result of significant hemolysis.

Table 2–7. Causes of pathologic unconjugated hyperbilirubinemia.

Overproduction of bilirubin
1. Hemolytic causes of increased bilirubin production (reticulocyte count elevated)
a. Immune-mediated: positive direct antibody (DAT, Coombs) test
• ABO blood group incompatibility, Rh incompatibility, minor blood group antigen incompatibility
b. Nonimmune: negative direct antibody (DAT, Coombs) test
• Abnormal red cell shapes: spherocytosis, elliptocytosis, pyknocytosis, stomatocytosis
• Red cell enzyme abnormalities: glucose-6-phosphate dehydrogenase deficiency, pyruvate kinase deficiency, hexokinase deficiency, other metabolic defects
c. Patients with bacterial or viral sepsis
2. Nonhemolytic causes of increased bilirubin production (reticulocyte count normal)
a. Extravascular hemorrhage: cephalohematoma, extensive bruising, intracranial hemorrhage
b. Polycythemia
c. Exaggerated enterohepatic circulation of bilirubin: bowel obstruction, functional ileus
d. Breast feeding–associated jaundice (inadequate intake of breast milk causing exaggerated enterohepatic circulation of bilirubin)
Decreased rate of conjugation
1. Crigler-Najjar syndrome (rare, severe)
a. Type I glucuronyl transferase deficiency, autosomal-recessive
b. Type II glucuronyl transferase deficiency, autosomal-dominant
2. Gilbert syndrome (common, milder)
3. Hypothyroidism

A. Increased Bilirubin Production

Increased bilirubin production is caused by excessive destruction of neonatal red blood cells. Destruction may be mediated by maternal antibodies (Coombs test–positive), or may be due to abnormal red cell membranes (spherocytosis), or abnormal red cell enzymes (glucose-6-phosphate dehydrogenase [G6PD] deficiency) causing decreased red cell life span not mediated by antibodies. Antibodies can be directed against the major blood group antigens (type A or type B infant of a type O mother) or the antigens of the Rh-system (D, E, C, d, e, c, Kell, Duffy, and others).

1. Antibody-mediated hemolysis (Coombs test–positive)

A. ABO BLOOD GROUP INCOMPATIBILITY—This finding can accompany any pregnancy in a type O mother. Hemolysis is usually mild, but the severity is unpredictable because of variability in the amount of naturally occurring maternal anti-A or anti-B IgG antibodies. Although 20% of pregnancies are "set-ups" for ABO incompatibility (mother O, infant A or B), only 33% of infants in such cases have a positive direct Coombs test and only 20% of these develop jaundice that requires therapy. Since maternal antibodies may persist for several months after birth, the newborn may become progressively more anemic over the first few weeks of life, occasionally to the point of requiring transfusion.

B. RH-ISOIMMUNIZATION—This hemolytic process is less common, more severe, and more predictable than ABO incompatibility. The severity increases with each immunized pregnancy because of an anamnestic maternal IgG antibody response. Most Rh-disease can be prevented by giving high-titer Rho (D) immune globulin to the Rh-negative woman after invasive procedures during pregnancy or after miscarriage, abortion, or delivery of an Rh-positive infant. Affected neonates are often anemic at birth, and continued hemolysis rapidly causes hyperbilirubinemia and more severe anemia. The most severe form of Rh-isoimmunization, erythroblastosis fetalis, is characterized by life-threatening anemia, generalized edema, and fetal or neonatal heart failure. Without ante-natal intervention, fetal or neonatal death often results. The cornerstone of antenatal management is transfusion of the fetus with Rh-negative cells, either directly into the umbilical vein or into the fetal abdominal cavity. Phototherapy is usually started in these infants upon delivery, with exchange transfusion frequently needed. Intravenous immune globulin (IVIG; 0.5–1 g/kg) given to the infant as soon as the diagnosis is made may decrease the need for exchange transfusion. Ongoing hemolysis occurs until all maternal antibodies are gone;

therefore, these infants require monitoring for 2–3 months for recurrent anemia severe enough to require transfusion.

2. Nonimmune hemolysis (Coombs test-negative)

A. HEREDITARY SPHEROCYTOSIS—This condition is the most common of the red cell membrane defects and causes hemolysis by decreasing red cell deformability. Affected infants may have hyperbilirubinemia severe enough to require exchange transfusion. Splenomegaly may be present. Diagnosis is suspected by peripheral blood smear and family history. See Chapter 30 for a more in-depth discussion.

B. G6PD DEFICIENCY—This condition is the most common **red cell enzyme defect** causing hemolysis, especially in infants of African, Mediterranean, or Asian descent. Onset of jaundice is often later than in isoimmune hemolytic disease, toward 1 week of age. The role of G6PD deficiency in neonatal jaundice is probably underestimated as up to 10%–13% of African Americans are G6PD-deficient. Although the disorder is X-linked, female heterozygotes are also at increased risk of hyperbilirubinemia due to X-chromosome inactivation. In most cases, no triggering agent for hemolysis is found in the newborn. Rather, some infants who develop severe jaundice with G6PD deficiency have been found also to have Gilbert syndrome (see below). Their increased bilirubin production is further exaggerated by a decreased rate of bilirubin conjugation. Since G6PD enzyme activity is high in reticulocytes, neonates with a large number of reticulocytes may have falsely normal enzyme tests. A low G6PD level should always raise suspicions. Repeat testing in suspect cases with initially normal results is indicated at 2–3 months of age. Please also see Chapter 30 for more details.

3. Nonhemolytic increased bilirubin production— **Enclosed hemorrhage**, such as cephalohematoma, intracranial hemorrhage, or extensive bruising in the skin, can lead to jaundice. **Polycythemia** leads to jaundice by increased red cell mass, with increased numbers of cells reaching senescence daily. Bowel obstruction, functional or mechanical, leads to an increased enterohepatic circulation of bilirubin.

B. Decreased Rate of Conjugation

1. UDPGT deficiency: Crigler-Najjar syndrome type I (complete deficiency, autosomal recessive) and type II (partial deficiency, autosomal dominant)—These rare conditions result from mutations in the exon or encoding region of the UDPGT gene that cause complete or nearly complete absence of enzyme activity. Both can cause severe unconjugated hyperbilirubinemia, bilirubin encephalopathy, and death if untreated. In type II, the enzyme can be induced with phenobarbital, which may lower bilirubin levels by 30%–80%. Liver transplantation is curative.

2. Gilbert syndrome—This is a common mild autosomal dominant disorder characterized by decreased hepatic UDPGT activity caused by genetic polymorphism at the promoter region of the UDPGT gene. Approximately 9% of the population is homozygous, and 42% is heterozygous for this abnormality, with a gene frequency of 0.3. Affected individuals tend to develop hyperbilirubinemia in the presence of conditions that increase bilirubin load, including G6PD deficiency. They are also more likely to have prolonged neonatal jaundice and breast-milk jaundice.

C. Hyperbilirubinemia Caused by Unknown or Multiple Factors

1. Racial differences—Asians (23%) are more likely than whites (10%–13%) or African Americans (4%) to have a peak neonatal TSB greater than 12 mg/dL (206 mmol/L). It is likely that these differences result from racial variations in prevalence of UDPGT gene polymorphisms or associated G6PD deficiency.

2. Prematurity—Premature infants often have poor enteral intake, delayed stooling, and increased enterohepatic circulation, as well as a shorter red cell life. Infants at 35–36 weeks' gestation are 13 times more likely than term infants to be readmitted for hyperbilirubinemia. Even early-term infants (37–38 weeks' gestation) are four times more likely than term neonates to have TSB greater than 13 mg/dL (224 mmol/L).

3. Breast feeding and jaundice

A. BREAST-MILK JAUNDICE—Unconjugated hyperbilirubinemia lasting until 2–3 months of age is common in breast-fed infants. An increased prevalence of the Gilbert syndrome promoter polymorphism is likely involved. Moderate unconjugated hyperbilirubinemia for 6–12 weeks in a thriving breast-fed infant without evidence of hemolysis, hypothyroidism, or other disease strongly suggests this diagnosis.

B. BREAST FEEDING–ASSOCIATED JAUNDICE—This common condition has also been called "lack-of-breast-milk" jaundice. Breast-fed infants have a higher incidence (9%) of unconjugated serum bilirubin levels greater than 13 mg/dL (224 mmol/L) than do formula-fed infants (2%) and are more likely to have TSB greater than 15 mg/dL (258 mmol/L) than formula-fed infants (2% vs 0.3%). The pathogenesis is probably poor enteral intake and increased enterohepatic circulation. There is no apparent increase in bilirubin production as measured by carbon monoxide exhalation. Although rarely severe enough to cause bilirubin encephalopathy, nearly 100% of the infants with kernicterus reported over the past 20 years were exclusively breast fed, and in 50%, breast feeding was the only known risk factor. Excessive jaundice should be considered a possible sign of failure to establish an adequate milk supply, and should prompt specific inquiries (Table 2–8). If intake is inadequate, the infant should receive supplemental formula and the mother should be instructed to nurse more frequently and to use an electric breast pump every 2 hours to enhance milk production. Consultation with a lactation specialist should be considered. Because hospital discharge of normal newborns occurs before the milk supply is established and before jaundice peaks, a follow-up visit 2 days

Table 2–8. Signs of inadequate breast-milk intake.

Weight loss of > 8%–10% from birth
Fewer than six noticeably wet diapers per 24 h by day 3–4
Fewer than four stools per day, or still meconium, by day 3–4
Nursing fewer than eight times per 24 h, or for less than 10 min each feeding

after discharge is recommended by the AAP to evaluate adequacy of intake and degree of jaundice.

3. Bilirubin Toxicity

Unconjugated bilirubin anion is the agent of bilirubin neurotoxicity. The anion binds to the phospholipids (gangliosides) of neuronal plasma membranes causing injury, which then allows more anion to enter the neuron. Intracellular bilirubin anion binds to the membrane phospholipids of subcellular organelles, causing impaired energy metabolism and cell death. The blood-brain barrier undoubtedly has a role in protecting the infant from brain damage, but its integrity is impossible to measure clinically. The amount of albumin available to bind the unconjugated bilirubin anion and the presence of other anions that may displace bilirubin from albumin-binding sites are also important. It is unknown whether there is a fixed level of bilirubin above which brain damage always occurs. The term *kernicterus* describes the pathologic finding of staining of basal ganglia and brainstem nuclei, as well as the clinical syndrome of chronic brain injury due to hyperbilirubinemia. The term *acute bilirubin encephalopathy* describes the signs and symptoms of evolving brain injury in the newborn.

The risk of bilirubin encephalopathy is small in healthy, term neonates even at bilirubin levels of 25–30 mg/dL (430–516 mmol/L). Risk depends on the duration of hyper-bilirubinemia, the concentration of serum albumin, associated illness, acidosis, and the concentrations of competing anions such as sulfisoxazole and ceftriaxone. Premature infants are at greater risk than term infants because of the greater frequency of associated illness affecting the integrity of the blood-brain barrier, reduced albumin levels, and decreased affinity of albumin-binding sites. For these reasons, the "exchange level" (the level at which bilirubin encephalopathy is thought likely to occur) in premature infants may be lower than that of a term infant.

4. Acute Bilirubin Encephalopathy

ESSENTIALS OF DIAGNOSIS & TYPICAL FEATURES

- Lethargy, poor feeding.
- Irritability, high-pitched cry.
- Arching of the neck (retrocollis) and trunk (opisthotonos).
- Apnea, seizures, coma (late).

Newborn infants with evolving acute bilirubin encephalopathy may be described as "sleepy and not interested in feeding." Although these symptoms are nonspecific, they are also the earliest signs of acute bilirubin encephalopathy and should trigger, in the jaundiced infant, a detailed evaluation of the birth and postnatal history, feeding and elimination history, an urgent assessment for signs of bilirubin-induced neurologic dysfunction (BIND), and a TSB and albumin measurement. A scoring system has been proposed (Table 2–9) to monitor the severity and progression of bilirubin encephalopathy. A score of 4–6 indicates progressive encephalopathy likely to be

Table 2–9. BIND scoring system.

	1 Point (Nonspecific, Subtle)	2 Points (Progressive Toxicity)	3 Points (Advanced Toxicity)
Mental status	Sleepy, poor feeding	Lethargy + irritability	Semi-coma, seizures, apnea
Muscle tone	Slight decrease	Hypertonia or hypotonia, depending on arousal state **or** Mild arching	Markedly increased (opisthotonus) or decreased **or** Bicycling
Cry	High-pitched	Shrill	Inconsolable

BIND, bilirubin-induced neurologic dysfunction.

Adapted, with permission, from Bhutani VK, Johnson LH, Keren R: Treating acute bilirubin encephalopathy—before it's too late. Contemp Pediatr 2005;22:57.

Correlation between TSB level and neurotoxicity is poor. Although 65% of recently reported cases of kernicterus had TSB levels above 35 mg/dL, 15% had levels below 30 mg/dL, and 8% were below 25 mg/dL. Measurement of free, unbound, unconjugated bilirubin (B_f) may be a more meaningful predictor of risk for brain injury, although this test is not yet clinically available. Currently the most sensitive means of assessing neurotoxicity may be the auditory brainstem evoked response, which shows predictable, early effects of bilirubin toxicity.

reversible with aggressive treatment, whereas a score of 7–9 represents advanced and possibly irreversible damage.

5. Chronic Bilirubin Encephalopathy (Kernicterus)

ESSENTIALS OF DIAGNOSIS & TYPICAL FEATURES

- Extrapyramidal movement disorder (choreoathetoid cerebral palsy).
- Gaze abnormality, especially limitation of upward gaze.
- Auditory disturbances (deafness, failed auditory brainstem evoked response with normal evoked otoacoustic emissions, auditory neuropathy, auditory dyssynchrony).
- Dysplasia of the enamel of the deciduous teeth.

Kernicterus is an irreversible brain injury characterized by choreoathetoid cerebral palsy and hearing impairment. Intelligence is probably normal but may be difficult to assess because of associated hearing, communication, and coordination problems. The diagnosis is clinical but is strengthened if audiologic testing shows auditory neuropathy and auditory dyssynchrony in which the otoacoustic emission test is normal but the auditory brainstem response is absent. Infants with such findings are usually deaf. Infants with milder kernicterus may have normal audiograms but abnormal auditory processing and subsequent problems with speech comprehension. Magnetic resonance imaging (MRI) scanning of the brain is nearly diagnostic if it shows abnormalities isolated to the globus pallidus or the subthalamic nuclei, or both.

Evaluation of Hyperbilirubinemia

Because most newborns are discharged at 24–48 hours of age, before physiologic jaundice peaks and before maternal milk supply is established, a predischarge TSB or a transcutaneous bilirubin measurement (TcB) may help predict which infants are at risk for severe hyperbilirubinemia. In all infants, an assessment of risk for severe hyperbilirubinemia should be performed before discharge (Table 2–10). As recommended by the AAP, follow-up within 24–48 hours for all infants discharged before 72 hours of age (depending on the number of risk factors present) is imperative. Although jaundice is usually visible above a TSB level of 5 mg/dL (86 mmol/L), visual estimation of the bilirubin level is inaccurate. TSB should be measured and interpreted based on the age of the infant in hours at the time of sampling. Term infants with a TSB level greater than the 95th percentile for age in hours have a 40% risk of developing significant hyperbilirubinemia (see Figure 2–2). Serial bilirubin levels should be obtained from a single laboratory whenever possible to make interpretation of serial measurements more meaningful. It is important to

Table 2–10. Factors affecting the risk of severe hyperbilirubinemia in infants 35 or more weeks' gestation (in approximate order of importance).

Major risk factors
Predischarge TSB or TcB level in the high-risk zone (> 95th percentile; see Figure 2-2)
Jaundice observed in the first 24 h
Blood group incompatibility with positive direct Coombs test, other known hemolytic disease (eg, G6PD deficiency), or elevated ETCO
Gestational age 35-36 wk
Previous sibling required phototherapy
Cephalohematoma or significant bruising
Exclusive breast feeding, particularly if weight loss is excessive
East Asian race[a]
Minor risk factors
Predischarge TSB or TcB level in the high-intermediate-risk zone (75-95th percentile)
Gestational age 37-38 wks
Jaundice observed before discharge
Previous sibling with jaundice
Macrosomic infant of a diabetic mother
Decreased risk (these factors are associated with decreased risk of significant jaundice, listed in order of decreasing importance)
TSB or TcB level in the low-risk zone (see Figure 2-2)
Gestational age ≥ 41 wk
Exclusive bottle feeding
Black race[a]
Discharge from hospital after 72 h

[a]Race as defined by mother's description.
ETCO, end-tidal carbon monoxide; G6PD, glucose-6-phosphate dehydrogenase; TcB, transcutaneous bilirubin; TSB, total serum bilirubin.

remember that these nomograms apply only to early-term and full-term infants, 36 weeks and older.

Infants with visible jaundice on the first day of life or who develop excessive jaundice require further evaluation. The minimal evaluation consists of the following:

- Feeding and elimination history.
- Birth weight and percent weight change since birth.
- Examination for sources of excessive heme breakdown.
- Assessment of blood type, Coombs testing, complete blood count (CBC) with smear, serum albumin, and TSB.
- G6PD test if jaundice is otherwise unexplained, and in African-American infants with severe jaundice.
- Fractionated bilirubin level in infants who appear ill, those with prolonged jaundice, acholic stool, hepatosplenomegaly, or dark urine.

Treatment of Indirect Hyperbilirubinemia

A. Phototherapy

Phototherapy is the most common treatment for indirect hyperbilirubinemia. It is relatively noninvasive and safe. Light of wavelength 425–475 nm (blue-green spectrum) is

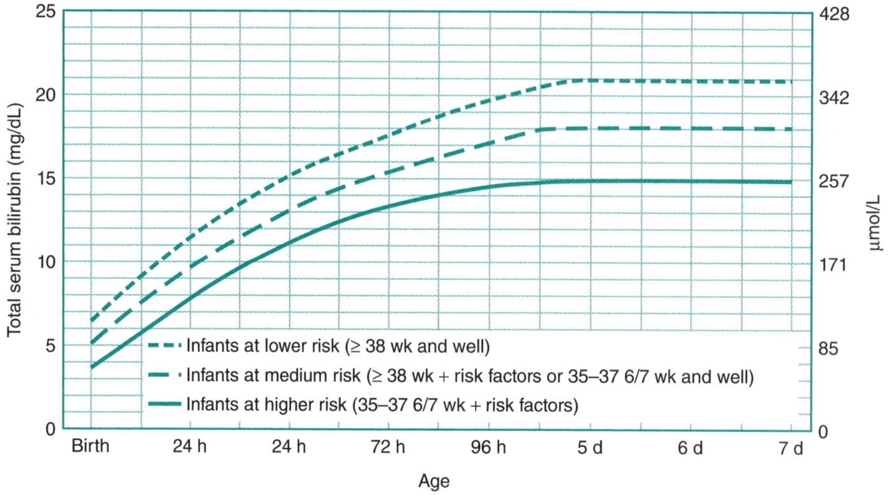

- Use total bilirubin. Do not subtract direct reacting of conjugated bilirubin.
- Risk factors = isoimmune hemolytic disease, G6PD deficiency, asphyxia, significant lethargy, temperature instability, sepsis, acidosis, or albumin < 3.0 g/dL (if measured).
- For well infants 35–37 6/7 wk can adjust TSB levels for intervention around the medium-risk line. It is an option to intervene at lower TSB levels for intants closer to 35 wk and at higher TSB levels for those closer to 37 6/7 wk.
- It is an option to provide conventional phototherapy in hospital or at home at TSB levels 2–3 mg/dL (35–50 mmol/L) below those shown but home phototherapy should not be used in any infant with risk factors.

▲ **Figure 2–3.** Guidelines for phototherapy in hospitalized infants of 35 or more weeks' gestation. These guidelines are based on limited evidence and levels shown are approximations. The guidelines refer to the use of intensive phototherapy (at least 30 μW/cm² in the blue-green spectrum), which should be used when the total serum bilirubin (TSB) exceeds the line indicated for each category. If TSB approaches the exchange level, the sides of the incubator or bassinet should be lined with aluminum foil or white material. (Reproduced, with permission, from the AAP Subcommittee on Hyperbilirubinemia: Management of hyperbilirubinemia in the newborn infant 35 or more weeks of gestation. Pediatrics 2004;114:297.)

absorbed by unconjugated bilirubin in the skin converting it to a water-soluble stereoisomer that can be excreted in bile without conjugation. The minimum effective light dose is 10–14 μW/cm² irradiance. Intensive phototherapy employs irradiance of 30 μW/cm² or higher. Irradiance can be increased by increasing the exposed body surface area or by moving the light source closer to the infant. Special blue fluorescent tubes labeled F20 T12/BB or TL52/20W are most commonly used. Fiberoptic blankets are useful as adjuncts but are not adequate as sole therapy for term infants because they do not cover sufficient surface area. Intensive phototherapy should decrease TSB by 30%–40% in the first 24 hours, most significantly in the first 4–6 hours. The infant's eyes should be shielded to prevent retinal damage. Diarrhea, which sometimes occurs during phototherapy, can be treated if necessary by feeding a nonlactose-containing formula.

Phototherapy is started electively when the TSB is approximately 6 mg/dL (102 mmol/L) lower than the predicted exchange level for that infant (eg, at 16–19 mg/dL [272–323 mmol/L] for a full-term infant for whom exchange transfusion would be considered at a TSB of approximately 22–25 mg/dL [374–425 mmol/L]). AAP guidelines for phototherapy and exchange transfusion in infants of 35 or more weeks' gestation are shown in ures 2–3 and 2–4. Hyperbilirubinemic infants should be fed by mouth if possible to decrease enterohepatic bilirubin circulation. Casein hydrolysate formula to supplement breast milk decreases enterohepatic circulation by inhibiting mucosal β-glucuronidase activity. IVIG (0.5–1.0 g/kg) in severe antibody-mediated hemolysis may interrupt the hemolytic process. Although phototherapy has been shown to decrease the need for exchange transfusion, its long-term benefits, if any, in infants with less severe jaundice are unknown.

B. Exchange Transfusion

Although most infants with indirect hyperbilirubinemia can be treated with phototherapy, extreme indirect

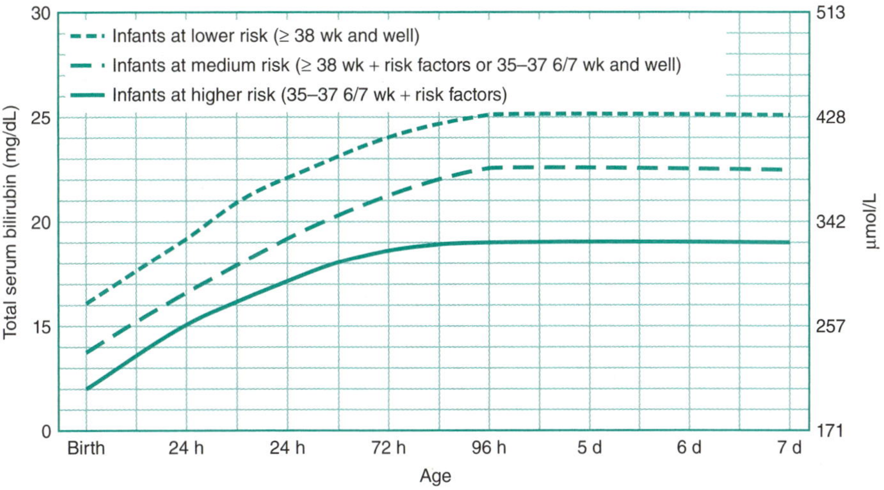

- The dashed lines for the first 24 hours indicate uncertainty due to a wide range of clinical circumstances and a range of responses to phototherapy.
- Immediate exchange transfusion is recommended if inflant shows signs of acute bilirubin encephalopathy (hypertonia, arching, retrocolitis, opisthotonos, fever, high pitched cry) or if TSB is ≥ 5 mg/dL (85 μmol/L) above these lines.
- Risk factors—isoimmune hemolytic disease, G6PD deficiency, asphyxia, significant lethargy, temperature instability, sepsis, acidosis.
- Measure serum albumin and calculate B/A ratio (see legend).
- Use total bilirubin. Do not subtract direct reading or conjugated bilirubin.
- If infant is well and 35–37 6/7 wk (median risk), individualize TSB levels for exchange based on actual gestational age.

▲ **Figure 2–4.** Guidelines for exchange transfusion in infants of 35 or more weeks' gestation. These guidelines represent approximations for which an exchange transfusion is indicated in infants treated with intensive phototherapy. For readmitted infants, if the total serum bilirubin (TSB) level is above the exchange level, repeat TSB measurement every 2–3 hours and consider exchange if the TSB remains above the level after 6 hours of intensive phototherapy. The total serum bilirubin/albumin ratio (TSB [mg/dL]/Alb [g/dL]; 8.0 for infants at lower risk, 7.2 for medium risk, and 6.8 for higher risk) can be used together with, but not in lieu of the TSB level as an additional factor in determining the need for transfusion. If the TSB is at or approaching exchange level, send blood for an immediate type and crossmatch. (Reproduced, with permission, from the AAP Subcommittee on Hyperbilirubinemia: Management of hyperbilirubinemia in the newborn infant 35 or more weeks of gestation. Pediatrics 2004;114:297.)

hyperbilirubinemia is a medical emergency. Infants should be admitted at once to a neonatal intensive care unit where exchange transfusion can be performed before irreversible neurologic damage occurs. Intensive phototherapy should be instituted immediately, during transport to the hospital if possible. As TSB nears the potentially toxic range, serum albumin should be determined. Albumin (1 g/kg) will aid in binding and removal of bilirubin during exchange transfusion, as well as afford some neuroprotection while preparing for the procedure. Table 2–11 illustrates the bilirubin/albumin ratios at which exchange transfusion should be considered.

Double-volume exchange transfusion (approximately 160–200 mL/kg body weight) is most often required in infants with extreme hyperbilirubinemia secondary to Rh isoimmunization, ABO incompatibility, or hereditary spherocytosis.

Table 2–11. Additional guidelines for exchange transfusion: effects of albumin.

Risk Category	Bilirubin/Albumin Ratio at Which to Consider Exchange Transfusion (TSB [mg/dL]:Albumin [g/dL])
Infants > 38 wk and well	8.0
Infants 35-38 wk and well, or > 38 wk with higher risk (hemolysis, G6PD deficiency, sepsis, acidosis)	7.2
Infants 35-38 wk with higher risk, as above	6.8

G6PD, glucose-6-phosphate dehydrogenase; TSB, total serum bilirubin.

The procedure decreases serum bilirubin acutely by approximately 50% and removes about 80% of sensitized or abnormal red blood cells and offending antibody so that ongoing hemolysis is decreased. Exchange transfusion is also indicated in any infant with TSB above 30 mg/dL, in infants with signs of encephalopathy, or when intensive phototherapy has not lowered TSB by at least 0.5 mg/dL/h after 4 hours. The decision to perform exchange transfusion should be based on TSB, not on the indirect fraction of bilirubin.

Exchange transfusion is invasive, potentially risky, and infrequently performed. It should therefore be performed at a referral center. Mortality is 1%–5% and is greatest in the smallest, most immature, and unstable infants. Sudden death during the procedure can occur in any infant. There is a 5%–10% risk of serious complications such as necrotizing enterocolitis (NEC), infection, electrolyte disturbances, or thrombocytopenia. Isovolemic exchange (withdrawal through an arterial line with infusion through a venous line) may decrease the risk of some complications.

C. Protoporphyrins

Tin and zinc protoporphyrin or mesoporphyrin (Sn-PP, Zn-PP; Sn-MP, Zn-MP) are inhibitors of heme oxygenase, the enzyme that initiates the catabolism of heme (iron protoporphyrin). Studies are underway involving a single injection of these substances shortly after birth to prevent the formation of bilirubin. Although results are promising, these drugs are not yet approved for use in the United States.

American Academy of Pediatrics Subcommittee on Hyperbilirubinemia: Clinical practice guideline: management of hyper-bilirubinemia in the newborn infant 35 or more weeks of gestation. Pediatrics 2004;114:297 [PMID: 15231951].

Engle WA et al: Committee on Fetus and Newborn: Late preterm infants: a population at risk. Pediatrics 2007;120:1390 [PMID: 18055691].

Maisels MJ et al: Hyperbilirubinemia in the newborn infant ≥ 35 weeks' gestation: An update with clarifications. Pediatrics 2009;124:1193 [PMID: 19786452].

Newman TB: Universal bilirubin screening, guidelines, and evidence. Pediatrics 2009;124:1199 [PMID: 19786453]

Preer GL, Philipp BL: Understanding and managing breast milk jaundice. Arch Dis Child Fetal Neonatal Ed 2010. Doi:10.1136/adc.2010.184416

Smits-Wintjens VEHJ et al: Intravenous immunoglobulin in neonates with rhesus hemolytic disease: A randomized controlled trial. Pediatrics 2011;127:680 [PMID: 21422084].

Watchko JF: Hyperbilirubinemia in African-American neonates: clinical issues and current challenges. Semin Fetal & Neonat Med 2010;15:176-82 [PMID: 19942984]

Watchko JF: Identification of neonates at risk for hazardous hyper-bilirubinemia: Emerging clinical insights. Pediatr Clin N Am 2009;56:671 [PMID: 19501698].

HYPOGLYCEMIA

ESSENTIALS OF DIAGNOSIS & TYPICAL FEATURES

- Blood glucose < 40 mg/dL at birth to 4 h, or < 45 mg/dL at 4–24 h of age.
- LGA, SGA, preterm, and stressed infants at risk.
- May be asymptomatic.
- Infants can present with lethargy, poor feeding, irritability, or seizures.

General Considerations

Blood glucose concentration in the fetus is approximately 15 mg/dL less than maternal glucose concentration. Glucose concentration decreases in the immediate postnatal period, to as low as 30 mg/dL in many healthy infants at 1–2 hours after birth. Concentrations below 40 mg/dL after the first feeding are considered hypoglycemic. By 3 hours, the glucose concentration in normal full-term infants stabilizes at ≥ 45 mg/dL. The two groups of full-term newborn infants at highest risk for hypoglycemia are infants of diabetic mothers (IDMs) and IUGR infants.

A. Infants of Diabetic Mothers

The Infant of a Diabetic Mother(IDM) has abundant glucose stores in the form of glycogen and fat but develops hypoglycemia because of hyperinsulinemia induced by maternal and fetal hyperglycemia. Increased energy supply to the fetus from the maternal circulation results in a macrosomic infant. The large infant is at increased risk for trauma during delivery. Some infants have cardiomyopathy (asymmetrical septal hypertrophy) which may present with murmur, respiratory distress, or cardiac failure. Microcolon is occasionally present in IDMs and causes symptoms of low intestinal obstruction similar to Hirschsprung disease. Other neonatal problems include hypercoagulability and polycythemia, a combination that predisposes the infant to large vein thromboses (especially the renal vein). IDMs are often somewhat immature for their gestational age and are at increased risk for hyaline membrane disease, hypocalcemia, and hyperbilirubinemia. Infants of mothers who were diabetic at conception have a higher incidence of congenital anomalies, probably related to first-trimester glucose control.

B. Intrauterine Growth-Restricted Infants

The Intrauterine Growth-Restricted (IUGR) infant has reduced glucose stores in the form of glycogen and body fat and is prone to hypoglycemia. In addition, marked hyperglycemia and a transient diabetes mellitus–like syndrome occasionally develops, particularly in the very premature IUGR infant. These problems usually respond to adjustment in glucose intake, although insulin is sometimes needed transiently. Some IUGR infants have hyperinsulinemia that persists for a week or more.

C. Other Causes of Hypoglycemia

Hypoglycemia occurs in disorders with islet cell hyperplasia including the Beckwith-Wiedemann syndrome, erythroblastosis fetalis, and genetic forms of hyperinsulinism. Hypoglycemia also occurs in certain inborn errors of metabolism such as glycogen storage disease and galactosemia, and with endocrine disorders such as panhypopituitarism, characterized by counterregulatory hormone deficiency. The combination of hypoglycemia and micropenis is very suggestive of this disorder. Hypoglycemia also occurs, probably secondary to stress, in infants with birth asphyxia, hypoxia, and bacterial and viral sepsis. Premature infants are at risk for hypoglycemia because of decreased glycogen stores.

Clinical Findings and Monitoring

The signs of hypoglycemia in the newborn infant may be nonspecific and subtle: lethargy, poor feeding, irritability, tremors, jitteriness, apnea, and seizures. Hypoglycemia due to increased insulin is the most severe and most resistant to treatment. Cardiac failure may occur in severe cases, particularly in IDMs with cardiomyopathy. Hypoglycemia in hyperinsulinemic states can develop within the first 30–60 minutes of life.

Blood glucose can be measured by heelstick using a bedside glucometer. All infants at risk should be screened, including IDMs, IUGR infants, premature infants, and any infant with suggestive symptoms. All low or borderline values should be confirmed by laboratory measurement of blood glucose concentration. It is important to continue surveillance of glucose concentration until the baby has been on full enteral feedings without intravenous supplementation for 24 hours, with a target of > 45 mg/dL before feeding. Relapse of hypoglycemia thereafter is unlikely.

Infants with hypoglycemia requiring IV glucose infusions for more than 5 days should be evaluated for less common disorders, including inborn errors of metabolism, hyperinsulinemic states, and deficiencies of counterregulatory hormones.

Treatment

Therapy is based on the provision of enteral or parenteral glucose. Treatment guidelines are shown in Table 2–12. In hyperinsulinemic states, glucose boluses should be avoided and a higher glucose infusion rate used. After initial correction with a bolus of 10% dextrose in water ($D_{10}W$; 2 mL/kg), glucose infusion should be increased gradually as needed from a starting rate of 6 mg/kg/min. IDMs and IUGR infants with polycythemia are at greatest risk for symptomatic hypoglycemia. In such infants, hypoglycemia and polycythemia should be treated with IV glucose and partial exchange transfusion, respectively.

Table 2–12. Hypoglycemia: suggested therapeutic regimens.

Screening Test[a]	Presence of Symptoms	Action
30–40 mg/dL	No symptoms of hypoglycemia	Draw blood glucose[b]; if the infant is alert and vigorous, feed; follow with frequent glucose monitoring.
		If the infant continues to have blood glucose < 40 mg/dL or is unable to feed, provide intravenous glucose at 6 mg/kg/min ($D_{10}W$ at 3.6 mL/kg/h).
< 40 mg/dL	Symptoms of hypoglycemia present	Draw blood glucose[b]; provide bolus of $D_{10}W$ (2 mL/kg) followed by an infusion of 6 mg/kg/min (3.6 mL/kg/h).
< 30 mg/dL	With or without symptoms of hypoglycemia	Draw blood glucose[b]; provide bolus of $D_{10}W$ followed by an infusion of 6 mg/kg/min.
		If IV access cannot be obtained immediately, an umbilical vein line should be used.

[a]Rapid bedside determination.
[b]Laboratory confirmation.

Prognosis

The prognosis of hypoglycemia is good if therapy is prompt. CNS sequelae are more common in infants with hypoglycemic seizures and in neonates with persistent hyperinsulinemic hypoglycemia. Hypoglycemia may also potentiate brain injury after perinatal depression or other insults, and should be avoided.

Adamkin DH, and Committee on Fetus and Newborn: Clinical Report – postnatal glucose homeostasis in late preterm and term infants. Pediatrics 2011;127:575 [PMID: 21357346].

Hay WW et al: Knowledge gaps and research needs for understanding and treating neonatal hypoglycemia: workshop report from Eunice Kennedy Shriver National Institute of Child Health and Human Development. J Pediatr 2009;155:612 [PMID: 19840614].

Rozance PJ, Hay WW Jr: Neonatal hypoglycemia. Neoreviews 2010;11:e681.

RESPIRATORY DISTRESS IN THE TERM NEWBORN INFANT

ESSENTIALS OF DIAGNOSIS & TYPICAL FEATURES

- Tachypnea, respiratory rate > 60 breaths/min.
- Intercostal and sternal retractions.
- Expiratory grunting.
- Cyanosis in room air.

General Considerations

Respiratory distress is one of the most common symptom complexes of the newborn. It may result from cardiopulmonary and noncardiopulmonary causes (Table 2–13). Chest radiography, arterial blood gases, and pulse oximetry are useful in assessing the cause and severity of the distress. It is important to consider the noncardiopulmonary causes (see Table 2–13), because the natural tendency is to focus on the heart and lungs. Most of the noncardiopulmonary causes can be ruled out by the history, physical examination, and a few simple laboratory tests. The most common pulmonary causes of respiratory distress in the full-term infant are transient tachypnea, aspiration syndromes, congenital pneumonia, and air leaks.

Table 2–13. Causes of respiratory distress in the newborn.

Noncardiopulmonary
Hypothermia or hyperthermia
Hypoglycemia
Polycythemia
Metabolic acidosis
Drug intoxications or withdrawal
Insult to the central nervous system
Asphyxia
Hemorrhage
Neuromuscular disease
Phrenic nerve injury
Skeletal dysplasia
Cardiovascular
Left-sided outflow tract obstruction
Hypoplastic left heart
Aortic stenosis
Coarctation of the aorta, interrupted aortic arch
Cyanotic lesions
Transposition of the great vessels
Total anomalous pulmonary venous return
Tricuspid atresia
Right-sided outflow obstruction
Respiratory Tract
Upper airway obstruction
Choanal atresia
Vocal cord paralysis
Lingual thyroid
Meconium aspiration
Clear fluid aspiration
Transient tachypnea
Pneumonia
Pulmonary hypoplasia
Hyaline membrane disease
Pneumothorax
Pleural effusions
Mass lesions
Lobar emphysema
Cystic adenomatoid malformation

Reproduced, with permission, from Rosenberg AA: The Neonate. In Gabbe SG, et al (editors): *Obstetrics: Normal and Problem Pregnancies.* Churchill Livingstone; 2007.

A. Transient Tachypnea (Retained Fetal Lung Fluid)

Respiratory distress is typically present at birth, usually associated with a mild-to-moderate oxygen requirement (25%–50% O_2). The infant is usually full term or late preterm, nonasphyxiated, and born following a short labor or cesarean section without labor. The pathogenesis of the disorder is related to delayed clearance of fetal lung fluid via the circulation and pulmonary lymphatics. The chest radiograph shows perihilar streaking and fluid in interlobar fissures. Resolution usually occurs within 12–24 hours. Nasal CPAP can be very helpful in the clearance of the fluid.

B. Aspiration Syndromes

The infant is typically full term or late preterm with fetal distress prior to delivery or depression at delivery. Blood or meconium is often present in the amniotic fluid. Aspiration of meconium most commonly occurs in utero as a stressed infant gasps. Delivery room management of these infants is discussed in the resuscitation section. Respiratory distress is present from birth, often accompanied by a barrel chest appearance and coarse breath sounds. Pneumonitis may cause an increasing O_2 need and may require intubation and ventilation. The chest radiograph shows coarse irregular infiltrates, hyperexpansion, and in the worst cases, lobar consolidation. In some cases, because of secondary surfactant deficiency, the radiograph shows a diffuse homogeneous infiltrate pattern. Infants who aspirate are at risk of pneumothorax because of uneven aeration with segmental overdistention and are at risk for persistent pulmonary hypertension (see section on Cardiac Problems in the Newborn Infant, later).

C. Congenital Pneumonia

The lungs are the most common site of infection in the neonate. Infections usually ascend from the genital tract before or during labor, with the vaginal or rectal flora the most likely agents (group B streptococci and *Escherichia coli*). Infants of any gestational age, with or without a history of prolonged rupture of membranes, chorioamnionitis, or maternal antibiotic administration, may be affected. Respiratory distress may begin at birth or may be delayed for several hours. The chest radiograph may resemble that of retained lung fluid or hyaline membrane disease. Rarely, there may be a lobar infiltrate.

Shock, poor perfusion, absolute neutropenia (< 2000/mL), and elevated C-reactive protein provide supportive evidence for pneumonia. Gram stain of tracheal aspirate may be helpful. Because no signs or laboratory findings can confirm a diagnosis of pneumonia, all infants with respiratory distress should have a blood culture performed and should receive broad-spectrum antibiotic therapy (ampicillin, 100 mg/kg in two divided doses, and gentamicin, 4 mg/kg q24h or 2.5 mg/kg q12h) until the diagnosis of bacterial infection is eliminated.

D. Spontaneous Pneumothorax

Spontaneous pneumothorax occurs in 1% of all deliveries. Risk is increased by manipulations such as positive-pressure ventilation (PPV) in the delivery room. Respiratory distress (primarily tachypnea) is present from birth and typically is not severe. Breath sounds may be decreased on the affected side; heart tones may be shifted toward the opposite side and may be distant. The chest radiograph shows pneumothorax or pneumomediastinum.

Treatment usually consists of supplemental O_2 and watchful waiting. Breathing 100% O_2 for a few hours may accelerate reabsorption of extrapulmonary gas by creating a diffusion gradient for nitrogen across the surface of the lung (nitrogen washout technique). This is effective only if the infant was breathing room air or a low O_2 concentration at the time of the pneumothorax; the long-term effects of the use of 100% O_2 in this way are unknown. Drainage by needle thoracentesis or tube thoracostomy is occasionally required. There is a slightly increased risk of renal abnormalities associated with spontaneous pneumothorax. Thus, careful physical examination of the kidneys and observation of urine output are indicated. If pulmonary hypoplasia with pneumothorax is suspected, renal ultrasound is also indicated.

E. Other Respiratory Tract Causes

Other respiratory tract causes of respiratory distress are rare. Bilateral choanal atresia should be suspected if there is no air movement when the infant breathes through the nose. These infants have good color and heart rate while crying at delivery but become cyanotic and bradycardiac when they resume normal nasal breathing. Other causes of upper airway obstruction usually produce some degree of stridor or poor air movement despite good respiratory effort. Pleural effusion is likely in hydropic infants. Space-occupying lesions cause a shift of the mediastinum with asymmetrical breath sounds and are apparent on chest radiographs. Many are associated with severe respiratory distress.

▶ Treatment

Whatever the cause, neonatal respiratory distress is treated with supplemental oxygen sufficient to maintain a $Pa{O_2}$ of 60–70 mm Hg and an oxygen saturation by pulse oximetry ($Sp{O_2}$) of 92%–96%. Oxygen should be warmed, humidified, and delivered through an air blender. Concentration should be measured with a calibrated oxygen analyzer. An umbilical or peripheral arterial line should be inserted in infants requiring more than 45% fraction of inspired oxygen ($FI{O_2}$) by 4–6 hours of life to allow frequent blood gas determinations. Noninvasive monitoring with pulse oximetry should be used.

Other supportive treatment includes IV glucose and water. Unless infection can be ruled out, blood cultures should be obtained and broad-spectrum antibiotics started. Volume expansion (normal saline) can be given in infusions of 10 mL/kg over 30 minutes for low blood pressure, poor perfusion, and metabolic acidosis. Other specific testing should be done as indicated by the history and physical examination. In most cases, a chest radiograph, blood gas measurements, CBC, and blood glucose determination allow a diagnosis.

Intubation and ventilation should be undertaken if there is respiratory failure ($Pa{O_2}$ < 60 mm Hg in > 60% $FI{O_2}$, $Pa{CO_2}$ > 60 mm Hg, or repeated apnea). Peak pressures should be adequate to produce chest wall expansion and audible breath sounds (usually 18–24 cm H_2O). Positive end-expiratory pressure (4–6 cm H_2O) should be used. Ventilation rates of 20–40 breaths/min are usually required. The goal is to maintain a $Pa{O_2}$ of 60–70 mm Hg and a $Pa{CO_2}$ of 45–55 mm Hg.

▶ Prognosis

Most respiratory conditions of the full-term infant are acute and resolve in the first several days. Meconium aspiration and congenital pneumonia carry a mortality rate of up to 10% and can produce significant long-term pulmonary morbidity. Mortality has been reduced by use of high-frequency oscillatory ventilation and inhaled nitric oxide for treatment of pulmonary hypertension. Only rarely is extracorporeal membrane oxygenation (ECMO) needed as rescue therapy.

Ramachandrappa A, Jain L: Elective cesarean section: its impact on neonatal respiratory outcome. Clin Perinatol 2008;35:373 [PMID: 18456075].

Hooper SB et al: Establishing functional residual capacity at birth. NeoReviews 2010;11:e474.

TePas AB et al: From liquid to air: Breathing after birth. J Pediatr 2008;152:607 [PMID: 18410760].

Warren JB, Anderson JM: Newborn respiratory disorders. Pediatr Rev 2010;31:487 [PMID: 21123510].

Yeh TF: Core concepts: Meconium aspiration syndrome: pathogenesis and current management. NeoReviews 2010;11:e503.

HEART MURMURS (SEE ALSO SECTION ON CARDIAC PROBLEMS IN THE NEWBORN INFANT)

Heart murmurs are common in the first days of life and do not usually signify structural heart problems. If a murmur is present at birth, it should be considered a valvular problem until proved otherwise because the common benign transitional murmurs (eg, patent ductus arteriosus) are not audible until minutes to hours after birth.

If an infant is pink, well-perfused, and in no respiratory distress, with palpable and symmetrical pulses (right brachial pulse no stronger than the femoral pulse), the murmur is most likely transitional. Transitional murmurs are soft (grade 1–3/6), heard at the left upper to midsternal border, and generally loudest during the first 24 hours. If the murmur persists beyond 24 hours of age, blood pressure in the right arm and a leg should be determined. If there is a difference of more than 15 mm Hg (arm > leg) or if the pulses in the lower extremities are difficult to palpate, a cardiologist should evaluate the infant for coarctation of the aorta. If there is no difference, the infant can be discharged home with follow-up in 2–3 days for auscultation and evaluation for signs of congestive failure. If signs of congestive failure or cyanosis are present, the infant should be referred for evaluation without delay. If the murmur persists without these signs, the infant can be referred for elective evaluation at age 2–4 weeks. Some centers now recommend routine pulse oximetry screening in the nursery to identify infants with serious congenital heart disease. Oxygen saturation less than 95% at sea level is evaluated by echocardiogram.

Frommelt MA: Differential diagnosis and approach to a heart murmur in term infants. Pediatr Clin North Am 2004;51:1023 [PMID: 15331284].

Mackie AS et al: Can cardiologists distinguish innocent from pathologic murmurs in neonates. J Pediatr 2009;154:150 [PMID: 18692204].

Mahle WT et al, on behalf of the American Heart Association Congenital Heart Defects Committee of the Council on Cardiovascular Disease in the Young, Council on Cardiovascular Nursing, and Interdisciplinary Council on Quality of Care and Outcomes Research, and the American Academy of Pediatrics Section on Cardiology and Cardiac Surgery, and Committee on Fetus and Newborn: Role of pulse oximetry in examining newborns for congenital heart disease: A scientific statement from the AHA and AAP. Pediatrics 2009;124:823 [PMID: 19581259].

BIRTH TRAUMA

Most birth trauma is associated with difficult delivery (eg, large fetus, abnormal presenting position, or fetal distress requiring rapid extraction). The most common injuries are soft tissue bruising, fractures (clavicle, humerus, or femur), and cervical plexus palsies. Skull fracture, intracranial hemorrhage (primarily subdural and subarachnoid), and cervical spinal cord injury can also occur.

Fractures are often diagnosed by the obstetrician, who may feel or hear a snap during delivery. Clavicular fractures may cause decreased spontaneous movement of the arm, with local tenderness and crepitus. Humeral or femoral fractures usually cause tenderness and swelling over the shaft with a diaphyseal fracture, and always cause limitation of movement. Epiphyseal fractures are harder to diagnose radiographically owing to the cartilaginous nature of the epiphysis. After 8–10 days, callus is visible on radiographs. Treatment in all cases is gentle handling, with immobilization for 8–10 days: the humerus against the chest with elbow flexed; the femur with a posterior splint from below the knee to the buttock.

Brachial plexus injuries may result from traction as the head is pulled away from the shoulder during delivery. Injury to the C5–C6 roots is most common (Erb-Duchenne palsy). The arm is limp, adducted, and internally rotated, extended and pronated at the elbow, and flexed at the wrist (so-called waiter's tip posture). Grasp is present. If the lower nerve roots (C8–T1) are injured (Klumpke palsy), the hand is flaccid. If the entire plexus is injured, the arm and hand are flaccid, with associated sensory deficit. Early treatment for brachial plexus injury is conservative, because function usually returns over several weeks. Referral should be made to a physical therapist so that parents can be instructed on range-of-motion exercises, splinting, and further evaluation if needed. Return of function begins in the deltoid and biceps, with recovery by 3 months in most cases.

Spinal cord injury can occur at birth, especially in difficult breech extractions with hyperextension of the neck, or in midforceps rotations when the body fails to turn with the head. Infants are flaccid, quadriplegic, and without respiratory effort at birth. Facial movements are preserved. The long-term outlook for such infants is poor.

Facial nerve palsy is sometimes associated with forceps use but more often results from in-utero pressure of the baby's head against the mother's sacrum. The infant has asymmetrical mouth movements and eye closure with poor facial movement on the affected side. Most cases resolve spontaneously in a few days to weeks.

Subgaleal hemorrhage into the large potential space under the scalp (Figure 2–5) is associated with difficult vaginal deliveries and repeated attempts at vacuum extraction. It can lead to hypovolemic shock and death from blood loss and coagulopathy triggered by consumption of clotting factors. This is an emergency requiring rapid replacement of blood and clotting factors.

Noetzel MJ: Perinatal trauma and cerebral palsy: Is there a link? Clin Perinatol 2006;33:355 [PMID: 16765729].

Sutcliffe TL: Brachial plexus injury in the newborn. NeoReviews 2007;8:e239.

Uhring MR: Management of birth injuries. Clin Perinatol 2005;32:19 [PMID: 15777819].

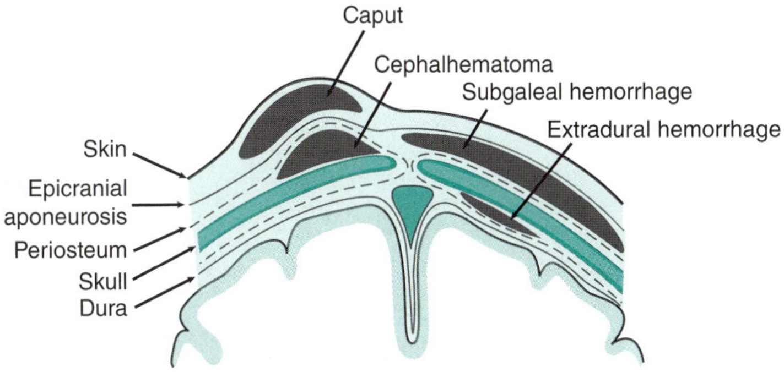

▲ **Figure 2–5.** Sites of extracranial bleeding in the newborn. (Adapted and reproduced, with permission, from Pape KE, Wigglesworth JS: *Haemorrhage Ischemia and the Perinatal Brain.* JB Lippincott, 1979.)

INFANTS OF MOTHERS WHO ABUSE DRUGS

Current studies estimate that up to 15% of women use alcohol and 5%–15% use illicit drugs during pregnancy, depending on the population studied and the methods of ascertainment. Drugs most commonly used are tobacco, alcohol, marijuana, cocaine, and methamphetamine. Because mothers may abuse many drugs and give an unreliable history of drug usage, it is difficult to pinpoint which drug is causing the morbidity seen in a newborn infant. Early hospital discharge makes recognition of these infants based on physical findings and abnormal behavior difficult. Except for alcohol, a birth defect syndrome has not been defined for any substance of abuse.

1. Cocaine & Methamphetamine

ESSENTIALS OF DIAGNOSIS & TYPICAL FEATURES

- Triad of no prenatal care, premature delivery, placental abruption.
- Possible IUGR.
- Irritability.

Cocaine and methamphetamine are currently the most common hard drugs used during pregnancy, often in association with other drugs such as tobacco, alcohol, and marijuana. These stimulants can cause maternal hypertension, decreased uterine blood flow, fetal hypoxemia, uterine contractions, and placental abruption. Rates of stillbirth, placental abruption, symmetric IUGR, and preterm delivery are increased two- to fourfold in users. In the high-risk setting of no prenatal care, placental abruption, and preterm labor, urine toxicology screens should be performed on the mother and infant; consent from the mother for testing her urine may be required. Meconium should be sent for drug screening as it enhances diagnosis by indicating cumulative drug exposure from the first trimester forward. Although no specific malformation complex or withdrawal syndrome is described for cocaine and methamphetamine abuse, infants may show irritability and growth restriction.

Children of mothers who use methamphetamines are at particularly high risk for neglect and abuse. Social services evaluation is especially important to assess the home environment for these risks. The risk of SIDS is three to seven times higher in infants of users than in those of nonusers (0.5%–1% of exposed infants). The risk may be lessened by environmental interventions such as avoidance of tobacco smoke and supine infant positioning.

2. Opioids

ESSENTIALS OF DIAGNOSIS & TYPICAL FEATURES

- CNS—irritability, hyperactivity, hypertonicity, incessant high-pitched cry, tremors, seizures.
- GI—vomiting, diarrhea, weight loss, poor feeding, incessant hunger, excessive salivation.
- Metabolic and respiratory—nasal stuffiness, sneezing, yawning, sweating, hyperthermia.
- Often IUGR.

Clinical Findings

The withdrawal signs seen in infants born to narcotic-addicted mothers, whether heroin, prescription narcotics, or methadone, are similar. The symptoms in infants born to methadone-maintained mothers may be delayed in onset, more severe, and more prolonged than those seen with heroin addiction. Symptoms usually begin within 1–3 days of life. The clinical picture is typical enough to suggest a diagnosis even if a maternal history of narcotic abuse has not been obtained. Confirmation should be made with urine and meconium toxicology screening.

Treatment

If opioid abuse or withdrawal is suspected, the infant is not a candidate for early discharge. A serial scoring system should be used. Supportive treatment includes swaddling the infant and providing a quiet, dimly lit environment, minimizing procedures, and disturbing the infant as little as possible. Specific treatment should be used when the infant has severe symptoms or excessive weight loss. No single drug has been identified as optimally effective. Occasional doses of phenobarbital 5 mg/kg orally may be used for irritability. If diarrhea and weight loss are prominent, or if adequate control of symptoms has not been achieved, oral morphine sulphate 0.1–0.5 mg/kg/dose q6–12h, titrated to improve symptoms, or methadone (0.05–0.1 mg/kg q6h) are more beneficial than phenobarbital alone. Treatment can be tapered over several days to 2 weeks, as tolerated. It is also important to review maternal tests for HIV, hepatitis B, and hepatitis C, as all are common in intravenous drug users.

Prognosis

These infants often have chronic neurobehavioral handicaps; however, it is difficult to distinguish the effects of in-utero drug exposure from those of the environment. Infants of opioid abusers have a four- to fivefold increased risk of SIDS.

3. Alcohol

Alcohol is the only recreational drug of abuse that is clearly teratogenic, and prenatal exposure to alcohol is the most common preventable cause of mental retardation. Prevalence estimates of fetal alcohol syndrome (FAS) in the United States range from 0.5 to 2 per 1000 live births with up to 1 in 100 having lesser effects (fetal alcohol spectrum disorders). The effects of alcohol on the fetus and newborn are determined by the degree and timing of ethanol exposure and by the maternal, fetal, and placental metabolism of ethanol, which is likely genetically determined. Although there is no clear evidence that minimal amounts of alcohol are harmful, there is no established safe dose. Fetal growth and development are adversely affected if drinking continues throughout the pregnancy, and infants can occasionally experience withdrawal similar to that associated with maternal opioid abuse. Clinical features of FAS that may be observed in the newborn period are listed in Table 2–14. This diagnosis is usually easier to recognize in older infants and children.

Table 2–14. Features observed in fetal alcohol syndrome in the newborn.

Craniofacial
Short palpebral fissures
Thin vermillion of upper lip
Flattened philtrum
Growth
Prenatal and postnatal growth deficiency (small for gestational age, failure to thrive)
Central nervous system
Microcephaly
Partial or complete agenesis of the corpus callosum
Optic nerve hypoplasia
Hypotonia, poor feeding

4. Tobacco Smoking

Smoking has a negative effect on fetal growth rate. The more the mother smokes, the greater is the degree of IUGR. There is a twofold increase in low birth weight even in light smokers (< 10 cigarettes per day). Smoking during pregnancy has been associated with mild neurodevelopmental handicaps. The possibility of multiple drug abuse also applies to smokers, and the potential interaction of multiple factors on fetal growth and development must be considered.

5. Toluene Embryopathy

Solvent toxicity may be intentional (paint, lacquer, or glue sniffing) or environmental (dry cleaning industry). The active organic solvent in these agents is toluene. Features attributable to in-utero toluene exposure are prematurity, IUGR, microcephaly, craniofacial abnormalities similar to those associated with in-utero alcohol exposure (see Table 2–14), large anterior fontanelle, hair patterning abnormalities, nail hypoplasia, and renal anomalies. Long-term effects include postnatal growth deficiency and developmental delay.

6. Marijuana

Marijuana is the most frequently used illegal drug. It does not appear to be teratogenic, and although a mild abstinence-type syndrome has been described, infants exposed to marijuana in utero rarely require treatment. Some long-term neurodevelopmental problems, particularly disordered sleep patterns, have been noted.

7. Other Drugs

Other drugs with potential effects on the newborn fall in two categories. First are drugs to which the fetus is exposed because of therapy for maternal conditions. The human placenta is relatively permeable, particularly to lipophilic solutes. If possible, maternal drug therapy should be postponed until after the first trimester to avoid teratogenic effects. Drugs with potential fetal toxicity include antineoplastics, antithyroid agents, warfarin, lithium, and angiotensin-converting enzyme inhibitors (eg, captopril and enalapril). Anticonvulsants, especially high-dose or multiple drug therapy, may be associated with craniofacial abnormalities. The use of selective serotonin reuptake inhibitors, benzodiazepines, and antipsychotic medications appears to be generally safe, and risk should be balanced against the risk of untreated psychiatric conditions in the mother. However, up to 33% of infants exposed to SSRI medications in utero experience signs of neonatal abstinence syndrome during the first days of life. Paroxetine seems to have the greatest propensity to cause abstinence symptoms. Phenobarbital may be used for severe irritability.

In the second category are drugs transmitted to the infant in breast milk. Most drugs taken by the mother achieve some concentration in breast milk, although they usually do not present a problem to the infant. If the drug is one that could have adverse effects on the infant, timing breast feeding to coincide with trough concentrations in the mother may be useful.

Ackerman JP et al: A review of the effects of prenatal cocaine exposure among school-aged children. Pediatrics 2010;125:554 [PMID: 20142293].

ACOG Committee on Health Care for Underserved Women: Committee Opinion #479: Methamphetamine abuse in women of reproductive age. Obstet Gynecol 2011;117:751 [PMID: 21343793].

Burgos AE, Burke BL: Neonatal abstinence syndrome. NeoReviews 2009;10:e222 [doi:10.1542/neo.10-5-e222].

Dannaway DC, Mulvihill JJ: Fetal alcohol spectrum disorder. NeoReviews 2009;10:e230 [doi:10.1542/neo.10-5-e230].

Jansson LM, Velez ML: Infants of drug dependent mothers. Pediatr Rev 2011;32:5 [PMID: 21196501].

O'Grady MF et al: Management of neonatal abstinence syndrome: a national survey and review of practice. Arch Dis Child Fetal Neonatal Ed 2009;94:F249 [PMID: 19174414].

Rayburn WF: Maternal and fetal effects from substance use. Clin Perinatol 2007;34:559 [PMID: 18063105].

Wong S et al and the Maternal-Fetal Medicine Committee, Family Physicians Advisory Committee, and Medicolegal Committee: Substance use in pregnancy. J Obstet Gynaecol Can 2011;33:367 [PMID: 21501542].

MULTIPLE BIRTHS

ESSENTIALS OF DIAGNOSIS & TYPICAL FEATURES

- Monochorial twins
  - Always monozygous (identical twins) and same sex.
  - Can be diamniotic or monoamniotic.
  - Risk for twin-to-twin transfusion and higher risk of congenital anomalies, neurodevelopmental problems, and cerebral palsy.
- Dichorial twins
  - Either dizygous (fraternal twins) or monozygous (identical twins); same sex or different sex.
  - Can have growth restriction due to abnormal placental implantation.
  - Not at risk for twin transfusion syndrome; less risk for anomalies and neurodevelopmental problems than monochorial twins.

Historically, twinning occurred at a rate of 1 in 80 pregnancies (1.25%). The incidence of twinning and higher-order multiple births in the United States has increased because of assisted reproductive technologies. In 2005, twins occurred in 3.2% of live births in the United States, a 70% increase since 1980.

A distinction should be made between dizygous (fraternal) and monozygous (identical) twins. Race, maternal parity, and maternal age affect the incidence of dizygous, but not monozygous, twinning. Drugs used to induce ovulation, such as clomiphene citrate and gonadotropins, increase the incidence of dizygotic or polyzygotic twinning. Monozygous twinning also seems to be more common after assisted reproduction. The incidence of malformations is also increased in identical twins and may affect only one of the twins. If a defect is found in one twin, the other should be examined carefully for lesser degrees of the same defect.

Early transvaginal ultrasound and examination of the placenta after birth can help establish the type of twinning. Two amnionic membranes and two chorionic membranes are found in all dizygous twins and in one-third of monozygous twins even when the placental disks appear to be fused into one. A single chorionic membrane always indicates monozygous twins. The rare monochorial, monoamniotic situation (1% of twins) is especially dangerous, with a high risk of antenatal cord entanglement and death of one or both twins. Close fetal surveillance is indicated, and preterm delivery is often elected.

Complications of Multiple Births

A. Intrauterine Growth Restriction

There is some degree of IUGR in most multiple pregnancies, especially after 32 weeks, although it is usually not clinically significant with two exceptions. First, in monochorial twin pregnancy an arteriovenous shunt may develop between the twins (twin-twin transfusion syndrome). The twin on the venous side (recipient) becomes plethoric and larger than the smaller anemic twin (donor), who may ultimately die or be severely growth restricted. The occurrence of polyhydramnios in the larger twin and severe oligohydramnios in the smaller may be the first sign of this problem. Second, discordance in size (birth weights that are significantly different) can also occur when separate placentas are present if one placenta develops poorly, because of a poor implantation site. In this instance, no fetal exchange of blood takes place but the growth rates of the two infants are different.

B. Preterm Delivery

Length of gestation tends to be inversely related to the number of fetuses. The mean age at delivery for singletons is 38.8 weeks, for twins 35.3 weeks, for triplets 32.2 weeks, and for quadruplets 29.9 weeks. The prematurity rate in multiple gestations is 5–10 times that of singletons, with 50% of twins and 90% of triplets born before 37 weeks. There is an increased incidence of cerebral palsy in multiple births, more so with monochorial than dichorial infants. Prematurity is the main cause of increased mortality and morbidity in twins, although in the case of monochorial twins, intravascular exchange through placental anastomoses, particularly after the death of one twin, also increases the risk substantially.

C. Obstetric Complications

Polyhydramnios, pregnancy-induced hypertension, premature rupture of membranes, abnormal fetal presentations, and prolapsed umbilical cord occur more frequently in women with multiple fetuses. Multiple pregnancy should always be identified prenatally with ultrasound examinations; doing so allows the obstetrician and pediatrician or neonatologist to plan management jointly. Because neonatal complications are usually related to prematurity, prolongation of pregnancy significantly reduces neonatal morbidity.

Cleary-Goldman J, D'Alton ME: Growth abnormalities and multiple gestations. Semin Perinatol 2008;32:206 [PMID: 18482623].
Habli M et al: Twin-to-twin transfusion syndrome: A comprehensive update. Clin Perinatol 2009;36:391 [PMID: 19559327].
Rand L, Lee H: Complicated monochorionic twin pregnancies: updates in fetal diagnosis and treatment. Clin Perinatol 2009;36: 417 [PMID: 19559328].

NEONATAL INTENSIVE CARE

PERINATAL RESUSCITATION

Perinatal resuscitation refers to the steps taken by the obstetrician to support the infant during labor and delivery and the resuscitative steps taken by the pediatrician after delivery. Intrapartum support includes maintaining maternal blood pressure, maternal oxygen therapy, positioning the mother to improve placental perfusion, readjusting oxytocin infusions or administering a tocolytic if appropriate, minimizing trauma to the infant, obtaining all necessary cord blood samples, and completing an examination of the placenta. The pediatrician or neonatologist focuses on temperature support, initiation and maintenance of effective ventilation, maintenance of perfusion and hydration, and glucose regulation.

A number of conditions associated with pregnancy, labor, and delivery place the infant at risk for birth asphyxia: (1) maternal diseases such as diabetes, pregnancy-induced hypertension, heart and renal disease, and collagen-vascular disease; (2) fetal conditions such as prematurity, multiple births, growth restriction, and fetal anomalies; and (3) labor and delivery conditions, including fetal distress with or without meconium in the amniotic fluid, and administration of anesthetics and opioid analgesics.

Physiology of Birth Asphyxia

Birth asphyxia can be the result of: (1) acute interruption of umbilical blood flow (eg, prolapsed cord with cord compression), (2) premature placental separation, (3) maternal hypotension or hypoxia, (4) chronic placental insufficiency, and (5) failure to perform resuscitation properly.

The neonatal response to asphyxia follows a predictable pattern (Figure 2–6). The initial response to hypoxia is an increase in respiratory rate and a rise in heart rate and blood pressure. Respirations then cease (primary apnea) as heart rate and blood pressure begin to fall. The initial period of apnea

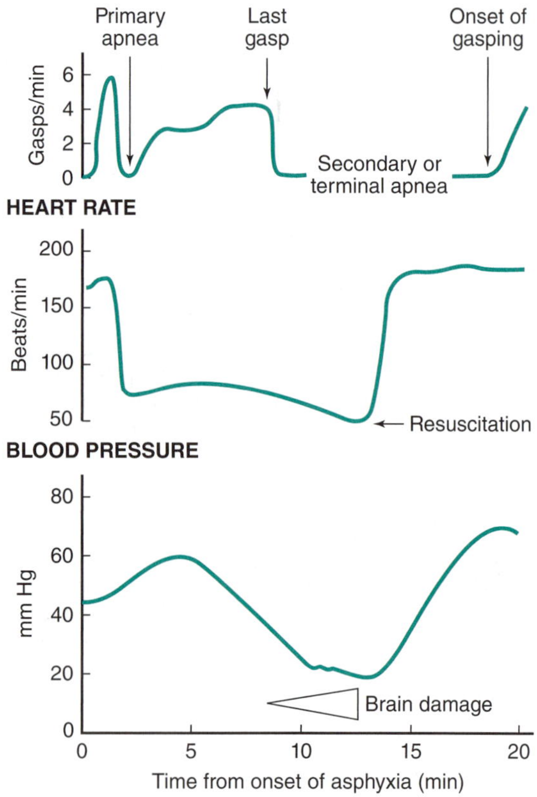

▲ **Figure 2–6.** Schematic depiction of changes in rhesus monkeys during asphyxia and on resuscitation by positive-pressure ventilation. The risk for permanent brain damage increases the longer effective resuscitation is delayed. (Adapted and reproduced, with permission, from Dawes GS: *Fetal and Neonatal Physiology*. Year Book, 1968.)

lasts 30–60 seconds. Gasping respirations (3–6 per minute) then begin, while heart rate and blood pressure gradually decline. Secondary or terminal apnea then ensues, with further decline in heart rate and blood pressure. The longer the duration of secondary apnea, the greater is the risk for hypoxic organ injury. A cardinal feature of the defense against hypoxia is the underperfusion of certain tissue beds (eg, skin, muscle, kidneys, and GI tract), which allows maintenance of perfusion to core organs (ie, heart, brain, and adrenals).

Response to resuscitation also follows a predictable pattern. During the period of primary apnea, almost any physical stimulus causes the infant to initiate respirations. Infants in secondary apnea require positive pressure ventilation (PPV). The first sign of recovery is an increase in heart rate, followed by an increase in blood pressure with improved perfusion. The time required for rhythmic, spontaneous respirations to occur is related to the duration of the secondary apnea. As a rough rule, for each minute past the last gasp, 2 minutes of PPV is required before gasping begins, and 4 minutes is required to reach rhythmic breathing. Not until sometime later do spinal and corneal reflexes return. Muscle tone gradually improves over the course of several hours.

Delivery Room Management

When asphyxia is anticipated, a resuscitation team of at least two persons should be present, one to manage the airway and one to monitor the heartbeat and provide assistance. The necessary equipment and drugs are listed in Table 2–15.

Table 2–15. Equipment for neonatal resuscitation.

Clinical Needs	Equipment
Thermoregulation	Radiant heat source with platform, mattress covered with warm sterile blankets, servocontrol heating, temperature probe, gallon size food-grade plastic bag or plastic wrap and an exothermic blanket (preterm)
Airway management	**Suction:** bulb suction, mechanical suction with sterile catheters (6F, 8F, 10F), meconium aspirator
	Ventilation: manual infant resuscitation bag connected to manometer or with a pressure-release valve, or T-piece resuscitator, capable of delivering 100% oxygen; appropriate masks for term and preterm infants, oral airways, stethoscope**, oxygen blender, pulse oximeter**
	Intubation: neonatal laryngoscope with No. 0 and No. 1 blades; endotracheal tubes (2.5, 3.0, 3.5 mm outer diameter with stylet): extra bulbs and batteries for laryngoscope; scissors, adhesive tape, gloves, end-tidal CO_2 detection device
Gastric decompression	Nasogastric tube: 8F with 20-mL syringe
Administration of drugs and volume replacement	Sterile umbilical catheterization tray, umbilical catheters (3.5F and 5F), normal saline, drug box[a] with appropriate neonatal vials and dilutions, sterile syringes, needles, and alcohol sponges
Transport	Warmed transport isolette with oxygen source

[a]Epinephrine 1:10,000; 10% dextrose.
Modified, with permission, from Rosenberg AA: The Neonate. In Gabbe SG et al (editors): Obstetrics: Normal and Problem Pregnancies. Churchill Livingstone; 2007.

A. Steps in the Resuscitative Process (Figure 2–7)

1. Dry the infant well, and place him or her under a radiant heat source. Do not allow the infant to become hyperthermic.
2. Position the infant to open the airway. Gently suction the mouth, then the nose.
3. Quickly assess the infant's condition. The best criteria are the infant's respiratory effort (apneic, gasping or, regular) and heart rate (> 100 or < 100 beats/min). A depressed heart rate—indicative of hypoxic myocardial depression—is the single most reliable indicator of the need for resuscitation.
4. Infants who are breathing and have heart rates more than 100 beats/min usually require no further intervention other than supplemental oxygen if persistently cyanotic. Infants with heart rates less than 100 beats/min and apnea or irregular respiratory efforts should be stimulated gently. The infant's back should be rubbed and/or heels flicked.
5. If the infant fails to respond to tactile stimulation within a few seconds, begin bag and mask ventilation, using a soft mask that seals well around the mouth and nose. For the initial inflations, pressures up to 30–40 cm H_2O may be necessary to overcome surface-active forces in the lungs. Adequacy of ventilation is assessed by observing expansion of the infant's chest accompanied by an improvement in heart rate, perfusion, and color. After the first few breaths, lower the peak pressure to 15–20 cm H_2O. The chest movement should resemble that of an easy breath rather than a deep sigh. The rate of bagging should be 40–60 breaths/min. An oximeter probe should be placed on the infant's right hand.
6. Most neonates can be resuscitated effectively with a bag and mask. If the infant does not respond to bag and mask ventilation, reposition the head (slight extension), reapply the mask to achieve a good seal, consider suctioning the mouth and the oropharynx, and try ventilating with the mouth open. An increase in peak pressure should also be attempted, but if the infant does not respond within 30 seconds, intubation is appropriate.

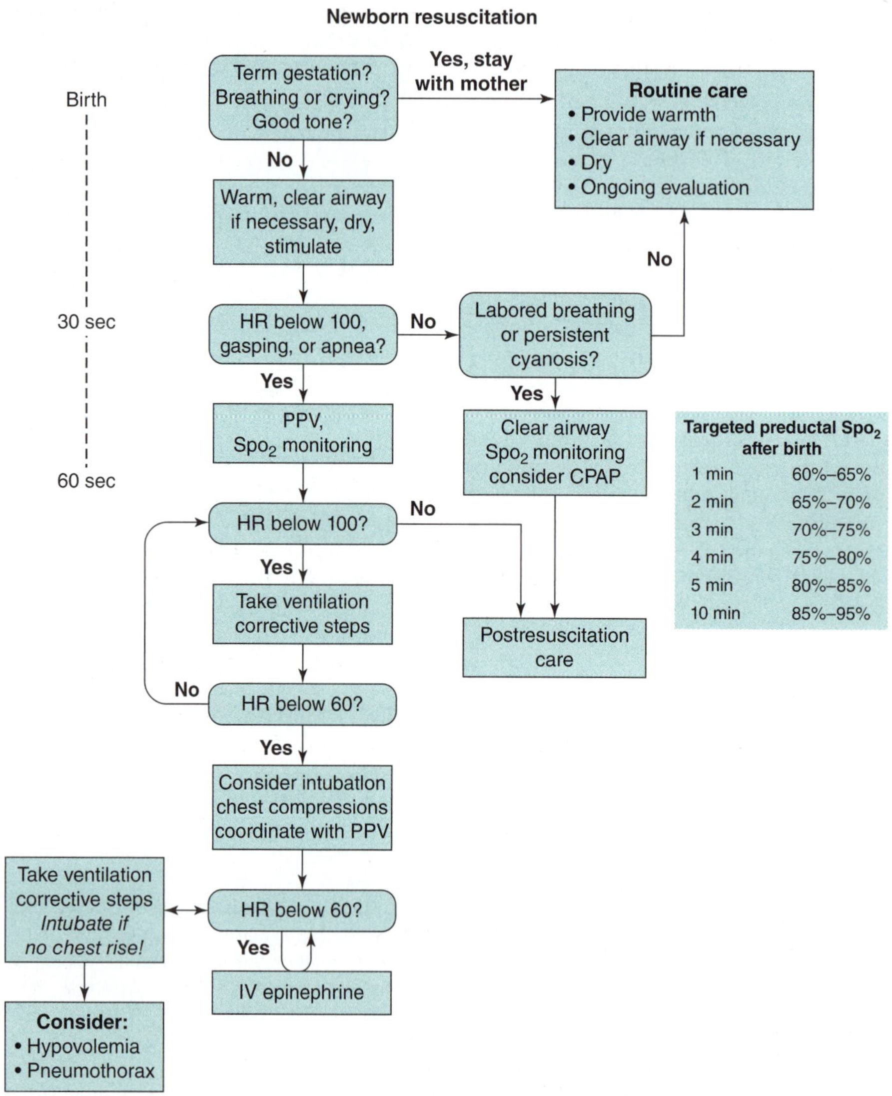

▲ **Figure 2–7.** Delivery room management. (Reproduced, with permission, from Kattwinkel J et al. Special Report: Neonatal Resuscitation: 2010 American Heart Association Guidelines for Cardiopulmonary Resuscitation and Emergency Cardiovascular Care. Pediatrics. 2010;126(5):e1400–e1413.)

Failure to respond to intubation and ventilation can result from (1) mechanical difficulties (Table 2–16), (2) profound asphyxia with myocardial depression, and (3) inadequate circulating blood volume.

Quickly rule out the mechanical causes listed in Table 2–16. Check to ensure that the endotracheal tube passes through the vocal cords. A CO_2 detector placed between the endotracheal tube and the bag can be helpful as a rapid confirmation of proper tube position in the airway. Occlusion of the tube should be suspected when there is resistance to bagging and no chest wall movement. Very few neonates (approximately 0.1%) require either cardiac compressions or drugs during resuscitation. Almost all newborns respond to ventilation if done effectively. All resuscitations in term infants should begin using room air. Oxygen concentration can be increased using an oxygen blender during positive pressure ventilation to achieve oxygen saturation targets (Figure 2-7). It is not expected for the preductal (right hand) oxygen saturation to reach 90% until 10 minutes of age. The use of 100% oxygen may increase the risk of postresuscitative oxidative injury without any improvement in efficacy.

Table 2–16. Mechanical causes of failed resuscitation.

Cause	Examples
Equipment failure	Malfunctioning bag, oxygen not connected or running
Endotracheal tube malposition	Esophagus, right main stem bronchus
Occluded endotracheal tube	
Insufficient inflation pressure to expand lungs	
Space-occupying lesions in the thorax	Pneumothorax, pleural effusions, diaphragmatic hernia
Pulmonary hypoplasia	Extreme prematurity, oligohydramnios

Reproduced with permission from Rosenberg AA: The Neonate. In Gabbe SG et al (editors): Obstetrics: Normal and Problem Pregnancies. Churchill Livingstone; 2007.

7. If mechanical causes are ruled out and the heart rate remains less than 60 beats/min after intubation and effective PPV for 30 seconds, cardiac compressions should be initiated. Chest compressions should be synchronized with ventilation at a 3:1 ratio (90 compressions and 30 breaths/min).
8. If drugs are needed, the drug and dose of choice is epinephrine 1:10,000 solution (0.1–0.3 mL/kg) given via an umbilical venous line. If volume loss is suspected, 10 mL/kg of normal saline should be administered through an umbilical vein line.

B. Continued Resuscitative Measures

The appropriateness of continued resuscitative efforts should be reevaluated in infants who do not respond to initial measures. In current practice, resuscitative efforts are made even in apparent stillbirths (ie, infants whose Apgar score at 1 minute is 0–1). Modern resuscitative techniques have led to improved survival in such infants, with 60% of survivors showing normal development. Although it is clear that resuscitation of these infants should be performed, subsequent continued support depends on the response to resuscitation. If the Apgar score does not improve markedly in the first 10 minutes of life, the mortality rate and the incidence of severe developmental handicaps among survivors are high.

C. Special Considerations

1. Preterm infants

A. Minimizing heat loss improves survival. Prewarmed towels should be available. The environmental temperature of the delivery suite should be raised to more than 25°C (especially for infants weighing < 1500 g). An occlusive skin cover such as a gallon-sized food-grade plastic bag with an opening to slip over the infant's head and an exothermic blanket should be used to minimize heat loss in the extremely low-birth-weight (< 1000 g) infant.

B. The lungs of preterm infants are especially prone to injury from PPV due to volutrauma. For this reason, if possible, the infant's respiratory efforts should be supported with nasal continuous positive airway pressure (CPAP) rather than PPV. If PPV is needed, a T-piece resuscitation device should be used to allow precise and consistent regulation of pressure delivery. Resuscitation in the preterm should begin with a blended oxygen concentration of 40% with titration to achieve target oxygen saturations (Figure 2–7).

C. In the infant of extremely low gestational age (< 27 weeks), immediate intubation for administration of surfactant should be considered.

D. Volume expanders should be infused slowly to minimize rapid swings in blood pressure, especially important in the ELBW infant.

2. Narcotic depression—In the case of opioid administration to the mother within 4 hours of delivery, institute resuscitation as described earlier. When the baby is stable with good heart rate, color, and perfusion, but still has poor respiratory effort, a trial of naloxone (0.1 mg/kg IV) may be indicated. Naloxone should not be administered in place of PPV. Naloxone should not be used in the infant of an opioid-addicted mother because it will precipitate withdrawal. Respiratory depression may recur over the next hours, requiring redosing of the antagonist.

3. Meconium-stained amniotic fluid

A. The obstetrician performs routine suctioning of the mouth and nose after birth.

B. If the infant is active and breathing, requiring no resuscitation, the airway need not be inspected—only further suctioning of the mouth and nasopharynx as required.

C. The airway of any depressed infant requiring ventilation must be checked and cleared (by passage of a tube below the vocal cords) before PPV is instituted. Special adapters are available for use with regulated wall suction to allow suction to be applied directly to the endotracheal tube.

D. Because most severe cases of meconium aspiration syndrome with pulmonary hypertension likely have their origins in utero, resuscitative efforts should not be excessively delayed with attempts to clear the airway of meconium.

4. Universal precautions—In the delivery suite, universal precautions should always be observed.

Treatment of the Asphyxiated Infant

Asphyxia is manifested by multiorgan dysfunction, seizures, neonatal encephalopathy, and metabolic acidemia. The infant with significant perinatal hypoxia and ischemia is at risk for dysfunction of multiple end organs (Table 2–17). The organ of greatest concern is the brain.

Table 2–17. Signs and symptoms caused by asphyxia.

Neonatal encephalopathy, seizures
Respiratory distress due to aspiration or secondary surfactant deficiency, pulmonary hemorrhage
Persistent pulmonary hypertension
Hypotension due to myocardial dysfunction
Transient tricuspid valve insufficiency
Anuria or oliguria due to acute tubular necrosis
Feeding intolerance; necrotizing enterocolitis
Elevated aminotransferases due to liver injury
Adrenal insufficiency due to hemorrhage
Disseminated intravascular coagulation
Hypocalcemia
Hypoglycemia
Persistent metabolic acidemia
Hyperkalemia

The features of neonatal encephalopathy are decreased level of consciousness, poor tone, decreased spontaneous movement, periodic breathing or apnea, and seizures. Brainstem signs (oculomotor and pupillary disturbances, absent gag reflex) may also be present. The severity and duration of clinical signs correlate with the severity of the insult. Other evaluations helpful in assessing severity in the full-term infant include electroencephalogram (EEG) and MRI which, particularly with diffusion-weighted imaging, is useful in the early evaluation of infants with perinatal asphyxia. A markedly abnormal EEG with voltage suppression and slowing evolving into a burst-suppression pattern is associated with severe clinical symptoms. MRI may show perfusion defects and areas of ischemic injury on diffusion weighted imaging.

Management is directed at supportive care and treatment of specific abnormalities. Fluids should be restricted initially to 60–80 mL/kg/d; oxygenation should be maintained with mechanical ventilation if necessary; blood pressure should be supported with judicious volume expansion (if hypovolemic) and pressors; and glucose should be in the normal range of 45–100 mg/dL. Hypocalcemia, coagulation abnormalities, and metabolic acidemia should be corrected and seizures treated with IV phenobarbital (20 mg/kg as loading dose, with total initial 24-hour dosing up to 40 mg/kg). Other anticonvulsants should be reserved for refractory seizures. Hypothermia, either selective head cooling with mild systemic hypothermia or whole body cooling, initiated within 6 hours of birth, has been shown to improve outcome at 18-month follow-up of infants with moderate neurologic symptoms and an abnormal amplitude-integrated EEG. Efficacy has not been proved in the most severe cases of neonatal encephalopathy.

Birth Asphyxia: Long-Term Outcome

Fetal heart rate tracings, cord pH, and 1-minute Apgar scores are imprecise predictors of long-term outcome. Apgar scores of 0–3 at 5 minutes in full-term infants are associated with an increased risk of death in the first year of life and an 8% risk of cerebral palsy among survivors. The risks of mortality and morbidity increase with more prolonged depression of the Apgar score. The single best predictor of outcome is the severity of clinical neonatal encephalopathy (severe symptomatology including coma carries a 75% chance of death and a 100% rate of neurologic sequelae among survivors). The major sequela of neonatal encephalopathy is cerebral palsy with or without mental retardation and epilepsy. Other prognostic features are prolonged seizures refractory to therapy, markedly abnormal EEG, and MRI scan with evidence of major ischemic injury. Other clinical features required to support perinatal hypoxia as the cause of cerebral palsy include the presence of fetal distress prior to birth, a low arterial cord pH of less than 7.00, evidence of other end-organ dysfunction, and absence of a congenital brain malformation.

American Heart Association and American Academy of Pediatrics: *Textbook of Neonatal Resuscitation,* 6th ed. American Heart Association/American Academy of Pediatrics, 2011.

Blackmon LR, Stark AR, Committee on Fetus and Newborn, American Academy of Pediatrics: Hypothermia: a neuroprotective therapy for neonatal hypoxic-ischemic encephalopathy. Pediatrics 2006;117:942 [PMID: 16510680].

Bry K: Newborn resuscitation and the lung. NeoReviews 2008;9:e506.

Carlo WA, Schelonka R: The outcome of infants with an Apgar score of zero at 10 minutes: Past and future. Am J Obstet Gynecol 2007;196:422 [PMID: 17466692].

Finer N et al: Use of oxygen for resuscitation of the extremely low birth weight infant. Pediatrics 2010;125:389 [PMID: 20100772].

Harrington DJ et al: The long-term outcome in surviving infants with Apgar zero at 10 minutes: A systematic review of the literature and hospital-based cohort. Am J Obstet Gynecol 2007;196:463.e1 [PMID: 17466703].

Lapointe A, Barrington KJ: Pulmonary hypertension and the asphyxiated newborn. J Pediatr 2011;158(supp):e19 [PMID: 21238701]

Nelson K: Causative factors in cerebral palsy. Clin Obstet Gynecol 2008;51:749 [PMID: 18981800].

Nuntnarumit P et al: Oxygen saturation trends in preterm infants during the first 15 minutes after birth. J Perinatol 2010;30:399 [PMID: 19890344].

Rutherford M et al: MRI of perinatal brain injury. Pediatr Radiol 2010;40:819 [PMID: 20432000].

Shankaran S: Neonatal encephalopathy: Treatment with hypothermia. NeoReviews 2010;11:e85.

Trevisanuto D et al: Heat loss prevention in very preterm infants in delivery rooms: A prospective, randomized, controlled trial of polyethylene caps. J Pediatr 2010;156:914 [PMID: 20227728].

THE PRETERM INFANT

Premature infants comprise the majority of high-risk newborns. The preterm infant faces a variety of physiologic handicaps:

1. The ability to coordinate sucking, swallowing, and breathing is not achieved until 34–36 weeks' gestation. Therefore, enteral feedings must be provided by gavage.

Further, preterm infants often have an immature gag reflex, which increases the risk of aspiration of feedings.

2. Lack of body fat stores causes decreased ability to maintain body temperature, and may predispose to hypoglycemia.
3. Pulmonary immaturity–surfactant deficiency is associated with structural immaturity in infants younger than 26 weeks' gestation. This condition is exacerbated by the combination of noncompliant lungs and an extremely compliant chest wall, causing inefficient respiratory mechanics.
4. Immature respiratory control leads to apnea and bradycardia.
5. Persistent patency of the ductus arteriosus compromises pulmonary gas exchange because of overperfusion and edema of the lungs.
6. Immature cerebral vasculature and structure predisposes to subependymal and intraventricular hemorrhage, and periventricular leukomalacia.
7. Impaired substrate absorption by the GI tract compromises nutritional management.
8. Immature renal function (including both filtration and tubular functions) complicates fluid and electrolyte management.
9. Increased susceptibility to infection.
10. Immaturity of metabolic processes predisposes to hypoglycemia and hypocalcemia.

1. Delivery Room Care

See section on Perinatal Resuscitation, earlier.

2. Care in the Nursery

A. Thermoregulation

Maintaining stable body temperature is a function of heat production and conservation balanced against heat loss. Heat production in response to cold stress occurs through voluntary muscle activity, involuntary muscle activity (shivering), and thermogenesis not caused by shivering. Newborns produce heat mainly through the last of these three mechanisms. This metabolic heat production depends on the quantity of brown fat, which is very limited in the preterm infant. Heat loss to the environment can occur through: (1) radiation—transfer of heat from a warmer to a cooler object not in contact; (2) convection—transfer of heat to the surrounding gaseous environment, influenced by air movement and temperature; (3) conduction—transfer of heat to a cooler object in contact; and (4) evaporation—cooling secondary to water loss through the skin. Heat loss in the preterm newborn is accelerated because of a high ratio of surface area to body mass, reduced insulation by subcutaneous tissue, and water loss through the immature skin.

The thermal environment of the preterm neonate must be regulated carefully. The infant can be kept warm in an isolette, in which the air is heated and convective heat loss is minimized. The infant can also be kept warm on an open bed with a radiant heat source. Although evaporative and convective heat losses are greater with radiant warmers, this system allows better access to an ill neonate. Ideally, the infant should be kept in a neutral thermal environment (Figure 2–8). The neutral thermal environment allows the infant to maintain a stable core body temperature with a minimum of metabolic heat production through oxygen consumption. The neutral thermal environment depends on the infant's size, gestational age, and postnatal age. The neutral thermal environment (for either isolette or radiant warmer care) can be obtained by maintaining an abdominal skin temperature of 36.5°C. Generally, when infants reach 1700–1800 g, they are able to maintain temperature while bundled in an open crib.

B. Monitoring the High-Risk Infant

At a minimum, equipment to monitor heart rate, respirations, and blood pressure should be available. Oxygen saturation is assessed continuously using pulse oximetry, correlated with arterial oxygen tension ($Pa{O_2}$) as needed. Transcutaneous $P{O_2}$ and $P{CO_2}$ can also be used to assess oxygenation and ventilation in sicker infants. Arterial blood gases, electrolytes, glucose, calcium, bilirubin, and other chemistries must be measured on small volumes of blood. Early in the care of a sick preterm infant, the most efficient

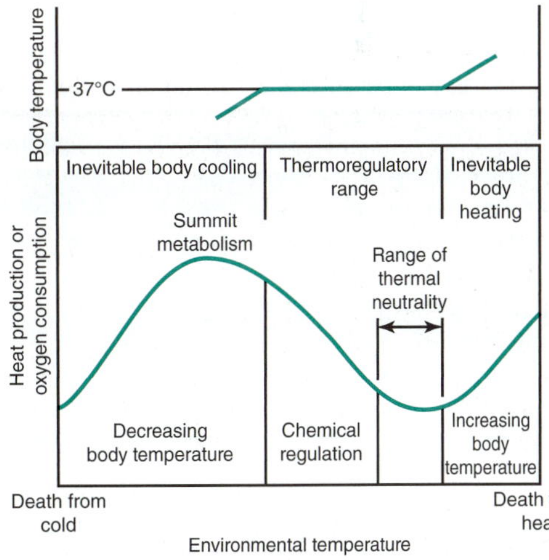

▲ **Figure 2–8.** Effect of environmental temperature on oxygen consumption and body temperature. (Adapted and reproduced, with permission, from Klaus MH, Fanaroff AA, Martin RJ: The physical environment. In: Klaus MH, Fanaroff AA eds.: *Care of the High-Risk Neonate*, 5th ed. WB Saunders, 2001.)

way to sample blood for tests as well as to provide fluids and monitor blood pressure is through an umbilical arterial line. Once the infant is stable and the need for frequent blood samples is reduced (usually 4–7 days), the umbilical line should be removed. All indwelling lines are associated with morbidity from thrombosis or embolism, infection, and bleeding.

C. Fluid and Electrolyte Therapy

Fluid requirements in preterm infants are a function of (1) insensible losses (skin and respiratory tract), (2) urine output, (3) stool output (< 5% of total), and (4) other losses, such as nasogastric losses. In most circumstances, the fluid requirement is determined largely by insensible losses plus urine losses. The major contribution to insensible water loss is evaporative skin loss. The rate of water loss is a function of gestational age (body weight, skin thickness, and maturity), environment (losses are greater under a radiant warmer than in an isolette), and the use of phototherapy. Respiratory losses are minimal when humidified oxygen is used. The renal contribution to water requirement is influenced by the limited ability of the preterm neonate either to concentrate the urine and conserve water, or to excrete a water load.

Electrolyte requirements are minimal for the first 24–48 hours until there is significant urinary excretion. Basal requirements thereafter are as follows: sodium, 3 mEq/kg/d; potassium, 2 mEq/kg/d; chloride, 2–3 mEq/kg/d; and bicarbonate, 2–3 mEq/kg/d. In the infant younger than 30 weeks' gestation, sodium and bicarbonate losses in the urine are often elevated, thereby increasing the infant's requirements.

Initial fluid management after birth varies with the infant's size and gestation. Infants of more than 1200 g should start at 80–100 mL/kg/d of $D_{10}W$. Those weighing less should start at 100–120 mL/kg/d of either $D_{10}W$ or D_5W (infants < 800 g and born before 26 weeks' gestation often become hyperglycemic on $D_{10}W$ at these infusion rates). The most critical issue in fluid management is monitoring. Monitoring body weight, urine output, fluid and electrolyte intake, serum and urine electrolytes, and glucose allows fairly precise determination of the infant's water, glucose, and electrolyte needs. Parenteral nutrition should be started early, preferably on the first day, and continued until an adequate enteral intake is achieved.

D. Nutritional Support

The average caloric requirement for the growing premature infant is 120 kcal/kg/d. Desired weight gain is 15–20 g/kg/d for infants younger than 35 weeks, and 15 g/kg/d for those older than 35 weeks; linear and head circumference growth should average 1 cm/week. Infants initially require IV glucose infusion to maintain blood glucose concentration in the range of 60–100 mg/dL. Infusions of 5–7 mg/kg/min (approximately 80–100 mL/kg/d of $D_{10}W$) are usually needed. Aggressive nutritional support in the very low-birth-weight infant should be started as soon as possible after birth, with parenteral alimentation solutions containing 3–4 g/kg/d of amino acids, given either peripherally or centrally via an umbilical vein line or percutaneous catheter (Table 2–18). Small-volume trophic feeds with breast milk

Table 2–18. Use of parenteral alimentation solutions.

	Volume (mL/kg/d)	Carbohydrate (g/dL)	Protein (g/kg)	Lipid (g/kg)	Calories (kcal/kg)
Peripheral: Short-term (7-10 d)					
Starting solution	100-150	$D_{10}W$	3	1	56-84
Target solution	150	$D_{12.5}W$	3-4	3	80-110
Central: Long-term (> 10 d)					
Starting solution	100-150	$D_{10}W$	3	1	56-84
Target solution	130	$D_{12.5}$-$D_{15}W$	3-4	3	80-110

Notes:

1. Advance dextrose in central hyperalimentation as tolerated per day as needed to achieve appropriate weight gain, as long as blood glucose remains normal, keeping glucose as 40%–60% of total calories administered.
2. Advance lipids by 0.5-1.0 g/kg/d as long as triglycerides are normal. Use 20% concentration.
3. Total water should be 100-150 mL/kg/d, depending on the child's fluid needs.

Monitoring:

1. Blood glucose two or three times a day when changing dextrose concentration, then daily.
2. Electrolytes daily, then twice a week when the child is receiving a stable solution.
3. Every 1-2 weeks: blood urea nitrogen and serum creatinine; total protein and serum albumin; serum calcium, phosphate, magnesium, direct bilirubin, and CBC with platelet counts.
4. Triglyceride level after 24 h at 2 g/kg/d and 24 h at 3 g/kg/d, then every other week.

or 20 kcal/oz premature formula should be started by gavage at 10% or less of the infant's nutritional needs (< 10 mL/kg/d) as soon as possible, generally within the first few days after birth. After several days of trophic feeds the infant can be slowly advanced to full caloric needs over 5–7 days. Even extremely small feedings can enhance intestinal readiness to accept larger feeding volumes. Intermittent bolus feedings are preferred because these appear to stimulate the release of gut-related hormones and may accelerate maturation of the GI tract, although in the extremely low-birth-weight infant (< 1000 g) or the postsurgical neonate, continuous-drip feeds are sometimes better tolerated. A more rapid advancement schedule is used for infants weighing more than 1500 g, and the slowest schedule for those weighing less than 1000 g.

In general, long-term nutritional support for infants of very low birth weight consists either of breast milk supplemented to increase protein, caloric density, and mineral content, or infant formulas modified for preterm infants. In these formulas, protein concentrations (approximately 2 g/dL) and caloric concentrations (approximately 24 kcal/oz) are relatively high. In addition, premature formulas contain some medium-chain triglycerides—which do not require bile for absorption—as an energy source. Increased calcium and phosphorus are provided to enhance bone mineralization. Formulas for both full-term and premature infants are enriched with long-chain polyunsaturated fatty acids in the hope of enhancing brain and retinal development. The infant should gradually be offered feedings of higher caloric density after a substantial volume (100–120 mL/kg/d) of 20 kcal/oz breast milk or formula is tolerated. Success of feedings is assessed by timely passage of feeds out of the stomach without emesis or large residual volumes, an abdominal examination free of distention, and a normal stool pattern.

When the preterm infant approaches term, the nutritional source for the bottle-fed infant can be changed to a transitional formula (22 kcal/oz) until age 6–9 months. Additional iron supplementation (2–4 mg/kg/d) is recommended for premature infants, beginning at 2 weeks to 2 months of age, depending on gestational age and number of previous transfusions. Infants who are treated with erythropoietin (epoetin alfa) for prevention or treatment of anemia of prematurity require a higher dosage of 4–6 mg/kg/d. Iron overload is a possibility in multiply-transfused sick preterm infants; such infants should be evaluated with serum ferritin levels prior to beginning iron supplementation.

Ehrenkranz RA: Early, aggressive nutritional management for very low birth weight infants: What is the evidence? Semin Perinatol 2007;31:48 [PMID: 17462488].

Rao R, Georgieff MK: Iron therapy for preterm infants. Clin Perinatol 2009;36:27 [PMID: 19161863].

Uhing MR, Das USG: Optimizing growth in the preterm infant. Clin Perinatol 2009;36:165 [PMID: 19161873].

3. Apnea in the Preterm Infant

ESSENTIALS OF DIAGNOSIS & TYPICAL FEATURES

- Respiratory pause of sufficient duration to result in cyanosis or bradycardia.
- Most common in infants born before 34 weeks' gestation; onset before 2 weeks of age.
- Methylxanthines (eg, caffeine) provide effective treatment.

General Considerations

Apnea is defined as a respiratory pause lasting more than 20 seconds—or any pause accompanied by cyanosis and bradycardia. Shorter respiratory pauses associated with cyanosis or bradycardia also qualify as significant apnea, whereas periodic breathing, which is common in full-term and preterm infants, is defined as regularly recurring ventilatory cycles interrupted by short pauses *not* associated with bradycardia or color change. By definition, apnea of prematurity is not associated with a predisposing factor, and is a diagnosis of exclusion. A variety of processes may precipitate apnea (Table 2–19) and should be considered before a diagnosis of apnea of prematurity is established.

Apnea of prematurity is the most frequent cause of apnea. Most apnea of prematurity is mixed apnea characterized by a centrally (brainstem) mediated respiratory pause preceded or followed by airway obstruction. Less common is pure central or pure obstructive apnea. Apnea of prematurity is the result of immaturity of both the central respiratory regulatory centers and protective mechanisms that aid in maintaining airway patency.

Table 2–19. Causes of apnea in the preterm infant.

Temperature instability—both cold and heat stress
Response to passage of a feeding tube
Gastroesophageal reflux
Hypoxemia
Pulmonary parenchymal disease
Patent ductus arteriosus
Anemia
Infection
Sepsis (viral or bacterial)
Necrotizing enterocolitis
Metabolic causes
Hypoglycemia
Intracranial hemorrhage
Posthemorrhagic hydrocephalus
Seizures
Drugs (eg, morphine)
Apnea of prematurity

Clinical Findings

Onset is typically during the first 2 weeks of life. The frequency of spells gradually increases with time. Pathologic apnea should be suspected if spells are sudden in onset, unusually frequent, or very severe. Apnea at birth or on the first day of life is unusual but can occur in the nonventilated preterm infant. In the full-term or late preterm infant, presentation at birth suggests neuromuscular abnormalities of an acute (asphyxia, birth trauma, or infection) or chronic (eg, congenital hypotonia or structural CNS lesion) nature.

All infants—regardless of the severity and frequency of apnea—require a minimum screening evaluation, including a general assessment of well-being (eg, tolerance of feedings, stable temperature, normal physical examination), a check of the association of spells with feeding, measurement of Pao_2 or Sao_2, blood glucose, hematocrit, and a review of the drug history. Infants with severe apnea of sudden onset require more extensive evaluation for primary causes, especially infection. Other specific tests are dictated by relevant signs, for example, evaluation for necrotizing enterocolitis (NEC) in an infant with apnea and abdominal distention or feeding intolerance.

Treatment

Any underlying cause should be treated. If the apnea is due simply to prematurity, symptomatic treatment is dictated by the frequency and severity of apneic spells. Spells frequent enough to interfere with other aspects of care (eg, feeding), or severe enough to cause cyanosis or bradycardia necessitating significant intervention or bag and mask ventilation require treatment. Caffeine citrate (20 mg/kg as loading dose and then 5–10 mg/kg/d) is the drug of choice. Side effects of caffeine are generally mild, and include tachycardia and occasional feeding intolerance. The dose used should be the smallest dose necessary to decrease the frequency of apnea and eliminate severe spells. Target drug level, if monitored, is usually 10–20 mcg/mL. Nasal continuous positive airway pressure (CPAP), by treating the obstructive component of apnea, is effective in some infants. Intubation and ventilation can eliminate apneic spells but carry the risks associated with endotracheal intubation. Although many preterm infants are treated medically for possible reflux-associated apnea, there is little evidence to support this intervention. If suspected, a trial of continuous drip gastric or transpyloric feedings can be helpful as a diagnostic and therapeutic intervention.

Prognosis

In most premature infants, apneic and bradycardiac spells cease by 34–36 weeks postmenstrual age. Spells that require intervention cease prior to self-resolving episodes. In infants born at less than 28 weeks' gestation, episodes may continue past term. Apneic and bradycardiac episodes in the nursery are not predictors of later SIDS, although the incidence of SIDS is slightly increased in preterm infants. Thus, home monitoring in infants who experienced apnea in the nursery is rarely indicated.

4. Hyaline Membrane Disease

ESSENTIALS OF DIAGNOSIS & TYPICAL FEATURES

- Tachypnea, cyanosis, and expiratory grunting.
- Poor air movement despite increased work of breathing.
- Chest radiograph showing hypoexpansion and air bronchograms.

General Considerations

The most common cause of respiratory distress in the preterm infant is hyaline membrane disease. The incidence increases from 5% of infants born at 35–36 weeks' gestation to more than 50% of infants born at 26–28 weeks' gestation. This condition is caused by a deficiency of surfactant production as well as surfactant inactivation by protein leak into airspaces. Surfactant decreases surface tension in the alveolus during expiration, allowing the alveolus to remain partly expanded and maintain a functional residual capacity. The absence or inactivation of surfactant results in poor lung compliance and atelectasis. The infant must expend a great deal of effort to expand the lungs with each breath, and respiratory failure ensues (Figure 2–9).

Clinical Findings

Infants with hyaline membrane disease show all the clinical signs of respiratory distress. On auscultation, air movement is diminished despite vigorous respiratory effort. The chest radiograph demonstrates diffuse bilateral atelectasis, causing

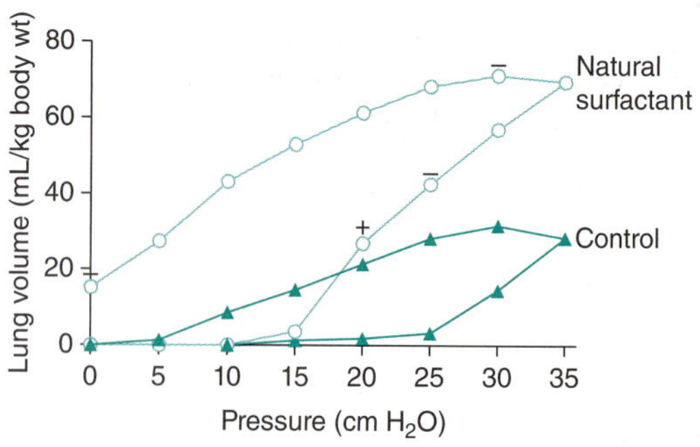

▲ **Figure 2–9.** Pressure–volume relationships for the inflation and deflation of surfactant-deficient and surfactant-treated preterm rabbit lungs. (Reproduced, with permission, from Jobe AH: The developmental biology of the lung. In: Fanaroff AA, Martin RJ editors: *Neonatal-Perinatal Medicine: Diseases of the Fetus and Infant*, 6th ed. Mosby, 1997.)

a ground-glass appearance. Major airways are highlighted by the atelectatic air sacs, creating air bronchograms. In the unintubated child, doming of the diaphragm and hypoinflation occur.

Treatment

Supplemental oxygen, nasal CPAP, early intubation for surfactant administration and ventilation, and placement of umbilical artery and vein lines are the initial interventions required. A ventilator that can deliver breaths synchronized with the infant's respiratory efforts (synchronized intermittent mandatory ventilation) and accurately deliver a preset tidal volume (5–6 mL/kg) should be used. Alternatively, pressure limited ventilation with measurement of exhaled tidal volumes can be used. High-frequency ventilators are available for rescue of infants doing poorly on conventional ventilation or who have air leak problems.

Surfactant replacement is used both in the delivery room as prophylaxis for infants born before 27 weeks' gestation and with established hyaline membrane disease as rescue, preferably within 2–4 hours of birth. Surfactant therapy decreases both the mortality rate in preterm infants and air leak complications of the disease. During the acute course, ventilator settings and oxygen requirements are significantly lower in surfactant-treated infants than in controls. The dose of the bovine-derived beractant (Survanta) is 4 mL/kg, the calf lung surfactant extract (Infasurf) is 3 mL/kg, and the porcine-derived poractant (Curosurf) is 1.25–2.5 mL/kg, given intratracheally. Repeat dosing is indicated in infants who remain on the ventilator in more than 30%–40% oxygen. A total of two to three doses given 8–12 hours apart may be administered. As the disease evolves, proteins that inhibit surfactant function leak into the air spaces, making surfactant replacement less effective. In stable infants, a trial of nasal CPAP at 5–6 cm H_2O pressure can be attempted prior to intubation and surfactant administration. For those who require mechanical ventilation, extubation to nasal CPAP should be done as early as possible to minimize lung injury and evolution of chronic lung disease. Nasal intermittent positive pressure ventilation (NIPPV) is another modality that may be attempted for ventilatory support of the VLBW infant, with potential for less morbidity. Antenatal administration of corticosteroids to the mother is an important strategy to accelerate lung maturation. Infants whose mothers were given corticosteroids more than 24 hours prior to preterm birth are less likely to have respiratory distress syndrome and have a lower mortality rate.

5. Chronic Lung Disease in the Premature Infant

General Considerations

Chronic lung disease, defined as respiratory symptoms, oxygen requirement, and chest radiograph abnormalities at 36 weeks postconception, occurs in about 20% of preterm infants ventilated for surfactant deficiency. The incidence is higher at lower gestational ages and in infants exposed to chorioamnionitis prior to birth. The development of chronic lung disease is a function of lung immaturity at birth, inflammation, and exposure to high oxygen concentrations and ventilator volutrauma. Surfactant-replacement therapy or early nasal CPAP has diminished the severity of chronic lung disease. The mortality rate from chronic lung disease is very low, but there is still significant morbidity secondary to reactive airway symptoms and hospital readmissions during the first 2 years of life for intercurrent respiratory infection.

Treatment

Long-term supplemental oxygen, mechanical ventilation, and nasal CPAP are the primary therapies for chronic lung disease of the premature. Diuretics (furosemide, 1–2 mg/kg/d, or hydrochlorothiazide-spironolactone, 1–2 mg/kg/d), inhaled β_2-adrenergics, inhaled corticosteroids (fluticasone or budesonide), and systemic corticosteroids (dexamethasone [0.2 mg/kg/d], prednisone [1–2 mg/kg/d] or hydrocortisone [4–5 mg/kg/d]) are used as adjunctive therapy. The use of systemic corticosteroids remains controversial. Although a decrease in lung inflammation can aid infants in weaning from ventilator support, there are data associating dexamethasone use in the first week of life with an increased incidence of cerebral palsy. This risk must be balanced against the higher risk of neurodevelopmental handicap in infants with severe chronic lung disease. There is likely a point in the course of these infants at which the benefit of using systemic corticosteroids for the shortest amount of time at the lowest dose possible outweighs the risk of continued mechanical ventilation. After hospital discharge, some of these infants will require oxygen at home. This can be monitored by pulse oximetry with a target Sao_2 of 94%–96%. Some will continue to manifest pulmonary symptomatology into adolescence.

AAP Committee on Fetus and Newborn: Hospital discharge of the high-risk neonate. Pediatrics 2008;122:1119 [PMID: 18977994].

Bhandari A, Bhandari V: Pitfalls, problems, and progress in bronchopulmonary dysplasia. Pediatrics 2009;123:1562 [PMID: 19482769].

Bhandari V et al: Synchronized nasal intermittent positive pressure ventilation and neonatal outcomes. Pediatrics 2009;124:517 [PMID: 19651577].

Engle JA, AAP Committee on Fetus and Newborn: Surfactant replacement therapy for respiratory distress in the preterm and term neonate. Pediatrics 2008;121:419 [PMID: 18245434].

Jobe AH: Postnatal corticosteroids for bronchopulmonary dysplasia. Clin Perinatol 2009;36:177 [PMID: 19161874].

Keszler M: State of the art in conventional mechanical ventilation. J Perinatol 2009;29:262 [PMID: 19242486].

Matthew OP: Apnea of prematurity: Pathogenesis and management strategies. J perinatol 2011;31:302 [PMID: 21127467].

Rojas MA et al: Very early surfactant without mandatory ventilation in premature infants treated with early continuous positive airway pressure: A randomized controlled trial. Pediatrics 2009;123:137 [PMID: 19117872].

Silvestri JM: Indications for home apnea monitoring (or not). Clin Perinatol 2009;36:87 [PMID: 19161867].

Warren JB, Anderson JM: Core concepts: Respiratory distress syndrome. NeoReviews 2009;10:e351.

Watterberg KL, and AAP Committee on Fetus and Newborn: Policy Statement—Postnatal corticosteroids to prevent or treat bronchopulmonary dysplasia. Pediatrics 2010;126:800 [PMID: 20819899].

6. Patent Ductus Arteriosus

ESSENTIALS OF DIAGNOSIS & TYPICAL FEATURES

- Hyperdynamic precordium.
- Widened pulse pressure.
- Hypotension.
- Presence of a systolic heart murmur in many cases.

General Considerations

Clinically significant patent ductus arteriosus usually presents on days 3–7 as the respiratory distress from hyaline membrane disease is improving. Presentation can be on days 1 or 2, especially in infants born before 28 weeks' gestation and in those who have received surfactant-replacement therapy. The signs include a hyperdynamic precordium, increased peripheral pulses, and a widened pulse pressure with or without a systolic machinery type heart murmur. Early presentations are sometimes manifested by systemic hypotension without a murmur or hyperdynamic circulation. These signs are often accompanied by an increased need for respiratory support and metabolic acidemia. The presence of patent ductus arteriosus is confirmed by echocardiography.

Treatment

Treatment of patent ductus arteriosus is by medical or surgical ligation. A clinically significant ductus can be closed with indomethacin (0.2 mg/kg IV q12h for three doses) in about two-thirds of cases. If the ductus reopens or fails to close completely, a second course of drug may be used or surgical ligation can be considered if the infant remains symptomatic. In addition, in the extremely low-birth-weight infant (< 1000 g) who is at very high risk of developing a symptomatic ductus, a prophylactic strategy of indomethacin (0.1 mg/kg q24h for 3–5 days) beginning on the first day of life may be used, with the possible additional benefit of decreasing the incidence of severe IVH, although there is no evidence of an effect on mortality or neurodevelopment. The most common side effect of indomethacin is transient oliguria, which can be managed by fluid restriction until urine output improves. Indomethacin should not be used if the infant is hyperkalemic, if the creatinine is higher than 2 mg/dL, or if the platelet count is less than 50,000/mL. There is an increased incidence of intestinal perforation if indomethacin is used concomitantly with hydrocortisone in extremely low-birth-weight infants (9% vs 2% for either drug alone). Ibuprofen lysine can be used as an alternative to indomethacin given every 24 hours as an initial dose of 10 mg/kg and then 5 mg/kg for two doses. Oliguria is less severe and less frequent than with indomethacin.

Benitz WE: Treatment of persistent patent ductus arteriosus in preterm infants: time to accept the null hypothesis? J Perinatol 2010;30:241 [PMID: 20182439].

Fowlie PW et al: Prophylactic intravenous indomethacin for preventing mortality and morbidity in preterm infants. Cochrane Database Syst Rev 2010;7:CD000174 [PMID: 20614421].

Gien J: Controversies in the management of patent ductus arteriosus. NeoReviews 2008;9:e477.

Hamrick SEG, Hansmann G: Patent ductus arteriosus of the preterm infant. Pediatrics 2010;125:1020 [PMID: 20421261].

Ohlsson A et al: Ibuprofen for the treatment of patent ductus arteriosus in preterm and/or low birth weight infants. Cochrane Database Syst Rev 2010 Apr 14;4:CD003481 [PMID: 20393936].

7. Necrotizing Enterocolitis

ESSENTIALS OF DIAGNOSIS & TYPICAL FEATURES

- Feeding intolerance with gastric residuals or vomiting.
- Bloody stools.
- Abdominal distention and tenderness.
- Pneumatosis intestinalis on abdominal radiograph.

General Considerations

NEC is the most common acquired GI emergency in the newborn. It is most common in preterm infants, with an incidence of 10% in infants less than 1500 g. In full-term infants, it occurs in association with polycythemia, congenital heart disease, and birth asphyxia. The pathogenesis of NEC is multifactorial. Ischemia, immaturity, microbial dysbiosis (proliferation of pathogenic bacteria with less colonization with beneficial or commensal bacteria), and genetics are all thought to play a role. In up to 20% of affected infants, the only risk factor is prematurity. IUGR infants with a history of absent or reversed end-diastolic flow in the umbilical artery prior to delivery have abnormalities of splanchnic flow after delivery and have an increased risk of NEC.

Clinical Findings

The most common presenting sign is abdominal distention. Other signs are vomiting, increased gastric residuals, heme-positive stools, abdominal tenderness, temperature instability, increased apnea and bradycardia, decreased urine output, and poor perfusion. There may be an increased white blood cell count with an increased band count or, as the disease progresses, absolute neutropenia. Thrombocytopenia often occurs along with stress-induced hyperglycemia and metabolic acidosis. Diagnosis is confirmed by the presence of pneumatosis intestinalis (air in the bowel wall) or biliary tract air on a plain abdominal radiograph. There is a spectrum of disease, and milder cases may exhibit only distention of bowel loops with bowel wall edema.

Treatment

A. Medical Treatment

NEC is managed by making the infant NPO, nasogastric decompression of the gut, maintenance of oxygenation, mechanical ventilation if necessary, and IV fluids to replace third-space GI losses. Enough fluid should be given to restore good urine output. Other measures include broad-spectrum antibiotics (usually ampicillin, a third-generation cephalosporin or an aminoglycoside, and possibly additional anaerobic coverage), close monitoring of vital signs, and serial physical examinations and laboratory studies (blood gases, white blood cell count, platelet count, and radiographs). Although there are no proven strategies to prevent NEC, use of trophic feedings, breast milk, and cautious advancement of feeds, as well as probiotic agents, may provide some protection, even though the optimal formulation and dose of probiotics for prevention are as yet unknown.

B. Surgical Treatment

Indications for surgery are evidence of perforation (free air present on a left lateral decubitus or cross-table lateral film), a fixed dilated loop of bowel on serial radiographs, abdominal wall cellulitis, or deterioration despite maximal medical support. All of these signs are indicative of necrotic bowel. In the operating room, necrotic bowel is removed and ostomies are created, although occasionally a primary end-to-end anastomosis may be performed. In extremely low-birth-weight infants, the initial surgical management may simply be the placement of peritoneal drains. Reanastomosis in infants with ostomies is performed after the disease resolves and the infant is bigger (usually > 2 kg and after 4–6 weeks).

Course & Prognosis

Infants treated medically or surgically should not be refed until the disease is resolved (normal abdominal examination and resolution of pneumatosis), usually after 7–10 days. Nutritional support during this time should be provided by total parenteral nutrition.

Death occurs in 10% of cases. Surgery is needed in fewer than 25% of cases. Long-term prognosis is determined by the amount of intestine lost. Infants with short bowel require long-term support with IV nutrition (see Chapter 21). Late strictures—about 3–6 weeks after initial diagnosis—occur in 8% of patients whether treated medically or surgically, and generally require operative management. Infants with surgically managed NEC have an increased risk of poor neurodevelopmental outcome.

Alfaleh K et al: Probiotics for prevention of necrotizing enterocolitis in preterm infants. Cochrane Database Syst Rev 2011 Mar 16;3:CD005496 [PMID: 21412889].

Deshpande G et al: Updated meta-analysis of probiotics for preventing necrotizing enterocolitis in preterm neonates. Pediatrics 2010;125:921 [PMID: 20403939].

Lin HC et al: Oral probiotics prevent necrotizing enterocolitis in very low birth weight preterm infants: a multicenter, randomized, controlled trial. Pediatrics 2008;122:693 [PMID: 18829790].

Neu J, Walker A: Necrotizing enterocolitis. N Engl J Med 2011;364:255 [PMID: 21247316].

Srinivasan PS et al: Necrotizing enterocolitis. Clin Perinatol 2008;35:251 [PMID: 18280885].

Young CM et al: Ischemia-reperfusion and neonatal intestinal injury. J Pediatr 2010;158(supp):e25 [PMID: 21238702].

8. Anemia in the Premature Infant

General Considerations

In the premature infant, the hemoglobin concentration reaches its nadir at about 8–12 weeks and is 2–3 g/dL lower than that of the full-term infant. The lower nadir in premature infants appears to be the result of decreased erythropoietin response to the low red cell mass. Symptoms of anemia include poor feeding, lethargy, increased heart rate, poor weight gain, and perhaps periodic breathing.

Treatment

Transfusion is not indicated in an asymptomatic infant simply because of a low hematocrit. Most infants become symptomatic if the hematocrit drops below 20%. Infants on ventilators and supplemental oxygen are usually maintained with hematocrits above 25%–30%. Alternatively, infants can be treated with erythropoietin (350 U/kg/d for 7–10 days for hematocrits < 28%). The therapeutic goal is to minimize blood draws and use conservative guidelines for transfusion. Delayed cord clamping 1–2 minutes after birth, if possible, can significantly decrease the need for future transfusion. Use of erythropoietin may increase the rate and severity of retinopathy of prematurity, and should be used judiciously.

Bishara N, Ohls RK: Current controversies in the management of the anemia of prematurity. Semin Perinatol 2009;33:29 [PMID: 19167579].

Crowley M, Kirpalani H: A rational approach to red blood cell transfusion in the neonatal ICU. Curr Opin Pediatr 2010;22:151 [PMID: 20087187].

Romagnoli C et al: Erythropoietin and retinopathy of prematurity. Early Hum Devel 2011;87S:S39 [PMID: 21303729].

Von Kohorn I, Ehrenkranz RA: Anemia in the preterm infant: Erythropoietin versus erythrocyte transfusion—it's not that simple. Clin Perinatol 2009;36:111 [PMID: 19161869].

9. Intraventricular Hemorrhage

ESSENTIALS OF DIAGNOSIS & TYPICAL FEATURES

- Large bleeds cause hypotension, metabolic acidosis, and altered neurologic status; smaller bleeds can be asymptomatic.
- Routine cranial ultrasound scanning is essential for diagnosis in infants born before 32 weeks' gestation.

General Considerations

Periventricular–intraventricular hemorrhage occurs almost exclusively in premature infants. The incidence is 15%–25% in infants born before 31 weeks' gestation and weighing less than 1500 g. The highest incidence occurs in infants of the lowest gestational age (< 26 weeks). Bleeding most commonly occurs in the subependymal germinal matrix (a region of undifferentiated cells adjacent to or lining the lateral ventricles). Bleeding can extend into the ventricular cavity. The proposed pathogenesis of bleeding is presented in Figure 2–10. The critical event is ischemia with reperfusion injury to the capillaries in the germinal matrix in the immediate perinatal period, in the face of immature cerebral pressure autoregulation. The actual amount of bleeding is also influenced by a variety of factors that affect the pressure gradient across the injured capillary wall, such as venous congestion. This pathogenetic scheme applies also to intraparenchymal bleeding (venous infarction in a region rendered ischemic) and to periventricular leukomalacia (ischemic white matter injury in a water-shed region of arterial supply). CNS complications in preterm infants are more frequent in infants exposed to intrauterine and postnatal infection, implying also the involvement of inflammatory mediators in the pathogenesis of brain injury.

Clinical Findings

Up to 50% of hemorrhages occur before 24 hours of age, and virtually all occur by the fourth day. The clinical syndrome ranges from rapid deterioration (coma, hypoventilation, decerebrate posturing, fixed pupils, bulging anterior fontanelle, hypotension, acidosis, or acute drop in hematocrit) to a more gradual deterioration with more subtle neurologic changes, to absence of any specific physiologic or neurologic signs.

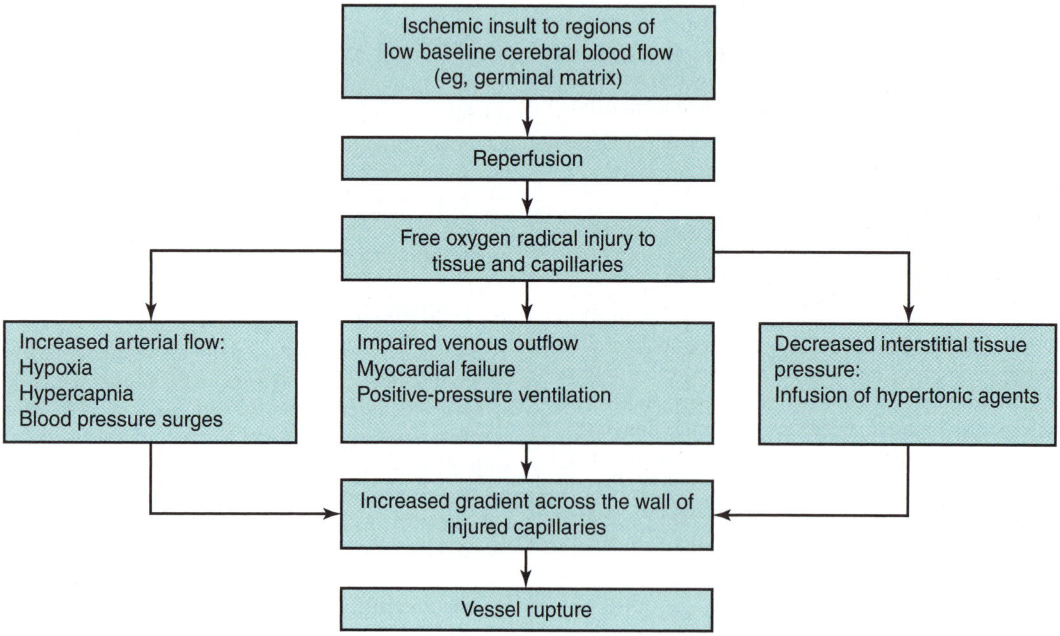

▲ **Figure 2–10.** Pathogenesis of periventricular and intraventricular hemorrhage.

The diagnosis can be confirmed by real-time ultrasound scan. Routine scanning should be done at 10–14 days in all infants born before 29 weeks' gestation. Hemorrhages are graded as follows: grade I, germinal matrix hemorrhage only; grade II, intraventricular bleeding without ventricular enlargement; grade III, intraventricular bleeding with ventricular enlargement; or grade IV, any intraparenchymal bleeding. The amount of bleeding is minor (grade I or II) in 75% of infants who bleed and major in the remainder. Follow-up ultrasound examinations are scheduled based on the results of the initial scan. Infants with no bleeding or germinal matrix hemorrhage require only a single follow- up scan at age 4–6 weeks to look for periventricular leukomalacia (PVL). An infant with blood in the ventricular system is at risk for posthemorrhagic ventriculomegaly. This is usually the result of impaired absorption of cerebrospinal fluid (CSF) but can also occur secondary to obstructive phenomena. An initial follow-up scan should be done 1–2 weeks after the initial scan. Infants with intraventricular bleeding and ventricular enlargement should be followed every 7–10 days until ventricular enlargement stabilizes or decreases. Infants born at 29–32 weeks' gestational age need only a single late scan done at 4–6 weeks of age to look for PVL or ventriculomegaly.

Treatment

During acute hemorrhage, supportive treatment (restoration of volume and hematocrit, oxygenation, and ventilation) should be provided to avoid further cerebral ischemia. Progressive posthemorrhagic hydrocephalus is treated initially with a subgaleal shunt. When the infant is large enough, this can be converted to a ventriculoperitoneal shunt.

Although the incidence and severity of intracranial bleeding in premature infants have decreased, strategies to prevent this complication are still needed. Maternal antenatal corticosteroids appear to decrease the risk of intracranial bleeding, and phenobarbital may have a role in the mother who has not been prepared with steroids and is delivering before 28 weeks' gestation. Magnesium sulfate administered to the mother appears to reduce the rate of cerebral palsy, although not the rate of IVH per se. The route of delivery may be important as infants delivered by cesarean section have a decreased rate of intracranial bleed. Postnatal strategies are less effective. Early indomethacin administration may have some benefit in minimizing bleeding, especially in males, with unclear influence on long-term outcome.

Prognosis

No deaths occur as a result of grade I and grade II hemorrhages. Grade III and grade IV hemorrhages carry a mortality rate of 10%–20%. Posthemorrhagic ventricular enlargement is rarely seen with grade I hemorrhages but is seen in 54%–87% of grade II–IV hemorrhages. Very few of these infants will require a ventriculoperitoneal shunt. Long-term neurologic sequelae are seen slightly more frequently in infants with grade I and grade II hemorrhages than in preterm infants without bleeding. In infants with grade III and grade IV hemorrhages, severe sequelae occur in 20%–25% of cases, mild sequelae in 35% of cases, but no sequelae in 40% of cases. Severe periventricular leukomalacia, large parenchymal bleeds, especially if bilateral, and progressive hydrocephalus increase the risk of neurologic sequelae. It is important to note that extremely low-birth-weight infants without major ultrasound findings also remain at increased risk for both cerebral palsy and cognitive delays. Recent reports using quantitative MRI scans demonstrate that subtle gray and white matter findings not seen with ultrasound are prevalent in preterm survivors and are predictive of neurodevelopmental handicap. This is especially true in infants born weighing less than 1000 g and before 28 weeks' gestation.

Aarnoudse-Moens CSH et al: Meta-analysis of neurobehavioral outcomes in very preterm and/or very low birth weight children. Pediatrics 2009;124:717[PMID: 19651588].

Ballabh P: Intraventricular hemorrhage in premature infants: mechanism of disease. Pediatr Res 2010;67:1 [PMID: 19816235].

Bass WT: Periventricular leukomalacia. NeoReviews 2011;12:e76.

Bassan H: Intracranial hemorrhage in the preterm infant: understanding it, preventing it. Clin Perinatol 2009;36:737 [PMID: 19944833].

McCrea HJ, Ment LR: The diagnosis, management, and prevention of intraventricular hemorrhage in the preterm neonate. Clin Perinatol 2008;35:777 [PMID: 19026340].

Volpe JJ: Brain injury in premature infants: A complex amalgam of destructive and developmental disturbances. Lancet Neurol 2009;8:110 [PMID: 19081519].

Whitelaw A: Core concepts: intraventricular hemorrhage. NeoReviews 2011;12:e94.

10. Retinopathy of Prematurity

ESSENTIALS OF DIAGNOSIS & TYPICAL FEATURES

- Risk of severe retinopathy is greatest in the most immature infants.
- Diagnosis depends on screening eye examinations in at-risk preterm infants.
- Examination evaluates stage of abnormal retinal vascular development, extent of retinal detachment, and distribution and amount of retina involved.

Retinopathy of prematurity occurs only in the incompletely vascularized premature retina. The incidence of retinopathy in infants weighing less than 1250 g is 66%, but only 6%

have retinopathy severe enough to warrant intervention. The incidence is highest in infants of the lowest gestational age. The condition appears to be triggered by an initial injury to the developing retinal vessels and low levels of insulin-like growth factor-1. After the initial injury, normal vessel development may follow or abnormal vascularization may occur due to excessive vascular endothelial growth factor (VEGF), with ridge formation on the retina. Lability in oxygen levels with periods of hypoxia/hyperoxia likely potentiate this progression. The frequency of retinopathy progressing to the need for treatment can be diminished by careful monitoring of the infant's oxygen saturation levels. The process can regress at this point or may continue, with growth of fibrovascular tissue into the vitreous associated with inflammation, scarring, and retinal folds or detachment. The disease is graded by stages of abnormal vascular development and retinal detachment (I–V), by the zone of the eye involved (1–3, with zone 1 being the posterior region around the macula), and by the amount of the retina involved, in "clock hours" (eg, a detachment in the upper, outer quadrant of the left eye would be defined as affecting the left retina from 12 to 3 o'clock).

Initial eye examination should be performed at 31 weeks postmenstrual age or at 4 weeks of age, whichever is earlier, in infants born at 30 weeks' gestation or less, as well as in infants up to 32 weeks' gestation with an unstable clinical course. Follow-up occurs at 1- to 3-week intervals, depending on the findings, until the retina is fully vascularized. Laser therapy is used in infants with progressive disease at risk for retinal detachment. Although this treatment does not always prevent retinal detachment, it reduces the incidence of poor outcomes based on visual acuity and retinal anatomy. A new form of therapy is intravitreal bevacizumab, an anti-VEGF monoclonal antibody, which may prove to be superior to laser therapy for severe Zone I and II retinopathy of prematurity.

American Academy of Pediatrics Section on Ophthalmology, American Academy of Ophthalmology and Association for Pediatric Ophthalmology and Strabismus: Screening examination of premature infants for retinopathy of prematurity. Pediatrics 2006;117:572 [PMID: 16452383].

Cole CH: Making sense of clinical determinants of retinopathy of prematurity. Pediatrics 2010;157:5 [PMID: 20547261].

Fleck BW, McIntosh N: Retinopathy of prematurity: Recent developments. NeoReviews 2009;10:e20.

Mintz-Hittner HA et al and the BEAT-ROP Cooperative Group: Efficacy of intravitreal bevacizumab for Stage 3+ retinopathy of prematurity. N Engl J Med 2011;364:603 [PMID: 21323540].

Salvin JH et al: Update on retinopathy of prematurity: treatment options and outcomes. Curr Opin Ophthalmol 2010;21:329 [PMID: 20634698].

SUPPORT Study Group of the Eunice Kennedy Shriver NICHD Neonatal Network: Target ranges of oxygen saturation in extremely preterm infants. N Engl J Med 2010;362:1959 [PMID: 20860514].

11. Discharge & Follow-Up of the Premature Infant

A. Hospital Discharge

Criteria for discharge of the premature infant include maintaining normal temperature in an open crib, adequate oral intake, acceptable weight gain, and absence of apnea and bradycardia spells requiring intervention. Infants going home on supplemental oxygen should not desaturate below 80% in room air or should demonstrate the ability to arouse in response to hypoxia. Factors such as support for the mother at home and the stability of the family situation play a role in the timing of discharge. Home nursing visits and early physician follow-up can be used to hasten discharge. Additionally, the American Academy of Pediatrics recommends that preterm infants have a period of observation in an infant car seat, preferably their own, before hospital discharge, with careful positioning to mimic optimal restraint as would occur in the car, to see that they do not have obstructive apnea or desaturation for periods up to 90–120 minutes.

B. Follow-Up

With advances in obstetric and maternal care, survival of infants born after 28 weeks' gestation or weighing as little as 1000 g at birth is now better than 90%. Seventy to 80% survive at 26–27 weeks' gestation and birth weights of 800–1000 g. Survival at gestational age 25 weeks and birth weight 700–800 g is 50%–70%, with a considerable drop-off below this level (Figure 2–11).

These high rates of survival come with some morbidity. Major neurologic sequelae, including cerebral palsy, cognitive delay, and hydrocephalus, occur in 10%–25% of survivors of birth weight less than 1500 g. The rate of these sequelae tends to be higher in infants with lower birth weights. Infants with birth weights less than 1000 g also have an increased rate of lesser disabilities, including learning, behavioral, and psychiatric problems. Risk factors for neurologic sequelae include seizures, grade III or IV intracranial hemorrhage, periventricular leukomalacia, ventricular dilation, white matter abnormalities on term-equivalent MRI examinations, severe IUGR, poor early head growth, need for mechanical ventilation, chronic lung disease, NEC, and low socioeconomic class. Maternal fever and chorioamnionitis are associated with an increased risk of cerebral palsy. Other morbidities include chronic lung disease and reactive airway disease, resulting in increased severity of respiratory infections and hospital readmissions in the first 2 years; retinopathy of prematurity with associated loss of visual acuity and strabismus; hearing loss; and growth failure. All of these issues require close multidisciplinary outpatient follow-up. Infants with residual lung disease are candidates for monthly palivizumab (Synagis) injections during their first winter after hospital discharge to prevent infection with

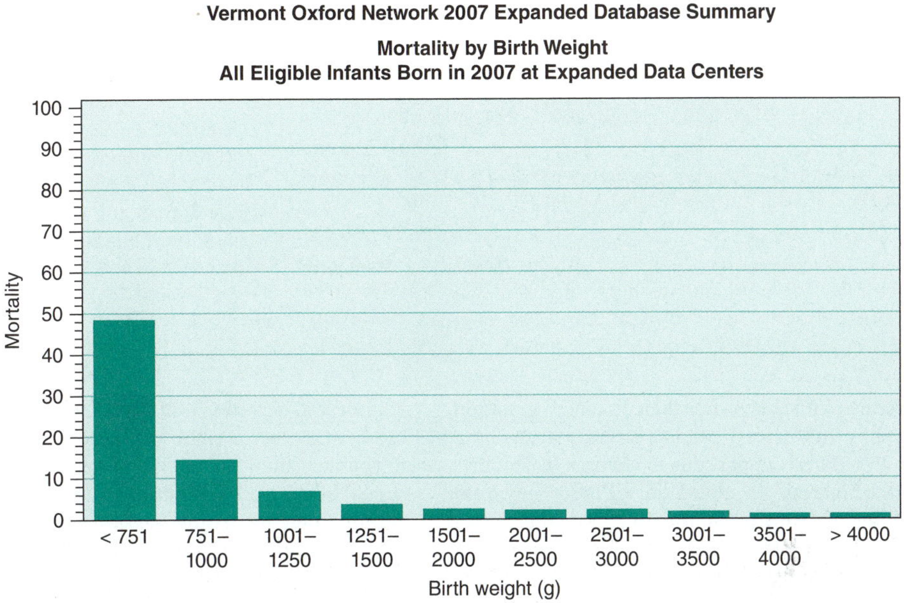

▲ **Figure 2–11.** Mortality rates before discharge by 100-g birth weight subgroups in 2007. (Reproduced, with permission, from the Vermont Oxford Network, 2008.)

respiratory syncytial virus. Routine immunizations should be given at the appropriate chronologic age and should not be age-corrected for prematurity.

Aarnoudse-Moens CSH et al: Meta-analysis of neurobehavioral outcomes in very preterm and/or very low birth weight children. Pediatrics 2009;124:77 [PMID: 19651588].

Aarnoudse-Moens CSH et al: Development of preschool and academic skills in children born very preterm. J Pediatr 2011;158:51 [PMID: 20708749].

Bull MJ, Engle WA, Committee on Injury, Violence and Poison prevention, and the Committee on Fetus and Newborn: Safe transportation of preterm and low birth weight infants at hospital discharge. Pediatrics 2009;123:1425 [PMID: 19596733].

Doyle LW, Saigal S: Long-term outcomes of very preterm or tiny infants. NeoReviews 2009;10:e130.

Ehrenkranz RA et al: Growth in the neonatal intensive care unit influences neurodevelopment and growth outcomes of extremely low birth weight infants. Pediatrics 2006;117:1253 [PMID: 16585322].

Hack M et al: Chronic conditions, functional limitations, and special healthcare needs of school-aged children born with extremely low-birth-weight in the 1990s. JAMA 2005;294:318 [PMID: 16030276].

Hintz SR et al: Early-childhood neurodevelopmental outcomes are not improving for infants born at < 25 weeks' gestational age. Pediatrics 2011;127:62 [PMID: 21187312].

Marlow N et al: Neurologic and developmental disability at six years of age after extremely preterm birth. N Engl J Med 2005;352:9 [PMID: 15635108].

Saigal S et al: Transition of extremely low-birth-weight infants from adolescence to young adulthood. Comparison with normal birth-weight controls. JAMA 2006;295:667 [PMID: 16467235].

Samara M et al: Pervasive behavior problems at 6 years of age in a total-population sample of children born at ≤ 25 weeks of gestation. Pediatrics 2008;122:562 [PMID: 18762527].

Stoll BG et al: Neonatal outcomes of extremely preterm infants from the NICHD neonatal research network. Pediatrics 2010;126:443 [PMID: 20732945].

Wilson-Costello D et al: Improved neurodevelopmental outcome for extremely low birth weight infants in 2000-2002. Pediatrics 2007;119:37 [PMID: 17200269].

Wolke D et al: Specific language difficulties and school achievement in children born at 25 weeks of gestation or less. J Pediatr 2008;152:256 [PMID: 18206699].

THE LATE PRETERM INFANT

The rate of preterm births in the United States has increased by more than 30% in the past 30 years, so that preterm infants now comprise 12.8% of all births. Late preterm births, those from 34 0/7 to 36 6/7 weeks' gestation (Figure 2–12), have increased the most, and now account for over 70% of

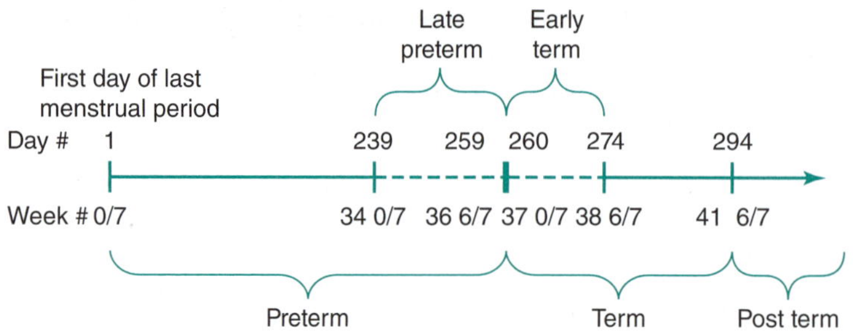

▲ **Figure 2–12.** Definitions of late preterm and early term infant. (Reproduced with permission from Engle WA, Kominiarek MA: Late preterm infants, early term infants, and timing of elective deliveries. Clin Perinatol 2008; 35:325.)

all preterm births. While births less than 34 weeks' gestation have increased by 10% since 1990, late preterm births have increased by 25%. This is in part due to changes in obstetric practice with an increase in inductions of labor (up from 9.5% in 1990 to 22.5% today), and an increase in cesarean sections (currently more than 30% of all births), as well as a rise in multiple births and an increasing demand for cesarean section "at maternal request."

Compared with term infants, late preterm infants have higher prevalence of acute neonatal problems including respiratory distress, temperature instability, hypoglycemia, kernicterus, apnea, seizures, feeding problems, and rehospitalization after hospital discharge. The respiratory issues are caused by delayed clearance of lung fluid or surfactant deficiency, or both, and can progress to respiratory failure requiring mechanical ventilation, persistent pulmonary hypertension, and even ECMO support. Feeding issues are caused by immature coordination of suck and swallow, which can interfere with bottle feeding and cause failure to establish successful breast feeding, putting the infant at risk for excessive weight loss and dehydration. These infants are nearly five times as likely as full-term infants to require either supplemental IV fluids, or gavage feedings. Related both to feeding issues and immaturity, late preterm infants have at least four times the risk of developing a bilirubin level above 20 mg/dL when compared with infants born after 40 completed weeks. As a consequence, late preterm gestation is a major risk factor for excessive hyperbilirubinemia and kernicterus. Rehospitalizations due to jaundice, proven or suspected infection, feeding difficulties, and failure to thrive are much more common than in term infants. Long-term development may also be adversely affected, with some large population-based studies showing a higher incidence of cerebral palsy, developmental delay, and behavioral and emotional disturbances compared with term infants.

Late preterm infants, even if similar in size to their term counterparts, should be considered preterm rather than near term, and require closer in-hospital monitoring after birth for complications. Although they may feed reasonably well for the first day or two, they often fail to increase feeding volume and become more sleepy and less interested in feeding as they lose weight and become jaundiced, especially if younger than 36 weeks. Discharge of these newborns should be delayed until they have demonstrated reliable and appropriately increasing intake despite the expected weight loss and jaundice, and absence of other issues such as hypothermia, hypoglycemia, or apnea. If nursing, use of a breast pump to assure adequate emptying of the breast and milk supply should also be instituted, along with supplementation of the infant's breast feeding with expressed milk by bottle or gavage. It is better to assure adequate feeding and mature behaviors for an extra day or two in the hospital than to have a readmission for "lethargy and poor feeding, possible sepsis" after premature discharge. Following nursery discharge, close outpatient follow-up is indicated, generally within 48–72 hours, to assure continued adequate intake and weight gain.

Bell EF et al, Committee on Fetus and Newborn: Hospital discharge of the high-risk neonate. Pediatrics 2008;122:1119 [PMID: 18977994].

Colin AA et al: Respiratory morbidity and lung function in preterm infants of 32 to 36 weeks' gestational age. Pediatrics 2010;126:115 [PMID: 20530073].

Engle WA et al, and the Committee on Fetus and Newborn: "Late-preterm" infants: a population at risk. Pediatrics 2007;120:1390 [PMID: 18055691].

Engle WA: Infants born late preterm: definition, physiologic and metabolic immaturity, and outcomes. NeoReviews 2009;10:e280.

Engle WA, Kominiarek MA: Late preterm infants, early term infants, and timing of elective deliveries. Clin Perinatol 2008;35:325 [PMID: 18456072].

McGowan JE et al: Early childhood development of late preterm infants: a systematic review. Pediatrics 2011;127:1111 [PMID: 21624885].

Ramachandrappa A, Jain L: Health issues of the late preterm infant. Ped Clin N Am 2009;56:565 [PMID: 19501692].

vanBaar et al: Functioning at school age of moderately preterm children born at 32 to 36 weeks' gestational age. Pediatrics 2009;124:251 [PMID: 19564307].

CARDIAC PROBLEMS IN THE NEWBORN INFANT

STRUCTURAL HEART DISEASE

1. Cyanotic Presentations

ESSENTIALS OF DIAGNOSIS & TYPICAL FEATURES

- Cyanosis, initially without associated respiratory distress.
- Failure to increase Pao_2 with supplemental oxygen.
- Chest radiograph with decreased lung markings suggests right heart obstruction, while increased lung markings suggest transposition or pulmonary venous obstruction.

General Considerations

The causes of cyanotic heart disease in the newborn are transposition of the great vessels, total anomalous pulmonary venous return, truncus arteriosus (some types), tricuspid atresia, and pulmonary atresia or critical pulmonary stenosis. Most are diagnosed antenatally by ultrasound.

Clinical Findings

Infants with these disorders present with early cyanosis. The hallmark of many of these lesions is cyanosis without associated respiratory distress. In most of these infants, tachypnea develops over time either because of increased pulmonary blood flow or secondary to metabolic acidemia from progressive hypoxemia. Diagnostic aids include comparing the blood gas or oxygen saturation in room air to that in 100% Fio_2. Failure of Pao_2 or Sao_2 to increase suggests cyanotic heart disease. ***Note:*** A Pao_2, if feasible, is the preferred measure. Saturation in the newborn may be misleadingly high despite pathologically low Pao_2 due to the left-shifted oxyhemoglobin dissociation curve seen with fetal hemoglobin. Other useful aids are chest radiography, electrocardiography, and echocardiography.

Transposition of the great vessels is the most common form of cyanotic heart disease presenting in the newborn. Examination generally reveals a systolic murmur and single S_2. Chest radiograph shows a generous heart size and a narrow mediastinum with normal or increased lung markings. There is little change in Pao_2 or Sao_2 with supplemental oxygen. Total anomalous pulmonary venous return, in which venous return is obstructed, presents early with severe cyanosis and respiratory failure because of severe pulmonary edema. The chest radiograph typically shows a small to normal heart size with marked pulmonary edema. Infants with right heart obstruction (pulmonary and tricuspid atresia, critical pulmonary stenosis, and some forms of truncus arteriosus) have decreased lung markings on chest radiographs and, depending on the severity of hypoxia, may develop metabolic acidemia. Those lesions with an underdeveloped right heart will have left-sided predominance on electrocardiography. Although tetralogy of Fallot is the most common form of cyanotic heart disease, the obstruction at the pulmonary valve is often not severe enough to result in cyanosis in the newborn. In all cases, diagnosis can be confirmed by echocardiography.

2. Acyanotic Presentations

ESSENTIALS OF DIAGNOSIS & TYPICAL FEATURES

- Most newborns with symptomatic acyanotic heart disease have left-sided outflow obstruction.
- Differentially diminished pulses (coarctation) or decreased pulses throughout (aortic atresia).
- Metabolic acidemia.
- Chest radiograph showing large heart and pulmonary edema.

General Considerations

Newborn infants who present with serious acyanotic heart disease usually have congestive heart failure secondary to left-sided outflow tract obstruction. Infants with left-to-right shunt lesions (eg, ventricular septal defect) may have murmurs in the newborn period, but clinical symptoms do not occur until pulmonary vascular resistance drops enough to cause significant shunting and subsequent congestive heart failure (usually at 3–4 weeks of age).

Clinical Findings

Infants with left-sided outflow obstruction generally do well the first day or so until the ductus arteriosus—the source of all or some of the systemic flow—narrows. Tachypnea, tachycardia, congestive heart failure, and metabolic acidosis develop. On examination, all of these infants have abnormalities of the pulses. In aortic atresia (hypoplastic left heart syndrome) and stenosis, pulses are all diminished, whereas in coarctation syndromes, differential pulses (diminished or absent in the lower extremities) are evident, and Spo_2 may be lower in the legs than in the right upper extremity. Chest radiographic films in these infants show a large heart and pulmonary edema. Diagnosis is confirmed with echocardiography.

3. Treatment of Cyanotic & Acyanotic Lesions

Early stabilization includes supportive therapy as needed (eg, IV glucose, oxygen, ventilation for respiratory failure, and pressor support). Specific therapy includes infusions of prostaglandin E_1 (0.0125–0.025 mcg/kg/min) to maintain ductal patency. In some cyanotic lesions (eg, pulmonary atresia, tricuspid atresia, and critical pulmonary stenosis) in which lung blood flow is ductus-dependent, this improves pulmonary blood flow and Pao_2 by allowing shunting through the ductus to the pulmonary artery. In left-sided outflow tract obstruction, systemic blood flow is ductus-dependent; prostaglandins improve systemic perfusion and resolve the acidosis. Further specific management—including palliative surgical and cardiac catheterization procedures—is discussed in Chapter 20. Neurodevelopmental outcome with congenital heart disease depends on the lesion, associated defects and syndromes, severity of neonatal presentation, and complications related to palliative and corrective surgery.

PERSISTENT PULMONARY HYPERTENSION

ESSENTIALS OF DIAGNOSIS & TYPICAL FEATURES

- Onset of symptoms on day 1 of life.
- Hypoxia with poor response to high concentrations of inspired oxygen.
- Right-to-left shunts through the foramen ovale, ductus arteriosus, or both.
- Most often associated with parenchymal lung disease.

General Considerations

Persistent pulmonary hypertension of the newborn (PPHN) results when the normal decrease in pulmonary vascular resistance after birth does not occur. Most affected infants are full term or postterm, and many have experienced perinatal asphyxia. Other clinical associations include hypothermia, meconium aspiration syndrome, hyaline membrane disease, polycythemia, neonatal sepsis, chronic intrauterine hypoxia, and pulmonary hypoplasia.

There are three underlying pathophysiologic mechanisms of PPHN: (1) vasoconstriction due to perinatal hypoxia related to an acute event such as sepsis or asphyxia; (2) prenatal increase in pulmonary vascular smooth muscle development, often associated with meconium aspiration syndrome; and (3) decreased cross-sectional area of the pulmonary vascular bed associated with lung hypoplasia (eg, diaphragmatic hernia).

Clinical Findings

Clinically, the syndrome is characterized by onset on the first day of life, usually from birth. Respiratory distress is prominent, and Pao_2 is usually poorly responsive to high concentrations of inspired oxygen. Many infants have associated myocardial depression with systemic hypotension. Echocardiography reveals right-to-left shunting at the level of the ductus arteriosus or foramen ovale, or both. The chest radiograph usually shows lung infiltrates related to associated pulmonary pathology (eg, meconium aspiration and hyaline membrane disease). If the majority of right-to-left shunting is at the ductal level, pre- and postductal differences in Pao_2 and Sao_2 will be observed.

Treatment

Therapy for PPHN involves treatment of other postasphyxia problems such as seizures, renal failure, hypoglycemia, and infection. Specific therapy is aimed at both increasing systemic arterial pressure and decreasing pulmonary arterial pressure to reverse the right-to-left shunting through fetal pathways. First-line therapy includes oxygen and ventilation (to reduce pulmonary vascular resistance) and crystalloid infusions (10 mL/kg, up to 30 mL/kg) to improve systemic pressure. Ideally, systolic pressure should be greater than 50–60 mm Hg. With compromised cardiac function, systemic pressors can be used as second-line therapy (eg, dopamine, 5–20 mcg/kg/min; dobutamine, 5–20 mcg/kg/min; or both). Metabolic acidemia should be corrected because acidemia exacerbates pulmonary vasoconstriction. Pulmonary vasodilation can be enhanced using inhaled nitric oxide, which is identical or very similar to endogenous endothelium-derived relaxing factor, at doses of 5–20 ppm. High-frequency oscillatory ventilation has proved effective in many of these infants, particularly those with severe associated lung disease, by improving lung expansion and recruitment. In cases in which conventional therapy is failing (poor oxygenation despite maximum support) extracorporeal membrane oxygenation (ECMO) is used. The lungs are essentially at rest during ECMO, and with resolution of pulmonary hypertension infants are weaned from ECMO back to ventilator therapy. Approximately 10%–15% of survivors of PPHN have significant neurologic sequelae, with cerebral palsy or cognitive delays. Other sequelae such as chronic lung disease, sensorineural hearing loss, and feeding problems have also been reported.

ARRHYTHMIAS

Irregularly irregular heart rates, commonly associated with premature atrial contractions and less commonly with premature ventricular contractions, are common in the first days of life in well newborns. These arrhythmias are benign. Clinically significant bradyarrhythmias are seen in association with congenital heart block. Heart block can be seen in an otherwise structurally normal heart (associated with maternal lupus) or with structural cardiac abnormalities. In the absence of fetal hydrops, the bradyarrhythmia is often well tolerated. Cardiac pacing may be required if there are symptoms of inadequate cardiac output.

Tachyarrhythmias can be either wide complex (ventricular tachycardia) or narrow complex (supraventricular tachycardia) on ECG. Supraventricular tachycardia is the most common neonatal tachyarrhythmia and may be a sign of structural heart disease, myocarditis, left atrial enlargement, and aberrant conduction pathways, or may be an isolated event. Acute treatment is ice to the face to induce a vagal response, and if unsuccessful, IV adenosine (50 mcg/kg). If there is no response, the dose can be increased every 2 minutes by 50 mcg/kg to a maximum dose of 250 mcg/kg. Long-term prophylactic antiarrhythmic therapy is generally indicated; cardiology consultation is suggested. Cardioversion is rarely needed for supraventricular tachycardia but is needed acutely for hemodynamically unstable ventricular tachycardia.

Lapointe A, Barrington KJ: Pulmonary hypertension and the asphyxiated newborn. J Pediatr 2011;158(supp):e19 [PMID: 21238701].

Silberbach M, Hannan D: Presentation of congenital heart disease in the neonate and young infant. Pediatr Rev 2007;28:123 [PMID: 17400823].

Tavera MC et al: Supraventricular tachyarrhythmic drug choice dilemma. J Matern Fetal Neonat Med 2011;24:541 [PMID: 20807153].

GASTROINTESTINAL & ABDOMINAL SURGICAL CONDITIONS IN THE NEWBORN INFANT (SEE ALSO CHAPTER 21)

ESOPHAGEAL ATRESIA & TRACHEOESOPHAGEAL FISTULA

ESSENTIALS OF DIAGNOSIS & TYPICAL FEATURES

- Polyhydramnios.
- Excessive drooling and secretions; choking with attempted feeding.
- Unable to pass an orogastric tube to the stomach.

General Considerations

Esophageal atresia is characterized by a blind esophageal pouch with or without a fistulous connection between the proximal or distal esophagus (or both) and the airway. In 85% of infants, the fistula is between the distal esophagus and the airway. Polyhydramnios is common because of high GI obstruction. Incidence is approximately 1 in 3000 births.

Clinical Findings

Infants present in the first hours of life with copious secretions, choking, cyanosis, and respiratory distress. Diagnosis is confirmed with chest radiograph after careful placement of a nasogastric (NG) tube to the point at which resistance is met. The tube will be seen radiographically in the blind pouch. If a tracheoesophageal fistula is present to the distal esophagus, gas will be present in the bowel. In esophageal atresia without tracheoesophageal fistula, there is no gas in the bowel.

Treatment

The NG tube in the proximal pouch should be placed on low intermittent suction to drain secretions and prevent aspiration. The head of the bed should be elevated to prevent reflux of gastric contents through the distal fistula into the lungs. IV glucose and fluids should be provided and oxygen administered as needed. Definitive treatment is surgical, and the technique used depends on the distance between the segments of esophagus. If the distance is not too great, the fistula can be ligated and the ends of the esophagus anastomosed. If the ends of the esophagus cannot be brought together, the initial surgery is fistula ligation and a feeding gastrostomy. Echocardiography should be performed prior to surgery to rule out a right-sided aortic arch (for which a left-sided thoracotomy would be preferred).

Prognosis

Prognosis is determined primarily by the presence or absence of associated anomalies, particularly cardiac, and low birth weight. Mortality is highest when the infant is less than 2000 g and has a serious associated cardiac defect. Vertebral, anal, cardiac, renal, and limb anomalies are the most likely to be observed (VACTERL association). Evaluation for associated anomalies should be initiated early.

Okamoto T et al: Esophageal atresia: Prognostic classification revisited. Surgery 2009;145:675 [PMID: 19486772].

INTESTINAL OBSTRUCTION

ESSENTIALS OF DIAGNOSIS & TYPICAL FEATURES

- Infants with high intestinal obstruction present soon after birth with emesis.
- Bilious emesis suggests intestinal malrotation with midgut volvulus until proved otherwise.
- Low intestinal obstruction is characterized by abdominal distention and late onset of emesis, often with delayed or absent stooling.

General Considerations

A history of polyhydramnios is common, and the fluid, if bile-stained, can easily be confused with thin meconium staining. The higher the location of the obstruction in the intestine, the earlier the infant will develop vomiting and the less prominent the abdominal distention will be. Lower intestinal obstruction presents with abdominal distention and later onset of emesis. Most obstructions are bowel atresias, believed to be caused by an ischemic event during development. Approximately 30% of cases of duodenal atresia are associated with Down syndrome. Meconium ileus is a distal small bowel obstruction caused by the viscous meconium produced in-utero by infants with pancreatic insufficiency secondary to cystic fibrosis. Hirschsprung disease is caused by a failure of neuronal migration to the myenteric plexus of the distal bowel. The distal bowel lacks ganglion cells, causing a lack of peristalsis in that region with a functional obstruction.

Malrotation with midgut volvulus is a surgical emergency that appears in the first days to weeks as bilious vomiting without distention or tenderness. If malrotation is not treated promptly, torsion of the intestine around the superior mesenteric artery will lead to necrosis of the entire small bowel. For this reason, bilious vomiting in the neonate always demands immediate attention and evaluation.

Clinical Findings

Diagnosis of intestinal obstructions depends on plain abdominal radiographs with either upper GI series (high obstruction suspected) or contrast enema (lower obstruction apparent) to define the area of obstruction. Table 2–20 summarizes the findings expected.

Infants with meconium ileus are presumed to have cystic fibrosis, although infants with pancolonic Hirschsprung disease, colon pseudo-obstruction syndrome, or colonic dysgenesis or atresia may also present with meconium impacted in the distal ileum. Definitive diagnosis of cystic fibrosis is by the sweat chloride test (Na^+ and Cl^- concentration > 60 mEq/L) or by genetic testing. Approximately 10%–20% of infants with cystic fibrosis have meconium ileus. Infants with cystic fibrosis and meconium ileus generally have a normal immunoreactive trypsinogen on their newborn screen because of the associated severe exocrine pancreatic insufficiency in utero.

Intestinal perforation in-utero results in meconium peritonitis with residual intra-abdominal calcifications. Many perforations are completely healed at birth. If the infant has no signs of obstruction or ongoing perforation, no immediate evaluation is needed. A sweat test to rule out cystic fibrosis should be done at a later date.

Low intestinal obstruction may present with delayed stooling (> 24 hours in term infants is abnormal) with mild distention. Radiographic findings of gaseous distention should prompt contrast enema to diagnose (and treat) meconium plug syndrome. If no plug is found, the diagnosis may be small left colon syndrome (occurring in IDMs) or Hirschsprung disease. Rectal biopsy will be required to clarify these two diagnoses. Imperforate anus is generally apparent on physical examination, although a rectovaginal fistula with a mildly abnormal-appearing anus can occasionally be confused with normal. High imperforate anus in males may be associated with rectourethral or rectovesical fistula, with meconium "pearls" seen along the median raphe of the scrotum, and meconium being passed via the urethra.

Table 2–20. Intestinal obstruction.

Site of Obstruction	Clinical Findings	Plain Radiographs	Contrast Study
Duodenal atresia	Down syndrome (30%–50%); early vomiting, sometimes bilious	"Double bubble" (dilated stomach and proximal duodenum, no air distal)	Not needed
Malrotation and volvulus	Bilious vomiting with onset anytime in the first few weeks	Dilated stomach and proximal duodenum; paucity of air distally (may be normal gas pattern)	UGI shows displaced duodenojejunal junction with "corkscrew" deformity of twisted bowel
Jejunoileal atresia, meconium ileus	Bilious gastric contents > 25 mL at birth; progressive distention and bilious vomiting	Multiple dilated loops of bowel; intra-abdominal calcifications if in-utero perforation occurred (meconium peritonitis)	Barium or osmotic contrast enema shows microcolon; contrast refluxed into distal ileum may demonstrate and relieve meconium obstruction (successful in about 50% of cases)
Meconium plug syndrome; Hirschsprung disease	Distention, delayed stooling (> 24 h)	Diffuse bowel distention	Barium or osmotic contrast enema outlines and relieves plug; may show transition zone in Hirschsprung disease; delayed emptying (> 24 h) suggests Hirschsprung disease

UGI, upper gastrointestinal contrast study.

Treatment

NG suction to decompress the bowel, IV glucose, fluid and electrolyte replacement, and respiratory support as necessary should be instituted. Antibiotics are usually indicated due to the bowel distention and possibility of translocation of bacteria. The definitive treatment for these conditions (with the exception of meconium plug syndrome, small left colon syndrome, and some cases of meconium ileus) is surgical.

Prognosis

Up to 10% of infants with meconium plug syndrome are subsequently found to have cystic fibrosis or Hirschsprung disease. For this reason, it is appropriate to obtain a sweat chloride test and rectal biopsy in all of these infants before discharge, especially the infant with meconium plug syndrome who is still symptomatic after contrast enema.

In duodenal atresia associated with Down syndrome, the prognosis depends on associated anomalies (eg, heart defects) and the severity of prestenotic duodenal dilation and subsequent duodenal dysmotility. Otherwise, these conditions usually carry an excellent prognosis after surgical repair.

ABDOMINAL WALL DEFECTS

1. Omphalocele

Omphalocele is a membrane-covered herniation of abdominal contents into the base of the umbilical cord; the incidence is 2 per 10,000 live births (0.02%). Over 50% of cases have either an abnormal karyotype or an associated syndrome. The sac may contain liver and spleen as well as intestine. Prognosis varies with the size of the lesion, with the presence of pulmonary hypoplasia and respiratory insufficiency, and with the presence of associated abnormalities.

At delivery, the omphalocele is covered with a sterile dressing soaked with warm saline to prevent fluid loss. NG decompression is performed, and IV fluids, glucose, and antibiotics are given. If the contents of the omphalocele will fit into the abdomen and can be covered with skin, muscle, or both, primary surgical closure is done. If not, staged closure is performed, with placement of a Gore-Tex patch over the exposed contents, and gradual coverage of the patch by skin over days to weeks. A large ventral hernia is left, which is repaired in the future.

2. Gastroschisis

In gastroschisis, the uncovered intestine extrudes through a small abdominal wall defect to the right of the umbilical cord. There is no membrane or sac and no liver or spleen outside the abdomen. Gastroschisis is associated with intestinal atresia in approximately 10%–20% of infants, and with intrauterine growth restriction (IUGR). The evisceration is thought to be related to abnormal involution of the right umbilical vein or a vascular accident involving the omphalomesenteric artery, although the exact cause is unknown. The prevalence of gastroschisis has been increasing worldwide over the past 20 years, from 0.03% to 0.1%. Environmental factors, including use of illicit drugs such as methamphetamine and cocaine, and cyclooxygenase inhibitors such as aspirin and ibuprofen taken during pregnancy, may be involved. Young maternal age is also strongly linked to the occurrence of gastroschisis.

Therapy initially involves placing the bowel or the lower half of the infant into a silastic bowel bag to decrease fluid and electrolyte losses as well as to conserve heat. IV fluids, antibiotics, and low intermittent gastric suction are required. The infant is placed right side down to preserve bowel perfusion. Subsequent therapy involves replacement of the bowel into the abdominal cavity. This is done as a single primary procedure if the amount of bowel to be replaced is small. If the amount of bowel is large or if the bowel is very dilated, staged closure with placement of a silastic silo and gradual reduction of the bowel into the underdeveloped abdominal cavity over several days is preferred. Postoperatively, third-space fluid losses may be extensive; fluid and electrolyte therapy, therefore, must be monitored carefully. Bowel motility, especially duodenal, may be slow to return if the bowel was dilated, thickened, matted together, and covered with a fibrinous "peel" at delivery. Prolonged intravenous nutrition is often required, but long-term outcome is very good.

Islam S: Clinical care outcomes in abdominal wall defects. Curr Opin Pediatr 2008;20:305 [PMID: 18475100].

Marven S, Owen A: Contemporary postnatal surgical management strategies for congenital abdominal wall defects. Seminars in Pediatric Surgery 2008;17:222 [PMID: 19019291].

DIAPHRAGMATIC HERNIA

ESSENTIALS OF DIAGNOSIS & TYPICAL FEATURES

- Respiratory distress from birth.
- Poor breath sounds; flat or scaphoid abdomen.
- Bowel loops seen in the chest with mediastinal shift to opposite side on chest radiograph.

This congenital malformation consists of herniation of abdominal organs into the hemithorax (usually left-sided) through a posterolateral defect in the diaphragm. The incidence overall is 1 in 2500 births. It is usually diagnosed antenatally by ultrasound, and, if so, delivery should occur at a perinatal center. If undiagnosed, it should be suspected in any infant with severe respiratory distress, poor breath sounds, and a scaphoid abdomen. The rapidity and severity of presentation depend on several factors: the degree of pulmonary hypoplasia resulting from lung compression by the intrathoracic abdominal contents in utero; degree of associated pulmonary hypertension; and associated anomalies, especially chromosomal abnormalities and congenital cardiac defects. Affected infants are prone to development of pneumothorax during attempts at ventilation of the hypoplastic lungs.

Treatment includes intubation, mechanical ventilation, and decompression of the GI tract with an NG tube. An IV infusion of glucose and fluid should be started. A chest radiograph confirms the diagnosis. Surgery to reduce the abdominal contents from the thorax and close the diaphragmatic defect is delayed until after the infant is stabilized and pulmonary hypertension and compliance have improved, usually after 24–48 hours. Both pre- and postoperatively, pulmonary hypertension may require therapy with high-frequency oscillatory ventilation, inhaled nitric oxide, or ECMO. The survival rate for infants with this condition is improving, and now approaches 80%. Use of a gentle ventilation style and permissive hypercarbia is recommended to avoid barotrauma and further lung injury. Many of these infants have ongoing problems with severe gastroesophageal reflux, and are at risk for neurodevelopmental problems, behavior problems, hearing loss, and poor growth.

Hedrick HL: Management of prenatally diagnosed congenital diaphragmatic hernia. Semin Fetal Neonat Med 2010;15:21 [PMID: 19884051].

Lally KP et al and the Section on Surgery and the Committee on Fetus and Newborn: Postdischarge follow-up of infants with congenital diaphragmatic hernia. Pediatrics 2008;121:627 [PMID: 18310215].

Van den Hout L et al: Actual outcome in infants with congenital diaphragmatic hernia: the role of a standardized postnatal treatment protocol. Fetal Diagn Ther 2011;29:55 [PMID: 21325859].

GASTROINTESTINAL BLEEDING

Upper Gastrointestinal Bleeding

Upper GI bleeding sometimes occurs in the newborn nursery, but is rarely severe. Old blood ("coffee-grounds" material) in the stomach of the newborn may be either swallowed maternal blood or infant blood from gastritis or stress ulcer. Bright red blood from the stomach is most likely from acute bleeding due to gastritis. Treatment generally consists of gastric lavage to obtain a sample for Apt testing or blood typing to determine if it is mother's or baby's blood, and antacid medication. If the volume of bleeding is large, intensive monitoring, fluid and blood replacement, and endoscopy are indicated. Coagulation studies should also be sent, and vitamin K administration confirmed or repeated.

Lower Gastrointestinal Bleeding

Rectal bleeding in the newborn is less common than upper GI bleeding and is associated with infections (eg, *Salmonella* acquired from the mother perinatally), milk protein intolerance (blood streaks with diarrhea), or, in ill infants, NEC. An abdominal radiograph should be obtained to rule out pneumatosis intestinalis or other abnormalities in gas pattern suggesting inflammation, infection, or obstruction. If the radiograph is negative and the examination is benign, a protein hydrolysate or elemental formula should be tried. The nursing mother should be instructed to avoid all cow milk protein products in her diet. If the amount of rectal bleeding is large or persistent, endoscopy may be needed.

Boyle JT: Gastrointestinal bleeding in infants and children. Pediatrics in Review 2008;29:39 [PMID: 18245300].

GASTROESOPHAGEAL REFLUX

Physiologic regurgitation is common in infants. Reflux is pathologic and should be treated when it results in failure to thrive owing to excessive regurgitation, poor intake due to dysphagia and irritability, apnea or cyanotic episodes, or chronic respiratory symptoms of wheezing and recurrent pneumonias. Diagnosis is clinical, with confirmation by pH probe or impedance study. Barium radiography is helpful to rule out anatomic abnormalities causing delayed gastric emptying, but is not diagnostic of pathologic reflux.

Most antireflux therapies have not been studied systematically in infants, especially in premature infants, and there is little correlation between clinical symptoms and documented gastroesophageal reflux events when studied. Treatment modalities have included thickened feeds (with cereal or guar gum) for those with frequent regurgitation and poor weight gain, and positioning in a prone or left side down position for 1 hour after a feeding, although this may increase risk for SIDS. Gastric acid suppressants such as ranitidine (2 mg/kg bid) or lansoprazole (1.5 mg/kg/d) can also be used, especially if there is associated irritability; however, these may be associated with an increased incidence of NEC and intestinal infections in the young and/or premature infant. Prokinetic agents such as erythromycin or metoclopramide are of little benefit and have significant side effects. Because most infants improve by 12–15 months of age, surgery is reserved for the most severe cases.

Tipnis NA, Tipnis SM: Controversies in the treatment of gastroesophageal reflux disease in preterm infants. Clin Perinatol 2009;36:153 [PMID: 19161872].

Vandenplas Y et al: Pediatric gastroesophageal reflux clinical practice guidelines: Joint recommendations of NASPGHAN and ESPGHAN. J Pediatr Gastroenterol Nutr 2009;49:498 [PMID: 19745761].

van der Pol RJ et al: Efficacy of proton-pump inhibitors in children with gastroesophageal reflux disease: A systematic review. Pediatrics 2011;127:925 [PMID: 21464183].

INFECTIONS IN THE NEWBORN INFANT

There are three major routes of perinatal infection: (1) blood-borne transplacental infection of the fetus (eg, cytomegalovirus [CMV], rubella, and syphilis); (2) ascending infection with disruption of the barrier provided by the amniotic membranes (eg, bacterial infections after 12–18 hours of ruptured membranes); and (3) infection on passage through an infected birth canal or exposure to infected blood at delivery (eg, herpes simplex, hepatitis B, HIV, and bacterial infections).

Susceptibility of the newborn infant to infection is related to immaturity of the immune system at birth. This feature applies particularly to the preterm neonate. Passive protection against some organisms is provided by transfer of IgG across the placenta, particularly during the third trimester of pregnancy. Preterm infants, especially those born before 30 weeks' gestation, do not have the full amount of passively acquired antibody.

BACTERIAL INFECTIONS

1. Bacterial Sepsis

ESSENTIALS OF DIAGNOSIS & TYPICAL FEATURES

- Most infants with early-onset sepsis present at < 24 hours of age.
- Respiratory distress is the most common presenting symptom.
- Hypotension, acidemia, and neutropenia are associated clinical findings.
- The presentation of late-onset sepsis is more subtle.

General Considerations

The incidence of early-onset (< 3 days) neonatal bacterial infection is 1–2 in 1000 live births. If rupture of the membranes occurs more than 24 hours prior to delivery, the infection rate increases to 1 in 100 live births. If early rupture of membranes with chorioamnionitis occurs, the infection rate increases further to 1 in 10 live births. Regardless of membrane rupture, infection rates are five times higher in preterm than in full-term infants.

Clinical Findings

Early-onset bacterial infections appear most commonly on day 1 of life, the majority by 12 hours of age. Respiratory distress due to pneumonia is the most common presenting sign. Other features include unexplained low Apgar scores without fetal distress, poor perfusion, and hypotension. Late-onset bacterial infection (> 3 days of age) presents in a more subtle manner, with poor feeding, lethargy, hypotonia, temperature instability, altered perfusion, new or increased oxygen requirement, and apnea. Late-onset bacterial sepsis is more often associated with meningitis or other localized infections.

Low total white count, absolute neutropenia (< 1000/mL), and elevated ratio of immature to mature neutrophils all suggest neonatal bacterial infection. Thrombocytopenia is another common feature. Other laboratory signs are hypoglycemia or hyperglycemia with no change in glucose administration, unexplained metabolic acidosis, and elevated C-reactive protein and procalcitonin. In early-onset bacterial infection, pneumonia is invariably present; chest radiography shows infiltrates, but these infiltrates cannot be distinguished from those resulting from other causes of neonatal lung disease. Presence of a pleural effusion makes a diagnosis of pneumonia more likely. Definitive diagnosis is made by positive cultures from blood, CSF, or other body fluids.

Early-onset infection is most often caused by group B β-hemolytic streptococci (GBS) and gram-negative enteric pathogens (most commonly *E coli*). Other organisms to consider are non-typeable *Haemophilus influenzae, Enterococcus, Staphylococcus aureus,* other streptococci and *Listeria monocytogenes.* Late-onset sepsis is caused by coagulase-negative staphylococci (most common in infants with indwelling central venous lines), *S aureus,* GBS, *Enterococcus,* and gram-negative organisms, in addition to Candida species (see Fungal Sepsis).

Treatment

A high index of suspicion is important in diagnosis and treatment of neonatal infection. Infants with risk factors (rupture of membranes > 18 hours, maternal chorioamnionitis, prematurity) need to be carefully observed for signs of infection. Evaluation with a CBC and differential, blood and cerebrospinal fluid cultures are indicated in infants with clinical signs of sepsis. Early-onset sepsis is usually caused by GBS or gram-negative enteric organisms; broad-spectrum coverage, therefore, should include ampicillin (100–150 mg/kg/d divided every 12 h) plus an aminoglycoside (3–4 mg/kg/dose every 24 hours based on gestational age at birth) or third-generation cephalosporin (cefotaxime 100 mg/kg/d divided every 12 h). Late-onset infections can also be caused by the same organisms, but coverage may need to be expanded to include staphylococci. In particular, the preterm infant with an indwelling line is at risk for infection with coagulase-negative staphylococci, for which vancomycin (10–15 mg/kg every 8–24 h based on gestational and postnatal age) is the drug of choice. Initial broad-spectrum coverage should also include a third-generation cephalosporin (cefotaxime or ceftazidime, if *Pseudomonas aeruginosa* is strongly suspected) or an aminoglycoside. To prevent the development of vancomycin-resistant organisms, vancomycin should be stopped as soon as cultures and sensitivities indicate that it is not needed. The

Intrapartum GBS prophylaxis indicated	Intrapartum GBS prophylaxis not indicated
• Previous infant with invasive GBS disease • GBS bacteriuria during any trimester of the current pregnancy[1] • Positive GBS vaginal-rectal screening culture in late gestation[2] during current pregnancy[1] • Unknown GBS status at the onset of lab or (culture not done, incomplete, or results unknown) and any of the following: - Delivery at <37 weeks' gestation - Amniotic membrane rupture ≥ 18 hours - Intrapartum temperature ≥ 100.4°F (≥ 38.0°C)[3] - Intrapartum NATT[4] positive for GBS	• Colonization with GBS during a previous pregnancy (unless an indication for GBS prophylaxis is present for current pregnancy) • GBS bacteriuria during previous pregnancy (unless an indication for GBS prophylaxis is present for current pregnancy) • Negative vaginal and rectal GBS screening culture in late gestation[2] during the current pregnancy, regardless of intrapartum risk factors • Cesarean delivery performed before onset of labor on a woman with intact amniotic membranes, regardless of GBS colonization status or gestational age

Abbreviation: NAAT Nucleic acid amplification tests

[1]Intrapartum antibiotic prophylaxis is not indicated in this circumstance if a cesarean delivery is performed before onset of labor on a woman with interact amniotic membranes.
[2]Optimal timing for prenatal GBS screening as at 35-37 weeks' gestation.
[3]If amnionitis is suspected, broad-spectrum antibiotic therapy that includes an agent known to be active against GBS should replace BGS prophylaxis.
[4]NAAT testing for GBS is optional and might not be available in all settings, if intrapartum NAAT is negative for GBS but any other intrapartum risk factor (delivery at ≤37 weeks' gestation, amniotic membrane rupture at ≥ 18 hours, or temperature ≥ 100.4°F (≥ 38.0°C) is present , then intrapartum antibiotic prophylaxis is indicated.

▲ **Figure 2–13.** Indications for intrapartum antimicrobial prophylaxis to prevent early-onset group B streptococcal (GBS) disease using a universal prenatal culture screening strategy at 35–37 weeks' gestation for all pregnant women. (Reproduced, with permission, from the Centers for Disease Control and Prevention: Prevention of perinatal group B streptococcal disease. *MMWR* 2010;59:RR-10.)

evaluation for late onset symptoms should include cultures of blood, urine, and cerebrospinal fluid. The duration of treatment for proven sepsis is 10–14 days of IV antibiotics. In sick infants, the essentials of good supportive therapy should be provided: IV glucose and nutritional support, volume expansion and pressors as needed, and oxygen and ventilator support.

Prevention

Prevention of early onset neonatal GBS infection has been achieved with intrapartum administration of penicillin given more than 4 hours prior to delivery, with overall rates of infection now at 0.3–0.4 cases per 1000 live births. The current guideline (Figure 2–13) is to perform a vaginal and rectal GBS culture at 35–37 weeks' gestation in all pregnant women. Prophylaxis with penicillin or ampicillin is given to GBS-positive women, to those who had GBS bacteriuria during the current pregnancy, to those who had a previous infant with invasive GBS disease, and to those who have unknown GBS status at delivery with risk factors for infection. Figure 2–14 presents an algorithm for secondary prevention of early onset GBS infections in newborns.

2. Meningitis

Any newborn with bacterial sepsis is at risk for meningitis. The incidence is low in infants presenting in the first day of life, and higher in infants with later-onset infection. The workup for any newborn with possible signs of CNS infection should include a lumbar puncture because blood cultures can be negative in neonates with meningitis. The presence of seizures should increase the suspicion for meningitis. Diagnosis is suggested by a CSF protein level higher than 150 mg/dL, glucose less than 30 mg/dL, leukocytes of more than 20/μL, and a positive Gram stain. The diagnosis is confirmed by culture. The most common organisms are GBS and gram-negative enteric bacteria. Although sepsis can be treated with antibiotics for 10–14 days, meningitis requires 14–21 days. Gram-negative infections, in particular, are difficult to eradicate, and may relapse. The mortality rate of neonatal meningitis is approximately 10%, with significant neurologic morbidity present in one-third of the survivors.

3. Pneumonia

The respiratory system can be infected in-utero, on passage through the birth canal, or postnatally. Early-onset neonatal infection is usually associated with pneumonia. Pneumonia should also be suspected in older neonates with a recent onset of tachypnea, retractions, and cyanosis. In infants already receiving respiratory support, an increase in the requirement for oxygen or ventilator support, perhaps with a change in the character of tracheal secretions, may indicate pneumonia. Not only common bacteria but also viruses (CMV, respiratory syncytial virus, adenovirus, influenza, herpes simplex, parainfluenza) and *Chlamydia* can cause pneumonia. In infants with preexisting respiratory disease, intercurrent pulmonary infections contribute to the development of chronic lung disease.

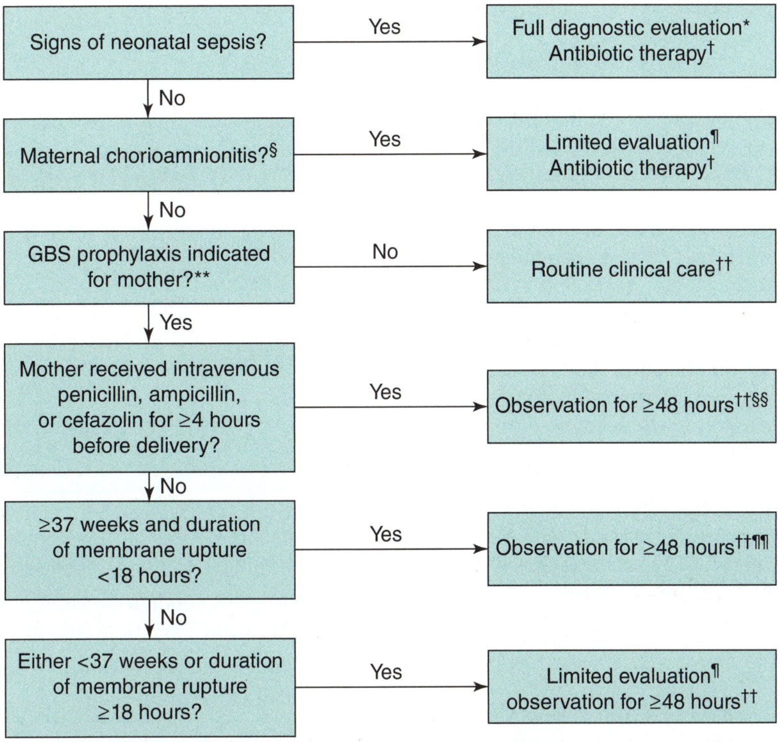

*Full diagnostic evaluation includes a blood culture, a complete blood count (CBC) including white blood cell differential and platelet counts, chest radiograph (*if* respiratory abnormalities are present), and lumbar puncture (if patient is stable enough to tolerate procedure and sepsis is suspected).

†Antibiotic therapy should be directed toward the most common causes of neonatal sepsis, including intravenous ampicillin for GBS and coverage for other organisms (including *Escherichia coli* and other gram-negative pathogens) and should take into account local antibiotic resistance patterns.

§Consultation with obstetric providers is important to determine the level of clinical suspicion for chorioamnionitis. Chorioamnionitis is diagnosed clinically and some of the signs are nonspecific.

¶Limited evaluation includes blood culture (at birth) and CBC with differential and platelets (at birth and/or at 6–12 hours of life).

**See Figure 2–13 for indications for intrapartum GBS prophylaxis.

††If signs of sepsis develop, a full diagnostic evaluation should be conducted and antibiotic therapy initiated.

§§If ≥37 weeks' gestation, observation may occur at home after 24 hours if other discharge criteria have been met, access to medical care is readily available, and a person who is able to comply fully with instructions for home observation will be present. If any of these conditions is not met, the infant should be observed in the hospital for at least 48 hours and until discharge criteria are achieved.

¶¶Some experts recommend a CBC with differential and platelets at age 6–12 hours.

▲ **Figure 2–14.** Algorithm for secondary prevention of early-onset group B streptococcal (GBS) disease among newborns. (Reproduced, with permission, from the Centers for Disease Control and Prevention: Prevention of perinatal group B streptococcal disease. MMWR 2010;59:RR-10)

4. Urinary Tract Infection

Infection of the urine is uncommon in the first days of life. Urinary tract infection in the newborn can occur in association with genitourinary anomalies and is usually caused by gram-negative enteric pathogens, or *Enterococcus*. Urine should always be evaluated as part of the workup for later-onset infection. Culture should be obtained either by suprapubic aspiration or bladder catheterization. Antibiotic IV therapy is continued for 3–5 days if the blood culture is negative and clinical signs resolve quickly, then completed with oral medications. Evaluation for genitourinary anomalies with an ultrasound examination and a voiding cystourethrogram should be done in most cases.

5. Omphalitis

A normal umbilical cord stump atrophies and separates at the skin level. A small amount of purulent material at the base of the cord is common and can be minimized by keeping the cord open to air and dry. The cord can become colonized with streptococci, staphylococci, or gram-negative organisms that can cause local infection. Infections are more common in cords manipulated for venous or arterial lines. Omphalitis is diagnosed when redness and edema develop in the soft tissues around the stump. Local and systemic cultures should be obtained. Treatment is with broad-spectrum IV antibiotics (usually nafcillin at 50–75 mg/kg/d divided every 8–12 h) or vancomycin and a third-generation cephalosporin. Complications are determined by the degree of infection of the cord vessels and include septic thrombophlebitis, hepatic abscess, necrotizing fasciitis, and portal vein thrombosis. Surgical consultation should be obtained because of the potential for necrotizing fasciitis. It is also prudent at this point to add anaerobic coverage with metronidazole (15 mg/kg/d divided every 12 h) as the infection may be polymicrobial.

6. Conjunctivitis

Neisseria gonorrhoeae may colonize an infant during passage through an infected birth canal. Gonococcal ophthalmitis presents at 3–7 days with copious purulent conjunctivitis. The diagnosis can be suspected when gram-negative intracellular diplococci are seen on a Gram-stained smear and confirmed by culture. Treatment for nondisseminated disease is with IV or IM ceftriaxone, 25–50 mg/kg (not to exceed 125 mg) given once. For disseminated disease (sepsis, arthritis, or meningitis) cefotaxime for 7–10 days is preferred. Prophylaxis at birth is with 0.5% erythromycin ointment. Infants born to mothers with known gonococcal disease should also receive a single dose of ceftriaxone. If significant hyperbilirubinemia is present, cefotaxime is preferred.

Chlamydia trachomatis is another important cause of conjunctivitis, appearing at 5 days to several weeks of age with conjunctival congestion, edema, and minimal discharge. The organism is acquired at birth after passage through an infected birth canal. Acquisition occurs in 50% of infants born to infected women, with a 25%–50% risk of conjunctivitis. Prevalence in pregnancy is over 10% in some populations. Diagnosis is by isolation of the organism or by rapid antigen detection tests. Treatment is with oral erythromycin (30 mg/kg/d in divided doses q8–12h) for 14 days. Topical treatment alone will not eradicate nasopharyngeal carriage, leaving the infant at risk for the development of pneumonitis.

Bentlin MR, Suppo de Souza Rugolo LM: Late-onset sepsis: epidemiology, evaluation, and outcome. NeoReviews 2010;11:e426.

Kestenbaum LA et al: Defining cerebrospinal fluid white blood cell count reference values in neonates and young infants. Pediatrics 2010;125:257 [PMID: 20064869].

Prevention of perinatal Group B Streptococcal disease revised guidelines from CDC, 2010. MMWR 2010;59:1-32.[PMID: 21088663].

Puopolo KM et al: Epidemiology of neonatal early-onset sepsis. NeoReviews 2008;9:e571.

Verani JR, Schrag SJ: Group B streptococcal disease in infants: progress in prevention and continued challenges. Clin Perinatol 2010;37:375 [PMID: 20569813].

FUNGAL SEPSIS

ESSENTIALS OF DIAGNOSIS & TYPICAL FEATURES

- Risk factors include low birth weight, indwelling central lines, and multiple antibiotic exposures.
- Colonization with *Candida* species is common; systemic infection occurs in 5%–7% of infants.
- Presents with often subtle clinical deterioration, thrombocytopenia, and hyperglycemia.

With the survival of smaller, sicker infants, infection with *Candida* species has become more common. Infants of extremely low birth weight with central lines who have had repeated exposures to broad-spectrum antibiotics are at highest risk. For infants of birth weight less than 1500 g, colonization rates of 27%–64% have been demonstrated. Many of these infants develop cutaneous lesions, with the GI tract as the initial site of colonization. A much smaller percentage develops systemic disease. The infection is more common in the smallest and least mature infants; up to 20% in infants 24 weeks' gestation, and 7% overall in those < 1000 g.

Clinical features of fungal sepsis can be indistinguishable from those of late-onset bacterial sepsis but are often more subtle. Thrombocytopenia may be the earliest and only sign. Deep organ involvement (renal, eye, or endocarditis) is commonly associated with systemic candidiasis. Treatment is with intravenous fluconazole (12 mg/kg loading dose followed by 6 mg/kg daily) or an amphotericin B lipid complex (5 mg/kg given daily). Prophylaxis for those infants at highest risk, for example, with central venous lines and receiving parenteral nutrition, is recommended. Prophylaxis with fluconazole diminishes intestinal colonization with yeast and decreases the frequency of systemic disease, with an overall reduction in invasive candidal disease of 83%, from 9% to 1.6%, without significant adverse effects, or resistance to fluconazole. Nystatin prophylaxis may also be effective, but has been less rigorously tested.

More rarely, *Malassezia furfur* is also seen in infants with central lines receiving IV fat emulsion. To eradicate this organism, as well as *Candida* species, it is necessary to remove the indwelling line.

Garland JS, Uhing MR: Strategies to prevent bacterial and fungal infection in the neonatal intensive care unit. Clin Perinatol 2009;36:1 [PMID: 19161861].

Kaufman DA, Manzoni P: Strategies to prevent invasive candidal infection in extremely preterm infants. Clin Perinatol 2010;37:611 [PMID: 20813274].

CONGENITAL INFECTIONS

ESSENTIALS OF DIAGNOSIS & TYPICAL FEATURES

- Can be acquired in utero, perinatally, and postnatally.
- Can be asymptomatic in the newborn period.
- Clinical symptom complexes include IUGR, chorioretinitis, cataracts, cholestatic jaundice, thrombocytopenia, skin rash, and brain calcifications.
- Diagnosis can be confirmed using polymerase chain reaction (PCR) testing, antigen and antibody studies, and culture.

1. Cytomegalovirus Infection (See also Chapter 40)

Cytomegalovirus (CMV) is the most common virus transmitted in utero, affecting approximately 1% of all newborns. Symptomatic disease in the newborn period occurs in 10% of these congenitally infected infants, with a spectrum of findings including hepatosplenomegaly, petechiae and blueberry muffin spots, growth restriction, microcephaly, direct hyperbilirubinemia, thrombocytopenia, intracranial calcifications, and chorioretinitis. More than half of these infants will develop long-term sequelae, including sensorineural deafness in 20%–30%. Sensorineural hearing loss is common even in asymptomatic infants, leading to deafness in another 10–15%. Transmission of CMV can occur during either primary or reactivated maternal infection; the risk of symptomatic neonatal disease is highest when the mother acquires a primary infection in the first half of pregnancy. Children, especially in the day care setting, are an important source of infection. Diagnosis in the neonate should be confirmed by culture of the virus from urine. Rapid diagnosis is possible with PCR testing of urine or saliva. Diagnosis can also be confirmed in utero from an amniocentesis specimen. Ganciclovir therapy (6 mg/kg IV q12h for 6 weeks) is recommended for neonates with symptomatic congenital infection affecting the central nervous system, in an attempt to prevent progression of hearing loss and neuronal damage. Trials with longer course therapy and oral valganciclovir are in progress.

Infection can also be acquired around the time of delivery, and postnatally through blood transfusion or ingestion of CMV-infected breast milk. These infections generally cause no symptoms or sequelae although hepatitis, pneumonia, and neurologic illness may occur in compromised seronegative premature infants. Transfusion risk can be minimized by using frozen, washed red blood cells; leukodepleted blood; or CMV antibody-negative donors.

2. Rubella (See also Chapter 40)

Congenital rubella infection occurs as a result of maternal rubella infection during pregnancy. The risk of fetal infection and congenital defects is as high as 80%–85% in mothers infected during the first trimester, but after 12 weeks' gestation, the risk of congenital malformation decreases markedly. Features of congenital rubella syndrome include microcephaly and encephalitis; cardiac defects (patent ductus arteriosus and pulmonary arterial stenosis and arterial hypoplasia); cataracts, retinopathy, and microphthalmia; growth restriction, hepatosplenomegaly, thrombocytopenia, and purpura; and deafness. Affected infants can be asymptomatic at birth but develop clinical sequelae during the first year of life as the viral infection is persistent due to an inadequate immune response. The diagnosis should be suspected in cases of a characteristic clinical illness in the mother (rash, adenopathy, and arthritis) confirmed by an increase in serum rubella-specific IgM or culture of pharyngeal secretions in the infant. Congenital rubella is now rare in industrialized countries because of widespread immunization, but is still possible due to the prevalence of unimmunized individuals in the population and widespread travel.

3. Varicella

Congenital varicella syndrome is rare (1%–2% after maternal varicella infection acquired during the first 20 weeks of pregnancy) and may include limb hypoplasia, cutaneous scars, microcephaly, cortical atrophy, chorioretinitis, and cataracts. Perinatal exposure (5 days before to 2 days after delivery) can cause severe to fatal disseminated varicella in the infant. If maternal varicella infection develops within this perinatal risk period, the newborn should receive varicella-zoster immune globulin. If varicella immune globulin is not available, IVIG can be used instead. If this has not been done, subsequent illness can be treated with IV acyclovir.

Hospitalized premature infants of at least 28 weeks' gestation whose mothers have no history of chickenpox—and all infants younger than 28 weeks' gestational age—should receive varicella immune globulin following any postnatal exposure.

4. Toxoplasmosis (See also Chapter 43)

Toxoplasmosis is caused by the protozoan *Toxoplasma gondii*. Maternal infection occurs in 0.1%–0.5% of pregnancies and is usually asymptomatic; it is estimated that between 1 in 1000 and 1 in 10,000 infants are infected, 70%–90% initially asymptomatic. These children may develop mental retardation, visual impairment and learning disabilities within months to years. The sources of infection include exposure to cat feces and ingestion of raw or undercooked meat. Although the risk of transmission increases to 90% near term, fetal damage is most likely to occur when maternal infection occurs in the second to sixth month of gestation.

Clinical findings may include growth restriction, chorioretinitis, seizures, jaundice, hydrocephalus, microcephaly, intracranial calcifications, hepatosplenomegaly, adenopathy, cataracts, maculopapular rash, thrombocytopenia, and pneumonia. The serologic diagnosis is based on a positive toxoplasma-specific IgA, IgE, or IgM in the first six months of life, a rise in serial IgG levels compared to the mother's, or a persistent IgG beyond 12 months. Infants with suspected infection should have eye and auditory examinations and a CT scan of the brain. Organism isolation from placenta or cord blood and PCR tests on amniotic fluid or CSF are also available for diagnosis.

Spiramycin (an investigational drug in the United States) treatment of primary maternal infection is used to try to reduce transmission to the fetus. Neonatal treatment using pyrimethamine and sulfadiazine with folinic acid can improve long-term outcome.

5. Parvovirus B19 Infection

Parvovirus B19 is a small, nonenveloped, single-stranded DNA virus that causes erythema infectiosum (fifth disease) in children, with a peak incidence at ages 6–7 years. Transmission to the mother is primarily by respiratory secretions. The virus replicates initially in erythroid progenitor cells and induces cell-cycle arrest, resulting in severe anemia, myocarditis, nonimmune hydrops, or fetal death in approximately 3%–6% of fetuses infected during pregnancy. Resolution of the hydrops may occur in utero, either spontaneously or after fetal transfusion. Mothers who have been exposed may have specific serologic testing, and serial ultrasound, Doppler examinations, and percutaneous umbilical cord blood sampling of the fetus to assess for anemia. If the fetus survives, the long-term outcome is good with no late effects from the infection.

6. Congenital Syphilis (See also Chapter 42)

Active primary and secondary maternal syphilis leads to transplacental passage of *Treponema pallidum* to the fetus in nearly 100% of affected pregnancies while latent maternal infection leads to transplacental infection of the fetus in 40% of cases, and late maternal infection in 10%. Fetal infection is rare before 18 weeks' gestation. Fetal infection can result in stillbirth or prematurity. Findings of early congenital syphilis (presentation before age 2 years) include mucocutaneous lesions, lymphadenopathy, hepatosplenomegaly, bony changes, and hydrops, although newborn infants are often asymptomatic. Late manifestations (after 2 years of age) in untreated infants involve the central nervous system, bones and joints, teeth, eyes and skin. An infant should be evaluated for congenital syphilis if he or she has proven or probable congenital syphilis, defined as a suggestive examination, serum quantitative nontreponemal titer more than fourfold the mother's, or positive darkfield or fluorescent antibody test of body fluids, or birth to a mother with positive nontreponemal tests confirmed by a positive treponemal test but without documented adequate treatment (parenteral penicillin G), including the expected fourfold decrease in nontreponemal antibody titer. Infants of mothers treated less than 1 month before delivery also require evaluation. Evaluation should include physical examination, a quantitative nontreponemal serologic test for syphilis, CBC, CSF examination for cell count and protein, Venereal Disease Research Laboratory testing, and long bone radiographs. Guidelines for therapy are presented in Table 2–21.

American Academy of Pediatrics: In Pickering LD et al (editors): *Red Book: 2009 Report of the Committee on Infectious Diseases.* 28th ed. American Academy of Pediatrics, 2009.

Bopanna SB, Ross SA, Shimamura M, Palmer AL et al: Saliva polymerase-chain-reaction assay for cytomegalovirus screening in newborns. N Engl J Med 2011;364:2111 [PMID: 21631323].

Cuixia T et al: Congenital infections, part I: CMV, toxoplasmosis, rubella and herpes simplex. NeoReviews 2010;11:e436.

Lombardi G et al: Congenital cytomegalovirus infection: treatment, sequelae and follow-up. J Matern Fetal Neonatal Med 2010;23(supp 3):45 [PMID: 20807160].

Nassetta L et al: Treatment of congenital cytomegalovirus infection: implications for future therapeutic strategies. J Antimicrob Chemother 2009;63:862 [PMID: 19287011].

PERINATALLY ACQUIRED INFECTIONS

1. Herpes Simplex (See also Chapter 40)

Herpes simplex virus infection is usually acquired at birth during transit through an infected birth canal. The mother may have either primary or reactivated secondary infection. Primary maternal infection, because of the high titer of organisms and the absence of antibodies, poses the greatest risk to the infant. The risk of neonatal infection with vaginal delivery in this setting is 25%–50%. Seventy percent of mothers with primary herpes at the time of delivery are asymptomatic. The risk to an infant born to a mother with recurrent herpes simplex is much lower (< 1%). Time of presentation of localized (skin, eye, or mouth) or disseminated disease (pneumonia, shock, or hepatitis) in the infant is usually 5–14 days of age. CNS disease usually presents later, at 14–28 days with lethargy, fever, and seizures. In rare cases, presentation is as early as day 1 of life, suggesting in-utero infection. In about 45% of patients, localized skin, eye, and mouth disease is the first indication of infection. Another

Table 2–21. Recommended management of neonates (1 month of age or younger) born to mothers with reactive serologic tests for syphilis.

Clinical Status	Evaluation (in Addition to Physical Examination and Quantitative Nontreponemal Testing)	Antimicrobial Therapy[a]
Proven or highly probable disease[b]	CSF analysis for VDRL, cell count, and protein CBC and platelet count Other tests as clinically indicated (eg, long-bone radiography, liver function tests, ophthalmologic examination)	Aqueous crystalline penicillin G, 100 000–150 000 U/kg/day, administered as 50 000 U/kg/dose, IV, every 12 h during the first 7 days of age and every 8 h thereafter for a total of 10 days **OR** Penicillin G procaine,[c] 50 000 U/kg/day, IM, in a single dose for 10 days
Normal physical examination and serum quantitative nontreponemal titer the same or less than fourfold the maternal titer:		
(a) (i) Mother was not treated or inadequately treated or has no documented Treatment; (ii) mother was treated with erythromycin or other nonpenicillin regimen; (iii) mother received Treatment 4 wk or less before delivery; (iv) maternal evidence of reinfection or relapse (less than fourfold decrease in titers)	CSF analysis for VDRL, cell count, and protein[d] CBC and platelet count[d] Long-bone radiography[d]	Aqueous crystalline penicillin G, IV, for 10 days[d] **OR** Penicillin G procaine,[c] 50 000 U/kg, IM, in a single dose for 10 days[d] **OR** Penicillin G benzathine,[c] 50 000 U/kg, IM, in a single dose[d]
(b) (i) Adequate maternal therapy given more than 4 wk before delivery; (ii) mother has no evidence of reinfection or relapse	None	Clinical, serologic follow-up, and penicillin G benzathine, 50 000 U/kg, IM, in a single dose[e]
(c) Adequate therapy before pregnancy and mother's nontreponemal serologic titer remained low and stable during pregnancy and at delivery	None	None[f]

CSF indicates cerebrospinal fluid; VDRL, Venereal Disease Research Laboratory; CBC, complete blood cell; IV, intravenously; IM, intramuscularly.
[a]If more than 1 day of therapy is missed, the entire course should be restarted.
[b]Abnormal physical examination, serum quantitative nontreponemal titer that is fourfold greater than the mother's titer, or positive result of darkfield or fluorescent antibody test of body fluid(s).
[c]Penicillin G benzathine and penicillin G procaine are approved for IM administration only.
[d]A complete evaluation (CSF analysis, bone radiography, CBC) is not necessary if 10 days of parenteral therapy is administered but may be useful to support a diagnosis of congenital syphilis. If a single dose of penicillin G benzathine is used, then the infant must be evaluated fully, results of the full evaluation must be normal, and follow-up must be certain. If any part of the infant's evaluation is abnormal or not performed or if the CSF analysis is uninterpretable, the 10-day course of penicillin is required.
[e]Some experts would not treat the infant but would provide close serologic follow-up.
[f]Some experts would treat with penicillin G benzathine, 50 000 U/kg, as a single IM injection, if follow-up is uncertain.
Reprinted, with permission, from Pickering LK, Baker CJ, Kimberlin DW, Long SS, eds. Red Book: 2009 Report of the Committee on Infectious Diseases. 28th ed. Elk Grove Village, IL: American Academy of Pediatrics; 2009.

30% present with CNS disease, whereas the remaining 25% have disseminated or multiorgan disease indistinguishable from bacterial sepsis. Herpes infection should be considered in neonates with sepsis syndrome, negative bacteriologic culture results, and severe liver dysfunction or coagulopathy. Herpes simplex virus also should be considered as a causative agent in neonates with fever, irritability, and abnormal CSF findings, especially in the presence of seizures. Viral culture from vesicles, usually positive in 24–72 hours, makes the definitive diagnosis. PCR can assist in diagnosis but may be falsely negative in the CSF early in the course. If a CSF PCR performed shortly after the onset of symptoms is negative, it should be repeated after several days if herpes simplex virus disease is considered a strong possibility.

Acyclovir (60 mg/kg/d divided q8h) is the drug of choice for neonatal herpes infection. Localized disease is treated for 14 days, and a 21-day course is used for disseminated or CNS disease. Treatment improves survival of neonates with CNS and disseminated disease and prevents the spread of localized disease. Prevention is possible by not allowing delivery through an infected birth canal (eg, by cesarean section within 6 hours after rupture of the membranes in the presence of known infection). However, antepartum cervical cultures are poor predictors of the presence of virus at the time of delivery. Furthermore, given the low incidence of infection in the newborn from recurrent maternal infection, cesarean delivery is not indicated for asymptomatic mothers with a history of recurrent herpes. Cesarean deliveries are performed in mothers with active lesions (either primary or recurrent) at the time of delivery. Infants born to mothers with a history of herpes simplex virus infection but no active lesions can be observed closely after birth, and do not need to be isolated. Cultures should be obtained and acyclovir treatment initiated only for clinical signs of herpes virus infection. In infants born to mothers with active lesions—regardless of the route of delivery—cultures of the eye, oropharynx, nasopharynx, and rectum should be performed 12–24 hours after delivery, and the infant should be in contact isolation or with the mother. If the infant is colonized (positive cultures) or if symptoms consistent with herpes infection develop, treatment with acyclovir should be started. In cases of primary maternal genital infection at the time of vaginal delivery, infant specimens should be obtained and some experts recommend that acyclovir be started pending the results of cultures. The major problem facing perinatologists is the high percentage of asymptomatic primary maternal infection. In these cases, infection in the neonate is not currently preventable. Cultures should be obtained and acyclovir started, pending the results of those cultures, in any infant who presents at the right age with symptoms consistent with neonatal herpes.

The prognosis is good for localized skin and mucosal disease that does not progress, although skin recurrences are common. The mortality rate for disseminated herpes is high (approximately 30%), with significant morbidity among survivors of both disseminated (20%) and CNS (80%) infections despite treatment. Cutaneous recurrences are common in all types, and examination of the CSF should be considered with skin recurrences. Infants with herpes encephalitis should receive long term oral acyclovir for 6 months after completion of intravenous treatment.

2. Hepatitis B & C

Infants become infected with hepatitis B at the time of birth; intrauterine transmission is rare. Clinical illness is rare in the neonatal period, but infants born to positive mothers are at risk of becoming chronic hepatitis B surface antigen (HBsAg) carriers and developing chronic active hepatitis, and even hepatocellular carcinoma. The presence of HBsAg should be determined in all pregnant women. If the result is positive, the infant should receive hepatitis B immune globulin (HBIG) and hepatitis B vaccine as soon as possible after birth, followed by two subsequent vaccine doses at 1 and 6 months of age. If HBsAg has not been tested prior to birth in a mother at risk, the test should be run after delivery and hepatitis B vaccine given within 12 hours after birth. If the mother is subsequently found to be positive, HBIG should be given as soon as possible (preferably within 48 hours, but not later than 1 week after birth). Subsequent vaccine doses should be given at 1 and 6 months of age. In premature infants born to HBsAg-positive mothers, vaccine and HBIG should be given at birth, but a three-vaccine hepatitis B series should be given beginning at 1 month of age.

Perinatal transmission of hepatitis C occurs in about 5% of infants born to mothers who carry the virus; maternal coinfection with HIV increases the risk of transmission. At present, no prevention strategies exist. Serum antibody to hepatitis C and hepatitis C RNA have been detected in colostrum, but the risk of hepatitis C transmission is similar in breast-fed and bottle-fed infants. Up to 12 months of age, the only reliable screen for hepatitis C infection is PCR. After that time, the presence of hepatitis C antibodies in the infant strongly suggests that infection has occurred.

3. Enterovirus Infection

Enterovirus infections occur most frequently in the late summer and early fall. Infection is usually acquired in the perinatal period. There is often a history of maternal fever, diarrhea, and/or rash in the week prior to delivery. The illness appears in the infant in the first 2 weeks of life and is most commonly characterized by fever, lethargy, irritability, diarrhea, and/or rash. More severe forms occasionally occur, especially if infection occurs before 1 week of age, including meningoencephalitis, myocarditis, hepatitis, pneumonia, shock, and disseminated intravascular coagulation. Diagnosis is best confirmed by PCR.

No therapy has proven efficacy. The prognosis is good in most cases, except those with severe hepatitis, myocarditis, or disseminated disease, which carry high mortality rates.

4. HIV Infection (See also Chapter 41)

HIV can be acquired in utero or at the time of delivery, or can be transmitted postpartum via breast milk. Testing for HIV should be performed in all pregnant women. Without treatment, transmission of virus occurs in 13%–39% of births to infected mothers, mostly at the time of delivery. Treating the mother with zidovudine therapy, starting as early as 14 weeks' gestation and intrapartum, and the infant for the first 6 weeks of life (zidovudine beginning within 12 hours of birth) decreases vertical transmission to 7%. Shorter courses of zidovudine and cesarean delivery before the onset of labor or rupture of membranes are also associated with decreased disease transmission. The combination of zidovudine treatment, elective cesarean delivery, and avoidance of breast feeding can lower transmission to 1%–2%. Treatment of the mother with highly active antiretroviral therapy during pregnancy coupled with intrapartum and neonatal prophylaxis further reduces the risk of ante- and intrapartum transmission to <1%. Current guidelines for antiretroviral drugs in pregnant HIV-infected women are similar to those for nonpregnant patients (eg, highly active antiretroviral combination therapy). In cases of unknown HIV status at presentation in labor, rapid HIV testing, and intrapartum treatment if positive should be offered. The risk of transmission is increased in mothers with advanced disease, high viral loads, low CD4 counts, and intrapartum events such as chorioamnionitis and prolonged membrane rupture that increase exposure of the fetus to maternal blood.

Newborns with congenitally acquired HIV are usually asymptomatic. Infants of HIV-infected women should be tested by HIV DNA PCR at less than 48 hours, at 2 weeks, at 1–2 months, and at 2–4 months. If an infant aged 4 months has a negative PCR result, infection can be reasonably excluded. HIV-positive mothers should be counseled not to breastfeed their infants if safe feeding alternatives are available.

American Academy of Pediatrics: In Pickering LD et al (editors) *Red Book: 2009 Report of the Committee on Infectious Diseases.* 28th ed. American Academy of Pediatrics, 2009.

Corey L, Wald A: Maternal and neonatal herpes simplex virus infections. N Engl J Med 2009;361:1376 [PMID: 19797284].

Havens PL, Mofenson LM, Committee on Pediatric AIDS: Evaluation and management of the infant exposed to HIV-1 in the United States. Pediatrics 2009;123:175 [PMID: 19117880].

Havens PL, Mofenson LM, Committee on Pediatric AIDS: HIV testing and prophylaxis to prevent mother-to-child transmission in the United States. Pediatrics 2008;122:1127 [PMID: 18977995].

Read JS: Prevention of mother-to-child transmission of HIV: Antiretroviral strategies. Clin Perinatol 2010;37:765 [PMID: 21078449].

HEMATOLOGIC DISORDERS IN THE NEWBORN INFANT

BLEEDING DISORDERS

Bleeding in the newborn infant may result from inherited clotting deficiencies (eg, factor VIII deficiency) or acquired disorders—hemorrhagic disease of the newborn (vitamin K deficiency), disseminated intravascular coagulation, liver failure, and isolated thrombocytopenia.

1. Vitamin K Deficiency Bleeding of the Newborn

ESSENTIALS OF DIAGNOSIS & TYPICAL FEATURES

- Frequently exclusively breast fed, otherwise clinically well infant.
- Bleeding from mucous membranes, GI tract, skin, or internal (intracranial).
- Prolonged prothrombin time (PT), relatively normal partial thromboplastin time (PTT), normal fibrinogen and platelet count.

Bleeding is caused by the deficiency of the vitamin K–dependent clotting factors (II, VII, IX, and X). Bleeding occurs in 0.25%–1.7% of newborns who do not receive vitamin K prophylaxis after birth, generally in the first 5 days to 2 weeks in an otherwise well infant. There is an increased risk in infants of mothers receiving therapy with anticonvulsants that interfere with vitamin K metabolism. Early vitamin K deficiency bleeding (0–2 weeks) can be prevented by either parenteral or oral vitamin K administration, whereas late disease (onset 2 weeks to 6 months) is most effectively prevented by administering parenteral vitamin K. Sites of ecchymoses and surface bleeding include the GI tract, umbilical cord, circumcision site, and nose, although devastating intracranial hemorrhage can occur. Bleeding from vitamin K deficiency is more likely to occur in exclusively breast-fed infants because of very low amounts of vitamin K in breast milk and slower and more restricted intestinal bacterial colonization. Differential diagnosis includes disseminated intravascular coagulation and hepatic failure (Table 2–22).

Table 2–22. Features of infants bleeding from vitamin K deficiency (VKDB), disseminated intravascular coagulation (DIC), or liver failure.

	VKDB	DIC	Liver Failure
Clinical	Well infant; no prophylactic vitamin K	Sick infant; hypoxia, sepsis, etc	Sick infant; hepatitis, inborn errors of metabolism, shock liver
Bleeding	GI tract, umbilical cord, circumcision, nose	Generalized	Generalized
Onset	2-3 d to 2 wk	Any time	Any time
Platelet count	Normal	Decreased	Normal or decreased
Prothrombin time	Prolonged	Prolonged	Prolonged
Partial thromboplastin time	Normal or prolonged	Prolonged	Prolonged
Fibrinogen	Normal	Decreased	Decreased

GI, gastrointestinal.

Treatment consists of 1 mg of vitamin K SC or IV. IM injections should be avoided in infants who are actively bleeding. Such infants may also require factor replacement in addition to vitamin K administration.

2. Thrombocytopenia

ESSENTIALS OF DIAGNOSIS & TYPICAL FEATURES

- Generalized petechiae; oozing at cord or puncture sites.
- Thrombocytopenia, often marked (platelets < 10,000–20,000/mL).
- In an otherwise well infant, suspect isoimmune thrombocytopenia.
- In a sick or asphyxiated infant, suspect disseminated intravascular coagulation.

Infants with thrombocytopenia have generalized petechiae (not just on the presenting part) and platelet counts less than 150,000/mL (usually < 50,000/mL; may be < 10,000/mL). Neonatal thrombocytopenia can be isolated in a seemingly well infant or may occur in association with a deficiency of other clotting factors in a sick infant. The differential diagnosis for thrombocytopenia is presented in Table 2–23. Treatment of neonatal thrombocytopenia is transfusion of platelets (10 mL/kg of platelets increases the platelet count by approximately 70,000/mL). Indications for transfusion in the full-term infant are clinical bleeding or a total platelet count less than 10,000–20,000/mL. In the preterm infant at risk for intraventricular hemorrhage, transfusion is indicated for counts less than 40,000–50,000/mL.

Isoimmune (alloimmune) thrombocytopenia is analogous to Rh-isoimmunization, with a human platelet antigen [HPA]-1a (in 80%)- or HPA-5b (in 15%)–negative mother and an HPA-1a– or HPA-5b–positive fetus. Transplacental passage of IgG antibody leads to platelet destruction. If platelet transfusion is required for acute bleeding, washed maternal platelets may be the most readily available antigen-negative platelet source, because 98% of the general population will also be HPA-1a– or HPA-5b–positive. Treatment with steroids has been disappointing. Treatment with IVIG infusion, 1 g/kg/d for 2–3 days, until the platelet count has doubled or is over 50,000/mL, is potentially beneficial. Twenty to thirty percent of infants with isoimmune thrombocytopenia will experience intracranial hemorrhage, half of them before birth. Antenatal therapy of the mother with IVIG with or without steroids may reduce this risk.

Infants born to mothers with idiopathic thrombocytopenic purpura are at low risk for serious hemorrhage despite the thrombocytopenia, and treatment is usually unnecessary. If bleeding does occur, IVIG can be used.

Table 2–23. Differential diagnosis of neonatal thrombocytopenia.

Disorder	Clinical Tips
Immune	
Passively acquired antibody; idiopathic thrombocytopenic purpura, systemic lupus erythematosus, drug-induced	Proper history, maternal thrombocytopenia
Isoimmune sensitization to HPA-1a antigen	No rise in platelet count from random donor platelet transfusion. Positive antiplatelet antibodies in baby's serum, sustained rise in platelets by transfusion of mother's platelets
Infections Bacterial infections Congenital viral infections	Sick infants with other signs consistent with infection
Syndromes Absent radii Fanconi anemia	Congenital anomalies, associated pancytopenia
Disseminated intravascular coagulation (DIC)	Sick infants, abnormalities of clotting factors
Giant hemangioma	
Thrombosis	Hyperviscous infants, vascular catheters
High-risk infant with respiratory distress syndrome, pulmonary hypertension, etc	Isolated decrease in platelets is not uncommon in sick infants even in the absence of DIC (localized trapping)

HPA, human platelet antigen.

ANEMIA

ESSENTIALS OF DIAGNOSIS & TYPICAL FEATURES

- Hematocrit < 40% at term birth.
- Acute blood loss—signs of hypovolemia, normal reticulocyte count.
- Chronic blood loss—pallor without hypovolemia, elevated reticulocyte count.
- Hemolytic anemia—accompanied by excessive hyperbilirubinemia.

The newborn infant with anemia from acute blood loss presents with signs of hypovolemia (tachycardia, poor perfusion, and hypotension), with an initially normal hematocrit that falls after volume replacement. Anemia from chronic blood loss is evidenced by pallor without signs of hypovolemia, with an initially low hematocrit and reticulocytosis.

Anemia can be caused by hemorrhage, hemolysis, or failure to produce red blood cells. Anemia occurring in the first 24–48 hours of life is the result of hemorrhage or hemolysis. Hemorrhage can occur in utero (fetoplacental, fetomaternal, or twin-to-twin), perinatally (cord rupture, placenta previa, placental abruption, or incision through the placenta at cesarean section), or internally (intracranial hemorrhage, cephalohematoma, or ruptured liver or spleen). Hemolysis is caused by blood group incompatibilities, enzyme or membrane abnormalities, infection, and disseminated intravascular coagulation, and is accompanied by significant hyperbilirubinemia.

Initial evaluation should include a review of the perinatal history, assessment of the infant's volume status, and a complete physical examination. A Kleihauer-Betke test for fetal cells in the mother's circulation should be done. A CBC, blood smear, reticulocyte count, and direct and indirect Coombs tests should be performed. This simple evaluation should suggest a diagnosis in most infants. Most infants tolerate anemia quite well due to the increased oxygen availability in the extrauterine environment; however, treatment with erythropoietin or transfusion might be needed if the infant fails to thrive or develops signs of cardiopulmonary compromise. Additionally, if blood loss is the cause of the anemia, early supplementation with iron will be needed. It is important to remember that hemolysis related to blood group incompatibility can continue for weeks after birth. Serial hematocrits should be followed, because late transfusion may be needed.

POLYCYTHEMIA

ESSENTIALS OF DIAGNOSIS & TYPICAL FEATURES

- Hematocrit > 65% (venous) at term.
- Plethora, tachypnea, retractions.
- Hypoglycemia, irritability, lethargy, poor feeding.

Polycythemia in the newborn is manifested by plethora, cyanosis, respiratory distress with tachypnea and oxygen need, hypoglycemia, poor feeding, emesis, irritability, and lethargy. Hyperbilirubinemia is expected. The consequence of polycythemia is hyperviscosity with decreased perfusion of the capillary beds. Clinical symptomatology can affect several organ systems (Table 2–24). Renal vein, other deep vein, or artery thrombosis is a severe complication. Screening can be done by measuring a capillary (heelstick) hematocrit. If the value is greater than 68%, a peripheral venous hematocrit should be measured. Values greater than 65% should be considered consistent with hyperviscosity.

Table 2–24. Organ-related symptoms of hyperviscosity.

Central nervous system	Irritability, jitteriness, seizures, lethargy
Cardiopulmonary	Respiratory distress secondary to congestive heart failure, or persistent pulmonary hypertension
Gastrointestinal	Vomiting, heme-positive stools, distention, necrotizing enterocolitis
Renal	Decreased urinary output, renal vein thrombosis
Metabolic	Hypoglycemia
Hematologic	Hyperbilirubinemia, thrombocytopenia

Elevated hematocrits occur in 2%–5% of live births. Delayed cord clamping is the most common cause of benign neonatal polycythemia. Although 50% of polycythemic infants are AGA, the prevalence of polycythemia is greater in the SGA and LGA populations. Other causes of increased hematocrit include (1) twin-twin transfusion, (2) maternal-fetal transfusion, and (3) chronic intrauterine hypoxia (SGA infants, and LGA infants of diabetic mothers).

Treatment is recommended for symptomatic infants. Treatment for asymptomatic infants based strictly on hematocrit is not indicated as there is no proven long term benefit for neurodevelopmental outcome. Treatment for symptomatic infants is isovolemic partial exchange transfusion with normal saline, effectively decreasing the hematocrit. The amount to exchange (in milliliters) is calculated using the following formula:

$$\text{Number of milliliters to exchange} = (\text{PVH} - \text{DH})/\text{PVH} \times \text{BV(mL/kg)} \times \text{Wt(kg)}$$

where PVH is peripheral venous hematocrit, DH is desired hematocrit, BV is blood volume in mL/kg, and Wt is weight in kilograms.

Blood is withdrawn at a steady rate from an umbilical venous line while the replacement solution is infused at the same rate through a peripheral IV line over 15–30 minutes. The desired hematocrit value is 50%–55%; the assumed blood volume is 80 mL/kg.

Hutton EK, Hassan ES: Late vs early clamping of the umbilical cord in full-term neonates. JAMA 2007;297:1241 [PMID: 17374818].

Manco-Johnson MJ: Bleeding disorders in the neonate. NeoReviews 2008;9:e162.

Manco-Johnson MJ: Hemostasis in the neonate. NeoReviews 2008;9:e119.

Ozek E et al: Partial exchange transfusion to prevent neurodevelopmental disability in infants with polycythemia. Cochrane Database Syst Rev 2010 Jan 20;(1):CD005089 [PMID: 20091569].

Remon JJ et al: Polycythemia in the newborn. NeoReviews 2011;12:e20.

Sarkar S, Rosenkrantz TS: Neonatal polycythemia and hyperviscosity. Semin Fetal Neonatal Med 2008;13:248 [PMID: 18424246].

RENAL DISORDERS IN THE NEWBORN INFANT (SEE ALSO CHAPTER 24)

Renal function depends on postmenstrual age. The glomerular filtration rate is 20 mL/min/1.73 m^2 in full-term neonates and 10–13 mL/min/1.73 m^2 in infants born at 28–30 weeks' gestation. The speed of maturation after birth also depends on postmenstrual age. Creatinine can be used as a clinical marker of glomerular filtration rate. Values in the first month of life are shown in Table 1–25. Creatinine at birth reflects the maternal level and should decrease slowly over the first 3–4 weeks. An increasing serum creatinine is never normal.

The ability to concentrate urine and retain sodium also depends on gestational age. Infants born before 28–30 weeks' gestation are compromised in this respect and can easily become dehydrated and hyponatremic. Preterm infants also have an increased bicarbonate excretion and a low tubular maximum for glucose (approximately 120 mg/dL).

RENAL FAILURE

ESSENTIALS OF DIAGNOSIS & TYPICAL FEATURES

- Clinical setting—birth depression, hypovolemia, hypotension, shock.
- Low or delayed urine output (< 1 mL/kg/h).
- Rising serum creatinine; hyperkalemia; metabolic acidosis; fluid overload.

Renal failure is most commonly seen in the setting of birth asphyxia, hypovolemia, or shock from any cause. The normal rate of urine flow is 1–3 mL/kg/h. After a hypoxic or ischemic insult, acute tubular necrosis may ensue. Typically, 2–3 days of anuria or oliguria is associated with hematuria, proteinuria, and a rise in serum creatinine. The period of anuria or oliguria is followed by a period of polyuria and then gradual recovery. During the polyuric phase, excessive urine sodium and bicarbonate losses may be seen.

Table 1–25. Normal values of serum creatinine (mg/dL).

Gestational Age at Birth (wk)	Postnatal Age (d)	
	0–2	28
< 28	1.2	0.7
29–32	1.1	0.6
33–36	1.1	0.45
36–42	0.8	0.3

The initial management is restoration of the infant's volume status. Thereafter, restriction of fluids to insensible water loss (40–60 mL/kg/d) without added electrolytes, plus milliliter-for-milliliter urine replacement, should be instituted. Serum and urine electrolytes and body weights should be followed frequently. These measures should be continued through the polyuric phase. After urine output has been reestablished, urine replacement should be decreased to between 0.5 and 0.75 mL for each milliliter of urine output to see if the infant has regained normal function. If that is the case, the infant can be returned to maintenance fluids.

Finally, many of these infants experience fluid overload and should be allowed to lose enough water through urination to return to birth weight. Hyperkalemia, which may become life-threatening, may occur in this situation despite the lack of added IV potassium. If the serum potassium reaches 7 mEq/L, therapy should be started with glucose and insulin infusion, giving 1 unit of insulin for every 3 g of glucose administered, in addition to binding resins per rectum. Calcium chloride (20 mg/kg bolus) and correction of metabolic acidosis with bicarbonate are also helpful in the acute management of arrhythmias resulting from hyperkalemia.

Peritoneal dialysis is occasionally needed for the management of neonatal acute renal failure and for removal of waste products and excess fluid. Hemodialysis, although possible, is difficult due to the small blood volume of the infant and problems with vascular access. Although most acute renal failure in the newborn resolves, ischemic injury severe enough to result in acute cortical necrosis and chronic renal failure can occur. Such infants are also at risk of developing hypertension.

URINARY TRACT ANOMALIES

Abdominal masses in the newborn are most frequently caused by renal enlargement. Most common is a multicystic or dysplastic kidney; congenital hydronephrosis is second in frequency. Chromosomal abnormalities and syndromes with multiple anomalies frequently include renal abnormalities. An ultrasound examination is the first step in diagnosis. In pregnancies complicated by oligohydramnios, renal agenesis or obstruction secondary to posterior urethral valves should be considered.

Only bilateral disease or disease in a solitary kidney is associated with oligohydramnios, significant morbidity, and death.

Such infants will generally also have pulmonary hypoplasia, and present with pulmonary rather than renal insufficiency.

Ultrasonography identifies many infants with renal anomalies (most often hydronephrosis) prior to birth. Postnatal evaluation of infants with hydronephrosis should include renal ultrasound and a voiding cystourethrogram at about 1 week of age, depending on the severity of the antenatal findings. Earlier postnatal ultrasound might underestimate the severity of the hydronephrosis due to low glomerular filtration rates in the first days of life, although cases in which oligohydramnios or severe renal abnormality are suspected will be accurately diagnosed even on the first day of life. Until the presence and severity of vesicoureteral reflux is evaluated, some experts recommend antibiotic prophylaxis with low-dose penicillin or amoxicillin. However, the necessity for prophylaxis in general is a controversial issue.

RENAL VEIN THROMBOSIS

ESSENTIALS OF DIAGNOSIS & TYPICAL FEATURES

- History of IDM, birth depression, dehydration.
- Hematuria, oliguria.
- Thrombocytopenia, polycythemia.
- Renal enlargement on examination.

Renal vein thrombosis occurs most often in dehydrated polycythemic newborns. At particular risk is the IDM with polycythemia. If fetal distress is superimposed on polycythemia and dehydration, prompt reduction in blood viscosity is indicated. Thrombosis is unilateral in 70%, usually begins in intrarenal venules, and can extend into larger veins and the vena cava. Hematuria, oliguria, thrombocytopenia, and possibly an enlarged kidney raise suspicion for this diagnosis. With bilateral renal vein thrombosis, anuria ensues. Diagnosis can be confirmed with an ultrasound examination that includes Doppler flow studies of the kidneys. Treatment involves correcting the predisposing condition; systemic heparinization or the use of thrombolytics for this condition is controversial. Prognosis for a full recovery is uncertain. Many infants will develop significant atrophy of the affected kidney, and some develop systemic hypertension. All require careful follow-up.

Askenazi DJ et al: Acute kidney injury in critically ill newborns: What do we know? What do we need to learn? Pediatr Nephrol 2009;24:265 [PMID: 19082634].

Estrada CR: Prenatal hydronephrosis: Early evaluation. Curr Opin Urol 2008;18:401 [PMID: 18520762].

Ringer SA: Acute renal failure in the neonate. NeoReviews 2010;11:e243.

NEUROLOGIC PROBLEMS IN THE NEWBORN INFANT

SEIZURES

ESSENTIALS OF DIAGNOSIS & TYPICAL FEATURES

- Usual onset at 12–48 hours.
- Seizure types include subtle (characterized by variable findings), tonic, and multifocal clonic.
- Most common causes include hypoxic-ischemic encephalopathy, intracranial bleeds, and infection.

Newborns rarely have well-organized tonic-clonic seizures because of their incomplete cortical organization and a preponderance of inhibitory synapses. The most common type of seizure is characterized by a constellation of findings, including horizontal deviation of the eyes with or without jerking; eyelid blinking or fluttering; sucking, smacking, drooling, and other oral-buccal movements; swimming, rowing, or paddling movements; and apneic spells. Strictly tonic or multifocal clonic episodes are also seen.

Clinical Findings

The differential diagnosis of neonatal seizures is presented in Table 2–26. Most neonatal seizures occur between 12 and 48 hours of age. Later-onset seizures suggest meningitis, benign familial seizures, or hypocalcemia. Information regarding antenatal drug use, the presence of birth asphyxia or trauma, and family history (regarding inherited disorders) should be obtained. Physical examination focuses on neurologic features, other signs of drug withdrawal, concurrent signs of infection, dysmorphic features, and intrauterine growth. Screening workup should include blood glucose, ionized calcium, and electrolytes in all cases. Further workup depends on diagnoses suggested by the history and physical examination. In most cases, a lumbar puncture should be done. Hemorrhages, perinatal stroke, and structural disease of the CNS can be addressed with ultrasound, CT, and MRI scans. Metabolic workup should be pursued when appropriate. EEG should be done; the presence of spike discharges must be noted and the background wave pattern evaluated. At times correlation between EEG changes and clinical seizure activity is absent making a prolonged EEG with video monitoring a useful tool.

Treatment

Adequate ventilation and perfusion should be ensured. Hypoglycemia should be treated immediately with a 2-mL/kg infusion of $D_{10}W$ followed by 6 mg/kg/min of

Table 2–26. Differential diagnosis of neonatal seizures.

Diagnosis	Comment
Hypoxic-ischemic encephalopathy	Most common cause (60%), onset in first 24 h
Intracranial hemorrhage	Up to 15% of cases, periventricular/intraventricular hemorrhage, subdural or subarachnoid bleeding, stroke
Infection	12% of cases
Hypoglycemia	Small for gestational age, IDM
Hypocalcemia, hypomagnesemia	Infant of low birth weight, IDM
Hyponatremia	Rare, seen with SIADH
Disorders of amino and organic acid metabolism, hyperammonemia	Associated acidosis, altered level of consciousness
Pyridoxine dependency	Seizures refractory to routine therapy; cessation of seizures after administration of pyridoxine
Developmental defects	Other anomalies, chromosomal syndromes
Drug withdrawal	
No cause found	10% of cases
Benign familial neonatal seizures	

IDM, infant of a diabetic mother; SIADH, syndrome of inappropriate secretion of antidiuretic hormone.

$D_{10}W$ (100 mL/kg/d). Other treatments such as calcium or magnesium infusion and antibiotics are indicated to treat hypocalcemia, hypomagnesemia, and suspected infection. Electrolyte abnormalities should be corrected. Phenobarbital (20 mg/kg IV) should be administered to stop seizures. Supplemental doses of 5 mg/kg can be used if seizures persist, up to a total of 40 mg/kg. In most cases, phenobarbital controls seizures.

If seizures continue, therapy with fosphenytoin or lorazepam may be indicated. For refractory seizures, a trial of pyridoxine is indicated.

Prognosis

Outcome is related to the underlying cause of the seizure. The outcomes for hypoxic-ischemic encephalopathy and intraventricular hemorrhage have been discussed earlier in this chapter. In these settings, seizures that are difficult to control carry a poor prognosis for normal development. Seizures resulting from hypoglycemia, infection of the CNS, some inborn errors of metabolism, and developmental defects also have a high rate of poor outcome. Seizures caused by hypocalcemia or isolated subarachnoid hemorrhage generally resolve without sequelae.

HYPOTONIA

One should be alert to the diagnosis of congenital hypotonia when a mother has polyhydramnios and a history of poor fetal movement. The newborn may present with poor respiratory effort and birth asphyxia. For a discussion of causes and evaluation, see Chapter 25.

INTRACRANIAL HEMORRHAGE[1]

1. Subdural Hemorrhage

Subdural hemorrhage is related to birth trauma; the bleeding is caused by tears in the veins that bridge the subdural space. Prospective studies relating incidence to specific obstetric complications are not available.

Most commonly, subdural bleeding is from ruptured superficial cerebral veins, with blood over the cerebral convexities. These hemorrhages can be asymptomatic or may cause seizures, with onset on days 2–3 of life, vomiting, irritability, and lethargy. Associated findings include retinal hemorrhages and a full fontanelle. The diagnosis is confirmed by CT scan.

Specific treatment entailing needle drainage of the subdural space is rarely necessary. Most infants survive; 75% are normal on follow-up.

2. Primary Subarachnoid Hemorrhage

Primary subarachnoid hemorrhage is the most common type of neonatal intracranial hemorrhage. In the full-term infant, it can be related to trauma of delivery, whereas subarachnoid hemorrhage in the preterm infant can be seen in association with germinal matrix hemorrhage. Clinically, these hemorrhages can be asymptomatic or can present with seizures and irritability on day 2, or rarely, a massive hemorrhage with a rapid downhill course. The seizures associated with subarachnoid hemorrhage are very characteristic—usually brief, with a normal examination interictally. Diagnosis can be suspected on lumbar puncture and confirmed with CT scan. Long-term follow-up is uniformly good.

3. Neonatal Stroke

Focal cerebral ischemic injury can occur in the context of intraventricular hemorrhage in the premature infant and hypoxic-ischemic encephalopathy. Neonatal stroke has also been described in the context of underlying disorders of thrombolysis, maternal drug use (cocaine), a history of infertility, preeclampsia, prolonged membrane rupture, and chorioamnionitis. In some cases, the origin is unclear. The

[1]Intraventricular hemorrhage is discussed earlier, in the section on The Preterm Infant.

injury often occurs antenatally. The most common clinical presentation of an isolated cerebral infarct is with seizures, and diagnosis can be confirmed acutely with diffusion-weighted MRI scan. The most frequently described distribution is that of the middle cerebral artery.

Treatment is directed at controlling seizures. Use of anticoagulants and thrombolytics are controversial. Long-term outcome is variable, ranging from near-normal to hemiplegias and cognitive deficits.

Barnette AR, Inder TE: Evaluation and management of stroke in the neonate. Clin Perinatol 2009;36:125 [PMID: 19161870].

Holmes GL: The long-term effects of neonatal seizures. Clin Perinatol 2009;36:901 [PMID: 19944841].

Jensen FE: Neonatal seizures: an update on mechanisms and management. Clin Perinatol 2009;36:881 [PMID: 19944840].

Lynch JK: Epidemiology and classification of perinatal stroke. Semin Fetal Neonatal Med 2009;14:245 [PMID: 19664976].

METABOLIC DISORDERS IN THE NEWBORN INFANT[2]

HYPERGLYCEMIA

Hyperglycemia may develop in preterm infants, particularly those of extremely low birth weight who are also SGA. Glucose concentrations may exceed 200–250 mg/dL, particularly in the first few days of life. This transient diabetes-like syndrome usually lasts approximately 1 week.

Management may include simply reducing glucose intake while continuing to supply IV amino acids to prevent protein catabolism with resultant gluconeogenesis and worsened hyperglycemia. Intravenous insulin infusions may be needed in infants who remain hyperglycemic despite glucose infusion rates of less than 5–6 mg/kg/min, but caution should be used as hypoglycemia is a frequent complication.

HYPOCALCEMIA (SEE ALSO CHAPTER 34)

ESSENTIALS OF DIAGNOSIS & TYPICAL FEATURES

- Irritability, jitteriness, seizures.
- Normal blood glucose.
- Possible dysmorphic features, congenital heart disease (DiGeorge syndrome).

Calcium concentration in the immediate newborn period decreases in all infants. The concentration in fetal plasma is higher than that of the neonate or adult. Hypocalcemia is usually defined as a total serum concentration less than 7 mg/dL (equivalent to a calcium activity of 3.5 mEq/L), although the physiologically active fraction, ionized calcium, should be measured whenever possible, and is usually normal even when total calcium is as low as 6–7 mg/dL. An ionized calcium level above 0.9 mmol/L (1.8 mEq/L; 3.6 mg/dL) is not likely to be detrimental.

Clinical Findings

The clinical signs of hypocalcemia and hypocalcemic tetany include a high-pitched cry, jitteriness, tremulousness, and seizures.

Hypocalcemia tends to occur at two different times in the neonatal period. Early-onset hypocalcemia occurs in the first 2 days of life and has been associated with prematurity, maternal diabetes, asphyxia, and rarely, maternal hypoparathyroidism. Late-onset hypocalcemia occurs at approximately 7–10 days and is observed in infants receiving modified cow's milk rather than infant formula (high phosphorus intake), in infants with hypoparathyroidism (DiGeorge syndrome, 22q11 deletion), or in infants born to mothers with severe vitamin D deficiency. Hypomagnesemia should be sought and treated in cases of hypocalcemia that are resistant to treatment.

Treatment

A. Oral Calcium Therapy

The oral administration of calcium salts, often along with vitamin D, is the preferred method of treatment for chronic forms of hypocalcemia resulting from hypoparathyroidism. (See Chapter 34.)

B. Intravenous Calcium Therapy

IV calcium therapy is usually needed for infants with symptomatic hypocalcemia or an ionized calcium level below 0.9 mmol/L. A number of precautions must be observed when calcium is given intravenously. The infusion must be given slowly so that there is no sudden increase in calcium concentration of blood entering the right atrium, which could cause severe bradycardia and even cardiac arrest. Furthermore, the infusion must be observed carefully, because an IV infiltrate containing calcium can cause full-thickness skin necrosis requiring grafting. For these reasons, IV calcium therapy should be given judiciously and through a central venous line if possible. IV administration of 10% calcium gluconate is usually given as a bolus of 100–200 mg/kg (1–2 mL/kg) over approximately 10–20 minutes, followed by a continuous infusion (0.5–1 g/kg/d) over 1–2 days, if central venous access is available. Ten percent calcium chloride (20 mg/kg or 0.2 mL/kg per dose) may result in a larger increment in ionized calcium and greater improvement in mean arterial blood pressure in sick hypocalcemic

[2]Hypoglycemia is discussed earlier, in the section on Common Problems in the Term Newborn.

infants and thus may have a role in the newborn. ***Note:*** Calcium salts cannot be added to IV solutions that contain sodium bicarbonate because they precipitate as calcium carbonate.

Prognosis

The prognosis is good for neonatal seizures entirely caused by hypocalcemia that is promptly treated.

INBORN ERRORS OF METABOLISM (SEE ALSO CHAPTER 36)

ESSENTIALS OF DIAGNOSIS & TYPICAL FEATURES

- Altered level of consciousness (poor feeding, lethargy, seizures) in a previously well-appearing infant.
- Tachypnea without hypoxemia or distress.
- Hypoglycemia, respiratory alkalosis, metabolic acidosis.
- Recurrent "sepsis" without proven infection.

Each individual inborn error of metabolism is rare, but collectively they have an incidence of 1 in 1000 live births. Expanded newborn genetic screening undoubtedly aids in the diagnosis of these disorders; however, many infants will present prior to these results being available. These diagnoses should be entertained when infants who were initially well present with sepsis-like syndromes, recurrent hypoglycemia, neurologic syndromes (seizures or altered levels of consciousness), or unexplained acidosis (suggestive of organic acidemias).

In the immediate neonatal period, urea cycle disorders present as an altered level of consciousness (coma) secondary to hyperammonemia. A clinical clue that supports this diagnosis is hyperventilation with primary respiratory alkalosis, along with a low blood urea nitrogen. The other major diagnostic category to consider consists of infants with severe and unremitting acidemia secondary to organic acidemias.

Kamboj M: Clinical approach to the diagnoses of inborn errors of metabolism. Pediatr Clin N Am 2008;55:1113 [PMID: 18929055].

Levy PA: Inborn errors of metabolism: part I: overview. Pediatr Rev 2009;30:131 [PMID: 19339386].

Marsden D, Larson C, Levy HL: Newborn screening for metabolic disorders. J Pediatr 2006;148:577 [PMID: 16737864].

Prasad AN, Hoffmann GF: Early onset epilepsy and inherited metabolic disorders: diagnosis and management. Can J Neurol Sci 2010;37:350 [PMID: 20481269].

QUALITY ASSESSMENT AND IMPROVEMENT IN THE NEWBORN NURSERY AND NICU

Quality improvement initiatives are a critical element to provide the best care possible for patients and their families. This involves recognition that there is a gap between care as it is and care as it could and should be. Clinical units either individually or as part of a consortium need to identify goals for improvement and carry out changes using a plan, do, study, act (PDSA) approach to rapid cycle improvements in care. This involves planning and enacting a change, studying and analyzing the data collected during the change and then acting to assess what changes are to be made for the next PDSA cycle. Individual units can benchmark their care through participation in multicenter databases such as the Vermont Oxford Network. Neonatal intensive care units from over 600 sites submit data on their care of infants born at less than 1500 g. An individual unit can track their outcomes compared to outcomes seen across the network. These data can form the framework for strategies to improve performance in areas in a unit that are below network standards. Examples of possible initiatives include lowering the incidence of central line-associated bacteremia, decreasing the incidence of ventilator-associated pneumonia or structured feeding protocols to decrease the incidence of necrotizing enterocolitis. There is currently a national collaborative through the Children's Hospitals National Consortium to reduce central line-associated blood stream infections in Children's hospitals neonatal intensive care units. This provides an example of a multicenter effort to determine best practices for line insertion and care.

Child Development & Behavior

3

Edward Goldson, MD
Ann Reynolds, MD

This chapter provides an overview of typical development, identifies developmental variations, and discusses several developmental disorders. This chapter does not cover typical development in the newborn period or adolescence (see Chapters 2 and 4, respectively). It will address behavioral variations that reflect the spectrum of normal development and not pathology along with developmental and behavioral disorders and their treatment. The developmental principle, that is, the concept of ongoing change and maturation, is integral to the daily practice of pediatrics. For example, we recognize that a 3-month-old infant is very different from a 3-year-old or a 13-year-old adolescent, not only with respect to what the child can do, but also in terms of the kind of illness he or she might have. From the perspective of the general pediatrician, all of these areas should be viewed in the context of a "medical home." The medical home is defined as the setting that provides consistent, continuous, culturally competent, comprehensive, and sensitive care to children and their families. It is a setting that advocates for all children, whether they are typical or have developmental challenges or disabilities. By incorporating the principles of child development—the concept that children are constantly changing—the medical home is the optimum setting to understand and enhance typical development and to address variations, delays, and deviations as they may occur in the life-trajectory of the child and family.

NORMAL DEVELOPMENT

Typical children follow a trajectory of increasing physical size (Figures 3–1 through 3–10) and increasing complexity of function (Figures 3–7 and 3–8 and Tables 3–1 and 3–2). Table 3–3 provides the theoretical perspectives of human behavior, taking into consideration the work of Freud, Erikson, and Piaget.

The first 5 years of life are a period of extraordinary physical growth and increasing complexity of function. The child triples his or her birth weight within the first year and achieves two-thirds of his or her brain size by age 2½–3 years. The child progresses from a totally dependent infant at birth to a mobile, verbal person who is able to express his or her needs and desires by age 2–3 years. In the ensuing 3 years the child further develops the capacity to interact with peers and adults, achieves considerable verbal and physical prowess, and becomes ready to enter the academic world of learning and socialization.

It is critical for the clinician to identify disturbances in development during these early years because there may be windows of time or sensitive periods when appropriate interventions may be instituted to effectively address developmental issues.

THE FIRST 2 YEARS

From a motor perspective, children develop in a cephalocaudal direction. They can lift their heads with good control at 3 months, sit independently at 6 months, crawl at 9 months, walk at 1 year, and run by 18 months. The child learning to walk has a wide-based gait at first. Next, he or she walks with legs closer together, the arms move medially, a heel-toe gait develops, and the arms swing symmetrically by 18–24 months.

Clinicians often focus on gross motor development, but an appreciation of fine motor development and dexterity, particularly the grasp, can be instructive not only in monitoring normal development but also in identifying deviations in development. The grasp begins as a raking motion involving the ulnar aspect of the hand at age 3–4 months. The thumb is added to this motion at about age 5 months as the focus of the movement shifts to the radial side of the hand. The thumb opposes the fingers for picking up objects just before age 7 months, and the neat pincer grasp emerges at about age 9 months. Most young children have symmetrical movements. Children should not have a significant hand preference before 1 year of age and typically develop handedness between 18 and 30 months.

Language is a critical area to consider as well. Communication is important from birth (Table 3–2 and

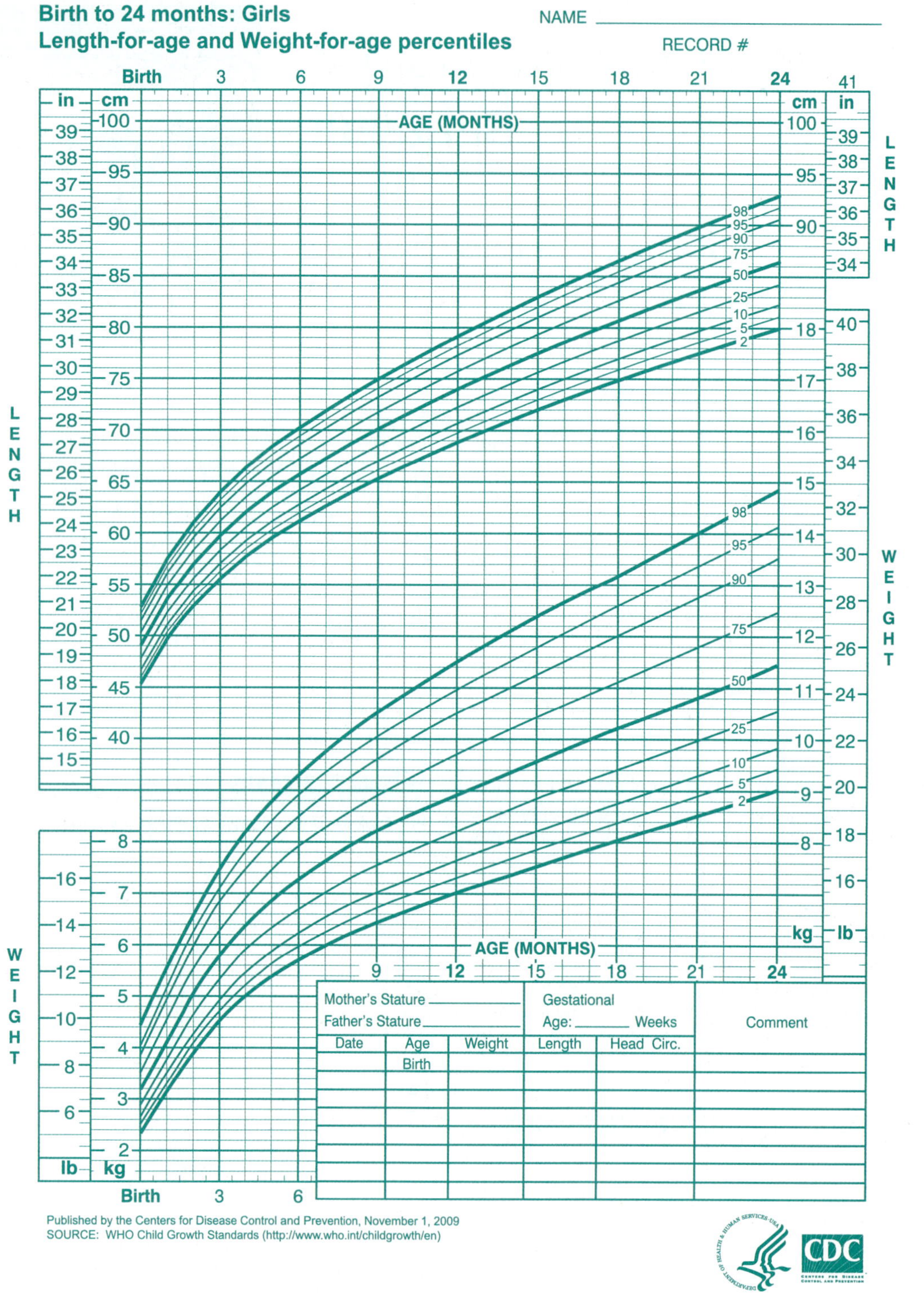

▲ **Figure 3–1.** Percentile standards for length for age and weight for age in girls, birth to age 36 months. (Centers for Disease Control and Prevention. November 1, 2009. Source: WHO Child Growth Standards—http://www.who.int/childgrowth/en.)

Birth to 24 months: Girls
Head circumference-for-age and
Weight-for-length percentiles

NAME ______________________

RECORD # __________

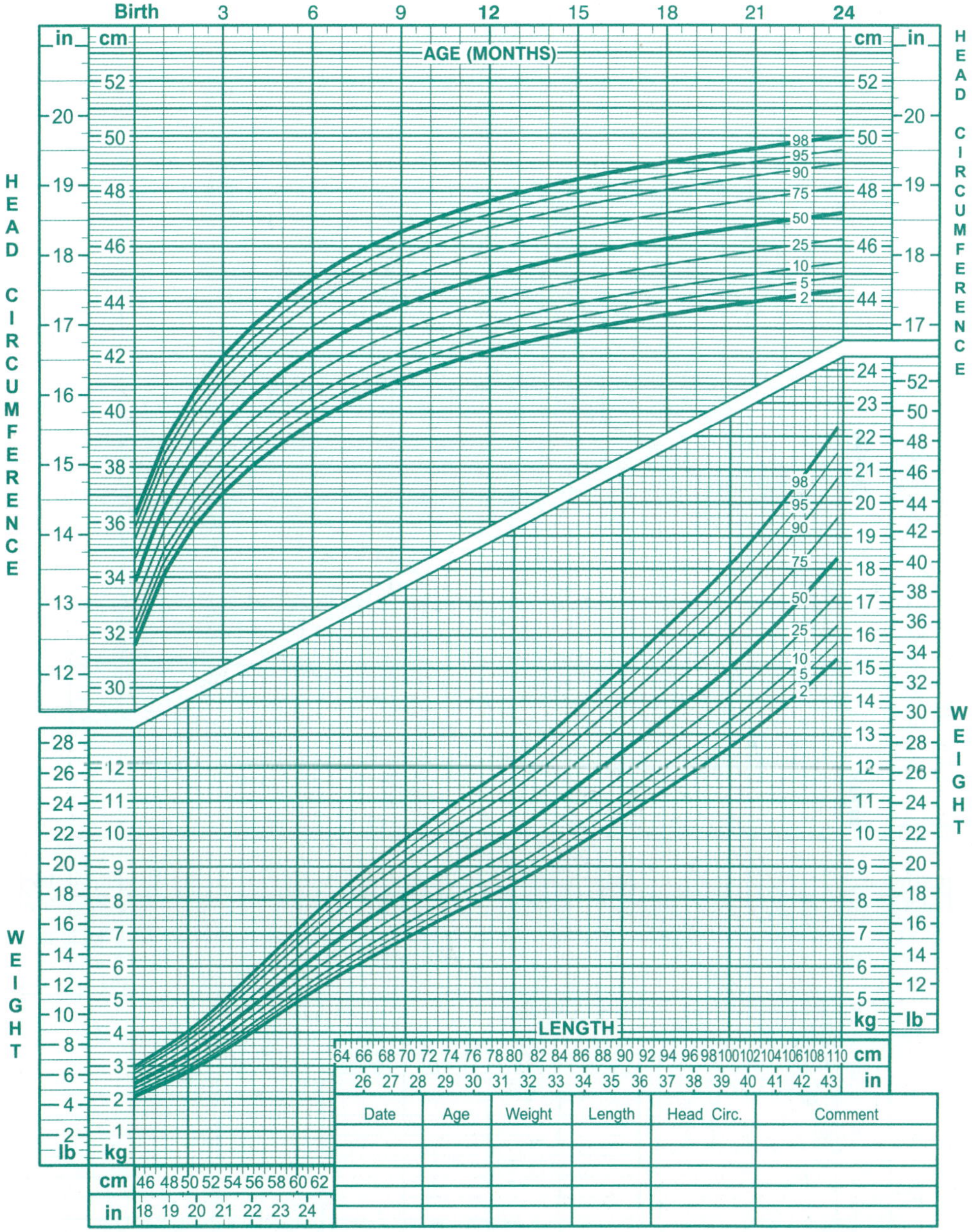

Published by the Centers for Disease Control and Prevention, November 1, 2009
SOURCE: WHO Child Growth Standards (http://www.who.int/childgrowth/en)

▲ **Figure 3–2.** Percentile standards for head circumference for age and weight for length in girls, birth to age 36 months. (Centers for Disease Control and Prevention. November 1, 2009. Source: WHO Child Growth Standards—http://www.who.int/childgrowth/en.)

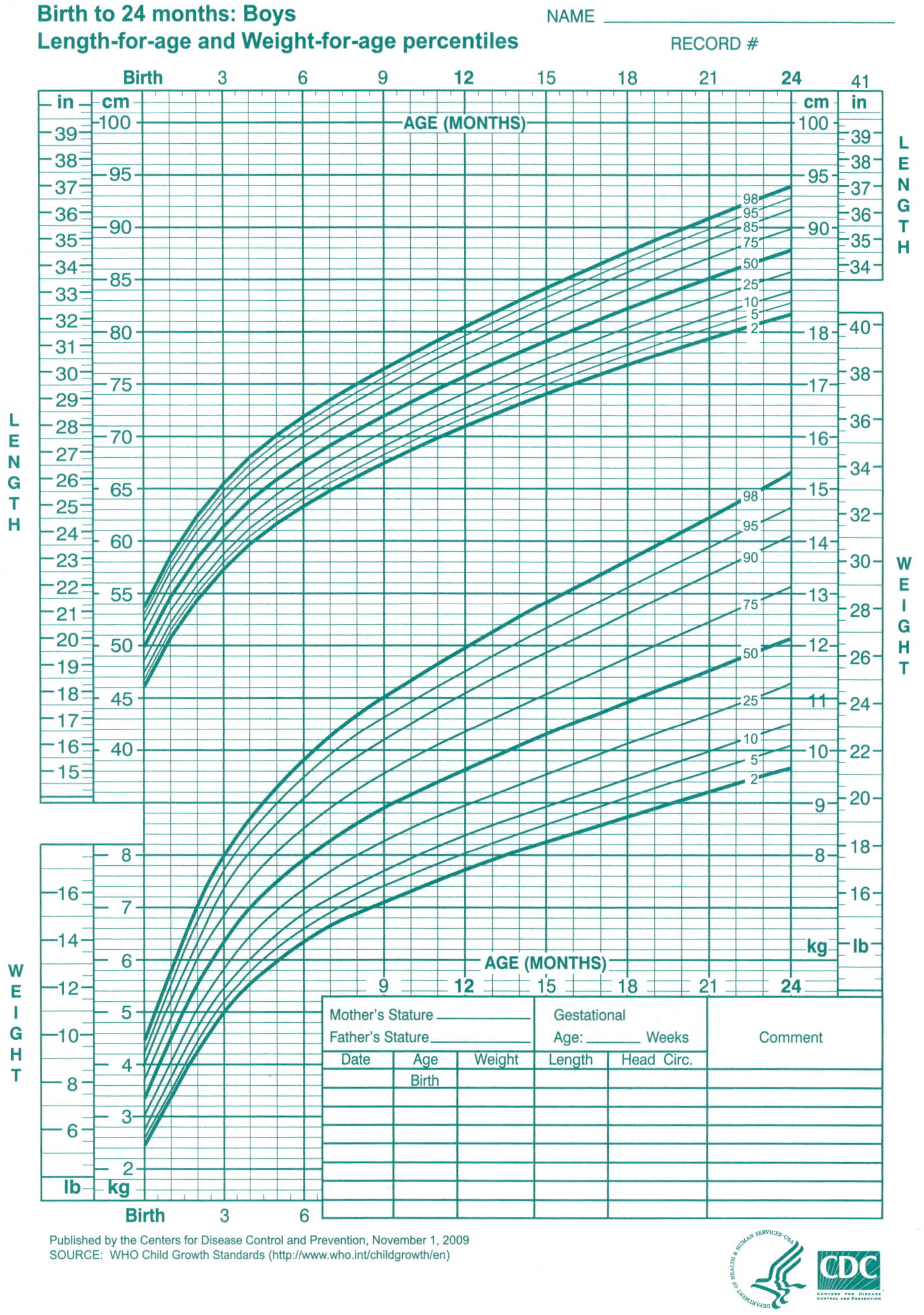

▲ **Figure 3–3.** Percentile standards for length for age and weight for age in boys, birth to age 36 months. (Centers for Disease Control and Prevention. November 1, 2009. Source: WHO Child Growth Standards—http://www.who.int/childgrowth/en.)

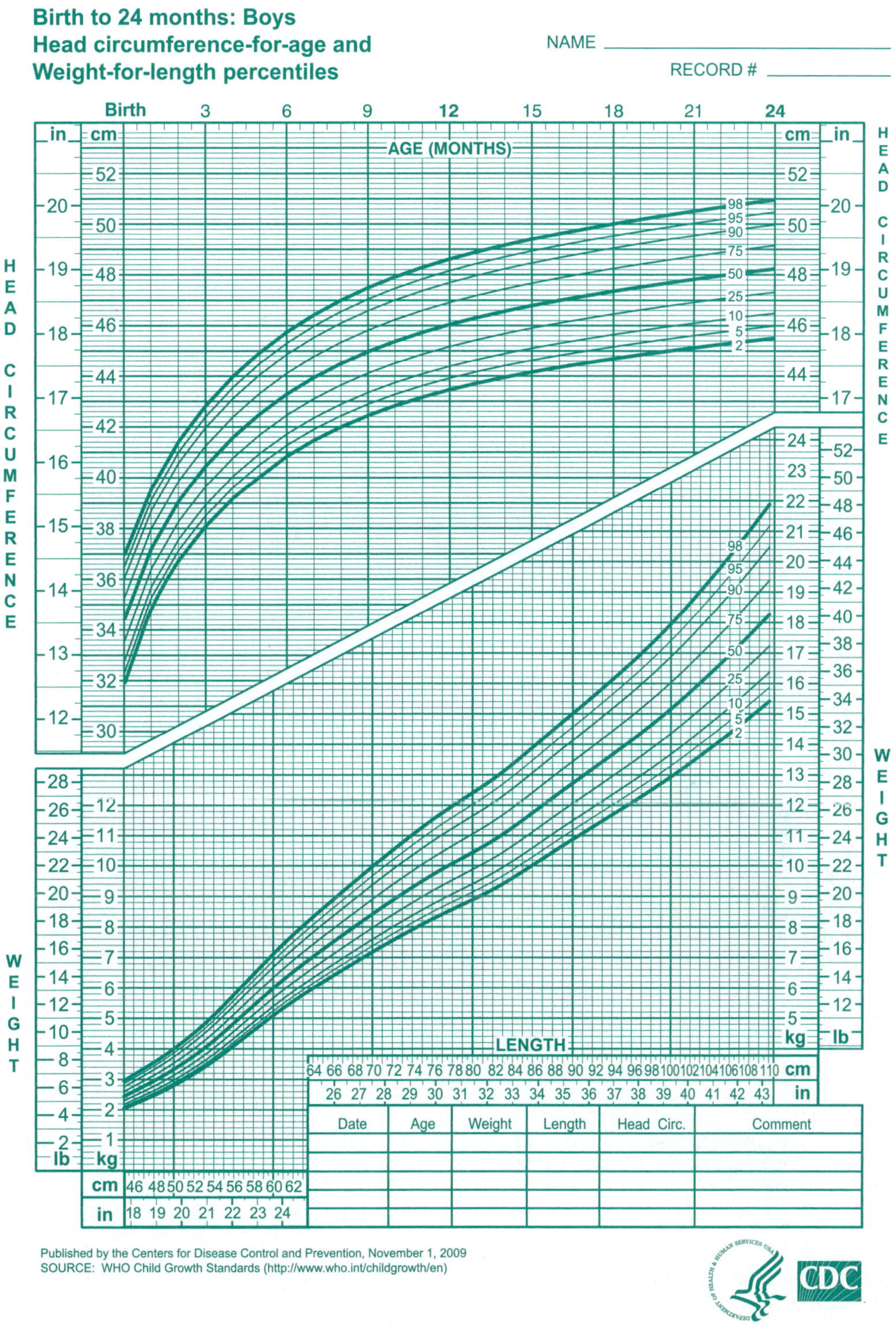

▲ **Figure 3–4.** Percentile standards for head circumference for age and weight for length in boys, birth to age 36 months. (Centers for Disease Control and Prevention. November 1, 2009. Source: WHO Child Growth Standards—http://www.who.int/childgrowth/en.)

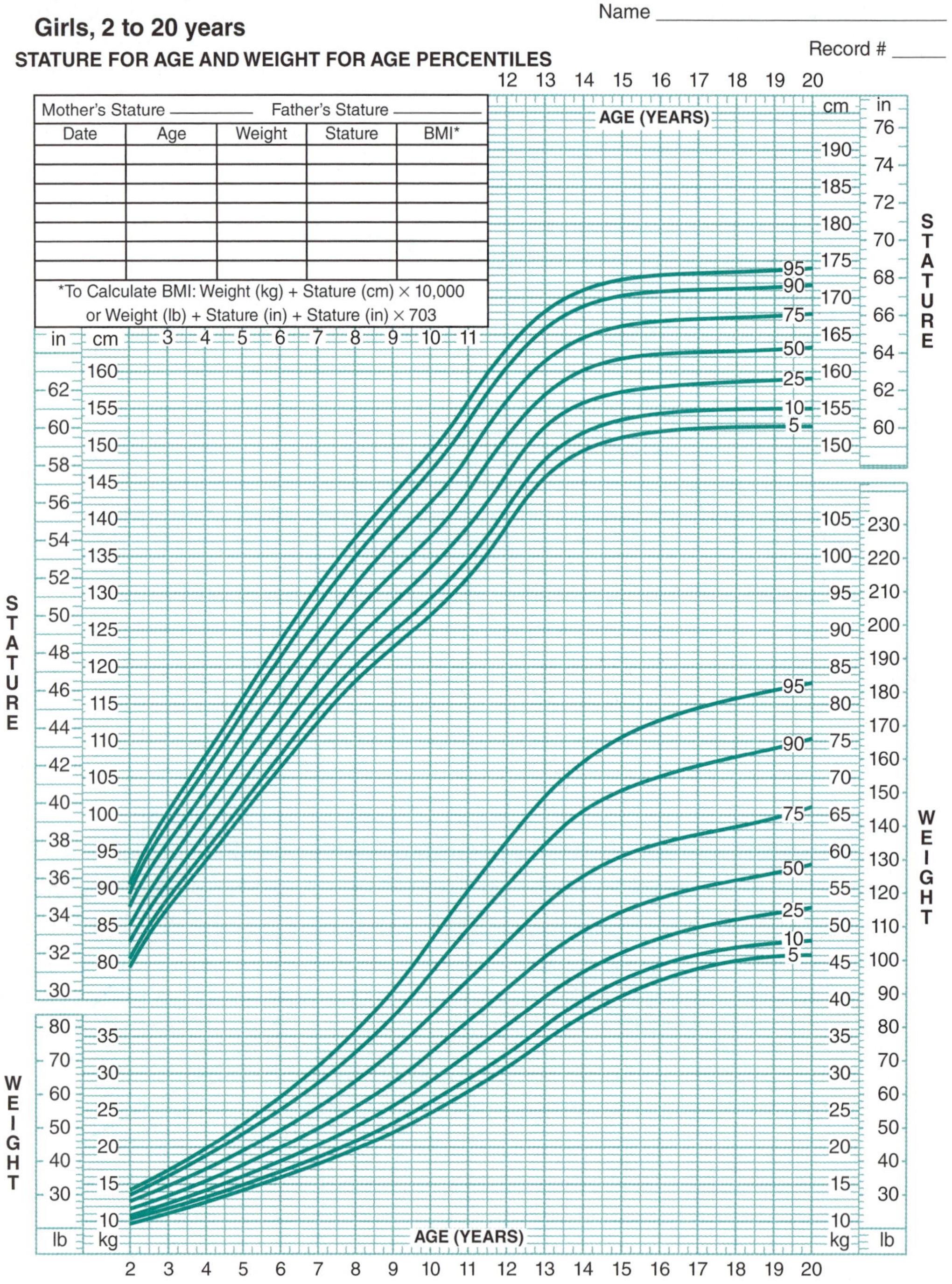

▲ **Figure 3–5.** Percentile standards for stature for age and weight for age in girls, 2–20 years. (Centers for Disease Control and Prevention.)

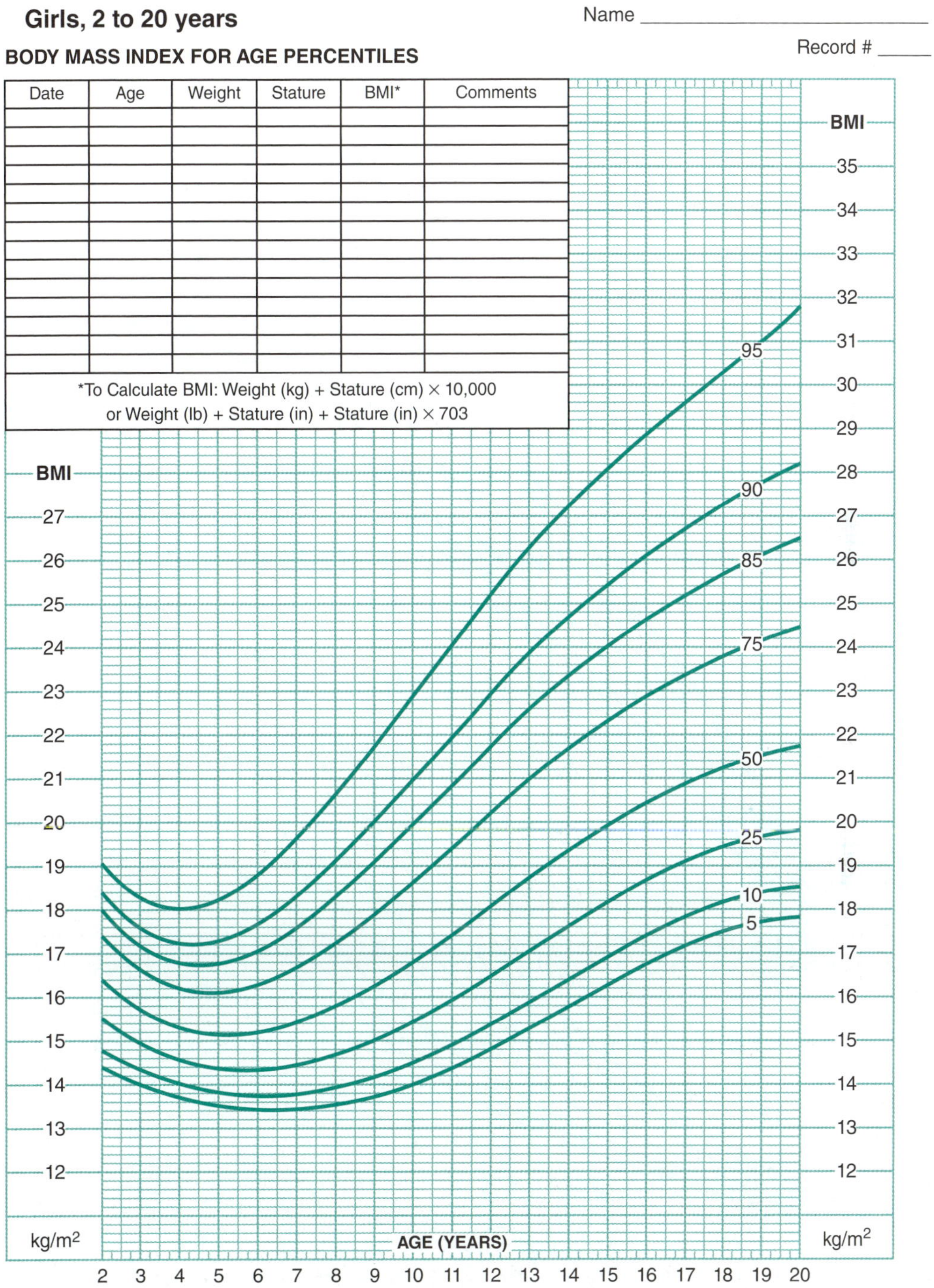

▲ **Figure 3–6.** Percentile standards for body mass index for age in girls, 2–20 years. (Centers for Disease Control and Prevention.)

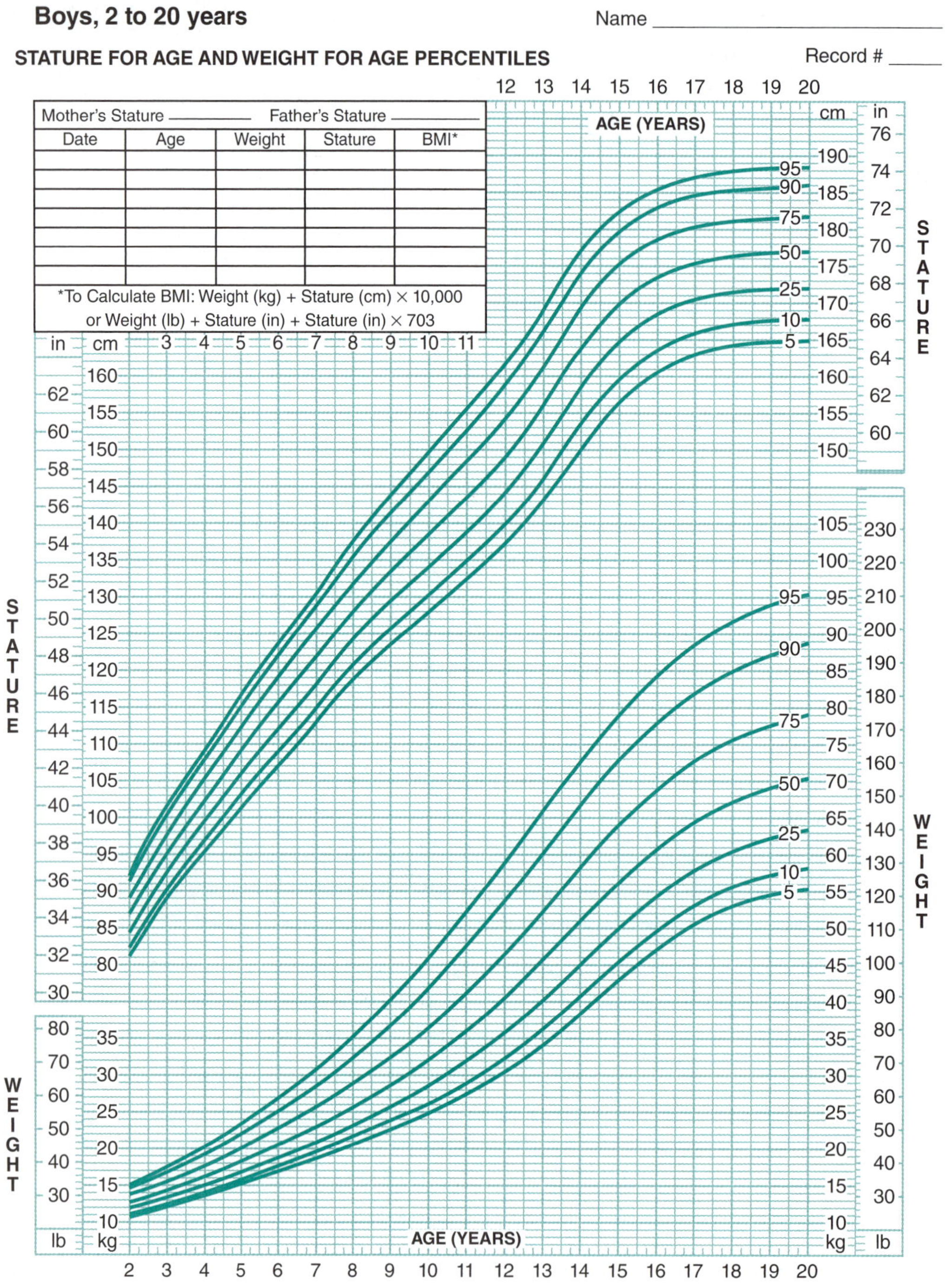

▲ **Figure 3-7.** Percentile standards for stature for age and weight for age in boys, 2–20 years. (Centers for Disease Control and Prevention.)

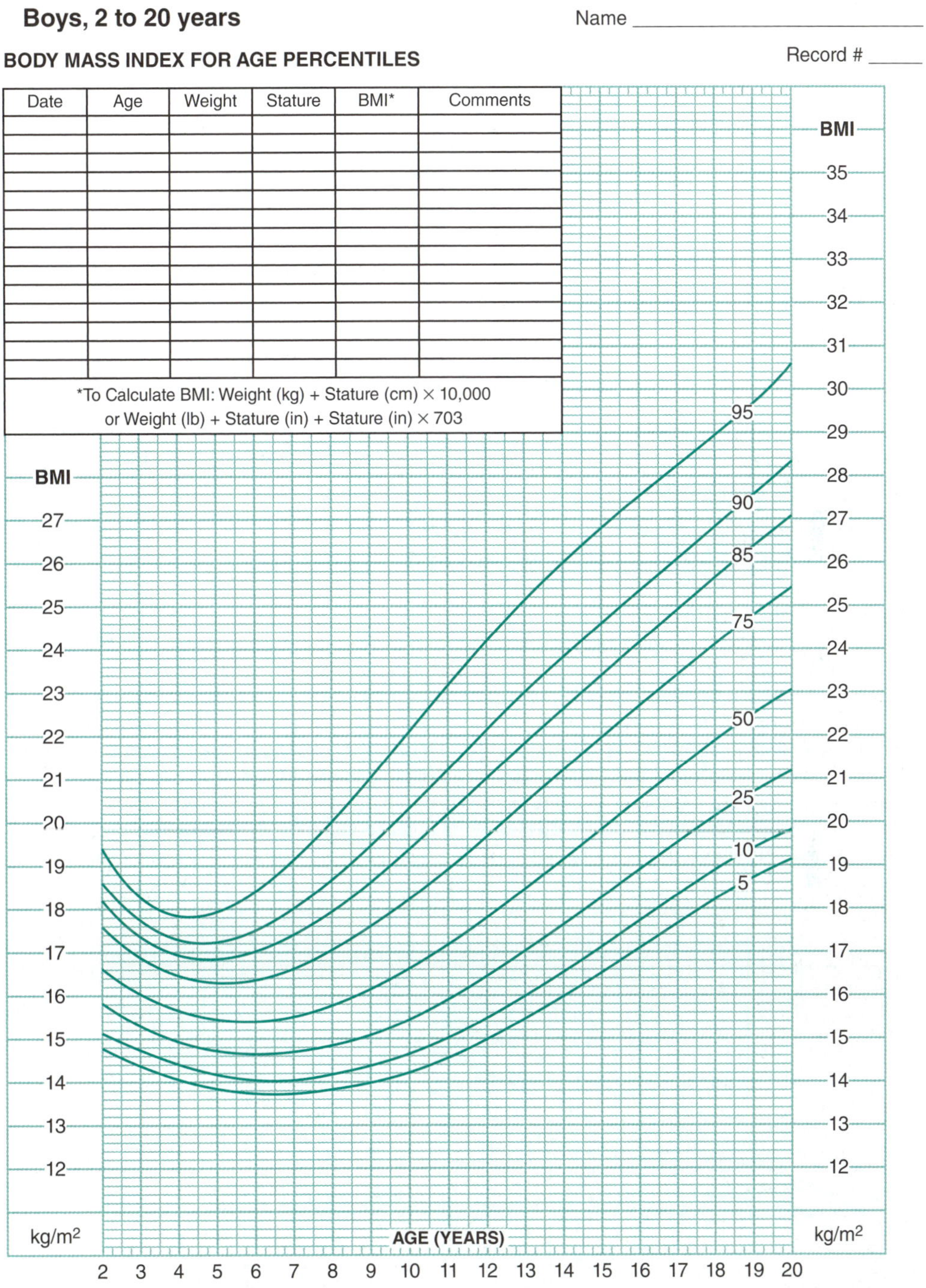

▲ **Figure 3–8.** Percentile standards for body mass index for age in boys, 2–20 years. (Centers for Disease Control and Prevention.)

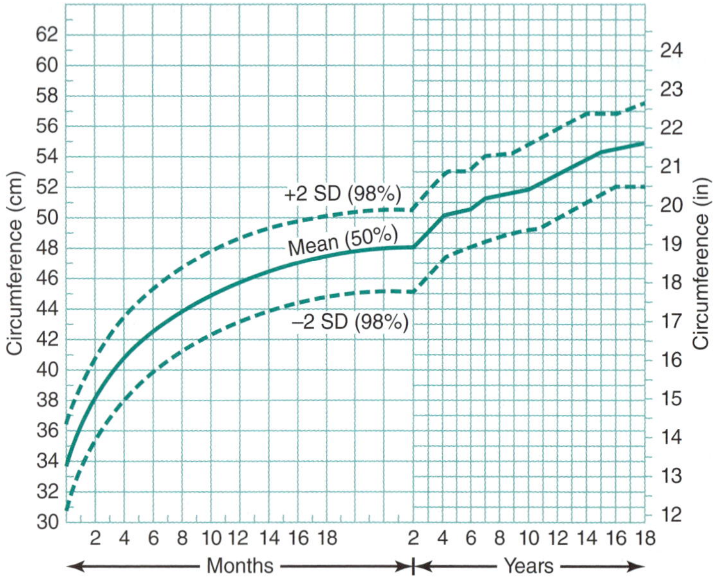

▲ **Figure 3–9.** Head circumference of girls. (Modified and reproduced, with permission, from Nelhaus G: Head circumference from birth to eighteen years. Practical composite international and interracial graphs. Pediatrics 1968;41:106.)

Figure 3–11), particularly the nonverbal, reciprocal interactions between infant and caregiver. By age 2 months, these interactions begin to include melodic vowel sounds called cooing and reciprocal vocal play between parent and child. Babbling, which adds consonants to vowels, begins by age 6–10 months, and the repetition of sounds such as "da-dada-da" is facilitated by the child's increasing oral muscular control. Babbling reaches a peak at age 12 months. The child then moves into a stage of having needs met by using individual words to represent objects or actions. It is common at this age for children to express wants and needs by pointing to objects or using other gestures. Children usually have 5–10 comprehensible words by 12–18 months; by age 2 years they are putting 2–3 words into phrases, 50% of which their care-givers can understand (see Tables 3–1 and 3–2 and Figure 3–11). The acquisition of expressive vocabulary varies greatly between 12 and 24 months of age. As a group, males and children who are bilingual tend to develop expressive language more slowly during that time. It is important to note, however, that for each individual, milestones should

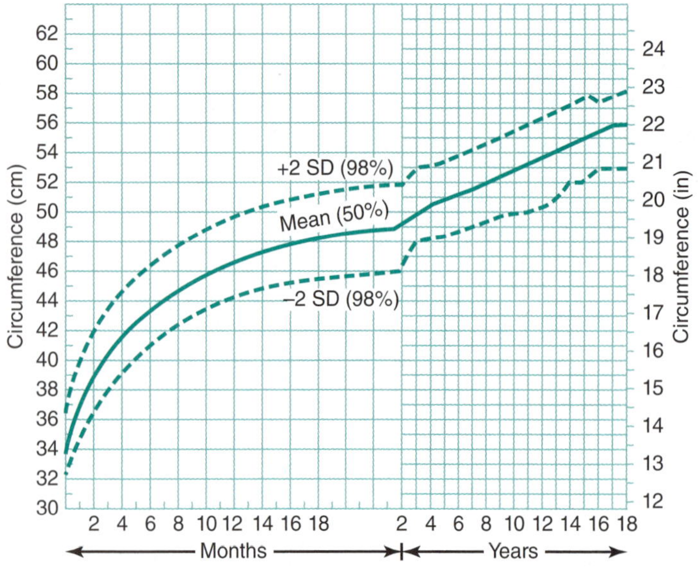

▲ **Figure 3–10.** Head circumference of boys. (Modified and reproduced, with permission, from Nelhaus G: Head circumference from birth to eighteen years. Practical composite international and interracial graphs. Pediatrics 1968;41:106.)

Table 3–1. Developmental charts.

1–2 mo

Activities to be observed:
- Holds head erect and lifts head.
- Turns from side to back.
- Regards faces and follows objects t hrough visual field.
- Drops toys.
- Becomes alert in response to voice.

Activities related by parent:
- Recognizes parents.
- Engages in vocalizations.
- Smiles spontaneously.

3–5 mo

Activities to be observed:
- Grasps cube—first ulnar then later thumb opposition.
- Reaches for and brings objects to mouth.
- Makes "raspberry" sound.
- Sits with support.

Activities related by parent:
- Laughs.
- Anticipates food on sight.
- Turns from back to side.

6–8 mo

Activities to be observed:
- Sits alone for a short period.
- Reaches with one hand.
- First scoops up a pellet then grasps it using thumb opposition.
- Imitates "bye-bye."
- Passes object from hand to hand in midline.
- Babbles.

Activities related by parent:
- Rolls from back to stomach.
- Is inhibited by the word *no*.

9–11 mo

Activities to be observed:
- Stands alone.
- Imitates pat-a-cake and peek-a-boo.
- Uses thumb and index finger to pick up pellet.

Activities related by parent:
- Walks by supporting self on furniture.
- Follows one-step verbal commands, eg, "Come here," "Give it to me."

1 y

Activities to be observed:
- Walks independently.
- Says "mama" and "dada" with meaning.
- Can use a neat pincer grasp to pick up a pellet.
- Releases cube into cup after demonstration.
- Gives toys on request.
- Tries to build a tower of 2 cubes.

Activities related by parent:
- Points to desired objects.
- Says 1 or 2 other words.

18 mo

Activities to be observed:
- Builds tower of 3–4 cubes.
- Throws ball.
- Seats self in chair.
- Dumps pellet from bottle.

Activities related by parent:
- Walks up and down stairs with help.
- Says 4–20 words.
- Understands a 2-step command.
- Carries and hugs doll.
- Feeds self.

24 mo

Activities to be observed:
- Speaks short phrases, 2 words or more.
- Kicks ball on request.
- Builds tower of 6–7 cubes.
- Points to named objects or pictures.
- Jumps off floor with both feet.
- Stands on either foot alone.
- Uses pronouns.

Activities related by parent:
- Verbalizes toilet needs.
- Pulls on simple garment.
- Turns pages of book singly.
- Plays with domestic mimicry.

30 mo

Activities to be observed:
- Walks backward.
- Begins to hop on one foot.
- Uses prepositions.
- Copies a crude circle.
- Points to objects described by use.
- Refers to self as I.
- Holds crayon in fist.

Activities related by parent:
- Helps put things away.
- Carries on a conversation.

3 y

Activities to be observed:
- Holds crayon with fingers.
- Builds tower of 9–10 cubes.
- Imitates 3-cube bridge.
- Copies circle.
- Gives first and last name.

Activities related by parent:
- Rides tricycle using pedals.
- Dresses with supervision.

(*Continued*)

Table 3–1. Developmental charts. (*Continued*)

3-4 y

Activities to be observed:

Climbs stairs with alternating feet.
Begins to button and unbutton.
"What do you like to do that's fun?" (Answers using plurals, personal pronouns, and verbs.)
Responds to command to place toy *in, on,* or *under* table.
Draws a circle when asked to draw a person.
Knows own sex. ("Are you a boy or a girl?")
Gives full name.
Copies a circle already drawn. ("Can you make one like this?")

Activities related by parent:

Feeds self at mealtime.
Takes off shoes and jacket.

4-5 y

Activities to be observed:

Runs and turns without losing balance.
May stand on one leg for at least 10 seconds.
Buttons clothes and laces shoes. (Does not tie.)
Counts to 4 by rote. "Give me 2 sticks." (Able to do so from pile of 4 tongue depressors.)
Draws a person. (Head, 2 appendages, and possibly 2 eyes. No torso yet.)
Knows the days of the week. ("What day comes after Tuesday?")
Gives appropriate answers to: "What must you do if you are sleepy? Hungry? Cold?"
Copies + in imitation.

Activities related by parent:

Self-care at toilet. (May need help with wiping.)
Plays outside for at least 30 minutes.
Dresses self except for tying.

5-6 y

Activities to be observed:

Can catch ball.
Skips smoothly.
Copies a + already drawn.
Tells age.
Concept of 10 (eg, counts 10 tongue depressors). May recite to higher number by rote.
Knows right and left hand.
Draws recognizable person with at least 8 details.
Can describe favorite television program in some detail.

Activities related by parent:

Does simple chores at home (eg, taking out garbage, drying silverware).
Goes to school unattended or meets school bus.
Good motor ability but little awareness of dangers.

6-7 y

Activities to be observed:

Copies a Δ.
Defines words by use. ("What is an orange?" "To eat.")
Knows if morning or afternoon.
Draws a person with 12 details.
Reads several one-syllable printed words. (My, dog, see, boy.)

7-8 y

Activities to be observed:

Counts by 2s and 5s.
Ties shoes.
Copies a ◊.
Knows what day of the week it is. (Not date or year.)
No evidence of sound substitution in speech (eg, *fr* for *thr*).
Draws a man with 16 details.
Reads paragraph #1 Durrell:

Reading:

Muff is a little yellow kitten. She drinks milk. She sleeps on a chair. She does not like to get wet.

Corresponding arithmetic:

$$\begin{array}{cccc} 7 & 6 & 6 & 8 \\ \underline{+4} & \underline{+7} & \underline{-4} & \underline{-3} \end{array}$$

Adds and subtracts one-digit numbers.

8-9 y

Activities to be observed:

Defines words better than by use. ("What is an orange?" "A fruit.")
Can give an appropriate answer to the following:
"What is the thing for you to do if . . .
—you've broken something that belongs to someone else?"
—a playmate hits you without meaning to do so?"
Reads paragraph #2 Durrell:

Reading:

A little black dog ran away from home. He played with two big dogs. They ran away from him. It began to rain. He went under a tree. He wanted to go home, but he did not know the way. He saw a boy he knew. The boy took him home.

Corresponding arithmetic:

$$\begin{array}{cccc} & 67 & & \\ 67 & 16 & 14 & 84 \\ \underline{+4} & \underline{+27} & \underline{-8} & \underline{-36} \end{array}$$

Is learning borrowing and carrying processes in addition and subtraction.

9-10 y

Activities to be observed:

Knows the month, day, and year.
Names the months in order. (15 s, 1 error.)
Makes a sentence with these 3 words in it: (1 or 2. Can use words orally in proper context.)
1. work . . . money . . . men
2. boy . . . river . . . ball
Reads paragraph #3 Durrell:

Reading:

Six boys put up a tent by the side of a river. They took things to eat with them. When the sun went down, they went into the tent to sleep. in the night, a cow came and began to eat grass around the tent. The boys were afraid. They thought it was a bear.

Should comprehend and answer the question: "What was the cow doing?"

Corresponding arithmetic:

$$\begin{array}{ccc} 5204 & 23 & 837 \\ \underline{-530} & \underline{\times 3} & \underline{\times 7} \end{array}$$

Learning simple multiplication.

(*Continued*)

Table 3–1. Developmental charts. (*Continued*)

10–12 y

Activities to be observed:

Should read and comprehend paragraph #5 Durrell:

Reading:

In 1807, Robert Fulton took the first long trip in a steamboat. He went one hundred and fifty miles up the Hudson River. The boat went five miles an hour. This was faster than a steamboat had ever gone before. Crowds gathered on both banks of the river to see this new kind of boat. They were afraid that its noise and splashing would drive away all the fish.

Answer: "What river was the trip made on?"

Ask to write the sentence: "The fishermen did not like the boat."

Corresponding arithmetic:

420×29 $\quad 9\overline{)72}$ $\quad 31\overline{)62}$

Should do multiplication and simple division.

12–15 y

Activities to be observed:

Reads paragraph #7 Durrell:

Reading:

Golf originated in Holland as a game played on ice. The game in its present form first appeared in Scotland. It became unusually popular and kings found it so enjoyable that it was known as "the royal game." James IV, however, thought that people neglected their work to indulge in this fascinating sport so that it was forbidden in 1457. James relented when he found how attractive the game was, and it immediately regained its former popularity. Golf spread gradually to other countries, being introduced in America in 1890. It has grown in favor until there is hardly a town that does not boast of a private or public course.

Ask to write a sentence: "Golf originated in Holland as a game played on ice."

Answers questions:

"Why was golf forbidden by James IV?"

"Why did he change his mind?"

Corresponding arithmetic:

$536\overline{)4762}$ $\quad \square + \square$ $\quad 7\frac{1}{6} - 3\frac{1}{6}$

Reduce fractions to lowest forms.

Does long division, adds and subtracts fractions.

Modified from Leavitt SR, Goodman H, Harvin D: Use of developmental charts in teaching well child care. Pediatrics 1963;31:499.

still fall within the expected range. Gender and exposure to two languages should never be used as an excuse for failing to refer a child who has significant delay in the acquisition of speech and language for further evaluation. It is also important to note that most children are not truly bilingual. Most children have one primary language, and any other languages are secondary.

Receptive language usually develops more rapidly than expressive language. Word comprehension begins to increase at age 9 months, and by age 13 months the child's receptive vocabulary may be as large as 20–100 words. After age 18 months, expressive and receptive vocabularies increase dramatically, and by the end of the second year there is typically a quantum leap in language development. The child begins to put together words and phrases and begins to use language to represent a new world, the symbolic world. Children begin to put verbs into phrases and focus much of their language on describing their new abilities, for example, "I go out." They begin to incorporate prepositions, such as "I" and "you" into speech and ask "why?" and "what?" questions more frequently. They also begin to appreciate time factors and to understand and use this concept in their speech (see Table 3–1).

The Early Language Milestone Scale-2 (see Figure 3–11) is a simple tool for assessing early language development in the pediatric office setting. It is scored in the same way as the Denver II (Figure 3–12) but tests receptive and expressive language areas in greater depth.

One may easily memorize the developmental milestones that characterize the trajectory of the typical child; however, these milestones become more meaningful and clinically useful if placed in empirical and theoretical contexts. The work of Piaget and others is quite instructive and provides some insight into behavioral and affective development (see Table 3–3). Piaget described the first 2 years of life as the sensorimotor period, during which infants learn with increasing sophistication how to link sensory input from the environment with a motor response. Infants build on primitive reflex patterns of behavior (termed schemata; sucking is an example) and constantly incorporate or assimilate new experiences. The schemata evolve over time as infants accommodate new experiences and as new levels of cognitive ability unfold in an orderly sequence. Enhancement of neural networks through dendritic branching and pruning (apoptosis) occurs.

In the first year of life, the infant's perception of reality revolves around itself and what it can see or touch. The infant follows the trajectory of an object through the field of vision, but before age 6 months the object ceases to exist once it leaves the infant's field of vision. At age 9–12 months, the infant gradually develops the concept of object permanence, or the realization that objects exist even when not seen. The development of object permanence correlates with enhanced frontal activity on the electroencephalogram (EEG). The concept attaches first to the image of the mother or primary caregiver because of his or her emotional importance and is a critical part of attachment behavior (discussed later). In the second year, children extend their ability to manipulate objects by using instruments, first by imitation and later by trial and error.

Table 3-2. Normal speech and language development.

Age	Speech	Language	Articulation
1 mo	Throaty sounds		Vowels: \ah\, \uh\, \ee\
2 mo	Vowel sounds ("eh"), coos		
2½ mo	Squeals		
3 mo	Babbles, initial vowels		
4 mo	Guttural sounds ("ah," "go")		Consonants: m, p, b
5 mo			Vowels: \o\, \u\
7 mo	Imitates speech sounds		
8 mo			Syllables: da, ba, ka
10 mo		"Dada" or "mama" nonspecifically	Approximates names: baba/bottle
12 mo	Jargon begins (own language)	One word other than "mama" or "dada"	Understandable: 2–3 words
13 mo		Three words	
16 mo		Six words	Consonants: t, d, w, n, h
18–24 mo		Two-word phrases	Understandable 2-word phrases
24–30 mo		Three-word phrases	Understandable 3-word phrases
2 y	Vowels uttered correctly	Approximately 270 words; uses pronouns	Approximately 270 words; uses phrases
3 y	Some degree of hesitancy and uncertainty common	Approximately 900 words; intelligible 4-word phrases	Approximately 900 words; intelligible 4-word phrases
4 y		Approximately 1540 words; intelligible 5-word phrases or sentences	Approximately 1540 words; intelligible 5-word phrases
6 y		Approximately 2560 words; intelligible 6- or 7-word sentences	Approximately 2560 words; intelligible 6- or 7-word sentences
7–8 y	Adult proficiency		

Data on articulation from Berry MF: *Language Disorders of Children*. Appleton-Century-Crofts, 1969; and from Bzoch K, League R: *Receptive-Expressive Emergent Language Scale*. University Park Press, 1970.

Freud described the first year of life as the oral stage because so many of the infant's needs are fulfilled by oral means. Nutrition is obtained through sucking on the breast or bottle, and self-soothing occurs through sucking on fingers or a pacifier. During this stage of symbiosis with the mother, the boundaries between mother and infant are blurred. The infant's needs are totally met by the mother, and the mother has been described as manifesting "narcissistic possessiveness" of the infant. This is a very positive interaction in the bidirectional attachment process called bonding. The parents learn to be aware of and to interpret the infant's cues, which reflect its needs. A more sensitive emotional interaction process develops that can be seen in the mirroring of facial expressions by the primary caregiver and infant and in their mutual engagement in cycles of attention and inattention, which further develop into social play. A parent who is depressed or cannot respond to the infant's expressions and cues can have a profoundly adverse effect on the child's future development. Erikson's terms of basic trust versus mistrust are another way of describing the reciprocal interaction that characterizes this stage. Turn-taking games, which occur between ages 3 and 6 months, are a pleasure for both the parents and the infant and are an extension of mirroring behavior. They also represent an early form of

Table 3–3. Perspectives of human behavior.

Age	Theories of Development			Skill Areas		Psychopathology
	Freud	Erikson	Piaget	Language	Motor	
Birth to 18 mo	Oral	Basic trust versus mistrust	Sensorimotor	Body actions; crying; naming; pointing	Reflex sitting, reaching, grasping, walking	Autism; anaclitic depression, colic; disorders of attachment; feeding, sleeping problems
18 mo–3 y	Anal	Autonomy versus shame, doubt	Symbolic (preoperational)	Sentences; telegraph jargon	Climbing, running	Separation issues; negativism; fearfulness; constipation; shyness, withdrawal
3–6 y	Oedipal	Initiative versus guilt	Intuition (preoperational)	Connective words; can be readily understood	Increased coordination; tricycle; jumping	Enuresis; encopresis; anxiety; aggressive acting out; phobias; nightmares
6–11 y	Latency	Industry versus inferiority	Concrete operational	Subordinate sentences; reading and writing; language reasoning	Increased skills; sports, recreational cooperative games	School phobias; obsessive reactions; conversion reactions; depressive equivalents
12–17 y	Adolescence (genital)	Identity versus role confusion	Formal operational	Reason abstract; using language; abstract manipulation	Refinement of skills	Delinquency; promiscuity; schizophrenia; anorexia nervosa; suicide

Adapted and reproduced, with permission, from Dixon S: Setting the stage: Theories and concepts of child development. In Dixon S, Stein M (editors): *Encounters with Children*, 2nd ed. Year Book, 1992.

imitative behavior, which is important in later social and cognitive development. More sophisticated games, such as peek-a-boo, occur at approximately age 9 months. The infant's thrill at the reappearance of the face that vanished momentarily demonstrates the emerging understanding of object permanence. Age 8–9 months is also a critical time in the attachment process because this is when separation anxiety and stranger anxiety become marked. The infant at this stage is able to appreciate discrepant events that do not match previously known schemata. These new events cause uncertainty and subsequently fear and anxiety. The infant must be able to retrieve previous schemata and incorporate new information over an extended time. These abilities are developed by age 8 months and give rise to the fears that may subsequently develop: stranger anxiety and separation anxiety. In stranger anxiety, the infant analyzes the face of a stranger, detects the mismatch with previous schemata or what is familiar, and responds with fear or anxiety, leading to crying. In separation anxiety, the child perceives the difference between the primary caregiver's presence and his or her absence by remembering the schema of the caregiver's presence. Perceiving the inconsistency, the child first becomes uncertain and then anxious and fearful. This begins at age 8 months, reaches a peak at 15 months, and disappears by the end of 2 years in a relatively orderly progression as central nervous system (CNS) maturation facilitates the development of new skills. A parent can put the child's understanding of object permanence to good use by placing a picture of the mother (or father) near the child or by leaving an object (eg, her sweater) where the child can see it during her absence. A visual substitute for the mother's presence may comfort the child.

Once the child can walk independently, he or she can move away from the parent and explore the environment. Although the child uses the parent, usually the mother, as "home base," returning to her frequently for reassurance, he or she has now taken a major step toward independence. This is the beginning of mastery over the environment and an emerging sense of self. The "terrible twos" and the frequent self-asserting use of "no" are the child's attempt to develop a better idea of what is or might be under his or her control. The child is starting to assert his or her autonomy. Ego development during this time should be fostered but with appropriate limits. As children develop a sense of self, they begin to understand the feelings of others and develop empathy. They hug another child who is in perceived distress or become concerned when one is hurt. They begin to understand how another child feels when he or she is harmed, and this realization helps them to inhibit their own aggressive behavior. Children also begin to understand

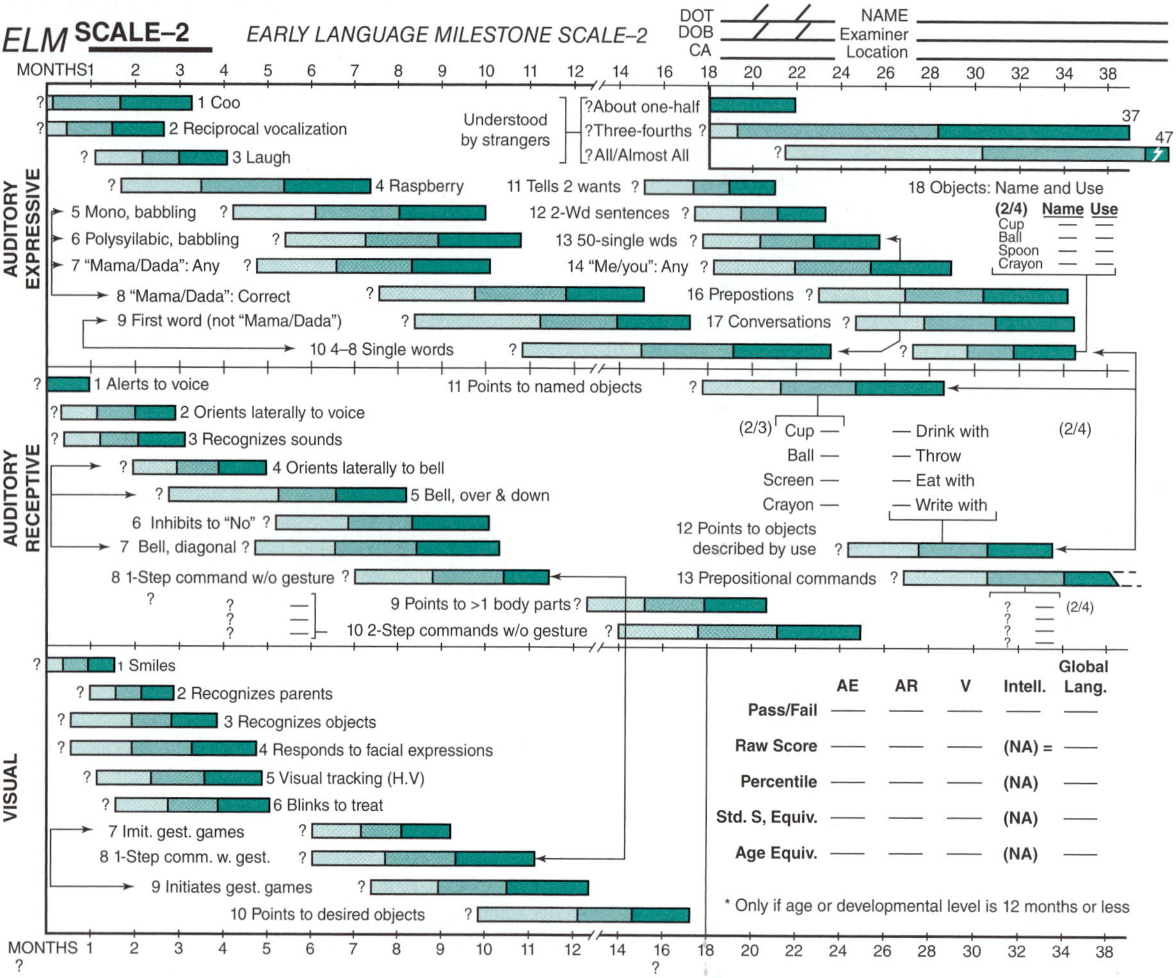

▲ Figure 3–11. Early Language Milestone Scale-2. (Reproduced, with permission, from Coplan J: *Early Language Milestone Scale*. Pro Ed, 1993.)

right and wrong and parental expectations. They recognize that they have done something "bad" and may signify that awareness by saying "uhoh" or with other expressions of distress. They also take pleasure in their accomplishments and become more aware of their bodies.

An area of child behavior that has often been overlooked is play. Play is the child's work and a significant means of learning. Play is a very complex process whose purpose can include the practice and rehearsal of roles, skills, and relationships; a means of revisiting the past; a means of actively mastering a range of experiences; and a way to integrate the child's life experiences. It involves emotional development (affect regulation and gender identification and roles), cognitive development (nonverbal and verbal function and executive functioning and creativity), and social/motor development (motor coordination, frustration tolerance, and social interactions such as turn-taking). Of interest is that play has a developmental progression. The typical 6- to 12-month-old engages in the game of peek-a-boo, which is a form of social interaction. During the next year or so, although children engage in increasingly complex social interactions and imitation, their play is primarily solitary. However, they do begin to engage in symbolic play such as by drinking from a toy cup and then by giving a doll a drink from a toy cup. By age 2–3 years children begin to engage in parallel play (engaging in behaviors that are imitative). This form of play gradually evolves into more interactive or collaborative play by age 3–4 years and is also more thematic in nature. There are of course wide variations in the development of play, reflecting cultural, educational, and

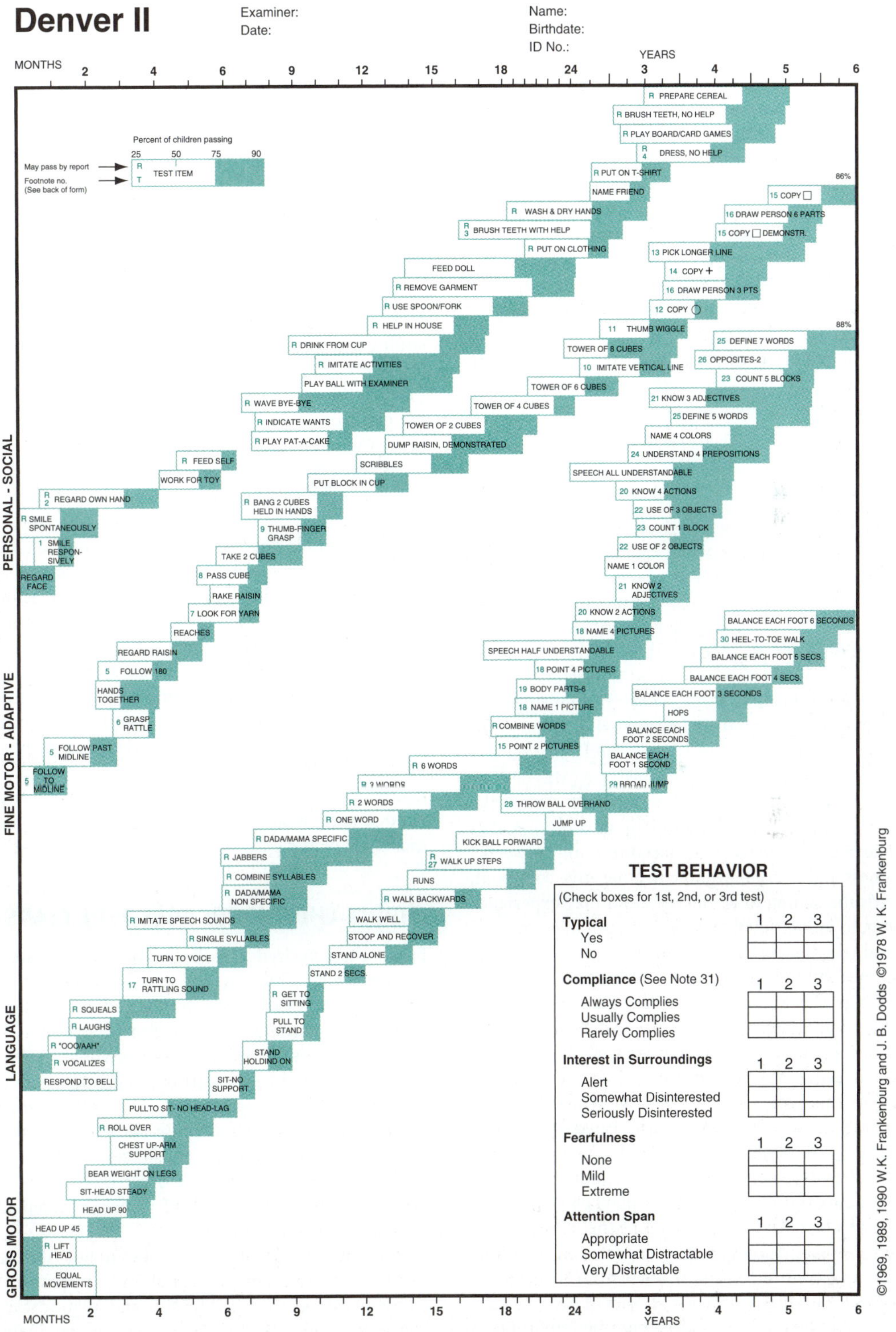

▲ **Figure 3–12.** Denver II. (Copyright © 1969, 1989, 1990 WK Frankenburg and JB Dodds. © 1978 WK Frankenberg.)

socioeconomic variables. Nevertheless, the development of play does follow a sequence that can be assessed and can be very informative in the evaluation of the child.

Brain maturation sets the stage for toilet training. After age 18 months, toddlers have the sensory capacity for awareness of a full rectum or bladder and are physically able to control bowel and urinary tract sphincters. They also take great pleasure in their accomplishments, particularly in appropriate elimination, if it is reinforced positively. Children must be given some control over when elimination occurs. If parents impose severe restrictions, the achievement of this developmental milestone can become a battle between parent and child. Freud termed this period the anal stage because the developmental issue of bowel control is the major task requiring mastery. It encompasses a more generalized theme of socialized behavior and overall body cleanliness, which is usually taught or imposed on the child at this age.

AGES 2–4 YEARS

Piaget characterized the 2- to 6-year-old stage as preoperational. This stage begins when language has facilitated the creation of mental images in the symbolic sense. The child begins to manipulate the symbolic world; sorts out reality from fantasy imperfectly; and may be terrified of dreams, wishes, and foolish threats. Most of the child's perception of the world is egocentric or interpreted in reference to his or her needs or influence. Cause-effect relationships are confused with temporal ones or interpreted egocentrically. For example, children may focus their understanding of divorce on themselves ("My father left because I was bad" or "My mother left because she didn't love me"). Illness and the need for medical care are also commonly misinterpreted at this age. The child may make a mental connection between a sibling's illness and a recent argument, a negative comment, or a wish for the sibling to be ill. The child may experience significant guilt unless the parents are aware of these misperceptions and take time to deal with them.

At this age, children also endow inanimate objects with human feelings. They also assume that humans cause or create all natural events. For instance, when asked why the sun sets, they may say, "The sun goes to his house" or "It is pushed down by someone else." Magical thinking blossoms between ages 3 and 5 years as symbolic thinking incorporates more elaborate fantasy. Fantasy facilitates development of role playing, sexual identity, and emotional growth. Children test new experiences in fantasy, both in their imagination and in play. In their play, children often create magical stories and novel situations that reflect issues with which they are dealing, such as aggression, relationships, fears, and control. Children often invent imaginary friends at this time, and nightmares or fears of monsters are common. At this stage, other children become important in facilitating play, such as in a preschool group. Play gradually becomes more cooperative; shared fantasy leads to game playing. Freud described the oedipal phase between ages 3 and 6 years, when there is strong attachment to the parent of the opposite sex. The child's fantasies may focus on play-acting the adult role with that parent, although by age 6 years oedipal issues are usually resolved and attachment is redirected to the parent of the same sex.

EARLY SCHOOL YEARS: AGES 5–7 YEARS

Attendance at kindergarten at age 5 years marks an acceleration in the separation-individuation theme initiated in the preschool years. The child is ready to relate to peers in a more interactive manner. The brain has reached 90% of its adult weight. Sensorimotor coordination abilities are maturing and facilitating pencil-and-paper tasks and sports, both part of the school experience. Cognitive abilities are still at the preoperational stage, and children focus on one variable in a problem at a time. However, most children have mastered conservation of length by age 5½ years, conservation of mass and weight by 6½ years, and conservation of volume by 8 years.

By first grade, there is more pressure on the child to master academic tasks—recognizing numbers, letters, and words and learning to write. Piaget described the stage of concrete operations beginning after age 6 years, when the child is able to perform mental operations concerning concrete objects that involve manipulation of more than one variable. The child is able to order, number, and classify because these activities are related to concrete objects in the environment and because these activities are stressed in early schooling. Magical thinking diminishes greatly at this time, and the reality of cause-effect relationships is better understood. Fantasy and imagination are still strong and are reflected in themes of play.

MIDDLE CHILDHOOD: AGES 7–11 YEARS

Freud characterized ages 7–11 years as the latency years, during which children are not bothered by significant aggressive or sexual drives but instead devote most of their energies to school and peer group interactions. In reality, throughout this period there is a gradual increase in sex drive, manifested by increasingly aggressive play and interactions with the opposite sex. Fantasy still has an active role in dealing with sexuality before adolescence, and fantasies often focus on movie and music stars. Organized sports, clubs, and other activities are other modalities that permit preadolescent children to display socially acceptable forms of aggression and sexual interest.

For the 7-year-old child, the major developmental tasks are achievement in school and acceptance by peers. Academic expectations intensify and require the child to concentrate on, attend to, and process increasingly complex auditory and visual information. Children with significant learning disabilities or problems with attention, organization, and impulsivity may have difficulty with academic tasks and subsequently may receive negative reinforcement from teachers, peers, and even parents. Such children may develop a poor self-image manifested as behavioral difficulties. The pediatrician must evaluate potential learning disabilities in any child who is not developing adequately at this stage or who presents with emotional or behavioral problems. The developmental status of school-aged children is not documented as easily as that of younger children because of the complexity of the milestones. In the school-aged child, the quality of the response, the attentional abilities, and the child's emotional approach to the task can make a dramatic difference in success at school. The clinician must consider all of these aspects in the differential diagnosis of learning disabilities and behavioral disorders.

Bjorklund FP: *Children's Thinking.* Brooks/Cole, 1995.

Dixon SD, Stein MT: *Encounters with Children: Pediatric Behavior and Development,* 4th ed. Mosby-Year Book, 2006.

Feldman HM: Evaluation and management of language and speech disorders in preschool children. Pediatr Rev 2005;26:131 [PMID: 15805236].

Frankenberg WK et al: The Denver II: A major revision and restandardization of the Denver Developmental Screening Test. Pediatrics 1992;89:91 [PMID: 1370185].

Glascoe FP, Dworkin PH: The role of parents in the detection of developmental and behavioral problems. Pediatrics 1995; 95:829 [PMID: 7539122].

Green M, Palfrey JS (editors): *Bright Futures: Guidelines for Health Supervision of Infants, Children, and Adolescents,* 2nd ed revised. National Center for Education in Maternal and Child Health Georgetown University, 2002.

BEHAVIORAL & DEVELOPMENTAL VARIATIONS

Behavioral and developmental variations and disorders encompass a wide range of issues of importance to pediatricians. Practitioners will be familiar with most of the problems discussed in this chapter; however, with increasing knowledge of the factors controlling normal neurologic and behavioral development in childhood, new perspectives on these disorders and novel approaches to their diagnosis and management are emerging.

Variations in children's behavior reflect a blend of intrinsic biologic characteristics and the environments with which the children interact. The next section focuses on some of the more common complaints about behavior encountered by those who care for children. These behavioral complaints are by and large normal variations in behavior, a reflection of each child's individual biologic and temperament traits and the parents' responses. There are no cures for these behaviors, but management strategies are available that can enhance the parents' understanding of the child and the child's relationship to the environment. These strategies also facilitate the parents' care of the growing infant and child.

The last section of this chapter discusses developmental disorders of cognitive and social competence. Diagnosis and management of these conditions requires a comprehensive and often multidisciplinary approach. The health care provider can play a major role in diagnosis, in coordinating the child's evaluation, in interpreting the results to the family, and in providing reassurance and support.

Capute AJ, Accardo PJ (editors): *Developmental Disabilities in Infancy and Childhood,* 2nd ed. Vol. 1, *Neurodevelopmental Diagnosis and Treatment.* Vol. 2, *The Spectrum of Developmental Disabilities.* Brookes/Cole, 1996.

Medical Home Initiatives for Children with Special Needs Project Advisory Committee, American Academy of Pediatrics: The medical home. Pediatrics 2002;110:184 [PMID: 12093969].

Wolraich ML et al (editors): *Developmental-Behavioral Pediatrics: Evidence and Practice.* Mosby/Elsevier, 2008.

Wolraich ML et al: *The Classification of Child and Adolescent Mental Diagnoses in Primary Care: Diagnostic and Statistical Manual for Primary Care (DSM-PC) Child and Adolescent Version.* American Academy of Pediatrics, 1996.

NORMALITY & TEMPERAMENT

The physician confronted by a disturbance in physiologic function rarely has doubts about what is abnormal. Variations in temperament and behavior are not as straightforward. Labeling such variations as disorders implies that a disease entity exists.

The behaviors described in this section are viewed as part of a continuum of responses by the child to a variety of internal and external experiences. Variations in temperament have been of interest to philosophers and writers since ancient times. The Greeks believed there were four temperament types: choleric, sanguine, melancholic, and phlegmatic. In more recent times, folk wisdom has defined temperament as a genetically influenced behavioral disposition that is stable over time. Although a number of models of temperament have been proposed, the one usually used by pediatricians in clinical practice is that of Thomas and Chess, who describe temperament as being the "how" of behavior as distinguished from the "why" (motivation) and the "what" (ability). Temperament is an independent psychological attribute that is expressed as a response to an external stimulus. The influence of temperament is bidirectional: The effect of a particular experience will be influenced by the child's temperament, and the child's temperament will influence the responses of others in the child's environment. Temperament is the style with which the child interacts with the environment.

The perceptions and expectations of parents must be considered when a child's behavior is evaluated. A child that one parent might describe as hyperactive might not be characterized as such by the other parent. This truism can be expanded to include all the dimensions of temperament. Thus, the concept of "goodness of fit" comes into play. For example, if the parents want and expect their child to be predictable but that is not the child's behavioral style, the parents may perceive the child as being bad or having a behavioral disorder rather than as having a developmental variation. An appreciation of this phenomenon is important because the physician may be able to enhance the parents' understanding of the child and influence their responses to the child's behavior. When there is goodness of fit, there will be more harmony and a greater potential for healthy development not only of the child but also of the family. When goodness of fit is not present, tension and stress can result in parental anger, disappointment, frustration, and conflict with the child.

Other models of temperament include those of Rothbart, Buss and Plomin, and Goldsmith and Campos (Table 3–4). All models seek to identify intrinsic behavioral characteristics that lead the child to respond to the world in particular ways. One child may be highly emotional and another less so (ie, calmer) in response to a variety of experiences, stressful or pleasant. The clinician must recognize that each child brings some intrinsic, biologically based traits to its environment and that such characteristics are neither good nor bad, right nor wrong, normal nor abnormal; they are simply part of the child. Thus, as one looks at variations in development, one should abandon the illness model and consider this construct as an aid to understanding the nature of the child's behavior and its influence on the parent-child relationship.

Barr RG: Normality: A clinically useless concept: The case of infant crying and colic. J Dev Behav Pediatr 1993;14:264 [PMID: 8408670].

Goldsmith HH et al: Roundtable: What is temperament? Four approaches. Child Dev 1987;58:505 [PMID: 3829791].

Nigg JT: Temperament and developmental psychopathology. J Child Psychol Psychiatr 2006;47:395–422.

Prior M: Childhood temperament. J Child Psychol Psychiatr 1992;33:249 [PMID: 1737829].

Thomas A, Chess S: *Temperament and Development.* Brunner/Mazel, 1977.

Table 3–4. Theories of temperament.

Thomas and Chess	Temperament is an independent psychologic attribute, biologically determined, which is expressed as a response to an external stimulus. It is the behavioral style: an interactive model.
Rothbart	Temperament is a function of biologically based individual differences in reactivity and self-regulation. It is subsumed under the concept of "personality" and goes beyond mere "behavioral style."
Buss and Plomin	Temperament is a set of genetically determined personality traits that appear early in life and are different from other inherited and acquired personality traits.
Goldsmith and Campos	Temperament is the probability of experiencing emotions and arousal.

ENURESIS & ENCOPRESIS

ESSENTIALS OF DIAGNOSIS & TYPICAL FEATURES

- A child who does not achieve urine and bowel continence by 5–6 years of age and generally has no underlying pathology to which the incontinence can be attributed.
- The child does not respond to a full bladder or rectum.
- The child is constipated and/or is withholding stools.

Enuresis and encopresis are common childhood problems encountered in the pediatric and family practitioner's office. Bedwetting is particularly common with about 20% of children in the first grade occasionally wetting the bed and 4% wetting the bed two or more times a week. Enuresis is more common in boys than in girls. In a recent large US study, the prevalence of enuresis among boys 7 and 9 years was 9% and 7%, respectively and among girls at those ages, 6% and 3%, respectively. The data on constipation and encopresis seem less clear with about 1%–3% of children experiencing this problem, but with anywhere from 0.3% to 29% of children worldwide experiencing constipation. Overall, encopresis/constipation accounts for 3% of referrals to pediatricians' offices. What is very striking, however, is that constipation and enuresis often co-occur; in such a case the constipation needs to be dealt with before the enuresis can be addressed.

ENURESIS

Enuresis is defined as repeated urination into the clothing during the day and into the bed at night by a child who is chronologically and developmentally older than 5 years; this pattern of urination must occur at least twice a week for 3 months. Enuresis has been categorized by the International Children's Continence Society as monosymptomatic or nonmonosymptomatic. Monosymptomatic enuresis is uncomplicated nocturnal enuresis (NE; must never have been dry at night for over 6 months with no daytime accidents); it is a reflection of a maturational disorder and there is no underlying organic problem. Complicated or nonmonosymptomatic enuresis often involves NE and daytime incontinence and often reflects an underlying disorder. The evaluation of both forms needs to take into consideration both the medical and psychological implications of these conditions.

Monosymptomatic enuresis reflects a delay in achieving nighttime continence and reflects a delay in the maturation of the urological and neurological systems. Both micturition and anorectal evacuation are dependent on neural connections and communications between the frontal lobes, locus ceruleus, mid pons, sacral voiding center, and the bladder and rectum. With respect to enuresis, most children are continent at night within 2 years of achieving daytime control. However, 15.5% of 7.5-year-old children wet the bed but only about 2.5% meet the criteria for enuresis. With each year of age the frequency of bedwetting decreases: by 15 years only about 1%–2% of children continue to wet. This occurs more commonly among boys than girls.

The causes for NE are varied and probably interact with one another. Genetic factors are strongly implicated, as enuresis tends to run in families. Many children with NE have a higher threshold for arousal and do not awake to the sensation of a full bladder. NE also can be a result of overproduction of urine from decreased production of desmopressin or a resistance to antidiuretic hormone. In such cases, the bladder has decreased functional capacity and empties before it is filled.

The evaluation of a child with NE involves a complete history and physical examination to rule out any anatomical abnormalities, underlying pathology, or the presence of constipation. In addition, every child with NE should undergo a urinalysis including a specific gravity. A urine culture should be obtained, especially in girls.

Treatment involves education and the avoidance of being judgmental and shaming the child. Most children feel ashamed and the goal of treatment is to help the child establish continence and maintain his or her self-esteem. A variety of behavioral strategies have been employed such as limiting liquids before sleep and awakening the child at night so that he/she can go to the toilet. Central to this simple strategy is consistency on the parents' part and the need for the child to be completely awake. If this simple approach is unsuccessful the use of bedwetting alarms is suggested. Every time the alarm goes off the child should go to the toilet and void. Therapy needs to be continued for at least 3 months and used every night. Critical to the success of therapy is that parents need to be active participants and get up with the child, as many children will just turn off the alarm and go back to sleep. The alarm system, which is a form of cognitive behavioral therapy, has been found to cure two-thirds of affected children and should be highly recommended to affected children and their parents as a safe, effective treatment for NE. The most common cause of failure of this intervention is that the child doesn't awaken or the parents do not wake the child.

While behavioral strategies should be the first-line of treatment, when these fail one may need to turn to medications. Desmopressin acetate (DDAVP), an antidiuretic hormone analogue, has been used successfully. DDAVP decreases urine production. Imipramine, a tricyclic antidepressant, also has been used successfully to control NE, although the mechanism of action is not understood. However, potential adverse side-effects, including the risk of death with an overdose, suggest that imipramine should be used only as a last resort. Unfortunately, when such medications are stopped there is a very high relapse rate.

Daytime incontinence or nonmonosymptomatic enuresis is more complicated than NE. Daytime continence is achieved by 70% of children by 3 years of age and by 90% of children by 6 years. When this is not the case one needs to consider underlying pathology, including cystitis; diabetes insipidus; diabetes mellitus; seizure disorders; neurogenic bladder; anatomical abnormalities of the urinary tract system such as urethral obstruction; constipation; and psychological stress and child maltreatment. A complete history and physical examination must be obtained, along with a diary that includes daily records of voiding and fecal elimination. Treatment must be directed at the underlying pathology and often requires the input of pediatric subspecialists. Following diagnosis, family support and education are essential.

ENCOPRESIS

Constipation (see Chapter 21) is defined by two or more of the following events for 2 months: (1) less than three bowel movements per week; (2) more than one episode of encopresis per week; (3) impaction of the rectum with stool; (4) passage of stool so large it obstructs the toilet; (5) retentive posturing and fecal withholding; and (6) pain with defecation.

Encopresis is defined in the *Diagnostic and Statistical Manual of Mental Disorders,* Fourth Edition, Text Revision (DSM-IV-TR) as the repeated passage of stool into inappropriate places (such as in the underpants) by child who is chronologically or developmentally > 4 years of age. Behavioral scientists often divide encopresis into (1) retentive encopresis, (2) continuous encopresis, and (3) discontinuous encopresis. In rare instances children have severe toilet phobia and so do not defecate into the toilet. It is critical to note that more than 90% of the cases of encopresis result from constipation. Thus, in the evaluation of a child with encopresis one must rule out underlying pathology associated with constipation (see Chapter 21) while at the same time addressing functional and behavioral issues. Conditions associated with constipation include metabolic disorders such as hypothyroidism, neurologic disorders such as cerebral palsy or tethered cord, and anatomical abnormalities of the anus. In addition, children who have been continent can also develop encopresis as a response to stress or child maltreatment.

The prevalence of encopresis is somewhat difficult to precisely ascertain as it is a subject often kept secret by the family and the child. However, some authors report that 1%–3% of children ages 4–11 years of age suffer from encopresis. The highest prevalence is between 5 and 6 years of age.

A complete history and meticulous physical examination must be performed, including a rectal examination, particularly looking for abnormalities around the anus and spine. An abdominal radiograph can be helpful in determining the degree of constipation, the appearance of the bowel, and whether there is obstruction. Assuming no gastrointestinal abnormalities, initial intervention starts with treatment of constipation. Subsequently education, support, and guidance around evacuation are essential, including behavioral strategies such as having the child sit on the toilet after meals to stimulate the gastrocolic reflex. It is most important to avoid punishing the child and making him or her feel guilty and ashamed. Helping the child to clean himself and his clothing in a nonjudgmental, nonpunitive manner are far more productive approaches than criticism and reproach. At the same time, if there is an underlying psychiatric disorder such as depression the child should be treated for the mental health problem along with the treatment of the constipation.

When medical management of constipation is indicated, oral medication or an enema for "bowel cleanout" followed by oral medications, should be used. Such treatment can be monitored by abdominal radiographs to be sure that the colon is clean. A bowel regimen needs to be established with the goal of the child achieving continence and defecating in the toilet bowl on a regular basis. The child should be encouraged to have a daily bowel movement and the use of fibre, some laxatives, and even mineral oil can be helpful. Consultation with a gastroenterologist should be considered in more refractory cases.

Culbert TP, Banez GA: Integrative approaches to childhood constipation and encopresis. Pediatr Clin North Am 2007;54(6).

Nijman, RJM: Diagnosis and management of urinary incontinence and functional fetal incontinence (encopresis) in children. Clin Gastroenterol 2008;37(3).

Reiner W: Pharmacotherapy in the management of voiding and storage disorders, including enuresis and encopresis. J Am Acad Child Adolesc Psychiatry 2008;47:491–498.

Robson WLM: Evaluation and management of enuresis. NEJM 2009;360:1429–1436.

Schonwald A, Rappaport LA: Elimination conditions. In Wolraich ML et al (editors): *Developmental-Behavioral Pediatrics: Evidence and Practice.* Mosby Elsevier, 2008: 791–804.

COMMON DEVELOPMENTAL CONCERNS

COLIC

ESSENTIALS OF DIAGNOSIS & TYPICAL FEATURES

- An otherwise healthy infant aged 2–3 months seems to be in pain, cries for > 3 hours a day, for > 3 days a week, for > 3 weeks ("rule of threes").

Infant colic is characterized by severe and paroxysmal crying that occurs mainly in the late afternoon. The infant's knees are drawn up and its fists are clenched, flatus is expelled, the facies has a pained appearance, and there is minimal response to attempts at soothing. Studies in the United States have shown that among middle-class infants, crying occupies about 2 hours per day at 2 weeks of age, about 3 hours per day by 6 weeks, and gradually decreases to about 1 hour per day by 3 months. The word "colic" is derived from Greek *kolikos* ("pertaining to the colon"). Although colic has traditionally been attributed to gastrointestinal disturbances, this has never been proved. Others have suggested that colic reflects a disturbance in the infant's sleep-wake cycling or an infant state regulation disorder. In any case, colic is a behavioral sign or symptom that begins in the first few weeks of life and peaks at age 2–3 months. In about 30%–40% of cases, colic continues into the fourth and fifth months.

A colicky infant, as defined by Wessel, is one who is healthy and well fed but cries for more than 3 hours a day, for more than 3 days a week, and for more than 3 weeks—commonly referred to as the "rule of threes." The important word in this definition is "healthy." Thus, before the diagnosis of colic can be made, the pediatrician must rule out diseases that might cause crying. With the exception of the few infants who respond to elimination of cow's milk from its own or the mother's diet, there has been little firm evidence of an association of colic with allergic disorders. Gastroesophageal reflux is often suspected as a cause of colicky crying in young infants. Undetected corneal abrasion, urinary tract infection, and unrecognized traumatic injuries, including child abuse, must be among the physical causes of crying considered in evaluating these infants. Some attempts have been made to eliminate gas with simethicone and to slow gut motility with dicyclomine. Simethicone has not been shown to ameliorate colic. Dicyclomine has been associated with apnea in infants and is contraindicated.

This then leaves characteristics intrinsic to the child (ie, temperament) and parental caretaking patterns as contributing to colic. Behavioral states have three features: (1) they are self-organizing—that is, they are maintained until it is necessary to shift to another one; (2) they are stable over several minutes; and (3) the same stimulus elicits a state-specific response that is different from other states. The behavioral states are (among others) a crying state, a quiet alert state, an active alert state, a transitional state, and a state of deep sleep. The states of importance with respect to colic are the crying state and the transitional state. During transition from one state to another, infant behavior may be more easily influenced. Once an infant is in a stable state (eg, crying), it becomes more difficult to bring about a change (eg, to soothe). How these transitions are accomplished is probably influenced by the infant's temperament and neurologic maturity. Some infants move from one state to another easily and can be diverted easily; other infants sustain a particular state and are resistant to change.

The other factor to be considered in evaluating the colicky infant is the feeding and handling behavior of the caregiver. Colic is a behavioral phenomenon that involves interaction between the infant and the caregiver. Different caregivers perceive and respond to crying behavior differently. If the caregiver perceives the crying infant as being spoiled and demanding and is not sensitive to or knowledgeable about the infant's cues and rhythms—or is hurried and "rough" with the infant—the infant's ability to organize and soothe him- or herself or respond to the caregiver's attempts at soothing may be compromised. Alternatively, if the temperament of an infant with colic is understood and the rhythms and cues deciphered, crying can be anticipated and the caregiver can intervene before the behavior becomes "organized" in the crying state and more difficult to extinguish.

Management

Several approaches can be taken to the management of colic.

1. Parents may need to be educated about the developmental characteristics of crying behavior and made aware that crying increases normally into the second month and abates by the third to fourth month.
2. Parents may need reassurance, based on a complete history and physical examination, that the infant is not sick. Although these behaviors are stressful, they are normal variants and are usually self-limited. This discussion can be facilitated by having the parent keep a diary of crying and weight gain. If there is a diurnal pattern and adequate weight gain, an underlying disease process is less likely to be present. Parental anxiety must be relieved, because it may be contributing to the problem.
3. For parents to effectively soothe and comfort the infant, they need to understand the infant's cues. The pediatrician (or nurse) can help by observing the infant's behavior and devising interventions aimed at calming both the infant and the parents. One should encourage a quiet environment without excessive handling. Rhythmic stimulation such as gentle swinging or rocking, soft music, drives in the car, or walks in the stroller may be helpful, especially if the parents are able to anticipate the onset of crying. Another approach is to change the feeding habits so that the infant is not rushed, has ample opportunity to burp, and if necessary can be fed more frequently so as to decrease gastric distention if that seems to be contributing to the problem.
4. Medications such as phenobarbital elixir and dicyclomine have been found to be somewhat helpful, but their use is to be discouraged because of the risk of adverse reactions and overdosage. A trial of ranitidine hydrochloride or other proton pump inhibitor might be of help if gastroesophageal reflux is contributing to the child's discomfort.
5. For colic that is refractory to behavioral management, a trial of changing the feedings, and eliminating cow's milk from the formula or from the mother's diet if she is nursing, may be indicated. The use of whey hydrolysate formulas for formula-fed infants has been suggested.

Barr RG: Colic and crying syndromes in infants. Pediatrics 1998;102:1282 [PMID: 9794970].

Barr RG et al (editors): *Crying as a Sign, a Symptom, and a Signal: Clinical, Emotional, and Developmental Aspects of Infant and Toddler Crying.* MacKeith Press, 2000.

Cohen-Silver J, Ratnapalan S: Management of infantile colic: A review. Clin Pediatr (Phil) 2009;48:14–17.

Dihigo SK: New strategies for the treatment of colic: Modifying the parent-infant interaction. J Pediatr Health Care 1998;12: 256 [PMID: 9987256].

Garrison MM, Christakis DA. A systematic review if treatments for infant colic. Pediatrics 2000;106:1563–1569.

Keefe MR et al. Effectives of an intervention for colic. Clin Pediatr (Phila) 2996:45:123–133.

Turner JL, Palamountain S: Clinical features and etiology of colic. In: Rose BD (editor): *UpToDate.* UpToDate, 2005.

Turner JL, Palamountain S: Evaluation and management of colic. In: Rose BD (editor): *UpToDate.* UpToDate, 2005.

FEEDING DISORDERS IN INFANTS & YOUNG CHILDREN

ESSENTIALS OF DIAGNOSIS & TYPICAL FEATURES

- Inadequate or disordered intake of food due to any of the following conditions:
  - Poor oral-motor coordination.
  - Fatigue resulting from a chronic disease.
  - Lack of appetite.
  - Behavioral issues relating to parent-child interaction.
  - Pain associated with feeding.

Children have feeding problems for various reasons including oral-motor dysfunction, cardiopulmonary disorders leading to fatigue, gastrointestinal disturbances causing pain, social or emotional issues, and problems with regulation. The common denominator, however, is usually food refusal. Infants and young children may refuse to eat if they find eating painful or frightening. They may have had unpleasant experiences (emotional or physiologic) associated with eating, they may be depressed, or they may be engaged in a developmental conflict with the caregiver that is being played out in the arena of feeding. The infant may refuse to eat if the rhythm of the feeding experience with the caregiver is not harmonious. The child who has had an esophageal atresia repair and has a stricture may find eating uncomfortable. The very young infant with severe oral candidiasis may refuse to eat because of pain. The child who has had a choking experience associated with feeding may be terrified to eat (oral-motor dysfunction or aspiration). The child who is forced to eat by a maltreating parent or an overzealous caregiver may refuse feeds. Children who have required nasogastric feedings or who have required periods of fasting and intravenous nutrition in the first 1–2 months of life are more likely to display food refusal behavior upon introduction of oral feedings.

Depression in children may be expressed through food refusal. Food refusal may develop when the infant's cues around feeding are not interpreted correctly by the parent. The infant who needs to burp more frequently or who needs time between bites but instead is rushed will often passively refuse to eat. Some will be more active refusers, turning their heads away to avoid the feeder, spitting out food, or pushing away food.

Chatoor and coworkers have proposed a developmental and interactive construct of the feeding experience. The stages through which the child normally progresses are establishment of homeostasis (0–2 months), attachment (2–6 months), and separation and individuation (6 months to 3 years). During the first stage, feeding can be accomplished most easily when the parent allows the infant to determine the timing, amount, pacing, and preference of food intake. During the attachment phase, allowing the infant to control the feeding permits the parent to engage the infant in a positive manner. This paves the way for the separation and individuation phase. When a disturbance occurs in the parent-child relationship at any of these developmental levels, difficulty in feeding may ensue, with both the parent and the child contributing to the dysfunctional interaction. One of the most striking manifestations of food refusal occurs during the stage of separation and individuation. Conflict may arise if the parent seeks to dominate the child by intrusive and controlling feeding behavior at the same time the child is striving to achieve autonomy. The scenario then observed is of the parent forcing food on the child while the child refuses to eat. This often leads to extreme parental frustration and anger, and the child may be inadequately nourished and developmentally and emotionally thwarted.

When the pediatrician is attempting to sort out the factors contributing to food refusal, it is essential first to obtain a complete history, including a social history. This should include information concerning the parents' perception of the child's behavior and their expectations of the child. Second, a complete physical examination should be performed, with emphasis on oral-motor behavior and other clues suggesting neurologic, anatomic, or physiologic abnormalities that could make feeding difficult. The child's emotional state and developmental level must be determined. This is particularly important if there is concern about depression or a history of developmental delays. If evidence of oral-motor difficulty is suspected, evaluation by an occupational therapist is warranted. Third, the feeding interaction needs to be observed live, if possible. Finally, the physician needs to help the parents understand that infants and children may have different styles of eating and different food preferences and may refuse foods they do not like. This is not necessarily abnormal but reflects temperamental differences and variations in the child's way of processing olfactory, gustatory, and tactile stimuli.

Management

The goal of intervention is to identify factors contributing to the disturbance and to work to overcome them. The parents may be encouraged to view the child's behavior differently and try not to impose their expectations and desires. Alternatively, the child's behavior may need to be modified so that the parents can provide adequate nurturing.

When the chief complaint is failure to gain weight, a different approach is required. The differential diagnosis should include not only food refusal but also medical disorders and maltreatment. The most common reason for failure to gain weight is inadequate caloric intake. Excessive weight loss may be due to vomiting or diarrhea, to malabsorption, or to a combination of these factors. In this situation more extensive diagnostic evaluation may be needed. Laboratory studies may include a complete blood count; erythrocyte sedimentation rate; urinalysis and urine culture; blood urea nitrogen; serum electrolytes and creatinine; and stool examination for fat, occult blood, and ova and parasites. Some practitioners also include liver and thyroid profiles. Occasionally an assessment of swallowing function or evaluation for the presence of gastroesophageal reflux may be indicated. Because of the complexity of the problem, a team approach to the diagnosis and treatment of failure to thrive, or poor weight gain, may be most appropriate. The team should include a physician, nurse, social worker, and dietitian. Occupational and physical therapists, developmentalists, and psychologists may be required.

The goals of treatment of the child with poor weight gain are to establish a normal pattern of weight gain and to establish better family functioning. Guidelines to accomplishing these goals include the following: (1) establish a comprehensive diagnosis that considers all factors contributing to poor weight gain; (2) monitor the feeding interaction and ensure appropriate weight gain; (3) monitor the developmental progress of the child and the changes in the family dynamics that facilitate optimal weight gain and psychosocial development; and (4) provide support to the family as they seek to help the child.

Benoit D: Phenomenology and treatment of failure to thrive. Child Adolesc Psychiatr Clin North Am 1993;2:61.

Chatoor I et al: Failure to thrive and cognitive development in toddlers with infantile anorexia. Pediatrics 2004;113:e440 [PMID: 15121987].

Krugman SD, Dubowitz H: Failure to thrive. Am Fam Physician 2003;68:879 [PMID: 13678136].

Macht J: *Poor Eaters*. Plenum, 1990.

Reilly SM et al: Oral-motor dysfunction in children who fail to thrive: Organic or non-organic? Dev Med Child Neurol 1999;41:115 [PMID: 10075097].

Skuse D: Epidemiologic and definitional issues in failure to thrive. Child Adolesc Psychiatr Clin North Am 1993;2:37.

SLEEP DISORDERS

ESSENTIALS OF DIAGNOSIS & TYPICAL FEATURES

- Children younger than age 12 years:
  - Difficulty initiating or maintaining sleep that is viewed as a problem by the child or caregiver.
  - May be characterized by its severity, chronicity, frequency, *and* associated impairment in daytime function in the child *or* family.
  - May be due to a primary sleep disorder or occur in association with other sleep, medical, or psychiatric disorders.
- Adolescents—difficulty initiating or maintaining sleep, or early morning awakening, or nonrestorative sleep, or a combination of these problems.

Sleep is a complex physiologic process influenced by intrinsic biologic properties, temperament, cultural norms and expectations, and environmental conditions. Between 20% and 30% of children experience sleep disturbances at some point in the first 4 years of life. The percentage decreases to 10%–12% in school-aged children. Sleep disorders fall into two categories. **Dyssomnias** refer to problems with initiating and maintaining sleep or to excessive sleepiness. **Parasomnias** refer to abnormalities of arousal, partial arousal, and transitions between stages of sleep.

Sleep is controlled by two different biologic clocks. The first is a circadian rhythm–daily sleep-wake cycle. The second is an ultradian rhythm that occurs several times per night—the stages of sleep. Sleep stages cycle every 50–60 minutes in infants to every 90 minutes in adolescents. The circadian clock is longer than 24 hours. Environmental cues entrain the sleep-wake cycle into a 24-hour cycle. The cues are light-dark, ambient temperature, core body temperature, noise, social interaction, hunger, pain, and hormone production. Without the ability to perceive these cues (ie, blindness) a child might have difficulty entraining a 24-hour sleep-wake cycle.

Two major sleep stages have been identified clinically and with the use of polysomnography: rapid eye movement (REM) and nonrapid eye movement (NREM) sleep. In REM sleep, muscle tone is relaxed, the sleeper may twitch and grimace, and the eyes move erratically beneath closed lids. REM sleep occurs throughout the night but is increased during the latter half of the night. NREM sleep is divided into four stages. In the process of falling asleep, the individual enters stage 1, light sleep, characterized by reduced bodily movements, slow eye rolling, and sometimes opening and closing of the eyelids. Stage 2 sleep is characterized by slowing of eye movements, slowing of respirations and heart rate, and relaxation of the muscles. Most mature individuals spend about half of their sleep time in this stage. Stages 3 and 4 (also called delta or slow-wave sleep) are the deepest NREM sleep stages, during which the body is relaxed, breathing is slow and shallow, and the heart rate is slow. The deepest NREM sleep occurs during the first 1–3 hours after going to sleep. Most parasomnias occur early in the night during deep NREM sleep. Dreams and nightmares that occur later in the night occur during REM sleep.

Sleep is clearly a developmental phenomenon. Infants are not born with a sleep-wake cycle. REM sleep is more common than NREM sleep in newborns and decreases by 3–6 months of age.

Sleep patterns slowly mature throughout infancy, childhood, and adolescence until they become adultlike. Newborns sleep 10–19 hours per day in 2- to 5-hour blocks. Over the first year of life the infant slowly consolidates sleep at night into a 9- to 12-hour block and naps gradually decrease to one per day by about 12 months. Most children stop napping between 3 and 5 years of age. School-aged children typically sleep 10–11 hours per night without a nap. Adolescents need 9–9½ hours per night but often only get 7–7¼ hours per night. This is complicated by an approximate 1- to 3-hour sleep phase delay in adolescence that is due to physiologic changes in hormonal regulation of the circadian system. Often adolescents are not tired until 2 hours after their typical bedtime but still must get up at the same time in the morning. Some school districts have implemented later start times for high-school students because of this phenomenon.

1. Parasomnias

Parasomnias include both NREM arousal disorders such as night terrors, sleeptalking, and sleepwalking (somnambulism), and REM associated sleep abnormalities which are beyond the scope of this chapter.

A. Night Terrors and Sleepwalking

Night terrors commonly occur within 2 hours after falling asleep, during the deepest stage of NREM sleep, and are often associated with sleepwalking. They occur in about 3% of children. During a night terror, the child may sit up in bed screaming, thrashing about, and exhibiting rapid breathing, tachycardia, and sweating. The child is often incoherent and unresponsive to comforting. The episode may last up to half an hour, after which the child goes back to sleep and has no memory of the event the next day. The parents must be reassured that the child is not in pain and that they should let the episode run its course.

Management of night terrors is by reassurance of the parents plus measures to avoid stress, irregular sleep schedule, or sleep deprivation, which prolongs deep sleep when night terrors occur. Scheduled awakening (awakening the child 30–45 minutes before the time the night terrors usually occur) has been used in children with nightly or frequent night terrors, but there is little evidence that this is effective.

Sleepwalking also occurs during slow-wave sleep and is common between 4 and 8 years of age. It is typically benign except that injuries can occur while the child is walking around. Steps should be taken to ensure that the environment is free of obstacles and that doors to the outside are locked. Parents may also wish to put a bell on their child's door to alert them that the child is out of bed. As with night terrors, steps should be taken to avoid stress and sleep deprivation. Scheduled awakenings may also be used if the child sleep walks frequently and at a predictable time.

B. Nightmares

Nightmares are frightening dreams that occur during REM sleep, typically followed by awakening, which usually occurs in the latter part of the night. The peak occurrence is between ages 3 and 5 years, with an incidence between 25% and 50%. A child who awakens during these episodes is usually alert. He or she can often describe the frightening images, recall the dream, and talk about it during the day. The child seeks and will respond positively to parental reassurance. The child will often have difficulty going back to sleep and will want to stay with the parents. Nightmares are usually self-limited and need little treatment. They can be associated with stress, trauma, anxiety, sleep deprivation that can cause a rebound in REM sleep, and medications that increase REM sleep.

2. Dyssomnias

The dyssomnias include difficulty initiating sleep, and nighttime awakenings. Although parasomnias are frightening, dyssomnias are frustrating. They can result in daytime fatigue for both the parents and the child, parental discord about management, and family disruption.

Several factors contribute to these disturbances. The quantity and timing of feeds in the first years of life will influence nighttime awakening. Most infants beyond age 6 months can go through the night without being fed. Thus, under normal circumstances, night waking for feeds is probably a learned behavior and is a function of the child's arousal and the parents' response to that arousal.

Bedtime habits can influence settling in for the night as well as nighttime awakening. If the child learns that going to sleep is associated with pleasant parental behavior such as rocking, singing, reading, or nursing, going back to sleep after nighttime arousal without these pleasant parental attentions may be difficult. This is called a sleep onset association disorder and usually is the reason for night waking. Every time that the child gets to the light sleep portion of the sleep-wake cycle he or she may wake up. This is usually brief and not remembered the next morning, but for the child who does not have strategies for getting to sleep, getting back to sleep may require the same interventions needed to get to sleep initially, such as rocking, patting, and drinking or sucking. Most of these interventions require a parent. Night waking occurs in 40%–60% of infants and young children. Parents need to set limits for the child while acknowledging the child's individual biologic rhythms. They should resist the child's attempts to put off bedtime or to engage them during nighttime awakenings. The goal is to establish clear bedtime rituals, to put the child to bed while still awake, and to create a quiet, secure bedtime environment.

The child's temperament is another factor contributing to sleep. It has been reported that children with low sensory thresholds and less rhythmicity (regulatory disorder) are more prone to night waking. Night waking often starts at about 9 months as separation anxiety is beginning. Parents should receive anticipatory guidance prior to that time so that they know to reassure their child without making the interaction prolonged or pleasurable.

Finally, psychosocial stressors and changes in routine can play a role in night waking.

3. Sleep-Disordered Breathing

Sleep-disordered breathing or obstructive sleep apnea is characterized by obstructed breathing during sleep accompanied by loud snoring, chest retractions, morning headaches and dry mouth, and daytime sleepiness. Obstructive sleep apnea occurs in 1%–3% of preschoolers. It has its highest peak in childhood between the ages of 2 and 6 years, which corresponds with the peak in adenotonsillar hypertrophy. It has been associated with daytime behavioral disorders, including attention-deficit/hyperactivity disorder (ADHD). A thorough physical examination is important to look for adenotonsillar hypertrophy, hypotonia, and facial anomalies that may predispose the child to obstruction during sleep. Lateral neck films may be helpful. The gold standard for diagnosis is polysomnography. (See also Chapter 18.)

4. Restless Legs Syndrome & Periodic Limb Movement Disorder

Restless legs syndrome and periodic limb movement disorder are common disorders in adults and frequently occur together. The frequency of these disorders in children is about 2%. Restless legs syndrome is associated with an uncomfortable sensation in the lower extremities that occurs at night when trying to fall asleep, is relieved by movement, and is sometimes described by children as "creepy-crawly" or "itchy bones." Periodic limb movement disorder is stereotyped, repetitive limb movements often associated with a partial arousal or awakening. The etiology of these disorders is unknown but there has been some association with iron deficiency. A diagnosis of restless legs syndrome is generally made by history and a diagnosis of periodic limb movement disorder can be made with a sleep study.

Management of Sleep Disorders

A complete medical and psychosocial history should be obtained and a physical examination performed. A detailed sleep history and diary should be completed and both parents should contribute. Assessment for allergies, lateral neck films, and polysomnography may be indicated to complete the evaluation, especially if sleep-disordered breathing is suspected. It is important to consider disorders such as gastroesophageal reflux, which may cause discomfort or pain when recumbent. Dental pain or eczema may cause nighttime awakening. It also is important to make sure that any medications that the child is taking do not interfere with sleep.

The key to treatment of children who have difficulty going to sleep or who awaken during the night and disturb others is for the physician and parents to understand normal sleep patterns, the parents' responses that inadvertently reinforce undesirable sleep behavior, and the child's individual temperament traits. Good sleep hygiene includes discontinuing any activities that are stimulating in the hour before bedtime. It is also important to dim lights during the "wind down" time. Television and video games are particularly stimulating.

There is little evidence regarding pharmacologic management of sleep disorders in children. While the role for melatonin in children with typical development is unclear, there is mounting evidence that it can be effective in children with visual impairments, developmental disabilities, and autism spectrum disorders. Medications such as clonidine are often used for sleep disorders, especially in children with ADHD and autistic spectrum disorder (ASD), but there is little data to support its use.

The June 2011 Pediatric Sleep Medicine Update in Pediatric Clinics of North America is a good resource for more in-depth information.

American Academy of Sleep Medicine sponsored web site. Available at: http://yoursleep.aasmnet.org/

Andersen IM et al: Melatonin for insomnia in children with autism spectrum disorders. J Child Neurol 2008;23(5):482–485.

Braam W, Smits MG, Didden R, Korzilius H, Van Geijlswijk IM, Curfs LM. Exogenous melatonin for sleep problems in individuals with intellectual disability: A meta-analysis. Dev Med Child Neurol 2009;51(5):340–349.

Buscemi N, Witmans M: What is the role of melatonin in the management of sleep disorders in children? Paediatr Child Health 2006;11:517–519.

Chervin RD et al: Inattention, hyperactivity, and symptoms of sleep-disordered breathing. Pediatrics 2002;109:449 [PMID: 11875140].

Ferber R: *Solve Your Child's Sleep Problems.* Simon & Schuster Adult Publishing Group, 2006.

Jan JE, Owens JA, Weiss MD, Johnson KP, Wasdell MB, Freeman RD, et al. Sleep hygiene for children with neurodevelopmental disabilities. Pediatrics 2008;122(6):1343–1350.

Mindel JA, Owens JA: *A Clinical Guide to Pediatric Sleep: Diagnosis and Management of Sleep Problems.* Lippincott Williams & Wilkins, 2003.

Moore BA, Friman PC, Fruzzetti AE, MacAleese K. Brief report: Evaluating the Bedtime Pass Program for child resistance to bedtime—a randomized, controlled trial. J Pediatr Psychol 2007;32(3):283–287.

National Sleep Foundation sponsored web site. Available at: http://www.sleepforkids.org/

Owens JA et al: The use of pharmacotherapy in the treatment of pediatric insomnia in primary care: Rational approaches. A consensus meeting summary. J Clin Sleep Med 2005;1:49 [PMID: 17561616].

Owens JA, Moturi S. Pharmacologic treatment of pediatric insomnia. Child Adolesc Psychiatr Clin N Am 2009;18(4): 1001–1016.

Pediatric Sleep Medicine Update, Editors Judith Owens, Jodi Mindell, Pediatric Clinics of North America, June 2011.

Reed HE, McGrew SG, Artibee K, Surdkya K, Goldman SE, Frank K, et al. Parent-based sleep education workshops in autism. J Child Neurol 2009;24(8):936–945.

Rhode Island Hospital-sponsored web site on sleep and sleep disorders in children: http://www.kidzzzsleep.org

Sheldon S, Ferber R: *Principles and Practice of Pediatric Sleep Medicine.* Elsevier Saunders, 2005.

Simakajornboon N, Kheirandish-Gozal L, Gozal D. Diagnosis and management of restless legs syndrome in children. Sleep Med Rev 2009;13(2):149–156.

TEMPER TANTRUMS & BREATH-HOLDING SPELLS

ESSENTIALS OF DIAGNOSIS & TYPICAL FEATURES

- Behavioral responses to stress, frustration, and loss of control.
- Tantrum—child may throw him- or herself on the ground, kick, scream, or strike out at others.
- Breath-holding spell—child engages in a prolonged expiration that is reflexive and may become pale or cyanotic.
- Rule out underlying organic disease in children with breath-holding spells (eg, CNS abnormalities, Rett syndrome, seizures).

1. Temper Tantrums

Temper tantrums are common between ages 12 months and 4 years, occurring about once a week in 50%–80% of children in this age group. The child may throw him- or herself down, kick and scream, strike out at people or objects in the room, and hold his or her breath. These behaviors may be considered normal as the young child seeks to achieve autonomy and mastery over the environment. They are often a reflection of immaturity as the child strives to accomplish age-appropriate developmental tasks and meets with difficulty because of inadequate motor and language skills, impulsiveness, or parental restrictions. In the home, these behaviors may be annoying. In public, they are embarrassing.

Some children tolerate frustration well, are able to persevere at tasks, and cope easily with difficulties; others have a much greater problem dealing with experiences beyond their developmental level. Parents can minimize tantrums by understanding the child's temperament and what he or she is trying to communicate. Parents must also be committed to supporting the child's drive to master his or her feelings.

Management

Appropriate intervention can provide an opportunity for enhancing the child's growth. The tantrum is a loss of control on the child's part that may be a frightening event and a blow to the child's self-image. The parents and the physician need to view these behaviors within the child's developmental context rather than from a negative, adversarial, angry perspective.

Several suggestions can be offered to parents and physicians to help manage tantrums:

1. Minimize the need to say "no" by "child-proofing" the environment so that fewer restrictions need to be enforced.
2. Use distraction when frustration increases; direct the child to other, less frustrating activities; and reward the positive response.
3. Present options within the child's capabilities so that he or she can achieve mastery and autonomy.
4. Fight only those battles that need to be won, and avoid those that arouse unnecessary conflict.
5. Do not abandon the preschool child when a tantrum occurs. Stay nearby during the episode without intruding. A small child may need to be restrained. An older child can be asked to go to his or her room. Threats serve no purpose and should not be used.
6. Do not use negative terms when the tantrum is occurring. Instead, point out that the child is out of control and give praise when he or she regains control.
7. Never let a child hurt him- or herself or others.
8. Do not "hold a grudge" after the tantrum is over, but do not grant the child's demands that led to the tantrum.
9. Seek to maintain an environment that provides positive reinforcement for desired behavior. Do not overreact to undesired behavior, but set reasonable limits and provide responsible direction for the child.
10. Approximately 5%–20% of young children have severe temper tantrums that are frequent and disruptive. Such tantrums may result from a disturbance in the parent-child interaction, poor parenting skills, lack of limit-setting, and permissiveness. They may be part of a larger behavioral or developmental disorder or may emerge under adverse socioeconomic conditions, in circumstances of maternal depression and family dysfunction, or when the child is in poor health. Referral to a psychologist or psychiatrist is appropriate while the pediatrician continues to support and work with the family.

2. Breath-Holding Spells

Whereas temper tantrums can be frustrating to parents, breath-holding spells can be terrifying. The name for this behavior may be a misnomer in that it connotes prolonged inspiration. In fact, breath-holding occurs during expiration and is reflexive—not volitional—in nature. It is a paroxysmal event occurring in 0.1%–5% of healthy children from age 6 months to 6 years. The spells usually start during the first year of life, often in response to anger or a mild injury. The child is provoked or surprised, starts to cry—briefly or for a considerable time—and then falls silent in the expiratory phase of respiration. This is followed by a color change. Spells have been described as either pallid (acyanotic) or cyanotic, with the latter usually associated with anger and the former with an injury such as a fall. The spell may resolve spontaneously, or the child may lose consciousness. In severe cases, the child may become limp and progress to opisthotonos, body jerks, and urinary incontinence. Only rarely does a spell proceed to asystole or a seizure.

Management

For the child with frequent spells, underlying disorders such as seizures, orthostatic hypotension, obstructive sleep apnea, abnormalities of the CNS, tumors, familial dysautonomia, and Rett syndrome need to be considered. An association exists among breath-holding spells, pica, and iron-deficiency anemia. These conditions can be ruled out on the basis of the history, physical examination, and laboratory studies. Once it has been determined that the child is healthy, the focus of treatment is behavioral. Parents should be taught to handle the spells in a matter-of-fact manner and monitor the child for any untoward events. The reality is that parents cannot completely protect the child from upsetting and frustrating experiences and probably should not try to do so. Just as in temper tantrums, parents need to help the child control his or her responses to frustration. Parents need to be careful not to be too permissive and submit to the child's every whim for fear the child might have a spell.

If loss of consciousness occurs, the child should be placed on his or her side to protect against head injury and aspiration. Maintaining a patent oral airway is essential, but cardiopulmonary resuscitation should be avoided. There are no prophylactic medications. Atropine, 0.01 mg/kg given subcutaneously, has been used with some benefit in spells accompanied by bradycardia or asystole.

Breningstall GN: Breath holding spells. Pediatr Neurol 1996;14:91 [PMID: 8703234].

DiMario FJ Jr: Breath-holding spells in childhood. Am J Dis Child 1992;146:125 [PMID: 1736640].

Greene RW: *The Explosive Child.* Quill, 2001.

Needleman R et al: Psychosocial correlates of severe temper tantrums. J Dev Behav Pediatr 1991;12:77.

Needleman R et al: Temper tantrums: When to worry. Contemp Pediatr 1989;6:12.

WELL CHILD SURVEILLANCE & SCREENING

The American Academy of Pediatrics (AAP) recently published guidelines for surveillance and screening at well child visits. Surveillance is a procedure for recognizing children at risk for a developmental disorder and involves asking parents if they have concerns about their child's development. The PEDS (Pediatric Evaluation of Developmental Status) can be used for this purpose. Screening involves use of a standardized tool to clarify identified risk. An evaluation would be done by a specialist and would involve a more definitive evaluation of a child's development.

Surveillance should occur at all well child visits. Screening of development should occur at 9, 18, and 30 months. Because a 30-month visit is not part of the standard well child visit schedule and may not be reimbursed, screening may occur at 24 months instead. It is also recommended that autism-specific screening should occur at the 18-month visit. Although an autism-specific screen was only recommended at the 18-month visit in the AAP guidelines, the Autism Workgroup of the AAP separately has recommended a second autism-specific screen at 24–30 months in order to pick up children missed at the 18-month screen. Because the average age of regression is 20 months, some children may be missed by a single screen at 18 months. Clinicians should keep in mind that if they are administering a screen because they are concerned and the child passes the screen, they should still schedule an early follow-up visit to ensure that appropriate progress has been made and that there are no further concerns.

Implementation of screening requires planning for timing of screening administration during office visits, defining the process for referral, and designing handouts prior to beginning screening. Screening is done to optimize the child's development. However, it also demonstrates to the parent the interest their caretaker has not only for the child's physical well-being but also for the child's developmental and psychosocial well-being. Parents of children who receive a developmental assessment express greater satisfaction with their care provider.

The Child Health and Development Interactive System (CHADIS) is an online system that allows parents and teachers to complete screening questionnaires online prior to the visit. It supports billing for 96,110 screening assessments and complex visits, and provides quality assurance documentation.

American Academy of Pediatrics: Identifying infants and young children with developmental disorders in the medical home: An algorithm for developmental surveillance and screening. Pediatrics 2006;118:405 [PMID: 1681859].

Dietz C et al: Screening for autistic spectrum disorder in children aged 14–15 months. II. Population screening with the Early Screening of Autism Traits Questionnaire (ESAT). Design and general findings. J Autism Dev Disord 2006;36:713 [PMID: 16644887].

Earls MF, Hay SS: Setting the stage for success: implementation of developmental and behavioral screening and surveillance in primary care practice—the North Carolina Assuring Better Child Health and Development (ABCD) Project. Pediatrics 2006;118(1):e183–e188.

Gupta VB et al: Identifying children with autism early? Pediatrics 2007;119:152 [PMID: 17200280].

Halfon N et al: Satisfaction with health care for young children. Pediatrics 2004;113:1926 [PMID: 15173468].

Luyster R et al: Early regression in social communication in autism spectrum disorders: A CPEA study. Dev Neuropsychol 2005;27:311 [PMID: 15843100].

Pinto-Martin JA et al: Developmental stages of developmental screening: Steps to implementation of a successful program. Am J Pub Health 2005;95:1928 [PMID: 16195523].

Reznick JS et al: A parent-report instrument for identifying one-year-olds at risk for an eventual diagnosis of autism: The first year inventory. J Autism Dev Disord 2007;37:1691 [PMID: 17180716].

Wiggins LD et al: The utility of the social communication questionnaire in screening for autism in children referred for early intervention. Focus on Autism and Developmental Disorders 2007;22(1): 33–38.

American Academy of Pediatrics: www.medicalhomeinfo.org/tools/Coding/Developmental%20Screening-Testing%20Coding%20Fact%20Sheet.doc

Child Health and Development Interactive System: www.CHADIS.com

DEVELOPMENTAL DISORDERS

Developmental disorders include abnormalities in one or more aspects of development, such as verbal, motor, visual-spatial, attentional, and social abilities. These problems are diagnosed by comparing the child's performance level with norms accumulated from observation and testing of children of the same age. Problems with development are often noted by parents when a child does not meet typical motor and language milestones. Developmental disorders may also include difficulties with behavior or attention. ADHD is the most common neurodevelopmental disorder. ADHD occurs in 2%–10% of school-aged children and may occur in combination with a variety of other learning or developmental issues. Mild developmental disorders are often not noted until the child is of school age.

Many biologic and psychosocial factors may influence a child's performance on developmental tests. In the assessment of the child, it is important to document adverse psychosocial factors, such as neglect or poverty, which can negatively influence developmental progress. Many of the biologic factors that influence development are genetic and are discussed throughout this section.

Evaluation

The neurodevelopmental evaluation must focus on (1) defining the child's level of developmental abilities in a variety of domains, including language, motor, visual-spatial, attentional, and social abilities; (2) attempting to determine the etiology for the child's developmental delays; and (3) planning a treatment program. These objectives are best achieved by a multidisciplinary team that includes the physician, a psychologist, a speech or language therapist, an occupational therapist, and an educational specialist. The psychologist will usually carry out standardized testing of intellectual ability appropriate to the child's age. The motor and language specialists will also carry out clinical testing to document the deficits in their areas and to organize a treatment program. The educational specialist will usually carry out academic testing for the school-aged child and plan a course of special education support through the school. The physician is usually the integrator of the information from the team and must also obtain a detailed medical and developmental history and conduct the physical and neurologic examinations.

Medical & Neurodevelopmental Examination

The medical history should begin with pregnancy, labor, and delivery to identify conditions that might compromise the child's CNS function. The physician must ask the child's parents about prenatal exposures to toxins, medications, alcohol, drugs, smoking, and infections; maternal chronic illness; complications of pregnancy or delivery; and neonatal course. Problems such as failure to thrive, chronic illnesses, hospitalizations, and abuse can interfere significantly with normal development. Major illnesses or hospitalizations should be discussed. Any CNS problems, such as trauma, infection, or encephalitis, should be documented. The presence of metabolic diseases, such as diabetes or phenylketonuria, and exposure to environmental toxins such as lead should be determined. Chronic diseases such as chronic otitis media, hyper- or hypothyroidism, and chronic renal failure can interfere with normal development. The presence of motor or vocal tics, seizures, or sleep disturbances should be documented. In addition, parents should be questioned about any motor, cognitive, or behavioral regression.

The physician should review and document the child's temperament, difficulties with feeding, and subsequent developmental milestones. The child's difficulties with tantrums, poor attention, impulsivity, hyperactivity, or aggression should be documented.

A detailed history of school-related events should be recorded, including previous special education support, evaluations through the school, history of repeating grades, difficulties with specific academic areas, problems with peers, and the teacher's impressions of the child's difficulties, particularly related to attentional problems, impulsivity, or hyperactivity. Input from teachers can be invaluable and should be sought prior to the evaluation.

Perhaps the most important aspect of the medical history is a detailed family history of learning strengths and weaknesses, emotional or behavioral problems, learning disabilities, intellectual disability, or psychiatric disorders. Parental learning strengths and weaknesses, temperament difficulties, or attentional problems may be passed on to the child. For instance, dyslexia (deficits in decoding skills that result in reading difficulties) is often inherited.

The neurodevelopmental examination should include a careful assessment of dysmorphic features such as epicanthal folds, palpebral fissure size, shape of the philtrum, low-set or posteriorly rotated ears, prominent ear pinnae, unusual dermatoglyphics (eg, a single palmar crease), hyperextensibility of the joints, syndactyly, clinodactyly, or other unusual features. A detailed physical and neurologic examination needs to be carried out with an emphasis on both soft and hard neurologic findings. Soft signs can include motor incoordination, which can relate to handwriting problems and academic delays in written language or drawing. Visual-motor coordination abilities can be assessed by having the child write, copy designs, or draw a person.

The child's growth parameters, including height, weight, and head circumference, need to be assessed, along with hearing and visual acuity. Cranial nerve abnormalities and oral-motor coordination problems need to be noted. The examiner should watch closely for motor or vocal tics. Both fine and gross motor abilities should be assessed. Dyspraxia (motor planning difficulties or imitating complex motor movements) and disorders of fine motor coordination are fairly common. Tandem walking, one-foot balancing, and coordinating a skip may often show surprising abnormalities. Tremors can be noted when watching a child stack blocks or draw.

The developmental aspects of the examination can include an assessment of auditory processing and perceptual ability with simple tasks, such as two- to fivefold directions, assessing right and left directionality, memory for a series of spoken words or digit span, and comprehension of a graded paragraph. In assessing expressive language abilities, the examiner should look for difficulties with word retrieval, formulation, and articulation, and adequacy of vocabulary. Visual-perceptual abilities can be assessed by simple visual memory tasks, puzzles, or object assembly, and evaluating the child's ability to decode words or organize math problems. Visual-motor integration and coordination can be assessed again with handwriting, design copying, and drawing a person. Throughout the assessment the clinician should pay special attention to the child's ability to focus attention and concentrate, and to other aspects of behavior such as evidence of depression or anxiety.

Additional questionnaires and checklists—such as the Child Behavior Checklist by Achenbach; ADHD scales such as the Conners' Parent/Teacher Rating Scale; and the Swanson, Nolan and Pelham Questionnaire-IV, which includes the DSM-IV-TR criteria for ADHD—can be used to help with this assessment.

Referral of family to community resources is critical, as is a medical home (described earlier in the chapter).

American Academy of Pediatrics Council on Children with Disabilities: Care coordination in the medical home: Integrating health and related systems of care for children with special health care needs. Pediatrics 2005;116:1238 [PMID: 16264016].

Medical Home Initiatives for Children with Special Needs Project Advisory Committee, American Academy of Pediatrics: The medical home. Pediatrics 2002;110:184 [PMID: 12093969].

Reynolds CR, Mayfield JW: Neuropsychological assessment in genetically linked neurodevelopmental disorders. In Goldstein S, Reynolds CR (editors): *Handbook of Developmental and Genetic Disorders in Children*. Guilford, 1999.

ATTENTION-DEFICIT/HYPERACTIVITY DISORDER

ADHD is a common neurodevelopmental disorder that may affect 2%–10% of school-aged children and may persist into adolescence and adulthood. It is associated with a triad of symptoms: impulsivity, inattention, and hyperactivity. DSMIV-TR has described three ADHD subtypes: hyperactive-impulsive, inattentive, and combined; the combined subtypes often do not appear until 7 years of age. To be classified according to either subtype, the child must exhibit six or more of the symptoms listed in Table 3–5.

The majority of children with ADHD have a combined type with symptoms of inattention as well as hyperactivity and impulsivity. Girls have a higher prevalence of the inattentive subtype; boys have a higher prevalence of the hyper-active subtype. Although symptoms begin in early childhood, they can diminish between ages 10 and 25 years. Hyperactivity declines more quickly, and impulsivity and inattentiveness often persist into adolescence and adulthood. ADHD may be combined with other psychiatric conditions, such as mood disorder in approximately 20% of patients, conduct disorders in 20%, and oppositional defiant disorder in up to 40%. Up to 25% of children with ADHD seen in a referral clinic have tics or Tourette syndrome. Conversely, well over 50% of individuals with Tourette syndrome also have ADHD.

Table 3–5. Attention-deficit/hyperactivity disorder subtypes.

Subtype	Symptoms[a]
Hyperactive-impulsive	Fidgetiness Difficulty remaining seated in the class Excessive running or climbing Difficulty in engaging in quiet activities Excessive talking and blurting out answers before questions have been completed Difficulty awaiting turns Interrupting and intruding on others
Inattentive	Failure to give close attention to detail Difficulty sustaining intention in task Failure to listen when spoken to directly Failure to follow instructions Difficulty organizing tasks and activities Reluctance to engage in tasks Losing utensils necessary for tasks or activities Easy distractibility Forgetfulness in daily activities

[a]The child must exhibit six or more of these symptoms.
Adapted, with permission, from American Psychiatric Association: *Diagnostic and Statistical Manual of Mental Disorders*, 4th ed. American Psychiatric Association, 2000.

ADHD has a substantial genetic component. Several candidate genes have been identified, although there is strong evidence that ADHD is a disorder involving multiple genes. ADHD is also associated with a variety of genetic disorders related to developmental disorders, including fragile X syndrome, Williams syndrome, Angelman syndrome, XXY syndrome (Klinefelter syndrome), and Turner syndrome. Fetal alcohol syndrome (FAS) is also strongly associated with ADHD. CNS trauma, CNS infections, prematurity, and a difficult neonatal course with brain injury can also be associated with later ADHD. Metabolic problems such as hyperthyroidism can sometimes cause ADHD. These organic causes of ADHD should be considered in the evaluation of any child presenting with attentional problems, hyperactivity, or impulsivity. However, in the majority of children who have ADHD the cause remains unknown.

Management

The treatment of ADHD varies depending on the complexity of the individual case, including comorbid disorders such as anxiety and learning disabilities. It is important to educate the family regarding the symptoms of ADHD and to clarify that it is a neurologic disorder which makes the symptoms difficult for the child to control. Despite that, behavior modification techniques usually help these children and should include structure with consistency in daily routine, positive reinforcement whenever possible, and time out for negative behaviors. A variety of educational interventions can be helpful, including preferential seating in the classroom, a system of consistent positive behavior reinforcement, consistent structure, the repetition of information when needed, and the use of instruction that incorporates both visual and auditory modalities. Many children with ADHD have significant social difficulties, and social skills training can be helpful. Individual counseling is beneficial in alleviating poor self-esteem, oppositional behavior, and conduct problems.

Stimulant medications (methylphenidate, dextroamphetamine, and lisdexamfetamine) are available in short- and long-acting preparations. A recently introduced methylphenidate preparation is delivered transdermally. Alternative medications for the treatment of ADHD include clonidine or guanfacine, which are α_2-adrenergic presynaptic agonists that decrease norepinephrine levels, and atomoxetinewhich is a norepinephrine reuptake inhibitor. They are particularly helpful for individuals who are hyperreactive to stimuli and may decrease motor tics in patients who have Tourette syndrome.

It is most important that, no matter what medication is used, the diagnosis is correct and the correct dosage is prescribed. A recent study has demonstrated that one of the major factors contributing to treatment failure is inadequate dosing or the failure to recognize the presence of comorbid conditions such as learning disability, anxiety disorders, and depression.

Seventy percent to ninety percent of children with normal intellectual abilities respond well to stimulant medications. Stimulants enhance both dopamine and norepinephrine neurotransmission, which seems to improve impulse control, attention, and hyperactivity. The main side effects of methylphenidate and dextroamphetamine include appetite suppression and resulting weight loss, as well as sleep disturbances. Atomoxetine is a selective inhibitor of the presynaptic norepinephrine transporter, which increases norepinephrine and dopamine, and has a similar side-effect profile to the stimulants as well as side effects associated with antidepressants. Cardiovascular effects of stimulant medications have undergone significant scrutiny over the past 2 years. It is unclear whether stimulants increase the risk of sudden death over the risk in the general population, especially in children without any underlying risk. Prior to beginning a stimulant medication, it is recommended that clinicians obtain any history of syncope, palpitations, chest pain, and family history of sudden death prior to age 30 that may predispose a child to sudden death. Some individuals experience increased anxiety, particularly with higher doses of stimulant medications. Children with autism and developmental disabilities may be at increased risk for side effects with stimulants. Stimulants may exacerbate psychotic symptoms. They may also exacerbate motor tics in 30% of patients, but in 10% motor tics may be improved.

American Academy of Pediatrics: Clinical practice guideline: Treatment of the school-aged child with attention-deficit/hyper-activity disorder. Pediatrics 2001;108:1033 [PMID: 11581465].

Brown RT et al: American Academy of Pediatrics Committee on Quality Improvement; American Academy of Pediatrics Subcommittee on Attention-Deficit/Hyperactivity Disorder: Treatment of attention-deficit/hyperactivity disorder: Overview of the evidence. Pediatrics 2005;115:e749 [PMID: 15930203].

Jensen PS et al: Findings from the NIMS Multimodal Treatment Study of ADHD (MTA): Implications and applications for primary care providers. J Develop Behav Pediatr 2001;22:60 [PMID: 11265923].

Krull KA: Evaluation and diagnosis of attention deficit hyperactivity disorders in children. In Rose BD (editor): *UpToDate*. UpToDate, 2005.

Krull KA: Treatment and prognosis of attention deficit hyperactivity disorders in children. In Rose BD (editor): *UpToDate*. UpToDate, 2005.

Reiff MI: *ADHD: A Compete Authoritative Guide*. American Academy of Pediatrics, 2004.

Reiff MI (ed): *ADHD: What Every Parent Needs to Know*. American Academy of Pediatrics, 2011.

Attention Deficit Disorder Association: http://www.add.org

Children and Adults with Attention Deficit/Hyperactivity Disorder: http://www.chadd.org

Questions and Answers: Safety of Pills For Treating ADHD: http://www.aap.org/healthtopics/adhd.cfm

AUTISM SPECTRUM DISORDERS

ESSENTIALS OF DIAGNOSIS & TYPICAL FEATURES

- Three core deficits:
  - Qualitative impairments in communication
  - Qualitative impairments in reciprocal social interaction
  - Presence of stereotypic, restrictive, and repetitive patterns of behavior, interests, and activities.

Autism is a neurologic disorder characterized by (1) qualitative impairments in social interaction; (2) qualitative impairments in communication; and (3) restricted repetitive and stereotyped patterns of behavior, interests, and activities. Autism is currently grouped under the pervasive developmental disorders in the DSM-IV with Asperger disorder, pervasive developmental disorder not otherwise specified, childhood disintegrative disorder, and Rett syndrome. Asperger disorder is characterized by impairment in social interaction and restricted interest/repetitive behaviors. Individuals with Asperger disorder should not have significant delays in cognitive, language, or self-help skills. Pervasive developmental disorder not otherwise specified is characterized by impairment in reciprocal social interaction along with impairment in communication skills, or restricted interest or repetitive behaviors. Children with pervasive developmental disorder not otherwise specified do not meet full criteria for autism. Childhood disintegrative disorder (CDD) is characterized by typical development for at least 2 years followed by a regression in at least two of the following three areas: social interaction, communication, and behavior (characterized by restricted interests or repetitive behaviors). Rett syndrome is a genetic syndrome caused by a mutation on the X chromosome that is characterized by regression in skills in the first year of life. Table 3–6 lists the DSM-IV-TR criteria for diagnosis of an autism spectrum disorder. DSM-V will likely not include CDD or Rett syndrome.

Table 3–6. Criteria for diagnosis of an autism spectrum disorder.

Qualitative impairment in social interaction (at least 2)
Impairment in nonverbal behaviors such as eye contact
Failure to develop peer
Lack of seeking to share enjoyment or interests
Lack of social or emotional reciprocity
Qualitative impairment in communication (at least 1)
Delay in or lack of spoken language
If speech is present, lack of ability to initiate or sustain conversation
Stereotyped and repetitive/idiosyncratic language
Lack of pretend/social imitative play
Restricted interests/repetitive behavior (at least 1)
Preoccupation with restricted interest
Inflexible adherence to nonfunctional routines or rituals
Stereotyped and repetitive motor mannerisms (hand flapping)
Persistent preoccupation with parts of objects

Reprinted, with permission, from American Psychiatric Association: *Diagnostic and Statistical Manual of Mental Disorders,* 4th ed, text revision. American Psychiatric Association, 2000.

Autism spectrum disorders are relatively common, occurring in approximately 1 in 150 children. Males are overrepresented 3–4:1, with reports as high as 9.5:1 (especially when higher functioning individuals are included). No known etiology can be found in 80%–90% of cases. A genetic syndrome such as fragile X syndrome or chromosome 15q duplication is found in 10%–20% of cases. There is a strong familial component. Parents of one child with autism of unknown etiology have a 2%–9% chance of having a second child with autism. The concordance rate among monozygotic twins is high but not absolute, and there is an increased incidence of speech, language, reading, attention, and affective disorders in family members of children with autism.

Evaluation & Management

Children with autism are often not diagnosed until age 3–4 years, when their disturbances in reciprocal social interaction and communication become more apparent. However, impairments in communication and behavior can often be recognized in the first 12–18 months of life. The most common characteristics during the first year are a consistent failure to orient to one's name, regard people directly, use gestures, and to develop speech. Even if one of these skills is present, it is often diminished in frequency, inconsistent, or fleeting. Every interaction should be an opportunity to engage socially. Sharing affect or enjoyment is an important precursor to social interaction. By 16–18 months a child should have "joint attention," which occurs when two people attend to the same thing at the same time. This is usually accomplished by shifting eye gaze, pointing, or saying "look." Toddlers should point to get needs met ("I want that") and to show ("look at that") by 1 year of age and they should do it regularly. By 18 months a toddler should be able to follow a point, imitate others, and engage in functional play (using toys in the way that they are intended to be used, such as rolling a car, throwing a ball, or feeding a baby doll). Restricted interests and repetitive behaviors sometimes do not emerge until after age 2, but usually are present before age 2.

There is mounting evidence that a diagnosis of autism spectrum disorder can be made reliably by age 2 years and is stable over time. Because there is evidence that early intervention is particularly important for children with autism, great interest has arisen in developing a screening instrument that can be used in very young children. The Modified Checklist for Autism in Toddlers (M-CHAT) is designed for children 16–30 months of age (Figure 3–13). It is a parent report measure with 23 yes/no questions. This test is still undergoing study to determine sensitivity and specificity but preliminary outcomes show good sensitivity and specificity. Specificity is greater if parents of children who screen positive on the M-CHAT receive a follow-up phone call asking for specific examples of failed items to confirm accuracy.

An autism-specific screen is recommended at 18 months. A second autism-specific screen has been recommended at 24–30 months. The second screen was recommended because some of the symptoms may be more obvious in an older child, and because about 30% of children with autism spectrum disorders experience a regression or plateau in skills between 12 and 24 months. Screening at 18 months could miss many of these children.

When behaviors raising concern for autism are noted, the child should be referred to a team of specialists experienced in the assessment of autism spectrum disorders. The child should also be referred to a local early intervention program and to a speech and language pathologist to begin therapy as soon as possible. All children with autism should have a formal audiology evaluation. Laboratory tests such as high-resolution chromosome analysis and fluorescence in situ hybridization (FISH) for 15q duplication, or an Array Comparative Genomic Hybridization (aCGH otherwise known as microarray) and a DNA for fragile X syndrome should be considered. Metabolic screening, lead level, thyroid studies, and a Wood lamp test for tuberous sclerosis may also be done if indicated by findings in the history and physical examination. Neuroimaging is not routinely indicated even in the presence of mild/relative macrocephaly because children with autism often have relatively large heads. Neuroimaging should be done if microcephaly or focal neurologic signs are noted.

Approximately 30% of children with autism demonstrate plateauing or loss of skills (usually language and social skills only) between 12 and 24 months of age. This regression/plateau in skills has been documented in prospective longitudinal studies of infant siblings of children with ASD. The loss is usually gradual. It can co-occur with atypical development

Instructions for Use

The M-CHAT is validated for screening toddlers between 16 and 30 months of age, to assess risk for autism spectrum disorders (ASD). The M-CHAT can be administered and scored as part of a well-child check-up, and also can be used by specialists or other professionals to assess risk for ASD. The primary goal of the M-CHAT was to maximize sensitivity, meaning to detect as many cases of ASD as possible. Therefore, there is a high false positive rate, meaning that not all children who score at risk for ASD will be diagnosed with ASD. To address this, we have developed a structured follow-up interview for use in conjunction with the M-CHAT; it is available at the two websites listed above. Users should be aware that even with the follow-up questions, a significant number of the children who fail the M-CHAT will not be diagnosed with an ASD; however, these children are at risk for other developmental disorders or delays, and therefore, evaluation is warranted for any child who fails the screening.

The M-CHAT can be scored in less than two minutes. Scoring instructions can be downloaded from **http://www2.gsu.edu/~wwwpsy/faculty/robins.htm or www.firstsigns.org**. We also have developed a scoring template, which is available on these websites; when printed on an overhead transparency and laid over the completed M-CHAT, it facilitates scoring. Please note that minor differences in printers may cause your scoring template not to line up exactly with the printed M-CHAT.

Children who fail more than 3 items total or 2 critical items (particularly if these scores remain elevated after the follow-up interview) should be referred for diagnostic evaluation by a specialist trained to evaluate ASD in very young children. In addition, children for whom there are physician, parent, or other professional's concerns about ASD should be referred for evaluation, given that it is unlikely for any screening instrument to have 100% sensitivity.

M-CHAT

Please fill out the following about how your child usually is. Please try to answer every question. If the behavior is rare (e.g., you've seen it once or twice), please answer as if the child does not do it.

1.	Does your child enjoy being swung, bounced on your knee, etc.?	Yes No
2.	Does your child take an interest in other children?	Yes No
3.	Does your child like climbing on things, such as up stairs?	Yes No
4.	Does your child enjoy playing peek-a-boo/hide-and-seek?	Yes No
5.	Does your child ever pretend, for example, to talk on the phone or take care of a doll or pretend other things?	Yes No
6.	Does your child ever use his/her index finger to point, to ask for something?	Yes No
7.	Does your child ever use his/her index finger to point, to indicate interest in something?	Yes No
8.	Can your child play properly with small toys (e.g. cars or blocks) without just mouthing, fiddling, or dropping them?	Yes No
9.	Does your child ever bring objects over to you (parent) to show you something?	Yes No
10.	Does your child look you in the eye for more than a second or two?	Yes No
11.	Does your child ever seem oversensitive to noise? (e.g., plugging ears)	Yes No
12.	Does your child smile in response to your face or your smile?	Yes No
13.	Does your child imitate you? (e.g., you make a face-will your child imitate it?)	Yes No
14.	Does your child respond to his/her name when you call?	Yes No
15.	If you point at a toy across the room, does your child look at it?	Yes No
16.	Does your child walk?	Yes No
17.	Does your child look at things you are looking at?	Yes No
18.	Does your child make unusual finger movements near his/her face?	Yes No
19.	Does your child try to attract your attention to his/her own activity?	Yes No
20.	Have you ever wondered if your child is deaf?	Yes No
21.	Does your child understand what people say?	Yes No
22.	Does your child sometimes stare at nothing or wander with no purpose?	Yes No
23.	Does your child look at your face to check your reaction when faced with something unfamiliar?	Yes No

▲ **Figure 3-13.** M-CHAT revisions and related materials are available for download at www.mchatscreen.com. (Reproduced, with permission, from Diana Robins, Deborah Fein, and Marianne Barton.)

and can be fluctuating. It usually occurs before the child attains a vocabulary of 10 words. If a child presents with regression, he or she should be referred to a child neurologist. An overnight EEG should be considered when there is a history of regression to rule out epileptiform discharges during sleep. It should be noted that the recommendations for treatment of EEG abnormalities are still being debated. Metabolic testing and a magnetic resonance imaging (MRI) of the brain should also be considered when there is a history of regression.

Early, intensive behavioral intervention for children with ASD is essential. The National Research Council reviewed the available literature in 2001 and recommended entry into treatment as soon as autism is suspected; 25 hours of intervention per week; parent training and involvement in treatment; ongoing assessment, program evaluation, and programmatic adjustment as needed; and intervention that focuses on communication, social interaction, and play skills that can be generalized in a naturalistic setting. Functional use of language leads to better behavioral and medical outcomes. Early detection and early intervention have a positive impact on children with ASDs. The National Research Council states: "A substantial subset of children with autistic spectrum disorders are able to make marked progress during the period that they receive intensive early intervention, and nearly all children with autistic spectrum disorders appear to show some benefit. Children with ASD who begin treatment before age 3–3½ years make the greatest gains with intervention." Naturalistic training models for children with autism implemented before age 3 result in 90% of children attaining functional use of language compared to 20% who begin intervention after age 5. There are many models for this type of intervention and much variability in what is available in different areas of the country. Families should be encouraged to find a model that best suits the needs of the child and the family.

One role of the primary care provider is to ensure that medical concerns such as sleep disorders, seizures, or gastrointestinal symptoms are addressed. Any worsening of behavior in a child with autism may be secondary to unrecognized medical issues such as pain from a dental abscess or esophagitis. Psychopharmacologic management is often needed to address issues with attention, hyperactivity, anxiety, aggression, and other behaviors that have a significant impact on daily function. Psychiatric comorbidities are common and should be addressed by the PCP or a specialist. The primary care provider also provides a medical home for children with ASD. This requires coordination of care.

Many complementary and alternative (CAM) treatments for autism have been proposed. As many as 33% of families use special diets and 54% of families use supplements for their child with ASD based on data from the Interactive Autism Network. The review of CAM prepared by the AAP Task Force on Complementary and Alternative Medicine and the Provisional Section on Complementary, Holistic, and Integrative Medicine is particularly valuable.

Autism and Developmental Disorders Monitoring Network Surveillance Year 2002 Principal Investigators; Centers for Disease Control and Prevention: Prevalence of autism spectrum disorders—Autism and Developmental Disabilities Monitoring Network, 14 Sites, United States, 2002. MMWR Surveill Summ 2007;56:12 [PMID: 17287715].

Chavez B et al: Atypical antipsychotics in children with pervasive developmental disorders. Paediatr Drugs 2007;9(4):249–266.

Chawarska K, Klin A, Volkmar F: *Autism Spectrum Disorders in Infants and Toddlers, Diagnosis, Assessment, and Treatment.* Guilford. 2008.

Dumont-Mathieu T, Fein D: Screening for autism in young children: The Modified Checklist for Autism in Toddlers (M-CHAT) and other measures. Ment Retard Dev Disabil Res Rev 2005;11:253.

Gabriels RL, Hill DE (editors): *Growing Up with Autism: Working with School-Age Children and Adolescents.* Guildford, 2007.

Goldson E: Autism spectrum disorders: An overview. Adv Pediatr 2004;51:63–109 [PMID: 15366771].

Johnson CP, Myers SM; American Academy of Pediatrics Council on Children with Disabilities: Identification and evaluation of children with autism spectrum disorders. Pediatrics 2007; 120(5):1183–1215.

Kemper KJ, Vohra S, Walls R; Task Force on Complementary and Alternative Medicine; Provisional Section on Complementary, Holistic, and Integrative Medicine: The use of complementary and alternative medicine in pediatrics. Pediatrics 2008;122;1374–1386.

Landa RJ et al: Social and communication development in toddlers with early and later diagnosis of autism spectrum disorders. Arch Gen Psychiatry 2007;64:853 [PMID: 17606819].

Lord C, McGee JP (editors): *Educating Children with Autism.* National Academy of Sciences Press, 2001.

Luyster R et al: Early regression in social communication in autism spectrum disorders: A CPEA Study. Dev Neuropsychol. 2005;27:311–336.

Malone R et al: Advances in drug treatments for children and adolescents with autism and other pervasive developmental disorders. CNS Drugs 2005;19(11):923–934.

Myers SM, Johnson CP; American Academy of Pediatrics Council on Children with Disabilities: Management of children with autism spectrum disorders. Pediatrics 2007;120(5):1162–1182.

Schaefer GB, Mendelsohn NJ, Professional Practice and Guidelines Committee: Clinical genetics evaluation in identifying the etiology of autism spectrum disorders. Genet Med 2008;10(4).

Volkman FR: *Autism and Pervasive Developmental Disorders,* 2nd ed. Cambridge University Press, 2007.

AAP Autism Tool Kit

Autism Speaks: http://www.autismspeaks.org

Division TEACCH (Treatment and Education of Autistic and Related Communication-handicapped Children): http://teacch.com

FDA Center for Safety and Applied Nutrition: http://www.cfsan.fda.gov/%7Edms/ds-warn.html

First Signs (educational site on autism): http://firstsigns.org

Hanen Centre (information on family-focused early intervention programs): http://www.hanen.org

Interactive Autism Network (based at Johns Hopkins, families complete questionnaires online regarding their child with autism): https://www.ianexchange.org

Learn the Signs, Act Early (website with resources and free handouts for families): www.cdc.gov/actearly

MCHAT with Phone Follow-up (free download of the MCHAT available): http://www2.gsu.edu/~wwwpsy/faculty/robins.htm

The National Center for Complementary and Alternative Medicine (NCCAM) was established in 1998. NCCAM sponsors and conducts research using scientific methods and advanced technologies: http://nccam.nih.gov/

INTELLECTUAL DISABILITY

The field of developmental disabilities has been evolving and redefining the constructs of disability and intellectual disability and thereby using new terms to reflect that evolution. The term *retardation* was first used in an educational context to describe educationally compromised students. Indeed, during the early 20th century, educators and psychologists struggled to identify the causes of the problems these students encountered. Interestingly, their "differential diagnoses" included biologic, environmental, and emotional etiologies, not dissimilar to those we deal with in the 21st century. In addition, it was—and continues to be—acknowledged that the term *mental retardation* and earlier terms such as *idiocy, feeblemindedness,* and *mental deficiency* are pejorative, demeaning, and dehumanizing.

Recently, a rethinking of the construct of disability has emerged that shifts the focus from limitations in intellectual functioning and adaptive capability (a person-centered trait) to a human phenomenon with its source in biologic or social factors and contexts. The current view is a social-ecological conception of disability that articulates the role of disease or disorder leading to impairments in structure and function, limitations in activities, and restriction in participation in personal and environmental interactions. The term *intellectual disability,* which is consistent with this broader view, is increasingly being used and reflects an appreciation of the humanness and potential of the individual. The diagnostic criteria currently remain the same; however, the construct and context has changed.

Having noted this, it is important to acknowledge that significant delays in the development of language, motor skills, attention, abstract reasoning, visual-spatial skills, and academic or vocational achievements are associated with intellectual disability (ID). Deficits on standardized testing in cognitive and adaptive functioning greater than two standard deviations below the mean for the population are considered to fall in the range of ID (Table 3–7). The most common way of reporting the results of these tests is by using an intelligence quotient. The intelligence quotient is a statistically derived number reflecting the ratio of age-appropriate cognitive function and the child's actual level of cognitive function. A number of accepted standardized measurement tools, such as the Wechsler Intelligence Scale for Children, third edition, can be used to assess these capacities. To receive a diagnosis of ID a child must not only have an intelligence quotient of less than 70, but also must demonstrate adaptive skills more than two standard deviations below the mean. Adaptive function refers to the child's ability to function in his or her environment and can be measured by a parent or teacher interview recorded using an instrument such as the Vineland Adaptive Behavior Scales.

Table 3–7. Categories of intellectual disability (ID).

Mental ID/MR Range	Intelligence Quotient (IQ)
Mild ID	50–69
Moderate ID	35–49
Severe ID	20–34
Profound ID	< 20

The prevalence of ID is approximately 3% in the general population, although some states have reported a prevalence of less than 2%. Mild levels of ID are more common and more likely to have a sociocultural cause than are more severe levels. Poverty, deprivation, or a lack of exposure to a stimulating environment can contribute to developmental delays and poor performance on standardized tests. In addition, physical problems such as hearing loss, blindness, and brain trauma can lead to developmental delays and low intelligence quotient test scores. Great strides in our identification of genetic causes of ID have been made since the 1990s because of the Human Genome Project. More than 750 genetic disorders have been associated with ID, and over 200 of those disorders are carried on the X chromosome alone. In approximately 60% of cases, the cause of the intellectual disability can be identified. Table 3–8 summarizes the findings of several studies examining the causes of intellectual disability.

Table 3–8. Causes of intellectual disability (ID).

Cause	Percentage of Cases
Chromosomal abnormalities	4–28
Fragile X syndrome	2–5
Monogenetic conditions	4–14
Structural CNS abnormalities	7–17
Complications of prematurity	2–10
Environmental or teratogenic causes	5–13
"Cultural-familial" ID	3–12
Metabolic or endocrine causes	1–5
Unknown	30–50

CNS, central nervous system.

Adapted from Curry CJ et al: Evaluation of mental retardation: Reco-mmendations of a consensus conference. Am J Med Genet 1997;72:468.

Evaluation

Children who present with developmental delays should be evaluated by a team of professionals as described at the beginning of this section. For children 0–3½ years of age, the Bayley Scales of Infant Development, second edition, is a well-standardized developmental test. For children older than 3 years of age standardized cognitive testing, such as the Wechsler Preschool and Primary Scale of Intelligence-Revised; the Wechsler Intelligence Scale for Children, third edition; the Stanford-Binet IV; or the Kaufman Assessment Battery for Children should be administered to assess cognitive function over a broad range of abilities, including verbal and nonverbal scales. For the nonverbal patient, a scale such as the Leiter-R will assess skills that do not involve language.

A full psychological evaluation in school-aged children should include an emotional assessment if psychiatric or emotional problems are suspected. Such problems are common in children with developmental delays or ID. A hearing test and a vision screening or ophthalmologic evaluation are important to determine whether hearing and vision are normal.

Diagnostic testing should be carried out in an effort to find the cause of ID. Because chromosomal abnormalities occur in 4%–28% of patients with ID, cytogenetic testing is important in cases without a known cause. A consensus panel has recommended a high-resolution karyotype so that small deletions or duplications can be visualized. In addition, FISH studies are available. These studies use a fluorescent DNA probe that hybridizes to a region of DNA where a deletion or duplication is suspected. Microdeletion syndromes—such as Prader-Willi syndrome or Angelman syndrome, caused by a deletion at 15q; velocardiofacial syndrome, caused by a deletion at 22q; Smith-Magenis syndrome, caused by a deletion at 17p; and Williams syndrome, caused by a 7p deletion—can be assessed with FISH studies. Sometimes the deletion is so small that it may not be visualized through the microscope even with high-resolution cytogenetic studies. If clinical features consistent with any of the microdeletion syndromes are present, then FISH studies should be ordered to look for a small deletion in a specific region. In addition, duplications may be present. For example, duplication at 15q has been associated with pervasive developmental disorder or autistic spectrum disorders and with ID. This duplication can be identified by FISH testing.

Structural abnormalities of the brain can occur in many individuals with ID. MRI is superior to computed tomography (CT) in identifying structural and myelination abnormalities. CT is the study of choice in evaluation of intracranial calcifications, such as those seen in congenital infections or tuberous sclerosis. The value of CT and MRI studies in a child with a normal-sized head and no focal neurologic signs is unclear, and they are not routinely carried out. Neuroimaging is important in patients with microcephaly, macrocephaly, seizures, loss of psychomotor skills, or specific neurologic signs such as spasticity, dystonia, ataxia, or abnormal reflexes. Neuroimaging is not routinely carried out in children with known genetic disorders such as Down syndrome, fragile X syndrome, or microdeletion syndromes because the CNS abnormalities have been well described and documentation of the abnormalities usually does not affect management.

Metabolic screening has a relatively low yield (0%–5%) in children who present with developmental delay or ID. Many patients with metabolic disorders such as hypothyroidism, phenylketonuria, and galactosemia are identified through newborn screening. Most patients with metabolic problems will present with specific indications for more focused testing, such as failure to thrive, recurrent unexplained illnesses, plateauing or loss of developmental skills, coarse facial features, cataracts, recurrent coma, abnormal sexual differentiation, arachnodactyly, hepatosplenomegaly, deafness, structural hair abnormalities, muscle tone changes, and skin abnormalities. Thyroid function studies should be carried out in any patient who has a palpably abnormal thyroid or exhibits clinical features associated with hypothyroidism. Serum amino acids, urine organic acid, and mucopolysaccharide screens should be considered in children with developmental delays and a suggestive history. Preliminary laboratory findings such as lactic acidosis, hyperuricemia, hyperammonemia, or a low or high cholesterol level require additional metabolic workup.

Serial follow-up of patients is important as the physical and behavioral phenotype changes over time and diagnostic testing improves with time. Although cytogenetic testing may have been negative 10 years earlier, advances in high-resolution techniques, FISH testing, and fragile X DNA testing may now reveal an abnormality that was not identified previously. A stepwise approach to diagnostic testing may also be more cost-effective, so that the test most likely to be positive is done first.

Management

Once a diagnosis of ID is made, treatment should include a combination of individual therapies, such as speech and language therapy, occupational therapy or physical therapy, special education support, behavioral therapy or counseling, and medical intervention, which may include psychopharmacology. To illustrate how these interventions work together, two disorders are described in detail in the next section.

Curry CJ et al: Evaluation of mental retardation: Recommendations of a consensus conference. Am J Med Genet 1997;72:468 [PMID: 9375733].

Hagerman RJ: *Neurodevelopmental Disorders: Diagnosis and Treatment*. Oxford University Press, 1999.

Schalock RL et al: The renaming of *mental retardation*: Understanding the change to the term *intellectual disability*. Intellect Dev Disab 2007;45:116 [PMID: 17428134].

Smith JD, Smallwood G: From whence came mental retardation? Asking why while saying goodbye. Intellect Dev Disab 2007;45:132 [PMID: 17428137].
The Arc of the United States (grassroots advocacy organization for people with disabilities): http://www.thearc.org

SPECIFIC FORMS OF INTELLECTUAL DISABILITY & ASSOCIATED TREATMENT ISSUES

1. Fragile X Syndrome

The most common inherited cause of ID is fragile X syndrome, which is caused by a trinucleotide expansion (CGG repeated sequence) within the fragile X mental retardation I (*FMR1*) gene. Individuals with ID of unknown origin should receive *FMR1* DNA testing to look for an expansion of the CGG repeats causing dysfunction of this gene. The CGG sequence at *FMR1* in the normal population includes 5–50 repeats. Carriers of the premutation have 54–200 repeats, and have been considered unaffected. However, there is mounting evidence for a specific phenotype in these individuals. Women with the premutation have a higher incidence of premature ovarian failure, anxiety, and mild facial dysmorphisms. Males with the premutation are at risk for developing fragile X tremor ataxia syndrome (FXTAS). Individuals with the premutation have normal levels of FMR1 protein but increased levels of mRNA. It should be noted that seemingly unaffected females can pass an expansion of the CGG repeat to the next generation. Approximately 1 in 250 women and 1 in 700 men in the general population are premutation carriers. When a premutation of more than 90 repeats is passed on by a female to her offspring, it will expand to a full mutation (more than 200 repeats) 100% of the time, which usually causes ID or learning disabilities. The full mutation is associated with methylation of the gene, which turns off transcription, resulting in a deficiency in the FMR1 protein. These deficiencies result in ID or significant learning and emotional issues.

Fragile X syndrome includes a broad range of symptoms. Patients can present with shyness, social anxiety, and learning problems, or they can present with ID. Girls are usually less affected by the syndrome because they have a second X chromosome that is producing FMR1 protein. Approximately 70% of girls with the full mutation have cognitive deficits in addition to emotional problems, such as mood lability, ADHD, anxiety, and shyness. Approximately 85% of males with the syndrome have ID and autistic-like features, such as poor eye contact, hand flapping, hand biting, and tactile defensiveness. About 20% of males with fragile X syndrome meet the criteria for autism.

Children with fragile X syndrome usually present with cognitive and language delays, hyperactivity, and difficult behavior in early childhood. Although prominent ears and hyperextensible finger joints are common, approximately 30% of children with the syndrome may not have these features. The diagnosis must be suspected because of behavioral problems and developmental delays alone. As the boys move into puberty, macro-orchidism develops with an average adult volume of 50 mL, or twice the normal volume. The child's face may become longer during puberty.

Management

A variety of therapies are helpful for individuals with fragile X syndrome. Speech and language therapy can decrease oral hypersensitivity, improve articulation, enhance verbal output and comprehension, and stimulate abstract reasoning skills. Because approximately 10% of boys with the syndrome will be nonverbal at age 5 years, the use of augmentative communication techniques—such as signing; the use of pictures to represent food, toys, or activities; or the use of computers that can be programmed for communication—are helpful. Tantrums and hyperarousal to stimuli, along with hyperactivity, are common. Occupational therapy can be helpful in calming hyperarousal to stimuli and in improving the child's fine and gross motor coordination and motor planning. If the behavioral problems are severe, it can be helpful to involve a behavioral psychologist who emphasizes positive reinforcement, time outs, consistency in routine, and the use of both auditory and visual modalities, such as a picture schedule, to help with transitions and new situations.

Psychopharmacology can also be useful to treat ADHD, aggression, anxiety, or severe mood instability. Clonidine or guanfacine may be helpful in low doses, beginning in the preschool period to treat hyperarousal, tantrums, or severe hyperactivity. Stimulant medications such as methylphenidate and dextroamphetamine are usually beneficial by age 5 years and occasionally earlier. Relatively low doses are used (eg, 0.2–0.3 mg/kg per dose of methylphenidate) because irritability is often a problem with higher doses.

Anxiety may also be a significant problem for boys with fragile X syndrome, and the use of a selective serotonin reuptake inhibitor (SSRI) such as fluoxetine is often helpful. SSRIs may also decrease aggression or moodiness, although in approximately 25% of cases, an increase in agitation or even hypomania may occur. Shyness and social anxiety combined with mild ADHD are commonly seen in girls who have fragile X syndrome. The social anxiety is sometimes so severe that selective mutism (refusal to speak in some environments, especially school) is seen in girls who have the full mutation. The treatment for selective mutism may include an SSRI, language therapy, and counseling.

Aggression may become a significant problem in childhood or adolescence for boys with fragile X syndrome. Counseling can often be helpful, although medication may be needed. Stimulants, clonidine, guanfacine, and an SSRI may decrease aggression, although sometimes an atypical antipsychotic may be needed. Clinical trials have begun in adults and adolescents with Fragile X syndrome to evaluate metabotropic glutamate receptor 5 antagonists and gaba agonists that have shown promising results in mouse models of fragile X syndrome.

An important component of treatment is genetic counseling. Parents should meet with a genetic counselor after the diagnosis of fragile X syndrome is made because there is a high risk that other family members are carriers or may be affected by the syndrome. A detailed family history is essential. Female carriers have a 50% risk of having a child with the fragile X mutation. Male carriers are at risk for developing FXTAS, a neurodegenerative disorder, as they age.

It is also helpful to refer a newly diagnosed family to a parent support group. Educational materials and parent support information may be obtained by calling the National Fragile X Foundation at 1-800-688-8765.

Hagerman RJ et al: Advances in the treatment of fragile X syndrome. Pediatrics 2009;123(1):378–390.

Fragile X Research Foundation: http://www.fraxa.org

National Fragile X Foundation: http://www.FragileX.org

2. Fetal Alcohol Spectrum Disorders

Alcohol exposure in utero is associated with a broad spectrum of developmental problems, ranging from learning disabilities to severe intellectual disability. Fetal alcohol spectrum disorders (FASD) is an umbrella term describing the range of effects that can occur in an individual exposed to alcohol prenatally. The Institute of Medicine in 1996 defined the diagnostic categories in individuals with documented prenatal maternal alcohol exposure as follows.

A. Fetal Alcohol Syndrome

FAS refers to the full syndrome associated with prenatal alcohol exposure. The diagnosis of FAS requires the presence of a characteristic pattern of facial abnormalities (short palpebral fissures, thin upper lip, and indistinct or smooth philtrum, for which there are standard measurements), growth deficiency, and evidence of CNS damage and neurodevelopmental abnormalities. This diagnosis can be made with or without confirmed maternal prenatal use of alcohol.

B. Partial Fetal Alcohol Syndrome

The diagnosis of partial FAS requires the presence of at least two of the facial anomalies as well as at least one of the following: growth retardation, CNS neurodevelopmental abnormalities, or behavioral or cognitive abnormalities that are inconsistent with the child's developmental level and cannot be explained by familial background or environment. This diagnosis can be made with or without confirmed maternal prenatal use of alcohol, although this can be difficult because of the subtle facial anomalies, and the lack of growth retardation in many of these children.

C. Alcohol-Related Neurodevelopmental Disorder

Alcohol-related neurodevelopmental disorder does not require the presence of dysmorphic facial features, but it does require the presence of neurodevelopmental abnormalities or evidence of a pattern of behavioral or cognitive abnormalities. These abnormalities may include learning disabilities; poor impulse control; and problems in memory, attention, and judgment. These characteristics must be inconsistent with the child's developmental level and cannot be explained by familial background or environment. This diagnosis requires confirmation of prenatal alcohol exposure.

D. Alcohol-Related Birth Defects

The diagnosis of alcohol-related birth defects requires a history of prenatal alcohol exposure, at least two characteristic facial features, and the presence of one or more congenital anomalies, including malformations and dysplasias in cardiac, skeletal, renal, ocular, or auditory areas (ie, sensorineural hearing loss) or two or more minor anomalies (ie, hypoplastic nails, clinodactyly).

Animal and human data support these diagnostic categories. The prevalence of FAS, partial FAS, and alcohol-related neurodevelopmental disorder combined is approximately 1 per 100 in the general population. These are common problems. Thus, the physician should always ask about alcohol (and other drug) intake during pregnancy. This is particularly true when evaluating a child presenting with developmental delays. The exact amount of alcohol consumption that leads to teratogenesis remains unclear.

Evaluation & Management

Essential to the evaluation of a child with FASD, or one suspected of having FASD, is an assessment by a multidisciplinary team. The evaluation should include examination of growth, facial and other dysmorphic features, developmental or cognitive abilities, behavioral function, and the documentation of prenatal alcohol exposure.

Individuals with FASD typically have significant difficulty with complex cognitive tasks and executive function (planning, conceptual set shifting, affective set shifting, response inhibition, and fluency). They process information slowly. They may do well with simple tasks but have difficulty with more complex tasks. They have difficulty with attention and short-term memory. They are also at risk for social difficulties and mood disorders. Functional classroom assessments can be a very helpful part of a complete evaluation. Structure is very important for individuals with FASD. Types of structure that may be helpful are visual structure (color code each content area), environmental structure (keep work area uncluttered, avoid decorations), and task structure (clear beginning, middle, and end). Psychopharmacologic intervention may be needed to address issues such as attention and mood.

American Academy of Pediatrics, Committee on Substance Abuse and Committee on Child with Disabilities: Fetal alcohol syndrome and alcohol-related neurodevelopmental disorders. Pediatrics 2000;106:358 [PMID: 10920168].

Astley SJ: Comparison of the 4-digit diagnostic code and the Hoyme diagnostic guidelines for fetal alcohol spectrum disorders. Pediatrics 2006;118:1532–1545.

Centers for Disease Control and Protection: Surveillance for fetal alcohol syndrome using multiple sources—Atlanta, Georgia, 1981–1989. MMWR 1997;46:1118–1120.

Hoyme HE et al: A practical clinical approach to diagnosis of fetal alcohol spectrum disorders: Clarification of the 1996 institute of medicine criteria. Pediatrics 2005;115:39–47.

Kalberg WO, Buckley D: FASD: What types of intervention and rehabilitation are useful? Neurosci Biobehav Rev 2007; 31:278–285.

Kodituwakku PW: Defining the behavioral phenotype in children with fetal alcohol spectrum disorders: A review. Neurosci Biobehav Rev 2007;31:192–201.

Manning MA, Eugene Hoyme H: Fetal alcohol spectrum disorders: A practical clinical approach to diagnosis. Neurosci Biobehav Rev 2007;31:230–238.

Paley B. Intervention for individuals with fetal alcohol spectrum disorders: Treatment approaches and case management. Dev Disabil Res Rev 2009:15:258–267.

Streissguth AP: *Fetal Alcohol Syndrome: A Guide for Families and Communities*. Brookes/Cole, 1997.

Center for Disease Control (fetal alcohol syndrome: guidelines for referral and diagnosis. July 2004): http://www.cdc.gov/ncbddd/fasd/documents/FAS_guidelines_accessible.pdf

National Organization on Fetal Alcohol Syndrome: http://www.nofas.org

REFERENCES

Print Resources

Levine MD, Carey WB, Crocker AC (editors): *Developmental Behavioral Pediatrics*, 3rd ed. WB Saunders, 1999.

Parker S, Zuckerman B (editors): *Behavioral and Developmental Pediatrics: A Handbook for Primary Care*. Lippincott Williams & Wilkins, 2005.

Wolraich ML et al: *Developmental-Behavioral Pediatrics: Evidence and Practice*. Mosby Elsevier, 2008.

Wolraich ML (editor): *Disorders of Development and Learning: A Practical Guide to Assessment and Management*, 3rd ed. BC Decker, 2003.

Web Resources

The Arc of the United States (grassroots advocacy organization for people with disabilities): http://www.thearc.org

American with Disabilities Act Information: National Access for Public Schools Project: http://www.adaptenv.org

Family Voices (web site devoted to children and youth with special health care needs): http://www.familyvoices.org

The Hanen Centre (information on family-focused early intervention programs): http://www.hanen.org

National Association of Developmental Disabilities Councils: http://www.naddc.org

National Dissemination Center for Children with Disabilities: http://www.nichcy.org

Parent Training and Information Centers: Alliance Coordinating Office: http://www.taalliance.org

Title V Program Information: Institute for Child Health Policy: http://www.ichp.edu

Adolescence

4

Amy E. Sass, MD, MPH
David W. Kaplan, MD, MPH

Adolescence is a period of rapid physical, emotional, cognitive, and social development. Generally, adolescence begins at age 11–12 years and ends between ages 18 and 21. Most teenagers complete puberty by age 16–18 years; in Western society, however, for educational and cultural reasons, the adolescent period is prolonged to allow for further psychosocial development before the individual assumes adult status. The developmental passage from childhood to adulthood includes the following steps: (1) completing puberty and somatic growth; (2) developing socially, emotionally, and cognitively, and moving from concrete to abstract thinking; (3) establishing an independent identity and separating from the family; and (4) preparing for a career or vocation.

DEMOGRAPHY

In the United States in 2009, there were 21.5 million adolescents aged 15–19 years and 21.5 million aged 20–24 years. Adolescents and young adults (ages 15–24 years) constitute 14% of the U.S. population. Between 1990 and 2006, the population 10–24 years of age increased from 40.1 to 63.3 million. In the next several decades, the proportion of racial and ethnic minority adolescents is expected to increase. It is projected that by 2040 the percentage of non-Hispanic whites will drop below 50% of the total adolescent population. Hispanics are becoming the second most populous racial and ethnic group of adolescents.

MORTALITY DATA

In adolescence, cultural and environmental rather than organic factors pose the greatest threats to life. The three leading causes of death in adolescents aged 15–19 years in 2007 were unintentional injury (48.8%), homicide (16.7 %), and suicide (11.1 %). Motor vehicle crashes are the leading cause of death among teens in the United States, accounting for approximately one-third of deaths in this age group. During 2004–2008, the annual population-based rate for drivers aged 16 or 17 years involved in fatal crashes declined 38%, from 27.1 per 100,000 population in 2004 to 16.7 in 2008. Much of the reduction is a result of states implementing graduated driver licensing (GDL) programs and vigorously enforcing laws on minimum legal drinking age, blood alcohol concentration (BAC), and safety belt use.

MORBIDITY DATA

Demographic and economic changes in the American family have had a profound effect on children and adolescents. The percentage of children and adolescents living in two-parent households has decreased significantly, from 79% in 1980 to 66% in 2009 (range: 80% in Asians, 60% in Hispanics, 33% in blacks). Between 2000 and 2007, the number of children living below the official poverty threshold increased by 14.7%. The rate of poverty varies significantly by race and family structure. In 2007, 34% of black children and 27% of Hispanic children lived in families with incomes below the official poverty threshold.

The major causes of morbidity during adolescence are psychosocial and often correlate with poverty: unintended pregnancy, sexually transmitted infection (STI), substance abuse, smoking, dropping out of school, depression, running away from home, physical violence, and juvenile delinquency. High-risk behavior in one area is frequently associated with problems in another (Figure 4–1). For example, teenagers who live in a dysfunctional family (eg, drinking, physical, or sexual abuse) are much more likely than other teenagers to be depressed. A depressed teenager is at greater risk for drug and alcohol abuse, academic failure, inappropriate sexual activity, STIs, pregnancy, and suicide.

Early identification of the teenager at risk for these problems is important in preventing immediate complications and future associated morbidities. Early indicators for problems related to depression include

1. Decline in school performance
2. Excessive school absences or cutting class
3. Frequent or persistent psychosomatic complaints

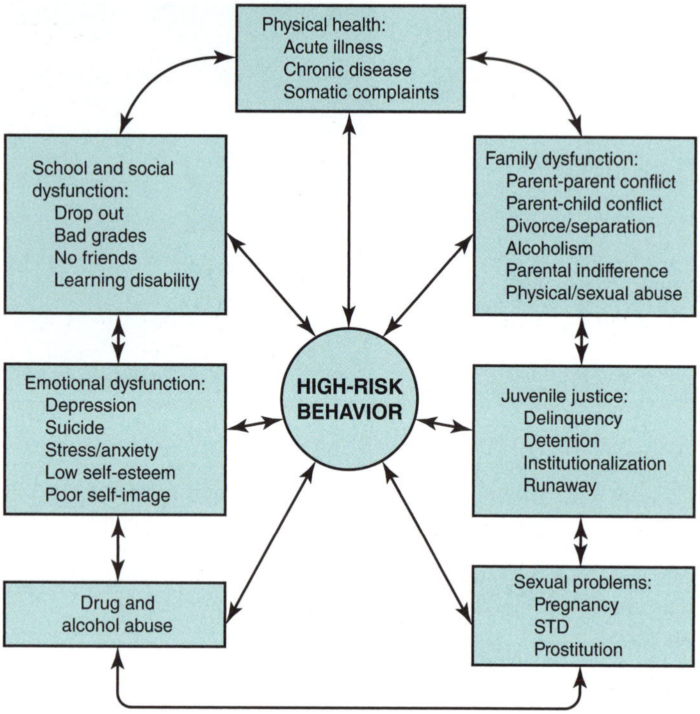

▲ **Figure 4–1.** Interrelation of high-risk adolescent behavior.

4. Changes in sleeping or eating habits
5. Difficulty in concentrating or persistent boredom
6. Signs or symptoms of depression, extreme stress, or anxiety
7. Withdrawal from friends or family or change to a new group of friends
8. Severe violent or rebellious behavior or radical personality change
9. Conflict with parents
10. Sexual acting-out
11. Conflicts with the law
12. Suicidal thoughts or preoccupation with themes of death
13. Drug and alcohol abuse
14. Running away from home

Centers for Disease Control and Prevention: Web-based Injury Statistics Query and Reporting System (WISQARS). Atlanta: U.S. Department of Health and Human Services, CDC; 2007. Available at: http://www.cdc.gov/injury/wisqars/index.html.

Drivers aged 16 or 17 years involved in fatal crashes—United States, 2004-2008. MMWR Morb.Mortal.Wkly.Rep. 2010;59(41): 1329–1334.

D'Angelo LJ, Halpern-Felsher BL et al: Adolescents and driving: a position paper of the Society for Adolescent Health and Medicine. J Adolesc Health 2010;47(2):212–214.

Chen LH et al: Graduated driver licensing programs and fatal crashes of 16-year-old drivers: A national evaluation. Pediatrics 2006;118:56 [PMID: 16818549].

Eaton DK et al: Youth risk behavior surveillance—United States, 2009. MMWR Surveill Summ 2009;59(SS-5):1.

Healthy People 2010: National Health Promotion and Disease Prevention Objectives. Washington, DC: U.S. Government Printing Office, 2000.

Mulye TP et al: Trends in adolescent and young adult health in the United States. J Adolesc Health 2009;45(1):8–24 [PMID: 19541245].

DELIVERY OF HEALTH SERVICES

How, where, why, and when adolescents seek health care depends on ability to pay, distance to health care facilities, availability of transportation, accessibility of services, time away from school, and privacy. Many common teenage health issues, such as unintended pregnancy, contraception, STI, substance abuse, depression, and other emotional problems have moral, ethical, and legal implications. Teenagers are often reluctant to confide in their parents for fear of punishment or disapproval. Recognizing this reality, health care providers have established specialized programs such as teenage family planning clinics, drop-in centers, STI clinics, hotlines, and adolescent clinics. Establishing a trusting and confidential relationship with adolescents is basic to meeting their health care needs. Patients who sense that the physician will inform their parents about a confidential problem may lie or fail to disclose information essential for proper diagnosis and treatment.

GUIDELINES FOR ADOLESCENT PREVENTIVE SERVICES

The American Medical Association guidelines for adolescent preventive services and the American Academy of Pediatrics' *Bright Futures: Guidelines for Health Supervision of Infants, Children, and Adolescents* cover health screening and guidance, immunization, and health care delivery. The goals of these guidelines are (1) to deter adolescents from participating in behaviors that jeopardize health; (2) to detect physical, emotional, and behavioral problems early and intervene promptly; (3) to reinforce and encourage behaviors that promote healthful living; and (4) to provide immunization against infectious diseases. The guidelines recommend that adolescents between ages 11 and 21 years have annual routine health visits. Health services should be developmentally appropriate and culturally sensitive. Confidentiality between patient and physician should be ensured.

RELATING TO THE ADOLESCENT PATIENT

Adolescence is one of the physically healthiest periods in life. The challenge of caring for most adolescents lies not in managing complex organic disease, but in accommodating the cognitive, emotional, and psychosocial changes that influence health behavior. The physician's initial approach to the adolescent may determine the success or failure of the visit. The physician should behave simply and honestly, without an authoritarian or excessively professional manner. Because the self-esteem of many young adolescents is fragile, the physician must be careful not to overpower and intimidate the patient. To establish a comfortable and trusting relationship, the physician should strive to present the image of an ordinary person who has special training and skills.

Because the onset and termination of puberty vary from child to child, chronologic age may be a poor indicator of physical, physiologic, and emotional maturity. In communicating with an adolescent, the physician must be sensitive to the adolescent's developmental level; recognizing that outward appearance and chronologic age may not be an accurate reflection of cognitive development.

Working with teenagers can be emotionally draining. Adolescents have a unique ability to identify hidden emotional vulnerabilities. The physician who has a personal need to control patients or foster dependency may be disappointed in caring for teenagers. Because teenagers are consumed with their own emotional needs, they rarely provide the physician with ego rewards as do younger or older patients.

The physician should be sensitive to the issue of countertransference—the emotional reaction elicited in the physician by the adolescent. How the physician relates to the adolescent patient often depends on the physician's personal characteristics. This is especially true of physicians who treat families that are experiencing parent-adolescent conflicts. It is common for young physicians to overidentify with the teenage patient and for older physicians to see the conflict from the parents' perspective.

Overidentification with parents is readily sensed by the teenager, who is likely to view the physician as just another authority figure who cannot understand the problems of being a teenager. Assuming a parental-authoritarian role may jeopardize the establishment of a working relationship with the patient. In the case of the young physician, overidentification with the teenager may cause the parents to become defensive about their parenting role and to discount the physician's experience and ability.

THE SETTING

Adolescents respond positively to settings and services that communicate sensitivity to their age. A pediatric waiting room with toddlers' toys and infant-sized examination tables makes adolescent patients feel they have outgrown the practice. A waiting room filled with geriatric or pregnant patients can also make a teenager feel out of place.

CONFIDENTIALITY

It is not uncommon that a teenage patient is brought to the office against his or her wishes, especially for evaluations of drug and alcohol use, parent-child conflict, school failure, depression, or a suspected eating disorder. Even in cases of acute physical illness, the adolescent may feel anxiety about having a physical examination. If future visits are to be successful, the physician must spend time on the first visit to foster a sense of trust and comfort.

It is helpful at the beginning of the visit to talk with the adolescent and the parents about what to expect. The physician should address the issue of confidentiality, telling the parents that two meetings—one with the teenager alone and one with only the parents—will take place. Adequate time must be spent with both patient and parents or important information may be missed. At the beginning of the interview with the patient, it is useful to say, "I am likely to ask you some personal questions. This is not because I am trying to pry into your personal affairs, but because these questions may be important to your health. I want to assure you that what we talk about is confidential, just between the two of us. If there is something I feel we should discuss with your parents, I will ask your permission first unless I feel it is life-threatening."

THE STRUCTURE OF THE VISIT

Caring for adolescents is time-intensive. In many adolescent practices, a 40%–50% no-show rate is not unusual. The stated chief complaint often conceals the patient's real concern.

For example, a 15-year-old girl may say she has a sore throat but actually may be worried about being pregnant.

By age 11 or 12 years, patients should be seen alone. This gives them an opportunity to ask questions they may be embarrassed to ask in front of a parent. Because of the physical changes that take place in early puberty, some adolescents are too self-conscious to undress in front of a parent. If an adolescent comes in willingly, for an acute illness or for a routine physical examination, it may be helpful to meet with the adolescent and parent together to obtain the history. For angry adolescents brought in against their will, it is useful to meet with the parents and patient for 3–5 minutes to allow the parents to describe the conflict and voice their concerns. The adolescent should then be seen alone. This approach conveys that the physician is primarily interested in the adolescent patient, yet gives the physician an opportunity to acknowledge parental concerns.

The Interview

The first few minutes may determine whether or not a trusting relationship can be established. A few minutes just getting to know the patient is time well spent. For example, immediately asking "Do you smoke marijuana?" when a teenager is brought in for suspected marijuana use confirms the adolescent's negative preconceptions about the physician and the purpose of the visit. It is preferable to spend a few minutes asking nonthreatening questions, such as "Tell me a little bit about yourself so I can get to know you," "What do you like to do most?" "Least?" and "What are your friends like?" Neutral questions help defuse some of the patient's anger and anxiety. Toward the end of the interview, the physician can ask more directed questions about psychosocial concerns.

Medical history questionnaires for the patient and the parents are useful in collecting historical data (Figure 4–2). The history should include an assessment of progress with psychodevelopmental tasks and of behaviors potentially detrimental to health. The review of systems should include questions about the following:

1. Nutrition: Number and balance of meals; calcium, iron, fiber, and cholesterol intake; body image.
2. Sleep: Number of hours, problems with insomnia or frequent waking.
3. Seat belt or helmet: Regularity of use.
4. Self-care: Knowledge of testicular or breast self-examination, dental hygiene, and exercise.
5. Family relationships: Parents, siblings, relatives.
6. Peers: Best friend, involvement in group activities, gangs, boyfriends, girlfriends.
7. School: Attendance, grades, activities.
8. Educational and vocational interests: College, career, short-term and long-term vocational plans.
9. Tobacco: Use of cigarettes, chewing and smokeless tobacco.
10. Substance abuse: Frequency, extent, and history of alcohol and drug use.
11. Sexuality: Sexual activity, contraceptive use, pregnancies, history of STI, number of sexual partners, risk for human immunodeficiency virus (HIV) infection.
12. Emotional health: Signs of depression, anxiety, and excessive stress.

The physician's personal attention and interest is likely to be a new experience for the teenager, who has probably received medical care only through a parent. The teenager should leave the visit with a sense of having a personal physician.

Physical Examination

During early adolescence, teenagers may be shy and modest, especially with a physician of the opposite sex. The examiner should address this concern directly, because it can be allayed by acknowledging the uneasiness verbally and by explaining the purpose of the examination. For example, "Many boys that I see who are your age are embarrassed to have their penis and testes examined. This is an important part of the examination for a couple of reasons. First, I want to make sure that there aren't any physical problems, and second, it helps me determine if your development is proceeding normally." This also introduces the subject of sexual development for discussion.

A pictorial chart of sexual development is useful for showing the patient how development is proceeding and what changes to expect. Figure 4–3 shows the relationship between height, penis and testes development, and pubic hair growth in the male, and Figure 4–4 shows the relationship between height, breast development, menstruation, and pubic hair growth in the female. Although teenagers may not admit that they are interested in this subject, they are usually attentive when it is raised. This discussion is particularly useful in counseling teenagers who lag behind their peers in physical development.

Because teenagers are sensitive about their changing bodies, it is useful to comment during the examination: "Your heart sounds fine. I feel a small lump under your right breast. This is very common during puberty in boys. It is called gynecomastia and should disappear in 6 months to a year."

Bright Futures: Guidelines for Health Supervision of Infants, Children, and Adolescents. American Academy of Pediatrics, 2007.

Ford C, English A, Sigman G: Confidential Health Care for Adolescents: Position paper for the Society for Adolescent Medicine. J Adolesc Health 2004;35:160 [PMID: 15298005].

CONFIDENTIAL

ADOLESCENT HEALTH HISTORY

This information is **CONFIDENTIAL**. Its purpose is to help your doctor give you better care. We request that you fill out the form completely, but you may skip any question that you do not wish to answer.

NAME ______________________________ DATE ______________

First   Middle Initial   Last

BIRTHDATE ______________ **AGE** ________ Name you like to be called ______________

1. Why did you come to the clinic today? ______________________________

MEDICAL HISTORY

2. Are you allergic to any medicines? .... YES NO
   If Yes: Name of Medicine ______________________________
3. Are you taking any medicines now? .... YES NO
   If Yes: Name of Medicine ______________________________
4. Were you born prematurely or did you have any serious problems as an infant? .... YES NO
5. Do you have any chronic health conditions? .... YES NO
   Condition ______________________________
6. Have you ever been hospitalized? .... YES NO
   Have you had any serious or sports related injuries? .... YES NO
   If YES to any of the above: Describe the reason/problem:

DATE	REASON/PROBLEM
______	______________________________
______	______________________________
______	______________________________

7. Have you ever had any of the following infections, illnesses or problems?
   If Yes: Write down your age when the infection, illness or problem started:

	Yes	No	Age		Yes	No	Age
Chickenpox	____	____	____	Pneumonia	____	____	____
Epilepsy/Seizures	____	____	____	Mononucleosis	____	____	____
Migraines	____	____	____	Tuberculosis	____	____	____
Heart Disease	____	____	____	Arthritis	____	____	____
Asthma	____	____	____	Scoliosis	____	____	____
Acne	____	____	____	Anemia	____	____	____
Stomach problems	____	____	____	Diabetes	____	____	____
Urine Infections	____	____	____	Thyroid Disease	____	____	____
Hepatitis	____	____	____	Cancer	____	____	____
Sexually Transmitted Diseases	____	____	____	Eczema	____	____	____
				Other____________			____

SCHOOL INFORMATION

8. Are you in school? .... YES NO
   If Yes: Name of school ______________________________
   a. What grade are you in, or the highest grade you completed? ______________
   (i.e.: 7th, 8th, 9th, 10th, 11th, 12th, College)
   b. What grade do you usually make in English? ________ (i.e.: A, B, C, D, E, F)
   c. What grade do you usually make in math? ________
   d. How many days were you absent from school last semester? ________
   If No: e. Why did you leave? ______________________________
9. Have you ever been suspended or expelled? .... YES NO

▲ **Figure 4–2.** Adolescent medical history questionnaire. (*Continued*)

10. Have you ever dropped out of school? .... YES NO

JOB/CAREER INFORMATION

11. Are you working? .... YES NO

If Yes, what is your job? ______
How many hours do you work each week? ______

12. What are your future plans or career goals? ______

FAMILY INFORMATION

13. Who do you live with? (Check all that apply)

_____ Both natural parents _____ Stepmother _____ Brother(s)/ages: ______
_____ Mother _____ Stepfather _____ Sister(s)/ages: ______
_____ Father _____ Guardian _____ Foster Home: ______
_____ Adoptive parents _____ Alone _____ Other: explain: ______

14. Were you adopted? .... YES NO
15. Have there been any changes in your family since your last visit here such as:

_____ Marriage _____ Serious illness _____ Births
_____ Separation _____ Loss of job _____ Deaths
_____ Divorce _____ Move to a new house _____ Other

If Checked: Please explain: ______

16. Father's/stepfather's occupation or job: ______
Mother's/stepmother's occupation or job: ______
17. How satisfied are you with how well you get along with your family?

_____ A lot _____ Somewhat _____ Not much _____ Not at all

18. How much tension or conflict is there in your family?

_____ None _____ A little _____ A fair amount _____ A Lot

19. Have you ever lived in foster care or an institution? .... YES NO

SELF-INFORMATION

20. What do you like about yourself? ______
21. What do you do best? ______
22. If you could, what would you like to change about your life or yourself? ______
______
______
23. List any habits you would like to break: ______
24. Have you lost or gained any weight in the last year? .... YES NO

If Yes: (circle) Gained **OR** Lost How much? ______

25. In the past year, have you tried to lose weight or control your weight by vomiting, taking diet pills or laxatives, or starving yourself? .... YES NO
26. Do you feel you have any friends you can count on? .... YES NO
27. Have you ever run away from home overnight? .... YES NO
28. Have you gotten into any trouble because of your anger/temper? .... YES NO
29. Have you been in a pushing/shoving fight during the past 6 months? .... YES NO
30. Is there a gun in your house? .... YES NO
31. Have you ever threatened or been threatened with a knife/gun/or other weapon? .... YES NO
32. Have you ever seen someone shot or stabbed? .... YES NO
33. Have you ever been physically or sexually abused? .... YES NO

▲ **Figure 4-2.** (*Continued*)

HEALTH CONCERNS

In the past two weeks, how often have you been bothered by each of the following symptoms:

PHQ-9	Not At All (0)	Several Days (1)	More Than Half the Days (2)	Nearly Every Day (3)
1. Feeling down, depressed, irritable, or hopeless?				
2. Little interest or pleasure in doing things?				
3. Trouble falling asleep, staying asleep, or sleeping too much?				
4. Poor appetite, weight loss, or overeating?				
5. Feeling tired, or having little energy?				
6. Feeling bad about yourself – or feeling that you are a failure, or that you have let yourself or your family down?				
7. Trouble concentrating on things like school work, reading, or watching TV?				
8. Moving or speaking so slowly that other people could have noticed? Or the opposite – being so fidgety or restless that you were moving around a lot more than usual?				
9. Thoughts that you would be better off dead, or of hurting yourself in some way?				

Kroenke K, Spitzer RL. The PHQ-9: A new depression and diagnostic severity measure. Psychiatric Annals 2002; 32: 509 – 521.

34. Do you have any questions or concerns about any of the following? (Check all that apply)

_____ Too tall
_____ Too short
_____ Overweight
_____ Underweight
_____ Blood pressure
_____ Headaches/migraines
_____ Dizziness/passing out
_____ Eyes/vision
_____ Ears/hearing/earaches
_____ Bloody nose
_____ Hay fever
_____ Frequent colds
_____ Mouth/teeth
_____ Neck/back
_____ Chest pain
_____ Wheezing

_____ Cough
_____ Breasts
_____ Heart
_____ Stomach pain
_____ Nausea/vomiting
_____ Diarrhea/Constipation
_____ Rash
_____ Acne/complexion
_____ Arms, legs/muscle or joint pain
_____ Frequent or painful urination
_____ Wetting the bed
_____ Sexual organs/genitals
_____ Trouble sleeping
_____ Tiredness
_____ Diet/food/appetite
_____ Eating disorder

_____ Smoking, drugs, alcohol
_____ Future plans/job
_____ Worried about parent(s)
_____ Family Violence/physical abuse
_____ Feeling down or depressed
_____ Dating
_____ Sex
_____ Worried about STD
_____ Masturbation
_____ Having children/ parenting/adoption
_____ Cancer or dying
_____ Other (explain) _____________
____

HEALTH BEHAVIOR INFORMATION

35. Do you wear a seatbelt every time you ride in a car? .... YES NO
36. Have you ever been the driver in an auto accident? .... YES NO
37. Have you ever driven after drinking alcohol or when high? .... YES NO
38. Do you ever smoke cigarettes or use snuff or chewing tobacco? .... YES NO
39. Do you ever use marijuana? .... YES NO
40. In the past month, did you get drunk or very high on beer, wine, or other alcohol? .... YES NO

▲ **Figure 4–2.** (*Continued*)

Revised 11/28/2011

41. Have you ever used street drugs (speed, cocaine, acid, crack, etc.)? .... YES NO
42. Does anyone in your household smoke? .... YES NO
43. Does anyone in your family have a problem with drugs or alcohol? .... YES NO
44. Have you ever been in trouble with the police or the law? .... YES NO
45. Have you begun dating? .... YES NO
46. Do you currently have a boyfriend or girlfriend? .... YES NO
    If Yes: How old is he/she? ________
47. Do you think you might be gay, lesbian, bisexual or transgender? .... YES NO
48. Have you ever had sex (sexual intercourse)? .... YES NO
    If Yes: Are you (or your partner) using any birth control to prevent pregnancy? .... YES NO
    Have you ever been treated for gonorrhea or chlamydia or other sexually transmitted diseases? .... YES NO
    During your life, with how many people have you had sexual intercourse?.......... ________
49. Have you been taught how to use a condom correctly? .... YES NO
50. Do you have any other personal problems that you would like to discuss with the doctor but would rather not write down? ... . YES NO

For males only

51. If you have had sex, do you use a condom every time? .... YES NO
52. Have you ever fathered a child? .... YES NO

For females only

53. How old were you when your periods began? ____________
54. What date did your last period start? ______________
55. Are your periods regular (once a month)?.......... YES NO
56. Do you have painful or excessively heavy periods? .... YES NO
57. Have you ever had a vaginal infection or been treated for a female disorder? .... YES NO
58. Do you think you might be pregnant? .... YES NO
59. Have you ever been pregnant? .... YES NO

FAMILY HISTORY

60. Have any of your relatives (parents, grandparents, uncles, aunts, brothers or sisters), living or deceased, had any of the following problems? If the answer is **YES**, please state their relationship to you.

	YES	RELATIONSHIP		YES	RELATIONSHIP
ADHD			High Blood Pressure		
Alcoholism			High Cholesterol		
Anemia			Kidney Disease		
Anxiety			Mental Retardation		
Asthma			Migraine Headaches		
Bipolar			Obesity		
Blood Clots			Seizure disorder/Epilepsy		
Cancer			Stomach Disorders		
Depression			Stroke		
Diabetes			Suicide		
Drug Problems			Thyroid Disease		
Eating Disorder			Tuberculosis		
Heart Attack			Other		

▲ **Figure 4-2.** (*Continued*)

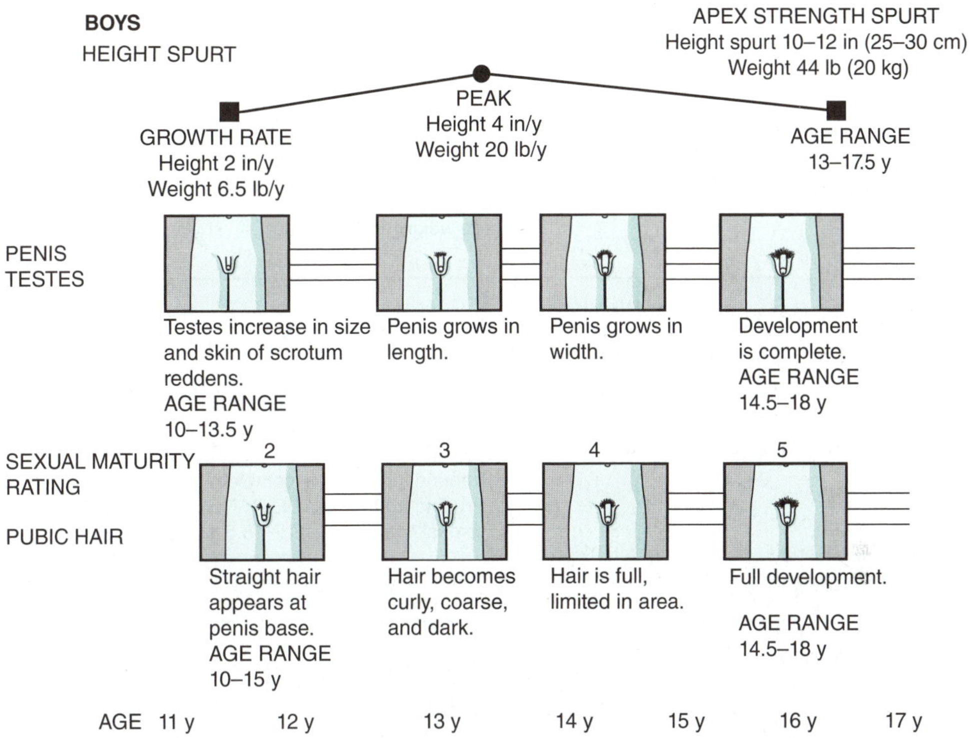

▲ **Figure 4–3.** Adolescent male sexual maturation and growth.

GROWTH & DEVELOPMENT

PUBERTY

Pubertal growth and physical development are a result of activation of the hypothalamic-pituitary-gonadal axis in late childhood. Before puberty, pituitary and gonadal hormone levels are low. At onset of puberty, the inhibition of gonadotropin-releasing hormone in the hypothalamus is removed, allowing pulsatile production and release of the gonadotropins, luteinizing hormone (LH), and follicle-stimulating hormone (FSH). In early to middle adolescence, pulse frequency and amplitude of LH and FSH secretion increase, stimulating the gonads to produce estrogen or testosterone. In females, FSH stimulates ovarian maturation, granulosa cell function, and estradiol secretion. LH is important in ovulation and also is involved in corpus luteum formation and progesterone secretion. Initially, estradiol inhibits the release of LH and FSH. Eventually, estradiol becomes stimulatory, and the secretion of LH and FSH becomes cyclic. Estradiol levels progressively increase, resulting in maturation of the female genital tract and breast development.

In males, LH stimulates the interstitial cells of the testes to produce testosterone. FSH stimulates the production of spermatocytes in the presence of testosterone. The testes also produce inhibin, a Sertoli cell protein that inhibits the secretion of FSH. During puberty, circulating testosterone levels increase more than 20-fold. Levels of testosterone correlate with the physical stages of puberty and the degree of skeletal maturation.

PHYSICAL GROWTH

A teenager's weight almost doubles in adolescence, and height increases by 15%–20%. During puberty, major organs double in size, except for lymphoid tissue, which decreases in mass. Before puberty, there is little difference in the muscular strength of boys and girls. The muscle mass and muscle strength both increase during puberty, with maximal strength lagging behind the increase in mass by many months. Boys attain greater strength and mass, and strength continues to increase into late puberty. Although motor coordination lags behind growth in stature and musculature, it continues to improve as strength increases.

The pubertal growth spurt begins nearly 2 years earlier in girls than in boys. Girls reach peak height velocity between ages 11½ and 12 years, and boys between ages 13½ and 14 years. Linear growth at peak velocity is 9.5 cm/y ± 1.5 cm in boys and 8.3 cm/y ± 1.2 cm in girls. Pubertal growth lasts

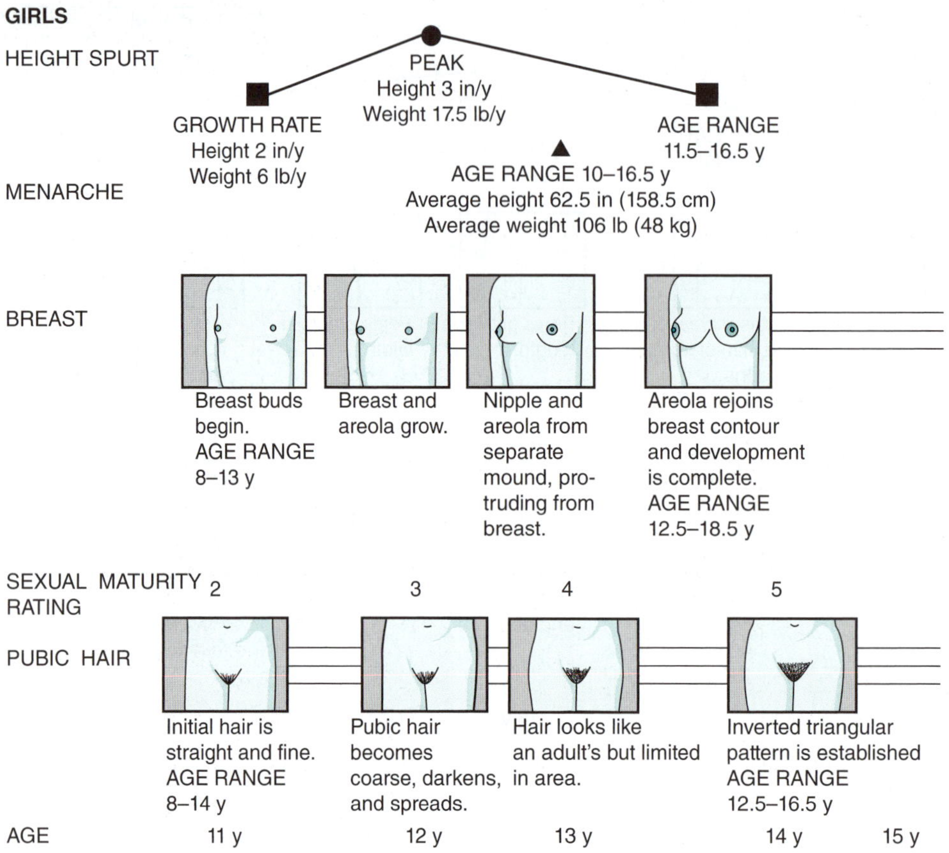

▲ **Figure 4–4.** Adolescent female sexual maturation and growth.

about 2–4 years and continues longer in boys than in girls. By age 11 years in girls and age 12 years in boys, 83%–89% of ultimate height is attained. An additional 18–23 cm in females and 25–30 cm in males is achieved during late pubertal growth. Following menarche, height rarely increases more than 5–7.5 cm.

In boys, the lean body mass increases from 80% to 85% to approximately 90% at maturity. Muscle mass doubles between 10 and 17 years. By contrast, in girls, the lean body mass decreases from approximately 80% of body weight in early puberty to approximately 75% at maturity.

SEXUAL MATURATION

Sexual maturity rating (SMR) is useful for categorizing genital development. SMR staging includes age ranges of normal development and specific descriptions for each stage of pubic hair growth, penis and testis development in boys, and breast maturation in girls. Figures 4–3 and 4–4 show this chronologic development. SMR 1 is prepuberty and SMR 5 is adult maturity. In SMR 2 the pubic hair is sparse, fine, nonpigmented, and downy; in SMR 3, the hair becomes pigmented and curly and increases in amount; and in SMR 4, the hair is adult in texture but limited in area. The appearance of pubic hair precedes axillary hair by more than 1 year. Male genital development begins with SMR 2 during which the testes become larger and the scrotal skin reddens and coarsens. In SMR 3, the penis lengthens; and in SMR 4, the penis enlarges in overall size and the scrotal skin becomes pigmented.

Female breast development follows a predictable sequence. Small, raised breast buds appear in SMR 2. In SMR 3, the breast and areolar tissue generally enlarge and become elevated. The areola and nipple form a separate mound from the breast in SMR 4, and in SMR 5 the areola assumes the same contour as the breast.

There is great variability in the timing and onset of puberty and growth, and psychosocial development does not always parallel physical changes. Chronologic age, therefore, may be a poor indicator of physiologic and psychosocial development. Skeletal maturation correlates well with growth and pubertal development.

Teenagers began entering puberty earlier in the last century because of better nutrition and socioeconomic conditions. In the United States, the average age at menarche is 12.53 years, but varies by race and ethnicity; 12.57 for non-Hispanic whites; 12.09 years in non-Hispanic blacks, and 12.09 for Mexican American girls. Among girls reaching menarche, the average weight is 48 kg, and the average height is 158.5 cm. Menarche may be delayed until age 16 years or may begin as early as age 10. Although the first measurable sign of puberty in girls is the beginning of the height spurt, the first conspicuous sign is usually the development of breast buds between 8 and 11 years. Although breast development usually precedes the growth of pubic hair, the sequence may be reversed. A common concern for girls at this time is whether the breasts will be of the right size and shape, especially because initial breast growth is often asymmetrical. The growth spurt starts at about age 9 years in girls and peaks at age 11½ years, usually at SMR 3–4 breast development and stage 3 pubic hair development. The spurt usually ends by age 14 years. Girls who mature early will reach peak height velocity sooner and attain their final height earlier. Girls who mature late will attain a greater final height because of the longer period of growth before the growth spurt ends. Final height is related to skeletal age at onset of puberty as well as genetic factors. The height spurt correlates more closely with breast developmental stages than with pubic hair stages.

The first sign of puberty in the male, usually between ages 10 and 12 years, is scrotal and testicular growth. Pubic hair usually appears early in puberty but may do so any time between ages 10 and 15 years. The penis begins to grow significantly a year or so after the onset of testicular and pubic hair development, usually between ages 10 and 13½ years. The first ejaculation usually occurs about 1 year after initiation of testicular growth, but its timing is highly variable. About 90% of boys have this experience between ages 11 and 15 years. Gynecomastia, a hard nodule under the nipple, occurs in a majority of boys, with a peak incidence between ages 14 and 15 years. Gynecomastia usually disappears within 6 months to 2 years. The height spurt begins at age 11 years but increases rapidly between ages 12 and 13 years, with the peak height velocity reached at age 13½ years. The period of pubertal development lasts much longer in boys and may not be completed until age 18 years. The height velocity is higher in males (8–11 cm/y) than in females (6.5–9.5 cm/y). The development of axillary hair, deepening of the voice, and the development of chest hair in boys usually occur in midpuberty, about 2 years after onset of growth of pubic hair. Facial and body hair begin to increase at age 16–17 years.

Anderson SE, Must A: Interpreting the continued decline in the average age at menarche: Results from two nationally representative surveys of U.S. girls studied 10 years apart. J Pediatr 2005;147(6):753–760.

Susman EJ, Houts RM et al: Longitudinal development of secondary sexual characteristics in girls and boys between ages 91/2 and 151/2 years. Arch Pediatr Adolesc Med 2010;164(2):166–173.

Rogol AD et al: Growth at puberty. J Adolesc Health 2002;31(Suppl): 192 [PMID: 12470915].

Rosen DS: Physiologic growth and development during adolescence. Pediatr Rev 2004;25:194 [PMID: 15173452].

PSYCHOSOCIAL DEVELOPMENT

Adolescence is a period of progressive individuation and separation from the family. Adolescents must learn who they are, decide what they want to do, and identify their personal strengths and weaknesses. Because of the rapidity of physical, emotional, cognitive, and social growth during adolescence, it is useful to divide it into three phases. Early adolescence is roughly from 10 to 13 years of age; middle adolescence is from 14 to 16 years; and late adolescence is from 17 years and later.

Early Adolescence

Early adolescence is characterized by rapid growth and development of secondary sex characteristics. Body image, self-concept, and self-esteem fluctuate dramatically. Concerns about how personal growth and development deviate from that of peers may be great, especially in boys with short stature or girls with delayed breast development or delayed menarche. Although there is a certain curiosity about sexuality, young adolescents generally feel more comfortable with members of the same sex. Peer relationships become increasingly important. Young teenagers still think concretely and cannot easily conceptualize about the future. They may have vague and unrealistic professional goals, such as becoming a movie star or a lead singer in a rock group.

Middle Adolescence

During middle adolescence, as rapid pubertal development subsides, teenagers become more comfortable with their new bodies. Intense emotions and wide swings in mood are typical. Although some teenagers go through this experience relatively peacefully, others struggle. Cognitively, the middle adolescent moves from concrete thinking to formal operations and abstract thinking. With this new mental power comes a sense of omnipotence and a belief that the world can be changed by merely thinking about it. Sexually active teenagers may believe they do not need to worry about using contraception because they can't get pregnant ("it won't happen to me"). Sixteen-year-old drivers believe they are the best drivers in the world and think the insurance industry is conspiring against them by charging high rates for automobile insurance. With the onset of abstract thinking, teenagers begin to see themselves as others see them and may become extremely self-centered. Because they are establishing their own identities, relationships with peers and others are narcissistic. Experimenting with different self-images is common. As sexuality increases in importance, adolescents may begin dating and experimenting with sex. Relationships tend to be one-sided and narcissistic. Peers determine the standards for identification, behavior, activities, and clothing and provide emotional support, intimacy, empathy, and the sharing of guilt and anxiety during the struggle for autonomy. The struggle for independence and autonomy is often a stressful period for both teenagers and parents.

Late Adolescence

During late adolescence, the young person generally becomes less self-centered and more caring of others. Social relationships shift from the peer group to the individual. Dating becomes much more intimate. By 10th grade, 40.9% of adolescents (41.9% of males and 39.6% of females) have had sexual intercourse, and by 12th grade, this has increased to 62.3% (59.6% of males and 65% of females). Abstract thinking allows older adolescents to think more realistically about their plans for the future. This is a period of idealism; older adolescents have rigid concepts of what is right or wrong.

Sexual Orientation

Sexual orientation develops during early childhood. Gender identity is established by age 2 years, and a sense of masculinity or femininity usually solidifies by age 5 or 6 years. Homosexual adults describe homosexual feelings during late childhood and early adolescence, years before engaging in overt homosexual acts.

Although only 5%–10% of American young people acknowledge having had homosexual experiences and only 5% feel that they are or could be gay, homosexual experimentation is common, especially during early and middle adolescence. Experimentation may include mutual masturbation and fondling the genitals and does not by itself cause or lead to adult homosexuality. Theories about the causes of homosexuality include genetic, hormonal, environmental, and psychological models.

The development of homosexual identity in adolescence commonly progresses through two stages. The adolescent feels different and develops a crush on a person of the same sex without clear self-awareness of a gay identity and then goes through a coming-out phase in which the homosexual identity is defined for the individual and revealed to others. The coming-out phase may be a difficult period for the young person and the family. The young adolescent is afraid of societal bias and seeks to reject homosexual feelings. The struggle with identity may include episodes of both homosexual and heterosexual promiscuity, STI, depression, substance abuse, attempted suicide, school avoidance and failure, running away from home, and other crises.

In a clinical setting, the issue of homosexual identity most often surfaces when the teenager is seen for an STI, family conflict, school problem, attempted suicide, or substance abuse rather than as a result of a consultation about sexual orientation. Pediatricians should be aware of the psychosocial and medical implications of homosexual identity and be sensitive to the possibility of these problems in gay adolescents. Successful management depends on the physician's ability to gain the trust of the gay adolescent and on the physician's knowledge of the wide range of medical and psychological problems for which gay adolescents are at risk. Pediatricians must be nonjudgmental in posing sexual questions if they are to be effective in encouraging the teenager to share concerns. Physicians who for religious or other personal reasons cannot be objective must refer the homosexual patient to another professional for treatment and counseling.

Eisenberg ME, Resnick MD: Suicidality among gay, lesbian and bisexual youth: The role of protective factors. J Adolesc Health 2006;39:662 [PMID: 17046502].

Frankowski BL: American Academy of Pediatrics Committee on Adolescence. Sexual orientation and adolescents. Pediatrics 2004;113:1827 [PMID: 15173519].

Gutgesell ME, Payne N: Issues of adolescent psychological development in the 21st century. Pediatr Rev 2004;25:79 [PMID: 14993515].

Silenzio VM et al: Sexual orientation and risk factors for suicidal ideation and suicide attempts among adolescents and young adults. Am J Public Health 2007;97(11):2017–2019.

BEHAVIOR & PSYCHOLOGICAL HEALTH

It is not unusual for adolescents to seek medical attention for apparently minor complaints. In early adolescence, teenagers may worry about normal developmental changes such as gynecomastia. They may present with vague symptoms, but have a hidden agenda of concerns about pregnancy or an STI. Adolescents with emotional disorders often present with somatic symptoms—abdominal pain, headaches, dizziness, syncope, fatigue, sleep problems, and chest pain—which appear to have no biologic cause. The emotional basis of such complaints may be varied: somatoform disorder, depression, or stress and anxiety.

PSYCHOPHYSIOLOGIC SYMPTOMS & CONVERSION REACTIONS

The most common somatoform disorder of adolescence is conversion disorder or conversion reaction. A conversion reaction is a psychophysiologic process in which unpleasant feelings, especially anxiety, depression, and guilt, are communicated through a physical symptom. Psychophysiologic symptoms result when anxiety activates the autonomic nervous system, causing symptoms such as tachycardia, hyperventilation, and vasoconstriction. The emotional feeling may be threatening or unacceptable to the individual, who expresses it as a physical symptom rather than verbally. The process is unconscious, and the anxiety or unpleasant feeling is dissipated by the somatic symptom. The degree to which the conversion symptom lessens anxiety, depression, or the unpleasant feeling is referred to as primary gain. Conversion symptoms not only diminish unpleasant feelings but also release the adolescent from conflict or an uncomfortable situation. This is called secondary gain. Secondary gain may intensify the symptoms, especially with increased attention from concerned parents and friends. Adolescents with conversion symptoms tend to have overprotective parents and become increasingly dependent on their parents as the symptom becomes a major focus of concern in the family.

Clinical Findings

Symptoms may appear at times of stress. Nervous, gastrointestinal, and cardiovascular symptoms are common and include paresthesias, anesthesia, paralysis, dizziness, syncope, hyperventilation, abdominal pain, nausea, and vomiting. Specific symptoms may reflect existing or previous illness (eg, pseudoseizures in adolescents with epilepsy) or modeling of a close relative's symptom (eg, chest pain in a boy whose grandfather died of a heart attack). Conversion symptoms are more common in girls than in boys. Although they occur in patients from all socioeconomic levels, the complexity of the symptom may vary with the sophistication and cognitive level of the patient.

History and physical findings are usually inconsistent with a physical cause of symptoms. Conversion symptoms occur most frequently during stress and in the presence of individuals meaningful to the patient. The common personality traits of these patients include egocentricity, emotional lability, and dramatic, attention-seeking behaviors.

Differential Diagnosis

Conversion reactions must be differentiated from hypochondriasis, which is a preoccupation with developing or having a serious illness despite medical reassurance that there is no evidence of disease. Over time, the fear of one disease may give way to concern about another. In contrast to patients with conversion symptoms, who seem relieved if an organic cause is considered, patients with hypochondriasis become more anxious when such a cause is considered.

Malingering is uncommon during adolescence. The malingering patient consciously and intentionally fabricates or exaggerates physical or psychological symptoms. Such patients are motivated by external incentives such as avoiding work, evading criminal prosecution, obtaining drugs, or obtaining financial compensation. These patients may be hostile and aloof. Parents of patients with conversion disorders and malingering have a similar reaction to illness. They have an unconscious psychological need to have sick children and reinforce their child's behavior.

Somatic delusions are physical symptoms, often bizarre, that accompany other signs of mental illness. Examples are visual or auditory hallucinations, delusions, incoherence or loosening of associations, rapid shifts of affect, and confusion.

Treatment

The physician must emphasize from the outset that both physical and emotional causes of the symptom will be considered. The relationship between physical causes of emotional pain and emotional causes of physical pain should be described to the family, using examples such as stress causing an ulcer or making a severe headache worse. The patient should be encouraged to understand that the symptom may persist and that at least a short-term goal is to continue normal daily activities. Medication is rarely helpful. If the family will accept it, psychological referral is often a good initial step toward psychotherapy. If the family resists psychiatric or psychological referral, the pediatrician may need to begin to deal with some of the emotional factors responsible for the symptom while building rapport with the patient and family. Regular appointments should be scheduled. During visits, the teenager should be seen first and encouraged to talk about school, friends, the relationship with the parents, and the stresses of life. Discussion of the symptom itself should be minimized; however, the physician should be supportive and must never suggest that the pain is not real. As parents gain insight into the cause of the symptom, they will become less indulgent and facilitate resumption of normal activities. If management is successful, the adolescent will gain coping skills and become more independent, while decreasing secondary gain.

If the symptom continues to interfere with daily activities and if the patient and parents feel that no progress is being made, psychological referral is indicated. A psychotherapist experienced in treating adolescents with conversion reactions is in the best position to establish a strong therapeutic relationship with the patient and family. After referral is made, the pediatrician should continue to follow the patient to ensure compliance with psychotherapy.

American Psychiatric Association: Diagnostic and Statistical Manual of Mental Disorders, 4th ed, text revision. American Psychiatric Press, 2000.

Kreipe RE: The biopsychosocial approach to adolescents with somatoform disorders. Adolesc Med Clin 2006;17:1 [PMID: 16473291].

Silber TJ: Somatization disorders: Diagnosis, treatment, and prognosis. Pediatr Rev 2011;32(2):56–63.

DEPRESSION (SEE ALSO CHAPTER 7)

Symptoms of clinical depression (lethargy, loss of interest, sleep disturbances, decreased energy, feelings of worthlessness, and difficulty concentrating) are common during adolescence. The intensity of feelings during adolescence, often in response to seemingly trivial events such as a poor grade on an examination or not being invited to a party, makes it difficult to differentiate severe depression from normal sadness or dejection. In less severe depression, sadness or unhappiness associated with problems of everyday life is generally short-lived. The symptoms usually result in only minor impairment in school performance, social activities and relationships. Symptoms respond to support and reassurance.

Clinical Findings

The presentation of serious depression in adolescence may be similar to that in adults, with vegetative signs—depressed mood, crying spells, inability to cry, discouragement, irritability, a sense of emptiness and futility, negative expectations of oneself and the environment, low self-esteem, isolation, helplessness, diminished interest or pleasure in activities, weight loss or weight gain, insomnia or hypersomnia, fatigue or loss of energy, feelings of worthlessness, and diminished ability to think or concentrate. In adolescents, it is not unusual for a serious depression to be masked because the teenager cannot tolerate the severe feelings of sadness. Such a teenager may present with recurrent or persistent psychosomatic complaints, such as abdominal pain, chest pain, headache, lethargy, weight loss, dizziness, syncope, or other nonspecific symptoms. Other behavioral manifestations of masked depression include truancy, running away from home, defiance of authorities, self-destructive behavior, vandalism, drug and alcohol abuse, sexual acting out, and delinquency.

Differential Diagnosis

A complete history and physical examination, and review of the past medical and psychosocial history should be performed. The family history should be explored for psychiatric problems. Early onset depression and bipolar illness are more likely to occur in families with a multigenerational history of early onset and chronic depression. The lifetime risk of depressive illness in first-degree relatives of adult depressed patients is between 18% and 30%.

The teenager should be questioned about the symptoms of depression and, specifically, about suicidal ideation or preoccupation with thoughts of death. The history should include an assessment of school performance, looking for signs of academic deterioration, excessive absence, cutting class, changes in work or other outside activities, and changes in the family (eg, separation, divorce, serious illness, loss of employment by a parent, recent move to a new school, increasing quarrels or fights with parents, or death of a close relative). The teenager may have withdrawn from friends or family or switched allegiance to a new group of friends. The physician should inquire about possible physical and sexual abuse, drug and alcohol abuse, conflicts with the police, sexual acting-out, running away from home, unusually violent or rebellious behavior, or radical personality changes. Patients with vague somatic complaints or concerns about having a fatal illness may have an underlying affective disorder.

Adolescents with symptoms of depression require a thorough medical evaluation to rule out contributing or underlying medical illness. Among the medical conditions associated with affective disorders are eating disorders, organic central nervous system disorders (tumors, vascular lesions, closed head trauma, and subdural hematomas), metabolic and endocrinologic disorders (hypothyroidism, hyperthyroidism, hyperparathyroidism, Cushing syndrome, Addison disease, or premenstrual syndrome), Wilson disease, systemic lupus erythematosus, infections (infectious mononucleosis or syphilis), and mitral valve prolapse. Marijuana use, phencyclidine abuse, amphetamine withdrawal, and excessive caffeine intake can cause symptoms of depression. Common medications, including birth control pills, anticonvulsants, and β-blockers, may cause depressive symptoms.

Some screening laboratory studies for organic disease are indicated, including complete blood count and erythrocyte sedimentation rate, urinalysis, serum electrolytes, blood urea nitrogen, serum calcium, thyroxine and thyroid-stimulating hormone (TSH), Venereal Disease Research Laboratory testing or rapid plasma reagin, and liver enzymes. Although metabolic markers such as abnormal secretion of cortisol, growth hormone, and thyrotropin-releasing hormone have been useful in confirming major depression in adults, these neurobiologic markers are less reliable in adolescents.

Treatment

The primary care physician may be able to counsel adolescents and parents if depression is mild or situational and the patient is not contemplating suicide or other life-threatening behaviors. If there is evidence of a long-standing depressive disorder, suicidal thoughts, or psychotic thinking, or if the physician does not feel prepared to counsel the patient, psychological referral should be made.

Counseling involves establishing and maintaining a positive supportive relationship; following the patient at least weekly; remaining accessible to the patient at all times; encouraging the patient to express emotions openly, defining the problem, and clarifying negative feelings, thoughts, and expectations; setting realistic goals; helping to negotiate interpersonal crises; teaching assertiveness and social skills; reassessing the depression as it is expressed; and staying alert to the possibility of suicide.

Patients with bipolar disease or those with depression that is unresponsive to supportive counseling should be referred to a psychiatrist for evaluation and antidepressant medication. The Food and Drug Administration has issued a "black box warning" alerting providers that using antidepressants in children and adolescents may increase the risk of suicidal thoughts and behavior. Adolescents taking these medications should be monitored closely.

Belmaker RH: Bipolar disorder. N Engl J Med 2004;351:476 [PMID: 15282355].

Brent DA, Birmaher B: Clinical practice. Adolescent depression. N Engl J Med 2002;347:667 [PMID: 12200555].

Mann JJ: The medical management of depression. N Engl J Med 2005; 353:1819 [PMID: 16251538].

March JS, Vitiello B: Clinical messages from the Treatment for Adolescents With Depression Study (TADS). Am J Psychiatry 2009; 166(10):1118–1123.

Simon GE: The antidepressant quandary—considering suicide risk when treating adolescent depression. N Engl J Med 2006;355: 2722 [PMID: 17192536].

Wilkinson P, Dubicka B et al: Treated depression in adolescents: Predictors of outcome at 28 weeks. Br J Psychiatry 2009;194(4): 334–341.

ADOLESCENT SUICIDE (SEE ALSO CHAPTER 7)

In 2007, 4140 adolescents and young adults 15–24 years committed suicide, including 1481 suicides among those aged 15–19 years, and 2659 among those aged 20–24 years. In the younger group, males had a suicide rate five times higher than females, and white males had the highest rate, 15.5 per 100,000. The incidence of unsuccessful suicide attempts is three times higher in females than in males. The estimated ratio of attempted suicides to actual suicides is estimated to be 100:1–50:1. Firearms account for 50% of suicide deaths in both males and females.

Mood swings are common in adolescence. Short periods of depression are common and may be accompanied by thoughts of suicide. Normal adolescent mood swings rarely interfere with sleeping, eating, or normal activities. Acute depressive reactions (transient grief responses) to the loss of a family member or friend may cause depression lasting for weeks or even months. An adolescent who is unable to work through this grief can become increasingly depressed. A teenager who is unable to keep up with schoolwork, does not participate in normal social activities, withdraws socially, has sleep and appetite disturbances, and has feelings of hopelessness and helplessness should be considered at increased risk for suicide.

Angry teenagers attempting to influence others by their actions may be suicidal. They may be only mildly depressed and may not have any long-standing wish to die. Teenagers in this group, usually females, may attempt suicide or make an impulsive suicidal gesture as a way of getting back at someone or gaining attention by frightening another person. Adolescents with serious psychiatric disease such as acute schizophrenia or psychotic depressive disorder are also at risk for suicide.

Risk Assessment

The physician must determine the extent of the teenager's depression and the risk that he or she might inflict self-injury. Evaluation should include interviews with both the teenager and the family. The history should include the medical, social, emotional, and academic background. The PHQ-9 is a nine item standardized depression questionnaire that is incorporated in the Adolescent Health Questionnaire in the section labeled 'Health Concerns'. (See Figure 4-2.)

Treatment

The primary care physician is often in a unique position to identify an adolescent at risk for suicide because many teenagers who attempt suicide seek medical attention in the weeks preceding the attempt. These visits are often for vague somatic complaints. If the patient shows evidence of depression, the physician must assess the severity of the depression and suicidal risk. The pediatrician should always seek emergency psychological consultation for any teenager who is severely depressed, psychotic, or acutely suicidal. It is the responsibility of the psychologist or psychiatrist to assess the seriousness of suicidal ideation and decide whether hospitalization or outpatient treatment is most appropriate. Adolescents with mild depression and low risk for suicide should be followed closely, and the extent of the depression should be assessed on an ongoing basis. If it appears that the patient is worsening or is not responding to supportive counseling, referral should be made.

Prager LM: Depression and suicide in children and adolescents. Pediatr Rev 2009;30(6):199–205.

Wilkinson P, Kelvin R et al: Clinical and psychosocial predictors of suicide attempts and nonsuicidal self-injury in the Adolescent Depression Antidepressants and Psychotherapy Trial (ADAPT). Am J Psychiatry 2011;168(5):495–501.

Brent DA, Greenhill LL, Compton S et al: The Treatment of Adolescent Suicide Attempters study (TASA): Predictors of suicidal events in an open treatment trial. J Am Acad Child Adolesc Psychiatry 2009;48(10):987–996.

Connor J, Rueter M: Predicting adolescent suicidality: Comparing multiple informants and assessment techniques. J Adolesc 2009; 32(3):619–631.

Kroenke K, Spitzer RL: The PHQ-9: A new depression and diagnostic severity measure. Psychiatric Annals 2002;32:509–521.

Williams SB, O'Connor EA et al: Screening for child and adolescent depression in primary care settings: A systematic evidence review for the US Preventive Services Task Force. Pediatrics 2009;123(4):e716–e735.

Richardson LP, McCauley E et al: Evaluation of the patient health questionnaire-9 item for detecting major depression among adolescents. Pediatrics 2010;126(6):1117–1123.

Centers for Disease Control and Prevention: Suicide trends among youths and young adults aged 10–24 years—United States, 1990–2004. MMWR Morb Mortal Wkly Rep 2007;56(35): 905–908 [PMID: 17805220].

SUBSTANCE ABUSE

Substance abuse is a complex problem for adolescents and the broader society. See Chapter 5 for an in-depth look at this issue.

EATING DISORDERS (SEE CHAPTER 6)

OVERWEIGHT AND OBESITY (SEE ALSO CHAPTER 11)

Background

The prevalence of obesity among adolescents 12–19 years has increased from 5% to 17% in the past 25 years, with higher rates in black and Hispanic youth. Obesity during adolescence is defined using the 2000 Centers for Disease Control growth charts as a body mass index (BMI) > 95th percentile for age and gender. Overweight is defined as BMI between 85th and 95th percentiles for age and gender. An overweight adolescent has a 70% chance of becoming an obese adult. Figure 4–5 illustrates the multiple morbidities related to overweight and obesity during adolescence and the risk of the additional comorbidities associated with obesity in adulthood. Perhaps the most common short-term morbidities for overweight and obese adolescents are psychosocial, including social marginalization, poor self-esteem, depression, and poor quality of life. Like physical comorbidities, these psychosocial complications can extend into adulthood. Recent data on adolescent dietary and physical activity behaviors that potentiate overweight and obesity indicate that almost 80% of teens have deficient fiber intake, 63% have less than the recommended level of physical activity (60 minutes per day, 5 days per week), 33% watch 3 or more hours of television per average school day, and 25% participate in nonacademic computer activities for more than 3 hours per average school day.

Evaluation

Regular screening for overweight and obesity by measuring BMI during routine visits and providing anticipatory guidance for the adolescent and family regarding healthy nutrition and physical activity are essential for early identification and prevention of overweight and related comorbidities. A family history of obesity, diabetes mellitus, hypertension, hyperlipidemia, and coronary heart disease places the overweight young person at even higher risk of developing these comorbidities. Details of individual and family dietary behaviors, assessment of physical activity and time spent with sedentary activities, previous efforts to lose weight, and current readiness to change can identify

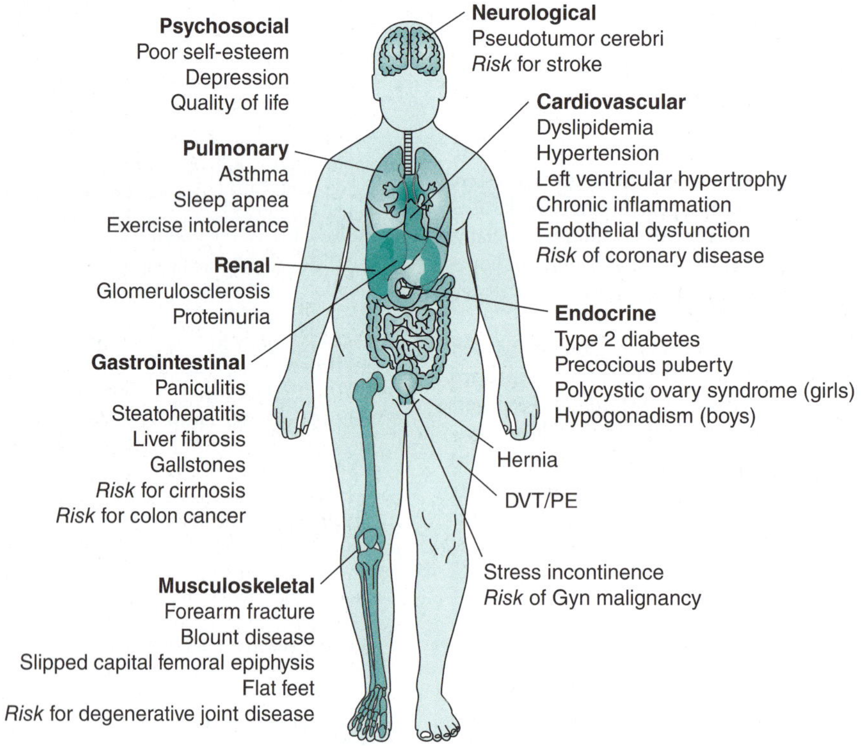

▲ **Figure 4–5.** Complications of obesity. DVT, Deep venous thrombosis; PE, pulmonary embolism. (Adapted and reproduced, with permission, from Xanthakos SA, Daniels SR, Inge TH: Bariatric surgery in adolescents: An update. Adolesc Med Clinics 2006;17.)

Table 4–1. Screening tests for overweight and obese adolescents in the primary care setting.

BMI	Risk Factors	Tests
85th–94th percentile	None	Fasting lipid levels
85th–94th percentile	Family history of obesity-related diseases; elevated blood pressure and/or lipid levels; tobacco use	Fasting lipid levels, AST and ALT, fasting serum glucose
≥ 95th percentile		Fasting lipid levels, AST and ALT, fasting serum glucose

ALT, alanine aminotransferase; AST, aspartate aminotransferase; BMI, body mass index.

areas for modifiable lifestyle behaviors to promote weight loss. The review of systems should include questions about symptoms associated with comorbid conditions including insulin resistance and diabetes, gallbladder disease or steatohepatitis, sleep dysfunction, and menstrual irregularities (female patients). If an overweight adolescent is otherwise healthy and has no delay in growth or sexual maturation, an underlying endocrinologic, neurologic, or genetic cause of overweight is unlikely. Key components of the history and physical evaluation of an overweight adolescent are outlined in Chapter 11. BMI percentile and the presence of risk factors for morbidities can serve as guides for laboratory evaluations of overweight adolescents in the primary care setting (Table 4–1).

Treatment

Comprehensive interventions that include both behavioral therapy and modifications in diet and physical activity seem to be the most successful approaches to obesity and its comorbidities, but clinical trials testing these interventions are limited. Several studies of childhood obesity treatment have confirmed the critical importance of parental participation in weight control programs. The greater independence of adolescents means that providers must discuss health behaviors directly with them while involving parents in the discussions and encouraging the whole family to make the home environment and family lifestyle a healthy one.

The most current evidence on obesity treatment in the pediatric population recommends a four-stage approach that includes (1) prevention plus (Table 4–2); (2) structured weight management; (3) comprehensive multidisciplinary intervention; and (4) tertiary care intervention. The treatment algorithm helps providers determine the appropriate weight management stage for each patient based on age, BMI percentile, comorbid disease, and past obesity treatment history. This approach is described further in Chapter 11

Table 4–2. Components of stage 1, "prevention plus" healthy lifestyle approach to weight management for adolescents.

Recommend ≥ 5 servings of fruits and vegetables per day.
No more than 2 h of screen time per day.
No television in room where teen sleeps.
Minimize or eliminate sugar-sweetened beverages.
Address eating behaviors (eg, avoid skipping breakfast).
Recommend ≥ 1 h of moderate intensity physical activity per day.[a]
Involve whole family in lifestyle changes and acknowledge cultural differences.

[a]Overweight teens will likely need to start with shorter periods of lower-intensity activity and gradually increase the time spent being active as well as the intensity of the activity.

and the detailed model can be found in the original publication, "Recommendations for Treatment of Child and Adolescent Overweight and Obesity in Pediatrics" by Spear and colleagues.

Providers caring for overweight and obese adolescents should identify comorbidities and treat them as indicated. For example, an overweight teen with daytime somnolence and disruptive snoring may need a sleep study to evaluate for obstructive sleep apnea. A nonpregnant overweight young woman with acanthosis nigricans and oligomenorrhea should be evaluated for polycystic ovary syndrome (PCOS). There are few guidelines regarding pharmacotherapy for obesity in the adolescent. Only two medications are currently approved. Sibutramine, a selective serotonin reuptake inhibitor (SSRI), is approved for patients age 16 and older. Orlistat, a lipase inhibitor, is approved for patients age 12 and older. In general, obese adolescents who might benefit from medication should be referred to a multidisciplinary weight loss program for evaluation and treatment as medication should only be used as part of a comprehensive program which includes diet, physical activity, and behavioral modifications. Bariatric surgery is reserved for severely obese adolescents who are physically mature, who have a BMI of 50 kg/m^2 or more (or ≥ 40 kg/m^2 with significant comorbidities), who have failed a structured 6 month weight loss program, and who are deemed by psychological assessment to be capable of adhering to the long-term lifestyle changes required after surgery.

Barlow SE: Expert committee recommendations regarding the prevention, assessment, and treatment of child and adolescent overweight and obesity: Summary report. Pediatrics 2007;120 (Suppl 4):S164–S192 [PMID: 18055651].

Daniels SR, Greer FR: Committee on Nutrition: Lipid screening and cardiovascular health in childhood. Pediatrics 2008;122(1): 198–208 [PMID: 18596007].

Davis MM et al: Recommendation for prevention of childhood obesity. Pediatrics 2007;120(Suppl 4):S229–S253 [PMID: 18055653].

Eaton DK et al: Youth risk behavior surveillance—United States, 2009. MMWR Surveill Summ 2010;59(5):1–142 [PMID 20520591]. Available at: http://www.cdc.gov/mmwr/pdf/ss/ss5905.pdf

Krebs NF et al: Assessment of child and adolescent overweight and obesity. Pediatrics 2007;120(Suppl 4):S193–S228 [PMID: 18055652].

Skelton JA et al: Prevalence and trends of severe obesity among US children and adolescents. Acad Pediatr 2009;9:322–329 [PMID: 19560993].

Spear BA et al: Recommendations for treatment of child and adolescent overweight and obesity. Pediatrics 2007;120(Suppl 4): S254–S288 [PMID: 18055654].

Xanthakos SA, Daniels SR, Inge TH: Bariatric surgery in adolescents: An update. Adolesc Med Clin 2006;17(3):589–612 [PMID: 17030281].

Growth charts are available at the Centers for Disease Control and Prevention web site, http://www.cdc.gov/growthcharts.

SCHOOL AVOIDANCE

A teenager who has missed more than 1 week of school for a physical illness or symptom and whose clinical picture is inconsistent with serious illness should be suspected of having primary or secondary emotional factors that contribute to the absence. Investigation of absences may show a pattern, such as missing morning classes or missing the same days at the beginning or end of the week.

School avoidance should be suspected in children who are consistently absent in spite of parental and professional attempts to encourage attendance. Adolescents with school avoidance often have a history of excessive school absences or separation difficulties as younger children. They may have a record of recurrent somatic complaints. Parents often feel helpless to compel their adolescent to attend school, may lack the sophistication to distinguish malingering from illness, or may have an underlying need to keep the teenager at home.

A complete history and physical examination should include a review of the patient's medical, educational, and psychiatric history. Any symptoms of emotional problems should be explored. After obtaining permission from the patient and parents, the physician may find it helpful to speak directly with school officials and some key teachers. The adolescent may be having problems with particular teachers or subjects or experiencing adversity at school (eg, bullying or an intimidating instructor). Some students get so far behind academically that they see no way of catching up and feel overwhelmed. Separation anxiety, sometimes of long duration, may be manifested in subconscious worries that something may happen to the mother while the teenager is at school.

The school nurse may have useful information on the frequency of nurse visits in past school years. It is important to determine the parent's typical responses to absences and somatic complaints. The parent(s) may be making subconscious attempts to keep the adolescent at home, which may in turn produce secondary gains for the patient that perpetuate the complaint.

Treatment

Returning to school quickly after a period of avoidance is key to recovery. The pediatrician should facilitate this process by offering to speak with school officials to excuse missed examinations, homework, and papers. The pediatrician should speak directly with teachers who are punitive with the objective of making the transition back to school as easy as possible. The longer adolescents stay out of school, the more anxious they may become about returning. If an illness or symptom becomes so severe that an adolescent cannot go to school, the patient and the parents must be informed that a visit to a medical office is necessary. The physician focuses visits on the parents as much as on the adolescent to alleviate parental guilt about sending the child to school. If the adolescent cannot stay in school, hospitalization should be recommended for in-depth medical and psychiatric evaluation. Parents should be cautioned about the possibility of relapse after school holidays, summer vacation, or an acute illness.

Hanna GL et al: Separation anxiety disorder and school refusal in children and adolescents. Pediatr Rev 2006;27:56 [PMID: 16452275].

Suveg C et al: Separation anxiety disorder, panic disorder, and school refusal. Child Adolesc Psychiatr Clin N Am 2005;14:773 [PMID: 16171702].

SCHOOL FAILURE

The amount and complexity of course work increase significantly in middle school at the same time as the rapid physical, social, and emotional changes of puberty. To perform well academically, young adolescents must have the necessary cognitive capacity, study habits, concentration, motivation, interest, and emotional focus. Academic failure presenting at adolescence has a broad differential:

1. Limited intellectual ability
2. Learning disabilities
3. Depression or emotional problems
4. Visual or hearing problems; other physical disability
5. Excessive school absenteeism secondary to chronic disease such as asthma or neurologic dysfunction
6. Inability to concentrate
7. Attention-deficit/hyperactivity disorder
8. Lack of motivation
9. Drug and alcohol use/abuse

Each of these causes must be explored. Evaluation requires a careful history, physical examination, appropriate laboratory tests, and standardized educational and psychological testing.

Treatment

Management must be individualized to fit the specific needs and foster the specific strengths of the patient. For children with learning disabilities, an individual prescription for special education courses, teachers, and extracurricular activities is important. Counseling helps these adolescents gain coping skills, raise self-esteem, and develop socialization skills. If the patient has hyperactivity or attention-deficit disorder causing poor ability to concentrate, a trial of stimulant medication (eg, methylphenidate or dextroamphetamine) may be useful. If the teenager is depressed or if other serious emotional problems are uncovered, psychological evaluation should be recommended.

Wilens TE et al: Attention-deficit/hyperactivity disorder in adults. JAMA 2004;292:619 [PMID: 15292088].

Wolraich ML et al: Attention-deficit/hyperactivity disorder among adolescents: A review of the diagnosis, treatment, and clinical implications. Pediatrics 2005;115:1734 [PMID: 15930238].

BREAST DISORDERS

The breast examination should be part of the routine physical examination in girls as soon as breast budding occurs. The preadolescent will thus accept breast examination as a routine part of health care, and the procedure can serve as an opportunity to offer reassurance and education. The breast examination begins with inspection of the breasts for symmetry and SMR stage. Asymmetrical breast development is common in young adolescents, and is generally transient, although 25% of women may continue to have asymmetry as adults. Organic causes of breast asymmetry include unilateral breast hypoplasia, amastia, absence of the pectoralis major muscle, and unilateral juvenile hypertrophy, in which there is rapid overgrowth of breast tissue usually immediately after thelarche.

The breast examination is performed with the patient supine and the ipsilateral arm placed behind the head. Using flat finger pads, the examiner palpates the breast tissue in concentric circles starting at the outer borders of the breast tissue along the sternum, clavicle, and axilla and then moving in toward the areola. The areola should be compressed gently to check for nipple discharge. Supraclavicular and infraclavicular and axillary regions should be palpated for lymph nodes.

Teaching adolescents to perform breast self-examinations is controversial. In the past, experts have recommended adolescent self-examination as a means of helping them develop comfort with their changing bodies and for future cancer detection. More recently, however, experts have questioned whether self-examination might in fact result in anxiety, increased physician visits, and unnecessary invasive procedures since the vast majority of breast masses in adolescents are benign. The U.S. Preventive Services Task Force found little evidence that teaching or performing routine breast self-examination in adolescents reduces breast cancer mortality. Despite the lack of data for or against teaching or performing breast self-examinations during adolescence, there is some consensus that young women at increased risk of breast cancer—adolescents with a history of malignancy, adolescents who are at least 10 years postradiation therapy to the chest, and adolescents 18–21 year s of age whose mothers carry the *BRCA 1* or *BRCA 2* gene—should perform monthly breast self-examinations after each menstrual period.

BREAST MASSES

The majority of breast masses in adolescents are benign (Table 4–3). The incidence of primary and secondary breast cancers in girls aged 15–19 years during 2004–2008 was 0.2 per 100,000. Rare malignancies of adolescent girls include juvenile secretory carcinoma, intraductal carcinoma, rhabdomyosarcoma, malignant cystosarcoma phylloides, and metastatic tumor. Retrospective studies indicate that biopsies of breast masses in adolescents most commonly show fibroadenoma (67%), fibrocystic change (15%), and abscess or mastitis (3%).

Table 4–3. Breast masses in adolescent females.

Common
Fibroadenoma
Fibrocystic changes
Breast cysts (including subareolar cysts)
Breast abscess or mastitis
Fat necrosis (after trauma)
Less common (benign)
Lymphangioma
Hemangioma
Intraductal papilloma
Juvenile papillomatosis
Giant fibroadenoma
Neurofibromatosis
Nipple adenoma or keratoma
Mammary duct ectasia
Intramammary lymph node
Lipoma
Hematoma
Hamartoma
Galactocele
Rare (malignant or malignant potential)
Juvenile secretory carcinoma
Intraductal carcinoma
Cystosarcoma phylloides
Sarcomas (fibrosarcoma, malignant fibrous histiocytoma, rhabdomyosarcoma)
Metastatic cancer (hepatocellular carcinoma, lymphoma, neuroblastoma, rhabdomyosarcoma)

1. Fibroadenoma

Fibroadenomas are the most common breast masses of adolescent girls. These and other breast lesions are listed in Tables 4–3 and 4–4. Fibroadenomas are composed of glandular and fibrous tissue. A fibroadenoma is typically nontender and diagnosed clinically with exam findings of a rubbery, smooth, well-circumscribed, mobile mass most often in the upper outer quadrant of the breast, although fibroadenomas can be found in any quadrant. Ten to twenty five percent of girls will have multiple or bilateral lesions. Fibroadenomas are typically slow growing with average size 2–3 cm. They may remain static in size for months to years with 10%–40% completely resolving during adolescence. The dense fibroglandular tissue of the adolescent breast may cause false-positive results on standard mammograms. Thus, ultrasonography is the best imaging modality with which to evaluate a breast mass in an adolescent if further evaluation beyond the clinical exam is necessary. Fibroadenomas less than 5 cm can be monitored for growth or regression over 3–4 months. Further evaluation will be dictated by the patient's course with semiannual clinical examinations for a few years followed by annual examinations for a mass that is regressing. Patients with concerning breast masses including fibroadenomas that are larger than 5 cm, undiagnosed breast masses that are enlarging or have overlying skin changes, and any suspicious breast mass in a patient with a history of previous malignancy should be referred to a breast care specialist.

Table 4–4. Characteristics and management of breast lesions in adolescent females.

Fibroadenoma	2- to 3-cm, rubbery, well circumscribed, mobile, nontender. Commonly found in upper outer quadrant of the breast. Management is observation.
Giant juvenile fibroadenoma	Large, >5 cm fibroadenoma with overlying skin stretching and dilated superficial veins. Benign but requires excision for confirmation of diagnosis and for cosmetic reasons.
Breast cysts	Usually caused by ductal ectasia or blocked Montgomery tubercles, both of which can have associated nipple discharge. Ultrasound can help differentiate from solid mass. Most resolve spontaneously.
Fibrocystic changes	More common with advancing age after adolescence. Mild swelling and palpable nodularity in upper outer quadrants. Associated with cyclic premenstrual mastalgia.
Abscess	Often associated with overlying mastitis and/or purulent nipple discharge. Culture abscess material and/or nipple discharge before starting antibiotics.
Cystosarcoma phyllodes	Large, rapidly growing tumor associated with overlying skin changes, dilated veins and skin necrosis. Requires excision. Most often benign but can be malignant.
Intraductal papilloma	Palpable intraductal tumor, which is often subareolar with associated nipple discharge, but may be in the periphery of the breast in adolescents. Requires surgical excision.
Juvenile papillomatosis	Rare breast tumor characterized by a grossly nodular breast mass described as having a "Swiss-cheese" appearance. Requires surgical excision.
Fat necrosis	Localized inflammatory process in the breast; typically follows trauma (sports or seat belt injuries). Subsequent scarring may be confused with changes similar to those associated with malignancy.

2. Fibrocystic Breast Changes

Fibrocystic breast changes are much more common in adults than adolescents. Symptoms include mild swelling and palpable nodularity most commonly in the upper outer quadrants. Mastalgia is typically cyclic, usually occurring just before menstruation. Reassuring the young woman about the benign nature of the process may be all that is needed. Nonsteroidal anti-inflammatory medications such as ibuprofen or naproxen sodium help alleviate symptoms. Oral contraceptive pills are also beneficial. Supportive bras may provide symptomatic relief. Studies have shown no association between methylxanthine and fibrocystic breasts; however, some women report reduced symptoms when they discontinue caffeine.

3. Breast Abscess

Although breast feeding is the most common cause of mastitis, shaving or plucking periareolar hair, nipple piercing, and trauma occurring during sexual activity are predisposing factors in teenagers. The most common causative organisms are normal skin flora. The female with a breast abscess usually complains of unilateral breast pain, and examination reveals overlying inflammatory changes. The examination may be misleading in that the infection may extend deeper into the breast than suspected. *Staphylococcus aureus* is the most common pathogen. β-Hemolytic streptococci, *Escherichia coli,* and *Pseudomonas aeruginosa* have also been implicated. Fluctuant abscesses should be incised and drained and fluid cultured. Antimicrobial coverage for *S aureus* (including methicillin-resistant strains) should be given initially (generally orally, unless infection is severe) and the patient should be monitored closely for response to therapy until culture and sensitivity results are available.

Healing time after nipple piercing is 3–6 months. Health risks associated with nipple piercing, in addition to breast abscess, include allergic reactions to the jewelry, keloid scar formation, and increased risk of hepatitis B and C and HIV. Complications associated with abscess formation secondary to nipple piercing include endocarditis, cardiac valve injury, cardiac prosthesis infection, metal foreign body reaction in the breast tissue, and recurrent infection.

NIPPLE DISCHARGE AND GALACTORRHEA

Ductal ectasia is a common cause of nipple discharge in the developing breast and is associated with dilation of the mammary ducts, periductal fibrosis, and inflammation. It can present with bloody, brown, or sticky multicolored nipple discharge and/or a cystic breast mass, which is usually in the subareolar region. Blocked ducts and fluid collections usually resolve spontaneously but can become infected, producing mastitis. Patients should look for erythema, warmth, and tenderness indicating mastitis. Oral antibiotics covering skin flora should be initiated if infection is suspected. Serous or serosanguineous nipple discharge is common and can be associated with fibrocystic breast changes. Montgomery tubercles are small glands located at the outer aspect of the areola that can drain clear or brownish fluid through an ectopic opening on the areola and may be associated with a small subareolar mass. These lesions and discharge typically resolve spontaneously. Intraductal papillomas arising from proliferation of ductal cells projecting into the duct lumen are a rare cause of bloody or serosanguineous nipple discharge and can also present with a subareolar or peripheral mass. These lesions are associated with increased risk of malignancy in adults.

Galactorrhea is distinguishable from other causes of nipple discharge by its milky character and tendency to involve both breasts. It is usually benign. The most common causes include chronic stimulation or irritation of the nipple, medications and illicit drugs (drugs causing galactorrhea are listed in Table 4–5), pregnancy, childbirth, or abortion. Prolactin-secreting tumors (prolactinomas) and hypothyroidism are common pathologic causes of galactorrhea during adolescence. Less common causes of hyperprolactinemia and galactorrhea include diseases in or near the hypothalamus or pituitary that interfere with the secretion of dopamine or its delivery to the hypothalamus. Included are tumors of the hypothalamus and/or pituitary, both benign (eg, craniopharyngiomas) and malignant (eg, metastatic disease), infiltrative diseases of the hypothalamus (eg, sarcoidosis), and pituitary stalk damage (eg, section due to head trauma or surgery or compression). Stimulation of the intercostal nerves (eg, chest wall surgery or herpes zoster infection), renal failure (decreased prolactin clearance), Polycystic Ovarian Syndrome, and emotional or physical stress can also cause hyperprolactinemia, which can induce galactorrhea.

Table 4–5. Medications and herbs associated with galactorrhea.

Anticonvulsants (valproic acid)
Antidepressants (selective serotonin reuptake inhibitors, tricyclic antidepressants)
Anxiolytics (alprazolam)
Antihypertensives (atenolol, methyldopa, reserpine, verapamil)
Antipsychotics
Typical (haloperidol, phenothiazine, pimozide)
Atypical (risperidone, olanzapine, molindone)
Antiemetics (prochlorperazine)
Herbs (anise, blessed thistle, fennel, fenugreek seed, nettle)
Hormonal contraceptives
Isoniazid
Illicit drugs (amphetamines, cannabis, opiates)
Motility agents (metoclopramide)
Muscle relaxants (cyclobenzaprine)

Clinical Findings

Breast ultrasonography can be helpful in determining the cause of nipple discharge and breast masses. Depending upon additional findings from the history and examination, evaluation of galactorrhea may include a pregnancy test, prolactin level, and thyroid function studies. If there is a question as to whether the discharge is true galactorrhea, fat staining of the discharge can be confirmatory. Elevated TSH confirms the diagnosis of hypothyroidism. Elevated prolactin and normal TSH, often accompanied by amenorrhea, in the absence of medication known to cause hyperprolactinemia suggests a hypothalamic or pituitary tumor. In such cases, magnetic resonance imaging (MRI) of the brain and consultation with a pediatric endocrinologist are indicated.

Treatment

Observation with serial examination is recommended for nipple discharge associated with breast mass unless a papilloma is suspected by the presence of bloody or serosanguineous nipple discharge with or without a subareolar or peripheral mass. This entity requires further evaluation and excision by a breast surgeon. Treating the underlying cause of galactorrhea is usually effective. Galactorrhea due to hypothyroidism should be treated with thyroid hormone replacement. An alternative medication can be prescribed in cases of medication-induced galactorrhea. Adolescents with galactorrhea without a breast mass who have normal prolactin and TSH levels can be followed clinically and counseled about supportive measures such as avoidance of nipple stimulation, stress reduction, and keeping a menstrual calendar to monitor for oligomenorrhea which might indicate a systemic hormonal problem such as hyperprolactinemia or thyroid disease. In many cases, symptoms resolve spontaneously and no underlying diagnosis is made. Medical management of prolactinomas with dopamine agonists such as bromocriptine is the favored approach.

GYNECOMASTIA

Gynecomastia, benign subareolar glandular breast enlargement, affects up to 65% of adolescent males. It typically appears at least 6 months after the onset of secondary sex characteristics with peak incidence during SMR stages 3 and 4. Breast tissue enlargement usually regresses within 1–3 years and persistence beyond age 17 years is uncommon. Approximately half of young men with gynecomastia have a positive family history of gynecomastia. The pathogenesis of pubertal gynecomastia has long been attributed to a transient imbalance between estrogens that stimulate proliferation of breast tissue and androgens which antagonize this effect. Leptin has recently been implicated in the development of gynecomastia, as levels are higher in healthy nonobese adolescent males with gynecomastia when compared to controls. There are several proposed mechanisms in which leptin acts biochemically to alter the estrogen-androgen ratio.

Clinical Findings

Palpation of the breasts is necessary to distinguish adipose tissue (pseudogynecomastia) from the glandular tissue found in true gynecomastia, which is palpable as a fibroglandular mass located concentrically beneath the nipple-areolar complex. Gynecomastia is bilateral in almost two-thirds of patients. Findings that indicate more serious disease include hard or firm breast tissue, unilateral breast growth, eccentric masses outside of the nipple-areolar complex, and overlying skin changes. A genitourinary examination is needed to evaluate pubertal SMR, testicular volume and masses, or irregularities of the testes.

In the absence of abnormalities on history or physical examination, clinical monitoring of male gynecomastia for 12–18 months is sufficient. Laboratory evaluation is warranted if the patient with gynecomastia is prepubertal, appears undervirilized, has an eccentric breast mass, has a rapid progression of breast enlargement, has a testicular mass, or has persistence of gynecomastia beyond the usual observation period. The initial laboratory evaluation includes thyroid function tests, testosterone, estradiol, human chorionic gonadotropin (hCG), and luteinizing hormone (LH). Additional studies depending on preliminary findings include karyotype, liver and renal function studies, dehydroepiandrosterone sulfate, and prolactin. Any patient with a testicular mass or laboratory results suggesting possible tumor, such as high serum testosterone, hCG, or estradiol, should have a testicular ultrasound. Further evaluation includes adrenal or brain imaging if a prolactin-secreting pituitary tumor or adrenal tumor is suspected.

Differential Diagnosis

Gynecomastia may be drug-induced (Table 4–6). Testicular, adrenal, or pituitary tumors, Klinefelter syndrome, secondary hypogonadism, partial or complete androgen insensitivity syndrome, hyperthyroidism, or chronic diseases (eg. cystic fibrosis, ulcerative colitis, liver disease, renal failure, and acquired immunodeficiency syndrome) leading to malnutrition may be associated with gynecomastia. Breast cancer in the adolescent male is extraordinarily rare.

Table 4–6. Drugs associated with gynecomastia.

	Examples
Antiandrogens	Cyproterone, finasteride, flutamide, ketoconazole, nilutamide, spironolactone
Antineoplastic and immunomodulators	Alkylating agents, bleomycin, cisplatin, cyclosporine, imatinib, methotrexate, nitrosurea, vincristine
Antiulcer drugs	Cimetidine, metoclopramide, omeprazole, ranitidine
Cardiovascular drugs	Amiodarone, angiotensin-converting enzyme inhibitors, calcium channel blockers, digitoxin, reserpine, spironolactone
Drugs of abuse	Alcohol, amphetamines, marijuana, opiates
Hormones	Anabolic androgenic steroids, estrogens, testosterone, chorionic gonadotropin
Infectious agents	Antiretrovirals, ketoconazole, isoniazid, metronidazole
Psychoactive medications	Diazepam, tricyclic antidepressants, haloperidol, atypical antipsychotics, phenothiazines

Treatment

If gynecomastia is idiopathic, reassurance about the common and benign nature of the process can be given. Resolution may take up to 2 years. Surgery is reserved for those with persistent severe breast enlargement and/or significant psychological trauma. In cases of drug-induced gynecomastia, the inciting agent should be discontinued if possible. The patient should be referred to an endocrinologist or oncologist if other pathologic etiologies are diagnosed.

ACOG Committee Opinion: Breast concerns in the adolescent. Obstet Gynecol 2006;108(5):1329–1336 [PMID: 17077268].

De Silva et al: Disorders of the breast in children and adolescents, part 2: Breast masses. J Pediatr Adolesc Gynecol 2006;19(6): 415–418 [PMID: 17174833].

Fallat ME, Ignacio RC: Breast disorders in children and adolescents. J Pediatr Adolesc Gynecol 2008;21(6):311–316 [PMID: 19064223].

Hagan JF, Shaw JS, Duncan PM: Bright Futures: Guidelines for Health Supervision of Infants, Children, and Adolescents, 3rd ed. American Academy of Pediatrics, 2008.

Howlader N et al (editors): SEER Cancer Statistics Review, 1975-2008, National Cancer Institute. Bethesda, MD. http://seer.cancer.gov/csr/1975_2008/. Based on November 2010 SEER data submission, posted to the SEER web site, 2011.

Jayasinghe Y, Simmons PS: Fibroadenomas in adolescence. Curr Opin Obstet Gynecol 2009;21(5):402–406 [PMID: 19606032].

Laufer MR, Goldstein DP: The breast: examination and lesions. In: Emans SJ, Laufer MR, Goldstein DP (editors): Pediatric and Adolescent Gynecology, 5th ed. Lippincott Williams & Wilkins, 2005:729–759.

Ma NS, Geffner ME: Gynecomastia in prepubertal and pubertal boys. Curr Opin Pediatr 2008;20(4):465–470 [PMID: 18622206].

GYNECOLOGIC DISORDERS IN ADOLESCENCE

PHYSIOLOGY OF MENSTRUATION

The ovulatory menstrual cycle is divided into three consecutive phases: follicular (days 1–14), ovulatory (midcycle), and luteal (days 16–28). During the follicular phase, pulsatile gonadotropin-releasing hormone from the hypothalamus stimulates anterior pituitary secretion of follicle stimulating hormone (FSH) and LH. Under the influence of FSH and LH, a dominant ovarian follicle emerges by day 5–7 of the menstrual cycle, and the other follicles become atretic. Rising estradiol levels produced by the maturing follicle cause proliferation of the endometrium. By the midfollicular phase, FSH begins to decline secondary to estradiol-mediated negative feedback, while LH continues to rise as a result of estradiol-mediated positive feedback.

Rising LH initiates progesterone secretion and luteinization of the granulosa cells of the follicle. Progesterone in turn further stimulates LH and FSH. This leads to the LH surge, which causes the follicle to rupture and expel the oocyte. During the luteal phase, LH and FSH gradually decline. The corpus luteum secretes progesterone. The endometrium enters the secretory phase in response to rising levels of estrogen and progesterone, with maturation 8–9 days after ovulation. If pregnancy and placental hCG release do not occur, luteolysis begins; estrogen and progesterone levels decline and the endometrial lining is shed as menstrual flow approximately 14 days after ovulation. In the first 2 years after menarche, the majority of cycles (50%–80%) are anovulatory. Between 10% and 20% of cycles are anovulatory for up to 5 years after menarche.

PELVIC EXAMINATION

Indications for a pelvic examination in an adolescent include abdominal or pelvic pain, intra-abdominal or pelvic mass, abnormal vaginal bleeding or other menstrual disorders, pathologic vaginal discharge, or need for cervical cytology screening. The American College of Obstetricians and Gynecologists advocates starting Papanicolaou (Pap) screening at age 21 years for both sexually experienced and sexually inexperienced women. This is based on the low incidence of cervical cancer in younger women and the potential for adverse effects associated with follow-up of young women with abnormal cytology screening results, regardless of type of test used. Pregnancy during adolescence does not alter screening guidelines. Recommendations for special populations, including sexually active adolescents newly diagnosed with HIV, include performing a Pap test twice in the first year after diagnosis and annually thereafter. In addition, adolescents who have been sexually active and are immunocompromised (eg, organ transplant recipient, long-term steroid use) should have Pap screening after the onset of sexual activity even if younger than 21 years of age. This screening should include Pap tests at 6 month intervals during the first year of screening and then annual Pap tests thereafter. Algorithms for managing abnormal cytology can be found at the American Society for Colposcopy and Cervical Pathology website, http://www.asccp.org/ConsensusGuidelines/tabid/7436/Default.aspx. Guidelines for management of abnormal cytology in HIV positive women can be obtained through the Centers for Disease Control at http://www.cdc.gov/mmwr/preview/mmwrhtml/rr5804a1.htm.

The adolescent may be apprehensive about the first pelvic examination. Sensitive counseling and age-appropriate education about the purpose of the examination, pelvic anatomy, and the components of the examination should occur in an unhurried manner. The use of diagrams and models may facilitate discussion. Time should be allotted for the adolescent to ask questions. Ideally, the examination should occur in a controlled and comfortable setting. The adolescent may request to have her mother or family member present during the examination for reassurance; however, in many instances an adolescent will request that the examination occur confidentially. Having another female staff present to support the adolescent in this setting may be helpful. A female staff chaperone should be present with male examiners.

The pelvic examination begins by placing the patient in the dorsal lithotomy position after equipment and supplies are ready (Table 4–7). Patients with orthopedic or other

Table 4–7. Items for pelvic examination.

General	Gloves, good light source, appropriate sized speculums, sterile cotton applicator swabs, large swabs to remove excess bleeding or discharge, patient labels, hand mirror for patient education
Wet prep of vaginal discharge	pH paper, microscope slides and cover slips, NaCl and KOH solutions
Pap smear	Pap smear liquid media or slides with fixative; cervical spatula and endocervical cytologic brush; or broom for collection
STI testing	Gonorrhea and Chlamydia test media with specific collection swabs
Bimanual examination	Gloves, water-based lubricant

physical disabilities require accommodation for proper positioning and comfort. The examiner inspects the external genitalia, noting sexually maturity rating, estrogenization of the vaginal mucosa (moist, pink, and more elastic mucosa), shape of the hymen, the size of the clitoris (2–5 mm wide is normal), any unusual rashes or lesions on the vulva such as folliculitis from shaving, warts or other skin lesions, and genital piercing or body art. It can be helpful to ask an adolescent if she has any questions about her body during the inspection as she might have concerns that she was too shy to ask (eg, normalcy of labial hypertrophy). In cases of alleged sexual abuse or assault, the presence of any lesions, including lacerations, bruises, scarring, or synechiae about the hymen, vulva, or anus, should be noted.

The patient should be prepared for insertion of the speculum to help her remain relaxed. The speculum should be inserted into the vagina posteriorly with a downward direction to avoid the urethra. A medium Pedersen speculum is most often used in sexually experienced patients; a narrow Huffman is used for virginal patients. In a virginal female prior to the speculum examination, a one-finger examination in the vagina can help the provider identify the position of the cervix and can give the patient an appreciation for the sensation she can expect with placement of the speculum. Warming the speculum with tap water prior to insertion can be more comfortable for the patient and also provide lubrication. Simultaneously touching the inner aspect of the patient's thigh or applying gentle pressure to the perineum away from the introitus while inserting the speculum helps distract attention from the placement of the speculum. The vaginal walls and cervix are inspected for anatomical abnormalities, inflammation, and lesions and the quantity and quality of discharge adherent to the vaginal walls and pooled in the vagina are noted. The presence of a cervical ectropion is commonly observed in adolescents as erythema surrounding the cervical os. The ectropion is the extension of the endocervical columnar epithelium outside the cervical os onto the face of the cervix.

Specimens are obtained in the following order: vaginal pH, saline and KOH wet preparations, cervical cytology (Pap) screening if indicated, and endocervical swabs for gonorrhea and *Chlamydia* (Table 4–8). Sexually transmitted infections are discussed in further detail in Chapter 44. The speculum is then removed, and bimanual examination is performed with one or two fingers in the vagina and the other hand on the abdomen to palpate the uterus and adnexa for size, position, and tenderness.

Table 4–8. Diagnostic tests and procedures performed during speculum vaginal examination.

Vaginal pH	Use applicator swab to sample vaginal discharge adherent to the wall or in the vaginal pool if a speculum is in place; immediately apply it to pH paper for reading.
Saline and KOH wet preparations	Sample discharge as above with different swabs, smear small sample on glass slide, apply small drop or saline or KOH and immediately cover with coverslip, and evaluate under microscope.
Pap smear[a]	Gently remove excessive discharge from surface of cervix. Exocervical cells are sampled with a spatula by applying gentle pressure on the cervix with the spatula while rotating it around the cervical os. Endocervical cells are sampled by gently inserting the cytologic brush into the cervical os and rotating it. Both cell types are collected by the broom when it is centered over the cervical os and rotated.
STI testing[a]	Insert specific test swabs (eg, Dacron for most *Chlamydia* test media) into the cervical os to obtain endocervical samples for *Chlamydia* and gonorrhea.

[a]Refer to manufacturer instructions for sample collection and processing. STI, sexually transmitted infections.

MENSTRUAL DISORDERS

1. Amenorrhea

Primary amenorrhea is defined as having no menstrual periods or secondary sex characteristics by age 13 years or no menses in the presence of secondary sex characteristics by age 15 years. In the adolescent who has achieved menarche, secondary amenorrhea is defined as the absence of menses for three consecutive cycles or for 6 months in a patient with irregular cycles.

A. Evaluation of Primary and Secondary Amenorrhea

In evaluating amenorrhea, it is helpful to consider anatomical levels of possible abnormalities from the hypothalamus to the genital tract (Table 4–9).

A stepwise approach, using clinical history, growth charts, physical examination, and appropriate laboratory studies will allow providers to determine the etiology of amenorrhea in most adolescents. Evaluation begins with a thorough developmental and sexual history. Establishing a pubertal timeline including age at thelarche, adrenarche, growth spurt, and menarche is helpful in evaluating pubertal development. Although there can be variations in the onset, degree, and timing of these stages, the progression of stages is predictable. Adrenal androgens are largely responsible for axillary and pubic hair. Estrogen is responsible for breast development; maturation of the external genitalia, vagina and uterus; and menstruation. Lack of development suggests pituitary or ovarian failure or gonadal dysgenesis. Determining the patient's gynecologic age (time in years and months since menarche) is helpful in assessing the maturity

Table 4–9. Differential diagnosis of amenorrhea by anatomic site of cause.

Hypothalamic-pituitary axis
Hypothalamic suppression
Chronic disease
Stress
Malnutrition
Strenuous athletics
Drugs (haloperidol, phenothiazines, atypical antipsychotics)
Central nervous system lesion
Pituitary lesion: adenoma, prolactinoma
Craniopharyngioma, brainstem, or parasellar tumors
Head injury with hypothalamic contusion
Infiltrative process (sarcoidosis)
Vascular disease (hypothalamic vasculitis)
Congenital conditions[a]
Kallmann syndrome (anosmia)
Ovaries
Gonadal dysgenesis[a]
Turner syndrome (XO)
Mosaic (XX/XO)
Injury to ovary
Autoimmune disease (oophoritis)
Infection (mumps)
Toxins (alkylating chemotherapeutic agents)
Irradiation
Trauma, torsion (rare)
Polycystic ovary syndrome
Ovarian failure
Uterovaginal outflow tract
Müllerian dysgenesis[a]
Congenital deformity or absence of uterus, uterine tubes, or vagina
Imperforate hymen, transverse vaginal septum, vaginal agenesis, agenesis of the cervix[a]
Androgen insensitivity syndrome (absent uterus)[a]
Uterine lining defect
Asherman syndrome (intrauterine synechiae postcurettage or endometritis)
Tuberculosis, brucellosis
Defect in hormone synthesis or action (virilization may be present)
Adrenal hyperplasia[a]
Cushing disease
Adrenal tumor
Ovarian tumor (rare)
Drugs (steroids, ACTH)

[a]Indicates condition that usually presents as primary amenorrhea.
ACTH, adrenocorticotropic hormone.

of the hypothalamic-pituitary-ovarian axis. A menstrual history includes date of last menstrual period (LMP), frequency and duration of periods, amount of bleeding, and premenstrual symptoms. Irregular menstrual cycles are common in the first 1–2 years after menarche. Two-thirds of adolescents with a gynecologic age more than 2 years have regular menstrual cycles.

Relevant components of the past medical and surgical histories include the neonatal history, treatment for malignancies, presence of autoimmune disorders or endocrinopathies, and current medications (prescribed and over-the-counter). Family history includes age at menarche of maternal relatives, familial gynecologic or fertility problems, autoimmune diseases, or endocrinopathies. A review of systems should focus on symptoms of hypothalamic-pituitary disease such as weight change, headache, visual disturbance, galactorrhea, polyuria, and/or polydipsia. A history of cyclic abdominal and/or pelvic pain in a mature adolescent with amenorrhea may indicate an anatomic abnormality such as an imperforate hymen. Acne and hirsutism are clinical markers of androgen excess. Both hypo- and hyperthyroidism can cause menstrual irregularities. Changes in weight, quality of skin and hair, and stooling pattern may indicate a thyroid problem. A confidential social history should include sexual activity, contraceptive use, the possibility of pregnancy, and use of tobacco, drugs, or alcohol. The patient should also be questioned about major stressors, symptoms of depression and anxiety, dietary habits including any disordered eating or weight-loss behaviors, and athletic participation.

A thorough physical examination should include the components listed in Table 4–10. If a patient cannot tolerate a pelvic or bimanual examination, the presence of the uterus can be assessed by rectoabdominal examination or ultrasonography. Ultrasound provides evaluation of pelvic anatomy and possible genital tract obstruction, measurement of the

Table 4–10. Components of the physical examination for amenorrhea.

General appearance	Syndromic features (eg, Turner syndrome with webbed neck, shield chest, widely spaced nipples, increased carrying angle of the arms)
Anthropometrics	Height, weight, BMI and percentiles for age, vital signs (HR, BP)
Ophthalmologic	Visual field cuts, papilledema
Neck	Thyromegaly
Breast	SMR staging, galactorrhea
Abdomen	Masses
Genital	SMR staging, estrogenization of vaginal mucosa (pink and moist vs thin red mucosa of hypoestrogenization), hymenal patency, clitoromegaly (width > 5 mm)
Pelvic and bimanual	Vaginal depth by insertion of a saline moistened applicator swab into the vagina or by bimanual examination (normal >2 cm); palpation of the uterus and ovaries by bimanual examination
Skin	Acne, hirsutism, acanthosis nigricans

BMI, body mass index; BP, blood pressure; HR, heart rate; SMR, sexual maturity rating endometrial stripe as an indicator of estrogen stimulation, and identification of ovarian cysts or masses.

Figure 4-6 illustrates an approach to the laboratory and radiologic evaluation of primary or secondary amenorrhea. Initial studies should include a urine pregnancy test, complete blood count, TSH, prolactin, and FSH. If there is evidence of hyperandrogenemia (acne, hirsutism) and PCOS is suspected, total and free testosterone and dehydroepiandrosterone sulfate (DHEAS) should be obtained. If systemic illness is suspected, a urinalysis and a chemistry

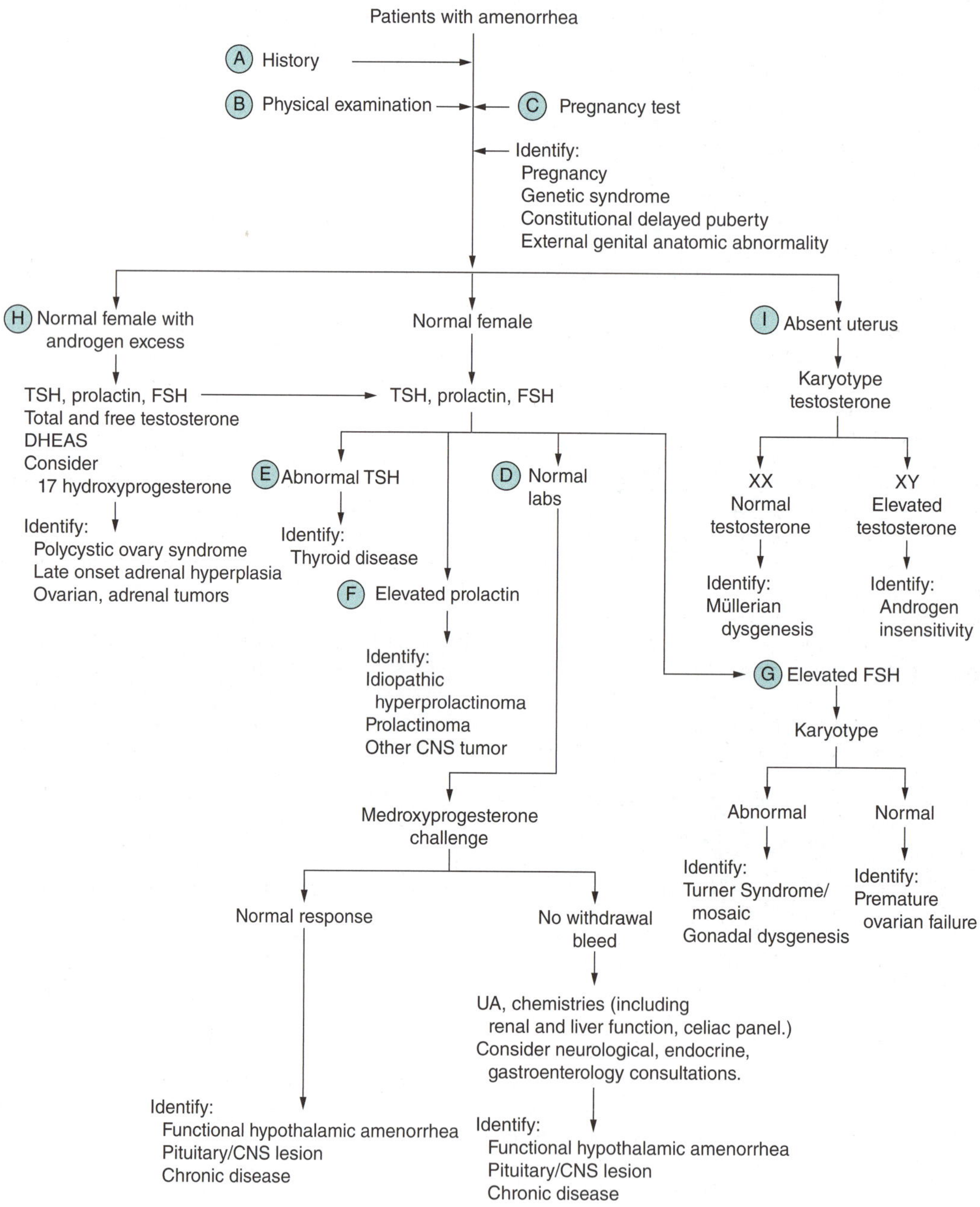

▲ **Figure 4–6.** Evaluation of primary amenorrhea and secondary amenorrhea. CNS, central nervous system; DHEAS, dehydroepiandrosterone sulfate; FSH, follicle-stimulating hormone; TSH, thyroid-stimulating hormone; UA, urine analysis.

panel (including renal and liver function tests) and erythrocyte sedimentation rate should be obtained. If short stature and delayed puberty are present, a bone age and karyotype should be done.

If pelvic examination or ultrasonography reveals normal female external genitalia and pelvic organs and the patient is not pregnant, the patient should be given a challenge of oral medroxyprogesterone, 10 mg daily for 10 days. Positive response to the progestin challenge with withdrawal bleeding is suggestive of the presence of a normal, estrogen-primed uterus.

Elevated serum prolactin indicates a possible prolactin secreting tumor. Prolactin testing is sensitive and can be elevated with stress, eating, or sexual intercourse. A mildly elevated test should be repeated prior to MRI of the brain for a prolactinoma. Elevated FSH indicates ovarian insufficiency or gonadal dysgenesis and a karyotype for Turner syndrome or Turner mosaic should be obtained. Autoimmune oophoritis should be assessed by antiovarian antibodies if the chromosome analysis is normal. Normal or low serum gonadotropins indicate hypothalamic suppression and functional amenorrhea if the patient's weight is normal and there is a reasonable explanation such as vigorous exercise. Functional amenorrhea, although relatively common, is a diagnosis of exclusion. Low serum gonadotropin concentration can also be caused by malnutrition as in anorexia nervosa, endocrinopathies, and chronic diseases or by a central nervous system tumor.

If the physical examination or ultrasound reveals an absent uterus, chromosomal analysis and serum testosterone should be obtained to differentiate between Mullerian dysgenesis and androgen insensitivity. Mullerian dysgenesis or Mayer-Rokitansky-Küster-Hauser (MRKH) syndrome is the congenital absence of the vagina with variable uterine development. These women have normal serum testosterone levels. Pelvic MRI is helpful to clarify the nature of the vaginal agenesis and to differentiate it from low-lying transverse vaginal septum, agenesis of the uterus and vagina, and imperforate hymen. Individuals with androgen insensitivity are phenotypically female but have an absent upper vagina, uterus, and fallopian tubes; a male karyotype; and an elevated serum testosterone (normal range for males).

The management of primary or secondary amenorrhea depends on the underlying pathology. Hormonal treatment is used in patients with hypothalamic, pituitary, and ovarian causes. Surgical repair may be required in patients with outflow tract anomalies.

B. Polycystic Ovary Syndrome

Polycystic Ovary Syndrome (PCOS) is the most common endocrine disorder of reproductive-aged women. It occurs in up to 6% of adolescents and 12% of adult women. PCOS is characterized by ovarian dysfunction, disordered gonadotropin secretion, and hyperandrogenism, which cause amenorrhea, hirsutism, and acne. Many adolescents with PCOS are overweight and the association of PCOS with insulin resistance is well established. Adolescents with PCOS are at increased risk for obesity-related morbidities including type 2 diabetes mellitus, dyslipidemia, and cardiovascular disease, low self-esteem, and adult reproductive health problems including infertility and endometrial cancer.

The adolescent with PCOS usually presents with overweight, oligomenorrhea or secondary amenorrhea, acne, and hirsutism. The most recent set of diagnostic criteria for PCOS from the Androgen Excess and Polycystic Ovary Syndrome Society include: (1) presence of hyperandrogenism (hirsutism and/or biochemical hyperandrogenemia), (2) ovarian dysfunction (oligo-anovulation and/or presence of polycystic ovaries by ultrasound), and (3) the exclusion of other androgen excess or related disorders.

Table 4–11 outlines a standard laboratory evaluation for PCOS. If other etiologies of virilization such as late onset congenital adrenal hyperplasia (history of premature pubarche, high DHEAS, clitoromegaly) are suspected, a first morning 17-hydroxyprogesterone should be collected to look for 21-hydroxylase deficiency. Urine cortisol or a dexamethasone suppression test is performed if Cushing syndrome is suspected. If the patient is overweight and/or has acanthosis nigricans, a fasting insulin, lipid panel, and 2-hour oral glucose challenge test are recommended. A simple fasting glucose is not sufficient, as women with PCOS can have normal fasting glucose but impaired postprandial tests. Consultation with a pediatric endocrinologist can assist in further evaluation and management of significantly elevated androgens and endocrinopathies.

Encouraging lifestyle changes that will promote weight loss is a primary goal of therapy for PCOS in adolescence. Weight loss is associated with improved menstrual regulation and decreased symptoms of hyperandrogenemia, obesity-related comorbidities, and infertility. Combination of estrogen/progesterone oral contraceptives may improve menstrual regularity, decrease ovarian and adrenal androgen production

Table 4–11. Laboratory evaluation for polycystic ovary syndrome (PCOS).

Pregnancy test	
Testosterone (total and free)	> 200 ng/dL suggests tumor
Sex hormone-binding globulin (SHBG)	
Dehydroepiandrosterone sulfate (DHEAS)	> 700 mcg/dL suggests tumor
Thyroid-stimulating hormone (TSH)	
Follicle-stimulating hormone (FSH)	
Luteinizing hormone (LH)	LH:FSH ratio is elevated if > 2.5:1

and increase sex hormone-binding globulin (SHBG). There are no current guidelines for the use of insulin sensitizing medications such as metformin to treat PCOS in adolescents.

2. Dysmenorrhea

Dysmenorrhea, or pain with menstrual periods is the most common gynecologic complaint of adolescent girls, with up to 90% of adolescent girls reporting some symptoms. Fifteen percent of adolescent women describe their symptoms as severe. The prevalence of dysmenorrhea increases with gynecologic age due to its association with ovulatory cycles. Dysmenorrhea can be designated as primary or secondary depending upon the absence or presence of underlying pelvic pathology (Table 4–12). Potent prostaglandins are the mediators of dysmenorrhea, producing uterine contractions, tissue ischemia, and hypersensitivity of pain fibers in the uterus.

In addition to taking a gynecologic and sexual history, an accurate characterization of the pain (timing with menses, intensity, duration, use of pain medications) is important in determining functional impairment. The pelvic examination can usually be deferred in nonsexually active adolescents with probable primary dysmenorrhea. Adolescents should be encouraged to keep track of their menstrual cycles using a calendar to predict when a period is imminent, thereby allowing for more proactive use of nonsteroidal anti-inflammatory drugs (NSAIDs) one to two days before the start of the anticipated period or with the first indication of discomfort. NSAIDs are typically continued for an additional 2–3 days after onset of pain. Recommended medications are ibuprofen 400–600 mg every 6 hours, or naproxen 500 mg twice a day. If the patient does not respond to NSAIDs, suppression of ovulation with oral contraceptive pills or other combined hormonal contraceptives such as the transdermal patch or intravaginal ring can be effective. These products can also be used continuously by skipping placebo pills or the fourth week off with the patch or ring when the menstrual period is expected to decrease the frequency of menstrual periods. Progestin-only medications such as depot medroxyprogesterone acetate (DMPA) are also options. If patients do not respond to these products and NSAIDs, further evaluation for secondary dysmenorrhea is indicated. A pelvic examination, pelvic imaging with ultrasonography or MRI, and diagnostic laparoscopy may be necessary for diagnosis. Secondary dysmenorrhea is more likely to be associated with chronic pelvic pain, midcycle pain, dyspareunia, and metrorrhagia.

3. Dysfunctional Uterine Bleeding

Dysfunctional uterine bleeding (DUB) results from irregular endometrial sloughing accompanying anovulatory cycles. It may be characterized by menorrhagia (prolonged bleeding that occurs at regular intervals) or menometrorrhagia (heavy prolonged bleeding that occurs irregularly and more frequently than normal). The differential diagnosis of common and less common etiologies in adolescences are listed in Table 4–13.

Evaluation

In addition to a menstrual and sexual history, the bleeding pattern should be characterized by cycle length, duration, and quantity of bleeding (eg, number of soaked pads or tampons in 24 hours, number of menstrual accidents). Bleeding for more than 10 days is usually considered abnormal. The patient should be assessed for symptoms of anemia including fatigue, lightheadedness, syncope, tachycardia, and for other abnormal bleeding (gingivae, stool, easy bruising). The physical examination includes an assessment of hemodynamic stability with orthostatic heart rate and blood pressure measurements. Mucous membranes and skin should be evaluated for pallor; the heart for tachycardia and murmur; the abdomen for organomegaly; and the external genitalia for signs of trauma or congenital anomalies. If the patient has never been sexually active, a pelvic examination is usually unnecessary. In a sexually experienced female, a pelvic and bimanual examination to examine the vagina, cervix, and adnexa may be helpful to elucidate the diagnosis. Laboratory studies should include a complete blood cell count, pregnancy test, reticulocyte count, prothrombin time, partial thromboplastin time, thyroid-stimulating hormone and iron studies. A von Willebrand panel and a platelet function analysis should be considered with a history of heavy menstrual bleeding from menarche and/or bleeding from other sources. For patients suspected of having PCOS, total and free testosterone and dehydroepiandrosterone sulfate should be obtained. For sexually experienced females, cervical or urine-based testing for chlamydia and gonorrhea should be obtained.

Treatment

The severity of DUB is determined by hemodynamic status and degree of anemia and classified as mild, moderate, or severe (Table 4–14). The goals of treatment include (1) establishment and/or maintenance of hemodynamic stability, (2) correction of acute or chronic anemia, (3) resumption of normal menstrual cycles, (4) prevention of recurrence, and (5) prevention of long-term consequences of anovulation. Management depends on the severity of the problem and its specific etiology (Table 4–14). Monophasic oral contraceptive pills containing a potent progestin such as norgestrel 0.3 mg/ethinyl estradiol 30 μg or levonorgestrel 0.15 mg/ethinyl estradiol 30 μg are frequently used for patients without medical contraindications to exogenous estrogens. The active pills in monophasic formulations contain the same concentration of progestins and estrogen and are preferred over multiphasic formulations which contain variable concentrations of estrogen which could potentially increase the risk of breakthrough bleeding. It is important

Table 4–12. Dysmenorrhea in the adolescent.

	Etiology	Onset and Duration	Symptoms	Pelvic Examination	Treatment
Primary Dysmenorrhea[a]					
Primary	Excessive amount of prostaglandin $F_2\alpha$, which attaches to myometrium, causing uterine contractions, hypoxia, and ischemia. Also, directly sensitizes pain receptors.	Begins just prior to or with the onset of menstrual flow and lasts 1–2 days. Typically does not start until 1–2 y after menarche, when cycles are more regularly ovulatory.	Lower abdominal cramps radiating to lower back and thighs. Associated nausea, vomiting, and diarrhea due to excess prostaglandins.	Normal. May wait to examine if never sexually active and history is consistent with primary dysmenorrhea.	Mild—menstrual calendar, start NSAIDs day before bleeding or at the onset of bleeding or pain if timing of cycle is difficult to predict. Moderate to severe—NSAIDs and OCPs or other birth control product to suppress ovulation.
Secondary Dysmenorrhea[b]					
Infection	Most often due to an STI such as Chlamydia or gonorrhea.	Recent onset of pelvic pain. Can also have chronic pain with prolonged untreated infection.	Pelvic pain, excessive or irregular menstrual bleeding, unusual vaginal discharge.	Mucopurulent or purulent discharge from cervical os, cervical friability, cervical motion, uterine or adnexal tenderness, positive wet prep for bacterial vaginosis, positive test for STI.	Appropriate antibiotics.
Endometriosis	Ectopic implants of endometrial tissue in pelvis or abdomen; may result from retrograde menstruation. Definitive diagnosis requires laparoscopy.	Generally starts more than 2 y after menarche, is not significantly responsive to standard NSAID and suppression of ovulation therapies, and worsens through time.	Cyclic or acyclic chronic pelvic pain.	Mild to moderate tenderness typically in the posterior vaginal fornix or along the uterosacral ligaments.	Suppression of ovulation with combined hormonal contraceptive methods. Continuous use may provide additional control. If pain persists, refer to a gynecologist for further evaluation of chronic pelvic pain and consideration of gonadotropin-releasing hormone agonists.
Complication of pregnancy	Spontaneous abortion, ectopic pregnancy.	Acute onset.	Pelvic or abdominal pain associated with vaginal bleeding following missed menstrual period.	Positive hCG, enlarged uterus, or adnexal mass.	Pelvic US if hemodynamically stable to evaluate for intrauterine pregnancy. Immediate obstetric or surgical consult with concern for ectopic pregnancy.
Congenital anomalies	Outflow tract anomalies: imperforate hymen, transverse or longitudinal vaginal septum, septate uterus.	Onset at menarche.	Cyclic pelvic or abdominal pain which can become chronic.	Imperforate hymen may be visible on external examination. Pelvic US for general anatomy. Pelvic MRI is most sensitive and specific test for septums.	Gynecology consult for further evaluation and management.
Pelvic adhesions	Previous abdominal surgery or pelvic inflammatory disease.	Delayed onset after surgery or PID.	Abdominal pain, may or may not be associated with menstrual cycles; possible alteration in bowel pattern.	Variable.	Gynecology consult for possible lysis of adhesion.

[a]No pelvic pathology.
[b]Underlying pathology present.
DMPA, depot medroxyprogesterone acetate; hCG, human chorionic gonadotropin; MRI, magnetic resonance imaging; NSAID, nonsteroidal anti-inflammatory drug; OCP, oral contraceptive pill; PID, pelvic inflammatory disease; STI, sexually transmitted infection; US, ultrasound.

Table 4–13. Differential diagnosis of dysfunctional uterine bleeding in adolescents.

Condition	Examples
Anovulation	
Sexually transmitted infections	Cervicitis, pelvic inflammatory disease
Pregnancy complications	Ectopic, miscarriage
Bleeding disorders	von Willebrand disease, platelet function abnormalities, thrombocytopenia, coagulopathy
Endocrine disorders	Hypo-/hyperthyroidism, hyperprolactinemia, adrenal insufficiency, PCOS
Anatomic abnormalities	Congenital anomalies, ovarian cysts or tumors, cervical polyps
Trauma	Vaginal laceration
Foreign body	Retained tampon
Chronic illness	Liver, renal, inflammatory bowel, lupus
Malignancy	Leukemia
Drugs	Contraception, anticoagulants

PCOS, polycystic ovary syndrome

to remind adolescents and their families that compliance with medications to control bleeding and treat anemia is imperative. Adolescents should be treated until the anemia is resolved and often for an additional 6 months or longer if there is an underlying problem such as platelet function abnormality or von Willebrand disease.

4. Mittelschmerz

Mittelschmerz is midcycle discomfort resulting from ovulation. The cause of the pain is unknown but irritation of the peritoneum due to spillage of fluid from the ruptured follicular cyst at the time of ovulation has been suggested. The patient presents with a history of midcycle, unilateral dull, or aching abdominal pain lasting a few minutes to as long as 8 hours. Rarely, the pain mimics that of acute appendicitis, torsion or rupture of an ovarian cyst, or ectopic pregnancy. The patient should be reassured and treated symptomatically.

5. Premenstrual Syndrome and Premenstrual Dysphoric Disorder

It is estimated that 51%–86% of adolescent women experience some premenstrual symptoms. Premenstrual syndrome (PMS) is a cluster of physical and psychological symptoms

Table 4–14. Management of dysfunctional uterine bleeding.

	Mild	Moderate	Severe
Hgb value	Hgb > 12 g/dL	Hgb 9–12 g/dL	Hgb < 9 g/dL
Acute treatment	Menstrual calendar; iron supplementation. NSAID with menses may help reduce flow. Consider OCPs if patient is sexually active and desires contraception.	OCP BID until bleeding stops, continue active pill QD for 21 days followed by 1 week of placebo pills.	Admit to hospital if Hgb < 7 g/dL or patient is hemodynamically unstable. Transfusion based on degree of hemodynamic instability and ability to control bleeding. OCP every 4 h until bleeding slows (usually 24–36 h). Antiemetic 2 h prior to OCPs as needed for nausea. Gynecology consultation for further evaluation and possible dilation and curettage. then OCP QID for 2–4 d then OCP TID for 3 d then OCP BID for total 21 d or until HCT >30% (Conjugated estrogens, 25 mg IV every 4 h for 2–3 doses can be used as an alternative to the PO q4h regimen.)
Long-term management	Monitor menstrual calendar and Hgb. Follow-up in 2–3 mo.	Iron supplementation. Monitor Hgb closely for improvement. May need to revert to BID dosing if bleeding persists. If bleeding controlled, cycle with OCPs (28 d pack) for 3–6 mo.	Iron supplementation. Serial hematocrits. If HCT >30%, cycle with OCPs (28 d pack) for 3–6 mo.

BID, twice daily; NSAID, nonsteroidal anti-inflammatory drug; OCP, oral contraceptive pill; Hgb, hemoglobin; HCT, hematocrit; PO, by mouth; QD, daily; QID, four times per day; TID, three times per day.

that occur during the luteal phase of the menstrual cycle and resolve with menstruation. Physical symptoms include bloating, breast tenderness, fatigue, headache, myalgia, increased appetite, and food craving. Premenstrual emotional symptoms may include fatigue, mood lability, anxiety, depression, irritability, hostility, sleep dysfunction, and impaired social function. PMS can be diagnosed when at least one disabling physical or psychological symptom is documented prospectively for at least two consecutive menstrual cycles, is restricted to the luteal phase of the menstrual cycle, resolves by the end of menses, results in functional impairment, and is not an exacerbation of another underlying disorder. Severe PMS with functional impairment affects 3%–5% of women of reproductive age and is classified in the *Diagnostic and Statistical Manual of Mental Disorders,* Fourth Edition, Text Revision as premenstrual dysphoric disorder (PMDD). The clinical diagnosis of PMDD requires five physical symptoms with at least one affective symptom occurring in the majority of cycles during the preceding year.

The pathophysiology of PMS is not well understood; however, there is some evidence of dysregulation of serotonergic activity and/or of GABAergic receptor functioning during the luteal phase of the menstrual cycle with heightened sensitivity to circulating progesterone metabolites. PMS and PMDD are highly associated with unipolar depressive disorder and anxiety disorders, such as obsessive-compulsive disorder, panic disorder, and generalized anxiety disorder. During adolescence, it may be difficult to determine if the affective symptoms represent a mood or anxiety disorder, a premenstrual exacerbation of a psychiatric disorder, or simple PMS.

Current treatment for PMS in adolescence is based on findings from adult studies and includes lifestyle recommendations and pharmacologic agents that suppress the rise and fall of ovarian steroids or augment serotonin. SSRIs are increasingly used as first-line therapy for PMS and PMDD in adults, and a recent Cochrane review of SSRIs in severe adult PMS determined that SSRIs administered continuously or during the luteal phase were effective in reducing premenstrual symptoms. Once a diagnosis is made, proven effective interventions including education about pathophysiology, lifestyle changes (eg, increasing physical activity and smoking cessation), stress reduction, cognitive behavioral therapy, and nutritional counseling to improve calcium intake and/or calcium supplementation should be attempted. If contraception or cycle control is important, a combined hormonal contraceptive pill may be beneficial. The pill containing 20 μg ethinyl estradiol and 3 mg drospirenone with a 24/4 formulation has been shown to be therapeutic in studies of adult women with PMDD. If these interventions do not adequately control symptoms, luteal phase or continuous administration of SSRIs can be considered. Case reports indicate that adolescents with PMDD respond well to luteal phase dosing of fluoxetine at the standard adult dosage of 20 mg/d. SSRIs are not formally approved by the Food and Drug Administration for treatment of PMS or PMDD in adolescents.

6. Ovarian Cysts

Functional cysts account for the majority of benign ovarian tumors in postpubertal adolescents and are a result of the normal process of ovulation. They may be asymptomatic or may cause menstrual irregularities or pelvic pain. Large cysts can cause constipation or urinary frequency. Follicular cysts are the most common functional cysts. They are usually unilateral, less than 3 cm in diameter, and resolve spontaneously in 1–2 months. Cyst pain occurs as the diameter of the cyst increases, stretching the overlying ovarian cortex and capsule. If the patient's discomfort is tolerable, she can be reexamined monthly and observed for resolution. Hormonal contraceptive products that suppress ovulation can be started to prevent additional cysts from forming. Patients with cysts should be counseled about the signs and symptoms of ovarian and/or tubal torsion, which are serious complications. Adnexal torsion presents with the sudden onset of pain, nausea, and vomiting. Low-grade fever, leukocytosis, and the development of peritoneal signs with rebound and guarding can be found. Torsion is a surgical emergency due to the risk of ischemia and death of the ovary. Patients should be referred to a gynecologist for potential laparoscopy if the cyst has a solid component, measures more than 6 cm by ultrasonography, if there are symptoms or signs of hemorrhage or torsion, or if the cyst fails to regress within 2 months. Corpus luteum cysts occur less commonly and may be large, 5–10 cm in diameter. The patient may have associated amenorrhea, or as the cyst becomes atretic, heavy vaginal bleeding. There may be bleeding into the cyst or rupture with intraperitoneal hemorrhage. To determine whether the bleeding is self-limited, serial hematocrit measurements and ultrasounds can be used. If the patient is stable, hormonal contraception that suppresses ovulation can be started to prevent additional cyst formation and the patient may be monitored for 3 months for resolution. Laparoscopy may be indicated if the cyst is larger than 6 cm or if there is severe pain or hemorrhage.

ACOG Committee Opinion No. 463: Cervical cancer in adolescents: screening, evaluation, and management. Obstet Gynecol 2010;116:469–472 [PMID 20664421].

American Psychiatric Association: Diagnostic and Statistical Manual of Mental Disorders, 4th ed, text revision. American Psychiatric Association, 2000.

Azziz R et al: Task force on the phenotype of the polycystic ovary syndrome of The Androgen Excess and PCOS Society. The Androgen Excess and PCOS Society criteria for the polycystic ovary syndrome: The complete task force report. Fertil Steril 2009;91(2):456–488.

Berlan ED, Emans SJ: Managing polycystic ovary syndrome in adolescent patients. J Pediatr Adolesc Gynecol 2009;22(2):137–140 [PMID: 19350748].

Bloomfield D: Secondary amenorrhea. Pediatr Rev 2006;27(3):113–114 [PMID: 16510552].

Braverman PK et al: Gynecologic examination for adolescents in the pediatric office setting. Pediatr 2010;126(3):583–590 [PMID: 20805151].

Brown J et al: Selective serotonin reuptake inhibitors for premenstrual syndrome. Cochrane Database Syst Rev 2009;15(2): CD001396 [PMID: 19370564].

Gray SH, Emans SJ: Abnormal vaginal bleeding in adolescents. Pediatr Rev 2007;28(5):175–182 [PMID 17473122].

Gordon CM: Clinical Practice. Functional hypothalamic amenorrhea. N Engl J Med 2010;363(4):365–371 [PMID 20660404].

Kaplan JE et al: Guidelines for prevention and treatment of opportunistic infections in HIV-infected adults and adolescents: Recommendations from CDC, the National Institutes of Health, and the HIV Medicine Association of the Infectious Diseases Society of America. MMWR Recomm Rep 2009; 58:1-207 [PMID 19357635].

LaCour DE at al: Dysfunctional uterine bleeding in adolescent females associated with endocrine causes and medical conditions. J Pediatr Adolesc Gynecol 2010;23(2):62–70 [PMID: 20347757].

Rapkin AJ, Mikacich JA: Premenstrual syndrome and premenstrual dysphoric disorder in adolescents. Curr Opin Obstet Gynecol 2008;20(5):455–463 [PMID: 18797268].

Sanfilippo JS, Lara-Torre E: Adolescent gynecology. Obstet Gynecol 2009;113(4):935–947 [PMID: 19305342].

CONTRACEPTION

According to the Centers for Disease Control 2009 Youth Risk Behavior Survey, almost half of high school students (46%) reported having had sexual experience and 34% reported being currently sexually active. Sixty-one percent reported using a condom at their latest intercourse. Most young people have sex for the first time at about the age of 17, but do not marry until their middle or late twenties. This means that young adults are at risk of unwanted pregnancy and STIs for nearly a decade. A sexually active female who does not use contraceptives has almost a 90% chance of becoming pregnant within a year.

Table 4–15. Contraceptive efficacy.

Method	Percentage of Women Experiencing an Unintended Pregnancy within the First Year of Use	
	Typical Use	Perfect Use
No method	85	85
Spermicides only	29	18
Withdrawal	27	4
Diaphragm	16	6
Condom		
Female	21	5
Male	15	2
Oral contraceptive pill	8	0.3
Evra Patch	8	0.3
NuvaRing	8	0.3
Depo-Provera	3	0.3
IUD		
ParaGard	0.8	0.6
Mirena	0.2	0.2
Implanon	0.05	0.05

IUD, intrauterine device.
Adapted from Trussell J: Contraceptive efficacy. In Hatcher RA et al (editors): *Contraceptive Technology,* 19th ed revised. Ardent Media, 2007.

Abstinence & Decision Making

Talking with teenagers about sexual intercourse and its implications can help teens make informed decisions regarding engaging in sexual activity. The American Academy of Pediatrics endorses a comprehensive approach to sexuality education that incorporates encouraging abstinence while providing appropriate risk reduction counseling regarding sexual behaviors. Counseling should include discussions about STI prevention and contraceptive methods including emergency contraception (Table 4–15). Encouraging adolescents to use contraception when they do engage in sexual intercourse does not lead to higher rates of sexual activity. Adolescents often delay seeing a clinician for contraceptive services after initiating sexual activity. Concern about lack of confidentiality is an important reason for this delay.

Methods Counseling

The goals of counseling adolescents about contraception include promoting safe and responsible sexual behavior through delaying the initiation of sexual activity, reinforcing consistent condom use for those who are sexually active, and discussing other contraceptive options to provide protection from unwanted pregnancy. Providers should familiarize themselves with their state policies regarding the ability of minors to consent for sexual and reproductive health care services. These data are accessible on the Internet from the Guttmacher Institute (http://www.guttmacher.org) and the Center for Adolescent Health and the Law (http://www.adolescenthealthlaw.org).

Providers should consider the adolescent's lifestyle, potential challenges to compliance, the patient's need for confidentiality around the use of contraception, previous experiences with contraception and reasons for discontinuation, and any misconceptions regarding contraceptive options. Barriers to health care access including transportation and financial limitations should be identified. Prescribing contraception for other medical reasons (eg, management of dysmenorrhea) can create opportunities for providers and adolescent patients to make parents aware of the use of the medication while maintaining confidentiality around the sexual behaviors.

Mechanism of Action

The primary mechanism of action for combined hormonal contraceptives containing estrogen and progestin (OCPs, transdermal patch, intravaginal ring) and the progestin-only methods (pills, DMPA, and the etonogestrel implant) is inhibition of ovulation. Thickening of the cervical mucus also makes sperm penetration more difficult, and atrophy of the endometrium diminishes the chance of implantation. Starting all birth control methods during the menstrual period (either first day of bleeding or first Sunday of bleeding) produces the most reliable suppression of ovulation. Conventional oral contraceptive pills, transdermal patches, and intravaginal rings typically require that the adolescent wait for her next period to begin before starting. Data show that many women who receive prescriptions or even samples of medication never begin the prescribed method. Furthermore, these women could become pregnant while waiting to start. "Quick start" is an alternative approach to starting contraception that allows the patient to begin contraception on the day of the appointment regardless of menstrual cycle day, following a negative pregnancy test. This approach has been studied in adolescent women and increases adherence with the method of choice. Unfortunately, these studies also highlight the generally poor long-term compliance with contraceptive treatment in this age group.

Medical Considerations

Evaluation of an adolescent female requesting contraception should include a review of current and past medical conditions, current medications and allergies, menstrual history, confidential social history including sexual history, and family medical history. Important components of a sexual history include age at first intercourse, number of partners in lifetime, history of STIs and pelvic inflammatory disease (PID), condom use, current and past use of other contraceptives and reasons for discontinuation, and pregnancy history and outcomes. It is helpful to have a baseline weight, height, BMI, and blood pressure. A pelvic examination is not necessary before initiating contraception. However, if the woman is sexually active and has missed menstrual periods or has symptoms of pregnancy, a pregnancy test is warranted. Screening for STIs should be offered if a sexually experienced woman is asymptomatic and testing for STIs is indicated if she is symptomatic.

The World Health Organization's publication, *Improving Access to Quality Care in Family Planning: Medical Eligibility Criteria for Contraceptive Use* is an evidence-based guide providing criteria for initiating and continuing contraceptive methods based on a risk assessment of an individual's characteristics or known preexisting medical condition.

Table 4–16. Contraindications to combined oral contraceptive (COC) pills.

Absolute contraindications
Pregnancy
Breast feeding (within 6 wk of childbirth)
Hypertension SBP > 160 mm Hg or DBP > 100 mm Hg
History of thrombophlebitis; current thromboembolic disorder, cerebrovascular disease, or ischemic heart disease
Known thrombogenic mutations (factor V Leiden; prothrombin mutation; protein S, protein C, and antithrombin deficiencies)
Systemic lupus erythematosus
Complicated valvular heart disease (with pulmonary hypertension; atrial fibrillation; history of bacterial endocarditis)
Diabetes with nephropathy; retinopathy; neuropathy
Liver disease: active viral hepatitis; severe cirrhosis; tumor (hepatocellular adenoma or hepatoma)
Breast cancer (current)
Migraine headaches with aura
Major surgery with prolonged immobilization
Relative contraindications
Postpartum (first 3 wk)
Breastfeeding (6 wk–6 mo following childbirth)
Hypertension (adequately controlled HTN; any history of HTN where BP cannot be evaluated; SBP 140–159 mm Hg or DPB 90–99 mm Hg)
Migraine headache without aura (for continuation of COC)
Breast cancer history with remission for 5 y
Active gallbladder disease or history of COC-induced cholestasis
Use of drugs that affect liver enzymes (rifampin, phenytoin, carbamazepine, barbiturates, primidone, topiramate, oxcarbazepine, lamotrigine, ritonavir-boosted protease inhibitors)

BP, blood pressure; DBP, diastolic blood pressure; HTN, hypertension; SBP, systolic blood pressure.

Table 4–16 lists absolute (a condition which represents an unacceptable health risk if the contraceptive method is used) and relative (a condition where the theoretical or proven risks usually outweigh the advantages of using the method) contraindications to using combined hormonal birth control pills. These contraindications can be extended to other combined hormonal products that contain estrogen and progestins including the transdermal patch and intravaginal ring. The Centers for Disease Control and Prevention has also published the *U.S. Medical Eligibility Criteria for Contraceptive Use* which was adapted from the WHO publication and allows the consideration of use of combined hormonal contraceptive products for women who are currently receiving anticoagulation therapy.

It is important to assess patients for possible risk factors for venous thromboembolic events (VTE) prior to initiating any contraceptive product containing estrogen. The risk of VTE for reproductive-aged women is extremely low (4 per 100,000 women per year for nonpregnant women not using contraceptive product containing estrogen). The use of estrogen increases the risk of VTE for nonpregnant women

Table. 4–17. Screening questions for inherited thrombophilia.

Have you or a first-degree relative...	...ever had blood clots in the legs or lungs? ... ever been hospitalized for blood clots in the legs or lungs?
What were the circumstances in which the blood clot took place?	Cancer, air travel, obesity, immobility, postpartum
Did you or a family member require blood thinning medication?	

(10–30 per 100,000 women per year); however, pregnancy itself markedly increases the risk of VTE (60 per 100,000 women per year). In light of the low population risk of VTE, it is not cost-effective to screen all reproductive-aged women for inherited thrombophilia (factor V Leiden, prothrombin mutation, protein S, protein C, and antithrombin deficiencies). Table 4–17 shows helpful screening questions for personal and family history of VTE. If a close relative had a VTE, determine whether testing for inherited thrombophilia was conducted. If a specific defect was identified, testing the patient for that defect prior to initiating a product containing estrogen is warranted. If testing is unknown but the family history is highly suggested of inherited thrombophilia, testing for all of the inherited thrombophilic disorders prior to initiating estrogen should be considered. Additionally, if testing is indicated but not possible, providers should consider alternative contraceptive products that do not contain estrogen.

Tips for Prescribing and Monitoring Contraceptive Use

It is important to thoroughly review the advantages, disadvantages, potential side effects, and instructions for use of contraceptive methods in a concise and age-appropriate manner with adolescent patients. Written instructions that are clear and at an appropriate educational level can also be helpful (www.youngwomenshealth.org is a useful source for instructions). Some offices utilize consent forms to further ensure that the adolescent has a full understanding of the chosen contraceptive method. Teens need to be reminded that hormonal contraception will not protect them from STI transmission (including HIV infection) and condoms need to be used consistently. Encouraging teens to be creative about personal reminders such as setting a cell phone alarm to take a pill can help with compliance. Teens often discontinue birth control for nonmedical reasons or minor side effects and should be encouraged to contact their providers if any questions or concerns about the chosen method arise to avoid unintentional pregnancy. Frequent follow-up visits every few months with a provider may also improve adherence. These visits also provide opportunities for further reproductive health education and STI screening.

Barrier Methods

Male condoms have been used more widely in the last several decades as a result of educational and marketing efforts driven by the AIDS epidemic. All sexually active adolescents should be counseled to use condoms correctly and consistently with all intimate behaviors (oral, vaginal, and anal intercourse). Condoms offer protection against STIs by providing a mechanical barrier. Polyurethane condoms can be used by adolescents with an allergy to latex. Spermicides containing nonoxynol-9 are no longer recommended, as exposure to spermicide can cause genital irritation which may facilitate the acquisition of STIs including HIV. Patients should be counseled to use water-based lubricants with condoms.

Vaginal barrier methods include the female condom, diaphragm, and cervical cap. The female condom is a polyurethane vaginal pouch that can be used as an alternative to the male condom. Female condoms have lower efficacy in preventing pregnancy and STIs and are more expensive than male condoms. Diaphragms and cervical caps may not be feasible for adolescents as they require prescription, professional fitting, and skill with insertion. They also have higher failure rates with typical use (20% and 40%, respectively; see Table 4–15).

Combined Hormonal Methods

Oral Contraceptive Pills, Transdermal Patch, and Intravaginal Ring

COCs are the most commonly used contraceptive method in the adolescent age group. COCs are also utilized for noncontraceptive indications (Table 4–18). All COCs contain estrogen (ethinyl estradiol or EE). "Low-dose" COCs contain 20–35 mcg of ethinyl estradiol per pill. There are a variety of progestins, most made from testosterone with differing androgenic profiles. Drospirenone is a newer progestin derived from spironolactone that possesses antiandrogenic and antimineralocorticoid activity. This formulation has appeal for use with patients who have PCOS but should not be prescribed for patients with risk of hyperkalemia (those who have renal, hepatic, or adrenal insufficiency or taking certain medications including angiotensin-converting enzyme inhibitors and angiotensin II receptor antagonists). Extended cycle regimens are available which allow women to decrease menstrual frequency from four menstrual cycles per year to formulations that provide hormonal pills daily for the whole year, eliminating menstrual periods altogether. New formulations with fewer placebo pills (4 vs the standard 7) decrease the duration of the menstrual period. There is also a chewable COC for those who cannot swallow pills.

Table 4–18. Noncontraceptive health benefits of oral contraceptive pills.

Protection against life-threatening conditions
Ovarian cancer
Endometrial cancer
Pelvic inflammatory disease
Ectopic pregnancy
Morbidity and mortality due to unintended pregnancies
Alleviate conditions affecting quality of life
Iron-deficiency anemia
Benign breast disease
Dysmenorrhea
Irregular menstrual cycles
Functional ovarian cysts
Premenstrual syndrome
Acne

In general, contraceptive side effects are mild and improve or lessen during the first 3 months of use. Table 4–19 shows the more common estrogenic, progestogenic, and combined (estrogenic and progestogenic) effects of combined oral contraceptive pills (COCs). In general, these symptoms can also be extended to the other combined hormonal methods. If a patient taking contraceptive pills has persistent minor side effects for more than 3 months, a different type of COC can be tried to achieve the hormonal effects desired (eg, decreasing the estrogen content or changing progestin). Breakthrough bleeding is a common side effect in the first few months of COC use and generally resolves without intervention. If breakthrough bleeding is persistent, the provider should rule out other possible etiologies such as missed pills, pregnancy, infection, or interaction with other medications. For women who have spotting or bleeding before completing the active hormonal pills, increasing the progestin content will provide more endometrial support. For those with continued spotting or bleeding after the period, increasing the estrogen content will provide more endometrial support.

Transdermal Patch

The transdermal patch, Ortho Evra, releases 20 mcg of ethinyl estradiol and 150 mcg of norelgestromin daily. One patch is worn for 7 days and changed weekly for 3 consecutive weeks. The patch is an attractive alternative to COCs for adolescents who have difficulty remembering to take a pill every day; however, the higher bioavailability of estrogens delivered transdermally (60% higher than with 35 mcg COCs) has raised concern that the patch might increase the risk of VTE over other estrogen-containing contraceptive products. Studies evaluating this risk have shown conflicting results. The Food and Drug Administration (FDA) updated the safety labeling for Ortho Evra in September 2009 to include its interpretation of these studies showing a zero to twofold increase in the risk of thromboembolic events. The

Table 4–19. Estrogenic, progestenic, and combined effects of COCs by system.

System	Estrogen Effects	Progestin Effects	Estrogen and Progestin Effects
General		Bloating	Cyclic weight gain due to fluid retention
Cardiovascular	Hypertension		Hypertension
Gastrointestinal	Nausea; hepatocellular adenomas	Increased appetite and weight gain; increased LDL cholesterol levels; decreased HDL cholesterol levels; decreased carbohydrate tolerance; increased insulin resistance	
Breast	Increased breast size	Increased breast tenderness or breast size	Breast tenderness
Genitourinary	Leukorrhea; cervical eversion or ectopy		
Hematologic	Thromboembolic complications, including pulmonary emboli (rare), deep venous thrombosis, cerebrovascular accident, or myocardial infarction (rare)		
Neurological			Headaches
Skin	Telangiectasia, melasma	Acne, oily skin	
Psychological		Depression, fatigue, decreased libido	

COC, combined oral contraceptive pill; HDL, high-density lipoprotein; LDL, low-density lipoprotein.
Adapted from Hatcher RA et al: *Contraceptive Technology,* 19th ed. Ardent Media, 2007.

FDA maintains that Ortho Evra is a well-tolerated and effective contraceptive for women with low-risk profile for VTE. As with other estrogen-containing contraceptive products, patients should be advised to avoid smoking and consider planned discontinuation of these methods around major surgery and prolonged immobilization. In clinical trials, the most common side effects included breast disorders (pain and swelling), headache, nausea, and skin irritation. The patch may be less effective in women weighing more than 90 kg and those with skin conditions preventing absorption.

Intravaginal Ring

The NuvaRing is a vaginal ring that releases 15 mcg of ethinyl estradiol and 120 mcg of etonogestrel per day. The patient places the ring inside the vagina for 3 weeks, and removes it the first day of the fourth week to allow for withdrawal bleeding. A new ring is inserted each month. In clinical trials, the most common side effects included vaginitis and vaginal discharge, headache, weight gain, and nausea.

Progestin-Only Methods

Oral Contraceptive Pills

Progestin-only pills (POPs) do not contain estrogen. They are used in women with contraindications to estrogen-containing products such as the presence of inherited risk factors for thrombophilia or unacceptable estrogen-related side effects with COCs. The efficacy of POPs in preventing pregnancy is slightly less than COCs. They require strict compliance and regular dosing schedule due to the shorter half-life of the progestin. A patient must take POPs daily at the same time (within 3 hours). The primary mechanisms by which pregnancy is prevented includes thickening cervical mucous and thinning the endometrial lining. Ovulation is inhibited in approximately 50% of women. The main side effect of POPs is unpredictable menstrual patterns. The need for strict compliance and the possibility of breakthrough bleeding may make POPs a less desirable method for teens.

Injectable Hormonal Contraceptives

Depot medroxyprogesterone acetate (DMPA), or DepoProvera, is a long-acting injectable progestin contraceptive. It is injected into the gluteal or deltoid muscle every 12 weeks at a dose of 150 mg. The first injection should be given during the first 5 days of the menstrual cycle to ensure immediate contraceptive protection. The quick-start method may also be used with DMPA following a negative pregnancy test. Adolescents who have been sexually active within the previous 2 weeks of administration of DMPA using the quick-start method should be informed of the chance of pregnancy and instructed to return for a repeat pregnancy test 2 weeks after receiving DMPA. With a failure rate of less than 0.3%, long-acting nature reducing compliance issues, reversibility, and lack of estrogen-related side effects, it is an attractive contraceptive option for many adolescents. The hypoestrogenic state that results from DMPA suppression of the hypothalamic-pituitary-ovarian axis reduces the normal effect of estrogen to inhibit bone resorption. The FDA issued a black box warning in 2004 that long-term (> 2 years) use of DMPA was a cause of decreased bone density. This factor is of particular concern as adolescence is the critical time of peak bone accretion. Current recommendations are that long-term use of DMPA should be limited to situations where other contraceptive methods are inadequate. Although DMPA use is associated with decreased bone density, there are studies showing that bone mineral density recovers after stopping DMPA. There are no studies to date that can answer the question of whether decreased bone density from adolescent DMPA use increases the risk of osteoporosis and fractures in adulthood. The consensus of experts in the field at this time is that the advantages of using DMPA generally outweigh the theoretical risks of fractures later in life. As with every other contraceptive method, providers need to help their patients weigh the pros and cons of initiating and continuing with this method of contraception. Adolescents using DMPA should be counseled to take adequate dietary calcium (1300 mg/d) and vitamin D (400 IU/d), to avoid tobacco smoking and to have regular weight-bearing physical activity for overall bone health. Other adverse effects of DMPA include unpredictable menstrual patterns, weight gain (typically 5 lb per year for the first two years of use), and mood changes.

Contraceptive Implant

Implanon is a single-rod implant containing the progestin, etonogestrel which is a metabolite of desogestrel. It is placed subdermally in the patient's nondominant upper arm and is effective for 3 years. It is a highly effective long-acting reversible contraceptive (LARC) with failure rates less than 1%. Implanon suppresses ovulation and thickens cervical mucous like DMPA, but does not suppress ovarian estradiol production or induce a hypoestrogenic state. The risk of decreased bone density is less than that associated with DMPA. Placement should occur during the first 5 days of the menstrual period, or any time if a woman is correctly using a different hormonal contraceptive method. Proper timing minimizes the likelihood that the implant is placed during an early pregnancy or in a nonpregnant woman too late to inhibit ovulation in the first cycle of use. Irregular menstrual bleeding is the single most common reason for stopping use in clinical trials. On average the volume of bleeding is similar to the woman's typical menstrual periods but the schedule of bleeding is irregular and unpredictable. Other side effects include headache, weight gain, acne, breast pain, and emotional lability. Return to fertility is rapid following removal. Implanon has not been tested in woman with a BMI greater than 130% ideal and could have decreased efficacy in these women. It is not recommended for women who chronically take drugs that are potent hepatic enzyme inducers because etonogestrel levels may be substantially reduced in these women. Insertion is a straightforward office-based procedure. Interested health care providers must complete formal training from the manufacturer to be able to insert Implanon.

Intrauterine Systems and Devices

Intrauterine systems (IUS) and devices (IUD) are not commonly chosen by adolescents for contraception despite their utility in nulliparous teens, high efficacy (failure rates <1%), and convenience. The levonorgestrel-releasing IUS, Mirena, releases 20 mcg of levonorgestrel per day and is approved for contraception for up to 5 years. It has many contraceptive actions including thickening of cervical mucous, inhibiting sperm capacitation and survival, suppressing the endometrium and suppression of ovulation in some women. Irregular bleeding is common in the first few months following insertion because endometrial suppression takes several months to evolve. Bleeding is then markedly decreased and secondary amenorrhea can occur. In addition to pregnancy prevention, women with the IUS report reduced symptoms of dysmenorrhea and reduced pain from endometriosis. Cramping is common during insertion and spontaneous expulsion can occur. Uterine perforation during insertion is an uncommon risk. The copper T 380A IUD, ParaGard, does not contain hormones and can provide contraception for up to 10 years. Its contraceptive actions include the release of copper ions which inhibit sperm migration and development of a sterile inflammatory reaction which is toxic to sperm and ova and prevents implantation. Menstrual pain and heavy bleeding are the most common reasons for discontinuation. A common misconception about IUS and IUD use is that they increase the risk of PID. Current research shows that the risk of PID is increased above baseline only at the time of insertion. IUS and IUD have also not been shown to increase the risk of tubal infertility or ectopic pregnancy. Contraindications for placement of IUS/IUD include pregnancy, PID, or postabortion sepsis within the past 3 months, current STI, purulent cervicitis, undiagnosed abnormal vaginal bleeding, malignancy of the genital tract, uterine anomalies, or leiomyomata distorting the uterine cavity making insertion incompatible. Allergy to any component of the IUS/IUD is a contraindication. Patients with disorders of copper metabolism (Wilson disease) should not use the copper-containing IUD. Adolescents should be screened for STIs prior to insertion of an IUS or IUD.

Emergency Contraception

Emergency contraception (EC) refers to the use of hormonal medications within 72 hours of unprotected or underprotected intercourse for the prevention of pregnancy (Table 4–20). EC has been studied up to 120 hours following unprotected intercourse; however, its efficacy diminishes with time from the event. EC is 90% effective if used within 24 hours, 75% effective if used within 72 hours, and approximately 60% effective if used within 60 hours. It is therefore important to counsel patients to take the medication as soon as possible following unprotected intercourse or contraception failure. EC could potentially prevent approximately 80% of unintended pregnancies and should be part of anticipatory guidance given to sexually active adolescents of both genders. Advanced prescription for EC at health maintenance visits should be considered in sexually active teens. Indications for EC include failure of contraceptive methods (condom breakage), missing two or more active COC pills, detached contraceptive patch, removed vaginal ring, or late DMPA injection. EC is also used following sexual assault. The exact mechanism of EC is unknown but is thought to disrupt follicular development or interfere with the maturation of the corpus luteum. EC is not teratogenic and does not interrupt a pregnancy that has already implanted in the uterine lining. Plan B is a two-pill progestin-only method delivering 0.75 mg of levonorgestrel per pill that causes significantly less nausea and vomiting than combined estrogen-progesterone methods. It was initially prescribed with instructions to take one pill immediately after unprotected intercourse, followed by a second pill 12 hours later. Current studies have shown that taking two pills simultaneously has the same efficacy. Plan B One-Step was approved in July 2009 and is a one-pill regimen that contains 1.5 mg of levonorgestrel. Both products are available over the counter for patients older than age 17 years. A prescription is required for adolescents younger than age 17. If Plan B is not available, certain COCs containing levonorgestrel or norgestrel can be used for

Table 4–20. Emergency contraception regimens.

Pill (progestin-only)	Dose: once
Plan B	2 pills
Plan B One-Step	1 pill
Pill (estrogen and progestin)	**Dose: repeat in 12 h**
Ovral, Ogestrel	2 white pills
Levlen, Nordette	4 orange pills
Lo/Ovral, Low-ogestrel, Levora, Quasence, Cryselle	4 white pills
Jolessa, Portia, Seasonale, Trivora	4 pink pills
Triphasil, Tri-leven	4 yellow pills
Seasonique	4 light blue-green pills
Empresse	4 orange pills
Alesse, Lessina, Levlite	5 pink pills
Aviane	5 orange pills
Lutera	5 white pills

EC in a two-dose regimen separated by 12 hours known as the Yuzpe method (see Table 4–20). An antiemetic drug take 30 minutes prior to pills containing estrogen may help control nausea. A pregnancy test is not required prior to prescription and administration of EC. A follow-up appointment should be held in 10–14 days for pregnancy testing, STI screening, and counseling regarding reproductive health and contraceptive use.

American College of Obstetricians and Gynecologists: ACOG Committee Opinion No. 392, December 2007. Intrauterine device and adolescents. Obstet Gynecol 2007;110(6):1493–1495 [PMID: 18055754].

Duffy K, Gould MA: Adolescents and emergency contraception: Update 2011. Curr opin Obstet Gynecol 2011;23(5):328–333 [PMID: 21836502].

Committee on Adolescence: Contraception and adolescents. Pediatr 2007;120(5):1135–1148 [PMID: 17974753].

Committee on Adolescence: Emergency contraception. Pediatr 2005;116(4):1026–1035 [PMID: 16147972].

Eaton DK et al: Centers for Disease Control and Prevention (CDC): Youth risk behavior surveillance—United States, 2009. MMWR Surveill Summ 2010;59(5):1–142 [PMID: 20520591]. Available at: http://www.cdc.gov/mmwr/pdf/ss/ss5905.pdf.

Farr S et al: U.S. medical eligibility criteria for contraceptive use, 2010: Adapted from the World Health Organization Medical Eligibility Criteria for Contraceptive Use, 4th ed. MMWR Recomm Rep 2010;59(RR-4):1–86 [PMID: 20559203]. Available at: http://www.cdc.gov/mmwr/preview/mmwrhtml/rr5904a1.htm?s_cid=rr5904a1_w.

Gupta N et al: Hormonal contraception for the adolescent. Pediatr Rev 2008;29(11):386–396 [PMID: 18977857].

Tolaymat LL, Kaunitz AM: Long-acting contraceptives in adolescents. Curr Opin Obstet Gynecol 2007:19:453–460 [PMID: 17885461].

Trenor CC et al: Hormonal Contraception and thrombotic risk: A multidisciplinary approach. Pediatr 2011:127(2):347–357 [PMID: 21199853].

Trussell J: Contraceptive efficacy. In: Hatcher RA et al (editors): Contraceptive Technology, 19th ed revised. Ardent Media, 2007.

World Health Organization: Improving Access to Quality care in Family Planning: Medical Eligibility Criteria for Contraceptive Use. World Health Organization, 2004. Available at: http://whqlibdoc.who.int/publications/2004/9241562668.pdf.

PREGNANCY

In the United States, approximately 740,000 adolescents younger than age 19 become pregnant every year. The majority of teen pregnancies are unintended. Fifty-seven percent of adolescent pregnancies result in live births; 27% end in abortion; and 16% in miscarriage. The United States has the highest rate of teen pregnancy in the developed world. Pregnancy rates for female Hispanic and non-Hispanic black adolescents aged 15–19 years are much higher (128.9 and 123.8 per 1000, respectively) than their non-Hispanic white peers (44 per 1000). Lower socioeconomic status and lower maternal education are risk factors for teen pregnancy regardless of racial or ethnic group. The birth rate for adolescents in 2009, 39.1 births per 1000 females aged 15–19 years, was the lowest it has ever been for all racial and ethnic groups since the historic high reached in 1957 (96.3).

Presentation

Pregnancy is the most common cause of secondary amenorrhea and should be considered as a cause of even one missed period. The level of denial about the possibility of pregnancy is high and adolescents with undiagnosed pregnancies may present with abdominal pain, nausea or vomiting, breast tenderness, urinary frequency, dizziness, or other nonspecific symptoms. In addition to denial, difficult social situations can delay diagnosis and contribute to delay in seeking prenatal care. Young newly pregnant adolescents may fear violence from their partner or abandonment by their family. Clinicians should have a low threshold for suspecting pregnancy and obtaining pregnancy tests.

Diagnosis

Pregnancies are dated from the first day of the LMP. The estimated due date can be calculated by adding 7 days to the LMP, subtracting 3 months and adding 1 year. Pregnancy dating calendars are widely available on the Internet. A speculum examination is not mandatory at the time of pregnancy diagnosis for an asymptomatic adolescent. If there is vaginal spotting or bleeding, unusual vaginal discharge, symptoms of STI, pelvic pain or abdominal pain, a speculum examination is required. The differential diagnostic possibilities include infection, miscarriage, ectopic pregnancy, and other disorders of early pregnancy. An 8-week gestational age uterus is about the size of an orange and a 12-week uterus is about the size of a grapefruit on bimanual examination. The uterine fundus is just palpable at the symphysis pubis at 12 weeks' gestational age, midway between the symphysis and umbilicus at 16 weeks and typically at the umbilicus at 20 weeks. If the uterus is smaller than expected for pregnancy dates, possible diagnoses include inaccurate dates, false-positive test, ectopic pregnancy, or incomplete or missed abortion. A uterus that is larger than expected may be caused by inaccurate dates, twin gestation, molar pregnancy, or a corpus luteum cyst of pregnancy. Enzyme-linked immunosorbent assay test kits specific for the β-hCG subunit and sensitive to less than 50 mIU/mL of serum hCG can be performed on urine (preferably the day's first voided specimen, because it is more concentrated) in less than 5 minutes and are accurate by the expected date of the missed period in almost all patients. Serum radioimmunoassay, also specific for the β-hCG subunit, is accurate within 7 days after fertilization and is helpful in ruling out ectopic pregnancy or threatened abortion. Serum hCG doubles approximately every 2 days in the first 6–7 weeks of the pregnancy and a gestational sac is identifiable using transvaginal ultrasonography at hCG levels of 1000–2000 mIU/mL. In the absence of an accurate

LMP, ultrasonography for confirmation of the presence of an intrauterine pregnancy and accurate dating can be obtained.

Management

A. Counseling at the Time of Pregnancy Testing

When an adolescent presents for pregnancy testing, it is helpful, before performing the test, to find out what she hopes the result will be and what she thinks she will do if the test is positive. The diagnosis of pregnancy may be met with shock, fear, anxiety, happiness, or most likely a combination of emotions. The clinician must discuss all pregnancy options with the patient including termination or continuing with the pregnancy and either placing the infant for adoption or raising the infant. Patients should be informed of the gestational age and time frames required for the different options. If providers are not comfortable discussing the option of termination, the adolescent should be referred to a provider who is comfortable with comprehensive options counseling. Many teenagers need help in telling and involving their parents. It is also important to ascertain the teen's safety and make appropriate referral to social services if there are legitimate concerns. If the patient knows what she wants to do, she should be referred to the appropriate resources. If a teenager is ambivalent about her plans, it is helpful to follow up in 1 week to be certain that a decision has been made. Avoiding a decision reduces the adolescent's options and may result in poor pregnancy outcomes. Providers can help ensure that the patient obtains prenatal care if she has chosen to continue the pregnancy. In addition, counseling about healthful diet; folic acid supplementation (400 mcg/d); and avoiding alcohol, tobacco, and other drugs is important.

B. Pregnancy Outcomes

Young maternal age, low maternal prepregnancy weight, poor weight gain, delay in prenatal care, maternal depression, exposure to domestic violence, and low socioeconomic status contribute to low birth weight and increased neonatal mortality. The poor nutritional status of some teenagers, substance abuse, and high incidence of STIs also play a role in poor outcomes. Teenagers are at greater risk than adults for preeclampsia, eclampsia, iron-deficiency anemia, cephalopelvic disproportion, prolonged labor, premature labor, and maternal death.

Good family support, early prenatal care, and good nutrition can make a difference with several of these problems. The psychosocial consequences for the teenage mother and her infant are listed in Table 4–21. Teenagers who are pregnant require additional support from their caregivers. Multidisciplinary clinics for young mothers, if available, may be the best providers for pregnant adolescents. Adolescent mothers tend to be more negative and authoritative when disciplining their children. They may have inadequate knowledge of normal behavior and development. Providers can help by educating the adolescent mother during routine visits regarding appropriate discipline and expectations of her child's behavior.

Table 4–21. Psychosocial consequences of pregnancy for the adolescent mother and her infant.

Mother	Infant
Increased morbidity related to pregnancy	**Greater health risks**
Greater risk of eclampsia, anemia, prolonged labor, premature labor	Increased chance of low birth weight or prematurity
Increased chance of miscarriages, stillbirths	Increased risk of infant death
Increased chance of maternal mortality	Increased risk of injury and hospitalization by age 5 y
Decreased academic achievement	**Decreased educational attainment**
Less likely to get high school diploma, go to college, or graduate	Lower cognitive scores
Delayed education (average 2 y)	Decreased development
Lower occupational attainment and prestige	Greater chance of being behind grade or needing remedial help
Less chance of stable employment (some resolution over time)	Lower chance of advanced academics
Lower job satisfaction	Lower academic aptitude as a teenager and perhaps a higher probability of dropping out of school
Lower income and wages	**Psychosocial consequences**
Greater dependence on public assistance	Greater risk of behavior problems
Less stable marital relationships	Poverty
Higher rates of single parenthood	Higher probability of living in a nonintact home while in high school
Earlier marriage (though less common than in the past)	Greater risk of adolescent pregnancy
Accelerated pace of marriage, separation, divorce, and remarriage	
Faster pace of subsequent childbearing	
High rate of repeat unintended pregnancy	
More births out of marriage	
Closer spacing of births	
Larger families	

Postpartum contraceptive counseling and follow-up may help prevent additional pregnancies. In untreated girls, the risk of a second unintended pregnancy within the next 2 years is approximately 30%. Combined hormonal contraceptive options can be started 6 weeks after delivery in non-breastfeeding adolescents; progestin-only methods can be started immediately postpartum, even in breastfeeding adolescents.

Ectopic Pregnancy

In the United States, approximately 2% of pregnancies are ectopic. Adolescents have the highest mortality rate from ectopic pregnancy, most likely related to delayed diagnosis. Risk factors include history of PID or STIs. Repeat infections with chlamydia increase risk for ectopic pregnancy, as does cigarette smoking. Conception while on progestin-only methods of contraception also increases the risk of ectopic pregnancy, because of the progestin-mediated decrease in tubal motility. The classic presentation is missed menstrual period, abdominal pain, and vaginal bleeding. A urine pregnancy test is usually positive by the time of presentation. The patient may have abdominal or pelvic tenderness, adnexal tenderness, and/or an adnexal mass on examination. The uterus is typically either normal sized or slightly enlarged. Diagnosis is based on serial serum quantitative hCG levels and transvaginal ultrasound. Patients should be referred urgently to an obstetrician gynecologist for management to avoid a ruptured ectopic pregnancy which is a surgical emergency. These patients often present in shock with an acute surgical abdomen.

Klein JD: Adolescent pregnancy: Current trends and issues. Pediatrics 2005;116(1):281–286 [PMID: 15995071].

Markovitz BP et al: Socioeconomic factors and adolescent pregnancy outcomes: Distinctions between neonatal and post-neonatal deaths? BMC Public Health 2005;5:79 [PMID: 16042801].

Mathews TJ et al: Annual summary of vital statistics: 2008. Pediatrics 2011;127(1):146–157 [PMID: 21173001].

Santelli JS et al: Changing behavioral risk for pregnancy among high school students in the United States, 1991–2007. J Adolesc Health 2009;45(1):25–32 [PMID: 19541246].

Seeber B, Barnhart K: Suspected ectopic pregnancy. Obstet Gynecol 2006;107(2 Pt 1):399–413 [PMID: 16449130].

Ventura SJ, Hamilton BE: U.S. teenage birth rate resumes decline. NCHS Data Brief 2011;58:1–8 [PMID: 21592421].

Adolescent Substance Abuse

5

Paritosh Kaul, MD

Substance abuse tends to be a chronic, progressive disease. The first or initiation stage—from nonuser to user—is such a common feature of becoming an American adult that many authorities call it normative behavior. At this stage, substance use is typically limited to experimentation with tobacco or alcohol (so-called gateway substances). During adolescence, young people are expected to establish an independent, autonomous identity. They try out a variety of behaviors within the safety of families and peer groups. This process often involves experimentation with psychoactive substances, usually in culturally acceptable settings. Progression to the second or continuation stage of substance abuse is a nonnormative risk behavior with the potential to compromise adolescent development. The American Psychiatric Association has outlined criteria to judge the severity of substance use that progresses beyond the experimentation stage to substance abuse or dependency. Progression within a class of substances (eg, from beer to liquor) and progression across classes of substances (eg, from alcohol to heroin) are the third and fourth stages of substance abuse. Individuals at these stages are polysubstance abusers, and most manifest one or more symptoms of dependency, such as tolerance or withdrawal. The transition from one stage to the next is often a cyclic process of regression, cessation, and relapse. Common physiologic effects and symptoms of intoxication (which can occur at any stage) and withdrawal (a symptom of dependency) for the major classes of substances are shown in Tables 5–1 and 5–2.

American Psychiatric Association: Diagnostic and Statistical Manual of Mental Disorders, 4th ed. Text Revision. American Psychiatric Association, 2000.

Briones DF et al: Risk factors and prevention in adolescent substance abuse: A biopsychosocial approach. Adolesc Med Clin 2006;17:335–352 [PMID: 16814697].

U.S. Department of Health and Human Services: Healthy People 2010, 2nd ed, with Understanding and Improving Health and Objectives for Improving Health (2 vols). U.S. Government Printing Office, 2000.

Meyers JL, Dick DM: Genetic and environmental risk factors for adolescent-onset substance use disorders. Child Adolesc Psychiatr Clin N Am 2010 Jul;19(3):465–477 [PMID: 20682215].

SCOPE OF THE PROBLEM

The best current source of information on the prevalence of substance abuse among American children and adolescents is the Monitoring the Future study (2010), which tracks health-related behaviors in a sample of approximately 50,000 8th, 10th, and 12th graders in the United States. This study probably understates the magnitude of the problem of substance abuse because it excludes high-risk adolescent groups—school dropouts, runaways, and those in the juvenile justice system. Substance abuse among American youth rose in the 1960s and 1970s, declined in the 1980s, peaked in the 1990s, and declined in the early 2000s. There was a decrease in substance use initiation between 1999 and 2008, but this trend reversed between 2008 and 2010 and substance use in adolescents continues to be a significant problem. The use of alcohol, tobacco, and illicit drugs doubles from 8th to 12th grade. The use of alcohol and cigarettes more than triples from adolescence (12–17 years) to young adulthood (18–25 years). Initiation of substance abuse is rare after age 20 years.

The Monitoring the Future survey and others show that alcohol is the most frequently abused substance in the United States. Experimentation with alcohol typically begins in or before middle school. It is more common among boys than girls. It is most common among Whites, less common among Hispanics and Native Americans, and least common among Blacks and Asians. Almost three-fourths (71%) of adolescents consume alcohol before graduating from high school. Approximately one-sixth (16%) of eighth graders and 54% of high school students report being drunk at least once in their life. Marijuana is the most commonly used illicit drug in the United States. First experiences with marijuana and the substances listed in Table 5–2 typically occur during middle

Table 5–1. Physiologic effects of commonly abused mood-altering substances by organ/system.

Eyes/pupils	
Mydriasis	Amphetamines, MDMA, or other stimulants; cocaine; glutethimide; jimson weed; LSD. Withdrawal from alcohol and opioids
Miosis	Alcohol, barbiturates, benzodiazepines, opioids, PCP
Nystagmus	Alcohol, barbiturates, benzodiazepines, inhalants, PCP
Conjunctival injection	LSD, marijuana
Lacrimation	Inhalants, LSD. Withdrawal from opioids
Cardiovascular	
Tachycardia	Amphetamines, MDMA, or other stimulants; cocaine; LSD; marijuana; PCP. Withdrawal from alcohol, barbiturates, benzodiazepines
Hypertension	Amphetamines, MDMA, or other stimulants; cocaine; LSD; marijuana; PCP. Withdrawal from alcohol, barbiturates, benzodiazepines
Hypotension	Barbiturates, opioids. Orthostatic: marijuana. Withdrawal from depressants
Arrhythmia	Amphetamines, MDMA, or other stimulants; cocaine; inhalants; opioids; PCP
Respiratory	
Depression	Opioids, depressants, GHB
Pulmonary edema	Opioids, stimulants
Core body temperature	
Elevated	Amphetamines, MDMA, or other stimulants; cocaine; PCP. Withdrawal from alcohol, barbiturates, benzodiazepines, opioids
Decreased	Alcohol, barbiturates, benzodiazepines, opioids, GHB
Peripheral nervous system response	
Hyperreflexia	Amphetamines, MDMA, or other stimulants; cocaine; LSD; marijuana; methaqualone; PCP. Withdrawal from alcohol, barbiturates, benzodiazepines
Hyporeflexia	Alcohol, barbiturates, benzodiazepines, inhalants, opioids
Tremor	Amphetamines or other stimulants, cocaine, LSD. Withdrawal from alcohol, barbiturates, benzodiazepines, cocaine
Ataxia	Alcohol, amphetamines, MDMA, or other stimulants; barbiturates; benzodiazepines; inhalants; LSD; PCP; GHB
Central nervous system response	
Hyperalertness	Amphetamines, MDMA, or other stimulants; cocaine
Sedation, somnolence	Alcohol, barbiturates, benzodiazepines, inhalants, marijuana, opioids, GHB
Seizures	Alcohol, amphetamines, MDMA, or other stimulants; cocaine; inhalants; methaqualone; opioids (particularly meperidine, propoxyphene). Withdrawal from alcohol, barbiturates, benzodiazepines
Hallucinations	Amphetamines, MDMA, or other stimulants; cocaine; inhalants; LSD; marijuana; PCP. Withdrawal from alcohol, barbiturates, benzodiazepines
Gastrointestinal	
Nausea, vomiting	Alcohol, amphetamines or other stimulants, cocaine, inhalants, LSD, opioids, peyote, GHB. Withdrawal from alcohol, barbiturates, benzodiazepines, cocaine, opioids

GHB, γ-hydroxybutyrate; LSD, lysergic acid diethylamide; MDMA, methylenedioxymethamphetamine (ecstasy); PCP, phencyclidine hydrochloride. Adapted, with permission, from Schwartz B, Alderman EM: Substance abuse. Pediatr Rev 1997;18:215.

Table 5–2. Effects of commonly abused mood-altering substances by agent.

Substance	Pharmacology	Intoxication	Withdrawal	Chronic Use
Alcohol (ethanol)	Depressant; 10 g/drink Drink: 12-oz beer, 4-oz wine, 1½-oz liquor; one drink increases blood level by approximately 0.025 g/dL (varies by weight)	Legal: 0.05–0.1 g/dL (varies by state) Mild (< 0.1 g/dL): disinhibition, euphoria, mild sedation, and Impaired coordination Moderate (0.1–0.2 g/dL): impaired mentation and judgment, slurred speech, ataxia Severe: > 0.3 g/dL: confusion, stupor > 0.4 g/dL: coma, Depressed respiration	Mild: headache, tremors, nausea and vomiting ("hangover") Severe: fever, sweaty, seizure, agitation, hallucination, hypertension, tachycardia Delirium tremens (chronic use)	Hepatitis, cirrhosis, cardiac disease, Wernicke encephalopathy, Korsakoff syndrome
Marijuana (cannabis)	δ-9-Tetrahydrocannabinol (THC); 4–6% in marijuana; 20–30% in hashish	Low: euphoria, relaxation, impaired thinking High: mood changes, depersonalization, hallucinations Toxic: panic, delusions, paranoia, psychosis	Irritability, disturbed sleep, tremor, nystagmus, anorexia, diarrhea, vomiting	Cough, gynecomastia, low sperm count, infertility, amotivational syndrome, apathy
Cocaine	Stimulant; releases biogenic amines; concentration varies with preparation and route of administration	Hyperalert, increased energy, confident, insomnia, anxiety, paranoia, dilated pupils, tremors, seizures, hypertension, arrhythmia, tachycardia, fever, dry mouth Toxic: coma, psychosis, seizure, myocardial infarction, stroke, hyperthermia, rhabdomyolysis	Drug craving, depression, dysphoria, irritability, lethargy, tremors, nausea, hunger	Nasal septum ulceration, epistaxis, lung damage, intravenous drug use
Opioids (heroin, morphine, codeine, methadone, opium, fentanyl, meperidine, propoxyphene)	Depressant; binds central opioid receptor; variable concentrations with substance	Euphoria, sedation, impaired thinking, low blood pressure, pinpoint pupil, urinary retention Toxic: hypotension, arrhythmia, depressed respiration, stupor, coma, seizure, death	Only after > 3 wk of regular use: drug craving, rhinorrhea, lacrimation, muscle aches, diarrhea, anxiety, tremors, hypertension, tachycardia	Intravenous drug use: cellulitis, endocarditis, embolisms, HIV
Amphetamines	Stimulant; sympathomimetic	Euphoria, hyperalert state, hyperactive, hypertension, arrhythmia, fever, flushing, dilated pupils, tremor, ataxia, dry mouth	Lethargy, fatigue, depression, anxiety, nightmares, muscle cramps, abdominal pain, hunger	Paranoia, psychosis
MDMA (ecstasy)	Stimulant, psychedelic; releases serotonin, dopamine, and norepinephrine; inhibits reuptake of neurotransmitters; increases dopamine synthesis; inhibits MAO	Enhanced empathy, euphoria, increased energy and self-esteem, tachycardia, hypertension, increased psychomotor drive, sensory enhancement, illusions, difficulty concentrating and retaining information, headaches, palpitations, flushing, hyperthermia Toxic: frank psychosis, coma, seizures, intracranial hemorrhage, cerebral infarction, asystole, pulmonary edema, multisystem organ failure, acute renal or hepatic failure, ARDS, DIC, SIADH, death	None	Paranoid psychosis

(*continued*)

Table 5–2. Effects of commonly abused mood-altering substances by agent. (*Continued*)

Substance	Pharmacology	Intoxication	Withdrawal	Chronic Use
GHB (liquid ecstasy)	Depressant, endogenous CNS transmitter; influences dopaminergic activity, higher levels of GABA-B activity	10 mg/kg: sleep 30 mg/kg: memory loss 50 mg/kg: general anesthesia Toxic: CNS and respiratory depression, aggressiveness, seizures, bradycardia, apnea	Only after chronic use with dosing every 3 h. Early: mild tremor, tachycardia, hyper-tension, diaphoresis, moderate anxiety, insomnia, nausea, vomiting Progressive: confusion, delirium, hallucinations, autonomic instability, death	Wernicke-Korsakoff syndrome
Sedative-hypnotics (barbiturates, benzodiazepines, methaqualone)	Depressant	Sedation, lethargy, slurred speech, pinpoint pupils, hypotension, psychosis, seizures Toxic: stupor, coma, cardiac arrest, seizure, pulmonary edema, death	Only after weeks of use: agitation, delirium, psychosis, hallucinations, fever, flushing, hyper-/hypotension, death	Paranoia
Hallucinogens (LSD, peyote, mescaline, mushrooms, nutmeg, jimson weed)	Inhibition of serotonin release	Illusions, depersonalization, hallucination, anxiety, paranoia, ataxia, dilated pupils, hypertension, dry mouth Toxic: coma, terror, panic, "crazy feeling"	None	Flashbacks
Phencyclidine	Dissociative anesthetic	Low dose (< 5 mg): illusions, hallucinations, ataxia, hypertension, flushing Moderate dose (5–10 mg): hyperthermia, salivation, myoclonus High dose (> 10 mg): rigidity, seizure, arrhythmia, coma, death	None	Flashbacks
Inhalants (toluene, benzene, hydrocarbons, and fluorocarbons)	Stimulation progressing to depression	Euphoria, giddiness, impaired judgment, ataxia, rhinorrhea, salivation, hallucination Toxic: respiratory depression, arrhythmia, coma, stupor, delirium, sudden death	None	Permanent damage to nerves, liver, heart, kidney, brain
Nicotine	Releases dopamine, 1 mg nicotine per cigarette	Relaxation, tachycardia, vertigo, anorexia	Drug craving, irritability, anxiety, hunger, impaired concentration	Permanent damage to lung, heart, cardiovascular system
Anabolic steroids[a]	Bind steroid receptor Stacking: use many types simultaneously Pyramiding: increase dosage	Increased muscle bulk, strength, endurance, increased drive, hypogonadism, low sperm count, gynecomastia, decreased libido, virilization, irregular menses, hepatitis, early epiphysial closure, aggressiveness	Drug craving, dysphoria, irritability, depression	Tendon rupture, cardiomyopathy, atherosclerosis, peliosis hepatis (orally active C17 derivatives of testosterone are especially hepatotoxic)

[a]Despite conventional assumptions, scientific studies show that anabolic steroids do not improve aerobic athletic performance and improve strength only in athletes trained in weight lifting before they begin using steroids and who continue to train and consume a high-protein diet.
ARDS, acute respiratory distress syndrome; CNS, central nervous system; DIC, disseminated intravascular coagulation; GABA, γ-aminobutyric acid; GHB, γ-hydroxybutyrate; HIV, human immunodeficiency virus; LSD, lysergic acid diethylamide; MAO, monoamine oxidase; MDMA, methylenedioxymethamphetamine; SIADH, syndrome of inappropriate secretion of antidiuretic hormone.

or early high school. Marijuana use continued to rise in 2010 among all students. The lifetime prevalence of marijuana use among 12th graders in 2010 was 43.8% and daily use of marijuana continued to increase, with one in sixteen (6.1%) high school seniors a daily or near daily user. In the past decade, LSD, and methamphetamine use has decreased while cocaine use has increased. Recently, ecstasy use has increased after a steady decline of several years. In the past 10 years, there has also been an increase in the recreational use of prescription medications and over-the-counter (OTC) cough and cold medications among adolescents. In one study, 1 in 10 high school seniors reported nonmedical use of prescription opioids, and almost half (45%) used opioids to "relieve physical symptoms" in the past year. Vicodin use decreased among 12th graders to 8% in 2010, but it remains one of the most widely used illicit drugs. Medication used in the management of chronic pain, depression, anxiety, and attention-deficit/hyper-activity disorder can all be drugs of abuse.

Studies indicate that variations in the popularity of a substance of abuse are influenced by changes in the perceived risks and benefits of the substance among adolescent users. For example, the use of inhalants was rising until 2006, when both experience and educational efforts resulted in a perception of these substances as being "dangerous." As the perception of danger decreases, old drugs may reappear in common use. This process is called "generational forgetting." Currently, use of LSD, inhalants, and ecstasy all reflect the effects of generational forgetting.

DiFranza JR et al: Let the children be heard: Lessons from studies of the early onset of tobacco addiction. Pediatrics 2008;121:623–624 [PMID: 18310213].

Johnston LD et al: Monitoring the Future national results on adolescent drug use: Overview of key findings, 2010. Ann Arbor: Institute for Social Research, The University of Michigan, 2011.

Mulye TP et al: Trends in adolescent and young adult health in the United States. J Adolesc Health 2009 Jul;45(1):8–24 [PMID: 19541245].

Substance Abuse and Mental Health Services Administration: Results from the 2010 National Survey on Drug Use and Health: Summary of National Findings, NSDUH Series H-41, HHS Publication No. (SMA) 11-4658. Rockville, MD: Substance Abuse and Mental Health Services Administration, 2011.

Boyd CJ et al: Non-medical use of prescription analgesics: A three-year national longitudinal study. J Addict Dis. 2009 Jul;28(3):232–242 [PMID: 20155592].

Latimer W et al: Epidemiologic trends of adolescent use of alcohol, tobacco, and other drugs. Child Adolesc Psychiatr Clin N Am. 2010 Jul;19(3):451–464 [PMID: 20682214].

MORBIDITY DATA

Use and abuse of alcohol or other mood-altering substances in adolescents in the United States are tightly linked to their leading causes of death, motor vehicle accidents, unintentional injury, homicide, and suicide. Substance abuse is also associated with physical and sexual abuse. Drug use and abuse contribute to other high-risk behaviors, such as unsafe sexual activity, unintended pregnancy, and sexually transmitted disease. Adolescents may also be involved with selling of drugs.

Risks associated with tobacco, alcohol, and cocaine are listed in Table 5–2. Less well known are the long- and short-term adolescent morbidities connected with the currently most popular illicit drugs, marijuana and ecstasy. The active ingredient in marijuana, δ-9-tetrahydrocannabinol (THC), transiently causes tachycardia, mild hypertension, and bronchodilation. Regular use can cause lung changes similar to those seen in tobacco smokers. Heavy use decreases fertility in both sexes and impairs immunocompetence. It is also associated with abnormalities of cognition, learning, coordination, and memory. It is possible that heavy marijuana use is the cause of the so-called amotivational syndrome, characterized by inattention to environmental stimuli and impaired goal-directed thinking and behavior. Analysis of confiscated marijuana recently has shown increasing THC concentration and adulteration with other substances.

The popularity and accessibility of ecstasy is again increasing among adolescents. Chronic use is associated with progressive decline of immediate and delayed memory, and with alterations in mood, sleep, and appetite that may be permanent. Even first-time users may develop frank psychosis indistinguishable from schizophrenia. Irreversible cardiomyopathy, noncardiogenic pulmonary edema, and pulmonary hypertension may occur with long-term use. Acute overdose can cause hyperthermia and multiorgan system failure.

Prenatal and environmental exposure to abused substances also carries health risks. Parental tobacco smoking is associated with low birth weight in newborns, sudden infant death syndrome, bronchiolitis, asthma, otitis media, and fire-related injuries. Maternal use of marijuana during pregnancy is associated with an increased risk of sudden infant death syndrome. In-utero exposure to alcohol may produce fetal malformations, intrauterine growth restriction, and brain injury.

Ellickson PL et al: Reducing early smokers' risk for future smoking and other problem behavior: Insights from a five-year longitudinal study. J Adolesc Health 2008;43:394–400 [PMID: 18809138].

Hanewinkel R et al: Longitudinal study of exposure to entertainment media and alcohol use among German adolescents. Pediatrics 2009;123:989–995 [PMID: 19255030].

Hingson RW et al: Age of drinking onset, alcohol use disorders, frequent heavy drinking, and unintentionally injuring oneself and others after drinking. Pediatrics 2009;123:1477–1484 [PMID: 19482757].

Kerr JM et al: Anabolic-androgenic steroids: Use and abuse in pediatric patients. Pediatr Clin North Am 2007;54:771–785 [PMID: 17723876].

Levine SB et al: Nonmedical use of prescription medications: An emerging risk behavior among rural adolescents. J Adolesc Health 2009;44:407–409 [Epub 2008] [PMID: 19306802].

Sherman SG et al: Patterns of risky behaviors associated with methamphetamine use among young Thai adults: A latent class analysis. J Adolesc Health 2009;44:169–175 [PMID: 19167666].

McCabe SE et al: Medical misuse of controlled medications among adolescents. Arch Pediatr Adolesc Med. 2011 Aug;165(8):729–735 [PMID: 21810634].

Goldsworthy RC et al: Recreational versus nonrecreational prescription borrowing: Time for an expanded conceptualization? J Adolesc Health 2009 Dec;45(6):539–540 [PMID: 20307833].

Taylor DJ et al: Patterns and consequences of inadequate sleep in college students: Substance use and motor vehicle accidents. J Adolesc Health 2010 Jun;46(6):610–612 [PMID: 20472221].

Walton MA et al: Sexual risk behaviors among teens at an urban emergency department: Relationship with violent behaviors and substance use. J Adolesc Health 2011 Mar;48(3):303–305 [PMID: 21338903].

Herrick AL et al: Sex while intoxicated: A meta-analysis comparing heterosexual and sexual minority youth. J Adolesc Health 2011 Mar;48(3):306–309 [PMID: 21338904].

Bailey JA: Addressing common risk and protective factors can prevent a wide range of adolescent risk behaviors. J Adolesc Health 2009 Aug;45(2):107–108 [PMID: 19628134].

Opioids: Nonmedical use and abuse in older children. Pediatr Rev 2011 Apr;32(4) [PMID: 21460089].

SUPPLEMENT USE & ABUSE

Use of supplements or special diets to enhance athletic performance dates to antiquity. Today, many elite and casual athletes use ergogenic (performance-enhancing) supplements in an attempt to improve performance. The most popular products used by adolescents are anabolic-androgenic steroids, steroid hormone precursors, creatine, human growth hormone, diuretics, and protein supplements. Anabolic-androgenic steroids increase strength and lean body mass and lessen muscle breakdown. However, they are associated with side effects including acne, liver tumors, hypertension, premature closure of the epiphysis, ligamentous injury, and precocious puberty. In females, they can cause hirsuitism, male pattern baldness, and virilization; in boys, they can cause gynecomastia and testicular atrophy. Creatine increases strength and improves performance but can cause dehydration, muscle cramps, and has potential for renal toxicity. Human growth hormone has no proven effects on performance although it decreases subcutaneous fat. Potential risks include coarsening of facial features and cardiovascular disease. Strength athletes (ie, weight lifters) use protein powders and shakes to enhance muscle repair and mass. The amount of protein consumed often greatly exceeds the recommended daily allowance for weight lifters and other resistance-training athletes (1.6–1.7 g/kg/d). Excess consumption of protein provides no added strength or muscle mass and can provoke renal failure in the presence of underlying renal dysfunction. The American Academy of Pediatrics (AAP) cautions against the use of performance-enhancing substances.

As the use of supplements and herbs increases, it is increasingly important for pediatric care providers to be familiar with their common side effects. The Internet has become a source for information about and distribution of these products. The easy accessibility, perceived low risk, and low cost of these products significantly increase the likelihood that they will become substances of abuse by adolescents.

Mulcahey MK et al: Anabolic steroid use in adolescents: Identification of those at risk and strategies for prevention. Phys Sportsmed 2010 Oct;38(3):105–113 [PMID: 20959703].

Harmer PA: Anabolic-androgenic steroid use among young male and female athletes: Is the game to blame? Br J Sports Med 2010 Jan;44(1):26–31 [PMID: 19919946].

Kaminer Y: Problematic use of energy drinks by adolescents. Child Adolesc Psychiatr Clin N Am 2010 Jul;19(3):643–650 [PMID: 20682226].

Casavant MJ et al: Consequences of use of anabolic androgenic steroids. Pediatr Clin North Am 2007;54:677 [PMID: 17723870].

Gregory AJM, Fitch RW: Sports medicine: Performance-enhancing drugs. Pediatr Clin North Am 2007;54:797 [PMID: 17723878].

Primack BA et al: Media exposure and marijuana and alcohol use among adolescents. Subst Use Misuse 2009;44:722–739 [PMID: 19306219].

VandenBerg P et al: Steroid use among adolescents: Longitudinal findings from Project EAT. Pediatrics 2007;119:476 [PMID: 17332200].

Morgenstern M et al: Exposure to alcohol advertising and teen drinking. Prev Med 2011 Feb 1;52(2):146–151 [PMID: 21130108].

McCool J et al: Do parents have any influence over how young people appraise tobacco images in the media? J Adolesc Health 2011 Feb;48(2):170 [PMID: 21257116].

BATH SALTS

Since 2010, there has been an increase in the use of a new drug of abuse called "bath salts." These products, which are not related to hygienic products, are also known as Vanilla Sky or Ivory Wave. They can be procured via the Internet. The main ingredient is 4-methylene-dioxypyrovalerone, a central nervous stimulant which acts by inhibiting norepinephrine-dopaminergic reuptake. Their effects are similar to those of stimulants like PCP, ecstasy, and LSD (see Tables 5–1 and 5–2). Overdoses can potentially be severe and lethal. In 2011, the number of calls to poison control centers increased 5-fold compared to 2010. These substances cannot be detected by routine drug screen, which may complicate management in the emergency department.

American Association of Poison Control Centers: U.S. poison centers raise alarm about toxic substance marketed as bath salts; states begin taking action. Alexandria, VA: American Association of Poison Control Centers; March 22, 2011. Available at http://www.aapcc.org/dnn/portals/0/prrel/bathsaltsmarch22.pdf

Centers for Disease Control and Prevention (CDC): Emergency department visits after use of a drug sold as "bath salts"—Michigan, November 13, 2010-March 31, 2011. MMWR Morb Mortal Wkly Rep. 2011 May 20;60(19):624–627 [PMID: 21597456].

Ross EA et al: "Bath salts" intoxication. N Engl J Med 2011 Sep 8; 365(10):967–968 [PMID: 21899474].

Spiller HA et al: Clinical experience with and analytical confirmation of "bath salts" and "legal highs" (synthetic cathinones) in the United States. Clin Toxicol (Phila) 2011 Jul;49(6):499–505 [PMID: 21824061].

PREDICTING THE PROGRESSION FROM USE TO ABUSE

Initially, most adolescents use mood-altering substances intermittently or experimentally. The challenge to pediatric health care providers is to recognize warning signs, identify potential abusers early, and intervene in an effective fashion before acute or chronic use produces morbidity. The prediction of progression from use to abuse is best viewed within the biopsychosocial model. Substance abuse is a symptom of personal and social maladjustment as often as it is a cause. Because there is a direct relationship between the number of risk factors listed in Table 5–3 and the frequency of substance abuse, a combination of risk factors is the best indicator of risk. Even so, most teenagers with multiple risk characteristics never progress to substance abuse. It is unclear why only a minority of young people exhibiting the high-risk characteristics listed in Table 5–3 go on to abuse substances, but presumably the protective factors listed in Table 5–3 give most adolescents the resilience to cope with stress in more socially adaptive ways. Being aware of the risk domains in Table 5–3 will help physicians identify youngsters most apt to need counseling about substance abuse.

Table 5–3. Factors that influence the progression from substance use to substance abuse.

Enabling Risk Factors	Potentially Protective Factors
Societal and community	
Experimentation encouraged by media Illicit substances available Extreme economic deprivation Neighborhood disorganization, crowding Tolerance of licit and illicit substance use	Regular involvement in church activities Support for norms and values of society Strict enforcement of laws prohibiting substance use among minors and abuse among adults Neighborhood resources, supportive adults
School	
Lack of commitment to school or education Truancy Academic failure Early, persistent behavior problems	Strong commitment to school or education Future-oriented goals Achievement oriented
Family	
Models of substance abuse and other unconventional behavior Dysfunctional parenting styles; excessive authority or permissiveness High family conflict; low bonding	Models of conventional behavior Attachment to parents Cohesive family Nurturing parenting styles
Peers	
Peer rejection in elementary grades Substance use prevalent among peers Peer attitudes favorable to substance abuse and unconventional behavior	Popular with peers Abstinent friends Peer attitudes favor conventional behavior
Individual	
Genetic predisposition Psychological diagnoses (attention-deficit/hyperactivity disorder; antisocial personality) Depression and low self-esteem Alienation and rebelliousness Sexual or physical abuse Early onset of deviant behavior or delinquency Early onset of sexual behavior Aggressive	Positive self-concept, good self-esteem Intolerance of deviance Internally motivated, takes charge of problems

Clark DB et al: Adolescent-onset substance use disorders predict young adult mortality. J Adolesc Health 2008;42:637–639 [PMID: 18486875].

Meyers JL et al: Genetic and environmental risk factors for adolescent-onset substance use disorders. Child Adolesc Psychiatr Clin N Am 2010 Jul;19(3):465–477 [PMID: 20682215].

Prado G et al: What accounts for differences in substance use among U.S.-born and immigrant Hispanic adolescents? Results from a longitudinal prospective cohort study. J Adolesc Health 2009 Aug;45(2):118–125 [PMID: 19628137].

Strachman A et al: Early adolescent alcohol use and sexual experience by emerging adulthood: A 10-year longitudinal investigation. J Adolesc Health 2009 Nov;45(5):478–482 [PMID: 19837354].

Chartier KG et al: Development and vulnerability factors in adolescent alcohol use. Child Adolesc Psychiatr Clin N Am 2010 Jul;19(3):493–504 [PMID: 20682217].

McCoy SI et al: A trajectory analysis of alcohol and marijuana use among Latino adolescents in San Francisco, California. J Adolesc Health 2010 Dec;47(6):564–574 [PMID: 21094433].

Cleveland MJ et al: The role of risk and protective factors in substance use across adolescence. J Adolesc Health 2008;43: 157–164 [PMID: 18639789].

Fisher LB et al: Predictors of initiation of alcohol use among US adolescents: Findings from a prospective cohort study. Arch Pediatr Adolesc Med 2007;161:959–966 [PMID: 17909139].

Fletcher A et al: How might schools influence young people's drug use? Development of theory from qualitative case-study research. J Adolesc Health 2009 Aug;45(2):126–132 [PMID: 19628138].

Rostosky SS et al: Is religiosity a protective factor against substance use in young adulthood? Only if you're straight! J Adolesc Health 2007;40:440–447 [PMID: 17448402].

Schinke SP et al: Substance use among early adolescent girls: Risk and protective factors. J Adolesc Health 2008;43:191–194 [PMID: 18639794].

Sutfin EL et al: Protective behaviors and high-risk drinking among entering college freshmen. Am J Health Behav 2009;33:610–619 [PMID: 19296751].

Wells K: Substance abuse and child maltreatment. Pediatr Clin North Am 2009;56:345–362 [PMID: 19358920].

Tobler AL et al: Trajectories or parental monitoring and communication and effects on drug use among urban young adolescents. J Adolesc Health 2010 Jun;46(6):560–568 [PMID: 20472213].

MANAGEMENT OF SUBSTANCE ABUSE

Office Screening

The AAP Committee on Substance Abuse recommends that pediatricians include discussions of substance abuse as part of their anticipatory care. This should include screening for substance abuse with parents at the first prenatal visit. Given the high incidence of substance abuse and the subtlety of its early signs and symptoms, a general psychosocial assessment is the best way to screen for substance abuse among adolescents. The universal screening approach outlined in the American Medical Association (AMA) Guidelines for Adolescent Preventive Services (GAPS) is a good guide for routine screening and diagnosis. Interviewing and counseling techniques and methods for taking a psychosocial history are discussed in Chapter 4. In an atmosphere of trust and confidentiality, physicians should ask routine screening questions of all patients and be alert for addictive diseases, recognizing the high level of denial often present in addicted patients. Clues to possible substance abuse include truancy, failing grades, problems with interpersonal relationships, delinquency, depressive affect, chronic fatigue, recurrent abdominal pains, chest pains or palpitations, headache, chronic cough, persistent nasal discharge, and recurrent complaints of sore throat. Substance abuse should be included in the differential diagnosis of all behavioral, family, psychosocial, and medical problems. A family history of drug addiction or abuse should raise the level of concern about drug abuse in the pediatric patient. Possession of promotional products such as T-shirts and caps with cigarette or alcohol logos should also be a red flag because teenagers who own these items are more likely to use the products they advertise. Pediatricians seeing patients in emergency departments, trauma units, or prison should have an especially high index of suspicion.

In the primary care setting, insufficient time and lack of training are the greatest barriers to screening adolescents for substance abuse. Brief questionnaires can be used if time does not allow for more detailed investigation. A screening instrument that has been rigorously studied in primary care settings is the CAGE questionnaire. CAGE is a mnemonic derived from the first four questions that asks the patient questions regarding their substance abuse. These are their need to reduce it, annoyance if asked about it, feeling guilty about the use, and the need of the drug/alcohol as an eye opener. A score of 2 or more is highly suggestive of substance abuse. Although constructed as a screening tool for alcohol abuse in adults, the CAGE questionnaire can be adapted to elicit information about use of other mood-altering substances by pediatric patients and their close contacts (eg, parents and older siblings). Clinicians may find it helpful to use such questionnaires to stimulate discussion of the patient's self-perception of his or her substance use. For example, if an adolescent admits to a previous attempt to cut down on drinking, this provides an opportunity to inquire about events that may have led to the attempt.

Ewing JA. Detecting alcoholism. The CAGE questionnaire. JAMA 1984 Oct;252(14):1905–1907 [PMID: 6471323].

Kokotailo B: Alcohol use by youth and adolescents: A pediatric concern. Pediatrics 2010 May;125(5):1078–1087 [PMID: 20385640].

Sims TH: Committee on Substance Abuse. From the American Academy of Pediatrics: Technical report—Tobacco as a substance of abuse. Pediatrics 2009 Nov;124(5):e1045–1053 [PMID: 19841120].

Strasburger VC: Policy statement—children, adolescents, substance abuse, and the media. Pediatrics 2010 Oct;126(4):791–799 [PMID: 20876181].

Hassan A et al: Primary care follow-up plans for adolescents with substance use problems. Pediatrics 2009;124:144–150 [PMID: 19564294].

Heyman RB: Screening for substance abuse in the office setting: A developmental approach. Adolesc Med State Art Rev 2009;20: 9–21 [PMID: 19492688].

Schydlower M (editor): Substance Abuse: A Guide for Health Professionals, 2nd ed. American Academy of Pediatrics, 2002.

Diagnosis

When the psychosocial history suggests the possibility of substance use, the primary tasks of the diagnostic interview are the same as for the evaluation of other medical problems (Table 5–4).

First, specific information about the extent and circumstances of the problem is gathered. Eliciting information through multiple-choice questions is a useful technique. For example, "Has anything really good ever happened to you when you are high? Some of my patients like to get high because they feel good; others find it helps them relax and be sociable with friends; and some find it helps them forget their problems. Are any of these things true for you?"

Second, the provider should determine why the patient has progressed from initiation to the continuation or maintenance phase of substance abuse. The cause may be different at different periods of development. Although peer group characteristics are one of the best predictors of substance use among early and middle adolescents, this is not so among older adolescents and young adults.

Table 5–4. Evaluation of positive psychosocial screens for substance abuse.

I. Define the extent of the problem by determining:
- Age at onset of substance use
- Which substances are being used
- Circumstances of use
  - Where?
  - When?
  - With whom?
- To what extent substances are being used
  - How frequently?
  - How much (quantity)?
  - With what associated symptoms (eg, tolerance, withdrawal)?
- With what result?
  - What does the patient gain from becoming high?
  - Does the patient get into risky situations while high?
  - Does the patient engage in behaviors while high that are later regretted?

II. Define the cause of the problem

Although few children and adolescents will have been abusing substances long enough to have developed overt signs and symptoms, it is important to look for them on physical examination. Positive physical findings can be a tool to penetrate a patient's denial and convince him or her of the significance of the alcohol or drug use.

Griffin KW et al: Evidence-based interventions for preventing substance use disorders in adolescents. Child Adolesc Psychiatr Clin N Am 2010 Jul;19(3):505–526 [PMID: 20682218].

Van Hook S et al: The "Six T's": Barriers to screening teens for substance abuse in primary care. J Adolesc Health 2007;40:456 [PMID: 17448404].

Comorbidity

Comorbidities, especially other psychiatric disorders, are common among substance-abusing patients (Table 5–5). Affective disorder, anxiety disorder, and mania are most strongly associated with alcohol and drug dependence. Attention-deficit/hyperactivity has also been closely linked with adolescent substance abuse. Adolescents with depression are likely to use drugs in an attempt to feel pleasure, but this type of self-medication may exacerbate their condition. Although it is often difficult to determine which diagnosis is primary, it is important for pediatric health care providers to recognize the possibility of a comorbid condition and provide appropriate treatment. Finally, in addition to identifying psychiatric comorbidities, it is imperative that providers look for medical conditions that mimic symptoms of drug withdrawal or intoxication.

Bukstein OG et al: Management of the adolescent with substance use disorders and comorbid psychopathology. Child Adolesc Psychiatr Clin N Am 2010 Jul;19(3):609–623 [PMID: 20682224].

Levy S et al: Screening adolescents for substance use-related high-risk sexual behaviors. J Adolesc Health 2009 Nov;45(5): 473–477 [PMID: 19837353].

Riggs P et al: Comorbid psychiatric and substance abuse disorders: Recent treatment research. Subst Abus 2008;29:51–63 [PMID: 19042206].

Riggs PD et al: A randomized controlled trial of fluoxetine and cognitive behavioral therapy in adolescents with major depression, behavior problems, and substance use disorders. Arch Pediatr Adolesc Med 2007;161:1026–1034 [PMID: 17984403].

Table 5–5. Common comorbid conditions associated with adolescent substance abuse.

1. Attention-deficit/hyperactivity disorder
2. Bipolar disorder
3. Depression disorder
4. Anxiety disorders (often with depressive disorders)

Pharmacologic Screening

The use of urine and blood testing for detecting substance abuse is controversial. The consensus is that pharmacologic screening should be reserved for situations in which behavioral dysfunction is of sufficient concern to outweigh the practical and ethical drawbacks of testing. The AAP recommends screening under certain circumstances (eg, an inexplicably obtunded patient in the emergency department) but discourages routine screening for the following reasons: (1) voluntary screening is rarely truly voluntary owing to the negative consequences for those who decline to participate; (2) infrequent users or individuals who have not used substances recently may be missed; (3) confronting substance-abusing individuals with objective evidence of their use has little or no effect on behavior; and (4) the role of health care providers is to provide counseling and treatment, not law enforcement, so drug testing should not be done for the purpose of detecting illegal use. If testing is to be performed, the provider should discuss the plan for screening with the patient, explain the reasons for it, and obtain informed consent. The AAP does not consider parental request and permission sufficient justification for involuntary screening of mentally competent minors.

If testing is to be performed, it is imperative that it be done accurately and that the limitations of testing be understood. Tests range from inexpensive, chromatographic spot tests, which can be performed in the office, to gas chromatography and mass spectrometry, which require specialized laboratory equipment and are usually reserved for forensic investigations. Most commercial medical laboratories use the enzyme multiplication immunoassay technique, in which a sample of the fluid to be tested is added to a test reagent containing a known quantity of the radiolabeled index drug under question. If the index drug is also present in the patient's urine or serum, it competes with the radiolabeled drug for binding sites on the test kit antibody. The unbound or excess drug can then be quantified with a spectrophotometer. Most of the commonly abused mood-altering substances, with the exception of solvents and inhalants, can be detected by this method.

Interpretation of results is complicated by false-positives resulting from antibody cross-reactions with some medications and substances (Table 5–6) or from a patient's passive exposure to illicit substances. The most common cause of false-negative tests is infrequent use. Table 5–7 shows the duration of detectability in the urine after last use by class of substance and duration of use. Detectability ranges from a few hours for alcohol to several weeks for regular marijuana use. False-negative results can also occur if the patient alters or adulterates the specimen. Some of the commercial products used to adulterate samples include glutaraldehyde, nitrite, pyridinium chlorochromate, peroxidate, and peroxide (stealth). Household products such as bleach, vinegar, Visine eye drops (for marijuana), strong alkali drain cleaners, and detergents are also used. (Teenagers should be advised that despite street lore, ingesting these compounds is an ineffective and potentially dangerous way to prevent drug detection in the urine.) Close observation during collection and testing the temperature, specific gravity, and pH of urine samples may detect attempts at deception.

Table 5–6. Causes of false-positive drug screens.

Opioids
Poppy seeds
Dextromethorphan
Chlorpromazine
Diphenoxylate
Amphetamines
Ephedrine
Phenylephrine
Pseudoephedrine
N-acetylprocainamide
Chloroquine
Procainamide
Phencyclidines
Dextromethorphan
Diphenhydramine
Chlorpromazine
Doxylamine
Thioridazine

Table 5–7. Duration of urine positivity for selected drugs.

Drug Class	Detection Time
Amphetamines	< 48 h
Barbiturates	Short-acting: 1 d Long-acting: 2–3 wk
Benzodiazepines	Single dose: 3 d Habitual use: 4–6 wk
Cocaine metabolites	Acute use: 2–4 d Habitual use: 2 wk
Ethanol	2–14 h
Methadone	Up to 3 d
Opioids	Up to 2 d
Propoxyphene	6–48 h
Cannabinoid	Moderate use: 5 d Habitual use: 10–20 d
Methaqualone	2 wk
Phencyclidine	Acute use: 1 wk Habitual use: 3 wk
Anabolic steroids	Days to weeks

Reprinted, with permission, from Woolf A, Shannon M: Clinical toxicology for the pediatrician. Pediatr Clin North Am 1995;42:317.

Home drug-testing products are available for parents and can be procured via the Internet; however, these products have limitations and potential risks. The AAP recommends that home and school-based drug testing not be implemented until the safety and efficacy of these procedures can be established. It further recommends that parents be encouraged to consult the adolescent's primary care provider rather than relying on home drug-testing products.

Levy S et al: Acceptability of drug testing in an outpatient substance abuse program for adolescents. J Adolesc Health 2011 Mar;48(3):229–233 [PMID: 21338892].

Committee on Substance Abuse, American Academy of Pediatrics; Council on School Health, American Academy of Pediatrics, Knight JR, Mears CJ: Testing for drugs of abuse in children and adolescents: Addendum—testing in schools and at home. Pediatrics 2007;119:627 [PMID: 17332219].

Goldberg L et al: Outcomes of a prospective trial of student-athlete drug testing: The Student Athlete Testing Using Random Notification (SATURN) study. J Adolesc Health 2007;41: 421–429 [PMID: 17950161].

Jaffee WB et al: Is this urine really negative? A systematic review of tampering methods in urine drug screening and testing. J Subst Abuse Treat 2007;33:33 [PMID: 17588487].

Table 5–8. Stages of change and intervention tasks.

Patient Stage	Motivation Tasks
Precontemplation	Create doubt, increase the patient's awareness of risks and problems with current patterns of substance use
Contemplation	Help the patient weigh the relative risks and benefits of changing substance use; evoke reasons to change and risks of not changing; strengthen the patient's self-efficacy for changing current use
Determination	Help the patient determine the best course of action to change substance use from among available alternatives
Action	Help the patient establish a clear plan of action toward changing substance use
Maintenance	Help the patient identify and use strategies to prevent relapse
Relapse	Help the patient renew the process of change starting at contemplation

Reprinted, with permission, from Werner MJ: Principles of brief intervention for adolescent alcohol, tobacco, and other drug use. Pediatr Clin North Am 1995;42:341.

TREATMENT & REFERRAL

Office-Based Treatment

The AMA and the AAP recommend that all children and adolescents receive counseling about the dangers of substance use and abuse from their primary care providers. By offering confidential health care services and routinely counseling about the risks associated with drug abuse, primary care providers can help most patients avoid the adverse consequences of experimentation with mood-altering substances. However, more intervention is required for youngsters in environments where substance abuse is regarded as acceptable recreational behavior. Counseling strategies appropriate for patients who wish to change their behavior may be ineffective for patients who do not consider use of mood-altering substances to be a problem. It may therefore be preferable to begin discussions about treatment by helping youngsters consider alternative ways of meeting the needs that substance use is currently providing. The clinician may in this way help the patient devise alternatives that are more attractive than substance use. Realistically, few substance-abusing teenagers will choose to quit because of a single conversation even with a highly respected health care provider. The message is most effective when offered repeatedly from many sources—family, peers, guidance counselors, and teachers. Brief interventions for adolescents have also shown some improvement among high-risk youth. Motivational interviewing for substance-abusing teens has shown some promise.

Assessment of the patient's readiness to change is the critical first step in office-based intervention. Clinicians should consider the construct presented in Table 5–8. In theory, individuals pass through this series of stages in the course of changing problem behaviors. Thus, to be maximally effective, providers should tailor their counseling messages to the patient's stage of readiness to change.

Once it has been established that a patient is prepared to act on information about treatment, the next step is to select the program that best fits his or her individual needs. Most drug treatment programs are not designed to recognize and act on the individual vulnerabilities that have predisposed the patient to substance abuse. When programs are individualized, even brief (5- to 10-minute) counseling sessions may promote reductions in cigarette smoking and drinking. This strategy appears to be most effective when the health care provider's message is part of an office-wide program so that the entire staff reinforces the cessation message with every patient.

Kaplan G et al: Pharmacotherapy for substance abuse disorders in adolescence. Pediatr Clin North Am 2011 Feb;58(1):243–258 [PMID: 21281859].

Simkin DR et al: Pharmacotherapies for adolescent substance use disorders. Child Adolesc Psychiatr Clin N Am 2010 Jul;19(3): 591–608 [PMID: 20682223].

Smoking Cessation in Pediatrics

Although more than half of adolescents who smoke regularly say they want to quit and have tried to quit, only a minority report that they have been advised or helped to do so by a health care provider. Practitioners unfamiliar with approaches to smoking cessation may feel that smoking cessation interventions are time-consuming, nonreimbursable, and impractical in a busy office. An easy guideline for health care providers is the "Five A's" for tobacco cessation (Table 5–9), published by the Public Health Service and endorsed by the AAP.

Smoking cessation is a process that takes time. Relapse must be regarded as a normal part of quitting rather than evidence of personal failure or a reason to forgo further attempts. Patients can actually benefit from relapses if they are helped to identify the circumstances that led to the relapse and to devise strategies to prevent subsequent relapses or respond to them in a different manner.

Nicotine is a physically and psychologically addictive substance. Providers should be aware that adolescents may not exhibit the same symptoms of nicotine dependence as adults and that dependence may be established within as little as 4 weeks. Replacement therapy improves smoking cessation rates and may relieve withdrawal symptoms. Both nicotine gum and transdermal nicotine patch replacement therapies are recommended for teens.

Those who are not comfortable prescribing and monitoring nicotine—replacement therapies should limit their involvement with patients who smoke to those who do not exhibit signs of nicotine dependency (eg, patients who smoke less than a pack of cigarettes a day or do not feel a craving to smoke their first cigarette within 30 minutes after waking). In addition to nicotine-replacement therapies, sustained-release forms of the antidepressants bupropion, clonidine, and nortriptyline have been shown in randomized trials to help smokers quit and to decrease relapse rates fivefold.

Cullen J et al: Depictions of tobacco use in 2007 broadcast television programming popular among US youth. Arch Pediatr Adolesc Med 2011 Feb;165(2):147–151 [PMID: 21300655].

Difranza JR: Which interventions against the sale of tobacco to minors can be expected to reduce smoking? Tob Control 2011 Oct 12 [PMID: 21994275].

Table 5–9. "Five A's" for tobacco cessation.

Ask about tobacco use from all patients
Advise all tobacco users to quit
Assess willingness and motivation for tobacco user to make a quit attempt
Assist in the quit attempt
Arrange for follow-up

Adapted from Fiore MC et al: *Treating Tobacco Use and Dependence. Clinical Practice Guidelines*. U.S. Department of Health and Human Services, Public Health Service, 2000.

DiFranza JR: Who are you going to believe? Adolescents and nicotine addiction. J Adolesc Health 2011 Jan;48(1):1–2 [PMID: 21185515].

Hanewinkel R et al: Cigarette advertising and teen smoking initiation. Pediatrics 2011 Feb;127(2):e271–e278 [PMID: 21242217].

Lewis TL et al: Internalizing problems: A potential pathway from childhood maltreatment to adolescent smoking. J Adolesc Health 2011 Mar;48(3):247–252 [PMID: 21338895].

Lessov-Schlaggar CN et al: Sensitivity to secondhand smoke exposure predicts future smoking susceptibility. Pediatrics 2011 Aug;128(2):254–262 [PMID: 21746728].

Rubinstein ML et al: Smoking-related cue-induced brain activation in adolescent light smokers. J Adolesc Health 2011 Jan;48(1): 7–12 [PMID: 21185518].

Adachi-Mejia AM et al: Influence of movie smoking exposure and team sports participation on established smoking. Arch Pediatr Adolesc Med 2009;163:638–643 [PMID: 19581547].

Kulig JW; American Academy of Pediatrics Committee on Substance Abuse: Tobacco, alcohol, and other drugs: The role of the pediatrician in prevention, identification, and management of substance abuse. Pediatrics 2005;115:816 [PMID: 15741395].

Referral

There is no consensus about which substance-abusing patients can be adequately treated in the office, which require referral, and which require hospitalization. Factors to be considered prior to referral are summarized in Table 5–10. When doubt exists about the seriousness of the problem or the advisability of office management, consultation with a specialist should be sought.

Although most primary pediatric providers will not assume responsibility for the treatment of substance-abusing

Table 5–10. Factors to consider prior to referral for substance abuse.

Duration and frequency of substance use
The type of substances being used
Presence of other psychological disorders
Attention-deficit/hyperactivity disorder
Depression
Antisocial personality disorder
Presence of other social morbidities
School failure
Delinquency
Homelessness
Ongoing or past physical or sexual abuse
Program evaluation
View on substance abuse as primary disorder vs symptom
Offers comprehensive evaluation of patient and can manage associated problems identified in initial assessment (eg, comorbid conditions)
Adherence to abstinence philosophy
Patient-staff ratios
Separate adolescent and adult treatment programs
Follow-up and continuing care

youngsters, clinicians can be instrumental in motivating patients to seek treatment and in guiding them to appropriate treatment resources. Substance-abusing teenagers are best treated in teen-oriented treatment facilities. Despite the similarities between adult and adolescent substance abuse, adult programs are usually developmentally inappropriate and ineffective for adolescents. Many adolescents are concrete thinkers and their inability to reason deductively, especially about emotionally charged issues, makes it difficult for them to understand the abstract concepts (such as denial) that are an integral component of most adult-oriented programs. This invariably frustrates counselors who misinterpret lack of comprehension as resistance to therapy and concrete responses as evidence of deceit.

Treatment programs range from low-intensity, outpatient, school-based student-assistance programs, which rely heavily on peers and nonprofessionals, to residential, hospital-based programs staffed by psychiatrists and other professionals. Outpatient counseling programs are most appropriate for motivated patients who do not have significant mental health or behavioral problems and are not at risk for withdrawal. Some investigators have raised the concern that in pediatric settings, low-problem users may actually experience a strengthening of the drug subculture by associating with high-problem users in group therapy. More intensive day treatment programs are available for those who require a structured environment. Inpatient treatment should be considered for patients who need medical care and detoxification in addition to counseling, education, and family therapy.

Finally, special dual-diagnosis facilities are available for substance-abusing patients who also have other psychological conditions. These patients are difficult to diagnose and treat because it is often unclear whether their symptoms are a consequence of substance use or a symptom of a comorbid psychological disorder. Recognition of such disorders is critical because they must be treated in programs that include psychiatric expertise.

Approaches to the treatment of substance abuse in children and adolescents are typically modeled after adult treatment programs. Key elements of an effective adolescent drug treatment program include: assessment and treatment matching, comprehensive and integrated treatment approach, family involvement, developmentally appropriate program, engagement and retention of teens, qualified staff, gender and cultural competence, continuing care, and treatment outcomes. Several studies of adolescent substance abuse treatment programs have shown that many do not adequately address all of the important components of therapy.

Fang L et al: Preventing substance use among early Asian-American adolescent girls: Initial evaluation of a web-based, mother-daughter program. J Adolesc Health 2010 Nov;47(5):529–532 [PMID: 20970090].

Kaminer Y et al: From assessment reactivity to aftercare for adolescent substance abuse: Are we there yet? Child Adolesc Psychiatr Clin N Am 2010 Jul;19(3):577–590 [PMID: 20682222].

Macgowan MJ et al: Evidence for optimism: Behavior therapies and motivational interviewing in adolescent substance abuse treatment. Child Adolesc Psychiatr Clin N Am 2010 Jul;19(3):527–545 [PMID: 20682219].

Rowe CL: Multidimensional family therapy: Addressing co-occurring substance abuse and other problems among adolescents with comprehensive family-based treatment. Child Adolesc Psychiatr Clin N Am 2010 Jul;19(3):563–576 [PMID: 20682221].

Stanger C et al: Contingency management approaches for adolescent substance use disorders. Child Adolesc Psychiatr Clin N Am 2010 Jul;19(3):547–562 [PMID: 20682220].

Tripodi SJ et al: Interventions for reducing adolescent alcohol abuse: A meta-analytic review. Arch Pediatr Adolesc Med 2010 Jan;164(1):85–91 [PMID: 20048247].

Williams JF: Adolescent substance abuse and treatment acceptability. J Adolesc Health 2011 Mar;48(3):217–219 [PMID: 21338890].

PREVENTION

Prevention of substance abuse has been a public health priority since the 1980s. Pediatric health care providers are important advocates and educators of the community and government on developmentally appropriate programs. *Primary level* programs focus on preventing the initiation of substance use. The Drug Awareness and Resistance Education (D.A.R.E.) program is a familiar example of a primary prevention program that attempts to educate elementary- and middle-school students about the adverse consequences of substance abuse and enable them to resist peer pressures.

Secondary level programs target populations at increased risk for substance use. Their aim is to prevent progression from initiation to continuance and maintenance, relying on individualized intervention to reduce the risk and enhance the protective factors listed in Table 5–3. This approach enables the provider to focus scarce resources on those who are most likely to benefit from them. Alateen, which supports the children of alcoholic parents, typifies secondary level prevention.

Tertiary level prevention programs target young people who have been identified as substance abusers. Their aim is to prevent the morbid consequences of substance use. One example is identifying adolescents who misuse alcohol and drugs at parties and providing them with a safe ride home. Because prevention is more effective when targeted at reducing the initiation of substance use than at decreasing use or associated morbidity, tertiary prevention is the least effective approach.

Very few population-based programs undergo rigorous scientific evaluation. It is the consensus among drug educators that primary prevention programs, such as D.A.R.E., have minimal effect in decreasing the use of illicit substances.

Parents and others should understand that most adolescents who abuse alcohol and drugs do not do so just for the high. Rather, these behaviors are often purposeful, developmentally appropriate coping strategies. To the extent that these behaviors meet young peoples' developmental needs, they are not apt to be abandoned unless equally attractive alternatives are available. For example, even though many teenagers cite stress and anxiety as reasons for smoking, teen-oriented smoking cessation programs rarely address the young smoker's need for alternative coping strategies by offering stress management training. Similarly, for the youngster growing up in an impoverished urban environment, the real costs of substance abuse may be too low and the rewards too high to be influenced by talk and knowledge alone. It is unreasonable to expect a talk-based intervention to change attitudes and behaviors in a direction that is opposite to that of the child's own social milieu. The efficacy of the most promising prevention models and interventions is apt to decay over time unless changes in the social environment provide substance-abusing children and adolescents with realistic alternative ways to meet their developmental needs.

Ellickson PL et al: Long-term effects of drug prevention on risky sexual behavior among young adults. J Adolesc Health 2009; 45:111–117 [PMID: 19628136].

Schinke SP et al: Longitudinal outcomes of an alcohol abuse prevention program for urban adolescents. J Adolesc Health 2010 May;46(5):451–457 [PMID: 20413081].

REFERENCES

Web Resources

American Lung Association (site for and by teens): http://www.lungusa.org/smokefreeclass

Monitoring the Future Study (detailed information and longitudinal data): http://www.monitoringthefuture.org

National Clearinghouse Drug and Alcohol Abuse (information and resources, including free publications for providers, parents, and adolescents): http://www.health.org

National Institute on Drug Abuse: http://www.nida.nih.gov

Substance Use and Mental Health Services Administration (SAMSA; resources for both substance use and mental health services): http://www.samhsa.gov

Eating Disorders

6

Eric J. Sigel, MD

Adolescents as well as younger children engage in disordered eating behavior at an alarming rate, and many develop partial or full-blown eating disorders (EDs). The spectrum of eating disorders includes anorexia nervosa (AN), bulimia nervosa (BN), binge-eating disorder (BED), and eating disorders not otherwise specified (EDNOS). These disorders are best defined in a biopsychosocial context. New diagnostic categories and criteria for EDs will be available upon release of DSM-V in 2013.

ETIOLOGY

There is strong evidence for a genetic basis for eating disorders. The incidence of AN is 7% in first-degree relatives of anorexic patients compared with 1%–2% in the general population. The concordance rate in monozygotic twins is 55% compared with 7% in dizygotic twins. Twin studies estimate the heritability of AN as 33%–84% and BN as 28%–83%. First-degree female relatives of males with AN have a 20-fold relative risk of AN. Most studies also find a higher incidence of eating disorders among first-degree relatives of bulimic patients. The family of neurotrophin proteins has been shown to be involved in the regulation of eating behavior and energy metabolism, and has been intensively studied to assess their potential role in the genetic susceptibility to EDs. In a study of European families with EDs, Mercader found a strong association between rs7180942, a neurotrophin protein encoded by the *NTRK3* gene and the presence of EDs, with an undertransmission of the heterozygous genotype and an overtransmission of the homozygous genotype associated with increased phenotypic expression of EDs.

There is evidence of altered serotonergic and dopaminergic function and alterations in neuropeptides and gut peptides in AN and BN. It remains unclear whether abnormalities of neurotransmitters contribute to the development of EDs or are a consequence of the physiologic changes associated with the disorders. Patients with BN or BED appear to have a blunted serotonin response to eating and satiety. With a decreased satiety response, patients continue to eat, leading to a binge. Treatment with selective serotonin reuptake inhibitors (SSRIs) tends to equilibrate satiety regulation. An alteration in dopamine has also been recognized, although its significance is not clear. Adiponectin is elevated in AN, although it is unclear whether this is merely secondary to the malnourished state. Cholecystokinin is decreased in BN, perhaps contributing to the lack of postingestion satiety that perpetuates a binge. Ghrelin, a gut peptide, is elevated in patients with AN, and does not decrease normally after a meal in these patients. Obestatin, a gut peptide that inhibits appetite, is elevated in AN as well.

Leptin physiology is deranged in patients with AN. Abnormalities of leptin may mediate energy changes that affect the hypothalamic-pituitary axis and play a role in perpetuating AN. Leptin levels increase excessively as individuals with AN regain weight. The abnormally high levels of leptin may contribute to the difficulty AN patients have when trying to regain weight, as higher leptin levels signal the body to decrease energy intake. Leptin also plays a significant role in some of the sequelae of AN, with low levels signaling the hypothalamus to inhibit reproductive hormone production.

Some experts have hypothesized that the intrauterine hormonal milieu may explain the differences in prevalence of ED between females and males. Procopio has studied the risk of developing AN in the same sex and opposite sex twin pairs when one twin has AN. There was approximately an eightfold risk of developing AN in males with a female twin with AN compared to the risk of developing AN in males who had a male twin with AN. Though the study could not separate environmental influences, evidence from animal models suggests that increased exposure to estrogen and/or decreased exposure to androgens influence brain development and may play a role in determining which individuals are at risk for AN. One study determined that season of birth actually influenced the rate of developing AN, with an excess in those born from March-June (OR 1.15, p = .01) and a deficit in those born September-October (OR 0.8, p < .001), suggesting an additional environmental effect.

Traditional psychological theory has suggested many environmental factors that might promote the development of eating disorders. Enmeshment of mother with daughter to the point that the teenager cannot develop her own identity (a key developmental marker of adolescence) may be a predisposing factor. The teenager may cope by asserting control over food, as she senses her lack of control in the developmental realm. A second theory involves father-daughter distancing. As puberty progresses and a girl's sexuality blossoms, a father may experience difficulty in dealing with his daughter as a sexual being and may respond by withdrawing emotionally and physically. The teenage girl may intuitively recognize this and subconsciously decrease her food intake in order to become prepubertal again. A third theory is related to puberty itself. Some teenagers may fear or dislike their changing bodies. By restricting food intake they lose weight, stop menstruating, and effectively reverse pubertal development.

Society has promoted the message that being thin or muscular is necessary for attractiveness and success. The ease of access to diet products—foods and diet pills—as well as Internet instructions (pro-anorexia sites) makes it simple for adolescents to embark on a quest for thinness or muscularity.

Genetic predisposition, environmental factors, and psychological factors likely combine to create a milieu that promotes development of eating disorders.

Bailer UF, Kaye WH: A review of neuropeptide and neuroendocrine dysregulation in anorexia and bulimia nervosa. Curr Drug Target CNS Neurol Disord 2003;2:53 [PMID: 12769812].

Bulik CM, Slof-Op't Landt MC, van Furth EF, Sullivan PF: The genetics of anorexia nervosa. Annu Rev Nutr 2007a;27:263–275.

Campbell IC, Mill J, Uher R, Schmidt U: Eating disorders, gene-environment interaction, and epigentics. Neuroscience and Biobehavioral Reviews 2011;35:784–793.

Disanto G, Handel AE, Pare AE et al: Season of birth and anorexia nervosa. Brit J Psych 2011;198(5):404–407 [PMID: 21415047].

Germain N et al: Ghrelin/obestatin ratio in two populations with low bodyweight: Constitutional thinness and anorexia nervosa. Psychoneuroendocrinology 2009;34(3):413–419 [PMID: 18995969].

Mercader JM et al: Association of NTRK3 and its interaction with NGF suggest an altered cross-regulation of the neurotrophin signaling pathway in eating disorders. Hum Mol Genet 2008;17(9):1234–1244.

Procopio M, Marriott P: Intrauterine hormonal environment and risk of developing anorexia nervosa. Arch Gen Psych 2007; 64(12):1402.

Strober M et al: Males with anorexia nervosa: A controlled study of eating disorders in first-degree relatives. Int J Eat Disord 2001;29:263 [PMID: 11262504].

Warren, MP: Endocrine manifestations of eating disorders. *J Clinical Endocrin Metabolism* 2011;96(2):333 [PMID: 21159848].

INCIDENCE

AN is the third most common chronic illness of adolescent girls in the United States. The incidence has been increasing steadily in the United States since the 1930s. Although ascertaining exact incidence is difficult, most studies show that 1%–2% of teenagers develop AN and 2%–4% develop BN. Adolescents outnumber adults 5 to 1, although the number of adults with eating disorders is rising. Incidence is also increasing among younger children. Prepubertal patients often have associated psychiatric diagnoses. Males comprise about 10% of patients with EDs, though this prevalence appears to be increasing as well, associated with the increased media emphasis on muscular, chiseled appearance as the male ideal.

Literature on preadolescents with EDs suggests that patients younger than 13 years are more likely to be male compared to teenagers and more likely to have EDNOS. Younger patients are less likely to engage in behaviors characteristic of BN. They present with more rapid weight loss and lower percentile body weight than adolescents.

Teenagers' self-reported prevalence of ED *behavior* is much higher than the official incidence of AN or BN. In the most recent Youth Risk Behavior Survey of US teenagers (2009), 59% of females and 31% of males had attempted to lose weight during the preceding 30 days. Eleven percent had fasted for more than 24 hours to lose weight, and 5% had used medications to lose weight (6.3% of girls and 3.8% of boys). Self-induced vomiting or laxative use was reported by 5.4% of females and 2.6% of males. Forty-six percent of females and 30% of males reported at least one binge episode during their lifetime. Although the number of youth with full-spectrum eating disorders is low, it is alarming that so many youth experiment with unhealthy weight control habits. These behaviors may be precursors to the development of eating disorders, and clinicians should explore these practices with all adolescent patients.

Center for Disease Control and Prevention: Youth Risk Behavior Surveillance: United States 2009. MMWR Surveill Summ June 4 2010;59(SS-5). http://www.cdc.gov/mmwr/pdf/ss/ss5905.pdf.

Halmi KA: Anorexia nervosa: An increasing problem in children and adolescents. Dialogues Clin Neurosci 2009;11(1):100–103 [PMID: 19432392].

Peebles R et al: How do children with eating disorders differ from adolescents with eating disorders at initial evaluation? J Adolesc Health 2006;39:800 [PMID: 17116508].

PREDISPOSING FACTORS & CLINICAL PROFILES

Children involved in gymnastics, figure skating, and ballet—activities that emphasize thin bodies—are at higher risk for AN than are children in sports that do not emphasize body image. Adolescents who believe that being thin represents the ideal frame for a female, those who are dissatisfied with their bodies, and those with a history of dieting are at increased risk for eating disorders. Sudden changes in dietary habits, such as becoming vegetarian, may be a first sign of anorexia, especially if the change is abrupt and without good reason.

The typical bulimic patient tends to be impulsive and to engage in risk-taking behavior such as alcohol use, drug use, and sexual experimentation. Bulimic patients are often an appropriate weight for height or slightly overweight. They have average academic performance. Some studies report that 50% of bulimic patients have been sexually abused. Youth with diabetes have an increased risk of BN. In males, wrestling predisposes to BN, and homosexual orientation is associated with binge eating.

Shaw H et al: Body image and eating disturbances across ethnic groups: More similarities than differences. Psychol Addict Behav 2004;18:8 [PMID: 15008651].

Striegel-Moore RH, Bulik CM: Risk factors for eating disorders. Am Psychol 2007;62:181 [PMID: 17469897].

ANOREXIA NERVOSA

Table 6–1 lists the diagnostic criteria for AN, according to the *Diagnostic and Statistical Manual of Mental Disorders*, Fourth Edition, Text Revision (DSM-IV-TR). There are two forms of AN. In the restricting type, patients do not regularly engage in binge eating or purging. In the purging type, AN is combined with binge eating or purging behavior, or both. Distinguishing between the two is important as they carry different implications for prognosis and treatment. There is ongoing debate about the diagnostic criteria for AN. Some experts suggest eliminating amenorrhea as a criterion. Although patients may not demonstrate all features of AN, they may still exhibit the deleterious symptoms associated with AN. DSM-V will contain significant changes to the diagnosis of AN, including the elimination of amenorrhea and weight of 85% of expected as specific criteria.

Clinical Findings

A. Symptoms and Signs

Clinicians should recognize the early symptoms and signs of AN because early intervention may prevent the full-blown syndrome from developing. Patients may show some of the behaviors and psychology of AN, such as reduction in dietary fat and intense concern with body image, even before weight loss or amenorrhea occurs.

Making the diagnosis of AN can be challenging because adolescents may try to conceal their illness. Assessing the patient's body image is essential to determining the diagnosis. Table 6–2 lists screening questions that help tease out a teenager's perceptions of body image. Other diagnostic screening tools (eg, Eating Disorders Inventory) assess a range of eating and dieting behaviors. Parental observations are critical in determining whether a patient has expressed dissatisfaction over body habitus and which weight loss techniques the child has used. If the teenager is unwilling to share his or her concerns about body image, the clinician may find clues to the diagnosis by carefully considering other presenting symptoms or signs. Weight loss from a baseline of normal body weight is an obvious red flag for the presence of an eating disorder. Additionally, AN should be considered in any girl with secondary amenorrhea who has lost weight.

Physical symptoms and signs are usually secondary to weight loss and proportional to the degree of malnutrition. The body effectively goes into hibernation, becoming functionally hypothyroid (euthyroid sick) to save energy. Body temperature decreases, and patients report being cold. Bradycardia develops, especially in the supine position. Dizziness, light-headedness, and syncope may occur

Table 6–1. Diagnostic criteria for anorexia nervosa.

A. Refusal to maintain body weight at or above the minimal normal weight for age and height (eg, weight loss leading to maintenance of body weight less than 85% of that expected; or failure to make expected weight gain during a period of growth, leading to body weight less than 85% of that expected).
B. Intense fear of gaining weight or becoming fat, even though underweight.
C. Disturbance in the way in which one's body weight or shape is experienced, undue influence of body weight or shape on self-evaluation, or denial of the seriousness of the current low body weight.
D. In postmenarchal females, amenorrhea, ie, the absence of at least three menstrual cycles. (A woman is considered to have amenorrhea if her periods occur only following hormone, eg, estrogen, administration.)

Table 6–2. Screening questions to help diagnose anorexia and bulimia nervosa.

How do you feel about your body?
Are there parts of your body you might change?
When you look at yourself in the mirror, do you see yourself as overweight, underweight, or satisfactory?
If overweight, how much do you want to weigh?
If your weight is satisfactory, has there been a time that you were worried about being overweight?
If overweight [underweight], what would you change?
Have you ever been on a diet?
What have you done to help yourself lose weight?
Do you count calories or fat grams?
Do you keep your intake to a certain number of calories?
Have you ever used nutritional supplements, diet pills, or laxatives to help you lose weight?
Have you ever made yourself vomit to get rid of food or lose weight?

as a result of orthostasis and hypotension secondary to impaired cardiac function. Left ventricular mass is decreased (as is the mass of all striated muscle), stroke volume is compromised, and peripheral resistance is increased, contributing to left ventricular systolic dysfunction. Patients can develop prolonged QTc syndrome and increased QT dispersion (irregular QT intervals), putting them at risk for cardiac arrhythmias. Peripheral circulation is reduced. Hands and feet may be blue and cool. Hair thins, nails become brittle, and skin becomes dry. Lanugo develops as a primitive response to starvation. The gastrointestinal tract may be affected; inability to take in normal quantities of food, early satiety, and gastroesophageal reflux can develop as the body adapts to reduced intake. The normal gastrocolic reflex may be lost due to lack of stimulation by food, causing bloating and constipation. Delayed gastric emptying may be present in restricting type and purging type AN. Nutritional rehabilitation improves gastric emptying and dyspeptic symptoms in AN restricting type, but not in those who vomit. Neurologically, patients may experience decreased cognition, inability to concentrate, increased irritability, and depression, which may be related to structural brain changes and decreased cerebral blood flow.

Nutritional assessment is vital. Often patients eliminate fat from their diets and may eat as few as 100–200 kcal/d. A gown-only weight after urination is the most accurate way to assess weight. Patients tend to wear bulky clothes and may hide weights in their pockets or drink excessive fluid (water-loading) to trick the practitioner. Assessing BMI is the standard approach to interpreting the degree of malnutrition. BMI below the 25th percentile indicates risk for malnutrition, and < 5th percentile indicates significant malnutrition. Median body weight should be calculated as it serves both as the denominator in determining what percent weight an individual is, as well as to provide a general goal weight during recovery. Median body weight (MBW) for height is calculated by using the 50th percentile of BMI for age.

A combination of malnutrition and stress causes hypothalamic hypogonadism. The hypothalamic-pituitary-gonadal axis shuts down as the body struggles to survive, directing finite energy resources to vital functions. This may be mediated by the effect of low serum leptin levels on the hypothalamic-pituitary axis. Pubertal development and skeletal growth may be interrupted, and adolescents may experience decreased libido.

Amenorrhea, although being eliminated as a diagnostic criterion, remains a hallmark of AN. It occurs for two reasons. The hypothalamic-pituitary-ovarian axis shuts down under stress, causing hypothalamic amenorrhea. In addition, adipose tissue is needed to convert estrogen to its activated form. When weight loss is significant, there is not enough substrate to activate estrogen. Resumption of menses occurs only when both body weight and body fat increase. Approximately, 73% of postmenarchal girls resume menstruating if they reach 90% of MBW. An adolescent female needs about 17% body fat to restart menses and 22% body fat to initiate menses if she has primary amenorrhea. Some evidence suggests that target weight gain for return of menses is approximately 1 kg higher than the weight at which menses ceased.

Table 6–3. Laboratory findings: anorexia nervosa.

Increased blood urea nitrogen and creatinine secondary to renal insufficiency
Decreased white blood cells, platelets, and less commonly red blood cells and hematocrit secondary to bone marrow suppression or fat atrophy of the bone marrow
Increased AST and ALT secondary to malnutrition
Increased cholesterol, thought to be related to altered fatty acid metabolism
Decreased alkaline phosphatase secondary to zinc deficiency
Low- to low-normal thyroid-stimulating hormone and thyroxine
Decreased follicle-stimulating hormone, luteinizing hormone, estradiol, and testosterone secondary to shutdown of hypothalamicpituitary-gonadal axis
Abnormal electrolytes related to hydration status
Decreased phosphorus
Decreased insulin-like growth factor
Increased cortisol
Decreased urine specific gravity in cases of intentional water intoxication

ALT, alanine aminotransferase; AST, aspartate aminotransferase.

B. Laboratory Findings

All organ systems may suffer some degree of damage in the anorexic patient, related both to severity and duration of illness (Table 6–3). Initial screening should include complete blood count with differential; serum levels of electrolytes, blood urea nitrogen, creatinine, phosphorus, calcium, magnesium, and thyroid-stimulating hormone; liver function tests; and urinalysis. Increase in lipids, likely due to abnormal liver function, is seen in 18% of those with AN, with subsequent return to normal once weight is restored. An electrocardiogram should be performed, because significant electrocardiographic abnormalities may be present, most importantly prolonged QTc syndrome. Bone densitometry should be done if illness persists for 6 months, as patients begin to accumulate risk for osteoporosis.

Differential Diagnosis

If the diagnosis is unclear (ie, the patient has lost a significant amount of weight but does not have typical body image distortion or fat phobia), then the clinician must consider the differential diagnosis for weight loss in adolescents. This includes inflammatory bowel disease, diabetes, hyperthyroidism, malignancy, depression, and chronic infectious disease such as HIV. Less common diagnoses include adrenal insufficiency and malabsorption syndromes such as celiac disease. The history and physical examination should direct specific laboratory and radiologic evaluation.

Complications (Table 6–4)

A. Short-Term Complications

1. Early satiety—Patients may have difficulty tolerating even modest quantities of food when intake increases; this usually resolves after the patients adjust to larger meals. Gastric emptying is poor. Pancreatic and biliary secretion is diminished.

2. Superior mesenteric artery syndrome—As patients become malnourished, the fat pad between the superior mesenteric artery and the duodenum shrinks and compression of the transverse duodenum may cause obstruction and vomiting, especially with solid foods. The upper GI series shows to-and-fro movement of barium in the descending and transverse duodenum proximal to the obstruction. Treatment involves a liquid diet or nasoduodenal feedings until restoration of the fat pad has occurred, coincident with weight gain.

3. Constipation—Patients may be very constipated. Two mechanisms contribute—loss of the gastrocolic reflex and loss of colonic muscle tone. Typically stool softeners are not effective because the colon has decreased peristaltic amplitude. Agents that induce peristalsis, such as bisacodyl, as well as osmotic agents, such as polyethylene glycol-electrolyte solution (MiraLax), are helpful. Constipation can persist for up to 6–8 weeks after refeeding. Occasionally enemas are required.

4. Refeeding syndrome—Described in the Treatment section.

B. Long-Term Complications

1. Osteoporosis—Approximately 50% of females with AN have reduced bone mass at one or more sites. The lumbar spine has the most rapid turnover, and is the area likely to be affected first. Teenagers are particularly at risk as they accrue 40% of their bone mineral during adolescence. Low body weight is most predictive of bone loss. The causes of osteopenia

Table 6–4. Complications of anorexia and bulimia nervosa, by mechanism.

Cardiovascular	**Hematologic**
Bradycardia (WL/MN)	Leukopenia (WL/MN)
Postural hypotension (WL/MN, SIV, LX)	Anemia (WL/MN)
Arrhythmia, sudden death (WL/MN, SIV, LX)	Thrombocytopenia (WL/MN)
Congestive heart failure (during refeeding) (WL/MN)	↓ ESR (WL/MN)
Pericardial effusion (WL/MN)	Impaired cell-mediated immunity (WL/MN)
Mitral valve prolapse (WL/MN)	**Metabolic**
ECG abnormalities (prolonged QT, low voltage, T-wave abnormalities, conduction defects) (WL/MN)	Dehydration (WL/MN, SIV, LXA, DU)
Endocrine	Acidosis (LXA)
↓ LH, FSH (WL/MN)	Alkolosis (SIV)
↓ T_3, ↑ rT_3, ↓ T_4, TSH (WL/MN)	Hypokalemia (SIV, LXA, DU)
Irregular menses (WL/MN, B/P)	Hyponatremia (SIV, LXA, DU, WL/MN)
Amenorrhea (WL/MN)	Hypochloremia (SIV)
Hypercortisolism (WL/MN)	Hypocalcemia (WL/MN, SIV)
Growth retardation (WL/MN)	Hypophosphatemia (WL/MN)
Delayed puberty (WL/MN)	Hypomagnesemia (WL/MN)
Decreased libido (WL/MN)	Hypercarotenemia (WL/MN)
Gastrointestinal	**Neurologic**
Dental erosion (SIV)	Cortical atrophy-white and gray matter (WL/MN)
Parotid swelling (SIV)	Peripheral neuropathy (WL/MN)
Esophagitis, esophageal tears (SIV)	Seizures (WL/MN, SIV, LXA)
Delayed gastric emptying (WL/MN, SIV)	Thermoregulatory abnormalities (WL/MN)
Gastric dilation (rarely rupture) (SIV)	↓ REM and slow-wave sleep (All)
Pancreatitis (WL/MN)	**Renal**
Constipation (WL/MN, LXA)	Hematuria (WL/MN)
Diarrhea (LXA)	Proteinuria (WL/MN)
Superior mesenteric artery syndrome (WL/MN)	↓ Renal concentrating ability (WL/MN, DU)
Hypercholesterolemia (WL/MN)	Enuresis (WL/MN)
↑ Liver function tests (fatty infiltration of the liver) (WL/MN)	**Skeletal**
	Osteopenia (WL/MN)
	Fractures (WL/MN)

WL/MN, weight loss/malnutrition; SIV, self-induced vomiting; LXA, laxative abuse; DU, diuretic abuse; B/P, binge-purge
ECG, electrocardiogram; ESR, erythrocyte sedimentation rate; FSH, follicle-stimulating hormone; LH, luteinizing hormone; REM, rapid eye movement; rT_3, resin triiodothyronine uptake; T_3, triiodothyronine; T_4, thyroxine; TSH, thyroid-stimulating hormone.

and osteoporosis are multiple. Estrogen and testosterone are essential to potentiate bone development. Bone minerals begin to resorb without estrogen. Elevated cortisol levels and decreased insulin-like growth factor-1 also contribute to bone resorption. Amenorrhea is highly correlated with osteoporosis. Studies show that as few as 6 months of amenorrhea is associated with osteopenia or osteoporosis. Males may also develop osteoporosis due to decreased testosterone and elevated cortisol.

The only proven treatment for bone loss in girls with AN is regaining sufficient weight and body fat to restart the menstrual cycle. Most studies do not support use of hormone replacement therapy to improve bone recovery; however, some evidence indicates that hormone replacement therapy may stop further bone loss and may be of particular benefit for patients with extremely low body weight (< 70% MBW). Some practitioners use hormone replacement therapy if amenorrhea has been present for more than 1 year and the patient is not able to achieve normal body weight. Bisphosphonates used to treat postmenopausal osteoporosis are currently being studied in adolescents. Two small randomized controlled trials have shown small positive effects on bone density with alendronate and risedronate, although clinical effectiveness has not yet been determined. Newer treatments with possible effectiveness, including recombinant insulin-like growth factor-1 injection and dehydroepiandrosterone, are under investigation.

2. Brain changes—As malnutrition becomes pronounced, brain tissue—both white and gray matter—is lost, with a compensatory increase in cerebrospinal fluid in the sulci and ventricles. Follow-up studies of weight-recovered anorexic patients show a persistent loss of gray matter, although white matter returns to normal. Functionally, there does not seem to be a direct relationship between cognition and brain tissue loss, although studies have shown a decrease in cognitive ability and decreased cerebral blood flow in very malnourished patients. Making patients and family aware that brain tissue can be lost may improve their perception of the seriousness of this disorder. There is a burgeoning literature on functional brain imaging. Neurochemical changes, including changes related to serotonin and dopamine systems, occur as a result of starvation and lead to altered metabolism in frontal, cingulate, temporal, and parietal regions (for a detailed review, see Kaye, 2009).

3. Effects on future children—This area has just recently been studied. Findings suggest that there may be feeding issues for infants who are born to mothers who have a history of either AN or BN. Infants born to mothers with a history of AN have more feeding difficulties at 0 and 6 months and tend to be lower weight (30th percentile on average). Infants born to mothers with current or past BN are more likely to be overweight and have faster growth rates than controls. Pediatricians should ascertain an eating disorders history from mothers of patients who are having feeding issues.

Asiero D, Frishman WH: Cardiovascular complications of eating disorders. Cardiol Rev 2006;14:227 [PMID: 16924163].

Golden NH et al: Treatment goal weight in adolescents with anorexia nervosa: Use of BMI percentiles. Int J Eat Disord 2008;41(4):301–306.

Kaye WH, Fudge JL, Paulus M: New insights into symptoms and neurocircuit function of anorexia nervosa. Nat Rev Neurosci 2009;10(8):573–584 [PMID: 19603056].

Micali N, Simonoff E, Treasure J: Infant feeding and weight in the first year of life in babies of women with eating disorders. J Pediatr 2009;154(1):55–60.e1 [PMID: 18783793].

C. Mortality

Patients with eating disorders are at a higher risk of death than the general population. Meta-analysis shows that the risk of dying from their illness is 5.9% in patients with AN. Mortality estimates vary between 0% and 18%, depending on the patient population and the duration of follow-up. One study showed the risk of dying to be 0.56% per year. Death in anorexic patients is due to suicide, abnormal electrolytes, and cardiac arrhythmias.

Treatment

A. General Approach

Factors that determine treatment interventions are severity of illness, duration of illness, specific manifestations of disease, previous treatment approaches and outcomes, program availability, financial resources, and insurance coverage. Treatment options include outpatient management, day treatment hospitalization, inpatient medical or psychiatric hospitalization, and residential treatment. The key to determining level of intervention is the degree of malnutrition, the rapidity of weight loss, the degree of medical compromise, and the presence of life-threatening electrolyte abnormalities. No absolute criteria determine level of intervention. The practitioner must examine the degree of medical compromise and consider immediate risks and the potential for an individual to reverse the situation on his or her own. Day treatment programs are a good intervention for patients who do not yet need inpatient care but who are not improving with outpatient management. Treatment is costly. Many patients do not have insurance benefits that adequately cover the cost of treatment, leaving parents and practitioners with profound dilemmas as to how to best provide treatment in the face of financial constraints. Legally, however, eating disorders are now recognized as a parity mental health diagnosis similar to the other biologically based mental health illnesses in many states, which has increased the ease of obtaining insurance coverage.

A multidisciplinary approach is most effective and should include medical monitoring, nutrition therapy, and individual and family psychotherapy by experienced practitioners. Family therapy is especially helpful with younger teenagers, whereas older teenagers tend to benefit more from individual therapy. Family therapy is an important means of helping families understand the development of the disease and addressing issues that may be barriers to recovery. Both types of psychotherapy are encouraged in most treatment programs, and recovery without psychotherapy is unusual. The average length of psychotherapy is roughly 6–9 months, although some individuals continue therapy for extended periods. Adjunctive modalities include art and horticulture therapy, therapeutic recreation, and massage therapy.

Manualized family therapy, developed in Britain by Maudsley and adapted by Lock and LeGrange, has shifted the therapeutic approach to adolescents with AN. Traditional therapy allowed the adolescent to control his or her eating and the parents to remain uninvolved with the food-portion of recovery. The manualized approach gives power and control back to parents. Treatment is prescribed for 20 weekly sessions. The first 10 weeks are devoted to empowering parents, putting them in control of their child's nutrition and exercise. Parents are educated about the dangers of malnutrition and are instructed to supervise each meal. The next phase, sessions 11–16, returns control over eating to the adolescent once he or she accepts the demands of the parents. The last phase of treatment, sessions 17–20, occurs when the patient is maintaining a healthy weight and shifts the focus away from the eating disorder, examining instead the impact that the eating disorder has had on establishing a healthy adolescent identity. This approach is reported to result in good or intermediate outcomes in 90% of treated adolescents.

Careful instruction in nutrition helps the teenager and family dispel misconceptions about nutrition, identify realistic nutritional goals, and normalize eating. Initially, nutrition education may be the most important intervention as the teenager slowly works through his or her fears of fat-containing foods and weight gain. The teenager begins to trust the nutrition therapist and restore body weight, eventually eating in a well-balanced, healthy manner.

B. Inpatient Treatment

Table 6–5 lists the criteria for hospital admission generally used in the medical community. It is usually quite difficult for a patient who is losing weight rapidly (> 2 lb/wk) to reverse the weight loss because the body is in a catabolic state.

Table 6–5. Criteria for inpatient treatment of anorexia nervosa.

Body weight < 75% of ideal body weight
Supine heart rate < 45/min
Symptomatic hypotension or syncope
Hypokalemia: K^+ < 2.5 mEq/L
Rapid weight loss that cannot be interrupted as outpatient
Failure of outpatient management
Acute food refusal

Goals of hospitalization include arresting weight loss and stabilizing hemodynamics. Nutrition is the most vital inpatient medicine. Clinicians can safely begin with a meal plan containing approximately 250 kcal more than the patient has been routinely eating, which can usually be accomplished orally. Patients should start with a well-balanced meal plan, with appropriate proportions of carbohydrate, protein, and fat. Oral meals are usually tolerated, although it is important to be supervised by medical staff. If the patient resists, nasogastric or intravenous alimentation can be used. Aside from caloric needs, the clinician needs to consider the patient's hydration and include the appropriate amount of fluid with the meal plan. Dehydration should be corrected slowly. The oral route is usually adequate. Aggressive intravenous fluid administration should be avoided because left ventricular mass is compromised and a rapid increase in volume may not be tolerated. Regulating fluid intake is important, because water intoxication can contribute to abnormal electrolytes and falsified weights.

During the initial introduction of food, the clinician should monitor the patient for refeeding syndrome, a phenomenon that occurs if caloric intake is increased too rapidly. Signs of refeeding syndrome are decreased serum phosphorus (as the body resumes synthesis of adenosine triphosphate), decreased serum potassium (as increased insulin causes K^+ to shift from extracellular fluid into K^+-depleted cells), and, rarely, edema related to fluid shifts or congestive heart failure.

Although specific guidelines do not exist, many practitioners begin phosphorus supplementation if patients are severely malnourished (< 70% MBW) or their intake has been consistently less than 500 kcal/d.

Caloric intake can be increased 250 kcal/per day as long as refeeding syndrome does not occur. Weight goals vary depending on programmatic approach. Typically intake is adjusted to reach a goal of 0.1–0.25 kg/d weight gain.

Overnight monitoring for bradycardia is helpful in assessing degree of metabolic compromise. Usually the more rapid and severe the weight loss, the worse the bradycardia. Improving bradycardia correlates with weight recovery. Orthostatic hypotension is most severe around hospital day 4, improving steadily and correcting by the third week of nutritional rehabilitation. An electrocardiogram should be obtained because the patient is at risk for prolonged QTc syndrome and junctional arrhythmias related to the severity of bradycardia.

It usually takes 2–3 weeks to reach the initial goals of hospitalization—steady weight gain, toleration of oral diet without signs of refeeding syndrome, corrected bradycardia (heart rate > 45 beats/min for three consecutive nights), and correction of orthostasis. Specific weight criteria are used by many programs when considering discharge. This depends partly on admission weight. Ideally a patient gains at least 5% of his or her MBW. Some programs set discharge at 80%, 85%, or 90% MBW. Patient outcomes are improved with discharge at a higher body weight. Some evidence exists that patients do better if discharged at 95% MBW. In many practitioners' experience, relapse rates are high if patients are discharged at less than 75% MBW. Frequently, insurance companies do not pay for hospital stays beyond strict medical stabilization (normal vital signs and normal electrolytes).

C. Pharmacotherapy

Practitioners frequently use psychotropic medications for treatment of AN, despite the lack of evidence supporting efficacy. Several open label trials suggest that atypical antipsychotics (risperidone olanzapine, quetiapine) may be helpful. One review found that olanzapine (2.5–15 mg/d) was associated with improved body weight, decreased delusional thinking, improvement in body image, and decreased agitation and premeal anxiety. However, a recent randomized controlled trial did not show any difference in outcomes between risperidone and placebo.

SSRIs repeatedly have been shown to not be helpful in the initial therapy of AN. However, once the patient has achieved approximately 85% MBW, then SSRIs (fluoxetine, citalopram, or sertraline) may help prevent relapse.

Zinc deficiency is common in AN, and several studies support its use as a supplement during the initial phases of treatment. Because zinc deficiency adversely affects neurotransmitters, administering zinc helps restore neurotransmitter action to baseline. Additionally zinc may restore appetite and improve depressive mood. Zinc should be administered for approximately 2 months from the beginning of therapy, with at least 14 mg of elemental zinc daily.

Because of global nutritional deficits, a multivitamin with iron is also recommended daily. Symptomatic treatment for constipation and reflux should be used appropriately until symptoms resolve.

D. Outpatient Treatment

Not all patients with AN require inpatient treatment, especially if parents and clinicians recognize the warning signs early. These patients can receive treatment as outpatients, employing the same multidisciplinary team approach. Manualized family-based treatment is ideal for the outpatient setting if a trained therapist is available. Appropriate nutrition counseling is vital in guiding a patient and family through the initial stages of recovery. As the nutrition therapist is working at increasing the patient's caloric intake, a practitioner needs to monitor the patient's weight and vital signs. Often activity level needs to be decreased to help reverse the catabolic state. A reasonable weight gain goal may be 0.2–0.5 kg/wk. If weight loss persists, careful monitoring of vital signs, including supine heart rate, is important in determining whether an increased level of care is needed. Concomitantly, the patient should be referred to a psychotherapist and, if indicated, assessed by a psychiatrist.

Birmingham CL, Gritzner S: How does zinc supplementation benefit anorexia nervosa? Eat Weight Disord 2006;11:e109 [PMID: 17272939].

Claudino AM et al: Antidepressants for anorexia nervosa. Cochrane Database Syst Rev 2006;(1):CD004365 [PMID: 16437485].

Dunican KC, DelDotto D: The role of olanzapine in the treatment of anorexia nervosa. Ann Pharmacother 2007;41:111 [PMID: 17190846].

Hagman J, Gralla J, Sigel E et al: A double-blind, placebo-controlled study of risperidone for the treatment of anorexia nervosa. J Am Acad Child Adolesc Psychiatry 2011;50(9):915–924.

LeGrange D et al: Manualized family-based treatment for anorexia nervosa: A case series. J Am Acad Child Adolesc Psychiatry 2005;44:41 [PMID: 15608542].

Swenne I: Weight requirements for return of menstruations in teenage girls with eating disorders, weight loss, and secondary amenorrhea. Acta Paediatr 2004;93:1449 [PMID: 08035253].

BULIMIA NERVOSA

Table 6–6 lists the diagnostic criteria for BN. Binge eating is either eating excessive amounts of food during a normal mealtime or having a meal that lasts longer than usual. Bulimic individuals feel out of control while eating, unable or unwilling to recognize satiety signals. Any type of food may be eaten in a binge, although typically it includes carbohydrates or junk food. Extreme guilt is often associated with the episode. At some point, either prior to or during a binge, bulimic individuals often decide to purge as a means of preventing weight gain. The most common ways to purge are self-induced vomiting, exercise, and laxative use. Some individuals will vomit multiple times during a purge

Table 6–6. Diagnostic criteria for bulimia nervosa.

A. Recurrent episodes of binge eating. An episode of binge eating is characterized by both of the following:
   (1) Eating, in a discrete period of time (eg, within any 2-hour period), an amount of food that is definitely larger than most people would eat during a similar period of time and under similar circumstances.
   (2) A sense of lack of control over eating during the episodes (eg, a feeling that one cannot stop eating or control what or how much one is eating).
B. Recurrent inappropriate compensatory behavior in order to prevent weight gain, such as self-induced vomiting; misuse of laxatives, diuretics, enemas, or other medications; fasting; or excessive exercise.
C. The binge eating and inappropriate compensatory behaviors both occur, on average, at least twice a week for 3 months.
D. Self-evaluation is unduly influenced by body shape and weight.
E. The disturbance does not occur exclusively during episodes of anorexia nervosa.

Reprinted, with permission, from the *Diagnostic and Statistical Manual of Mental Disorders*, 4th ed. Text Revision. Copyright 2000. American Psychiatric Association.

episode, after using large amounts of water to cleanse their system. This can induce significant electrolyte abnormalities such as hyponatremia and hypokalemia, which may put the patient at acute risk for arrhythmia or seizure. Other methods of purging include diuretics, diet pills, cathartics, and nutritional supplements that promote weight loss, such as Metabolife or Sensa.

Diagnosing BN can be difficult unless the teenager is forthcoming or parents or caregivers can supply direct observations. Bulimic patients are usually average or slightly above average in body weight and have no physical abnormalities. Screening all teenagers for body image concerns is crucial. If the teenager expresses concern about being overweight, then the clinician needs to screen the patient about dieting methods. Asking whether patients have binged, feel out of control while eating, or whether they cannot stop eating can clarify the diagnosis. Parents may report that significant amounts of food are missing or disappearing more quickly than normal. If the physician is suspicious, direct questioning about all the ways to purge should follow. Indicating first that the behavior is not unusual can make questioning less threatening and more likely to elicit a truthful response. For example, the clinician might say, "Some teenagers who try to lose weight make themselves vomit after eating. Have you ever considered or done that yourself?" (See Table 6–2 for additional screening questions.)

Clinical Findings

A. Symptoms and Signs

Symptoms are related to the mechanism of purging. GI problems are most prominent. Abdominal pain is common. Gastroesophageal reflux occurs as the lower esophageal sphincter becomes compromised due to repetitive vomiting. Frequent vomiting may also cause esophagitis or gastritis, as the mucosa is irritated by acid exposure. Early satiety, involuntary vomiting, and complaints that food is "coming up" on its own are frequent. Hematemesis and esophageal rupture have been reported. Patients may report diarrhea or constipation, especially if laxatives have been used. Sialadenitis (parotid pain and enlargement) may be caused by frequent vomiting. Erosion of dental enamel results from increased oral acid exposure during vomiting. Because comorbid depression is common in BN, patients may report difficulty sleeping, decreased energy, decreased motivation, and headaches. Lightheadedness or syncope may develop secondary to dehydration.

It is important to note that most purging methods are ineffective. When patients binge, they may consume thousands of calories. Digestion begins rapidly. Although the patient may be able to vomit some of the food, much is actually digested and absorbed. Laxatives work in the large intestine, leading to fluid and electrolyte loss, but consumed calories are still absorbed from the small intestine. Use of diuretics may result in decreased fluid weight and electrolyte imbalance.

On physical examination, bulimic patients may be dehydrated and have orthostatic hypotension. Sialadenitis, tooth enamel loss, dental caries, and abdominal tenderness are the most common findings. Abrasion of the proximal interphalangeal joints may occur secondary to scraping the fingers against teeth while inducing vomiting. Rarely, a heart murmur is heard which may be due to mitral valve prolapse. Irreversible cardiomyopathy can develop secondary to ipecac use. Tachycardia and hypertension may occur secondary to caffeine and diet pill use.

B. Laboratory Findings

Electrolyte disturbances are common in bulimic patients. The method of purging results in specific abnormalities. Vomiting causes metabolic alkalosis, hypokalemia, and hypochloremia. If laxatives are used, then a metabolic acidosis develops with hypokalemia and hypochloremia. Diuretic use may lead to hypokalemia, hyponatremia, hypocalcemia, and metabolic alkalosis. Amylase may be increased secondary to chronic parotid stimulation.

Complications

A. Short-Term Complications

Complications in normal-weight bulimic patients are related to the mechanisms of purging, and many of these complications are listed under Symptoms and Signs. If the bulimic patient is significantly malnourished, complications may be the same as those encountered in the anorexic patient. Other complications of bulimia include esophageal rupture, acute or chronic esophagitis, and, rarely, Barrett's esophogitis. Chronic vomiting can lead to metabolic alkalosis, and laxative abuse may cause metabolic acidosis. Patients may develop aspiration pneumonia from vomiting. Diet pill use can cause insomnia, hypertension, tachycardia, palpitations, seizures, and sudden death.

Patients who stop taking laxatives can have severe constipation. Treating constipation can be difficult psychologically, because the practitioner may need to prescribe agents similar to the drugs of abuse used during the eating disorder.

B. Mortality

The mortality rate in bulimic patients is similar to that in anorexic patients. Death usually results from suicide or electrolyte derangements.

Treatment

Treatment of BN depends on the frequency of bingeing and purging and the severity of biochemical and psychiatric derangement. If K^+ is less than 3.0 mEq/L, inpatient medical admission is warranted. Typically extracellular K^+ is spared at the expense of intracellular K^+, so a patient may become hypokalemic several days after the serum K^+ concentration appears to be corrected. Usually cessation of purging is sufficient to correct K^+ concentration and is the recommended intervention for K^+ above 3.0 mEq/L. If K^+ is 2.5–2.9 mEq/L, oral supplementation is suggested. If K^+ is less than 2.5 mEq/L, then intravenous therapy is recommended. Supplements can be stopped once K^+ levels are more than 3.5 mEq/L. Total body K^+ can be assumed to be normal when serum K^+ corrects and remains normal 2 days after supplements are stopped. Continued hospitalization depends on the patient's psychological status.

Some bulimic patients who abuse laxatives may become chronically dehydrated. The renin-angiotensin-aldosterone axis is activated and the antidiuretic hormone level may be elevated to compensate. These systems do not shut down automatically when laxatives are stopped, and fluid retention of up to 10 kg/wk may result. This puts patients at risk for congestive heart failure and can scare them as their weight increases dramatically. Diuresis often occurs after 7–10 days. Parents and patients should be advised of this possible complication of initial therapy to help maintain their confidence in the care plan.

Hospitalization of bulimic patients is also recommended if there has been failure of outpatient management. The binge-purge cycle is addictive and can be difficult for patients to interrupt on their own. Hospitalization can offer a forced break from the cycle, allowing patients to normalize their eating, interrupt the addictive behavior, and regain the ability to recognize satiety signals.

Outpatient management can be pursued if patients are medically stable. Cognitive-behavioral therapy is crucial to help bulimic patients understand their disease and to offer suggestions for decreasing bingeing and purging. Nutrition therapy offers patients ways to regulate eating patterns so that they can avoid the need to binge. Medical monitoring should be done to check electrolytes periodically, depending on the purging method used.

SSRIs are generally helpful in treating the binge-purge cycle. Fluoxetine has been studied most extensively; a dose of 60 mg/d is most efficacious in teenagers. Other SSRIs appear to be effective as well and may be used in patients experiencing side effects of fluoxetine. Treatment for gastroesophageal reflux and gastritis should be used when appropriate. The pain and swelling of enlarged parotid glands can be helped by sucking on tart candy and by the application of heat.

American Psychiatric Association: Diagnostic and Statistical Manual of Mental Disorders, 4th ed, text revision. American Psychiatric Association, 2000.

Bacaltchuk J et al: Antidepressant versus placebo for the treatment of bulimia nervosa: A systematic review. Aust N Z J Psychiatry 2000;34:310 [PMID: 10789536].

Benini LT et al: Gastric emptying in patients with restricting and binge/purging subtypes of anorexia nervosa. Am J Gastroenterol 2004;99:1448 [PMID: 15307858].

Mehler PS: Medical complications of bulimia nervosa and their treatments. Int J Eat Disord (0276-3478) 2011,Mar;44(2):95 [PMID: 21312201].

Sysko R, Sha N, Wang W: Early response to antidepressant treatment in bulimia nervosa. Psychological Medicine 2010;40(6):999 [PMID: 20441691].

Panagiotopoulos C et al: Electrocardiographic findings in adolescents with eating disorders. Pediatrics 2000;105:1100 [PMID: 10790469].

Steinhausen HC, Weber S: The outcome of bulimia nervosa: Findings from one-quarter century of research. Am J Psychiatry 2009;166:1331–1341 [PMID: 19884225].

BINGE-EATING DISORDER

The diagnostic category of binge-eating disorder (BED) was created in DSM-IV, but it is still considered a research diagnosis. Studies show that most adults who have BED (a prevalence of 2%–4%) develop symptoms during adolescence. Table 6–7 lists the diagnostic criteria.

Clinical Findings

A. Symptoms and Signs

BED most often occurs in overweight or obese individuals. Eighteen percent of such patients report bingeing at least once in the past year. Patients with BED have an increased

Table 6–7. Diagnostic criteria for binge-eating disorder.

A. Recurrent episodes of binge eating. An episode of binge eating is characterized by both of the following:
  (1) Eating, in a discrete period of time (eg, within any 2-hour period), an amount of food that is definitely larger than most people would eat in a similar period of time under similar circumstances.
  (2) A sense of lack of control over eating during the episode (eg, a feeling that one cannot stop eating or control what or how much one is eating).
B. The binge-eating episodes are associated with three (or more) of the following:
  (1) Eating much more rapidly than normal
  (2) Eating until feeling uncomfortably full
  (3) Eating large amounts of food when not feeling physically hungry
  (4) Eating alone because of being embarrassed by how much one is eating
  (5) Feeling disgusted with oneself, depressed, or very guilty after overeating
C. Marked distress regarding binge eating.
D. The binge eating occurs, on average, at least 2 days a week for 6 months.
E. The binge eating is not associated with regular use of inappropriate compensatory behaviors (eg, purging, fasting, excessive exercise) and does not occur exclusively during the course of anorexia nervosa or bulimia nervosa.

incidence of depression and substance abuse. Using the DSM-IV-TR diagnostic criteria as a guide for evaluation, the possibility of BED should be raised for any significantly overweight patient. Specific questionnaires are available for evaluating patients suspected of BED.

B. Laboratory Findings

The clinician should assess causes and complications of obesity, and laboratory evaluation should include thyroid function tests and measurement of cholesterol and triglyceride levels.

Treatment

A combination of cognitive-behavioral therapy and antidepressant medication has been helpful in treating BED in adults. Use of SSRIs for BED in adolescents has not been studied, but in adults, fluoxetine and citalopram help decrease binge episodes, improve depressive symptoms, and possibly decrease appetite. This evidence suggests that SSRIs in adolescents with BED may be helpful as well. BED has been recognized only recently, and outcomes have not been studied. Little is known regarding long-term prognosis.

Fairburn CG et al: The natural course of bulimia nervosa and binge eating disorder in young women. Arch Gen Psychiatry 2000;57:659 [PMID: 10891036].

Johnson WG et al: Measuring binge eating in adolescents: Adolescent and parent versions of the questionnaire of eating and weight patterns. Int J Eat Disord 1999;26:301 [PMID: 10441246].

McElroy SL et al: Citalopram in the treatment of binge-eating disorder: A placebo-controlled trial. J Clin Psychiatry 2003;64:807 [PMID: 12934982].

Schneider M: Bulimia nervosa and binge eating disorder in adolescents. Adolesc Med State Art Rev 2003;14:119 [PMID: 12529196].

EATING DISORDER NOT OTHERWISE SPECIFIED

Eating Disorder Not Otherwise Specificed (EDNOS) is the most common eating disorder diagnosis, but least studied. Patients do not meet all the criteria for either AN or BN, but have features of either or both. Table 6–8 lists the diagnostic criteria. This has become a "catch-all" category and some researchers describe this as an atypical eating disorder or partial syndrome eating disorder. EDNOS is estimated to affect 0.5%–14% of the general adolescent population, and accounts for about 50% of all ED diagnoses. The incidence of EDNOS will decrease dramatically with DSM-V, as the definition of AN will broaden to include some patients characterized as having EDNOS in DSM IV-TR. Regardless of specific diagnostic criteria, it is imperative for the clinician to pay careful attention to patient concerns about body weight and dieting behaviors to facilitate recognition of eating disorder behavior. Symptoms and sequelae depend on specific behaviors. Some patients with EDNOS will go on to develop full-blown AN or BN, and early recognition and treatment may decrease further complications.

Table 6–8. Diagnostic criteria for eating disorder not otherwise specified.

The eating disorder not otherwise specified category is for disorders of eating that do not meet the criteria for any specific eating disorder. Examples include

1. For females, all of the criteria for anorexia nervosa are met except that the individual has regular menses.
2. All of the criteria for anorexia nervosa are met except that, despite significant weight loss, the individual's current weight is in the normal range.
3. All of the criteria for bulimia nervosa are met except that the binge eating and inappropriate compensatory mechanisms occur at a frequency of less than twice a week or for a duration of less than 3 months.
4. The regular use of inappropriate compensatory behavior by an individual of normal body weight after eating small amounts of food (eg, self-induced vomiting after the consumption of two cookies).
5. Repeatedly chewing and spitting out, but not swallowing, large amounts of food.

PROGNOSIS

Outcome in eating disorders, especially AN, has been studied extensively. Unfortunately, most studies have focused on specific inpatient treatment programs, and few have evaluated less ill patients who do not need hospitalization. About 40%–50% of patients receiving treatment recover; 20%–30% have intermittent relapses; and 20% have chronic, unremitting illness. As time from initial onset lengthens, the recovery rate decreases and mortality associated with AN and BN increases.

The course of AN often includes significant weight fluctuations over time, and it may be a matter of years until recovery is certain. The course of BN often includes relapses of bingeing and purging, although bulimic patients initially recover faster than do anorexic patients. Up to 50% of anorexic patients may develop bulimia, as well as major psychological complications, including depression, anxiety, and substance abuse disorders. Bulimic patients also develop similar psychological illness but rarely develop anorexia. Long-term medical sequelae, aside from low body weight and amenorrhea, have not been systematically studied, although AN is known to have multiple medical consequences, including osteoporosis and structural brain changes.

It is unclear whether age at onset affects outcome, but shorter length of time between symptom onset and therapy tends to improve outcome. Various treatment modalities can prove effective. Favorable outcomes have been found with brief medical hospitalization and long psychiatric or residential hospitalization. Higher discharge weight, as well as more rapid weight gain during inpatient treatment (> 0.8 kg/wk) seems to improve the initial outcome. It is difficult to compare treatment regimens, because numbers are small and the type of patient and illness varies among studies. No existing studies compare outpatient to inpatient treatment or the effects of day treatment on recovery.

Chamay-Weber C et al: Partial eating disorders among adolescents: A review. J Adolesc Health 2005;37:417 [PMID: 16227132].

Eddy KT et al: Eating disorder not otherwise specified in adolescents. J Am Acad Child Adolesc Psychiatry 2008;47(2):156–164.

Lund BC et al: Rate of inpatient weight restoration predicts outcome in anorexia nervosa. Int J Eat Disord 2009;42(4):301–305 [PMID: 19107835].

Steinhausen HC: Outcome of eating disorders. Child Adolesc Psychiatr Clin N Am 2009;18(1):225–242 [PMID: 19014869].

RESOURCES FOR PRACTIONERS AND FAMILIES

Web Resources:

National Eating Disorders Association: (Information available to help individuals/families locate resources and treatment for eating disorders around the world) http://www.nationaleating-disorders.org/

Academy for Eating Disorders: (The Academy for Eating Disorders (AED) is a global, multidisciplinary professional organization that provides cutting-edge professional training and education, inspires new developments in eating disorders research, prevention, and clinical treatments, and is the international source for state-of-the-art information in the field of eating disorders.) www.aedweb.org

Child & Adolescent Psychiatric Disorders & Psychosocial Aspects of Pediatrics

7

Brian Stafford, MD, MPH
Ayelet Talmi, PhD
Adam Burstein, DO

Mental illness affects between 14% and 20% of children and adolescents. The prevalence is higher for those juveniles living in poor socioeconomic circumstances. Unfortunately, the shortage of mental health providers, stigma attached to receiving mental health services, chronic underfunding, institutional barriers of the public mental health system, and disparate insurance benefits have contributed to the fact that only 2% of these children are actually seen by mental health specialists. About 75% of children with psychiatric disturbances are seen in primary care settings, and half of all pediatric office visits involve behavioral, psychosocial, or educational concerns. Parents and children often prefer discussing these issues with someone they already know and trust. As a result, pediatric primary care physicians and providers are compelled to play an important role in the prevention, identification, initiation, management, and coordination of mental health care in children and adolescents.

Despite being strategically positioned as the gatekeeper for identifying these concerns, primary care physicians identify fewer than 20% of children with emotional and behavioral problems during health supervision visits when these concerns are also present. In addition, these problems are not identified when they begin (and are more readily amenable to treatment). This gatekeeper role has become more important over the past decade as advances in mental health awareness and treatment have improved opportunities for early identification and intervention. This role is especially critical since child psychiatry remains an underserved medical specialty, with only 7000 board-certified child and adolescent psychiatrists in the United States. In contrast, the more than 50,000 board-certified pediatricians and innumerable mid-level pediatric providers in the United States are in a unique position to identify issues affecting the emotional health of children and to initiate treatment or referrals to other providers.

Emotional problems that develop during childhood and adolescence can have a significant impact on development and may continue into adulthood; in fact, most "adult" psychiatric disorders have their onset during childhood. Most disorders do not present as an "all-or-none" phenomenon; rather, they progress from adjustment concerns to perturbations in functioning to significant disturbances and severe disorders. Pediatricians have the capacity to manage emotional problems and behavioral conditions early on, when improvement can be achieved with less intensive interventions. If pediatricians and schools do not appropriately identify mental health problems, provide education about the benefits of intervention, and encourage and initiate intervention, childhood-onset disorders are more likely to persist, cause worsening impairment, and lead to a downward spiral of school and social difficulties, poor employment opportunities, and poverty in adulthood, as well as increased health care utilization and costs as adults.

Pediatricians and other pediatric care providers may be the first or sometimes only medical professional in a position to identify a mental health problem. This chapter reviews prevention, surveillance, and screening for mental illness; situations that may arise in the context of such assessments; illnesses that are often diagnosed during childhood or adolescence; current recommendations for interventions and use of psychotropic medications; and indications for referral to mental health professionals.

Belfer ML: Child and adolescent mental disorders: The magnitude of the problem across the globe. J Child Psychol Psychiatry 2008 Mar;49(3):226–236 [PMID: 18221350].

Costello EJ, Egger H, Angold A: 10-year research update review: The epidemiology of child and adolescent psychiatric disorders: I. Methods and public health burden. J Am Acad Child Adolesc Psychiatry 2005;44:972–986 [PMID: 16175102].

Costello EJ, Foley DL, Angold A: 10-year research update review: The epidemiology of child and adolescent psychiatric disorders: II. Developmental epidemiology. J Am Acad Child Adolesc Psychiatry 2006 Jan;45(1):8–25 [PMID: 16327577].

Roberts RE, Roberts CR, Xing Y: Prevalence of youth-reported DSM-IV psychiatric disorders among African, European, and Mexican American adolescents. J Am Acad Child Adolesc Psychiatry 2006 Nov;45(11):1329–1337 [PMID: 17075355].

MODELS OF CARE ENCOMPASSING MENTAL HEALTH IN THE PRIMARY CARE SETTING

Given the many barriers to receiving mental health care, new approaches to identifying concerns and providing mental health professional services have been recently explored.

Usual or typical pediatric care of emotional and behavioral problems is related to the comfort level of the individual pediatric provider and available resources. The efficacy of surveillance in the form of developmentally appropriate anticipatory guidance and counseling is variable; the average time spent is 2.5 minutes. However, as stated earlier, the majority of emotional and behavioral problems are not identified in this model of care. In addition, when they are identified, the logistics of referral can be problematic. Although pediatricians often refer to mental health providers, only 50% of families will actually attend an appointment and the average number of appointments attended is only slightly greater than one. Based on level of comfort and training, the primary clinician in this model is more likely to be responsible for psychiatric medications if prescribed.

Among the technological interventions that can enhance identification of problems and target specific symptoms for assessment is the **Child Health and Interactive Developmental System (CHADIS)** (http://www.childhealthcare.org). In this system, parents use a computer kiosk to note their level of concern about various behaviors, which triggers algorithmic interviews for each concern based on psychiatric diagnostic criteria. The CHADIS system provides an electronic worksheet of analyzed results, school communication tools, as well as other resources.

Enhanced care is a model of care in which a pediatric developmental or behavioral specialist is embedded in the clinic, thus making for improved referral and communication and management. This "co-location" creates easier access for patients and improved communication with mental health professionals.

Telephonic consultation or **telepsychiatry** with mental health consultation teams in a stepped care approach allows enhanced access to mental health providers, especially for children in rural communities. The provision of consultation to pediatric care providers also allows pediatric providers ongoing education with the eventual goal of pediatric providers learning to manage these concerns on their own.

Collaborative care provides high-quality, multidisciplinary, and collaborative care through the co-location of educators, consultants, or direct service mental health providers in the clinic. Successful collaborative care results in greater specialist involvement by negating identification and referral and other system-of-care barriers. Successful components include a leadership team, primary clinicians, mental health and developmental specialists, administrators, clinical informatics specialists, and care managers. Collaborative care implies that nearly all visits are done jointly and that mental health professionals are always available for consultation, in contrast to the approach in the enhanced care model, which requires the scheduling of an appointment with a mental health specialist in the practice. These interventions can be accomplished through collaboration among mental health and primary care providers, mental health systems and primary care practices, and in academic settings with interdepartmental collaboration. Typically, philanthropic or other foundation grants are necessary to start a collaborative program so that reimbursement and sustainability concerns can be identified and remedied.

American Academy of Child and Adolescent Psychiatry Committee on Health Care Access and Economics Task Force on Mental Health: Improving mental health services in primary care: reducing administrative and financial barriers to access and collaboration. Pediatrics 2009 Apr;123(4):1248–1251 [PMID: 19336386].

Brito A et al: Bridging mental health and medical care in underserved pediatric populations: three integrative models. Adv Pediatr 2010;57(1):295–313 [PMID: 21056744].

Chenven M: Community systems of care for children's mental health. Child Adolesc Psychiatr Clin N Am 2010 Jan;19(1):163–174 [PMID: 19951815].

Committee on Psychosocial Aspects of Child and Family Health and Task Force on Mental Health: Policy statement—the future of pediatrics: Mental health competencies for pediatric primary care. Pediatrics 2009 Jul;124(1):410–421 [PMID: 19564328].

Connor DF et al: Targeted child psychiatric services: A new model of pediatric primary clinician—child psychiatry collaborative care. Clin Pediatr 2005;45:423 [PMID: 16891275].

Kelleher KJ et al: Management of pediatric mental disorders in primary care: Where are we now and where are we going? Curr Opin Pediatr 2006;18:649 [PMID: 17099365].

Kelleher KJ, Stevens J: Evolution of child mental health services in primary care. Acad Pediatr 2009 Jan–Feb;9(1):7–14 [PMID: 19329085].

Williams J et al: Co-location of mental health professionals in primary care settings: Three North Carolina models. Clin Pediatr (Phila) 2006;45;537 [PMID: 16893859].

Yellowlees PM et al: A retrospective analysis of a child and adolescent eMental Health program. J Am Acad Child Adolesc Psychiatry 2008 Jan;47(1):103–107 [PMID: 18174831].

EARLY IDENTIFICATION & PREVENTION OF DEVELOPMENTAL & SOCIOEMOTIONAL PROBLEMS

The role of the primary care pediatrician continues to expand to include public health, mental health, and community concerns. The American Academy of Pediatrics (AAP) Policy Statement on Community Pediatrics addresses the fact that today's children and families live in a period of rapid social change and declining economic circumstances. In addition, the economic organization of the health care and social service systems in the United States is undergoing profound changes. For many pediatric providers, efforts to promote the health of children have been directed at attending to the needs of particular children in a practice setting, on an individual basis, and providing them with a medical home. This approach, in combination with pediatricians' own personal community interests and commitments, has been dramatically successful. Increasingly, however, the major threats to the health of U.S. children—the new morbidity—arise from problems that cannot be adequately addressed by the practice model alone. These problems include unacceptably high infant mortality rates in certain communities, extraordinary levels of intentional and unintentional injuries, chemical dependency, behavioral and developmental consequences of inappropriate care and experience, family dysfunction, sexually transmitted diseases, unplanned pregnancies and out-of-wedlock births, and lack of a medical home. The Policy Statement concludes that "We must become partners with others, or we will become increasingly irrelevant to the health of children."

Today's community pediatrician seeks to provide a far more realistic and complete clinical picture by taking responsibility for all children in a community, providing preventive and curative services, and understanding the determinants and consequences of child health and illness, as well as the effectiveness of services provided.

Bright Futures

Bright Futures is a national health promotion and disease prevention initiative that addresses children's health needs in the context of family and community. In addition to use in pediatric practice, many states implement Bright Futures principles, guidelines, and tools to strengthen the connections between state and local programs, pediatric primary care, families, and local communities. The *Bright Futures Guidelines*, now in its third edition, was developed to provide comprehensive health supervision guidelines, including recommendations on immunizations, routine health screenings, and anticipatory guidance. In addition, Bright Futures for Mental Health provides numerous guidelines, tools, and strategies for improving mental health identification, assessment, initiation, management, and coordination.

Surgeon General's National Action Plan

The U.S. Surgeon General also recommends that pediatrics continue to evolve and include lifestyle, health system, and other psychosocial areas. The U.S. Surgeon General's National Action Agenda on Mental Health includes several calls to primary care pediatricians, including the following: engage other professional organizations in educating new frontline providers in various systems (eg, teachers, physicians, nurses, hospital emergency personnel, day care providers, probation officers, and other child health care providers) in child development; equip them with skills to address and enhance children's mental health; and train them to recognize early symptoms of emotional or behavioral problems for proactive intervention. Such training must focus on developmental and cultural differences in cognitive, social, emotional, and behavioral functioning, and understanding these issues in familial and ecological context.

Rushton FE Jr: American Academy of Pediatrics Committee on Community Health Services: The pediatrician's role in community pediatrics. Pediatrics 2005;115:1092 [PMID: 15805396].

Sheldrick RC, Merchant S, Perrin EC: Identification of developmental-behavioral problems in primary care: A systematic review. Pediatrics 2011 Aug;128(2):356–363 [Epub 2011 Jul 4] [PMID: 2172710].

Hacker KA, Arsenault LN, Williams S, Digirolamo: Mental and behavioral health screening at preventive visits: Opportunities for follow-up of patients who are nonadherent with the next preventive visit. AMJ Pediatr. 2011 Apr;158(4):666–671.e2 [Epub 2010 Nov 11] [PMID: 21074180].

American Academy of Pediatrics: Children's Mental Health in Primary Care. Available at: http://www.aap.org/mentalhealth/index.html

Bright Futures Mental Health. Available at: http://www.brightfutures.org/mentalhealth/pdf/index.html;

http://www.brightfutures.org/mentalhealth/pdf/tools.html

Massachusetts Child Psychiatry Access Project. Available at: http://mcpap.typepad.com

U.S. Surgeon General's National Action Agenda. Available at: http://www.surgeongeneral.govlcmh/childreport.htm

Zero to Three. Available at: http://www.zerotothree.org

Summary of the Pediatrician's Role

Given these calls for a new pediatric role as the gatekeeper for socioemotional health, the expanding role of the primary care pediatric provider encompasses the following broad categories: prevention, identification, assessment, initiation, management, coordination, and collaboration (Table 7–1).

Table 7–1. The pediatric primary care provider's role in mental health.

Role	Specific Activities
Prevention	Screen and address social risk factors on intake Screen and refer for early socioemotional risk
Identification	Shared family concern Surveillance Screening
Assessment	Interview and Physical Assessment tools Comorbid conditions
Initiation	Psychoeducation about condition and treatment options • Wait and watch • Refer to mental health for further evaluation • Refer for therapy • Start medication
Management	Monitor condition for improvement Monitor for side effects
Coordination	With social work, therapist, psychologist, or psychiatrist
Collaboration	With mental health service providers With child protection With local schools

IDENTIFICATION & ASSESSMENT DURING HEALTH MAINTENANCE VISITS

Most families seek help from their primary care providers when they are concerned about a child's health, growth, or development. Historically, the most efficient indicator in eliciting psychosocial problems is the history provided by parents or guardians, and interview and observation of the child. The possible approaches to identification of problems include surveillance, screening, and assessment.

Surveillance consists of the following elements: checking in, eliciting concerns, asking open-ended questions, watching and waiting, listening for red flags, identifying risk factors, and monitoring closely over time. Like vital signs, which represent an essential component of the physical evaluation, the essential components of the primary care surveillance for mental health concerns should generally include a review of the youth's general functioning in different aspects of their life. Five questions forming the mnemonic **PSYCH** can be addressed to parents and youth as a surveillance means of uncovering areas of concern.

1. **P**arent-child interaction: How are things going with you and your parents? Or you and your infant (or toddler)?
2. **S**chool: How are things going in school (or child care; academically, behaviorally, and socially)?
3. **Y**outh: How are things going with peer relationships/ friendships (how does child get along with same-aged peers)?
4. **C**asa: How are things going at home (including siblings, family stresses, and relationship with parents)?
5. **H**appiness: How would you describe your mood? How would you describe your child's mood?

Many pediatric practices are hampered by lack of continuity and not enough time for in-depth surveillance. In addition, surveillance is notoriously tied to office and provider characteristics. Given current time constraints for current pediatric visits, and the fact that only 18% of parents reporting elevated behavior problems in children actually told their providers about it, surveillance is currently considered nonoptimal. Although part of the clinical interview with families, surveillance is not a separate and billable service under current Medicaid and insurance reimbursement plans, whereas formal screening is.

Screening is the process of using standardized instruments to identify areas of risk, delay, or concern. Newborn, hearing, vision, and developmental screenings are common in today's pediatric practice. However, the morbidity associated with developmental, emotional, and psychosocial problems requires that socioemotional screening to identify the presence of symptoms of emotional, behavioral, or relationship disorders also be performed. Screening tools are brief, easy to use, and can be administered as a questionnaire or using an interview format. A positive screen warrants a more complete assessment. The use of screening tools can also lead to early identification and interrupt the adjustment-perturbation-disturbance-disorder pathway. Newer methods of eliciting socioemotional and behavior concerns have been developed (see next sections). Helpful information can also be obtained from broad screening checklists and symptom-specific questionnaires (such as depression or anxiety self-report inventories). Questions can be incorporated into the general pediatric office screening forms, or specific questionnaires can be used.

Tools for Mental Health Screening in the Office Setting

Given the low rates of identification of psychosocial problems by pediatric surveillance, the use of standardized screening tools has become standard practice. Typically, broad screeners that elicit information regarding multiple domains are employed first and are followed by targeted screens to address symptomatology, severity, impairment, and context of specific psychosocial problems.

Multiple Screening Tools. Available at: http://mcpap.typepad.com/

http://www.schoolpsychiatry.org

http://www.wpic.pitt.edu/research

http://www.brightfutures.org/mentalhealth/pdf/tools.html

A. General or Broad Screening Tools

1. Strengths and Difficulties Questionnaires (SDQs)—The SDQs are brief behavioral screening questionnaires targeting patients 3–16 years old with parent, teacher, and child self-report versions available. Several versions are available and can readily be used by researchers, clinicians, and educators. They have been well validated and are available on the Internet without cost. The SDQs are available in over 40 languages. The domains assessed include: emotional problems, conduct problems, hyperactivity/inattention, peer relationship problems, and prosocial behaviors. For further information, refer to the following web site: http://www.sdqinfo.org.

Vostanis P: Strengths and Difficulties Questionnaire: Research and clinical applications. Curr Opin Psychiatry 2006 Jul;19(4): 367–372 [PMID: 16721165].

2. Pediatric Symptoms Checklist (PSC)—The PSC is a one-page questionnaire listing a broad range of children's emotional and behavioral problems that reflects parents' impressions of their children's psychosocial functioning. An adolescent self-report version is also available for children ages 11 and older. The PSC was developed initially for children older than age 5, but cutoff scores for preschool and school-aged children indicating clinical levels of dysfunction have been empirically derived. The questionnaire is easy to score, is free of charge, and is available in English and

Spanish from the following web sites: http://brightfutures.org/mentalhealth/pdf/professionals/ped_symptom_chklst.pdf; http://psc.partners.org/psc_order.htm.

Kostanecka A et al: Behavioral health screening in urban primary care settings: Construct validity of the PSC-17. J Dev Behav Pediatr 2008 Apr;29(2):124–128 [PMID: 18408533].

3. Parents Evaluation of Developmental Status (PEDS)—The PEDS is a validated screener for socioemotional, developmental, and behavioral concerns in children aged 1 month to 8 years. Parents answer yes/no about their concerned in various areas of their child's development. Scoring the PEDS is more labor intensive than other general screeners and the instrument must be purchased. Its benefits include extensive validity data and useful pathways for level of concern and referral. It is available in English, Vietnamese, and Spanish. For further information, see the following web site: http://www.pedstest.com.

Brothers KT et al: PEDS: Developmental milestones—an accurate brief tool for surveillance and screening. Clin Pediatr (Phila) 2007 Dec;5 [Epub ahead of print] [PMID: 18057141].

4. Ages and Stages, Socioemotional (SE)—The Ages and Stages, SE is a companion to the Ages and Stages Developmental Screen. It is an easy-to-use tool with a deep, exclusive focus on infant, toddlers, and younger children's social and emotional behavior. After a one-time cost, the instrument is reproducible, making it cost-effective. It is culturally sensitive for use across diverse pediatric populations. Screens are available for the 6, 12, 18, 24, 36, 48, and 60 month visits, and in English, French, Spanish, and Korean.

Briggs-Gowan MJ, Carter AS: Social-emotional screening status in early childhood predicts elementary school outcomes. Pediatrics 2008 May;121(5):957–962 [PMID: 18450899].

Ages and Stages, SE (technical data): http://www.brookespublishing.com/store/books/bricker-asq/asq-technical.pdf

5. Family Psychosocial Screen—(Kemper KJ, Kelleher KJ 1996). Available at: http://www.brightfutures.org/mentalhealth/pdf/professionals/ped_intake_form.pdf Family psychosocial screening.

6. WE CARE—Available in appendix of article. (Garg A et al: Improving the management of family psychosocial problems at low-income children's well-child care visits: The WE CARE Project. Pediatrics 2007 Sep;120(3):547–558 [PMID: 17766528].)

Assessment of Behavioral & Emotional Signs & Symptoms

When an emotional problem or mental illness is mentioned by the patient or parents, elicited by an interview, or identified by a screening instrument, a thorough evaluation is indicated. At least 30 minutes should be scheduled, and additional appointments may be necessary to gather information or perform tests to determine a mental health diagnosis. Examples of more thorough questions and observation are given in Table 7–2. Targeted assessment screening tools are also useful in determining severity, comorbidity, and context of impairment.

It is useful to see both parents and the child first together, then the parents alone, and then the child alone (for school age children and adolescents). This sequence enables the physician to observe interactions among family members, allows the child to feel more comfortable with the provider, and offers the parents and the child an opportunity to talk confidentially about their concerns. Parents and children often feel shame and guilt about some personal inadequacy they perceive to be causing the problem. The physician can facilitate the assessment by acknowledging that the family is trying to cope and that the ultimate task of assessment is to seek solutions and not to assign blame. An attitude of nonjudgmental inquiry can be communicated with supportive statements such as, "Let's see if we can figure out what might be happening here and find some ways to make things better."

A. History of the Presenting Problem

First, obtain a detailed description of the problem.

- When did it start?
- Where and with whom does it occur?
- Were there unusual stresses, changes, or life events at that time?
- How is the child's life and the family's functioning affected?
- What does the child say about the problem?
- What attempts have been made to alleviate the problem?
- Do the parents have any opinions about the cause of the problem?

B. Techniques for Interviewing Children and Adolescents

1. Interviewing the preschool child—Preschool children should be interviewed with their parents. As the parents discuss their concerns, the physician can observe the child's behavior, including their activity level and any unusual behaviors or symptoms. It is helpful to have toy human figures, animals, or puppets, and crayons and paper available that the child can use to express him- or herself. After hearing the history from the parents and observing and talking with the child, the physician can begin to develop an impression about the problem and formulate a treatment plan to discuss with the family.

2. Interviewing the school-aged child—Most school-aged children have mastered separation anxiety sufficiently to tolerate at least a brief interview alone with the physician.

Table 7–2. Assessment of psychosocial problems.

Developmental history

1. Review the landmarks of psychosocial development
2. Summarize the child's temperamental traits
3. Review stressful life events and the child's reactions to them
   a. Separations from primary caregivers or close family members
   b. Losses
   c. Marital conflict, family violence, divorce
   d. Illnesses, injuries, and hospitalizations
   e. Moves, household changes
   f. School transitions
   g. Traumatic events
   h. Financial changes that impact daily living environment
4. Obtain details of past mental health problems and their treatment

Family history

1. Marital/relationship history
   a. Overall satisfaction with the marriage/partnership
   b. Conflicts or disagreements within the relationship
   c. Quantity and quality of time together away from children
   d. Whether the child comes between or is a source of conflict between the parents
   e. Marital history prior to having children
2. Parenting history
   a. Feelings about parenthood
   b. Whether parents feel united in dealing with the child
   c. "Division of labor" in parenting
   d. Parental energy or stress level
   e. Sleeping arrangements
   f. Privacy
   g. Attitudes about discipline
   h. Interference with discipline from outside the family (eg, ex-spouses, grandparents)
3. Stresses on the family
   a. Problems with employment
   b. Financial problems
   c. Changes of residence or household composition
   d. Illness, injuries, and deaths
4. Family history of mental health problems and treatment
   a. Depression? Who?
   b. Suicide attempts? Who?
   c. Psychiatric hospitalizations? Who?
   d. "Nervous breakdowns"? Who?
   e. Substance abuse or problems? Who?
   f. Nervousness or anxiety? Who?

Observation of the parents

1. Do they agree on the existence of the problem or concern?
2. Are they uncooperative or antagonistic about the evaluation? (temperamental traits)
3. Do the parents appear depressed or overwhelmed? (reactions to them)
4. Can the parents present a coherent picture of the problem and their family life?
5. Do the parents accept some responsibility for the child's problems, or do they blame forces outside the family and beyond their control?
6. Do they appear burdened with guilt about the child's problem?

Observation of the child

1. Does the child acknowledge the existence of a problem or concern?
2. Does the child want help?
3. Is the child uncooperative or antagonistic about the assessment?
4. What is the child's predominant mood or attitude?
5. What does the child wish could be different (eg, "three wishes")?
6. Does the child display unusual behavior (activity level, mannerisms, fearfulness)?
7. What is the child's apparent cognitive level?

Observation of parent-child interaction

1. Do the parents show concern about the child's feelings?
2. Does the child control or disrupt the joint interview?
3. Does the child respond to parental limits and control?
4. Do the parents inappropriately answer questions addressed to the child?
5. Is there obvious tension between family members?

Data from other sources

1. Waiting room observations by office staff
2. School (teacher, nurse, social worker, counselor, day care provider)
3. Department of social services
4. Other caregivers: grandparents, etc

In addition, they may have important information to share about their own worries. The child should be told beforehand by the parents or physician (or both) that the doctor will want to talk to the child about his or her feelings. School-aged children understand and even appreciate parental concern about unhappiness, worries, and difficulty in getting along with people. At the outset, it is useful to explore the child's thoughts about certain issues raised by the parents and ask whether the child thinks that a problem exists (eg, unhappiness, anxiety, or sleep disturbance) and any other concerns the child may have. The physician should ask the child to describe the problem in his or her own words and ask what he or she thinks is causing the problem. It is important to ask the child how the problem affects the child and the family. At the end of the interview with the child, it is important to share or reiterate the central points derived from the interview and to state that the next step is to talk with the parents about ways to make things better for the child. At that time, it is good to discuss any concerns or misgivings the child might have about sharing information with parents so that the child's right to privacy is not arbitrarily violated. Most children want to make things better and thus will allow the physician to share appropriate concerns with the parents.

3. Interviewing the adolescent—The physician usually begins by meeting briefly with the parents and adolescent together to define the concerns. Because the central developmental task of adolescence is to create an identity separate from that of the parents, the physician must show respect for the teen's point of view. The physician should then meet alone with the adolescent or, at least, give the teen the option. After the physician has interviewed the adolescent and talked further with the parents, he or she should formulate thoughts and recommendations. Whenever possible, it is helpful to discuss these with the adolescent before presenting them to the parents and teen together. The issue of confidentiality must be discussed early in the interview: "What we talk about today is between you and me unless we decide together that someone should know or unless it appears to me that you might be in a potentially dangerous situation."

The interview with the adolescent alone might start with a restatement of the parents' concerns. The teen should be encouraged to describe the situation in his or her own words and say what he or she would like to be different. The physician should ask questions about the adolescent's primary concerns, predominant mood state, relationships with family members, level of satisfaction with school and peer relationships, plans for the future, drug and alcohol use, and sexual activity.

In concluding the interview, the physician should summarize his or her thoughts and develop a plan with the teenager to present to the parents. If teenagers participate in the solution, they are more likely to work with the family to improve the situation. This should include a plan either for further investigation or for ways of dealing with the problem and arranging subsequent appointments with the physician or an appropriate referral to a mental health care provider.

C. Targeted Screening Tools and Assessment Measures

As with broad screening tools, targeted screening tools or assessment instruments can be very valuable in the clinic since they are standardized and allow for the assessment of current symptoms and severity. They can also be useful for following or reassessing a patient's progress after initiation of treatment.

1. Vanderbilt Assessment Scales for Attention-Deficit/Hyperactivity Disorder—These scales are included in the American Academy of Pediatrics/National Initiative for Children's Health Quality (AAP/NICHQ) Attention-Deficit/Hyperactivity Disorder Practitioner's Toolkit, available at: http://www.nichq.org/resources/toolkit/ or http://www.schoolpsychiatry.org.

2. Center for Epidemiologic Scales Depression Scale for Children (CESD-C)—Available at: http://www.brightfutures.org/mentalhealth/pdf/tools.html.

3. Self-Report for Childhood Anxiety Related Emotional Disorders (SCARED)—Available at: http://www.wpic.pitt.edu/research/.

4. PHQ-9—Available at: http://www.depression-primarycare.org/clinicians/toolkits/materials/forms/phq9/

Also at http://www.teenscreen.org/images/stories/PDF/PHQ-9Padreadonly2.11.pdf

5. Other Tools

A. **Bright futures**—The Bright Futures Tool Kit has numerous guidelines, tools, and other resources for identifying mental health concerns. Available at: http://www.brightfutures.org/mentalhealth/pdf/tools.html.

B. **Chaddis**—See earlier discussion of models of health care.

C. **Disorder-specific screening tools**—Useful tools for evaluating other mental health concerns, such as obsessive-compulsive disorder (OCD), post-traumatic stress disorder (PTSD), and pervasive developmental disorder (PDD), can be found at the following web sites: http://www.schoolpsychiatry.org and http://mcpap.typepad.com/.

Diagnostic Formulation & Interpretation of Findings

Diagnosis, the final product of the assessment, starts with a description of the presenting problem, which is then evaluated within the context of the child's age, developmental needs, the stresses and strains on the child and the family, and the functioning of the family system.

The physician's first task is to decide whether a problem exists. For example, how hyperactive must a 5-year-old child be before he or she is too hyperactive? When a child's functioning is impaired in major domains of life, such as learning, peer relationships, family relationships, authority relationships, and recreation, or when a substantial deviation from the trajectory of normal developmental tasks occurs, a differential diagnosis should be sought based on the symptom profile. The physician then develops an etiologic hypothesis based on the information gathered:

1. The behavior falls within the range of normal given the child's developmental level.
2. The behavior is a temperamental variation.
3. The behavior is related to central nervous system impairment (eg, prematurity, exposure to toxins in utero, seizure disorder, or genetic disorders).
4. The behavior is a normal reaction to stressful circumstances (eg, medical illness, change in family structure, or loss of a loved one).
5. The problem is primarily a reflection of family dysfunction (eg, the child is the symptom bearer, scapegoat, or the identified patient for the family).
6. The problem indicates a possible psychiatric disorder.
7. The problem is complicated by an underlying medical condition.
8. Some combination of the above.

Sharing of the diagnosis is also the beginning of initiating treatment. The physician's interpretation of the complaint and diagnosis is then presented to the family. The interpretive process includes the following components:

1. Psychoeducation: An explanation of how the presenting problem or symptom is a reflection of a suspected cause and typical outcomes both with and without intervention.
2. A discussion of possible interventions, including the following options:
   a. Close monitoring.
   b. Counseling provided by the primary care provider.
   c. Referral to a mental health professional.
   d. Initiation of medication.
   e. Some combination of the above.
3. A discussion of the parent's and adolescent's response to the diagnosis and potential interventions.

A joint plan involving the physician, parents, and child is then negotiated to address the child's symptoms and developmental needs in light of the family structure and stresses. If an appropriate plan cannot be developed, or if the physician feels that further diagnostic assessment is required, referral to a mental health practitioner should be recommended.

Kelleher KJ et al: Management of pediatric mental disorders in primary care: Where are we now and where are we going? Curr Opin Pediatr 2006;18:649 [PMID: 17099365].

Richardson LP, Katzenellenbogen R: Childhood and adolescent depression: The role of primary care providers in diagnosis and treatment. Curr Probl Pediatr Adolesc Health Care 2005;35:6 [PMID: 15611721].

Situations Requiring Emergent or More Extensive Psychiatric Assessment

If there is any concern about the child's safety, the provider must also evaluate the risk of danger to self (suicidal attempts or ideation), danger to others (assault, aggression, or homicidal ideation), and screen for other factors that could heighten the risk of danger to self or others, such as physical or sexual abuse or illicit substance use or abuse. The presence of drug or alcohol abuse in adolescent patients may require referral to community resources specializing in the treatment of these addictive disorders.

The following questions should be asked of the youth. The parents should be asked similar questions about what they have observed. Specific details about the circumstances should be asked if any question below is answered with "yes."

1. Have you ever been sad for more than a few days at a time such that it affected your sleep or appetite?
2. Have you ever been so sad that you wished you weren't alive?
3. Have you ever thought of ways of killing yourself or made a suicide attempt?
4. Have you ever thought about killing someone else, or tried to kill someone?
5. Has anyone ever hit you and left marks? (If yes, ask who, when, and under what circumstances, and if it was reported.)
6. Has anyone ever touched your private areas when they weren't supposed to, or in a way that made you feel uncomfortable? (If yes, ask who, when, and under what circumstances, and if it was reported.)
7. Do you use alcohol, tobacco, or illicit drugs? (If yes, ask what, when, with whom, and how much.)

A. Civil Commitment and Involuntary Mental Health "Holds"

If further assessment indicates a need for inpatient hospitalization, it is optimal if the patient and guardian give consent for this care. In a situation in which the guardian is unwilling or unable to give consent for emergency department–based assessment or inpatient hospitalization of a child or adolescent, an involuntary mental health "hold" may become necessary.

The term involuntary mental health "hold" refers to a legal process that can be initiated by physicians, police officers, and certified mental health professionals, which allows the individual to be prevented from leaving the emergency department or hospital for up to 72 hours. This allows the physician to establish a safe environment and prevent the individual from harming themselves or others, and allows sufficient time to determine if the individual is a risk to him- or herself or others due to mental illness. Each state has laws specifying rules and regulations that must be followed as part of this process. A specific form must be completed and the patient and family informed of their rights. As this involves revoking the civil rights of a patient or their guardian, it is critical to implement the procedure correctly. All physicians should be familiar with their state laws regulating this process.

Although the precise wording and conditions of involuntary mental health holds may vary slightly from state to state, they are generally quite similar. A 72-hour involuntary mental health hold is obtained for the purpose of acute evaluation and determination of the patient's safety when the evaluator elicits sufficient information to confirm a significant risk exists of danger to self or others. Additional criteria for involuntary psychiatric admission include a determination that the patient is "gravely disabled" by virtue of impaired judgment, which renders the patient unable to provide food, clothing, or shelter for him- or herself, or in the case of a child or adolescent, that he or she is unable to eat and perform normal activities of daily living. In addition, patients that have a medical condition(s) requiring urgent or emergent treatment do not require a mental health hold. In this case, the primary team/physician should conduct a capacity evaluation.

Baren JM et al: Children's mental health emergencies—part 1: Challenges in care: Definition of the problem, barriers to care, screening, advocacy, and resources. Pediatr Emerg Care 2008 Jun;24(6):399–408 [PMID: 18562887].

Baren JM et al: Children's mental health emergencies—part 2: Emergency department evaluation and treatment of children with mental health disorders. Pediatr Emerg Care 2008 Jul;24(7):485–498.

Baren JM, Mace SE, Hendry PL: Children's mental health emergencies—part 3: Special situations: Child maltreatment, violence, and response to disasters. Pediatr Emerg Care 2008 Aug;24(8):569–577 [PMID: 18708906].

Dolan MA, Fein JA: Committee on Pediatric Emergency Medicine. Pediatric and adolescent mental health emergencies in the emergency medical services system. Pediatrics 2011 May;127(5):e1356–e1366 [Epub 2011 Apr 25] [PMID: 21518712].

B. Mandatory Reporting of Abuse or Neglect or Threat to Others

Mandatory reporting by a physician of suspicion of physical or sexual abuse or neglect to the local human services agency is discussed in greater detail in Chapter 8. The "Tarasoff Rule" refers to a California legal case that led to a "duty to warn": Physicians are mandated to warn potential victims of harm when plans are disclosed to them about serious threats to harm specific individuals. Documentation of a phone call and registered letter to the individual being threatened are mandated. Under such circumstances, arrangement for the involuntary civil commitment of the potential perpetrator of harm is likely to be in order as well.

C. Referral of Patients to Mental Health Care Professionals

Primary care physicians often refer patients to a child and adolescent psychiatrist or other qualified child mental health professional when the diagnosis or treatment plan is uncertain, or when medication is indicated and the pediatrician prefers that a specialist initiate or manage treatment of the mental illness (Table 7–3). For academic difficulties not associated with behavioral difficulties, a child educational psychologist may be most helpful in assessing patients for learning disorders and potential remediation. For cognitive difficulties associated with head trauma, epilepsy, or brain tumors, a referral to a pediatric neuropsychologist may be indicated.

Table 7–3. When to consider consultation or referral to a child and adolescent psychiatrist.

The diagnosis is not clear
The pediatrician feels that further assessment is needed
The pediatrician believes medication may be needed, but will not be prescribing it
The pediatrician has started medications and needs further psychopharmacologic consultation
Individual, family, or group psychotherapy is needed
Psychotic symptoms (hallucinations, paranoia) are present
Bipolar affective disorder is suspected
Chronic medical regimen nonadherence has a risk of lethality
Delirium is suspected

Patients with private mental health insurance need to contact their insurance company for a list of local mental health professionals trained in the assessment and treatment of children and adolescents who are on their insurance panel. Patients with Medicaid or without mental health insurance coverage can usually be assessed and treated at their local mental health care center. The referring pediatrician or staff should assist the family by providing information to put them in touch with the appropriate services. Personal relationships with community mental health administrators and clinicians improve the success of referrals. Additionally, new delivery systems in which mental health professionals are "co-located" in the clinic remove barriers and improve access and care (see earlier discussion). In addition, the distant poles of involuntary inpatient psychiatric hospitalization and outpatient treatment have been filled in by other levels of treatment to provide a spectrum of care and include the following: inpatient psychiatric hospitalization, day treatment hospitalization, residential treatment, home-based care, intensive outpatient, outpatient treatment, primary care management.

Pediatricians who feel comfortable implementing the recommendations of a mental health professional with whom they have a collaborative relationship should consider remaining involved in the management and coordination of treatment of mental illness in their patients. The local branches of the American Academy of Child and Adolescent Psychiatry and the American Psychological Association should be able to provide a list of mental health professionals who are trained in the evaluation and treatment of children and adolescents.

CONSULTATION-LIAISON PSYCHIATRY

The field of consultation-liaison psychiatry was developed to address the need for mental health assessment and intervention of medically hospitalized pediatric patients. Psychiatric consultation on the medical floor and in the intensive care units can be complex and often requires assessment and intervention beyond the individual patient. The psychiatric consultation, in addition to evaluating the patient's symptom presentation, should also include assessment of family dynamics as related to the patient, and may include evaluation of how the medical team is addressing care of the patient and family. The psychiatric consultation focuses on the various hierarchies related to the interaction of the patient and staff, or staff and staff, in addition to the patient per se; this evaluation can be quite enlightening and may lead to more productive interventions.

When requesting a psychiatric consultation, as with any medical specialty, it is critical that the concern and focus of the consultation request be as specific as possible. The liaison role of the psychiatrist is to often assist in clarifying or formulating the specific reason for the consult. Psychiatric consultation on the medical floor is often requested when the patient's emotional state is affecting his or her response to medical care, or when an underlying mental illness may be contributing to the presenting symptoms. Patients admitted to the intensive care unit or a medical floor after a suicide attempt or supposed unintentional overdose should be evaluated by a psychiatric consultant before discharge.

Another common reason for requesting a psychiatric consultation on the medical floor is change in mental status. Be alert to the likelihood that acute mental status changes in the medical setting can represent delirium, as this has significant assessment and treatment implications. Delirium is defined as an acute and fluctuating disturbance of the sensorium (ie, alertness and orientation). Delirium can be manifested by a variety of psychiatric symptoms including paranoia, hallucinations, anxiety, and mood disturbances. However, aside from dementia and possibly dissociation and malingering, primary psychiatric presentations do not typically involve disturbances of alertness and orientation that are, by definition, always present in delirium.

Shaw RJ et al: Practice patterns in pediatric consultation-liaison psychiatry: A national survey. Psychosomatics 2006 Jan–Feb; 47(1):43–49 [PMID: 16384806].

Hindley PJ: Pediatric consultation-liaison psychiatry. Psychosom Res 2010 Apr;68(4):325-327 [PMID: 20307698].

THE CHRONICALLY ILL CHILD

Advances in the treatment of pediatric and adolescent illness have transformed several previously fatal conditions into life-threatening but potentially survivable conditions. These include advances in the fields of neonatal medicine, cardiac surgery, and hematology-oncology, including bone marrow transplantation. Additionally, solid organ transplantation, including heart, liver, kidney, and lung, among others, has revolutionized the potential treatment options for a whole host of once-fatal illnesses.

However, the intensity of treatment can in itself be highly stressful and even traumatic physically, financially, and psychologically, for children as well as their parents and siblings. Survivors are at risk of long-term medical and psychological sequelae. Those who are fortunate enough to survive the initial treatment of a potentially life-threatening condition often exchange a life-threatening biologic illness for a chronic emotional condition and physical disability.

Phase-Oriented Intervention

Psychosocial interventions should vary, depending on the developmental level of the patient, siblings, and family, and the phase of the illness. A first crisis is dealt with differently than interventions made during a long course of illness, or a period of stabilization or remission. With this in mind, the Organ Procurement and Transplantation Network/United Network for Organ Sharing established new by-laws in August 2004 which set minimum requirements for the psychosocial services available as part of an accredited solid organ transplant program. These guidelines include: (1) the establishment of a team comprising a transplantation psychiatrist, psychologist, nurse practitioner, and psychiatric social worker; (2) a formal psychiatric and substance abuse evaluation of prospective transplantation candidates; (3) evaluation of any potential renal or hepatic living donors; and (4) the availability of individual supportive counseling, crisis intervention, support groups, and death, dying, and bereavement counseling to transplantation patients and their families.

Reactions to Chronic Physical or Mental Illness & Disability

Between 5% and 10% of individuals experience a prolonged period of medical illness or disability during childhood and another 5%–10% experience the onset of mental illness in childhood. The psychosocial effects for the child and the family are often profound. Although the specific effect of illness on children and their families depends on the characteristics of the illness, the age of the child, and premorbid functioning, it can be expected that both the child and the parents will go through stages toward eventual acceptance of the disease state. It may take months for a family to accept the diagnosis, to cope with the stresses, and to resume normal life to the extent possible. These stages resemble those that follow the loss of a loved one. If anxiety and guilt remain prominent within the family, a pattern of overprotection can evolve. Likewise, when the illness is not accepted as a reality to be dealt with, a pattern of denial may become prominent. The clinical manifestations of these patterns of behavior are presented in Table 7–4.

Children are very observant and intuitive when it comes to understanding their illness and its general prognosis. At the same time, their primary concerns usually are the effects of the illness on everyday life (eg, routines), feeling sick, and limitations on normal, age-appropriate activities. Children are also keenly aware of the family's reactions and may be

Table 7–4. Patterns of coping with chronic illness.

Overprotection
Persistent anxiety or guilt
Few friends and peer activities
Poor school attendance
Overconcern with somatic symptoms
Secondary gain from the illness
Effective coping
Realistic acceptance of limits imposed by illness
Normalization of daily activities with peers, play, and school
Denial
Lack of acceptance of the illness
Poor medical compliance
Risk-taking behaviors
Lack of parental follow-through with medical instructions
General pattern of acting-out behavior

reluctant to bring up issues they know are upsetting to their parents. Whenever possible, parents should be encouraged to discuss the child's illness and to answer questions openly and honestly, including exploration of the child's fears and fantasies. Such interactions promote closeness and relieve the child's sense of isolation. Even with these active attempts to promote effective sharing between the child and the family, ill children frequently experience fear, anxiety, irritability, and anger over their illness, and guilt over causing family distress. Sleep disturbances, tears, and clinging, dependent behavior are not infrequent or abnormal. Parents frequently need support in an individual or group format to help them cope with the diagnosis and stress caused by the disease, its treatments, and its affect on the afflicted child and other family members.

The Vicious Cycle of Disease Empowerment

Submission to the power of illness, resulting, for example, in staying in bed longer than strictly necessary or withdrawing from friends and family, reduces a variety of opportunities to experience normal life. When reinforced by further relapses, increased helplessness and apprehension about symptoms raise the idea that symptoms and relapse strike unpredictably and cannot be influenced by the patient. Consequently, the patient experiences an increase in fear of illness and a reduction of activity because it can be interrupted at any time by unpredictable relapse. This submission to fear of illness by waiting for relapse reinforces the status of the chronically ill with increased helplessness. Both cycles result in lowering of self-esteem and disempowerment.

Families of chronically ill patients sometimes continue to use the same behavior and strategies, favoring rigidity and predictable long-standing habits. Although such rigidity is constraining, families often consider change as being unsafe. Past, present, and future collapse into a timeless dimension under the tyranny of illness. Rituals and metaphors serve the purpose of introducing distinctions in time. Rituals have always been used to demarcate different phases in life and to celebrate significant moments. Introducing different rituals that are consistent with family growth and helping the family to seek out their developmental priorities can represent an important intervention.

Discussions and interventions that take into account both emotional and medical symptoms will help the child and family better understand their experiences and attitude toward illness and life. The family and child will benefit from discussions about such questions as "What is the real nature of this illness? Why has it affected us? What will be our future? What does the treatment do to me?" Such discussions can be quite enlightening and empowering, as they encourage open discussion for the child and parents and an active role in treatment.

Patient- and parent-reported outcome tools, known either as Health Status or Health Related Quality of Life (HRQOL) measures, can also be routinely used in pediatric specialty clinics. These measures adopt the World Health Organization's definition of health as "a state of complete physical, mental, and social well-being and not merely the absence of disease." Health-related quality of life refers to the subjective and objective impact of dysfunction associated with an illness or injury and is multidimensional, including four core domains: disease state and physical symptoms, functional status, psychological functioning, and social functioning. A team approach is often necessary when providing care to complex and chronically ill children. Including these measures during annual visits and incorporating a mental health professional on the team can improve overall adjustment and quality of care.

Davis E et al: Paediatric quality of life instruments: A review of the impact of the conceptual framework on outcomes. Dev Med Child Neurol 2006 Apr;48(4):311–318 [Review] [PMID: 16542522].

THE TERMINALLY ILL CHILD

The diagnosis of a potentially fatal illness in a child is a severe blow even to families who have reason to suspect that outcome. The discussion with parents and the child about terminal illness is one of the most difficult tasks for a physician working with children and adolescents. Although parents want and need to know the truth, they are best told in stepwise fashion beginning with temporizing phrases such as "The news is not good" and "This is a life-threatening illness." The parents' reactions and questions can then be observed for clues about how much they want to be told at any one time. The physician must also attempt to gauge how much of the information the parents are able to comprehend during the initial discussion and consider involvement of appropriate support services. Some parents may dissociate during the sharing of frightening and overwhelming news, and crucial information may need to be addressed again when the parents are less shocked or traumatized and in a more receptive state. Parents may prefer to discuss difficult news when supportive people in their lives are present for the conversation as these supportive others can often retain information, ask clarifying questions, and review it with parents at a later point in time. Parents' reactions may follow a grief sequence, including initial shock and disbelief lasting days to weeks, followed by anger, despair, and guilt over weeks to months, and ending in acceptance of the reality of the situation. These responses vary in their expression, intensity, and duration for each member of the family. Even when the illness is cured, some parents may continue to suffer from post-traumatic stress symptoms related to the diagnosis and treatment.

Developmental and phase-oriented perspectives of patients, siblings, parents, and caretakers are reviewed in Table 7–5. Although most children do not fully understand the permanency of death until about age 8, most ill children experience a sense of danger and doom that is associated with death before that age. Even so, the question of whether

Table 7–5. Children's response to death.

	Before			During				After		
	Developmental Concerns			Sudden	Acute	Chronic				
Child										
0-5 y	Ideas on death Abandonment; punishment	Death and stage anxieties Fear of loss of love			Avoidance of pain; need for love	Withdrawal; separation anxiety				
5-10 y	Concepts of inevitability; confusion	Castration anxiety			Guilt (bad), regression, denial	Guilt (religious), regression, denial				
10-15 y	Reality	Control of body and other developmental tasks			Depression; despair for future	Depression; despair, anxiety, anger				
	Sudden	Acute	Chronic					Sudden	Acute	Chronic
Parents		Anxiety; concern; hopefulness	Premature mourning, guilt, anticipatory grief, reaction formation and displacements, need for information		Disbelief; displaced rage; accelerate grief; prolonged numbness	Desperate concern; denial; guilt	Denial; remorse; resurgence of love	Guilt; mourning	Anger at doctors; need for follow-up, overidealizing, fantasy loss	Remorse; relief and guilt
Siblings										
0-5 y		Reactions to changes in parents (sense of loss of love and withdrawal)						1. Respond to reaction of parents		
5-10 y		Concern about their implications; fearful for themselves						2. Survivor guilt		
10-15 y		Generally supportive								
Staff		Anxiety; conspiracy of silence			Reaction: withdraw Tasks: 1. Correct distortions (eg, "Am I safe?"; "Will someone be with me?"; "Will I be helped to feel better?") 2. Comfort parents 3. Allow hope and promote feeling of actively coping 4. Protect dignity of patient			Need for aftercare of survivors; autopsy request tactful; accurate information regarding disposal of body; delay billing		

Adapted, with permission, from Lewis M: *Clinical Aspects of Child and Adolescent Development*, 3rd ed. Lea & Febiger, 1990.

to tell a child about the fatal nature of a disease should in most cases be answered in the affirmative unless the parents object. When the parents object, this should alert the physician to involve the unit social worker, who can work with the family to ensure their decision is in the best interest of the child. Refusal of the adults to tell the child, especially when the adults themselves are very sad, leads to a conspiracy of silence that increases fear of the unknown in the child and leads to feelings of loneliness and isolation at the time of greatest need. In fact, children who are able to discuss their illness with family members are less depressed, have fewer behavior problems, have higher self-esteem, feel closer to their families, and adapt better to the challenges of their disease and its treatment.

The siblings of dying children are also significantly affected. They may feel neglected and deprived because of the time their parents must spend with the sick child. Anger and jealousy may then give rise to feelings of guilt over having such feelings about their sick sibling. Awareness of the emotional responses, coping abilities, and available resources for support of other family members can diminish these feelings and make a significant difference in the family's overall ability to cope with the illness.

After the child dies, the period of bereavement may last indefinitely. Family members may need help in dealing with their grief through supportive counseling services or peer-support groups. Bereavement usually does not substantially interfere with overall life functioning for more than 2–3 months. Most parents and siblings are able to return to work and school within a month, although their emotional state and thoughts may continue to be dominated by the loss for some time. Grief responses may resurface around anniversaries (eg, of the diagnosis, medical procedure, death) or birthdays of the deceased child. When the individual is unable to function in his or her societal and family role beyond this time frame, a diagnosis of complicated bereavement, major depression, post-traumatic stress disorder (PTSD), or adjustment disorder should be considered and appropriate interventions recommended, such as referral for counseling or psychotherapy and possibly antidepressant medication.

Long-Term Coping

The process of coping with a chronic or terminal illness is complex and varies with the dynamics of each individual child and family. Each change in the course of illness and each new developmental stage may present different challenges for the child and family. It is important for health care providers to continually assess the family's and child's needs and coping abilities over time and to provide appropriate support, information, and access to interventions.

Assistance from Health Care Providers

A. Educate the Patient and Family

Children and their families should be given information about the illness, including its course and treatment, at frequent intervals. Factual, open discussions minimize anxieties. The explanation should be comprehensible to all, and time should be set aside for questions and answers. The setting can be created with an invitation such as "Let's take some time together to review the situation again."

B. Prepare the Child for Changes and Procedures

The physician should explain, in an age-appropriate manner, what is expected with a new turn in the illness or with upcoming medical procedures. This explanation enables the child to anticipate and in turn to master the new development and promotes trust between the patient and the health care providers.

C. Encourage Normal Activities

The child should attend school and play with peers as much as the illness allows. Individual education plans should be requested from the school if accommodation beyond the regular classroom is necessary. At the same time, parents should be encouraged to apply the same rules of discipline and behavior to the ill child as to the siblings.

D. Encourage Compensatory Activities, Interests, and Skill Development

Children who experience disability or interruption of their usual activities and interests should be encouraged to explore new interests, and the family should be supported in adapting the child's interests for their situation, and in presenting new opportunities.

E. Promote Self-Reliance

Children often feel helpless when others must do things for them, or assist with their daily needs. The health care provider should guide and encourage parents in helping ill children assume responsibility for some aspects of their medical care and continue to experience age-appropriate independence and skills whenever possible.

F. Periodically Review Family Coping

Families are often so immersed in the crisis of their child's illness that they neglect their own needs or the needs of other family members. From time to time, the physician should ask "How is everyone doing?" The feelings of the patient, the parents, and other children in the family are explored. Parents should be encouraged to stay in touch with people in their support system, and to encourage their children in such efforts as well. Feelings of fear, guilt, anger, and grief should be monitored and discussed as normal reactions to difficult circumstances. If these experiences are interfering with the family's functioning, involvement of the pediatric social worker or a therapist can be helpful.

Appropriate lay support groups for the patient and family should be recommended. Many hospitals have such groups, and hospital social workers can facilitate participation for the patient and family.

Lewis M, Vitulano LA: Biopsychosocial issues and risk factors in the family when the child has a chronic illness. Child Adolesc Psychiatr Clin N Am 2003 Jul;12(3):389–399 [PMID: 12910814].

Pao M, Bosk A: Anxiety in medically ill children/adolescents. Depress Anxiety 2011 Jan;28(1):40–49 doi: 10.1002/da.20727 [Epub 2010 Aug 18] [PMID: 20721908].

Vitulano LA: Psychosocial issues for children and adolescents with chronic illness: Self-esteem, school functioning and sports participation. Child Adolesc Psychiatr Clin N Am 2003 Jul;12(3):585–592 [PMID: 12910824].

Pediatric Medical Traumatic Stress Toolkit. Available at: http://www.nctsn.org/nccts/nav.do?pid=typ_mt

PSYCHIATRIC DISORDERS OF CHILDHOOD & ADOLESCENCE

A psychiatric disorder is defined as a characteristic cluster of signs and symptoms (emotions, behaviors, thought patterns, and mood states) that are associated with subjective distress or maladaptive behavior. This definition presumes that the individual's symptoms are of such intensity, persistence, and duration that the ability to adapt to life's challenges is compromised.

Psychiatric disorders have their origins in neurobiologic, genetic, psychological (life experience), or environmental sources. The neurobiology of childhood disorders is one of the most active areas of investigation in child and adolescent psychiatry. Although much remains to be clarified, data from genetic studies point to heritable transmission of attention-deficit/hyperactivity disorder (ADHD), schizophrenia, mood and anxiety disorders, eating disorders, pervasive developmental disorders, learning disorders, and tic disorders, among others. About 3%–5% of children and 10%–15% of adolescents will experience psychiatric disorders.

The *Diagnostic and Statistical Manual of Mental Disorders*, Fourth Edition, Text Revision (DSM-IV-TR) is the formal reference text for psychiatric disorders and includes the criteria for each of the mental illnesses, including those that begin in childhood and adolescence. Psychiatric diagnoses are given on five axes to allow the physician to address the developmental, medical, psychosocial, and overall adaptive issues that contribute to the primary diagnosis on axis I or II.

Axis I: Clinical disorders

Axis II: Personality disorders, mental retardation, learning disabilities

Axis III: General medical conditions

Axis IV: Psychosocial and environmental problems

Axis V: Global assessment of functioning (on a scale of 0–100, with 100% being the highest level of functioning)

Unfortunately, available mental health classification systems are infrequently used in pediatric primary care settings since they address the more severe and extensive conditions. As previously stated, primary care providers frequently see a spectrum of disturbances in their clinical practice, many not achieving full DSM-IV-TR criteria. In order to combat the fact that current nosologies do not provide enough detail about common problems and situations that primary care pediatric providers come across, the AAP and the American Psychiatric Association (APA) collaboratively developed the DSM-IV Primary Care (DSM-PC), including a child and adolescent version. The key assumptions of the DSM-PC (C&A) are based on the fact that children's environments have an impact on their mental health, and that children demonstrate a continuum of symptoms from normality to severe disorders. The DSM-PC is compatible with the DSMIV-TR, is clear and concise, and is available for research testing and subsequent refinement. It is organized into sections covering environmental situations, child manifestations, and severity (Table 7–6). Categories of the major environmental factors that may affect a child, ranging from economic issues to family violence, are described and given V codes. Specific behavioral manifestations are listed under broad groupings and include complaints, definitions, symptoms, differential diagnosis, developmental variation, and etiology. Severity, in the DSM-PC, has several dimensions, including symptoms, functioning, burden of suffering, and risk and protective factors. The DSM-PC has a great deal of promise, not only as a mechanism to classify the complexities of children's behavior problems, but also as a mechanism for the future to facilitate financial reimbursement for early identification of and intervention for children's behavioral problems. Pediatricians should find this manual to be a valuable tool in the care of children and their families.

Table 7–6. Areas of focus in the Diagnostic and Statistical Manual, Primary Care (DSM-PC).

DSM-PC Section	Area of Focus
Environmental situations	Challenges to primary support group Changes in caregiving Community or social changes Educational challenges Parent or adolescent occupational challenges Housing challenges Economic challenges Inadequate access to health or mental health services Legal system or crime problem Other environmental situations Health-related situations
Child manifestations	Developmental competencies Impulsive, hyperactive, and inattentive behaviors Negative and antisocial behaviors Substance use and abuse Emotions and moods, and emotional behaviors Somatic behaviors Feeding, eating, and elimination Illness-related behaviors Sexual behaviors Atypical behaviors
Severity of disorder	
Mild	Unlikely to cause serious developmental difficulties or impairment in functioning
Moderate	May cause, or is causing, some developmental difficulties or impairment. Further evaluation and intervention planning are warranted.
Severe	Is causing serious developmental difficulties and dysfunction in one or more key areas of the child's life. Mental health referral and comprehensive treatment planning are often indicated, possibly on an urgent basis.

The descriptions of disorders in this chapter follow the DSM-IV-TR nosology rather than the DSM-PC criteria. Pediatricians are encouraged to become familiar with the DSM-PC, perhaps mastering one section at a time. A revised DSM-PC is being developed.

American Academy of Pediatrics: *Diagnostic and Statistical Manual for Primary Care (DSM-PC), Child and Adolescent Version.* American Academy of Pediatrics, 1996.

American Psychiatric Association: *Diagnostic and Statistical Manual of Mental Disorders*, 4th ed, text revision. American Psychiatric Association, 2000.

MOOD DISORDERS

1. Depression in Children & Adolescents

ESSENTIALS OF DIAGNOSIS & TYPICAL FEATURES

- Dysphoric mood, mood lability, irritability, or depressed appearance, persisting for days to months at a time.
- Characteristic neurovegetative signs and symptoms (changes in sleep, appetite, concentration, and activity levels).
- Suicidal ideation, feeling of hopelessness.

General Considerations

The incidence of depression in children increases with age, from 1% to 3% before puberty to around 8% for adolescents. The rate of depression in females approaches adult levels by age 15. The lifetime risk of depression ranges from 10% to 25% for women and 5% to 12% for men. The incidence of depression in children is higher when other family members have been affected by depressive disorders. The sex incidence is equal in childhood, but with the onset of puberty the rates of depression for females begin to exceed those for males by 5:1.

Clinical Findings

Clinical depression can be defined as a persistent state of unhappiness or misery that interferes with pleasure or productivity. The symptom of depression in children and adolescents is as likely to be an irritable mood state accompanied by tantrums or verbal outbursts as it is to be a sad mood. Typically, a child or adolescent with depression begins to look unhappy and may make comments such as "I have no friends," "Life is boring," "There is nothing I can do to make things better," or "I wish I were dead." A change in behavior patterns usually takes place that includes social isolation, deterioration in schoolwork, loss of interest in usual activities, anger, and irritability. Sleep and appetite patterns commonly change, and the child may complain of tiredness and nonspecific pain such as headaches or stomach aches (Table 7–7).

Table 7–7. Clinical manifestations of depression in children and adolescents.

Depressive Symptom	Clinical Manifestations
Anhedonia	Loss of interest and enthusiasm in play, socializing, school, and usual activities; boredom; loss of pleasure
Dysphoric mood	Tearfulness; sad, downturned expression; unhappiness; slumped posture; quick temper; irritability; anger
Fatigability	Lethargy and tiredness; no play after school
Morbid ideation	Self-deprecating thoughts, statements; thoughts of disaster, abandonment, death, suicide, or hopelessness
Somatic symptoms	Changes in sleep or appetite patterns; difficulty in concentrating; bodily complaints, particularly headache and stomach ache

Differential Diagnosis

Clinical depression can usually be identified simply by asking about the symptoms. Children are often more accurate than their caregivers in describing their own mood state. When several depressive symptoms cluster together over time, are persistent (2 weeks or more), and cause impairment, a major depressive disorder may be present. When depressive symptoms are of lesser severity but have persisted for 1 year or more, a diagnosis of dysthymic disorder should be considered. Milder symptoms of short duration in response to some stressful life event may be consistent with a diagnosis of adjustment disorder with depressed mood.

The Center for Epidemiologic Study of Depression–Child Version (CESD-C), Child Depression Inventory (CDI), Beck Depression Rating Scale, and Reynolds Adolescent Depression Scale are self-report rating scales that are easily used in primary care to assist in assessment and monitoring response to treatment.

Depression often coexists with other mental illnesses such as ADHD, conduct disorders, anxiety disorders, eating disorders, and substance abuse disorders. Medically ill patients also have an increased incidence of depression. Every child and adolescent with a depressed mood state should be asked directly about suicidal ideation and physical and sexual abuse. Depressed adolescents should also be screened for hypothyroidism and substance abuse.

Complications

The risk of suicide is the most significant risk associated with depressive episodes. In addition, adolescents are likely to self-medicate their feelings through substance abuse, or indulge in self-injurious behaviors such as cutting or burning themselves (without suicidal intent). School performance usually suffers during a depressive episode, as children are unable to concentrate or motivate themselves to complete homework or projects. The irritability, isolation, and withdrawal that often result from the depressive episode can lead to loss of peer relationships and tense dynamics within the family.

Treatment

Treatment includes developing a comprehensive plan to treat the depressive episode and help the family to respond more effectively to the patient's emotional needs. Referrals should always be made for individual and family therapy. Cognitive-behavioral therapy has been shown to effectively improve depressive symptoms in children and adolescents. Cognitive-behavioral therapy includes a focus on building coping skills to change negative thought patterns that predominate in depressive conditions. It also helps the young person to identify, label, and verbalize feelings and misperceptions. In therapy, efforts are also made to resolve conflicts between family members and improve communication skills within the family.

When the symptoms of depression are moderate to severe and persistent, and have begun to interfere with relationships and school performance, antidepressant medications may be indicated (Table 7–8). Mild depressive symptoms often do not require antidepressant medications and may improve with psychotherapy alone. A positive family history of depression increases the risk of early-onset depression in children and adolescents and the chances of a positive response to antidepressant medication. Depression in toddlers and young children is best approached with parent-child relational therapies.

Controversy continues regarding the efficacy and safety of antidepressants in children and adolescents. (See Psychopharmacology section, later.) Following the addition of a "black box warning" for all antidepressants in October 2005, a 20% decrease in prescriptions for those younger than age 20 was noted with a corresponding 18% increase in suicides. Also supporting treatment is the finding that suicide rates in children and adolescents were lowest in areas of the country that had the highest rate of selective serotonin reuptake inhibitor (SSRI) prescriptions. These debates will continue, but best practice is to educate the family and monitor carefully, especially in the first 4 weeks and subsequent 3 months, watching carefully for any increase in suicidal ideation or self-injurious urges, as well as improvement in target symptoms of depression.

Table 7–8. Interventions for the treatment of depression.

Disorder	Interventions	
Adjustment disorder with depressed mood	Refer for psychotherapy	Medications usually not needed
Mild depression	Refer for psychotherapy	Medications may not be needed
Moderate depression	Refer for psychotherapy	Consider antidepressant medication
Severe depression	Refer for psychotherapy	Strongly encourage antidepressant medication

Prognosis

A comprehensive treatment intervention, including psychoeducation for the family, individual and family psychotherapy, medication assessment, and evaluation of school and home environments, often leads to complete remission of depressive symptoms over a 1- to 2-month period. If medications are started and prove effective, they must be continued for 6–9 months after remission of symptoms to prevent relapse. Early-onset depression (before age 15) is associated with increased risk of recurrent episodes and the potential need for longer term treatment with anti-depressants. Education of the family and child (or adolescent) will help them identify depressive symptoms sooner and limit the severity of future episodes with earlier interventions. Some studies suggest that up to 30% of preadolescents with major depression manifest bipolar disorder at 2-year follow-up. It is important to reassess the child or adolescent with depressive symptoms regularly for at least 6 months and to maintain awareness of the depressive episode in the course of well-child care.

Cheung AH et al: GLAD PC Steering Committee Expert survey for the management of adolescent depression in primary care. Pediatrics 2008 Jan;121(1):e101–e107 [PMID: 18166529].

Cheung AH et al: GLAD-PC Steering Group. Guidelines for Adolescent Depression in Primary Care (GLAD-PC): II. Treatment and ongoing management. Pediatrics 2007 Nov;120(5):e1313–e1326. Erratum in: Pediatrics 2008 Jan;121(1):227 [PMID: 17974724].

Cheung AH et al: Pediatric depressive disorders: Management priorities in primary care. Curr Opin Pediatr 2008 Oct;20(5):551–559 [Review] [PMID: 18781118].

Richardson L, McCauley E, Katon W: Collaborative care for adolescent depression: A pilot study. Gen Hosp Psychiatry 2009 Jan–Feb;31(1):36–45 [Epub 2008 Nov 18] [PMID: 19134509].

Richardson LP et al: Evaluation of the Patient Health Questionnaire-9 Item for detecting major depression among adolescents. Pediatrics 2010 Dec;126(6):1117–1123 [Epub 2010 Nov 1] [PMID: 21041282].

US Preventive Services Task Force Screening and treatment for major depressive disorder in children and adolescents: US Preventive Services Task Force Recommendation Statement. Pediatrics 2009 Apr;123(4):1223–1228. Erratum in: Pediatrics. 2009 Jun;123(6):1611 [PMID: 19336383].

Williams SB et al: Screening for child and adolescent depression in primary care settings: A systematic evidence review for the US Preventive Services Task Force. Pediatrics 2009 Apr;123(4):e716–e735 [Review] [PMID: 19336361].

Zuckerbrot RA et al: GLAD-PC Steering Group. Guidelines for Adolescent Depression in Primary Care (GLAD-PC): I. Identification, assessment, and initial management. Pediatrics 2007 Nov;120(5):e1299–e1312 [PMID: 17974723].

The Guidelines for Adolescent Depression in Primary Care Toolkit. Available at: http://www.thereachinstitute.org/guidelines-for-adolescent-depression-in-primary-care-glad-pc.html

http://www.thereachinstitute.org/files/documents/GLAD-PCToolkit.pdf

2. Bipolar Affective Disorder

ESSENTIALS OF DIAGNOSIS & TYPICAL FEATURES

- Periods of abnormally and persistently elevated, expansive, or irritable mood, and heightened levels of energy and activity.
- Associated symptoms: grandiosity, diminished need for sleep, pressured speech, racing thoughts, impaired judgment.
- Not caused by prescribed or illicit drugs.

General Considerations

Bipolar affective disorder (previously referred to as manic-depressive disorder) is an episodic mood disorder manifested by alternating periods of mania and major depressive episodes or, less commonly, manic episodes alone. Children and adolescents often exhibit a variable course of mood instability combined with aggressive behavior and impulsivity. At least 20% of bipolar adults experience onset of symptoms before age 20 years. Onset of bipolar disorder before puberty is uncommon; however, symptoms often begin to develop and may be initially diagnosed as ADHD or other disruptive behavior disorders. The lifetime prevalence of bipolar disorder in middle to late adolescence approaches 1%.

Clinical Findings

In about 70% of patients, the first symptoms are primarily those of depression; in the remainder, manic, hypomanic, or mixed states dominate the presentation. Patients with mania display a variable pattern of elevated, expansive, or irritable mood along with rapid speech, high energy levels, difficulty in sustaining concentration, and a decreased need for sleep. The child or adolescent may also have hypersexual behavior, usually in the absence of a history or sexual abuse. (It is critical to rule out abuse, or be aware of abuse factors contributing to the clinical presentation.) Patients often do not acknowledge any problem with their mood or behavior. The clinical picture can be quite dramatic, with florid psychotic symptoms of delusions and hallucinations accompanying extreme hyperactivity and impulsivity. Other illnesses on the bipolar spectrum are bipolar type II, which is characterized by recurrent major depressive episodes alternating with hypomanic episodes (lower intensity manic episodes that do not cause social impairment and do not typically last as long as manic episodes) and cyclothymic disorder, which is diagnosed when the child or adolescent has had 1 year of hypomanic symptoms alternating with depressive symptoms that do not meet criteria for major depression.

It is also common for individuals diagnosed with bipolar spectrum disorders to have a history of attentional and hyperactivity problems in childhood, and some will have a diagnosis of ADHD as well. ADHD and bipolar disorder are highly comorbid; however, it is also felt that attentional and hyperactivity problems accompanied by mood swings can be an early sign of bipolar disorder before full criteria for the disorder have emerged and clustered together in a specific pattern.

Differential Diagnosis

Differentiating ADHD, bipolar disorder, and major depressive disorder can be a challenge even for the seasoned clinician, and confusion about the validity of the disorder in younger children still exists. The situation is further complicated by the potential for the coexistence of ADHD and mood disorders in the same patient.

A history of the temporal course of symptoms can be most helpful. ADHD is typically a chronic disorder of lifelong duration. However, it may not be a problem until the patient enters the classroom setting. Mood disorders are typically characterized by a normal baseline followed by an acute onset of symptoms usually associated with acute sleep, appetite, and behavior changes. If inattentive, hyperactive, or impulsive behavior was not a problem a year ago, it is unlikely to be ADHD. Typically, all of these disorders are quite heritable, so a positive family history for other affected individuals can be enlightening. Successful treatment of relatives can offer guidance for appropriate treatment.

In prepubescent children, mania may be difficult to differentiate from ADHD and other disruptive behavior disorders. In both children and adolescents, preoccupation with violence, decreased need for sleep, impulsivity, poor judgment, intense and prolonged rages or dysphoria, hypersexuality, and some cycling of symptoms suggest bipolar disorder. Table 7–9 further defines points of differentiation between ADHD, conduct disorder, and bipolar disorder.

Physical or sexual abuse and exposure to domestic violence can also cause children to appear mood labile, hyperactive, and aggressive, and PTSD should be considered by reviewing the history for traumatic life events in children with these symptoms. Diagnostic considerations should also include substance abuse disorders, and an acute organic process,

Table 7–9. Differentiating behavior disorders.

	ADHD	Conduct Disorder	Bipolar Disorder
School problems	Yes	Yes	Yes
Behavior problems	Yes	Yes	Yes
Defiant attitude	Occasional	Constant	Episodic
Motor restlessness	Constant	May be present	May wax and wane
Impulsivity	Constant	May be present	May wax and wane
Distractibility	Constant	May be present	May wax and wane
Anger expression	Short-lived (minutes)	Plans revenge	Intense rages (minutes to hours)
Thought content	May be immature	Blames others	Morbid or grandiose ideas
Sleep disturbance	May be present	No	May wax and wane
Self-deprecation	Briefly, with criticism	No	Prolonged, with or without suicidal ideation
Obsessed with ideas	No	No	Yes
Hallucinations	No	No	Diagnostic, if present
Family history	May be a history of school problems	May be a history of antisocial behavior	May be a history of mood disorders

ADHD, attention-deficit/hyperactivity disorder.

especially if the change in personality has been relatively sudden, or is accompanied by other neurologic changes. Individuals with manic psychosis may resemble those with schizophrenia. Psychotic symptoms associated with bipolar disorder should clear with resolution of the mood symptoms, which should also be prominent. Hyperthyroidism should be ruled out. The Young Mania Rating Scale and The Child Mania Rating Scale may be helpful in eliciting concerning symptoms and educating families and patients, and in aiding timely referral to local mental health resources.

Complications

Children and adolescents with bipolar disorder are more likely to be inappropriate or aggressive toward peers and family members. Their symptoms almost always create significant interference with academic learning and peer relationships. The poor judgment associated with manic episodes predisposes to dangerous, impulsive, and sometimes criminal activity. Legal difficulties can arise from impulsive acts, such as excessive spending, and acts of vandalism, theft, or aggression, that are associated with grandiose thoughts. Affective disorders are associated with a 30-fold greater incidence of successful suicide. Substance abuse may be a further complication, often representing an attempt at self-medication for the mood problem.

Treatment & Prognosis

Most patients with bipolar disorder respond to pharmacotherapy with either mood stabilizers, such as lithium, or atypical antipsychotics. The recent data on the mood stabilizers carbamazepine and valproate have been less promising. The atypical neuroleptics are increasingly being used as primary mood stabilizers to treat bipolar disorder as primary agents, and olanzapine, risperidone, quetiapine, aripiprazole, and ziprasidone have been approved by the Food and Drug Administration (FDA) for the treatment of bipolar affective disorder in adults. If the individual is being treated primarily for manic episodes with a non-antipsychotic mood stabilizer (such as lithium), the addition of a neuroleptic medication may be necessary if psychotic symptoms (hallucinations, paranoia, or delusions) or significant aggression is also present. In cases of severe impairment, hospitalization is required to maintain safety and initiate treatment. Dual use of mood stabilizers and antipsychotics is still used in most settings, although the only approved medication for treatment of acute mania in youth aged 12 and older is lithium. It is often possible to discontinue the antipsychotic after remission of psychotic symptoms; it is usually necessary to continue treatment with a mood stabilizer for at least a year, and longer if the individual has had recurrent episodes. It is not uncommon for the patient to need lifelong medication. Supportive psychotherapy for the patient and family and education about the recurrent nature of the illness are critical. Family therapy should also include improving skills for conflict management and appropriate expression of emotion.

In its adult form, bipolar disorder is an illness with a remitting course of alternating depressive and manic episodes. The time span between episodes can be years or months depending on the severity of illness and ability to comply with medication interventions. In childhood, the symptoms may be more pervasive and not fall into the intermittent episodic pattern until after puberty.

Chang K: Challenges in the diagnosis and treatment of pediatric bipolar depression. Dialogues Clin Neurosci 2009;11(1):73–80 [PMID: 19432389].

Cummings CM, Fristad MA: Pediatric bipolar disorder: Recognition in primary care. Curr Opin Pediatr 2008 Oct;20(5):560–565 [PMID: 18781119].

Demeter CA et al: Current research in child and adolescent bipolar disorder. Dialogues Clin Neurosci 2008;10(2):215–228 [PMID: 18689291].

Miklowitz DJ, Chang KD: Prevention of bipolar disorder in at-risk children: Theoretical assumptions and empirical foundations. Dev Psychopathol 2008 Summer;20(3):881–897 [PMID: 18606036].

Miklowitz DJ et al: Family-focused treatment for adolescents with bipolar disorder: Results of a 2-year randomized trial. Arch Gen Psychiatry 2008 Sep;65(9):1053–1061 [PMID: 18762591].

Youngstrom EA, Birmaher B, Findling RL: Pediatric bipolar disorder: Validity, phenomenology, and recommendations for diagnosis. Bipolar Disord 2008 Feb;10(1 Pt 2):194–214 [PMID: 18199237].

SUICIDE IN CHILDREN & ADOLESCENTS

The suicide rate in young people has remained high for several decades. In 2007, suicide was the third leading cause of death among children and adolescents aged 10–24 years in the United States. The suicide rate among adolescents aged 15–19 years quadrupled from approximately 2.7 to 11.3 per 100,000 since the 1960s. It is estimated that each year, approximately 2 million U.S. adolescents attempt suicide, yet only 700,000 receive medical attention for their attempt. Suicide and homicide rates for children in the United States are two to five times higher than those for the other 25 industrialized countries combined, primarily due to the prevalence of firearms in the United States. For children younger than 10 years, the rate of completed suicide is low, but from 1980 to 1992, it increased by 120%, from 0.8 to 1.7 per 100,000.

Adolescent girls make three to four times as many suicide attempts as boys of the same age, but the number of completed suicides is three to four times greater in boys. Firearms are the most commonly used method in successful suicides, accounting for 40%–60% of cases; hanging, carbon monoxide poisoning, and drug overdoses each account for approximately 10%–15% of cases.

Suicide is almost always associated with a psychiatric disorder and should not be viewed as a philosophic choice about life or death or as a predictable response to overwhelming stress. Most commonly it is associated with a mood disorder and the hopelessness that accompanies a severe depressive episode. Suicide rates are higher for Native American and Native Alaskan populations than for white, black, and Latinos/Hispanic populations. Although suicide attempts are more common in individuals with a history of behavior problems and academic difficulties, other suicide victims are high achievers who are temperamentally anxious and perfectionistic and who commit suicide impulsively after a failure or rejection, either real or perceived. Mood disorders (in both sexes, but especially in females), substance abuse disorders (especially in males), and conduct disorders are commonly diagnosed at psychological autopsy in adolescent suicide victims. Some adolescent suicides reflect an underlying psychotic disorder, with the young person usually committing suicide in response to auditory hallucinations or psychotic delusions.

The vast majority of young people who attempt suicide give some clue to their distress or their tentative plans to commit suicide. Most show signs of dysphoric mood (anger, irritability, anxiety, or depression). Over 60% make comments such as "I wish I were dead" or "I just can't deal with this any longer" within the 24 hours prior to death. In one study, nearly 70% of subjects experienced a crisis event such as a loss (eg, rejection by a girlfriend or boyfriend), a failure, or an arrest prior to completed suicide.

Assessment of Suicide Risk

Any clinical assessment for depression must include direct questions about suicidal ideation. If a child or adolescent expresses suicidal thinking, the physician must ask if he or she has an active plan, intends to complete that plan, and has made previous attempts. Suicidal ideation accompanied by any plan warrants immediate referral for a psychiatric crisis assessment. This can usually be accomplished at the nearest emergency department.

Assessment of suicide risk calls for a high index of suspicion and a direct interview with the patient and his or her parents or guardians. The highest risk of suicide is among white adolescent boys. High-risk factors include previous suicide attempts, a suicide note, and a viable plan for suicide with the availability of lethal means, close personal exposure to suicide, conduct disorder, and substance abuse. Other risk factors are signs and symptoms of major depression or dysthymia, a family history of suicide, a recent death in the family, and a view of death as a relief from the pain in the patient's life.

Intervention

Suicidal ideation and any suicide attempt must be considered a serious matter. The patient should not be left alone, and the physician should express concern and convey a desire to help. The physician should meet with the patient and the family, both alone and together, and listen carefully to their problems and perceptions. It should be made clear that with the assistance of mental health professionals, solutions can be found.

The majority of patients who express suicidal ideation and all who have made a suicide attempt should be referred for psychiatric evaluation and possible hospitalization. Most providers feel uncomfortable and have little experience in evaluating suicidality and risk. In addition, this evaluation frequently takes considerable time and requires contact with multiple informants. The physician should err on the side of caution as referral for further assessment is always appropriate when there is concern about suicidal thinking and behavior.

An evaluation in a psychiatrist's office or the emergency department will help determine level of risk and disposition. If the patient has suicidal ideation without a plan, has a therapist he or she can see the next day, is able to "contract for safety," and the family is able to provide supervision and support, then the evaluating physician can consider sending the patient and family home that day from the office or emergency department without need for hospitalization. If there appears to be potential for suicide as determined by suicidal ideation with a plan, there are no available resources for therapy, and the patient is not able to cooperate with a plan to ensure safety; if the patient is severely depressed or intoxicated; if the family does not appear to be appropriately concerned; or if there are practical limitations on providing supervision and support to ensure safety, the individual should be hospitalized on an inpatient psychiatric unit. Any decision to send the patient home from the emergency department without hospitalization should be made only after consultation with a mental health expert. The decision should be based on lessening of the risk of suicide and assurance of the family's ability to follow through with outpatient therapy and provide appropriate support and supervision. Guns, knives, and razor blades should be removed from the home, and, as much as possible, access to them outside the home must be denied. Medications and over-the-counter drugs should be kept locked in a safe place with all efforts made to minimize the risk of the patient having access (eg, key kept with a parent, or use of combination lock on the medicine chest). The patient should be restricted from driving for at least the first 24 hours to lessen the chance of impulsive motor vehicle crashes. Instructions and phone numbers for crisis services should be given, and the family must be committed to a plan for mental health treatment.

Suicide prevention efforts include heightened awareness in the community and schools to promote identification of at-risk individuals and increasing access to services, including hotlines and counseling services. Restricting young people's access to firearms is also a critical factor, as firearms are responsible for 85% of deaths due to suicide or homicide in youth in the United States.

Finally, the physician should be aware of his or her own emotional reactions to dealing with suicidal adolescents and their families. Because the assessment can require considerable time and energy, the physician should be on guard against becoming tired, irritable, or angry. The physician should not be afraid of precipitating suicide by direct and frank discussions of suicidal risk. Reviewing difficult cases with colleagues, developing formal or informal relationships with psychiatrists, and attending workshops on assessment and management of depression and suicidal ideation can decrease the anxiety and improve competence for primary care providers.

Bursztein C, Apter A: Adolescent suicide. Curr Opin Psychiatry 2009 Jan;22(1):1–6 [PMID: 19122527].

Carballo JJ et al: The role of the pediatrician in preventing suicide in adolescents with alcohol use disorders. Int J Adolesc Med Health 2007 Jan–Mar;19(1):61–65 [PMID: 17458325].

Dervic K, Brent DA, Oquendo MA: Completed suicide in childhood. Psychiatr Clin North Am 2008 Jun;31(2):271–291 [PMID: 18439449].

Dudley M et al: New-generation antidepressants, suicide and depressed adolescents: How should clinicians respond to changing evidence? Aust N Z J Psychiatry 2008 Jun;42(6):456–466 [PMID: 18465372].

Gardner W, Klima J, Chisolm D, Feehan H, Bridge J, Campo J, Cunningham N, Kelleher K: Screening, triage, and referral of patients who report suicidal thought during a primary care visit. Pediatrics 2010 May;125(5):945–952 [Epub 2010 Apr 12] [PMID: 20385642].

Greydanus D, Patel D, Pratt H: Suicide risk in adolescents with chronic illness: Implications for primary care and specialty pediatric practice: A review. Dev Med Child Neurol 2010 Dec;52(12):1083–1087 [Epub 2010 Aug 31] [PMID: 20813018].

Goldstein TR: Suicidality in pediatric bipolar disorder. Child Adolesc Psychiatr Clin N Am 2009 Apr;18(2):339–352, viii [PMID: 19264267].

Kim YS, Leventhal B: Bullying and suicide. Int J Adolesc Med Health 2008 Apr–Jun;20(2):133–154 [PMID: 18714552].

Prager LM: Depression and suicide in children and adolescents. Pediatr Rev 2009 Jun;30(6):199–205; quiz 206 [PMID: 19487428].

Steele MM, Doey T: Suicidal behaviour in children and adolescents. Part 1: Etiology and risk factors. Can J Psychiatry 2007 Jun;52(6 Suppl 1):21S–33S [PMID: 17824350].

Steele MM, Doey T: Suicidal behaviour in children and adolescents. Part 2: Treatment and prevention. Can J Psychiatry 2007 Jun;52(6 Suppl 1):35S–45S [PMID: 17824351].

Wintersteen MB, Diamond GS, Fein JA: Screening for suicide risk in the pediatric emergency and acute care setting. Curr Opin Pediatr 2007 Aug;19(4):398–404 [PMID: 17630602].

ADJUSTMENT DISORDERS

The most frequent and most disturbing stresses for children and adolescents are marital discord, separation and divorce, family illness, the loss of a loved one, a change of residence, and, for adolescents, peer relationship problems. When faced with stress, children can experience many different symptoms, including changes in mood, changes in behavior, anxiety symptoms, and physical complaints. Key findings for the diagnosis of an adjustment disorder include the following:

- The precipitating event or circumstance is identifiable.
- The symptoms have appeared within 3 months after the occurrence of the stressful event.
- Although the child experiences distress or some functional impairment, the reaction is not severe or disabling.
- The reaction does not persist more than 6 months after the stressor has terminated.

Differential Diagnosis

When symptoms are a reaction to an identifiable stressor but are severe, persistent, or disabling, depressive disorder, anxiety disorder, and conduct disorders must be considered.

Treatment

The mainstay of treatment is the physician's genuine empathy and assurance to the parents and the patient that the emotional or behavioral change is a predictable consequence of the stressful event. This validates the child's reaction and encourages the child to talk about the stressful occurrence and its aftermath. Parents are encouraged to help the child with appropriate verbal expression of feelings, while defining boundaries for behavior that prevent the child from feeling out of control.

Prognosis

The duration of symptoms in adjustment reactions depends on the severity of the stress; the child's personal sensitivity to stress and vulnerability to anxiety, depression, and other psychiatric disorders; and the available support system.

SCHIZOPHRENIA

The incidence of schizophrenia is about 1 per 10,000 per year. The onset of schizophrenia is typically between the middle to late teens and early 30s, with onset before puberty being relatively rare. Symptoms usually begin after puberty, although a full "psychotic break" may not occur until the young adult years. Childhood onset (before puberty) of psychotic symptoms due to schizophrenia is uncommon and usually indicates a more severe form of the spectrum of schizophrenic disorders. Childhood-onset schizophrenia is more likely to be found in boys.

Schizophrenia is a biologically based disease with a strong genetic component. Other psychotic disorders that may be encountered in childhood or adolescence include schizoaffective disorder and psychosis not otherwise specified (psychosis NOS). Psychosis NOS may be used as a differential diagnosis when psychotic symptoms are present, but the cluster of symptoms is not consistent with a schizophrenia diagnosis.

ESSENTIALS OF DIAGNOSIS & TYPICAL FEATURES

- Delusional thoughts.
- Disorganized speech (rambling or illogical speech patterns).
- Disorganized or bizarre behavior.
- Hallucinations (auditory, visual, tactile, olfactory).
- Paranoia, ideas of reference.
- Negative symptoms (ie, flat affect, avolition, alogia).

Clinical Findings

Children and adolescents display many of the symptoms of adult schizophrenia. Hallucinations or delusions, bizarre and morbid thought content, and rambling and illogical speech are typical. Affected individuals tend to withdraw into an internal world of fantasy and may then equate fantasy with external reality. They generally have difficulty with schoolwork and with peer relationships. Adolescents may have a prodromal period of depression prior to the onset of psychotic symptoms. The majority of patients with childhood-onset schizophrenia have had nonspecific psychiatric symptoms or symptoms of delayed development for months or years prior to the onset of their overtly psychotic symptoms.

Differential Diagnosis

Obtaining the family history of mental illness is critical when assessing children and adolescents with psychotic symptoms. Psychological testing is often helpful in identifying or ruling out psychotic thought processes. Psychotic symptoms in children younger than age 8 years must be differentiated from manifestations of normal vivid fantasy life or abuse-related symptoms. Children with psychotic disorders often have learning disabilities and attention difficulties in addition to disorganized thoughts, delusions, and hallucinations. In psychotic adolescents, mania is differentiated by high levels of energy, excitement, and irritability. Any child or adolescent exhibiting new psychotic symptoms requires a medical evaluation that includes physical and neurologic examinations (including consideration of magnetic resonance imaging and electroencephalogram), drug screening, and metabolic screening for endocrinopathies, Wilson disease, and delirium.

Treatment

The treatment of childhood and adolescent schizophrenia focuses on four main areas: (1) decreasing active psychotic symptoms, (2) supporting development of social and cognitive skills, (3) reducing the risk of relapse of psychotic symptoms, and (4) providing support and education to parents and family members. Antipsychotic medications (neuroleptics) are the primary psychopharmacologic intervention. In addition, a supportive, reality-oriented focus in relationships can help to reduce hallucinations, delusions, and frightening thoughts. A special school or day treatment environment may be necessary, depending on the child's or adolescent's ability to tolerate the school day and classroom activities. Support for the family emphasizes the importance of clear, focused communication and an emotionally calm climate in preventing recurrences of overtly psychotic symptoms.

Prognosis

Schizophrenia is a chronic disorder with exacerbations and remissions of psychotic symptoms. It is generally believed that earlier onset (prior to age 13 years), poor premorbid functioning (oddness or eccentricity), and predominance of negative symptoms (withdrawal, apathy, or flat affect) over positive symptoms (hallucinations or paranoia) predict more severe disability, while later age of onset, normal social and school functioning prior to onset, and predominance of positive symptoms are generally associated with better outcomes and life adjustment to the illness.

Bhangoo RK, Carter RS: Very early interventions in psychotic disorders. Psychiatr Clin North Am 2009 Mar;32(1):81–94 [DOI: 10.1016].

Cantor-Graae E: The contribution of social factors to the development of schizophrenia: A review of recent findings. Can J Psychiatry 2007 May;52(5):277–286 [PMID: 17542378].

Carlisle LL, McClellan J: Psychopharmacology of schizophrenia in children and adolescents. Pediatr Clin North Am 2011 Feb;58(1):205–218, xii [PMID: 21281857].

Kennedy E, Kumar A, Datta SS: Antipsychotic medication for childhood-onset schizophrenia. Cochrane Database Syst Rev 2007 Jul 18;(3):CD004027 [PMID: 17636744].

Masi G, Mucci M, Pari C: Children with schizophrenia: Clinical picture and pharmacological treatment. CNS Drugs 2006;20(10):841–866 [PMID: 16999454].

Sprong M et al: Pathways to psychosis: A comparison of the pervasive developmental disorder subtype Multiple Complex Developmental Disorder and the "At Risk Mental State." Schizophr Res 2008 Feb;99(1–3):38–47 [PMID: 18055179].

Thomas LE, Woods SW: The schizophrenia prodrome: A developmentally informed review and update for psychopharmacologic treatment. Child Adolesc Psychiatr Clin N Am 2006 Jan;15(1):109–133 [PMID: 16321727].

Family resources. Available at: http://www.nami.org/template.cfm? section=your_local_nami http://www.mentalhealthamerica.net/go/faqs

CONDUCT DISORDERS

ESSENTIALS OF DIAGNOSIS & TYPICAL FEATURES

- A persistent pattern of behavior that includes the following:
  - Defiance of authority.
  - Violating the rights of others or society's norms.
  - Aggressive behavior toward persons, animals, or property.

General Considerations

Disorders of conduct affect approximately 9% of males and 2% of females younger than 18 years. This is a very heterogeneous population, and overlap occurs with ADHD, substance abuse, learning disabilities, neuropsychiatric disorders, mood disorders, and family dysfunction. Many of these individuals come from homes where domestic violence, child abuse, drug abuse, shifting parental figures, and poverty are environmental risk factors. Although social learning partly explains this correlation, the genetic heritability of aggressive conduct and antisocial behaviors is currently under investigation.

Clinical Findings

The typical child with conduct disorder is a boy with a turbulent home life and academic difficulties. Defiance of authority, fighting, tantrums, running away, school failure, and destruction of property are common symptoms. With increasing age, fire-setting and theft may occur, followed in adolescence by truancy, vandalism, and substance abuse. Sexual promiscuity, sexual perpetration, and other criminal behaviors may develop. Hyperactive, aggressive, and uncooperative behavior patterns in the preschool and early school years tend to predict conduct disorder in adolescence with a high degree of accuracy, especially when ADHD goes untreated. A history of reactive attachment disorder is an additional childhood risk factor. The risk for conduct disorder increases with inconsistent and severe parental disciplinary techniques, parental alcoholism, and parental antisocial behavior.

Differential Diagnosis

Young people with conduct disorders, especially those with more violent histories, have an increased incidence of neurologic signs and symptoms, psychomotor seizures, psychotic symptoms, mood disorders, ADHD, and learning disabilities. Efforts should be made to identify these associated disorders (see Table 7–9) because they may suggest specific therapeutic interventions. Conduct disorder is best conceptualized as a final common pathway emerging from a variety of underlying psychosocial, genetic, environmental, and neuropsychiatric conditions.

Treatment

Effective treatment can be complicated by the psychosocial problems often found in the lives of children and adolescents with conduct disorders, and the related difficulty achieving compliance with treatment recommendations. Efforts should be made to stabilize the environment and improve functioning within the home, particularly as it relates to parental functioning and disciplinary techniques. Identification of learning disabilities and placement in an optimal school environment is also critical. Any associated neurologic and psychiatric disorders should be addressed.

Residential treatment may be needed for some individuals whose symptoms do not respond to lower level interventions, or whose environment is not able to meet their needs for supervision and structure. It is not unusual for the juvenile justice system to be involved when conduct disorder behaviors lead to illegal activities, theft, or assault.

Medications such as mood stabilizers, neuroleptics, stimulants, and antidepressants have all been studied in youth with conduct disorders, yet none has been found to be consistently effective in this population. Early involvement in programs such as Big Brothers, Big Sisters, scouts, and team sports in which consistent adult mentors and role models interact with youth decreases the chances that the youth with conduct disorders will develop antisocial personality disorder. Multisystemic therapy (MST) is being used increasingly as an intervention for youth with conduct disorders and involvement with the legal system. Multisystemic therapy is an intensive home-based model of care that seeks to stabilize and improve the home environment and to strengthen the support system and coping skills of the individual and family.

Prognosis

The prognosis is based on the ability of the child's support system to mount an effective treatment intervention consistently over time. The prognosis is generally worse for children in whom the disorder presents before age 10 years; those who display a diversity of antisocial behaviors across multiple settings; and those who are raised in an environment characterized by parental antisocial behavior, alcoholism or other substance abuse, and conflict. Nearly half of individuals with a childhood diagnosis of conduct disorder develop antisocial personality disorder as adults.

1. Oppositional Defiant Disorder

ESSENTIALS OF DIAGNOSIS & TYPICAL FEATURES

- A pattern of negativistic, hostile, and defiant behavior lasting at least 6 months.
- Loses temper, argues with adults, defies rules.
- Blames others for own mistakes and misbehavior.
- Angry, easily annoyed, vindictive.
- Does not meet criteria for conduct disorder.

Oppositional defiant disorder usually is evident before 8 years of age and may be an antecedent to the development of conduct disorder. The symptoms usually first emerge at home, but then extend to school and peer relationships. The disruptive behaviors of oppositional defiant disorder are generally less severe than those associated with conduct disorder and do not include hurting other individuals or animals, destruction of property, or theft.

Oppositional defiant disorder is more common in families in whom caregiver dysfunction is present, and in children with a history of multiple changes in caregivers; inconsistent, harsh, or neglectful parenting; or serious marital discord.

Interventions include careful assessment of the psychosocial situation and recommendations to support parenting skills and optimal caregiver functioning. Assessment for comorbid psychiatric diagnoses such as learning disabilities, depression, and ADHD should be pursued and appropriate interventions recommended.

2. Violent Behavior in Youth

Of particular concern to physicians today, as well as to society at large, is the tragic increase in teen violence, including school shootings. There is strong evidence that screening and initiation of interventions by primary care providers can make a significant difference in violent behavior in youth. Although the prediction of violent behavior remains a difficult and imprecise endeavor, physicians can support and encourage several important prevention efforts.

- The vast majority of the increase in youth violence including suicides and homicides involves the use of firearms. Thus, the presence of firearms in the home, the method of storage and safety measures taken when present, and access to firearms outside the home should be explored regularly with all adolescents as part of their routine medical care.
- Violent behavior is often associated with suicidal impulses. In the process of screening for violent behavior, suicidal ideation should not be overlooked. In general, the suicidal youth is somewhat easier to identify than the homicidal youth, and in many cases may be one and the same (see the section on Suicide in Children & Adolescents, earlier). Any comment about wishes to be dead or hopelessness should be taken seriously and help sought.
- Parents and guardians should be aware of their child's school attendance and performance and peer groups. They should know their children's friends and be aware of who they are going out with, where they will be, what they will be doing, and when they will be home. Any concerns should be discussed with the teen and interventions sought if necessary.
- Most students involved in school violence could have benefited from earlier interventions to address problems in social and educational functioning in the school environment. Many communities and school districts have increased their efforts to identify and intervene with students whom teachers, peers, or parents recognize as having difficulty.
- Suicidal and homicidal ideation are co-occurring conditions. A pediatrician should remember to screen for and be aware of both concurrently.

Barker ED, Maughan B: Differentiating early-onset persistent versus childhood-limited conduct problem youth. Am J Psychiatry 2009 Aug;166(8):900–908 [Epub 2009 Jul 1] [PMID: 19570930].

Boylan K et al: Comorbidity of internalizing disorders in children with oppositional defiant disorder. Eur Child Adolesc Psychiatry 2007 Dec;16(8):484–494 [Epub 2007 Sep 24] [PMID: 17896121].

Dretzke J et al: The effectiveness and cost-effectiveness of parent training/education programmes for the treatment of conduct disorder, including oppositional defiant disorder, in children. Health Technol Assess 2005 Dec;9(50):iii, ix–x, 1–233 [PMID: 16336845].

Eyberg SM, Nelson MM, Boggs SR: Evidence-based psychosocial treatments for children and adolescents with disruptive behavior. J Clin Child Adolesc Psychol 2008 Jan;37(1):215–237 [PMID: 18444059].

Fazel S, Doll H, Långström N: Mental disorders among adolescents in juvenile detention and correctional facilities: A systematic review and metaregression analysis of 25 surveys. J Am Acad Child Adolesc Psychiatry 2008 Sep;47(9):1010–1019 [PMID: 18664994].

Hamilton SS, Armando J: Oppositional defiant disorder. Am Fam Physician 2008 Oct 1;78(7):861–866 [PMID: 18841736].

Henggeler SW et al: Mediators of change for multisystemic therapy with juvenile sexual offenders. J Consult Clin Psychol 2009 Jun;77(3):451–462 [PMID: 19485587].

Jensen PS: The role of psychosocial therapies in managing aggression in children and adolescents. J Clin Psychiatry 2008;69(Suppl 4):37–42 [PMID: 18533767].

Loeber R, Burke J, Pardini DA: Perspectives on oppositional defiant disorder, conduct disorder, and psychopathic features. J Child Psychol Psychiatry 2009 Jan;50(1–2):13342 [PMID: 19220596].

Moffitt TE et al: DSM-V conduct disorder: Research needs for an evidence base. J Child Psychol Psychiatry 2008 Jan;49(1):3–33 [PMID: 18181878].

Ogden T, Amlund HK: What works for whom? Gender differences in intake characteristics and treatment outcomes following Multisystemic Therapy. J Adolesc 2009 Jul;18 [PMID: 19619894].

Turgay A: Psychopharmacological treatment of oppositional defiant disorder. CNS Drugs 2009;23(1):1–17 [PMID: 19062772].

ANXIETY DISORDERS

1. Anxiety-Based School Refusal (School Avoidance)

ESSENTIALS OF DIAGNOSIS & TYPICAL FEATURES

- A persistent pattern of school avoidance related to symptoms of anxiety.
- Somatic symptoms on school mornings, with symptoms resolving if the child is allowed to remain at home.
- No organic medical disorder that accounts for the symptoms.
- High levels of parental anxiety are commonly observed.

General Considerations

Anxiety-based school refusal should be considered if a child presents with a medically unexplained absence from school for more than 2 weeks. Anxiety-based school refusal is a persistent behavioral symptom rather than a diagnostic entity. It refers to a pattern of school nonattendance resulting from anxiety, which may be related to a dread of leaving home (separation anxiety), a fear of some aspect of school, or a fear of feeling exposed or embarrassed at school (social phobia). In all cases, a realistic cause of the fear (eg, an intimidating teacher or a playground bully) should be ruled out. In most cases, anxiety-based school refusal is related to developmentally inappropriate separation anxiety. The incidence between males and females is about equal, and there are peaks of incidence at ages 6–7 years, again at ages 10–11 years, and in early adolescence.

Clinical Findings

In the preadolescent years, school refusal often begins after some precipitating stress in the family. The child's anxiety is then manifested either as somatic symptoms or in displacement of anxiety onto some aspect of the school environment. The somatic manifestations of anxiety include dizziness, nausea, and stomach distress. Characteristically, the symptoms become more severe as the time to leave for school approaches and then remit if the child is allowed to remain at home for the day. In older children, the onset is more insidious and often associated with social withdrawal and depression. The incidence of anxiety and mood disorders is increased in these families.

Differential Diagnosis

The differential diagnosis of school nonattendance is presented in Table 7–10. Medical disorders that may be causing the somatic symptoms must be ruled out. Children with learning disorders may wish to stay home to avoid the sense of failure they experience at school. Children may also have transient episodes of wanting to stay at home during times of significant family stress or loss. The onset of school avoidance in middle or late adolescence may be related to the onset of schizophrenia. Children who are avoiding school for reasons related to oppositional defiant disorder or conduct disorder can be differentiated on the basis of their chronic noncompliance with adult authority and their preference for being with peers rather than at home.

Complications

The longer a child remains out of school, the more difficult it is to return and the more strained the relationship between child and parent becomes. Many parents of nonattending children feel tyrannized by their defiant, clinging child. Children often feel accused of making up their symptoms, leading to further antagonism between the child, parents, and medical caregivers.

Table 7–10. Differential diagnosis of school nonattendance.[a]

I. Emotional or anxiety-based refusal[b]
A. Separation anxiety disorder (50%–80% of anxious refusers)
B. Generalized anxiety disorder
C. Mood or depressive disorder (with or without combined anxiety)
D. Social phobia
E. Specific phobia
F. Panic disorder
G. Psychosis
II. Truancy[c] behavior disorders
A. Oppositional defiant disorder, conduct disorder
B. Substance abuse disorders
III. Situation-specific school refusal
A. Learning disability, unaddressed or undetected
B. Bullying or gang threat
C. Psychologically abusive teacher
D. Family-sanctioned nonattendance
1. For companionship
2. For child care
3. To care for the parent (role-reversal)
4. To supplement family income
E. Socioculturally sanctioned nonattendance (school is not valued)
F. Gender concerns
IV. Undiagnosed medical condition (including pregnancy)

[a]Medically unexplained absence of more than 2 weeks.
[b]Subjectively distressed child who generally stays at home.
[c]Nonsubjectively distressed and not at home.

Treatment

Once the comorbid diagnoses and situations related to school avoidance or refusal have been identified and interventions begun (ie, educational assessment if learning disabilities are suspected, medication if necessary for depression or anxiety, or addressing problems in the home), the goal of treatment is to help the child confront anxiety and overcome it by returning to school. This requires a strong alliance between the parents and the health care provider. The parent must understand that no underlying medical disorder exists, that the child's symptoms are a manifestation of anxiety, and that the basic problem is anxiety that must be faced to be overcome. Parents must be reminded that being good parents in this case means helping a child cope with a distressing experience. Children must be reassured that their symptoms are caused by worry and that they will be overcome on return to school.

A plan for returning the child to school is then developed with parents and school personnel. Firm insistence on full compliance with this plan is essential. The child is brought to school by someone not likely to give in, such as the father or an older sibling. If symptoms develop at school, the child should be checked by the school nurse and then returned to class after a brief rest. The parents must be reassured that school staff will handle the situation at school and that school personnel can reach the primary health care provider if any questions arise.

If these interventions are ineffective, increased involvement of a therapist and consideration of a day treatment program may be necessary. For children with persistent symptoms of separation that do not improve with behavioral interventions, medications such as SSRIs should be considered. Comorbid diagnoses of panic disorder, generalized anxiety disorder, or major depression should be carefully screened for, and if identified, treated appropriately.

Prognosis

The vast majority of preadolescent children improve significantly with behavioral interventions and return to school. The prognosis is worsened by the length of time the child remains out of school. Long-term outcomes are influenced by comorbid diagnoses and responsiveness to behavioral or medication interventions. A history of school refusal is more common in adults with panic and anxiety disorders and agoraphobia than in the general population.

Bailey KA et al: Brief measures to screen for social phobia in primary care pediatrics. J Pediatr Psychol 2006 Jun;31(5):512–521 [PMID: 16034004].

Bowen R et al: Nature of anxiety comorbid with attention deficit hyperactivity disorder in children from a pediatric primary care setting. Psychiatry Res 2008 Jan 15;157(1–3):201–209 [Epub 2007 Nov 19] [PMID: 18023880].

Chavira DA et al: Child anxiety in primary care: Prevalent but untreated. Depress Anxiety 2004;20(4):155–164 [PMID: 15643639].

Gardner W et al: Comparison of the PSC-17 and alternative mental health screens in an at-risk primary care sample. J Am Acad Child Adolesc Psychiatry 2007 May;46(5):611–618 [PMID: 17450052].

Khalid-Khan S et al: Social anxiety disorder in children and adolescents: Epidemiology, diagnosis, and treatment. Paediatr Drugs 2007;9(4):227–237 [PMID: 17705562].

Ross WJ, Chan E, Harris SK, Goldman SJ, Rappaport LA: Pediatrician-psychiatrist collaboration to care for children with attention deficit hyperactivity disorder, depression, and anxiety. Clin Pediatr (Phila) 2011 Jan;50(1):37–43 [2010 Aug 19] [PMID: 20724316].

Sakolsky D, Birmaher B: Pediatric anxiety disorders: Management in primary care. Curr Opin Pediatr 2008 Oct;20(5):538–543 [PMID: 18781116].

Wren FJ, Bridge JA, Birmaher B: Screening for childhood anxiety symptoms in primary care: Integrating child and parent reports. J Am Acad Child Adolesc Psychiatry 2004 Nov;43(11):1364–1371 [PMID: 15502595].

2. Generalized Anxiety Disorder & Panic Disorder

General Considerations

Anxiety can be manifested either directly or indirectly, as shown in Table 7–11. The characteristics of anxiety disorders in childhood are listed in Table 7–12. Community-based

Table 7–11. Signs and symptoms of anxiety in children.

Psychological
Fears and worries
Increased dependence on home and parents
Avoidance of anxiety-producing stimuli
Decreased school performance
Increased self-doubt and irritability
Frightening themes in play and fantasy
Psychomotor
Motoric restlessness and hyperactivity
Sleep disturbances
Decreased concentration
Ritualistic behaviors (eg, washing, counting)
Psychophysiologic
Autonomic hyperarousal
Dizziness and lightheadedness
Palpitations
Shortness of breath
Flushing, sweating, dry mouth
Nausea and vomiting
Panic
Headaches and stomach aches

studies of school-aged children and adolescents suggest that nearly 10% of children have some type of anxiety disorder. The differential diagnosis of symptoms of anxiety is presented in Table 7–13.

The evaluation of anxiety symptoms in children must consider the age of the child, the developmental fears that can normally be expected at that age, the form of the symptoms and their duration, and the degree to which the symptoms disrupt the child's life. The family and school environment should be evaluated for potential stressors, marital discord, family violence, harsh or inappropriate disciplinary methods, sexual abuse, neglect, and emotional overstimulation. The child's experience of anxiety and its relationship to life events should be explored.

Table 7–12. Anxiety disorders in children and adolescents.

Disorder	Major Clinical Manifestations
Generalized anxiety disorder	Intense, disproportionate, or irrational worry, often about future events
Panic disorder	Unprovoked, intense fear with sympathetic hyperarousal, and often palpitations or hyper-ventilation
Post-traumatic stress disorder	Fear of a recurrence of an intense, anxiety-provoking traumatic experience, causing sympathetic hyperarousal, avoidance of reminders, and the reexperiencing of aspects of the traumatic event
Separation anxiety disorder	Developmentally inappropriate wish to maintain proximity with caregivers; morbid worry of threats to family integrity or integrity of self upon separation; intense homesickness
Social phobia	Painful shyness or self-consciousness; fear of humiliation with public scrutiny
Specific phobia	Avoidance of specific feared stimuli

Table 7–13. Differential diagnosis of symptoms of anxiety.

I. Normal developmental anxiety
A. Stranger anxiety (5 mo–2½ years, with a peak at 6–12 mo)
B. Separation anxiety (7 mo–4 y, with a peak at 18–36 mo)
C. The child is fearful or even phobic of the dark and monsters (3–6 y)
II. "Appropriate" anxiety
A. Anticipating a painful or frightening experience
B. Avoidance of a reminder of a painful or frightening experience
C. Child abuse
III. Anxiety disorder (see Table 7–12), with or without other comorbid psychiatric disorders
IV. Substance abuse
V. Medications and recreational drugs
A. Caffeinism (including colas and chocolate)
B. Sympathomimetic agents
C. Idiosyncratic drug reactions
VI. Hypermetabolic or hyperarousal states
A. Hyperthyroidism
B. Pheochromocytoma
C. Anemia
D. Hypoglycemia
E. Hypoxemia
VII. Cardiac abnormality
A. Dysrhythmia
B. High-output state
C. Mitral valve prolapsed

Treatment

Therapy to incorporate specific cognitive and behavioral techniques to diminish the anxiety should be recommended for children and adolescents struggling with both generalized anxiety as well as panic disorder. Cognitive, behavioral, environmental, and virtual treatments are typically available in both the privately insured as well as in community mental health settings. When panic attacks or anxiety symptoms do not remit with cognitive, behavioral, and environmental interventions, and they significantly affect life functioning, psychopharmacologic agents may be helpful. SSRIs may be effective across a broad spectrum of anxiety symptoms including panic and generalized anxiety, although no SSRIs are approved for this indication. Occasionally, short-term use of benzodiazapines can be helpful for severe impairment and for treatment relief while waiting for the SSRI to achieve benefit (usually within 3-4 weeks).

Complications

Some adolescents with panic disorder can develop agoraphobia, a subsequent fear that a panic attack may occur in public or other places where help or escape may not be available.

Prognosis

The average age of onset for an anxiety disorder is 5 years of age. In addition, there is continuity between high levels of childhood anxiety and anxiety disorders in adulthood. Anxiety disorders are thus likely to be lifelong conditions, yet with effective interventions, individuals can minimize their influence on overall life functioning.

Alfano CA, Ginsburg GS, Kingery JN: Sleep-related problems among children and adolescents with anxiety disorders. J Am Acad Child Adolesc Psychiatry 2007 Feb;46(2):224–232 [PMID: 17242626].

Ipser JC et al: Pharmacotherapy for anxiety disorders in children and adolescents. Cochrane Database Syst Rev 2009 Jul 8;(3):CD005170 [PMID: 19588367].

Keeton CP, Kolos AC, Walkup JT: Pediatric generalized anxiety disorder: Epidemiology, diagnosis, and management. Paediatr Drugs 2009;11(3):171–183 [PMID: 19445546].

Lavigne JV et al: The prevalence of ADHD, ODD, depression, and anxiety in a community sample of 4-year-olds. J Clin Child Adolesc Psychol 2009 May;38(3):315–328 [PMID: 19437293].

Manassis K: Silent suffering: Understanding and treating children with selective mutism. Expert Rev Neurother 2009 Feb; 9(2):235–243 [PMID: 19210197].

Roy AK et al: The CAMS Team: Attention bias toward threat in pediatric anxiety disorders. J Am Acad Child Adolesc Psychiatry 2008 Aug 8;47(10):1189–1196 [PMID: 18698266].

Rynn MA et al: Efficacy and safety of extended-release venlafaxine in the treatment of generalized anxiety disorder in children and adolescents: Two placebo-controlled trials. Am J Psychiatry 2007 Feb;164(2):290–300 [PMID: 17267793].

OBSESSIVE-COMPULSIVE DISORDER

ESSENTIALS OF DIAGNOSIS & TYPICAL FEATURES

- Recurrent obsessive thoughts, impulses, or images that are not simply excessive worries about real-life problems.
- Obsessions and compulsions cause marked distress, are time-consuming, and interfere with normal routines.
- Repetitive compulsive behaviors or mental acts are performed to prevent or reduce distress stemming from obsessive thoughts.

Obsessive-compulsive disorder (OCD) is an anxiety disorder that often begins in early childhood but may not be diagnosed until the teen or even young adult years. The essential features of OCD are recurrent obsessions or compulsions that are severe enough to be time-consuming or cause marked distress and functional impairment. Obsessions are persistent ideas, thoughts, or impulses that are intrusive and often inappropriate. Children may have obsessions about contamination or cleanliness; ordering and compulsive behaviors will follow, such as frequent hand washing, counting, or ordering objects. The goal of the compulsive behavior for the individual with OCD is to reduce anxiety and distress. There may be significant avoidance of situations due to obsessive thoughts or fears of contamination. OCD is often associated with major depressive disorder. OCD is a biologically based disease and has a strong genetic/familial component. Pediatric autoimmune disorders associated with group B streptococci have also been implicated in the development of OCD for some children. The prevalence of OCD is estimated to be around 2%, and the rates are equal between males and females.

Trichotillomania, while technically classified as an impulse disorder, is also thought to be related to OCD. It involves the recurrent pulling out of hair, often to the point of bald patches, and can also involve pulling out eyelashes, eyebrows, and hair from any part of the body. Trichotillomania should be considered in the differential diagnosis for any patient with alopecia. Treatment often includes the same medications used to treat OCD, and behavior therapy to decrease hair pulling and restore normal social functioning.

Treatment

OCD is best treated with a combination of cognitive-behavioral therapy specific to OCD and medications in more severe cases. SSRIs are effective in diminishing OCD symptoms. Fluvoxamine and sertraline have FDA approval for the treatment of pediatric OCD. The tricyclic antidepressant (TCA) clomipramine has FDA approval for the treatment of OCD in adults.

Prognosis

Although OCD is usually a lifelong condition, most individuals can achieve significant remission of symptoms with the combination of cognitive-behavioral therapy and medications. A minority of individuals with OCD are completely disabled by their symptoms.

Gilbert AR, Maalouf FT: Pediatric obsessive-compulsive disorder: Management priorities in primary care. Curr Opin Pediatr 2008 Oct;20(5):544–550 [PMID: 18781117].

Reinblatt SP, Walkup JT: Psychopharmacologic treatment of pediatric anxiety disorders. Child Adolesc Psychiatr Clin N Am 2005 Oct;14(4):877–908 [PMID: 16171707].

Seidel L, Walkup JT: Selective serotonin reuptake inhibitor use in the treatment of the pediatric non-obsessive-compulsive disorder anxiety disorders. J Child Adolesc Psychopharmacol 2006 Feb–Apr;16(1–2):171–179 [PMID: 16553537].

Stafford B, Troha C, Gueldner BA: Intermittent abdominal pain in a 6-year-old child: The psycho-social-cultural evaluation. Curr Opin Pediatr 2009 Oct;21(5):675–677 [PMID: 19521239].

Storch EA et al: Family-based cognitive-behavioral therapy for pediatric obsessive-compulsive disorder: Comparison of intensive and weekly approaches. J Am Acad Child Adolesc Psychiatry 2007 Apr;46(4):469–478 [PMID: 17420681].

POST-TRAUMATIC STRESS DISORDER

ESSENTIALS OF DIAGNOSIS & TYPICAL FEATURES

- Signs and symptoms of autonomic hyperarousal such as easy startle, increased heart rate, and hypervigilance.
- Avoidant behaviors and numbing of responsiveness.
- Flashbacks to a traumatic event such as nightmares and intrusive thoughts.
- Follows traumatic events such as exposure to violence, physical or sexual abuse, natural disasters, car accidents, dog bites, and unexpected personal tragedies.

General Considerations

Factors that predispose individuals to the development of post-traumatic stress disorder (PTSD) include proximity to the traumatic event or loss, a history of exposure to trauma, preexisting depression or anxiety disorder, and lack of an adequate support system. PTSD can develop in response to natural disasters, terrorism, motor vehicle crashes, and significant personal injury, in addition to physical, sexual, and emotional abuse. Natural disasters such as hurricanes, fires, flooding, and earthquakes, for example, can create situations in which large numbers of affected individuals are at heightened risk for PTSD. Individuals who have a previous history of trauma, or an unstable social situation are at greatest risk of PTSD.

Long overdue, attention is now being paid to the substantial effects of family and community violence on the psychological development of children and adolescents. Abused children are most likely to develop PTSD and to suffer wide-ranging symptoms and impaired functioning. As many as 25% of young people exposed to violence develop symptoms of PTSD.

Heightened concern about terrorism in the United States has created increased awareness of PTSD and community-based interventions to decrease the risk of PTSD. Studies after the terrorist attacks of September 11, 2001, and the Oklahoma City bombing reported up to 40% of children and adolescents experienced PTSD symptoms. Studies after Hurricane Katrina also identified PTSD rates up to 60% in young children after the disaster.

Clinical Findings

Children and adolescents with PTSD show persistent evidence of fear and anxiety and are hypervigilant to the possibility of repetition. They may regress developmentally and experience fears of strangers, of the dark, and of being alone, and avoid reminders of the traumatic event. Children also frequently reexperience elements of the events in nightmares and flashbacks. In their symbolic play, one can often notice a monotonous repetition of some aspect of the traumatic event. Children with a history of traumatic experiences or neglect in infancy and early childhood are likely to show signs of reactive attachment disorder and have difficulty forming relationships with caregivers.

Treatment

The cornerstone of treatment for PTSD is education of the child and family regarding the nature of the disorder so that the child's emotional reactions and regressive behavior are not mistakenly viewed as crazy or manipulative. Support, reassurance, and repeated explanations and understanding are needed. It is critical that the child be living in a safe environment, and if caregivers have been abusive, concerns must be reported to social services. Efforts should be made to establish or maintain daily routines as much as possible, especially after a trauma or disaster that interrupts the family's environment. In the case of media coverage of a disaster or event, children's viewing should be avoided or limited. Interventions to maintain safety of the child are imperative. Individual and family psychotherapy are central features of treatment interventions. Specific fears usually wane with time, and behavioral desensitization may help. Cognitive-behavioral therapy is considered first-line treatment for PTSD, and there is some preliminary evidence that eye movement desensitization and reprocessing (EMDR) may also be useful.

A supportive relationship with a caregiving adult is essential. Frequently caregivers also have PTSD and need referral for treatment so that they can also assist in their child's recovery.

For children with more severe and persistent symptoms, assessment for treatment with medication is indicated. Sertraline has approval for the treatment of PTSD in adults. Target symptoms (eg, anxiety, depression, nightmares, and aggression) should be clearly identified and appropriate medication trials initiated with close monitoring. Some of the medications used to treat children with PTSD include clonidine or guanfacine (Tenex), mood stabilizers, antidepressants, and neuroleptics. Children who have lived for an extended time in abusive environments or who have been exposed to multiple traumas are more likely to require treatment with medications. Occupational therapy for sensory integration can also be effective in decreasing reactivity to stimuli and helping the child and caregivers develop and implement self-soothing skills. Individuals who have suffered single-episode traumas usually benefit significantly from psychotherapy and may require limited treatment with medication to address symptoms of anxiety, nightmares, and sleep disturbance.

Prognosis

At 4- to 5-year follow-up investigations, many children who have been through a traumatic life experience continue to have vivid and frightening memories and dreams and a pessimistic view of the future. The effects of traumatic experiences can be far-reaching. The ability of caregivers to provide a safe, supportive, stable, empathic environment enhances the prognosis for individuals with PTSD. Timely access to therapy and use of therapy over time to work through symptoms also enhance prognosis. Evidence is growing to support a connection between victimization in childhood and unstable personality and mood disorders in later life.

Banh MK et al: Physician-reported practice of managing childhood posttraumatic stress in pediatric primary care. Gen Hosp Psychiatry 2008 Nov–Dec;30(6):536–545 [PMID: 19061680].

Cohen JA, Kelleher KJ, Mannarino AP: Identifying, treating, and referring traumatized children: The role of pediatric providers. Arch Pediatr Adolesc Med 2008 May;162(5):447–452 [PMID: 18458191].

Cohen JA, Scheeringa MS: Post-traumatic stress disorder diagnosis in children: Challenges and promises. Dialogues Clin Neurosci 2009;11(1):91–99 [PMID: 19432391].

Kirsch V, Wilhelm FH, Goldbeck L: Psychophysiological characteristics of PTSD in children and adolescents: A review of the literature. J Trauma Stress 2011 Apr;24(2):146–154. [doi: 10.1002/jts.20620] [Epub 2011 Mar 24] [Review] Erratum in: J Trauma Stress. 2011 Jun;24(3):370–372 [PMID: 21438015].

Scheeringa MS, Zeanah CH: Reconsideration of harm's way: Onsets and comorbidity patterns of disorders in preschool children and their caregivers following Hurricane Katrina. J Clin Child Adolesc Psychol 2008 Jul;37(3):508–518 [PMID: 18645742].

National Child Traumatic Stress Network. Multiple invaluable resources available at: http://www.nctsn.org

SOMATOFORM DISORDERS

ESSENTIALS OF DIAGNOSIS & TYPICAL FEATURES

- A symptom suggesting physical dysfunction.
- No physical disorder accounting for the symptom.
- Symptoms causing distress, dysfunction, or both.
- Symptoms not voluntarily created or maintained, as in malingering.

Clinical Findings

Hypochondriasis, somatization, and conversion disorders involve an unhealthy overemphasis and preoccupation with somatic experiences and symptoms. Somatoform disorders are defined by the presence of physical illness or disability for which no organic cause can be identified, although neither the patient nor the caregiver is consciously fabricating the symptoms. The category includes body dysmorphic disorder, conversion disorder, hypochondriasis, somatization disorder, and somatoform pain disorder (Table 7–14).

Table 7–14. Somatoform disorders in children and adolescents.

Disorder	Major Clinical Manifestations
Body dysmorphic disorder	Preoccupation with an imagined defect in personal appearance
Conversion disorder	Symptom onset follows psychologically stressful event; symptoms express unconscious feelings and result in secondary gain
Hypochondriasis	Preoccupation with worry that physical symptoms manifest unrecognized and threatening condition; medical assurance does not provide relief from worry
Somatization disorder	Long-standing preoccupation with multiple somatic symptoms
Somatoform pain disorder	Preoccupation with pain that results in distress or impairment beyond what would be expected from physical findings

Conversion symptoms most often occur in school-aged children and adolescents. The exact incidence is unclear, but in pediatric practice they are probably seen more often as transient symptoms than as chronic disorders requiring help from mental health practitioners. A conversion symptom is thought to be an expression of underlying psychological conflict. The specific symptom may be symbolically determined by the underlying conflict; the symptom may resolve the dilemma created by the underlying wish or fear (eg, a seemingly paralyzed child need not fear expressing his or her underlying rage or aggressive retaliatory impulses). Although children can present with a variety of symptoms, the most common include neurologic and gastrointestinal complaints. Children with conversion disorder may be surprisingly unconcerned about the substantial disability deriving from their symptoms. Symptoms include unusual sensory phenomena, paralysis, vomiting, abdominal pain, intractable headaches, and movement or seizure-like disorders.

In the classic case of conversion disorder, the child's symptoms and examination findings are not consistent with the clinical manifestations of any organic disease process. The physical symptoms often begin within the context of a family experiencing stress, such as serious illness, a death, or family discord. On closer examination, the child's symptoms are often found to resemble symptoms present in other family members. Children with conversion disorder may have some secondary gain associated with their symptoms. Several reports have pointed to the increased association of conversion disorder with sexual overstimulation or sexual abuse. As with other emotional and behavioral problems, health care providers should always screen for physical and sexual abuse.

Differential Diagnosis

It is sometimes not possible to rule out medical disease as a source of the symptoms. Medical follow-up is required to monitor for changes in symptoms and response to recommended interventions.

Somatic symptoms are often associated with anxiety and depressive disorders (see Tables 7–7 and 7–11). Occasionally, psychotic children have somatic preoccupations and even somatic delusions.

Treatment & Prognosis

In most cases, conversion symptoms resolve quickly when the child and family are reassured that the symptom is a way of reacting to stress. The child is encouraged to continue with normal daily activities, knowing that the symptom will abate when the stress is resolved. Treatment of conversion disorders includes acknowledging the symptom rather than telling the child that the symptom is not medically justified and responding with noninvasive interventions such as physical therapy while continuing to encourage normalization of the symptoms. If the symptom does not resolve with reassurance, further investigation by a mental health professional is indicated. Comorbid diagnoses such as depression and anxiety disorders should be addressed, and treatment with psychopharmacologic agents may be helpful.

Patients presenting with somatoform disorders are often resistant to mental health treatment, in part fearing that any distraction from their vigilance will put them at greater risk of succumbing to a medical illness. Psychiatric consultation is often helpful and for severely incapacitated patients, referral psychiatric consultation is always indicated.

Somatoform disorder is not associated with the increased morbidity and mortality associated with other psychiatric disorders such as mood disorders or psychotic illness. Somatoform patients are best treated with regular, short, scheduled medical appointments to address the complaints at hand. In this way they do not need to precipitate emergencies to elicit medical attention. Avoid invasive procedures unless clearly indicated and offer sincere concern and reassurance. Avoid telling the patient "it's all in your head" and do not abandon or avoid the patient, as somatoform patients are at great risk of seeking multiple alternative treatment providers and potentially unnecessary treatments.

Andresen JM, Woolfolk RL, Allen LA, Fragoso MA, Youngerman NL, Patrick-Miller TJ, Gara MA: Physical symptoms and psychosocial correlates of somatization in pediatric primary care. Clin Pediatr (Phila) 2011 May;16 [PMID: 21576182].

Campo JV et al: Physical and emotional health of mothers of youth with functional abdominal pain. Arch Pediatr Adolesc Med 2007 Feb;161(2):131–137 [PMID: 17283297].

Ginsburg GS, Riddle MA, Davies M: Somatic symptoms in children and adolescents with anxiety disorders. J Am Acad Child Adolesc Psychiatry 2006 Oct;45(10):1179–1187 [PMID: 17003663].

Goldbeck L, Bundschuh S: Illness perception in pediatric somatization and asthma: Complaints and health locus of control beliefs. Child Adolesc Psychiatry Ment Health 2007 Jul 16;1(1):5 [PMID: 17678524].

Kozlowska K et al: A conceptual model and practice framework for managing chronic pain in children and adolescents. Harv Rev Psychiatry 2008;16(2):136–150 [PMID: 18415885].

Kozlowska K et al: Conversion disorder in Australian pediatric practice. J Am Acad Child Adolesc Psychiatry 2007 Jan;46(1):68–75 [PMID: 17195731].

Masia WC et al: CBT for anxiety and associated somatic complaints in pediatric medical settings: An open pilot study. J Clin Psychol Med Settings 2009 Jun;16(2):169–177 [PMID: 19152057].

Mulvaney S et al: Trajectories of symptoms and impairment for pediatric patients with functional abdominal pain: A 5-year longitudinal study. J Am Acad Child Adolesc Psychiatry 2006 Jun;45(6):737–744 [PMID: 16721324].

Plioplys S et al: Multidisciplinary management of pediatric nonepileptic seizures. J Am Acad Child Adolesc Psychiatry 2007 Nov;46(11):1491–1495 [PMID: 18049299].

Seshia SS, Phillips DF, von Baeyer CL: Childhood chronic daily headache: A biopsychosocial perspective. Dev Med Child Neurol 2008 Jul;50(7):541–545 [PMID: 18611206].

Walker LS et al: Appraisal and coping with daily stressors by pediatric patients with chronic abdominal pain. J Pediatr Psychol 2007 Mar;32(2):206–216 [PMID: 16717138].

OTHER PSYCHIATRIC CONDITIONS

Several psychiatric conditions are covered elsewhere in this book. Refer to the following chapters for detailed discussion:

- Attention-deficit/hyperactivity disorder (ADHD): see Chapter 3.
- Autism and pervasive developmental disorders: see Chapter 3
- Enuresis and encopresis: see Chapter 3
- Eating disorders: see Chapter 6.
- Intellectual disability/mental retardation: see Chapter 3.
- Substance abuse: see Chapter 5.
- Sleep disorders: see Chapter 3.
- Tourette syndrome: see Chapter 25.

PEDIATRIC PRIMARY CARE BEHAVIORAL HEALTH SERVICES

Delivering mental health and behavioral services in the context of pediatric primary care provides a mechanism for improving access, quality, and effectiveness of services (Guevara & Forrest, 2006; Trupin, 2011) within a medical home for children. In the ideal, medical homes provide children and families with comprehensive, coordinated, individualized, strength-based, culturally sensitive, and family-centered care that is inclusive of physical, mental, and oral health (Strickland, Jones, Ghandour, Kogan, & Newacheck, 2011). Mental health and behavioral services span the continuum from co-locating a behavioral health provider within a primary care setting and offering traditional outpatient mental health services in isolation of primary care services but at the same clinic to integrating of behavioral health clinicians into the routine practice of a pediatric primary care clinic. Behavioral health services include direct clinical interventions, consultation to pediatric providers on challenging cases, joint visits, and trainings (Strohm et al., 2005). Co-located services primarily target children and families while integrated services target children, families, pediatric providers, and systems of care in which services are being delivered.

Behavioral health providers working in pediatric primary care settings must be prepared to address a wide range of presenting problems, health conditions, and family circumstances. Difficulties span daily routine disruptions (eg, eating and sleeping), developmental delays, management of chronic illness (eg, asthma, obesity), adjustment to life events and stressors (eg, moving, divorce), acute traumas (eg, accidents, episodes of abuse), chronic family circumstances (eg, family violence, financial hardship, parental mental illness), academic challenges, relationship disruptions, and mental health disorders. Consequently, behavioral health providers utilize numerous strategies to address the varied and often complex presentations.

First and foremost, behavioral health providers strive to establish a relationship with the child and family. Rapport and relationship building are essential to engaging families in treatment and, importantly, to having families return to the primary care setting for ongoing treatment and support. Once a strong relationship is established, behavioral health providers strive to identify challenges and concerns through screening and assessment, diagnose and treat those issues that can be managed in primary care, triage and refer families to external resources, and ultimately, improve child and family outcomes. In integrated models, behavioral health providers work collaboratively with pediatric primary care providers to develop and implement care plans.

Interventions that have successfully addressed development, psychosocial factors, and to a more limited extent, mental health and behavioral issues in pediatric primary care settings, have typically targeted specific behavioral concerns including sleep disruptions, discipline techniques, obesity, and pain (Allen, Elliott, & Arndorfer, 2002) with the goals of symptom reduction, improved adaptive behaviors and functioning, decreased family distress, and increased adherence to medical regimens. Behavioral health clinicians frequently manage prevalent mental health disorders including anxiety (Saklosky & Birmaher, 2008), depression, and attention deficit/hyperactivity by adapting outpatient treatments for use in primary care. Exposures, relaxation techniques, and cognitive skills are among the many that can be readily taught. Educational interventions including counseling sessions, written information, and videotapes have been used to enhance parent-child interactions and bolster parental confidence (Pinilla & Birch, 1993; Wolfson, Lacks & Futterman, 1992). Behavioral health clinicians often coordinate screening and identification efforts (Simonian, 2006; Weitzman & Leventhal, 2006) by implementing procedures and developing protocols for successful screening, identification, referral, and feedback.

The Healthy Steps for Young Children Program incorporated developmental specialists and enhanced developmental services into pediatric primary care settings. Findings from an evaluation of the program suggest that participating families received more developmental services, were more satisfied with the quality of care provided, were more likely to attend well-child visits and receive vaccinations on time, and were less likely to use severe discipline techniques with their children (Minkovitz, et al., 2003). Participation in the program also increased the likelihood that mothers at risk for depression would discuss their sadness with someone in the pediatric setting.

In reviewing the literature, Regalado and Halfon (2001) found that methods of identifying children with developmental difficulties in primary care settings were not adequate and assessment approaches for behavioral problems in the first three years of life were particularly lacking. This review also noted that physicians underestimate the extent of psychosocial challenges faced by families and their impact on behavior problems in children. Although a compelling case can be made for providing access to behavioral health services in pediatric primary care, particularly in infancy and early childhood (Talmi, Stafford, & Buchholz, 2009; Zeanah & Gleason, 2009), little evidence exists regarding the use of interventions with respect to their role in preventing mental health issues and long term developmental sequellae. Importantly, without behavioral health supports in pediatric primary care settings, the burden of addressing mental health, developmental, and behavioral issues falls on the pediatric provider who has neither adequate time (Cooper et al., 2006) nor the ability to bill and receive reimbursement for such services (Meadows et al., 2011). Moreover, despite the recognition that clinical skills are needed to identify and address children's and parent's complex behavioral health needs, developmental and psychosocial issues have only recently become more central in pediatric training (American Academy of Pediatrics, 2009).

REFERENCES

American Academy of Pediatrics: Committee on Psychosocial Aspects of Child and Family Health and Task Force on Mental Health. The future of pediatrics: Mental health competencies for pediatric primary care. Pediatrics 2009;124:410–421 [PMID: 19564328].

Anstiss Tim: Motivational interviewing in primary care. Journal of Clinical Psychology in Medical Settings (1068–9583) 2009;16(1):87 [PMID: 19253016].

Cooper S, Valleley R J, Polaha J, Begeny J, Evans J H: Running out of time: Physician management of behavioral health concerns in rural pediatric primary care. Pediatrics 2006;118(1):e132 [PMID: 16818528].

Dilallo JJ, Weiss G: Motivational interviewing and adolescent psychopharmacology. Journal of the American Academy of Child and Adolescent Psychiatry (0890-8567) 2009;48(2):108 [PMID: 20040823].

Guevara JP, Forrest CB: Modernizing pediatric primary care to better manage children's behavioral health. Current Opinion in Pediatrics 2006;18(6):639 [PMID: 17099363].

Meadows T, Valleley R, Haack MK, Thorson R, Evans J: Physician "costs" in providing behavioral health in primary care. Clinical Pediatrics 2011;50(5):447 [PMID: 21196418].

Pinilla T, Birch LL: Help me make it through the night: Behavioral entrainment of breast-fed infants' sleep patterns. Pediatrics 1993;91:436–444 [PMID: 8424024].

Regalado M, Halfon N: Primary care services promoting optimal child development from birth to age 3 years. Archives of Pediatric and Adolescent Medicine 2001;155:1311–1322 [PMID: 11732949].

Strickland B, Jones J, Ghandour R, Kogan M, Newacheck P: The medical home: Health care access and impact for children and youth in the United States. Pediatrics 2011;127:604–611 [PMID: 21402643].

Strohm J, Campo JV, Shafer S, Lucas A, Altman H, Cassesse CG, Shaeffer D: Pediatric Behavioral Health in Primary Care: A Collaborative Approach 2009.

Talmi A, Stafford B, Buchholz M: Providing perinatal mental health services in pediatric primary care. Zero to Three 2009 May;10–16.

Trupin E: Behavioral health screening and intervention in primary care. Archives of Pediatrics & Adolescent Medicine 2011;165(7):669 [PMID: 21383257].

Weitzman CC, Leventhal JM: Screening for behavioral health problems in primary care. Current Opinion in Pediatrics 2006;18(6):641–648 [PMID: 17099364].

Whitlock EP, Orleans CT, Pender N, Allan J: Evaluating primary care behavioral counseling interventions. American Journal of Preventative Medicine 2002;22(4):267–284 [PMID: 11988383].

Zeanah PD, Gleason MM: Handbook of Infant Mental Health: Third Edition. New York, NY: Guilford Publications; 2009.

OVERVIEW OF PEDIATRIC PSYCHOPHARMACOLOGY

Pediatric psychopharmacology has improved significantly over the past decade with increasing study of the effect of psychoactive medications on mental illness in childhood and adolescence. Although relatively few medications are approved for use in children, many of the same psychopharmacologic agents used in adults are used in children and adolescents.

As with any medication, the risks as well as the benefits of administering psychoactive medications must be discussed with the child's parent or guardian and with the child or adolescent, as is age-appropriate. A recommendation for medication is warranted if the symptoms observed and reported by the child or family are associated with a psychiatric diagnosis known to respond to a particular medication or class of medications. Medication is more likely to be recommended if the disorder is interfering with psychosocial development, interpersonal relationships, daily functioning, or the patient's sense of personal well-being, and if there is significant potential for benefit with the medication and relatively low risk of harm. Informed consent should be given by the parent or guardian and noted in the record. The recommendation and target symptoms for medication should be discussed with both children and adolescents, and adolescents should also provide informed consent for treatment. In some states, adolescents aged 15 and older must give informed consent. Informed consent includes a discussion of the diagnosis, target symptoms, possible common side effects, any side effects that should be closely monitored, potential benefits associated with the medication, and documentation of informed consent in the medical record. Psychopharmacologic agents are seldom the only treatment for a psychiatric disorder. They are best used in combination with other interventions such as individual therapy, family psychotherapy, and other psychosocial interventions, including assessment of school functioning and special needs.

When considering the use of psychoactive medications, specific target symptoms of the medication should be identified and followed to evaluate the efficacy of treatment. These symptoms should be also measured either by self-report rating scales (child, family, or both) or by clinician-rated scales. When initiating treatment, start with low doses and increase slowly (in divided doses, if indicated) while monitoring for side effects along with therapeutic effects. When a medication is discontinued, it should usually be tapered over 2–4 weeks to minimize withdrawal effects. When multiple choices exist, one should select the medication that has a pediatric FDA approval (Table 7–15), or has been studied for the specific indication for which it is being prescribed, ideally in the age range of the patient. The side-effect profile of each option should be carefully considered, and the medication selected with the fewest and least serious risks and side effects. Polypharmacy should be avoided by choosing one drug that might diminish most or all of the target symptoms before considering the simultaneous administration of two or more agents. General guidelines regarding comfort level for pediatric providers in initiating and managing psychotropic classes of medications are outlined in Table 7–16.

In the text that follows, the major classes of psychopharmacologic agents with clinical indications in child and adolescent psychiatry are represented. The more commonly prescribed drugs from each class are reviewed with reference to indications, relative contraindications, initial medical screening procedures (in addition to a general pediatric examination), dosage, adverse effects, drug interactions, and medical follow-up recommendations. This is meant to be a brief reference guide, and the physician should consult a child and adolescent psychopharmacology textbook for additional information on specific medications.

Table 7–15. Psychoactive medications approved by the FDA for use in children and adolescents.[a]

Drug	Indication	Age for Which Approved (y)
Mixed amphetamine salts (Adderall)	ADHD	3 and older
Dextroamphetamine (Dexedrine, Dextrostat)	ADHD	3 and older
Methylphenidate (Concerta, Ritalin, others)	ADHD	6 and older
Atomoxetine (Straterra) Guanfacine ER (Intuniv) Clomipramine (Anafranil)	ADHD ADHD OCD	6 and older 6 and older 10 and older
Fluvoxamine (Luvox)	OCD	8 and older
Sertraline (Zoloft)	OCD Aggression and autism Schizophrenia and mania	6 and older 5 and older 10 and older
Pimozide (Orap)[b]	Tourette syndrome	12 and older
Lithium (Eskalith, Lithobid, Lithotabs)	Bipolar disorder	12 and older
Fluoxetine (Prozac)	Depression OCD	12 and older 6 and older
Escitalopram (Lexapro)	Depression	12 and older
Imipramine (Norpramin)	Enuresis	6 and older
Aripiprazole (Abilify)	Bipolar Disorder Schizophrenia Aggression and Autism	10 and older 13 and older 6 and older
Risepridone (Risperdal)	Bipolar Disorder Schizophrenia Aggression and Autism	10 and older 13 and older 6 and older
Quetiapine (Seroquel, XR)	Bipolar Disorder Schizophrenia	10 and older 13 and older
Ziprasidone (Geodon)	Bipolar Disorder Schizophrenia	10 and older 13 and older
Olanzapine (Zyprexa)	Bipolar Disorder Schizophrenia	10 and older 13 and older

[a]Haloperidol and chlorpromazine have an indication for use in psychotic disorders. Their use in children, however, is not currently recommended.

[b]Use of pimozide in the treatment of movement disorders is discussed in Chapter 25.

ADHD, attention-deficit/hyperactivity disorder; FDA, Food and Drug Administration; OCD, obsessive-compulsive disorder.

Table 7–16. Guidelines for management of psychiatric medications by the pediatrician.

Drug or Class	Comfort Initiating	Comfort Managing
Stimulants	+++	+++
α-Agonists	++	+++
Antidepressants	+	++
Atypical antipsychotics	Recommend psychiatrist involvement	++
Typical antipsychotics	Requires psychiatrist involvement	+/−
Clozapine (Clozaril)	Requires psychiatrist involvement	Requires psychiatrist involvement
Mood stabilizers	Recommend psychiatrist involvement	+
Lamotrigine (Lamictal)	Requires psychiatrist involvement	++
Sleep medicines	+	++
Tricyclic antidepressants	+	++

Symbols: +++, high comfort; ++, comfort; +, mild caution; +/−, caution required.
Dexmethylphenidate (Focalin, Focalin XR)
Clonidine (Catapres, Clonipress); guanfacine; (Tenex, Intuniv);
Atomoxetine (Strattera)

MEDICATIONS FOR ATTENTION-DEFICIT/ HYPERACTIVITY DISORDER

Dextroamphetamine (Dexedrine, Dextrostat)

Mixed amphetamine salts (Adderall, Adderall XR)

Lisdexamfetamine (Vyvanse)

Methylphenidate (Concerta, Metadate, Methylin, Ritalin, Ritalin LA, Ritalin SR, Daytrana, Transdermal)

1. Indications—Approximately 75% of children with ADHD experience improved attention span, decreased hyperactivity, and decreased impulsivity when given stimulant medications. Children with ADHD who do not respond favorably to one stimulant may respond well to another. Children and adolescents with ADHD without prominent hyperactivity (ADHD, predominantly inattentive type) are also likely to be responsive to stimulant medications. Atomoxetine (Strattera) and bupropion (Wellbutrin) are nonstimulant medications used to treat ADHD. Atomoxetine has FDA approval for the treatment of ADHD and is a selective noradrenergic reuptake inhibitor. Bupropion is primarily used as an antidepressant, and blocks dopamine reuptake.

2. Contraindications—Reports in the medical literature and to the FDA of sudden death and reports to the FDA of serious cardiovascular adverse events among children taking concern about the safety of these medications. In fact, the labels for methylphenidate and amphetamine medications were changed in 2006 to note reports of stimulant-related deaths in patients with heart problems and advised against using these products in individuals with known serious structural abnormalities of the heart, cardiomyopathy, or serious heart rhythm abnormalities. There continues to be, however, insufficient data to confirm whether taking stimulant medication causes cardiac problems or sudden death. The FDA is advising physicians and other providers to conduct a thorough physical examination, paying close attention to the cardiovascular system, and to collect information about the patient's history and any family history of cardiac problems. If these examinations indicate a potential problem, providers may want to consider a screening electrocardiogram (ECG) or an echocardiogram. In addition, stimulants should also be used cautiously in individuals with a personal or family history of motor tics or Tourette syndrome, as these medications may cause or worsen motor tics. Caution should also be taken if there is a personal or family history of substance abuse or addictive disorders, as these medications can be abused or sold as drugs of abuse. Stimulants are also contraindicated for individuals with psychotic disorders, as they can significantly worsen psychotic symptoms. Stimulants should be used with caution in individuals with comorbid bipolar affective disorder and ADHD and consideration of concurrent mood stabilization is critical.

FDA Statement. Available at: http://www.fda.gov/Drugs/DrugSafety/PostmarketDrugSafetyInformationforPatientsandProviders/DrugSafetyInformationforHeathcareProfessionals/ucm165858.htm

3. Initial medical screening—The child should be observed for involuntary movements. Height, weight, pulse, and blood pressure should be recorded. (See also Chapter 3.)

4. Adverse effects—These are often dose-related and time-limited.

A. COMMON ADVERSE EFFECTS—Anorexia, weight loss, abdominal distress, headache, insomnia, dysphoria and tearfulness, irritability, lethargy, mild tachycardia, and mild elevation in blood pressure.

B. LESS COMMON EFFECTS—Interdose rebound of ADHD symptoms, emergence of motor tics or Tourette syndrome, behavioral stereotypy, tachycardia or hypertension, depression, mania, and psychotic symptoms. Reduced growth velocity occurs only during active administration. Growth rebound occurs during periods of discontinuation. Ultimate height is not usually noticeably compromised. Treatment with stimulant medications does not predispose to future substance abuse.

5. Drug interactions—Additive stimulant effects are seen with sympathomimetic amines (ephedrine and pseudoephedrine).

6. Medical follow-up—Pulse, blood pressure, height, and weight should be recorded every 3–4 months and at times of dosage increases. Assess for abnormal movements such as motor tics at each visit.

7. Dosage

A. METHYLPHENIDATE—The usual starting dose is 5 mg once or twice a day, before school and at noon (or 2.5 mg twice a day for children aged 4–6 years), gradually increasing as clinically indicated. The maximum daily dose should not exceed 60 mg, and a single dose should not exceed 0.7 mg/kg. Administration on weekends and during vacations is determined by the need at those times. The duration of action is approximately 3–4 hours. Extended-release forms can prevent the need for taking medication at school and most families and schools prefer that longer acting preparations are prescribed for optimal adherence and decreased logistical problems. Dexmethylphenidate (Focalin) is typically administered at a dose of 2.5 mg twice a day (eg, 8 AM and noon), to a maximum of 20 mg.

B. DEXTROAMPHETAMINE SULFATE—The dose is 2.5–10 mg twice daily, before school and at noon, with or without another dose at 4 PM. A sustained-release preparation may have clinical effects for up to 8 hours. There is also an extended-release form. As with methylphenidate-based preparations, most families prefer longer-acting preparations.

C. PEMOLINE—Pemoline is generally not recommended for the treatment of ADHD due to a significant risk of liver failure.

D. ATOMOXETINE HYDROCHLORIDE—The starting dose for children and adolescents up to 70 kg is 0.5 mg/kg, with titration to a maximum dose of 1.2 mg/kg, in single or divided dosing.

ANTIDEPRESSANTS

The "black box warning" that was issued in October 2005 for all antidepressants continues to have a significant impact on prescription of these medications for children. The black box warning reads "Pooled analysis of short term (4–16 weeks) placebo-controlled trials of antidepressant drugs (SSRIs and others) in children and adolescents with Major Depressive Disorder (MDD), Obsessive-Compulsive Disorder (OCD), and other psychiatric disorders (a total of 24 trials involving more than 4400 patients) has revealed a greater risk of adverse events representing suicidal thinking or behavior (suicidality) during the first few months of treatment in those receiving antidepressants.

The average risk of such events was 4%, twice the placebo risk of 2%. No suicides occurred in these trials." Since these guidelines were published, prescribing and use of antidepressants has decreased. Unfortunately, suicide completion in adolescents has increased as a result.

The "medication guide" created for consumers along with the black box warning that now appears in all antidepressant packaging recommends the following monitoring schedule for health care providers when starting an antidepressant:

- Once every week for the first 4 weeks.
- Every 2 weeks for the next 4 weeks.
- After taking the antidepressant for 12 weeks.
- After 12 weeks, follow your health care provider's advice on how often to come back.

The Treatment of Adolescent Depression Study found that cognitive-behavioral therapy combined with fluoxetine led to the best outcomes in the treatment of pediatric depression. Escitalopram recently received FDA approval for the treatment of adolescent depression.

It is important to be cognizant of evidence-based medical practice when prescribing for any indication. Target symptoms should be carefully monitored for improvement or worsening, and it is important to ask and document the responses about any suicidal thinking and self-injurious behaviors. When recommending an antidepressant, the physician should also firmly recommend cognitive-behavioral or interpersonal therapy and discuss the options for medication treatment, including which medications have FDA approval for pediatric indications (see Table 7–15). Recent findings suggest that fluoxetine has the best evidence for improvement in depressive symptoms.

1. Selective Serotonin Reuptake Inhibitors

Fluoxetine (Prozac)

Citalopram, escitalopram (Celexa, Lexapro), Fluvoxamine (Luvox)

Paroxetine (Paxil)

Sertraline (Zoloft)

1. Indications—The SSRIs have become the agents of first choice for the treatment of depression and anxiety. Fluvoxamine and sertraline both have approval from the FDA for treatment of pediatric OCD and fluoxetine and escitalopram have approval for pediatric and adolescent depression. Although no other SSRIs have FDA approval for pediatric indications, some published studies support the efficacy of SSRIs for the treatment of depression, anxiety, and OCD in pediatric populations. Each SSRI has different FDA indications. However, once an indication is obtained for one SSRI, it is widely believed that other SSRIs are likely to be effective as well for the same indication. The FDA-approved indications for SSRIs are the following:

Major depression: fluoxetine (age 6 years and older); escitalopram (age 12 and older); paroxetine, citalopram, sertraline (18 and older).

Panic disorder: sertraline (18 and older), paroxetine (18 and older).

OCD: fluvoxamine (6 and older), sertraline (6 and older).

Bulimia: fluoxetine (18 and older).

PTSD: sertraline (18 and older).

Premenstrual dysphoric disorder: fluoxetine (18 and older).

2. Contraindications—Caution should be used in cases of known liver disease or chronic or severe illness where multiple medications may be prescribed, because all SSRIs are metabolized in the liver. Caution should be used when prescribing for an individual with a family history of bipolar disorder, or when the differential diagnosis includes bipolar disorder, because antidepressants can induce manic or hypomanic symptoms.

3. Initial medical screening—General medical examination.

4. Adverse effects—Often dose-related and time-limited: gastrointestinal (GI) distress and nausea (can be minimized by taking medication with food), headache, tremulousness, decreased appetite, weight loss, insomnia, sedation (10%), sexual dysfunction (25%). Irritability, social disinhibition, restlessness, and emotional excitability can occur in approximately 20% of children taking SSRIs. Monitor for improvement and onset or worsening of suicidal or self-injurious thinking, in addition to other target symptoms.

5. Drug interactions—All SSRIs inhibit the efficiency of the hepatic microsomal enzyme system. The order of inhibition is: fluoxetine > fluvoxamine > paroxetine > sertraline > citalopram > escitalopram. This can lead to higher-than-expected blood levels of other drugs, including antidepressants, antiarrhythmics, antipsychotics, β-blockers, opioids, and antihistamines. Taking tryptophan while on an SSRI may result in a serotonergic syndrome of psychomotor agitation and GI distress. A potentially fatal interaction that clinically resembles neuroleptic malignant syndrome may occur when SSRIs are administered concomitantly with monoamine oxidase inhibitors. Fluoxetine has the longest half-life of the SSRIs and should not be initiated within 14 days of the discontinuation of a monoamine oxidase inhibitor, or a monoamine oxidase inhibitor initiated within at least 5 weeks of the discontinuation of fluoxetine. One should be cautious of Fluoxetine and Ibuprofen and other NSAIDs for concerns of GI bleeding.

6. Dosage (Table 7–17)—Therapeutic response should be expected 4–6 weeks after a therapeutic dose has been reached. The starting dose for a child younger than 12 years old is generally half the starting dose for an adolescent.

A. SSRIs—The SSRIs are usually given once a day, in the morning with breakfast. One in ten individuals may experience sedation and prefer to take the medication at bedtime. Fluoxetine and escitalopram are the only SSRIs with FDA approval and replicable efficacy.

Table 7–17. Medications used to treat depression in adolescents.

Generic	Trade Name	Adolescent Starting Dose	Target Dose (Average Effective Dose)	Maximum Dose
Selective serotonin reuptake inhibitors				
Citalopram[a]	Celexa	20 mg q AM	20 mg q AM	40–60 mg q AM
Escitalopram	Lexapro	10 mg	10 mg	30 mg
Fluoxetine[a]	Prozac	10 mg q AM	20 mg q AM	60 mg q AM
Fluvoxamine	Luvox	50 mg qhs	100–150 mg qd	100 mg bid
Paroxetine	Paxil	10 mg q AM	20 mg q AM	60 mg q AM
Paroxetine CR	Paxil CR	25 mg	25 mg	50 mg
Sertraline	Zoloft	25 mg q AM	50 mg q AM	150 mg q AM
Other antidepressants				
Bupropion	Wellbutrin	75 mg q AM	150 mg bid	200 mg bid
Bupropion SR	Wellbutrin SR	100 mg q AM	100 mg bid	150 mg bid
Bupropion XL	Wellbutrin Xl	150 mg q AM	150–300 q AM	450 q AM
Duloxetine	Cymbalta	20 mg bid	20 mg bid	60 mg qd
Mirtazapine	Remeron	7.5 mg qhs	15 mg qhs	30 mg qhs
Venlafaxine	Effexor	37.5 mg q AM	75 mg bid	150 mg bid
Venlafaxine XR	Effexor XR	37.5 mg q AM	150 mg qd	225 mg qd
Desvenlafaxine ER	Pristiq	50 mg q AM	50 mg q AM	100 mg qd
Olanzapine and fluoxetine HCl	Symbyax	3 mg/25 mg qhs	6 mg/25 mg/h	12 mg/50 mg/h

[a]FDA approved for depression in children older than age 12 years.
bid, twice a day; q AM, every morning; qd, every day; qhs, every night at bedtime.

B. Alternative antidepressants and fluvoxamine—The alternative antidepressants (see below) and fluvoxamine are usually given in twice-daily dosing. Paroxetine, bupropion, and venlafaxine are now available in a sustained- and extended-release form.

2. Other Antidepressants

Bupropion (Wellbutrin), bupropion SR (sustained-release), bupropion XL (extended-release)

Duloxetine (Cymbalta)

Mirtazapine (Remeron)

Venlafaxine (Effexor), venlafaxine XR (extended-release), desvenlafaxine ER (Pristiq)

A. Bupropion

1. Indications—Bupropion is an antidepressant that inhibits reuptake of primarily serotonin, but also norepinephrine and dopamine. It is approved for treatment of major depression in adults, but is receiving favorable attention for its therapeutic effects in adolescents with major depressive disorder and in children and adolescents with ADHD. Like the SSRIs, bupropion has very few anticholinergic or cardiotoxic effects. The IR is usually dosed BID or TID, SR is dosed BID, and XL preparations are most frequently used given once a day dosing. Buproprion can interfere with sleep, so dosing earlier in the day is paramount to adherence and to eliminate side effects.

2. Contraindications—History of seizure disorder or bulimia nervosa.

3. Initial medical screening and follow-up—General medical examination.

4. Adverse effects—Psychomotor activation (agitation or restlessness), headache, GI distress, nausea, anorexia with weight loss, insomnia, tremulousness, precipitation of mania, and induction of seizures with doses above 450 mg/d.

B. Venlafaxine

Venlafaxine is an antidepressant that primarily inhibits reuptake of serotonin and norepinephrine.

Desvenlafaxine is the major active metabolite of the antidepressant venlafaxine.

1. Indications—It is approved for the treatment of major depression in adults.

2. Contraindications—Hypertension.

3. Initial medical screening and follow-up—General medical examination.

4. Adverse effects—The most common adverse effects are nausea, nervousness, and sweating. Hypertension is likely with doses over 300 mg or over 225 mg of the extended-release version. Venlafaxine must be discontinued slowly to minimize withdrawal symptoms: severe headaches, dizziness, and significant flulike symptoms. It is also available in an extended-release form.

C. Mirtazapine

Mirtazapine is an α_2-antagonist that enhances central noradrenergic and serotonergic activity.

1. Indications—It is approved for the treatment of major depression in adults.

2. Contraindications—Mirtazapine should not be given in combination with monoamine oxidase inhibitors. Very rare side effects are acute liver failure (1 case per 250,000–300,000), neutropenia, and agranulocytosis.

3. Initial medical screening and follow-up—General medical examination.

4. Adverse effects—Dry mouth, increased appetite, constipation, weight gain.

D. Duloxetine

Duloxetine is a selective serotonin and norepinephrine reuptake inhibitor.

1. Indications—It is approved for the treatment of major depression, generalized anxiety disorder, and diabetic peripheral neuropathic pain in adults.

2. Contraindications—Duloxetine should not be given in combination with monoamine oxidase inhibitors. Very rare side effects are orthostatic hypotension and liver toxicity.

3. Initial medical screening and follow-up—General medical examination.

4. Adverse effects—Nausea, dizziness, dry mouth, and fatigue.

E. Olanzapine and Fluoxetine HCl Capsules (Symbyax)

Symbyax (olanzapine and fluoxetine HCl capsules) combines an atypical antipsychotic (olanzapine) and an SSRI (fluoxetine hydrochloride).

1. Indications—It is approved for the treatment of bipolar depression and treatment-resistant depression in adults.

2. Contraindications—It should not be given in combination with monoamine oxidase inhibitors. Other contraindications are consistent with SSRIs and atypical antipsychotics.

3. Initial medical screening and follow-up—General medical examination. See SSRIs and Atypical Antipsychotics sections.

4. Adverse effects—Nausea, dizziness, dry mouth, and fatigue.

3. Tricyclic Antidepressants

Imipramine
Desipramine
Clomipramine
Nortriptyline
Amitriptyline

With the introduction of the SSRIs and alternative antidepressants, use of the TCAs has become uncommon for the treatment of depression and anxiety disorders. The TCAs have more significant side-effect profiles, require more substantial medical monitoring, and are quite cardiotoxic in overdose. For these reasons, in general, SSRIs or alternative antidepressants should be considered before recommending a TCA. In some countries, where access to newer and more costly medications is difficult, TCAs are still frequently employed for certain behavioral, emotional, and functional conditions.

1. Indications—TCAs have been prescribed for chronic pain syndromes, migraines, headache, depression, anxiety, enuresis, bulimia nervosa, OCD, and PTSD in children and adolescents. Imipramine and desipramine have FDA approval for the treatment of major depression in adults and for enuresis in children age 6 years and older. Some published studies have demonstrated clinical efficacy in the treatment of ADHD, panic disorder, anxiety-based school refusal, separation anxiety disorder, bulimia, night terrors, and sleepwalking. But as yet, the FDA has not approved their use for these indications. Studies have not supported efficacy in major depression in children and adolescents. Nortriptyline has FDA approval for the treatment of major depression in adults. Clomipramine has FDA approval for the treatment of depression and OCD in adults and may be helpful for obsessive symptoms in autism.

2. Contraindications—Known cardiac disease or arrhythmia, undiagnosed syncope, known seizure disorder, family history of sudden cardiac death or cardiomyopathy, known electrolyte abnormality (with bingeing and purging).

3. Initial medical screening—The family history should be examined for sudden cardiac death; the patient's history for cardiac disease, arrhythmias, syncope, seizure disorder, or congenital hearing loss (associated with prolonged QT interval). Other screening procedures include serum electrolytes and blood urea nitrogen in patients who have eating disorders, cardiac examination, and a baseline ECG.

4. Medical follow-up—Measure pulse and blood pressure (monitor for tachycardia and orthostatic hypotension) with each dosage increase, and obtain an ECG to monitor for arteriovenous block with each dosage increase; after reaching steady state, record pulse, blood pressure, and ECG every 3–4 months.

5. Adverse effects

A. CARDIOTOXIC EFFECTS—The cardiotoxic effects of TCAs appear to be more common in children and adolescents than in adults. In addition to anticholinergic effects, TCAs have quinidine-like effects that result in slowing of cardiac conduction. Increased plasma levels appear to be weakly associated with an increased risk of cardiac conduction abnormalities. Steady-state plasma levels of desipramine or of desipramine plus imipramine should therefore not exceed 300 ng/mL. In addition, for each dosage increase above 3 mg/kg/d, pulse and blood pressure must be carefully checked and repeated ECGs be obtained to monitor for arteriovenous block. Upper limits for cardiovascular parameters when administering TCAs to children and adolescents are listed in Table 7–18.

B. ANTICHOLINERGIC EFFECTS—Tachycardia, dry mouth, stuffy nose, blurred vision, constipation, sweating, vasomotor instability, withdrawal syndrome (GI distress and psychomotor activation).

C. OTHER EFFECTS—Orthostatic hypotension and dizziness, lowered seizure threshold, increased appetite and weight gain, sedation, irritability and psychomotor agitation, rash (often associated with yellow dye No. 5), headache, abdominal complaints, sleep disturbance and nightmares, mania.

6. Drug interactions—TCAs may potentiate the effects of central nervous system depressants and stimulants; barbiturates and cigarette smoking may decrease plasma levels; phenothiazines, methylphenidate, and oral contraceptives may increase plasma levels; SSRIs given in combination with TCAs will result in higher TCA blood levels due to inhibition of TCA metabolism by liver enzymes (eg, cytochrome P-450 isoenzymes).

7. Dosage—Refer to a pediatric psychopharmacology text for dosages. Daily dosage requirements vary considerably with different clinical disorders.

Table 7–18. Upper limits of cardiovascular parameters with tricyclic antidepressants.

Heart rate	130/min
Systolic blood pressure	130 mm Hg
Diastolic blood pressure	85 mm Hg
PR interval	0.2 s
QRS interval	0.12 s, or no more than 30% over baseline
QT corrected	0.45 s

MOOD STABILIZERS AND ATYPICAL ANTIPSYCHOTICS

Mood Stabilizers

Carbamazepine (Tegretol), oxcarbazepine (Trileptal)

Gabapentin (Neurontin)

Lamotrigine (Lamictal)

Lithium carbonate (Eskalith, Eskalith CR, Lithobid, Lithotabs)

Valproic acid (Depakote, Depakote ER)

Atypical Antipsychotics

Aripiprazole (Abilify)

Olanzapine (Zyprexa)

Risperidone (Risperdal) (Risperdal Consta [IM]); paliperidone (Invega)

Quetiapine (Seroquel) (Seroquel XR)

Ziprasidone (Geodon)

Lithium and antiepileptic medications have historically been the drugs of choice for mood stabilization in bipolar mood disorder. New research also finds that the atypical antipsychotic medications are also effective. Lithium, valproic acid, olanzapine, risperidone, aripiprazole, and ziprasidone are FDA approved for the treatment of adult bipolar disorder. Carbamazepine and oxcarbazepine, although not FDA approved for treatment of bipolar disorder, may also be effective and carry less risk of weight gain. Lamotrigine (Lamictal) was recently approved for the treatment of bipolar depression in adults. Other antiepileptic medications, such as gabapentin and topiramate, have also been used with varying efficacy. Medications that are effective as mood stabilizers may be helpful also in the treatment of severe aggressive symptoms.

A. Lithium

1. Indications—Lithium remains a front-line drug in the treatment of bipolar disorder and has been shown to have an augmenting effect when combined with SSRIs for treatment-resistant depression and OCD.

2. Contraindications—Lithium is contraindicated in patients with known renal, thyroid, or cardiac disease; those at high risk for dehydration and electrolyte imbalance (eg, vomiting and purging); and those who may become pregnant (teratogenic effects).

3. Initial medical screening—General medical screening with pulse, blood pressure, height, and weight; complete blood cell count (CBC); serum electrolytes, blood urea nitrogen, and creatinine; and thyroid function tests, including thyroid-stimulating hormone levels.

4. Dosage—For children the starting dose is usually 150 mg once or twice a day, with titration in 150- to 300-mg increments. (Dose may vary with the brand of lithium used; consult a psychopharmacology textbook for medication-specific information.) Oral doses of lithium should be titrated to maintain therapeutic blood levels of 0.8–1.2 mEq/L. The drug is generally given in two doses. Blood samples should be drawn 12 hours after the last dose.

5. Adverse effects

A. LITHIUM TOXICITY—Lithium has a narrow therapeutic index. Blood levels required for therapeutic effects are close to those associated with toxic symptoms. Mild toxicity may be indicated by increased tremor, GI distress, neuromuscular irritability, and altered mental status (confusion), and can occur when blood levels exceed 1.5 mEq/L. Moderate to severe symptoms of lithium toxicity are associated with blood levels above 2 mEq/L. Acute renal failure can occur at levels over 2.5–3 mEq/L. Given its low therapeutic index, a provider should be cautious in patients with a known overdose history or current risk. Lithium toxicity is a medical emergency and hemodialysis may be indicated for supertoxic levels.

B. SIDE EFFECTS—Lithium side effects include intention tremor, GI distress (including nausea and vomiting and sometimes diarrhea), hypothyroidism, polyuria and polydipsia, drowsiness, malaise, weight gain, acne, and granulocytosis.

6. Drug interactions—Excessive salt intake and salt restriction should be avoided. Thiazide diuretics and nonsteroidal anti-inflammatory agents (except aspirin and acetaminophen) can lead to increased lithium levels. Ibuprofen should be avoided by individuals who take lithium due to combined renal toxicity. Precautions against dehydration are required in hot weather and during vigorous exercise.

7. Medical follow-up—Serum lithium levels should be measured 5–7 days following a change in dosage and then quarterly at steady state; serum creatinine and thyroid-stimulating hormone concentrations should be determined every 3–4 months.

B. Valproic Acid

1. Indications—Valproate has FDA approval for the treatment of bipolar disorder in adults. Its efficacy in acute mania equals that of lithium, but it is generally better tolerated. Valproate is more effective than lithium in patients with rapid-cycling bipolar disorder (more than four cycles per year) and in patients with mixed states (coexisting symptoms of depression and mania). Valproate may be more effective than lithium in adolescents with bipolar disorder because they often have rapid cycling and mixed states.

2. Contraindications—Liver dysfunction.

3. Initial medical screening—CBC and liver function tests (LFTs).

4. Dosage—The starting dose is usually 15 mg/kg/d. This is increased in increments of 5–10 mg/kg/d every 1–2 weeks to a range of 500–1500 mg/d in two or three divided doses. Trough levels in the range of 80–120 mg/mL are thought to be therapeutic.

5. Adverse effects—Between 10% and 20% of patients experience sedation or anorexia, especially early in treatment or if the dose is increased too rapidly. GI upset occurs in 25% of patients, and when severe, can usually be treated with cimetidine. Increased appetite and weight gain can be troublesome for children and adolescents. Blurred vision, headache, hair loss, and tremor occur occasionally. Slight elevations in aminotransferases are frequent. Severe idiosyncratic hepatitis, pancreatitis, thrombocytopenia, and agranulocytosis occur only rarely.

6. Medical follow-up—LFTs should be checked monthly for 3–4 months; subsequently, LFTs, a CBC, and trough valproate levels should be obtained every 3–4 months.

C. Carbamazepine/Oxcarbazepine

1. Indications—Similar to lithium and valproate, carbamazepine may be effective for treating bipolar disorder or for the target symptoms of mood instability, irritability, or behavioral dyscontrol. Some data suggest that it is more effective than valproate for the depressive phases of bipolar disorder. A new form of carbamazepine—oxcarbazepine (Trileptal)—is also rarely being used for pediatric mood disorders; however, its efficacy has not been established. Reportedly, it does not have the worrisome side effects of bone marrow suppression and liver enzyme induction. Blood levels cannot be monitored, and the dose range is similar to that of carbamazepine.

2. Contraindications—History of previous bone marrow depression or adverse hematologic reaction to another drug; history of sensitivity to a TCA.

3. Initial medical screening—Obtain a CBC with platelets, reticulocytes, serum iron, and blood urea nitrogen; LFTs; urinalysis.

4. Dosage—The drug is usually started at 10–20 mg/kg/d, in two divided doses, in children younger than 6 years; 100 mg twice daily in children aged 6–12 years; and 200 mg twice daily in children older than 12 years. Doses may be increased weekly until there is effective symptom control. Total daily doses should not exceed 35 mg/kg/d in children younger than 6 years; 1000 mg/d in children aged 6–15 years; and 1200 mg/d in adolescents older than 15 years. Plasma levels in the range of 4–12 mg/mL are thought to be therapeutic.

5. Adverse effects—Nausea, dizziness, sedation, headache, dry mouth, diplopia, and constipation reflect the drug's mild anticholinergic properties. Rashes are more common with carbamazepine than with other mood stabilizers. Aplastic anemia and agranulocytosis are rare. Leukopenia and thrombocytopenia are more common, and if present, should be monitored closely for evidence of bone marrow depression. These effects usually occur early and transiently and then spontaneously revert toward normal. Liver enzyme induction may significantly change the efficacy of medications given concurrently.

6. Medical follow-up—Hematologic, hepatic, and renal parameters should be followed at least every 3 months for the first year. White blood cell counts (WBCs) below 3000/mL and absolute neutrophil counts below 1000/mL call for discontinuation of the drug and referral for hematology consultation.

D. Lamotrigine

Lamotrigine is approved for the treatment of bipolar depression in adults. The most concerning side effects of this medication are serious rashes that can require hospitalization and can include Stevens-Johnson syndrome (0.8% incidence). Lamotrigine should be used very carefully. The starting dose is 25 mg, with a slow titration of increasing the dose by 25 mg/wk to a target dose (as clinically indicated) of 300 mg/d.

E. Gabapentin

Like valproate and carbamazepine, gabapentin is an anticonvulsant that has been used as a mood stabilizer in some adult populations. It may be used along with either valproate or carbamazepine in individuals with treatment-resistant disorders. The usual adult dose range for seizure disorders is 900–1800 mg/d in three divided doses and may need to be adjusted downward in individuals with renal impairment. Although its use among adolescents and even children is increasing, gabapentin is not approved for this indication, and reports of its efficacy remain largely anecdotal. Some reports suggest it may worsen behavioral parameters in children with underlying ADHD.

ANTIPSYCHOTICS

Atypical Antipsychotics

Aripiprazole (Abilify)

Clozapine (Clozaril)

Olanzapine (Zyprexa)

Risperidone (Risperdal), Risperidone Consta (IM), Paliperidone (Invega)

Quetiapine (Seroquel), Quetiapine XR (Seroquel XR)

Ziprasidone (Geodon)

Conventional Neuroleptics

Chlorpromazine

Haloperidol

Molindone

Perphenazine

Thioridazine

Thiothixene

Trifluoperazine

The antipsychotics, formerly known as neuroleptics, are indicated for psychotic symptoms in patients with schizophrenia. Some now have an FDA-approved indication for bipolar affective disorder in adults (risperidone and olanzapine). They are also used for acute mania and as adjuncts to antidepressants in the treatment of psychotic depression (with delusions or hallucinations). The antipsychotics may be used cautiously in refractory PTSD, in refractory OCD, and in individuals with markedly aggressive behavioral problems unresponsive to other interventions. They may also be useful for the body image distortion and irrational fears about food and weight gain associated with anorexia nervosa.

The "atypical antipsychotics" differ from conventional antipsychotics in their receptor specificity and effect on serotonin receptors. Conventional antipsychotics are associated with a higher incidence of movement disorders and extrapyramidal symptoms (EPS) due to their wider effect on dopamine receptors. The introduction of the atypical antipsychotics has significantly changed neuroleptic prescribing patterns. The atypical antipsychotics have a better side-effect profile for most individuals and comparable efficacy for the treatment of psychotic symptoms and aggression. Atypical antipsychotics have a decreased incidence of EPS and tardive dyskinesia (TD). Significant side effects can include substantial weight gain and sedation. Because of their increased use over conventional antipsychotics, this section focuses primarily on the atypical antipsychotics.

A. Aripiprazole

Aripiprazole (Abilify) is the newest atypical neuroleptic and is indicated for the treatment of adults with schizophrenia and bipolar disorder. It is a partial dopamine blocker and a serotonin agonist. Side effects include nausea and vomiting and fatigue. It is associated with minimal weight gain. Doses over 30 mg are more likely to be associated with EPS. The dose range is 5–30 mg, and pills can be split.

B. Olanzapine

The FDA has approved this agent for the treatment of schizophrenia and bipolar disorder in adults. Olanzapine (Zyprexa) has greater affinity for type 2 serotonin receptors than dopamine-2 receptors and also has an effect on muscarinic, histaminic, and α-adrenergic receptors. As with the other atypical antipsychotics, it may be more helpful for treating the negative symptoms of schizophrenia (flat affect, isolation and withdrawal, and apathy) than conventional antipsychotics. Anecdotal and case report data support its utility in child and adolescent psychotic disorders. The adult dose range of 5–15 mg/d administered in a single bedtime dose is probably applicable to adolescents as well. Weight gain can be a significant side effect. The starting dose for children is usually 1.25 mg.

C. Quetiapine

Quetiapine (Seroquel) is an antagonist at multiple receptor sites, including serotonin (5-HT_{1A} and 5-HT_2), dopamine (D_1 and D_2), histamine, and adrenergic receptors. Quetiapine is given in 25- to 50-mg increments up to 800 mg for the treatment of psychotic symptoms. It is thought to be a weight-neutral medication, and the primary side effect is sedation. It also comes in an extended-release preparation (XR).

D. Risperidone

Risperidone (Risperdal) blocks type 2 dopamine receptors (similarly to haloperidol) and type 2 serotonin receptors. It is approved for the treatment of schizophrenia and bipolar affective disorder in adults. Risperidone has also demonstrated clinical efficacy in the treatment of Tourette syndrome. The initial dose is 1–2 mg/d. It is typically titrated up in 0.5- to 1-mg increments to a maximum dose of 4–10 mg for psychotic disorders. Side effects include weight gain and sedation. A dissolvable tablet (m-tab) and a long-acting OROS version of the major active metabolite of risperidone is also available (paliperidone). An intramuscular injectable form (Consta) is available for long-term management of bipolar disorder and schizophrenia in adults and is given every 2 weeks.

E. Ziprasidone

Ziprasidone (Geodon) has affinity for multiple serotonin receptors (5-HT_2, 5-HT_{1A}, 5-HT_{1D}, and 5-HT_{2C}) and dopamine-2 receptors, and it moderately inhibits norepinephrine and serotonin reuptake. It also has moderate affinity for H_1 and α_1 receptors. Ziprasidone has a greater effect on cardiac QT intervals and requires a baseline ECG and ECG monitoring when a dose of 80 mg is reached and with each dose change above 80 mg to monitor for QT prolongation. Ziprasidone is reported to cause minimal weight gain. The initial dose is 20 mg, with dose changes in 20-mg increments to a total daily dose of 140 mg for the treatment of psychotic symptoms in adults. There are no studies of ziprasidone in children and adolescents at this time.

F. Clozapine

Clozapine (Clozaril) is usually reserved for individuals who have not responded to multiple other antipsychotics due to its side effect of agranulocytosis. Clozapine blocks type 2 dopamine receptors weakly and is virtually free of EPS, apparently including TD. It was very effective in about 40% of adult patients with chronic schizophrenia who did not respond to conventional antipsychotics.

Non-dose-related agranulocytosis occurs in 0.5–2% of subjects. Some case reports note benefit from clozapine in child and adolescent schizophrenic patients who were resistant to other treatment. Contraindications are concurrent treatment with carbamazepine and any history of leukopenia. Initial medical screening should include a CBC and LFTs. The daily dose is 200–600 mg in two divided doses. Because of the risk of neutropenia, patients taking clozapine must be registered with the Clozapine Registry and a WBC must be obtained biweekly before a 2-week supply of the drug is dispensed. If the white count falls below 3000/mL, clozapine is usually discontinued. Other side effects include sedation, weight gain, and increased salivation. The incidence of seizures increases with doses above 600 mg/d.

General Antipsychotic Information

The following adverse effects of antipsychotics apply to both typical and atypical antipsychotics, but are thought to have a significantly lower incidence with the atypical antipsychotics.

1. Initial medical screening—One should observe and examine for tremors and other abnormal involuntary movements and establish baseline values for CBC and LFTs. An ECG should be obtained if there is a history of cardiac disease or arrhythmia, and to establish a baseline QT interval (cardiac repolarization) prior to initiation of the antipsychotics that have a greater effect on the QT interval (eg, ziprasidone and thioridazine). Antipsychotics can cause QT prolongation leading to ventricular arrhythmias, such as torsades de pointes. Medications that affect the cytochrome P-450 isoenzyme pathway (including SSRIs) may increase the neuroleptic plasma concentration and increase risk of QTc prolongation.

2. Adverse effects—The most troublesome adverse effects of the atypical antipsychotics are cognitive slowing, sedation, orthostasis, and weight gain. The conventional antipsychotics have an increased incidence of EPS and TD. Sedation, cognitive slowing, and EPS all tend to be dose-related. Because of the risk of side effects, neuroleptic medications should be used with caution and monitored regularly. The risk-benefit ratio of the medication for the identified target symptom should be carefully considered and reviewed with the parent or guardian.

A. Weight gain, hyperglycemia, hyperlipidemia, and diabetes mellitus—In postmarketing clinical use, there have been significant reports of weight gain, hyperglycemia, and diabetes mellitus. This led to a consensus statement by concerned professional societies about how best to monitor and manage these significant side effects.

Table 7–19. Health monitoring and antipsychotics.

	After Initiation			Thereafter[a]		
Baseline	**4 wk**	**8 wk**	**12 wk**	**Quarterly**	**Annually**	**q5y**
Personal/ family history					✓	
Weight (BMI)	✓	✓	✓	✓		
Waist circumference					✓	
BP			✓		✓	
Fasting blood sugar			✓		✓	
Fasting lipid profile			✓			✓

[a]More frequent assessments may be warranted based on clinical status.

Table 7–19 presents the currently recommended monitoring calendar. Baseline and ongoing evaluations of significant markers are considered standard clinical practice.

B. Extrapyramidal side effects—EPS and acute dystonic reactions are tonic muscle spasms, often of the tongue, jaw, or neck. EPS symptoms can be mildly uncomfortable or may result in such dramatically distressing symptoms as oculogyric crisis, torticollis, and even opisthotonos. Onset is usually within days after a dosage change and symptoms may occur in up to 25% of children treated with conventional antipsychotics. Acute neuroleptic-induced dystonias are quickly relieved by anticholinergics such as benztropine (Cogentin) and diphenhydramine.

C. Tardive dyskinesias—TDs are involuntary movement disorders that are often irreversible and may appear after long-term use of neuroleptic medications. Choreoathetoid movements of the tongue and mouth are most common, but the extremities and trunk may also be involved. The risk of TD is small in patients on atypical antipsychotics, and those on conventional antipsychotics for less than 6 months. There is no universally effective treatment.

D. Pseudoparkinsonism—Pseudoparkinsonism is usually manifested 1–4 weeks after the start of treatment. It presents as muscle stiffness, cogwheel rigidity, masklike facial expression, bradykinesia, drooling, and occasionally pill-rolling tremor. Anticholinergic medications or dosage reductions are helpful.

E. Akathisia—Akathisia is usually manifested after 1–6 weeks of treatment. It presents as an unpleasant feeling of driven motor restlessness that ranges from vague muscular discomfort to a markedly dysphoric agitation with frantic pacing. Anticholinergic agents or β-blockers are sometimes helpful.

F. Neuroleptic malignant syndrome—Neuroleptic malignant syndrome is a very rare medical emergency associated primarily with the conventional antipsychotics, although it has also been reported with atypical antipsychotics. It is manifested by severe muscular rigidity, mental status changes, fever, autonomic lability, and myoglobinemia. Neuroleptic malignant syndrome can occur without muscle rigidity in patients taking atypical antipsychotics and should be considered in the differential diagnosis of any patient on antipsychotics who presents with high fever and altered mental status. Mortality as high as 30% has been reported. Treatment includes immediate medical assessment, withdrawal of the neuroleptic, and may require transfer to an intensive care unit.

G. Withdrawal dyskinesias—Withdrawal dyskinesias are reversible movement disorders that appear following withdrawal of neuroleptic medications. Dyskinetic movements develop within 1–4 weeks after withdrawal of the drug and may persist for months.

H. Other adverse effects—These include cardiac arrhythmias, irregular menses, gynecomastia, and galactorrhea due to increased prolactin, sexual dysfunction, photosensitivity, rashes, lowered seizure threshold, hepatic dysfunction, and blood dyscrasias.

3. Drug interactions—Potentiation of central nervous system depressant effects or the anticholinergic effects of other drugs may occur, as well as increased plasma levels of antidepressants.

4. Medical follow-up—The patient should be examined at least every 3 months for signs of the side effects listed. An Abnormal Involuntary Movement Scale can be used to monitor for TD in patients taking antipsychotics. Most antipsychotic treatments seem to be associated with relevant weight gain, which increases the risk of the development of metabolic syndrome and future cardiovascular morbidity and mortality. New recommendations include quarterly monitoring of blood pressure, weight gain, abdominal circumference, dietary and exercise habits, and, if indicated, fasting blood glucose and lipid panels. In cases of significant weight gain or abnormal laboratory values, patients should either be switched to an agent with a decreased risk for these adverse events or should receive additional treatments to reduce specific adverse events in cases in which discontinuation of the offending agent is clinically contraindicated or unfeasible.

ADRENERGIC AGONISTS

Clonidine (Catapres) & Guanfacine (Tenex)

1. Indications—Clonidine is a nonselective α-adrenergic agonist that is clinically useful in decreasing states of hyperarousal seen in children and adolescents with PTSD and ADHD. Guanfacine is a selective agonist for α_2-adrenergic receptors with advantages over the nonselective agonist clonidine. Guanfacine is less sedating and less hypotensive than clonidine and has a longer half-life, allowing for twice-daily dosing. Case reports find guanfacine effective in ADHD and in Tourette syndrome with comorbid ADHD. Bedtime doses of adrenergic agonists can be helpful for the delayed onset of sleep and nightmares that can occur with PTSD, for the difficulty settling for sleep seen in ADHD, or for ameliorating the side effects of stimulant medications. These agents are also effective in the treatment of tics in Tourette syndrome.

2. Contraindications—Adrenergic agonists are contraindicated in patients with known renal or cardiovascular disease and in those with a family or personal history of depression.

3. Initial medical screening—The pulse and blood pressure should be recorded prior to starting an adrenergic agonist.

4. Dosage—The initial dosage of clonidine is usually 0.025–0.05 mg at bedtime. The dosage can be increased after 3–5 days by giving 0.05 mg in the morning. Further dosage increases are made by adding 0.05 mg first in the morning, then at noon, and then in the evening every 3–5 days to a maximum total daily dose of 0.3 mg in three or four divided doses per day. The half-life of clonidine is in the range of 3–4 hours. Although a clinical response generally becomes apparent by about 4 weeks, treatment effects may increase over 2–3 months. Therapeutic doses of methylphenidate can frequently be decreased by 30%–50% when used in conjunction with clonidine. Transdermal administration of clonidine using a skin patch can be quite effective but may result in skin irritation in 40% of patients. Patches are generally changed every 5 days.

The starting dosage of guanfacine is usually 0.5–1 mg once a day, increasing as clinically indicated after 3–5 days to 2–4 mg/d in two or three divided doses per day. The new longer acting preparation, Intuniv, is dosed once daily from 1 mg to 4 mg per day and is FDA approved for the treatment of ADHD in children older than 6 years of age. Adverse effects include transient headaches and stomach aches in 25% of patients. Sedation and hypertension are mild. For medical follow-up, pulse and blood pressure should be checked every 1–2 weeks for 2 months and then at 3-month intervals.

5. Adverse effects—Sedation can be prominent. Side effects include fatigability, dizziness associated with hypotension, increased appetite and weight gain, headache, sleep disturbance, GI distress, skin irritation with transdermal clonidine administration, and rebound hypertension with abrupt withdrawal. Bradycardia can occasionally be marked.

6. Drug interactions—Increased sedation with central nervous system depressants; possible increased anticholinergic toxicity. Several case reports have mentioned cardiac toxicity with clonidine when combined with methylphenidate, although other medications and clinical factors were present in each case.

7. Medical follow-up—Pulse and blood pressure should be recorded every 2 weeks for 2 months and then every 3 months. The discontinuation of clonidine or guanfacine should occur gradually, with stepwise dosage decreases every 3–5 days to avoid rebound hypertension. Blood pressure should be monitored during withdrawal.

Antonuccio D: Treating depressed children with antidepressants: More harm than benefit? J Clin Psychol Med Settings 2008 Jun;15(2):92–97. Erratum in: J Clin Psychol Med Settings 2008 Sep;15(3):260 [PMID: 19104973].

Apter A et al: Evaluation of suicidal thoughts and behaviors in children and adolescents taking paroxetine. J Child Adolesc Psychopharmacol 2006 Feb–Apr;16(1–2):77–90 [PMID: 16553530].

Armenteros JL, Davies M: Antipsychotics in early onset Schizophrenia: Systematic review and meta-analysis. Eur Child Adolesc Psychiatry 2006 Mar;15(3):141–148 [Epub 2006 Feb 9] [PMID: 16470340].

Azorin JM, Findling RL: Valproate use in children and adolescents with bipolar disorder. CNS Drugs 2007;21(12):1019–1033 [PMID: 18020481].

Barzman DH, Findling RL: Pharmacological treatment of pathologic aggression in children. Int Rev Psychiatry 2008 Apr;20(2):151–157 [Review] [PMID: 18386205].

Biederman J et al: Treatment of ADHD with stimulant medications: Response to Nissen perspective in the New England Journal of Medicine. J Am Acad Child Adolesc Psychiatry 2006 Oct;45(10):1147–1150 [PMID: 16840880].

Bridge JA et al: Placebo response in randomized controlled trials of antidepressants for pediatric major depressive disorder. Am J Psychiatry 2009 Jan;166(1):42–49 [PMID: 19047322].

Chang KD: The use of atypical antipsychotics in pediatric bipolar disorder. J Clin Psychiatry 2008;69(Suppl 4):4–8 [PMID: 18533762].

Correll CU: Assessing and maximizing the safety and tolerability of antipsychotics used in the treatment of children and adolescents. J Clin Psychiatry 2008;69(Suppl 4):26–36 [PMID: 18533766].

Correll CU, Kratochvil CJ, March JS. Developments in pediatric psychopharmacology: Focus on stimulants, antidepressants, and antipsychotics. J Clin Psychiatry 2011 May;72(5):655–670 [PMID: 21658348].

Daughton JM, Kratochvil CJ: Review of ADHD pharmacotherapies: Advantages, disadvantages, and clinical pearls. J Am Acad Child Adolesc Psychiatry 2009 Mar;48(3):240–248 [PMID: 19242289].

Dudley M et al: New-generation antidepressants, suicide and depressed adolescents: How should clinicians respond to changing evidence? Aust N Z J Psychiatry 2008 Jun;42(6): 456–466 [PMID: 18465372].

Findling RL et al: Is there a role for clozapine in the treatment of children and adolescents? J Am Acad Child Adolesc Psychiatry 2007 Mar;46(3):423–428 [PMID: 17314729].

Correll CU, Kratochvil CJ, March JS: Developments in pediatric psychopharmacology: Focus on stimulants, antidepressants, and antipsychotics. J Clin Psychiatry 2011 May;72(5):655–670 [PMID: 21658348].

Gilbert D: Treatment of children and adolescents with tics and Tourette syndrome. J Child Neurol 2006 Aug;21(8):690–700 [PMID: 16970870].

Hammerness P, McCarthy K, Mancuso E, Gendron C, Geller D: Atomoxetine for the treatment of attention-deficit/hyperactivity disorder in children and adolescents: A review. Neuropsychiatr Dis Treat 2009;5:215–226 [PMID:19557116].

Henry K, Harris CR: Deadly ingestions. Pediatr Clin North Am 2006 Apr;53(2):293–315 [PMID: 16574527].

Hughes CW et al: Texas Children's Medication Algorithm Project: Update from Texas Consensus Conference Panel on Medication Treatment of Childhood Major Depressive Disorder. Texas Consensus Conference Panel on Medication Treatment of Childhood Major Depressive Disorder. J Am Acad Child Adolesc Psychiatry 2007 Jun;46(6):667–686 [PMID: 17513980].

Jensen PS et al: Management of psychiatric disorders in children and adolescents with atypical antipsychotics: A systematic review of published clinical trials. Eur Child Adolesc Psychiatry 2007 Mar;16(2):104–120 [Epub 2006 Oct 30] [PMID: 17075688].

Lopez-Larson M, Frazier JA: Empirical evidence for the use of lithium and anticonvulsants in children with psychiatric disorders. Harv Rev Psychiatry 2006 Nov–Dec;14(6):285–304 [PMID: 17162653].

Mancuso E, Faro A, Joshi G, Geller DA: Treatment of pediatric obsessive-compulsive disorder: A review. J Child Adolesc Psychopharmacol 2010 Aug;20(4):299–308 [PMID: 20807068].

McVoy M, Findling R: Child and adolescent psychopharmacology update. Psychiatr Clin North Am 2009 Mar;32(1):111–133 [PMID: 19248920].

Moreno C, Roche AM, Greenhill LL: Pharmacotherapy of child and adolescent depression. Child Adolesc Psychiatr Clin N Am 2006 Oct;15(4):977–998, x [PMID: 16952771].

Nevels RM, Dehon EE, Alexander K, Gontkovsky ST: Psychopharmacology of aggression in children and adolescents with primary neuropsychiatric disorders: A review of current and potentially promising treatment options. Exp Clin Psychopharmacol 2010 Apr;18(2):184–201 [PMID: 20384430].

Posey DJ, McDougle CJ: Guanfacine and guanfacine extended release: Treatment for ADHD and related disorders. CNS Drug Rev 2007 Winter;13(4):465–474 [PMID: 18078429].

Thomas T, Stansifer L, Findling RL: Psychopharmacology of pediatric bipolar disorders in children and adolescents. Pediatr Clin North Am 2011 Feb;58(1):173–187, xii [PMID: 21281855].

Tsapakis EM et al: Efficacy of antidepressants in juvenile depression: Meta-analysis. Br J Psychiatry 2008 Jul;193(1):10–17 [PMID: 18700212].

Usala T et al: Randomised controlled trials of selective serotonin reuptake inhibitors in treating depression in children and adolescents: A systematic review and meta-analysis. Eur Neuropsychopharmacol 2008 Jan;18(1):62–73 [PMID: 17662579].

Vitiello B: An international perspective on pediatric psychopharmacology. Int Rev Psychiatry 2008 Apr;20(2):121–126 [PMID: 18386201].

Handout for monitoring side effects of Atypical Antipsychotics. Available at: http://webspace.psychiatry.wisc.edu/walaszek/geropsych/docs/atypical-antipsychotic.doc

Child Abuse & Neglect

8

Antonia Chiesa, MD
Andrew P. Sirotnak, MD

ESSENTIALS OF DIAGNOSIS

- Forms of maltreatment:
  - Physical abuse.
  - Sexual abuse.
  - Emotional abuse and neglect.
  - Physical neglect.
  - Medical care neglect.
  - Munchausen syndrome by proxy (medical child abuse).
- Common historical features in child physical abuse cases:
  - Implausible mechanism provided for an injury.
  - Discrepant, evolving, or absent history.
  - Delay in seeking care.
  - Event or behavior by a child that triggers a loss of control by the caregiver.
  - History of abuse in the caregiver's childhood.
  - Inappropriate affect of the caregiver.
  - Pattern of increasing severity or number of injuries if no intervention.
  - Social or physical isolation of the child or the caregiver.
  - Stress or crisis in the family or the caregiver.
  - Unrealistic expectations of caregiver for the child.
  - Behavior changes of child.

In 2009, an estimated 3.3 million referrals were made to child protective service agencies, involving the alleged maltreatment of approximately 6.0 million children. The total number of children confirmed as maltreated by child protective services was 702,000 in 2009, yielding an abuse victimization rate of 9.3 per 1000 American children. (This statistic is referred to as the "unique count" where a child is counted only once regardless of the number of times the child is substantiated as a victim.) This is the lowest victimization rate over the previous five year period. There were 1676 victims of fatal child abuse in 2009 from 49 states, resulting in a rate of 2.34 child abuse deaths per 100,000 children. Based on this information, it is estimated that nationally 1770 children died from abuse and neglect. While rates of physical and sexual abuse have declined recently, fatalities from abuse have not.

Substance abuse, poverty and economic strains, parental capacity and skills, and domestic violence are cited as the most common presenting problems in abusive families. Abuse and neglect of children are best considered in an ecological perspective, which recognizes the individual, family, social, and psychological influences that come together to contribute to the problem. Kempe and Helfer termed this the *abusive pattern*, in which the child, the crisis, and the caregiver's potential to abuse are components in the event of maltreatment. This chapter focuses on the knowledge necessary for the recognition, intervention, and follow-up of the more common forms of child maltreatment and highlights the role of pediatric professionals in prevention.

U.S. Department of Health and Human Services: Administration for Children, Youth, and Families. Child Maltreatment 2009. Available at: http://www.acf.hhs.gov/programs/cb/pubs/cmo9/index.htm. Accessed August 2, 2010.

PREVENTION

Physical abuse is preventable in many cases. Extensive experience with and evaluation of high-risk families have shown that the home visitor services to families at risk can prevent abuse and neglect of children. These services can be provided by public health nurses or trained paraprofessionals, although more data are available describing public health nurse intervention. The availability of these services could make it as easy for a family to pick up the telephone and ask for help before they abuse a child as it is for a neighbor or physician to report an episode of abuse after it has occurred. Parent education and anticipatory guidance are also helpful, with attention to handling situations that stress parents (eg, colic, crying behavior, and toilet training), age-appropriate discipline, and general developmental issues. Prevention of abusive injuries perpetrated by nonparent caregivers (eg, babysitters, nannies, and unrelated adults in the home) may be addressed by education and counseling of mothers about safe child care arrangements and choosing safe life partners. Promising new data suggest the efficacy of hospital-based programs that teach parents about the dangers of shaking an infant and how to respond to a crying infant.

The prevention of sexual abuse is more difficult. Most efforts in this area involve teaching children to protect themselves and their "private parts" from harm or interference. The age of toilet training is a good time to provide anticipatory guidance to encourage parents to begin this discussion. The most rational approach is to place the burden of responsibility of prevention on the adults who supervise the child and the medical providers rather than on the children themselves. Knowing the parents' own history of any victimization is important, as the ability to engage in this anticipatory guidance discussion with a provider and their child may be affected by that history. Promoting Internet safety and limiting exposure to sexualized materials and media should be part of this anticipatory guidance. Finally, many resource books on this topic for parents can be found in the parenting and health sections of most bookstores.

Efforts to prevent emotional abuse of children have been undertaken through extensive media campaigns. No data are available to assess the effectiveness of this approach. The primary care physician can promote positive, nurturing, and nonviolent behavior in parents. The message that they are role models for a child's behavior is important. Screening for domestic violence during discussions on discipline and home safety can be effective in identifying parents and children at risk.

Augustyn M, McAlister B: If we don't ask, they aren't going to tell: Screening for domestic violence. Contemp Pediatr 2005;22:43.

Cahill L, Sherman P: Child abuse and domestic violence. Pediatr Rev 2006;27:339–345 [PMID: 16950939].

Dias MS et al: Preventing abusive head trauma among infants and young children: A hospital-based, parent education program. Pediatrics 2005;115:e470 [PMID: 15805350].

Olds DL, Sadler L, Kitzman H: Programs for parents of infants and toddlers: Recent evidence from randomized trials. J Child Psychol Psychiatry 2007;48:355 [PMID: 17355402].

CLINICAL FINDINGS

Child maltreatment may occur either within or outside the family. The proportion of intrafamilial to extrafamilial cases varies with the type of abuse as well as the gender and age of the child. Each of the following conditions may exist as separate or concurrent diagnoses. Neglect is the most commonly reported and substantiated form of child maltreatment annually.

Recognition of any form of abuse and neglect of children can occur only if child abuse is considered in the differential diagnosis of the child's presenting medical condition. The approach to the family should be supportive, nonaccusatory, and empathetic. The individual who brings the child in for care may not have any involvement in the abuse. Approximately one-third of child abuse incidents occur in extrafamilial settings. Nevertheless, the assumption that the caregiver is "nice," combined with the failure to consider the possibility of abuse, can be costly and even fatal. Raising the possibility that a child has been abused is not the same as accusing the caregiver of being the abuser. The health professional who is examining the child can explain to the family that several possibilities might explain the child's injuries or abuse-related symptoms. If the family or presenting caregiver is not involved in the child's maltreatment, they may actually welcome the necessary report and investigation.

In all cases of abuse and neglect, a detailed psychosocial history is important because psychosocial factors may indicate risk for or confirm child maltreatment. This history should include information on who lives in the home, other caregivers, domestic violence, substance abuse, and prior family history of physical or sexual abuse. Inquiring about any previous involvement with social services or law enforcement can help to determine risk.

Physical Abuse

Physical abuse of children is most often inflicted by a caregiver or family member but occasionally by a stranger. The most common manifestations include bruises, burns, fractures, head trauma, and abdominal injuries. A small but significant number of unexpected pediatric deaths, particularly in infants and very young children (eg, sudden unexpected infant death), are related to physical abuse.

A. History

The medical diagnosis of physical abuse is based on the presence of a discrepant history, in which the history offered by the caregiver is not consistent with the clinical findings. The discrepancy may exist because the history is absent, partial, changing over time, or simply illogical or improbable. A careful past medical, birth, and family history should also be obtained in order to assess for any other medical condition that might affect the clinical presentation. The presence of a discrepant history should prompt a request for consultation with a multidisciplinary child protection team or a report to the child protective services agency. This agency is mandated by state law to investigate reports of suspected child abuse and neglect. Investigation by social services and possibly law enforcement officers, as well as a home visit, may be required to sort out the circumstances of the child's injuries.

B. Physical Findings

The findings on examination of physically abused children may include abrasions, alopecia (from hair pulling), bites, bruises, burns, dental trauma, fractures, lacerations, ligature marks, or scars. Injuries may be in multiple stages of healing. Bruises in physically abused children are sometimes patterned (eg, belt marks, looped cord marks, or grab or pinch marks) and are typically found over the soft tissue areas of the body. Toddlers or older children typically sustain accidental bruises over bony prominences such as shins and elbows. Any bruise in an infant not developmentally mobile should be viewed with concern. Of note, the dating of bruises is not reliable and should be approached cautiously. (Child abuse emergencies are listed in Table 8–1.) Lacerations of the frenulum or tongue and bruising of the lips may be associated with force feeding or blunt force trauma. Pathognomonic burn patterns include stocking or glove distribution; immersion burns of the buttocks, sometimes with a "doughnut hole" area of sparing; and branding burns such as with cigarettes or hot objects (eg, grill, curling iron, or lighter). The absence of splash marks or a pattern consistent with spillage may be helpful in differentiating accidental from nonaccidental scald burns.

Head and abdominal trauma may present with signs and symptoms consistent with those injuries. Inflicted head trauma (eg, shaken baby syndrome) and abdominal injuries may have no visible findings on examination. Symptoms can be subtle and may mimic other conditions such as gastroenteritis. Studies have documented that cases of inflicted head injury will be missed when practitioners fail to consider the diagnosis. The finding of retinal hemorrhages in an infant without an appropriate medical condition (eg, leukemia, congenital infection, or clotting disorder) should raise concern about possible inflicted head trauma. Retinal hemorrhages are not commonly seen after cardiopulmonary resuscitation in either infants or children.

Table 8–1. Potential child abuse medical emergencies.

Any infant with bruises (especially head, facial, or abdominal), burns, or fractures
Any infant or child younger than 2 years with a history of suspected "shaken baby" head trauma or other inflicted head injury
Any child who has sustained suspicious or known inflicted abdominal trauma
Any child with burns in stocking or glove distribution or in other unusual patterns, burns to the genitalia, and any unexplained burn injury
Any child with disclosure or sign of sexual assault within 48-72 h after the alleged event if the possibility of acute injury is present or if forensic evidence exists

C. Radiologic and Laboratory Findings

Certain radiologic findings are strong indicators of physical abuse. Examples are metaphyseal "corner" or "bucket handle" fractures of the long bones in infants, spiral fracture of the extremities in nonambulatory infants, rib fractures, spinous process fractures, and fractures in multiple stages of healing. Skeletal surveys in children aged 3 years or younger should be performed when a suspicious fracture is diagnosed. Computed tomography or magnetic resonance imaging findings of subdural hemorrhage in infants—in the absence of a clear accidental history—are highly correlated with abusive head trauma. Abdominal computed tomography is the preferred test in suspected abdominal trauma. Any infant or very young child with suspected abuse-related head or abdominal trauma should be evaluated immediately by an emergency physician or trauma surgeon.

Coagulation studies and a complete blood cell count with platelets are useful in children who present with multiple or severe bruising in different stages of healing. Coagulopathy conditions may confuse the diagnostic picture but can be excluded with a careful history, examination, laboratory screens, and hematologic consultation, if necessary.

American Academy of Pediatrics: *Visual Diagnosis of Child Abuse* [CD ROM]. 3rd ed. American Academy of Pediatrics, 2008.

American Academy of Pediatrics Section on Radiology: Diagnostic imaging of child abuse. Pediatrics 2009;123(5):1430–1435 [PMID: 19403511].

Christian CW, Block R: American Academy of Pediatrics Committee on Child Abuse and Neglect: Abusive head trauma in infants and children. Pediatrics 2009;123(5):1409–1411 [PMID: 19403508].

Hymel KP: American Academy of Pediatrics Committee on Child Abuse and Neglect; National Association of Medical Examiners: Distinguishing sudden infant death syndrome from child abuse fatalities. Pediatrics 2006;118:421 [PMID: 16818592].

Kempe AM et al: Patterns of skeletal fractures in child abuse: Systematic review. BMJ 2008;337:a1518 [PMID: 18832412].

Sirotnak AP et al: Physical abuse of children. Pediatr Rev 2004;25: 264 [PMID: 15286272].

Sexual Abuse

Sexual abuse is defined as the engaging of dependent, developmentally immature children in sexual activities that they do not fully comprehend and to which they cannot give consent, or activities that violate the laws and taboos of a society. It includes all forms of incest, sexual assault or rape, and pedophilia. This includes fondling, oral-genital-anal contact, all forms of intercourse or penetration, exhibitionism, voyeurism, exploitation or prostitution, and the involvement of children in the production of pornography. Although over the past decade there has been a small downward trend nationally in total reports of sexual abuse cases, exploitation and enticement of children and adolescents via the Internet remains a growing trend.

A. History

Sexual abuse may come to the clinician's attention in different ways: (1) The child may be brought in for routine care or for an acute problem, and sexual abuse may be suspected by the medical professional as a result of the history or the physical examination. (2) The parent or caregiver, suspecting that the child may have been sexually abused, may bring the child to the health care provider and request an examination to rule in or rule out abuse. (3) The child may be referred by child protective services or the police for an evidentiary examination following either disclosure of sexual abuse by the child or an allegation of abuse by a parent or third party. Table 8–2 lists the common presentations of child sexual abuse. It should be emphasized that with the exception of acute trauma, certain sexually transmitted infections (STIs), or forensic laboratory evidence, none of these presentations is specific. The presentations listed should arouse suspicion of the possibility of sexual abuse and lead the practitioner to ask the appropriate questions—again, in a compassionate and nonaccusatory manner. Asking the child nonleading, age-appropriate questions is important and is often best handled by the most experienced interviewer after a report is made. Community agency protocols may exist for child advocacy centers that help in the investigation of these reports. Concerns expressed about sexual abuse in the context of divorce and custody disputes should be handled in the same manner, with the same objective, nonjudgmental documentation. The American Academy of Pediatrics has published guidelines for the evaluation of child sexual abuse as well as others relating to child maltreatment.

Table 8–2. Presentations of sexual abuse.

General or direct statements about sexual abuse
Sexualized knowledge, play, or behavior in developmentally immature children
Sexual abuse of other children by the victim
Behavioral changes
Sleep disturbances (eg, nightmares and night terrors)
Appetite disturbances (eg, anorexia, bulimia)
Depression, social withdrawal, anxiety
Aggression, temper tantrums, impulsiveness
Neurotic or conduct disorders, phobias or avoidant behaviors
Guilt, low self-esteem, mistrust, feelings of helplessness
Hysterical or conversion reactions
Suicidal, runaway threats or behavior
Excessive masturbation
Medical conditions
Recurrent abdominal pain or frequent somatic complaints
Genital, anal, or urethral trauma
Recurrent complaints of genital or anal pain, discharge, bleeding
Enuresis or encopresis
Sexually transmitted infections
Pregnancy
Promiscuity or prostitution, sexual dysfunction, fear of intimacy
School problems or truancy
Substance abuse

B. Physical Findings

The genital and anal findings of sexually abused children, as well as the normal developmental changes and variations in prepubertal female hymens, have been described in journal articles and visual diagnosis guides. To maintain a sense of comfort and routine for the patient, the genital examination should be conducted in the context of a full body checkup. For nonsexually active, prepubertal girls, an internal speculum examination is rarely necessary unless there is suspicion of internal injury. The external female genital structures can be well visualized using labial separation and traction with the child in the supine frog leg or knee-chest position. The majority of victims of sexual abuse exhibit no physical findings. The reasons for this include delay in disclosure by the child, abuse that may not cause physical trauma (eg, fondling, oral-genital contact, or exploitation by pornographic photography), or rapid healing of minor injuries such as labial, hymenal, or anal abrasions, contusions, or lacerations. Nonspecific abnormalities of the genital and rectal regions such as erythema, rashes, and irritation may not suggest sexual abuse in the absence of a corroborating history, disclosure, or behavioral changes.

Certain STIs should strongly suggest sexual abuse. *Neisseria gonorrhoeae* infection or syphilis beyond the perinatal period is diagnostic of sexual abuse. *Chlamydia trachomatis*, herpes simplex virus, trichomoniasis, and human papillomavirus are all sexually transmitted, although the course of these potentially perinatally acquired infections may be protracted. Herpes simplex can be transmitted by other means; however, the presence of an infection should prompt a careful assessment for sexual abuse. Risk is higher in children older than five with isolated genital lesions or with herpes simplex type 2 infections. In the case of human papillomavirus, an initial appearance of venereal warts beyond the toddler age should prompt a discussion regarding concerns of sexual abuse. Human papillomavirus is a ubiquitous virus and can be spread innocently by caregivers with hand lesions; biopsy and viral typing is rarely indicated and often of limited availability. Finally, sexual abuse must be considered with the diagnosis of *Chlamydia trachomatis* or human immunodeficiency virus (HIV) infections when other modes of transmission (eg, transfusion or perinatal acquisition) have been ruled out. Postexposure prophylaxis medications for HIV in cases of acute sexual assault should be considered only after assessment of risk of transmission and consultation with an infectious disease expert.

Although sensitivity and specificity of nonculture tests such as nucleic acid amplification tests (NAATs) have improved, they have not yet been approved for the screening of STIs in sexual abuse victims or for children younger than 12 years of age. If an NAAT is positive, a second confirmatory NAAT test that analyzes an alternate target of the genetic material in the sample or a standard culture is needed. Finally, the Centers for Disease Control and Prevention and many sexual abuse atlases list guidelines for the screening and treatment of STIs in the context of sexual abuse.

C. Examination, Evaluation, and Management

The forensic evaluation of sexually abused children should be performed in a setting that prevents further emotional distress. All practitioners should have access to a rape kit, which guides the practitioner through a stepwise collection of evidence and cultures. This should occur in an emergency department or clinic where chain of custody for specimens can be assured. The most experienced examiner (pediatrician, nurse examiner, or child advocacy center) is preferable. For cases of adolescent abuse or rape that occurred in the preceding 120 hours, most states require for legal purposes that a rape kit be used. If the history indicates that the adolescent may have had contact with the ejaculate of a perpetrator within 120 hours, a cervical examination to look for semen or its markers (eg, acid phosphatase) should be performed according to established protocols. Prior to any speculum exam of an assault victim, it is important to consider the child's physiologic and emotional maturation, and whether she has been sexually active or had a speculum exam in the past. A speculum exam in a prepubertal child is rarely indicated unless there is concern for internal injury and in those cases it is generally advised to perform the exam under anesthesia and with the assistance of gynecology. More important, if there is a history of possible sexual abuse of any child within the past several days, and the child reports a physical complaint or a physical sign is observed (eg, genital or anal bleeding or discharge), the child should be examined for evidence of trauma. Colposcopic examination may be critical for determining the extent of the damage and providing documentation for the legal system.

All the components of a forensic evidence collection kit may not be indicated in the setting of child sexual abuse (as opposed to adult rape cases); the clinical history and exposure risk should guide what specimens are collected. Beyond 120 hours, evaluation is tailored to the history provided. The involved orifices should be cultured for *N gonorrhoeae* and *C trachomatis*, and vaginal secretions evaluated for *Trichomonas*. These infections and bacterial vaginosis are the most frequently diagnosed infections among older girls who have been sexually assaulted. RPR, hepatitis B, and HIV serology should be drawn at baseline and repeated in 3 months. Pregnancy testing should be done as indicated.

Acute sexual assault cases that involve trauma or transmission of body fluid should have STI prophylaxis. Using adult doses of ceftriaxone (125 mg IM in a single dose), metronidazole (2 g orally in a single dose), and either azithromycin (1 g orally in a single dose) or doxycycline (100 mg orally twice a day for 7 days) should be offered when older or adolescent patients present for evaluation. (Pediatric dosing is calculated by weight and can be found in standard references.) Hepatitis B vaccination should be administered to patients if they have not been previously vaccinated. No effective prophylaxis is available for hepatitis C. Evaluating the perpetrator for a sexually transmitted infection, if possible, can help determine risk exposure and guide prophylaxis. HIV prophylaxis should be considered in certain circumstances (see Chapter 44). For postpubertal girls, contraception should be given if rape abuse occurred within 120 hours.

Although it is often difficult for persons to comply with follow-up examinations weeks after an assault, such examinations are essential to detect new infections, complete immunization with hepatitis B vaccination if needed, and continue psychological support.

Adams JA et al: Guidelines for medical care of children who may have been sexually abused. J Pediatr Adolesc Gynecol 2007;20:163 [PMID: 17561184].

American Academy of Pediatrics Clinical Report: The evaluation of sexual abuse of children. Pediatrics 2005;116:506 [PMID: 16061610].

Berkoff MC et al: Has this prepubertal girl been sexually abused? JAMA 2008;300:2779 [PMID: 19088355].

Black CM et al: Multicenter study of nucleic acid amplification tests for detection of *Chlamydia trachomatis* and *Neisseria gonorrhoeae* in children being evaluated for sexual abuse. Pediatr Infect Dis 2009;28(7):608–613 [PMID: 19451856].

Centers for Disease Control and Prevention: Sexually Transmitted Diseases Treatment Guidelines 2010. Available at: http://www.cdc.gov/std/treatment/2010/sexual-assault.htm.

Girardet RG et al: Collection of forensic evidence from pediatric victims of sexual assault. Pediatrics 2011;128:233–238 [PMID: 21788219].

Girardet RG et al: HIV post-exposure prophylaxis in children and adolescents presenting for reported sexual assault. Child Abuse Negl 2009;33:173 [PMID: 19324415].

Kellogg N: American Academy of Pediatrics Committee on Child Abuse and Neglect: The evaluation of sexual abuse in children. Pediatrics 2007;119(6):1232–1241 [PMID: 17545397].

McCann J et al: Healing of hymenal injuries in prepubertal and adolescent girls: A descriptive study. Pediatrics 2007;119:e1094 [PMID: 17420260].

Thackeray et al: Forensic evidence collection and DNA identification in acute child sexual assault. Pediatrics 2011;128:227–232 [PMID: 21788217].

Woods CR: Sexually transmitted diseases in prepubertal children: Mechanisms of transmission, evaluation of sexually abused children, and exclusion of chronic perinatal viral infections. Sem Pediatr Infect Dis 2005;16:317 [PMID: 16210111].

Emotional Abuse & Neglect

Emotional or psychological abuse has been defined as the rejection, ignoring, criticizing, isolation, or terrorizing of children, all of which have the effect of eroding their self-esteem. The most common form is verbal abuse or denigration. Children who witness domestic violence should be considered emotionally abused, as a growing body of literature has shown the negative effects of intimate partner violence on child development.

The most common feature of emotional neglect is the absence of normal parent-child attachment and a subsequent inability to recognize and respond to an infant's or child's needs. A common manifestation of emotional neglect in infancy is nutritional (nonorganic) failure to thrive. Emotionally neglectful parents appear to have an inability to recognize the physical or emotional states of their children. For example, an emotionally neglectful parent may ignore an infant's cry if the cry is perceived incorrectly as an expression of anger. This misinterpretation leads to inadequate nutrition and failure to thrive.

Emotional abuse may cause nonspecific symptoms in children. Loss of self-esteem or self-confidence, sleep disturbances, somatic symptoms (eg, headaches and stomach aches), hypervigilance, or avoidant or phobic behaviors (eg, school refusal or running away) may be presenting complaints. These complaints may also be seen in children who experience domestic violence. Emotional abuse can occur in the home or day care, school, sports team, or other settings.

Physical Neglect & Failure to Thrive

Physical neglect is the failure to provide the necessary food, clothing, and shelter and a safe environment in which children can grow and develop. Although often associated with poverty or ignorance, physical neglect involves a more serious problem than just lack of resources. There is often a component of emotional neglect and either a failure or an inability, intentionally or otherwise, to recognize and respond to the needs of the child.

A. History

Even though in 2009 neglect was confirmed for in over three-quarters of all victims, neglect is not easily documented on history. Physical neglect—which must be differentiated from the deprivations of poverty—will be present even after adequate social services have been provided to families in need. The clinician must evaluate the psychosocial history and family dynamics when neglect is a consideration, and a careful social services investigation of the home and entire family may be required.

The history offered in cases of growth failure (failure to thrive) is often discrepant with the physical findings. Infants who have experienced a significant deceleration in growth are probably not receiving adequate amounts or appropriate types of food despite the dietary history provided. Medical conditions causing poor growth in infancy and early childhood can be ruled out with a detailed history and physical examination with minimal laboratory tests. A psychosocial history may reveal maternal depression, family chaos or dysfunction, or other previously unknown social risk factors (eg, substance abuse, violence, poverty, or psychiatric illness). Placement of the child with another caregiver is usually followed by a dramatic weight gain. Hospitalization of the severely malnourished patient is sometimes required, but most cases are managed on an outpatient basis.

B. Physical Findings

Infants and children with nonorganic failure to thrive have a relative absence of subcutaneous fat in the cheeks, buttocks, and extremities. Other conditions associated with poor nutrient and vitamin intake may be present. If the condition has persisted for some time, these patients may also appear and act depressed. Older children who have been chronically emotionally neglected may also have short stature (ie, deprivation dwarfism). The head circumference is usually normal in cases of nonorganic failure to thrive. Microcephaly may signify a prenatal condition, congenital disease, or chronic nutritional deprivation and increases the likelihood of more serious and possibly permanent developmental delay.

C. Radiologic and Laboratory Findings

Children with failure to thrive or malnutrition may not require an extensive workup. Assessment of the patient's growth curve, as well as careful plotting of subsequent growth parameters after treatment, is critical. Complete blood cell count, urinalysis, electrolyte panel, and thyroid and liver function tests are sufficient screening. Newborn screening should be documented as usual. Other tests should be guided by any aspect of the clinical history that points to a previously undiagnosed condition. A skeletal survey and head computed tomography scan may be helpful if concurrent physical abuse is suspected. The best screening method, however, is placement in a setting in which the child can be fed and monitored. Hospital or foster care placement may be required. Weight gain may not occur for several days to a week in severe cases.

Medical Care Neglect

Medical care neglect is failure to provide the needed treatment to infants or children with life-threatening illness or other serious or chronic medical conditions. Many states have repealed laws that supported religious exemptions as reason for not seeking medical care for sick children.

Medical Child Abuse

Previously referred to as Munchausen syndrome by proxy, medical child abuse is the preferred term for a relatively unusual clinical scenario in which a caregiver seeks inappropriate and unnecessary medical care for a child. Oftentimes, the caregiver either simulates or creates the symptoms or signs of illness in a child. However, the use of the term medical child abuse emphasizes harm caused to the child as opposed to the psychopathology or motivation of the caregiver. Cases can be complicated and a detailed review of all medical documentation and a multidisciplinary approach is required. Fatal cases have been reported.

A. History

Children may present with the signs and symptoms of whatever illness is factitiously produced or simulated. The child can present with a long list of medical problems or often bizarre, recurrent complaints. Persistent doctor shopping and enforced invalidism (eg, not accepting that the child is healthy and reinforcing that the child is somehow ill) are also described in the original definition of Munchausen syndrome by proxy.

B. Physical Findings

They may be actually ill or, more often, are reported to be ill and have a normal clinical appearance. Among the most common reported presentations are recurrent apnea, dehydration from induced vomiting or diarrhea, sepsis when contaminants are injected into a child, change in mental status, fever, gastrointestinal bleeding, and seizures.

C. Radiologic and Laboratory Findings

Recurrent polymicrobial sepsis (especially in children with indwelling catheters), recurrent apnea, chronic dehydration of unknown cause, or other highly unusual unexplained laboratory findings should raise the suspicion of Munchausen syndrome by proxy. Toxicological testing may also be useful.

Black MM et al: Failure to thrive as distinct from child neglect. Pediatrics 2006;117:1456–1457.

Block RW, Krebs NF: Failure to thrive as a manifestation of child neglect. Pediatrics 2005;116:1234–1237.

DeBellis MD: The psychobiology of neglect. Child Maltreat 2005;10:150 [PMID: 15798010].

Hymel KP; American Academy of Pediatrics Committee on Child Abuse and Neglect: When is lack of supervision neglect? Pediatrics 2006;118:1296 [PMID: 16951030].

Roesler T, Jenny C: *Medical Child Abuse: Beyond Munchausen Syndrome by Proxy.* American Academy of Pediatrics, 2009.

Shaw RJ et al: Factitious disorder by proxy: Pediatric condition falsification. Harv Rev Psychiatry 2008;16:215–224 [PMID 18661364].

DIFFERENTIAL DIAGNOSIS

The differential diagnosis for abuse and neglect may be straightforward (ie, traumatic vs nontraumatic injury). It can also be more elusive as in the case of multiple injuries that may raise concern for an underlying medical condition or in situations where complex, but nonspecific behavior changes or physical symptoms reflect the emotional impact of maltreatment.

The differential diagnosis of all forms of physical abuse can be considered in the context of a detailed trauma history, family medical history, radiographic findings, and laboratory testing. The diagnosis of osteogenesis imperfecta or other collagen disorders, for example, may be considered in the child with skin and joint findings or multiple fractures with or without the classic radiographic presentation and is best made in consultation with a geneticist, an orthopedic surgeon, and a radiologist. Trauma—accidental or inflicted—leads the differential diagnosis list for subdural hematomas. Coagulopathy; disorders of copper, amino acid, or organic acid metabolism (eg, Menkes syndrome and glutaric acidemia type 1); chronic or previous central nervous system infection; birth trauma; or congenital central nervous system malformation (eg, arteriovenous malformations or cerebrospinal fluid collections) may need to be ruled out in some cases. It should be recognized, however, that children with these rare disorders can also be victims of abuse or neglect.

There are medical conditions that may be misdiagnosed as sexual abuse. When abnormal physical examination findings are noted, knowledge of these conditions is imperative to avoid misinterpretation. The differential diagnosis includes vulvovaginitis, lichen sclerosus, dermatitis, labial adhesions, congenital urethral or vulvar disorders, Crohn's disease, and accidental straddle injuries to the labia. In most circumstances, these can be ruled out by careful history and examination.

TREATMENT

A. Management

Physical abuse injuries, STIs, and medical sequelae of neglect should be treated immediately. Children with failure to thrive related to emotional and physical neglect need to be placed in a setting in which they can be fed and cared for. Likewise, the child in danger of recurrent abuse or neglect needs to be placed in a safe environment. Cases can be complicated and psychosocial difficulties are common; therefore, a multidisciplinary approach to cases is helpful. Cooperation and coordination with social work and mental health colleagues are key. Given the developmental and emotional implications, prompt referral to mental health resources for any patient with a history of child abuse or neglect is crucial. There has been significant progress made in identifying, researching, and implementing effective, evidence-based treatment of child maltreatment. Pediatricians should be aware of community partners and resources to help families in need of services.

B. Reporting

In the United States, clinicians and many other professionals who come in contact with or care for children are mandated reporters. If abuse or neglect is suspected, a report must be made to the local or state agency designated to investigate such matters. In most cases, this will be the child protective services agency. Law enforcement agencies may also receive such reports. The purpose of the report is to permit professionals to gather the information needed to determine whether the child's environment (eg, home, school, day care setting, or foster home) is safe. Recent studies document physician barriers to reporting, but practioners should be mindful that good faith reporting is a legal requirement for any suspicion of abuse. Failure to report concerns may have legal ramifications for the provider or serious health and safety consequences for the patient. Many hospitals and communities make child protection teams or consultants available when there are questions about the diagnosis and management in a child abuse case. A listing of pediatric consultants in child abuse is available from the American Academy of Pediatrics.

Except in extreme cases, the reporting of emotional abuse is not likely to generate an immediate response from child protection agencies. This should not deter reporting, especially if there is also concern for domestic violence or other forms of abuse or neglect. Practitioners can encourage parents to become involved with parent effectiveness training programs (eg, Healthy Families America or Parents Anonymous) or to seek mental health consultation. Support for the child may also include mental health counseling or age-appropriate peer and mentoring activities in school or the community. Finally, communication with social services, case management, and careful follow-up by primary care providers is crucial to ensuring ongoing safety of child.

American Humane Society: Protecting children. Available at: http://www.americanhumane.org/children/. Accessed August 3, 2011.

American Professional Society on the Abuse of Children. Available at: http://www.apsac.org/. Accessed August 3, 2011.

Jones R et al: Clinicians' description of factors influencing their reporting of suspected child abuse: Report of the Child Abuse Reporting Experience Study Research Group. Pediatrics 2008 Aug;122(2):259–266 [PMID: 18676541].

PROGNOSIS

Depending on the extent of injury resulting from physical or sexual abuse, the prognosis for complete recovery varies. Serious physical abuse that involves head injury, multisystem trauma, severe burns, or abdominal trauma carries significant morbidity and mortality risk. Hospitalized children with a diagnosis of child abuse or neglect have longer stays and are more likely to die. Long-term medical and developmental consequences are common. For example, children who suffer brain damage related to abusive head injury can have significant neurologic impairment, such as cerebral palsy, vision problems, epilepsy, microcephaly, and learning disorders. Other injuries like minor bruises or burns, fractures, and even injuries resulting from penetrating genital trauma can heal well and with no sequelae.

The emotional and psychological outcomes for child victims are often more detrimental than the physical injuries. Research demonstrates that there are clear neurobiologic effects of child maltreatment and other types of early childhood stress. Physiologic changes to the brain can adversely affect the mental and physical health development of children for decades. Long-standing concerns have been validated; victims have increased rates of childhood and adult health problems, adolescent suicide, alcoholism and drug abuse, anxiety and depression, criminality and violence, and learning problems.

Centers for Disease Control and Prevention: Adverse childhood experiences study. Available at: http://www.cdc.gov/ace/index.htm. Accessed August 4, 2011.

Child Welfare Information Gateway: Long-term consequences of child abuse and neglect. Available at: http://www.childwelfare.gov/pubs/factsheets/long_term_consequences.cfm. Accessed August 4, 2011.

Stirling J, American Academy of Pediatrics Committee on Child Abuse and Neglect and Section on Adoption and Foster Care; Amaya-Jackson L, American Academy of Child and Adolescent Psychiatry; Amaya-Jackson L, National Center for Child Traumatic Stress: Understanding the behavioral and emotional consequences of child abuse. Pediatrics 2008;122(3):667–673 [PMID: 18762538].

Ambulatory & Office Pediatrics

9

Maya Bunik, MD, MSPH
Meghan Treitz, MD
David Fox, MD

Pediatric ambulatory outpatient services provide children and adolescents with preventive health care and acute and chronic care management services and consultations. In this chapter, special attention is given to the pediatric history and physical examination, normal developmental stages, screening laboratories, and a number of common pediatric issues.

The development of a physician-patient-parent relationship is crucially important if the patient and parent are to effectively confide their concerns. This relationship develops over time, with increasing numbers of visits, and is facilitated by the continuity of clinicians and other staff members. This clinical relationship is based on trust that develops as a result of several experiences in the context of the office visit. Perhaps the greatest factor facilitating the relationship is for patients or parents to experience advice as valid and effective. Anticipatory guidance should be age-appropriate and timely in order to be most helpful. Important skills include choosing vocabulary that communicates understanding and competence, demonstrating commitment of time and attention to the concern, and showing respect for areas that the patient or parent does not wish to address (assuming there are no concerns relating to physical or sexual abuse or neglect). Parents and patients expect that their concerns will be managed confidentially and that the clinician understands and sympathizes with those concerns. The effective physician-patient-parent relationship is one of the most satisfying aspects of ambulatory pediatrics.

Tanner JL, Stein MT, Olson LM, Frintner MP, Radecki L: Reflections on well-child care practice: A national study of pediatric clinicians. Pediatrics 2009 Sep;124(3):849–857 [Epub 2009 Aug 10] [PMID: 19706587].

PEDIATRIC HISTORY

A unique feature of pediatrics is that the history represents an amalgam of parents' objective reporting of facts (eg, fever for 4 days), parents' subjective interpretation of their child's symptoms (eg, infant crying interpreted by parents as abdominal pain), and for older children their own history of events. Parents and patients may provide a specific and detailed history, or a vague history that necessitates more focused probing. Parents may or may not be able to distinguish whether symptoms are caused by organic illness or a psychological concern. Understanding the family and its hopes for and concerns about the child can help in the process of distinguishing organic, emotional, and/or behavioral conditions, thus minimizing unnecessary testing and intervention.

Although the parents' concerns need to be understood, it is essential also to obtain as much of the history as possible directly from the patient. Direct histories not only provide firsthand information but also give the child a degree of control over a potentially threatening situation and may reveal important information about the family.

Obtaining a comprehensive pediatric history is time-consuming. Many offices provide questionnaires for parents to complete before the clinician sees the child. Data from questionnaires can make an outpatient visit more productive, allowing the physician to address problems in detail while more quickly reviewing areas that are not of concern. Questionnaires may be more productive than face-to-face interviews in revealing sensitive parts of the history. Developmental and mental health screening saves provider time and the results when reviewed with the parent or family member can yield critical information. However, failure to review and assimilate this information prior to the interview may cause a parent or patient to feel that the time and effort have been wasted.

Elements of the history that will be useful over time should be readily accessible in the medical record. In absence of an electronic medical record, such information can be accumulated on a summary sheet, as illustrated in Figure 9–1. Demographic data; a problem list; information about chronic medications, allergies, and previous hospitalizations; and the names of other physicians providing care for the patient are commonly included. Documentation of immunizations,

Name ______________________ Nickname ______________________ D.O.B. __________
Mother/parent (1)______________ Father/parent (2)______________ Sibs __________
S.S.# ______________________ Insurance ______________________

Problems		
Date of onset	Description	Date resolved

Chronic Medications		
Start date		Stop date

Allergies	
Date	

Date	Hospitalizations/Injuries/Procedures

Date	Consultants

▲ **Figure 9–1.** Use of a summary sheet such as this at the front of the chart or the electronic medical record facilitates reorienting the caregiver and his or her partners to the patient. Some practices keep track of health supervision visits on this sheet to tell the physician whether the child is likely to have received the appropriate preventive services. A second page documenting immunizations should record data required by the National Childhood Vaccine Injury Act. When an allergy with potential for anaphylaxis is identified, the patient should wear a medical alert bracelet and obtain an epinephrine kit, if appropriate.

including all data required by the National Childhood Vaccine Injury Act, should be kept on a second page.

The components of a comprehensive pediatric history are listed in Table 9–1. The information should, ideally, be obtained at the first office visit. The first seven items may be included on a summary sheet at the front of the medical record. Items 8 and 9, and a focused review of systems, are dealt with at each acute or chronic care visit. The entire list should be reviewed and augmented with relevant updates at each health supervision visit.

PEDIATRIC PHYSICAL EXAMINATION

During the pediatric physical examination, time must be taken to allow the patient to become familiar with the examiner. Interactions and instructions help the child understand what is occurring and what is expected. A gentle, friendly manner and a quiet voice help establish a setting that yields a nonthreatening physical examination. The examiner should take into consideration the need for a quiet child, the extent of trust established, and the possibility of an emotional

Table 9–1. Components of the pediatric historical database.[a]

1. Demographic data	Patient's name and nickname, date of birth, social security number, sex, race, parents' names (first and last), siblings' names, and payment mechanism.
2. Problem list	Major or significant problems, including dates of onset and resolution.
3. Allergies	Triggering allergen, nature of the reaction, treatment needed, and date allergy was diagnosed.
4. Chronic medications	Name, concentration, dose, and frequency of chronically used medications.
5. Birth history	Maternal health during pregnancy such as bleeding, infections, smoking, alcohol and any medications, complications of pregnancy; duration of labor; form of delivery; and labor complications. Infant's birth weight, gestational age, Apgar scores, and problems in the neonatal period.
6. Screening procedures	Results of newborn screening, vision and hearing screening, any health screen, or screening laboratory tests. (Developmental screening results are maintained in the development section; see item 14, below.)
7. Immunizations	Antigen(s), date administered, vaccine manufacturer and lot number, and name and title of the person administering the vaccine; site, previous reaction and contraindications (eg, immunodeficiency or an evolving neurologic problem), date on vaccine information statement (VIS), and date VIS was provided.
8. Reasons for visit	The patient's or parents' concerns, stated in their own words, serve as the focus for the visit.
9. Present illness	A concise chronologic summary of the problems necessitating a visit, including the duration, progression, exacerbating factors, ameliorating interventions, and associations.
10. Medical history	A statement regarding the child's functionality and general well-being, including a summary record of significant illnesses, injuries, hospitalizations, and procedures.
11. Diet	Eating patterns, likes and dislikes, use of vitamins, and relative amounts of carbohydrates, fat, and protein in the diet, percentage of fat of milk provided. Inquiry about intake of fast food, candy and sugar drinks.
12. Family history	Information about the illnesses of relatives, preferably in the form of a family tree.
13. Social history	Family constellation, relationships, parents' educational background, religious preference, and the role of the child in the family; socioeconomic profile of the family to identify resources available to the child, access to services that may be needed, and anticipated stressors.
14. Development	(1) Attainment of developmental milestones (including developmental testing results); (2) social habits and milestones (toilet habits, play, major activities, sleep patterns, discipline, peer relationships); (3) school progress and documentation of specific achievements and grades.
15. Sexual history	Family's sexual attitudes, sex education, sexual development sexual secondary characteristics, activity, sexually transmitted diseases, menstruation onset and characteristics and birth control measures.
16. Review of systems (ROS)	Common symptoms in each major body system.

[a]The components of this table should be included in a child's medical record and structured to allow easy review and modification. The practice name and address should appear on all pages.

response (crying!) when deciding the order in which the child's organ systems are examined. Painful or unpleasant procedures (eg, otoscopic examinations) should be deferred until the end of the examination. Whether or not the physician can establish rapport with the child, the process should proceed efficiently and systematically.

Because young children may fear the examination and become fussy, simple inspection is important. For example, during an acute-care visit for fever, the examiner should observe the child's skin color and work of breathing prior to beginning the examination. During a health supervision visit, observation will provide the examiner with an opportunity to assess parent-child interactions.

Clothing should be removed slowly and gently to avoid threatening the child. A parent or the child is usually the best person to do this. Modesty should always be respected, and gown or drapes should be provided. Examinations of adolescents should be chaperoned whenever a pelvic examination or a stressful or painful procedure is performed.

Examination tables are convenient, but a parent's lap is a comfortable location for a young child. For most purposes, an adequate examination can be conducted on a "table" formed by the parent's and examiner's legs as they sit facing each other.

Although a thorough physical examination is important at every age, at some ages the examination tends to focus on specific issues and concerns. At any age, an astute clinician can detect signs of important clinical conditions in an asymptomatic child. In infancy, for example, physical examination can reveal the presence of craniosynostosis, congenital heart disease, or developmental dysplasia of the hip. Similarly, examination of a toddler may reveal pallor (possible iron-deficiency anemia) or strabismus. The routine examination of an adolescent may reveal scoliosis or acanthosis nigricans (a finding associated with insulin resistance).

HEALTH SUPERVISION VISITS

One of several timetables for recommended health supervision visits is illustrated in Figure 9–2. (***Note***: A PDF printable format of this figure is available from the American Academy of Pediatrics [AAP].) The federal Maternal and Child Health Bureau has developed comprehensive health supervision guidelines through their Bright Futures program. In areas where evidence-based information is lacking, expert opinion has been used as the basis for these plans. Recently revised *Bright Futures Guidelines* emphasizes working collaboratively with families, recognizing the need for attention toward children with special health care needs, gaining cultural competence, and addressing complementary and alternative care, as well as integrating mental health care into the primary care setting. Practitioners should remember that guidelines are not meant to be rigid; services should be individualized according to the child's needs.

During health supervision visits, the practitioner should review child development and acute and chronic problems, conduct a complete physical examination, order appropriate screening tests, and anticipate future developments. New historical information should be elicited through an interval history. For example, "Since your last visit have there been any changes in your child and family's life that I should be aware of?" Development should be assessed by parental report and clinician observation at each visit. Developmental surveillance is augmented with systematic use of parent-directed questionnaires or screening tests. Growth parameters should be carefully recorded and weight, length or height, head circumference (up to age 3), and body mass index (BMI) (for > 2 years) should be plotted and evaluated using established growth charts (see Chapter 3). Vision and hearing should be assessed subjectively at each visit, with objective assessments at intervals beginning after the child is old enough to cooperate with the screening test, usually at 3–4 years of age. Various laboratory screening tests may also be part of the visit.

Because fewer than 4% of asymptomatic children have physical findings on routine health maintenance visits, a major portion of the health supervision visit is devoted to anticipatory guidance. This portion of the visit enables the health care provider to address behavioral, developmental, injury prevention, and nutritional issues; school problems; and other age-appropriate issues that will arise before the next well-child visit.

American Academy of Pediatrics Committee on Practice and Ambulatory Medicine: Recommendations for preventive pediatric health care. Pediatrics 2007;120:1376.

Dinkevich E, Ozuah PO: Well-child care: Effectiveness of current recommendations. Clin Pediatr 2002;41:211 [PMID:12041716].

Bright Futures Guidelines, 3rd ed. Available at: http://brightfutures.aap.org/3rd_Edition_Guidelines_and_Pocket_Guide.html. Assessed August 24, 2009.

DEVELOPMENTAL & BEHAVIORAL ASSESSMENT

Addressing developmental and behavioral problems is one of the central features of pediatric primary care. The term *developmental delay* refers to the circumstance in which a child has not demonstrated a developmental skill (such as walking independently) by an age at which the vast majority of normally developing children have accomplished this task. Developmental delays are, in fact, quite common: approximately 18% of children younger than age 18 years either have developmental delays or have conditions that place them at risk of developmental delays.

Pediatric practitioners are in a unique position to assess the development of their patients. This developmental assessment should ideally take the form of *developmental surveillance*, in which a skilled individual monitors development in multiple domains (gross motor, fine motor, language, and personal/social) over time as part of providing routine care. Developmental surveillance includes several key elements: listening to parent concerns; obtaining a developmental history; making careful observations during office visits; periodically screening all infants and children for delays using validated screening tools; recognizing conditions and circumstances that place children at increased risk of delays; and referring children who fail screening tests for further evaluation and intervention.

The prompt recognition of children with developmental delays is important for several reasons. The presence of delays may lead practitioners to diagnose unsuspected but important conditions, such as genetic syndromes or metabolic disorders. Children with delays can be referred for a wide range of developmental therapies, such as those provided by physical, speech/language, and/or educational therapists. Children with delays, regardless of the cause, make better developmental progress if they receive appropriate developmental therapies than if they do not. Many infants and toddlers younger than age 3 years with delays are eligible to receive a range of therapies and other services, often provided in the home, at no cost to families. Children

Recommendations for Preventive Pediatric Health Care

Each child and family is unique; therefore, these **Recommendations for Preventive Pediatric Health Care** are designed for the care of children who are receiving competent parenting, have no manifestations of any important health problems, and are growing and developing in satisfactory fashion. **Additional visits may become necessary** if circumstances suggest variations from normal.

Developmental, psychosocial, and chronic disease issues for children and adolescents may require frequent counseling and treatment visits separate from preventive care visits.

These guidelines represent a consensus by the American Academy of Pediatrics (AAP) and Bright Futures. The AAP continues to emphasize the great importance of **continuity of care** in comprehensive health supervision and the need to avoid **fragmentation of care.**

The recommendations in this statement do not indicate an exclusive course of treatment or standard of medical care. Variations, taking into account individual circumstances, may be appropriate.

	INFANCY								EARLY CHILDHOOD							MIDDLE CHILDHOOD						ADOLESCENCE										
Age[a]	Prenatal[b]	Newborn[c]	3–5 d[d]	By 1 mo	2 mo	4 mo	6 mo	9 mo	12 mo	15 mo	18 mo	24 mo	30 mo	3 y	4 y	5 y	6 y	7 y	8 y	9 y	10 y	11 y	12 y	13 y	14 y	15 y	16 y	17 y	18 y	19 y	20 y	21 y
HISTORY																																
Initial/interval	●	●	●	●	●	●	●	●	●	●	●	●	●	●	●	●	●	●	●	●	●	●	●	●	●	●	●	●	●	●	●	●
MEASUREMENTS																																
Length/height and weight		●	●	●	●	●	●	●	●	●	●	●	●	●	●	●	●	●	●	●	●	●	●	●	●	●	●	●	●	●	●	●
Head circumference		●	●	●	●	●	●	●	●	●	●	●																				
Weight for length		●	●	●	●	●	●	●	●	●	●																					
Body mass index												●	●	●	●	●	●	●	●	●	●	●	●	●	●	●	●	●	●	●	●	●
Blood pressure[e]		★	★	★	★	★	★	★	★	★	★	★	★	●	●	●	●	●	●	●	●	●	●	●	●	●	●	●	●	●	●	●
SENSORY SCREENING																																
Vision		★	★	★	★	★	★	★	★	★	★	★	★	●[f]	●	●	●	★	●	★	●	★	●	★	●	●	★	●	★	★	★	★
Hearing		●[g]	★	★	★	★	★	★	★	★	★	★	★	★	●	●	●	★	●	★	●	★	★	★	★	★	★	★	★	★	★	★
DEVELOPMENTAL/BEHAVIORAL ASSESSMENT																																
Developmental screening[h]								●			●		●																			
Autism screening[i]											●	●																				
Developmental surveillance[h]		●	●	●	●	●	●		●	●		●		●	●	●	●	●	●	●	●	●	●	●	●	●	●	●	●	●	●	●
Psychosocial/behavioral assessment		●	●	●	●	●	●	●	●	●	●	●	●	●	●	●	●	●	●	●	●	●	●	●	●	●	●	●	●	●	●	●
Alcohol and drug use assessment																						★	★	★	★	★	★	★	★	★	★	★
PHYSICAL EXAMINATION[j]		●	●	●	●	●	●	●	●	●	●	●	●	●	●	●	●	●	●	●	●	●	●	●	●	●	●	●	●	●	●	●
PROCEDURES[k]																																
Newborn metabolic/hemoglobin screening[l]		←	●	→	→																											
Immunization[m]		●	●	●	●	●	●	●	●	●	●	●	●	●	●	●	●	●	●	●	●	●	●	●	●	●	●	●	●	●	●	●
Hematocrit or hemoglobin[n]						★			●		★	★		★	★	★	★	★	★	★	★	★	★	★	★	★	★	★	★	★	★	★
Lead screening[o]							★	★	●or★[p]		★	●or★[p]		★	★	★	★															
Tuberculin test[q]				★			★		★		★	★		★	★	★	★	★	★	★	★	★	★	★	★	★	★	★	★	★	★	★
Dyslipidemia screening[r]												★			★		★	★	★		★	★	★	★	★	★	★	★	←	→	●	→
STI screening[s]																						★	★	★	★	★	★	★	★	★	★	★
Cervical dysplasia screening[t]																						★	★	★	★	★	★	★	★	★	★	★
ORAL HEALTH[u]							★	★	●or★[u]		●or★[u]	●or★[u]	●or★[u]	●[v]			●[v]															
ANTICIPATORY GUIDANCE[w]	●	●	●	●	●	●	●	●	●	●	●	●	●	●	●	●	●	●	●	●	●	●	●	●	●	●	●	●	●	●	●	●

▲ **Figure 9–2.** Recommendations for preventive health care. (Hagen JF, Shaw JS, Duncan PM, eds. *Bright Futures: Guidelines for Health Supervision of Infants, Children, and Adolescents,* 3rd ed. American Academy of Pediatrics, 2008.)

● = to be performed ★ = risk assessment to be performed, with appropriate action to follow, if positive ←●→ = range during which a service may be provided, with the symbol indicating the preferred age

a If a child comes under care for the first time at any point on the schedule, or if any items are not accomplished at the suggested age, the schedule should be brought up to date at the earliest possible time.

b A prenatal visit is recommended for parents who are at high risk, for first-time parents, and for those who request a conference. The prenatal visit should include anticipatory guidance, pertinent medical history, and a discussion of benefits of breast feeding and planned method of feeding per AAP statement "The Prenatal Visit" (2001) [URL:http://aappolicy.aappublications.org/cgi/content/full/pediatrics;107/6/1456].

c Every infant should have a newborn evaluation after birth, breast feeding encouraged, and instruction and support offered.

d Every infant should have an evaluation within 3–5 days of birth and within 48–72 hours after discharge from the hospital, to include evaluation for feeding and jaundice. Breast feeding infants should receive formal breast-feeding evaluation, encouragement, and instruction as recommended in AAP statement "Breast feeding and the Use of Human Milk" (2005) [URL:http://aappolicy.aappublications.org/cgi/content/full/pediatrics;115/2/496]. For newborns discharged in less than 48 hours after delivery, the infant must be examined within 48 hours of discharge per AAP statement "Hospital Stay for Healthy Term Newborns" (2004) [URL: http://aappolicy.aappublications.org/cgi/content/full/pediatrics;113/5/1434].

e Blood pressure measurement in infants and children with specific risk conditions should be performed at visits before age 3 years.

f If the patient is uncooperative, rescreen within 6 months per AAP statement "Eye Examination and Vision Screening in Infants, Children, and Young Adults" (1996) [URL:http://aappolicy.aappublications.org/cgi/reprint/pediatrics;98/1/153.pdf].

g All newborns should be screened per AAP statement "Year 2000 Position Statement: Principles and Guidelines for Early Hearing Detection and Intervention Programs" (2000) [URL: http://aappolicy.aappublications.org/cgi/content/full/pediatrics;106/4/798]. Joint Committee on Infant Hearing. Year 2007 position statement: principles and guidelines for early hearing detection and intervention programs. *Pediatrics*. 2007;120;898–921.

h AAP Council on Children With Disabilities, AAP Section on Developmental Behavioral Pediatrics, AAP Bright Futures Steering Committee. AAP Medical Home Initiatives for Children With Special Needs Project Advisory Committee. Identifying infants and young children with developmental disorders in the medical home: an algorithm for developmental surveillance and screening. *Pediatrics*. 2006;118:405–420 [URL:http://aappolicy.aappublications.org/cgi/content/full/pediatrics;118/1/405].

i Gupta VB, Hyman SL, Johnson CP, et al. Identifying children with autism early? *Pediatrics*, 2007;119:152–153 [URL:http://pediatrics. aappublications.org/cgi/content/full/119/1/152].

j At each visit, age-appropriate physical examination is essential, with infant totally unclothed, older child undressed and suitably draped.

k These may be modified, depending on entry point into schedule and individual need.

l Newborn metabolic and hemoglobinopathy screening should be done according to state law. Results should be reviewed at visits and appropriate retesting or referral done as needed.

m Schedules per the Committee on Infectious Diseases, published annually in the January issue of *Pediatrics*. Every visit should be an opportunity to update and complete a child's immunizations.

n See AAP *Pediatric Nutrition Handbook*, 5th Edition (2003) for a discussion of universal and selective screening options. See also Recommendations to prevent and control iron deficiency in the United States. *MMWR Recomm Rep*. 1998; 47(RR-3):1–36.

o For children at risk of lead exposure, consult the AAP statement "Lead Exposure in Children: Prevention, Detection, and Management" (2005) [URL:http://aappolicy.aappublications.org/cgi/content/full/pediatrics;116/4/1036]. Additionally, screening should be done in accordance with state law where applicable.

p Perform risk assessments or screens as appropriate, based on universal screening requirements for patients with Medicaid or high prevalence areas.

q Tuberculosis testing per recommendations of the Committee on Infectious Diseases, published in the current edition of *Red Book: Report of the Committee on Infectious Diseases*. Testing should be done in recognition of high-risk factors.

r "Third Report of the National Cholesterol Education Program (NCEP) Expert Panel on Detection, Evaluation, and Treatment of High Blood Cholesterol in Adults (Adult Treatment Panel III) Final Report" (2002) [URL:http://circ.ahajournals.org/cgi/content/full/106/25/3143] and "The Expert Committee Recommendations on the Assessment, Prevention, and Treatment of Child and Adolescent Overweight and Obesity." Supplement to *Pediatrics*, In press.

s All sexually active patients should be screened for sexually transmitted infections (STIs).

t All sexually active girls should have screening for cervical dysplasia as part of a pelvic examination beginning within 3 years of onset of sexual activity or age 21 (whichever comes first).

u Referral to dental home, if available. Otherwise, administer oral health risk assessment. If the primary water source is deficient in fluoride, consider oral fluoride supplementation.

v At the visits for 3 years and 6 years of age, it should be determined whether the patient has a dental home. If the patient does not have a dental home, a referral should be made to one. If the primary water source is deficient in fluoride, consider oral fluoride supplementation.

w Refer to the specific guidance by age as listed in Bright Futures Guidelines. (Hagan JF, Shaw JS, Duncan PM, eds. *Bright Futures: Guidelines for Health Supervision of Infants, Children, and Adolescents,* 3rd ed. Elk Grove Village, IL: American Academy of Pediatrics: 2008.)

▲ **Figure 9–2.** *(Continued)*

aged 3 years and older with delays are eligible for developmental services through the local school system.

Although the benefits of early detection of developmental delays are clear, it is often difficult to incorporate developmental surveillance into busy outpatient practice. Only 30% of pediatricians routinely use formal screening tests; most rely on clinical judgment alone. However, when screening tests are not used, delays are often not detected until school age, particularly when the delays are not severe. There are several practical barriers to performing routine surveillance using standardized screening tools: perceived lack of time to screen all children at every well-child visit; lack of familiarity with the various screening tools; not wanting to concern parents by identifying a possible delay; and not knowing where in the community to refer patients with suspected delays. There are some solutions to these barriers, such as using parent developmental questionnaires rather than provider-administered tests to save time, become familiar with one or two screening tests, and making use of Internet-based resources. For example, the National Dissemination Center for Children with Disabilities maintains a web site with links to a wide variety of resources in each state (http://www.nichcy.org).

Several parent-administered and physician-administered developmental screening tools are available. The Parents' Evaluation of Developmental Status (PEDS), the Ages and Stages Questionnaires (ASQ), and the Child Development Inventories (CDI) are screening tests that rely on parent report. Other screening tools, such as the Denver II screening test (reproduced in Chapter 3, Figure 3–12), the Early Language Milestone Scale (see Chapter 3, Figure 3–11), and the Bayley Infant Neurodevelopmental Screener, involve the direct observation of a child's skills by a care provider. All developmental screening tests have their strengths and weaknesses. The Denver II is familiar to many pediatric providers and is widely used. However, whereas the Denver II has relatively high sensitivity for detecting possible developmental delays, the specificity is poorer, and this may lead to the over-referral of normal children for further developmental testing.

In addition to general developmental screening, autism-specific screens (such as the Modified Checklist for Autism in Toddlers, MCHAT) should be administered at the 18- and 24-month health supervision visits.

Regardless of the approach taken to developmental screening, there are a number of important considerations: (1) the range of normal childhood development is broad, and therefore a child with a single missing skill in a single developmental area is less likely to have a significant developmental problem than a child showing multiple delays in several developmental areas (eg, gross motor *and* language delays); (2) continuity of care is important, because development is best assessed over time; (3) it is beneficial to routinely use formal screening tests to assess development; (4) if developmental delays are detected in primary care, these patients need referral for further testing and likely will benefit from receiving developmentally focused therapies; (5) parents appreciate when attention is paid to their child's development, and generally react positively to referrals for appropriate developmental therapies.

Several developmental charts with age-based expectations for normal development are presented in Chapter 3 (see Tables 3–1, 3–2, and 3–3), as well as a discussion of the recommended medical and neurodevelopmental evaluation of a child with a suspected developmental disorder.

In addition to developmental issues, pediatric providers are an important source of information and counseling for parents regarding a broad range of behavioral issues. The nature of the behavioral problems, of course, varies with the child's age. Some common issues raised by parents, discussed in detail in Chapter 3, include colic, feeding disorders, sleep problems, temper tantrums, breath-holding spells, and noncompliance. Behavioral issues in adolescents are discussed in Chapter 4.

American Academy of Pediatrics Council on Children with Disabilities: Identifying infants and young children with developmental disorders in the medical home: An algorithm for develop-mental surveillance and screening. Pediatrics 2006; 118:1808 [PMID: 168118591].

GROWTH PARAMETERS

Monitoring appropriate growth is pivotal in ambulatory pediatric practice. Centers for Disease Control (CDC) recently recommended use of the World Health Organization (WHO) growth standards to monitor growth for infants and children ages 0 to 2 in the United States, in lieu of its own growth charts because the WHO standards are based on a sample of 8500 babies (from Brazil, Ghana, India, Norway, Oman, and the United States) who were predominantly breastfed for at least four months, still nursing at one year, and living in nonsmoking households. The methods used to create the CDC growth charts and the WHO growth charts are similar for children 2 and above.

The 2- to 18-year growth charts include a chart of BMI for age, which is a measure that correlates well with adiposity- and obesity-related comorbidities. The BMI is calculated as the weight (in kilograms) divided by the squared height (in meters). The BMI is useful for determining obesity (BMI ≥ 95th percentile for age) and at risk for overweight (BMI between 85th and 95th percentiles), as well as underweight status (BMI ≤ 5th percentile for age).

Height, weight, and head circumference are carefully measured and plotted at each visit at each well-child examination. To ensure accurate weight measurements for longitudinal comparisons, infants should be undressed completely, and young children should be wearing underpants only. Recumbent length is plotted on the chart and when the child is old enough to be measured upright, height should be plotted on the charts for ages 2–20 years. If circumferential head growth has been steady for the first 2 years, routine measurements may be suspended. However, if a central nervous system problem exists or develops, or if the child has growth deficiency, this measurement continues to be useful. Tracking the growth velocity for each of these parameters allows early recognition of deviations from normal.

American Academy of Pediatrics: Prevention of pediatric overweight and obesity. Pediatrics 2003 Aug;112(2):424–430, Reaffirmed February 1, 2007.

WHO Growth Standards. Available at: www.who.int/childgrowth/standards/en

http://www.cdc.gov/growthcharts/data/who/GrChrt_Boys_24LW_9210.pdf

http://www.cdc.gov/growthcharts/data/who/GrChrt_Girls_24LW_9210.pdf.Assessed July 18, 2011.

Kuczmarski RJ et al: *CDC Growth Charts: United States. Advance Data from Vital and Health Statistics*, No. 314. National Center for Health Statistics, 2000. Available at: http://www.cdc.gov/growthcharts/default.htm

BLOOD PRESSURE

Blood pressure screening at well-child visits starts at age 3 years. There are some conditions that warrant blood pressure monitoring at an earlier age:

- History of prematurity, very low birthweight, or other neonatal complication requiring intensive care
- Congenital heart disease (repaired or nonrepaired)
- Recurrent urinary tract infections, hematuria, or proteinuria
- Known renal disease or urologic malformations
- Family history of congenital renal disease
- Solid organ transplant
- Malignancy or bone marrow transplant
- Treatment with drugs known to raise BP
- Other systemic illnesses associated with hypertension (neurofibromatosis, tuberous sclerosis, etc.)
- Evidence of elevated intracranial pressure

Accurate determination of blood pressure requires proper equipment (stethoscope, manometer and inflation cuff, or an automated system) and a cooperative, seated subject in a quiet room. Although automated blood pressure instruments are widely available and easy to use, blood pressure readings from these devices are typically 5 mm Hg higher for diastolic and 10 mm Hg higher for systolic blood pressure compared with auscultatory techniques. Therefore, the diagnosis of hypertension should not be made on the basis of automated readings alone. Additionally, blood pressure varies somewhat by the height and weight of the individual. Consequently, hypertension is diagnosed as a systolic or diastolic blood pressure greater than the 95th percentile based on the age and height (or weight) percentile of the patient.

The width of the inflatable portion of the cuff should be 40%–50% of the circumference of the limb. Obese children need a larger cuff size to avoid a falsely elevated blood pressure reading. Cuffs that are too narrow will overestimate and those that are too wide will underestimate the true blood pressure. Hypertension should not be diagnosed based upon readings at one visit, but rather three separate occasions of hypertension are required. Repeated measurements at different visits over time should be tracked using flow charts in an electronic medical record or equivalent in a paper chart. Children with repeated blood pressure readings from the 90th to the 95th percentile may be classified as having prehypertension. Those with greater than between the 95th and 99th percentile plus 5 mm of Hg are classified as Stage 1 hypertension, and those greater than the 99th percentile plus 5 mm of Hg are termed Stage 2 hypertension. National High Blood Pressure Education Program recommends that all children with blood pressure of greater than or equal to 95% should have a complete blood count, serum nitrogen, creatinine, electrolytes, fasting lipid panel, glucose, urinalysis, urine culture, renal ultrasound, echocardiogram, and retinal examination. Nonpharmacologic interventions include diet, exercise, and weight management. Indications for pharmacologic therapy may include:

- Symptomatic hypertension
- Secondary hypertension
- Hypertensive target-organ damage
- Diabetes (types 1 and 2)
- Persistent hypertension despite nonpharmacologic measures

National High Blood Pressure Education Program Working Group in High Blood Pressure in Children and Adolescents: The fourth report on diagnosis, evaluation and treatment of high blood pressure in children and adolescents. Revised 2005. Available at: http://www.nhlbi.nih.gov/health/prof/heart/hbp/hbp_ped.pdf

Park MK et al: Comparison of auscultatory and oscillometric blood pressures. Arch Pediatr Adolesc Med 2001;155:50 [PMID: 11177062].

Wiesen J et al: Evaluation of pediatric patients with mild to moderate hypertension: Yield of diagnostic testing. Pediatrics 2008;122:e988–e993 [PMID: 18977966].

VISION & HEARING SCREENING

Examination of the eyes and an assessment of vision should be performed at every health supervision visit. Eye problems are relatively common in children: refractive errors (including myopia, hyperopia, and astigmatism), amblyopia (loss of visual acuity from cortical suppression of the vision of the eye), and/or strabismus (misalignment of the eyes) occur in 5%–10% of preschoolers. Assessment of vision should include visual inspection of the eyes and eyelids, alignment of eyes, and visual acuity.

From birth to 3 years of age, the movement and alignment of the eyes should be assessed and the pupils and red reflexes examined. The red reflex, performed on each pupil individually and then on both eyes simultaneously, is used to detect eye opacities (eg, cataracts or corneal clouding) and retinal abnormalities (eg, retinal detachment or retinoblastoma). By three months of age, an infant should be able to track, or visually follow a moving object, with both eyes.

Starting at age 3, formal testing of visual acuity should be done. This can be performed in the office with a variety of tests, including the tumbling E chart or picture tests such as Allen cards. In these tests, each eye is tested separately, with the nontested eye completely covered. Credit is given for any line on which the child gets more than 50% correct. Children 4 years of age and older who are unable to cooperate should be retested, ideally within 1 month, and those who cannot cooperate with repeated attempts should be referred to an ophthalmologist. Because visual acuity improves with age, results of the test are interpreted using the cutoff values in Table 9–2. However, any two-line discrepancy between the two eyes, even within the passing range (eg, 20/20 in one eye, 20/30 in the other in a child aged 6 years or older) should be referred to an ophthalmologist.

Throughout childhood, clinicians should screen for undetected strabismus (ocular misalignment). The corneal light reflex test can be used starting at 3 months and the cover test can be used beginning at 6 months to assess for strabismus. The random dot E test may also be used for detecting strabismus. The corneal light reflex test, the cover test, and visual acuity test are described further in Chapter 16.

Recommendations for vision screening and indications for referral are listed in Table 9-3. Referral to an ophthalmologist is also recommended for preterm infants for evaluation of retinopathy of prematurity (ROP), as well as children with a family history of amblyopia, strabismus, retinoblastoma, or retinal degeneration. Children with Down syndrome should be referred to an ophthalmologist at 6 months of age given their increased risk for refractive error, strabismus, and cataracts.

Hearing loss, if undetected, can lead to substantial impairments in speech, language, and cognitive development.

Table 9–2. Age-appropriate visual acuity.[a]

Age (y)	Minimal Acceptable Acuity
3-5	20/40
6 and older	20/30

[a]Refer to an ophthalmologist if minimal acuity is not met at a given age or if there is a difference in scores of two or more lines between the eyes.

Table 9-3. Recommended vision screening in the primary care office.

Test	Age for Screening	Indication(s) for Referral
Inspection of eyes and lids	All	
Red reflex	Birth until child can read eye chart	Abnormal red reflex, asymmetry of the red reflexes, or partially obscured red reflex
Assessment of fixation and following	Starting at 2 months	Poor fixation/following by 3 months
Corneal Light Reflex for assessing strabismus	3 months to 5 years	Asymmetry of light reflex (in relation to iris and pupil)
Cover testing for assessing strabismus	6 months to 5 years	Presence of refixation movement
Fundoscopic examination	Starting at 3 years	
Preliterate eye chart testing	Starting at 3-4 years	Unable to pass 20/40 for ages 3-5 or 20/30 for 6 and older. Also refer if there is a difference of two or more lines between the eyes.

Because significant bilateral hearing loss is one of the more common major anomalies found at birth, and early detection and intervention of hearing loss leads to better outcomes for children, universal hearing screening is provided to newborns in most parts of the United States. Hearing in infants is assessed using either evoked otoacoustic emissions or auditory brain stem-evoked responses. Because universal newborn hearing screening is sometimes associated with false-positive test results, confirmatory audiology testing is required for abnormal tests.

Informal behavioral testing of hearing, such as observing an infant's response to a shaken rattle, may be unreliable. In fact, parental concerns about hearing are of greater predictive value than the results of informal tests, and such concerns should be taken seriously. Prior to age 4, infants should be referred to an audiologist for testing if a concern arises. Conventional screening audiometry, in which a child raises her hand when a sound is heard, can be performed starting at age 4. Each ear should be tested at 500, 1000, 2000, and 400 Hz and referred at threshold levels of greater than 20 dB at any of these frequencies. Any evidence of hearing loss should be substantiated by repeated testing, and if still abnormal, a referral for a formal hearing evaluation should be made.

The AAP periodicity schedule recommends routine hearing screening at 4, 5, 6, 8, and 10 years of age. Children with any risk factors for hearing loss should be closely followed and receive more frequent screening. A number of inherited or acquired conditions increase the risk of hearing loss. Sometimes hearing loss can be mistaken for inattention, and so hearing screening should be part of workup for attention problems. Additional details regarding hearing assessment are provided in Chapter 18.

American Academy of Pediatrics et al: Eye examination in infants, children, and young adults by pediatricians. Pediatrics 2003;111:902 [PMID: 12671132].

American Academy of Pediatrics et al: Red reflex examination in neonates, infants, and children. Pediatrics 2008;122:1401.

Harlor AD et al. American Academy of Pediatrics Committee on Practice and Ambulatory Medicine, Section of Otolaryngology. Hearing assessment in infants and children: Recommendations beyond neonatal screening. Pediatrics 2009;124:1253.

Katbamna B, Crumpton T, Patel DR: Hearing impairment in children. Pediatr Clin North Am 2008;55:1175.

Tingley DH: Vision screening essentials: Screening today for eye disorders in the pediatric patient. Pediatr Rev 2007;28:54.

SCREENING

Newborn Screening

Newborn screening involves population-wide testing for metabolic and genetic diseases. It has become an essential component in a public health program that screens over 4 million newborns every year. Blood samples are collected by heelstick from newborns before hospital discharge, and results are usually available within 1 week. Some states routinely repeat blood testing between 7 and 14 days of life, while others recommend it if the child is discharged in less than 24 hours. The state-to-state variation seen in newborn screen panels has begun to diminish thanks to national recommendations. In 2010, the Secretary Advisory Committee on Heritable Disorders in Newborns and Children recommended screening for 30 core conditions with another 26 detectable through differential diagnosis. Most states have adopted these guidelines.

Infants with a positive screening result should receive close follow-up, with additional confirmatory studies performed at a center with experience in doing these tests. Screening tests are usually accurate, but the sensitivity and specificity of a particular screening test must be carefully considered. If symptoms of a disease are present despite a negative result on a screening test, the infant should be tested further. Newborn screening has benefited thousands of infants and their families, preventing and diminishing the morbidity of many diseases. At the same time, the emotional cost of false-positive screening is a continuing challenge. Parents report high levels of stress during the evaluation process. Recommendations for useful resources, given the variability of information on the Internet, and prompt clinical services can help reduce this distress.

National Newborn Screening by State. Available at: http://genes-r-us.uthscsa.edu/nbsdisorders.pdf. Assessed July 19,2011.

Deluca JM, Kearney MH, Norton SA, Arnold GL: Parents' experiences of expanded newborn screening evaluations. Pediatrics 2011 Jul;128(1):53–61 [Epub 2011 Jun 27] [PMID: 21708804].

Committee report: Method for evaluating conditions nominated for population-based screening of newborns and children. Calonge N et al: Advisory Committee on Heritable Disorders in Newborns and Children. Genet Med 2010 Mar;12(3):153–159 [PMID: 20154628].

Fernoff PM: Newborn screening for genetic disorders. Pediatr Clin North Am 2009 Jun;56(3):505–513.

Lead Screening

The developing infant and child are at risk of lead poisoning or toxicity because of their propensity to place objects in the mouth and their efficient absorption of this metal. Children with lead toxicity are typically asymptomatic. High blood levels (> 70 mcg/dL) can cause severe health problems such as seizures and coma. Numerous neuropsychological deficits have been associated with increased lead levels. Blood lead levels less than 10 mcg/dL have been correlated with lower intelligence quotients. The primary source of lead exposure in this country remains lead-based paint, even though most of its uses have been banned since 1977. Lead levels have declined nationally from a mean of 16 mcg/dL in 1976 to 2 mcg/dL in 2001. However, considerable variation in lead levels exists in different regions of the United States, and a majority of children at risk of lead toxicity are not currently screened. Despite the wide variation in the prevalence of lead toxicity, the CDC recommends universal lead screening for children at ages 1 and 2 and targeted screening for older children living in communities with a high percentage of old housing (> 27% of houses built before 1950) or a high percentage of children with elevated blood lead levels (> 12% of children with levels above 10 mcg/dL). Previously, all Medicaid-enrolled children were screened, but now the recommendation is to screen those at risk because of local variations in lead exposure.

Communities with inadequate data regarding local blood lead levels should also undergo universal screening. Caregivers of children between 6 months and 6 years of age may be interviewed by questionnaire about environmental risk factors for lead exposure (Table 9–4), although the data to support the use of this screening are inconclusive. If risk factors are present, a blood lead level should be obtained.

A venous blood sample is preferred over a capillary specimen. An elevated capillary (fingerstick) blood sample should always be confirmed by a venous sample. No action is required for blood lead levels less than 10 mcg/dL. The cognitive development of children with confirmed blood levels higher than 14 mcg/dL should be evaluated and attempts

Table 9–4. Elements of a lead risk questionnaire.

Recommended questions
1. Does your child live in or regularly visit a house built before 1950? This could include a day care center, preschool, the home of a baby-sitter or relative, and so on.
2. Does your child live in or regularly visit a house built before 1978 with recent, ongoing, or planned renovation or remodeling?
3. Does your child have a sister or brother, housemate, or playmate being followed for lead poisoning?
Questions that may be considered by region or locality
1. Does your child live with an adult whose job (eg, at a brass/copper foundry, firing range, automotive or boat repair shop, or furniture refinishing shop) or hobby (eg, electronics, fishing, stained-glass making, pottery making) involves exposure to lead?
2. Does your child live near a work or industrial site (eg, smelter, battery recycling plant) that involves the use of lead?
3. Does your child use pottery or ingest medications that are suspected of having a high lead content?
4. Does your child have exposure to old, nonbrand-type toys or burning lead-painted wood?
5. Does your child play on an athletic field with artificial turf?

made to identify the environmental source. Iron deficiency should be treated if present. Chelation of lead is indicated for levels of 45 mcg/dL and higher and is urgently required for levels above 70 mcg/dL. All families should receive education to decrease the risk of lead exposure. With any elevated lead level (> 10 mcg/dL), rescreening should be performed at recommended intervals.

Iron Deficiency

Iron deficiency is the most common nutritional deficiency in the United States. Severe iron deficiency causes anemia, behavioral problems, and cognitive effects, but recent evidence suggests that even iron deficiency without anemia may cause behavioral and cognitive difficulties. Some effects, such as the development of abnormal sleep cycles, may persist even if iron deficiency is corrected in infancy.

Risk factors for iron deficiency include preterm or low-birth-weight births, multiple pregnancy, iron deficiency in the mother, use of nonfortified formula or cow's milk before age 12 months, and an infant diet that is low in iron-containing foods. Infants and toddlers consuming more than 24 oz/d of cow's milk are at risk, as are children with chronic illness, restricted diet, or extensive blood loss.

Primary prevention of iron deficiency should be achieved through dietary means, including feeding iron-containing cereals by age 6 months, avoiding low-iron formula during infancy, and limiting cow's milk to 24 oz/d in children aged 1–5 years.

Universal screening for anemia should occur at approximately 12 months of age by obtaining a hemoglobin or hematocrit. Premature and low-birth-weight infants may need testing before 6 months of age.

A full CBC to look at MCV can aid in the evaluation. Serum ferritin is a useful test to evaluate iron deficiency anemia, but can also pick up iron deficiency in the absence of anemia. Because ferritin is an acute-phase reactant and can be falsely reassuring in the presence of inflammation, infection, or malignancy, some experts recommend obtaining a concurrent CRP for accurate interpretation of the ferritin level. Other biochemical tests of iron deficiency include transferrin saturation (low) and erythrocyte protoporphyrin (elevated), which are sensitive measures, but are more costly. Lead poisoning can cause iron-deficiency anemia and should be explored as a cause for at-risk infants and children.

Management of iron deficiency with or without anemia includes treatment doses of iron, which is different than the supplementation dose found in multivitamins. The treatment dose is 3–6 mg/kg body weight of *elemental* iron.

Baker RD et al: American Academy of Pediatrics, Committee on Nutrition: Diagnosis and prevention and iron-deficiency anemia in infants and young children (0–3 years of age). Pediatrics 2010;126:1040.

Hypercholesterolemia & Hyperlipidemia

Cardiovascular disease is the leading cause of death in the United States and research has documented that the atherosclerotic process begins in childhood. Genetic factors, diet, and physical activity all play a role in the disease process. Fasting lipid screening is recommended for children between the ages of 2 and 10 if certain risk factors are present: family history of dyslipidemia, family history of early cardiovascular heart disease, obesity (95th > BMI ≥ 85th percentile), overweight (BMI ≥ 85th < 95th percentile), hypertension, or diabetes mellitus. Diet and weight management strategies are the primary interventions. However, for severe dyslipidemia (LDL ≥ 190 mg/dL), pharmacologic therapy should be considered. Consideration of pharmacotherapy should be made at 160 mg/dL if there is a family history of heart disease or there are two or more risk factors present. The presence of diabetes should lower the threshold for pharmacotherapy to 130 mg/dL. Patients who screen negative should be retested in 3–5 years.

Daniels SR, Greer FR; Committee on Nutrition: Lipid screening and cardiovascular health in childhood. Pediatrics 2008 Jul; 122(1):198–208.

Tuberculosis

According to the CDC, 13,299 cases of tuberculosis were reported in the United States in 2007. Risk of tuberculosis should be assessed at well-child visits, and screening should be based on high-risk status. High risk is defined as contact with a person with known or suspected tuberculosis; having symptoms or radiographic findings suggesting tuberculosis; birth, residence, or travel to a region with high tuberculosis prevalence (Asia, Middle East, Africa, Latin America); contact with a person with AIDS or HIV; or contact with a prisoner, migrant farm worker, illicit drug user, or a person who is or has been recently homeless. The Mantoux test (5 tuberculin units of purified protein derivative) is the only recommended screening test. It can be done as early as 3 months of age and should be repeated annually if the risk persists. The tine test should not be used. Previous vaccination with bacille Calmette-Guérin (BCG) is not a contraindication to tuberculosis skin testing.

Screening of Adolescent Patients

Adolescents may present with chief complaints that are not the true concern for the visit. Repeating the question 'Is there anything else you would like to discuss?' should be considered. Since suicide is a leading cause of morbidity and mortality in this age group, screening with the Pediatric Symptom Checklist for Youth or TeenScreen® for depression is recommended (http://www.teenscreen.org/resources/providers/).

Testing adolescents for blood cholesterol, tuberculosis, and HIV should be offered based on high-risk criteria outlined in this chapter and in Chapter 41. Females should have a screening hematocrit once after the onset of menses. During routine visits, adolescents should be questioned sensitively about risk factors (eg, multiple partners; early onset of sexual activity, including child sexual abuse) and symptoms (eg, genital discharge, infectious lesions, pelvic pain) of sexually transmitted diseases (STDs). An annual dipstick urinalysis for leukocytes is recommended for sexually active adolescents. Current guidelines recommend that the first Papanicolaou (Pap) test should be performed at age 21 years, regardless of onset of sexual activity. A complete pelvic exam should be performed when evaluating lower abdominal pain in an adolescent. See Chapter 3 for additional details. Because females with STDs are often not symptomatic, gonococcal and chlamydial urine test for Polymerase Chain Reaction (PCR) and screening tests for syphilis and trichomoniasis are appropriate at the time of each pelvic examination.

American Academy of Pediatrics: Tuberculosis. In Pickering LK (editor): *2009 Red Book: Report of the Committee on Infectious Diseases*, 28th ed. American Academy of Pediatrics, 2009.

American Academy of Pediatrics 2006:678. American Academy of Pediatrics, Committee on Environmental Health: Lead exposure in children: Prevention, detection, and management. Pediatrics 2005;116:1036 [PMID: 16199720].

Centers for Disease Control and Prevention lead fact sheet (English and Spanish). Available at: http://www.atsdr.cdc.gov/csem/lead/pbpated_sheet2.html

Centers for Disease Control and Prevention, National Center for HIV, STD and TB Prevention: Tuberculosis Surveillance Reports. Available at: http://www.cdc.gov/tb/surv/surv2006/default.htm

Haney EM et al: Screening and treatment for lipid disorders in children and adolescents: Systematic evidence for the US Preventive Services Task Force. Pediatrics 2007;120:e189 [PMID: 17606543].

ANTICIPATORY GUIDANCE

An essential part of the health supervision visit is anticipatory guidance. During this counseling, the clinician directs the parent's or the older child's attention to issues that may arise in the future. Guidance must be appropriate to age, focus on concerns expressed by the parent and patient, and address issues in depth rather than run through a number of issues superficially. Both oral and printed materials are used. When selecting written materials, providers should be sensitive to issues of literacy and primary language spoken by the family members. Areas of concern include diet, injury prevention, developmental and behavioral issues, and health promotion.

Injury Prevention

Injuries are the leading cause of death in children and adolescents after the first year of life. For young people aged 15–19 years, injuries are responsible for more than half of all deaths. In every age category, males are at higher risk than females for unintentional injury (Figure 9–3).

Injury prevention counseling is an important component of each health supervision visit and can be reinforced during all visits. Counseling should focus on problems that are frequent and age appropriate. Passive strategies of prevention should be emphasized, because these are more effective than active strategies; for example, placing chemicals out of reach in high, locked cupboards to prevent poisoning will be more effective than instructing parents to watch their children closely.

Informational handouts about home safety, such as The Injury Prevention Program (TIPP; available from the AAP), can be provided in the waiting room. Advice can then be tailored to the specific needs of each family, with reinforcement from age-specific TIPP handouts.

A. Motor Vehicle Injuries

The primary cause of death of children in the United States is motor vehicle injuries. In 2008, about 46% of children aged 14 years or younger who were killed in motor vehicle accidents were unrestrained.

The type and positioning of safety seats are confusing. While car seat and booster seat laws differ by state, a recent AAP policy statement describes the best practice

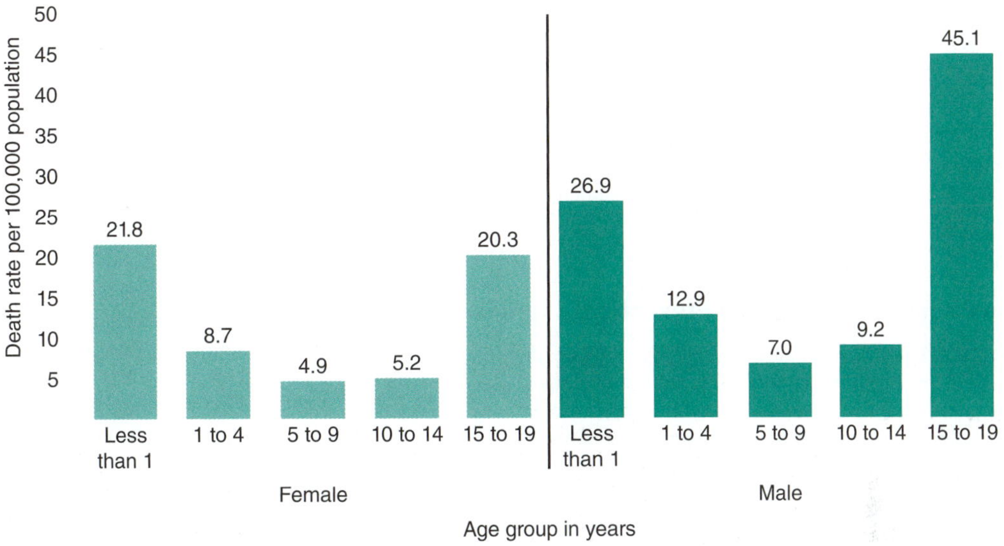

▲ **Figure 9–3.** Unintentional injury death rates among children 0–19 years, by sex for 2000–2005. (National Center for Health Statistics.)

recommendations. All infants and toddlers should ride in a rear-facing car safety seat until 2 years of age or until they reach the weight and height limits for convertible car safety seats (usually 35 pounds). Infants may ride in infant-only seats (which often have a carrying handle and snap into a base that is secured in the car) until they reach the height and weight limit for that seat, and then transition to a convertible car seat. Once a child reaches 2 years old (or younger than 2 if outgrown the weight and height limit of a convertible car seat), he can be in a forward-facing car safety seat with a harness. The safest scenario is for a child to remain in a car safety seat with a harness as long as possible. Once a child reaches the weight or height limits of a forward-facing seat, he may be transitioned to a belt-positioning booster until the vehicle's lap-and-shoulder belt fits properly (child can sit with his back against the vehicle seat, bend his knees at the edge of the seat, have the belt positioned in the center of the shoulder and across the chest, and have the lap belt touching the thighs). These criteria are generally met once a child reaches 4′9″ height and is between the ages of 8 and 12 years. All children under 13 years of age should be restrained in the rear seats of the vehicle.

A rear-facing car seat should never be used in a seat with a passenger air bag. Unfortunately, restraint use shows a decreasing trend with advancing age: children from 1 to 8 years of age use restraints over 90% of the time, but those 8–12 years of age use restraints less than 85% of the time. African American and Hispanic children use child safety seats less often than white children.

When a child is a passenger in a car crash, the case fatality rate is 1%; for children on the street who are hit by cars, the risk of fatality increases threefold. Pedestrian safety skills should be taught to children early in childhood; however, parental supervision of children near roadways continues to be required for many years.

A final motor vehicle risk for health involves the use of portable electronic devices. Using a cell phone while driving is associated with a fourfold increase in motor vehicle accidents. Texting while driving poses an even greater danger. Parents and teenage drivers should avoid these risks.

B. Bicycle Injuries

Each year, an average of nearly 400 children die from bicycle crashes, and over 450,000 are treated for bicycle-riding injuries. Over 150,000 children are treated annually in emergency departments for head injuries sustained while riding a bicycle. Many observational studies have shown a decreased risk of head injury with the use of bicycle helmets. Community-based interventions, especially those that provide free helmets, have been shown to increase observed bike helmet wearing. Counseling by physicians in various settings has also been shown to increase bike helmet use. While there is no federal law mandating bicycle helmets, some states have passed legislation requiring bicycle helmets, though most laws are limited to children under 18 years old. Proponents point out that studies show increased use of helmets, but others have raised concern that bike helmet laws may discourage bike riding and its beneficial effects on weight control.

C. Skiing and Snowboarding Injuries

Recent studies have suggested that the burden of skiing injuries is high among children, and that children have the highest rate of injury of any age group: approximately three injuries per 1000 skier days. Traumatic brain injuries are the leading cause of death for pediatric age skiers. Case control studies have shown a decrease in head injuries associated with helmet use. Appropriate counseling of helmet use is a reasonable strategy to increase helmet use in children.

D. Firearm Injuries and Violence Prevention

The United States has a higher rate of firearm-related death than any other industrialized country. For children younger than 15, the death rate from firearm-related injuries is nearly 12 times greater than that of 25 other industrialized nations. Some gun deaths may be accidental, but most are the result of homicide or suicide. A gun in the home doubles the likelihood of a lethal suicide attempt. Although handguns are often kept in homes for protection, a gun is more likely to kill a family member or a friend than an intruder. Adolescents with a history of depression or violence are at higher risk with a gun in the home. The most effective way to prevent firearm injuries is to remove guns from the home. Families who keep firearms at home should lock them in a cabinet or drawer and store ammunition in a separate locked location.

E. Drowning and Near Drowning

Drowning is the second leading cause of injury-related death in children, and those aged 1–3 years have the highest rate of drowning. For every death by drowning, six children are hospitalized for near drowning, and up to 10% of survivors experience severe brain damage. Children younger than 1 year of age are most likely to drown in the bathtub. Buckets filled with water also present a risk of drowning to the older infant or toddler. For children aged 1–4 years, drowning or near drowning occurs most often in home swimming pools; and for school-aged children and teens, drowning occurs most often in large bodies of water (eg, swimming pools or open water). Parents should be cautioned that inflatable swimming devises are not a substitution for approved live vests or close supervision and can give a false sense of security. School-aged children should be taught to swim, and recreational swimming should always be supervised. Home pools must be fenced securely, and parents should know how to perform cardiopulmonary resuscitation.

F. Fire and Burn Injuries

Fires and burns are the leading cause of injury-related deaths in the home. Categories of burn injury include smoke inhalation; flame contact; scalding; and electrical, chemical, and ultraviolet burns. Scalding is the most common type of burn in children. Most scalds involve foods and beverages, but nearly one-fourth of scalds are with tap water, and for that reason it is recommended that hot water heaters be set to a maximum of 120°F. Most fire-related deaths result from smoke inhalation. Smoke detectors can prevent 85% of the injuries and deaths caused by fires in the home. Families should discuss a fire plan with children and practice emergency evacuation from the home.

Sunburn is a common thermal injury, perhaps because symptoms of excessive sun exposure do not begin until after the skin has been damaged. Sunburn and excessive sun exposure are associated with skin cancers. Prevention of sunburn is best achieved by sun avoidance, particularly during the midday hours of 10 AM to 4 PM. A sunscreen with a minimum sun protection factor (SPF) of 15 that protects against UVA and UVB rays should be used on sunny and cloudy days to help protect against sunburn. Hats and sunglasses are also important aspects of safe sun exposure. The safety of sunscreen is not established for infants younger than 6 months; thus, sun avoidance, appropriate clothing, and hats are recommended for this age group. In extreme circumstances in which shade is not available, a minimal amount of sunscreen can be applied to small areas, including the face and back of the hands.

G. Choking

Choking is a leading cause of injury and death in young children. Choking hazards include food and small objects. Children under the age of three are particularly at risk because they do not have fully coordinated chewing and swallowing, and they are more apt to put small objects in their mouths. Foods that are commonly associated with choking include hot dogs, hard candy, nuts, popcorn, raw vegetables, and chunks of meat, fruit, or cheese. Common nonfood items that pose a risk for choking include coins, latex balloons, button batteries, marbles, small toys, and small toy parts. While being mindful of choking hazards is important, accidents can still occur. Parents and caregivers should be trained in CPR and choking first aid.

American Academy of Pediatrics, Committee on Injury and Poison Prevention: Bicycle helmets. Pediatrics 2001;108:1030 [PMID: 11581464].

American Academy of Pediatrics, Committee on Injury and Poison Prevention: Firearm-related injuries affecting the pediatric population. Pediatrics 2000;105:888 [PMID: 10742344].

American Academy of Pediatrics, Committee on Injury and Poison Prevention: Reducing the number of deaths and injuries from residential fires. Pediatrics 2000;105:1355 [PMID: 10835082].

American Academy of Pediatrics, Committee on Injury and Poison Prevention: Prevention of choking among children. Pediatrics 2010;125:601.

American Academy of Pediatrics, Committee on Injury, Violence, and Poison Prevention: Prevention of Drowning. Pediatrics 2011;126:e253.

American Academy of Pediatrics, Committee on Injury, Violence, and Poison Prevention: Child Passenger Safety. Pediatrics 2011; 127:788.

Centers for Disease Control and Prevention (CDC). WISQARS (Web-based Injury Statistics Query and Reporting System). Available at: www.cdc.gov/injury/wisqars/index.html. Accessed July 27, 2011.

Gardner HG; American Academy of Pediatrics Committee on Injury, Violence, and Poison Prevention: Office-based counseling for unintentional injury prevention. Pediatrics 2007 Jan; 119(1):202–206 [PMID: 17200289].

Parkin PC, Howard AW: Advances in the prevention of children's injuries: An examination of four common outdoor activities. Curr Opin Pediatr 2008 Dec;20(6):719–723.

NUTRITION COUNSELING

Screening for nutritional problems and guidance for age-appropriate dietary choices should be part of every health supervision visit. Overnutrition, undernutrition, and eating disorders can be detected by a careful analysis of dietary and activity patterns interpreted in the context of a child's growth pattern.

Human milk feeding is species-specific and is the preferred method for infant feeding for the first year of life. Pediatricians should assist mother-infant dyads with latch, and help manage breastfeeding difficulties in the early newborn period. For exclusively breastfed infants, vitamin D supplementation should be given. Iron-fortified formula should be used in situations when breastfeeding is contraindicated such as HIV, illicit drug use in the mother, active untreated tuberculosis, galactosemia, and certain medications. After the first year, breastfeeding may continue or whole cow's milk can be given because of continued rapid growth and high energy needs. After 2 years of life, milk with 2% fat or lower may be offered. Baby foods are generally introduced at about 6 months of age and self-feeding with finger foods encouraged at 7–8 months of age.

When obtaining a dietary history, it is helpful to assess the following: who purchases and prepares food; who feeds the child; whether meals and snacks occur at consistent times and in a consistent setting; whether children are allowed to snack or "graze" between meals; the types and portion sizes of food and drinks provided; the frequency of eating meals in restaurants or eating take-out food; and whether the child eats while watching television.

For children 2 years of age and older, a prudent diet consists of diverse food sources, encourages high-fiber foods (eg, fruits, vegetables, grain products), and limits sodium and fat intake. Since obesity is becoming increasingly prevalent, foods to be avoided or limited include processed foods, soft drinks, and candy. Parents should be gently reminded that they are modeling for a lifetime of eating behaviors in their children, both in terms of the types of foods they provide and the structure of meals (eg, the importance of the family eating together). For additional information on nutritional guidelines, undernutrition, and obesity, see Chapter 11; for eating disorders, see Chapter 6; for adolescent obesity, see Chapter 4.

As of 2009, the revised new Women, Infants, and Children (WIC) food packages will reflect the recommendations above and include provision of more fruits and vegetables, whole grains, yogurt and soy products, low-fat milk, and limitations on juice. Breastfeeding mothers will receive more food as part of their package, less formula supplementation, and breastfed infants will receive baby food meats as a first food (because of more iron and zinc).

American Academy of Pediatrics, Committee on Nutrition: Prevention of pediatric overweight and obesity. Pediatrics 2003; 112:424 [PMID: 12897303].

American Academy of Pediatrics Section on Breastfeeding Policy Statement: Breastfeeding and the use of human milk. Pediatrics 2005 Feb;115:496–506 [PMID: 15687461].

New WIC Food Packages. Available at: http://www.fns.usda.gov/wic/benefitsandservices/foodpkgallowances.HTM. Accessed August 24, 2009.

COUNSELING ABOUT TELEVISION & OTHER MEDIA

The average child in the United States watches approximately 3 hours of television per day, and this does not include time spent watching videotapes or DVDs, playing video games, or playing on computers. Having a television set in the bedroom is associated with watching more television as well as sleep disturbances. Up to 32% of 2- to 7-year-olds and 65% of 8- to 18-year-olds have a bedroom television set.

Watching television may have both positive and negative effects. Programs directed toward early childhood may increase knowledge and imaginativeness. Excessive television viewing of programs with inappropriate content has been shown to have negative effects with respect to violence, sexuality, substance abuse, nutrition, social skills, and body self-image. More recent data suggest that excessive viewing in childhood may have a long-lasting negative effect on cognitive development and academic achievement.

Clinicians should assess media exposure in their patients, and offer parents concrete advice. There should be limits on when and how much television is watched. The AAP recommends that children younger than 2 years of age should not watch any television, and that children 2 years and older be limited to 2 hours total time each day for all media. The television should not be on during mealtimes, night, or naptimes. Parents should themselves watch sensibly, monitor the program content to which their children are exposed, watch programs and discuss interesting content with children, remove television sets from all bedrooms, and encourage alternative activities.

Social networking sites are becoming increasingly popular and clinicians need to encourage parents to monitor participation and be aware of potential problems with cyberbullying, "Facebook depression," sexting, and exposure to inappropriate content on sites such as You Tube.

Hancox RJ et al: Association of television viewing during childhood with poor educational achievement. Arch Pediatr Adolesc Med 2005;159:614 [PMID: 15996992].

Jordan A: The role of media in children's development: An ecological perspective. J Dev Behav Pediatr 2004;25:196 [PMID: 15194905].

O'Keeffe Gwenn Schurgin, Clarke-Pearson Kathleen, and Council on Communications and Media. Clinical Report: The Impact of Social Media on Children, Adolescents, and Family. Pediatrics 2011;127(4):800–804 [published ahead of print March 28, 2011, doi:10.1542/peds.2011-0054].

IMMUNIZATIONS

A child's immunization status should be assessed at every visit and every opportunity should be taken to vaccinate. Even though parents may keep an immunization record, it is critical that providers also keep an accurate record of a child's immunizations. This information should be written in a prominent location in the paper or electronic chart or kept in an immunization registry.

Despite high overall national immunization coverage levels, areas of under immunization continue to exist in the United States. An understanding of true contraindications (vs "false contraindications") and a "no missed opportunities" approach to immunization delivery has been shown to successfully increase immunization levels. Therefore, it is important that clinicians screen records and administer required immunizations at all types of visits, and administer all needed vaccinations simultaneously. Additionally, clinicians should operate reminder/recall systems, in which parents of underimmunized children are prompted by mail, telephone, and text messages (particularly with adolescents) to visit the clinic for immunization. The assessment of clinic-wide immunization levels and feedback of these data to providers have also been shown to increase immunization rates.

A wealth of information for parents and providers about immunizations is also available at the National Immunization Program's web site (www.cdc.gov/vaccines).

Santoli JM et al: Immunization pockets of need: Science and practice. Am J Prev Med 2000;19(1S):89 [PMID: 11024333].

Task Force on Community Preventive Services: Recommendations regarding interventions to improve vaccination coverage in children, adolescents, and adults. Am J Prev Med 2000;18(1S):92 [PMID: 10806981].

Other Types of General Pediatric Service

ACUTE-CARE VISITS

Acute-care visits account for 30% or more of the general pediatrician's office visits. These visits are conducted in an efficient, structured way. Office personnel should determine the reason for the visit and whether it is an emergent situation, obtain a brief synopsis of the child's symptoms, carefully document vital signs, and list known drug allergies. The pediatric clinician should document the events related to the presenting problem and carefully describe them in the medical record. The record should include supporting laboratory data and a diagnosis. Treatments and follow-up instructions must be recorded, including when to return to the office if the problem is not ameliorated. Immunization status should be screened, as previously discussed. Depending on the severity of illness, this may also be an opportunity for age-appropriate health maintenance screenings and anticipatory guidance. This may be particularly true with older school-aged children or adolescents who may be seen more rarely for routine health maintenance visits.

PRENATAL VISITS

Ideally, a couple's first trip to a physician's office should take place before the birth of their baby. A prenatal visit goes a long way toward establishing trust and enables a pediatric provider to learn about a family's expectations, concerns, and fears regarding the anticipated birth. If the infant develops a problem during the newborn period, a provider who has already met the family is in a better position to maintain rapport and communication with the new parents.

In addition to helping establish a relationship between parents and pediatric providers, the prenatal visit can be used to gather information about the parents and the pregnancy, provide information and advice, and identify high-risk situations. A range of information can be provided to parents regarding feeding choices and the benefits of breastfeeding; injury prevention, including sleeping position and the appropriate use of car seats; and techniques for managing colic. Potential high-risk situations that may be identified include mental health issues in the parents, a history of domestic violence, or maternal medical problems that may affect the infant.

Serwint JR: The prenatal pediatric visit. Pediatr Rev 2003;24:31 [PMID: 12509543].

SPORTS PHYSICALS

The goal of the sports physical is to identify medical conditions that would make sports participation unsafe, screen for underlying illness through a traditional history and physical, and recognize preexisting injuries or medical problems that have affected previous sports seasons. As part of the history, the particular sport being played should be discussed. Different sports have different potentials for injury and prevention methods will differ. All patients should be asked about previous cardiac, respiratory, musculoskeletal, or neurologic problems associated with activity. Particular attention should be drawn to any suspicion of cardiac syncope, asthma symptoms, past concussions, or history of unilateral organs, such as kidneys or testicles. Anabolic steroid and nutritional supplement discussion should be detailed and explored. Any relevant family history of cardiac death younger than age 50 is important to document.

The physical examination obviously starts with vital signs, including accurate blood pressure screening and examination for obesity. Highlights of the examination include a careful respiratory and cardiac examination, looking for evidence of exercise-induced bronchospasm or anatomic heart disease. Electrocardiogram (ECG) or pulmonary function tests can be considered for suspected abnormalities. The skin examination should look for evidence of potentially contagious skin infections like impetigo or molluscum. The musculoskeletal examination should include all major muscle groups, as well as range of motion and stability testing of the neck, back, shoulder, hips, knees, and ankles. Any pain or limitation should prompt consideration of further investigation or therapy.

A few specific conditions bear mentioning during the counseling phase of the sports participation. A review of cardiac, respiratory, or musculoskeletal complaints that should prompt a return visit should be reviewed. The risks and danger of concussions and performance-enhancing drugs should be highlighted. Appropriate protective equipment should be encouraged.

Metzl JD et al: Preparticipation examination of the adolescent athlete: Parts 1 and 2. Pediatr Rev 2001;22:199–204, 227–239.

CHRONIC DISEASE MANAGEMENT

Chronic disease in pediatrics is defined as illness that has been present for more than 3 months. Twenty-five percent of children and 35% of adolescents have illnesses that meet the definition of a chronic illness. The most common chronic conditions in pediatric practice include asthma, obesity/overweight, attention-deficit/hyperactivity disorder, and allergic diseases, but also include congenital anomalies and other conditions. Many patients with chronic conditions are cared for only by a primary care provider. However, when subspecialist care is required, the primary care provider plays an integral part of the care to deal with the complexity of these conditions, which also includes understanding the child's growth and development, routine health promotion and anticipatory guidance, evaluating for social issues, advocating for children and their families, and care coordination.

The goal of chronic disease management is to optimize quality of life while minimizing the side effects of treatment interventions. The child and family's emotional responses to chronic illness should be addressed, and referrals to counselors should be offered if needed. Nutrition and the management of medical devices (eg, catheters, gastrostomy tubes) may need to be addressed, and care coordinated with appropriate specialists. Pediatric subspecialty referrals need to be arranged and monitored and results recorded in the chart in an organized manner. Problem lists in the chart should be used to document the chronic problems and monitor associated medications. A care plan should be created that includes basic health information and recommendations. Specific care plans have been developed for some diagnoses (such as the Asthma Action Plan). An example of a general healthcare plan can be downloaded from the AAP at www.aap.org/advocacy/blankform.pdf.

As a child with a chronic condition reaches 18–21 years of age, coordination of transition from child- to adult-oriented health care needs to occur. This transition should be specific to the individual patient and their family and should be planned well in advance. In children with special healthcare needs, discussions about transition should be initiated when the patient turns 12.

Ludder-Jackson P, Vessey JA: *Primary Care of the Child with a Chronic Condition*, 5th ed. Mosby-Year Book, 2010.

American Academy of Pediatrics; American Academy of Family Physicians; American College of Physicians, Transitions Clinic Report Authoring Group: Supporting the health care transition from adolescence to adulthood in the medical home. Pediatrics 2011;128:183.

MEDICAL HOME

The medical home is a concept in which children and their families have an identified, easily accessible primary care provider or group of primary care providers within an office. The American Academy of Pediatrics has identified seven characteristics of a medical home. The medical home must be (1) accessible, meaning that it must be within the child's community, physically accessible, and all insurances accepted; (2) family centered, with mutual responsibility and decision making between the patient/family and medical provider, and the family is recognized as an expert of the child; (3) continuous, in that the same medical professionals provide the continuity of care; (4) comprehensive, with provisions made such that ambulatory and inpatient care are available 24 hours per day, 7 days a week, for 52 weeks of the year; (5) coordinated, with a plan of care developed by the physician and family that is communicated to other providers and agencies as needed; (6) compassionate, meaning that concern is expressed and efforts are made to understand the patient's and family's perspective; and (7) culturally effective, in that the cultural background of the patient and family is respected and incorporated into care, and services are provided in the family's primary language or through a trained medical interpreter.

All children should have a medical home, but it is particularly crucial for children with special healthcare needs. A primary care provider through a medical home should be the center of healthcare for children to assist families with the amalgamation of consultant recommendations and development of a care plan to implement recommendations.

American Academy of Pediatrics. The medical home. Pediatrics 2002;110:184.

COUNSELING

Psychological disturbances are produced by physical or emotional stresses, injuries, inconsistent or overindulgent parenting practices, marital conflicts, child abuse and neglect, and school achievement problems. Topics amenable to office counseling include behavioral issues such as negativism and noncompliance, temper tantrums, oppositional behavior, and biting; childhood fears and feeding disorders; school problems; family upheavals such as separation, divorce, or remarriage; attention-deficit/hyperactivity disorder; and deaths of family members or close friends. Forty-five minutes is usually enough time for the therapeutic process to evolve, and this time should be protected from interruption. The young child is usually interviewed with the parent; school-aged children and adolescents benefit from time alone with the physician. After assessing the situation in one or two sessions, the primary care physician must decide whether the child's and family's needs are within his or her area of expertise or whether referral to another professional such as a psychologist or an education specialist would be appropriate. The pediatrician should know the warning signs of childhood depression and bipolar disorder and have a low threshold for referral of these concerns to the appropriate mental health professional. Ideally, mental health services not provided by the clinician are available in the same setting where physical health services are obtained (see later).

CONSULTATIONS

Physicians, other professionals, and parents may initiate consultations with a general pediatrician. Parents, subspecialists, family physicians, or professionals such as school officials, psychologists, or social workers may all seek medical consultation. Finally, an insurance company representative may want a second opinion before authorizing a set of services.

The types of consultations the general pediatrician may be asked to do include an evaluation only, an evaluation and interpretation, or an evaluation and treatment of an isolated problem. The type of consultation being requested should be clearly determined at the time of referral of the patient. This understanding should be clarified with the patient's insurance company so that appropriate authorization and reimbursement for the visit can occur.

Integrated Mental & Behavioral Health in the Primary Care Setting

In the United States, approximately 20% of school-age children suffer from a diagnosable emotional impairment. Prevalence is higher for children living in poor socioeconomic circumstances. About 75% of all children with psychiatric disturbances are seen in primary care settings, and half of all pediatric office visits involve behavioral, psychosocial, or educational concerns.

Child and family concerns routinely manifest in the context of visits with pediatric primary care providers. However, many pediatric providers in community settings do not feel equipped to address the growing mental health and behavioral needs of the populations they serve due to lack of training and perceived lack of support from mental health providers and systems. Parents are most likely to turn to their health care provider for information regarding parenting and child development than to another specialist.

Recent studies have shown that improved detection of mental health conditions is best done when there is a true partnership between clinical providers and families. A small number of clinic settings have moved forward with providing integrated behavior, development, and mental health training for physicians. The Healthy Steps for Young Children Program provides an example of training pediatric providers and delivering enhanced developmental services in pediatric primary care settings. Families participating in Healthy Steps received more developmental services, were more satisfied with the quality of care provided, were more likely to attend well-child visits and receive vaccinations on time, and were less likely to use severe discipline techniques with their children. Participation in the program also increased the likelihood that mothers at risk for depression would discuss their sadness with someone in the pediatric setting.

The primary care medical home is the ideal setting to engage families in efforts to address mental health care. Mental health has been brought to the forefront as a priority of the AAP in their April 2009 Call for Action "encourage the integration of mental health care into the primary medical home" as well as in the American Recovery and Reinvestment Act (ARRA) making mental health a priority in comparative effectiveness research. Moreover, improved detection of mental health conditions is best done when there is a true partnership between clinical providers and families.

American Academy of Pediatrics, Committee on Psychosocial Aspects of Child and Family Health and Task Force on Mental Health: The future of pediatrics: Mental health competencies for pediatric primary care. Pediatrics 2009 Jul;124:410–421 [PMID: 19564328].

Kelleher KJ et al: Management of pediatric mental disorders in primary care: Where are we now and where are we going? Curr Opin Pediatr 2006;18:649 [PMID: 17099365].

Williams J et al: Co-location of mental health professionals in primary care settings: Three North Carolina models. Clin Pediatr (Phila) 2006;45:537 [PMID: 16893859].

TELEPHONE MANAGEMENT & WEB-BASED INFORMATION

Providing appropriate, efficient, and timely clinical advice over the telephone is a critical element of pediatric primary care in the office setting. An estimated 20%–30% of all clinical care delivered by general pediatric offices is provided by telephone. Telephone calls to and from patients occur both during regular office hours and after the office has closed (termed after-hours), and the personnel and systems in place to handle office-hours versus before- and after-hours calls may differ. In either circumstance, several principles are important: (1) advice is given only by clinicians or other staff with formal medical education (eg, nurse, medical assistant), (2) staff is given additional training in providing telephone care, (3) documentation is made of all pertinent information from calls, (4) standardized protocols covering the most common pediatric symptoms are used, and (5) a physician is always available to handle urgent or difficult calls.

During routine office hours, approximately 20%–25% of all telephone calls to pediatric offices involve clinical matters. Many of these calls, however, are routine in nature, and an experienced nurse within the office can screen calls and provide appropriate advice by telephone. Calls from inexperienced or anxious parents about simple concerns should be answered with understanding and respect. Certain types of calls received during office hours should be promptly transferred to a physician: (1) true emergencies, (2) calls regarding hospitalized patients, (3) calls from other medical professionals, and (4) calls from parents who demand to speak with a physician. Nurses should also seek help from a clinician whenever they are uncertain about how to handle a particular call. When in doubt about the diagnosis or necessary treatment, nurses giving telephone advice should err on the side of having the patient seen in the office.

After-hours telephone answering services are available to many clinicians. Pediatric call centers, although not available in all communities, have certain benefits. Calls are managed using standardized protocols, the call centers are typically staffed by nurses with abundant pediatric experience, the calls are well-documented, and call centers often perform ongoing quality assurance. Extensive research on pediatric call centers has revealed a high degree of appropriate referrals to emergency departments, safety in terms of outcomes, parent satisfaction with the process, and savings to the health care system.

In general, after-hours pediatric telephone calls tend to be more serious than calls made during regular office hours. Deciding which patients need to be seen, and how urgently, are the most important aspects of these after-hours telephone "encounters." Several factors influence this final patient disposition: (1) the age of the patient, (2) the duration and type of symptom, (3) the presence of any underlying chronic condition, (4) whether the child appears "very sick" to the caller, and (5) the anxiety level of the caller. Once all the pertinent medical information is gathered, a decision is made about whether the child should be seen immediately (by ambulance versus car), seen in the office later (today versus tomorrow), or whether the illness can be safely cared for at home. At the end of the call, it should be confirmed that parents understand and feel comfortable with the plan for their child.

The Internet has become a common tool used in pediatric office settings. Information about the practice and providers, the care of common minor problems, scheduling of appointments, insurance issues, prescription refills, and laboratory test results are often available using the web. Pertinent health information, with appropriate permissions and authority, can often be provided via the Internet to other locations such as hospitals and pharmacies. A well-functioning Internet site is now a crucial service of a pediatric practice.

Bunik M et al: Pediatric telephone call centers—how do they affect health care utilization and costs? Pediatrics 2007;119:e1 [PMID:17272593].

Kempe A et al: How safe is triage by an after-hours telephone call center? Pediatrics 2006;118:457 [PMID: 16882795].

Liederman EM, Morefield CS: Web messaging: A new tool for patient-physician communication. J Am Med Inform Assoc 2003;10:260 [PMID: 12626378].

ADVOCACY & COMMUNITY PEDIATRICS

Community pediatrics is "a perspective that enlarges the pediatrician's focus from one child to all children in the community." Pediatricians have historically been very involved in supporting and developing services for vulnerable children in their communities. As a group, pediatricians recognize that communities are integral determinants of a child's health and that the synthesis of public health and personal health principles and practices is important in the practice of community pediatrics. As well, pediatricians have long been committed to working with other professionals in the community and advocating for the needs of all children. For example, pediatricians have been instrumental in the passage of laws requiring car seats and bicycle helmets, as well as expanded health care coverage through State Children's Health Insurance Program (SCHIP) working with legislators on both local and federal levels.

Advocacy refers to the act of representing or pleading a cause on behalf of another. Physicians have a unique position to champion the rights of their patients. Pediatricians and other providers who care for children have an added responsibility to be a voice for a population who cannot vote or advocate for themselves very effectively. Advocacy can be broken down into three categories: individual (patient-based), community, and legislative (policy-based).

Pediatricians in practice are frequently instrumental in one-on-one advocacy, which may take the form of writing a letter of medical necessity or referring children and families to valuable services and resources. Pediatricians must be familiar with programs in the community. For example, children with special health care needs may be eligible for services typically funded through state health departments and through programs such as those provided based on the Individuals with Disabilities Education Act (IDEA). A variety of community-based immunization programs can provide access to needed immunizations for eligible children. Food and nutrition programs such as the federally funded WIC program provide sources of food at no cost to eligible families. Finally, subsidized preschool and child care services such as the federally funded Head Start program provide preschool programs for qualifying children.

Community advocacy goes beyond the walls of the office or hospital. Pediatricians can become involved with local organizations that help children in the community. Pediatricians and other child advocates can work with community partners to address issues that influence child health. Community advocacy might focus on a particular condition (such as obesity) or environmental factors (such as exposure to violence) or improving health prevention (such as promoting programs to incorporate oral health into well child visits). Finally, pediatricians can learn about issues that affect children and work to affect change at a local, state, or national level. Physician advocates may write or call their legislators, educate the public and disseminate information by writing letters or opinion pieces, provide expert testimony for legislative committees, or even help to draft laws.

American Academy of Pediatrics: The pediatrician's role in community pediatrics. Pediatrics 2005;115:1092 [PMID: 15805396].

Duggan A et al: The essential role of research in community pediatrics. Pediatrics 2005;115(Suppl):1195 [PMID: 15821310].

Earnest MA et al: Physician Advocacy: What is it and why do we do it? Academic Medicine 2010;85:63.

Satcher D et al: The expanding role of the pediatrician in improving child health in the 21st century. Pediatrics 2005;115(Suppl):1124 [PMID: 15821293].

COMMON GENERAL PEDIATRIC ISSUES

FEVER

General Considerations

Fever is one of the most common reasons for pediatric office visits, emergency department encounters, and after-hours telephone calls. Several different definitions of fever exist, but most experts define fever as a rectal temperature of 38°C or above. Temperature in pediatric patients can be measured in a variety of manners: rectal (using a mercury or digital thermometer), oral (mercury or digital), axillary (mercury, digital, or liquid crystal strip), forehead (liquid crystal strip), or tympanic (using a device that measures thermal infrared energy from the tympanic membrane). Tympanic measurement of temperature is quick and requires little patient cooperation. Several cautions apply to the use of this technique: tympanic temperatures have been shown to be less accurate in infants younger than 3 months of age and are subject to false readings if the instrument is not positioned properly or the external ear canal is occluded by wax.

Causes

Fever occurs when there is a rise in the hypothalamic set-point in response to endogenously produced pyrogens. Among the broad range of conditions that cause fever are infections, malignancies, autoimmune diseases, metabolic diseases, chronic inflammatory conditions, medications (including immunizations), central nervous system abnormalities, and exposure to excessive environmental heat. In most settings, the majority of fevers in pediatric patients are caused by self-limiting viral infections. Teething does not cause fever over 38.4°C.

Clinical Findings

A. Initial Evaluation

When evaluating a child with fever, one should elicit from the parents information about the duration of fever, how the temperature was taken, the maximum height of fever documented at home, all associated symptoms, any chronic medical conditions, any medications taken, medication allergies, fluid intake, urine output, exposures and travel, and any additional features of the illness that concern the parents (Table 9–5). In the office, temperature, heart rate, respiratory rate, and blood pressure should be documented, as well as an oxygen saturation if the child has any increased work of breathing. A complete physical examination, including a neurologic examination, should then be performed, with particular attention paid to the child's degree of toxicity and hydration status. A well-appearing, well-hydrated child with evidence of a routine viral infection can be safely sent home with symptomatic treatment and careful return precautions.

Depending on patient age, presence of underlying conditions, type of infection, and the provider's assessment of toxicity and hydration, many children with focal bacterial

Table 9–5. Guidelines for evaluating children with fever.

A. See immediately if:

1. Child is < age 3 months with fever >100.4
2. Fever is > 40.6°C.
3. Child is crying inconsolably or whimpering
4. Child is crying when moved or even touched
5. Child is difficult to awaken
6. Child's neck is stiff
7. Purple spots or dots are present on the skin
8. Child's breathing is difficult and not better after nasal passages are cleared
9. Child is drooling saliva and is unable to swallow anything
10. A convulsion has occurred
11. Child has sickle cell disease, spenectomy, HIV, chemotherapy, organ transplant, chronic steroids
12. Child acts or looks "very sick"

B. See within 24 h if:

1. Child is 3–6 mo old (unless fever occurs within 48 h after a diphtheria-tetanus-pertussis vaccination and infant has no other serious symptoms)
2. Fever exceeds 40°C (especially if child is < age 3 y)
3. Burning or pain occurs with urination
4. Fever has been present for > 24 h without an obvious cause or identified site of infection
5. Fever has subsided for > 24 h and then returned
6. Fever has been present > 72 h

infections can also be treated as outpatients, with appropriate oral antibiotics as discussed in Chapter 42.

B. Fever Without a Focus of Infection

Children who present with fever but without any symptoms or signs of a focal infection are often a diagnostic and management challenge. When assessing a child with fever but no apparent source of infection on examination, the provider needs to carefully consider the likelihood of a serious but "hidden" or occult bacterial infection. With the widespread use of effective vaccines against *Haemophilus influenzae* type b and *Streptococcus pneumoniae*, two of the most common causes of invasive bacterial infections in unimmunized children, the incidence of occult bacterial infections has declined. However, vaccines are not 100% effective, and other organisms cause serious occult infections in children; therefore, febrile children will always demand careful evaluation and observation. Appropriate choices for empiric antibiotic therapy of children with fever without focus are discussed in Chapter 39.

Febrile infants 28 days old or younger, because of their likelihood of serious disease, including sepsis, should always be treated conservatively. Hospitalization and parenteral antibiotics should be strongly considered in all circumstances. An initial diagnostic evaluation should include complete blood count; blood culture; urinalysis; urine culture; and Gram stain, cerebrospinal fluid protein and glucose tests, as well as culture of the cerebrospinal fluid. Consideration should also be given to the possibility of a perinatal herpes simplex virus infection (neonatal herpes is described in more detail in Chapter 40). A chest radiograph should be obtained for any infant with increased work of breathing.

Infants aged 29–90 days are at risk of developing a variety of invasive bacterial infections, including perinatally acquired organisms (eg, group B streptococci) or infections acquired in the household (eg, pneumococci or meningococci). Febrile infants without a focus of infection can be divided into those who appear toxic versus nontoxic, and those at low risk versus higher risk of invasive bacterial disease. As with febrile neonates, toxic children in this age group should be admitted to the hospital for parenteral antibiotics and close observation. Viral illness is the most common cause of fever in this age group; if there is evidence of viral disease (upper respiratory infection, bronchiolitis), further workup may not be necessary. Urinary tract infection is the most common bacterial cause of infection in this age group. In nontoxic infants, low risk has been defined as previously healthy; no focal infection on examination; peripheral white blood cell (WBC) count between 5000 and 15,000/mm^3; band cells less than 1500/mm^3; normal urinalysis; and, when diarrhea is present, less than 5 WBCs per high-power field and negative gram stain on stool sample. Nontoxic low-risk infants in this age group are typically treated as outpatients with close follow-up. Clinicians should be confident that lumbar puncture is unnecessary if they decide not to perform this procedure.

In an era of increasing immunization coverage against the most commonly invasive pneumococcal serotypes, it is difficult to estimate the risk of occult bacteremia in febrile 3- to 36-month-olds with no focus of infection. Nevertheless, when assessing children aged 3–36 months with temperatures of 39°C or higher, urine cultures should be considered in all male children younger than 6 months of age and in all females younger than 2 years of age. Chest radiographs should be performed in any child with increased work of breathing and should also be considered in children with high (20,000/mm^3) WBC counts but no respiratory symptoms. Depending on the child's appearance, underlying medical condition, and height of fever, blood cultures should also be obtained. Empiric antibiotic therapy may be considered, particularly for children with temperature of 39°C and WBC count of 15,000/mm^3. However, in previously healthy, well-appearing, fully immunized children with reassuring laboratory studies, observation without antibiotics is appropriate.

Treatment

Fever phobia is a term that describes parents' anxious response to the fevers that all children experience. In a recent study, 91% of caregivers thought that a fever could cause harmful effects. Seven percent of parents thought that if they did not treat the fever, it would keep going higher. Parents need to be reassured that fevers lower than 41.7°C do not cause brain damage. They should be counseled that, although fevers can occasionally cause seizures—in which case their child needs to be seen—febrile seizures are generally harmless and likewise do not cause brain damage.

Several safe and effective medications are available for the treatment of fever. Acetaminophen is indicated in children older than 2 months of age who have fever of 39°C or are uncomfortable. Acetaminophen is given in a dosage of 15 mg/kg of body weight per dose and can be given every 4–6 hours. The other widely used antipyretic is ibuprofen, which can be used in children 6 months and older. Ibuprofen is given in a dosage of 10 mg/kg of body weight per dose and can be given every 6–8 hours. Ibuprofen and acetaminophen are similar in safety and their ability to reduce fever; however, ibuprofen is longer lasting. Aspirin should not be used for treating fever in any child or adolescent, because of its association with the development of Reye syndrome (particularly during infections with varicella and influenza). With all antipyretics, parents should be counseled to be very careful with dosing and frequency of administration as poisoning can be dangerous.

Avner JR: Acute Fever. Pediatr Rev 2009;30:5.

Crocetti M et al: Fever phobia revisited: Have parental misconceptions about fever changed in 20 years? Pediatrics 2001;107:1241 [PMID: 11389237].

Klein JO: Management of the febrile child without a focus of infection in the era of universal pneumococcal immunization. Pediatr Infect Dis J 2002;21:584 [PMID: 12182394].

McCarthy PL: Fever without apparent source on clinical examination. Curr Opin Pediatr 2002;14:103 [PMID: 11880744].

Rehm KP: Fever in infants and children. Curr Opin Pediatr 2001;13:83 [PMID: 11216593].

Sullivan JE et al: American Academy of Pediatrics Clinical Report–Fever and antipyretic use in children. Pediatrics 2011;127:580.

GROWTH DEFICIENCY

Growth deficiency—formerly termed failure to thrive—is deceleration of growth velocity resulting in crossing two major percentile lines on the growth chart. The diagnosis also is warranted if a child younger than age 6 months has not grown for 2 consecutive months or if a child older than age 6 months has not grown for 3 consecutive months. Growth deficiency occurs in about 8% of children.

Patterns of growth deficiency suggest, but are not specific for, different causes. In type I growth deficiency, the head circumference is preserved and the weight is depressed more than the height. This most common type results from inadequate caloric intake, excessive loss of calories, or inability to use calories peripherally. Most cases of type I deficiencies are the result of poverty, lack of caregiver understanding, poor caregiver-child interaction, abnormal feeding patterns, or a combination of factors. Type II growth deficiency, which is associated with genetically determined short stature, endocrinopathies, constitutional growth delay, heart or renal disease, or various forms of skeletal dysplasias, is characterized by normal head circumference and proportionate diminution of height and weight. In type III growth deficiency, all three parameters of growth—head circumference, weight, and height—are lower than normal. This pattern is associated with central nervous system abnormalities, chromosomal defects, and in utero or perinatal insults.

Just because an infant crosses a growth percentile does not mean an infant necessarily has a problem. Infants can cross growth curves normally, either "lagging down" or "shooting up." This crossing of growth percentiles is usually normal if it meets the following criteria: change in body weight and length are symmetrical, the size of the infant parallels the midparental weight and stature, the development remains normal, and a new growth curve is subsequently established, usually around 15 months of age; this also can be seen in the exclusively breastfed infants at 6 months and it can be reassuring to plot such infants on the new WHO curves that are based on children who were exclusively or primarily breastfed in the first 4 months of life.

Clinical Findings

A. Initial Evaluation

The history and physical examination will identify the cause of growth reduction in the vast majority of cases (Table 9–6).

Table 9–6. Components of initial evaluation for growth deficiency.

Birth history: newborn screening result; rule out intrauterine growth retardation, anoxia, congenital infections
Feeding and nutrition: difficulty sucking, chewing, swallowing
Feeding patterns: intake of formula, milk, juice, solids
Stooling and voiding of urine: diarrhea, constipation, vomiting, poor urine stream
Growth pattern: several points on the growth chart are crucial
Recurrent infections
Hospitalizations
HIV risk factors
Developmental history
Social and family factors: family composition, financial status, supports, stresses; heritable diseases, heights and weights of relatives
Review of system

The physical examination should focus on signs of organic disease or evidence of abuse or neglect: dysmorphic features, skin lesions, neck masses, adventitial breath sounds, heart murmurs, abdominal masses, and neuromuscular tone and strength. Throughout the evaluation, the physician should observe the caregiver-child interaction and the level of family functioning. Developmental screening and laboratory screening tests (complete blood count, blood urea nitrogen, creatinine, electrolytes, urinalysis, and urine culture) complete the initial office evaluation.

B. Further Evaluation

A prospective 3-day diet record should be a standard part of the evaluation. Occasionally an infant or child may need to be hospitalized to obtain an accurate assessment of intake. This is useful in assessing undernutrition even when organic disease is present. The diet history is evaluated by a pediatric dietitian for calories, protein, and micronutrients as well as for the pattern of eating. Additional laboratory tests should be ordered based on the history and physical examination. For example, stool collection for fat determination is indicated if a history of diarrhea suggests malabsorption. Moderate or high amounts of proteinuria should prompt workup for nephrotic syndrome. Vomiting should suggest a gastrointestinal, metabolic, neurologic, infectious, or renal cause. The tempo of evaluation should be based on the severity of symptoms and the magnitude of growth failure.

Treatment

A successful treatment plan addresses the child's diet and eating patterns, the child's development, caregiver skills, and any organic disease. High-calorie diets in the form of higher calorie formula or liquid supplement and frequent monitoring (every 1 or 2 weeks initially) are essential. Acceptable weight gain varies by age (Table 9–7).

Table 9–7. Acceptable weight gain by age.

Age (mo)	Weight Gain (g/d)
Birth to 3	20–30
3–6	15–20
6–9	10–15
9–12	6–11
12–18	5–8
18–24	3–7

The child with growth deficiency may also be developmentally delayed because of living in an environment that fails to promote development or from the effect on the brain of nutrient deprivation. Restoring nutrition does not fully reverse the deficit but does reduce the long-term consequences.

Education in nutrition, child development, and behavioral management as well as psychosocial support of the primary caregiver is essential. If family dysfunction is mild, behavior modification and counseling will be useful. Day care may benefit the child by providing a structured environment for all activities, including eating. If family dysfunction is severe, the local department of social services can help provide structure and assistance to the family. Rarely, the child may need to be temporarily or permanently removed from the home. Hospitalization is reserved for management of dehydration, for cases in which home therapy has failed to result in expected growth, for children who show evidence of abuse or willful neglect, for management of an illness that compromises a child's ability to eat, or for care pending foster home placement.

Weston JA: Growth deficiency. In Berman S (editor): *Pediatric Decision Making*, 4th ed. Mosby-Year Book, 2003.

Web Resources

American Academy of Pediatrics: http://www.aap.org

American Heart Association: http://americanheart.org

Bright Futures National Health Promotion Initiative: http://www.brightfutures.org

Centers for Disease Control and Prevention: Vaccines and immunizations home page: http://www.cdc.gov/vaccines

Healthy People 2020: http://www.healthypeople.gov

National Information Center for Children and Youth with Disabilities: http://www.nichcy.org

National Newborn Screening Status Report (2005): http://genes-r-us.uthscsa.edu

10 Immunization

Matthew F. Daley, MD
Sean T. O'Leary, MD, MPH
Ann-Christine Nyquist, MD, MSPH

Immunization is widely recognized as one of the greatest public health achievements of the past century. Largely as a consequence of immunization, the annual incidences of diphtheria, paralytic poliomyelitis, measles, mumps, rubella, and *Haemophilus influenzae* type b (Hib) in the United States have fallen by more than 99% compared with the average annual incidences of these diseases in the 20th century. Invasive pneumococcal disease in children less than 5 years of age has declined by 76% since routine pneumococcal vaccination began in 2000. Similarly, rotavirus vaccination has been associated with substantial declines in hospitalizations and emergency department visits for diarrheal illnesses in young children. Through routine vaccination, children and adolescents can now receive protection against at least 16 different diseases, and many new vaccines are under development.

Every year, roughly 4 million children are born in the United States, and successful immunization of each birth cohort requires the concerted effort of health care providers, public health officials, vaccine manufacturers, and the public. Public perceptions about immunizations, particularly routine childhood immunizations, are generally positive. However, parent concerns about the safety of vaccines have risen in recent years, in part fueled by unfounded speculation about an association between various vaccines or vaccine components and autism. Modern vaccines have a high degree of safety, and serious adverse events following vaccination are rare. Nonetheless, health care providers need to be prepared to discuss the benefits and risks of vaccination with uncertain parents, providing factual information in a clear and empathic fashion.

This chapter starts with general principles regarding immunizations and the recommended pediatric and adolescent vaccination schedules, followed by a discussion of vaccine safety. Each routinely recommended vaccine is then discussed further. Vaccines that are only given in special circumstances are discussed in the final section. Several abbreviations that are commonly used in this and other vaccine-related publications are summarized in the accompanying box.

Because the field of immunizations is rapidly changing, it is important for health care providers to seek the most up-to-date information available. The immunization recommendations outlined in this chapter are current but will change as technology evolves and our understanding of the epidemiology of vaccine-preventable diseases changes. The most useful sources for regularly updated information about immunization are the following:

1. National Center for Immunization and Respiratory Diseases at the Centers for Disease Control and Prevention (CDC). Maintains a web site with extensive vaccine-related resources, including the recommendations of the Advisory Committee on Immunization Practices (ACIP), vaccination schedules, Vaccine Information Statements, information for the public and providers, and links to other vaccine materials. Available at: http://www.cdc.gov/vaccines.
2. CDC Contact Center. The CDC-INFO contact center provides services to the public and health care professionals regarding a variety of health-related issues, including immunizations; available 24 hours a day, 7 days a week, at 1-800-232-4636 (English and Spanish).
3. *The Red Book: Report of the Committee on Infectious Diseases.* Published at 2- to 3-year intervals by the American Academy of Pediatrics (AAP). The 2009 *Red Book* is available from the AAP. Updates are published in the journal *Pediatrics* and can also be accessed at http://aapredbook.aappublications.org.
4. Immunization Action Coalition. This nonprofit organization creates and distributes educational materials for health care providers and the public related to vaccines. All materials are provided free of charge and can be accessed at http://www.immunize.org.
5. *Morbidity and Mortality Weekly Report* (MMWR). Published weekly by the CDC. Available at: http://www.cdc.gov/mmwr.

STANDARDS FOR PEDIATRIC IMMUNIZATION PRACTICES

In the United States, every infant requires more than 25 doses of vaccine by age 18 months to be protected against 14 or more childhood diseases. In 2010, immunization coverage rates for children aged 19–35 months were greater than 90% for poliovirus, measles-mumps-rubella, varicella, and hepatitis B vaccines, and were steadily increasing for more recently recommended vaccines such as pneumococcal conjugate and hepatitis A vaccines. However, data from the Vaccine Safety Datalink (VSD) project show that only 36% of children younger than age 2 years were completely compliant with vaccination recommendations: 30% had a missed opportunity for immunization; 20% had an invalid immunization; and 12% received unnecessary immunization (costing an estimated $26.5 million). The AAP recommends the following specific proven practices to improve these vaccination outcomes: (1) sending caretakers reminder and recall notices, (2) using prompts in patient medical records during all visits, (3) periodic measurement of immunization rates, and (4) having standing orders for vaccines.

Vaccine-related abbreviations

ACIP	Advisory Committee on Immunization Practices
BCG	Bacillus Calmette-Guérin vaccine against tuberculosis
CDC	Centers for Disease Control and Prevention
CISA	Clinical Immunization Safety Assessment Network
DT	Pediatric diphtheria and tetanus toxoids
DTaP	Pediatric diphtheria and tetanus toxoids and acellular pertussis vaccine
DTP	Pediatric diphtheria and tetanus toxoids and whole-cell pertussis vaccine
HBIG	Hepatitis B immune globulin
HBsAg	Hepatitis B surface antigen
HepA	Hepatitis A vaccine
HepB	Hepatitis B vaccine
Hib	*Haemophilus influenzae* type b
HIV	Human immunodeficiency virus
HPV	Human papillomavirus
HPV2	HPV vaccine, bivalent
HPV4	HPV vaccine, quadrivalent
IPV	Inactivated poliovirus vaccine
LAIV	Live attenuated influenza vaccine
MCV4	Meningococcal conjugate vaccine
MMR	Measles-mumps-rubella vaccine
MMRV	Measles-mumps-rubella-varicella vaccine
MPSV4	Meningococcal polysaccharide vaccine
OPV	Oral poliovirus vaccine
PCV	Pneumococcal conjugate vaccine
PCV7	Pneumococcal conjugate vaccine, 7-valent
PCV13	Pneumococcal conjugate vaccine, 13-valent
PPSV23	Pneumococcal polysaccharide vaccine, 23-valent
RV1	Rotavirus vaccine, monovalent
RV5	Rotavirus vaccine, pentavalent
TB	Tuberculosis
Td	Adult tetanus and diphtheria toxoid
Tdap	Tetanus and reduced diphtheria and acellular pertussis vaccine for adolescents and adults
TIV	Trivalent inactivated influenza vaccine
VAERS	Vaccine Adverse Events Reporting System
VAR	Varicella virus vaccine
VIS	Vaccine Information Statement
VSD	Vaccine Safety Datalink
VariZIG	Varicella-zoster immune globulin
VZV	Varicella-zoster virus

The National Childhood Vaccine Injury Act of 1986 requires that for each vaccine covered under the Vaccine Injury Compensation Program, caretakers should be advised about the risks and benefits of vaccination in a standard manner, using Vaccine Information Statements (VIS) produced by the CDC. Each time a Vaccine Injury Compensation Program–covered vaccine is administered, the current version of the VIS must be provided to the nonminor patient or legal caretaker. Vaccination documentation that is required in the medical record includes the vaccine manufacturer, lot number, and date of administration and expiration. The VIS version and date, and site and route of administration should also be recorded.

Needles used for vaccination should be sterile and disposable to minimize the opportunity for contamination. A 70% solution of alcohol is appropriate for disinfection of the stopper of the vaccine container and of the skin at the injection site. A 5% topical emulsion of lidocaine-prilocaine applied to the site of vaccination for 30–60 minutes prior to the injection minimizes the pain, especially when multiple vaccines are administered.

Compliance with the manufacturer's recommendations for route and site of administration of injectable vaccines are critical for safety and efficacy. All vaccines containing an adjuvant must be administered intramuscularly to avoid granuloma formation or necrosis. With the exception of Bacillus Calmette-Guérin (BCG) vaccine, which is used rarely in the United States, all vaccines are given either intramuscularly or subcutaneously. Intramuscular injections are given at a 90-degree angle to the skin, using a needle that is sufficiently long to reach the muscle tissue, but not so long as to injure underlying nerves, blood vessels, or bones. The anterolateral thigh is the preferred site of vaccination in newborns and children up to 2 years of age, and the deltoid muscle of the arm is the preferred site for children aged 3–18 years. Needle length and location should be as follows: ⅝ inch in newborn infants in the thigh; 1 inch in infants 1- to 12-month-olds (thigh), 1–1¼ inches in 1- to 18-year-olds (thigh), and ⅝–1 inch in 1- to 18-year-olds (deltoid). Subcutaneous injections should be administered at a 45-degree angle into the anterolateral aspect of the thigh (for infants younger than 12 months) or the upper outer triceps area (for children 12 months and older) using a 23- or 25-gauge, ⅝-inch needle. Pulling back on the syringe prior to vaccine injection (aspiration) is not required in CDC recommendations. A separate syringe and needle should be used for each vaccine.

Many combinations of vaccines can be administered simultaneously without increasing the risk of adverse effects or compromising immune response. Inactivated vaccines can be given simultaneously with, or at any time after, a different vaccine. Injectable or nasally given live-virus vaccines, if not administered on the same day, should be given at least 4 weeks apart (eg, measles-mumps-rubella [MMR] and varicella [VAR]). Lapses in the immunization schedule do not call for reinstitution of the series. Extra doses of hepatitis B (HepB), Hib, MMR, and VAR are not harmful, but repetitive exposure to tetanus vaccine beyond the recommended intervals can result in hypersensitivity reactions and should be avoided. If an immunoglobulin (Ig) or blood product has been administered, live-virus vaccination should be delayed 3 to 11 months, depending on the product, to avoid interference with the immune response (eg, 3 months for tetanus Ig, hepatitis B Ig, and pooled Ig for hepatitis A; 5–6 months for measles Ig or cytomegalovirus Ig; and 11 months for intravenous Ig for Kawasaki disease).

With the large number of vaccine preparations available, interchangeability of vaccines is an issue. All brands of Hib conjugate, HepB, and hepatitis A (HepA) vaccines are interchangeable. For vaccines containing acellular pertussis antigens, it is recommended that the same brand be used, but when the brand is unknown or the same brand is unavailable, any vaccine with diphtheria and tetanus toxoids and acellular pertussis should be used to continue vaccination. Longer than recommended intervals between vaccinations does not reduce final antibody titers, and lapsed schedules do not require restarting the series.

The numerous vaccines and other immunologic substances used by the practitioner vary in the storage temperatures required. The majority of vaccines should never be subjected to freezing temperatures. Vaccines that require routine freezing are MMRV, VAR, and herpes zoster vaccines. Yellow fever vaccine may also be stored frozen. Product package inserts should be consulted for detailed information on vaccine storage conditions and shelf life.

Vaccines very rarely cause acute anaphylactic-type reactions. All vaccine providers should have the equipment, medications, staff, established protocols, and training to manage emergencies that may occur following vaccination.

CDC: General recommendations on immunization: Recommendations of the Advisory Committee on Immunization Practices (ACIP). MMWR 2011;60(RR-02):1 [PMID: 21293327].

CDC: National and state vaccination coverage among children aged 19-35 months—United States, 2010. MMWR 2011;60:1157 [PMID: 21881546].

Mell LK et al: Compliance with national immunization guidelines for children younger than 2 years, 1996–1999. Pediatrics 2005; 115:461 [PMID: 15687456].

ROUTINE CHILDHOOD & ADOLESCENT IMMUNIZATION SCHEDULES

Each year, the CDC recommends immunization schedules for children and adolescents. While variation from these schedules may be necessitated by epidemiologic or individual clinical circumstances, these schedules are an important guide for vaccination providers. Vaccines in the schedules are roughly ordered by the age at which the vaccines are first given. For example, HepB is given to newborn infants at birth, followed at 2 months of age by rotavirus, diphtheria-tetanus-acellular pertussis (DTaP), Hib, pneumococcal conjugate 13-valent (PCV13), and inactivated poliovirus (IPV) vaccines. Table 10–1 sets forth the 2012 schedule of routine immunizations for normal infants and children from birth to 6 years. Table 10–2 presents the 2012 schedule of routine immunization for persons aged 7–18 years. Table 10–3 presents the 2012 schedule for children who did not start vaccination at the recommended time during the first year of life. Updated immunization schedules are available at http://www.cdc.gov/vaccines

Combination vaccines help solve the problem of large numbers of injections during a clinic visit. Currently available combination vaccines include MMR, measles-mumps-rubella-varicella (MMRV), and various combinations of Hib, HepB, IPV, and DTaP, including DTaP-HepB-IPV and DTaP-IPV-Hib combination vaccines. Separate vaccines should not be combined into one syringe by the provider unless approved by the Food and Drug Administration (FDA), because this could decrease the efficacy of components in the vaccine.

VACCINE SAFETY

Vaccine Safety Monitoring

The United States has a sophisticated, multi-faceted system to monitor the safety of licensed vaccines. The Vaccine Adverse Events Reporting System (VAERS), the Vaccine Safety Datalink (VSD), and the Clinical Immunization Safety Assessment (CISA) Network each provide distinct contributions to the ongoing monitoring of vaccine safety. VAERS is a national passive surveillance system administered jointly by the FDA and CDC. VAERS accepts reports from health care providers and the public about possible vaccine-related adverse events. Reports of adverse events possibly related to vaccination may be made via the Internet (http://vaers.hhs.gov) or by telephone (1-800-822-7967). As a passive surveillance system, VAERS is subject to certain limitations, including underreporting, overreporting, the reporting of events that are temporally but not causally related to vaccination, and the lack of denominator data. The VSD, in comparison, is an active surveillance system with continuous safety monitoring of vaccines in defined patient populations. The VSD can conduct timely investigations of

Table 10–1. Recommended immunization schedule for persons aged 0 through 6 years, United States, 2012 (for those who fall behind or start late, see the catch-up schedule, Table 10–3).

Vaccine ▼ Age ▶	Birth	1 month	2 months	4 months	6 months	9 months	12 months	15 months	18 months	19–23 months	2–3 years	4–6 years
Hepatitis B[1]	Hep B	HepB			HepB							
Rotavirus[2]			RV	RV	RV[2]							
Diphtheria, tetanus, pertussis[3]			DTaP	DTaP	DTaP		see footnote[3]	DTaP				DTaP
Haemophilus influenzae type b[4]			Hib	Hib	Hib[4]		Hib					
Pneumococcal[5]			PCV	PCV	PCV		PCV				PPSV	
Inactivated poliovirus[6]			IPV	IPV	IPV							IPV
Influenza[7]					Influenza (Yearly)							
Measles, mumps, rubella[8]							MMR			see footnote[8]		MMR
Varicella[9]							Varicella			see footnote[9]		Varicella
Hepatitis A[10]							Dose 1[10]				HepA Series	
Meningococcal[11]						MCV4 — see footnote[11]						

Range of recommended ages for all children

Range of recommended ages for certain high-risk groups

Range of recommended ages for all children and certain high-risk groups

This schedule includes recommendations in effect as of December 23, 2011. Any dose not administered at the recommended age should be administered at a subsequent visit, when indicated and feasible. The use of a combination vaccine generally is preferred over separate injections of its equivalent component vaccines. Vaccination providers should consult the relevant Advisory Committee on Immunization Practices (ACIP) statement for detailed recommendations, available online at http://www.cdc.gov/vaccines/pubs/acip-list.htm. Clinically significant adverse events that follow vaccination should be reported to the Vaccine Adverse Event Reporting System (VAERS) online (http://www.vaers.hhs.gov) or by telephone (800-822-7967).

1. **Hepatitis B (HepB) vaccine.** (Minimum age: birth)
   At birth:
   - Administer monovalent HepB vaccine to all newborns before hospital discharge.
   - For infants born to hepatitis B surface antigen (HBsAg)–positive mothers, administer HepB vaccine and 0.5 mL of hepatitis B immune globulin (HBIG) within 12 hours of birth. These infants should be tested for HBsAg and antibody to HBsAg (anti-HBs) 1 to 2 months after completion of at least 3 doses of the HepB series, at age 9 through 18 months (generally at the next well-child visit).
   - If mother's HBsAg status is unknown, within 12 hours of birth administer HepB vaccine for infants weighing ≥2,000 grams, and HepB vaccine plus HBIG for infants weighing <2,000 grams. Determine mother's HBsAg status as soon as possible and, if she is HBsAg-positive, administer HBIG for infants weighing ≥2,000 grams (no later than age 1 week).

   Doses after the birth dose:
   - The second dose should be administered at age 1 to 2 months. Monovalent HepB vaccine should be used for doses administered before age 6 weeks.
   - Administration of a total of 4 doses of HepB vaccine is permissible when a combination vaccine containing HepB is administered after the birth dose.
   - Infants who did not receive a birth dose should receive 3 doses of a HepB-containing vaccine starting as soon as feasible (Figure 3).
   - The minimum interval between dose 1 and dose 2 is 4 weeks, and between dose 2 and 3 is 8 weeks. The final (third or fourth) dose in the HepB vaccine series should be administered no earlier than age 24 weeks and at least 16 weeks after the first dose.
2. **Rotavirus (RV) vaccines.** (Minimum age: 6 weeks for both RV-1 [Rotarix] and RV-5 [Rota Teq])
   - The maximum age for the first dose in the series is 14 weeks, 6 days; and 8 months, 0 days for the final dose in the series. Vaccination should not be initiated for infants aged 15 weeks, 0 days or older.
   - If RV-1 (Rotarix) is administered at ages 2 and 4 months, a dose at 6 months is not indicated.
3. **Diphtheria and tetanus toxoids and acellular pertussis (DTaP) vaccine.** (Minimum age: 6 weeks)
   - The fourth dose may be administered as early as age 12 months, provided at least 6 months have elapsed since the third dose.
4. ***Haemophilus influenzae* type b (Hib) conjugate vaccine.** (Minimum age: 6 weeks)
   - If PRP-OMP (PedvaxHIB or Comvax [HepB-Hib]) is administered at ages 2 and 4 months, a dose at age 6 months is not indicated.
   - Hiberix should only be used for the booster (final) dose in children aged 12 months through 4 years.
5. **Pneumococcal vaccines.** (Minimum age: 6 weeks for pneumococcal conjugate vaccine [PCV]; 2 years for pneumococcal polysaccharide vaccine [PPSV])
   - Administer 1 dose of PCV to all healthy children aged 24 through 59 months who are not completely vaccinated for their age.
   - For children who have received an age-appropriate series of 7-valent PCV (PCV7), a single supplemental dose of 13-valent PCV (PCV13) is recommended for:
     — All children aged 14 through 59 months
     — Children aged 60 through 71 months with underlying medical conditions.
   - Administer PPSV at least 8 weeks after last dose of PCV to children aged 2 years or older with certain underlying medical conditions, including a cochlear implant. See *MMWR* 2010:59(No. RR-11), available at http://www.cdc.gov/mmwr/pdf/rr/rr5911.pdf.
6. **Inactivated poliovirus vaccine (IPV).** (Minimum age: 6 weeks)
   - If 4 or more doses are administered before age 4 years, an additional dose should be administered at age 4 through 6 years.
   - The final dose in the series should be administered on or after the fourth birthday and at least 6 months after the previous dose.
7. **Influenza vaccines.** (Minimum age: 6 months for trivalent inactivated influenza vaccine [TIV]; 2 years for live, attenuated influenza vaccine [LAIV])
   - For most healthy children aged 2 years and older, either LAIV or TIV may be used. However, LAIV should not be administered to some children, including 1) children with asthma, 2) children 2 through 4 years who had wheezing in the past 12 months, or 3) children who have any other underlying medical conditions that predispose them to influenza complications. For all other contraindications to use of LAIV, see *MMWR* 2010;59(No. RR-8), available at http://www.cdc.gov/mmwr/pdf/rr/rr5908.pdf.
   - For children aged 6 months through 8 years:
     — For the 2011–12 season, administer 2 doses (separated by at least 4 weeks) to those who did not receive at least 1 dose of the 2010–11 vaccine. Those who received at least 1 dose of the 2010–11 vaccine require 1 dose for the 2011–12 season.
     — For the 2012–13 season, follow dosing guidelines in the 2012 ACIP influenza vaccine recommendations.
8. **Measles, mumps, and rubella (MMR) vaccine.** (Minimum age: 12 months)
   - The second dose may be administered before age 4 years, provided at least 4 weeks have elapsed since the first dose.
   - Administer MMR vaccine to infants aged 6 through 11 months who are traveling internationally. These children should be revaccinated with 2 doses of MMR vaccine, the first at ages 12 through 15 months and at least 4 weeks after the previous dose, and the second at ages 4 through 6 years.
9. **Varicella (VAR) vaccine.** (Minimum age: 12 months)
   - The second dose may be administered before age 4 years, provided at least 3 months have elapsed since the first dose.
   - For children aged 12 months through 12 years, the recommended minimum interval between doses is 3 months. However, if the second dose was administered at least 4 weeks after the first dose, it can be accepted as valid.
10. **Hepatitis A (HepA) vaccine.** (Minimum age: 12 months)
    - Administer the second (final) dose 6 to18 months after the first.
    - Unvaccinated children 24 months and older at high risk should be vaccinated. See *MMWR* 2006;55(No. RR-7), available at http://www.cdc.gov/mmwr/pdf/rr/rr5507.pdf.
    - A 2-dose HepA vaccine series is recommended for anyone aged 24 months and older, previously unvaccinated, for whom immunity against hepatitis A virus infection is desired.
11. **Meningococcal conjugate vaccines, quadrivalent (MCV4).** (Minimum age: 9 months for Menactra [MCV4-D], 2 years for Menveo [MCV4-CRM])
    - For children aged 9 through 23 months 1) with persistent complement component deficiency; 2) who are residents of or travelers to countries with hyperendemic or epidemic disease; or 3) who are present during outbreaks caused by a vaccine serogroup, administer 2 primary doses of MCV4-D, ideally at ages 9 months and 12 months or at least 8 weeks apart.
    - For children aged 24 months and older with 1) persistent complement component deficiency who have not been previously vaccinated; or 2) anatomic/functional asplenia, administer 2 primary doses of either MCV4 at least 8 weeks apart.
    - For children with anatomic/functional asplenia, if MCV4-D (Menactra) is used, administer at a minimum age of 2 years and at least 4 weeks after completion of all PCV oses.
    - See *MMWR* 2011;60:72–6, available at http://www.cdc.gov/mmwr/pdf/wk/mm6003. pdf, and Vaccines for Children Program resolution No. 6/11-1, available at http://www. cdc.gov/vaccines/programs/vfc/downloads/resolutions/06-11mening-mcv.pdf, and *MMWR* 2011;60:1391–2, available at http://www.cdc.gov/mmwr/pdf/wk/mm6040. pdf, for further guidance, including revaccination guidelines.

This schedule is approved by the Advisory Committee on Immunization Practices (http://www.cdc.gov/vaccines/recs/acip), the American Academy of Pediatrics (http://www.aap.org), and the American Academy of Family Physicians (http://www.aafp.org).
Department of Health and Human Services • Centers for Disease Control and Prevention

Reproduced from CDC, Recommended immunization schedules for persons aged 0-18 years, United States, 2012. MMWR 2012;61(5)

Table 10–2. Recommended immunization schedule for persons aged 7 through 18 years, United States, 2012 (for those who fall behind or start late, see the schedule below and the catch-up schedule, Table 10–3).

Vaccine ▼ Age ►	7–10 years	11–12 years	13–18 years
Tetanus, diphtheria, pertussis[1]	1 dose (if indicated)	1 dose	1 dose (if indicated)
Human papillomavirus[2]	*see footnote*[2]	3 doses	Complete 3-dose series
Meningococcal[3]	See footnote[3]	Dose 1	Booster at 16 years old
Influenza[4]	Influenza (yearly)		
Pneumococcal[5]	See footnote[5]		
Hepatitis A[6]	Complete 2-dose series		
Hepatitis B[7]	Complete 3-dose series		
Inactivated poliovirus[8]	Complete 3-dose series		
Measles, mumps, rubella[9]	Complete 2-dose series		
Varicella[10]	Complete 2-dose series		

Legend:
- Range of recommended ages for all children
- Range of recommended ages for catch-up immunization
- Range of recommended ages for certain high-risk groups

This schedule includes recommendations in effect as of December 23, 2011. Any dose not administered at the recommended age should be administered at a subsequent visit, when indicated and feasible. The use of a combination vaccine generally is preferred over separate injections of its equivalent component vaccines. Vaccination providers should consult the relevant Advisory Committee on Immunization Practices (ACIP) statement for detailed recommendations, available online at http://www.cdc.gov/vaccines/pubs/acip-list.htm. Clinically significant adverse events that follow vaccination should be reported to the Vaccine Adverse Event Reporting System (VAERS) online (http://www.vaers.hhs.gov) or by telephone (800-822-7967).

1. **Tetanus and diphtheria toxoids and acellular pertussis (Tdap) vaccine.** (Minimum age: 10 years for Boostrix and 11 years for Adacel)
   - Persons aged 11 through 18 years who have not received Tdap vaccine should receive a dose followed by tetanus and diphtheria toxoids (Td) booster doses every 10 years thereafter.
   - Tdap vaccine should be substituted for a single dose of Td in the catch-up series for children aged 7 through 10 years. Refer to the catch-up schedule if additional doses of tetanus and diphtheria toxoid–containing vaccine are needed.
   - Tdap vaccine can be administered regardless of the interval since the last tetanus and diphtheria toxoid–containing vaccine.
2. **Human papillomavirus (HPV) vaccines (HPV4 [Gardasil] and HPV2 [Cervarix]).** (Minimum age: 9 years)
   - Either HPV4 or HPV2 is recommended in a 3-dose series for females aged 11 or 12 years. HPV4 is recommended in a 3-dose series for males aged 11 or 12 years.
   - The vaccine series can be started beginning at age 9 years.
   - Administer the second dose 1 to 2 months after the first dose and the third dose 6 months after the first dose (at least 24 weeks after the first dose).
   - See *MMWR* 2010;59:626–32, available at http://www.cdc.gov/mmwr/pdf/wk/mm5920.pdf.
3. **Meningococcal conjugate vaccines, quadrivalent (MCV4).**
   - Administer MCV4 at age 11 through 12 years with a booster dose at age 16 years.
   - Administer MCV4 at age 13 through 18 years if patient is not previously vaccinated.
   - If the first dose is administered at age 13 through 15 years, a booster dose should be administered at age 16 through 18 years with a minimum interval of at least 8 weeks after the preceding dose.
   - If the first dose is administered at age 16 years or older, a booster dose is not needed.
   - Administer 2 primary doses at least 8 weeks apart to previously unvaccinated persons with persistent complement component deficiency or anatomic/functional asplenia, and 1 dose every 5 years thereafter.
   - Adolescents aged 11 through 18 years with human immunodeficiency virus (HIV) infection should receive a 2-dose primary series of MCV4, at least 8 weeks apart.
   - See *MMWR* 2011;60:72–76, available at http://www.cdc.gov/mmwr/pdf/wk/mm6003.pdf, and Vaccines for Children Program resolution No. 6/11-1, available at http://www.cdc.gov/vaccines/programs/vfc/downloads/resolutions/06-11mening-mcv.pdf, for further guidelines.
4. **Influenza vaccines (trivalent inactivated influenza vaccine [TIV] and live, attenuated influenza vaccine [LAIV]).**
   - For most healthy, nonpregnant persons, either LAIV or TIV may be used, except LAIV should not be used for some persons, including those with asthma or any other underlying medical conditions that predispose them to influenza complications. For all other contraindications to use of LAIV, see *MMWR* 2010;59(No.RR-8), available at http://www.cdc.gov/mmwr/pdf/rr/rr5908.pdf.
   - Administer 1 dose to persons aged 9 years and older.
   - For children aged 6 months through 8 years:
     — For the 2011–12 season, administer 2 doses (separated by at least 4 weeks) to those who did not receive at least 1 dose of the 2010–11 vaccine. Those who received at least 1 dose of the 2010–11 vaccine require 1 dose for the 2011–12 season.
     — For the 2012–13 season, follow dosing guidelines in the 2012 ACIP influenza vaccine recommendations.
5. **Pneumococcal vaccines (pneumococcal conjugate vaccine [PCV] and pneumococcal polysaccharide vaccine [PPSV]).**
   - A single dose of PCV may be administered to children aged 6 through 18 years who have anatomic/functional asplenia, HIV infection or other immunocompromising condition, cochlear implant, or cerebral spinal fluid leak. See *MMWR* 2010:59(No. RR-11), available at http://www.cdc.gov/mmwr/pdf/rr/rr5911.pdf.
   - Administer PPSV at least 8 weeks after the last dose of PCV to children aged 2 years or older with certain underlying medical conditions, including a cochlear implant. A single revaccination should be administered after 5 years to children with anatomic/functional asplenia or an immunocompromising condition.
6. **Hepatitis A (HepA) vaccine.**
   - HepA vaccine is recommended for children older than 23 months who live in areas where vaccination programs target older children, who are at increased risk for infection, or for whom immunity against hepatitis A virus infection is desired. See *MMWR* 2006;55(No. RR-7), available at http://www.cdc.gov/mmwr/pdf/rr/rr5507.pdf.
   - Administer 2 doses at least 6 months apart to unvaccinated persons.
7. **Hepatitis B (HepB) vaccine.**
   - Administer the 3-dose series to those not previously vaccinated.
   - For those with incomplete vaccination, follow the catch-up recommendations (Figure 3).
   - A 2-dose series (doses separated by at least 4 months) of adult formulation Recombivax HB is licensed for use in children aged 11 through 15 years.
8. **Inactivated poliovirus vaccine (IPV).**
   - The final dose in the series should be administered at least 6 months after the previous dose.
   - If both OPV and IPV were administered as part of a series, a total of 4 doses should be administered, regardless of the child's current age.
   - IPV is not routinely recommended for U.S. residents aged18 years or older.
9. **Measles, mumps, and rubella (MMR) vaccine.**
   - The minimum interval between the 2 doses of MMR vaccine is 4 weeks.
10. **Varicella (VAR) vaccine.**
    - For persons without evidence of immunity (see *MMWR* 2007;56[No. RR-4], available at http://www.cdc.gov/mmwr/pdf/rr/rr5604.pdf), administer 2 doses if not previously vaccinated or the second dose if only 1 dose has been administered.
    - For persons aged 7 through 12 years, the recommended minimum interval between doses is 3 months. However, if the second dose was administered at least 4 weeks after the first dose, it can be accepted as valid.
    - For persons aged 13 years and older, the minimum interval between doses is 4 weeks.

This schedule is approved by the Advisory Committee on Immunization Practices (http://www.cdc.gov/vaccines/recs/acip), the American Academy of Pediatrics (http://www.aap.org), and the American Academy of Family Physicians (http://www.aafp.org).
Department of Health and Human Services • Centers for Disease Control and Prevention

Reproduced from CDC, Recommended immunization schedules for persons aged 0-18 years, United States, 2012. MMWR 2012;61(5).

Table 10–3. Catch-up immunization schedule for persons aged 4 months through 18 years who start late or who are more than 1 month behind, United States, 2012.

Vaccine	Minimum Age for Dose 1	Minimum Interval Between Doses			
		Dose 1 to dose 2	Dose 2 to dose 3	Dose 3 to dose 4	Dose 4 to dose 5
Persons aged 4 months through 6 years					
Hepatitis B	Birth	4 weeks	8 weeks and at least 16 weeks after first dose; minimum age for the final dose is 24 weeks		
Rotavirus[1]	6 weeks	4 weeks	4 weeks[1]		
Diphtheria, tetanus, pertussis[2]	6 weeks	4 weeks	4 weeks	6 months	6 months[2]
Haemophilus influenzae type b[3]	6 weeks	4 weeks if first dose administered at younger than age 12 months 8 weeks (as final dose) if first dose administered at age 12–14 months No further doses needed if first dose administered at age 15 months or older	4 weeks[3] if current age is younger than 12 months 8 weeks (as final dose)[3] if current age is 12 months or older and first dose administered at younger than age 12 months and second dose administered at younger than 15 months No further doses needed if previous dose administered at age 15 months or older	8 weeks (as final dose) This dose only necessary for children aged 12 months through 59 months who received 3 doses before age 12 months	
Pneumococcal[4]	6 weeks	4 weeks if first dose administered at younger than age 12 months 8 weeks (as final dose for healthy children) if first dose administered at age 12 months or older or current age 24 through 59 months No further doses needed for healthy children if first dose administered at age 24 months or older	4 weeks if current age is younger than 12 months 8 weeks (as final dose for healthy children) if current age is 12 months or older No further doses needed for healthy children if previous dose administered at age 24 months or older	8 weeks (as final dose) This dose only necessary for children aged 12 months through 59 months who received 3 doses before age 12 months or for children at high risk who received 3 doses at any age	
Inactivated poliovirus[5]	6 weeks	4 weeks	4 weeks	6 months[5] minimum age 4 years for final dose	
Meningococcal[6]	9 months	8 weeks[6]			
Measles, mumps, rubella[7]	12 months	4 weeks			
Varicella[8]	12 months	3 months			
Hepatitis A	12 months	6 months			
Persons aged 7 through 18 years					
Tetanus, diphtheria/ tetanus, diphtheria, pertussis[9]	7 years[9]	4 weeks	4 weeks if first dose administered at younger than age 12 months 6 months if first dose administered at 12 months or older	6 months if first dose administered at younger than age 12 months	
Human papillomavirus[10]	9 years	Routine dosing intervals are recommended[10]			
Hepatitis A	12 months	6 months			
Hepatitis B	Birth	4 weeks	8 weeks (and at least 16 weeks after first dose)		
Inactivated poliovirus[5]	6 weeks	4 weeks	4 weeks[5]	6 months[5]	
Meningococcal[6]	9 months	8 weeks[6]			
Measles, mumps, rubella[7]	12 months	4 weeks			
Varicella[8]	12 months	3 months if person is younger than age 13 years 4 weeks if person is aged 13 years or older			

1. **Rotavirus (RV) vaccines (RV-1 [Rotarix] and RV-5 [Rota Teq]).**
   - The maximum age for the first dose in the series is 14 weeks, 6 days; and 8 months, 0 days for the final dose in the series. Vaccination should not be initiated for infants aged 15 weeks, 0 days or older.
   - If RV-1 was administered for the first and second doses, a third dose is not indicated.
2. **Diphtheria and tetanus toxoids and acellular pertussis (DTaP) vaccine.**
   - The fifth dose is not necessary if the fourth dose was administered at age 4 years or older.
3. ***Haemophilus influenzae* type b (Hib) conjugate vaccine.**
   - Hib vaccine should be considered for unvaccinated persons aged 5 years or older who have sickle cell disease, leukemia, human immunodeficiency virus (HIV) infection, or anatomic/functional asplenia.
   - If the first 2 doses were PRP-OMP (PedvaxHIB or Comvax) and were administered at age 11 months or younger, the third (and final) dose should be administered at age 12 through 15 months and at least 8 weeks after the second dose.
   - If the first dose was administered at age 7 through 11 months, administer the second dose at least 4 weeks later and a final dose at age 12 through 15 months.
4. **Pneumococcal vaccines.** (Minimum age: 6 weeks for pneumococcal conjugate vaccine [PCV]; 2 years for pneumococcal polysaccharide vaccine [PPSV])
   - For children aged 24 through 71 months with underlying medical conditions, administer 1 dose of PCV if 3 doses of PCV were received previously, or administer 2 doses of PCV at least 8 weeks apart if fewer than 3 doses of PCV were received previously.
   - A single dose of PCV may be administered to certain children aged 6 through 18 years with underlying medical conditions. See age-specific schedules for details.
   - Administer PPSV to children aged 2 years or older with certain underlying medical conditions. See *MMWR* 2010:59(No. RR-11), available at http://www.cdc.gov/mmwr/pdf/rr/rr5911.pdf.
5. **Inactivated poliovirus vaccine (IPV).**
   - A fourth dose is not necessary if the third dose was administered at age 4 years or older and at least 6 months after the previous dose.
   - In the first 6 months of life, minimum age and minimum intervals are only recommended if the person is at risk for imminent exposure to circulating poliovirus (i.e., travel to a polio-endemic region or during an outbreak).
   - IPV is not routinely recommended for U.S. residents aged 18 years or older.
6. **Meningococcal conjugate vaccines, quadrivalent (MCV4).** (Minimum age: 9 months for Menactra [MCV4-D]; 2 years for Menveo [MCV4-CRM])
   - See Figure 1 ("Recommended immunization schedule for persons aged 0 through 6 years") and Figure 2 ("Recommended immunization schedule for persons aged 7 through 18 years") for further guidance.
7. **Measles, mumps, and rubella (MMR) vaccine.**
   - Administer the second dose routinely at age 4 through 6 years.
8. **Varicella (VAR) vaccine.**
   - Administer the second dose routinely at age 4 through 6 years. If the second dose was administered at least 4 weeks after the first dose, it can be accepted as valid.
9. **Tetanus and diphtheria toxoids (Td) and tetanus and diphtheria toxoids and acellular pertussis (Tdap) vaccines.**
   - For children aged 7 through 10 years who are not fully immunized with the childhood DTaP vaccine series, Tdap vaccine should be substituted for a single dose of Td vaccine in the catch-up series; if additional doses are needed, use Td vaccine. For these children, an adolescent Tdap vaccine dose should not be given.
   - An inadvertent dose of DTaP vaccine administered to children aged 7 through 10 years can count as part of the catch-up series. This dose can count as the adolescent Tdap dose, or the child can later receive a Tdap booster dose at age 11–12 years.
10. **Human papillomavirus (HPV) vaccines (HPV4 [Gardasil] and HPV2 [Cervarix]).**
    - Administer the vaccine series to females (either HPV2 or HPV4) and males (HPV4) at age 13 through 18 years if patient is not previously vaccinated.
    - Use recommended routine dosing intervals for vaccine series catch-up; see Figure 2 ("Recommended immunization schedule for persons aged 7 through 18 years").

Clinically significant adverse events that follow vaccination should be reported to the Vaccine Adverse Event Reporting System (VAERS) online (http://www.vaers.hhs.gov) or by telephone (800-822-7967). Suspected cases of vaccine-preventable diseases should be reported to the state or local health department. Additional information, including precautions and contraindications for vaccination, is available from CDC online (http://www.cdc.gov/vaccines) or by telephone (800-CDC-INFO [800-232-4636]).

Reproduced from CDC, Recommended immunization schedules for persons aged 0-18 years, United States, 2012. MMWR 2012;61(5).

newly licensed vaccines or emerging vaccine safety concerns. The CISA Network is designed to develop protocols for the evaluation, diagnosis, and treatment of adverse events following immunization, and to provide a better understanding of adverse events following immunization at the individual level. Patients with rare and serious adverse events following immunization can be referred to the CISA Network for evaluation.

Baggs J et al: The Vaccine Safety Datalink: A model for monitoring immunization safety. Pediatrics 2011;127 (Suppl 1):S45 [PMID: 21502240].

Freed GL et al: Parental vaccine safety concerns in 2009. Pediatrics 2010;125:654 [PMID: 20194286].

Omer SB et al: Vaccine refusal, mandatory immunization, and the risks of vaccine-preventable diseases. N Engl J Med 2009;360:1981 [PMID: 19420367].

Vaccine Risk-Benefit Communication

Most parents in the United States choose to vaccinate their children: in 2009, less than 1% of young children had received no vaccines. However, parents' concerns about vaccines are on the rise, and an increasing number of parents are choosing to delay or decline vaccination for their children. While there are myriad reasons why some parents may not vaccinate, several themes recur. Some parents do not believe their children are at risk for diseases such as poliomyelitis, measles, and tetanus. Other parents do not believe that certain vaccine-preventable diseases, such as varicella and pertussis, are particularly serious. There are also widespread concerns about the safety of vaccines. In a recent survey of more than 1500 parents, one-quarter believed that vaccines can cause autism in healthy children (despite no scientific evidence to support this claim), and more than one in 10 parents had refused at least one recommended vaccine. Health care providers have a critically important role in discussing the known risks and benefits of vaccination with parents. In this context, it is important that providers recognize that parent decisions are often based on inaccurate information about vaccine risk provided by the media or Internet sources. Parents with questions about vaccine safety should be directed to trusted web sites, such as those of the AAP, the American Academy of Family Physicians (AAFP), the CDC (http://www.cdc.gov/vaccines), and the Immunization Action Coalition (http://www.immunize.org).

Vaccine Contraindications and Precautions

All vaccines have certain contraindications and precautions that guide their administration. A contraindication indicates that the potential vaccine recipient is at increased risk of a serious adverse event. A vaccine should not be given when a contraindication to that vaccine is present, whereas a precaution indicates a circumstance that might increase the risk of adverse events or diminish the effectiveness of the vaccine. In the setting of precautions, the risks and benefits of vaccination must be carefully weighed prior to a decision regarding vaccination. Precautions are often temporary, in which case vaccination can resume once the precaution no longer applies. Contraindications and precautions are listed below with each vaccine. Additional, more detailed, information is available from the CDC (http://www.cdc.gov/vaccines), in the AAP's *Red Book*, and in vaccine package inserts.

VACCINATION IN SPECIAL CIRCUMSTANCES

Minor Acute Illnesses

Minor acute illnesses, with or without low-grade fever, are not contraindications to vaccination, because there is no evidence that vaccination under these conditions increases the rate of adverse effects or decreases efficacy. A moderate to severe febrile illness may be a reason to postpone vaccination. Routine physical examination and temperature assessment are not necessary before vaccinating healthy infants and children.

Children with Chronic Illnesses

Most chronic diseases are not contraindications to vaccination; in fact, children with chronic diseases may be at greater risk of complications from vaccine-preventable diseases, such as influenza and pneumococcal infections. Premature infants are a good example. They should be immunized according to their chronologic, not gestational, age. Vaccine doses should not be reduced for preterm or low-birth-weight infants. One exception to this rule is children with progressive central nervous system disorders. Vaccination with DTaP should be deferred until the child's neurologic status has been clarified and is stable.

Immunodeficient Children

Congenitally immunodeficient children should not be immunized with live-virus vaccines (oral polio vaccine [OPV, available only in developing countries], MMR, VAR, MMRV, yellow fever, or live-attenuated influenza vaccine [LAIV]) or live-bacteria vaccines (BCG or live typhoid fever vaccine). Depending on the nature of the immunodeficiency, other vaccines are safe, but may fail to evoke an immune response. Children with cancer and children receiving high-dose corticosteroids or other immunosuppressive agents should not be vaccinated with live-virus or live-bacteria vaccines. This contraindication does not apply if the malignancy is in remission and chemotherapy has not been administered for at least 90 days. Live-virus vaccines may also be administered to previously healthy children receiving low to moderate doses of corticosteroids (defined as up to 2 mg/kg/d of prednisone or prednisone equivalent, with a 20 mg/d maximum) for less than 14 days; children receiving short-acting alternate-day corticosteroids; children being maintained on physiologic corticosteroid therapy without other immunodeficiency; and children receiving only topical, inhaled, or intraarticular corticosteroids.

Contraindication of live-pathogen vaccines also applies to children with HIV infection who are severely immunosuppressed. In general those who receive MMR should have at least 15% CD4 cells, a CD4 lymphocyte count equivalent to CDC immunologic class 2, and be asymptomatic from their HIV. MMR for these children is recommended at 12 months of age (after 6 months during an epidemic). For HIV-infected children, a booster MMR dose may be given at least one month after the initial dose; in fact, giving this booster dose earlier than at 4 to 6 years of age is often encouraged. The booster dose may be given as early as 1 month later, but doses given before 1 year of age should not be considered part of a complete series. VAR vaccination is also recommended for HIV-infected children with CD4 cells preserved as listed above. The ACIP recommends only IPV routine vaccination for all children. Thus, immunodeficient children should no longer be exposed to OPV through household contacts. MMR and VAR are not contraindicated in household contacts of immunocompromised children. The recommended immunization schedule for immunocompromised children is available at http://www.cdc.gov/vaccines/pubs/pinkbook/.

Allergic or Hypersensitive Children

Hypersensitivity reactions are rare following vaccination (1.53 cases per 1 million doses). They are generally attributable to a trace component of the vaccine other than to the antigen itself; for example, MMR, IPV, and VAR contain microgram quantities of neomycin, and IPV also contains trace amounts of streptomycin and polymyxin B. Children with known anaphylactic responses to these antibiotics should not be given these vaccines. Trace quantities of egg antigens may be present in both inactivated and live influenza and yellow fever vaccines. Guidelines for influenza vaccination in children with egg allergies have recently changed. Children with only hives following exposure to egg can be vaccinated, as long as TIV is used as opposed to LAIV, vaccination is by a health care provider experienced in recognizing allergic reactions, and the child is observed for 30 minutes following vaccination. Children with more serious allergic reactions to egg, such as angioedema, respiratory symptoms, or anaphylaxis, may be eligible for TIV, but should be referred to an allergist for an assessment of vaccination risk. Some vaccines (MMR, MMRV, and VAR) contain gelatin, a substance to which persons with known food allergy may develop an anaphylactic reaction. For any persons with a known history of anaphylactic reaction to any component contained in a vaccine, the vaccine package insert should be reviewed and additional consultation sought, such as from a pediatric allergist. Some tips and rubber plungers of vaccine syringes contain latex. These vaccines should not be administered to individuals with a history of severe anaphylactic allergy to latex, but may be administered to people with less severe allergies. Thimerosal is an organic mercurial compound used as a preservative in vaccines since the 1930s. While there is no evidence that thimerosal has caused serious allergic reactions or autism, all routinely recommended vaccines for infants have been manufactured without thimerosal since mid-2001. Thimerosal-free formulations of TIV are available, and LAIV does not contain thimerosal.

Other Circumstances

Detailed recommendations for preterm low-birth-weight infants; pediatric transplant recipients; Alaskan Natives/American Indians; children in residential institutions or military communities; or refugees, new immigrants, or travelers are available from the CDC (at http://www.cdc.gov/vaccines) and from the AAP's *Red Book*.

CDC: General recommendations on immunization: Recommendations of the Advisory Committee on Immunization Practices (ACIP). MMWR 2011;60(RR-02):1 [PMID: 21293327].

Greenhawt MJ et al: Administering influenza vaccine to egg allergic recipients: A focused practice parameter update. Ann Allergy Asthma Immunol 2011;106:11 [PMID: 1195939].

HEPATITIS B VACCINATION

The incidence of reported cases of acute hepatitis B has declined dramatically in the United States, largely attributable to vaccination. Based on surveillance data from 2007, acute hepatitis B incidence has declined by 82% since 1990, to the lowest rate ever measured. The greatest declines have been seen in children younger than 15 years of age, in whom rates have decreased by 98%.

Successes in reducing the burden of hepatitis B in the United States are due, in large part, to a comprehensive hepatitis B prevention strategy initiated in 1991. The four central elements of this approach are (1) immunization of all infants beginning at birth; (2) routine screening of all pregnant women for hepatitis B infection, and provision of hepatitis B immune globulin (HBIg) to all infants born to infected mothers; (3) routine vaccination of previously unvaccinated children and adolescents; and (4) vaccination of adults at increased risk of hepatitis B infection.

While high immunization rates have been achieved in young children (more than 92% were fully immunized in 2009), there has been less success in identifying hepatitis B-infected mothers and at immunizing high-risk adults. Of the estimated 23,000 mothers who deliver each year who are hepatitis B surface antigen (HBsAg) positive, only 9000 are identified through prenatal screening. While there are an average of 90 cases of perinatally acquired hepatitis B infection reported to the CDC every year, the actual number of perinatal HBV infection cases is estimated to be 10 to 20 times higher than the number currently detected and reported. This circumstance represents a significant missed opportunity for prevention, given that administration of hepatitis B vaccine (HepB) in conjunction with HBIg is 95% effective at preventing mother-to-infant transmission of the virus. Further, many hospitals do not routinely offer HepB to all newborns, despite ACIP recommendations for universal newborn HepB vaccination. Similarly, while HepB alone is 90%–95% effective at preventing hepatitis B infection, only 45% of high-risk adults have been vaccinated.

All pregnant women should be routinely screened for HBsAg. Infants born to HBsAg-positive mothers should receive both HepB and HBIg immediately after birth. Infants for whom the maternal HBsAg status is unknown should receive vaccine (but not HBIg) within 12 hours of birth. In such circumstances, the mother's HBsAg status should be determined as soon as possible during her hospitalization, and the infant given HBIg if the mother is found to be HBsAg-positive. For all infants, the hepatitis B immunization series should be started at birth, with the first dose given prior to discharge from the hospital. The ACIP has recommended that any decision to defer the birth dose require an explanation in the medical record, accompanied by a copy of the mother's negative HBsAg test during the current pregnancy. In 2009, 61% of infants nationally received HepB within 3 days after birth.

Routine immunization with three doses of HepB is recommended for all infants and all previously unvaccinated children aged 0–18 years. A two-dose schedule is available for adolescents as well. In addition, persons 19 years and older with an increased risk of exposure to hepatitis B virus should be vaccinated. This includes men who have sex with men, persons with multiple sexual partners, intravenous and injection drug users, recipients of clotting factor concentrates, hemodialysis patients, household contacts and sexual contacts of persons with chronic hepatitis B infection, long-term international travelers to endemic areas, and all health care personnel. HepB is also recommended for persons with chronic liver disease or HIV. Screening for markers of past infection before vaccinating is generally not indicated for children and adolescents, but may be considered for high-risk adults. Because HepB vaccines consist of an inactivated subunit of the virus, the vaccines are not infectious and are not contraindicated in immunosuppressed individuals or pregnant women.

Vaccines Available

1. Hepatitis B vaccine (Recombivax HB, Merck) contains recombinant HepB only.
2. Hepatitis B vaccine (Engerix-B, GlaxoSmithKline) contains recombinant HepB only.
3. Hepatitis B-Hib (Comvax, Merck) contains vaccines against hepatitis B and Hib.
4. DTaP-HepB-IPV (Pediarix, GlaxoSmithKline) contains vaccines against diphtheria, tetanus, pertussis, hepatitis B, and poliovirus.

Only the noncombination vaccines (Recombivax HB and Engerix-B) can be given between birth and 6 weeks of age. Any single or combination vaccine listed above can be used to complete the hepatitis B vaccination series. Thimerosal has been removed from all pediatric HepB formulations. A combination vaccine against hepatitis A and hepatitis B (Twinrix, GlaxoSmithKline) is available, but is only licensed in the United States for persons 18 years and older.

Dosage Schedule of Administration

HepB is recommended for all infants and children in the United States. Table 10–4 presents the vaccination schedule for newborn infants, dependent on maternal HBsAg status. Infants born to mothers with positive or unknown HBsAg status should receive HepB vaccine within 12 hours of birth. Infants born to HBsAg-negative mothers should receive the vaccine prior to hospital discharge.

For children younger than 11 years of age not previously immunized, three intramuscular doses of HepB are needed. Adolescents aged 11–15 years have two options: the standard pediatric three-dose schedule or two doses of adult Recombivax HB (1.0 mL dose), with the second dose administered 4–6 months after the first dose. Simultaneous administration with other vaccines at different anatomic sites is safe and effective. The vaccine should be given intramuscularly in either the anterolateral thigh or deltoid, depending on the age and size of the patient.

Certain patients may have reduced immune response to HepB vaccination, including preterm infants weighing less than 2000 g at birth, the elderly; immunosuppressed patients, and those receiving dialysis. Preterm infants whose mothers are HBsAg-positive or with unknown HBsAg status should receive both HepB and HBIg within 12 hours of birth. For preterm infants whose mothers are known to be HBsAg-negative, initiation of the vaccination series should be delayed until 30 days of chronologic age if the infant is medically stable or prior to hospital discharge if the infant is discharged before 30 days of age. Pediatric hemodialysis patients and immunocompromised persons may require larger doses or an increased number of doses, with dose amounts and schedules available in the most recent CDC hepatitis B recommendations (see references).

Contraindications & Precautions

HepB should not be given to persons with a serious allergic reaction to yeast or to any vaccine components. Individuals with a history of serious adverse events, such as anaphylaxis, after receiving HepB should not receive additional doses. Vaccination is not contraindicated in persons with a history of Guillain-Barré syndrome, multiple sclerosis, autoimmune disease, or other chronic conditions. Pregnancy is also not a contraindication to vaccination.

Table 10–4. Hepatitis B vaccine schedules for newborn infants, by maternal hepatitis B surface antigen (HBsAg) status.[a]

Maternal HBsAg Status	Single Antigen Vaccine		Single Antigen Followed by Combination Vaccine	
	Dose	Age	Dose	Age
Positive[b]	1[c]	Birth (≤ 12 h)	1[c]	Birth (≤ 12 h)
	HBIg[d]	Birth (≤ 12 h)	HBIg	Birth (≤ 12 h)
	2	1–2 mo	2	2 mo
			3	4 mo
	3[e]	6 mo	4[e]	6 mo (Pediarix) or 12–15 mo (Comvax)
Unknown[f]	1[c]	Birth (≤ 12 h)	1[c]	Birth (≤ 12 h)
	2	1–2 mo	2	2 mo
			3	4 mo
	3[e]	6 mo	4[e]	6 mo (Pediarix) or 12–15 mo (Comvax)
Negative	1[c,g]	Birth (before discharge)	1[c,g]	Birth (before discharge)
	2	1–2 mo	2	2 mo
			3	4 mo
	3[e]	6–18 mo	4[e]	6 mo (Pediarix) or 12–15 mo (Comvax)

[a]See text for vaccination of preterm infants weighing less than 2000 g.
[b]Infants born to HBsAg-positive mothers should be tested at one year after completion of the immunization series for anti-HBs and HBsAg.
[c]Recombivax HB or Engerix-B should be used for the birth dose. Comvax and Pediarix cannot be administered at birth or before age 6 weeks.
[d]Hepatitis B immune globulin (HBIg) (0.5 mL) administered intramuscularly in a separate site from vaccine.
[e]The final dose in the vaccine series should not be administered before age 24 weeks (164 days).
[f]Mothers should have blood drawn and tested for HBsAg as soon as possible after admission for delivery; if the mother is found to be HBsAg-positive, the infant should receive HBIg as soon as possible, but no later than age 7 days.
[g]On a case-by-case basis and only in rare circumstances, the first dose may be delayed until after hospital discharge for an infant who weighs ≥ 2000 g and whose mother is HBsAg-negative, but only if a physician's order to withhold the birth dose and a copy of the mother's original HBsAg-negative laboratory report are documented in the infant's medical record.
Reproduced, with permission, from CDC: A comprehensive immunization strategy to eliminate transmission of hepatitis B virus infection in the United States, part 1: Immunization of infants, children, and adolescents. MMWR Recomm Rep 2005;54(RR-16):1.

Adverse Effects

The overall rate of adverse events following vaccination is low. Those reported are minor, including fever (1%–6%) and pain at the injection site (3%–29%). There is no evidence of an association between vaccination and sudden infant death syndrome, multiple sclerosis, autoimmune disease, or chronic fatigue syndrome.

Postexposure Prophylaxis

Postexposure prophylaxis is indicated for unvaccinated persons with perinatal, sexual, household, percutaneous, or mucosal exposure to hepatitis B virus. When prophylaxis is indicated, unvaccinated individuals should receive HBIg (0.06 mL/kg) and the first dose of HepB at a separate anatomic site. For sexual contact or household blood exposure to an acute case of hepatitis B, HBIg and HepB should be given. Sexual and household contacts of someone with chronic infection should receive HepB (but not HBIg). For individuals with percutaneous or permucosal exposure to blood, HepB should be given, and HBIg considered depending on the HBsAg status of the person who was the source of the blood and on the vaccination response status of the exposed person. All previously vaccinated persons exposed to hepatitis B should be retested for anti-HBs. If antibody levels are adequate (≥ 10 mIU/mL), no treatment is necessary. If levels are inadequate and the exposure was to HBsAg-positive blood, HBIg and vaccination are required.

Antibody Preparations

HBIg is prepared from HIV-negative and hepatitis C virus-negative donors with high titers of hepatitis B surface antibody. The process used to prepare this product inactivates or eliminates any undetected HIV and hepatitis C virus. The uses of HBIg are described earlier in this section.

CDC: A comprehensive immunization strategy to eliminate transmission of hepatitis B virus infection in the United States, part 1: Immunization of infants, children, and adolescents. MMWR Recomm Rep 2005;54(RR-16):1 [PMID: 16371945].

CDC: Assessing completeness of perinatal hepatitis B virus infection reporting through comparison of immunization program and surveillance data—United States. MMWR 2011; 60(13):410–413 [PMID: 21471948].

Van Herck K et al: Benefits of early hepatitis B immunization programs for newborns and infants. Pediatr Infect Dis J 2008;27:861 [PMID: 18776823].

Wasley A et al: The prevalence of hepatitis B virus infection in the United States in the era of vaccination. J Infect Dis 2010;202:192 [PMID: 20533878].

Willis BC et al: Gaps in hospital policies and practices to prevent perinatal transmission of hepatitis B virus. Pediatrics 2010;125:704 [PMID: 20211952].

ROTAVIRUS VACCINATION

Rotavirus is the leading cause of hospitalization and death from acute gastroenteritis in young children worldwide. The burden of rotavirus is particularly severe in the developing world, where as many as 500,000 children die each year from rotavirus-associated dehydration and other complications. While deaths from rotavirus were uncommon in the United States (20–60 deaths per year), prior to the introduction of rotavirus vaccine rotavirus infections caused substantial morbidity annually with an estimated 2.7 million diarrheal illnesses, 410,000 office visits, and 55,000–70,000 hospitalizations.

A rhesus-based rotavirus vaccine (RotaShield, Wyeth-Lederle) was licensed by the FDA and recommended for routine use by the ACIP in 1998 but was withdrawn from the market within one year after it was noted that there was an increased risk of intussusception after the first dose. Two other rotavirus vaccines were in development at the time, and underwent extensive prelicensure testing. No association with intussusception was found in prelicensure studies for either new rotavirus vaccine. The ACIP made a recommendation to include pentavalent rotavirus vaccine (RV5; RotaTeq) in the routine infant series in February 2006, a recommendation that was updated in June 2008 to include the monovalent rotavirus vaccine (RV1; Rotarix).

Since the introduction of these vaccines, use in routine practice by pediatricians occurred relatively rapidly and to a lesser extent with family physicians. Vaccination coverage in 2009 in the United States for ≥2 doses of rotavirus vaccine was 44%. Despite this relatively low coverage, the impact of the vaccines has been substantial, reducing both hospitalizations and outpatient visits. Death from rotavirus disease was a rare occurrence in the United States prior to licensure, but rotavirus vaccine has had a profound impact on deaths in the developing countries where it has been introduced.

However, there were two recent findings that raised concern about the safety of the newer rotavirus vaccines. In March 2010, the FDA recommended temporarily suspending use of RV1 due to the detection of porcine circovirus, a nonhuman pathogen, in the vaccine. This recommendation was lifted 2 months later after investigations showed that there was likely no threat to human health. Shortly thereafter, in August 2010, the Global Advisory Committee on Vaccine Safety of the World Health Organization reviewed preliminary data from postmarketing studies that showed a possible increased risk of intussusception for RV1 in Mexico. On September 22, 2010, the FDA recommended a label change for RV1 advising providers of the new data.

Vaccines Available

1. RV5 (Rotateq, Merck) is a pentavalent, live, oral, human-bovine reassortant rotavirus vaccine. The vaccine is a liquid, does not require any reconstitution, and does not contain any preservatives. The dosing tube is latex-free.
2. RV1 (Rotarix, GlaxoSmithKline) is a monovalent, live, oral, attenuated human rotavirus vaccine. The vaccine needs to be reconstituted with 1 mL of diluent using a prefilled oral applicator. The vaccine does not contain any preservatives. The oral applicator contains latex.

Dosage & Schedule of Administration

Either RV5 or RV1 can be used to prevent rotavirus gastroenteritis. RV5 should be administered orally, as a three-dose series, at 2, 4, and 6 months of age. RV1 should be administered orally, as a two-dose series, at 2 and 4 months of age. For both rotavirus vaccines, the minimum age for dose 1 is 6 weeks, and the maximum age for dose 1 is 14 weeks and 6 days. The vaccination series should not be started at 15 weeks of age or older, because of the lack of safety data around administering dose 1 to older infants. The minimum interval between doses is 4 weeks. All doses should be administered by 8 months and 0 days of age. While the ACIP recommends that the vaccine series be completed with the same product (RV5 or RV1) used for the initial dose, if this is not possible, providers should complete the series with whichever product is available.

Either rotavirus vaccine can be given simultaneously with all other recommended infant vaccines. Rotavirus vaccine can be given to infants with minor acute illness. No restrictions are placed on infant feeding before or after receiving rotavirus vaccine. Infants readily swallow the vaccine in most circumstances; however, if an infant spits up or vomits after a dose is administered, the dose should not be readministered; the infant can receive the remaining doses at the normal intervals.

Contraindications & Precautions

Rotavirus vaccine should not be given to infants with a severe hypersensitivity to any components of the vaccine, or to infants who had a serious allergic reaction to a previous dose of the vaccine. Because the RV1 oral applicator contains latex rubber, RV1 should not be given to infants with a severe latex allergy; RV5 is latex-free. Both vaccines are contraindicated in infants with severe combined immunodeficiency (SCID). Vaccination should be deferred in infants with acute moderate or severe gastroenteritis. Limited data suggest that rotavirus vaccination is safe and effective in premature infants. A small trial in South Africa also demonstrated that RV1 was well tolerated and immunogenic in HIV-infected children. However, vaccine safety and efficacy in infants with immunocompromising conditions other than SCID, preexisting chronic gastrointestinal conditions (eg, Hirschsprung disease or short-gut syndrome), or a prior episode of intussusception, has not been established. Clinicians should weigh the potential risks and benefits of vaccination in such circumstances. Infants living in households with pregnant women or immunocompromised persons can be vaccinated.

Adverse Effects

Because of new information regarding a possible increased risk of intussusception after the first dose from postmarketing surveillance done in Mexico, the FDA recently recommended a change to the labeling of RV1 (Rotarix), but not RV5 (Rotateq), informing providers of the possible increased risk.

Data from a large study in Mexico and Brazil found that there may be a small increase in the risk of intussusception in the 1–7 day time frame after the first dose of RV1 in Mexico (incident rate ratio of 5.3 with a 95% confidence interval of 3.0 to 9.3), but not in Brazil (incident rate ratio of 1.1 with a 95% confidence interval of 0.3 to 3.3). A possible explanation for the discrepancy is that live oral poliovirus vaccine is given in Brazil, but not in Mexico, where inactivated poliovirus vaccine is given. It is important to note that the same study showed that the benefits of rotavirus vaccination far exceeded any possible risk, and recommendations for use of RV1 have not changed in Mexico or elsewhere. Also, the background rate of intussusception in Mexico, between 60 and 90 per 100,000 children per year, is higher than in the United States. Active surveillance conducted in the United States has not shown an increased risk of intussusception following RV5 vaccination; comparable data are not yet available for RV1 vaccination.

CDC: Prevention of rotavirus gastroenteritis among infants and children. MMWR Recomm Rep 2009;58(RR-2):1 [PMID: 19194371].

CDC. Reduction in rotavirus after vaccine introduction—United States, 2000-2009. MMWR 2009;58:1146 [PMID: 19847149].

CDC. Addition of severe combined immunodeficiency as a contraindication for administration of rotavirus vaccine. MMWR 2010;59:687 [PMID: 20535093].

Haber P et al: Postlicensure monitoring of intussusception after RotaTeq vaccination in the United States, February 1, 2006, to September 25, 2007. Pediatrics 2008;121:1206 [PMID: 18519491].

Patel MM et al: Intussusception risk and health benefits of rotavirus vaccination in Mexico and Brazil. N Engl J Med 2011; 364:2283 [PMID: 21675888].

Staat MA et al: Effectiveness of pentavalent rotavirus vaccine against severe disease. Pediatrics 2011;128:e267 [PMID: 21768317].

Yen C et al: Diarrhea-associated hospitalizations among US children over 2 rotavirus seasons after vaccine introduction. Pediatrics 2011;127:e9 [PMID: 21172995].

DIPHTHERIA-TETANUS-ACELLULAR PERTUSSIS VACCINATION

Diphtheria, tetanus, and pertussis (DTP) vaccines have been given in a combined vaccine for many decades, and have dramatically reduced each of these diseases. The efficacy with antigens in the combined vaccine is similar to that with antigens in single component vaccines. The pertussis component of DTP vaccines contains whole-cell pertussis antigens. Although these vaccines are used widely in the world, DTP vaccines have been entirely replaced in the United States with DTaP vaccines, which are acellular pertussis vaccines made with purified, inactivated components of the bacterium.

Diphtheria is caused by a gram-positive bacillus, *Corynebacterium diphtheriae*. It is a toxin-mediated disease, with diphtheria toxin causing local tissue destruction, as in pharyngeal and tonsillar diphtheria, as well as systemic disease, particularly myocarditis and neuritis. The overall case fatality rate is between 5% and 10%, with higher death rates in persons younger than 5 years, or older than 40 years, of age. As many as 200,000 cases of diphtheria occurred each year in the 1920s in the United States. Largely because of successful vaccination programs, only five cases of diphtheria have been reported in the United States since 2000, and a confirmed case has not been reported since 2003. In the last several decades, the majority of diphtheria cases in the United States have been in unimmunized or inadequately immunized persons. The clinical efficacy of diphtheria vaccine is not precisely known, but has been estimated to be greater than 95%.

The anaerobic gram-positive rod *Clostridium tetani* causes tetanus, usually through infection of a contaminated wound. When *C tetani* colonizes devitalized tissue, the exotoxin tetanospasmin is disseminated to inhibitory motor neurons, resulting in generalized rigidity and spasms of skeletal muscles. Tetanus-prone wounds include (1) puncture wounds, including those acquired due to body piercing, tattooing, and intravenous drug abuse; (2) animal bites; (3) lacerations and abrasions; and (4) wounds resulting from nonsterile delivery and umbilical cord care (neonatal tetanus). In persons who have completed the primary vaccination series and have received a booster dose within the past 10 years, vaccination is virtually 100% protective. In 2008, 19 cases of tetanus occurred in the United States with almost all cases in persons who have had inadequate, distant (> 10 years) or no tetanus immunization. Pertussis is also primarily a toxin-mediated disease. Called whooping cough because of the high-pitched inspiratory whoop that can follow intense paroxysms of cough, pertussis is caused by the bacterium *Bordetella pertussis*. Complications from pertussis include death, often from associated pneumonia, seizures, and encephalopathy. Eighty-two deaths from pertussis were reported to the CDC in 2004–2006; 84% were in children 3 months of age or younger. Prior to the widespread use of pertussis vaccines in the 1940s, roughly 1 million pertussis cases were reported over a 6-year period. Pertussis incidence in the United States declined dramatically between the 1940s and 1980s, but beginning in the early 1980s, incidence has been slowly increasing, with adolescents and adults accounting for a greater proportion of reported cases. Generally there is a significant degree of underreporting of pertussis with enhanced awareness occurring during localized outbreaks of pertussis. In 2010, 27,550 cases of pertussis were reported in the United States with many localized outbreaks necessitating enhanced vaccination programs. California had the highest incidence since 1958 when a rate of 26.0 cases/100,000 was reported with over 9143 cases, including ten infant deaths.

A single booster dose of a different formulation, Tdap, is now recommended for all adolescents and adults, as is discussed in more detail later in this chapter. Providing a booster dose of pertussis-containing vaccine should prevent adolescent and adult pertussis cases, and also has the potential to reduce the spread of pertussis to infants, who are most susceptible to complications from the disease.

Vaccines Available

Diphtheria, Tetanus, and Acellular Pertussis Combinations

1. DTaP (Daptacel, sanofi pasteur; Infanrix, GlaxoSmithKline; Tripedia, sanofi pasteur) contains tetanus toxoid, diphtheria toxoid, and acellular pertussis vaccine. This DTaP is licensed for ages 6 weeks through 6 years and can be used for doses 1 through 5.
2. Tdap (Boostrix, GlaxoSmithKline) is a tetanus-reduced dose diphtheria-acellular pertussis vaccine formulated for persons 10 years of age and older, including adults and the elderly.
3. Tdap (Adacel, sanofi pasteur) is a tetanus-diphtheria-acellular pertussis vaccine approved for persons 11 through 64 years of age.

DTaP Combined with Other Vaccines

1. DTaP-Hib (TriHIBit, sanofi pasteur) contains an Hib vaccine reconstituted with Tripedia. It is licensed for the fourth dose of the DTaP and Hib vaccination series, but not for doses 1 through 3.
2. DTaP-IPV-Hepatitis B (Pediarix, GlaxoSmithKline) contains DTaP combined with poliovirus and HepB vaccines. It is approved for the first three doses of the DTaP and IPV series, given at 2, 4, and 6 months of age. Although it is approved for use through age 6 years, it is not licensed for booster doses. It cannot be used, for example, as the fourth dose of DTaP (the dose typically given at 15–18 months of age).
3. DTaP-IPV-Hib (Pentacel, sanofi pasteur) contains DTaP, IPV, and Hib vaccines. The Hib component is Hib capsular polysaccharide bound to tetanus toxoid. This vaccine is approved for use as doses 1 through 4 of the DTaP series among children 6 weeks to 4 years of age. It is typically given at 2, 4, 6, and 15–18 months of age, and should not be used as the fifth dose in the DTaP series.
4. DTaP-IPV (Kinrix, GlaxoSmithKline) contains DTaP and IPV vaccines. The vaccine is licensed for children 4–6 years of age, for use as the fifth dose of the DTaP vaccine series and the fourth dose of the IPV series. Using this vaccine would reduce by one the number of injections a 4- to 6-year-old child would receive.

Diphtheria and Tetanus Combinations

1. DT (generic, sanofi pasteur) contains tetanus toxoid and diphtheria toxoid to be used only in children younger than age 7 years with a contraindication to pertussis vaccination.
2. Td (Decavac, sanofi pasteur; generic, Massachusetts Biological Labs) contains tetanus toxoid and a reduced quantity of diphtheria toxoid, which is typically used for adults requiring tetanus prophylaxis.

Tetanus Only

TT (generic, sanofi pasteur) contains tetanus toxoid only, and can be used for adults or children. However, the use of this single-antigen vaccine is generally not recommended, because of the need for periodic boosting for both diphtheria and tetanus.

Dosage & Schedule of Administration

Although several different vaccines are available, a few general considerations can help guide their use in specific circumstances. DTaP (alone or combined with other vaccines) is used for infants and children between 6 weeks and 6 years of age. Children 7 to 10 years of age not fully immunized against pertussis (meaning those who have not received 5 prior doses of DTaP, or 4 doses of DTaP if the fourth dose was given on or after the fourth birthday), who have no contraindications to pertussis immunization, should receive a single dose of Tdap for pertussis protection. For adolescents and adults, a single dose of Tdap is used, followed by booster doses of Td every 10 years; a detailed description of Tdap use is provided later in this chapter.

The primary series of DTaP vaccination should consist of four doses, given at 2, 4, 6, and 15–18 months of age. The fourth dose may be given as early as 12 months of age if 6 months have elapsed since the third dose. Giving the fourth dose between 12 and 15 months of age is indicated if the provider thinks the child is unlikely to return for a clinic visit between 15 and 18 months of age. Children should receive a fifth dose of DTaP at 4–6 years of age. However, a fifth dose of DTaP is not needed if the fourth dose was given after the child's fourth birthday. The same brand of DTaP should be used for all doses if feasible.

Contraindications & Precautions

DTaP vaccines should not be used in individuals who have had an anaphylactic-type reaction to a previous vaccine dose or to a vaccine component. DTaP should not be given to children who developed encephalopathy, not attributable to another identified cause, within 7 days of a previous dose of DTaP or DTP. DTaP vaccination should also be deferred in individuals with progressive neurologic disorders, such as infantile spasms, uncontrolled epilepsy, or progressive encephalopathy, until their neurologic status is clarified and stabilized.

Precautions to DTaP vaccination include: high fever (≥ 40.5°F), persistent inconsolable crying, or shock-like state within 48 hours of a previous dose of DTP or DTaP; seizures within 3 days of a previous dose of DTP or DTaP; Guillain-Barré syndrome less than 6 weeks after a previous tetanus-containing vaccine; or incident moderate or severe acute illness with or without a fever.

Adverse Effects

Local reactions, fever, and other mild systemic effects occur with one-fourth to two-thirds the frequency noted following whole-cell DTP vaccination. Moderate to severe systemic effects, including fever of 40.5°C, persistent inconsolable crying lasting 3 hours or more, and hypotonic-hyporesponsive episodes, are less frequent than with whole-cell DTP. These are without sequelae. Severe neurologic effects have not been temporally associated with DTaP vaccines in use in the United States. A recent study from Canada showed no evidence of encephalopathy related to pertussis vaccine (< 1 case per 3 million doses of DTP and < 1 per 3.5 million doses of DTaP). Data are limited regarding differences in reactogenicity among currently licensed DTaP vaccines. With all currently licensed DTaP vaccines, reports of substantial local reactions at injection sites have increased with increasing dose number (including swelling of the thigh or entire upper arm after receipt of the fourth and fifth doses).

Diphtheria Antibody Preparations

Diphtheria antitoxin is manufactured in horses. Dosage depends on the size and location of the diphtheritic membrane and an estimate of the patient's level of intoxication. Sensitivity to diphtheria antitoxin must be tested before it is given. Consultation on the use of diphtheria antitoxin is available from the CDC's National Center for Immunization and Respiratory Diseases. Diphtheria antitoxin is not commercially available in the United States and must be obtained from the CDC.

Tetanus Antibody Preparations

Human tetanus immune globulin (TIg) is indicated in the management of tetanus-prone wounds in individuals who have had an uncertain number or fewer than three tetanus immunizations. Persons fully immunized with at least three doses do not require TIg, regardless of the nature of their wounds (Table 10–5). The optimal dose of TIg has not been established, but some sources recommend 3000–5000 units as a single dose, with part of the dose infiltrated around the wound.

Table 10–5. Recommendations for the use of tetanus prophylaxis after a wound.

	Clean, Minor Wounds		All Other Wounds	
History of Tetanus Toxoid–Containing Vaccines[a]	DTaP, DT, Td, or Tdap[b]	TIg	DTaP, DT, Td, or Tdap[b]	TIg
< 3 doses or unknown vaccine status[a,b]	Yes	No	Yes	Yes
≤ 3 doses and 5–9 y since last tetanus toxoid-containing vaccine[c]	No	No	Yes[d]	No
≤ 3 doses and > 10 y since last tetanus toxoid-containing vaccine[c]	Yes[c]	No	Yes[c]	No

[a]For infants younger than age 6 months who have not received three doses of tetanus-containing vaccine, use maternal tetanus immunization history at the time of delivery and apply the guidelines in the table above.
[b]If tetanus immunization is not complete at the time of the wound treatment, a dose of age-appropriate tetanus-containing vaccine should be given. Children younger than age 7 years should receive DTaP or DT. Children 7 to 10 years of age should receive Tdap if pertussis immunization is also needed. Tdap is preferred (over Td) for adolescents who have never previously received Tdap. Tdap is licensed for one dose only. Adolescents who have previously received a dose of Tdap and who need additional tetanus toxoid–containing vaccine, should receive Td.
[c]Persons who have received at least three doses of tetanus toxoid–containing vaccines, but have not received a tetanus toxoid-containing vaccine for more than 10 years, should receive an age-appropriate tetanus toxoid-containing vaccine regardless of the nature of the wound.
[d]Persons who received at least three doses of tetanus toxoid-containing vaccines, but have not received a tetanus toxoid-containing vaccine for more than 5 years, should receive an age-appropriate tetanus toxoid-containing vaccine unless the wounds are clean and minor.
Recommendations based on American Academy of Pediatrics: Tetanus. In Pickering LK et al (editors): *Red Book, 2009 Report of the Committee on Infectious Diseases*, 28th ed. American Academy of Pediatrics 2009:657.

CDC: Updated recommendations for the use of tetanus toxoid, reduced diphtheria toxoid and acellular pertussis (Tdap) vaccine from the Advisory Committee on Immunization Practices, 2011. MMWR 2011; 60:13 [PMID: 21228763].

CDC: Diphtheria. In: Atkinson W et al (editors): *Epidemiology and Prevention of Vaccine-Preventable Diseases*, 12th ed. Public Health Foundation, 2011: 75.

CDC: Pertussis. In: Atkinson W et al (editors): *Epidemiology and Prevention of Vaccine-Preventable Diseases*, 12th ed. Public Health Foundation, 2011: 215.

CDC: Tetanus. In: Atkinson W et al (editors): *Epidemiology and Prevention of Vaccine-Preventable Diseases*, 12th ed. Public Health Foundation, 2011: 291.

Roper MH et al: Maternal and neonatal tetanus. Lancet 2007; 370:1947 [PMID: 17854885].

HAEMOPHILUS INFLUENZAE TYPE B VACCINATION

H influenzae type b (Hib) causes a wide spectrum of serious bacterial illnesses, particularly in young children, including meningitis, epiglottitis, pneumonia, septic arthritis, and cellulitis. Before the introduction of effective vaccines, Hib was the leading cause of invasive bacterial disease in children younger than 5 years of age in the United States. Nearly all Hib disease occurred in this age group, and two-thirds of cases occurred in children younger than 18 months of age.

Hib is surrounded by a polysaccharide capsule (polyribosyl ribitol phosphate [PRP]) that contributes to virulence, and antibodies to this polysaccharide confer immunity to the disease. When Hib polysaccharide was chemically bonded (conjugated) to certain protein carriers, the conjugate induced long-term T-cell dependent immune memory and was highly effective in young children. All current Hib vaccines are based on this polysaccharide-protein conjugate technology.

Describing the epidemiology of invasive Hib disease is difficult because bacterial serotyping is required to differentiate Hib-caused infections from those caused by other encapsulated and nonencapsulated *H influenzae* species. However, it has been estimated that roughly 20,000 cases of invasive Hib disease occurred each year in the United States in the early 1980s. Since the introduction of Hib vaccines, disease incidence has declined by more than 99%. In the United States in 2009, 35 cases of invasive Hib disease occurred in children younger than age 5 years. An additional 178 cases were caused by *H influenzae* species in which the serotype was not reported. Current Hib vaccine supplies are sufficient for all children to receive a full vaccine series, including the booster dose, despite a recent history of Hib vaccine shortages.

Vaccines Available

Six vaccines against Hib disease are available in the United States; three are Hib-only vaccines, and three are combination vaccines. Each vaccine contains Hib polysaccharide conjugated to a protein carrier, but different protein carriers are used. The Hib conjugate vaccine that uses a meningococcal outer membrane protein carrier is abbreviated PRP-OMP; and PRP-T vaccine uses a tetanus toxoid carrier.

Hib-Only Vaccines

1. Hib (PedvaxHIB, Merck, uses PRP-OMP), for use at 2, 4, and 12–15 months of age.
2. Hib (ActHIB, sanofi pasteur, uses PRP-T), for use at 2, 4, 6, and 12–15 months of age.
3. Hib (Hiberix, GlaxoSmithKline, uses PRP-T), for use as the booster (final) dose in the Hib vaccine series for children 15 months of age and older; it is not licensed for the primary series.

Hib Combined with Other Vaccines

1. DTaP-Hib (TriHIBit, uses PRP-T reconstituted with Tripedia brand of DTaP, sanofi pasteur). It is licensed for the booster (final) dose of the Hib vaccination series, but not for doses 1 through 3.
2. Hepatitis B-Hib (Comvax, uses PRP-OMP, Merck), for use at 2, 4, and 12–15 months of age. It should not be given prior to 6 weeks of age.
3. DTaP-IPV-Hib (Pentacel, sanofi pasteur, uses PRP-T) contains DTaP, IPV, and Hib vaccines. This vaccine is approved for use in children 6 weeks to 4 years of age.

Dosage & Schedule of Administration

Hib vaccination is recommended for all infants in the United States. The vaccine dose is 0.5 mL given intramuscularly. As shown in Table 10–6, the vaccination schedule depends on which type of Hib vaccine is used. The recommended interval between doses in the primary series is 8 weeks, but a minimal interval of 4 weeks is permitted. For infants who missed the primary vaccination series, a catch-up schedule is used (see Table 10–3). Hib vaccine is not generally recommended for children 5 years of age or older.

Contraindications & Precautions

Hib vaccine should not be given to anyone who has had a severe allergic reaction to a prior Hib vaccine dose or to any vaccine components. Hib vaccine should not be given to infants before 6 weeks of age.

Adverse Effects

Adverse reactions following Hib vaccination are uncommon. Between 5% and 30% of vaccine recipients experience swelling, redness, or pain at the vaccination site. Systemic reactions such as fever and irritability are rare.

Table 10–6. Schedule for *Haemophilus influenzae* type b (Hib) vaccination depending on type of protein conjugate used.

Conjugate Type	Trade Name	Age			
		2 mo	4 mo	6 mo	12–15 mo
PRP-T[a]	ActHIB, TriHIBit, Hiberix, Pentacel	Dose 1	Dose 2	Dose 3	Booster dose
PRP-OMP[b]	PedvaxHIB, Comvax[c]	Dose 1	Dose 2		Booster dose

[a]Tetanus toxoid carrier.
[b]Meningococcal outer membrane protein.
[c]See Table 10–4 for the use of Comvax in infants born to mothers with positive or unknown hepatitis B surface antigen status.

CDC: Invasive *Haemophilus influenzae* type B disease in five young children-Minnesota, 2008. MMWR 2009;58:58 [PMID: 19177041].

Watt JP et al: Burden of disease caused by *Haemophilus influenzae* type b in children younger than 5 years: Global estimates. Lancet 2009;374:903 [PMID: 19748399].

PNEUMOCOCCAL VACCINATION

Before the routine use of pneumococcal conjugate vaccines in infants, *Streptococcus pneumoniae* (pneumococcus) was the leading cause of invasive bacterial disease in children. Pneumococcus remains a leading cause of febrile bacteremia, bacterial sepsis, meningitis, and pneumonia in children and adults in the United States and worldwide. It is also a common cause of otitis media and sinusitis. At least 90 different serotypes of pneumococcus have been identified, and immunity to one serotype does not confer immunity to other serotypes.

A conjugate vaccine against 7 pneumococcal serotypes (PCV7) was first licensed in the United States in 2000. This vaccine was composed of the capsular polysaccharides from 7 serotypes (4, 6B, 9V, 14, 18C, 19F, and 23F) coupled to a nontoxic modified diphtheria protein. Similar to current Hib vaccines, the conjugation to another protein created a highly immunogenic vaccine in infants and children. In a large clinical trial, PCV7 reduced the incidence of invasive pneumococcal disease caused by vaccine serotypes by 97%.

The routine use of PCV7 led to a dramatic decrease in pneumococcal disease in the United States. By 2008, invasive pneumococcal disease in children <5 years old decreased by 79% compared to the years preceding PCV7 use. Rates of invasive pneumococcal disease in adults and especially the elderly has also decreased, indicating some protection of the unimmunized through herd immunity. There have also been reductions in other diseases such as otitis media and pneumonia, and a reduced rate of infection and colonization by antibiotic-resistant pneumococcal strains. However, as disease from PCV7 serotypes has declined greatly, disease caused by pneumococcal serotypes not included in this vaccine, particularly serotype 19A, has increased.

In 2010, a 13-valent pneumococcal conjugate vaccine (PCV13) was licensed for use in the United States. Made by the same manufacturer and using the same processes as for PCV7 development, the vaccine contains the seven serotypes included in PCV7 as well as six additional pneumococcal serotypes (1, 3, 5, 6A, 7F, and 19A). PCV13 has replaced PCV7 in the United States, and PCV7 is no longer available. In 2008, 61% of all invasive pneumococcal disease in children < 5 years old was caused by serotypes covered by PCV13 vaccine.

An older, 23-valent pneumococcal vaccine (PPSV23) is also available in the United States, but its use in children is limited to enhancing pneumococcal immunity in children with certain chronic medical conditions. PPSV23 is a polysaccharide vaccine and protects against 23 serotypes. However, the vaccine does not induce robust immunologic memory and does not reduce nasopharyngeal carriage, and therefore does not appear to reduce disease in the unimmunized public by a herd immunity effect.

While all children and adults are at risk of pneumococcal disease, certain children are at particularly high risk of invasive pneumococcal disease. As seen in Table 10–7, these include children with congenital or acquired immunodeficiency, those without a functioning spleen, and immunocompetent children with certain chronic conditions. These children need enhanced protection against pneumococcal disease, with a more extensive vaccination schedule than healthy children, including the use of PPSV23.

Vaccines Available

1. PCV13 (Prevnar13, Wyeth). It contains the capsular polysaccharide antigens of 13 serotypes, each individually conjugated to a nontoxic diphtheria carrier protein. The vaccine contains an aluminum phosphate adjuvant, and does not contain thimerosal preservative. It is licensed for use in children 6 weeks to 71 months of age.
2. PPSV23 (Pneumovax23, Merck). It contains the capsular polysaccharide antigens of 23 pneumococcal serotypes. It contains phenol as a preservative. It is licensed for children 2 years of age and older, and for adults.

TABLE 10–7. Chronic medical conditions that are indications for enhanced pneumococcal vaccination among children, by risk group.

Risk Group	Condition
Immunocompetent children	Chronic heart disease[a] Chronic lung disease[b] Diabetes mellitus Cerebrospinal fluid leaks Cochlear implant
Children with functional or anatomic asplenia	Sickle cell disease and other hemoglobinopathies Congenital or acquired asplenia, or splenic dysfunction
Children with immunocompromising conditions	HIV infection Chronic renal failure and nephrotic syndrome Diseases associated with treatment with immunosuppressive drugs or radiation therapy, including malignant neoplasms, leukemias, lymphomas and Hodgkin disease; or solid organ transplantation Congenital immunodeficiency[c]

Source: Advisory Committee on Immunization Practices, 2010.
[a]Particularly cyanotic congenital heart disease and cardiac failure.
[b]Including asthma if treated with high-dose oral corticosteroid therapy.
[c]Includes B- (humoral) or T-lymphocyte deficiency; complement deficiencies, particularly C1, C2, C3, and C4 deficiency; and phagocytic disorders (excluding chronic granulomatous disease).

Dosage & Schedule of Administration

PCV13 is given as a 0.5 mL intramuscular dose. PPSV23 is given as a 0.5 mL dose by either the intramuscular or subcutaneous route.

The recommended immunization schedule for infants and children is complicated by several factors, including the age at first vaccination, the transition from PCV7 to PCV13, and the need to provide enhanced protection to children at an increased risk of pneumococcal disease (Table 10–8). Updated and detailed schedule information is available from the CDC (at http://www.cdc.gov/vaccines) and the Immunization Action Coalition (at http://www.immunize.org).

PCV13 is routinely recommended for infants at 2, 4, 6, and 12–15 months of age. For children < 24 months of age who did not receive PCV13 on this schedule, the recommended number and spacing of doses is given in Table 10–8. The dosing schedule for children 24–71 months of age is shown in Table 10–9. These tables highlight several important features of pneumococcal vaccination recommendations. Healthy children 24–59 months of age who completed a 4-dose PCV7 series should nonetheless receive a single dose of PCV13, to provide them with protection against additional serotypes contained in PCV13. Children 24–71 months of age with certain underlying medical conditions (Table 10–7) should also receive additional PCV13 doses. Children 6–18 years of age may also receive a single dose of PCV13, if PCV13 had not been given previously (although PCV13 is not licensed in this age group).

TABLE 10–8. Recommended schedule for administering doses of 13-valent pneumococcal conjugate vaccine (PCV13) to children aged < 24 months by PCV vaccination history and age.

Age at This Visit (mo)	Vaccination History: Total Number of PCV7 and/or PCV13 Doses Received Previously	Recommended PCV13 Regimen[a]
2-6 mo	0 doses	3 doses, 8 wks apart; fourth dose at age 12-15 mo
	1 dose	2 doses, 8 wks apart; fourth dose at age 12-15 mo
	2 doses	1 dose, 8 wks after the most recent dose; fourth dose at age 12-15 mo
7-11 mo	0 doses	2 doses, 8 wks apart; third dose at 12-15 mo
	1 or 2 doses before age 7 mo	1 dose at age 7-11 mo, with a second dose at 12-15 mo, ≥ 8 wks later
12-23 mo	0 doses	2 doses, ≥ 8 wks apart
	1 dose before age 12 mo	2 doses, ≥ 8 wks apart
	1 dose at ≥ 12 mo	1 dose, ≥ 8 wks after the most recent dose†
	2 or 3 doses before age 12 mo	1 dose, ≥ 8 wks after the most recent dose[b]
	4 doses of PCV7 or other age-appropriate, complete PCV7 schedule	1 supplemental dose ≥ 8 wks after the most recent dose

Source: Advisory Committee on Immunization Practices, 2010.
[a]Minimum interval between doses is 8 weeks except for children vaccinated at age < 1 year, for whom minimum interval between doses is 4 weeks.
[b]No additional PCV13 doses are indicated for children aged 12–23 months who have received 2 or 3 doses of PCV7 before age 12 months and at least 1 dose of PCV13 at age ≥ 12 months.

TABLE 10–9. Recommended schedule for administering doses of 13-valent pneumococcal conjugate vaccine (PCV13) to children aged ≥ 24 months by PCV vaccination history and age.

Age at This Visit (mo)	Vaccination History: Total Number of PCV7 and/or PCV13 Doses Received Previously Before Age 24 mo	Recommended PCV13 Regimen[a]
24-59 mo in healthy children	Unvaccinated or any incomplete schedule	1 dose, ≥ 8 wks after the most recent dose
	4 doses of PCV7 or other age-appropriate, complete PCV7 schedule	1 supplemental dose, ≥ 8 wks after the most recent dose
24-71 mo in children with underlying medical conditions[b]	Unvaccinated or any incomplete schedule of < 3 doses	2 doses, the first dose ≥ 8 wks after the most recent dose and a second dose ≥ 8 wks later
	Any incomplete schedule of 3 doses	1 dose, ≥ 8 wks after the most recent dose
	4 doses of PCV7 or other age-appropriate complete PCV7 schedule	1 supplemental dose, ≥ 8 wks after the most recent dose

Source: Advisory Committee on Immunization Practices, 2010.
[a]Minimum interval between doses is 8 weeks.
[b]For list of conditions, see Table 10–7.

Children with certain chronic medical conditions (Table 10–7) should receive PPSV23 in addition to PCV13. The rationale for this recommendation is that, while less immunogenic than PCV13, PPSV23 covers additional serotypes that may cause significant disease in this population. For children ≥ 2 years of age with chronic medical conditions, 1 dose of PPSV23 should be given at least 8 weeks after the most recent PCV13 dose. Children 24–71 months of age with chronic medical conditions with any incomplete PCV7 series should receive PCV13 (see Table 10–9), followed ≥ 8 weeks later by PPSV23 vaccination. A second dose of PPSV23 is recommended 5 years after the first dose of PPSV23 for children with anatomic or functional asplenia, HIV infection, or immunocompromising conditions. Immunocompetent children with chronic illness should receive the first dose of PPSV23, but are not recommended for PPSV23 revaccination after 5 years.

Contraindications & Precautions

For both PCV13 and PPSV23, vaccination is contraindicated in individuals who suffered a severe allergic reaction such as anaphylaxis after a previous vaccine dose or to a vaccine component (including to any diphtheria toxoid-containing vaccine). PCV13 and PPV23 vaccination should be deferred during moderate or severe acute illness, with or without fever. A history of invasive pneumococcal disease is not a contraindication to vaccination.

Adverse Effects

The most common adverse effects associated with PCV13 administration are fever, injection site reactions, irritability, and increased or decreased sleep. With PPSV23, 50% of vaccine recipients develop pain and redness at the injection site. Fewer than 1% develop systemic side effects such as fever and myalgia. Anaphylaxis is rare. PPSV23 appears to be safe and immunogenic during pregnancy, although safety data are lacking regarding vaccination during the first trimester of pregnancy.

CDC: Prevention of pneumococcal disease among infants and children—use of 13-valent pneumococcal conjugate vaccine and 23-valent pneumococcal polysaccharide vaccine—recommendations of the Advisory Committee on Immunization Practices (ACIP). MMWR 2010;59:1 [PMID: 21150868].

CDC: Invasive pneumococcal disease in young children before licensure of 13-valent pneumococcal conjugate vaccine—United States, 2007. MMWR 2010;59:253 [PMID: 20224541].

Glanz JM et al: Parental decline of pneumococcal vaccination and risk of pneumococcal related disease in children. Vaccine 2011;29:994 [PMID: 21145372].

Pilishvili T et al: Sustained reductions in invasive pneumococcal disease in the era of conjugate vaccine. J Infect Dis 2010;201:32 [PMID: 19947881].

Yeh SH et al: Immunogenicity and safety of 13-valent pneumococcal conjugate vaccine in infants and toddlers. Pediatrics 2010; 126:e493 [PMID: 20732948].

POLIOMYELITIS VACCINATION

The polioviruses are highly infectious, spread primarily by a fecal-oral route, and cause acute flaccid paralysis via destruction of motor neurons. Poliomyelitis can be prevented by vaccination, and in 1988 the World Health Assembly resolved to eradicate poliomyelitis from the world by the year 2000. While that goal was not met, the global incidence of polio has decreased from roughly 350,000 cases annually to 1291 cases reported in 2010. While polio cases have declined dramatically in polio-endemic countries (Afghanistan, India, Nigeria, and Pakistan), polio transmission has become reestablished in Angola, Chad, and the Democratic Republic of the Congo, and 15 other countries have suffered polio outbreaks. In 2011, over 80% of all cases of poliomyelitis have come from Chad, the Democratic Republic of the Congo, and Pakistan.

The worldwide polio eradication program has encountered a number of challenges. Wild-type polioviruses can spread to previously polio-free countries, and sustained transmission can occur in areas with low vaccination coverage rates. In India, oral poliovirus vaccines (OPV) have been less effective than originally anticipated, likely because of the high incidence of diarrheal diseases, malnutrition, and overcrowded living conditions. In other polio-endemic countries, armed conflict and limited infrastructure have led to serious limitations in the ability of public health officials to access and vaccinate susceptible children. Finally, vaccine-derived pathogenic polioviruses can revert from OPV and spread in poorly vaccinated populations. OPV can also persist in immunodeficient patients for years, so any pathogenic revertants that emerge may be shed for extended periods. Updates on the worldwide polio eradication program can be found at www.polioeradication.org.

An injectable poliovirus vaccine of enhanced potency, which has a higher content of antigens than prior vaccines, IPV is an inactivated vaccine. It is the only vaccine against poliomyelitis available in the United States, and cannot cause poliomyelitis, whereas OPV can do so rarely.

Completely immunized adult visitors to areas of continuing wild-type poliovirus circulation should receive a booster dose of IPV. Unimmunized or incompletely immunized adults and children should have received two (preferably three) doses of the vaccine prior to travel to these and other areas with circulation of wild-type or vaccine-type virus.

Vaccines Available

1. IPV (IPOL, sanofi pasteur) is given subcutaneously.
2. DTaP-HepB-IPV (Pediarix, GlaxoSmithKline) contains diphtheria and tetanus toxoids and acellular pertussis adsorbed, hepatitis B, and inactivated poliovirus vaccine. Approved for use at 2, 4, and 6 months of age; not approved for use as the fourth dose of IPV or the fourth or fifth doses of DTaP; given intramuscularly.
3. DTaP-IPV-Hib (Pentacel, sanofi pasteur) contains DTaP, IPV, and Hib vaccines. Approved for use at 2, 4, 6, and 15–18 months of age; not approved for use as the final 4- to 6-year-old booster dose of IPV; given intramuscularly.
4. DTaP-IPV (Kinrix, GlaxoSmithKline) contains DTaP and IPV vaccines. The vaccine is licensed for children 4–6 years of age, for use as a final booster dose of IPV; given intramuscularly.

Dosage & Schedule of Administration

In the United States, all children without contraindications should receive an IPV-containing vaccine at 2 months, 4 months, 6–18 months, and 4–6 years of age. A dose of IPV should be given at 4 years of age or older, regardless of the number of prior doses of IPV. For example, if four doses of DTaP-IPV-Hib are given prior to 4 years of age, a fifth dose of IPV (in the form of IPV-only or DTaP-IPV) is still needed at 4–6 years of age.

Contraindications & Precautions

IPV vaccination is contraindicated in individuals who suffered a severe allergic reaction such as anaphylaxis after a previous vaccine dose or to a vaccine component. IPV vaccination should be deferred during moderate or severe acute illness with or without fever. Pregnancy is also a precaution to IPV vaccination. Receipt of previous doses of OPV is not a contraindication to IPV.

Adverse Effects

Minor local reactions, such as pain or redness at the injection site, may occur following IPV vaccination. No serious adverse reactions following IPV vaccination have been described.

Aylward B, Yamada T: The polio endgame. N Engl J Med 2011;364:2273 [PMID: 21675884].

CDC: Updated recommendations of the Advisory Committee on Immunization Practices (ACIP) regarding routine poliovirus vaccination. MMWR 2009;58:829 [PMID: 19661857].

CDC: Progress toward interruption of wild poliovirus transmission—worldwide, January 2010-March 2011. MMWR 2011;60:582 [PMID: 21566559].

Duintjer Tebbens RJ et al: Economic analysis of the global polio eradication initiative. Vaccine 2010;29:334 [PMID: 21029809].

INFLUENZA VACCINATION

Influenza occurs each winter-early spring period, often associated with significant morbidity and mortality in certain high-risk persons. Up to 36,000 deaths per year in the United States are attributable to influenza, and global epidemics (pandemics) can occur. In April 2009, a pandemic H1N1 strain began circulation and infected millions throughout the world with varying degrees of morbidity and mortality. In the United States, there were an estimated more than 60 million ill, more than 270,000 hospitalizations, and a decreased mortality rate with 12,500 deaths. A monovalent vaccine was produced and given throughout the nation and subsequently incorporated into the seasonal trivalent vaccine. Each year, recommendations are formulated in the spring regarding the constituents of influenza vaccine for the coming season. These recommendations are based on the results of surveillance in Asia and the southern hemisphere during the preceding 6 months. The vaccine each year is a trivalent vaccine containing antigens from two strains of influenza A and one strain of influenza B, which are chosen as being likely to circulate in the United States during the upcoming season. Children at high risk of seasonal influenza-related complications include those with hemoglobinopathies or with chronic cardiac, pulmonary (including asthma), metabolic, renal, and immunosuppressive diseases (including immunosuppression caused by medications or by HIV); and those with any condition (eg, cognitive dysfunction, spinal cord injuries, seizure disorders, or other neuromuscular disorders) that can compromise respiratory function or the handling of respiratory secretions, or that can increase the risk of aspiration. Children and adolescents receiving long-term aspirin therapy are also at risk of influenza-related Reye syndrome. Healthy children aged 6–23 months are at substantially increased risk of influenza-related hospitalizations, and children aged 24–59 months (ie, 2–4 years) are at increased risk of influenza-related clinic and emergency department visits and hospitalizations, but less than younger children.

Annual influenza vaccination is routinely recommended for all persons older than 6 months of age. Physicians should identify high-risk children in their practices and encourage parents to seek influenza vaccination for them as soon as influenza vaccine is available. Influenza prevention will help prevent lower respiratory tract disease or other secondary complications in high-risk groups, thereby decreasing hospitalizations and deaths.

Vaccines Available

The trivalent inactivated influenza vaccine virus (TIV) is grown in eggs, formalin-inactivated, and may contain trace quantities of thimerosal as a preservative. Only split-virus or purified surface antigen preparations are available in the United States. Several manufacturers produce similar vaccines each year. Fluzone split-virus (sanofi pasteur) is approved for children 6 months and older; Fluvirin (Novartis) is approved only for children 4 years and older, Fluarix (GlaxoSmithKline) is approved for children 3 years and older, and Afluria (CSL Biotherapies) is recommended for children 9 years and older. Additional manufacturers (ID Biomedical Corporation) produce influenza vaccines approved for adults.

To eliminate the need for injections, and potentially to enhance mucosal and systemic immune response to vaccination, a live attenuated intranasal vaccine has been developed. This vaccine consists of cold-adapted and temperature-sensitive viruses that replicate poorly in the lower respiratory tract, but well in the nasal mucosa (thereby producing immunity). The intranasal trivalent live attenuated influenza virus vaccine (LAIV [FluMist, MedImmune]) is also a trivalent formulation using the virus strains present in the inactivated vaccine. It is also made in eggs and comes in a single-use prefilled sprayer that should be stored refrigerated at 2–8°C.

Dosage & Schedule of Administration

Inactivated Influenza Virus Vaccine

Because influenza can circulate yearly from November through early March in the United States, the key time to initiate vaccination is as soon as vaccine is available in the early fall. However, providers should continue vaccinating individuals as long as vaccine is available and there is still influenza activity in the community. Children younger than age 6 months should not be immunized. Two doses are recommended for children younger than age 9 years who did not receive a priming pandemic H1N1-containing vaccine in the recent season. Older children receiving vaccine for the first time require only a single dose. The dose for children aged 6–35 months is 0.25 mL given intramuscularly; for older children the dose is 0.5 mL given intramuscularly. The recommended site of vaccination is the anterolateral aspect of the thigh for younger children and the deltoid for older children. Pregnancy is not a contraindication to use of inactivated vaccine, and vaccine is recommended for all pregnant women and those contemplating pregnancy during the influenza season. Simultaneous administration with other routine vaccines is acceptable.

Live Attenuated Influenza Virus Vaccine

This vaccine is supplied in a prefilled single-use sprayer containing 0.2 mL of the vaccine, approximately half of which is sprayed into each nostril. A dose divider clip is provided to assist in dividing the dose. If the patient sneezes during administration, the dose should not be repeated. It can be administered to children with minor illnesses, but should not be given if significant nasal congestion is present. Because it is a live vaccine it should be administered 48 hours after cessation of therapy in children receiving anti-influenza antiviral drugs, and antivirals should not be given for 2 weeks after vaccination. Two doses are recommended for children younger than age 9 years who did not receive at least 1 dose of the 2010–11 seasonal influenza vaccine. One dose is recommended for individuals 9–49 years of age.

Contraindications & Precautions

Inactivated Influenza Virus Vaccine

TIV is contraindicated in individuals with a severe allergic reaction, such as anaphylaxis, to a previous dose or to a TIV vaccine component. However, guidelines for influenza vaccination in children with egg allergies have recently changed. Children with only hives following exposure to egg can be vaccinated, as long as TIV is used as opposed to LAIV, vaccination is by a health care provider experienced in recognizing and treating allergic reactions, and the child is observed for 30 minutes following vaccination. Children with more serious allergic reactions to egg, such as angioedema, respiratory symptoms, or anaphylaxis, may be eligible for TIV, but should be referred to an allergist for an assessment of vaccination risk.

Live Attenuated Influenza Virus Vaccine

LAIV is contraindicated in individuals with history of hypersensitivity to eggs, egg proteins, gentamicin, gelatin, or arginine, or with life-threatening reactions to previous influenza vaccinations, and in children and adolescents receiving concomitant aspirin or aspirin-containing therapy. LAIV should not be administered to the following persons: (1) children younger than 24 months of age, because of an increased risk of hospitalization and wheezing that was observed in clinical trials; (2) any individual with asthma or children younger than age 5 years with recurrent wheezing unless the potential benefit outweighs the potential risk; (3) individuals with severe asthma or active wheezing; or (4) within 48 hours of influenza antiviral therapy. Health care providers should wait 2 weeks after antiviral therapy to administer LAIV unless medically necessary.

All health care workers, including those with asthma and other underlying health conditions (except severe immune compromise), can administer LAIV. Health care workers who are vaccinated with LAIV can safely provide care to patients within a hospital or clinic, except for severely immunosuppressed patients that require a protected environment (ie, bone marrow transplant patients). In this instance, there should be a 7-day interval between receiving LAIV and care for these patients.

Adverse Effects

Inactivated Influenza Virus Vaccine

Injection site reactions are the most common adverse events after TIV administration. A small proportion of children will experience some systemic toxicity, consisting of fever, malaise, and myalgias. These symptoms generally begin 6–12 hours after vaccination and may last 24–48 hours. Cases of Guillain-Barré syndrome followed the swine influenza vaccination program in 1976–1977, but careful study by the Institute of Medicine showed no association with that vaccine in children and young adults—nor in any age group that received vaccines in subsequent years.

Live Attenuated Influenza Virus Vaccine

The most common adverse reactions (occurring at < 10% in individuals receiving LAIV and at least 5% greater than in placebo) are runny nose or nasal congestion in recipients of all ages and fever higher than 37.7°C in children 2–6 years of age. These reactions were reported more frequently with the first dose and were all self-limited.

AAP Committee on Infectious Diseases: Policy statement-recommendations for prevention and control of influenza in children, 2011–2012. Pediatrics 2011;128:1 [PMID: 20805143].

CDC: Prevention and control of influenza. Recommendations of the Advisory Committee on Immunization Practices (ACIP). MMWR Recomm Rep 2010;59(RR-8):1 [PMID: 20689501].

CDC: Prevention and control of influenza with vaccines: Recommendations of the Advisory Committee on Immunization Practices (ACIP), 2011. MMWR 2011;60:1128 [PMID: 21866086].

Fiore AE, Bridges CB, Cox NJ: Seasonal influenza vaccines. Curr Top Microbiol Immunol 2009;333:43 [PMID: 19768400].

Glezen WP: Clinical practice. Prevention and treatment of seasonal influenza. N Eng J Med 2008;359:2579 [PMID: 19073977].

Greenhawt MJ et al: Administering influenza vaccine to egg allergic recipients: A focused practice parameter update. Ann Allergy Asthma Immunol 2011;106:11 [PMID: 1195939].

MEASLES, MUMPS, & RUBELLA VACCINATION

Prior to introduction of the measles vaccine in 1963, there were approximately 500,000 reported cases per year, with 450 deaths and 4000 cases of encephalitis. Within 20 years of introduction, there were less than 1500 cases per year. However, there was resurgence of measles between 1989 and 1991, with 50,000 cases reported. Factors involved included underimmunization in children with inadequate access to health care and primary vaccine failure in 2%–10% of those vaccinated. Therefore, recommendations were made to change from a one-dose to a two-dose vaccination schedule at 12–15 months and at 4–6 years of age. Shortly thereafter, measles rates declined dramatically, and the disease was declared eliminated from the United States in the year 2000.

Since 2000, there have been sporadic importations of measles from countries with lower vaccination rates. Because measles is one of the first diseases to reappear when vaccination coverage falls, since 2008 there have been numerous outbreaks of measles, primarily from viral transmission within the United States after initial exposure to imported cases. In the first 8 months of 2011, there were 198 cases and 15 outbreaks of measles confirmed in the United States, the highest number reported for the same period since 1996. Of these cases, the vast majority was unvaccinated and 90% were associated with United States residents traveling internationally.

In the United States, after the introduction of mumps vaccine in 1967 and the recommendation for its use in 1977, there was a 99% decline in mumps from 185,691 cases reported in 1968 to fewer than 300 cases each year between 2001 and 2003. However, between 2005 and 2006, there was a large multistate outbreak of mumps with almost 6000 confirmed or probable mumps cases reported to the CDC. Six states—Iowa, Kansas, Wisconsin, Illinois, Nebraska, and South Dakota—recorded 85% of the cases. This outbreak occurred mostly on college campuses, but also involved high schools and middle schools. Several factors may have contributed to the outbreaks: conditions on college and high school campuses may be conducive to spread of respiratory infections; two doses of MMR vaccine may not be 100% effective in preventing mumps and even less effective in preventing asymptomatic infection; and waning immunity may have occurred in young adults who had last received mumps-containing vaccine 6–17 years earlier.

The rubella vaccine is not primarily intended to protect individuals from rubella infection, but rather to prevent the serious consequences of rubella infection in pregnant women: miscarriage, fetal demise, and congenital rubella syndrome. Congenital rubella syndrome is a group of birth defects including deafness, cataracts, heart defects, and mental retardation. In the United States and the United Kingdom, the approach has been to vaccinate young children. The intent is to reduce transmission to susceptible women of childbearing age via a herd immunity effect. Although immunity typically wanes after approximately 15 years, there is likely some residual immunity among vaccinated women that also helps prevent congenital rubella syndrome. With the use of rubella vaccines since 1970, rubella incidence rates have declined more than 99% and rubella is now essentially eliminated in the United States with less than 10 cases per year. However, approximately 10% of persons older than 5 years remain susceptible to rubella. Currently most cases of rubella are seen in foreign-born adults, and outbreaks have occurred in poultry- and meat-processing plants that employ many foreign-born workers. There were only two cases of congenital rubella syndrome in the United States between 2004 and 2010.

Although recent measles and mumps outbreaks have not changed the recommendations for two doses of MMR vaccination for all children, in May 2006 the ACIP redefined evidence of immunity to mumps as follows: one dose of a live mumps virus vaccine for preschool children and adults not at high risk; and two doses for children in grades K–12 and adults at high risk (health care workers, international travelers, and students at post-high school level educational facilities). Other evidence of immunity is birth before 1957, documentation of physician-diagnosed mumps, or laboratory evidence of immunity. A recent change (currently a provisional recommendation from the ACIP) is that for unvaccinated health care personnel born before 1957 who lack laboratory evidence of measles, mumps, and/or rubella immunity or laboratory confirmation of disease, health care facilities should *consider* vaccinating personnel with two doses of MMR vaccine at the appropriate interval, and in the event of an outbreak of measles or mumps, that two doses of MMR vaccine *should* be given. During an outbreak of rubella, only one dose of MMR is recommended.

Despite many reports in the lay press and on the Internet of a link between MMR and autism, there is overwhelming evidence in the scientific literature that there is no causal association between the two. There is also no evidence that separation of MMR into its individual component vaccines lessens the risk of any vaccine adverse event, and such practice is not recommended.

It has been known for some time that there is a small but increased risk of febrile seizures after MMR. A recent study found that in 12- to 23-month-old children, the risk for febrile seizures with the MMRV preparation appears to be twice that of MMR and VAR given separately, resulting in one additional febrile seizure per 2300–2600 children vaccinated with MMRV.

Vaccines Available

1. Measles-mumps-rubella (MMR II, Merck): MMR II is a lyophilized preparation of measles, mumps, and rubella vaccines. The measles and mumps portions are prepared using chick embryo tissue cultures and rubella is grown in human diploid cells. There is no adjuvant and no preservative. It does contain small amounts of gelatin, sorbitol, and neomycin. The individual components of MMR II are no longer available.
2. MMRV: In September 2005, the FDA licensed a combined live attenuated measles, mumps, rubella, and varicella vaccine (ProQuad, Merck) for use in children 1–12 years of age. The measles, mumps, and rubella components are identical to MMR II. The varicella component has a higher varicella zoster virus titer than the varicella-only (VAR) vaccine. MMRV is currently not available in the United States due to supply problems, and while the manufacturer intends to continue to produce the vaccine, currently there is no timeline on its availability.

Dosage & Schedule of Administration

Routine Vaccination

Measles, mumps, and rubella vaccinations should be given as MMR or MMRV at 12–15 months and again at 4–6 years of age. Both MMR and MMRV can cause febrile seizures, although uncommonly. Because febrile seizures following MMRV occur at a rate twice that of MMR (see "Adverse Effects"), the ACIP recommends that after a discussion of the benefits and risks of both vaccination options with the parents or caregivers, either MMR or MMRV may be given at 12–15 months of age. MMRV is the preferred vaccine at 4–6 years of age if available. A personal or family history of febrile seizures in an infant is considered a precaution for the use of MMRV, and MMR and VAR given separately is preferred. A dose of 0.5 mL should be given subcutaneously. The second dose of MMR or MMRV is recommended at school entry to help prevent school-based measles and mumps outbreaks. Children not reimmunized at school entry should receive their second dose by age 11–12 years. If an infant receives the vaccine before 12 months of age, two doses are required to complete the series, the first after at least 12 months of age and the second at least 1 month later. Ig interferes with the immune response to the attenuated vaccine strains of MMR and MMRV. Therefore, after Ig administration MMR and MMRV immunization should be deferred by 3–11 months, depending on the type of Ig product received. Consult the AAP's 2009 *Red Book* for specific recommendations.

A person can be considered immune to rubella only with documentation of either serologic immunity to rubella or vaccination with at least one dose of rubella vaccine after age 1 year, or if born before 1957. A clinical diagnosis of rubella is unacceptable. Susceptible pubertal girls and postpubertal women identified by prenatal screening should also be immunized. Whenever rubella vaccination is offered to a woman of childbearing age, pregnancy should be ruled out and the woman advised to prevent conception for 3 months following vaccination. If a pregnant woman is vaccinated or becomes pregnant within 3 weeks of vaccination, she should be counseled regarding the risk to her fetus, although no cases of rubella vaccine-related fetal anomalies have been reported. The risk of congenital rubella syndrome after wild-type maternal infection in the first trimester of pregnancy is 20%–85%. All susceptible adults in institutional settings (including colleges), day care center personnel, military personnel, and hospital and health care personnel should be immunized.

Vaccination of Travelers

People traveling abroad should be immune to measles and mumps. Infants 6–11 months of age traveling to high-risk areas should receive one dose of MMR prior to travel followed by either MMR or MMRV at 12–15 months of age (given at least 4 weeks after the initial dose) and either MMR or MMRV at 4–6 years of age to complete the series. Children over 12 months of age who are traveling to high-risk areas should receive two doses separated by at least 4 weeks. Children traveling internationally to lower-risk areas should be immunized as soon as possible after their first birthday and complete the series at 4–6 years of age in the usual fashion.

Revaccination Under Other Circumstances

Persons entering college and other institutions for education beyond high school, medical personnel beginning employment, and persons traveling abroad should have documentation of immunity to measles and mumps, defined as receipt of two doses of measles vaccine after their first birthday, birth before 1957, or a documented measles or mumps history or immunity.

Outbreak Control of Measles

A community outbreak is defined as a single documented case of measles. Control depends on immediate protection of all susceptible persons (defined as persons who have no documented immunity to measles in the affected community). In the case of unvaccinated individuals, the following recommendations hold: (1) age 6–11 months, MMR if cases are occurring in children younger than age 1 year, followed by two doses of MMR or MMRV at age 12–15 months and again at age 4–6 years; and (2) age 12 months or older, MMR or MMRV followed by revaccination at age 4–6 years. A child with an unclear or unknown vaccination history should be reimmunized with MMR or MMRV. Anyone with a known exposure who is not certain of having previously received two doses of MMR should receive an additional dose. Unimmunized persons who are not immunized within 72 hours of exposure, which is the acceptable interval for postexposure prophylaxis, should be excluded from contact with potentially infected persons until at least 2 weeks after the onset of rash of the last case of measles.

Contraindications & Precautions

MMR and MMRV vaccines are contraindicated in pregnant women, women intending to become pregnant within the next 28 days, immunocompromised persons (except those with asymptomatic HIV who have age-specific $CD4^+$ lymphocytes counts > 15%), and persons with anaphylactic egg or neomycin allergy. It is also contraindicated in children receiving high-dose corticosteroid therapy (≥ 2 mg/kg/d, or 20 mg/d total, for longer than 14 days) with the exception of those receiving physiologic replacement doses. In these patients, an interval of 1 month between cessation of steroid therapy and vaccination is sufficient. Leukemic patients who have been in remission and off chemotherapy for at least 3 months can receive MMR and MMRV safely. Children with minor acute illnesses (including febrile illnesses), non-anaphylactic egg allergy, or a history of tuberculosis should be immunized. MMR and MMRV may be safely administered simultaneously with other routine pediatric immunizations. A personal or family history of febrile seizures in an infant is considered a precaution for the use of MMRV, and MMR and VAR separately is preferred.

Adverse Effects

Between 5% and 15% of vaccinees receiving MMR become febrile to 39.5°C or higher about 6–12 days following vaccination, lasting approximately 1–2 days, and 5% may develop a transient morbilliform rash. Transient thrombocytopenia occurs at a rate of 1 per 40,000 vaccine recipients. Encephalitis and other central nervous system conditions, such as aseptic meningitis and Guillain-Barré syndrome, are reported to occur at a frequency of 1 case per 3 million doses in the United States. This rate is lower than the rate of these conditions in unvaccinated children, implying that the relationship between them and MMR vaccination is not causal. Reactions after mumps vaccination are rare and include parotitis, low-grade fever, and orchitis. In children, adverse effects from rubella vaccination are very unusual. Between 5% and 15% of vaccinees develop rash, fever, or lymphadenopathy 5–12 days after rubella vaccination. Rash also occurs alone or as a mild rubella illness in 2–4% of adults. Arthralgia and arthritis occur in 10–25% of adult vaccinees, as opposed to only 0–2% of 6- to 16-year-old vaccinees. Chronic arthritis, which may be causally related to rubella vaccination, occurs more often in women aged 45 or older, starting 10–11 days after vaccination and lasting for up to

1 year. Possible rare complications include peripheral neuritis and neuropathy, transverse myelitis, and diffuse myelitis.

MMR vaccination is associated with an increased risk of febrile seizures 8–14 days after vaccination with the first dose, but no subsequent long-term complications have been seen. The risk associated for febrile seizures in children 12–23 months old with MMRV appears to be twice that of MMR and VAR given separately, resulting in one additional febrile seizure per 2300–2600 children vaccinated with MMRV.

Antibody Preparations Against Measles

If a child is seen within 72 hours after exposure to measles, vaccination is the preferred method of postexposure protection. If vaccine is contraindicated, Ig, given intramuscularly at a dose of 0.25 mL/kg (0.5 mL/kg in immunocompromised patients; maximum dose in either circumstance is 15 mL), is effective in preventing or modifying measles if it is given within 6 days after exposure. MMR or MMRV vaccine should be given 5 months later to children receiving the 0.25-mL/kg dose and 6 months later for the higher dose. For children receiving regular intravenous immune globulin, a dose of 100–400 mg/kg should be adequate for measles prophylaxis for exposures occurring within 3 weeks of the last dose.

CDC: Update: Recommendations from the Advisory Committee on Immunization Practices (ACIP) regarding administration of combination MMRV vaccine. MMWR 2008;57:258 [PMID: 18340332].

CDC: Notes from the field: Measles outbreak—Indiana, June–July 2011. MMWR 2011;60:1169 [PMID: 21881549].

CDC: Measles: United States, January–May 20, 2011. MMWR 2011;60:666 [PMID: 21617634].

France EK et al: Risk of immune thrombocytopenic purpura after measles-mumps-rubella immunization in children. Pediatrics 2008;121:e687 [PMID: 18310189].

Omer SB et al: Vaccine refusal, mandatory immunization, and the risks of vaccine-preventable diseases. N Engl J Med 2009; 360:1981 [PMID: 19420367].

VARICELLA VACCINATION

Prior to the availability of vaccine, about 4 million cases of varicella-zoster virus (VZV) infection occurred annually in the United States, mostly in children younger than 10 years old. This resulted in 11,000 hospitalizations and 100 deaths per year due to severe complications such as secondary bacterial infections, pneumonia, encephalitis, hepatitis, and Reye syndrome.

A live, attenuated varicella vaccine (VAR) has been licensed in the United States since 1995 and routine immunization of children 12 months of age and older has been recommended since then. The vaccine is more than 95% effective at preventing severe disease. The morbidity, mortality, and medical costs associated with varicella infection have significantly declined since VAR was first licensed. While there is no national system of surveillance for varicella disease in place, a variety of data sources have shown a consistent pattern of more than 85% reduction in varicella-associated disease. Evaluation of the impact of the one-dose varicella vaccination program documented a decline of 88% overall in varicella mortality

Once the routine use of VAR was achieved, it became apparent that there is "breakthrough" (usually very mild) varicella occurring in about 15% of immunized patients. Outbreaks of wild-type infectious VZV have been reported in schools with high one-dose VAR vaccination coverage (96%–100%). The vaccine efficacy in those outbreaks against any disease was similar (72%–85%) to that previously observed. Varicella attack rates among these children varied between 11% and 17% and thus, it was concluded that a single VAR dose could not prevent varicella outbreaks completely.

A second dose of VAR vaccine in children, when given 3 months or 4–6 years after the initial dose, greatly increased the anti-VZV antibody response, which is a correlate of vaccine efficacy. A combination MMRV vaccine has also been shown to be immunologically noninferior to the individual components administered compared with MMR and VAR vaccines administered concomitantly, either as primary immunization or as a booster administered to children age 4–6 years. The two-dose regimen is 97%–100% effective against severe varicella, and the risk of breakthrough varicella is threefold less than the risk with a one-dose regimen. Therefore, in 2006 and 2007, the ACIP and the AAP changed the recommendation from one to two doses of VAR vaccine for children older than 12 months of age, and for adolescents and adults without evidence of immunity.

Data from the United States and Japan suggest that the vaccine is also effective in preventing or modifying VZV severity in susceptible individuals exposed to VZV if used within 3 days of exposure. A study in the United States suggests that the efficacy of postexposure vaccination is 95% for prevention of any disease and 100% for prevention of moderate or severe disease. There is no evidence that postexposure prophylaxis will increase the risk of vaccine-related adverse events or interfere with development of immunity.

VACCINES AVAILABLE

1. A cell-free preparation of Oka strain VZV is produced and marketed in the United States as Varivax (Merck). Each dose of VAR contains not less than 1350 plaque-forming units of VZV and trace amounts of neomycin, fetal bovine serum, and gelatin. There is no preservative. Storage in a freezer at a temperature of −15°C or colder provides a shelf life of 15 months. VAR may be stored for 72 hours at refrigerator temperature in its lyophilized state, but it must be administered within 30 minutes after thawing and reconstitution.

2. MMRV (measles-mumps-rubella-varicella, ProQuad, Merck) is licensed for use in children 1–12 years of age. MMRV is well-tolerated and provides adequate immune response to all of the antigens it contains. In MMRV, the varicella component is present in higher titer than in the VAR vaccine. Concomitant administration of MMRV with DTaP, Hib, and HepB vaccines is acceptable. MMRV should be stored in a freezer at a temperature of −15°C or colder. MMRV is currently not available. The manufacturer intends to continue to produce the vaccine, but currently there is no timeline on its availability.

Dosage & Schedule of Administration

Two doses (0.5 mL) of VAR vaccine are recommended for immunization of all healthy children aged 12 months and older, and for adolescents and adults without evidence of immunity. For children aged 12 months to 12 years the immunization interval is 3 months, and for persons 13 years or older it is 4 weeks. MMRV is approved only for healthy children aged 12 months to 12 years. A second dose of catch-up vaccination is required for children, adolescents, and adults who previously received one dose of VAR vaccine. All children should have received two doses of vaccine before prekindergarten or school. Asymptomatic or mildly symptomatic HIV-infected children (≥ 15% $CD4^+$ cells) should receive two doses of the single-antigen vaccine (with a 3-month interval between doses).

VAR may be given simultaneously with MMR at separate sites. If not given simultaneously, the interval between administration of VAR and MMR must be greater than 28 days. Simultaneous VAR administration does not appear to affect the immune response to other childhood vaccines. VAR should be delayed 5 months after receiving intravenous immune globulin, blood, or plasma. In addition, persons who received a VAR should not be administered an antibody-containing product or an antiviral medication active against varicella for at least 2 weeks, and if needed in that interval, the individual may need to be tested for immunity or revaccinated. After a discussion of the benefits and risks of both vaccination options with the parents or caregivers (see below, "Adverse Effects"), either MMR or MMRV may be given at 12–15 months. MMRV is the preferred vaccine if available at 4–6 years of age.

Contraindications & Precautions

Contraindications to VAR vaccination include a severe allergic reaction after a previous vaccine dose or to a vaccine component. Because VAR and MMRV are live-virus vaccines, they are also contraindicated in children who have cellular immunodeficiencies, including those with leukemia, lymphoma, other malignancies affecting the bone marrow or lymphatic systems, and congenital T-cell abnormalities (although VAR vaccine administration to children with acute lymphocytic leukemia is under investigation). The exception to this rule is the recommendation that VAR be administered to HIV-infected children who are not severely immunosuppressed. Children receiving immunosuppressive therapy, including high-dose steroids, should not receive VAR or MMRV. Household contacts of immunodeficient patients should be immunized. VAR should not be given to pregnant women; however, the presence of a pregnant mother in the household is not a contraindication to immunization of a child within that household. A personal or family history of febrile seizures in an infant is considered a precaution for the use of MMRV; administration of MMR and VAR separately is preferred for the first dose.

Adverse Events

Since the approval of VAR in 1995, more than 50 million doses have been distributed in the United States. The most commonly recognized adverse reactions, occurring in approximately 20% of vaccinees, are minor injection site reactions. Additionally, 3%–5% of patients will develop a rash at the injection site, and an additional 3%–5% will develop a sparse varicelliform rash outside of the injection site. These rashes typically consist of two to five lesions and may appear 5–26 days after immunization. The two-dose vaccine regimen is generally well tolerated with a safety profile comparable to that of the one-dose regimen. The incidence of fever and varicelliform rash is lower after the second dose than the first. Although VAR is contraindicated in pregnancy, there have now been several hundred inadvertent administrations of vaccine to pregnant women tracked by the "Pregnancy Registry for Varivax" with no known cases of congenital varicella syndrome.

Studies comparing MMRV to MMR and VAR administered concomitantly showed more systemic adverse events following MMRV (fever 21.5% vs 14.9% and measles-like rash 3% vs 2.1%, respectively). The risk of febrile seizures in children 12–23 months old with the MMRV preparation is twice that of MMR and VAR given separately, resulting in one additional febrile seizure per 2300–2600 children vaccinated with MMRV.

Transmission of vaccine virus from healthy vaccinees to other healthy persons is very rare, has never been documented in the absence of a rash in the index case, and has only resulted in mild disease. Herpes zoster infection has occurred in recipients of VAR in immunocompetent and immunocompromised persons within 25–722 days after immunization. Many of these cases were due to presumably unappreciated latent wild-type virus. Vaccine-strain varicella does cause herpes zoster in children, but the age-specific risk of herpes zoster infection seems lower in children following VAR immunization than after natural infection, and it is also tends to be milder.

Antibody Preparations

In the event of an exposure to varicella, there are currently two antibody preparations potentially available in the United States for postexposure prophylaxis, VariZIG and intravenous Ig. Exposure is defined as a household contact or playmate contact (> 1 h/d), hospital contact (in the same or contiguous room or ward), intimate contact with a person with herpes zoster deemed contagious, or a newborn contact. Susceptibility is defined as the absence of a reliable history of varicella or varicella vaccination. Uncertainty in this diagnosis can be resolved with an appropriate test for anti-VZV antibody.

A Canadian preparation (VariZIG, Cangene Corporation) can be obtained from FFF Enterprises, Temecula, CA (1-800-843-7477). If VariZig is not available, it is recommended that intravenous Ig be used in its place. The dose is 400 mg/kg administered once. A subsequent exposure does not require additional prophylaxis if this occurs within 3 weeks of intravenous Ig administration. Varicella-zoster immune globulin (VZIg) was a preparation used for postexposure prophylaxis that is no longer available in the United States.

AAP Committee on Infectious Diseases: Prevention of varicella: Recommendations for use of quadrivalent and monovalent varicella vaccines in children. Pediatrics 2011;128:630 [PMID: 21873692].

CDC: Prevention of varicella: Recommendations of the Advisory Committee on Immunization Practices (ACIP). MMWR Recomm Rep 2007;56(RR-4):1 [PMID: 17585291].

CDC: Update: Recommendations from the Advisory Committee on Immunization Practices (ACIP) regarding administration of combination MMRV vaccine. MMWR 2008;57:258 [PMID: 18340332].

Marin M, Zhang JX, Seward JF: Near elimination of varicella deaths in the US after implementation of the vaccination program. Pediatrics 2011;128:214 [PMID: 21788222].

HEPATITIS A VACCINATION

The incidence of hepatitis A in the United States has decreased dramatically in recent years. An average of 28,000 cases was reported annually in the years prior to availability of a hepatitis A vaccine. Hepatitis A infection rates are now at historical lows, with fewer than 2000 reported cases annually.

Hepatitis A vaccines first became available in the United States in 1995. Initially, vaccination was recommended for certain high-risk groups, such as international travelers, users of illegal drugs, and men who have sex with men. Children, who are more likely than adults to be asymptomatic while infected, have often contributed to the spread of hepatitis A through households and communities. Therefore, since 2006 hepatitis A vaccination has been routinely recommended for all children 12–23 months of age. The widespread use of the vaccine in children has been associated with a distinct change in the epidemiology of hepatitis A infection: in a recent investigation, more than 40% of cases were associated with international travel, often in foreign-born persons returning to their countries of origin.

In addition to routine immunization of all children 12–23 months of age, hepatitis A vaccination is indicated for the following groups: (1) travelers to countries with moderate to high rates of hepatitis A, (2) children with chronic hepatitis B or hepatitis C infections or other chronic liver disease, (3) children with clotting factor disorders, (4) adolescent and adult males who have sex with men, (5) persons with an occupational exposure to hepatitis A, (6) illegal drug users, and (7) all previously unvaccinated persons who anticipate close personal contact (such as household contact or babysitting) with an international adoptee from countries with moderate to high rates of hepatitis A. Vaccination should also be considered in previously unimmunized children 2–18 years old, even if none of the above risk factors are present.

Vaccines Available

Two inactivated hepatitis A vaccines are available for children: Havrix (GlaxoSmithKline) and Vaqta (Merck). Neither vaccine contains a preservative. Both vaccines contain an aluminum adjuvant. Both vaccines are approved for children 12 months and older. A combination vaccine against hepatitis A and hepatitis B (Twinrix, GlaxoSmithKline) is also available, but is only licensed in the United States for persons 18 years and older.

Dosage & Schedule of Administration

Havrix is available in two formulations. For individuals between the ages of 1 and 18 years, 720 ELU (enzyme-linked immunosorbent assay [ELISA] units) per dose is administered intramuscularly in two doses of 0.5 mL, separated by 6–12 months. For persons older than 18 years, a higher dose (1440 ELU per dose) is recommended, also in two doses of 1 mL.

Vaqta also has two formulations. For persons aged 1–18 years, two doses of 25 units per dose (0.5 mL) are given, separated by 6–18 months. Individuals 19 years of age and older are given 50 units per dose (1.0 mL) in a two-dose schedule.

Both vaccines should be shipped and stored at 2–8°C and should not be frozen. Hepatitis A vaccines are given intramuscularly, and may be given simultaneously with other vaccines, including HepB.

Contraindications & Precautions

Hepatitis A vaccine should not be given to anyone with a prior severe allergic reaction, such as anaphylaxis, after a previous vaccine dose or to a vaccine component. Precautions to vaccination include pregnancy and moderate or severe acute illness. The vaccine should not be administered to children with hypersensitivity to neomycin (in the case of Havrix) or alum (for both preparations).

Adverse Effects

Adverse reactions, which are uncommon and mild, consist of pain, swelling, and induration at the injection site

(10%–15%), headache, and loss of appetite. There have been no reports of serious adverse events attributed definitively to hepatitis A vaccine.

Postexposure Prophylaxis

Postexposure prophylaxis is recommended for household or sexual contacts of persons with serologically confirmed hepatitis A, and for daycare staff and attendees in outbreak situations. Postexposure prophylaxis may also be recommended in food-borne outbreaks, depending on the extent and timing of exposure. Postexposure prophylaxis of unimmunized persons who are exposed to hepatitis A should consist of either a single dose of hepatitis A vaccine or Ig (0.02 mL/kg), given as soon as possible after exposure. For healthy people 12 months through 40 years of age, hepatitis A vaccine is preferred to Ig for postexposure prophylaxis because of the advantages of vaccination, including long-term protection and ease of administration. For those over 40 years of age, Ig is preferred, although the vaccine should be used if Ig is not available. Ig should also be used for children < 12 months of age, immunocompromised persons, those with chronic liver disease, and anyone for whom vaccination is contraindicated. People who are given Ig, and for whom hepatitis A vaccine is recommended for other reasons, should receive a dose of vaccine simultaneously with Ig. If given at the same time, the vaccine and Ig should be administered at different anatomic injection sites. The efficacy of Ig when given more than 2 weeks after exposure has not been established.

Antibody Preparations

Ig is effective against hepatitis A infection through the passive transfer of antibodies. Ig can be used as preexposure as well as postexposure prophylaxis. Ig is indicated as preexposure prophylaxis in children younger than age 12 months at increased risk of hepatitis A infection (eg, those traveling to endemic areas, or those with clotting factor disorders). For preexposure prophylaxis, recommended dosages are 0.02 mL/kg in a single intramuscular dose if the duration of exposure is likely to be less than 3 months and 0.06 mL/kg if exposure is likely to be more than 3 months. For long-term prophylaxis of persons not eligible for vaccination, prophylactic doses can be repeated every 5 months.

Byrd KK et al: Predictors of hepatitis A vaccination among young children in the United States. Vaccine 2011;29:3254 [PMID: 21352942].

CDC: Prevention of hepatitis A through active or passive immunization: Recommendations of the Advisory Committee on Immunization Practices (ACIP). MMWR Recomm Rep 2006; 55(RR-7):1 [PMID: 16708058].

CDC: Updated recommendations from the Advisory Committee on Immunization Practices (ACIP) for use of hepatitis A vaccine in close contacts of newly arriving international adoptees. MMWR 2009;58:1006 [PMID: 19763077].

CDC: Update: Prevention of hepatitis A after exposure to hepatitis A virus and in international travelers. Updated recommendations of the Advisory Committee on Immunization Practices (ACIP). MMWR 2007;56:1080 [PMID: 17947967].

CDC (hepatitis A vaccine information): Available at: http://www.cdc.gov/hepatitis/HAV.htm

Klevens RM et al: The evolving epidemiology of hepatitis A in the United States: Incidence and molecular epidemiology from population-based surveillance, 2005-2007. Arch Intern Med 2010; 170:1811 [PMID: 21059974].

MENINGOCOCCAL VACCINATION

Infections with *Neisseria meningitidis* cause significant morbidity and mortality, with an estimated 1400–2800 cases of meningococcal disease occurring in the United States annually. Even with appropriate treatment, meningococcal disease has an estimated case-fatality rate of 10%–14%, and up to 19% of survivors are left with serious disabilities, such as neurologic deficits, loss of limbs or limb function, or hearing loss. Five serogroups of meningococcus (A, B, C, W-135, and Y) cause the vast majority of disease worldwide. Serogroups B, C, and Y are the predominant causes of invasive meningococcal disease in the United States, while serogroups A and C cause most disease in developing countries. Intensive research efforts have been made to develop an effective vaccine against serogroup B, which causes more than 50% of cases among children younger than 1 year of age. However, the bacterial capsule proteins of serogroup B are poorly immunogenic in humans, presenting a significant obstacle to vaccine development.

There are two tetravalent meningococcal polysaccharide-protein conjugate vaccines (MCV4) available, Menactra, licensed in 2005, and Menveo, licensed in 2010. Both vaccines are recommended by the ACIP and are indicated for use in persons 2–55 years of age. MCV4 is recommended for all persons 11 to 18 years of age, as well as for persons 2–55 years who are at increased risk of meningococcal disease. Persons at increased risk include college freshmen living in dormitories, microbiologists who are routinely exposed to isolates of *Neisseria meningitidis*, military recruits, persons who travel to or reside in countries where meningococcal disease is hyperendemic or epidemic, persons with persistent complement component deficiencies, and persons with anatomic or functional asplenia.

Because of mounting evidence of waning immunity by 5 years postvaccination, a booster dose is now recommended for adolescents aged 16 years and older who received their first dose at ages 11 to 15 years. A booster dose is not recommended for persons who received their first dose at age 16 years or older. A 2 dose *primary* series administered 2 months apart is indicated for persons age 2 through 55 years with persistent complement component deficiency, functional or anatomic asplenia, and for adolescents 11 to 18 years with human immunodeficiency virus (HIV) infection. Whenever meningococcal vaccination is indicated, MCV4 is preferred for persons 2–55 years old, while tetravalent meningococcal polysaccharide vaccine (MPSV4, Menomume) should be used for persons older than 55 years. If MCV4 is not available, MPSV4 is an appropriate alternative for persons 2–55 years old for the initial dose. For a booster dose, MPSV4 is not recommended and either MCV4 product may be used (Menactra or Menveo). There are limited data available on the interchangeability of MCV4 products, and whenever feasible the same brand of vaccine should be used for all doses of the vaccine series. However, providers should use every opportunity to provide the booster dose when indicated, regardless of the vaccine brand used (Menactra or Menveo) for previous doses.

Vaccines Available

1. MCV4 (Menactra, sanofi pasteur): A single 0.5-mL dose contains 4 mcg each of capsular polysaccharide from serogroups A, C, Y, and W-135 conjugated to 48 mcg of diphtheria toxoid. Available in single-dose vials only.
2. MCV4 (Menveo, Novartis): A single 0.5-mL dose contains 10 mcg of serogroup A capsular polysaccharide and 5 mcg each of serogroups C, Y, and W-135 capsular polysaccharide, all of which is conjugated to CRM_{197}, a nontoxic mutant of diphtheria toxoid.
3. MPSV4 (Menomune-A/C/Y/W-135, sanofi pasteur): Each dose consists of 50 mcg each of the four bacterial capsular polysaccharides. Available in 1- and 10-dose vials.

Dosage & Schedule of Administration

1. MCV4 is given as a single intramuscular dose of 0.5 mL. If a dose is inadvertently administered subcutaneously, it does not need to be repeated.
2. MPSV4 is administered as a single subcutaneous dose of 0.5 mL.

MCV4 and MPSV4 can be given at the same time as other vaccines, at a different anatomic site. Protective antibody levels are typically achieved within 10 days of vaccination.

Contraindications & Precautions

MCV4 and MPSV4 are contraindicated in anyone with a known severe allergic reaction to any component of the vaccine, including diphtheria toxoid (for MCV4) and rubber latex. Although MCV4 vaccination is not contraindicated in someone with a prior history of Guillain-Barré syndrome, providers should discuss the possible risks and benefits of vaccination in anyone with a history of Guillain-Barré syndrome. Both MCV4 and MPSV4 can be given to individuals who are immunosuppressed. MPSV4 is thought to be safe during pregnancy; no information is available regarding the safety of MCV4 during pregnancy.

Adverse Effects

Both MCV4 products and MPSV4 are generally well tolerated in adolescent patients. Local vaccination reactions (redness, swelling, or induration) occur in 11%–16% of persons 11–18 years old receiving MCV4 and in 4%–6% of persons the same age receiving MPSV4. The most common solicited complaints among children aged 2–10 years were injection site pain and irritability. More severe systemic reactions (presence of any of the following: fever of 39.5°C or above; headache, fatigue, malaise, chills, or arthralgias requiring bed rest; anorexia; multiple episodes of vomiting or diarrhea; rash; or seizures) occur in 4.3% of MCV4 recipients and 2.6% of MPSV4 recipients. Although cases of Guillain-Barré syndrome, a rare neurologic disorder, have been reported after MCV4, the current data does not suggest that the rate is above that which would be expected in the absence of vaccination. Any cases of suspected Guillain-Barré syndrome after vaccination should be reported to VAERS.

Postexposure Prophylaxis

Close contacts of a patient with invasive meningococcal disease should receive antimicrobial prophylaxis to prevent infection. Because the rate of disease among close contacts is highest immediately after exposure, postexposure prophylaxis should be started as soon as possible, ideally within 24 hours of exposure. Close contacts are defined as (1) household members, (2) daycare center contacts, and (3) anyone encountering an infected patient's secretions, such as through kissing, mouth-to-mouth resuscitation, or endotracheal intubation. Rifampin or ceftriaxone are used for chemoprophylaxis in children; rifampin, ceftriaxone, or ciprofloxacin may be used for adults.

CDC: Prevention and control of meningococcal disease—recommendations of the Advisory Committee on Immunization Practices (ACIP). MMWR 2005;54(RR-7):1 [PMID: 15917737].

CDC: Updated Recommendation from the Advisory Committee on Immunization Practices (ACIP) for revaccination of persons at prolonged increased risk for meningococcal disease. MMWR 2009;58:1042 [PMID: 19779400].

CDC: Licensure of a meningococcal conjugate vaccine for children aged 2 through 10 years and updated booster dose: Guidance for adolescents and other persons at increased risk for meningococcal disease—Advisory Committee on Immunization Practices (ACIP), 2011. MMWR 2011;60:1018 [PMID: 21814165].

CDC: Updated recommendations for use of meningococcal conjugate vaccines—Advisory Committee on Immunization Practices (ACIP), 2010. MMWR 2011;60:72 [PMID: 21270745].

CDC: Licensure of a meningococcal conjugate vaccine (Menveo) and guidance for use—Advisory Committee on Immunization Practices (ACIP), 2010. MMWR 2010;59(9):273 [PMID: 20224545].

Poland GA: Prevention of meningococcal disease: Current use of polysaccharide and conjugate vaccines. Clin Infect Dis 2010;50 (Suppl 2):S45 [PMID: 20144016].

TETANUS-REDUCED DIPHTHERIA-ACELLULAR PERTUSSIS VACCINATION (ADOLESCENTS & ADULTS)

Pertussis is increasingly recognized as a disease affecting older children and adults, including fully vaccinated persons with waning immunity. In the United States, the most dramatic increases in pertussis incidence are among adolescents and young adults, prompting development of booster pertussis vaccines for this population. FDA approval in 2005 of the tetanus-reduced dose diphtheria-acellular pertussis (Tdap) vaccine was based on comparable seroresponse to pertussis antigens and a safety profile similar to control Td. Adolescent, adult, and elderly immunization not only has the capacity to protect adolescents from pertussis, but also should limit spread of pertussis from adults to infants and decrease overall pertussis endemicity.

Vaccines Available

1. Tdap (Boostrix, GlaxoSmithKline) contains tetanus toxoid, diphtheria toxoid, and three acellular pertussis antigens (detoxified pertussis toxin [PT], filamentous hemagglutinin [FHA], and pertactin) and is licensed for use in persons aged 10 years and older; this vaccine can be used in adults and the elderly.
2. Tdap (Adacel, sanofi pasteur) contains tetanus toxoid, diphtheria toxoid, and five acellular pertussis antigens (PT, FHA, pertactin, and fimbriae types 2 and 3) and is licensed for use in persons aged 11–64 years.

Dosage & Schedule of Administration

Adolescents 11–18 years of age should receive a 0.5-mL dose of Tdap intramuscularly in the deltoid, instead of the tetanus and diphtheria toxoids (Td) vaccine for booster immunization. The preferred age for Tdap immunization is 11–12 years. Adults 19 to 64 years of age should receive a single dose of Tdap. Adults 65 years of age and older should receive a single dose of Tdap if they have not previously received Tdap and if they anticipate close contact with an infant less than 12 months of age. Tdap can be administered regardless of the interval since the last tetanus- or diphtheria-toxoid containing vaccine. Tdap and MCV4 should be administered during the same visit if both vaccines are indicated. If not administered at the same time, a minimum interval of 1 month between vaccines is suggested.

Contraindications & Precautions

Contraindications to Tdap include severe allergic reaction to any vaccine component and encephalopathy (eg, coma, prolonged seizures) not attributable to an identifiable cause within 7 days of administration of a vaccine with pertussis components. Precautions for Tdap administration include Guillain-Barré syndrome occurring within 6 weeks of a previous dose of a tetanus toxoid-containing vaccine, a progressive neurologic disorder, uncontrolled epilepsy, or progressive encephalopathy until the condition has stabilized. If there is a history of a severe Arthus reaction after a previous tetanus toxoid-containing or diphtheria toxoid-containing vaccine, Tdap should be deferred for at least 10 years.

Adverse Effects

Pain at the injection site was the most frequently reported local adverse event among adolescents. Headache and fatigue were the most frequently reported systemic adverse events.

AAP, Committee on Infectious Diseases: Prevention of pertussis among adolescents: Recommendations for use of tetanus toxoid, reduced diphtheria toxoid, and acellular pertussis (Tdap). Pediatrics 2006;117:965 [PMID: 16382131].

CDC: Updated recommendations for the use of tetanus toxoid, reduced diphtheria toxoid and acellular pertussis (Tdap) vaccine from the Advisory Committee on Immunization Practices, 2011. MMWR 2011; 60:13 [PMID: 21228763].

Yih WK et al. An assessment of the safety of adolescent and adult tetanus-diphtheria-acellular pertussis (Tdap) vaccine, using active surveillance for adverse events in the Vaccine Safety Datalink. Vaccine 2009;27:4257 [PMID: 19486957].

HUMAN PAPILLOMAVIRUS VACCINATION

Genital human papillomavirus (HPV) is the most common sexually transmitted infection in the United States. Most of the estimated 6.2 million persons newly infected every year have no symptoms. Up to 75% of new infections occur among persons 15–24 years of age. Over 40% of the 100 HPV types identified can infect the genital area. Approximately 70% of cervical cancers are caused by the high cancer risk types 16 and 18. Over 90% of genital warts are caused by low cancer risk types 6 and 11.

Two HPV vaccines are currently licensed in the United States. Quadrivalent HPV vaccine (HPV4) types 6, 11, 16, and 18 (Gardasil, Merck) is approved for females and males 9 through 26 years of age. Bivalent HPV (HPV2) types 16 and 18 vaccine (Cervarix, GlaxoSmithKline) is approved for females 10 through 25 years of age. Routine vaccination of females and males aged 11–12 years is recommended. Catch-up vaccination for females aged 13–26 years and males aged 13–21 years who were not previously vaccinated or have not completed the full vaccine series is also recommended. Females who might have been exposed to HPV, or who have an equivocal or abnormal Pap test or a positive hybrid capture II high-risk test, should be vaccinated and are still likely to benefit from HPV vaccine. Routine use of HPV4 in males has been recommended since October 2011.

Vaccines Available

1. Quadrivalent HPV vaccine (Gardasil, Merck), an inactivated vaccine; a 0.5-mL dose contains 20 mcg each of

HPV-6 and HPV-18 L1 proteins, and 40 mcg each of HPV-11 and HPV-16 L1 proteins.

2. Bivalent HPV vaccine (Cervarix, GlaxoSmithKline), an inactivated vaccine is a 0.5-mL dose that contains 40 mcg HPV-16 L1 protein and 20 mcg HPV-18 L1 protein.

Dosage & Schedule of Administration

HPV vaccine is administered intramuscularly as three separate 0.5-mL doses. The second dose should be administered 1–2 months after the first dose and the third dose 6 months after the first dose. The minimum interval between the first and second dose is 4 weeks; the minimum recommended interval between the second and third doses of vaccine is 12 weeks. HPV vaccine may be administered with other vaccines. Each vaccine should be administered using a separate syringe at a different anatomic site. If the vaccine schedule is interrupted, the series need not be restarted.

Contraindications & Precautions

HPV vaccine is contraindicated in persons with a history of anaphylaxis to any vaccine component. HPV vaccine is not recommended for use in pregnancy. The vaccine can be administered to persons with minor acute illnesses and to immunocompromised persons.

Adverse Effects

Injection site pain (83.9%) and mild to moderate swelling and erythema were the most common adverse events reported by vaccine recipients. Fever (10.3%), nausea (4.2%), and dizziness (2.8%) were reported as systemic adverse events. Postmarketing reports of syncope, which were reported after vaccination with HPV vaccine, may follow any vaccination, so vaccine recipients should be observed for 15 minutes after vaccination.

CDC: Quadrivalent human papillomavirus vaccine: Recommendations of the Advisory Committee on Immunization Practices (ACIP). MMWR 2007;56(RR-2):1 [PMID: 17380109].

CDC: FDA licensure of bivalent human papillomavirus vaccine (HPV2, Cervarix) for use in females and updated HPV vaccination recommendations from the Advisory Committee on Immunization Practices (ACIP). MMWR 2010;59:626 [PMID: 20508593].

CDC: Recommendations on the use of quadrivalent human papillomavirus vaccine in males: Advisory Committee on Immunization Practices (ACIP). MMWR 2011;60:1705 [PMID: 22189893].

Gee J et al: Monitoring the safety of quadrivalent human papillomavirus vaccine: Findings from the Vaccine Safety Datalink. Vaccine 2011; [Epub ahead of print] [PMID: 21907257].

Jenson HB: Human papillomavirus vaccine: A paradigm shift for pediatricians. Curr Opin Pediatr 2009;21:112 [PMID: 19242247].

VACCINATIONS FOR SPECIAL SITUATIONS

RABIES VACCINATION

After symptoms of infection develop, rabies is almost invariably fatal in humans. Only seven persons are known to have recovered from rabies infection, five of whom had either been vaccinated prior to infection or received some form of postexposure prophylaxis. While animal rabies in the United States is common, the incidence of human rabies is very low, with fewer than three cases per year. Although dogs represent the most important vector for human rabies worldwide, in the United States, because of widespread vaccination of dogs and cats the most common rabies virus variants responsible for human rabies are bat-related. Rabies is also common in skunks, raccoons, and foxes; it is uncommon in rodents.

Human rabies is preventable with appropriate and timely postexposure prophylaxis. Postexposure care consists of local wound care, passive immunization, and active immunization. Immediately after an animal bite, all wounds should be flushed and aggressively cleaned with soap and water. If possible, the wound should not be sutured. Passive immunization after high-risk exposure consists of the injection of human rabies immune globulin (RIG) near the wound, as described later. Active immunization is accomplished by completing a schedule of immunization with one of the two available rabies vaccines licensed in the United States. Because bites from bats are often unrecognized, prophylaxis should be given if a bat is found indoors even if there is no history of contact, especially if found in the same room with a sleeping or unattended child or with an intoxicated or otherwise incapacitated individual.

Local public health officials should be consulted before postexposure rabies prophylaxis is started to avoid unnecessary vaccination and to assist in the proper handling of the animal (if confinement or testing of the animal is appropriate). To facilitate consultation, the health care provider should know the species of animal, its availability for testing or confinement, the nature of the attack (provoked or unprovoked), and the nature of the exposure (bite, scratch, lick, or aerosol of saliva). Preexposure prophylaxis is indicated for veterinarians, animal handlers, and any persons whose work or home environment potentially places them in close contact with animal species in which rabies is endemic. Rabies immunization should also be considered for children traveling to countries where rabies is endemic; this is particularly important for travelers to rural areas where there is no prompt access to medical care should an exposure occur.

Vaccines Available

Rabies vaccines stimulate immunity after 7–10 days, and the immunity persists for 2 years or more postvaccination. Two inactivated preparations are licensed in the United States.

1. Imovax Rabies (sanofi pasteur) human diploid cell vaccine (HDCV)
2. RabAvert (Novartis) purified chick embryo cell vaccine (PCEC)

Dosage & Schedule of Administration

The two rabies vaccines available in the United States are equally safe and efficacious for both preexposure and postexposure prophylaxis. For each vaccine, 1 mL is given intramuscularly in the deltoid (for adults and older children) or anterolateral thigh (for infants and young children). The volume of the dose is not reduced for children. Vaccine should not be given in the gluteal region.

Primary Preexposure Vaccination

Preexposure rabies immunization should be considered for individuals at high risk of exposure to rabies (eg, veterinarians, animal handlers, spelunkers, and people moving to or extensively traveling in areas with endemic rabies). Three intramuscular injections in the deltoid area of 1 mL of any vaccine are given on days 0, 7, and 21 or 28.

Postexposure Prophylaxis

After an individual has possibly been exposed to rabies, decisions about whether to initiate postexposure prophylaxis need to be made urgently, in consultation with local public health officials.

1. In previously unvaccinated individuals—After prompt and thorough wound cleansing, an individual exposed to rabies should receive rabies vaccination and RIG. Vaccination is given on the day of exposure (day 0) and on days 3, 7, and 14 following exposure. Immune suppressed individuals should receive five doses of vaccine, on days 0, 3, 7, 14, and 28, in addition to testing for rabies virus neutralizing antibody during the vaccination course to assess immune response. RIG should also be given as soon as possible after exposure, ideally on the day of exposure, in a recommended dose of 20 IU/kg. If anatomically possible, the entire dose of RIG should be infiltrated into and around the wound. Any remaining RIG should be administered intramuscularly at an anatomic site distant from the location used for rabies vaccination. If RIG was not administered when vaccination was begun, it can be administered up to 7 days after the first dose of vaccine. Postexposure failures have occurred only when some deviation from the approved protocol occurred (eg, no cleansing of the wound, less than usual amount of RIG, no RIG at the wound site, or vaccination in the gluteal area).

2. In previously vaccinated individuals—RIG should not be administered, and only two doses of vaccine on days 0 and 3 after exposure are needed.

Booster Vaccination

Previously vaccinated individuals with potential continued exposure to rabies should have a serum sample tested for rabies antibody every 2 years. If the titer is less than 1:5 for virus neutralization, a booster dose of rabies vaccine should be administered.

Adverse Effects

The rabies vaccines are relatively free of serious reactions and rates of adverse reactions may differ between the vaccines. Local reactions at the injection site such as pain, swelling, induration, or erythema range in frequency from 11% to 89% of vaccinees. These are more common than mild systemic reactions, such as headache, nausea, muscle aches, and dizziness, which range from 6% to 55% of vaccinees. An immune complex-like reaction occurs in about 6% of persons 2–21 days after receiving booster doses of the rabies vaccine.

Travelers to countries where rabies is endemic may need immediate postexposure prophylaxis and may have to use locally available vaccines and RIG. In many developing countries, the only vaccines readily available may be nerve tissue vaccines derived from the brains of adult animals or suckling mice, and the RIG may be of equine origin. Although adverse reactions to RIG are uncommon and typically mild, the nervous tissue vaccines may induce neuroparalytic reactions in 1:200–1:8000 vaccinees; this is a significant risk and is another justification for preexposure vaccination prior to travel in areas where exposure to potentially rabid animals is likely.

Antibody Preparations

In the United States, RIG is prepared from the plasma of human volunteers hyperimmunized with rabies vaccine. The recommended dose is 20 IU/kg body weight. The rabies-neutralizing antibody content is 150 IU/mL, supplied in 2- or 10-mL vials. It is very safe.

CDC: Use of a reduced (4-dose) vaccine schedule for postexposure prophylaxis to prevent human rabies: Recommendations of the Advisory Committee on Immunization Practices. MMWR 2010; 59(RR-2):1 [PMID: 20300058].

CDC (rabies information page): http://www.cdc.gov/rabies/

Leung AKC, Davies HD, Hon KLE: Rabies: Epidemiology, pathogenesis, and prophylaxis. Adv Ther 2007;24:1340 [PMID: 18165217].

Manning SE et al: CDC: Human rabies prevention—United States, 2008: Recommendations of the Advisory Committee on Immunization Practices. MMWR 2008;57(RR-3):1 [PMID: 18496505].

TYPHOID FEVER VACCINATION

Globally, the burden of typhoid fever is substantial, causing an estimated 22 million illnesses and 200,000 deaths each year. In the United States, typhoid fever is relatively uncommon, with approximately 150–300 laboratory-confirmed cases each year, the majority acquired abroad. In a review of typhoid fever cases reported to the CDC, 79% of patients reported recent travel outside the United States, only 5% of whom had received typhoid vaccination.

Two vaccines against *Salmonella enterica typhi,* the bacterium that causes typhoid fever, are available in the United States: a live attenuated vaccine given orally (Ty21a), and an inactivated vaccine composed of purified capsular polysaccharide (ViCPS) given parenterally. Both vaccines protect 50%–80% of vaccine recipients. The oral vaccine is most commonly used because of its ease of administration. However, noncompliance with the oral vaccine dosing schedule occurs frequently, and correct usage should be stressed or the parenteral ViCPS vaccine used.

Routine typhoid vaccination is recommended only for children who are traveling to typhoid-endemic areas or who reside in households with a documented typhoid carrier. While CDC recommendations emphasize typhoid vaccination for travelers expected to have long-term exposure to potentially contaminated food and drink, vaccination should also be considered for short-term travel to high-risk countries. Although typhoid fever occurs throughout the world, areas of highest incidence include southern Asia and southern Africa. Travelers should be advised that because the typhoid vaccines are not fully protective, and because of the potential for other food- and water-borne illnesses, careful selection of food and drink and appropriate hygiene remain necessary when traveling internationally.

Vaccines Available

1. Parenteral ViCPS (Typhim Vi, sanofi pasteur) is for intramuscular use.
2. Oral live attenuated Ty21a vaccine (Vivotif Berna Vaccine, Swiss Serum and Vaccine Institute) is supplied as enteric-coated capsules.

Dosage & Schedule of Administration

ViCPS is administered as a single intramuscular dose (0.5 mL) in the deltoid muscle, with boosters needed every 3 years if exposure continues. It is approved for children aged 2 years and older.

The dose of the oral preparation is one capsule every 2 days for a total of four capsules, taken 1 hour before meals. The capsules should be taken with cool liquids and should be kept refrigerated. All doses should be administered at least 1 week prior to potential exposure. A full course of four capsules is recommended every 5 years if exposure continues. Mefloquine and proguanil may decrease the effect of the live vaccine, and the vaccine should be given at least 1 day or 10 days after a dose of mefloquine or proguanil, respectively. This vaccine is not approved for children younger than age 6 years. As with all live attenuated vaccines, Ty21a should not be given to immunocompromised patients.

Adverse Reactions

Both the oral and parenteral vaccines are well tolerated, and adverse reactions are uncommon and usually self-limited. The oral vaccine may cause gastroenteritis-like illness, fatigue, and myalgia, whereas the parenteral vaccine may cause injection site pain, abdominal pain, dizziness, and pruritus.

Fraser A et al: Typhoid fever vaccines: Systematic review and meta-analysis of randomized controlled trials. Vaccine 2007;25:7848 [PMID: 17928109].

Lynch MF et al: Typhoid fever in the United States, 1999–2006. JAMA 2009;302:859 [PMID: 19706859].

Sur D et al: A cluster-randomized effectiveness trial of Vi typhoid vaccine in India. N Engl J Med 2009;361:335 [PMID: 19625715].

JAPANESE ENCEPHALITIS VACCINATION

Japanese encephalitis virus (JE) is a mosquito-borne flavivirus that carries a high morbidity and mortality for those infected. It is endemic in parts of Asia, although the risk to most travelers to Asia is low. Travel to rural areas and extended travel in endemic areas may increase the risk. There are two safe and effective vaccines, only one of which is licensed for use in children. The ACIP recently released recommendations regarding prevention of JE infection in travelers. Travelers to JE-endemic countries should be advised of risks of JE and the importance of measures to reduce mosquito bites. Vaccination is recommended for travelers who plan to spend more than 1 month in endemic areas during the JE transmission season. Vaccination should be *considered* for short-term travelers to endemic areas during the JE transmission season if they will travel outside of an urban area *and* their activities will increase the risk of JE exposure. It should also be considered for travelers to an area with an ongoing JE outbreak. Vaccination is not recommended for short-term travelers whose visit will be restricted to urban areas or outside of a well-defined JE transmission season.

Vaccines Available and Schedule of Administration

1. JE-VAX (sanofi pasteur) is an inactivated mouse brain-derived JE vaccine first licensed in the United States in 1992. It is licensed for use in children aged 1 year or older and adults. It contains thimerosal as a preservative. It is given subcutaneously as a three-dose primary series on days 0, 7, and 30. JE-VAX is no longer produced, although the manufacturer has reserved a stockpile to be used only in children 1–16 years. It is unknown how long this supply will last.
2. Ixiaro (Novartis) is an inactivated Vero cell-derived JE vaccine licensed in March 2009. It is licensed for persons aged 17 or older. It contains aluminum hydroxide as an adjuvant and has no preservative. It is given intramuscularly in a two-dose series at 0 and 28 days.

CDC: Japanese encephalitis among three U.S. travelers returning from Asia, 2003–2008. MMWR 2009;58:737 [PMID: 19609246].

Erlanger TE et al: Past, present, and future of Japanese encephalitis. Emerg Infect Dis 2009;15:1 [PMID: 19116041].

CDC: Japanese encephalitis vaccines: recommendations of the Advisory Committee on Immunization Practices (ACIP). MMWR 2010;59(RR-1):1 [PMID: 20224546].

TUBERCULOSIS VACCINATION

Approximately one-third of the world's population is infected with *Mycobacterium tuberculosis,* which is a leading cause of death in low- and middle-income nations, killing approximately 2 million people annually. It is relatively uncommon in the United States, and most cases occur in persons born in other countries or their close contacts. Bacille Calmette-Guérin vaccine (BCG) consists of live attenuated *Mycobacterium bovis.* BCG is the most widely used vaccine in the world and has been administered to over 3 billion people with a low incidence of adverse events following immunization. Nearly 80% of the world's population has been vaccinated with BCG. BCG vaccine is inexpensive, can be given any time after birth, sensitizes the vaccinated individual for 5–50 years, and stimulates both B-cell and T-cell immune responses. BCG reduces the risk of tuberculous meningitis and disseminated TB in pediatric populations by 50%–100% when administered in the first month of life. Efficacy against pulmonary tuberculosis has been variable (0%–80%) depending on the study setting and other factors.

BCG is indicated for use in the United States in two circumstances: (1) in tuberculin-negative infants or older children residing in households with untreated or poorly treated individuals with active infection with isoniazid- and rifampin-resistant *M tuberculosis,* and (2) in infants or children that live under constant exposure without the possibility of removal or access to prophylaxis and treatment. It is not recommended for travel.

The two currently licensed BCG vaccines in the United States are produced by Organon Teknika Corporation (Tice BCG) and sanofi pasteur (Mycobax). They are given intradermally in a dose of 0.05 mL for newborns and 0.1 mL for all other children. Tuberculin skin testing (TST) is advised 2–3 months later, and revaccination is advised if the TST result is negative. Adverse effects occur in 1%–10% of healthy individuals, including local ulceration, regional lymph node enlargement, and very rarely lupus vulgaris. The vaccine is contraindicated in pregnant women and in immunocompromised individuals, including those with HIV infection, because it has caused extensive local adenitis and disseminated or fatal infection.

BCG almost invariably causes its recipients to be tuberculin-positive (5–7 mm), but the reaction often becomes negative after 3–5 years. Thus, a positive TST test in a child with a history of BCG vaccination who is being investigated for TB as a case contact should be interpreted as indicating infection with *M tuberculosis.* There are several interferon release tests useful for the diagnosis of *M tuberculosis* infection in adults. These tests may be useful in the future for distinguishing BCG reaction from infection in children as they should be negative in BCG recipients. However, currently this area has not been well studied in children.

Bergamini BM et al: Performance of commercial blood tests for the diagnosis of latent tuberculosis infection in children and adolescents. Pediatrics 2009;123:e419 [PMID: 19254978].

CDC: Controlling tuberculosis in the United States of America. Recommendations from the American Thoracic Society, CDC and the Infectious Diseases Society of America. MMWR 2005;54(RR-12):1 [PMID: 16267499].

CDC: Trends in tuberculosis—United States, 2010. MMWR 2011;60:333 [PMID: 21430636].

Maartens G, Wilkinson RJ: Tuberculosis. Lancet 2007;370:2030 [PMID: 17719083].

YELLOW FEVER VACCINATION

A live, attenuated vaccine against yellow fever is available for use in the United States. However, the vaccine is available only at official yellow fever vaccination locations (typically public health departments), and should only be given after consultation with travel medicine specialists or public health officials. Immunization against yellow fever is indicated for children age 9 months and older traveling to endemic areas or to countries that require it for entry. Yellow fever vaccine is made from the 17D yellow fever attenuated virus strain grown in chick embryos. It is contraindicated in infants younger than age 6 months, in persons with anaphylactic egg allergy, and in immunocompromised individuals or individuals with a history of thymus disease. In children 6 to 8 months of age, the vaccine risks and benefits should be weighed on an individual basis. When yellow fever vaccine is indicated, a single subcutaneous injection of 0.5 mL of reconstituted vaccine is administered. The International Health Regulations require revaccination at 10-year intervals, although immunity following vaccination may be lifelong. Adverse reactions are generally mild, consisting of low-grade fever, mild headache, and myalgia 5–10 days after vaccination, occurring in fewer than 25% of vaccinees. Although relatively uncommon, several types of severe adverse reactions can occur following vaccination. Serious allergic reactions occur in roughly 1 case per every 55,000 vaccine recipients. The risk of vaccine-associated neurotropic disease within 30 days following vaccination has been estimated to be 4–6 cases per 1 million doses. The risk of severe multiple organ system failure following vaccination has been estimated at 1 case per every 250,000 vaccine recipients. Health care providers should be careful to administer yellow fever vaccine only to persons truly at risk of exposure to yellow fever. There is no contraindication to giving other live-virus vaccines simultaneously with yellow fever vaccine.

CDC: Yellow fever vaccine: recommendations of the Advisory Committee on Immunization Practices (ACIP). MMWR 2010;59(RR-7):1 [PMID: 20671663].

Hayes EB: Is it time for a new yellow fever vaccine? Vaccine 2010;28:8073 [PMID: 20971115].

Thomas RE et al: Active and passive surveillance of yellow fever vaccine 17D or 17DD-associated serious adverse events: Systematic review. Vaccine 2011;29:4544 [PMID: 21549787].

PASSIVE PROPHYLAXIS

1. Intramuscular & Specific Intravenous Immune Globulin

Ig may prevent or modify infection with hepatitis A virus if administered in a dose of 0.02 mL/kg within 14 days after exposure. Measles infection may be prevented or modified in a susceptible person if Ig is given in a dose of 0.25 mL/kg within 6 days after exposure. Special forms of Ig include tetanus Ig (TIg), hepatitis B Ig (HBIg), rabies Ig (RIg), rubella Ig, CMV Ig (IV), botulism Ig (IV), and varicella-zoster Ig (VariZig). These are obtained from donors known to have high titers of antibody against the organism in question. Ig must be given only in the manner for which it is recommended (ie, IM must be given intramuscularly, IV must be given intravenously). The dose varies depending on the clinical indication. Adverse reactions include pain at the injection site, headache, chills, dyspnea, nausea, and anaphylaxis, although all but the first are rare.

Prophylaxis to prevent respiratory syncytial virus (RSV) in infants and children at increased risk of severe disease is available as an intramuscular immune globulin. Palivizumab (Synagis, MedImmune) is a humanized monoclonal antibody against RSV that is used to prevent RSV infection in high-risk populations with monthly doses during RSV season. Palivizumab should be considered for (1) infants and children younger than age 2 years with chronic lung disease who have required medical therapy (supplemental oxygen, bronchodilator, diuretic, or corticosteroid therapy) for their disease within 6 months before the anticipated RSV season; (2) infants born between 32 weeks 0 days and 34 weeks 6 days gestation or earlier without chronic lung disease with at least one out of two of the following risk factors: child care attendance *or* siblings under age 5 years (this recommendation is for those infants who are born during or within 3 months of the onset of RSV season); prophylaxis for these infants should be discontinued once they reach 3 months of age; (3) infants with congenital airway abnormalities or severe neuromuscular disease up to age 12 months; (4) infants born at less than 32 weeks' gestation; and (5) infants and children who are 24 months old or younger with hemodynamically significant cyanotic or acyanotic congenital heart disease.

Palivizumab is administered in a dose of 15 mg/kg once a month beginning with the onset of the RSV season and continuing until the end of the season, regardless of breakthrough RSV illness during that RSV season. The maximum number of doses recommended in any one season is five (the maximum is three doses for 32- to 35-week premature infants without chronic lung disease). Palivizumab is packaged in 50- and 100-mg vials. Palivizumab does not interfere with response to routine childhood vaccinations.

Environmental tobacco smoke is no longer considered a specific risk factor when considering RSV prophylaxis. Due to a lack of data, there are no specific recommendations for palivizumab prophylaxis in infants with immune deficiencies or cystic fibrosis. However, prophylaxis may be considered in these patients in certain circumstances (severe immune compromise such as severe combined immunodeficiency syndrome).

2. Intravenous Immune Globulin

The primary indications for IVIg are for replacement therapy in antibody-deficient individuals; for the treatment of Kawasaki disease, immune thrombocytopenic purpura, Guillain-Barré syndrome, and other autoimmune diseases; and replacement therapy in chronic B-cell lymphocytic leukemia. IVIg may be beneficial in some children with HIV infection, toxic shock syndrome, and for anemia caused by parvovirus B19. It may also be used as postexposure prophylaxis for varicella in at-risk persons when VariZIG is not available.

AAP: Policy Statement—Modified recommendations for use of palivizumab for prevention of respiratory syncytial virus infections. Pediatrics 2009;124:1694 [PMID: 19736258].

CDC: Respiratory syncytial virus activity—United States, July 2007–December 2008. MMWR 2008;57:1355 [PMID: 19092759].

Frogel M et al: Improved outcomes with home-based administration of palivizumab: Results from the 2000–2004 Palivizumab Outcomes Registry. Pediatr Infect Dis J 2008;27:870 [PMID: 18776822].

Hall CB et al: The burden of respiratory syncytial virus infection in young children. N Engl J Med 2009;360:588 [PMID: 19196675].

11 Normal Childhood Nutrition & Its Disorders

Matthew Haemer, MD
Laura E. Primak, RD, CNSD, CSP
Nancy F. Krebs, MD, MS

NUTRITIONAL REQUIREMENTS

NUTRITION & GROWTH

The nutrient requirements of children are influenced by (1) growth rate, (2) body composition, and (3) composition of new growth. These factors vary with age and are especially important during early postnatal life. Growth rates are higher in early infancy than at any other time, including the adolescent growth spurt (Table 11–1). Growth rates decline rapidly starting in the second month of postnatal life (proportionately later in the premature infant). Nutrient requirements also depend on body composition. In the adult, the brain, which accounts for only 2% of body weight, contributes 19% to the total basal energy expenditure. In contrast, in a full-term neonate, the brain accounts for 10% of body weight and for 44% of total energy needs under basal conditions. Thus, in the young infant, total basal energy expenditure and the energy requirement of the brain are relatively high.

Composition of new tissue is a third factor influencing nutrient requirements. For example, fat accounts for about 40% of weight gain between birth and 4 months but for only 3% between 24 and 36 months. The corresponding figures for protein are 11% and 21%; for water, 45% and 68%. The high rate of fat deposition in early infancy has implications not only for energy requirements but also for the optimal composition of infant feedings.

Because of the high nutrient requirements for growth and the body composition, the young infant is especially vulnerable to undernutrition. Slowed physical growth rate is an early and prominent sign of undernutrition in the young infant. The limited fat stores of the very young infant mean that energy reserves are unusually modest. The relatively large size and continued growth of the brain render the central nervous system (CNS) especially vulnerable to the effects of malnutrition in early postnatal life.

ENERGY

The major determinants of energy expenditure are (1) basal metabolism, (2) metabolic response to food, (3) physical activity, and (4) growth. The efficiency of energy use may be a significant factor, and thermoregulation may contribute in extremes of ambient temperature if the body is inadequately clothed. Because adequate data on requirements for physical activity in infants and children are unavailable and because individual growth requirements vary, recommendations have been based on calculations of actual intakes by healthy subjects. Suggested guidelines for energy intake of infants and young children are given in Table 11–2. Also included in this table are calculated energy intakes of infants who are exclusively breast-fed, which have been verified in a number of centers. Growth velocity of breast-fed infants during the first 3 months equals and may exceed that of formula-fed infants, but from 6 to 12 months breast-fed infants typically weigh less than formula-fed babies and may show a decrease in growth velocity. The World Health Organization has developed growth standards derived from an international sample of healthy breast-fed infants and young children raised in environments that do not constrain growth. These are considered to represent physiologic growth for infants and young children. (See also section on Pediatric Undernutrition.)

After the first 4 years, energy requirements expressed on a body weight basis decline progressively. The estimated daily energy requirement is about 40 kcal/kg/d at the end of adolescence. Approximate daily energy requirements can be calculated by adding 100 kcal/y to the base of 1000 kcal/d at age 1 year. Appetite and growth are reliable indices of caloric needs in most healthy children, but intake also depends to some extent on the energy density of the food offered. Individual energy requirements of healthy infants and children vary considerably, and malnutrition and disease increase the variability. Premature infant energy requirements can exceed 120 kcal/kg/d, especially during illness or when catch-up growth is desired.

Table 11–1. Changes in growth rate, energy required for growth, and body composition in infants and young children.

Age (mo)	Growth Rate (g/d)			Energy Requirements for Growth (kcal/kg/d)	Body Composition (%)		
	Male	Both	Female		Water	Protein	Fat
0–0.25		0[a]			75	11.5	11
0.25–1	40		35	50			
1–2	35		30	25			
2–3	28		25	16			
3–6		20		10	60	11.5	26
6–9		15					
9–12		12					
12–18		8					
18–36		6		2	61	16	21

[a]Birth weight is regained by 10 days. Weight loss of more than 10% of birth weight indicates dehydration or malnutrition; this applies to both formula- and breast-fed infants.
Data reprinted with permission, from Fomon SJ (editor): *Infant Nutrition*, 2nd ed. WB Saunders, 1974.

One method of calculating requirements for malnourished patients is to base the calculations on the ideal body weight (ie, 50th percentile weight for the patient's length-age, 50th percentile weight-for-length, or weight determined from current height and the 50th percentile body mass index [BMI] for age), rather than actual weight.

World Health Organization: Report of a Joint FAO/WHO/UNO Expert Consultation: Energy and Protein Requirements. WHO Tech Rep Ser No. 724, 1985;724.

Grummer-Strawn LM et al: Use of World Health Organization and CDC growth charts for children aged 0–59 months in the United States. Centers for Disease Control and Prevention (CDC). MMWR Recomm Rep. 2020 Sep 10;59(RR-9):1–15 [PMID: 20829749].

Table 11–2. Recommendations for energy and protein intake.

Age	Energy (kcal/kg/d)			Protein (g/kg/d)	
	Based on Measurements of Energy Expenditure	Intake from Human Milk	Guidelines for Average Requirements	Intake from Human Milk	Guidelines for Average Requirements
10 d–1 mo	—	105	120	2.05	2.5
1–2 mo	110	110	115	1.75	2.25
2–3 mo	95	105	105	1.36	2.25
3–4 mo	95	75–85	95	1.20	2.0
4–6 mo	95	75–85	95	1.05	1.7
6–12 mo	85	70	90	—	1.5
1–2 y	85	—	90	—	1.2
2–3 y	85	—	90	—	1.1
3–5 y	—	—	90	—	1.1

Data reprinted with permission, from Krebs NF et al: Growth and intakes of energy and zinc in infants fed human milk. J Pediatr 1994;124:32; Garza C, Butte NF: Energy intakes of human milk-fed infants during the first year. J Pediatr 1990;117:(S)124.

PROTEIN

Only amino acids and ammonium compounds are usable as sources of nitrogen in humans. Amino acids are provided through the digestion of dietary protein. Nitrogen is absorbed from the intestine as amino acids and short peptides. Absorption of nitrogen is more efficient from synthetic diets that contain peptides in addition to amino acids. Some intact proteins are absorbed in early postnatal life, a process that may be important in the development of protein tolerance or allergy.

Because there are no major stores of body protein, a regular dietary supply of protein is essential. In infants and children, optimal growth depends on an adequate dietary protein supply. Relatively subtle effects of protein deficiency are now recognized, especially those affecting tissues with rapid protein turnover rates, such as the immune system and the gastrointestinal (GI) mucosa.

Relative to body weight, rates of protein synthesis and turnover and accretion of body protein are exceptionally high in the infant, especially the premature infant. Eighty percent of the dietary protein requirement of a premature infant is used for growth, compared with only 20% in a 1-year-old child. Protein requirements per unit of body weight decline rapidly during infancy as growth velocity decreases. The recommendations in Table 11–2 are derived chiefly from the Joint FAO/WHO/UNO Expert Committee and are similar to the Recommended Dietary Allowances (RDAs). They deliver a protein intake above the quantity provided in breast milk. The protein intake required to achieve protein deposition equivalent to the in utero rate in very low-birth-weight infants is 3.7–4.0 g/kg/d simultaneously with adequate energy intake. Protein requirements increase in the presence of skin or gut losses, burns, trauma, and infection. Requirements also increase during times of catch-up growth accompanying recovery from malnutrition (approximately 0.2 g of protein per gram of new tissue deposited). Young infants experiencing rapid recovery may need as much as 1–2 g/kg/d of extra protein. By age 1 year, the extra protein requirement is unlikely to be more than 0.5 g/kg/d.

The quality of protein depends on its amino acid composition. Infants require 43% of protein as essential amino acids, and children require 36%. Adults cannot synthesize eight essential amino acids: isoleucine, leucine, lysine, methionine, phenylalanine, threonine, tryptophan, and valine. Histidine may be added to this list. Cysteine and tyrosine are considered partially essential because their rates of synthesis are limited and may be inadequate in certain circumstances. In young infants, synthetic rates for cysteine, tyrosine, and perhaps taurine are insufficient for needs. Taurine, an amino acid used to conjugate bile acids, may also be conditionally essential in infancy. Lack of an essential amino acid leads to weight loss within 1–2 weeks. Wheat and rice are deficient in lysine, and legumes are deficient in methionine. Appropriate mixtures of vegetable protein are therefore necessary to achieve high protein quality.

Because the mechanisms for removal of excess nitrogen are efficient, moderate excesses of protein are not harmful and may help to ensure an adequate supply of certain micronutrients. Adverse effects of excessive protein intake may include increased calcium losses in urine and, over a life span, increased loss of renal mass. Excessive protein intake may also cause elevated blood urea nitrogen, acidosis, hyperammonemia, and, in the premature infant, failure to thrive, lethargy, and fever. In a randomized large-scale trial of formula-fed infants, a higher protein content was associated with higher weight (but not length) in the first 2 years of life.

Hay WW Jr: Strategies for feeding the preterm infant. Neonatology 2008;94(4):245–254 [PMID: 18836484].

Koletzko B et al: Lower protein in infant formula is associated with lower weight up to age 2 yr: A randomized clinical trial. Am J Clin Nutr 2009;89:1836–1845 [PMID: 19386747].

LIPIDS

Fats are the main dietary energy source for infants and account for up to 50% of the energy in human milk. Over 98% of breast milk fat is triglyceride (TG), which has an energy density of 9 kcal/g. Fats can be stored efficiently in adipose tissue with a minimal energy cost of storage. This is especially important in the young infant. Fats are required for the absorption of fat-soluble vitamins and for myelination of the central nervous system. Fat also provides essential fatty acids (EFAs) necessary for brain development, for phospholipids in cell membranes, and for the synthesis of prostaglandins and leukotrienes. The EFAs are polyunsaturated fatty acids, linoleic acid (18:2ω6) and linolenic acid (18:3ω3). Arachidonic acid (20:4ω6) is derived from dietary linoleic acid and is present primarily in membrane phospholipids. Important derivatives of linolenic acid are eicosapentaenoic acid (20:6ω3) and docosahexaenoic acid (DHA, 22:6ω3) found in human milk and brain lipids. Visual acuity and possibly psychomotor development of formula-fed premature infants is improved in formulas supplemented with DHA (22:6ω3) and ARA (20:4ω6). The benefits of long-chain polyunsaturated fatty acid supplementation in formulas for healthy term infants are unclear (though safety has been established).

Clinical features of EFA ω6 deficiency include growth failure, erythematous and scaly dermatitis, capillary fragility, increased fragility of erythrocytes, thrombocytopenia, poor wound healing, and susceptibility to infection. The clinical features of deficiency of ω3 fatty acids are less well defined, but dermatitis and neurologic abnormalities including blurred vision, peripheral neuropathy, and weakness have been reported. Fatty fish are the best dietary source of ω3 fatty acids. A high intake of fatty fish is associated with decreased platelet adhesiveness and decreased inflammatory response.

Up to 5%–10% of fatty acids in human milk are polyunsaturated, with the specific fatty acid profile reflective of maternal dietary intake. Most of these are ω6 series with smaller amounts of long-chain ω3 fatty acids. About 40% of breast milk fatty acids are monounsaturates, primarily oleic acid (18:1), and up to 10% of total fatty acids are medium-chain triglycerides (MCTs) (C_8 and C_{10}) with a calorie density of 7.6 kcal/g. In general, the percentage of calories derived from fat is a little lower in infant formulas than in human milk.

The American Academy of Pediatrics recommends that infants receive at least 30% of calories from fat, with at least 2.7% of total fat as linoleic acid, and 1.75% of total fatty acids as linolenic. It is appropriate that 40%–50% of energy requirements be provided as fat during at least the first year of life. Children older than 2 years should be switched gradually to a diet containing approximately 30% of total calories from fat, with no more than 10% of calories either from saturated fats or polyunsaturated fats.

β-Oxidation of fatty acids occurs in the mitochondria of muscle and liver. Carnitine is necessary for oxidation of the fatty acids, which must cross the mitochondrial membranes as acylcarnitine. Carnitine is synthesized in the human liver and kidneys from lysine and methionine. Carnitine needs of infants are met by breast milk or infant formulas. In the liver, substantial quantities of fatty acids are converted to ketone bodies, which are then released into the circulation as an important fuel for the brain of the young infant.

MCTs are sufficiently soluble that micelle formation is not required for transport across the intestinal mucosa. They are transported directly to the liver via the portal circulation. MCTs are rapidly metabolized in the liver, undergoing β-oxidation or ketogenesis. They do not require carnitine to enter the mitochondria. MCTs are useful for patients with luminal phase defects, absorptive defects, and chronic inflammatory bowel disease. The potential side effects of MCT administration include diarrhea when given in large quantities; high octanoic acid levels in patients with cirrhosis; and, if they are the only source of lipids, deficiency of EFA.

Belkind-Gerson J et al: Fatty acids and neurodevelopment. J Pediatr Gastroenterol Nutr 2008 Aug;47(Suppl 1):S7–S9 [PMID: 18667917].

CARBOHYDRATES

The energy density of carbohydrate is 4 kcal/g. Approximately 40% of caloric intake in human milk is in the form of lactose, or milk sugar. Lactose supplies 20% of the total energy in cow's milk. The percent of total energy in infant formulas from carbohydrate is similar to that of human milk.

The rate at which lactase hydrolyzes lactose to glucose and galactose in the intestinal brush border determines how quickly milk carbohydrates are absorbed. Lactase levels are highest in young infants, and decline with age depending on genetic factors. About 20% of nonwhite Hispanic and black children younger than 5 years of age have lactase deficiency. White children typically do not develop symptoms of lactose intolerance until they are at least 4 or 5 years of age, while nonwhite Hispanic, Asian-American, and black children may develop these symptoms by 2 or 3 years of age. Lactose-intolerant children have varying symptoms depending on the specific activity of their intestinal lactase and the amount of lactose consumed. Galactose is preferentially converted to glycogen in the liver prior to conversion to glucose for subsequent oxidation. Infants with galactosemia, an inborn metabolic disease caused by deficient galactose-1-phosphate uridyltransferase, require a lactose-free diet starting in the neonatal period.

After the first 2 years of life, 50%–60% of energy requirements should be derived from carbohydrates, with no more than 10% from simple sugars. These dietary guidelines are, unfortunately, not reflected in the diets of North American children, who typically derive 25% of their energy intake from sucrose and less than 20% from complex carbohydrates.

Children and adolescents in North America consume large quantities of sucrose and high-fructose corn syrup in soft drinks and other sweetened beverages, candy, syrups, and sweetened breakfast cereals. A maximum intake of 10% of daily energy from sucrose has been recommended by the World Health Organization, but typical intakes have been reported to far exceed this recommended level. A high intake of these sugars, especially in the form of sweetened beverages, may predispose to obesity and insulin resistance, is a major risk factor for dental caries, and may be associated with an overall poorer quality diet, including high intake of saturated fat. Sucrase hydrolyzes sucrose to glucose and fructose in the brush border of the small intestine. Fructose absorption through facilitated diffusion occurs more slowly than glucose absorption through active transport. Fructose does not stimulate insulin secretion or enhance leptin production. Since both insulin and leptin play a role in regulation of food intake, consumption of fructose (eg, as high-fructose corn syrup) may contribute to increased energy intake and weight gain. Fructose is also easily converted to hepatic triglycerides, which may be undesirable in patients with insulin resistance/metabolic syndrome and cardiovascular disease risk.

Dietary fiber can be classified in two major types: nondigested carbohydrate (β1–4 linkages) and noncarbohydrate (lignin). Insoluble fibers (cellulose, hemicellulose, and lignin) increase stool bulk and water content and decrease gut transit time. Soluble fibers (pectins, mucilages, oat bran) bind bile acids and reduce lipid and cholesterol absorption. Pectins also slow gastric emptying and the rate of nutrient absorption. Few data regarding the fiber needs of children are available. The Dietary Reference Intakes recommend 14 g of fiber per 1000 kcal consumed. The American Academy of Pediatrics recommends that children older than 2 years consume in grams per day an amount of fiber equal to 5 plus the age in years. Fiber intakes are often low in North America. Children who have higher dietary fiber intakes have been found to consume more nutrient-dense diets than children with low-fiber intakes. In general, higher fiber diets are associated with lower risk of chronic diseases such as obesity, cardiovascular disease, and diabetes.

Brannon PM et al: Lactose intolerance and health. NIH Consens State Sci Statements 2010 Feb 24;27(2) [PMID: 20186234]. Available at: http://consensus.nih.gov.

Johnson L et al: Energy-dense, low-fiber, high-fat dietary pattern is associated with increased fatness in childhood. Am J Clin Nutr 2008 Apr;87(4):846–857 [PMID: 18400706].

Ruottinen S et al: High sucrose intake is associated with poor quality of diet and growth between 13 months and 9 years of age: The Special Turku Coronary Risk Factor Intervention Project. Pediatrics 2008;121:e1676–11685 [PMID: 18519471].

MAJOR MINERALS

Dietary sources, absorption, metabolism, and deficiency of the major minerals are summarized in Table 11–3. Recommended intakes are provided in Table 11–4.

TRACE ELEMENTS

Trace elements with a recognized role in human nutrition are iron, iodine, zinc, copper, selenium, manganese, molybdenum, chromium, cobalt (as a component of vitamin B_{12}), and fluoride. Information on food sources, functions, and deficiencies of the trace elements is summarized in Table 11–5. Supplemental fluoride recommendations are listed in Table 11–6. Dietary reference intakes of trace elements are summarized in Table 11–4. Iron deficiency is discussed in Chapter 30.

Brown KH et al: Dietary intervention strategies to enhance zinc nutrition: Promotion and support of breastfeeding for infants and young children. Food Nutr Bull 2009 Mar;30(Suppl 1):S144–S171 [PMID: 19472605].

VITAMINS

1. Fat-Soluble Vitamins

Because they are insoluble in water, the fat-soluble vitamins require digestion and absorption of dietary fat and a carrier system for transport in the blood. Deficiencies in these vitamins develop more slowly than deficiencies in water-soluble vitamins because the body accumulates stores of fat-soluble vitamins; but prematurity and some childhood conditions can place infants and children at risk (Table 11–7). Excessive intakes carry a considerable potential for toxicity (Table 11–8). A summary of reference intakes for select vitamins is found in Table 11–9. Dietary sources of the fat-soluble vitamins, absorption and metabolism, and deficiency and treatment information are summarized in Tables 11–10 and 11–11. Although the RDA for vitamin D has not been revised, recent recognition of low levels of 25-OH-vitamin D in a relatively large percentage of the population and the broad range of functions beyond calcium absorption have led many experts to recommend a daily intake of at least 400 IU (10 mcg)/d for all infants, including those who are breast-fed, beginning shortly after birth.

Boy E et al: Achievements, challenges, and promising new approaches in vitamin and mineral deficiency control. Nutr Rev 2009 May;67(Suppl 1):S24–S30 [PMID: 19453674].

Cesur Y et al: Evaluation of children with nutritional rickets. J PediatrEndocrinolMetab 2011;24(1-2):35–43 [PMID: 21528813].

Pludowski P et al: Vitamin d supplementation and status in infants: A prospective cohort observational study. J Pediatr Gastroenterol Nutr 2011 Jul;53(1):93–99 [PMID: 21694542].

Taylor CE, Camargo CA Jr: Impact of micronutrients on respiratory infections. Nutr Rev 2011 May;69(5):259–269 [PMID: 21521228].

IOM: Dietary reference intakes for calcium and vitamin D.

Washington, DC: The National Academies Press; 2011.

Wagner CL et al: Prevention of rickets and vitamin D deficiency in infants, children, and adolescents. Pediatrics 2008;122:1142 [PMID: 18977996].

2. Water-Soluble Vitamins

Deficiencies of water-soluble vitamins are generally uncommon in the United States because of the abundant food supply and fortification of prepared foods. Cases of deficiencies (eg, scurvy) in children with special needs have been reported in the context of sharply restricted diets. Most bread and wheat products are fortified with B vitamins, including the mandatory addition of folic acid to enriched grain products since January 1998. There is conclusive evidence that folic acid supplements (400 mcg/d) during the periconceptional period protect against neural tube defects. Dietary intakes of folic acid from natural foods and enriched products also are protective. Biological roles of water-soluble vitamins are listed in Table 11–12.

The risk of toxicity from water-soluble vitamins is not as great as that associated with fat-soluble vitamins because excesses are excreted in the urine. However, deficiencies of these vitamins develop more quickly than deficiencies in fat-soluble vitamins because of limited stores, with the exception of Vitamin B_{12}.

Major dietary sources of the water-soluble vitamins are listed in Table 11–13. Additional salient details are summarized in Tables 11–7, 11–14, and 11–15.

Table 11–3. Summary of major minerals.

Mineral	Absorption/Metabolism	Deficiency: Causes	Deficiency: Clinical Features
Calcium *Dietary sources*: dairy products, legumes, broccoli, green leafy vegetables.	20%–30% from diet; 60% from HM. Enhanced by lactose, glucose, protein; impaired by phytate, fiber, oxalate, unabsorbed fat. Absorption is regulated by serum calcitriol, which increases when PTH is secreted in response to low plasma-ionized calcium. PTH also promotes release of calcium from bone. Renal excretion.	Can occur in premature infants without adequate supplementation and in lactating adolescents with limited calcium intake or in patients with steatorrhea.	Osteopenia or osteoporosis, tetany.
Phosphorus *Dietary sources*: meats, eggs, dairy products, grains, legumes, and nuts; high in processed foods and sodas.	80% from diet. PTH decreases tubular resorption of phosphorus in kidneys; homeostasis is maintained by GI tract and kidneys.	Rare, but can occur in premature infants fed unfortified HM (results in osteoporosis and rickets, sometimes hypercalcemia). Also seen in patients with protein-energy malnutrition.	Muscle weakness, bone pain, rhabdomyolysis, osteomalacia, and respiratory insufficiency.
Magnesium *Dietary sources*: vegetables, cereals, nuts.	Kidneys regulate homeostasis by decreasing excretion when intake is low.	Occurs as part of refeeding syndrome with protein-energy malnutrition. Renal disease, malabsorption, or magnesium wasting medications may lead to depletion. May cause secondary hypocalcemia.	Neuromuscular excitability, muscle fasciculation, neurologic abnormalities, ECG changes.
Sodium *Dietary sources*: processed foods, table salt.	Hypo- and hypernatremic dehydration are discussed in Chapter 23. Kidneys are primary site of homeostatic regulation.	Results from excess losses associated with diarrhea and vomiting.	Anorexia, vomiting, hypotension, and mental apathy. Severe malnutrition, stress, and hypermetabolism may lead to excess intracellular sodium, affecting cellular metabolism.
Chloride *Dietary sources*: table salt or sea salt, seaweed, many vegetables.	Homeostasis is closely linked to sodium. Plays an important role in physiologic mechanisms of kidneys and gut.	Can occur in infants fed low chloride-containing diets, or in children with cystic fibrosis, vomiting, diarrhea, chronic diuretic therapy, or Bartter syndrome.	Associated with failure to thrive and especially poor head growth; anorexia, lethargy, muscle weakness, vomiting, dehydration, hypovolemia. *Laboratory findings*: may include hypochloremia, hypokalemia, metabolic alkalosis, hyperreninemia.
Potassium *Dietary sources*: nuts, whole grains, meats, fish, beans, fruits and vegetables, especially bananas, orange juice.	Kidneys control potassium homeostasis via the aldosteronerenin-angiotensin endocrine system. Amount of total body potassium depends on lean body mass.	Occurs in protein-energy malnutrition (eg, refeeding syndrome) and can cause cardiac failure and sudden death if not treated aggressively. With loss of lean body mass, excessive potassium is excreted in urine in any catabolic state. Can also occur during acidosis, from diarrhea, and from diuretic use. Hyperkalemia may result from renal insufficiency.	Muscle weakness, mental confusion, arrhythmias.

ECG, electrocardiogram; GI, gastrointestinal; HM, human milk; PTH, parathyroid hormone.

Table 11–4. Summary of dietary reference intakes for selected minerals and trace elements.

	0–6 mo	7–12 mo	1–3 y	4–8 y	9–13 y	14–18 y male	14–18 y female
Calcium (mg/d)	210[a]	270[a]	500[a]	800[a]	1300[a]	1300[a]	1300[a]
Phosphorus (mg/d)	100[a]	275[a]	460[a]	500	1250	1250	1250
Magnesium (mg/d)	30[a]	75[a]	80	130	240	410	360
Iron (mg/d)	0.27[a]	11	7	10	8	11	15
Zinc (mg/d)	2[a]	3	3	5	8	11	9
Copper (mcg/d)	200[a]	220[a]	340	440	700	890	890
Selenium (mcg/d)	15[a]	20[a]	20	30	40	55	55

[a]Adequate Intakes (AI). All other values represent the recommended Dietary Allowances (RDAs). Both the RDA and AI may be used as goals for individual intakes.

Carnitine is synthesized in the liver and kidneys from lysine and methionine. In certain circumstances (see Table 11–14), synthesis is inadequate, and carnitine can then be considered a vitamin. A dietary supply of other organic compounds, such as inositol, may also be required in certain circumstances.

INFANT FEEDING

BREAST FEEDING

Breast feeding provides optimal nutrition for the normal infant during the early months of life. The World Health Organization recommends exclusive breast feeding for approximately the first 6 months of life, with continued breast feeding along with appropriate complementary foods through the first 2 years of life. Numerous immunologic factors in breast milk (including secretory immunoglobulin A [IgA], lysozyme, lactoferrin, bifidus factor, and macrophages) provide protection against GI and upper respiratory infections.

In developing countries, lack of refrigeration and contaminated water supplies make formula feeding hazardous. Although formulas have improved progressively and are made to resemble breast milk as closely as possible, it is impossible to replicate the nutritional or immune composition of human milk. Additional differences of physiologic importance continue to be identified. Furthermore, the relationship developed through breast feeding can be an important part of early maternal interactions with the infant and provides a source of security and comfort to the infant.

Breast feeding has been reestablished as the predominant initial mode of feeding young infants in the United States. Unfortunately, breast-feeding rates remain low among several subpopulations, including low-income, minority, and young mothers. Many mothers face obstacles in maintaining lactation once they return to work, and rates of breast feeding at 6 months are considerably less than the goal of 50%. Skilled use of a breast pump, particularly an electric one, can help to maintain lactation in these circumstances.

Absolute contraindications to breast feeding are rare. They include tuberculosis (in the mother) and galactosemia (in the infant). Breast feeding is associated with maternal-to-child transmission of human immunodeficiency virus (HIV), but the risk is influenced by duration and pattern of breast-feeding and maternal factors, including immunologic status and presence of mastitis. Complete avoidance of breast feeding by HIV-infected women is presently the only mechanism to ensure prevention of maternal–infant transmission. Current recommendations are that HIV-infected mothers in developed countries refrain from breast feeding if safe alternatives are available. In developing countries, the benefits of breast feeding, especially the protection of the child against diarrheal illness and malnutrition, outweigh the risk of HIV infection via breast milk. In such circumstances, mixed feeding should be avoided because of the increased risk of HIV transmission with mixed feeds.

In newborns less than 1750 g, human milk should be fortified to increase protein, calcium, phosphorus, and micronutrient content as well as caloric density. Breast-fed infants with cystic fibrosis can be breast-fed successfully if exogenous pancreatic enzymes are provided. If normal growth rates are not achieved in breast-fed infants with cystic fibrosis, energy or specific macronutrient supplements may be necessary. All infants with cystic fibrosis should receive supplemental vitamins A, D, E, K, and sodium chloride.

Agostoni C et al: Breast-feeding: A commentary by the ESPGHAN Committee on nutrition. J Pediatr Gastroenterol Nutr 2009 Jul;49(1):112–125 [PMID: 19502997].

Table 11–5. Summary of trace elements.

Mineral	Deficiency		Treatment
	Causes	Clinical Features	
Zinc *Dietary sources*: human milk, meats, shellfish, legumes, nuts, and whole-grain cereals. *Functions*: component of many enzymes and gene transcription factors; plays critical roles in nucleic acid metabolism, protein synthesis, and gene expression; supports membrane structure and function.	Diets low in available zinc (high phytate), unfortified synthetic diets; malabsorptive diseases (enteritis, celiac disease, cystic fibrosis); excessive losses (chronic diarrhea); inborn errors of zinc metabolism (acrodermatitis enteropathica, mammary gland zinc secretion defect). Inadequate intake in breast-fed infants after age 6 mo. Prematurity and low birth weight are risk factors.	Mild: impaired growth, poor appetite, impaired immunity. Moderate–severe: mood changes, irritability, lethargy, impaired immune function, increased susceptibility to infection; acro-orificial skin rash, diarrhea, alopecia. Response to zinc supplement is gold standard for diagnosis of deficiency; plasma zinc levels are lowered by acute phase response.	1 mg/kg/d of elemental zinc for 3 mo (eg, 4.5 mg/kg/d of zinc sulfate salt), given separately from meals and iron supplements. With acrodermatitis enteropathica, 30–50 mg Zn^{2+} per day (or more) sustains remission.
Copper *Dietary sources*: human milk, meats, shellfish, legumes, nuts, and whole-grain cereals. *Functions*: vital component of several oxidative enzymes: cytochrome c oxidase (electron transport chain), cytosolic and mitochondrial superoxide dismutase (free radical defense), lysyl oxidase (cross-linking of elastin and collagen), ferroxidase (oxidation of ferrous storage iron prior to transport to bone marrow).	Generalized malnutrition, prolonged PN without supplemental copper, malabsorption, or prolonged diarrhea. Prematurity is a risk factor.	Osteoporosis, enlargement of costochondral cartilages, cupping and flaring of long bone metaphyses, spontaneous rib fractures. Neutropenia and hypochromic anemia resistant to iron therapy. Defect of copper metabolism (Menkes kinky hair syndrome) results in severe CNS disease. Low plasma levels help to confirm deficiency; levels are normally very low in young infants. Age-matched normal data are necessary for comparison. Plasma levels are raised by acute phase response.	1% copper sulfate solution (2 mg of salt) or 500 mcg/d elemental copper for infants.
Selenium *Dietary sources*: seafood, meats, garlic (geochemical distribution affects levels in foods). *Function*: essential component of glutathione peroxidase (reduction of hydrogen peroxide to water in the cell cytosol).	Inadequate dietary intake; can occur with selenium-deficient PN. Renal disease.	Skeletal muscle pain and tenderness, macrocytosis, loss of hair pigment. Keshan disease, an often fatal cardiomyopathy in infants and children.	Minimum recommended selenium content for full-term infant formulas is 1.5 mcg/100 kcal, and for preterm formulas, 1.8 mcg/100 kcal. PN should be supplemented.
Iodine *Dietary source*: iodized salt. *Functions*: essential component of thyroid hormones; regulates metabolism, growth, and neural development.	Inadequate dietary intake. Maternal iodine deficiency causes endemic neonatal hypothyroidism in 5%–16% of neonates who may have goiter at birth.	Neurologic endemic cretinism (severe mental retardation, deafmutism, spastic diplegia, and strabismus) occurs with severe deficiency. Myxedematous endemic cretinism occurs in some central African countries where signs of congenital hypothyroidism are present.	Use of iodized salt is effective in preventing goiter. Injections of iodized oil can also be used for prevention.
Fluoride *Function*: incorporated into the hydroxyapatite matrix of dentin.	Inadequate intake (unfluoridated water supply).	Low intake increases incidence of dental caries.	See Table 11–6 for supplementation guidelines. Excess fluoride intake results in fluorosis.

CNS, central nervous system; PN, parenteral nutrition.

Table 11–6. Supplemental fluoride recommendations (mg/d).

Age	Concentration of Fluoride in Drinking Water		
	< 0.3 ppm	0.3–0.6 ppm	> 0.6 ppm
6 mo–3 y	0.25	0	0
3–6 y	0.5	0.25	0
6–16 y	1	0.5	0

Reproduced, with permission, from Centers for Disease Control and Prevention: Recommendations for using fluoride to prevent and control dental caries in the United States. MMWR Morb Mortal Wkly Rep 2001;50(RR-14):8.

Buchanan AM, Cunningham CK: Advances and failures in preventing perinatal human immunodeficiency virus infection. Clin Microbiol Rev 2009 Jul;22(3):493–507 [PMID: 19597011].

Jansson LM: Academy of Breastfeeding Medicine Protocol Committee ABM clinical protocol #21: Guidelines for breastfeeding and the drug-dependent woman. Breastfeed Med 2009 Dec; 4(4):225–228 [PMID: 19835481].

Zachariassen G et al: Nutrient enrichment of mother's milk and growth of very preterm infants after hospital discharge. Pediatrics 2011 Apr;127(4):e995–e1003 [Epub 2011 Mar 14] [PMID: 21402642].

Table 11–7. Circumstances associated with risk of vitamin deficiencies.

Circumstance	Possible Deficiency
Prematurity	All vitamins
Protein-energy malnutrition	B_1, B_2, folate, A
Synthetic diets without adequate fortification (including total parenteral nutrition)	All vitamins
Vitamin-drug interactions	Folate, B_{12}, D, B_6
Fat malabsorption syndromes	Fat-soluble vitamins
Breast feeding	B_1,[a] folate,[b] B_{12},[c] D,[d] K[e]
Periconceptional	Folate
Bariatric surgery (all types)	B vitamins

[a]Alcoholic or malnourished mother.
[b]Folate-deficient mother.
[c]Vegan mother or maternal pernicious anemia.
[d]Infant not exposed to sunlight and mother's vitamin D status suboptimal.
[e]Maternal status poor; neonatal prophylaxis omitted.

Table 11–8. Effects of vitamin toxicity.

Pyridoxine
Sensory neuropathy at doses > 500 mg/d

Niacin
Histamine release → cutaneous vasodilation; cardiac arrhythmias; cholestatic jaundice; gastrointestinal disturbance; hyperuricemia; glucose intolerance

Folic acid
May mask B_{12} deficiency, hypersensitivity

Vitamin C
Diarrhea; increased oxalic acid excretion; renal stones

Vitamin A
(> 20,000 IU/d): Vomiting, increased intracranial pressure (pseudotumor cerebri); irritability; headaches; insomnia; emotional lability; dry, desquamating skin; myalgia and arthralgia; abdominal pain; hepatosplenomegaly; cortical thickening of bones of hands and feet

Vitamin D
(> 50,000 IU/d): Hypercalcemia; vomiting; constipation; nephrocalcinosis

Vitamin E
(> 25–100 mg/kg/d intravenously): Necrotizing enterocolitis and liver toxicity (but probably due to polysorbate 80 used as a solubilizer)

Vitamin K
Lipid-soluble vitamin K: Very low order of toxicity
Water-soluble, synthetic vitamin K: Vomiting; porphyrinuria; albuminuria; hemolytic anemia; hemoglobinuria; hyperbilirubinemia (do not give to neonates)

Support of Breast Feeding

In developed countries, health professionals are now playing roles of greater importance in supporting and promoting breast feeding. Organizations such as the American Academy of Pediatrics and La Leche League have initiated programs to promote breast feeding and provide education for health professionals and mothers.

Perinatal hospital routines and early pediatric care have a great influence on the successful initiation of breast feeding by promoting prenatal and postpartum education, frequent mother-baby contact after delivery, one-on-one advice about breast-feeding technique, demand feeding, rooming-in, avoidance of bottle supplements, early follow-up after delivery, maternal confidence, family support, adequate maternity leave, and advice about common problems such as sore nipples. A 2011 CDC Morbidity and Mortality Report found that most U.S. hospitals do not have policies that optimally support breast feeding. Medical providers can modify their own practice patterns and advocate for hospital policies that support breast feeding.

Very few women are unable to nurse their babies. The newborn is generally fed ad libitum every 2–3 hours, with longer intervals (4–5 hours) at night. Thus, a newborn infant nurses at least 8–10 times a day, so that a generous milk

Table 11–9. Summary of dietary reference intakes for select vitamins.

	0–6 mo	7–12 mo	1–3 y	4–8 y	9–13 y	14–18 y male	14–18 y female
Thiamin (mg/d)	0.2[a]	0.3[a]	0.5	0.6	0.9	1.2	1.0
Riboflavin (mg/d)	0.3[a]	0.4[a]	0.5[a]	0.6[a]	0.9[a]	1.3[a]	1.0[a]
Pyridoxine (mg/d)	0.1[a]	0.3[a]	0.5	0.6	1.0	1.3	1.2
Niacin (mg/d)	2[a]	4[a]	6	8	12	16	14
Pantothenic acid (mg/d)	1.7[a]	1.8[a]	2[a]	3[a]	4[a]	5[a]	5[a]
Biotin (mcg/d)	5[a]	6[a]	8[a]	12[a]	20[a]	25[a]	25[a]
Folic acid (mcg/d)	65[a]	80[a]	150	200	300	400	400
Cobalamin (mcg/d)	0.4[a]	0.5[a]	0.9	1.2	1.8	2.4	2.4
Vitamin C (mg/d)	40[a]	50[a]	15	25	45	75	65
Vitamin A (mcg/d)	400[a]	500[a]	300	400	600	900	700
Vitamin D (IU/d)	200[ab]	200[ab]	200[ab]	200[ab]	200[ab]	200[ab]	200[ab]
Vitamin E (mg/d)	4[a]	5[a]	6	7	11	15	15
Vitamin K (mcg/d)	2[a]	2.5[a]	30[a]	55[a]	60[a]	75[a]	75[a]

[a]Adequate Intakes (AI). All other values represent the Recommended Dietary Allowances (RDAs). Both the RDA and AI may be used as goals for individual intakes.
[b]American Academy of Pediatrics in 2008 recommended 400 IU/d vitamin D for infants, children, and adolescents.
Data from National Academy of Sciences, Food and Nutritional Board, Institute of Medicine: *Dietary Reference Intakes, Applications in Dietary Assessment*. National Academy Press, 2000:287. Available online at: http://www.nap.edu

supply is stimulated. This frequency is not an indication of inadequate lactation. In neonates, a loose stool is often passed with each feeding; later (at age 3–4 months), there may be an interval of several days between stools. Failure to pass several stools a day in the early weeks of breast feeding suggests inadequate milk intake and supply.

Expressing milk may be indicated if the mother returns to work or if the infant is premature, cannot suck adequately, or is hospitalized. Electric breast pumps are very effective and can be borrowed or rented.

Technique of Breast Feeding

Breast feeding can be started after delivery as soon as both mother and baby are stable. Correct positioning and breast-feeding technique are necessary to ensure effective nipple stimulation and optimal breast emptying with minimal nipple discomfort.

If the mother wishes to nurse while sitting, the infant should be elevated to the height of the breast and turned completely to face the mother, so that their abdomens touch. The mother's arms supporting the infant should be held tightly at her side, bringing the baby's head in line with her breast. The breast should be supported by the lower fingers of her free hand, with the nipple compressed between the thumb and index fingers to make it more protractile. The infant's initial licking and mouthing of the nipple helps make it more erect. When the infant opens its mouth, the mother should rapidly insert as much nipple and areola as possible.

The most common early cause of poor weight gain in breast-fed infants is poorly managed mammary engorgement, which rapidly decreases milk supply. Unrelieved engorgement can result from inappropriately long intervals between feeding, improper infant suckling, a nondemanding infant, sore nipples, maternal or infant illness, nursing from only one breast, and latching difficulties. Poor maternal feeding technique, inappropriate feeding routines, and inadequate amounts of fluid and rest all can be factors. Some infants are too sleepy to do well on an ad libitum regimen and may need waking to feed at night. Primary lactation failure occurs in less than 5% of women.

A sensible guideline for duration of feeding is 5 minutes per breast at each feeding the first day, 10 minutes on each side at each feeding the second day, and 10–15 minutes per side thereafter. A vigorous infant can obtain most of the available milk in 5–7 minutes, but additional sucking time ensures breast emptying, promotes milk production, and satisfies the infant's sucking urge. The side on which feeding

Table 11–10. Summary of fat-soluble vitamins.

Vitamin	Absorption/Metabolism	Deficiency: Causes	Deficiency: Clinical Features
Vitamin A *Dietary sources*: dairy products, eggs, liver, meats, fish oils. Precursor β-carotene is abundant in yellow and green vegetables. *Functions*: has critical role in vision, helping to form photosensitive pigment rhodopsin; modifies differentiation and proliferation of epithelial cells in respiratory tract; and is needed for glycoprotein synthesis.	Retinol is stored in liver and from there is exported, attached to RBP and prealbumin. RBP may be decreased in liver disease or in protein energy malnutrition. Circulating RBP may be increased in renal failure.	Occurs in premature infants, in association with inadequately supplemented PN; protein-energy malnutrition (deficiency worsened by measles); dietary insufficiency and fat malabsorption.	Night blindness, xerosis, xerophthalmia, Bitot spots, keratomalacia, ulceration and perforation of cornea, prolapse of lens and iris, and blindness; follicular hyperkeratosis; pruritus; growth retardation; increased susceptibility to infection.
Vitamin K *Dietary sources*: leafy vegetables, fruits, seeds; synthesized by intestinal bacteria. *Functions*: necessary for the maintenance of normal plasma levels of coagulation factors II, VII, IX, and X; essential for maintenance of normal levels of the anticoagulation protein C; essential for osteoblastic activity.	Absorbed in proximal small intestine in micelles with bile salts; circulates with VLDL.	Occurs in newborns, especially those who are breast-fed and who have not received vitamin K prophylaxis at delivery; in fat malabsorption syndromes; and with use of unabsorbed antibiotics and anticoagulant drugs (warfarin).	Bruising or bleeding in GI tract, genitourinary tract, gingiva, lungs, joints, and brain.
Vitamin E *Dietary sources*: vegetable oils, some cereals, dairy, wheat germ, eggs. *Functions*: α-tocopherol has highest biologic activity; as a free-radical scavenger, stops oxidation reactions. Located at specific sites in cell membrane to protect polyunsaturated fatty acids in membrane from peroxidation and to protect thiol groups and nucleic acids; also acts as cell membrane stabilizer; may function in electron transport chain; may modulate chromosomal expression.	Emulsified in intestinal lumen with bile salts; absorbed via passive diffusion; transported by chylomicrons and VLDL.	May occur with prematurity, cholestatic liver disease, pancreatic insufficiency, abetalipoproteinemia, and short bowel syndrome. Isolated inborn error of vitamin E metabolism. May result from increased consumption during oxidant stress.	Hemolytic anemia; progressive neurologic disorder with loss of deep tendon reflexes, loss of coordination, vibratory and position sensation, nystagmus, weakness, scoliosis, and retinal degeneration.
Vitamin D *Dietary sources*: fortified milk and formulas, egg yolk, fatty fish. *Functions*: calcitriol, the biologically active form of vitamin D, stimulates intestinal absorption of calcium and phosphate, renal reabsorption of filtered calcium, and mobilization of calcium and phosphorus from bone.	Normally obtained primarily from cholecalciferol (D_3) produced by UV radiation of dehydrocholesterol in skin. Ergocalciferol (D_2) is derived from UV irradiation of ergosterol in skin. Vitamin D is transported from skin to liver, attached to a specific carrier protein.	Results from a combination of inadequate sunlight exposure, dark skin pigmentation, and low dietary intake. Breast-fed infants are at risk because of low vitamin D content of human milk. Cow's milk and infant formulas are routinely supplemented with vitamin D. Deficiency also occurs in fat malabsorption syndromes. Hydroxylated vitamin D may be decreased by CYP-450–stimulating drugs, hepatic or renal disease, and inborn errors of metabolism.	Osteomalacia (adults) or rickets (children), in which osteoid with reduced calcification accumulates in bone. *Clinical findings*: craniotabes, rachitic rosary, pigeon breast, bowed legs, delayed eruption of teeth and enamel defects, Harrison groove, scoliosis, kyphosis, dwarfism, painful bones, fractures, anorexia, and weakness. *Radiographic findings*: cupping, fraying, flaring of metaphyses.

CYP, cytochrome P; GI, gastrointestinal; PN, parenteral nutrition; PTH, parathyroid hormone; RBP, retinol-binding protein; UV, ultraviolet; VLDL, very low-density lipoproteins.

Table 11–11. Evaluation and treatment of deficiencies of fat-soluble vitamins.

Vitamin Deficiency	Diagnostic Laboratory Findings and Treatment
Vitamin A	*Laboratory findings*: serum retinol < 20 mcg/dL; molar ratio of retinol:RBP < 0.7 is also diagnostic. *Treatment*: xerophthalmia requires 5000–10,000 IU/kg/d for 5 d PO or IM; with fat malabsorption, standard dose is 2500–5000 IU. Toxicity effects are listed in Table 11–8.
Vitamin K	*Laboratory findings*: assess plasma levels of PIVKA or PT. *Treatment*: Oral: 2.5–5.0 mg/d or IM/IV: 1–2 mg/dose as single dose.
Vitamin E	*Laboratory findings*: normal serum level is 3–15 mg/mL for children. Ratio of serum vitamin E to total serum lipid is normally ≥ 0.8 mg/g. *Treatment*: large oral doses (up to 100 IU/kg/d) correct deficiency from malabsorption; for abetalipoproteinemia, 100–200 IU/kg/d are needed.
Vitamin D	*Laboratory findings*: low serum phosphorus and calcium, high alkaline phosphatase, high serum PTH, low 25-OH-cholecalciferol. American Academy of Pediatrics recommends supplementation, as follows: 400 IU/d for all breast-fed infants, beginning in first 2 months of life and continuing until infant is receiving ≥ 500 mL/d of vitamin D-fortified formula or cow's milk. *Treatment*: 1600–5000 IU/d of vitamin D_3 for rickets. If poorly absorbed, give 0.05–0.2 mcg/kg/d of calcitriol.

IM, intramuscular; IV, intravenous; PIVKA, protein-induced vitamin K absence; PO, by mouth; PT, prothrombin time; PTH, parathyroid hormone; RBP, retinol-binding protein.

Table 11–12. Summary of biologic roles of water-soluble vitamins.

B vitamins involved in production of energy

Thiamin (B_1)
- Thiamin pyrophosphate is a coenzyme in oxidative decarboxylation (pyruvate dehydrogenase, α-ketoglutarate dehydrogenase, and transketolase).

Riboflavin (B_2)
- Coenzyme of several flavoproteins (eg, flavin mononucleotide [FMN] and flavin adenine dinucleotide [FAD]) involved in oxidative/electron transfer enzyme systems.

Niacin
- Hydrogen-carrying coenzymes: nicotinamide-adenine dinucleotide (NAD), nicotinamide-adenine dinucleotide phosphate (NADP); decisive role in intermediary metabolism.

Pantothenic acid
- Major component of coenzyme A.

Biotin
- Component of several carboxylase enzymes involved in fat and carbohydrate metabolism.

Hematopoietic B vitamins

Folic acid
- Tetrahydrofolate has essential role in one-carbon transfers. Essential role in purine and pyramidine synthesis; deficiency → arrest of cell division (especially bone marrow and intestine).

Cobalamin (B_{12})
- Methyl cobalamin (cytoplasm): synthesis of methionine with simultaneous synthesis of tetrahydrofolate (reason for megaloblastic anemia in B_{12} deficiency). Adenosyl cobalamin (mitochondria) is coenzyme for mutases and dehydratases.

Other B vitamins

Pyridoxine (B_6)
- Prosthetic group of transaminases, etc, involved in amino acid interconversions; prostaglandin and heme synthesis; central nervous system function; carbohydrate metabolism; immune development.

Other water-soluble vitamins

l-Ascorbic acid (C)
- Strong reducing agent—probably involved in all hydroxylations. Roles include collagen synthesis; phenylalanine → tyrosine; tryptophan → 5-hydroxytryptophan; dopamine → norepinephrine; Fe^{3+}; folic acid → folinic acid; cholesterol → bile acids; leukocyte function; interferon production; carnitine synthesis. Copper metabolism; reduces oxidized vitamin E.

is commenced should be alternated. The mother may break suction gently after nursing by inserting her finger between the baby's gums.

Follow-Up

Individualized assessment before discharge should identify mothers and infants needing additional support. All mother–infant pairs require early follow-up. The onset of copious milk secretion between the second and fourth postpartum days is a critical time in the establishment of lactation. Failure to empty the breasts during this time can cause engorgement, which quickly leads to diminished milk production.

Common Problems

Nipple tenderness requires attention to proper positioning of the infant and correct latch-on. Ancillary measures include nursing for shorter periods, beginning feedings on the less sore side, air drying the nipples well after nursing, and use of lanolin cream. Severe nipple pain and cracking usually indicate improper infant attachment. Temporary pumping may be needed.

Breast-feeding jaundice is exaggerated physiologic jaundice associated with inadequate intake of breast milk, infrequent stooling, and unsatisfactory weight gain. (See Chapter 2.) If possible, the jaundice should be managed by increasing the frequency of nursing and, if necessary, augmenting the infant's sucking with regular breast pumping. Supplemental

Table 11–13. Major dietary sources of water-soluble vitamins.

Thiamin (B_1)	Whole and enriched grains, lean pork, legumes
Riboflavin (B_2)	Dairy products, meat, poultry, wheat germ, leafy vegetables
Niacin (B_3)	Meats, poultry, fish, legumes, wheat, all foods except fats; synthesized in body from tryptophan
Pyridoxine (B_6)	Animal products, vegetables, whole grains
Pantothenic acid	Ubiquitous
Biotin	Yeast, liver, kidneys, legumes, nuts, egg yolks (synthesized by intestinal bacteria)
Folic acid	Leafy vegetables (easily destroyed in cooking), fruits, whole grains, wheat germ, beans, nuts
Cobalamin (B_{12})	Eggs, dairy products, liver, meats; *none in plants*
Vitamin C	Fruits and vegetables
Carnitine	Meats, dairy products; *none in plants*

Table 11–14. Causes of deficiencies in water-soluble vitamins.

Thiamin	Beriberi: in infants breast-fed by mothers with history of alcoholism or poor diet; has been described as complication of parenteral nutrition (PN); protein-energy malnutrition; following bariatric surgery of all types—reported in adults and adolescents
Riboflavin	General undernutrition; inactivation in TPN solutions exposed to light
Niacin	Maize- or millet-based diets (high-leucine and low-tryptophan intakes); carcinoid tumors
Pyridoxine	Prematurity (these infants may not convert pyridoxine to pyridoxal-5-P); B6 dependency syndromes; drugs (isoniazid)
Biotin	Suppressed intestinal flora and impaired intestinal absorption; regular intake of raw egg whites
Folic acid	Breast-fed infants whose mothers are folate-deficient; term infants fed unsupplemented processed cow's milk or goat's milk; kwashiorkor; chronic overcooking of food sources; malabsorption of folate because of a congenital defect; celiac disease; drugs (phenytoin)
	Increased requirements: chronic hemolytic anemias, diarrhea, malignancies, extensive skin disease, cirrhosis, pregnancy
Cobalamin (B_{12})	Breast-fed infants of mothers with latent pernicious anemia or who are on an unsupplemented vegan diet; absence of luminal proteases; short gut syndrome (absence of stomach or ileum); congenital malabsorption of B_{12}
Vitamin C	Maternal megadoses during pregnancy → deficiency in infants (rebound); diet without fruits or vegetables; seen in infants fed formula based on pasteurized cow's milk (historical)
Carnitine	Premature infants fed unsupplemented formula or fed intravenously; dialysis; inherited deficits in carnitine synthesis; organic acidemias; infants receiving valproic acid

feedings may be necessary, but care should be taken not to decrease breast milk production further.

In a small percentage of breast-fed infants, breast milk jaundice is caused by an unidentified property of the milk that inhibits conjugation of bilirubin. In severe cases, interruption of breast feeding for 24–36 hours may be necessary. The mother's breast should be emptied with an electric breast pump during this period.

The symptoms of mastitis include flulike symptoms with breast tenderness, firmness, and erythema. Antibiotic therapy covering β-lactamase–producing organisms should be given for 10 days. Analgesics may be necessary, but breast feeding should be continued. Breast pumping may be helpful adjunctive therapy.

Centers for Disease Control and Prevention (CDC): HIV-2 Infection Surveillance—United States, 1987–2009. MMWR Morb Mortal Wkly Rep 2011 Aug 5 30;60:1009-1044 [PMID: 21796096].

http://www.cdc.gov/vitalsigns/Breastfeeding/index.html

Keister D et al: Strategies for breastfeeding success. Am Fam Physician 2008 Jul 15;78(2):225–232 [PMID: 18697506].

Maternal Drug Use

Factors playing a role in the transmission of drugs in breast milk include the route of administration, dosage, molecular weight, pH, and protein binding. Generally, any drug prescribed to a newborn can be consumed by the breast-feeding mother without ill effect. Very few drugs are absolutely contraindicated in breast-feeding mothers; these include radioactive compounds, antimetabolites, lithium, diazepam, chloramphenicol, antithyroid drugs, and tetracycline. For up-to-date information, a regional drug center should be consulted.

Maternal use of illicit or recreational drugs is a contraindication to breast feeding. Expression of milk for a feeding or two after use of a drug is not an acceptable compromise. The breast-fed infants of mothers taking methadone (but not alcohol or other drugs) as part of a treatment program have generally not experienced ill effects when the daily maternal methadone dose is less than 40 mg.

Table 11–15. Clinical features of deficiencies in water-soluble vitamins.

Thiamin (B_1)	
	"Dry" Beriberi (paralytic or nervous): peripheral neuropathy, with impairment of sensory, motor, and reflex functions
	"Wet" Beriberi: high output congestive heart failure ± signs of dry beriberi
	Cerebral Beriberi: ophthalmoplegia, ataxia, mental confusion, memory loss
Riboflavin	
	Cheilosis; angular stomatitis; glossitis; soreness and burning of lips and mouth; dermatitis of nasolabial fold and genitals; ± ocular signs (photophobia → indistinct vision)
Niacin	
	Pellagra (dermatitis, especially on sun-exposed areas; diarrhea; dementia)
Pyridoxine (B_6)	
	Listlessness; irritability; seizures; anemia; cheilosis; glossitis
Biotin	
	Scaly dermatitis; alopecia; irritability; lethargy
Folic acid	
	Megaloblastic anemia; neutropenia; growth retardation; delayed maturation of central nervous system in infants; diarrhea (mucosal ulcerations); glossitis; neural tube defects
Cobalamin (B_{12})	
	Megaloblastic anemia; hypersegmented neutrophils; neurologic degeneration: paresthesias, gait problems, depression
Ascorbic acid (C)	
	Irritability, apathy, pallor; increased susceptibility to infections; hemorrhages under skin, petechiae in mucous membranes, in joints and under periosteum; long-bone tenderness; costochondral beading
Carnitine	
	Increased serum triglycerides and free fatty acids; decreased ketones; fatty liver; hypoglycemia; progressive muscle weakness, cardiomyopathy, hypoglycemia

Case Western Reserve University. Available at: http://www.breastfeedingbasics.org

United States National Library of Medicine Drugs and Lactation Database (Lactmed). Available at: http://toxnet.nlm.nih.gov/cgi-bin/sis/htmlgen?LACT

Nutrient Composition

The nutrient composition of human milk is summarized and compared with that of cow's milk and formulas in Table 11–16. Outstanding characteristics include (1) relatively low but highly bioavailable protein content, which is adequate for the normal infant; (2) generous but not excessive quantity of essential fatty acids; (3) long-chain polyunsaturated fatty acids, of which DHA is thought to be especially important; (4) relatively low sodium and solute load; and (5) lower concentration of highly bioavailable minerals, which are adequate for the needs of normal breast-fed infants for approximately 6 months.

Complementary Feeding

The American Academy of Pediatrics and the World Health Organization recommend the introduction of solid foods in normal infants at about 6 months of age. Gradual introduction of a variety of foods including fortified cereals, fruits, vegetables, and meats should complement the breast milk diet. Meats provide an important dietary source of iron and zinc, both of which are low in human milk by 6 months, and pureed meats may be introduced as an early complementary food. Single-ingredient complementary foods are introduced one at a time at 3–4 day intervals before a new food is given. Fruit juice is not an essential part of an infant diet. Juice should not be introduced until after 6 months; should only be offered in a cup; and the amount should be limited to 4 oz/d. Delaying the introduction of complementary foods beyond 6 months has not been shown to prevent atopic disease. Breast feeding should ideally continue for at least 12 months, and thereafter for as long as mutually desired. Whole cow's milk can be introduced after the first year of life.

Krebs NF et al: Complementary feeding: A Global Network cluster randomized controlled trial. BMC Pediatr 2011 Jan 13;11:4. [Epub 2011 Jan 13] [PMID: 21232139].

SPECIAL DIETARY PRODUCTS FOR INFANTS

Soy Protein Formulas

Historically, a common rationale for the use of soy protein formulas was the transient lactose intolerance after acute gastroenteritis. Lactose-free cow's milk protein-based formulas are also now available. These formulas are also useful for infants with galactosemia and with hereditary lactase deficiency, and they provide an option when a vegetarian diet is preferred. Soy protein formulas are often used in cases of suspected intolerance to cow's milk protein. Although infants with true cow's milk protein intolerance may also be intolerant of soy protein, those with documented IgE-mediated allergy to cow's milk protein usually do well on soy formula.

Semi-Elemental & Elemental Formulas

Semi-elemental formulas include protein hydrolysate formulas. The major nitrogen source of most of these products is casein hydrolysate, supplemented with selected amino acids, but partial hydrolysates of whey are also available. These formulas contain an abundance of EFA from vegetable oil; certain brands also provide substantial amounts of MCTs. Elemental formulas are available with free amino acids and varying levels and types of fat components.

Semi-elemental and elemental formulas are invaluable for infants with a wide variety of malabsorption syndromes. They are also effective in infants who cannot tolerate cow's

Table 11–16. Composition of human and cow's milk and typical infant formula (per 100 kcal).

Nutrient (unit)	Minimal Level Recommended[a]	Mature Human Milk	Typical Commercial Formula	Cow's Milk (mean)
Protein (g)	1.8[b]	1.3–1.6	2.3	5.1
Fat (g)	3.3[c]	5	5.3	5.7
Carbohydrate (g)	—	10.3	10.8	7.3
Linoleic acid (mg)	300	560	2300	125
Vitamin A (IU)	250	250	300	216
Vitamin D (IU)	40	3	63	3
Vitamin E (IU)	0.7/g linoleic acid	0.3	2	0.1
Vitamin K (mcg)	4	2	9	5
Vitamin C (mg)	8	7.8	8.1	2.3
Thiamin (mcg)	40	25	80	59
Riboflavin (mcg)	60	60	100	252
Niacin (mcg)	250	250	1200	131
Vitamin B_6 (mcg)	15 mcg of protein	15	63	66
Folic acid (mcg)	4	4	10	8
Pantothenic acid (mcg)	300	300	450	489
Vitamin B_{12} (mcg)	0.15	0.15	0.25	0.56
Biotin (mcg)	1.5	1	2.5	3.1
Inositol (mg)	4	20	5.5	20
Choline (mg)	7	13	10	23
Calcium (mg)	5	50	75	186
Phosphorus (mg)	25	25	65	145
Magnesium (mg)	6	6	8	20
Iron (mg)	1	0.1	1.5	0.08
Iodine (mcg)	5	4–9	10	7
Copper (mcg)	60	25–60	80	20
Zinc (mg)	0.5	0.1–0.5	0.65	0.6
Manganese (mcg)	5	1.5	5–160	3
Sodium (mEq)	0.9	1	1.7	3.3
Potassium (mEq)	2.1	2.1	2.7	6
Chloride (mEq)	1.6	1.6	2.3	4.6
Osmolarity (mOsm)	—	11.3	16–18.4	40

[a]Committee on Nutrition, American Academy of Pediatrics.
[b]Protein of nutritional quality equal to casein.
[c]Includes 300 mg of essential fatty acids.

milk and soy protein. Controlled trials suggest that for infants with a family history of atopic disease, partial hydrolysate formulas may delay or prevent atopic disease. For specific product information, consult standard pediatric reference texts, formula manufacturers, or a pediatric dietitian.

Bhatia J et al: Use of soy protein-based formulas in infant feeding. Pediatrics 2008;121:1062 [PMID: 18450914].

Greer FR et al: Effects of early nutritional interventions on the development of atopic disease in infants and children: The role of maternal dietary restriction, breastfeeding, timing of complementary foods, and hydrolyzed formulas. Pediatrics 2008;121:183 [PMID: 18166574].

Formula Additives

Occasionally it may be necessary to increase the caloric density of an infant feeding to provide more calories or restrict fluid intake. Concentrating formula to 24–26 kcal/oz is usually well tolerated, delivers an acceptable renal solute load, and increases the density of all the nutrients. Beyond this, individual macronutrient additives (Table 11–17) are usually employed to achieve the desired caloric density (up to 30 kcal/oz) based on the infant's needs and underlying condition(s). A pediatric nutrition specialist can be helpful in formulating calorically dense infant formula feedings. The caloric density of breast milk can be increased by adding infant formula powder or any of the additives used with infant formula. Human milk fortifiers are generally used only for premature infants because of their specialized nutrient composition.

Special Formulas

Special formulas are those in which one component, often an amino acid, is reduced in concentration or removed for the dietary management of a specific inborn metabolic disease. Also included under this heading are formulas designed for the management of specific disease states, such as hepatic failure, pulmonary failure with chronic carbon dioxide retention, and renal failure. These condition-specific formulas were formulated primarily for critically ill adults and are even used sparingly in those populations; thus, their use in pediatrics should only be undertaken with clear indication and caution.

Complete information regarding the composition of these special formulas, the standard infant formulas, specific metabolic disease formulas, and premature infant formulas can be found in standard reference texts and in the manufacturers' literature.

NUTRITION FOR THE OLDER CHILD

Because of the association of diet with the development of such chronic diseases as diabetes, obesity, and cardiovascular disease, learning a healthy eating behavior at a young age is an important preventative measure.

Salient features of the diet for children older than 2 years include the following:

1. Consumption of three regular meals per day, and two or three healthful snacks according to appetite, activity, and growth needs.
2. Inclusion of a variety of foods. Diet should be nutritionally complete and promote optimal growth and activity.
3. Fat less than 35% of total calories (severe fat restriction may result in an energy deficit and growth failure). Saturated fats should provide less than 10% of total calories. Monounsaturated fats should provide 10% or more of caloric intake. Trans-fatty acids, found in stick margarine and shortening, and in many processed foods, should provide less than 1% of total calories.
4. Cholesterol intake less than 100 mg/1000 kcal/d, to a maximum of 300 mg/d.

Table 11–17. Common infant formula additives.

Additive	Kcal/g	Kcal/Tbsp	Kcal/mL	Comments
Dry rice cereal	3.75	15	—	Thickens formula but not breast milk
Polycose (Abbott Nutrition)	3.8	23	2	Glucose polymers
MCT oil (Mead Johnson)	8.3	116	7.7	Not a source of essential fatty acids
Microlipid (Mead Johnson)	9	68.5	4.5	Safflower oil emulsion with 0.4 g linoleic acid/mL
Vegetable oil	9	124	8.3	Does not mix well
Beneprotein (Nestle)	3.6	16.7 (4 g protein)	—	Whey protein
Duocal (SHS)	4.9	42	—	Protein-free mix of hydrolyzed corn starch (60% kcal) and fat (35% MCT)

MCT, medium-chain triglyceride.

5. Carbohydrates should provide 45%–65% of daily caloric intake, with no more than 10% in the form of simple sugars. A high-fiber, whole-grain-based diet is recommended.
6. Limitation of grazing behavior, eating while watching television, and the consumption of soft drinks and other sweetened beverages.
7. Limitation of sodium intake by choosing fresh over-processed foods and limiting added salt.
8. Consumption of lean cuts of meats, poultry, and fish should be encouraged. Skim or low-fat milk, and vegetable oils (especially canola or olive oil) should be used. Whole-grain bread and cereals and plentiful amounts of fruits and vegetables are recommended. The consumption of processed foods, juice drinks, soft drinks, desserts, and candy should be limited. The American Academy of Pediatrics has endorsed use of low-fat milk in children after 12 months of age.

Lifestyle counseling for children should also include maintenance of a desirable BMI; regular physical activity, limiting sedentary behaviors; avoidance of smoking; and screening for hypertension. The optimal target populations for cholesterol screening in childhood are somewhat controversial. Current recommendations are to routinely screen those children who have diabetes, smoke, are overweight or obese, or have a positive family history of premature cardiovascular disease. If the result of random total cholesterol is high (≥ 200 mg/dL), a fasting lipoprotein analysis should be obtained.

Daniels SR et al: Lipid screening and cardiovascular health in childhood. Pediatrics 2008;122:198–208 [PMID: 18596007].

Lee JM et al: Poor performance of body mass index as a marker for hypercholesterolemia in children and adolescents. Arch Pediatr Adolesc Med 2009;163:716 [PMID: 19652103].

Szymlek-Gay EA et al: Food-based strategies improve iron status in toddlers: A randomized controlled trial 12. Am J Clin Nutr 2009 Dec;90(6):1541–1551 [Epub 2009 Oct 14] [PMID: 19828711].

Wu TC, Chen PH: Health consequences of nutrition in childhood and early infancy. Pediatr Neonatol 2009 Aug;50(4):135–142 [PMID: 19750886].

PEDIATRIC UNDERNUTRITION

ESSENTIALS OF DIAGNOSIS & TYPICAL FEATURES

- Poor weight gain or weight loss.
- Loss of subcutaneous fat, temporal wasting.
- Most commonly related to inadequate caloric intake.
- Often associated in toddlers with marginal or low iron and zinc status.

General Considerations

Pediatric undernutrition is usually multifactorial in origin, and successful treatment depends on accurate identification and management of those factors. The terms "organic" and "nonorganic" failure to thrive, though still used by many medical professionals, are not helpful because any systemic illness or chronic condition can cause growth impairment and yet may also be compounded by psychosocial problems.

Clinical Findings

A. Definitions

Failure to thrive is a term used to describe growth faltering in infants and young children whose weight curve has fallen by two major percentile channels from a previously established rate of growth, or whose weight for length decreases below the 5th percentile. (See Chapter 9.) The World Health Organization growth charts (http://www.who.int/childgrowth/en/) should be used to evaluate the growth of breast-fed infants, as these charts reflect the slower velocity of weight gain for healthy breast-fed infants without formula supplementation. Differences in weight gain are particularly notable after 6 months of age, and a lower weight for age on the Centers for Disease Control growth references should not necessarily be interpreted to reflect undernutrition. The acute loss of weight, or failure to gain weight at the expected rate, produces a condition of reduced weight for height known as *wasting*. The reduction in height for age, as is seen with more chronic malnutrition, is termed *stunting*.

The typical pattern for mild pediatric undernutrition is decreased weight, with normal height and head circumference. In more chronic malnutrition, linear growth will slow relative to the standard for age, although this should also prompt consideration of nonnutritional etiologies. Significant calorie deprivation produces severe wasting, called *marasmus*. Significant protein deprivation in the face of adequate energy intake, possibly with additional insults such as infection, may produce edematous malnutrition called *kwashiorkor*.

B. Risk Factors

A discussion of the multiple medical conditions that can cause pediatric undernutrition is beyond the scope of this chapter. However, the most common cause is inadequate dietary intake. In young but otherwise healthy breast- or bottle-fed infants, a weak or uncoordinated suck may be the causative factor; evaluation for congenital heart disease, breathing problems (eg, laryngomalacia), and other physical problems that may interfere with normal feeding. Inappropriate formula mixing or a family's dietary beliefs may lead to hypocaloric or unbalanced dietary intakes. Diets restricted because of suspected food allergies or intolerances may result in inadequate intake of calories, protein, or specific micronutrients. Iron and zinc are micronutrients that are marginal in many older infants and young children with undernutrition. Deficiencies occur in older breast-fed infants whose diets are low in meats, and in toddlers who are not on any fortified formula and also do not consume good dietary sources. Cases of severe malnutrition and kwashiorkor have occurred in infants of well-intentioned parents who substitute "health food" milk alternatives (eg, rice milk or unfortified soy milk) for infant formula.

C. Assessment

1. Measurement of weight for age; length/height for age; occipital frontal circumference (OFC) for age (for < 2 years age), weight for length; and calculation of percent ideal body weight (current weight/median [50th percentile] weight for current length). Assess for downward crossing of growth percentiles (acute malnutrition) and for linear growth stunting (chronic malnutrition).
2. History should include details of diet intake and feeding patterns (including restrictive intake, grazing feeding pattern, inappropriate foods for age and development, excessive juice, sugar-sweetened beverages, or water intake); past medical history, including birth and developmental history; family history; social history; and review of systems.
3. Physical examination should include careful examination of skin (for rashes), mouth, eyes, nails, and hair for signs of micronutrient and protein deficiencies, as well as for abnormal neurologic function (eg, loss of deep tendon reflexes, abnormal strength and tone).
4. Laboratory studies are generally of low yield for diagnosis for growth faltering in the absence of other findings, and should be reserved for moderately severe cases of malnutrition. In such cases, risk of and suspicion for nutrient deficiencies and systemic pathology should guide studies ordered. Typical screening laboratories include chemistry panel; complete blood count; and iron panel, including ferritin. Thyroid function testing is indicated with linear growth faltering. Serology for celiac disease may also be warranted for toddlers. Guidelines for screening for inborn errors of metabolism have recently been published.
5. Some infants are naturally small and have weight for age percentile values below the 5th percentile and may have length and head circumferences at higher percentiles. Such infants are often called "constitutionally small" as their thinness was present from birth, there was no evidence of intrauterine growth restriction, their mothers had small stature and usually thinness, and the family growth pattern is similar. Mothers of such normally small children should not be discouraged from breast feeding and should not be counseled to prematurely add food supplements. Workup for failure to thrive is not indicated in these infants and evaluations or referrals for growth failure or child abuse from underfeeding are not warranted.

When providing nutritional rehabilitation to infants/children with severe malnutrition, refeeding syndrome may occur. Monitoring for hypophosphatemia, hypokalemia, hypomagnesemia, and hyperglycemia is prudent, and calorie intake should be slowly increased to avoid metabolic instability.

▶ Treatment

Poor eating is often a learned behavior. Families should be counseled regarding choices of foods that are appropriate for the age and developmental level of the child. Increasing the caloric density of foods is associated with increased daily caloric intake and improved weight gain, but such weight gain usually is due to fat gain unless the calorie supplements include significant protein. Micronutrient deficiencies should be corrected. For repletion of iron, 2–4 mg/kg/d, divided BID, can be initiated. For zinc, 1 mg/kg/d for 1–2 months, administered several hours apart from iron supplement is typically adequate. Children should have structured meal times (eg, three meals and two to three snacks during the day), ideally at the same time other family members eat. Consultation with a pediatric dietitian can be helpful for educating the families. Poor feeding may be related to family dysfunction. Children whose households are chaotic and children who are abused, neglected, or exposed to poorly controlled mental illness may be described as poor eaters, and may fail to gain. Careful assessment of the social environment of such children is critical, and disposition options may include support services, close medical follow-up visits, family counseling, and even foster placement while a parent receives therapy.

Ficicioglu C, Haack K: Failure to thrive: When to suspect inborn errors of metabolism. Pediatrics 2009;124:972–979.

Jaffe AC: Failure to thrive: current clinical concepts. Pediatr Rev 2011 Mar;32(3):100–107; quiz 108 [No abstract available] [PMID: 21364013].

PEDIATRIC OVERWEIGHT AND OBESITY (SEE ALSO CHAPTER 4 FOR SPECIFICS ON ADOLESCENT OBESITY)

ESSENTIALS OF DIAGNOSIS & TYPICAL FEATURES

- Excessive rate of weight gain; upward change in BMI percentiles.
- BMI for age between the 85th and 95th percentiles indicates overweight.
- BMI for age > 95th percentile indicates obesity and is associated with increased risk of secondary complications.
- BMI for age > 99th percentile indicates severe obesity and a higher risk of complications.

General Considerations

The prevalence of childhood and adolescent obesity has increased rapidly in the United States and many other parts of the world. Currently in the United States, approximately 17% of 6- to 19-year-olds are obese, with even higher rates among subpopulations of minority and economically disadvantaged children. The increasing prevalence of childhood obesity is related to a complex combination of socioeconomic, genetic, and biologic factors.

Childhood obesity is associated with significant comorbidities, which, if untreated, are likely to persist into adulthood. The probability of obesity persisting into adulthood has been estimated to increase from 20% at 4 years to 80% by adolescence. Obesity is associated with cardiovascular and endocrine abnormalities (eg, dyslipidemia, insulin resistance, and type 2 diabetes), orthopedic problems, pulmonary complications (eg, obstructive sleep apnea), and mental health problems (Table 11–18).

Huang TT et al: Pediatricians' and family physicians' weight-related care of children in the U.S. Am J Prev Med 2011 Jul;41(1):24–32 [PMID: 21665060].

Krebs NF et al: Assessment of child and adolescent overweight and obesity. Pediatrics 2007;120 (Suppl 4):S193–S228 [PMID: 18055652].

Nadeau KJ, Maahs DM, Daniels SR, Eckel RH: Childhood obesity and cardiovascular disease: Links and prevention strategies. Nat Rev Cardiol 2011 Jun 14 [PMID: 21670745].

Ross MM et al: Multidisciplinary treatment of pediatric obesity: Nutrition evaluation and management. Nutr Clin Pract 2010 Aug;25(4):327–334 [PMID: 20702836].

Clinical Findings

A. Definitions

BMI is the standard measure of obesity in adults and children. BMI is correlated with more accurate measures of body fatness and is calculated with readily available information: weight and height (kg/m^2). Routine plotting of the BMI on age- and gender-appropriate charts (http://www.cdc.gov/growthcharts) can identify those with excess weight. Definitions were outlined in 2007 by an Expert Committee (www.ama-assn.org/ped_obesity_recs.pdf). BMI between the 85th and 95th percentiles for age and sex identifies those who are overweight. Obese is defined as BMI at or above 95% and is associated with increased risk of secondary complications. Severe obesity is characterized by BMI for age and sex at or above the 99th percentile. An upward change in BMI percentiles in any range should prompt evaluation and possible treatment. An annual increase of more than 2 kg/m^2 is almost always an indicator of a rapid increase in body fat. For children younger than 2 years, weight for length greater than 95th percentile indicates overweight and warrants further assessment, especially of energy intake and feeding behaviors.

B. Risk Factors

There are multiple risk factors for developing obesity, reflecting the complex relationships between genetic and environmental factors. Family history is a strong risk factor. If one parent is obese, the odds ratio is approximately 3 for obesity in adulthood, but if both parents are obese, the odds ratio increases to greater than 10 compared to children with two nonobese parents.

Risk factors in the home environment offer targets for intervention. Consumption of sugar-sweetened beverages, lack of family meals, large portion sizes, foods prepared outside the home, television viewing, video gaming, poor sleep, and lack of activity are all associated with risk of excessive weight gain.

C. Assessment

Early recognition of rapid weight gain or high-risk behaviors is essential. Anticipatory guidance or intervention before weight gain becomes severe is more likely to be successful than delayed intervention. Routine evaluation at well-child visits should include

1. Measurement of weight and height, calculation of BMI, and plotting all three parameters on age- and sex-appropriate growth charts (http://www.cdc.gov/growthcharts). Evaluate for upward crossing of BMI percentile channels.
2. History regarding diet and activity patterns (Table 11–19); family history, and review of systems. Physical examination should include careful blood pressure measurement, distribution of adiposity (central vs generalized); markers of comorbidities, such as acanthosis nigricans, hirsutism, hepatomegaly, orthopedic abnormalities; and physical stigmata of genetic syndrome (eg, Prader-Willi syndrome).
3. Laboratory studies are recommended as follows for children older than 2 years:

Overweight—fasting lipid profile (cholesterol, low-density lipoprotein [LDL], high-density lipoprotein [HDL], triglyceride [TG]).

Overweight with personal or family history of heart disease risk factors—fasting lipid profile, fasting glucose, alanine aminotransferase (ALT).

Obese—fasting lipid profile, fasting glucose, ALT.

Other studies should be guided by findings in the history and physical.

Barton M: Screening for obesity in children and adolescents: US Preventive Services Task Force recommendation statement. Pediatrics 2010 Feb;125(2):361–367 [PMID: 20083515].

Treatment

Treatment should be based on risk factors, including age, severity of obesity, and comorbidities, as well as family history and support. For children with uncomplicated obesity,

Table 11–18. Selected complications of childhood obesity.

System	Condition	Note	Review of Systems
Pulmonary	Obstructive sleep apnea	13%–33% of obese youth	Snoring, apnea, poor sleep, nocturnal enuresis, AM headaches, fatigue, poor school performance
	Obesity-hypoventilation syndrome	Severe obesity, restrictive lung disease, may lead to right heart failure	Dyspnea, edema, somnolence
Cardiovascular	Hypertension	3 occasions > 95th percentile on National Heart, Lung, and Blood Institute (NHLBI) tables for gender, age, and height	
	Lipid abnormalities	Total cholesterol 170–199 borderline, > 200 high Low-density lipoprotein (LDL) 110–129 borderline, > 130 high High-density lipoprotein (HDL) < 40 low	
		Triglycerides (TG) > 150 high	Assess for pancreatitis if TG > 400, nausea, vomiting, abdominal pain
GI	Nonalcoholic fatty liver disease (NAFLD)	10%–25% of obese youth; elevated alanine aminotransferase (ALT); rule out other liver disease; steatohepatitis may progress to fibrosis, cirrhosis	Commonly asymptomatic; rarely abdominal pain: vague, recurrent,
	Gastroesophageal reflux disease (GERD)	Increased abdominal pressure	Abdominal pain: heartburn
	Gallstones	Associated with rapid weight loss	Abdominal pain: right upper or epigastric
	Constipation	Associated with inactivity, r/o encopresis	Abdominal pain: distension, hard infrequent stools, soiling/incontinence
Endocrine	Impaired glucose metabolism	Elevated fasting glucose = 100–125	Acanthosis nigricans
		Impaired glucose tolerance = 2 h OGGT 140–199	
	Type 2 diabetes (T2DM)	Random glucose > 200 with symptoms; Fasting glucose > 126, 2 h OGTT > 200, HgA1c > 6.5	Polyuria and polydipsia, unintentional weight loss
	Polycystic ovarian syndrome (PCOS)	Two of three: 1. Hyperandrogenism 2. Oligomenorrhea 3. Polycystic ovaries; insulin resistance; risk of infertility and endometrial cancer	Oligomenorrhea (< 9 menses/y), hyperandrogenism: hirsuitism, acne
	Hypothyroid	Associated with poor linear growth	Asymptomatic until uncompensated: linear growth failure, cold intolerance, decline in school performance, coarse features, thin hair
Neurology/ ophthalmology	Psuedotumor cerebri	Papilledema, vision loss possible, consult neuro/ ophthalmology	Headaches (severe, recurrent), often worse in AM
Orthopedic	Blount disease	Stress injury to medial tibial growth plate, often painless	Bowed legs, ± knee pain
	Slipped capital femoral epiphysis (SCFE)	More likely to progress to bilateral disease in obese	Hip, groin, or knee pain; limp with leg held in external rotation
Dermatology	Acanthosis nigricans	Secondary effect of elevated insulin	Darkening of skin on neck, axillae, groin, ± skin tags
	Intertrigo/furunculosis/panniculitis	Examine skin folds, pannus; bacteria, and/or yeast	Rash/infection in skin folds, inflammatory papules
	Hydradenitis suppurativa	Draining cysts in axillae or groin	Rash/infection in skin folds, blocked glands, recurrent and unrelenting
Psychiatric	Depression/anxiety	May lead to worsening obesity if untreated	Full psycho/social review, including mood, school performance, peer and family relationships
	Eating disorder	Assess for binging ± purging behavior	
	History of abuse	Increases risk of severe obesity	

OGTT, Oral Glucose Tolerance Test.

Table 11–19. Suggested areas for assessment of diet and activity patterns.

Diet
- Portion sizes: adult portions for young children
- Frequency of meals away from home (restaurants or take out)
- Frequency/amounts of sugar-sweetened beverages (soda, juice drinks)
- Meal and snack pattern: structured vs grazing, skipping meals
- Frequency of eating fruits and vegetables
- Frequency of family meals
- Television viewing while eating

Activity
- Time spent in sedentary activity: television, video games, computer
- Time spent in vigorous activity: organized sports, physical education, free play
- Activities of daily living: walking to school, chores, yard work
- Sleep duration: risk of obesity is increased with inadequate sleep

the primary goal is to achieve healthy eating and activity patterns, not necessarily to achieve ideal body weight. For children with a secondary complication, improvement of the complication is an important goal. In general, weight loss goals for obese children range from 1 lb/mo for those younger than 12 years to 2 lb/wk for those older than 12 years. More rapid weight loss should be monitored for pathologic causes that may be associated with nutrient deficiencies and linear growth stunting (Table 11–20).

Treatment focused on behavior changes in the context of family involvement has been associated with sustained weight loss and decreases in BMI. Clinicians should assess the family's readiness to take action, employing motivational interviewing techniques to promote readiness, including open-ended questioning, exploring and resolving the family's ambivalence toward changes, and accepting the family's resistance nonjudgmentally. Providers should engage the family in collaborative decision making about which behavior change goals will be targeted. Improving dietary habits and activity levels concurrently is desirable for successful weight management. The entire family should adopt healthy eating patterns, with parents modeling healthy food choices, controlling foods brought into the home, and guiding appropriate portion sizes. The American Academy of Pediatrics recommends no television for children younger than 2 years old, a maximum of 2 h/d of television and video games for older children, with lower levels recommended for children during attempts at BMI reduction.

A "staged approach" for treatment has been proposed, with the initial level depending on the severity of overweight, the age of the child, the readiness of the family to implement changes, the preferences of the parents and child, and the skills of the health care provider.

1. **Prevention plus:** Counseling regarding problem areas identified by screening questions (see Table 11–19); emphasis on lifestyle changes, including healthy eating and physical activity patterns.
2. **Structured weight management:** Provides more specific and structured dietary pattern, such as meal planning, exercise prescription, and behavior change goals. This may be done in the primary care setting. Generally referral to at least one ancillary health professional will be required: dietitian, behavior specialist, and/or physical therapist. Monitoring is monthly or tailored to patient and family's needs.
3. **Comprehensive multidisciplinary:** This level further increases the structure of therapeutic interventions and support, employs a multidisciplinary team, and may involve weekly group meetings.
4. **Tertiary care intervention:** This level is for patients who have not been successful at the other intervention levels or who are severely obese. Interventions are prescribed by a multidisciplinary team, and may include intensive behavior therapy, specialized diets, medications, and surgery.

Pharmacotherapy can be an adjunct to dietary, activity, and behavioral treatment, but by itself it is unlikely to result in significant or sustained weight loss. Only one medication is approved for obesity treatment in adolescents: orlistat, a lipase inhibitor, is approved for patients older than 12 years. For severely obese adolescents, particularly with comorbidities, bariatric surgery is performed in some centers. There is emerging evidence that in carefully selected and closely monitored patients, surgery can result in significant weight loss with a reduction in comorbidities.

Barlow SE: Expert Committee recommendations regarding the prevention, assessment, and treatment of child and adolescent overweight and obesity: Summary report. Pediatrics 2007;120(Suppl 4):S164 [PMID: 18055651].

Table 11–20. Weight management goals.

Age	BMI	Weight Change Goal to Achieve BMI < 85%
2–5 y	85%–94%	Maintain weight
	95%–98%	Maintain weight, or if complications lose 1 lb/mo
	99%	Lose 1 lb/mo
6–11 y	85%–94%	Maintain weight
	95%–98%	Lose 1 lb/mo
	99%	Lose 2 lb/wk
12–18 y	85%–95%	Maintain weight
	95%–98%	Lose 2 lb/wk
	99%	Lose 2 lb/wk

Homer CJ: Responding to the childhood obesity epidemic: From the provider visit to health care policy-steps the health care sector can take. Pediatrics 2009 Jun;123(Suppl 5):S253–S257 [PMID: 19470600].

Pratt JS et al: Best practice updates for pediatric/adolescent weight loss surgery. Obesity (Silver Spring) 2009 May;17(5):901–910 [PMID: 19396070].

NUTRITION SUPPORT

1. ENTERAL

Indications

Enteral nutrition support is indicated when a patient cannot adequately meet nutritional needs by oral intake alone and has a functioning GI tract. This method of support can be used for short- and long-term delivery of nutrition. Even when the gut cannot absorb 100% of nutritional needs, some enteral feedings should be attempted. Enteral nutrition, full or partial, has many benefits:

1. Maintaining gut mucosal integrity
2. Preserving gut-associated lymphoid tissue
3. Stimulation of gut hormones and bile flow

Access Devices

Nasogastric feeding tubes can be used for supplemental enteral feedings, but generally are not used for more than 6 months because of the complications of otitis media and sinusitis. Initiation of nasogastric feeding usually requires a brief hospital stay to ensure tolerance to feedings and to allow for parental instruction in tube placement and feeding administration.

If long-term feeding support is anticipated, a more permanent feeding device, such as a gastrostomy tube, may be considered. Referral to a home care company is necessary for equipment and other services such as nursing visits and dietitian follow-up.

Table 11–21 suggests appropriate timing for initiation and advancement of drip and bolus feedings, according to a child's age. Clinical status and tolerance to feedings should ultimately guide their advancement.

Monitoring

Monitoring the adequacy of enteral feeding depends on nutritional goals. Growth should be frequently assessed, especially for young infants and malnourished children. Hydration status should be monitored carefully at the initiation of enteral feeding. Either constipation or diarrhea can be problems, and attention to stool frequency, volume, and consistency can help guide management. When diarrhea occurs, factors such as infection, hypertonic enteral medications, antibiotic use, and alteration in normal gut flora should be addressed.

In medically stable patients, the enteral feeding schedule should be developmentally appropriate (eg, 5–6 small feedings/d for a toddler). When night drip feedings are used in conjunction with daytime feeds, it is suggested that less than 50% of goal calories be delivered at night so as to maintain a daytime sense of hunger and satiety. This will be especially important once a transition to oral intake begins. Children who are satiated by tube feedings will be less likely to take significant amounts of food by mouth, thus possibly delaying the transition from tube to oral nutrition.

ASPEN Board of Directors: Clinical guidelines for the use of enteral nutrition in adult and pediatric patients 2009. JPEN 2009 May–Jun;33(3):255–259 [PMID: 19398611].

2. PARENTERAL NUTRITION

Indications

A. Peripheral Parenteral Nutrition

Peripheral parenteral nutrition is indicated when complete enteral feeding is temporarily impossible or undesirable.

Table 11–21. Guidelines for the initiation and advancement of tube feedings.

	Drip Feeds		Bolus Feeds	
Age	Initiation	Advancement	Initiation	Advancement
Preterm	1-2 mL/kg/d	5-10 mL q8-12h over 5-7 d as tolerated	5-20 mL	5-10 mL as tolerated
Birth-12 mo	5-10 mL/h	5-10 mL q2-8h	10-60 mL	20-40 mL q3-4h
1-6 y	10-15 mL/h	10-15 mL q2-8h	30-90 mL	30-60 mL q feed
6-14 y	15-20 mL/h	10-20 mL q2-8h	60-120 mL	60-90 mL q feed
> 14 y	20-30 mL/h	20-30 mL q2-8h	60-120 mL	60-120 mL q feed

Short-term partial intravenous (IV) nutrition via a peripheral vein is a preferred alternative to administration of dextrose and electrolyte solutions alone. Because of the osmolality of the solutions required, it is usually impossible to achieve total calorie and protein needs with parenteral nutrition via a peripheral vein.

B. Total Parenteral Nutrition

Total parenteral nutrition (TPN) should be provided only when clearly indicated. Apart from the expense, numerous risks are associated with this method of feeding (see section on Complications). Even when TPN is indicated, every effort should be made to provide at least a minimum of nutrients enterally to help preserve the integrity of the GI mucosa and of GI function.

The primary indication for TPN is the loss of function of the GI tract that prohibits the provision of required nutrients by the enteral route. Important examples include short bowel syndrome, some congenital defects of the GI tract, and prematurity.

Catheter Selection & Position

An indwelling central venous catheter is preferred for long-term IV nutrition. For periods of up to 3–4 weeks, a percutaneous central venous catheter threaded into the superior vena cava from a peripheral vein can be used. For the infusion of dextrose concentrations higher than 12.5%, the tip of the catheter should be located in the superior vena cava. Catheter positioning in the right atrium has been associated with complications, including arrhythmias and right atrial thrombus. After placement, a chest radiograph must be obtained to check catheter position. If the catheter is to be used for nutrition and medications, a double-lumen catheter is preferred.

Complications

A. Mechanical Complications

1. Related to catheter insertion or to erosion of catheter through a major blood vessel—Complications include trauma to adjacent tissues and organs, damage to the brachial plexus, hydrothorax, pneumothorax, hemothorax, and cerebrospinal fluid penetration. The catheter may slip during dressing or tubing changes, or the patient may manipulate the line.

2. Clotting of the catheter—Addition of heparin (1000 U/L) to the solution is an effective means of preventing this complication. If an occluded catheter does not respond to heparin flushing, filling the catheter with recombinant tissue plasminogen activator may be effective.

3. Related to composition of infusate—Calcium phosphate precipitation may occur if excess amounts of calcium or phosphorus are administered. Factors that increase the risk of calcium phosphate precipitation include increased pH and decreased concentrations of amino acids. Precipitation of medications incompatible with TPN or lipids can also cause clotting.

> Doellman D: Prevention, assessment, and treatment of central venous catheter occlusions in neonatal and young pediatric patients. J Infus Nurs 2011 Jul-Aug;34(4):251–258 [PMID: 21734521].

B. Septic Complications

Septic complications are the most common cause of nonelective catheter removal, but strict use of aseptic technique and limiting entry into the catheter can reduce the rates of line sepsis. Fever over 38–38.5°C in a patient with a central catheter should be considered a line infection until proved otherwise. Cultures should be obtained and IV antibiotics empirically initiated. Removing the catheter may be necessary with certain infections (eg, fungal), and catheter replacement may be deferred until infection is treated.

C. Metabolic Complications

Many of the metabolic complications of IV nutrition are related to deficiencies or excesses of nutrients in administered fluids. These complications are less common as a result of experience and improvements in nutrient solutions. However, specific deficiencies still occur, especially in the premature infant. Avoidance of deficiencies and excesses and of metabolic disorders requires attention to the nutrient balance, electrolyte composition, and delivery rate of the infusate and careful monitoring, especially when the composition or delivery rate is changed.

Currently the most challenging metabolic complication is cholestasis, particularly common in premature infants of very low birth weight. The cause of cholestasis associated with TPN is unknown. Patient and medical risk factors include prematurity, sepsis, hypoxia, major surgery (especially GI surgery), absence of enteral feedings, and small bowel bacterial overgrowth. Risk factors related to IV nutrition include amino acid excess or imbalance, use of IV soybean oil-based lipid emulsions, and prolonged duration of PN administration. Amino acid solutions with added cysteine decrease cholestasis. Practices that may minimize cholestasis include initiating even minimal enteral feedings as soon as feasible, avoiding sepsis by meticulous line care, avoiding overfeeding, using cysteine- and taurine-containing amino acid formulations designed for infants, preventing or treating small bowel bacterial overgrowth, protecting TPN solutions from light, and avoiding hepatotoxic medications.

> Gura KM et al: Safety and efficacy of a fish oil based fat emulsion in the treatment of PN associated liver disease. Pediatrics 2008 Mar;121(3):e678–e686 [PMID: 18310188].

Kurvinen A et al: Effects of long-term parenteral nutrition on serum lipids, plant sterols, cholesterol metabolism, and liver histology in pediatric intestinal failure. J Pediatr Gastroenterol Nutr 2011 Apr 30 [PMID: 21543999].

Nehra D et al: The prevention and treatment of intestinal failure-associated liver disease in neonates and children. Surg Clin North Am 2011 Jun;91(3):543–563 [PMID: 21621695].

NUTRIENT REQUIREMENTS & DELIVERY

Energy

When patients are fed intravenously, no fat and carbohydrate intakes are unabsorbed, and no energy is used in nutrient absorption. These factors account for at least 7% of energy in the diet of the enterally fed patient. The intravenously fed patient usually expends less energy in physical activity because of the impediment to mobility. Average energy requirements may therefore be lower in children fed intravenously, and the decrease in activity probably increases this figure to a total reduction of 10%–15%. Caloric guidelines for the IV feeding of infants and young children are outlined below.

The guidelines are averages, and individuals vary considerably. Factors significantly increasing the energy requirement estimates include exposure to cold environment, fever, sepsis, burns, trauma, cardiac or pulmonary disease, and catch-up growth after malnutrition.

With few exceptions, such as some cases of respiratory insufficiency, at least 50%–60% of energy requirements are provided as glucose. Up to 40% of calories may be provided by IV fat emulsions.

Dextrose

The energy density of IV dextrose (monohydrate) is 3.4 kcal/g. Dextrose is the main exogenous energy source provided by total IV feeding. IV dextrose suppresses gluconeogenesis and provides a substrate that can be oxidized directly, especially by the brain, red and white blood cells, and wounds. Because of the high osmolality of dextrose solutions ($D_{10}W$ yields 505 mOsm/kg H_2O), concentrations greater than 10%–12.5% cannot be delivered via a peripheral vein or improperly positioned central line.

Dosing guidelines: The standard initial quantity of dextrose administered will vary by age (Table 11–22). Tolerance to IV dextrose normally increases rapidly, due primarily to suppression of hepatic production of endogenous glucose. Dextrose can be increased by 2.5 g/kg/d, by 2.5%–5%/d, or by 2–3 mg/kg/min/d if there is no glucosuria or hyperglycemia. Standard final infusates for infants via a properly positioned central venous line usually range from 15% to 25% dextrose, though concentrations of up to 30% dextrose may be used at low flow rates. Tolerance to IV dextrose loads is markedly diminished in the premature neonate and in hypermetabolic states.

Problems associated with IV dextrose administration include hyperglycemia, hyperosmolality, and glucosuria (with osmotic diuresis and dehydration). Possible causes of unexpected hyperglycemia include the following: (1) inadvertent infusion of higher glucose concentrations than ordered, (2) uneven flow rate, (3) sepsis, (4) a stress situation, and (5) pancreatitis. IV insulin reduces hyperglycemia by suppressing hepatic glucose production and increasing glucose uptake by muscle and fat tissues. It usually increases plasma

Table 11–22. Pediatric macronutrient guidelines for total parenteral nutrition.

Age	Dextrose		Amino acids	Lipid
	mg/kg/min	g/kg/d	g/kg/d	g/kg/d
	50%–60% kcal		10%–20% kcal	30%–40% kcal
Preterm	Initial 5-8 Max 11-12.5	Initial 7-11 Max 16-18	Initial 1.5-2 Max 3-4	Initial 0.5-1 Max 2.5-3.5
Birth-12 mo	Initial 6-8 Max 11-15	Initial 9-11 Max 16-21.5	Initial 1.5-2 Max 3	Initial 1 Max 2.5-3.5
1-6 y	Initial 6-7 Max 10-12	Initial 8-10 Max 14-17	Initial 1-1.5 Max 2-2.5	Initial 1 Max 2.5-3.5
> 6 y	Initial 5-7 Max 9	Initial 8-10 Max 13	Initial 1 Max 1.5-2	Initial 1 Max 3
> 10 y	Initial 4-5 Max 6-7	Initial 5-7 Max 8-10	Initial 1 Max 1.5-2	Initial 1 Max 2-3
Adolescents	Initial 2-3 Max 5-6	Initial 3-4 Max 7-8	Initial 1 Max 1.5-2	Initial 0.5-1 Max 2

lactate concentrations, but does not necessarily increase glucose oxidation rates; it may also decrease the oxidation of fatty acids, resulting in less energy for metabolism. Hence, insulin should be used very cautiously. A standard IV dose is 1 U/4 g of carbohydrate, but much smaller quantities may be adequate and, usually, one starts with 0.2–0.3 U/4 g of carbohydrate.

Hypoglycemia may occur after an abrupt decrease in or cessation of IV glucose. When cyclic IV nutrition is provided, the IV glucose load should be decreased steadily for 1–2 hours prior to discontinuing the infusate. If the central line must be removed, the IV dextrose should be tapered gradually over several hours.

Maximum oxidation rates for infused dextrose decrease with age. It is important to note that the ranges for dextrose administration provided in Table 11–22 are guidelines and that individual patient tolerance and clinical circumstances may warrant administration of either less or more dextrose. Quantities of exogenous dextrose in excess of maximal glucose oxidation rates are used initially to replace depleted glycogen stores; hepatic lipogenesis occurs thereafter. Excess hepatic lipogenesis may lead to a fatty liver. Lipogenesis results in release of carbon dioxide, which when added to the amount of carbon dioxide produced by glucose oxidation (which is 40% greater than that produced by lipid oxidation) may elevate the $PaCO_2$ and aggravate respiratory insufficiency or impede weaning from a respirator.

Lipids

The energy density of lipid emulsions (20%) is 10 kcal/g of lipid or 2 kcal/mL of infusate. The lipids are derived from either soybean or safflower oil. All commonly available formulations consist of more than 50% linoleic acid and 4%–9% linolenic acid. It is recognized that this high level of linoleic acid is not ideal due to the proinflammatory potential of omega-6 fatty acids, except when small quantities of lipid are being given to prevent an EFA deficiency. Ultimately, improved emulsions are anticipated, including an omega-3 fish oil based product that is currently available in Europe and in clinical trials or available for compassionate use for children with TPN-associated cholestatic liver disease in the US. Because 10% and 20% lipid emulsions contain the same concentrations of phospholipids, a 10% solution delivers more phospholipid per gram of lipid than a 20% solution. Twenty percent lipid emulsions are preferred. IV lipid is often used to provide 30%–40% of calorie needs for infants and up to 30% of calorie needs in older children and teens.

The level of lipoprotein lipase (LPL) activity is the rate-limiting factor in the metabolism and clearance of fat emulsions from the circulation. LPL activity is inhibited or decreased by malnutrition, leukotrienes, immaturity, growth hormone, hypercholesterolemia, hyperphospholipidemia, and theophylline. LPL activity is enhanced by glucose, insulin, lipid, catecholamines, and exercise. Heparin releases LPL from the endothelium into the circulation and enhances the rate of hydrolysis and clearance of triglycerides. In small premature infants, lowdose heparin infusions may increase tolerance to IV lipid emulsion.

In general, adverse effects of IV lipid can be avoided by starting with modest quantities and advancing cautiously in light of results of triglyceride monitoring and clinical circumstances. In cases of severe sepsis, special caution is required to ensure that the lipid is metabolized effectively. Monitoring with long-term use is also essential.

IV lipid dosing guidelines: Check serum triglycerides before starting and after increasing the dose. Commence with l g/kg/d, given over 12–20 hours or 24 hours in small preterm infants. Advance by 0.5–1.0 g/kg/d, every 1–2 days, up to goal (see Table 11–22).

As a general rule, do not increase the dose if the serum triglyceride level is above 250 mg/dL during infusion (150 mg/dL in neonates) or if the level is greater than 150 mg/dL 6–12 hours after cessation of the lipid infusion.

Serum triglyceride levels above 400–600 mg/dL may precipitate pancreatitis. In patients for whom normal amounts of IV lipid are contraindicated, 4%–8% of calories as IV lipid should be provided (300 mg linoleic acid/100 kcal) to prevent essential fatty acid deficiency. Neonates and malnourished pediatric patients receiving lipid-free parenteral nutrition are at high risk for EFA deficiency because of limited adipose stores.

Park KT, Nespor C, Kerner J Jr: The use of Omegaven in treating parenteral nutrition-associated liver disease. J Perinatol 2011 Apr;31(Suppl 1):S57–S60 [PMID: 21448206].

Nitrogen

One gram of nitrogen is yielded by 6.25 g of protein (1 g of protein contains 16% nitrogen). Caloric density of protein is equal to 4 kcal/g.

A. Protein Requirements

Protein requirements for IV feeding are the same as those for normal oral feeding (see Table 11–2).

B. Intravenous Amino Acid Solutions

Nitrogen requirements can be met by one of the commercially available amino acid solutions. For older children and adults, none of the standard preparations has a clear advantage over the others as a source of amino acids. For infants, however, including premature infants, accumulating evidence suggests that the use of TrophAmine (McGaw) is associated with a normal plasma amino acid profile, superior nitrogen retention, and a lower incidence of cholestasis. TrophAmine contains 60% essential amino acids, is relatively high in branched-chain amino acids, contains taurine, and is compatible with the addition of cysteine within 24–48 hours after administration. The dose of added cysteine is 40 mg/g of TrophAmine. The relatively low pH of TrophAmine is also advantageous for solubility of calcium and phosphorus.

C. Dosing Guidelines

Amino acids can be started at 1–2 g/kg/d in most patients (see Table 11–22). In severely malnourished infants, the initial amount should be 1 g/kg/d. Even in infants of very low birth weight, there is evidence that higher initial amounts of amino acids are tolerated with little indication of protein "toxicity." Larger quantities of amino acids in relation to calories can minimize the degree of negative nitrogen balance even when the infusate is hypocaloric. Amino acid intake can be advanced by 0.5–1.0 g/kg/d toward the goal. Normally the final infusate will contain 2%–3% amino acids, depending on the rate of infusion. Concentration should not be advanced beyond 2% in peripheral vein infusates due to osmolality.

D. Monitoring

Monitoring for tolerance of the IV amino acid solutions should include routine blood urea nitrogen. Serum alkaline phosphatase, γ-glutamyltransferase, and bilirubin should be monitored to detect the onset of cholestatic liver disease.

Minerals & Electrolytes

A. Calcium, Phosphorus, and Magnesium

Intravenously fed premature and full-term infants should be given relatively high amounts of calcium and phosphorus. Current recommendations are as follows: calcium, 500–600 mg/L; phosphorus, 400–450 mg/L; and magnesium, 50–70 mg/L. After 1 year of age, the recommendations are as follows: calcium, 200–400 mg/L; phosphorus, 150–300 mg/L; and magnesium, 20–40 mg/L. The ratio of calcium to phosphorous should be 1.3:1.0 by weight or 1:1 by molar ratio. These recommendations are deliberately presented as milligrams per liter of infusate to avoid inadvertent administration of concentrations of calcium and phosphorus that are high enough to precipitate in the tubing. During periods of fluid restriction, care must be taken not to inadvertently increase the concentration of calcium and phosphorus in the infusate. These recommendations assume an average fluid intake of 120–150 mL/kg/d and an infusate of 25 g of amino acid per liter. With lower amino acid concentrations, the concentrations of calcium and phosphorus should be decreased.

B. Electrolytes

Standard recommendations are given in Table 11–23. After chloride requirements are met, the remainder of the anion required to balance the cation should be given as acetate to avoid the possibility of acidosis resulting from excessive chloride. The required concentrations of electrolytes depend to some extent on the flow rate of the infusate and must be modified if flow rates are unusually low or high and if there are specific indications in individual patients. IV sodium should be administered sparingly in the severely malnourished patient because of impaired membrane function and high intracellular sodium levels. Conversely, generous quantities of potassium are indicated. Replacement electrolytes and fluids should be delivered via a separate infusate.

C. Trace Elements

Recommended IV intakes of trace elements are as follows: zinc 100 mcg/kg, copper 20 mcg/kg, manganese 1 mcg/kg, chromium 0.2 mcg/kg, selenium 2 mcg/kg, and iodide 1 mcg/kg. Of note, IV zinc requirements may be as high as 400 mcg/kg for premature infants and can be up to 250 mcg/kg for infants with short bowel syndrome and significant GI losses of zinc. When IV nutrition is supplemental or limited to fewer than 2 weeks, and preexisting nutritional deficiencies are absent, only zinc need routinely be added.

IV copper requirements are relatively low in the young infant because of the presence of hepatic copper stores. These are significant even in the 28-week fetus. Circulating levels of copper and manganese should be monitored in the presence of cholestatic liver disease. If monitoring is not feasible, temporary withdrawal of added copper and manganese is advisable.

Copper and manganese are excreted primarily in the bile, but selenium, chromium, and molybdenum are excreted primarily in the urine. These trace elements, therefore, should be administered with caution in the presence of renal failure.

Vitamins

Two vitamin formulations are available for use in pediatric parenteral nutrition: MVI Pediatric and MVI-12 (Astra-Zeneca). MVI Pediatric contains the following: vitamin A, 0.7 mg;

Table 11–23. Electrolyte requirements for parenteral nutrition.

Electrolyte	Preterm Infant	Full-Term Infant	Child	Adolescent
Sodium	2-5 mEq/kg	2-3 mEq/kg	2-3 mEq/kg	60-150 mEq/d
Chloride	2-5 mEq/kg	2-3 mEq/kg	2-3 mEq/kg	60-150 mEq/d
Potassium	2-3 mEq/kg	2-3 mEq/kg	2-3 mEq/kg	70-180 mEq/d

vitamin D, 400 IU; vitamin E, 7 mg; vitamin K, 200 mcg; ascorbic acid, 80 mg; thiamin, 1.2 mg; riboflavin, 1.4 mg; niacinamide, 17 mg; pyridoxine, 1 mg; vitamin B_{12}, 1 mcg; folic acid, 140 mcg; pantothenate, 5 mg; and biotin, 20 mcg. Recommended dosing is as follows: 5 mL for children weighing more than 3 kg, 3.25 mL for infants 1–3 kg, and 1.5 mL for infants weighing less than 1 kg. Children older than 11 years can receive 10 mL of the adult formulation, MVI-12, which contains the following: vitamin A, 1 mg; vitamin D, 200 IU; vitamin E, 10 mg; ascorbic acid, 100 mg; thiamin, 3 mg; riboflavin, 3.6 mg; niacinamide, 40 mg; pyridoxine, 4 mg; vitamin B_{12}, 5 mcg; folic acid, 400 mcg; pantothenate, 15 mg; and biotin, 60 mcg. MVI-12 contains no vitamin K.

IV lipid preparations contain enough tocopherol to affect total blood tocopherol levels. The majority of tocopherol in soybean oil emulsion is α-tocopherol, which has substantially less biologic activity than the α-tocopherol present in safflower oil emulsions.

A dose of 40 IU/kg/d of vitamin D (maximum 400 IU/d) is adequate for both full-term and preterm infants.

Fluid Requirements

The initial fluid volume and subsequent increments in flow rate are determined by basic fluid requirements, the patient's clinical status, and the extent to which additional fluid administration can be tolerated and may be required to achieve adequate nutrient intake. Calculation of initial fluid volumes to be administered should be based on standard pediatric practice. Tolerance of higher flow rates must be determined on an individual basis. If replacement fluids are required for ongoing abnormal losses, these should be administered via a separate line.

Monitoring

Vital signs should be checked on each shift. With a central catheter in situ, a fever of more than 38.5°C requires that peripheral and central-line blood cultures, urine culture, complete physical examination, and examination of the IV entry point be made. Instability of vital signs, elevated white blood cell count with left shift, and glycosuria

Table 11–24. Summary of suggested monitoring for parenteral nutrition.

Variables	Acute Stage	Long-Term[b]
Growth	Daily	Weekly
Weight	Weekly	
Length	Weekly	
Head circumference		
Urine		
Glucose (dipstick)	With each void	With changes in intake or status
Specific gravity	Void	
Volume	Daily	
Blood		
Glucose	4 h after changes,[a] then daily × 2 d	Weekly
Na^+, K^+, Cl^-, CO_2, blood urea nitrogen	Daily for 2 d after changes,[a] then twice weekly	Weekly
Ca^{2+}, Mg^{2+}, P	Initially, then twice weekly	Weekly
Total protein, albumin, bilirubin, aspartate transaminase, and alkaline phosphatase	Initially, then weekly	Every other week
Zinc and copper	Initially according to clinical indications	Monthly
Triglycerides	Initially, 1 d after changes,[a] then weekly	Weekly
Compete blood count	Initially, then twice weekly; according to clinical indications (see text)	Twice weekly

[a]Changes include alterations in concentration or flow rate.
[b]Long-term monitoring can be tapered to monthly or less often, depending on age, diagnosis, and clinical status of patient.

suggest sepsis. Removal of the central venous catheter should be considered if the patient is toxic or unresponsive to antibiotics.

A. Physical Examination

Monitor especially for hepatomegaly (differential diagnoses include fluid overload, congestive heart failure, steatosis, and hepatitis) and edema (differential diagnoses include fluid overload, congestive heart failure, hypoalbuminemia, and thrombosis of superior vena cava).

B. Intake and Output Record

Calories and volume delivered should be calculated from the previous day's intake and output records (that which was delivered rather than that which was ordered). The following entries should be noted on flow sheets: IV, enteral, and total fluid (mL/kg/d); dextrose (g/kg/d or mg/kg/min); protein (g/kg/d); lipids (g/kg/d); energy (kcal/kg/d); and percent of energy from enteral nutrition.

C. Growth, Urine, and Blood

Routine monitoring guidelines are given in Table 11–24. These are minimum requirements, except in the very long-term stable patient. Individual variables should be monitored more frequently as indicated, as should additional variables or clinical indications. For example, a blood ammonia analysis should be ordered for an infant with lethargy, pallor, poor growth, acidosis, azotemia, or abnormal liver test results.

Greene HL et al: Guidelines for the use of vitamins, trace elements, calcium, magnesium, and phosphorus in infants and children receiving total parenteral nutrition: Report of the Subcommittee on Pediatric Parenteral Nutrient Requirements from the Committee on Clinical Practice Issues of the American Society for Clinical Nutrition. Am J Clin Nutr 1988;48:1324 [PMID: 3142247].

Joffe A et al: Nutritional support for critically ill children. Cochrane Database Syst Rev 2009 Apr 15;(2):CD005144 [Review] [PMID: 19370617].

Skillman HE, Wishmeyer PE: Nutrition therapy in critically ill infants and children. JPEN 2008 Sept–Oct;32(5):520–534 [PMID: 18753390].

12 Emergencies & Injuries

Maria J. Mandt, MD
Joseph A. Grubenhoff, MD

ASSESSMENT AND MANAGEMENT OF THE ACUTELY ILL INFANT OR CHILD

When faced with a seriously ill or injured child, a systematic approach and rapid determination of the child's physiologic status with concurrent initiation of resuscitative measures is imperative. Initial management must be directed at correcting any physiologic derangement. Specifically, one must evaluate the airway for any obstruction, assess ventilatory status, and evaluate for shock. Intervention to correct any abnormalities in these three parameters must be undertaken immediately. Following this initial intervention, the provider must then carefully consider the underlying cause, focusing on those that are treatable or reversible. Specific diagnoses can then be made, and targeted therapy (eg, intravenous [IV] glucose for hypoglycemia) can be initiated.

Pediatric cardiac arrest more frequently represents progressive respiratory deterioration or shock, also called asphyxial arrest, rather than primary cardiac etiologies. Unrecognized deterioration may lead to bradycardia, agonal breathing, hypotension, and ultimately asystole. Resulting hypoxic and ischemic insult to the brain and other vital organs make neurologic recovery extremely unlikely, even in the doubtful event that the child survives the arrest. Children who respond to rapid intervention with ventilation and oxygenation alone or to less than 5 minutes of advanced life support are much more likely to survive neurologically intact. In fact, >70% of children with respiratory arrest who receive rapid and effective bystander resuscitation survive with good neurologic outcomes. Therefore, it is essential to recognize the child who is at risk for progressing to cardiopulmonary arrest and to provide aggressive intervention before asystole occurs.

When cardiopulmonary arrest does occur, survival is rare and most often associated with significant neurological impairment. Current data reflect a 6% survival rate for out-of-hospital cardiac arrest, 8% for those who receive prehospital intervention, and 27% survival rate for in-hospital arrest.

The following discussion details care of the critically ill pediatric patient who does not require cardiopulmonary resuscitation (CPR). Detailed information regarding the 2010 Guidelines for Pediatric Basic (BLS) and Advanced Life Support (PALS) can be found under Statements & Guidelines at http://myamericanheart.org/professional. ***Note:*** Standard precautions (personal protective equipment) must be maintained during resuscitation efforts.

THE ABCS OF RESUSCITATION

Any severely ill child should be rapidly evaluated in a deliberate sequence of *a*irway patency, *b*reathing adequacy, and *c*irculation integrity. Derangement at each point must be corrected before proceeding. Thus, if a child's airway is obstructed, the airway must be opened (eg, by head positioning and the chin lift maneuver) before breathing and circulation are assessed.

Airway

Look for evidence of spontaneous breathing effort. Adventitious breath sounds such as stridor, stertor, or gurgling, or increased work of breathing without air movement is suggestive of airway obstruction. Significant airway obstruction often is associated with altered level of consciousness, including agitation or lethargy. During this rapid assessment, if the patient is noted to be apneic or producing only gasping (agonal) breaths, chest compressions should be initiated immediately in accordance with pediatric advanced life support guidelines.

The airway is managed initially by noninvasive means such as oxygen administration, chin lift, jaw thrust, suctioning, or bag-valve-mask ventilation. Invasive maneuvers such as endotracheal intubation, laryngeal mask insertion, or rarely, cricothyroidotomy are required if the aforementioned maneuvers are unsuccessful. If neck injury is suspected, the cervical spine must be immobilized and kept from extension or flexion. (See section on Approach to the Pediatric Trauma

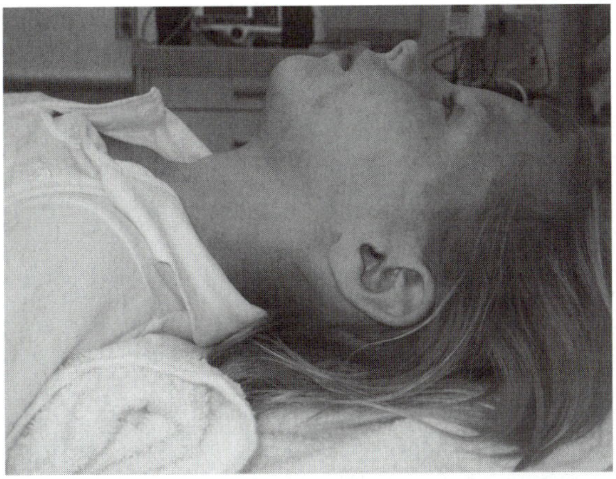

▲ **Figure 12–1.** Correct positioning of the child younger than age 8 years for optimal airway alignment: a folded sheet or towel is placed beneath the shoulders to accommodate the occiput and align the oral, pharyngeal, and tracheal airways.

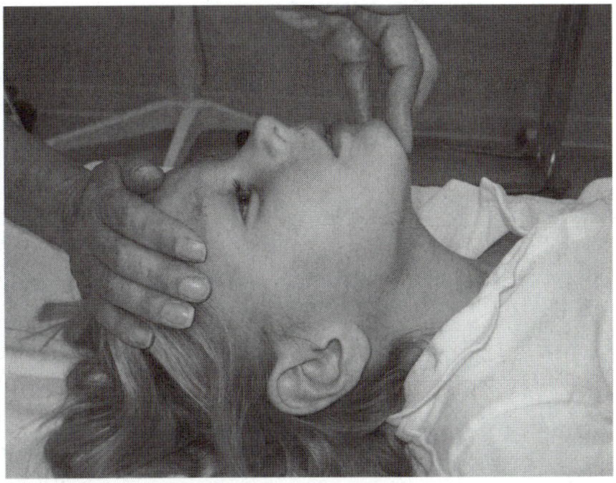

A

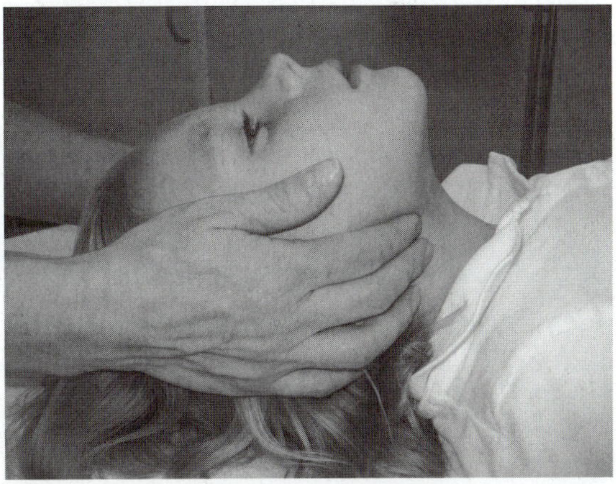

B

▲ **Figure 12–2.** **A:** Opening the airway with the head tilt and chin lift in patients without concern for spinal trauma: gently lift the chin with one hand and push down on the forehead with the other hand. **B:** Opening the airway with jaw thrust in patients with concern for spinal trauma: lift the angles of the mandible; this moves the jaw and tongue forward and opens the airway without bending the neck.

Patient, later.) The following discussion assumes that basic life support has been instituted.

Knowledge of pediatric anatomy is important for airway management. Children's tongues are large relative to their oral cavities, and the larynx is high and anteriorly located. Infants are obligate nasal breathers; therefore, secretions, blood, or foreign bodies in the nasopharynx can cause significant distress.

A. Place the head in the sniffing position. The neck should be slightly flexed and the head gently extended so as to bring the face forward. This position aligns the oral, pharyngeal, and tracheal planes. Reposition the head if airway obstruction persists after head tilt and jaw thrust. In infants and children younger than about 8 years of age, the relatively large occiput causes significant neck flexion and poor airway positioning. This is relieved by placing a towel roll under the shoulders, thus returning the child to a neutral position (Figure 12–1). In an older child, slightly more head extension is necessary. Avoid hyperextension of the neck, especially in infants.

B. Perform the chin lift or jaw thrust maneuver (Figure 12–2). Lift the chin upward while avoiding pressure on the submental triangle, or lift the jaw by traction upward on the angle of the jaw. **Head tilt must not be done if cervical spine injury is possible.**

C. Suction the mouth of any foreign material.

D. Remove visible foreign bodies, using fingers or a Magill forceps. Visualize by means of a laryngoscope if necessary. Blind finger sweeps should not be done.

E. Insertion of an airway adjunct, such as the oropharyngeal or nasopharyngeal airway (Figure 12–3), relieves upper airway obstruction due to prolapse of the tongue into the posterior pharynx. This is the most common cause of airway obstruction in unconscious children. The correct size for an oropharyngeal airway is obtained by measuring from the upper central gumline to the angle of the jaw (Figure 12–4) and should be used only in the unconscious victim. Proper sizing is paramount, as an oropharyngeal airway that is too small will push the tongue further into the airway while one that is too large will mechanically obstruct the airway. Nasopharyngeal airways should fit snugly within the

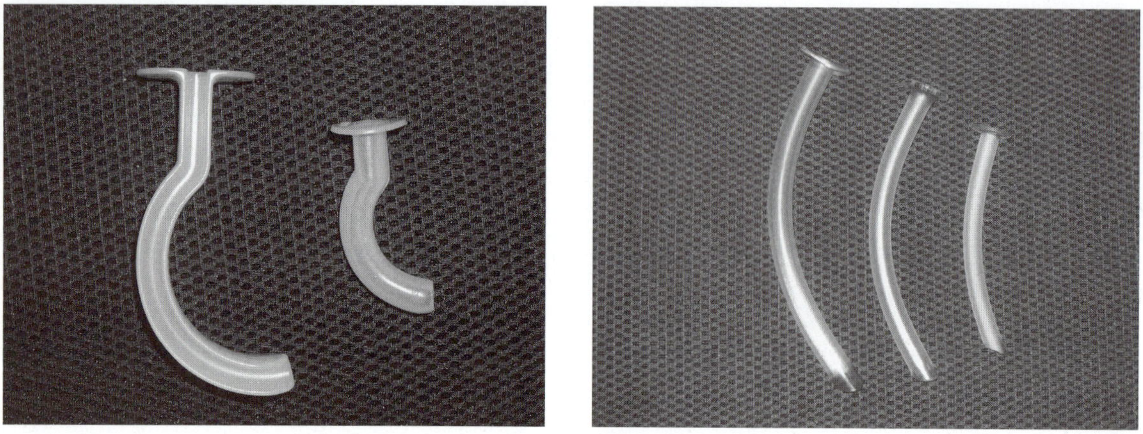

A

B

▲ **Figure 12–3.** **A:** Oropharyngeal airways of various sizes. **B:** Nasopharyngeal airways of different sizes.

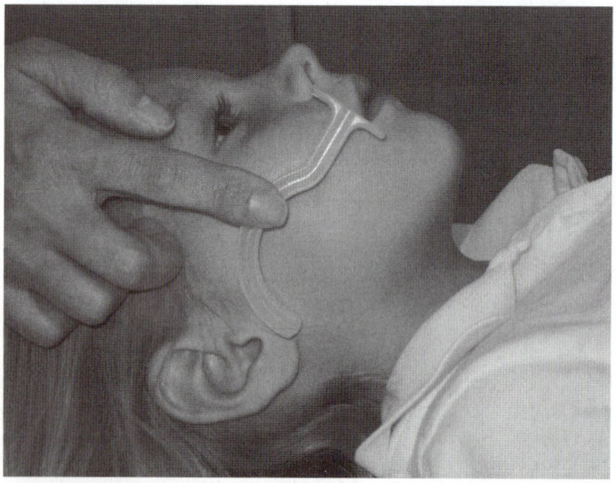

▲ **Figure 12–4.** Size selection for the oropharyngeal airway: hold the airway next to the child's face and estimate proper size by measuring from the upper central gumline to the angle of the jaw.

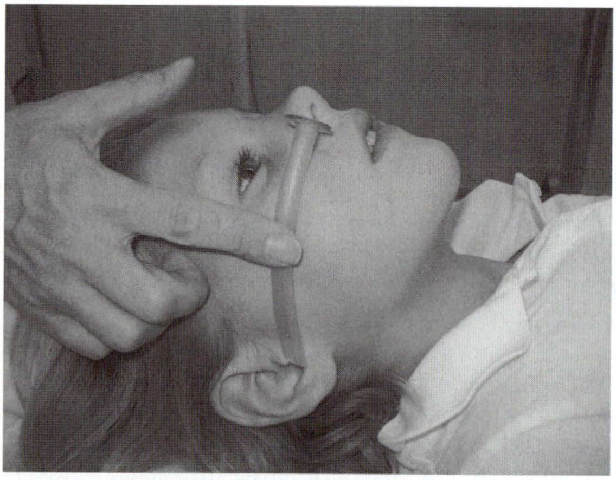

▲ **Figure 12–5.** Size selection for the nasopharyngeal airway: hold the airway next to the child's face and estimate proper size by measuring from the nares to the tragus.

nares and should be equal in length to the distance from the nares to the tragus (Figure 12–5). This airway adjunct should be avoided in children with significant injuries to the midface due to the risk of intracranial perforation through a damaged cribriform plate.

Breathing

Assessment of respiratory status is largely accomplished by inspection. *Look* for adequate and symmetrical chest rise and fall, rate and work of breathing (eg, retractions, flaring, and grunting), accessory muscle use, skin color, and tracheal deviation. Note the mental status. Pulse oximetry measurement and end-tidal CO_2 determination, if available, are highly desirable. *Listen* for adventitious breath sounds such as wheezing. Auscultate for air entry, symmetry of breath sounds, and rales. *Feel* for subcutaneous crepitus.

If spontaneous breathing is inadequate, initiate positive-pressure ventilation with bag-valve mask ventilation (BMV) and 100% oxygen. Assisted ventilations should be coordinated with the patient's efforts, if present. Effective BMV is a difficult skill which requires training and practice. To begin, ensure a proper seal by choosing a mask that encompasses the area from the bridge of the nose to the cleft of the chin. Form an E–C clamp around the mask to seal the mask tightly to the child's face. The thumb and index finger form the "C" surrounding the mask, while the middle, ring, and small fingers lift the jaw into the mask (Figure 12–6). Use only enough force and volume to make the chest rise visibly. In the patient with a perfusing rhythm, administer one breath every 3–5 seconds (12–20 breaths per minute). To more easily achieve this rate, recite the pneumonic "squeeze-release-release" in a normal speaking voice. Two-person ventilation using this technique is optimal. When proper technique is used, BMV is effective in the vast majority of cases.

Adequacy of ventilation is reflected in adequate chest movement and auscultation of good air entry bilaterally. Take care to avoid hyperventilation. Excessive ventilation leads to barotrauma, increased risk of aspiration, and a decreased likelihood that return of spontaneous circulation will be achieved during cardiac arrest. If the chest does not rise and fall easily with bagging, reposition the airway as previously described. Perform airway foreign body extraction maneuvers if the airway remains obstructed, including visualizing the airway with a laryngoscope and using Magill forceps. The presence of asymmetrical breath sounds in a child in shock or in severe distress suggests pneumothorax and is an indication for needle thoracostomy. In small children, the transmission of breath sounds throughout the chest may impair the ability to auscultate the presence of a pneumothorax. ***Note:*** Effective oxygenation and ventilation are the keys to successful resuscitation.

Cricoid pressure (Sellick maneuver) during positive-pressure ventilation may decrease gastric inflation; however, it has not been shown to reduce the risk of aspiration and should only be used if it does not interefere with ventilation or the speed and ease of intubation. Intubate or use an alternative advanced airway, such as a supraglottic device, in patients who are unresponsive to bag-mask ventilation, those in coma, those who require airway protection, or those who will require prolonged ventilation. Cricothyroidotomy is rarely necessary. Advanced airway management techniques are described in the references accompanying this section. (See also section on Approach to the Pediatric Trauma Patient, later.)

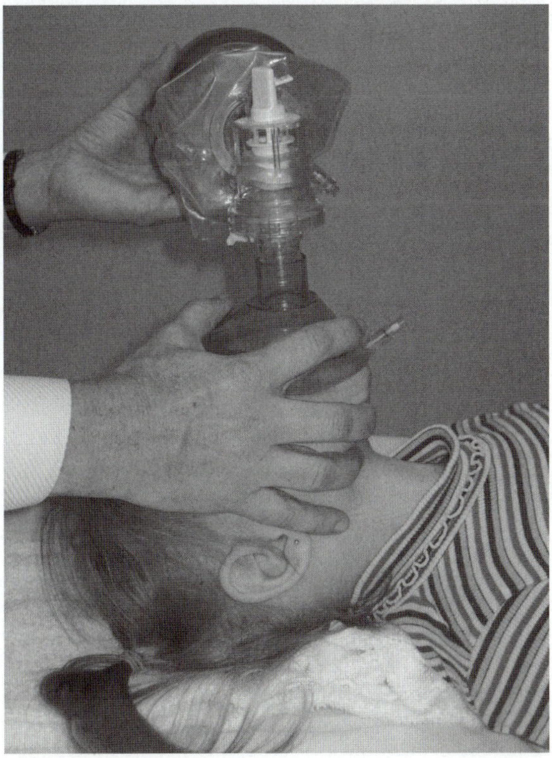

A

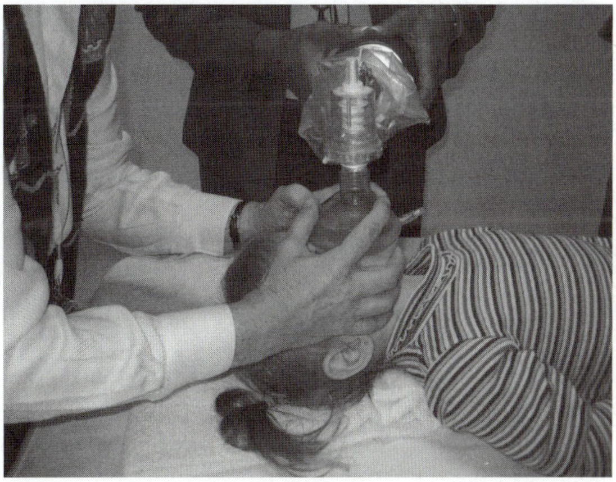

B

▲ **Figure 12–6.** **A:** Bag-valve-mask ventilation, one-person technique: the thumb and index finger form the "C" surrounding the mask, while the middle, ring, and little fingers lift the jaw into the mask. **B:** Bag-valve-mask ventilation, two-person technique: the first rescuer forms the "C" and "E" clamps with both hands; the second rescuer provides ventilation.

Circulation

The diagnosis of shock can and should be made by clinical examination, and must be done rapidly. Clinical assessments A–F aid in assessing perfusion.

A. Pulses

Check adequacy of peripheral pulses. Pulses become weak and thready only with severe hypovolemia. Compare peripheral pulses with central pulses. In the infant, central pulses should be checked at the brachial artery.

B. Heart Rate

Compare with age-specific norms. Tachycardia can be a nonspecific sign of distress; bradycardia for age is a prearrest sign and necessitates aggressive resuscitation.

C. Extremities

As shock progresses, extremities become cooler from distal to proximal. A child whose extremities are cool distal to the elbows and knees is in severe shock.

D. Capillary Refill Time

When fingertip pressure is applied to a patient's distal extremity and then released, blood should refill the area in less than 2 seconds. A prolonged capillary refill time in the setting of other signs of shock indicates a compensated shock state. It is important to recognize that capillary refill time is influenced by ambient temperature, limp position, site, age of the patient, and room lighting. These factors must be taken into consideration when measuring capillary refill time.

E. Mental Status

Hypoxia, hypercapnia, or ischemia will result in altered mental status. Other important treatable conditions may also result in altered mental status, such as intracranial hemorrhage, meningitis, and hypoglycemia.

F. Skin Color

Pallor, gray, mottled, or ashen skin colors all indicate compromised circulatory status.

G. Blood Pressure

It is important to remember that shock (inadequate perfusion of vital organs) may be present before the blood pressure falls below the normal limits for age. As intravascular volume falls, peripheral vascular resistance increases. Blood pressure is maintained until there is 35%–40% depletion of blood volume, followed by precipitous and often irreversible deterioration. Shock that occurs with any signs of decreased perfusion but normal blood pressure is **compensated** shock. When blood pressure also falls, **hypotensive** (decomensated) shock is present. Blood pressure determination should be done manually, using an appropriately sized cuff, because automated machines can give erroneous readings in children.

MANAGEMENT OF SHOCK

IV access is essential but can be difficult to establish in children with shock. Peripheral access, especially via the antecubital veins, should be attempted first, but central cannulation should follow quickly if peripheral access is unsuccessful. Alternatives are percutaneous cannulation of femoral, subclavian, or internal or external jugular veins; cutdown at antecubital, femoral, or saphenous sites; or intraosseous (IO) lines (Figure 12–7). Consider IO needle placement in any severely ill child when venous access cannot be established rapidly. Decisions on more invasive access should be

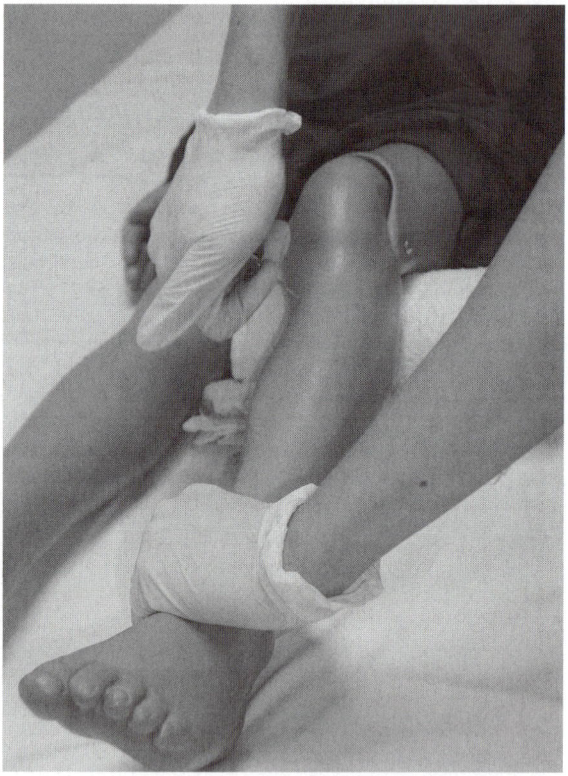

▲ **Figure 12–7.** Interosseous (IO) cannulation technique. The IO line is inserted by grasping the needle hub firmly with the palm of the hand and angling the needle tip perpendicular to the anterior tibial surface approximately two fingerbreadths distal to the tibial plateau. With a firm, twisting motion, advance the needle until a sudden lessening of resistance is felt as the needle enters the marrow space. Aspiration of blood and marrow confirms IO placement.

based on individual expertise as well as urgency of obtaining access. Use short, wide-bore catheters to allow maximal flow rates. Two IV lines should be started in severely ill children. In newborns, the umbilical veins may be cannulated. Consider arterial access if beat-to-beat monitoring or frequent laboratory tests will be needed.

Differentiation of Shock States & Initial Therapy

Therapy for inadequate circulation is determined by the cause of circulatory failure.

A. Hypovolemic Shock

The most common type of shock in the pediatric population is hypovolemia. Frequent causes include dehydration, diabetes, heat illness, hemorrhage, and burns. Normal saline or lactated Ringer solution (isotonic crystalloid) is given as initial therapy in shock and should be initiated even in normotensive patients. There is no advantage to the early administration of colloid (albumin). Give 20 mL/kg body weight, repeat as necessary, until perfusion normalizes. Children tolerate large volumes of fluid replacement and frequent reassessment is necessary. Typically, in hypovolemic shock, no more than 60 mL/kg is needed, but more may be required if ongoing losses are severe. Appropriate monitoring and reassessment will guide your therapy. Packed red blood cell transfusion is indicated in trauma patients not responding to initial crystalloid bolus fluid replacement; however, there is insufficient evidence to determine the volume required. Pressors are not required in simple hypovolemic states.

B. Distributive Shock

Distributive shock results from increased vascular capacitance with normal circulating volume. Examples are sepsis, anaphylaxis, and spinal cord injury. Initial therapy is again isotonic volume replacement with crystalloid, but pressors may be required if perfusion does not normalize after delivery of two or three 20-mL/kg boluses of crystalloid. If necessary, pressors may be initiated through a peripheral line until central access is obtained. Children in distributive shock must be admitted to a pediatric intensive care unit.

C. Cardiogenic Shock

Cardiogenic shock can occur as a complication of congenital heart disease, myocarditis, dysrhythmias, ingestions (eg, clonidine, cyclic antidepressants), or as a complication of prolonged shock due to any cause. The diagnosis is suggested by any of the following signs: abnormal cardiac rhythm, distended neck veins, rales, abnormal heart sounds such as an S_3 or S_4, friction rub, narrow pulse pressure, rales, or hepatomegaly. Chest radiographs may show cardiomegaly and pulmonary edema. An initial bolus of crystalloid may be given, but pressors, and possibly afterload reducers, are necessary to improve perfusion. Giving multiple boluses of fluid is deleterious. Comprehensive cardiopulmonary monitoring is essential. Children in cardiogenic shock must be admitted to a pediatric intensive care unit.

Observation & Further Management

Clinically reassess physiologic response to each fluid bolus to determine additional needs. Serial central venous pressure determinations or a chest radiograph may help determine volume status. Place an indwelling urinary catheter to monitor urine output.

Caution must be exercised with volume replacement if intracranial pressure is potentially elevated, as in severe head injury, diabetic ketoacidosis, or meningitis. Even in such situations, however, normal intravascular volume must be restored in order to achieve adequate mean arterial pressure and, thus, cerebral perfusion pressure.

SUMMARY OF RESUSCITATING THE ACUTELY ILL INFANT OR CHILD

Assess the ABCs in sequential fashion and, before assessing the next system, immediately intervene if physiologic derangement is detected. It is essential that each system be reassessed after each intervention to ensure improvement and prevent failure to recognize clinical deterioration.

ECC Committee, Subcommittes and Task Forces of the American Heart Association: Part 13: Pediatric Basic Life Support: 2010 American Heart Association Guidelines for Cardiopulmonary Resuscitation and Emergency Cardiovascular Care. Circulation 2010; 122:S862–S875.

ECC Committee, Subcommittees and Task Forces of the American Heart Association: Part 14: Pediatric Advanced Life Support: 2010 American Heart Association guidelines for Cardiopulmonary Resuscitation and Emergency Cardiovascular Care. Circulation 2010; 122;S876–S908.

Brierley J, Carcillo JA, Choong K et al: Clinical practice parameters for hemodynamic support of pediatric and neonatal septic shock: 2007 update from the American College of Critical Care Medicine. Crit Care Med 2009; 37(2):666–688.

Hazinski MF et al (editors): *PALS Provider Manual.* American Heart Association, 2006.

APLS (the pediatric emergency medicine resource). Available at: http://www.aplsonline.com

EMERGENCY PEDIATRIC DRUGS

Although careful attention to airway and breathing remains the mainstay of pediatric resuscitation, medications are often needed. Rapid delivery to the central circulation, which can be via peripheral IV catheter, is essential. Infuse medications close to the catheter's hub and flush with saline to achieve the most rapid systemic effects. In the rare instance that no IV or IO access is achievable, some drugs may be given by endotracheal tube (Table 12–1). However, the dose,

Table 12–1. Emergency drugs that may be given by endotracheal tube.

Lidocaine
Epinephrine
Atropine
Naloxone

absorption, and effectivity of drugs given via this route are either unknown or controversial. The use of length-based emergency measuring tapes that contain preprinted drug dosages, equipment sizes, and IV fluid amounts (Broselow tapes) or preprinted resuscitation drug charts is much more accurate than estimation formulas and helps minimize dosing errors. Selected emergency drugs used in pediatrics are summarized in Table 12–2.

APPROACH TO THE ACUTELY ILL INFANT OR CHILD

An unstable patient may present with a known diagnosis (asthma with status asthmaticus and respiratory failure; complications of known congenital heart disease) or in cardiorespiratory failure of unknown cause. The initial approach must rapidly identify the injuries, prioritize management, and reverse life-threatening conditions. Children with chronic disease may present with an acute exacerbation or a new, unrelated problem. Maintaining a broad differential diagnosis is essential to thorough assessment and management.

PREPARATION FOR EMERGENCY MANAGEMENT

Resuscitation occurs simultaneously at two levels: rapid cardiopulmonary assessment, with indicated stabilizing measures, while venous access is gained and cardiopulmonary

Table 12–2. Emergency pediatric drugs.

Drug	Indications	Dosage and Route	Comment
Atropine	1. Bradycardia, especially cardiac in origin 2. Vagally mediated bradycardia, eg, during laryngoscopy and intubation 3. Anticholinesterase poisoning	0.02 mg/kg IV/IO 0.04–0.06 mg/kg ET Minimum dose 0.1 mg; Maximum single dose 0.5 mg May repeat once if needed.	Atropine may be useful in hemodynamically significant primary cardiac-based bradycardias. Because of paradoxic bradycardia sometimes seen in infants, a minimum dose of 0.1 mg is recommended by the American Heart Association. Epinephrine is the first-line drug in pediatrics for bradycardia caused by hypoxia or ischemia.
Bicarbonate	1. Documented metabolic acidosis 2. Hyperkalemia	1 mEq/kg IV or IO; by arterial blood gas: 0.3 × kg × base deficit. May repeat every 5 min.	Infuse slowly. Sodium bicarbonate will be effective only if the patient is adequately oxygenated, ventilated, and perfused. Some adverse side effects.
Calcium chloride 10%	1. Documented hypocalcemia 2. Calcium channel blocker overdose 3. Hyperkalemia, hypermagnesemia	20 mg/kg slowly IV, preferably centrally, or IO with caution. Maximum single dose 2g.	Calcium is no longer indicated for asystole. Potent tissue necrosis results if infiltration occurs. Use with caution and infuse slowly.
Epinephrine	1. Bradycardia, especially hypoxic-ischemic 2. Hypotension (by infusion) 3. Asystole 4. Fine ventricular fibrillation refractory to initial defibrillation 5. Pulseless electrical activity 6. Anaphylaxis	*Bradycardia and cardiac arrest*: 0.01 mg/kg of 1:10,000 solution IV/IO: 0.1 mg/kg of 1:1,000 solution ET Anaphylaxis: 0.01 mg/kg of 1:1000 solution SC/IM Maximum dose: 0.3 mg. May repeat every 3–5 min. Constant infusion by IV drip: 0.1–1 mcg/kg/min.	Epinephrine is the single most important drug in pediatric resuscitation. Recent pediatric studies have shown no added advantage to high-dose epinephrine in terms of survival to discharge or neurologic outcome. Because other studies have indicated adverse effects, including increased myocardial oxygen consumption during resuscitation and worsened postarrest myocardial dysfunction, high-dose epinephrine is no longer recommended.
Glucose	1. Hypoglycemia 2. Altered mental status (empirical) 3. With insulin, for hyperkalemia	0.5–1 g/kg IV/IO. Continuous infusion may be necessary.	2–4 mL/kg $D_{10}W$, 1–2 mL/kg $D_{25}W$.
Naloxone	1. Opioid overdose 2. Altered mental status (empirical)	0.1 mg/kg IV/IO/ET; Maximum single dose, 2 mg. May repeat as necessary.	Side effects are few. A dose of 2 mg may be given in children ≥ 5 years or > 20 kg. Repeat as necessary, or give as constant infusion in opioid overdoses.

D_5W, 5% glucose in water; ET, endotracheally; IO, intraosseously; IV, intravenously; SC, subcutaneously.

monitoring initiated. The technique of accomplishing these concurrent goals is outlined as follows:

A. If advance notice of the patient's arrival has been received, prepare a resuscitation room and summon appropriate personnel as needed, such as a neurosurgeon for an unresponsive child after severe head injury or a radiology technician for imaging studies.

B. Assign team responsibilities, including a team leader plus others designated to manage the airway, perform chest compressions, achieve access, draw blood for laboratory studies, place monitors, gather additional historical data, and provide family support. The team approach is invaluable.

C. Age-appropriate equipment (including laryngoscope blade, endotracheal tubes, nasogastric or orogastric tubes, IV lines, and an indwelling urinary catheter) and monitors (cardiorespiratory monitor, pulse oximeter, and appropriate blood pressure cuff) should be assembled and readily available. Use a length-based emergency tape if available. See Table 12–3 for endotracheal tube sizes. Cuffed endotracheal tubes are acceptable during the inpatient setting for children and infants beyond the newborn period. Cuff inflation pressures must be carefully monitored and maintained below 20 cm H_2O. In certain circumstances, such as poor lung compliance or high airway resistance, the use of cuffed tubes may be preferable in controlled settings.

RECEPTION & ASSESSMENT

Upon patient arrival, the team leader begins a rapid assessment as team members perform their preassigned tasks. If the patient is received from prehospital care providers, careful attention must be paid to their report, which contains information that they alone have observed. Interventions and medications should be ordered only by the team leader to avoid confusion. The leader should refrain from personally performing procedures, which may distract him or her from optimal direction of the resuscitation. A complete timed record should be kept of events, including medications, interventions, and response to intervention.

All Cases

In addition to cardiac compressions and ventilation, ensure that the following are instituted:

1. Hundred percent high-flow oxygen.
2. Cardiorespiratory monitoring, pulse oximetry, and endtidal CO_2 if the patient is intubated.
3. Vascular (peripheral, IO, or central) access; two lines preferred.

Table 12–3. Equipment sizes and estimated weight by age.

Age (y)	Weight (kg)	Endotracheal Tube Size (mm)[a,b]	Laryngoscope Blade (Size)	Chest Tube (Fr)	Foley (Fr)
Premature	1-2.5	2.5 (uncuffed only)	0	8	5
Term newborn	3	3.0 (uncuffed only)	0–1	10	8
1	10	3.5–4.0	1	18	8
2	12	4.5	1	18	10
3	14	4.5	1	20	10
4	16	5.0	2	22	10
5	18	5.0–5.5	2	24	10
6	20	5.5	2	26	12
7	22	5.5–6.0	2	26	12
Age (y)	**Weight (kg)**	**Cuffed Endotracheal Tube Size (mm)[a,b]**	**Laryngoscope Blade (Size)**	**Chest Tube (Fr)**	**Foley (Fr)**
8	24	6.0	2	28	14
10	32	6.0–6.5	2–3	30	14
Adolescent	50	7.0	3	36	14
Adult	70	8.0	3	40	14

[a]Internal diameter.
[b]Decrease tube size by 0.5 mm if using a cuffed tube.

4. Blood drawn and sent. Bedside blood glucose determination is essential.
5. Full vital signs.
6. Clothes removed.
7. Foley catheter and nasogastric or orogastric tube inserted.
8. Complete history.
9. Notification of needed consultants.
10. Family support.
11. Law enforcement or security activation and emergency unit lockdown for cases involving potential terrorism, gang violence, or threats to staff or family.

As Appropriate

1. Immobilize neck.
2. Obtain chest radiograph (line and tube placement).
3. Insert central venous pressure and arterial line.

Kleinman ME, de Caen AR, Chameides L et al: Pediatric basic and advanced life support: 2010 international consensus on cardiopulmonary resuscitation and emergency cardiovascular care science with treatment recommendations. Pediatrics 2010;126(5):e1261–e1318.

Mandt MJ, Rappaport LD: Update in pediatric resuscitation. Adv Pediatr 2009;56:359–385.

Waltzman ML, Mooney DP: Chapter 105: Major Trauma. In Fleisher GR et al (editors): *Textbook of Pediatric Emergency Medicine,* 6th ed. Lippincott Williams & Wilkins, 2010:1244–1255.

Weiss M, Gerber AC: Cuffed tracheal tubes in children—things have changed. Pediatric Anesthesia 2006;16:1005 [PMID: 16972827].

APPROACH TO THE PEDIATRIC TRAUMA PATIENT

Traumatic injuries including motor vehicle crashes, falls, burns, and immersions, account for the greatest number of deaths among children older than age 1 year and exceeds all other causes of death combined. All providers of pediatric care must be cognizant of this sobering statistic. Cooperative efforts between injury prevention specialists, prehospital providers, and emergency, critical care, and rehabilitation physicians and nurses will help reduce these terrible losses.

A team approach to the severely injured child, using assigned roles as outlined in the preceding section, will optimize outcomes. A calm atmosphere in the receiving area will contribute to thoughtful care. Conscious children are terribly frightened by serious injury; reassurance can help alleviate anxiety. Analgesia and sedation must be given to stable patients. It is unconscionable to let children suffer pain needlessly. Treat pain expeditiously using oral or parenteral analgesics with ongoing monitoring. Parents are often anxious, angry, or guilty, requiring ongoing support from staff, social workers, or child life workers (therapists knowledgeable about child development). To provide optimal multidisciplinary care, regional pediatric trauma centers provide dedicated teams of pediatric specialists in emergency pediatrics, trauma surgery, orthopedics, neurosurgery, and critical care. However, most children with severe injuries are not seen in these centers. Primary care providers must be able to provide initial assessment and stabilization of the child with life-threatening injuries before transport to a verified pediatric trauma center.

MECHANISM OF INJURY

Document the time of occurrence, the type of energy transfer (eg, hit by a car, rapid deceleration), secondary impacts (if the child was thrown by the initial impact), appearance of the child at the scene, interventions performed, and clinical condition during transport. The report of emergency service personnel is invaluable. Forward all of this information with the patient to the referral facility if secondary transport occurs.

Trauma in children is predominantly blunt, with penetrating trauma occurring in 10% of cases. Head and abdominal injuries are particularly common and important.

INITIAL ASSESSMENT & MANAGEMENT

The vast majority of children who reach a hospital alive survive to discharge. As most deaths from trauma in children are due to head injuries, cerebral resuscitation must be the foremost consideration when treating children with serious injuries. The ultimate measure of outcome is the child's eventual level of functioning. Strict attention to the ABCs ensures optimal oxygenation, ventilation, and perfusion, and ultimately, cerebral perfusion.

The primary and secondary survey is a method for evaluating and treating injured patients in a systematic way that provides a rapid assessment and stabilization phase, followed by a head-to-toe examination and definitive care phase.

PRIMARY SURVEY

The primary survey is designed to immediately identify and treat all physiologic derangements resulting from trauma. It is the resuscitation phase. Priorities are still airway, breathing, and circulation, but with important further considerations in the trauma setting:

*A*irway, with cervical spine control

*B*reathing

*C*irculation, with hemorrhage control

*D*isability (neurologic deficit)

*E*xposure (maintain a warm *E*nvironment, undress the patient completely, and *E*xamine)

Evaluation and treatment of the ABCs are discussed earlier in this chapter. Remember that if the patient is apneic or has agonal breaths, the sequence becomes the *CABs* (chest compressions, open the airway, provide 2 rescue breaths). Please refer to pediatric advanced life support guidelines for further information. Modifications in the trauma setting are added in the sections that follow.

Airway

Failure to manage the airway appropriately is the most common cause of preventable morbidity and death. Administer 100% high-flow oxygen to all patients. During assessment and management of the airway, provide cervical spine protection, initially by manual inline immobilization, not traction. A hard cervical spine collar is then applied. The head and body are secured to a backboard, surrounded by a lightweight means of cushioning (eg, rolled blankets) to further immobilize the head and body and allow log-rolling of the child in case of vomiting. Assess the airway for patency. Use jaw thrust rather than chin lift during intubation to avoid flexion or extension of the neck. Suction the mouth and pharynx free of blood, foreign material, or secretions, and remove loose teeth. Insert an oropharyngeal airway if upper airway noises are heard or obstruction from posterior prolapse of the tongue occurs. A child with a depressed level of consciousness (Glasgow Coma Scale score < 9), a need for prolonged ventilation or hyper-ventilation, severe head trauma, or an impending operative intervention requires endotracheal intubation after bag-mask preoxygenation. Orotracheal intubation is the route of choice and is possible without cervical spine manipulation. Nasotracheal intubation may be possible in children 12 years of age or older who have spontaneous respirations—if not contraindicated by midfacial injury with the possibility of cribriform plate disruption.

Supraglottic devices, such as the laryngeal mask airway (LMA), are being used with increasing frequency, in both the prehospital and hospital settings. The device consists of a flexible tube attached to an inflatable rubber mask (Figure 12–8). The LMA is inserted blindly into the hypopharynx and is seated over the larynx, occluding the esophagus. Advantages to its use include ease of insertion, lower potential for airway trauma, and higher success rates. Patients remain at higher risk for aspiration with LMA use compared with orotracheal intubation; therefore, the LMA should not be used for prolonged, definitive airway management. Rarely, if tracheal intubation cannot be accomplished—particularly in the setting of massive facial trauma—cricothyroidotomy may be necessary. Needle cricothyroidotomy using a large-bore catheter through the cricothyroid membrane is the procedure of choice in patients younger than age 12 years. Operative revision will be needed for formal controlled tracheostomy.

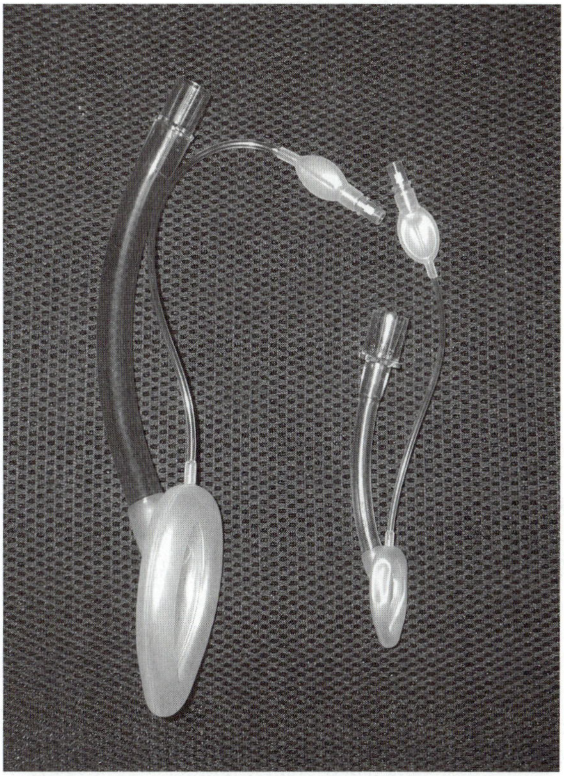

▲ **Figure 12–8.** Laryngeal mask airways of various sizes.

Breathing

Most ventilatory problems are resolved adequately by the airway maneuvers described earlier in this chapter and by positive-pressure ventilation. Breathing assessment is as described previously: Assess for an adequate rate and for symmetrical chest rise and breath sounds, work of breathing, color, tracheal deviation, crepitus, flail segments, deformity, or penetrating wounds. Sources of traumatic pulmonary compromise include pneumothorax, hemothorax, pulmonary contusion, flail chest, and central nervous system (CNS) depression. Asymmetrical breath sounds, particularly with concurrent tracheal deviation, cyanosis, or bradycardia, suggest pneumothorax, possibly under tension. To evacuate a tension pneumothorax, insert a large-bore catheter-over-needle assembly attached to a syringe through the second intercostal space in the midclavicular line into the pleural cavity and withdraw air. If a pneumothorax or hemothorax is present, place a chest tube in the fourth or fifth intercostal space in the anterior axillary line. Connect to water seal. Insertion should be over the rib to avoid the neurovascular bundle that runs below the rib margin. Open pneumothoraces can be treated temporarily by taping petrolatum-impregnated gauze on three sides over the wound, creating a flap valve.

Circulation

In addition to the circulatory assessment previously discussed, evaluation for ongoing external or internal hemorrhage is important in the trauma evaluation. Large-bore IV access should be obtained early during the assessment, preferably at two sites. If peripheral access is not readily available, a central line, cutdown, or IO line is established. A cardiorespiratory monitor and oximeter is applied, usually at patient arrival. Peripheral perfusion and blood pressure should be assessed and recorded at frequent intervals. Determine hematocrit and urinalysis in all patients. Blood type and cross-match should be obtained in the hypotensive child unresponsive to isotonic fluid boluses or with known hemorrhage. Consider coagulation studies, chemistry panel, liver transaminases, amylase, and toxicologic screening as clinically indicated.

External hemorrhage can be controlled by direct pressure. To avoid damage to adjacent neurovascular structures, avoid placing hemostats on vessels, except in the scalp. Determination of the site of internal hemorrhage can be challenging. Sites include the chest, abdomen, retroperitoneum, pelvis, and thighs. Bleeding into the intracranial vault rarely causes shock in children except in infants. Evaluation by an experienced clinician with adjunctive computed tomography (CT) or ultrasound will localize the site of internal bleeding.

Suspect cardiac tamponade after penetrating or blunt injuries to the chest if shock, pulseless electrical activity, narrowed pulse pressure, distended neck veins, hepatomegaly, or muffled heart sounds are present. Ultrasound may be diagnostic if readily available. Diagnose and treat with pericardiocentesis and rapid volume infusion.

Trauma ultrasonography, or the focused assessment with sonography for trauma (FAST), is routinely used in the adult trauma population. The purpose of the four-view examination (Morison pouch, splenorenal pouch, pelvic retrovesical space, and subcostal view of the heart) is to detect free fluid or blood in dependent spaces. In adults, such detection indicates clinically significant injury likely to require surgery. Accuracy and indications in children are much less clear. Solid organ injuries are more frequently missed and much of the pediatric trauma management is nonoperative. As a result, detection of free fluid by ultrasound in children is less likely to lead to surgery or result in a change in management.

Treat signs of poor perfusion vigorously: A tachycardic child with a capillary refill time of 3 seconds, or other evidence of diminished perfusion, is in *shock* and is sustaining vital organ insults. Recall that hypotension is a late finding. Volume replacement is accomplished initially by rapid infusion of normal saline or lactated Ringer solution at 20 mL/kg of body weight. If perfusion does not normalize after two crystalloid bolus infusions, 10 mL/kg of packed red blood cells is infused.

Rapid reassessment must follow each bolus. If clinical signs of perfusion have not normalized, repeat the bolus. Lack of response or later or recurring signs of hypovolemia suggest the need for blood transfusion and possible surgical exploration. For every milliliter of external blood loss, 3 mL of crystalloid solution should be administered.

A common problem is the brain-injured child who is at risk for intracranial hypertension and who is also hypovolemic. In such cases, circulating volume must be restored to ensure adequate cerebral perfusion; therefore, fluid replacement is required until perfusion normalizes. Thereafter provide maintenance fluids with careful serial reassessments. **Do not restrict fluids** for children with head injuries.

Table 12–4. AVPU system for evaluation of level of consciousness.

A	Alert
V	Responsive to Voice
P	Responsive to Pain
U	Unresponsive

Disability–Neurologic Deficit

Assess pupillary size and reaction to light and the level of consciousness. The level of consciousness can be reproducibly characterized by the AVPU system (Table 12–4). Pediatric Glasgow Coma Scale (GCS) assessments can be done as part of the secondary survey (Table 12–5).

Table 12–5. Glasgow Coma Scale.[a]

Eye opening response	
Spontaneous	4
To speech	3
To pain	2
None	1
Verbal response: Child (*Infant modification*)[b]	
Oriented (*Coos, babbles*)	5
Confused conversation (*Irritable cry, consolable*)	4
Inappropriate words (*Cries to pain*)	3
Incomprehensible sounds (*Moans to pain*)	2
None	1
Best upper limb motor response: Child (*Infant modification*)[b]	
Obeys commands (*Normal movements*)	6
Localizes pain (*Withdraws to touch*)	5
Withdraws to pain	4
Flexion to pain	3
Extension to pain	2
None	1

[a]The appropriate number from each section is added to total between 3 and 15. A score less than 8 usually indicates CNS depression requiring positive-pressure ventilation.

[b]If no modification is listed, the same response applies for both infants and children.

Exposure & Environment

Significant injuries can be missed unless the child is completely undressed and examined fully, front and back. Cutting away clothing can minimize movement. Within hours, pressure sores may develop on the buttocks and heels of an immobilized patient. Therefore, any patient transported on a backboard should be removed as soon as possible.

Because of their high ratio of surface area to body mass, infants and children cool rapidly. Hypothermia compromises outcome except with isolated head injuries; therefore, continuously monitor the body temperature and use warming techniques as necessary. Hyperthermia can adversely affect outcomes in children with acute brain injuries, so maintain normal body temperatures.

Monitoring

Cardiopulmonary monitors, pulse oximetry, and end-tidal CO_2 monitors should be put in place immediately. At the completion of the primary survey, additional "tubes" should be placed.

A. Nasogastric or Orogastric Tube

Children's stomachs should be assumed to be full. Gastric distention from positive-pressure ventilation increases the chance of vomiting and aspiration. The nasogastric route should be avoided in patients with significant midface injuries to avoid the increased risk of intracranial placement.

B. Urinary Catheter

An indwelling urinary bladder catheter should be placed to monitor urine output. Contraindications are based on the risk of urethral transection; signs include blood at the meatus or in the scrotum or a displaced prostate detected on rectal examination. Urine should be tested for blood. After the initial flow of urine with catheter placement, the urine output should exceed 1 mL/kg/h.

SECONDARY SURVEY

After the resuscitation phase, a focused history and a head-to-toe examination should be performed to reveal all injuries and determine priorities for definitive care.

History

Obtain a rapid, focused history from the patient (if possible), available family members or prehospital personnel. The AMPLE mneumonic is frequently used:

- A-Allergies
- M-Medications
- P-Past medical history/pregnancy
- L-Last meal
- E-Events/environment leading to the injury

Physical Examination

Skin

Search for lacerations, hematomas, burns, swelling, and abrasions. Remove foreign material, and cleanse as necessary. Cutaneous findings may indicate underlying pathology (eg, a flank hematoma overlying a renal contusion), although surface signs may be absent even with significant internal injury. Make certain the child's tetanus immunization status is current. Consider tetanus immune globulin for incompletely immunized children.

Head

Check for hemotympanum and for clear or bloody cerebrospinal fluid leak from the nares. Battle sign (hematoma over the mastoid) and raccoon eyes are late signs of basilar skull fracture. Explore wounds, evaluating for foreign bodies and defects in galea or skull. CT scan of the head is an integral part of evaluation for altered level of consciousness, posttraumatic seizure, or focal neurologic findings (see section on Head Injury, later). Pneumococcal vaccine may be considered for basilar skull fractures.

Spine

Cervical spine injury must be excluded in all children. This can be done clinically in children older than 4 or 5 years of age with normal neurologic findings on examination (including voluntary movement of all extremities) who are able to deny midline neck pain or midline tenderness on palpation of the neck and who have no other painful distracting injuries that might obscure the pain of a cervical spine injury. If radiographs are indicated, a cross-table lateral neck view is obtained initially followed by anteroposterior, odontoid, and in some cases, oblique views. Normal studies do not exclude significant injury, either bony or ligamentous, or involving the spinal cord itself. Therefore, an obtunded child should be maintained in cervical spine immobilization until the child has awakened and an appropriate neurologic examination can be performed. The entire thoracolumbar spine must be palpated and areas of pain or tenderness examined by radiography.

Chest

Children may sustain significant internal injury without outward signs of trauma. Pneumothoraces are detected and decompressed during the primary survey. Hemothoraces can occur with rib fractures or with injury to intercostal vessels, large pulmonary vessels, or lung parenchyma. Tracheobronchial disruption is suggested by large continued air leak despite chest tube decompression. Pulmonary contusions may require ventilatory support. Myocardial contusions and aortic injuries are unusual in children.

Abdomen

Blunt abdominal injury is common in multisystem injuries. Significant injury may exist without cutaneous signs or instability of vital signs. Abdominal pain and tenderness coupled with a linear contusion across the abdomen ("seat belt sign") increases the risk of intraabdominal injury threefold. Tenderness, guarding, distention, diminished or absent bowel sounds, or poor perfusion mandates immediate evaluation by a pediatric trauma surgeon. Injury to solid viscera frequently can be managed nonoperatively in stable patients; however, intestinal perforation or hypotension necessitates operative treatment. Serial examinations, ultrasound, and CT scan provide diagnostic help. Intra-abdominal injury is highly likely if the AST > 200 U/L or the ALT > 125 U/L; however, elevated levels that are below these thresholds do not exclude significant injury if a significant mechanism has occurred. When measured serially, a hematocrit < 30% also may suggest intra-abdominal injury in blunt trauma patients. Coagulation studies are rarely beneficial if no concomitant closed head injury is present. Obtaining a serum amylase immediately postinjury is controversial, as recent studies have shown variable correlation between elevated levels and pancreatic injury.

Pelvis

Pelvic fractures are classically manifested by pain, crepitus, and abnormal motion. Pelvic fracture is a relative contraindication to urethral catheter insertion. Many providers perform a rectal examination, noting tone, tenderness, and in boys, prostate position. If this is done, stool should be tested for blood.

Genitourinary System

If urethral transection is suspected (see earlier discussion), perform a retrograde urethrogram before catheter placement. Diagnostic imaging of the child with hematuria > 50 red blood cells per high-powered field often includes CT scan or occasionally, IV urograms. Management of kidney injury is largely nonoperative except for renal pedicle injuries.

Extremities

Long bone fractures are common but rarely life-threatening. Test for pulses, perfusion, and sensation. Neurovascular compromise requires immediate orthopedic consultation. Delayed diagnosis of fracture may occur when children are comatose; reexamination is necessary to avoid overlooking previously missed fractures. Treatment of open fractures includes antibiotics, tetanus prophylaxis, and orthopedic consultation.

Central Nervous System

Most deaths in children with multisystem trauma are from head injuries, so optimal neurointensive care is important. Significant injuries include diffuse axonal injury; cerebral edema; subdural, subarachnoid, and epidural hematomas; and parenchymal hemorrhages. Spinal cord injury occurs less commonly. Level of consciousness by the AVPU system (see Table 12–4) or Glasgow Coma Scale (see Table 12–5) should be assessed serially. A full sensorimotor examination should be performed. Deficits require immediate neurosurgical consultation and should be considered for a patient with a GCS < 12. Extensor or flexor posturing represents intracranial hypertension, not seizure activity, until proven otherwise. If accompanied by a fixed, dilated pupil, such posturing indicates that a herniation syndrome is present, and mannitol or 3% hypertonic saline should be given if perfusion is normal. Treatment goals include aggressively treating hypotension to optimize cerebral perfusion, providing supplemental oxygen to keep saturations above 90%, achieving eucapnia (end-tidal CO_2 35–40 mm Hg), avoiding hyperthermia, and minimizing painful stimuli. Early rapid sequence intubation, sedation, and paralysis should be considered. Mild prophylactic hyperventilation is no longer recommended, although brief periods of hyperventilation are still indicated in the setting of acute herniation. Seizure activity warrants exclusion of significant intracranial injury. In the trauma setting, seizures are frequently treated with fosphenytoin. The use of high-dose corticosteroids for suspected spinal cord injury has not been prospectively evaluated in children and is not considered standard of care. Corticosteroids are not indicated for head trauma.

Avarello JT, Cantor RM: Pediatric major trauma: An approach to evaluation and management. Emerg Med Clin North Am 2007;25:803 [PMID: 17826219].

Capraro AJ et al: The use of routine laboratory studies as screening tools in pediatric abdominal trauma. Pediatr Emerg Care 2006;22:480.

Eppich WJ, Zonfrillo MR: Emergency department evaluation and management of blunt abdominal trauma in children. Curr Opin Pediatr 2007;19:265–269.

Holmes JF et al: Performance of abdominal ultrasonography in pediatric blunt trauma patients: a meta-analysis. J Pediatr Surg 2007;42(9):1588.

Kellogg ND: Committee on Child Abuse and Neglect: Evaluation of suspected child physical abuse. Pediatrics 2007;119:1232 [PMID: 17545397].

Mendelson KG, Fallat ME: Pediatric Injuries: Prevention to resolution. Surg Clin N Am 2007;87:207–228.

Orenstein JB: Prehospital pediatric airway management. Clin Ped Emerg Med 2006;7:31.

Sayer FT et al: Methylprednisolone treatment in acute spinal cord injury: The myth challenged through a structured analysis of published literature. Spine J 2006;6:335 [PMID: 16651231].

Advanced Trauma Life Support: Available at: http://www.facs.org/trauma/atls/information.html

HEAD INJURY

Closed head injuries range in severity from minor asymptomatic trauma without sequelae to those leading to death.

Even following minor closed head injury, long-term disability and neuropsychiatric sequelae can occur.

ESSENTIALS OF DIAGNOSIS

- Traumatic brain injury is the most common injury in children.
- Rapid acceleration-deceleration forces (eg, the shaken infant) as well as direct trauma to the head can result in brain injury.
- Rapid assessment can be made by evaluating mental status with the Glasgow Coma Scale score and assessing pupillary light response.
- Minor head injuries require a screening evaluation with symptom inventory and complete neurologic examination.

Prevention

Wearing helmets properly during snowsports or while riding bicycles, scooters, skateboards, in-line skates, and horses is a simple preventative strategy. Chlidren as young as 8–9 years old can be taught to do this without parental assistance. The use of all-terrain vehicles (ATVs) is increasing rapidly among. Forty percent of children ride without helmets and 60% without adult supervision while < 5% received safety instruction. Thirty-five percent of all ATV-related deaths occur in children under 16 years old. Restricting use of ATVs by children should prevent head injuries. Counseling families not to use rolling infant walkers is a third important prevention strategy.

Clinical Findings

The history should include the time, mechanism, and details of the injury. Distance of the fall, landing surface, level of consciousness at event, subsequent mental status and activity, amnesia, and vomiting are important details. Physical examination, including a detailed neurologic examination, should be complete and mindful of the mechanism of injury. Look for associated injuries such as mandible fracture, scalp or skull injury, or cervical spine injury. Cerebrospinal fluid or blood from the ears or nose, hemotympanum or the later appearance of periorbital hematomas (raccoon eyes) or Battle sign implies a basilar skull fracture, an indication for pneumococcal vaccine. Obtain vital signs and assess the child's level of consciousness by the AVPU system (see Table 12–4) or Glasgow Coma Scale (see Table 12–5), noting irritability or lethargy; pupillary equality, size, and reaction to light; funduscopic examination; reflexes; body posture; and rectal tone. Always consider child abuse; the injuries observed should be consistent with the history, the child's developmental level, and the mechanism of injury.

Radiographic studies may be indicated. Plain films are not generally indicated. Major morbidity does not result directly from skull fractures, but rather from the associated intracranial injury. A recent multicenter investigation of head injured patients presenting to the ED derived and validated a decision rule for identifying those children at very low risk of clinically important traumatic brain injuries (Figure 12–9). In infants, a normal neurologic examination does not exclude significant intracranial hemorrhage; scalp findings such as large hematomas or concerns of non-accidental trauma should prompt the clinician to consider obtaining imaging.

Differential Diagnosis

In young infants when no history is available, consider sepsis. CNS infection, intoxication, or other medical causes of altered mental status may present similarly to head injuries which often have no external signs of injury.

CONCUSSION (MILD TRAUMATIC BRAIN INJURY)

A concussion is a brief alteration of mental status with or without loss of consciousness and most patients will have a GCS of 15. Somatic, cognitive, and emotional affects may be seen. Headache, amnesia, nausea, and vomiting are common. Ataxia is not uncommon but there are no focal findings on detailed neurologic examination. A CT scan will be normal. Disposition is based on the clinical course and availability of follow-up. The patient may be discharged after a period of observation once a clear trend of improving symptoms is documented. Parents may observe the child at home and return if the child exhibits altered level of consciousness, persistent vomiting, new or worsening symptoms.

Complications

Central Nervous System Infection

Open head injuries (fractures with overlying lacerations) are at risk of infection due to direct contamination. Basilar skull fractures that involve the cribriform plate or middle ear cavity may allow a portal of entry for *Streptococcus pneumoniae.*

Acute Intracranial Hypertension

Close observation will detect early signs and symptoms of intracranial pressure elevation. Early recognition is essential to avoid disastrous outcomes. In addition to traumatic causes, intracranial pressure elevation with or without herniation syndromes may be seen in spontaneous intracranial hemorrhage, CNS infection, hydrocephalus, ruptured arteriovenous malformation, metabolic derangement (eg, diabetic ketoacidosis), ventriculoperitoneal shunt obstruction, or tumor. Symptoms include headache, vision changes, vomiting, gait difficulties, and a progressively decreasing

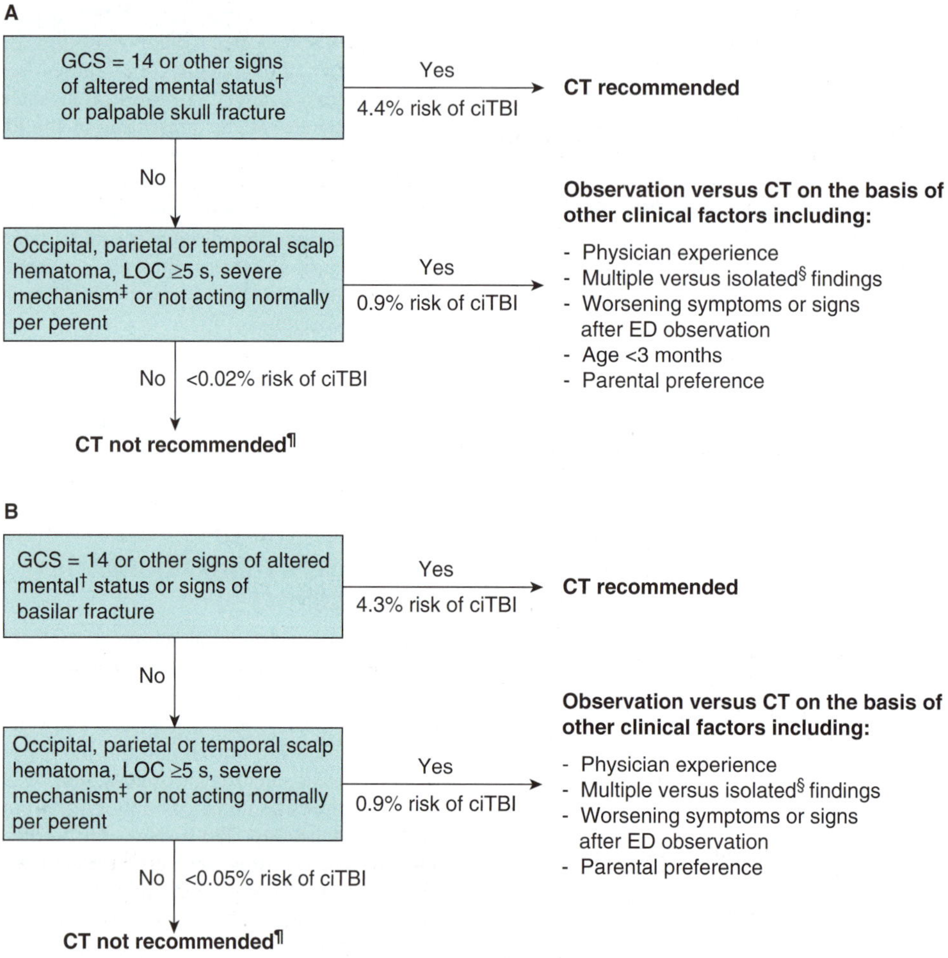

GCS = Glasgow Coma Scale. ciTBI = clinically important traumatic brain injury. LOC = loss of consciousness.
†Other signs of altered mental status: agitation, somnolence repetitive questioning, or slow response to verbal communication.
‡Severe mechanism of injury: motor vehicle crash with patient ejection, death of another passenger, or rollover; pedestrian or bicyclist without helmet struck by motorized vehicle; falls of more than 3 feet (or more than 5 feet for panel B); or head struck by a high-impact object.
§Patients with certain isolated findings (ie, with no other findings suggestive of traumatic brain injury), such as isolated LOC, isolated headache, isolated vomiting, and certain type of isolated scalp hematomas in infants older than 3 months, have a risk of ciTBI substantially lower than 1%.
¶Risk of ciTBI exceedingly low, generally lower than risk of CT-induced malignancies. Therefore, CT scans are not indicated for most patients in this group.

Adapted from *The Lancet* 374, Kuppermann et al, Identification of children at very low risk of clinically-important brain injuries after head trauma: a prospective cohort study. pp1160-1170. © 2009 with permission from Elsevier.

▲ **Figure 12–9.** Suggested CT algorithm for children younger than 2 years (A) and for those aged 2 years and older (B) with GCS scores 14–15 after head trauma.

level of consciousness. Papilledema is a cardinal sign of increased intracranial pressure. Other signs may include stiff neck, cranial nerve palsies, and progressive hemiparesis. Cushing triad (bradycardia, hypertension, and irregular respirations) is a late and ominous finding. Consider CT scan before lumbar puncture if there is concern about intracranial pressure elevation because of the risk of precipitating herniation. Lumbar puncture should be deferred if the patient is unstable.

Treatment—Therapy for elevated intracranial pressure must be swift and aggressive. Strict attention to adequate oxygenation, ventilation, and perfusion is paramount. Controlled rapid sequence intubation with appropriate sedation, muscle relaxation, agents to reduce the intracranial pressure elevation that accompanies intubation, and avoidance of hypoperfusion and hypoxemia are all important aspects of treatment. Brief periods of hyperventilation are reserved for acute herniation. Mannitol (0.5 g/kg IV), an osmotic diuretic, will reduce brain water. Hypertonic saline (3%; 4–6 mL/kg bolus doses or 1–2 mL/kg/hr infusion) also may be used. These measures may acutely lower intracranial pressure. Fluid infusion and, ultimately, pressors should be used to maintain normal arterial blood pressure and peripheral perfusion, if necessary. Adjunctive measures include elevating the head of the bed 30 degrees, treating hyperpyrexia and pain, and maintaining the head in a midline position. Obtain immediate neurosurgical evaluation. Further details about management of intracranial hypertension, (cerebral edema) are presented in Chapter 14.

Prognosis

Patients with mild traumatic brain injury may be discharged with detailed written instructions, if the examination remains normal after a period of observation, parental supervision and follow-up are appropriate. Children should not return to athletics until free of symptoms at rest and have progressed through a graduated return-to-play protocol. Most children recover fully. Persistent symptoms should prompt referral for rehabilitation and/or neuropsychological evaluation.

The prognosis for children with moderate to severe injuries depends on many factors including severity of initial injury, presence of hypoxia or ischemia, development and subsequent management of intracranial hypertension, and associated injuries.

Blake G, Velikonja D, Pepper V, Jilderda I, Georgiou G: Evaluating an in-school injury prevention programme's effect on children's helmet wearing habits. Brain Inj 2008;22(6)501–507 [PMID: 18465391].

Campbell BT, Kelliher KM, Borrup K, Corsi J, Saleheen H, Bourque MD, Lapidus G: All-terrain vehicle riding among youth: how do they fair? J Ped Surg 2010;45(5):925–929 [PMID: 20438928].

Dias MS: Traumatic brain and spinal cord injury. Pediatr Clin North Am 2004;51:271 [PMID: 15062672].

Kuppermann N, Holmes JF, Dayan PS, Hoyle JD Jr, Atabaki SM, Holubkov R et al: Identification of children at very low risk of clinically-important brain injuries after head trauma: A prospective cohort study. Lancet 2009;374(9696):1160–1170 [PMID: 19758692].

McCrory P et al: Consensus statement on concussion in sport: The 3rd international conference on concussion in sport. Neurosurgery 2009;44(4):434 [PMID: 19593427].

Mendelson KG: Pediatric injuries: Prevention to resolution. Surg Clin North Am 2007;87(1):207–228 [PMID: 17127129].

Pardes Berger R, Adelson PD: Evaluation and management of pediatric head trauma in the emergency department: Current concepts and state-of-the-art research. Clin Ped Emerg Med 2005;6:8.

BURNS

THERMAL BURNS

ESSENTIALS OF DIAGNOSIS & TYPICAL FEATURES

- Burn classification depends on location and extent of injury.
- Burns of the hands, feet, face, eyes, ears, and perineum are always considered to be major burns.

Thermal injury is a major cause of accidental death and disfigurement in children. Pain, morbidity, the association with child abuse, and the preventable nature of burns constitute an area of major concern in pediatrics. Common causes include hot water or food, appliances, flames, grills, vehicle-related burns, and curling irons. Burns occur commonly in toddlers—in boys more frequently than in girls.

Prevention

The vast majority of burns are preventable. Containers of hot liquids should be placed as far as possible from counter edges. Water heater thermostats should be turned to less than 120°F (49°C). Chemicals and electrical cords should be kept out of reach. Home visitation programs have been shown to reduce rates of electrical burns. Sunscreen should be applied and hats worn in children over 6 months old when participating in outdoor activities. Overall sun exposure should be minimized in this population.

Clinical Findings

Burns are classified clinically according to the nature of the burn and the extent and thickness. Superficial burns are painful, dry, red, and hypersensitive. Sunburn is a common example. Healing occurs with minimal damage to epidermis. Partial-thickness burns are subgrouped as superficial or deep, depending on appearance and healing time. Superficial partial-thickness burns are red and often blister. Deep partial-thickness burns are white and dry, blanch with pressure, and the involved skin has decreased sensitivity to pain. Full-thickness burns affect all epidermal and dermal elements, leaving devascularized skin. The wound is white or black, dry, depressed, leathery in appearance, and insensate. Unless skin grafting is provided, the scar will be hard, uneven, and fibrotic. Deep full-thickness, or subdermal, burns are the most severe, extending through all layers of skin as well as into the underlying fascia, muscle, and possibly bone. Singing of nasal or facial hair, carbonaceous material of the nose and mouth, and stridor may be present with inhalational burns that may herald critical airway compromise.

Differential Diagnosis

The differential diagnosis of burns is limited when a history is provided. In the preverbal child when no history is available, the primary alternate consideration is cellulitis.

Complications

Superficial and superficial partial-thickness burns typically heal well. Deep partial- and full-thickness burns are at risk of scarring. Loss of barrier function predisposes to infection. Damage to deeper tissues in full-thickness burns may result in loss of function, contractures, and in the case of circumferential burns, compartment syndrome. Renal failure secondary to myoglobinuria or microangiopathic hemolysis and hyperkalemia from rhabdomyolysis is a concern.

Treatment

Management depends on the depth and extent of injury. Burn extent can be classified as major or minor. Minor burns are less than 10% of the body surface area (BSA) for superficial and partial-thickness burns, or less than 2% for full-thickness burns. Partial- or full-thickness burns of the hands, feet, face, eyes, ears, and perineum are considered major.

A. Superficial and Partial-Thickness Burns

These injuries can generally be treated in the outpatient setting. Effective analgesia should be provided, and repeated as indicated by the child. Oral codeine or parenteral narcotics are indicated. Superficial burns are treated with cool compresses and analgesia. Treatment of partial-thickness burns with blisters consists of antiseptic cleansing, topical antimicrobial coverage, and observation for infection. Blisters appear early in deeper partial-thickness burns and, if open, may be debrided. Alternatively, the blister may be used as a protective flap after cleaning and dressing. After debridement, the wound should be cleansed with dilute (1%–5%) povidone-iodine solution, thoroughly washed with normal saline, and covered with topical antibiotic. The wound should be protected with a bulky dressing and reexamined within 24 hours and serially thereafter. Wounds with a potential to cause disfigurement or functional impairment—especially wounds of the face, hands, digits, or perineum—should be referred promptly to a burn surgeon. Outpatient analgesia should be provided on discharge.

B. Full-Thickness, Deep or Extensive Partial-Thickness, and Subdermal Burns

Major burns require particular attention to the ABCs of trauma management. Early establishment of an artificial airway is critical with oral or nasal burns because of their association with inhalation injuries and critical airway narrowing.

The protocol for the primary survey should be followed (see earlier discussion). There may be inhalation injury from carbon monoxide, cyanide, or other toxic products. A nasogastric tube and bladder catheter should be placed. The secondary survey should ascertain whether any other injuries are present, including those suggestive of abuse.

Fluid resuscitation should be based upon clinical assessment of volume status. Greater fluid losses are expected due to increased capillary permeability and denuded skin. Once adequate intravascular volume is achieved, appropriate fluids that account for increased losses are required. Fluid needs are based on examination findings, percentage of body surface area burned, depth, and age. Maintaining normal intravascular pressure and replacing fluid losses are essential. Figure 12–10 shows percentages of body surface area by body part in infants and children. The Parkland formula for fluid therapy is 4 mL/kg/% body surface area burned for the first 24 hours, with half administered in the first 8 hours, in addition to maintenance rates.

Indications for admission include major burns as previously defined, uncertainty of follow-up, suspicion of abuse, presence of upper airway injury, explosion, inhalation, electrical or chemical burns, burns associated with fractures, or the need for parenteral pain control. Children with chronic metabolic or connective tissue diseases and infants deserve hospitalization. Children with subdermal burns require immediate hospitalization at a burn center under the care of a burn specialist, fluid resuscitation, debridement of the wound, and placement of temporary wound coverage. Intensive insulin therapy can reduce morbidity in patients with > 30% BSA involvement.

Prognosis

Outcome depends on many factors. In general, the greater the surface area and depth of burn injury, the greater the risk of long-term morbidity and mortality.

ELECTRICAL BURNS

Even brief contact with a high-voltage source will result in a contact burn. These may be treated according to the above guidelines. When an infant or toddler bites an electric cord, burns to the commissure of the lips occur that appear gray

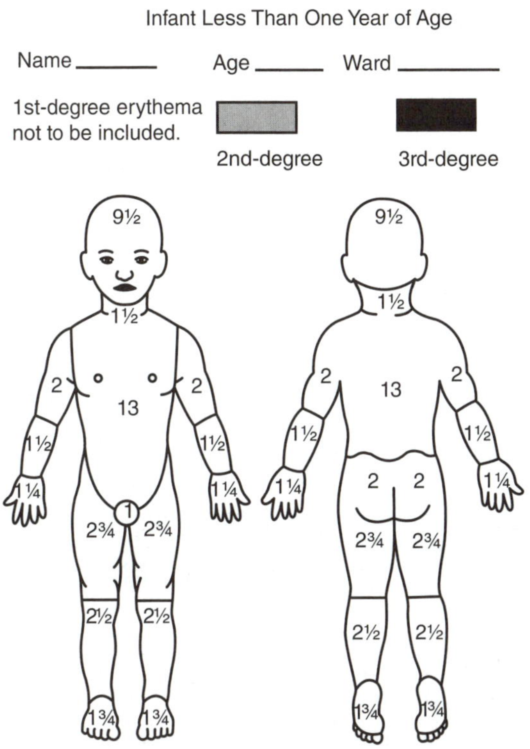

Variations From Adults Distribution in Infants and Children (in Percent).

	Newborn	1 Year	5 Years	10 Years
Head	19	17	13	11
Both thighs	11	13	16	17
Both lower legs	10	10	11	12
Neck	2			
Anterior trunk	13			
Posterior trunk	13			
Both upper arms	8			
Both lower arms	6			
Both hands	5			
Both buttocks	6			
Both feet	7			
Genitalia	1			
	100			

(Neck through Genitalia: These percentages remain constant at all ages)

▲ **Figure 12–10.** Lund and Browder modification of Berkow scale for estimating extent of burns. (The table under the illustration is after Berkow.)

and necrotic, with surrounding erythema. A late complication of this injury is labial artery hemorrhage. If an arc is created with passage of current through the body, the pattern of the thermal injury will depend on the path of the current; therefore, search for an exit wound and internal injuries. Extensive damage to deep tissues may occur. Current traversing the heart may cause nonperfusing arrhythmias. Neurologic effects of electrical burns can be immediate (eg, confusion, disorientation, peripheral nerve injury), delayed (eg, nerve damage in the thrombosed limb after compartment syndrome), or late (eg, impaired concentration or memory).

Duffy BJ et al: Assessment, triage, and early management of burns in children. Clin Ped Emerg Med 2006;7:82.

Jeschke MG, Kulp GA, Kraft R, Finnerty CC, Mlcak R et al: Intensive insulin therapy in severely burned pediatric patients: A prospective randomized trial. Am J Respir Crit Care Med 2010;182(3):351–359 [PMID: 20395554].

Odendaal W, van Niekerk A, Jordaan E, Seedat M: The impact of a home visitation programme on household hazards associated with unintentional childhood injuries: A randomised controlled trial. Accid Anal Prev 2009;41(1):183–190 [PMID: 19114153].

DISORDERS DUE TO ALTERED ENVIRONMENTAL TEMPERATURE

HEAT-RELATED ILLNESSES & HEAT STROKE

ESSENTIALS OF DIAGNOSIS

- Children are at increased risk due to unique responses to heat stress.
- Heat illness is a spectrum ranging from heat cramps to life-threatening heat stroke.
- A high index of suspicion is required to make the diagnosis given the lack of specific symptoms and a usually normal or only slightly elevated temperature.

Prevention

Exposure to extremes of temperature for extended periods should be avoided. Plan athletic activities for early morning or late afternoon and evening to avoid the hottest part of the days. Providing adequate water, shade, and rest periods is crucial.

Clinical Findings

Heat cramps are characterized by brief, severe cramping (not rigidity) of skeletal or abdominal muscles following exertion. Core body temperature is normal or slightly elevated. There may be associated hyponatremia, hypochloremia, and rarely, hypokalemia but laboratory evaluation is not routinely necessary.

Heat exhaustion includes multiple and often vague constitutional symptoms manifesting after heat exposure. Patients continue to sweat and have varying proportions of salt and water depletion. Core temperatures should be monitored frequently and are often normal or slightly increased. Presenting symptoms and signs include weakness, fatigue, headache, disorientation, pallor, thirst, nausea and vomiting, and occasionally muscle cramps without CNS dysfunction. Shock may be present.

Heat stroke represents failure of thermoregulation and is life-threatening. Diagnosis is based on a rectal temperature above 40.6°C with associated neurologic signs in a patient with an exposure history. Lack of sweating is **not** a necessary criterion. Symptoms are similar to those of heat exhaustion, but CNS dysfunction is more prominent. Patients with heat stroke are often incoherent and combative. In more severe cases, vomiting, shivering, coma, seizures, nuchal rigidity, and posturing may be present. Cardiac output may be high, low, or normal. Cellular hypoxia, enzyme dysfunction, and disrupted cell membranes lead to global end-organ derangements: rhabdomyolysis, myocardial necrosis, electrolyte abnormalities, acute tubular necrosis and renal failure, hepatic degeneration, acute respiratory distress syndrome, and disseminated intravascular coagulation.

Differential Diagnosis

Viral gastroenteritis, sepsis and other infectious processes, neuroleptic malignant syndrome, malignant hyperthermia, and anticholinergic poisoning may present similarly.

Treatment

Removal from a hot environment and removing clothing is the first step in managing any heat-related illness. **Heat cramps** typically respond to rest and rehydration with electrolyte solutions. More severe cramping and **heat exhaustion** should prompt evaluation of electrolytes to guide IV fluid rehydration. Heat cramps and heat exhaustion can be prevented by acclimatization and liberal water and salt intake during exercise.

Heat Stroke Management

1. Address the ABCs (airway, breathing, circulation), and administer 100% oxygen.
2. Administer IV fluids: isotonic crystalloid for hypotension, 5% dextrose normal saline for maintenance. Consider central venous pressure monitoring.
3. Once resuscitative efforts have begun, cool the patient by removing clothing; misting with cool water; applying ice at neck, groin, and axillae; fanning; and other cooling devices. Active cooling measures should be discontinued once core temperature reaches 39°C to prevent shivering.
4. Place monitors, check rectal temperatures continuously, and place a Foley catheter and nasogastric tube.
5. Order laboratory tests: complete blood count; electrolytes; glucose; creatinine; prothrombin time and partial thromboplastin time; creatine kinase; liver function tests; arterial blood gases; urinalysis; and serum calcium, magnesium, and phosphate.
6. Admit to the pediatric intensive care unit.

Prognosis

The prognosis for heat cramps and heat exhaustion is excellent. A full recovery is the rule. Patients with heat stroke are at risk of end organ damage due to volume depletion, rhabdomyolysis, direct renal injury, hepatocellular injury, and disseminated intravascular coagulation (DIC); however, even in this critically ill population, some children recover fully with intensive management.

HYPOTHERMIA

ESSENTIALS OF DIAGNOSIS

- Hypothermia is defined as a core temperature of < 35°C.
- Children are at increased risk due to a greater body surface area-weight ratio.
- In children, hypothermia is most commonly associated with water submersion.

Prevention

Given the high association with submersion injuries, children should be carefully monitored around water. Proper use of life vests is critical.

Clinical Findings

Clinical manifestations of hypothermia vary with severity of body temperature depression. As core temperature falls, a variety of mechanisms begin to conserve and produce heat. Peripheral vasoconstriction allows optimal maintenance of core temperature. Heat production can be increased by a hypothalamic-mediated increase in muscle tone and metabolism. Shivering increases heat production to two to four times the basal levels. Severe cases (< 28°C) mimic death: patients are pale or cyanotic, pupils may be fixed and dilated, muscles are rigid, and there may be no palpable pulses. Heart rates as low as 4–6 beats/min may provide adequate perfusion, because of lowered metabolic needs in severe hypothermia. Besides cold exposure, disorders that cause incidental hypothermia include sepsis, metabolic derangements, ingestions, CNS disorders, and endocrinopathies. Neonates, trauma victims, intoxicated patients, and the chronically disabled are particularly at risk. Mortality rates are high and are related to the underlying disorder. Because findings resulting from primary hypothermia may be easily confused with those of postmortem changes, death is not pronounced until the patient has been rewarmed and remains unresponsive to resuscitative efforts. Children with a core temperature as low as 19°C have survived neurologically intact.

Treatment

Seriously ill children should have core temperature quickly determined. Conversely, moderate therapeutic hypothermia (32–34°C) following hypoxic-ischemic CNS insult and isolated traumatic brain injury is now recommended as potentially beneficial for CNS recovery.

A. General Supportive Measures

Management of hypothermia is largely supportive. Core body temperature must be continuously documented; monitor with a low-reading indwelling rectal thermometer. Patients must be handled gently, because the hypothermic myocardium is exquisitely sensitive and prone to arrhythmias. Ventricular fibrillation may occur spontaneously or as a result of minor handling or invasive procedures. If asystole or ventricular fibrillation is present on the cardiac monitor, perform chest compressions and use standard pediatric advanced life support techniques as indicated. Defibrillation and pharmacologic therapy should be initiated as appropriate but may not be successful until core rewarming has occurred. Spontaneous reversion to sinus rhythm at 28–30°C may take place as rewarming proceeds.

B. Rewarming

Remove wet clothing. Rewarming techniques are categorized as passive external, active external, or active core rewarming. The method chosen is based on the degree of hypothermia. Passive rewarming, such as covering with blankets, is appropriate only for mild cases (> 33°C). Active external rewarming methods include warming lights, thermal mattresses or electric warming blankets, immersion in warm baths, and hot water bottles or warmed bags of IV solutions. One must be aware of the potential for core temperature depression after rewarming has begun, as vasodilation allows cooler peripheral blood to be distributed to the core circulation. This phenomenon is called afterdrop.

Active core rewarming techniques are used alone or in combination with active external warming for moderate to severe hypothermia. The techniques include the delivery of warmed, humidified oxygen and the use of warmed (to 40°C) fluids for IV replacement, peritoneal dialysis, and mediastinal lavage. Bladder and bowel irrigation are not generally effective because of low surface areas for temperature exchange. Extracorporeal blood rewarming achieves controlled core rewarming, can stabilize volume and electrolyte disturbances, and is maximally effective (Table 12–6). An established protocol for use of this technique will likely increase the chances of neurologically intact survival.

Prognosis

As with all trauma, recovery of the hypothermia victim is multifactorial. If associated with submersion injury (see next), the CNS anoxic injuries and lung injury play a major role.

Table 12–6. Management of hypothermia.

General measures
Remove wet clothing.
Administer warmed and humidified 100% oxygen.
Monitor core temperature, heart and respiratory rates, and blood pressure continuously.
Consider central venous pressure determination for severe hypothermia.
Laboratory studies
Complete blood count and platelets.
Serum electrolytes, glucose, creatinine, amylase.
Prothrombin time, partial thromboplastin time.
Arterial blood gases.
Consider toxicology screen.
Treatment
Correct hypoxemia, hypercapnia, pH < 7.2, clotting abnormalities, and glucose and electrolyte disturbances.
Start rewarming techniques: passive, active (core and external), depending on degree of hypothermia.
Replace intravascular volume with warmed intravenous crystalloid infusion at 42°C.
Treat asystole and ventricular fibrillation per PALS protocols. Continue cardiac massage at least until core temperature reaches 30°C, when defibrillation is more likely to be effective.

PALS, pediatric advanced life support.

Grubenhoff JA et al: Heat-related illnesses. Clin Ped Emerg Med 2007;8:59.

Scaife ER, Connors RC, Morris SE, Nichol PF, Black RE, Matlak ME et al: An established extracorporeal membrane oxygenation protocol promotes survival in extreme hypothermia. J Pediatr Surg 2007;42(12):2012–2016 [PMID: 18082698].

Trujillo MH, Bellorin-Font E, Fragachan CF, Perret-Gentil R: Multiple organ failure following near fatal exertional heat stroke. J Intensive Care Med 2009;24(1):72–78 [PMID: 19017664].

Ulrich AS, Rathlev NK: Hypothermia and localized cold injuries. Emerg Med Clin North Am 2004;22:281 [PMID: 15163568].

SUBMERSION INJURIES

ESSENTIALS OF DIAGNOSIS

- CNS and pulmonary injuries account for major morbidity.
- Child may appear well at presentation, but late CNS and pulmonary changes can occur hours later.
- Minimum observation period is 8–12 hours.

Prevention

Recently the World Health Organization redefined drowning as the process of experiencing respiratory impairment from submersion/immersion in liquid. The terms wet or dry drowning, near-drowning and others suffer from vagueness and cause difficulty when collecting injury surveillance data; thus, these terms are no longer used. Water hazards are ubiquitous including lakes and streams, swimming pools, bathtubs, and even toilets, buckets, and washing machines. Risk factors include epilepsy, alcohol, and lack of supervision. Males predominate in submersion deaths, as in most other nonintentional deaths. Prevention is paramount; fencing around public pools, use of life vests, avoiding swimming alone, and adequate supervision are important. Swim lessons may have a role in a comprehensive prevention strategy, even for children 1–4 years of age.

Pathogenesis

Major morbidity stems from CNS and pulmonary insult. Laryngospasm or breath-holding may lead to loss of consciousness and cardiovascular collapse before aspiration can occur (dry drowning). Anoxia from laryngospasm or aspiration leads to irreversible CNS damage after only 4–6 minutes. A child must fall through ice or directly into icy water for cerebral metabolism to be slowed sufficiently by hypothermia to provide protection from anoxic damage.

Clinical Findings

Depending on the duration of submersion and any protective hypothermia effects, children may appear clinically dead or completely normal. Cough, nasal flaring, grunting, retractions, wheezes and/or rales, and cyanosis may be present. Observation over time assists with prognosis. The child who has been rewarmed to at least 33°C and is still apneic and pulseless will probably not survive to discharge or will be left with severe neurologic deficits. Until a determination of brain death can be made, however, aggressive resuscitation should be continued in a patient with return of circulation. Cardiovascular changes include myocardial depression and arrhythmias. Electrolyte alterations are generally slight. Unless hemolysis occurs, hemoglobin concentrations also change only slightly. Chest radiographs may be normal or may show signs of pulmonary edema. Over time, children may develop acute respiratory distress syndrome (ARDS).

Treatment

Consider possible associated injuries, including head or neck trauma. For children who appear well initially, observation for 8–12 hours will detect late pulmonary compromise or changes in neurologic status. Respiratory distress, an abnormal chest radiograph, abnormal arterial blood gases, or hypoxemia by pulse oximetry indicates the need for treatment with supplemental oxygen, cardiopulmonary monitoring, and frequent reassessment. Serially assess respiratory distress and mental status. Signs of pulmonary infection may appear many hours after the submersion event.

Patients who are in coma and who require mechanical ventilation have a high risk of anoxic encephalopathy. The value of therapy with hyperventilation, corticosteroids, therapeutic hypothermia, and barbiturates remains unproved.

Prognosis

Survival of the near-drowning victim depends on the duration of anoxia and the degree of lung injury. Children experiencing brief submersion with effective, high quality resuscitation are likely to recover without sequelae.

Brenner RA, Taneja GS, Haynie DL, Trumble AC, Qian C et al: Association between swimming lessons and drowning in childhood: A case-control study. Arch Pediatr Adolesc Med 2009;163(3):203–210 [PMID: 19255386].

Weiss, J and The committee on injury, violence, and poison prevention: American Academy of Pediatrics. Technical Report—Prevention of Drowning. Pediatrics 2010;126(1):e253–e262 [PMID: 20498167].

ANIMAL & HUMAN BITES

Bites account for a large number of visits to the emergency department. Most fatalities are due to dog bites. However, human and cat bites cause the majority of infected bite wounds.

DOG BITES

Boys are bitten more frequently than girls, and the dog is known by the victim in most cases. Younger children have a higher incidence of head and neck wounds, whereas school-age children are bitten most often on the upper extremities.

Dog bites are treated similarly to other wounds: high-pressure, high-volume (> 1 L) irrigation with normal saline, debridement of any devitalized tissue, removal of foreign matter, and tetanus prophylaxis. The risk of rabies from dogs is low in developed countries, but rabies prophylaxis should be considered when appropriate. Wounds should be sutured only if necessary for cosmetic reasons because wound closure increases the risk of infection. Do not use tissue adhesives for closure. Prophylactic antibiotics have not been proven to decrease rates of infection in low-risk dog bite wounds not involving the hands or feet. If a bite involves a joint, periosteum, or neurovascular bundle, prompt orthopedic surgery consultation should be obtained.

Pathogens that infect dog bites include *Pasteurella canis* and *Pasteurella multocida*, streptococci, staphylococci, and anaerobes. Infected dog bites can be treated with penicillin for *P multocida*, and broad-spectrum coverage can be provided by amoxicillin and clavulanic acid or cephalexin (see dose for cat bites in the next section). Complications of dog bites include scarring, CNS infections, septic arthritis, osteomyelitis, endocarditis, and sepsis.

CAT BITES

Cat-inflicted wounds occur more frequently in girls, and their principal complication is infection. The infection risk is higher in cat bites than dog bites because cat bites produce a puncture wound. Management is similar to that for dog bites. Cat wounds should *not* be sutured except when absolutely necessary for cosmetic reasons. *P multocida* is the most common pathogen. Cat bites create a puncture-wound inoculum, and prophylactic antibiotics (penicillin plus cephalexin, or amoxicillin and clavulanic acid) are recommended. The dose of amoxicillin trihydrate and clavulanic acid should be on the high side of recommended dosage in order to ensure adequate tissue penetration both in dog and cat bites. The dosage of the amoxicillin component should be 80 mg/kg/24 h in three divided doses. The maximum dosage is 2 g/24 h. Scratches or bites from cats may also result in cat scratch disease. Strongly consider admission and IV antibiotics for infected wounds especially on the hands and feet.

HUMAN BITES

Most human bites occur during fights. *P multocida* is not a known pathogen in human bites; cultures most commonly grow streptococci, staphylococci, anaerobes, and *Eikenella corrodens*. Hand wounds and deep wounds should be treated with antibiotic coverage against *E corrodens* and gram-positive pathogens by a penicillinase-resistant antibiotic. Wound management is the same as for dog bites. Only severe lacerations involving the face should be sutured. Other wounds can be managed by delayed primary closure or healing by secondary intention. A major complication of human bite wounds is infection of the metacarpophalangeal joints. A hand surgeon should evaluate clenched-fist injuries from human bites. Operative debridement is followed in many cases by IV antibiotics.

Younggren BN: Emergency management of difficulty wounds: Part I. Emerg Med Clin North Am 2007;25:101 [PMID: 17400075].

PROCEDURAL SEDATION & ANALGESIA (PSA)

Relief of pain and anxiety is a paramount concept in the provision of acute care pediatrics, and should be considered at all times. Many agents also have amnestic properties. Parenteral agents can be effective and safe and produce few side effects if used judiciously.

Conditions such as fracture reduction, laceration repair, burn care, sexual assault examinations, lumbar puncture, and diagnostic procedures such as CT and magnetic resonance imaging may all be performed more effectively and compassionately if effective sedation or analgesia is used. The clinician should decide whether procedures will require sedation, analgesia, or both, and then choose agents accordingly.

Safe and effective sedation requires thorough knowledge of the selected agent and its side effects, as well as suitable monitoring devices, resuscitative medications, equipment, and personnel. The decision to perform PSA must be patient-oriented and tailored to specific procedural needs, while ensuring the child's safety throughout the procedure. In order to successfully complete this task, a thorough preprocedural assessment should be completed, including a directed history and physical examination. Risks, benefits, and limitations of the procedure should be discussed with the parent or guardian and informed; verbal consent must be obtained. PSA then proceeds as follows:

1. Choose the appropriate medication(s).
2. Ensure appropriate NPO (nothing-by-mouth) status for 2–6 hours, depending on age and type of intake. For certain emergency procedures, suboptimal NPO status may be allowed, with attendant risks identified.
3. Establish vascular access as required.
4. Ensure that resuscitative equipment and personnel are readily available. Attach appropriate monitoring devices, as indicated.
5. Give the agent selected, with continuous monitoring for side effects. A dedicated observer, usually a nurse, should monitor the patient at all times. Respiratory effort, perfusion, and mental status should be assessed and documented serially.
6. Titrate the medication to achieve the desired sedation level. The ideal level depends on sedation goals and procedure type. PSA goals in the emergency department setting usually involve minimal or moderate sedation. Minimal sedation is a state in which the patient's sensorium is dulled, but he is still responsive to verbal stimuli. Moderate sedation is a depression of consciousness in which the child responds to tactile stimuli. In both cases, airway reflexes are preserved. It is important to remember that sedation is a continuum and the child may drift to deeper, unintended levels of sedation.
7. Continue monitoring the patient after the procedure has finished and the child has returned to baseline mental status. Once a painful stimulus has been corrected, mental status and respiratory drive can decrease.
8. Criteria for discharge include the child's ability to sit unassisted, take oral fluids, and answer verbal commands. A PSA discharge handout should be given, with precautions for close observation and avoidance of potentially dangerous activities.

The following are some commonly used sedatives and analgesics:

1. Midazolam—This agent has particular usefulness in pediatrics due to its safety, rapid onset, and short half-life. Administration may be oral, rectal, intranasal, intramuscular, or IV. When given slowly intranasally, the drug's kinetics are similar as when given intravenously, although many patients report a burning sensation with administration. Oral or rectal administration results in relatively delayed onset, and titration is difficult. Intramuscular injections can be combined with opioid analgesics if systemic analgesia is desired. IV administration allows optimal ability to titrate dosing to the desired sedation level. It is best to place an IV for complicated or prolonged procedures to facilitate redosing, which also provides IV access if resuscitation becomes necessary. Potential side effects of midazolam include cardiorespiratory depression.

2. Barbiturates—This class of agents (eg, pentobarbital) has the benefit of minimizing movement during procedures, which makes them advantageous for diagnostic studies such as CT or magnetic resonance imaging. Rectal administration of thiopental is safe and effective. Onset of action with IV administration is rapid. Potential side effects, although uncommon, include cardiorespiratory depression and laryngospasm.

3. Narcotics—Agents such as fentanyl and morphine have powerful analgesic and sedative effects and can be combined with anxiolytics such as benzodiazepines. Desired and adverse effects, such as respiratory depression, are potentiated when benzodiazepines and narcotics or barbiturates are given together. Therefore, sedative doses should be reduced when sedatives and analgesics are given together.

4. Ketamine—A commonly used drug in the emergency department, ketamine provides analgesia, anxiolysis, and amnesia while allowing the child to retain protective airway reflexes and cardiovascular stability. In addition to providing "dissociative sedation," this sympathomimetic drug also increases heart rate and blood pressure. Side effects include salivation (therefore, it is usually given with glycopyrrolate as an antisalivation agent), laryngospasm (rarely), nystagmus, emergence reactions, and vomiting. With comprehensive knowledge of this medication, its use can be a significant advantage to children.

5. Propofol—Propofol is a nonopioid, nonbarbiturate sedative that is highly effective. It is finding increased use as an adjunct to analgesia for painful procedures in the emergency department. Onset of action and recovery are rapid. Side effects include transient hypotension and dose-dependent respiratory depression or apnea. Careful monitoring is essential. New research indicates that the combination of ketamine and propofol (ketofol) may be beneficial in children, allowing for faster recovery times, less vomiting and similar efficacy and adverse event profile than use of either agent alone.

American Academy of Pediatrics; American Academy of Pediatric Dentistry; Coté CJ et al: Guidelines for monitoring and management of pediatric patients during and after sedation for diagnostic and therapeutic procedures: An update. Pediatrics 2006;18:2587 [PMID: 17142550].

Doyle L, Colletti JE: Pediatric procedural sedation and analgesia. Pediatr Clin North Am 2006;53:279 [PMID: 16574526].

Godwin SA et al: Clinical policy: Procedural sedation and analgesia in the emergency department. Ann Emerg Med 2005;45:177 [PMID: 15671976].

Krauss B, Green SM: Procedural sedation and analgesia in children. Lancet 2006;367:766 [PMID: 16517277].

Meyer S et al: Sedation and analgesia for brief diagnostic and therapeutic procedures in children. Eur J Pediatr 2007;166:291 [PMID: 17205245].

Roback MG et al: Adverse events associated with procedural sedation and analgesia in a pediatric emergency department: A comparison of common parenteral drugs. Acad Emerg Med 2005;12:508 [PMID: 15930401].

Shah A et al: A blinded, randomized control trial to evaluate ketamine/propofol versus ketamine alone for procedural sedation in children. Ann Emerg Med 2011;57(5):425–433.

Poisoning

13

Barry H. Rumack, MD
Richard C. Dart, MD, PhD

Accidental and intentional exposures to toxic substances occur in children of all ages. Children younger than age 6 years are primarily involved in accidental exposures, with the peak incidence in 2-year-olds. Of the more than 2.5 million exposures reported by the American Association of Poison Control Centers' National Poison Data System in 2008, 51% occurred in children aged 5 years and younger, 6% in those aged 6–12 years, and 7% in those aged 13–19 years. Young children are occasionally exposed to intentional poisoning through the actions of parents or caregivers. Administration of agents such as diphenhydramine to induce sleep in a day-care setting, Munchausen syndrome by proxy to obtain parental secondary gain, or deliberate harm should be suspected when the history is not consistent. Involvement of child abuse specialists is very helpful in these cases. (See Chapter 8.) Adolescents are involved in intentional episodes when attempting suicide or experimenting with various drugs and agents. In some locales, small-scale industrial or manufacturing processes may be associated with homes and farms, and exposures to hazardous substances should be considered in the history.

Bronstein AC et al: 2008 Annual Report of the American Association of Poison Control Centers' National Poison Data System (NPDS). Clin Toxicol (Phila) 2007;45:815 [PMID: 18163234].

PHARMACOLOGIC PRINCIPLES OF TOXICOLOGY

In the evaluation of the poisoned patient, it is important to compare the anticipated pharmacologic or toxic effects with the patient's clinical presentation. If the history is that the patient ingested a tranquilizer 30 minutes ago, but the clinical examination reveals dilated pupils, tachycardia, dry mouth, absent bowel sounds, and active hallucinations—clearly anticholinergic toxicity—diagnosis and therapy should proceed accordingly.

LD_{50}

Estimates of the LD_{50} (the amount per kilogram of body weight of a drug required to kill 50% of a group of experimental animals) or median lethal dose are of little clinical value in humans. It is usually impossible to determine with accuracy the amount swallowed or absorbed, the metabolic status of the patient, or in which patients the response to the agent will be atypical. Furthermore, these values are often not valid in humans even if the history is accurate.

Half-Life ($t_{1/2}$)

The $t_{1/2}$ of an agent must be interpreted carefully. Most published $t_{1/2}$ values are for therapeutic dosages. The $t_{1/2}$ may increase as the quantity of the ingested substance increases for many common intoxicants such as salicylates. One cannot rely on the published $t_{1/2}$ for salicylate (2 hours) to assume rapid elimination of the drug. In an acute salicylate overdose (150 mg/kg), the apparent $t_{1/2}$ is prolonged to 24–30 hours.

Volume of Distribution

The volume of distribution (Vd) of a drug is determined by dividing the amount of drug absorbed by the blood level. With theophylline, for example, the Vd is 0.46 L/kg body weight, or 32 L in an average adult. In contrast, digoxin distributes well beyond total body water. Because the calculation produces a volume above body weight, this figure is referred to as an "apparent volume of distribution" (Table 13–1).

Body Burden

Using the pharmacokinetic principles permits a practical determination of the absorbed dose and permits an understanding of the patients status as to whether a therapeutic administration or an overdose has occurred. A 20-kg child with an acetaminophen blood level reported as 200 mcg/mL (equivalent to 200 mg/L) would have a body burden of 4000 mg of acetaminophen. This is ascertained by taking the volume

Table 13–1. Some examples of pK_a and Vd.[a]

Drug	pK_a	Diuresis	Dialysis	Apparent Vd
Amobarbital	7.9	No	No	200–300% body weight
Amphetamine	9.8	No	Yes	60% body weight
Aspirin	3.5	Alkaline	Yes	15–40% body weight
Chlorpromazine	9.3	No	No	40–50 L/kg (2800–3500% body weight)
Codeine	8.2	No	No	5–10 L/kg (350–700% body weight)
Desipramine	10.2	No	No	30–40 L/kg (2100–2800% body weight)
Ethchlorvynol	8.7	No	No	5–10 L/kg (350–700% body weight)
Glutethimide	4.5	No	No	10–20 L/kg (700–1400% body weight)
Isoniazid	3.5	Alkaline	Yes	61% body weight
Methadone	8.3	No	No	5–10 L/kg (350–700% body weight)
Methicillin	2.8	No	Yes	60% body weight
Phenobarbital	7.4	Alkaline	Yes	75% body weight
Phenytoin	8.3	No	No	60–80% body weight
Tetracycline	7.7	No	No	200–300% body weight

[a]Comprehensive listings of pharmacokinetic data for a large number of drugs are included just prior to the index in each edition of *Goodman & Gilman's The Pharmacological* Basis of *Therapeutics* (see reference list).

of distribution of 1 L times the weight of the child times the blood level in milligram per liter. This would be consistent with an overdose history of having consumed eight extrastrength 500-mg tablets but would not be consistent with a history of therapeutic administration of 15 mg/kg for four doses. Such a therapeutic administration would have a maximum administered dose of 1200 mg (20 kg times 15 mg/kg times four doses), which is well under the calculated body burden. Given metabolism of the drug with a normal half-life of 2 hours, it is apparent that much of the first doses would have been metabolized further adding to an understanding that this must not have been a therapeutic dose. While patients who develop hepatic toxicity from acetaminophen might have a prolonged half-life later in the course, it would certainly not occur with early therapeutic doses.

Metabolism & Excretion

The route of excretion or detoxification is important for planning treatment. Methanol, for example, is metabolized to the toxic product, formic acid. This metabolic step may be blocked by the antidote fomepizole or ethanol.

Blood Levels

Care of the poisoned patient should never be guided solely by laboratory measurements. Treatment should be directed first by the clinical signs and symptoms, followed by more specific therapy based on laboratory determinations. Clinical information may speed the identification of a toxic agent by the laboratory.

PREVENTING CHILDHOOD POISONINGS

Inclusion of poison prevention as part of routine well-child care should begin at the 6-month well-baby visit. The poison prevention handout included as Table 13–2 may be copied and distributed to parents. It contains poison prevention information as well as first-aid actions that should be taken in the event of an exposure. All poison control centers in the United States can be reached by dialing 1-800-222-1222; the call will be automatically routed to the correct regional center.

GENERAL TREATMENT OF POISONING

The telephone is often the first contact in pediatric poisoning. Some patients may contact their pediatrician's office first. Proper telephone management can reduce morbidity and prevent unwarranted or excessive treatment. The decision to refer the patient is based on the identity and dose of the ingested agent, the age of the child, the time of day, the reliability of the parent, and whether child neglect or endangerment is suspected. Poison control centers are the source

Table 13–2. Poison prevention and emergency treatment handout.

Poison safety tips	
If you or your child has come in contact with poison, call the Poison Center (1-800-222-1222). Nurses and pharmacists (that are poison experts) will answer your call. In most cases, they can help you take care of the problem right at home. When you need to get to the hospital, they will call ahead with detailed information to help doctors treat you or your child quickly and correctly.	
How people get poisoned	
People can breathe poison, eat or drink it, or get it on the skin or in the eyes. You probably know that antifreeze, bleach, and bug spray are poisonous. But did you know that vitamins, perfume, and makeup can be dangerous? Eating some plants can be toxic. Some spider bites can be dangerous. Taking medicine that is too old or not prescribed for you can make you sick. Also, mixing different kinds of medicine can be dangerous.	
Poison safety "do's" and "don'ts"	
DO:	***DON'T:***
1. Ask for "safety-lock" tops on all prescription drugs.	1. Don't store food and household cleaners together.
2. Keep cleaners, bug sprays, medicines, and other harmful products out of the reach and sight of children. If possible, keep the products locked up.	2. Don't take medicine in front of children; children love to imitate "mommy" and "daddy."
3. Store medicine in original containers.	3. Don't call medicine candy.
4. Read the label before taking medicine; don't take medicine that doesn't have a label.	4. Don't take medicine that is not for you. Never take medicine in the dark.
5. Follow the directions for all products.	5. Don't put gasoline, bug spray, antifreeze, or cleaning supplies in soft-drink bottles, cups, or bowls. Always keep them in their original containers.
Kids can get into things at any age!	
Children aged 0–6 mo	***Children aged 1–3 y***
Learn to roll over and reach for things.	Have the highest accident rate of any group.
Learn about their environment by putting things in their mouths.	Begin to imitate parents and other adults.
Children aged 7–12 mo	Put things in their mouths.
Start to get curious and explore.	Start to climb on things.
Learn to crawl, pull up to stand, and walk holding on.	
Put everything in their mouths.	
Pull things down.	
Different dangers at different times of the year	
Spring and summer dangers	***Fall and winter dangers***
Pesticides	Antifreeze
Fertilizers	Carbon monoxide
Outdoor plants and mushrooms	Black widow spider bites
Snake, spider, and other insect bites	Plants and autumn berries
Bee stings	Holly, mistletoe, and other holiday decorations
Ticks	
Charcoal lighter fluid	

(*Continued*)

Table 13–2. Poison prevention and emergency treatment handout. (*Continued*)

Follow this checklist to make sure your home is safe
Kitchen
__Remove products like detergent, drain cleaner, and dishwashing liquid from under the sink.
__Remove medicines from counters, tables, refrigerator top, or window sills.
__Put child safety latches on all drawers and cabinets that contain harmful products.
__Store harmful products away from food.
Bathroom
__Regularly clean out your medicine cabinet. *Do not* flush medicines down the toilet. Contact a pharmacy to see if they have a take-back program. If a take-back program is not available, then securely wrap the medication bottle/package in newspaper and duct tape before disposing of in household garbage.
__Keep all medicine in original safety-top containers.
__Keep medicine, hair spray, powder, makeup, fingernail polish, hair-care products, and mouthwash out of reach.
Bedroom
__Don't keep medicine in or on dresser or bedside table.
__Keep perfume, makeup, aftershave, and other products out of reach.
Laundry Area
__Keep bleach, soap, fabric softener, starch, and other supplies out of reach.
__Keep all products in their original containers.
Garage/Basement
__Keep bug spray, weed killers, gasoline, oil, paint, and other supplies in locked area.
__Keep all products in their original containers.
General household
__Keep beer, wine, and liquor out of reach.
__Keep ashtrays clean and out of reach.
__Keep plants out of reach.
__Keep paint in good repair.
Emergency action in case your child . . .
Breathes poison
Get child to fresh air right away. Open doors and windows. Always call the Poison Center.
Gets poison on the skin
Remove clothes that have poison on them. Rinse skin with lukewarm water for 10 minutes. Wash gently with soap and water and rinse. Always call the Poison Center.
Gets poison in the eye
Gently pour lukewarm water over the eye from a large glass 2 or 3 inches from the eye. Repeat for 15 minutes. Have child blink as much as possible while pouring water in the eye. Do not force the eyelid open. Always call the Poison Center.
Swallows poison
Medicines: Do not give child **anything** until you talk with the poison center or your doctor.
Chemicals or household products: Unless your child has passed out or cannot swallow, give milk or water right away. Always call the Poison Center.
Pediatrician: ______________________________(Tel): ____________________
National Toll Free Number which connects with your local Poison Center: **1-800-222-1222**

Information adapted from, and used, courtesy of the Rocky Mountain Poison Center, Denver Health and Hospital Authority, Denver, CO of expert telephone advice and have excellent follow-up programs to manage patients in the home as well as provide further poison prevention information.

INITIAL TELEPHONE CONTACT

Basic information obtained at the first telephone contact includes the patient's name, age, weight, address, and telephone number; the agent and amount of agent ingested; the patient's present condition; and the time elapsed since ingestion or other exposure. Use the history to evaluate the urgency of the situation and decide whether immediate emergency transportation to a health facility is indicated. An emergency exists if the ingestant is high risk (caustic solutions, hydrogen fluoride, drugs of abuse, or medications such as a calcium channel blocker, opioid, hypoglycemic agent, or antidepressant) or if the self-poisoning was intentional. If immediate danger does not exist, obtain more details about the suspected toxic agent. If the child requires transport to a health facility, instruct parents that everything in the vicinity of the child that may be a cause of poisoning should be brought to the health care facility.

It may be difficult to obtain an accurate history. Obtain names of drugs or ingredients, manufacturers, prescription numbers, names and phone numbers of prescribing physician and pharmacy, and any other pertinent information. Find out whether the substance was shared among several children, whether it had been recently purchased, who had last used it, how full the bottle was, and how much was spilled. Determine if this occurred in the home, school, or elsewhere. If unsure of the significance of an exposure, consult with a poison control center.

Each year, children are accidentally poisoned by medicines, polishes, insecticides, drain cleaners, bleaches, household chemicals, and materials commonly stored in the garage. It is the responsibility of adults to make sure that children are not exposed to potentially toxic substances.

Obtaining Information About Poisons

Current data on ingredients of commercial products and medications can be obtained from a certified regional poison center. It is important to have the actual container at hand when calling. Caution: Antidote information on labels of commercial products or in the *Physicians' Desk Reference* may be incorrect or inappropriate.

Follow-Up

In over 95% of cases of ingestion of potentially toxic substances by children, a trip to the hospital is not required. In these cases, it is important to call the parent at 1 and 4 hours after ingestion. If the child has ingested an additional unknown agent and develops symptoms, a change in management may be needed, including transportation to the hospital. An additional call should be made 24 hours after the ingestion to begin the process of poison prevention.

INITIAL EMERGENCY DEPARTMENT CONTACT

Make Certain the Patient Is Breathing

As in all emergencies, the principles of treatment are attention to airway, breathing, and circulation. These are sometimes overlooked under the stressful conditions of a pediatric poisoning.

Treat Shock

Initial therapy of the hypotensive patient should consist of laying the patient flat or head down and administering intravenous (IV) isotonic solutions. Vasopressors should be reserved for poisoned patients in shock who do not respond to these standard measures.

Treat Burns & Skin Exposures

Burns may occur following exposure to strongly acidic or strongly alkaline agents or petroleum distillates. Burned areas should be decontaminated by flooding with sterile saline solution or water. A burn unit should be consulted if more than minimal burn damage has been sustained. Skin decontamination should be performed in a patient with cutaneous exposure. Emergency department personnel in contact with a patient who has been contaminated (with an organophosphate insecticide, for example) should themselves be decontaminated if their skin or clothing becomes contaminated.

Take a Pertinent History

The history should be taken from the parents and all individuals present at the scene. It may be crucial to determine all of the kinds of poisons in the home. These may include drugs used by family members, chemicals associated with the hobbies or occupations of family members, or the purity of the water supply. Unusual dietary or medication habits or other clues to the possible cause of poisoning should also be investigated.

DEFINITIVE THERAPY OF POISONING

Treatment of poisoning or potential poisoning has evolved over time, and general measures such as prevention of absorption and enhancement of excretion are only instituted when specifically indicated. Specific therapy is directed at each drug, chemical, or toxin as described in the management section that follows.

Prevention of Absorption

A. Emesis and Lavage

These measures are rarely used in pediatric patients and should be performed only in consultation with a poison center.

B. Charcoal

The dose of charcoal is 1–2 g/kg (maximum, 100 g) per dose. Repeating the dose of activated charcoal may be useful for those agents that slow passage through the gastrointestinal (GI) tract. When multiple doses of activated charcoal are given, repeated doses of sorbitol or saline cathartics must not be given. Repeated doses of cathartics may cause electrolyte imbalances and fluid loss. Charcoal dosing is repeated every 2–6 hours until charcoal is passed through the rectum.

C. Catharsis

Despite their widespread use, cathartics do not improve outcome. The use of cathartics should therefore be avoided.

D. Whole Gut Lavage

Whole bowel lavage uses an orally administered, nonabsorbable hypertonic solution such as CoLyte or GoLYTELY. The use of this procedure in poisoned patients remains controversial. Preliminary recommendations for use of whole bowel irrigation include poisoning with sustained-release preparations, mechanical movement of items through the bowel (eg, cocaine packets, iron tablets), and poisoning with substances that are poorly absorbed by charcoal (eg, lithium, iron). Underlying bowel pathology and intestinal obstruction are relative contraindications to its use. Consultation with a certified regional poison center is recommended.

American Academy of Clinical Toxicology, European Association of Poisons Centers and Clinical Toxicologists: Position paper: Ipecac syrup. J Toxicol Clin Toxicol 2004;42:133 [PMID: 15214617].

American Academy of Clinical Toxicology, European Association of Poisons Centers and Clinical Toxicologists: Position statement and practice guidelines on the use of multidose activated charcoal in the treatment of acute poisoning. J Toxicol Clin Toxicol 1999;37:731 [PMID: 10584586].

Gielen AC et al: Effects of improved access to safety counseling, products, and home visits on parents' safety practices: Results of a randomized trial. Arch Pediatr Adolesc Med 2002;156:33 [PMID: 11772188].

Thummel KE, Shen DD: Design and optimization of dosage regimens: Pharmacokinetic data. In Goodman LS et al (editors): *Goodman & Gilman's The Pharmacological Basis of Therapeutics*. McGraw-Hill, 2001:1917.

Enhancement of Excretion

Excretion of certain substances can be hastened by urinary alkalinization or dialysis and is reserved for very special circumstances. It is important to make certain that the patient is not volume depleted. Volume-depleted patients should receive a normal saline bolus of 10–20 mL/kg, followed by sufficient IV fluid administration to maintain urine output at 2–3 mL/kg/h.

A. Urinary Alkalinization

1. Alkaline diuresis—Urinary alkalinization should be chosen on the basis of the substance's pK_a, so that ionized drug will be trapped in the tubular lumen and not reabsorbed (see Table 13–1). Thus, if the pK_a is less than 7.5, urinary alkalinization is appropriate; if it is over 8.0, this technique is not usually beneficial. The pK_a is sometimes included along with general drug information. Urinary alkalinization is achieved with sodium bicarbonate. It is important to observe for hypokalemia, caused by the shift of potassium intracellularly. Follow serum K^+ and observe for electrocardiogram (ECG) evidence of hypokalemia. If complications such as renal failure or pulmonary edema are present, hemodialysis or hemoperfusion may be required.

B. Dialysis

Hemodialysis (or peritoneal dialysis if hemodialysis is unavailable) is useful in the treatment of a few poisons and in the general management of a critically ill patient. Dialysis should be considered part of supportive care if the patient satisfies any of the following criteria:

1. Clinical criteria

A. Potentially life-threatening toxicity that is caused by a dialyzable drug and cannot be treated by conservative means.

B. Hypotension threatening renal or hepatic function that cannot be corrected by adjusting circulating volume.

C. Marked hyperosmolality or severe acid-base or electrolyte disturbances not responding to therapy.

D. Marked hypothermia or hyperthermia not responding to therapy.

2. Immediate dialysis—Immediate dialysis should be considered in ethylene glycol and methanol poisoning only if acidosis is refractory, the patient does not respond to fomepizole treatment, or blood levels of ethanol of 100 mg/dL are consistently maintained. Refractory salicylate intoxication may benefit from dialysis.

MANAGEMENT OF SPECIFIC COMMON POISONINGS

ACETAMINOPHEN (PARACETAMOL)

Overdosage of acetaminophen is the most common pediatric poisoning and can produce severe hepatotoxicity. The incidence of hepatotoxicity in adults and adolescents has been reported to be 10 times higher than in children younger than age 5 years. In the latter group, fewer than 0.1% develop hepatotoxicity after acetaminophen overdose. In children, toxicity most commonly results from repeated overdosage arising from confusion about the age-appropriate dose, use of multiple products that contain acetaminophen, or use of adult suppositories.

Acetaminophen is normally metabolized in the liver. A small percentage of the drug goes through a pathway leading to a toxic metabolite. Normally, this electrophilic reactant is removed harmlessly by conjugation with glutathione. In overdosage, the supply of glutathione becomes exhausted, and the metabolite may bind covalently to components of liver cells to produce necrosis. Some authors have proposed that therapeutic doses of acetaminophen may be toxic to children with depleted glutathione stores. However, there is no evidence that administration of therapeutic doses can cause toxicity, and only a few inadequate case reports have been made in this regard.

Treatment

Treatment is to administer acetylcysteine. It may be administered either orally or intravenously. Consultation on difficult cases may be obtained from your regional poison control center or the Rocky Mountain Poison and Drug Center (1-800-525-6115). Blood levels should be obtained 4 hours after ingestion or as soon as possible thereafter and plotted on Figure 13–1. The nomogram is used only for acute ingestion, not repeated supratherapeutic ingestions. If the patient has ingested acetaminophen in a liquid preparation, blood levels obtained 2 hours after ingestion will accurately reflect the toxicity to be expected relative to the standard nomogram (see Figure 13–1). Acetylcysteine is administered to patients whose acetaminophen levels plot in the toxic range on the nomogram. Acetylcysteine is effective even when given more than 24 hours after ingestion, although it is most effective when given within 8 hours postingestion.

The oral (PO) dose of acetylcysteine is 140 mg/kg, diluted to a 5% solution in sweet fruit juice or carbonated soft drink. The primary problems associated with administration are nausea and vomiting. After this loading dose, 70 mg/kg should be administered orally every 4 hours for 72 hours.

For children weighing 40 kg or more, IV acetylcysteine (Acetadote) should be administered as a loading dose of 150 mg/kg administered over 15–60 minutes; followed by a second infusion of 50 mg/kg over 4 hours, and then a third infusion of 100 mg/kg over 16 hours (a dosage calculator is available at http://www.acetadote.com) (Table 13–3).

For patients weighing less than 40 kg, IV acetylcysteine must have less dilution to avoid hyponatremia (Table 13–4).

Patient-tailored therapy is critical when utilizing the IV "20-hour" protocol and those patients who still have acetaminophen measurable and/or elevated aspartate transaminase/alanine transaminase (AST/ALT) may need treatment beyond the 20 hours called for in the product insert.

AST–serum glutamic oxaloacetic transaminase (AST–SGOT), ALT–serum glutamic pyruvic transaminase (ALT–SGPT), serum bilirubin, and plasma prothrombin time should be followed daily. Significant abnormalities of liver function may not peak until 72–96 hours after ingestion.

Repeated miscalculated overdoses given by parents to treat fever are the major source of toxicity in children younger than age 10 years, and parents are often unaware of the significance of symptoms of toxicity, thus delaying its prompt recognition and therapy.

Bond GR: Reduced toxicity of acetaminophen in children: It's the liver. J Toxicol Clin Toxicol 2004;42:149 [PMID: 15214619].

Dart RC, Rumack BH: Patient-tailored acetylcysteine administration. Ann Emerg Med 2007;50:280–281 [PMID: 17418449].

Marzullo L: An update of *N*-acetylcysteine treatment for acute acetaminophen toxicity in children. Curr Opin Pediatr 2005;17:239 [PMID: 15800420].

Rumack BH: Acetaminophen hepatotoxicity: The first 35 years. J Toxicol Clin Toxicol 2002;40:3 [PMID: 11990202].

Yarema MC et al: Comparison of the 20-hour intravenous and 72-hour oral acetylcysteine protocols for the treatment of acute acetaminophen poisoning. Ann Emerg Med 2009;54(4):606–614 [PMID: 19556028].

ALCOHOL, ETHYL (ETHANOL)

Alcoholic beverages, tinctures, cosmetics, mouthwashes, and rubbing alcohol are common sources of poisoning in children. Concomitant exposure to other depressant drugs increases the seriousness of the intoxication. In most states, alcohol levels of 50–80 mg/dL are considered compatible with impaired faculties, and levels of 80–100 mg/dL are considered evidence of intoxication. (Blood levels cited here are for adults; comparable figures for children are not available.)

Recent erroneous information regarding hand sanitizers has indicated that a "lick" following application on the hand could cause toxicity in children. In fact this is not the case, but because these hand sanitizers contain 62% ethanol, toxicity following ingestion is very possible. Potential blood ethanol concentration following consumption of a 62% solution in a 10-kg child is calculated as follows:

$$1 \text{ oz} = 30 \text{ mL} \times 62\% = 18.6 \text{ mL of pure ethanol}$$

$$18.6 \text{ mL} \times 0.79 \text{ (the specific gravity)} = 14.7 \text{ g of ethanol, or } 14{,}700 \text{ mg}$$

In a patient weighing 10 kg, the distribution into total body water (Vd) will be 6 L—this is the amount of the body water into which the ethanol will be distributed.

$$14{,}700 \text{ mg} \div 6 \text{ L} = 2450 \text{ mg/L}$$

$$2450 \text{ mg/L} \div 10 = 245 \text{ mg/dL}$$

Based on these calculations, a 10-kg child consuming 0.5 oz would have a concentration of 122.5 mg/dL; a 20-kg child

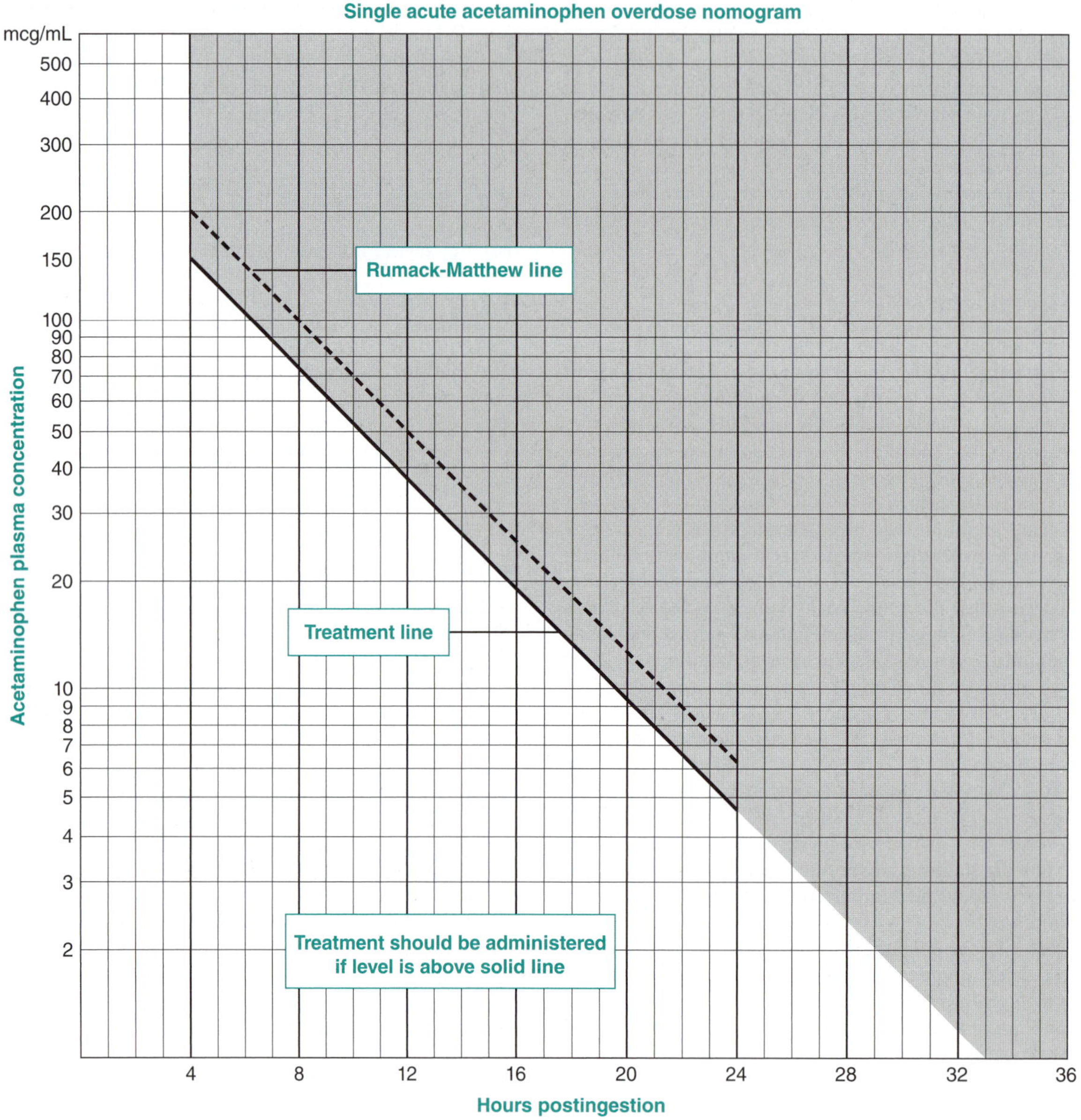

Nomogram: Acetaminophen plasma concentration vs time after acetaminophen ingestion (adapted with permission from Rumack and Matthew. *Pediatrics*. 1975;55:871–876).
The nomogram has been developed to estimate the probability of whether a plasma acetaminophen concentration in relation to the interval postingestion will result in hepatotoxicity and, therefore, whether acetylcysteine therapy should be administered.

Cautions for use of this chart:

1. Time coordinates refer to time postingestion.
2. Graph relates only to plasma concentrations following a single, acute overdose ingestion.
3. The Treatment line is plotted 25% below the Rumack-Matthew line to allow for potential errors in plasma acetaminophen assays and estimated time from ingestion of an overdose (Rumack et al. *Arch Intern Med*. 1981;141(suppl):380-385).

▲ **Figure 13–1.** Semi-logarithmic plot of plasma acetaminophen levels versus time. (Modified and reproduced, with permission, from Rumack BH, Matthew H: Acetaminophen poisoning and toxicity. Pediatrics 1975;55:871.)

Table 13–3. Intravenous acetylcysteine administration for children weighing 40 kg or more.

Body Weight		FIRST 150 mg/kg in 200 mL 5% Dextrose in 15 min	SECOND 50 mg/kg in 500 mL 5% Dextrose in 4 h	THIRD 100 mg/kg in 1000 mL 5% Dextrose in 16 h
(kg)	(lb)	Acetadote (mL)	Acetadote (mL)	Acetadote (mL)
100	220	75	25	50
90	198	67.5	22.5	45
80	176	60	20	40
70	154	52.5	17.5	35
60	132	45	15	30
50	110	37.5	12.5	25
40	88	30	10	20

Table 13–4. Intravenous acetylcysteine administration for children weighing less than 40 kg.

Body Weight		Loading Infusion (15 min)—150 mg/kg		
(kg)	(lb)	NAC 20% (mL)	Diluent Volume D_5W (mL)	Final Volume (mL)
30	66	22.5	90	112.5
25	55	18.75	75	93.75
20	44	15	60	75
15	33	11.25	45	56.25
10	22	7.5	30	37.5
Body Weight		Second Infusion (4 h)—50 mg/kg		
(kg)	(lb)	NAC 20% (mL)	Diluent Volume D_5W (mL)	Final Volume (mL)
30	66	7.5	30	37.5
25	55	6.25	25	31.25
20	44	5	20	25
15	33	3.75	15	18.75
10	22	2.5	10	12.5
Body Weight			Third Infusion (16 h)—100 mg/kg	
(kg)	(lb)	NAC 20% (mL)	Diluent Volume D_5W (mL)	Final Volume (mL)
30	66	15	60	75
25	55	12.5	50	62.5
20	44	10	40	50
15	33	7.5	30	37.5
10	22	5	20	25

consuming 1 oz would have a concentration of 122.5 mg/dL; a 30-kg child consuming 1 oz would have a concentration of 81.7 mg/dL; and a 70-kg adult consuming 1 oz would have a concentration of 35 mg/dL.

One "pump" from a hand sanitizer bottle dispenses approximately 2.5 mL of the product. If ingested, this amount (containing 62% ethanol) would create a blood ethanol concentration as follows:

1. In a 10-kg child: 23.1 mg/dL.
2. In a 20-kg child: 11.6 mg/dL.
3. In a 30-kg child: 7.7 mg/dL.

Children show a change in sensorium with blood levels as low as 10–20 mg/dL and any child displaying such changes should be seen immediately. Although a "lick" or a "drop" is unlikely to produce toxicity, the accuracy of the history should be considered when determining whether or not to see a child.

Complete absorption of alcohol requires 30 minutes to 6 hours, depending on the volume, the presence of food, and the time spent in consuming the alcohol. The rate of metabolic degradation is constant (about 20 mg/h in an adult). Absolute ethanol, 1 mL/kg, results in a peak blood level of about 100 mg/dL in 1 hour after ingestion. Acute intoxication and chronic alcoholism increase the risk of subarachnoid hemorrhage.

Treatment

Management of hypoglycemia and acidosis is usually the only measure required. Start an IV drip of D_5W or $D_{10}W$ if blood glucose is less than 60 mg/dL. Fructose and glucagon have been suggested but are no longer used. Death is usually caused by respiratory failure. In severe cases, cerebral edema may occur and should be appropriately treated.

AMPHETAMINES & RELATED DRUGS (METHAMPHETAMINE)

Clinical Presentation

A. Acute Poisoning

Amphetamine and methamphetamine poisoning is common because of the widespread availability of "diet pills" and the use of "speed," "crank," "crystal," and "ice" by adolescents. (Care must be taken in the interpretation of slang terms because they have multiple meanings.) A new cause of amphetamine poisoning is drugs for treating attention-deficit/hyperactivity disorder, such as methylphenidate. Symptoms include central nervous system (CNS) stimulation, anxiety, hyperactivity, hyperpyrexia, hypertension, abdominal cramps, nausea and vomiting, and inability to void urine. Severe cases often include rhabdomyolysis. A toxic psychosis indistinguishable from paranoid schizophrenia may occur. Methamphetamine laboratories in homes are a potential cause of childhood exposure to a variety of hazardous and toxic substances. Maternal use and the effect on the fetus as well as exposures of young children are a continuing problem.

B. Chronic Poisoning

Chronic amphetamine users develop tolerance; more than 1500 mg of IV methamphetamine can be used daily. Hyperactivity, disorganization, and euphoria are followed by exhaustion, depression, and coma lasting 2–3 days. Heavy users, taking more than 100 mg/d, have restlessness, incoordination of thought, insomnia, nervousness, irritability, and visual hallucinations. Psychosis may be precipitated by the chronic administration of high doses. Depression, weakness, tremors, GI complaints, and suicidal thoughts occur frequently.

Treatment

The treatment of choice is diazepam, titrated in small increments to effect. Very large total doses may be needed. In cases of extreme agitation or hallucinations, droperidol (0.1 mg/kg per dose) or haloperidol (up to 0.1 mg/kg) parenterally has been used. Chronic users may be withdrawn rapidly from amphetamines. If amphetamine–barbiturate combination tablets have been used, the barbiturates must be withdrawn gradually to prevent withdrawal seizures. Psychiatric treatment should be provided.

Schwartz RH, Miller NS: MDMA (ecstasy) and the rave: A review. Pediatrics 1997;100:705 [PMID: 9310529].

Smith LM et al: The infant development, environment, and lifestyle study: Effects of prenatal methamphetamine exposure, polydrug exposure, and poverty on intrauterine growth. Pediatrics 2006;118:1149–1156 [PMID: 16951010].

ANESTHETICS, LOCAL

Intoxication from local anesthetics may be associated with CNS stimulation, acidosis, delirium, ataxia, shock, convulsions, and death. Methemoglobinuria has been reported following local dental analgesia. The maximum recommended dose for subcutaneous (SQ) infiltration is 4.5 mg/kg. The temptation to exceed this dose in procedures lasting a long time is great and may result in inadvertent overdosage. PO application of viscous lidocaine may produce toxicity. Hypercapnia may lower the seizure threshold to locally injected anesthetics.

Local anesthetics used in obstetrics cross the placental barrier and are not efficiently metabolized by the fetal liver. Mepivacaine, lidocaine, and bupivacaine can cause fetal bradycardia, neonatal depression, and death. Prilocaine causes methemoglobinemia, which should be treated if levels in the blood exceed 40% or if the patient is symptomatic.

Accidental injection of mepivacaine into the head of the fetus during paracervical anesthesia has caused neonatal asphyxia, cyanosis, acidosis, bradycardia, convulsions, and death.

Treatment

If the anesthetic has been ingested, mucous membranes should be cleansed carefully and activated charcoal may be administered. Oxygen administration is indicated, with assisted ventilation if necessary. Methemoglobinemia is treated with methylene blue, 1%, 0.2 mL/kg (1–2 mg/kg per dose, IV) over 5–10 minutes; this should promptly relieve the cyanosis. Acidosis may be treated with sodium bicarbonate, seizures with diazepam, and bradycardia with atropine. Therapeutic levels of mepivacaine, lidocaine, and procaine are less than 5 mg/mL.

Spiller HA et al: Multi-center retrospective evaluation of oral benzocaine exposure in children. Vet Hum Toxicol 2000;42:228 [PMID: 10928690].

ANTIHISTAMINES & COUGH & COLD PREPARATIONS

The use of cough and cold preparations in young children has recently been called into question due to potential toxicity. In 2007, manufacturers voluntarily removed preparations intended for use in children younger than the age of 4 from the market. Considerable controversy remains as to the toxicity of these medications if they are used according to labeled directions and an evaluation of the cases on file at FDA stated, "In the cases judged to be therapeutic intent or unknown intent, several factors appeared to contribute to the administration of an overdosage: administration of 2 medicines containing the same ingredients, failure to use a measuring device, use of an adult product, use of the wrong product because of product misidentification, and 2 or more caregivers administering the same medication. In the cases of non-therapeutic intent, circumstances involved attempts at sedation and several included apparent attempts of overt child abuse and were under investigation by law enforcement authorities."

Medications included in this area are: antihistamine (brompheniramine, chlorpheniramine, diphenhydramine, doxylamine), antitussive (dextromethorphan), expectorant (guaifenesin), and decongestant (pseudoephedrine, phenylephrine). Although antihistamines typically cause CNS depression, children often react paradoxically with excitement, hallucinations, delirium, ataxia, tremors, and convulsions followed by CNS depression, respiratory failure, or cardiovascular collapse. Anticholinergic effects such as dry mouth, fixed dilated pupils, flushed face, fever, and hallucinations may be prominent.

They are absorbed rapidly and metabolized by the liver, lungs, and kidneys. A potentially toxic dose is 10–50 mg/kg of the most commonly used antihistamines, but toxic reactions have occurred at much lower doses.

Treatment

Activated charcoal should be used to reduce drug absorption. Whole bowel irrigation may be useful for sustained-release preparations. Physostigmine (0.5–2.0 mg IV, slowly administered) dramatically reverses the central and peripheral anticholinergic effects of antihistamines, but it should be used only for diagnostic purposes. Diazepam (0.1–0.2 mg/kg IV) can be used to control seizures. Cardiac dysrhythmias and hypotension should be treated with normal saline at a dose of 10–20 mg/kg and a vasopressor if necessary. Sodium bicarbonate may be useful if there is QRS widening at a dose of 1–2 mEq/kg, making certain that the arterial pH does not exceed 7.55. Forced diuresis is not helpful. Exchange transfusion was reported to be effective in one case.

Dart RC et al: Pediatric fatalities associated with over the counter nonprescription) cough and cold medications. Ann Emerg Med 2009;53:411–417 [PMID: 19101060].

Sharfstein JM, North M, Serwint JR: Over the counter but no longer under the radar—pediatric cough and cold medications. N Engl J Med 2007;357:2321–2324 [PMID: 18057333].

ARSENIC

Arsenic is used in some insecticides (fruit tree or tobacco sprays), rodenticides, weed killers, and wood preservatives. It is well absorbed primarily through the GI and respiratory tracts, but skin absorption may occur. Arsenic can be found in the urine, hair, and nails by laboratory testing.

Highly toxic soluble derivatives of this compound, such as sodium arsenite, are frequently found in liquid preparations and can cause death in as many as 65% of victims. The organic arsenates found in persistent or preemergence weed killers are relatively less soluble and less toxic. Poisonings with a liquid arsenical preparation that does not contain alkyl methanearsonate compounds should be considered potentially lethal. Patients exhibiting clinical signs other than gastroenteritis should receive treatment until laboratory tests indicate that treatment is no longer necessary.

Clinical Findings

A. Acute Poisoning

Abdominal pain, vomiting, watery and bloody diarrhea, cardiovascular collapse, paresthesias, neck pain, and garlic odor on the breath occur as the first signs of acute poisoning. Convulsions, coma, anuria, and exfoliative dermatitis are later signs. Inhalation may cause pulmonary edema. Death is the result of cardiovascular collapse.

B. Chronic Poisoning

Anorexia, generalized weakness, giddiness, colic, abdominal pain, polyneuritis, dermatitis, nail changes, alopecia, and anemia often develop.

Treatment

In acute poisoning, administer activated charcoal. Then immediately give dimercaprol (commonly known as BAL), 3–5 mg/kg intramuscularly (IM), and follow with 2 mg/kg IM every 4 hours. The dimercaprol–arsenic complex is dialyzable. A second choice is succimer. The initial dose is 10 mg/kg every 8 hours for 5 days. A third choice is penicillamine, 100 mg/kg PO to a maximum of 1 g/d in four divided doses.

Chronic arsenic intoxication should be treated with succimer or penicillamine. Collect a 24-hour baseline urine specimen and then begin chelation. If the 24-hour urine arsenic level is greater than 50 mg, continue chelation for 5 days. After 10 days, repeat the 5-day cycle once or twice, depending on how soon the urine arsenic level falls below 50 mg/24 h.

Abernathy CO et al: Arsenic: Health effects, mechanisms of actions, and research issues. Environ Health Perspect 1999;107:593 [PMID: 10379007].

BARBITURATES

The toxic effects of barbiturates include confusion, poor coordination, coma, miotic or fixed dilated pupils, and respiratory depression. Respiratory acidosis is commonly associated with pulmonary atelectasis, and hypotension occurs frequently in severely poisoned patients. Ingestion of more than 6 mg/kg of long-acting or 3 mg/kg of short-acting barbiturates is usually toxic.

Treatment

Activated charcoal should be administered. Careful, conservative management with emphasis on maintaining a clear airway, adequate ventilation, and control of hypotension is critical. Urinary alkalinization and the use of multiple-dose charcoal may decrease the elimination half-life of phenobarbital but have not been shown to alter the clinical course. Hemodialysis is not useful in the treatment of poisoning with short-acting barbiturates. Analeptics are contraindicated.

Cote CJ et al: Adverse sedation events in pediatrics: Analysis of medications used for sedation. Pediatrics 2000;4:633 [PMID: 11015502].

BELLADONNA ALKALOIDS (ATROPINE, JIMSONWEED, POTATO LEAVES, SCOPOLAMINE, STRAMONIUM)

The effects of anticholinergic compounds include dry mouth; thirst; decreased sweating with hot, dry, red skin; high fever; and tachycardia that may be preceded by bradycardia. The pupils are dilated, and vision is blurred. Speech and swallowing may be impaired. Hallucinations, delirium, and coma are common. Leukocytosis may occur, confusing the diagnosis.

Atropinism has been caused by normal doses of atropine or homatropine eye drops, especially in children with Down syndrome. Many common plants and over-the-counter medications contain belladonna alkaloids.

Treatment

If the patient is awake and showing no signs or symptoms, administer activated charcoal. Gastric emptying is slowed by anticholinergics, so that gastric decontamination may be useful even if delayed. Physostigmine (0.5–2.0 mg IV, administered slowly) dramatically reverses the central and peripheral signs of atropinism but should be used only as a diagnostic agent. High fever must be controlled. Catheterization may be needed if the patient cannot void.

Burns MJ et al: A comparison of physostigmine and benzodiazepines for the treatment of anticholinergic poisoning. Ann Emerg Med 2000;35:374 [PMID: 10736125].

CARBON MONOXIDE

The degree of toxicity correlates well with the carboxyhemoglobin level taken soon after acute exposure but not after oxygen has been given or when there has been some time since exposure. Onset of symptoms may be more rapid and more severe if the patient lives at a high altitude, has a high respiratory rate (ie, infants), is pregnant, or has myocardial insufficiency or lung disease. Normal blood may contain up to 5% carboxyhemoglobin (10% in smokers).

The most prominent early symptom is headache. Other effects include confusion, unsteadiness, and coma. Proteinuria, glycosuria, elevated serum aminotransferase levels, or ECG changes may be present in the acute phase. Permanent cardiac, liver, renal, or CNS damage occurs occasionally. The outcome of severe poisoning may be complete recovery, vegetative state, or any degree of mental injury between these extremes. The primary mental deficits are neuropsychiatric.

Treatment

The biologic half-life of carbon monoxide on room air is approximately 200–300 minutes; on 100% oxygen, it is 60–90 minutes. Hyperbaric oxygen therapy at 2.0–2.5 atm of oxygen shortens the half-life to 30 minutes. After the level has been reduced to near zero, therapy is aimed at the nonspecific sequelae of anoxia. Dexamethasone (0.1 mg/kg IV or IM every 4–6 hours) should be added if cerebral edema develops.

Chou KJ: Characteristics and outcome of children with carbon monoxide poisoning with and without smoke exposure referred for hyperbaric oxygen therapy. Pediatr Emerg Care 2000;3:151 [PMID: 10888449].

CAUSTICS

1. Acids (Hydrochloric, Hydrofluoric, Nitric, & Sulfuric Acids; Sodium Bisulfate)

Strong acids are commonly found in metal and toilet bowl cleaners, batteries, and other products. Hydrofluoric acid is the most toxic and hydrochloric acid the least toxic of these household substances. However, even a few drops can be fatal if aspirated into the trachea.

Painful swallowing, mucous membrane burns, bloody emesis, abdominal pain, respiratory distress due to edema of the epiglottis, thirst, shock, and renal failure can occur. Coma and convulsions sometimes are seen terminally. Residual lesions include esophageal, gastric, and pyloric strictures as well as scars of the cornea, skin, and oropharynx.

Hydrofluoric acid is a particularly dangerous poison. Dermal exposure creates a penetrating burn that can progress for hours or days. Large dermal exposure or ingestion may produce life-threatening hypocalcemia abruptly as well as burn reactions.

Treatment

Emetics and lavage are contraindicated. Water or milk (< 15 mL/kg) is used to dilute the acid, because a heat-producing chemical reaction does not occur. Take care not to induce emesis by excessive fluid administration. Alkalies should not be used. Burned areas of the skin, mucous membranes, or eyes should be washed with copious amounts of warm water. Opioids for pain may be needed. An endotracheal tube may be required to alleviate laryngeal edema. Esophagoscopy should be performed if the patient has significant burns or difficulty in swallowing. Acids are likely to produce gastric burns or esophageal burns. Evidence is not conclusive, but corticosteroids have not proved to be of use.

Hydrofluoric acid burns on skin are treated with 10% calcium gluconate gel or calcium gluconate infusion. Severe exposure may require large doses of IV calcium. Therapy should be guided by calcium levels, the ECG, and clinical signs.

2. Bases (Clinitest Tablets, Clorox, Drano, Liquid-Plumr, Purex, Sani-Clor—Examine the Label or Call a Poison Center to Determine Contents)

Alkalies produce more severe injuries than acids. Some substances, such as Clinitest tablets or Drano, are quite toxic, whereas the chlorinated bleaches (3–6% solutions of sodium hypochlorite) are usually not toxic. When sodium hypochlorite comes in contact with acid in the stomach, hypochlorous acid, which is very irritating to the mucous membranes and skin, is formed. Rapid inactivation of this substance prevents systemic toxicity. Chlorinated bleaches, when mixed with a strong acid (toilet bowl cleaners) or ammonia, may produce irritating chlorine or chloramine gas, which can cause serious lung injury if inhaled in a closed space (eg, bathroom).

Alkalies can burn the skin, mucous membranes, and eyes. Respiratory distress may be due to edema of the epiglottis, pulmonary edema resulting from inhalation of fumes, or pneumonia. Mediastinitis or other intercurrent infections or shock can occur. Perforation of the esophagus or stomach is rare.

Treatment

The skin and mucous membranes should be cleansed with copious amounts of water. A local anesthetic can be instilled in the eye if necessary to alleviate blepharospasm. The eye should be irrigated for at least 20–30 minutes. Ophthalmologic consultation should be obtained for all alkaline eye burns.

Ingestions should be treated with water as a diluent. Routine esophagoscopy is no longer indicated to rule out burns of the esophagus due to chlorinated bleaches unless an unusually large amount has been ingested or the patient is symptomatic. The absence of oral lesions does not rule out the possibility of laryngeal or esophageal burns following granular alkali ingestion. The use of corticosteroids is controversial, but has not been shown to improve long-term outcome except possibly in partial-thickness esophageal burns. Antibiotics may be needed if mediastinitis is likely, but they should not be used prophylactically. (See Caustic Burns of the Esophagus section in Chapter 21.)

Hamza AF et al: Caustic esophageal strictures in children: 30 years' experience. J Pediatr Surg 2003;338:828 [PMID: 12778375].

Lovejoy FH Jr: Corrosive injury of the esophagus in children: Failure of corticosteroid treatment reemphasizes prevention. N Engl J Med 1990;323:668 [PMID: 2385270].

Tiryaki T et al: Early bougienage for relief of stricture formation following caustic esophageal burns. Pediatr Surg Intl 2005;21:78 [PMID: 15619090].

COCAINE

Cocaine is absorbed intranasally or via inhalation or ingestion. Effects are noted almost immediately when the drug is taken intravenously or smoked. Peak effects are delayed for about an hour when the drug is taken orally or nasally. Cocaine prevents the reuptake of endogenous catecholamines, thereby causing an initial sympathetic discharge, followed by catechol depletion after chronic abuse.

Clinical Findings

A local anesthetic and vasoconstrictor, cocaine is also a potent stimulant to both the CNS and the cardiovascular system. The initial tachycardia, hyperpnea, hypertension, and stimulation of the CNS are often followed by coma, seizures, hypotension, and respiratory depression. In severe cases of overdose, various dysrhythmias may be seen, including sinus tachycardia, atrial arrhythmias, premature ventricular contractions, bigeminy, and ventricular fibrillation. If large doses are taken intravenously, cardiac failure, dysrhythmias, rhabdomyolysis, or hyperthermia may result in death.

In addition to those poisoned through recreational use of cocaine, others are at risk of overdose. A "body stuffer" is one who quickly ingests the drug, usually poorly wrapped, to avoid discovery. A "body packer" wraps the drug carefully for prolonged transport. A stuffer typically manifests toxicity within hours of ingestion; a packer is asymptomatic unless the package ruptures, usually days later. Newborns of cocaine using mothers may continue to have seizures for months after birth.

Treatment

Except in cases of body stuffers or body packers, decontamination is seldom possible. Activated charcoal should be administered, and whole bowel irrigation may be useful in selected cases. Testing for cocaine in blood or plasma is generally not clinically useful, but a qualitative analysis of the urine may aid in confirming the diagnosis. For severe cases, an ECG is indicated. In suspected cases of body packing, radiographs of the GI tract may show multiple packets. Radiographic films are usually not helpful for identifying stuffers. Seizures are treated with IV diazepam titrated to response. Hypotension is treated with standard agents. Because cocaine abuse may deplete norepinephrine, an indirect agent such as dopamine may be less effective than a direct agent such as norepinephrine. Agitation is best treated with a benzodiazepine.

Delaney-Black V: Prenatal cocaine exposure as a risk factor for later developmental outcomes. JAMA 2001;286:46 [PMID: 11434823].

Qureshi AI et al: Cocaine use and the likelihood of nonfatal myocardial infarction and stroke: Data from the Third National Health and Nutrition Examination Survey. Circulation 2001;103:502 [PMID: 11157713].

CONTRACEPTIVE PILLS

The only known toxic effects following acute ingestion of oral contraceptive agents are nausea, vomiting, and vaginal bleeding in girls.

COSMETICS & RELATED PRODUCTS

The relative toxicities of commonly ingested products in this group are listed in Table 13–5. Permanent wave neutralizers may contain bromates, peroxides, or perborates. Bromates have been removed from most products because they can cause nausea, vomiting, abdominal pain, shock, hemolysis, renal failure, and convulsions.

Table 13–5. Relative toxicities of cosmetics and similar products.

High toxicity	**Low toxicity**
Permanent wave neutralizers	Perfume
Moderate toxicity	Hair removers
Fingernail polish	Deodorants
Fingernail polish remover	Bath salts
Metallic hair dyes	**No toxicity**
Home permanent wave lotion	Liquid makeup
Bath oil	Vegetable hair dye
Shaving lotion	Cleansing cream
Hair tonic (alcoholic)	Hair dressing (nonalcoholic)
Cologne, toilet water	Hand lotion or cream
	Lipstick

Perborates can cause boric acid poisoning. Four grams of bromate salts is potentially lethal.

Poisoning is treated by gastric lavage with 1% sodium thiosulfate. Sodium bicarbonate, 2%, in the lavage fluid may reduce hydrobromic acid formation. Sodium thiosulfate, 25%, 1.65 mL/kg, can be given intravenously, but methylene blue should not be used to treat methemoglobinemia in this situation because it increases the toxicity of bromates. Dialysis is indicated in renal failure but does not enhance excretion of bromate.

Fingernail polish removers used to contain toluene but now usually have an acetone base, which does not require specific treatment other than monitoring CNS status.

Cobalt, copper, cadmium, iron, lead, nickel, silver, bismuth, and tin are sometimes found in metallic hair dyes. In large amounts they can cause skin sensitization, urticaria, dermatitis, eye damage, vertigo, hypertension, asthma, methemoglobinemia, tremors, convulsions, and coma. Treatment for ingestions is to administer demulcents and, only with large amounts, the appropriate antidote for the heavy metal involved.

Home permanent wave lotions, hair straighteners, and hair removers usually contain thioglycolic acid salts, which cause alkaline irritation and perhaps CNS depression.

Shaving lotion, hair tonic, hair straighteners, cologne, and toilet water contain denatured alcohol, which can cause CNS depression and hypoglycemia.

Deodorants usually consist of an antibacterial agent in a cream base. Antiperspirants are aluminum salts, which frequently cause skin sensitization. Zirconium oxide can cause granulomas in the axilla with chronic use.

CYCLIC ANTIDEPRESSANTS

Cyclic antidepressants (eg, amitriptyline, imipramine) have a very low ratio of toxic to therapeutic doses, and even a moderate overdose can have serious effects.

Cyclic antidepressant overdosage causes dysrhythmias, coma, convulsions, hypertension followed by hypotension, and hallucinations. These effects may be life-threatening and require rapid intervention. One agent, amoxapine, differs in that it causes fewer cardiovascular complications, but it is associated with a higher incidence of seizures.

Treatment

Decontamination should include administration of activated charcoal unless the patient is symptomatic.

An ECG should be obtained in all patients. A QRS interval greater than 100 ms specifically identifies patients at risk to develop dysrhythmias. If dysrhythmias are demonstrated, the patient should be admitted and monitored until free of irregularity for 24 hours. Another indication for monitoring is persistent tachycardia of more than 110 beats/min. The onset of dysrhythmias is rare beyond 24 hours after ingestion.

Alkalinization with sodium bicarbonate (0.5–1.0 mEq/kg IV) or hyperventilation may dramatically reverse ventricular dysrhythmias and narrow the QRS interval. Lidocaine may be added for treatment of arrhythmias. Bolus administration of sodium bicarbonate is recommended for all patients with QRS widening to above 120 ms and for those with significant dysrhythmias, to achieve a pH of 7.5–7.6. Forced diuresis is contraindicated. A benzodiazepine should be given for convulsions.

Hypotension is a major problem. Cyclic antidepressants block the reuptake of catecholamines, thereby producing initial hypertension followed by hypotension. Treatment with physostigmine is contraindicated. Vasopressors are generally effective. Dopamine is the agent of choice because it is readily available. If dopamine is ineffective, norepinephrine (0.1–1 mcg/kg/min, titrated to response) should be added. Diuresis and hemodialysis are not effective.

Kerr GW et al: Tricyclic antidepressant overdose: A review. Emerg Med J 2001;18:236 [PMID: 11435353].

DIGITALIS & OTHER CARDIAC GLYCOSIDES

Toxicity is typically the result of incorrect dosing or unrecognized renal insufficiency. Clinical features include nausea, vomiting, diarrhea, headache, delirium, confusion, and, occasionally, coma. Cardiac dysrhythmias typically involve bradydysrhythmias, but every type of dysrhythmia has been reported in digitalis intoxication, including atrial fibrillation, paroxysmal atrial tachycardia, and atrial flutter. Death usually is the result of ventricular fibrillation. Transplacental intoxication by digitalis has been reported.

Treatment

Administer activated charcoal. Potassium is contraindicated in acute overdosage unless there is laboratory evidence of hypokalemia. In acute overdosage, hyperkalemia is more common. Hypokalemia is common in chronic toxicity.

The patient must be monitored carefully for ECG changes. The correction of acidosis better demonstrates the degree of potassium deficiency present. Bradycardias have been treated with atropine. Phenytoin, lidocaine, magnesium salts (not in renal failure), amiodarone, and bretylium have been used to correct arrhythmias.

Definitive treatment is with digoxin immune Fab (ovine) (Digibind). Indications for its use include hypotension or any dysrhythmia, typically ventricular dysrhythmias and progressive bradydysrhythmias that produce clinical concern. Elevated T waves indicate high potassium and may be an indication for digoxin immune Fab (Digibind, DigiFab) use. Techniques of determining dosage and indications related to levels, when available are described in product literature.

Eyal D, Molczan KA, Carroll LS: Digoxin toxicity: Pediatric survival after asystolic arrest. Clin Toxicol (Phila) 2005;43:51–54 [PMID: 15732447].

Woolf AD et al: The use of digoxin-specific Fab fragments for severe digitalis intoxication in children. N Engl J Med 1992;326:1739 [PMID: 1997016].

DIPHENOXYLATE WITH ATROPINE (LOMOTIL) & LOPERAMIDE (IMODIUM)

Loperamide (Imodium) has largely replaced Lomotil and does not produce significant toxicity. Ingestions of up to 0.4 mg/kg can safely be managed at home.

Lomotil is still widely available and contains diphenoxylate hydrochloride, a synthetic narcotic, and atropine sulfate. Small amounts are potentially lethal in children; it is contraindicated in children younger than age 2 years. Early signs of intoxication with this preparation result from its anticholinergic effect and consist of fever, facial flushing, tachypnea, and lethargy. However, the miotic effect of the narcotic predominates. Later, hypothermia, increasing CNS depression, and loss of the facial flush occur. Seizures are probably secondary to hypoxia.

Treatment

Prolonged monitoring (24 hours) with pulse oximetry and careful attention to airway is sufficient in most cases.

Naloxone hydrochloride (0.4–2.0 mg IV in children and adults) should be given. Repeated doses may be required because the duration of action of diphenoxylate is considerably longer than that of naloxone.

McCarron MM et al: Diphenoxylate-atropine (Lomotil) overdose in children: An update. Pediatrics 1991;87:694 [PMID: 2020516].

DISINFECTANTS & DEODORIZERS

1. Naphthalene

Naphthalene is commonly found in mothballs, disinfectants, and deodorizers. Naphthalene's toxicity is often not fully appreciated. It is absorbed not only when ingested but also through the skin and lungs. It is potentially hazardous to store baby clothes in naphthalene, because baby oil is an excellent solvent that may increase dermal absorption. ***Note:*** Most mothballs contain *para*-dichlorobenzene and not naphthalene (see next section). Metabolic products of naphthalene may cause severe hemolytic anemia, similar to that due to primaquine toxicity, 2–7 days after ingestion. Other physical findings include vomiting, diarrhea, jaundice, oliguria, anuria, coma, and convulsions. The urine may contain hemoglobin, protein, and casts.

Treatment

Administer activated charcoal. Urinary alkalinization may prevent blocking of the renal tubules by acid hematin crystals. Anuria may persist for 1–2 weeks and still be completely reversible.

Siegel E, Wason S: Mothball toxicity. Pediatr Clin North Am 1986;33:369 [PMID: 3515301].

2. *P*-Dichlorobenzene, Phenolic Acids, & Others

Disinfectants and deodorizers containing *p*-dichlorobenzene or sodium sulfate are much less toxic than those containing naphthalene. Disinfectants containing phenolic acids are highly toxic, especially if they contain a borate ion. Phenol precipitates tissue proteins and causes respiratory alkalosis followed by metabolic acidosis. Some phenols cause methemoglobinemia.

Local gangrene occurs after prolonged contact with tissue. Phenol is readily absorbed from the GI tract, causing diffuse capillary damage and, in some cases, methemoglobinemia. Pentachlorophenol, which has been used in terminal rinsing of diapers, has caused infant fatalities.

The toxicity of alkalies, quaternary ammonium compounds, pine oil, and halogenated disinfectants varies with the concentration of active ingredients. Wick deodorizers are usually of moderate toxicity. Iodophor disinfectants are the safest. Spray deodorizers are not usually toxic, because a child is not likely to swallow a very large dose.

Signs and symptoms of acute quaternary ammonium compound ingestion include diaphoresis, strong irritation, thirst, vomiting, diarrhea, cyanosis, hyperactivity, coma, convulsions, hypotension, abdominal pain, and pulmonary edema. Acute liver or renal failure may develop later.

Treatment

Activated charcoal may be used. Castor oil dissolves phenol and may retard its absorption. This property of castor oil, however, has not been proved clinically. Mineral oil and alcohol are contraindicated because they increase the gastric absorption of phenol. The metabolic acidosis must be managed carefully. Anticonvulsants or measures to treat shock may be needed.

Because phenols are absorbed through the skin, exposed areas should be irrigated copiously with water. Undiluted polyethylene glycol may be a useful solvent as well.

Van Berkel M, de Wolff FA: Survival after acute benzalkonium chloride poisoning. Hum Toxicol 1988;7:191 [PMID: 3378808].

DISK-SHAPED BATTERIES

Small, flat, smooth disk-shaped batteries measure between 10 and 25 mm in diameter. About 69% of them pass through the GI tract in 48 hours and 85% in 72 hours. Some may become entrapped. These batteries contain caustic materials and heavy metals.

Batteries impacted in the esophagus may cause symptoms of refusal to take food, increased salivation, vomiting with or without blood, and pain or discomfort. Aspiration into the trachea may also occur. Fatalities have been reported in association with esophageal perforation.

When a history of disk battery ingestion is obtained, radiographs of the entire respiratory tract and GI tract should be taken so that the battery can be located and the proper therapy determined.

Treatment

If the disk battery is located in the esophagus, it must be removed immediately. If the battery has been in the esophagus for more than 24 hours, the risk of caustic burn is greater.

Location of the disk battery below the esophagus has been associated with tissue damage, but the course is benign in most cases. Perforated Meckel diverticulum has been the major complication. It may take as long as 7 days for spontaneous passage to occur, and lack of movement in the GI tract may not require removal in an asymptomatic patient.

Some researchers have suggested repeated radiographs and surgical intervention if passage of the battery pauses, but this approach may be excessive. Batteries that have opened in the GI tract have been associated with some toxicity due to mercury, but the patients have recovered.

Emesis is ineffective. Asymptomatic patients may simply be observed and stools examined for passage of the battery. If the battery has not passed within 7 days or if the patient becomes symptomatic, radiographs should be repeated. If the battery has come apart or appears not to be moving, a purgative, enema, or nonabsorbable intestinal lavage solution should be administered. If these methods are unsuccessful, surgical intervention may be required. Levels of heavy metals (mainly mercury) should be measured in patients in whom the battery has opened or symptoms have developed.

Dane S: A truly emergent problem: Button battery in the nose. Acad Emerg Med 2000;7:204 [PMID: 10691084].

Litovitz TL, Schmitz BF: Ingestion of cylindrical and button batteries: An analysis of 2382 cases. Pediatrics 1992;89:747 [PMID: 2304794].

ETHYLENE GLYCOL & METHANOL

Ethylene glycol and methanol are the toxic alcohols. The primary source of ethylene glycol is antifreeze, whereas methanol is present in windshield wiper fluid and also as an ethanol denaturant. Ethylene glycol causes severe metabolic acidosis and renal failure. Methanol causes metabolic acidosis and blindness. Onset of symptoms with both agents occurs within several hours after ingestion, longer if ethanol was ingested simultaneously.

Treatment

The primary treatment is to block the enzyme alcohol dehydrogenase, which converts both agents to their toxic metabolites. This is accomplished with fomepizole (loading dose of 15 mg/kg) or ethanol. Fomepizole is preferred for children, due to its reduced side effects in this age group.

Caravati EM et al: Ethylene glycol exposure: An evidence-based consensus guideline for out-of-hospital management. Clin Toxicol (Phila) 2005;43:327–345 [PMID: 16235508].

γ-HYDROXYBUTYRATE, γ-BUTYROLACTONE, & BUTANEDIOL

γ-Hydroxybutyrate (GHB), γ-butyrolactone (GBL), and butanediol have become popular drugs of abuse in adolescents and adults. GHB is a CNS depressant that is structurally similar to the inhibitory neurotransmitter γ-aminobutyric acid. GBL and butanediol are converted in the body to GHB. These drugs cause deep but short-lived coma; the coma often lasts only 1–4 hours. Treatment consists of supportive care with close attention to airway and endotracheal intubation if respiratory depression or decreased gag reflex complicates the poisoning. Atropine has been used successfully for symptomatic bradycardia.

Withdrawal from GHB, GBL, or butanediol can cause several days of extreme agitation, hallucination, or tachycardia. Treatment with high doses of benzodiazepines or with butyrophenones (eg, haloperidol or droperidol) or secobarbital may be needed for several days.

Dyer JE et al: Gamma-hydroxybutyrate withdrawal syndrome. Ann Emerg Med 2001;37:147 [PMID: 11174231].

Sporer KA et al: Gamma-hydroxybutyrate serum levels and clinical syndrome after severe overdose. Ann Emerg Med 2003;42:3 [PMID: 12827115].

HYDROCARBONS (BENZENE, CHARCOAL LIGHTER FLUID, GASOLINE, KEROSENE, PETROLEUM DISTILLATES, TURPENTINE)

Ingestion of hydrocarbons may cause irritation of mucous membranes, vomiting, blood-tinged diarrhea, respiratory distress, cyanosis, tachycardia, and fever. Although a small amount (10 mL) of certain hydrocarbons is potentially fatal, patients have survived ingestion of several ounces of other petroleum distillates. The more aromatic a hydrocarbon is and the lower its viscosity rating, the more potentially toxic it is. Benzene, gasoline, kerosene, and red seal oil furniture polish are the most dangerous. A dose exceeding 1 mL/kg is likely to cause CNS depression. A history of coughing or choking, as well as vomiting, suggests aspiration with resulting hydrocarbon pneumonia. This is an acute hemorrhagic necrotizing disease that usually develops within 24 hours of the ingestion and resolves without sequelae in 3–5 days. However, several weeks may be required for full resolution of hydrocarbon pneumonia. Pneumonia may be caused by the aspiration of a few drops of petroleum distillate into the lungs or by absorption from the circulatory system. Pulmonary edema and hemorrhage, cardiac dilation and dysrhythmias, hepatosplenomegaly, proteinuria, and hematuria can occur following large overdoses. Hypoglycemia is occasionally present. A chest radiograph may reveal pneumonia within hours after the ingestion. An abnormal urinalysis in a child with a previously normal urinary tract suggests a large overdose.

Treatment

Both emetics and lavage should be avoided. Mineral oil should not be given, because it can cause a low-grade lipoid pneumonia.

Epinephrine should not be used with halogenated hydrocarbons because it may affect an already sensitized myocardium. The usefulness of corticosteroids is debated, and antibiotics should be reserved for patients with infections. Oxygen and mist are helpful. Extracorporeal membrane oxygenation has been successful in at least two cases of failure with standard therapy.

Lifshitz M et al: Hydrocarbon poisoning in children: A 5-year retrospective study. Wilderness Environ Med 2003;14:78 [PMID: 12825880].

Lorenc JD: Inhalant abuse in the pediatric populations: A persistent challenge. Curr Opin Pediatr 2003;15:204 [PMID: 12640280].

IBUPROFEN

Most exposures in children do not produce symptoms. In one study, for example, children ingesting up to 2.4 g remained asymptomatic. When symptoms occur, the most common are abdominal pain, vomiting, drowsiness, and lethargy. In rare cases, apnea (especially in young children), seizures, metabolic acidosis, and CNS depression leading to coma have occurred.

Treatment

If a child has ingested less than 100 mg/kg, dilution with water or milk may be all that is necessary to minimize the GI upset. In children, the volume of liquid used for dilution should be less than 4 oz. When the ingested amount is more than 400 mg/kg, seizures or CNS depression may occur; therefore, gastric lavage may be preferred to emesis. Activated charcoal may also be of value. There is no specific antidote. Neither alkalinization of the urine nor hemodialysis is helpful.

Cuzzolin L et al: NSAID-induced nephrotoxicity from the fetus to the child. Drug Safety 2001;242:9 [PMID: 11219488].

Marciniak KE et al: Massive ibuprofen overdose requiring extracorporeal membrane oxygenation for cardiovascular support. Pediatr Crit Care Med 2007;8:180–182 [PMID: 17273120].

Oker EE et al: Serious toxicity in a young child due to ibuprofen. Acad Emerg Med 2000;7:821 [PMID: 10917334].

INSECT STINGS (BEE, WASP, & HORNET)

Insect stings are painful but not usually dangerous; however, death from anaphylaxis may occur. Bee venom has hemolytic, neurotoxic, and histamine-like activities that can on rare occasion cause hemoglobinuria and severe anaphylactoid reactions. Massive envenomation from numerous stings may cause hemolysis, rhabdomyolysis, and shock leading to multiple-organ failure.

Treatment

The physician should remove the stinger, taking care not to squeeze the attached venom sac. For allergic reactions, epinephrine 1:1000 solution, 0.01 mL/kg, should be administered IV or SQ above the site of the sting. Three to four whiffs from an isoproterenol aerosol inhaler may be given at 3- to 4-minute intervals as needed. Corticosteroids (hydrocortisone; 100 mg IV) and diphenhydramine (1.5 mg/kg IV) are useful ancillary drugs but have no immediate effect. Ephedrine or antihistamines may be used for 2 or 3 days to prevent recurrence of symptoms.

A patient who has had a potentially life-threatening insect sting should be desensitized against the Hymenoptera group, because the honey bee, wasp, hornet, and yellow jacket have common antigens in their venom. For the more usual stings, cold compresses, aspirin, and diphenhydramine (1 mg/kg PO) are sufficient.

Ross RN et al: Effectiveness of specific immunotherapy in the treatment of hymenoptera venom hypersensitivity: A meta-analysis. Clin Ther 2000;22:351 [PMID: 10963289].

Vetter RS et al: Mass envenomations by honey bees and wasps. West J Med 1999;170:223 [PMID: 10344177].

INSECTICIDES

The petroleum distillates or other organic solvents used in these products are often as toxic as the insecticide itself. Decontamination may be performed by aspirating the stomach with a nasogastric tube.

1. Chlorinated Hydrocarbons (eg, Aldrin, Carbinol, Chlordane, DDT, Dieldrin, Endrin, Heptachlor, Lindane, Toxaphene)

Signs of intoxication include salivation, GI irritability, abdominal pain, vomiting, diarrhea, CNS depression, and convulsions. Inhalation exposure causes irritation of the eyes, nose, and throat; blurred vision; cough; and pulmonary edema.

Chlorinated hydrocarbons are absorbed through the skin, respiratory tract, and GI tract. Decontamination of skin with soap and evacuation of the stomach contents are critical. All contaminated clothing should be removed. Castor oil, milk, and other substances containing fats or oils should not be left in the stomach because they increase absorption of the chlorinated hydrocarbons. Convulsions should be treated with diazepam (0.1–0.3 mg/kg IV). Epinephrine should not be used because it may cause cardiac arrhythmias.

2. Organophosphate (Cholinesterase-Inhibiting) Insecticides (eg, Chlorothion, Co-Ral, DFP, Diazinon, Malathion, Paraoxon, Parathion, Phosdrin, TEPP, Thio-TEPP)

Dizziness, headache, blurred vision, miosis, tearing, salivation, nausea, vomiting, diarrhea, hyperglycemia, cyanosis, sense of constriction of the chest, dyspnea, sweating, weakness, muscular twitching, convulsions, loss of reflexes and sphincter control, and coma can occur.

The clinical findings are the result of cholinesterase inhibition, which causes an accumulation of acetylcholine. The onset of symptoms occurs within 12 hours of the exposure. Red cell cholinesterase levels should be measured as soon as possible. (Some normal individuals have a low serum cholinesterase level.) Normal values vary in different laboratories. In general, a decrease of red cell cholinesterase to below 25% of normal indicates significant exposure.

Repeated low-grade exposure may result in sudden, acute toxic reactions. This syndrome usually occurs after repeated household spraying rather than agricultural exposure.

Although all organophosphates act by inhibiting cholinesterase activity, they vary greatly in their toxicity. Parathion, for example, is 100 times more toxic than malathion. Toxicity is influenced by the specific compound, type of formulation (liquid or solid), vehicle, and route of absorption (lungs, skin, or GI tract).

Treatment

Decontamination of skin, nails, hair, and clothing with soapy water is extremely important. Atropine plus a cholinesterase reactivator, pralidoxime, is an antidote for organophosphate insecticide poisoning. After assessment and management of the ABCs, atropine should be given and repeated every few minutes until airway secretions diminish. An appropriate starting dose of atropine is 2–4 mg IV in an adult and 0.05 mg/kg in a child. The patient should receive enough atropine to stop secretions (mydriasis in not an appropriate stopping point). Severe poisoning may require gram quantities of atropine administered over 24 hours.

Because atropine antagonizes the muscarinic parasympathetic effects of the organophosphates but does not affect the nicotinic receptor, it does not improve muscular weakness. Pralidoxime should also be given immediately in more severe cases and repeated every 6–12 hours as needed (25–50 mg/kg diluted to 5% and infused over 5–30 minutes at a rate of no more than 500 mg/min). Pralidoxime should be used in addition to—not in place of—atropine if red cell cholinesterase is less than 25% of normal. Pralidoxime is most useful within 48 hours after the exposure but has shown some effects 2–6 days later. Morphine, theophylline, aminophylline, succinylcholine, and tranquilizers of the reserpine and phenothiazine types are contraindicated. Hyperglycemia is common in severe poisonings.

Eisenstein EM, Amitai Y: Index of suspicion: Case 1. Organophosphate intoxication. Pediatr Rev 2000;21:205 [PMID: 10854316].

3. Carbamates (eg, Carbaryl, Sevin, Zectran)

Carbamate insecticides are reversible inhibitors of cholinesterase. The signs and symptoms of intoxication are similar to those associated with organophosphate poisoning but are generally less severe. Atropine titrated to effect is sufficient treatment. Pralidoxime should not be used with carbaryl poisoning but is of value with other carbamates. In combined exposures to organophosphates, give atropine but reserve pralidoxime for cases in which the red cell cholinesterase is depressed below 25% of normal or marked effects of nicotinic receptor stimulation are present.

4. Botanical Insecticides (eg, Black Flag Bug Killer, Black Leaf CPR Insect Killer, Flit Aerosol House & Garden Insect Killer, French's Flea Powder, Raid)

Allergic reactions, asthma-like symptoms, coma, and convulsions have been reported. Pyrethrins, allethrin, and rotenone do not commonly cause signs of toxicity. Antihistamines, short-acting barbiturates, and atropine are helpful as symptomatic treatment.

IRON

Five stages of intoxication may occur in iron poisoning: (1) Hemorrhagic gastroenteritis, which occurs 30–60 minutes after ingestion and may be associated with shock, acidosis, coagulation defects, and coma. This phase usually lasts 4–6 hours. (2) Phase of improvement, lasting 2–12 hours, during which patient looks better. (3) Delayed shock, which may occur 12–48 hours after ingestion. Metabolic acidosis, fever, leukocytosis, and coma may also be present. (4) Liver damage with hepatic failure. (5) Residual pyloric stenosis, which may develop about 4 weeks after the ingestion.

Once iron is absorbed from the GI tract, it is not normally eliminated in feces but may be partially excreted in the urine, giving it a red color prior to chelation. A reddish discoloration of the urine suggests a serum iron level greater than 350 mg/dL.

Treatment

GI decontamination is based on clinical assessment. The patient should be referred to a health care facility if symptomatic or if the history indicates toxic amounts. Gastric lavage and whole bowel irrigation should be considered in these patients.

Shock is treated in the usual manner. Sodium bicarbonate and Fleet Phospho-Soda left in the stomach to form the insoluble phosphate or carbonate have not shown clinical benefit and have caused lethal hypernatremia or hyperphosphatemia. Deferoxamine, a specific chelating agent for iron, is a useful adjunct in the treatment of severe iron poisoning. It forms a soluble complex that is excreted in the urine. It is contraindicated in patients with renal failure unless dialysis can be used. IV deferoxamine chelation therapy should be instituted if the patient is symptomatic and a serum iron determination cannot be obtained readily, or if the peak serum iron exceeds 400 mcg/dL (62.6 μmol/L) at 4–5 hours after ingestion.

Deferoxamine should not be delayed until serum iron levels are available in serious cases of poisoning. IV administration is indicated if the patient is in shock, in which case it should be given at a dosage of 15 mg/kg/h. Infusion rates up to 35 mg/kg/h have been used in life-threatening poisonings. Rapid IV administration can cause hypotension, facial flushing, urticaria, tachycardia, and shock. Deferoxamine, 90 mg/kg IM every 8 hours (maximum, 1 g), may be given if IV access cannot be established, but the procedure is painful. The indications for discontinuation of deferoxamine have not been clearly delineated. Generally, it can be stopped after 12–24 hours if the acidosis has resolved and the patient is improving.

Hemodialysis, peritoneal dialysis, or exchange transfusion can be used to increase the excretion of the dialyzable complex. Urine output should be monitored and urine sediment examined for evidence of renal tubular damage. Initial laboratory studies should include blood typing and cross-matching; total protein; serum iron, sodium, potassium, and chloride; PCO_2; pH; and liver function tests. Serum iron levels fall rapidly even if deferoxamine is not given.

After the acute episode, liver function studies and an upper GI series are indicated to rule out residual damage.

Black J et al: Child abuse by intentional iron poisoning presenting as shock and persistent acidosis. Pediatrics 2003;111:197 [PMID: 12509576].

Juurlink DN et al: Iron poisoning in young children: Association with the birth of a sibling. CMAJ 2003;165:1539 [PMID: 12796332].

LEAD

Lead poisoning (plumbism) causes vague symptoms, including weakness, irritability, weight loss, vomiting, personality changes, ataxia, constipation, headache, and colicky abdominal pain. Late manifestations consist of retarded development, convulsions, and coma associated with increased intracranial pressure, which is a medical emergency.

Plumbism usually occurs insidiously in children younger than age 5 years. The most likely sources of lead include flaking leaded paint, artist's paints, fruit tree sprays, solder, brass alloys, home-glazed pottery, and fumes from burning batteries. Only paint containing less than 1% lead is safe for interior use (eg, furniture, toys). Repetitive ingestions of small amounts of lead are far more serious than a single massive exposure. Toxic effects are likely to occur if more than 0.5 mg of lead per day is absorbed.

Blood lead levels are used to assess the severity of exposure. A complete blood count and serum ferritin concentration should be obtained; iron deficiency increases absorption of lead. Glycosuria, proteinuria, hematuria, and aminoaciduria occur frequently. Blood lead levels usually exceed 80 mcg/dL in symptomatic patients. Abnormal blood lead levels should be repeated in asymptomatic patients to rule out laboratory error. Specimens must be meticulously obtained in acid-washed containers. A normocytic, slightly hypochromic anemia with basophilic stippling of the red cells and reticulocytosis may be present in plumbism. Stippling of red blood cells is absent in cases involving only recent ingestion.

The cerebrospinal fluid (CSF) protein is elevated, and the white cell count usually is less than 100 cells/mL. CSF pressure may be elevated in patients with encephalopathy; lumbar punctures must be performed cautiously to prevent herniation.

Treatment

Succimer is an orally administered chelator approved for use in children and reported to be as efficacious as calcium edetate. Treatment for blood lead levels of 20–45 mcg/dL in children has not been determined. Succimer should be initiated at blood lead levels over 45 mcg/dL. The initial dose is 10 mg/kg (350 mg/m^2) every 8 hours for 5 days. The same dose is then given every 12 hours for 14 days. At least 2 weeks should elapse between courses. Blood lead levels increase somewhat (ie, rebound) after discontinuation of therapy. Courses of dimercaprol (4 mg/kg per dose) and calcium edetate may still be used but are no longer the preferred method, except in cases of lead encephalopathy.

Anticonvulsants may be needed. Mannitol or corticosteroids and volume restriction are indicated in patients with encephalopathy. A high-calcium, high-phosphorus diet and large doses of vitamin D may remove lead from the blood by depositing it in the bones. A public health team should evaluate the source of the lead. Necessary corrections should be completed before the child is returned home.

Markowitz M: Lead poisoning. Pediatr Rev 2000;21:327 [PMID: 11010979].

Rogan WJ et al: Treatment of Lead-Exposed Children Trial Group: The effect of chelation therapy with succimer on neuropsychological development in children exposed to lead. N Engl J Med 2001;344:1421 [PMID: 11346806].

MAGNETS

Although not strictly toxic, small magnets have been found to cause bowel obstructions in children. Recent cases have resulted in warnings and a recall by the Consumer Product Safety Commission following intestinal perforation and death in a 20-month-old child. Obstruction may occur following ingestion of as few as two magnets.

Alzahem AM et al: Ingested magnets and gastrointestinal complications. J Paediatr Child Health 2007:43:497 [PMID: 17535185].

Consumer Product Safety Commission: http://www.cpsc.gov/CPSCPUB/PREREL/prhtml07/07163.html 2007

MUSHROOMS

Toxic mushrooms are often difficult to distinguish from edible varieties. Contact a poison control center to obtain identification assistance. Symptoms vary with the species ingested, time of year, stage of maturity, quantity eaten, method of preparation, and interval since ingestion. A mushroom that is toxic to one individual may not be toxic to another. Drinking alcohol and eating certain mushrooms may cause a reaction similar to that seen with disulfiram and alcohol. Cooking destroys some toxins but not the deadly one produced by *Amanita phalloides*, which is responsible for 90% of deaths due to mushroom poisoning. Mushroom toxins are absorbed relatively slowly. Onset of symptoms within 2 hours of ingestion suggests muscarinic toxin, whereas a delay of symptoms for 6–48 hours after ingestion strongly suggests *Amanita* (amanitin) poisoning. Patients who have ingested *A phalloides* may relapse and die of hepatic or renal failure following initial improvement.

Mushroom poisoning may produce muscarinic symptoms (salivation, vomiting, diarrhea, cramping abdominal pain, tenesmus, miosis, and dyspnea), coma, convulsions, hallucinations, hemolysis, and delayed hepatic and renal failure.

Treatment

Administer activated charcoal. If the patient has muscarinic signs, give atropine, 0.05 mg/kg IM (0.02 mg/kg in toddlers), and repeat as needed (usually every 30 minutes) to keep the patient atropinized. Atropine, however, is used only when cholinergic effects are present and not for all mushrooms. Hypoglycemia is most likely to occur in patients with delayed onset of symptoms. Try to identify the mushroom if the patient is symptomatic. Consultation with a certified poison center is recommended. Local botanical gardens, university departments of botany, and societies of mycologists may be able to help. Supportive care is usually all that is needed; however, in the case of *A phalloides*, penicillin, silibinin, or hemodialysis may be indicated.

Lampe KF, McCann MA: Differential diagnosis of poisoning by North American mushrooms, with particular emphasis on *Amanita phalloides*-like intoxication. Ann Emerg Med 1987;16:956 [PMID: 3631682].

Pawlowska J et al: Liver transplantation in three family members after *Amanita phalloides* mushroom poisoning. Transplant Proc 2002;34:3313 [PMID: 12493457].

NITRITES, NITRATES, ANILINE, PENTACHLOROPHENOL, & DINITROPHENOL

Nausea, vertigo, vomiting, cyanosis (methemoglobinemia), cramping, abdominal pain, tachycardia, cardiovascular collapse, tachypnea, coma, shock, convulsions, and death are possible manifestations of nitrite or nitrate poisoning.

Nitrite and nitrate compounds found in the home include amyl nitrite, butyl nitrates, isobutyl nitrates, nitroglycerin, pentaerythritol tetranitrate, sodium nitrite, nitrobenzene, and phenazopyridine. Pentachlorophenol and dinitrophenol, which are found in wood preservatives, produce methemoglobinemia and high fever because of uncoupling of oxidative phosphorylation. Headache, dizziness, and bradycardia have been reported. High concentrations of nitrites in well water or spinach have been the most common cause of nitrite-induced methemoglobinemia. Symptoms do not usually occur until 15%–50% of the hemoglobin has been converted to methemoglobin. A rapid test is to compare a drop of normal blood with the patient's blood on a dry filter paper. Brown discoloration of the patient's blood indicates a methemoglobin level of more than 15%.

Treatment

Administer activated charcoal. Decontaminate affected skin with soap and water. Oxygen and artificial respiration may be needed. If the blood methemoglobin level exceeds 30%, or if levels cannot be obtained and the patient is symptomatic, give a 1% solution of methylene blue (0.2 mL/kg IV) over 5–10 minutes. Avoid perivascular infiltration, because it causes necrosis of the skin and subcutaneous tissues. A dramatic change in the degree of cyanosis should occur. Transfusion is occasionally necessary. Epinephrine and other vasoconstrictors are contraindicated. If reflex bradycardia occurs, atropine should be used.

Kennedy N et al: Faulty sausage production causing methaemoglobinaemia. Arch Dis Child 1997;76:367 [PMID: 9166036].

OPIOIDS (CODEINE, HEROIN, METHADONE, MORPHINE, PROPOXYPHENE)

Opioid-related medical problems may include drug addiction, withdrawal in a newborn infant, and accidental overdoses. Unlike other narcotics, methadone is absorbed readily from the GI tract. Most opioids, including heroin, methadone, meperidine, morphine, and codeine, are excreted in the urine within 24 hours and can be detected readily.

Narcotic-addicted adolescents often have other medical problems, including cellulitis, abscesses, thrombophlebitis, tetanus, infective endocarditis, human immunodeficiency virus (HIV) infection, tuberculosis, hepatitis, malaria, foreign body emboli, thrombosis of pulmonary arterioles, diabetes mellitus, obstetric complications, nephropathy, and peptic ulcer.

Treatment

A. Overdose

Opioids can cause respiratory depression, stridor, coma, increased oropharyngeal secretions, sinus bradycardia, and urinary retention. Pulmonary edema rarely occurs in children; deaths usually result from aspiration of gastric contents, respiratory arrest, and cerebral edema. Convulsions may occur with propoxyphene overdosage.

Although suggested doses for naloxone hydrochloride range from 0.01 to 0.1 mg/kg, it is generally unnecessary to calculate the dosage on this basis. This extremely safe antidote should be given in sufficient quantity to reverse opioid-binding sites. For children younger than age 1 year, 1 ampoule (0.4 mg) should be given initially; if there is no response, 5 more ampoules (2 mg) should be given rapidly. Older children should be given 0.4–0.8 mg, followed by 2–4 mg if there is no response. An improvement in respiratory status may be followed by respiratory depression, because the antagonist's duration of action is less than 1 hour. Neonates poisoned in utero may require 10–30 mg/kg to reverse the effect.

B. Withdrawal in the Addict

Diazepam (10 mg every 6 hours PO) has been recommended for the treatment of mild narcotic withdrawal in ambulatory adolescents. Management of withdrawal in the confirmed addict may be accomplished with the administration of clonidine, by substitution with methadone, or with reintroduction of the original addicting agent, if available through a supervised drug withdrawal program. A tapered course over 3 weeks will accomplish this goal. Death rarely, if ever, occurs. The abrupt discontinuation of narcotics (cold turkey method) is not recommended and may cause severe physical withdrawal signs.

C. Withdrawal in the Newborn

A newborn infant in opioid withdrawal is usually small for gestational age and demonstrates yawning, sneezing, decreased Moro reflex, hunger but uncoordinated sucking action, jitteriness, tremor, constant movement, a shrill protracted cry, increased tendon reflexes, convulsions, vomiting, fever, watery diarrhea, cyanosis, dehydration, vasomotor instability, seizure, and collapse.

The onset of symptoms commonly begins in the first 48 hours but may be delayed as long as 8 days, depending on the timing of the mother's last fix and her predelivery medication. The diagnosis can be confirmed easily by identifying the narcotic in the urine of the mother and the newborn.

Several treatment methods have been suggested for narcotic withdrawal in the newborn. Phenobarbital (8 mg/kg/d IM or PO in four doses for 4 days and then reduced by one-third every 2 days as signs decrease) may be continued for as long as 3 weeks. Methadone may be necessary in those infants with congenital methadone addiction who are not controlled in their withdrawal by large doses of phenobarbital. Dosage should be 0.5 mg/kg/d in two divided doses but can be increased gradually as needed. After control of the symptoms is achieved, the dose may be tapered over 4 weeks.

It is unclear whether prophylactic treatment with these drugs decreases the complication rate. The mortality rate of untreated narcotic withdrawal in the newborn may be as high as 45%.

Bailey JE, Campagna E, Dart RC: The underrecognized toll of prescription opioid abuse on young children. Ann Emerg Med 2009;53:419–424 [PMID: 18774623].

PHENOTHIAZINES (CHLORPROMAZINE, PROCHLORPERAZINE, TRIFLUOPERAZINE)

Clinical Findings

A. Extrapyramidal Crisis

Episodes characterized by torticollis, stiffening of the body, spasticity, poor speech, catatonia, and inability to communicate although conscious are typical manifestations. These episodes usually last a few seconds to a few minutes but have rarely caused death. Extrapyramidal crises may represent idiosyncratic reactions and are aggravated by dehydration. The signs and symptoms occur most often in children who have received prochlorperazine. They are commonly mistaken for psychotic episodes.

B. Overdose

Lethargy and deep prolonged coma commonly occur. Promazine, chlorpromazine, and prochlorperazine are the drugs most likely to cause respiratory depression and precipitous drops in blood pressure. Occasionally, paradoxic hyperactivity and extrapyramidal signs as well as hyperglycemia and acetonemia are present. Seizures are uncommon.

C. Neuroleptic Malignant Syndrome

Neuroleptic malignant syndrome is a rare idiosyncratic complication of phenothiazine use that may be lethal. It is a syndrome involving mental status change (confusion, coma), motor abnormalities (lead pipe rigidity, clonus), and autonomic dysfunction (tachycardia, hyperpyrexia).

Treatment

Extrapyramidal signs are alleviated within minutes by the slow IV administration of diphenhydramine, 1–2 mg/kg (maximum, 50 mg), or benztropine mesylate, 1–2 mg IV (1 mg/min). No other treatment is usually indicated.

Patients with overdoses should receive conservative supportive care. Activated charcoal should be administered. Hypotension may be treated with standard agents, starting with isotonic saline administration. Agitation is best treated with diazepam. Neuroleptic malignant syndrome is treated by discontinuing the drug, giving aggressive supportive care, and administering dantrolene or bromocriptine.

O'Malley GF et al: Olanzapine overdose mimicking opioid intoxication. Ann Emerg Med 1999;34:279 [PMID: 10424936].

PLANTS

Many common ornamental, garden, and wild plants are potentially toxic. Only in a few cases will small amounts of a plant cause severe illness or death. Table 13–6 **lists the most toxic plants, symptoms and signs of poisoning, and treatment.** Contact your poison control center for assistance with identification.

PSYCHOTROPIC DRUGS

Psychotropic drugs consist of four general classes: stimulants (amphetamines, cocaine), depressants (eg, narcotics, barbiturates), antidepressants and tranquilizers, and hallucinogens (eg, lysergic acid diethylamide [LSD], phencyclidine [PCP]).

Table 13–6. Poisoning due to plants.[a]

	Symptoms and Signs	Treatment
Arum family: *Caladium*, *Dieffenbachia*, callalily, dumb cane (oxalic acid)	Burning of mucous membranes and airway obstruction secondary to edema caused by calcium oxalate crystals.	Accessible areas should be thoroughly washed. Corticosteroids relieve airway obstruction. Apply cold packs to affected mucous membranes.
Castor bean plant (ricin—a toxalbumin) Jequinty bean (abrin—a toxalbumin)	Mucous membrane irritation, nausea, vomiting, bloody diarrhea, blurred vision, circulatory collapse, acute hemolytic anemia, convulsions, uremia.	Fluid and electrolyte monitoring. Saline cathartic. Forced alkaline diuresis will prevent complications due to hemagglutination and hemolysis.
Foxglove, lily of the valley, and oleander[b]	Nausea, diarrhea, visual disturbances, and cardiac irregularities (eg, heart block).	See treatment for digitalis drugs in text.
Jimsonweed: See Belladonna Alkaloids section in text	Mydriasis, dry mouth, tachycardia, and hallucinations.	Activated charcoal.
Larkspur (ajacine, *Delphinium*, delphinine)	Nausea and vomiting, irritability, muscular paralysis, and central nervous system depression.	Symptomatic. Atropine may be helpful.
Monkshood (aconite)	Numbness of mucous membranes, visual disturbances, tingling, dizziness, tinnitus, hypotension, bradycardia, and convulsions.	Activated charcoal, oxygen. Atropine is probably helpful.
Poison hemlock (coniine)	Mydriasis, trembling, dizziness, bradycardia. Central nervous system depression, muscular paralysis, and convulsions. Death is due to respiratory paralysis.	Symptomatic. Oxygen and cardiac monitoring equipment are desirable. Assisted respiration is often necessary. Give anticonvulsants if needed.
Rhododendron (grayanotoxin)	Abdominal cramps, vomiting, severe diarrhea, muscular paralysis. Central nervous system and circulatory depression. Hypertension with very large doses.	Atropine can prevent bradycardia. Epinephrine is contraindicated. Antihypertensives may be needed.
Yellow jessamine (active ingredient, geisemine, is related to strychnine)	Restlessness, convulsions, muscular paralysis, and respiratory depression.	Symptomatic. Because of the relation to strychnine, activated charcoal and diazepam for seizures are worth trying.

[a]Many other plants cause minor irritation but are not likely to cause serious problems unless large amounts are ingested. Data from Lampe KF, McCann MA: *AMA Handbook of Poisonous and Injurious Plants.* American Medical Association, 1985.
[b]Done AK: Ornamental and deadly. Emerg Med 1973;5:255.

Clinical Findings

The following clinical findings are commonly seen in patients abusing drugs. See also other entries discussed in alphabetic order in this chapter.

A. Stimulants

Agitation, euphoria, grandiose feelings, tachycardia, fever, abdominal cramps, visual and auditory hallucinations, mydriasis, coma, convulsions, and respiratory depression.

B. Depressants

Emotional lability, ataxia, diplopia, nystagmus, vertigo, poor accommodation, respiratory depression, coma, apnea, and convulsions. Dilation of conjunctival blood vessels suggests marijuana ingestion. Narcotics cause miotic pupils and, occasionally, pulmonary edema.

C. Antidepressants and Tranquilizers

Hypotension, lethargy, respiratory depression, coma, and extrapyramidal reactions.

D. Hallucinogens and Psychoactive Drugs

Belladonna alkaloids cause mydriasis, dry mouth, nausea, vomiting, urinary retention, confusion, disorientation, paranoid delusions, hallucinations, fever, hypotension, aggressive behavior, convulsions, and coma. Psychoactive drugs such as LSD cause mydriasis, unexplained bizarre behavior, hallucinations, and generalized undifferentiated psychotic behavior.

Treatment

Only a small percentage of the persons using drugs come to the attention of physicians; those who do are usually experiencing adverse reactions such as panic states, drug psychoses, homicidal or suicidal thoughts, or respiratory depression.

Even with cooperative patients, an accurate history is difficult to obtain. A drug history is most easily obtained in a quiet spot by a gentle, nonthreatening, honest examiner, and without the parents present. The user often does not really know what drug has been taken or how much. Street drugs are almost always adulterated with one or more other compounds. Multiple drugs are often taken together. Friends may be a useful source of information.

The patient's general appearance, skin, lymphatics, cardiorespiratory status, GI tract, and CNS should be focused on during the physical examination, because they often provide clues suggesting drug abuse.

Hallucinogens are not life-threatening unless the patient is frankly homicidal or suicidal. A specific diagnosis is usually not necessary for management; instead, the presenting signs and symptoms are treated. Does the patient appear intoxicated? In withdrawal? "Flashing back?" Is some illness or injury (eg, head trauma) being masked by a drug effect? (Remember that a known drug user may still have hallucinations from meningoencephalitis.)

The signs and symptoms in a given patient are a function not only of the drug and the dose but also of the level of acquired tolerance, the "setting," the patient's physical condition and personality traits, the potentiating effects of other drugs, and many other factors.

A common drug problem is the "bad trip," which is usually a panic reaction. This is best managed by "talking the patient down" and minimizing auditory and visual stimuli. Allowing the patient to sit with a friend while the drug effect dissipates may be the best treatment. This may take several hours. The physician's job is not to terminate the drug effect but to help the patient through the bad experience.

Drug therapy is often unnecessary and may complicate the clinical course of a drug-related panic reaction.

Although phenothiazines have been commonly used to treat bad trips, they should be avoided if the specific drug is unknown, because they may enhance toxicity or produce unwanted side effects. Diazepam is the drug of choice if a sedative effect is required. Physical restraints are rarely indicated and usually increase the patient's panic reaction.

For treatment of life-threatening drug abuse, consult the section on the specific drug elsewhere in this chapter and the section on general management at the beginning of the chapter.

After the acute episode, the physician must decide whether psychiatric referral is indicated; in general, patients who have made suicidal gestures or attempts and adolescents who are not communicating with their families should be referred.

Weir E: Raves: A review of the culture, the drugs and the prevention of harm. CMAJ 2000;162:1843 [PMID: 10906922].

SALICYLATES

The use of childproof containers and publicity regarding accidental poisoning have reduced the incidence of acute salicylate poisoning. Nevertheless, serious intoxication still occurs and must be regarded as an emergency. In recent years, the frequency of poisoning has begun to rise again.

Salicylates uncouple oxidative phosphorylation, leading to increased heat production, excessive sweating, and dehydration. They also interfere with glucose metabolism and may cause hypo- or hyperglycemia. Respiratory center stimulation occurs early.

Patients usually have signs of hyperventilation, sweating, dehydration, and fever. Vomiting and diarrhea sometimes occur. In severe cases, disorientation, convulsions, and coma may develop.

The severity of acute intoxication can, in some measure, be judged by serum salicylate levels. High levels are always dangerous irrespective of clinical signs, and low levels may be misleading in chronic cases. Other laboratory values usually indicate metabolic acidosis despite hyperventilation, low serum K^+ values, and often abnormal serum glucose levels.

In mild and moderate poisoning, stimulation of the respiratory center produces respiratory alkalosis. In severe intoxication (occurring in severe acute ingestion with high salicylate levels and in chronic toxicity with lower levels), respiratory response is unable to overcome the metabolic overdose.

Once the urine becomes acidic, progressively smaller amounts of salicylate are excreted. Until this process is reversed, the half-life will remain prolonged, because metabolism contributes little to the removal of salicylate.

Chronic severe poisoning may occur as early as 3 days after a regimen of salicylate is begun. Findings usually include vomiting, diarrhea, and dehydration.

Treatment

Charcoal binds salicylates well and should be given for acute ingestions. Mild poisoning may require only the administration of oral fluids and confirmation that the salicylate level is falling. Moderate poisoning involves moderate dehydration and depletion of potassium. Fluids must be administered at a rate of 2–3 mL/kg/h to correct dehydration and produce urine with a pH of greater than 7.0. Initial IV solutions should be isotonic, with sodium bicarbonate constituting half the electrolyte content. Once the patient is rehydrated, the solution can contain more free water and approximately 40 mEq/L of K^+.

Severe toxicity is marked by major dehydration. Symptoms may be confused with those of Reye syndrome, encephalopathy, and metabolic acidosis. Salicylate levels may even be in the therapeutic range. Major fluid correction of dehydration is required. Once this has been accomplished, hypokalemia must be corrected and sodium bicarbonate given. Usual requirements are sodium bicarbonate, 1–2 mEq/kg/h over the first 6–8 hours, and K^+, 20–40 mEq/L. A urine flow of 2–3 mL/kg/h should be established. Despite this treatment some patients will develop the paradoxical aciduria of salicylism. This is due to hypokalemia and the saving of K^+ and excretion of H^+ in the renal tubule. Correction of K^+ will allow the urine to become alkaline and ionize the salicylate, resulting in excretion rather than reabsorption of nonionized salicylate in acid urine.

Renal failure or pulmonary edema is an indication for dialysis. Hemodialysis is most effective and peritoneal dialysis is relatively ineffective. Hemodialysis should be used in all patients with altered mental status or deteriorating clinical status. Acetazolamide should not be used.

Yip L et al: Concepts and controversies in salicylate toxicity. Emerg Med Clin North Am 1994;12:351 [PMID: 8187688].

SCORPION STINGS

Scorpion stings are common in arid areas of the southwestern United States. Scorpion venom is more toxic than most snake venoms, but only minute amounts are injected. Although neurologic manifestations may last a week, most clinical signs subside within 24–48 hours.

The most common scorpions in the United States are *Vejovis*, *Hadrurus*, *Androctonus*, and *Centruroides* species. Stings by the first three produce edema and pain. Stings by *Centruroides* (the Bark scorpion) cause tingling or burning paresthesias that begin at the site of the sting; other findings include hypersalivation, restlessness, muscular fasciculation, abdominal cramps, opisthotonos, convulsions, urinary incontinence, and respiratory failure.

Treatment

Sedation is the primary therapy. Antivenom is reserved for severe poisoning. In severe cases, the airway may become compromised by secretions and weakness of respiratory muscles. Endotracheal intubation may be required. Patients may require treatment for seizures, hypertension, or tachycardia.

The prognosis is good as long as the patient's airway is managed appropriately.

Boyer LV et al: Antivenom for critically ill children with neurotoxicity from scorpion stings. N Engl J Med 2009;360:2090–2098 [PMID: 19439743].

LoVecchio F et al: Incidence of immediate and delayed hypersensitivity to *Centruroides* antivenom. Ann Emerg Med 1999;34:615 [PMID: 10533009].

SEROTONIN REUPTAKE INHIBITORS

Fluoxetine (Prozac), paroxetine (Paxil), sertraline (Zoloft), and many other agents comprise this class of drugs. Adverse effects in therapeutic dosing include suicidal thoughts, aggressive behavior, extrapyramidal effects, and cardiac dysrhythmias, and in overdose may include vomiting, lethargy, seizures, hypertension, tachycardia, hyperthermia, and abdominal pain. The findings in overdose are included in the serotonin syndrome due to the action of these drugs, which results in an increase of serotonin (5-hydroxytryptamine [5-HT]). Despite the degree of toxicity these agents generally are not life-threatening and intervention usually is not necessary.

Emptying the stomach is not helpful, but activated charcoal may be useful. Laboratory measurements of the drugs are not of benefit other than to establish their presence.

Treatment with benzodiazepines is most beneficial. Hypotension may be treated with fluids or norepinephrine. Cyproheptadine is an antagonist of serotonin, but its use has been limited. A dose of 0.25 mg/kg/d divided every 6 hours to a maximum of 12 mg/d may be useful in treating the serotonin syndrome. Adults and older adolescents have been treated with 12 mg initially followed by 2 mg every 2 hours to a maximum of 32 mg/d.

Boyer EW, Shannon M: The serotonin syndrome. N Engl J Med 2005;352:1112 [PMID: 15784664].

SNAKEBITE

Despite the lethal potential of venomous snakes, human morbidity and mortality rates are surprisingly low. The outcome depends on the size of the child, the site of the bite, the degree of envenomation, the type of snake, and the effectiveness of treatment.

Nearly all poisonous snakebites in the United States are caused by pit vipers (rattlesnakes, water moccasins, and copperheads). A few are caused by elapids (coral snakes), and occasional bites occur from cobras and other nonindigenous exotic snakes kept as pets. Snake venom is a complex mixture of enzymes, peptides, and proteins that may have predominantly cytotoxic, neurotoxic, hemotoxic, or cardiotoxic effects but other effects as well. Up to 25% of bites by pit vipers do not result in venom injection. Pit viper venom causes predominantly local injury with pain, discoloration, edema, and hemorrhage.

Swelling and pain occur soon after rattlesnake bite and are a certain indication that envenomation has occurred. During the first few hours, swelling and ecchymosis extend proximally from the bite. The bite is often obvious as a double puncture mark surrounded by ecchymosis. Hematemesis, melena, hemoptysis, and other manifestations of coagulopathy develop in severe cases. Respiratory difficulty and shock are the ultimate causes of death. Even in fatal rattlesnake bites, a period of 6–8 hours usually elapses between the bite and death; as a result, there is usually enough time to start effective treatment.

Coral snake envenomation causes little local pain, swelling, or necrosis, and systemic reactions are often delayed. The signs of coral snake envenomation include bulbar paralysis, dysphagia, and dysphoria; these signs may appear in

5–10 hours and may be followed by total peripheral paralysis and death in 24 hours.

Treatment

Children in snake-infested areas should wear boots and long trousers, should not walk barefoot, and should be cautioned not to explore under ledges or in holes.

A. Emergency (First-Aid) Treatment

The most important first-aid measure is transportation to a medical facility. Splint the affected extremity and minimize the patient's motion. Tourniquets and ice packs are contraindicated. Incision and suction are not useful for either crotalid or elapid snake bite.

B. Definitive Medical Management

Blood should be drawn for hematocrit, clotting time and platelet function, and serum electrolyte determinations. Establish two secure IV sites for the administration of antivenom and other medications.

Specific antivenom is indicated when signs of progressive envenomation are present. Two antivenoms are available for treating pit viper envenomation: polyvalent pit viper antivenom and polyvalent Crotalidae Fab (CroFab). Both are effective, but their indications differ. For coral snake bites, an eastern coral snake antivenom (Wyeth Laboratories) is available. Patients with pit viper bites should receive antivenom if progressive local injury, coagulopathy, or systemic signs (eg, hypotension, confusion) are present. (Antivenom should not be given IM or SQ.) See package labeling or call your certified poison center for details of use. Hemorrhage, pain, and shock diminish rapidly with adequate amounts of antivenom. For coral snake bites, give three to five vials of antivenom in 250–500 mL of isotonic saline solution. An additional three to five vials may be required. While generally considered best if administered within the first 6 hours, recent evidence demonstrates that delayed use may be therapeutic.

To control pain, administer a narcotic analgesic, such as meperidine (0.6–1.5 mg/kg per dose, given PO or IM). Cryotherapy is contraindicated because it commonly causes additional tissue damage. Early physiotherapy minimizes contractures. In rare cases, fasciotomy to relieve pressure within muscular compartments is required. The evaluation of function and of pulses will better predict the need for fasciotomy. Antihistamines and corticosteroids (hydrocortisone, 1 mg/kg, given PO for a week) are useful in the treatment of serum sickness or anaphylactic shock. Antibiotics are not needed unless clinical signs of infection occur. Tetanus status should be evaluated and the patient immunized, if needed.

Bebarta V, Dart RC: Effectiveness of delayed use of crotalidae polyvalent immune FAB (ovine) antivenoms. J Toxicol Clin Toxicol 2004;42:321–324 [PMID: 15362603].

Dart RC, McNally J: Efficacy, safety, and use of snake antivenoms in the United States. Ann Emerg Med 2001;37:181 [PMID: 11174237].

Offerman SR et al: Crotaline Fab antivenom for the treatment of children with rattle snake envenomation. Pediatrics 2002;110:968 [PMID: 12415038].

SOAPS & DETERGENTS

1. Soaps

Soap is made from salts of fatty acids. Some toilet soap bars contain both soap and detergent. Ingestion of soap bars may cause vomiting and diarrhea, but they have a low toxicity. Induced emesis is unnecessary.

2. Detergents

Detergents are nonsoap synthetic products used for cleaning purposes because of their surfactant properties. Commercial products include granules, powders, and liquids. Dishwasher detergents are very alkaline and can cause caustic burns. Low concentrations of bleaching and antibacterial agents as well as enzymes are found in many preparations. The pure compounds are moderately toxic, but the concentration used is too small to alter the product's toxicity significantly, although occasional primary or allergic irritative phenomena have been noted in persons who frequently use such products and in employees manufacturing these products.

A. Cationic Detergents (Ceepryn, Diaparene Cream, Phemerol, Zephiran)

Cationic detergents in dilute solutions (0.5%) cause mucosal irritation, but higher concentrations (10%–15%) may cause caustic burns to mucosa. Clinical effects include nausea, vomiting, collapse, coma, and convulsions. As little as 2.25 g of some cationic agents have caused death in an adult. In four cases, 100–400 mg/kg of benzalkonium chloride caused death. Cationic detergents are rapidly inactivated by tissues and ordinary soap.

Because of the caustic potential and rapid onset of seizures, emesis is not recommended. Activated charcoal should be administered. Anticonvulsants may be needed.

B. Anionic Detergents

Most common household detergents are anionic. Laundry compounds have water softener (sodium phosphate) added, which is a strong irritant and may reduce ionized calcium. Anionic detergents irritate the skin by removing natural oils. Although ingestion causes diarrhea, intestinal distention, and vomiting, no fatalities have been reported.

The only treatment usually required is to discontinue use if skin irritation occurs and replace fluids and electrolytes. Induced vomiting is not indicated following ingestion of automatic dishwasher detergent, because of its alkalinity. Dilute with water or milk.

C. Nonionic Detergents (Brij Products; Tritons X-45, X-100, X-102, and X-144)

These compounds include lauryl, stearyl, and oleyl alcohols and octyl phenol. They have a minimal irritating effect on the skin and are almost always nontoxic when swallowed.

Klasaer AE et al: Marked hypocalcemia and ventricular fibrillation in two pediatric patients exposed to a fluoride-containing wheel cleaner. Ann Emerg Med 1996;28:713 [PMID: 8953969].

Vincent JC, Sheikh A: Phosphate poisoning by ingestion of clothes washing liquid and fabric conditioner. Anesthesiology 1998;53:1004 [PMID: 9893545].

SPIDER BITES

Most medically important bites in the United States are caused by the black widow spider (*Latrodectus mactans*) and the North American brown recluse (violin) spider (*Loxosceles reclusa*). Positive identification of the spider is helpful, because many spider bites may mimic those of the brown recluse spider.

1. Black Widow Spider

The black widow spider is endemic to nearly all areas of the United States. The initial bite causes sharp fleeting pain. Local and systemic muscular cramping, abdominal pain, nausea and vomiting, and shock can occur. Convulsions occur more commonly in small children than in older children. Systemic signs of black widow spider bite may be confused with other causes of acute abdomen. Although paresthesias, nervousness, and transient muscle spasms may persist for weeks in survivors, recovery from the acute phase is generally complete within 3 days. In contrast to popular opinion, death is extremely rare.

Most authors recommend calcium gluconate as initial therapy (50 mg/kg IV per dose, up to 250 mg/kg/24 h), although it is often not effective and the effects are of short duration. Methocarbamol (15 mg/kg PO) or diazepam titrated to effect is useful. Morphine or barbiturates may occasionally be needed for control of pain or restlessness, but they increase the possibility of respiratory depression. Antivenom is available but should be reserved for severe cases in which the previously mentioned therapies have failed. Local treatment of the bite is not helpful.

2. Brown Recluse Spider (Violin Spider)

The North American brown recluse spider is most commonly seen in the central and Midwestern areas of the United States. Its bite characteristically produces a localized reaction with progressively severe pain within 24 hours. The initial bleb on an erythematous ischemic base is replaced by a black eschar within 1 week. This eschar separates in 2–5 weeks, leaving an ulcer that heals slowly. Systemic signs include cyanosis, morbilliform rash, fever, chills, malaise, weakness, nausea and vomiting, joint pains, hemolytic reactions with hemoglobinuria, jaundice, and delirium. Fatalities are rare. Fatal disseminated intravascular coagulation has been reported.

Although of unproved efficacy, the following therapies have been used: dexamethasone, 4 mg IV four times a day, during the acute phase; polymorphonuclear leukocyte inhibitors, such as dapsone or colchicine, and oxygen applied to the bite site; and total excision of the lesion to the fascial level.

Clark RF et al: Clinical presentation and treatment of black widow spider envenomation: A review of 163 cases. Ann Emerg Med 1992;21:782 [PMID: 1351707].

Sams HH et al: Nineteen documented cases of *Loxosceles reclusa* envenomation. J Am Acad Dermatol 2001;44:603 [PMID: 11260528].

THYROID PREPARATIONS (THYROID DESICCATED, SODIUM LEVOTHYROXINE)

Ingestion of the equivalent of 50–150 g of desiccated thyroid can cause signs of hyperthyroidism, including irritability, mydriasis, hyperpyrexia, tachycardia, and diarrhea. Maximal clinical effect occurs about 9 days after ingestion—several days after the protein-bound iodine level has fallen dramatically.

Administer activated charcoal. If the patient develops clinical signs of toxicity, propranolol, 0.01–0.1 mg/kg (maximum, 1 mg), is useful because of its antiadrenergic activity.

Brown RS et al: Successful treatment of massive acute thyroid hormone poisoning with iopanoic acid. J Pediatr 1998;132:903 [PMID: 9602214].

VITAMINS

Accidental ingestion of excessive amounts of vitamins rarely causes significant problems. Occasional cases of hypervitaminosis A and D do occur, however, particularly in patients with poor hepatic or renal function. The fluoride contained in many multivitamin preparations is not a realistic hazard, because a 2- or 3-year-old child could eat 100 tablets, containing 1 mg of sodium fluoride per tablet, without experiencing serious symptoms. Iron poisoning has been reported with multivitamin tablets containing iron. Pyridoxine abuse has caused neuropathies; nicotinic acid has resulted in myopathy.

Dean BS, Krenzelok EP: Multiple vitamins and vitamins with iron: Accidental poisoning in children. Vet Hum Toxicol 1988;30:23 [PMID: 3354178].

Fraser DR: Vitamin D. Lancet 1995;345:104 [PMID: 7815853].

WARFARIN (COUMADIN)

Warfarin is used as a rodenticide. It causes hypoprothrombinemia and capillary injury. It is absorbed readily from the GI tract but is absorbed poorly through the skin. A dose of 0.5 mg/kg of warfarin may be toxic in a child. A prothrombin time is helpful in establishing the severity of the poisoning.

If bleeding occurs or the prothrombin time is prolonged, give 1–5 mg of vitamin K_1 (phytonadione) IM or SQ. For large ingestions with established toxicity, 0.6 mg/kg may be given.

Another group of long-acting anticoagulant rodenticides (brodifacoum, difenacoum, bromadiolone, diphacinone, pinene, valone, and coumatetralyl) have been a more serious toxicologic problem than warfarin. They also cause hypoprothrombinemia and a bleeding diathesis that responds to phytonadione, although the anticoagulant activity may persist for periods ranging from 6 weeks to several months. Treatment with vitamin K_1 may be needed for weeks.

Isbister GK, Whyte IM: Management of anticoagulant poisoning. Vet Hum Toxicol 2001;43:117 [PMID: 11308119].

Critical Care

14

Joseph A. Albietz III, MD
Todd C. Carpenter, MD
Angela S. Czaja, MD, MSc
Emily L. Dobyns, MD, FCCM
Jennifer Exo, DO
Eva N. Grayck, MD
Peter M. Mourani, MD
Kathleen Ventre, MD

INTRODUCTION

The care of patients with life-threatening conditions requires a detailed understanding of human physiology and the pathophysiology of major illnesses, as well as an understanding of and experience with the rapidly changing technologies available in a modern intensive care unit (ICU). The science of caring for the critically ill patient has evolved rapidly over the past decade as the molecular mediators of illness have become better defined and new therapies have been devised based on those advances. As a result, critical care is a multidisciplinary field that requires a team-oriented approach, including critical care physicians and nursing staff, pharmacists, referring physicians, consulting specialists, and social services specialists.

Durbin CG Jr: Team model: Advocating for the optimal method of care delivery in the intensive care unit. Crit Care Med 2006;34(Suppl):S12 [PMID: 16477198].

ACUTE RESPIRATORY FAILURE

ESSENTIALS OF DIAGNOSIS & TYPICAL FEATURES

- Inability to deliver oxygen or remove carbon dioxide.
- PaO_2 is low while $PaCO_2$ is normal in type I respiratory failure (V/Q mismatch, diffusion defects, and intrapulmonary shunt).
- PaO_2 is low and $PaCO_2$ is high in type II respiratory failure (alveolar hypoventilation seen in CNS dysfunction, over-sedation, neuromuscular disorders).

Pathogenesis

Acute respiratory failure, defined as the inability of the respiratory system to adequately deliver oxygen or remove carbon dioxide, contributes significantly to the morbidity and mortality of critically ill children, accounting for approximately 50% of deaths in children younger than 1 year of age. Anatomic and developmental differences place infants at higher risk than adults for respiratory failure. An infant's thoracic cage is more compliant than that of the adult or older child. The intercostal muscles are poorly developed and unable to achieve the "bucket-handle" motion characteristic of adult breathing. Furthermore, the diaphragm is shorter and relatively flat with fewer type I muscle fibers, making it less effective and more easily fatigued. The infant's airways are smaller in caliber than those in older children and adults, resulting in greater resistance to inspiratory and expiratory airflow and greater susceptibility to occlusion by mucus plugging and mucosal edema. Compared with adults, the alveoli of children are smaller and have less collateral ventilation, resulting in a greater tendency to collapse and develop atelectasis. Finally, young infants may have an especially reactive pulmonary vascular bed, impaired immune system, or residual effects from prematurity, all of which increase the risk of respiratory failure.

Respiratory failure can be classified into two types, which usually coexist in variable proportion. Hypoxemia occurs in both, whereas hypercapnia occurs only in patients with type II respiratory failure (Table 14–1). ***Type I respiratory failure*** is a failure of oxygenation and occurs in three situations: (1) *V/Q mismatch*, which occurs when blood flows to parts of the lung that are inadequately ventilated, or when ventilated areas of the lung are inadequately perfused; (2) *diffusion defects*, caused by thickened alveolar membranes or excessive interstitial fluid at the alveolar-capillary junction; and (3) *intrapulmonary shunt*, which occurs when structural anomalies in the lung allow blood to flow through the lung without participating in gas exchange. ***Type II respiratory failure*** generally results from alveolar hypoventilation and is usually secondary to situations such as CNS dysfunction, over-sedation, or neuromuscular disorders (see Table 14–1).

Table 14–1. Types of respiratory failure.

Findings	Causes	Examples
Type I PaO_2 low $PaCO_2$ normal	Ventilation-perfusion (V/Q) defect	Positional (supine in bed), acute respiratory distress syndrome (ARDS), atelectasis, pneumonia, pulmonary embolus, bronchopulmonary dysplasia
	Diffusion impairment	Pulmonary edema, ARDS, interstitial pneumonia
	Shunt	Pulmonary arteriovenous malformation, congenital adenomatoid malformation
Type II PaO_2 low $PaCO_2$ high	Hypoventilation	Neuromuscular disease (polio, Guillain-Barré syndrome), head trauma, sedation, chest wall dysfunction (burns), kyphoscoliosis, severe reactive airways

Clinical Findings

The clinical findings in respiratory failure are the result of hypoxemia, hypercapnia, and arterial pH changes and are summarized in Table 14–2. Features of respiratory failure are not always clinically evident, however, and some signs or symptoms may have nonrespiratory causes. As a result, a strictly clinical assessment of arterial hypoxemia or hypercapnia is not reliable and precise assessment of the adequacy of oxygenation and ventilation must be based on both clinical and laboratory data.

Table 14–2. Clinical features of respiratory failure.

Respiratory
Wheezing
Expiratory grunting
Decreased or absent breath sounds
Flaring of alae nasi
Retractions of chest wall
Tachypnea, bradypnea, or apnea
Cyanosis
Neurologic
Restlessness
Irritability
Headache
Confusion
Convulsions
Coma
Cardiac
Bradycardia or excessive tachycardia
Hypotension or hypertension
General
Fatigue
Sweating

Laboratory Findings

Laboratory findings are helpful in assessing the severity and acuity of respiratory failure and in determining specific treatment. Arterial oxygen saturation (SaO_2) can be measured continuously and noninvasively by ***pulse oximetry***, a technique that should be used in the assessment and treatment of all patients with potential for respiratory failure. Pulse oximetry readings become markedly less accurate assessments of arterial oxygen content in patients with saturations below approximately 85% or with poor skin perfusion. Consequently, ***arterial blood gas (ABG)*** analysis remains the gold standard for assessment of acute respiratory failure. ABGs provide assessments of the patient's acid-base status (with a measured pH and calculated bicarbonate level) as well as Pao_2 and $Paco_2$ levels. Although measurement of capillary or venous blood gases may provide some reassurance regarding the adequacy of ventilation and can be useful for following trends, they yield virtually no useful information regarding oxygenation and may generate highly misleading information about the ventilatory status of patients who have poor perfusion or who had difficult blood draws. As a result, ABG analysis is important for all patients with suspected respiratory failure, particularly those with abnormal venous or capillary gases. ***End-tidal CO_2 ($ETCO_2$) monitoring*** provides a continuous noninvasive means of assessing the adequacy of ventilation. The $ETCO_2$ level closely approximates the alveolar CO_2 level (P_ACO_2), which should equal the arterial CO_2 level ($PaCO_2$) because carbon dioxide diffuses freely across the alveolar-capillary barrier. Though useful for following trends in ventilation, this technique is susceptible to significant error, particularly with patients who have rapid, shallow breathing or increased dead space ventilation.

Knowing the ABG values and the inspired oxygen concentration also enables one to calculate the ***alveolar-arterial oxygen difference*** (A–aDO_2, or A–a gradient, Table 14–10). The A–a gradient is less than 15 mm Hg under normal conditions, though it widens with increasing inspired oxygen concentrations to about 100 mm Hg in normal patients breathing 100% oxygen. This number has prognostic value in severe hypoxemic respiratory failure, with A–a gradients over 400 mm Hg being strongly associated with mortality. Diffusion impairment, shunts, and V/Q mismatch all increase the A–a gradient. In addition to the calculation of the A–a gradient, assessment of intrapulmonary shunting (the percentage of pulmonary blood flow that passes through nonventilated areas of the lung) may be helpful. Normal individuals have less than a 5% physiologic shunt from bronchial, coronary, and thebesian (cardiac intramural) circulations. ***Shunt fractions*** greater than 15% usually indicate the need for aggressive respiratory support. When intrapulmonary shunt reaches 50% of pulmonary blood flow, Pao_2 does not significantly increase regardless of the amount of supplemental oxygen used. Calculation of the shunt fraction (Table 14–10) requires a pulmonary arterial catheter for measurement of mixed venous blood gases. For patients without pulmonary artery catheters, the A–a gradient is a good surrogate measure of intrapulmonary shunting.

Treatment

Patients with hypoxemia induced by respiratory failure may respond to ***supplemental oxygen*** administration alone (Table 14–3). Those with hypoventilation and diffusion defects respond better than do patients with shunts or V/Q mismatch. Severe V/Q mismatch generally responds only to aggressive airway management and mechanical ventilation. Patients with severe hypoxemia, hypoventilation, or apnea require assistance with bag and mask ventilation until the airway is successfully intubated and controlled mechanical ventilation can be provided. Ventilation may be maintained for some time with a mask of the proper size, but gastric distention, emesis, and inadequate tidal volumes are possible complications.

For patients with respiratory failure not responding adequately to supplemental oxygen and treatment of their underlying condition, mechanical ventilation can be lifesaving. Mechanical ventilation can be provided either noninvasively via a face mask or via an endotracheal tube. These techniques are discussed in greater detail in the next section.

Endotracheal intubation in infants and children requires experienced personnel and the right equipment. A patient in respiratory failure whose airway must be stabilized should first be positioned properly to facilitate air exchange while supplemental oxygen is given. The sniffing position is used in infants. Head extension with jaw thrust is used in older children without neck injuries. If obstructed by secretions or vomitus, the airway must be cleared by suction. When not obstructed and properly positioned, the airway should be patent and easily visualized, allowing the placement of an oral or nasopharyngeal airway of the correct size. Patients with a normal airway may be intubated under intravenous (IV) anesthesia by experienced personnel (Table 14–4). While intubating patients with obstructed upper airways (eg, patients with croup, epiglottitis, foreign bodies, or subglottic stenosis), minimal sedation should be used and paralytic agents should be avoided unless trained airway specialists decide otherwise.

The size of the endotracheal tube (ETT) is of critical importance in pediatrics. An inappropriately large endotracheal tube can cause pressure necrosis of the tissues in the subglottic region, potentially leading to scarring and subglottic stenosis requiring surgical repair. An inappropriately small endotracheal tube can result in inadequate pulmonary toilet and excessive air leak around the endotracheal tube, making optimal ventilation and oxygenation difficult. Two useful methods for calculating the correct size of endotracheal tube for a child are (1) measuring the child's height with a Broselow Tape and then reading the corresponding endotracheal tube size on the tape, or (2) in children older than age 2 years, choosing a tube size using the formula ETT size = (16 + age in years) ÷ 4. Approximate proper insertion depth (in cm) as measured at the teeth can be estimated by tripling the size of the ETT. Correct placement of the endotracheal tube should be confirmed by auscultation for the presence of equal bilateral breath sounds *and* by the use of a colorimetric filter (pH-sensitive indicator that changes from purple to yellow when exposed to carbon dioxide) to

Table 14–3. Supplemental oxygen therapy.

Source	Maximum % O_2 Delivered	Range of Rates (L/min)	Advantages	Disadvantages
Nasal cannula	35%–40%	0.125–4	Easily applied, relatively comfortable	Uncomfortable at higher flow rates, requires open nasal airways, easily dislodged, lower % O_2 delivered, nosebleeds
Simple mask	50%–60%	5–10	Higher % O_2, good for mouth breathers	Uncomfortable, dangerous for patients with poor airway control and at risk for emesis, hard to give airway care, unsure of % O_2
Face tent	40%–60%	8–10	Higher % O_2, good for mouth breathers, less restrictive	Uncomfortable, dangerous for patients with poor airway control and at risk for emesis, hard to give airway care, unsure of % O_2
Nonrebreathing mask	80%–90%	5–10	Highest O_2 concentration, good for mouth breathers	Uncomfortable, dangerous for patients with poor airway control and at risk for emesis, hard to give airway care, unsure of % O_2
Oxyhood	90%–100%	5–10 (mixed at wall)	Stable and accurate O_2 concentration	Difficult to maintain temperature, hard to give airway care

Table 14–4. Drugs commonly used for controlled intubation.

Drug	Class of Agent	Dose	Advantages	Disadvantages
Atropine	Anticholinergic	0.02 mg/kg IV, minimum of 0.1 mg	Prevents bradycardia, dries secretions	Tachycardia, fever; seizures and coma with high doses
Fentanyl	Opioid (sedative)	1-3 mcg/kg IV	Rapid onset, hemodynamic stability	Respiratory depression, chest wall rigidity with rapid administration in neonates
Midazolam	Benzodiazepine (sedative)	0.1–0.2 mg/kg IV	Rapid onset, amnestic	Respiratory depression, hypotension
Thiopental	Barbiturate (anesthetic)	3-5 mg/kg IV	Rapid onset, lowers ICP	Hypotension, decreased cardiac output, no analgesia provided
Ketamine	Dissociative anesthetic	1-2 mg/kg IV 2-4 mg/kg IM	Rapid onset, bronchodilator, hemodynamic stability	Increases oral and airway secretions, may increase ICP and pulmonary artery pressure
Rocuronium	Nondepolarizing muscle relaxant	1 mg/kg	Rapid onset, suitable for rapid sequence intubation, lasts 30 min	Requires refrigeration
Pancuronium	Nondepolarizing muscle relaxant	0.1 mg/kg	Longer duration of action (40–60 min)	Tachycardia, slow onset (2-3 min)

ICP, intracranial pressure; IM, intramuscularly; IV, intravenously.

detect carbon dioxide. An assessment of air leakage around the endotracheal tube is an important measure of the appropriateness of endotracheal tube size. To assess the airway pressure required to generate an air leak around the ETT, connect an anesthesia bag and pressure manometer to the endotracheal tube and allow it to inflate, creating positive pressure. Check for leakage by auscultating over the throat, noting the pressure at which air audibly escapes around the endotracheal tube. A leak noted at pressures of 15–20 cm H_2O indicates acceptable ETT size. Higher leak pressures are acceptable only in patients who have poor lung compliance and as a result require higher airway pressures to effectively ventilate and oxygenate. Low leak pressures may lead to ineffective ventilation and can require changing to a larger or cuffed ETT. A chest radiograph is necessary for final assessment of endotracheal tube placement. A correctly positioned ETT will terminate in the mid-trachea between the thoracic inlet and the carina, at approximately the level of the second thoracic vertebrae.

Bledsoe GH, Schexnayder SM: Pediatric rapid sequence intubation: A review. Pediatr Emerg Care 2004;20:339 [PMID: 15123910].

Carroll CL et al: Emergent endotracheal intubations in children: Be careful if it's late when you intubate. Pediatr Crit Care Med 2010 May;11(3):343–348 [PMID: 20464775].

Nava S et al: Non-invasive ventilation in acute respiratory failure. Lancet 2009;18;374(9685):250–259 [PMID: 19616722].

Santillanes G, Guasche-Hill M: Pediatric airway management. Emerg Med Clin North Am 2008 Nov;26(4):961–975 [PMID: 19059095].

Trachsel D et al: Oxygenation index predicts outcome in children with acute hypoxemic respiratory failure. Am J Respir Crit Care Med 2005;172:206–211 [PMID: 15817802].

West JB: Pulmonary Pathophysiology, The Essentials 7th Edition: Chapter 8: Respiratory Failure. Lippincott Williams & Wilkinson, 2008.

MECHANICAL VENTILATION

ESSENTIALS OF DIAGNOSIS & TYPICAL FEATURES

- Understand the indications for mechanical ventilation (MV) and the goals.
- Choose settings that best achieve these goals with the least risk of complications.
- Constantly assess the patient and equipment for changes in status.
- Lung disease is a dynamic process, so the degree of respiratory support should be as well.

Indications

The principal indications for institution of mechanical ventilation are acute and chronic respiratory failure, or an airway rendered unstable either by illness, injury, or treatment with sedating medications. Examples of these conditions include pneumonia, sepsis, trauma, neuromuscular disease, and procedural sedation. The goals of mechanical ventilation are to facilitate the movement of gas into and out of the lungs (ventilation) and to improve oxygen uptake into the bloodstream (oxygenation). While life-saving in many situations, recent work has improved our understanding of the ways in which positive pressure ventilation can also be harmful. As a result, mechanical ventilation strategies must be adapted to achieve these goals in a way that minimizes further injury to the lung. The overriding principles of this "lung protective ventilation strategy" are to safely recruit underinflated lung, sustain lung volume, minimize phasic overdistention, and decrease lung inflammation. This strategy requires adjustment of ventilator settings with an understanding of the difference between the gas exchange that is permissible and that which is normal or optimal.

Terminology

Understanding the terminology used to operate mechanical ventilators is critical to understanding how they work and how to adjust the settings. Although many concepts are similar between different ventilator manufacturers, the terminology to describe the concepts may vary considerably among manufacturers.

The parameters used to control the delivery of positive pressure breaths are the trigger, cycle, control, and limit variables. The ***trigger variable*** describes how breaths are initiated, either by the patient or by the ventilator. Common triggers are time (breaths delivered at regular timed intervals regardless of patient demand) or patient effort (sensed as a drop in return pressure or gas flow to the ventilator). Most modern ventilators use flow triggers because they are more sensitive, especially in infants and small children. A newer trigger method, neurally adjusted ventilatory assist (NAVA), requires the introduction of an esophageal catheter to measure the electrical activity of the diaphragm to adjust the ventilator breaths to meet the patient's neural activity. While NAVA holds promise for improved patient-ventilator synchrony and improved weaning, there is little evidence to date showing superiority of NAVA for clinically relevant end points. The ***cycle variable*** describes how the inspiratory phase is terminated, either by the patient or by the ventilator. Most ventilator modes cycle according to a set inspiratory time (I-time) though flow-cycled modes can be used in spontaneously breathing patients. The ***control variable*** determines whether a machine breath is targeted to deliver a specific tidal volume (volume-controlled modes) or a specific pressure (pressure-controlled modes). Limit variables are parameters whose magnitude is constrained during inspiration (eg, pressure or tidal volumes) in order to prevent excessive pressure or volume from being delivered by the ventilator.

Breaths can also be classified as *spontaneous* or *mandatory*. ***Spontaneous*** breaths are those in which inspiration is triggered and cycled by the patient, who controls the timing and size of the breath. ***Mandatory*** breaths are triggered or cycled, or both, by the ventilator independent of patient activity. The ventilator also controls the timing and/or size of mandatory breaths. The breathing pattern can be set to one of three configurations; some modes use a combination of these. The first is ***continuous mandatory ventilation*** (CMV). All breaths are mandatory in this pattern, meaning that the ventilator determines the size and duration of the breath regardless of whether the breath is triggered by the machine or the patient. The second is called ***intermittent mandatory ventilation (IMV).*** In this configuration, mandatory breaths are set the same as CMV, but additional spontaneous breaths between and during mandatory breaths are accommodated and may be supported. The third is ***continuous spontaneous ventilation (CSV).*** All breaths in this configuration must be spontaneously generated, but may be supported.

A ***ventilator mode*** consists of a specific control variable (pressure or volume), a specific pattern of breathing (CMV, IMV, or CSV), and a specific set of phase variables (trigger, limit, and cycle). Initiation of breaths and the length of exhalation are controlled by setting the ***respiratory rate***. In time-cycled modes of ventilation, the ***inspiratory time (I-time)*** determines the length of inspiration and when to allow exhalation. Finally, the minimum distending pressure applied to the lung during the respiratory cycle is determined by setting the ***positive end-expiratory pressure (PEEP).*** All mechanical ventilators open their expiratory limbs at the end of inspiration allowing gas release until a preset pressure is achieved; this is the PEEP value. Conceptually, PEEP levels prevent the collapse of units opened during lung inflation. During ventilation of normal lungs, physiologic PEEP is in the range of 2–4 cm H_2O pressure. This pressure helps to prevent the end-expiratory collapse of open lung units, thus preventing atelectasis and shunting. In disease states such as pulmonary edema, pneumonia, or ARDS, a higher PEEP (10–15 cm H_2O) may increase the patient's functional residual capacity, help to keep open previously collapsed alveoli, increase MAP, and improve oxygenation. High levels of PEEP, although often valuable in improving oxygenation, may also cause gas trapping and CO_2 retention, barotrauma with resultant air leaks, decreased central venous return and resulting decline in cardiac output, and increased intracranial pressure (ICP).

Modes of Mechanical Ventilation

Most modern ventilators can deliver either a pressure-targeted or a volume-targeted breath in several manners. Control modes deliver breaths in a CMV pattern. In strict pressure-controlled or volume-controlled modes, the ventilator initiates all breaths and patient respiratory efforts are ignored. In ***assist control***, breaths are delivered in IMV pattern with mandatory breaths delivered independent of patient effort. However, the patient may initiate full ventilator-supported breaths with every respiratory effort that meets the set trigger requirement. ***Synchronized intermittent mandatory ventilation (SIMV)*** is a mode that delivers breaths in an IMV pattern but the ventilator allows a window of time around each mandatory breath to permit the patient to make an inspiratory effort. The machine breaths are then synchronized with the patient's efforts; if the patient does not make adequate respiratory effort, the ventilator will deliver a mandatory breath at the end of the window. In SIMV, the window for a synchronized ventilator breath is determined in part by the set ventilator *rate*, and the ventilator will not deliver more than one breath in each window regardless of whether the patient generates extra respiratory efforts. In ***pressure-support ventilation***, a CSV pattern is employed, and the patient's own efforts are assisted by the delivery of gas flow to achieve a targeted peak airway pressure. Pressure-support ventilation allows the patient to determine the rate and I-time of breaths, thus improving patient comfort and decreasing the work of breathing. The most commonly used mode of ventilation in most PICUs is ***synchronized intermittent mandatory ventilation with pressure support (SIMV+PS)***, a mixed mode allowing pressure-supported breaths between the synchronized machine breaths.

One of the ongoing controversies in critical care medicine surrounds the relative benefits of volume- vs pressure-controlled modes of ventilation. In ***pressure-controlled ventilation***, air flow begins at the start of the inspiratory cycle and continues until a preset airway pressure is reached. That airway pressure is then maintained until, at the end of the set I-time, the exhalation valve on the ventilator opens and gas exits into the machine. Because airway pressure is the controlling variable with this mode of ventilation, changes in the compliance of the respiratory system will lead to fluctuations in the actual tidal volume delivered to the patient. The advantage of pressure-targeted ventilation lies primarily in the avoidance of high airway pressures that might cause lung overdistention injury or barotrauma, particularly in patients with fragile lung parenchyma, such as premature infants. The main disadvantage of pressure-controlled ventilation is the possibility of delivering either inadequate or excessive tidal volumes during periods of changing lung compliance. In ***volume-controlled ventilation,*** the machine delivers a set tidal volume to the patient. Changes in lung compliance will lead to fluctuations in the peak airway pressure generated by the breath. The main advantage of volume ventilation is more reliable delivery of the desired tidal volume and thus better control of ventilation. More reliable tidal volume delivery may also help prevent atelectasis due to hypoventilation. Disadvantages of volume ventilation include the risk of barotrauma from excessive airway pressures and difficulties overcoming leaks in the ventilator circuit. In either pressure- or volume-controlled modes, alarm limits can be set in order to restrict changes in either tidal volume or airway pressure with changing lung compliance, though interpreting those alarms and adjusting the ventilator require the ICU clinician to understand the ventilator mode in use.

Setting and Adjusting the Ventilator

When initiating ***volume-controlled modes*** of ventilation, the ICU clinician must choose a set tidal volume, I-time, rate, and level of PEEP. A typical initial tidal volume is 6–10 mL/kg, as long as that volume does not cause excessive airway pressures (> 30 cm H_2O). The I-time is typically set at 1 second or 33% of the respiratory cycle, whichever is shorter. Rate can be adjusted to patient comfort and blood gas measurements, but generally patients starting on mechanical ventilation require full support at least initially with a rate of 20–30 breaths/min. ***Pressure-controlled ventilation*** is set up in a similar fashion, although the adequacy of the inspiratory pressure is assessed by observing the patient's chest rise and by measuring the delivered tidal volume. Typically, patients without lung disease require pressures of 15–20 cm H_2O, and patients with respiratory illnesses initially require 20–30 cm H_2O pressure to provide adequate ventilation. In general, PEEP should be set at 3–5 cm H_2O initially and titrated up to maintain adequate oxygenation at acceptable fractional inspired oxygen concentrations (FIO_2) while watching carefully for adverse effects.

Ventilated patients require careful ***monitoring*** for the efficacy of gas exchange, including respiratory rate and activity, chest wall movement, and quality of breath sounds. Oxygenation should be measured either by ABGs or by continuous pulse oximetry. Ventilation should be assessed by blood gas analysis or by noninvasive means, such as transcutaneous monitoring or $ETCO_2$ sampling. Transcutaneous PO_2 or PCO_2 measurements are most useful with younger patients who have good skin perfusion, but they become problematic with poorly perfused or obese patients. $ETCO_2$ monitoring is done by placing a gas-sampling port on the endotracheal tube and analyzing expired gas for CO_2. This technique is more valuable for patients with large tidal volumes, lower respiratory rates, and without leaks around the endotracheal tube. In practice, $ETCO_2$ values may differ significantly (usually lower) from measured $Paco_2$ values and thus are most useful for following relative fluctuations in ventilation. Frequent, preferably continuous, CVP and systemic blood pressure monitoring is also necessary for patients ventilated with high PEEP levels, given the risk of adverse cardiovascular effects.

Ventilator settings can be adjusted to optimize both ventilation (PCO_2) and oxygenation (PO_2). ***Ventilation*** is most closely associated with the delivered minute volume, or the tidal volume multiplied by the respiratory rate. As a result, abnormal PCO_2 values can be most effectively addressed by changes in the respiratory rate or the tidal volume. Increased respiratory rate or tidal volume should increase minute volume and thus decrease PCO_2 levels; decreases in respiratory rate or tidal volume should act in the opposite fashion. In some circumstances, additional adjustments may also be necessary. For example, for patients with disease characterized by extensive alveolar collapse, increasing PEEP may improve ventilation by helping to keep open previously collapsed lung units. Also, for patients with disease characterized by significant airway obstruction, decreases in respiratory rate may allow more time for exhalation and improve ventilation despite an apparent decrease in the minute volume provided.

The variables most closely associated with ***oxygenation*** are the inspired oxygen concentration and the mean airway pressure (MAP) during the respiratory cycle. Increases in inspired oxygen concentration will generally increase arterial oxygenation, unless right-to-left intracardiac or intrapulmonary shunting is a significant component of the patient's illness. Concentrations of inspired oxygen above 60%–65%, however, may lead to hyperoxic lung injury. Patients with hypoxemic respiratory failure requiring those levels of oxygen or higher to maintain adequate arterial saturations should have their hypoxemia addressed by increases in MAP to recruit underinflated lung units. MAP is affected by PEEP, peak inspiratory pressure, and I-time. Increases in any one of those factors will increase MAP and should improve arterial oxygenation. It is important to bear in mind, however, that increases in MAP may also lead to decreases in cardiac output, primarily by transmission of pressure to the thoracic cage, thus decreasing venous return to the heart. In this circumstance, raising MAP may increase arterial oxygenation, but actually compromise oxygen delivery to the tissues. For patients with severe hypoxemic respiratory failure, these tradeoffs highlight the need for careful monitoring by experienced personnel.

Mechanical ventilation can be associated with several complications, including ventilator-associated pneumonia. Thus, mechanical ventilation should be weaned and discontinued as soon as the patient is capable of spontaneous breathing. Premature extubation can also be problematic, resulting in additional complications. Extubation failure rates have been estimated between 4% and 20%. Therefore, considerable effort has been devoted to identifying predictors of extubation readiness and success. Unfortunately, the available literature does not support any specific weaning protocol or the use of any extubation readiness test that are consistently reliable and superior to clinical judgment alone. Successful extubation requires adequate gas exchange, adequate respiratory muscle strength, and the ability to protect the airway. If those conditions can be met, most practitioners as a test of extubation readiness will perform a trial of spontaneous breathing in which the patient, while remaining intubated, breathes either without assistance (through a t-piece) or with a low level of pressure support (through the ventilator) for a defined period of time, usually 1–2 hours. The patient is observed carefully for signs of rapid shallow breathing or worsened gas exchange during this trial, and if neither is observed, the patient can generally be safely extubated.

Management of the Mechanically Ventilated Patient

Patients undergoing mechanical ventilation require meticulous supportive care. Since mechanical ventilation is often frightening and uncomfortable for patients, leading to dyssynchrony with the ventilator and impaired ventilation and oxygenation, careful attention must be directed toward optimizing comfort and decreasing anxiety. Sedative-anxiolytics are typically provided as intermittent doses of benzodiazepines, with or without opioids. Some patients respond better to the steady state of sedation provided by continuous infusion of these agents, although oversedation of the ventilated patient may lead to longer duration of ventilation, difficulty with weaning from the ventilator, and other complications. It is beneficial to use standardized assessments of sedation level and target the minimum sedation level necessary to maintain endotracheal tube control and adequate gas exchange.

For a patient with severe respiratory illness, even small movements by the patient may compromise ventilation and oxygenation. In such cases, muscle paralysis may facilitate oxygenation and ventilation. Nondepolarizing neuromuscular blocking agents are most commonly used for this purpose, given as intermittent doses or as continuous infusions. When muscle relaxants are given, extra care must be taken to ensure that levels of sedation are adequate, as many of the usual signs of patient discomfort are masked by the paralytics.

It is important to provide adequate nutrition to mechanically ventilated patients. Mechanically ventilated patients can often be fed enterally with the use of nasogastric feeding tubes. However, reflux aspiration leading to ventilator-associated pneumonia can be a concern. In patients where reflux or emesis is a major concern, transpyloric feeding or parenteral nutrition should be considered.

Ventilator-associated pneumonia (VAP) is a significant complication of mechanical ventilation, leading to longer ICU stays and increased hospital costs. As a result, many local and national quality improvement initiatives have focused on minimizing the risks of VAP. These preventative measures include proper hand-washing, elevation of the head of the bed to 30 degrees to prevent reflux, frequent turning of the patient, proper oral care, the use of closed suction circuits on all ventilated patients and avoidance of breaking the closed suction system, sedation protocols to minimize sedation administration, and daily assessment of extubation readiness.

Troubleshooting

Troubleshooting problems in the mechanically ventilated patient should follow basic resuscitation ABCs. First, assess the airway. Determine whether the endotracheal tube is still in place using direct laryngoscopy or $ETCO_2$ measurements if necessary. Determine whether the ETT is patent and in the correct position by attempting to pass a suction catheter and by obtaining a chest x-ray if necessary. Second, assess the effectiveness of breathing. Ascertain whether there is adequate chest rise, present and equal breath sounds, and any changes in the examination that suggest atelectasis, bronchospasm, pneumothorax (consider needle thoracentesis), or pneumonia. Next, establish whether hemodynamic deterioration could be underlying acute respiratory compromise (shock or sepsis). If the problem cannot be readily identified, take the patient off the ventilator and begin manual ventilation by hand-bagging while the ventilator is checked for malfunction. Hand-bagging the patient can also determine the root of the problem if it lies within the patient, and can help determine the next ventilator adjustments.

Alternative Forms of Ventilation

High frequency oscillatory ventilation (HFOV) is an alternate mode of mechanical ventilation in which the ventilator provides very small, very rapid tidal volumes at high rates. Respiratory rates used during oscillatory ventilation typically range from 5 to 10 Hz (rates of 300–600 breaths/min) in most PICU patients. This mode of ventilation has been used successfully for neonates, older pediatric patients, and adults; and for diseases as diverse as pneumonia, pulmonary contusion, ARDS, and asthma. HFOV is most widely used in severe, diffuse lung diseases, such as ARDS, which require high MAP to maintain lung expansion and oxygenation. The advantage of HFOV is that high levels of MAP can be achieved without high peak inspiratory pressures or large tidal volumes, thus theoretically protecting the lung from ventilator-induced lung injury. Disadvantages of HFOV include general poor tolerance by patients who are not heavily sedated or paralyzed, the risk of cardiovascular compromise due to high MAP, and the risk of gas-trapping and barotrauma in patients with highly heterogeneous lung disease. Although HFOV clearly may be useful for selected patients, it remains unclear whether HFOV provides any benefit compared with carefully managed conventional modes of ventilation.

Noninvasive ventilation (NIV) refers to the administration of ventilatory support without using an invasive artificial airway (endotracheal tube or tracheostomy tube). The use of NIV has become an integral tool in the management of both acute and chronic respiratory failure. NIV can be used to avoid endotracheal intubation for milder cases of respiratory failure and as a bridge to extubation in mechanically ventilated patients with marginal lung function and respiratory mechanics. Ventilatory support can be achieved through a variety of interfaces (mouth piece or nasal, face, or helmet mask), using a variety of ventilatory modes, including continuous positive airway pressure (CPAP), bilevel positive airway pressure (BiPAP), volume ventilation, and pressure support. Ventilators dedicated to NIV exist, and many standard ventilators are capable of providing support through a mask with the appropriate adapters. Most current NIV ventilator models incorporate oxygen blenders for precise delivery of the fraction of inspired oxygen (FIO_2).

Successful application of NIV requires careful patient selection. Patients in the recovery phases of their illness or with primarily type 2 respiratory failure are the best candidates; controversy still exists as to the advisability of NIV in patients with acute hypoxemic respiratory failure. Patients suffering from coma, cardiac or respiratory arrest, or any other condition requiring immediate intubation are not candidates for NIV. BiPAP and CPAP are the most frequent modes of NIV utilized in the PICU. Initial settings for BiPAP focus on achieving adequate tidal volumes, usually in the range of 5–7 mL/kg. Initial settings for the inspiratory positive airway pressure (IPAP) are 10–12 cm H_2O and 6 cm H_2O for the expiratory positive airway pressure (EPAP). Additional support is provided to reduce the respiratory rate to a more comfortable range for the patient. Oxygen is adjusted on the basis of pulse oximetry to achieve adequate oxygenation. Serial blood gas measurements are essential to monitor the response to therapy and to guide further ventilator adjustments.

Girard TD, Bernard GR: Mechanical ventilation in ARDS: A state-of-the-art review. Chest 2007 Mar;131(3):921–929 [PMID: 17356115].

Haitsma JJ: Physiology of mechanical ventilation. Crit Care Clin 2007 Apr;23(2):117–134, vii [PMID: 17368160].

Khemani RG, Newth CJ: The design of future pediatric mechanical ventilation trials for acute lung injury. Am J Respir Crit Care Med 2010 Dec 15;182(12):1465–1474 [PMID: 20732987].

Kissoon N, Rimensberger PC, Bohn D: Ventilation strategies and adjunctive therapy in severe lung disease. Pediatr Clin North Am 2008;55(3):709–733, xii [PMID: 18501762].

Mesiano G, Davis GM: Ventilatory strategies in the neonatal and pediatric intensive care units. Paediatr Respir Rev 2008;9(4):281–288; quiz 288–289 [Epub 2008 Nov 6] [PMID: 19026369].

Newth CJ et al: Eunice Shriver Kennedy National Institute of Child Health and Human Development Collaborative Pediatric Critical Care Research Network: Weaning and extubation readiness in pediatric patients. Pediatr Crit Care Med 2009 Jan;10(1):1–11 [PMID: 19057432].

ACUTE LUNG INJURY AND THE ACUTE RESPIRATORY DISTRESS SYNDROME

ESSENTIALS OF DIAGNOSIS & TYPICAL FEATURES

- The acute respiratory distress syndrome (ARDS) is a severe form of acute lung injury (ALI), with $PaO_2/FIO_2 \leq 200$, bilateral pulmonary infiltrates, and no clinical evidence of left atrial hypertension.
- Extravascular lung water accumulates in ALI and ARDS principally as a result of increased capillary permeability, not elevated hydrostatic pressure.
- ALI and ARDS can arise as a consequence of either direct pulmonary injury or systemic conditions that are nonpulmonary in origin.

ARDS is a syndrome of acute respiratory failure characterized by increased pulmonary capillary permeability resulting in bilateral diffuse alveolar infiltrates on chest radiography, decreased lung compliance, and hypoxemia that is usually refractory to supplemental oxygen alone. Mortality rates for pediatric ARDS have fluctuated over time, depending on the criteria used to diagnose the disease, the presence of important co-existing conditions, and the quality and consistency of supportive care provided in the ICU. Mortality rates as high as 60%–75% were reported in the 1980s and early 1990s, before consensus diagnostic criteria were established. Since that time, there has been a trend toward decreased mortality in pediatric ARDS, ranging from 8% in a recent trial that excluded immunocompromised patients to nearly 40% in contemporary trials that do include immunocompromised patients, with mortality among the immunocompromised cohort approaching 60%. Across all subpopulations of pediatric ALI and ARDS patients, nonpulmonary organ failure remains an important cause of mortality.

In 1994, the American-European Consensus Conference established uniform diagnostic criteria for ALI and ARDS. Consensus diagnostic criteria for ARDS include (1) acute onset; (2) bilateral pulmonary infiltrates on chest radiograph; (3) pulmonary artery occlusion pressure (PAOP) ≤ 18 mm Hg or no clinical evidence of left atrial hypertension; and (4) severe hypoxemia in which the ratio of the arterial oxygen level (Pao_2) to inspired oxygen concentration (FIO_2) is ≤ 200. When the Pao_2:FIO_2 ratio is between 200 and 300 and the other criteria are met, consensus criteria define the case as ***acute lung injury***. While these criteria remain controversial because of their lack of specificity, they helped to usher in a new era of clinical research that has contributed greatly to what we now know about the pathophysiology of ALI and ARDS, and factors influencing their outcomes in children.

Presentation and Pathophysiology

ARDS may be precipitated by a variety of insults (Table 14–5). Pneumonia accounts for 35% of ALI and ARDS cases in children and appears to have overtaken sepsis as the most common cause of pediatric ARDS. Despite the diversity of potential causes, the clinical presentation is remarkably similar in most cases. ARDS can be divided roughly into four clinical phases (Table 14–6). In the earliest phase, the patient may have dyspnea and tachypnea with a relatively normal PaO_2 and hyperventilation-induced respiratory alkalosis. No significant abnormalities are noted on physical or radiologic examination of the chest. Experimental studies suggest that neutrophils accumulate in the lungs at this stage and that their products damage lung endothelium.

Table 14–5. Acute respiratory distress syndrome risk factors.

Direct Lung Injury	Indirect Lung Injury
Pneumonia Aspiration of gastric contents Inhalation injury (heat or toxin) Pulmonary contusion Hydrocarbon ingestion or aspiration Near-drowning	Sepsis Shock Burns Trauma Fat embolism Drug overdoses (including aspirin, opioids, barbiturates, tricyclic antidepressants) Transfusion of blood products Pancreatitis

Over the next few hours, hypoxemia worsens and respiratory distress becomes clinically apparent, with cyanosis, tachycardia, irritability, and dyspnea. Early radiographic changes include the appearance of increasingly confluent alveolar infiltrates initially appearing in dependent lung fields, in a pattern suggestive of pulmonary edema. The edema fluid typically has a high concentration of protein (75%–95% of plasma protein concentration), which is characteristic of edema due to increased vascular permeability edema and differs from the low protein concentration of hydrostatic pulmonary edema. Proteinaceous exudates in the alveolar space and direct injury to type II alveolar pneumocytes produce both quantitative and qualitative surfactant deficiency. As a result, the injured lung requires high inflation pressures to achieve lung opening, and increased positive end expiratory pressure (PEEP) to maintain end expiratory volume.

Besides interfering with surfactant production, injury to the alveolar type II cell also reduces the capacity for alveolar fluid clearance. Under normal conditions, sodium is taken up by channels on the apical surface of type II cells. Subsequently, Na^+/K^+-ATPases located on the basolateral cell membrane actively transport sodium back into the interstitial space, which creates the gradient for passive movement of water across the alveolar epithelium and back into the interstitium. In ARDS, this mechanism becomes overwhelmed as direct lung injury depopulates the alveolar epithelium, creating conditions that favor alveolar fluid accumulation. Pulmonary hypertension, reduced lung compliance, and increased airways resistance are also commonly observed. Clinical studies suggest that airways resistance may be increased in up to 50% of patients with ARDS, likely as a result of airway damage or inflammation-induced bronchospasm, though this increased resistance is only rarely clinically important.

Computer tomography (CT) studies of adult patients in the acute phases of ARDS demonstrate a heterogeneous pattern of lung involvement that is distributed along the gravitational axis. The most dependent lung regions remain consolidated throughout the respiratory cycle, and can only be recruited using exceedingly high inflation pressures. The most nondependent regions are overinflated throughout the respiratory cycle. Between these two zones lies a region that is either normally inflated or repetitively cycles between inflation and collapse. These observations suggest that it is most helpful to view the ARDS lung as smaller in volume than normal. Attempts to improve oxygenation by

Table 14–6. Pathophysiologic changes of acute respiratory distress syndrome.

Radiography	Symptoms	Laboratory Findings	Pathophysiology
Phase 1 (early changes)			
Normal radiograph	Dyspnea, tachypnea, normal chest examination	Mild pulmonary hypertension, normoxemic or mild hypoxemia, hypercapnia	Neutrophil sequestration, no clear tissue damage
Phase 2 (onset of parenchymal changes)[a]			
Patchy alveolar infiltrates beginning in dependent lung; normal heart size	Dyspnea, tachypnea, cyanosis, tachycardia, coarse rales	Moderate to severe hypoxemia, increasing shunt, decreased lung compliance, pulmonary hypertension, normal wedge pressure	Neutrophil infiltration, vascular congestion, increased lung permeability, pulmonary edema, fibrin strands, platelet clumps, type I epithelial cell damage
Phase 3 (acute respiratory failure with progression, 2–10 d)			
Diffuse alveolar infiltrates; air bronchograms; decreased lung volume; normal heart size	Tachypnea, tachycardia, hyper-dynamic state, sepsis syndrome, signs of consolidation, diffuse rhonchi	Progression of phase 2 abnormalities, increasing shunt fraction, further decrease in compliance, increased minute ventilation, impaired oxygen extraction of hemoglobin	Increased interstitial and alveolar inflammatory exudate with neutrophils and mononuclear cells, type II cell proliferation, beginning fibroblast proliferation, thromboembolic occlusion
Phase 4 (pulmonary fibrosis, pneumonia with progression, > 10 d)[b]			
Persistent diffuse infiltrates; superimposed new pneumonic infiltrates; air leak; normal heart size or enlargement due to cor pulmonale	Symptoms as above, recurrent sepsis, evidence of multiple organ system failure	Phase 3 changes persist; recurrent pneumonia, progressive lung restriction, impaired tissue oxygenation, impaired oxygen extraction; multiple organ system failure	Type II cell hyperplasia, interstitial thickening; infiltration of lymphocytes, macrophages, fibroblasts; loculated pneumonia or interstitial fibrosis; medial thickening and remodeling of arterioles

[a]The process is readily reversible at this stage if the initiating factor is controlled.
[b]Multiple organ system failure is common. The mortality rate is greater than 80% at this stage, since resolution is more difficult.
Data from Demling RH: Adult respiratory distress syndrome: Current concepts. New Horiz 1993;1:388.

recruiting the collapsed dependent lung regions occur at the expense of damaging nondependent regions by profound hyperinflation. This process, termed ***volutrauma***, incites a potent inflammatory response that is capable of worsening nonpulmonary organ dysfunction. Appreciation for this phenomenon has prompted a shift toward ventilating ARDS patients with smaller tidal volumes and a tolerance for the relative hypercarbia that typically ensues. Even in normal lungs, ventilation with large tidal volumes and low positive end-expiratory pressure (PEEP) levels can produce a lung injury that is histologically indistinguishable from ARDS. This phenomenon is called ***ventilator-induced lung injury***. Taken together, these findings suggest that mechanical injury from positive pressure ventilation is superimposed on the initial insult and is an integral part of the pathogenesis of ARDS. This concept has placed tremendous focus on how to ventilate ARDS patients in a way that limits ventilator-induced injury. Published evidence currently supports using PEEP levels sufficient to stabilize those alveoli with tendency to collapse at end-expiration but below a threshold level that would overdistend nondependent lung regions at end-inspiration. Volutrauma is then mitigated by tidal volume reduction and/or peak pressure limitation. This approach is termed the "open-lung strategy" of mechanical ventilation.

The **subacute phase** of ARDS (2–10 days after lung injury) is characterized by type II pneumocyte and fibroblast proliferation in the interstitium of the lung. This results in decreased lung volumes and signs of consolidation that are noted clinically and radiographically. Worsening of the hypoxemia with an increasing shunt fraction occurs, as well as a further decrease in lung compliance. Some patients develop an accelerated fibrosing alveolitis. The mechanisms responsible for these changes are unclear. Current investigation centers on the role of growth and differentiation factors, such as transforming growth factor-β and platelet-derived growth factor released by resident and nonresident lung cells, such as alveolar macrophages, mast cells, neutrophils, alveolar type II cells, and fibroblasts. During the chronic phase of ARDS (10–14 days after lung injury), fibrosis, emphysema, and pulmonary vascular obliteration occur. During this phase of the illness, oxygenation defects generally improve, and the lung becomes more fragile and susceptible to barotrauma. Air leak is common among patients ventilated with high airway pressures at this late stage. Also, patients have increased dead space and difficulties with ventilation are common. Airway compliance remains low because of ongoing pulmonary fibrosis and insufficient surfactant production.

Secondary infections are common in the subacute and chronic phases of ARDS and can impact clinical outcomes. The mechanisms responsible for increased host susceptibility to infection during this phase are not well understood. Mortality in the late phase of ARDS can exceed 80%. Death is usually caused by multiorgan failure and systemic hemodynamic instability rather than by hypoxemia, an observation further emphasizing the need for clinicians to provide meticulous monitoring and supportive care to patients with ALI and ARDS.

Treatment

Contemporary ***ventilator management*** of ARDS is directed at protecting vulnerable lung regions from cyclic alveolar collapse at end expiration and protecting overinflated lung regions from hyperinflation at end inspiration. The actual mode of ventilation (eg, volume limited vs pressure limited) employed for ARDS is ultimately not as important as limiting phasic alveolar stretch and stabilizing lung units that are prone to repetitive end expiratory collapse. Over a decade ago, the landmark multicenter trial conducted by the ARDSNet investigators established that adult ARDS patients who were ventilated using a 6 mL/kg (ideal body weight) tidal volume had a 22% mortality reduction and fewer extrapulmonary organ failures relative to those randomized to receive tidal volumes of 12 mL/kg. The trial also demonstrated a greater reduction in plasma levels of pro-inflammatory cytokines among those in the lower tidal volume group, a finding suggesting that appropriate ventilator strategies can actually reduce the systemic inflammatory response. Though this trial has never been replicated in pediatric patients, application of these same management principles has gained widespread acceptance among pediatric ICU clinicians.

Since an FIO_2 greater than 0.6 can cause additional injury to the lung within 24 hours, mean airway pressure (MAP) should be increased to a level that allows maintenance of arterial saturations ≥ 88%–90% and a Pao_2 between 60 and 80 mm Hg using an FIO_2 of 0.6 or less. In general, this can be accomplished by small incremental increases in PEEP until adequate oxygenation is achieved or until a limiting side effect of the PEEP is reached. Whenever escalating mechanical ventilator settings, clinicians should minimize the endotracheal tube cuff leak (if possible), ensure an appropriate plane of patient sedation, and optimize the ventilation to perfusion relationship by verifying that the patient's intravascular volume status is appropriate.

Given the large body of evidence supporting the benefits of low tidal volume ventilation, we suggest that mechanical ventilation of pediatric ALI and ARDS patients be initiated using a tidal volume of 6–8 mL/kg (ideal body weight), combined with PEEP sufficient to produce target arterial saturations (≥88%–90%) using an FIO_2 of ≤0.6. Permissive hypercapnia should be used unless a clear contraindication exists (eg, increased intracranial pressure). If adequate ventilation cannot be achieved (pH remains below 7.25 due to hypercapnia), the ventilator rate can then be increased, provided the patient has time to adequately exhale before the next breath. Subsequently, tidal volume can then be increased as necessary toward 8 mL/kg (ideal body weight), monitoring again for adequacy of expiratory time. Throughout the course, efforts should be made to limit the alveolar plateau pressure (pressure at end-inspiration) to 20–25 cm H_2O or less.

Fluid management is an important element of the care of patients with ARDS. Given the increased pulmonary capillary permeability in ARDS, further pulmonary edema accumulation is likely with any elevation in pulmonary hydrostatic pressures. Evidence in adults has shown that a "conservative" fluid strategy targeting lower cardiac filling pressures (CVP < 4 mm Hg, or, if a pulmonary artery catheter is used, pulmonary artery occlusion pressure < 8 mm Hg) is associated with better oxygenation and a shorter duration of mechanical ventilation compared to a "liberal" fluid strategy targeting CVP 10–14 mm Hg (or PAOP 14–18 mm Hg). It is important to emphasize that fluid restriction should only be implemented after hemodynamic variables stabilize and volume resuscitation should not be denied to hemodynamically unstable patients with ARDS.

Hemodynamic support is directed toward increasing perfusion and oxygen delivery. Patients should be given adequate intravascular volume resuscitation using either crystalloid or colloid solutions to restore adequate circulating volume, and inotropes or vasopressors should be titrated to achieve adequate end-organ perfusion and oxygen delivery. While blood transfusions are excellent volume expanders and should theoretically increase oxygen-carrying capacity, transfusion incurs the risks of volume overload and transfusion-related lung injury. Moreover, banked red blood cells are less deformable and have less 2,3-diphosphoglycerate and S-nitrosohemoglobin, qualities which can produce abnormal vascular responses to hypoxia. There is no evidence to support transfusion above a normal hemoglobin level in ARDS patients.

Patients with ARDS require careful invasive ***monitoring***. Given the risks of ventilator-induced lung injury and the inherent limitations of pulse oximetry and capnography, arterial blood gas analysis is strongly preferred for accurate assessment of oxygenation and ventilation and careful titration of mechanical ventilation. Indwelling arterial catheters are useful for continuous blood pressure monitoring and frequent laboratory sampling. Many clinicians advocate the use of CVP measurements to help determine the level of cardiac preload, although it is important to emphasize that the CVP value must be interpreted in the context of surrounding compartment pressure (ie, intrathoracic pressure) and myocardial compliance. For patients with severe disease or concurrent cardiac dysfunction, consideration can be given to pulmonary artery catheterization in order to guide fluid management and to allow assessment of mixed venous oxygen saturation as an index of overall tissue oxygenation. Obtaining chest films daily is important to monitor endotracheal tube placement, evaluate for development of air leak, and track the overall response to therapy. Since secondary infections are common and contribute to increased mortality rates, surveillance for infection is important, by obtaining appropriate cultures and following the temperature curve and white blood cell count. Renal, hepatic, and GI function should be watched closely because of the prognostic implications of multiorgan dysfunction in ARDS.

Additional Therapies

High-frequency oscillatory ventilation (HFOV) has been used successfully for many years in pediatric patients with ARDS. In theory, HFOV provides the ultimate "open lung" ventilation strategy by allowing maintenance of lung recruitment throughout the respiratory cycle, and by achieving alveolar ventilation using very small (subphysiologic) tidal volumes that are delivered at high frequency. No studies to date have compared HFOV to a modern lung protective conventional ventilation strategy, and whether HFOV provides any advantage over conventional ventilation for pediatric ARDS remains unknown. Earlier studies have demonstrated that pediatric ARDS patients treated with HFOV can demonstrate rapid and sustained improvements in oxygenation without adverse effects on ventilation, and have suggested that HFOV patients showed a reduced incidence of chronic lung injury, as evidenced by a decreased need for supplemental oxygen at 30 days. At present, whether HFOV is best used as a first-line ventilator strategy or as a rescue therapy for patients failing conventional ventilation remains a matter of institutional and clinician preference.

Prone positioning is a technique of changing the patient's position in bed from supine to prone, with the goal of reducing chest wall compliance and improving ventilation of collapsed dependent lung units via postural drainage and improved ventilation-perfusion matching. This technique can dramatically improve gas exchange in the short term, particularly for patients early in the course of ARDS, but the gains are often not sustained. To date, clinical trials examining the role of prone positioning in both adults and children with ALI and ARDS have not shown any improvement in mortality or in duration of mechanical ventilation.

Based on the ability of inhaled ***nitric oxide (iNO)*** to reduce pulmonary artery pressure and to improve the matching of ventilation with perfusion without producing systemic vasodilation, iNO can be used as a therapy for refractory ARDS. Several multicenter trials of iNO in the treatment of ARDS, both in adults and in children, showed acute improvements in oxygenation in subsets of patients, but no significant improvement in overall survival. As a result, iNO cannot be recommended as a standard therapy for ARDS. ***Surfactant-replacement*** therapy is also not routinely recommended for children with ARDS, as the data regarding its efficacy remain mixed. To date, it has been difficult to draw meaningful conclusions from the completed surfactant trials because they differ so greatly with respect to surfactant composition, dosing regimen, study population, and mechanical ventilation strategy. A recent review of published pediatric studies suggests a decrease in mortality and length of ventilation with the use of surfactant, and there are ongoing trials evaluating various surfactant formulations.

The intense alveolar inflammation observed in ARDS has led to the suggestion that immune modulation with ***corticosteroids*** might improve outcomes. Early trials did not demonstrate that high-dose glucocorticoids provide any survival benefit in ARDS patients and even suggested an increase in life-threatening infections. More recent clinical data on low-dose, prolonged glucocorticoid treatment of ARDS showed significant improvement in inflammation and lung physiology with a more favorable benefit-risk profile. A recent large multicenter trial of methylprednisolone in the late phase of adult ARDS (> 7 days after onset) showed no difference in mortality rates compared with placebo, despite corticosteroid-associated improvements in short-term measures such as hemodynamics, oxygenation, and respiratory system compliance. Compared with placebo, methylprednisolone did not increase the rate of infectious complications, but was associated with a higher rate of neuromuscular weakness. In addition, starting steroids more than 2 weeks after the onset of ARDS was associated with an increased risk of death. There are no definitive studies evaluating the role of corticosteroids in the management of children with ARDS. Given the conflicting literature, the routine use of corticosteroids in pediatric ARDS is not recommended.

ECMO has been used to support pediatric patients with severe ARDS, but not with the same success that this therapy has seen for neonates with respiratory failure. Recent registry data suggest the overall survival rate for children who require ECMO for ARDS is around 40%–50%. To date, the efficacy of ECMO has not been evaluated against lung sparing ventilation strategies for pediatric ARDS in a prospective randomized trial. In addition, recent improvements in outcome for pediatric ARDS patients receiving "conventional" therapies have made the role of ECMO less clear and have made further prospective randomized studies of ECMO difficult to complete. For now, ECMO remains a viable rescue therapy for patients with severe ARDS that is unresponsive to other modalities.

Outcomes

Information regarding the long-term outcome of pediatric patients with ARDS remains limited. One report of 10 children followed 1–4 years after severe ARDS showed three still symptomatic and seven with hypoxemia at rest. Until further information is available, all patients with a history of ARDS need close follow-up of pulmonary function.

Arnold JH, Hanson JH et al: Prospective, randomized comparison of high-frequency oscillatory ventilation and conventional mechanical ventilation in pediatric respiratory failure. Crit Care Med 1994;22(10):1530–1539 [PMID: 7924362].

Bernard GR, Artigas A, Brigham KL et al: The American-European Consensus Conference on ARDS. Definitions, mechanisms, relevant outcomes, and clinical trial coordination. Am J Respir Crit Care Med 1994;149:818–824 [PMID: 8199655].

Curley MA, Hibberd PL, Fineman LD et al: Effect of prone positioning on clinical outcomes in children with acute lung injury: A randomized controlled trial. JAMA 2005;294:229–237 [PMID: 16014597].

Duffett M et al: Surfactant therapy for acute respiratory failure in children: A systematic review and meta-analysis. Crit Care 2007;11:R66 [PMID: 17573963].

Flori HR, Glidden DV, Rutherford GW et al: Pediatric acute lung injury: Prospective evaluation of risk factors associated with mortality. Am J Respir Crit Care Med 2005;171:995–1001 [PMID: 15618461].

LaCroix J, Hebert PC, Hutchison JS et al: Transfusion strategies for patients in pediatric intensive care units. New Engl J Med 2007;356:1609–1619 [PMID: 17442904].

Peter JV et al: Corticosteroids in the prevention and treatment of acute respiratory distress syndrome (ARDS) in adults: Meta-analysis. BMJ 2008;336:1006–1009 [PMID: 18434379].

Randolph AG: Management of acute lung injury and acute respiratory distress syndrome in children. Crit Care Med 2009;37:2448–2454 [PMID: 19531940].

Willson DF, Thomas NJ, Markovitz BP et al: Effect of exogenous surfactant (calfactant) in pediatric acute lung injury: A randomized controlled trial. JAMA 2005;293:470–476 [PMID: 15671432].

STATUS ASTHMATICUS

ESSENTIALS OF DIAGNOSIS & TYPICAL FEATURES

- Status asthmaticus is reversible small airway obstruction that is refractory to sympathomimetic and anti-inflammatory agents and that may progress to respiratory failure without prompt and aggressive intervention.
- Dyspnea at rest that interferes with the ability to speak.
- Absence of wheezing may be misleading because, in order to produce a wheezing sound, the patient must take in sufficient air.
- Peak expiratory flow < 25% predicted or personal best.
- Patients with severe respiratory distress, signs of exhaustion, alterations in consciousness, elevated $Paco_2$, or acidosis should be admitted to the PICU.

Pathogenesis

Life-threatening asthma exacerbations are caused by severe bronchospasm, excessive mucus secretion, inflammation, and edema of the airways (see Chapter 38). Reversal of these mechanisms is key to successful treatment. Several structural and mechanical features of the lungs of infants and children place them at increased risk for respiratory failure from severe asthma exacerbations, including less elastic recoil than the adult lung, thicker airway walls which lead to greater peripheral airway resistance for any degree of bronchoconstriction, increased airway reactivity to bronchoconstrictors, fewer collateral channels of ventilation, and a more compliant chest wall which can lead to increased work of breathing with airway obstruction. In addition, some individual patients display a pattern of recurrent life-threatening asthma exacerbations. These patients will often have a history of previous ICU admissions or intubations; obesity, lower socioeconomic status, and non-Caucasian race are additional risk factors for severe asthma exacerbations.

Early treatment is the best strategy for management of acute asthma exacerbations. Patients who are at high risk for asthma-related death require special attention, particularly intensive education, monitoring, and care. Such patients should be counseled to seek medical care early during an exacerbation and instructed about the availability of ambulance services.

Clinical Findings

1. General—Patients with severe asthma exacerbations may display signs of panic or exhaustion and alterations in level of consciousness. Pulse oximetry should be performed on presentation. Saturations less than 90% on room air can be indicative of severe airway obstruction, especially in infants.

2. Respiratory—Patients are often tachypneic and may have trouble speaking. Dyspnea at rest that interferes with the ability to speak can be an ominous sign of severe airflow obstruction. Accessory muscle use (sternocleidomastoid) correlates well with expiratory flow rates less than 50% of normal predicted values. Inspiratory and expiratory wheezing, paradoxical breathing, cyanosis, and a respiratory rate more than 60 are all important signs of serious distress. Particular attention should be paid to the degree of aeration. Diffuse wheezing is typically appreciated, but if severe airway obstruction reduces airflow enough, wheezing may be absent.

3. Cardiovascular—Patients are typically tachycardic secondary to stress, dehydration, and β-agonist therapy. A pulsus paradoxus of over 22 mm Hg correlates with elevated $Paco_2$ levels. Diastolic blood pressure may be low secondary to dehydration and β-agonist use. Diastolic pressures less than 40 mm Hg in conjunction with extreme tachycardia may impair coronary artery filling and predispose to cardiac ischemia, especially in teenagers.

4. Neurological—Agitation, drowsiness, and confusion can be signs of elevated $Paco_2$ levels and may signify impending respiratory failure. Likewise, gasping respirations or frank apnea are indications for intubation.

Laboratory Findings

Blood gas measurements should be made on all patients with severe asthma exacerbations. Venous blood gas measurements may serve as a screening test for acidosis and hypercapnia but cannot substitute for arterial blood gas measurements in critically ill asthmatics. Patients with severe asthma exacerbations typically have increased minute ventilation and should be expected to have $Paco_2$ less than 40 mm Hg. Normal to elevated $Paco_2$ levels suggest respiratory failure. Metabolic acidosis may be due to relative dehydration, inadequate cardiac output, or underlying infection. Hypoxemia (Pao_2 < 60 mm Hg) on room air may be a sign of impending respiratory failure or significant ventilation/perfusion mismatch caused by pneumonia or atelectasis. Ventilation/perfusion mismatching also can be exacerbated by β-agonist therapy due to the effects on both the airway and vascular smooth muscle.

Monitoring of serum electrolytes may reveal decreased serum potassium, magnesium, and/or phosphate, especially in patients with prolonged β-agonist use. Blood count measurements are not required routinely. Leukocytosis is common in asthma exacerbations and corticosteroid treatment causes demargination of polymorphonuclear leukocytes within a few hours of administration. Differentiating infection from stress demargination as causes of leukocytosis can be difficult and measurement of other inflammatory markers such as C-reactive protein levels should be considered in those circumstances.

Imaging Studies

Chest x-rays are not recommended for routine exacerbations, but should be obtained in severe exacerbations to evaluate for bronchiolitis, pneumonia, foreign body, suspected air leak, or a chest mass (in patients without previous asthma history). Pneumothorax and pneumomediastinum are common complications of severe asthma exacerbations and may occur in nonintubated patients.

Special Studies

Measurement of *forced expiratory volume in 1 second* (FEV1) or *peak expiratory flow* (PEF) is recommended in the urgent or emergency care setting, though patients with life-threatening asthma exacerbation are often unable to cooperate with testing. Values of less than 40% of predicted indicate a severe exacerbation and values less than 25% of predicted indicate imminent respiratory arrest. Repeated measures of pulmonary function in very severe exacerbations are of limited value.

Electrocardiograms are not routinely recommended but may be indicated to rule out cardiac ischemia, especially in patients with known cardiac disease, extreme tachycardia and low diastolic blood pressure, or complaints of chest pain.

Differential Diagnosis

In patients with severe wheezing without previous asthma history, other diagnoses such as foreign body aspiration, congestive heart failure, pulmonary infections, or mediastinal mass should be entertained. Chest x-rays are useful to identify these conditions. An expiratory chest film is particularly helpful in identifying foreign bodies. Vocal cord dysfunction may also mimic severe asthma exacerbation and can be present in patients with true asthma. Laryngoscopy may be indicated to rule out this condition.

Treatment

Much of the morbidity associated with the treatment of severe asthma is related to the complications of providing mechanical ventilation in patients with severe airflow obstruction. As a result, the goal of initial treatment of patients with life-threatening status asthmaticus is to improve their ability to ventilate without resorting to intubation and MV. The medical therapies described in the following discussion should be undertaken swiftly and aggressively with the goal of reversing the bronchospasm before respiratory failure necessitates invasive ventilation.

Close monitoring of gas exchange, cardiovascular status, and mental status are crucial to assessing response to therapy and determining the appropriate interventions. Children with status asthmaticus require IV access, continuous pulse oximetry and cardiorespiratory monitoring. Due to inadequate minute ventilation and V/Q mismatching, patients with severe asthma are almost always hypoxemic and should receive supplemental humidified oxygen immediately to maintain saturations more than 90%.

The repetitive or continuous administration of a ***selective short-acting β_2-agonist*** is the most effective means of rapidly reversing airflow obstruction. Treatment with agents such as albuterol remains the first-line therapy for these patients. If the patient is in severe distress and has poor inspiratory flow rates, thus preventing adequate delivery of nebulized medication, subcutaneous injection of epinephrine or terbutaline may be considered. The frequency of β_2-agonist administration varies according to the severity of the patient's symptoms and the occurrence of adverse side effects. Nebulized albuterol may be given intermittently at a dose of 0.1 mg/kg per nebulization up to 5.0 mg every 10 to 15 minutes, or it can be administered continuously at a dose of 0.5 mg/kg/h to a maximum of 20 mg/h, usually without serious side effects. IV β-agonists should be considered in patients with severe bronchospasm unresponsive to inhaled bronchodilators. The agent most commonly used in the United States is terbutaline, a relatively specific β_2-agonist, which can be given as a bolus dose or as a continuous infusion. Owing to its relative specificity for β_2-receptors, terbutaline has fewer cardiac side effects than previously available IV β-agonists such as isoproterenol. Terbutaline is given as a bolus or loading dose of 10 mcg/kg followed by a continuous infusion of 0.5–5 mcg/kg/min. The heart rate and blood pressure should be monitored closely, because excessive tachycardia, ventricular ectopy, and diastolic hypotension may occur in patients receiving either inhaled or IV β_2-agonist therapy. In general, patients receiving IV therapy should have indwelling arterial lines for continuous blood pressure and blood gas monitoring.

Immediate administration of ***systemic corticosteroids*** is critical to the early management of life-threatening status asthmaticus. Although oral systemic corticosteroids are generally recommended, consideration should be given to IV steroid administration in critically ill patients secondary to frequent intolerance of enterally administered medications. A dose of 2 mg/kg/d of methylprednisolone is generally prescribed for the critical care setting.

Infants and children with status asthmaticus may become dehydrated as a result of increased respiratory rate and decreased oral intake. In these patients, clinicians should make an assessment of fluid status and provide appropriate corrections. Fluid replacement should be aimed toward restoration of euvolemia while avoiding overhydration. The hemodynamic effects of high dose β_2-agonist therapy (peripheral dilation, diastolic hypotension) may require some fluid resuscitation to maintain cardiac output and avoid metabolic acidosis. Antibiotics are generally not recommended for treatment of status asthmaticus unless a co-existing infection is identified or suspected.

Adjunctive Therapies

For severe exacerbations unresponsive to the initial treatments listed above, adjunctive treatments may be considered to avoid intubation. ***Ipratropium bromide***, an inhaled anticholinergic bronchodilator, is a reasonable intervention given its low side-effect profile, though two controlled clinical trials failed to detect a significant benefit from its addition to standard therapy in preventing hospitalization due to asthma.

Magnesium sulfate is reported to be an effective bronchodilator in adult patients with severe status asthmaticus when given in conjunction with steroids and β_2-agonists and may be considered for patients with impending respiratory failure or who have a life-threatening exacerbations that does not respond well to the first 1 hour of intensive conventional therapy. The mechanism of action of magnesium is unclear, but its smooth muscle relaxation properties are probably caused by interference with calcium flux in the bronchial smooth muscle cell. Magnesium sulfate is given IV at a dose of 25–50 mg/kg per dose. Although usually well tolerated, hypotension and flushing can be side effects of IV magnesium administration.

Heliox-driven albuterol nebulization can also be considered for patients refractory to conventional therapy. Heliox is a mixture of helium and oxygen that is less viscous than ambient air and can improve airway delivery of albuterol and gas exchange. Clear evidence of clinical efficacy is lacking for young patients, and heliox requires a mixture containing at least 60%–70% helium to alter viscosity sufficiently to significantly improve air flow, limiting its use in patients requiring higher concentrations of supplemental oxygen.

Theophylline is a methylxanthine that remains controversial in the management of severe asthma. Clinical studies have yielded a mixed verdict on its benefit when given with steroids and β_2-agonists for children with asthma. This uncertainty, together with its high side-effect profile, led to the general recommendation against the use of theophylline for asthma exacerbations, though it may still have a role in severe exacerbations as a means to prevent intubation. The theoretical benefit of theophylline is relaxation of airway smooth muscle by preventing degradation of cyclic guanosine monophosphate, which is a separate mechanism from β_2-agonists. Besides causing bronchodilation, this agent decreases mucociliary inflammatory mediators and reduces microvascular permeability. However, the pharmacokinetics of theophylline are erratic and therapeutic levels can be difficult to manage. It is also associated with serious side effects, such as seizures and cardiac arrhythmias that can occur with high drug levels. Theophylline is given IV as *aminophylline*. Each 1 mg/kg of aminophylline given as a loading dose will increase the serum level by approximately 2 mg/dL. For a patient who has not previously received aminophylline or oral theophylline preparations, load with 7–8 mg/kg of aminophylline in an attempt to achieve a level of 10–15 mg/dL; then start a continuous infusion of aminophylline at a dosage of 0.8–1 mg/kg/h. A postbolus level and steady-state level should be drawn with the initiation of the medication. Watch closely for toxicity (gastric upset, tachycardia, and seizures) and continue to monitor steady-state serum levels closely, trying to maintain steady-state levels of 12–14 mg/dL.

Leukotriene receptor antagonists (LTRAs) theoretically may provide another pathway to bronchodilation for status asthmaticus. A randomized trial of IV montelukast in moderate and severe exacerbations demonstrated significant improvement in pulmonary function within 10 minutes of administration. The oral formulation LTRA would take much longer to demonstrate benefit and has not been shown to be beneficial for status asthmaticus.

Noninvasive ventilation (NIV) is another approach for treatment of respiratory failure due to severe asthma exacerbation that may help avoid the need for intubation and mechanical ventilation. During acute asthma episodes, airways resistance and expiratory time constants are increased. Positive pressure may help to avoid airway collapse during exhalation as well as to unload fatigued respiratory muscles by reducing the force required to initiate each breath. Because of its noninvasive interface, spontaneous breathing and upper airway function are preserved, allowing the patient to provide their own airway clearance. Data on the effectiveness of NIV for acute severe asthma in children are limited to small studies and case series but have shown an improvement in gas exchange and respiratory effort.

If aggressive management fails to result in significant improvement, ***mechanical ventilation*** may be necessary. Patients who present with apnea or coma should be intubated immediately. Otherwise, if there is steady deterioration despite intensive therapy for asthma, the patient should be intubated and ventilated mechanically. Intubation should occur semi-electively, before acute respiratory arrest, because the procedure can be dangerous in patients with severe asthma given the high risk of barotrauma and cardiovascular collapse. Mechanical ventilation for patients with asthma is difficult because the severe airflow obstruction often leads to very high airway pressures, air trapping, and resultant barotrauma. The goal of mechanical ventilation for an intubated asthma patient is to maintain adequate oxygenation and ventilation with the least amount of barotrauma until other therapies become effective. Worsening hypercarbia following intubation is typical and aggressive efforts to normalize blood gases may only lead to complications. Due to the severe airflow obstruction, these patients will require long inspiratory times to deliver a breath and long expiratory times to avoid air trapping. In general, the ventilator rate should be decreased until the expiratory time is long enough to allow emptying prior to the next machine breath. Ventilator rates of 8–12 breaths/min are typical initially. Either volume- or pressure-targeted modes of ventilation can be used effectively, although tidal volume and pressure limits should be closely monitored. As a patient moves toward extubation, a support mode of ventilation is useful, as the patient can set his or her own I-time and flow rate. Due to air trapping, patients can have significant auto-PEEP. The level of PEEP on the ventilator is usually set low (0–5 cm H_2O) to minimize air trapping and high peak pressures. Isolated reports have noted patients who respond to greater PEEP, but these are exceptions.

These ventilator strategies and resulting hypercarbia typically are uncomfortable, requiring that patients be heavily sedated and often medically paralyzed. Fentanyl and midazolam are good choices for sedation. Ketamine is a dissociative anesthetic that can be used to facilitate intubation and also as a sedative infusion for intubated patients. Ketamine has bronchodilatory properties, although it also increases bronchial secretions. Barbiturates should be avoided as well as morphine, both of which can increase histamine release and worsen bronchospasm. Most patients, at least initially, will also require neuromuscular blockade to optimize ventilation and minimize airway pressures. In intubated patients not responding to the preceding strategies, inhaled anesthetics, such as isoflurane, should be considered. These agents act not only as anesthetics but also cause airway smooth muscle relaxation; they must be used with caution, however, as they can also cause significant hypotension due to vasodilation and myocardial depression.

Prognosis

Status asthmaticus remains among the most common reasons for admission to the PICU. It is associated with surprisingly high mortality rate (1%–3%), especially in patients with a previous PICU admission. As many as 75% of patients admitted to the PICU with life-threatening asthma flares will be readmitted with a future exacerbation, emphasizing the need for careful outpatient follow-up of this high-risk population.

Carroll CL et al: Identifying an at-risk population of children with recurrent near-fatal asthma exacerbations. J Asthma 2010 May;47(4):460–464 [PMID: 20528602].

Mitra A et al: Intravenous aminophylline for acute severe asthma in children over two years receiving inhaled bronchodilators. Cochrane Database Syst Rev 2005;(2):CD001276 [PMID: 15846615].

National Asthma Education and Prevention Program: Expert Panel Report 3: Guidelines for the Diagnosis and Management of Asthma—Summary Report 2007, Section 5, Managing Exacerbations of Asthma. Available at: http://www.nhlbi.nih.gov/guidelines/asthma/asthgdln.htm.

Ram FS et al: Non-invasive positive pressure ventilation for treatment of respiratory failure due to severe acute exacerbations of asthma. Cochrane Database Syst Rev 2005;(1):CD004360 [PMID: 15674944].

SHOCK

ESSENTIALS OF DIAGNOSIS & TYPICAL FEATURES

- Shock is defined as the inadequate delivery of oxygen and nutrients to tissues to meet metabolic needs.
- Shock can result from decreased delivery of oxygen (cardiovascular failure, hypovolemia, abnormal hemoglobin-carrying capacity) or from inadequate utilization of oxygen (distributive shock).
- Shock can be categorized as compensated, uncompensated, and irreversible.
- Early recognition and intervention are key to improving patient outcome.

Pathogenesis

Shock is a syndrome characterized by inadequate oxygen delivery that can complicate multiple different disease processes. Shock can be categorized by the primary physiologic disturbance (Table 14–7), though many of these conditions

Table 14–7. Categories of shock.

Type of Shock	Examples
Hypovolemic	Dehydration due to vomiting and/or diarrhea Trauma with severe hemorrhage Vasodilation secondary to anaphylaxis
Cardiogenic	Viral myocarditis Postoperative cardiac patient with poor heart function
Distributive	Septic shock
Dissociative	Carbon monoxide poisoning

overlap in severely ill patients as organ injury progresses. The key concept in shock is that the metabolic needs of the tissues are not met. This metabolic failure may occur as a result of increased tissue demand (as in infection or other major physiologic stresses), reduced oxygen delivery (as in lung or cardiac disease), or impaired oxygen utilization (as in severe sepsis). The failure of oxygen delivery leads to anaerobic metabolism in cells and ultimately to irreversible cellular damage. In patients with a cardiogenic component to their shock, heart failure activates the renin-angiotensin-aldosterone and adrenergic sympathetic systems, and decreases parasympathetic stimulation leading to sodium and water retention, increased afterload, increased energy expenditure, myocyte death, and progressive ventricular dysfunction. Persistent activation of the sympathetic nerves results in adrenergic receptor downregulation, which is further complicated in the neonatal heart by baseline decreased β-adrenergic receptor expression and limits the response to inotropic agents. The etiology of the impaired oxygen utilization seen in septic shock is not well understood but is likely multifactorial and includes maldistribution of blood flow in the microcirculation as well as mitochondrial dysfunction. Dissociative shock is a term referring to abnormalities of hemoglobin-oxygen dissociation that lead to impaired oxygen availability to the tissues, typically as a result of abnormal hemoglobin function due to poisoning. In all cases of shock, the defects in oxygen delivery and utilization lead to anaerobic metabolism, hypoxia, and lactic acidosis.

Shock can also be categorized into a series of recognizable stages: compensated, uncompensated, and irreversible. Patients in ***compensated shock*** have relatively normal cardiac output and normal blood pressures but have alterations in the microcirculation that increase flow to some organs and reduce flow to others. As shock progresses, cardiac output increases in order to meet the tissue demand for oxygen delivery. In infants, a compensatory increase in cardiac output is achieved primarily by tachycardia rather than by an increase in stroke volume. In older patients, cardiac contractility (stroke volume) and heart rate both increase to improve cardiac output. Blood pressure remains normal initially because of peripheral vasoconstriction and increased systemic vascular resistance. Thus, hypotension occurs late and is characteristic of ***uncompensated shock***. In this stage, the oxygen and nutrient supply to the cells deteriorates further with subsequent cellular breakdown and release of toxic substances, causing further redistribution of flow. Patients in uncompensated shock are at risk of developing multiorgan system failure (MOSF), which carries a high risk of mortality. In extreme cases, organ damage can progress to the point that restoration of oxygen delivery will not improve organ function, a condition known as ***irreversible shock***.

Shock can be best understood by examining the factors responsible for oxygen delivery to the tissues and the factors influencing utilization of oxygen by tissues (oxygen consumption). Oxygen delivery (DO_2) is the product of the ability of the heart to pump blood to the organs, that is, ***cardiac output (CO)*** and the ***oxygen content of the arterial blood*** (CaO_2) delivered by the heart and so can be expressed mathematically as $CO \times CaO_2$. ***Cardiac output*** in turn is determined by ventricular stroke volume (SV) and heart rate (HR) and is calculated as $SV \times HR$. Stroke volume is influenced by preload, afterload, contractility, and cardiac rhythm. Numerous different conditions can disrupt one or more of these factors. For example, ***preload*** can be decreased as a result of hypovolemia due to hemorrhage or dehydration, or of vasodilation due to anaphylaxis, medications, or septic shock. Impaired ***contractility*** can lead to shock in conditions such as cardiomyopathy, myocardial ischemia/reperfusion following a cardiac arrest postcardiac surgery, and sepsis. Age-dependent differences in myocardial physiology can also affect systolic performance and contractility. For example, in the infant heart the sarcolemma, sarcoplasmic reticulum, and T-tubules are less well developed than in older children, resulting in a greater dependency on transsarcolemma Ca^2_+ flux (ie, extracellular serum Ca^2_+) for contraction. ***Afterload*** can be increased, as seen in late septic shock and cardiac dysfunction, or decreased, as in "warm" septic shock. Cardiac dysrhythmias can also alter cardiac output and contribute to inadequate oxygen delivery. One common example is supraventricular tachycardia, in which reduced time for ventricular filling can lead to reduced stroke volume and cardiac output.

The ***oxygen content of the arterial blood*** comprises of the oxygen *bound* to hemoglobin and the oxygen *dissolved* in the blood. The bound oxygen is determined by the hemoglobin concentration and the percent of the hemoglobin saturated by oxygen. The dissolved oxygen is calculated from the partial pressure of oxygen in the arterial blood (Pao_2). Under most conditions, the main determinant of arterial oxygen content is the bound oxygen. As a result, both illnesses that affect oxygen saturation and illnesses that alter hemoglobin concentration can impair oxygen delivery. Abnormal hemoglobins can also impair oxygen delivery, since carboxyhemoglobin (formed in carbon monoxide poisoning) or methemoglobin, have different oxygen-carrying capacities than normal hemoglobin, resulting in impaired oxygen delivery and dissociative shock.

Clinical Findings

Symptoms and Signs (see Table 14–8)

1. Vitals and General Appearance—Rapid assessment of a child in shock is essential to determine the need for resuscitation. Alterations in pulse, blood pressure, respiratory rate, temperature, and mental status are important in assessing the severity of illness.

2. Skin and Extremities—One should note the color of the skin, temperature, capillary refill, and quality of pulses. In patients with impaired cardiac output and peripheral vasoconstriction, the skin will be cool and pale with delayed capillary refill (> 3 seconds) and the pulse thready. Additionally, the skin may appear gray or ashen, particularly in newborns, mottled or cyanotic in patients with certain congenital heart lesions.

Table 14–8. Clinical features of shock.

General
Fatigue
Altered mental status
Cardiac
Tachycardia
+/– Hypotension
Weak pulses
Bounding pulses (warm septic shock)
Delayed capillary refill
Brisk capillary refill (warm septic shock)
Active precordium
Gallop rhythm
Skin/extremities
Decreased turgor
Hyper- or hypothermia
Color (pale, cyanotic)
Rash (eg, purpura with meningococcus)
Respiratory
Tachypnea
Signs of lung disease (eg, diminished breath sounds, crackles, rales)
Increased work of breathing
GI/GU
Decreased urine output
Diarrhea/vomiting (etiology of dehydration)
Hepatomegaly (eg, heart failure)
Abdominal distension
Musculoskeletal
Hypotonia
Flaccidity
Neurologic
Confusion
Coma
Weakness

GI/GU, gastrointestinal/genitourinary.

In contrast, patients with early or warm septic shock can present with warm skin with brisk capillary refill and bounding pulses. The detection of peripheral edema is a worrisome sign; in a patient with shock this may reflect severe vascular leak due to sepsis or poor cardiac output with fluid and sodium retention. The skin examination can provide insight into the diagnosis; the presence of rash such as purpura fulminans may indicate an infectious etiology, or reveal the site and extent of traumatic injury. Cracked parched lips and dry mucous membranes may indicate severe volume depletion.

3. Cardiovascular System—Tachycardia, which is an important sign of impaired cardiac output, is generally apparent before there is a change in blood pressure. Not all patients can mount an appropriate increase in heart rate, so the presence of bradycardia in a patient with shock is particularly ominous. Hypotension occurs late in pediatric shock (median systolic blood pressure for a child older than age 2 years can be estimated by adding 70 mm Hg to twice the age in years). The simultaneous palpation of distal and proximal pulses is important. An increase in the amplitude difference of pulses between proximal arteries (carotid, brachial, and femoral) and distal arteries (radial, posterior tibial, and dorsalis pedis) can be palpated in early shock and reflects increased systemic vascular resistance. A discrepancy in pulses between lower extremities and upper extremities may indicate a critical coarctation of the aorta leading to shock, particularly in an infant with closure of the ductus arteriosus. A gallop cardiac rhythm can indicate heart failure, while a pathologic murmur suggests the possibility of congenital heart disease or valvular dysfunction. A rub or faint distant heart sounds may indicate a pericardial effusion.

4. Respiratory—The respiratory examination includes observation of the respiratory rate and work of breathing, and quality of breath sounds. A patient with severe metabolic acidosis due to shock will have a compensatory tachypnea and respiratory alkalosis. Rales, hypoxia, and increased work of breathing can be seen in patients with shock from heart failure or acute lung injury.

5. Gastrointestinal/Genitourinary (GI/GU)—Urine output is directly proportionate to renal blood flow and the glomerular filtration rate, and therefore is a good reflection of cardiac output. (Normal urine output is > 1 mL/kg/h; output < 0.5 mL/kg/h is considered significantly decreased.) Catheterization of the bladder is necessary to give accurate and continuous information. Hepatomegaly may suggest heart failure or fluid overload, while splenomegaly may suggest an oncologic process, and abdominal distension may suggest obstruction or perforated viscus as the etiology of shock.

6. Musculoskeletal System—Decreased oxygen delivery to the musculoskeletal system produces hypotonia, resulting in decreased spontaneous motor activity, flaccidity, and prostration.

7. Central Nervous System (CNS)—The level of consciousness reflects the adequacy of cortical perfusion. When cortical perfusion is severely impaired, the infant or child first fails to respond to verbal stimuli, then to light touch, and finally to pain. Lack of motor response and failure to cry in response to venipuncture or lumbar puncture is ominous. In uncompensated shock with hypotension, brain stem perfusion may be decreased. Poor thalamic perfusion can result in loss of sympathetic tone. Finally, poor medullary flow produces irregular respirations followed by gasping, apnea, and respiratory arrest.

Laboratory studies (Table 14–9) outlines studies necessary to evaluate the etiology of shock, assess the extent of impaired oxygen delivery, and determine end-organ functions. Assessments of oxygen delivery require measurement of oxygen saturation and hemoglobin concentration. Pulse oximetry is adequate to measure oxygen saturation in patients with low oxygen requirements. Arterial blood gas (ABG) analyses provide more accurate oxygen measurements, which are important for optimizing mechanical ventilation in patients with significant hypoxemia, as well as measurements of arterial pH, which can reflect the adequacy of tissue perfusion. A central venous or, if possible, mixed venous (pulmonary

Table 14–9. Laboratory studies in the case of shock.

Evaluation for infectious etiology
Sources include blood, urine, tracheal secretions, CSF, wound, pleural fluid, or stool
Stains, cultures, and other microbiologic tests (PCR, immunofluorescent antibody stains) for bacteria, fungus, viruses
Evaluation of organ function
Pulmonary: ABG (evaluate acid-base status, evaluation of oxygen delivery/consumption)
Cardiac: ABG, mixed venous saturation, lactate
Liver: LFTs, coagulation studies
Renal (and hydration status): BUN, creatinine, bicarbonate, serum sodium
Adrenal function (stress response): cortisol, ACTH stimulation test
Hematology: WBC count with differential, hemoglobin, hematocrit, platelet count
Evaluation for DIC: PT, PTT, fibrinogen, D-dimer
Extent of inflammatory state: CRP, WBC, ESR, procalcitonin
Additional studies
Electrolytes
Ionized calcium
Magnesium
Phosphate

ABG, arterial blood gas; ACTH, adrenocorticotropic hormone; BUN, blood urea nitrogen; CRP, C-reactive protein; CSF, cerebrospinal fluid; DIC, disseminated intravascular coagulation; LFTs, liver function tests; PCR, polymerase chain reaction; PT, prothrombin time; PTT, partial thromboplastin time; WBC, white blood cell.

artery) blood gas, can be used to determine central venous saturation and also by extension measure the adequacy of overall oxygen delivery. If oxygen delivery is inadequate for the needs of the tissues a greater portion of that oxygen will be consumed and the mixed venous saturation will be lower than normal (< 70% in a patient without cyanotic heart disease). In contrast, patients with septic shock may have an elevated mixed venous saturation due to impaired oxygen utilization by the tissues (> 80%).

Other laboratory studies should be directed at identifying signs of end-organ dysfunction due to inadequate oxygen delivery. These include evidence of anaerobic metabolism such as acidemia and elevated arterial lactate. Laboratory signs of organ dysfunction include increased serum creatinine, or abnormal liver function tests such as elevated transaminases or reduced production of clotting factors. Blood chemistry measurements are also essential in patients with shock. Hypo- or hypernatremia are common, as are potential life-threatening abnormalities in potassium levels, particularly hyperkalemia. Patients in shock may have decreased ionized calcium, which will adversely impact cardiac function, particularly in young patients, who have an increased dependence on extracellular calcium. Calcium homeostasis also requires normal magnesium levels and renal failure may disrupt phosphorus levels. Evaluation of a coagulation panel is required to detect disseminated intravascular coagulation (DIC), particularly in patients with purpura fulminans, petechiae, or those at risk for thrombosis.

The selection of ***imaging studies***, similar to laboratory studies, should be guided by the presumed etiology of shock. For patients presenting with shock secondary to trauma, standard trauma protocols to evaluate organ damage and potential sites of hemorrhage are indicated. Chest x-rays are routinely performed for critically ill patients to check endotracheal tube or central-line placement, to evaluate the extent of airspace disease, presence of pleural effusions or pneumothorax, and to evaluate for pulmonary edema and cardiomegaly. Computed tomography (CT) of the chest or abdomen may be indicated to better evaluate sites of infection in septic shock, and echocardiography can provide useful information about cardiac anatomy and function.

Patients with shock often need ***invasive hemodynamic monitoring*** for diagnostic and therapeutic reasons. ***Arterial catheters*** provide constant blood pressure readings, and to an experienced interpreter, the shape of the waveform is helpful in evaluating cardiac output. ***Central venous pressure (CVP)*** monitoring gives useful information about relative changes in volume status as therapy is given. CVP monitoring does not provide information about absolute volume status, as decreased right ventricular compliance will produce a higher CVP for the same volume status as a normally compliant ventricle. Intravascular volume can be assessed more accurately by monitoring pulmonary capillary wedge pressure or left atrial pressure using a ***pulmonary artery catheter***. The pulmonary artery catheter also provides valuable information on cardiac status and vascular resistance, and enables calculations of oxygen delivery and consumption (Table 14–10), but is associated with a higher complication rate than CVP lines. Most patients can be monitored using alternative strategies to pulmonary artery catheters.

Treatment

Regardless of the etiology, the end result of shock is organ dysfunction, which if untreated can lead to irreversible multiorgan system failure (MOSF). Therefore, early recognition of uncompensated shock, coupled with early intervention, is necessary to minimize end-organ injury and improve survival. *Airway, breathing, and circulation* should be rapidly assessed according to the guidelines established in Pediatric Advanced Life Support (PALS) by the American Heart Association, with appropriate stabilization of the airway, support of breathing, and stabilization of circulation. Indications for intubation and mechanical ventilation include altered mental status, significant hemodynamic instability, inability to protect the airway, poor respiratory effort, high work of breathing, or poor gas exchange. In addition, patients in shock who will require surgery or other interventions requiring general anesthesia will also require mechanical ventilation. A temporary interosseous line should be placed if IV access cannot be rapidly obtained for resuscitation fluids and medications. A central venous line should be considered in

Table 14–10. Hemodynamic parameters.

Oxygen delivery DO_2 (mL/min/m²)	$CaO_2 \times CI \times 10$
Oxygen content of arterial blood CaO_2 (mL/dL)	$(1.34 \times \text{hemoglobin} \times SaO_2) + (0.003 \times Pao_2)$
Partial pressure of oxygen PiO_2	(Barometric pressure − 47) × % inspired oxygen concentration
Alveolar-arterial oxygen difference A-aDO_2	$Pio_2 - (Paco_2/R) - Pao_2$ [normal = (5 − 15) mm Hg]
Cardiac output (L/min)	CO = HR × SV
Cardiac index (L/min/m²)	CI = CO/BSA
Oxygen consumption (Cvo_2) (mL/min/m²)	$(CaO_2 - Cvo_2) \times CI \times 10$
Intrapulmonary shunt fraction $\frac{Qs}{Qt}$	$\frac{Cco_2 - Cao_2}{Cco_2 - Cvo_2}$ (normal < 5%)
Cco_2	Oxygen content of pulmonary capillary blood
Cvo_2	Oxygen content of mixed venous blood (mL/dL)
$Paco_2$	Partial pressure of carbon dioxide in arterial blood (mm Hg)
Pao_2	Partial pressure of oxygen in arterial blood (mm Hg)
$Pcco_2$	Partial pressure of carbon dioxide in capillary blood (mm Hg)
Pio_2	Partial pressure of oxygen in inspired air (mm Hg)
R	Respiratory quotient (usually 0.8)
Systemic vascular resistance (dyn × s/cm⁵/m²)	$SVR = 79.9\frac{(MAP - CVP)}{CI}$
Pulmonary vascular resistance (dyn × s/cm⁵/m²)	$PVR = 79.9\frac{(MPAP - PCWP)}{CI}$
VO_2	Oxygen consumption per minute

patients with hemodynamic instability, particularly if they require ongoing resuscitation and infusions of vasoactive medications. While femoral venous lines are simpler and safer to place, they do not provide as accurate a measurement of CVP and are at higher risk of infection. Subclavian and internal jugular lines are preferred for CVP monitoring, but they do carry the additional risk of pneumothorax. The rapidity and accuracy of placing central venous lines may be improved with the use of ultrasound guidance.

Fluid resuscitation should start with 20 mL/kg boluses titrated to clinical measures of cardiac output (heart rate, urine output, capillary refill, and level of consciousness). Continuous pulse oximetry, heart rate, respiratory rate, and blood pressure should be closely monitored. Patients who do not respond rapidly to 40- to 60-mL/kg of fluid should be monitored in an intensive care setting and considered for invasive hemodynamic monitoring (placement of a CVP monitor, arterial line, and rarely pulmonary artery catheter). Initially, most patients tolerate crystalloid (salt solution), which is readily available and inexpensive. The indications for colloid infusions remain controversial. Patients with serious capillary leaks and ongoing plasma losses (eg, burn cases) should initially receive crystalloid, because in these cases colloid (protein and salt solution) leaks into the interstitium. Patients with hypoalbuminemia or those with intact capillaries who need to retain volume in the intravascular space (eg, patients at risk for cerebral edema) may benefit from colloid infusions. Experience with dextran (a starch compound dissolved in salt solution) is limited. Large volumes of fluid for acute stabilization in children with shock may be necessary to restore adequate oxygen delivery and do not increase the incidence of acute respiratory distress syndrome (ARDS) or cerebral edema. Increased fluid requirements may persist for several days. Patients in cardiogenic shock, however, may not tolerate aggressive fluid loading as well as patients with normal heart function and will require careful monitoring and titration of therapy to optimize oxygen delivery.

Empiric ***antibiotics*** are chosen according to the most likely cause of infection. Early administration of antibiotics is a key factor in improving outcome from serious bacterial infections. While it is highly desirable to obtain cultures prior to initiation of antibiotics in order to guide the choice and duration of antibiotic coverage, the acquisition of cultures should never delay antibiotic administration.

Inotropic and vasopressor agents should be considered for patients who continue to have clinical evidence of decreased cardiac output after receiving 60 mL/kg of fluid resuscitation (Table 14–11). ***Dopamine*** remains the first-line vasopressor, although norepinephrine or vasopressin may be considered early in patients with low systemic vascular resistance (SVR) and hypotension. Dopamine causes vasoconstriction by stimulating the release of norepinephrine from sympathetic nerves. Dopamine is also an α- and β-agonist that at moderate doses (3–10 mcg/kg/min) improves myocardial contractility. At higher doses (generally > 10 mcg/kg/min) the α-receptor effects predominate, with vasoconstriction increasing SVR and pulmonary vascular resistance (PVR). Lower doses (< 3 mcg/kg/min) may increase blood flow to the renal, coronary, and splanchnic beds via specific D_1 dopamine receptors in normal volunteers. Of note, no evidence exists to support the use of "renal-dose" dopamine to augment urine output or preserve renal function in critically ill patients and this approach is now widely discouraged. Newer agents (eg, fenoldopam) that are selective for dopaminergic receptors have

Table 14–11. Pharmacologic support of the patient with shock.

Drug	Dose	α-Adrenergic Effect[a]	β-Adrenergic Effect[a]	Vasodilator Effect	Actions and Advantages	Disadvantages
Dopamine	1–20 mcg/kg/min	+ to +++ (dose-related)	+ to +++ (dose-related)		Moderate inotrope, wide and safe dosage range, short half-life.	May cause worsening of pulmonary vasoconstriction
Dobutamine	1–10 mcg/kg/min	0	+++	β_2 vasodilation	Moderate inotrope, less chronotropic, fewer dysrhythmias than isoproterenol or epinephrine.	Marked variation among patients, tachycardia
Epinephrine	0.05–1 mcg/kg/min	++ to +++ (dose-related)	+++		Significant increases in inotropy, chronotropy, and SVR.	Tachycardia, dysrhythmias, renal ischemia, systemic and PVR
Isoproterenol	0.05–1 mcg/kg/min	0	+++	Peripheral vasodilation	Significant increase in inotropy and chronotropy. SVR can drop, and PVR should not increase and may decrease.	Significant myocardial oxygen consumption increases, tachycardia, dysrhythmias
Norepinephrine	0.05–1 mcg/kg/min	+++	+++		Potent vasoconstrictor (systemic and pulmonary); used in patients with low SVR.	Reduced cardiac output if afterload is too high, renal ischemia
Nitroprusside	0.05–8 mcg/kg/min	0	0	Arterial and venous dilation (smooth muscle relaxation)	Decreases SVR and PVR, very short-acting. Blood pressure returns to previous levels within 1–10 min after infusion is stopped.	Toxicities (thiocyanates and cyanide), increased intracranial pressure, ventilation-perfusion mismatch, methemoglobinemia
Milrinone	0.25–0.75 mcg/kg/min	0	0		Phosphodiesterase III inhibition. Decreases SVR and PVR, increases myocardial contractility with only mild increase in myocardial O_2 consumption. Usually used with low-dose dopamine or dobutamine.	

[a]0, no effect; +, small effect; ++, moderate effect; +++, potent effect. PVR, pulmonary vascular resistance; SVR, systemic vascular resistance.

been used to selectively improve renal blood flow and urine output in patients with heart failure, but again no evidence suggests that this approach is useful in pediatric patients with shock-induced renal failure. Infants younger than 6 months of age may not have fully developed sympathetic vesicles and may therefore be resistant to dopamine and more responsive to norepinephrine. ***Dobutamine*** is a synthetic β-agonist that may be used to improve myocardial contractility and reduce afterload. Children younger than 12 months of age, however, may be less responsive and more likely to develop hypotension and significant tachycardia with dobutamine. For patients with hypotension and low cardiac output states, epinephrine is another front-line agent that can be used alone or in conjunction with dopamine. ***Epinephrine*** is an α- and β-agonist that causes the greatest increase in myocardial O_2 consumption of all inotropes. At a low dose (< 0.05 mcg/kg/min), it increases heart rate and contractility and decreases SVR (β-receptor). At higher doses the α-receptor effects predominate, increasing SVR. Despite the drawbacks of increased cardiac afterload and increased myocardial oxygen consumption, epinephrine can be useful as a second-line agent in cases unresponsive to dopamine. In patients with heart failure, a vasodilator is often administered in combination with epinephrine to offset the drug's α-receptor effects. ***Milrinone*** (0.25–0.75 mcg/kg/min) is a useful phosphodiesterase inhibitor, preventing degradation of both cyclic guanosine monophosphate and cyclic adenosine monophosphate. Its beneficial effects include a limited increase in myocardial O_2 consumption, decreased SVR and PVR, increased contractility, and improved lusitropy. It is frequently used as a first-line drug for patients in cardiogenic shock, often in combination with dopamine or epinephrine. Calcium and diuretics can also be useful treatments for cardiogenic shock. Hypocalcemia is often a contributor to cardiac dysfunction in shock. ***Calcium*** replacement should be given to normalize ionized calcium levels. Cardiogenic failure is associated with elevated ventricular filling pressures (> 20 mm Hg). Thus, although increasing preload can result in augmented cardiac output (to a degree), volume should be administered cautiously as improvement may occur at the expense of elevated pulmonary venous pressure with resultant pulmonary edema. ***Diuretics*** can be administered in this situation to reduce pulmonary edema and improve pulmonary compliance, the work of breathing, and oxygenation.

Adjunctive Therapies

Corticosteroids may be of benefit in some forms of shock. The role of corticosteroids in septic shock is discussed in greater detail in the next section, but in brief hydrocortisone should be considered for children at risk for adrenal insufficiency—those with purpura fulminans or pituitary or adrenal abnormalities, those receiving steroids for chronic illness, and those with septic shock and multiorgan system dysfunction not responding to traditional inotropic therapy.

Blood products can be important supportive therapies in patients with shock. *Red blood cells* can be administered to patients with shock to improve oxygen-carrying capacity. In hemodynamically stable patients, hemoglobin levels should be maintained between 7 and 9 g/dL, while the transfusion threshold can be increased to 10 g/dL in unstable patients. DIC is common in shock, particularly septic shock, due to endothelial damage, formation of microvascular emboli, and consumptive coagulopathy. Thus, a process beginning as increased coagulation leads to a bleeding diathesis. *Platelets* are generally transfused when platelet counts are less than 20,000/μL, or less than 40,000–60,000/μL in a patient with bleeding or requiring surgical intervention. The presence of antiplatelet antibodies may modify these transfusion criteria. For severe coagulopathies associated with bleeding in the setting of shock, the standard treatment is *fresh frozen plasma* or, for fibrinogen replacement, *cryoprecipitate* with close monitoring of prothrombin time (PT), international normalized ratio (INR), and partial thromboplastin time (PTT). *Activated factor VII* is available for severe bleeding with liver failure or major trauma, but should be used with caution and appropriate input from a pediatric hematologist. Protein C is a primary regulator of coagulation, fibrinolysis, and coagulation-induced inflammation. Deficits in protein C activation correlate with morbidity and mortality in septic shock and have been found in children and adults with sepsis. ***Recombinant activated protein C*** reduced mortality in a large randomized, double-blind, placebo-controlled trial in adults with severe sepsis. A similarly designed trial of activated protein C in pediatric patients with severe sepsis was halted early due to concern over hemorrhagic complications and the absence of any clear clinical benefit. Finally, ***extracorporeal membrane oxygenation (ECMO)*** can be used as a life-saving measure in the treatment of severe shock in patients with recoverable cardiac and pulmonary function who have failed conventional management.

Annane D et al: Corticosteroids in the treatment of severe sepsis and septic shock in adults: A systematic review. JAMA 2009;301(22):2362–2375 [PMID: 19509383].

de Oliveira CF et al: ACCM/PALS haemodynamic support guidelines for paediatric septic shock: An outcomes comparison with and without monitoring central venous oxygen saturation. Intensive Care Med 2008;34(6):1065–1075 [PMID: 18369591].

Trzeciak S et al: Early increases in microcirculatory perfusion during protocol-directed resuscitation are associated with reduced multi-organ failure at 24 h in patients with sepsis. Intensive Care Med 2008;34(12):2210–2217 [PMID: 18594793].

SEPSIS

ESSENTIALS OF DIAGNOSIS & TYPICAL FEATURES

- Sepsis and septic shock remain major causes of death in children worldwide.
- The innate immune system plays a critical role in mediating the inflammatory responses to infection and tissue injury that lead to sepsis.
- Early recognition and aggressive fluid therapy titrated to physiologic end points lead to earlier reversal of septic shock and improved outcomes.
- Organized systematic approaches to the treatment of sepsis within an institution can improve survival.

Sepsis is one of the major illnesses leading to admission to the pediatric intensive care unit. Worldwide, an estimated 18 million patients develop sepsis each year, with 750,000 of those cases in North America. Sepsis is the tenth leading cause of death in the United States and accounts for approximately 40% of intensive care unit expenditures in the United States and Europe. Among children, an estimated 42,000 cases of severe sepsis occur annually in the United States, accompanied by a mortality rate of nearly 10%. The incidence of severe sepsis is highest in infancy, remains relatively low from age 1 to mid-life, then rises again in later life.

Published literature regarding sepsis uses a number of overlapping and sometimes confusing terminologies. The ***systemic inflammatory response syndrome (SIRS)*** refers to a nonspecific syndrome of systemic inflammation typically associated with fever, tachycardia, tachypnea, and an abnormal white blood cell count. ***Sepsis*** is defined as a clinical syndrome characterized by a documented or suspected infection, accompanied by clinical and laboratory signs of systemic inflammation (SIRS). Though the criteria used to define sepsis in adults and children differ in published guidelines (Table 14–12), the more specific adult criteria provide a useful framework for thinking about sepsis-related organ dysfunction. ***Severe sepsis*** is defined as sepsis along with evidence of at least 1 sepsis-induced major organ dysfunction such as hypotension, hypoxemia, lactic acidosis, oliguria, renal failure, thrombocytopenia, coagulopathy, or hyperbilirubinemia. Of note, the number of organ systems affected by severe sepsis is an important prognostic factor. The risk of death from sepsis rises with the number of organ failures, with a mortality rate of 7%–10% with single organ failure and up to 50% mortality with 4 organ failures. ***Septic shock*** is defined as severe sepsis associated with impaired oxygen delivery, often accompanied by hypotension unresponsive to fluids.

Table 14–12. Diagnostic criteria for sepsis in adult patients.

Infection, documented or suspected, and some of the following:
General signs and symptoms
• Fever (> 38.3°C)
• Hypothermia (core temperature < 36°C)
• Heart rate 90/min or > 2 SD above the normal value for age
• Tachypnea
• Altered mental status
• Significant edema or positive fluid balance (> 20 mL/kg over 24 h)
• Hyperglycemia (plasma glucose > 140 mg/dL or 7.7 mmol/L) in the absence of diabetes
Evidence of inflammation
• Leukocytosis (WBC count > 12,000/ul)
• Leukopenia (WBC count < 4000/ul)
• Normal WBC count with > 10% immature forms
• Plasma C-reactive protein > 2 SD above the normal value
• Plasma procalcitonin > 2 SD above the normal value
Hemodynamics
• Arterial hypotension (SBP < 90 mm Hg; MAP < 70 mm Hg; or an SBP decrease 40 mm Hg in adults or > 2 SD below normal for age)
Organ dysfunction
• Arterial hypoxemia ($PaO_2/FIO_2 < 300$)
• Acute oliguria (urine output < 0.5 mL/kg/h for at least 2 h, despite adequate fluid resuscitation)
• Creatinine increase > 0.5 mg/dL or 44.2 umol/L
• Coagulation abnormalities (INR > 1.5 or a PTT > 60 s)
• Ileus (absent bowel sounds)
• Thrombocytopenia (platelet count < 100,000/ul)
• Hyperbilirubinemia (plasma total bilirubin > 4 mg/dL or 70 umol/L)
Tissue perfusion
• Hyperlactatemia (upper limit of lab normal)
• Decreased capillary refill or mottling
Diagnostic criteria for sepsis in the pediatric population
Signs and symptoms of inflammation plus infection with hyper- or hypothermia (rectal temperature > 38.5°C or < 35°C), tachycardia (may be absent in hypothermic patients), and at least one of the following indications of altered organ function: altered mental status, hypoxemia, increased serum lactate level, or bounding pulses.

WBC, white blood cell; SBP, systolic blood pressure; MAP, mean arterial blood pressure; INR, international normalized ratio; aPTT, activated partial thromboplastin time. (Adapted from Dellinger et al 2008.)

Pathophysiology

The pathophysiology of sepsis is highly complex and still poorly understood. Recent work has brought to light the critical role of the innate immune system in the pathogenesis of sepsis. Infectious agents release ***pathogen associated molecular patterns (PAMPs)*** such as lipopolysaccharide or peptidoglycans, and damaged tissues release endogenous molecular triggers such as HMGB1, heat shock proteins, and nucleic acids, collectively referred to as ***damage-associated molecular patterns (DAMPs)***. These molecules are recognized by pattern recognition receptors of the innate immune system, most prominently the ***Toll-like receptors***, which then trigger inflammatory cascades throughout the body. Derangements of adaptive immunity also contribute to the pathogenesis of sepsis. Toll-like receptor signaling may activate subsets of regulatory T-cells in septic patients, leading to either immune paralysis or uncontrolled inflammation depending on the pathophysiologic setting. Cytokine production and leukocyte activation lead to endothelial damage and activation of the clotting system. Microvascular thrombi lead to impaired tissue perfusion, which leads to further tissue damage, which in turn leads to further activation of the immune system. The end result of these processes is impaired oxygen delivery to the tissues, impaired oxygen utilization and metabolic downregulation, leading to end-organ dysfunction and ultimately to death if the process is not reversed.

Treatment

Much attention has been directed in recent years to the role of standardized treatment guidelines in improving outcomes from sepsis, and detailed guidelines are now available from several professional organizations. Key principles are that early recognition and treatment of sepsis, preferably stemming from a consistent organized clinical approach, improve outcomes in all age ranges.

An important element of the treatment of sepsis is early aggressive ***fluid resuscitation*** targeted to measurable physiologic endpoints of organ perfusion, so-called "early goal directed therapy." Once sepsis is recognized, fluid resuscitation should begin in 20 mL/kg increments administered rapidly and repeated as necessary to total as much as 60 mL/kg or more until perfusion and tachycardia improve or until evidence of pulmonary edema or heart failure develops. Studies in adult patients with septic shock have reported improved survival using a combination of blood transfusions and crystalloid fluids to achieve a central venous oxygen saturation

($ScvO_2$) of greater than 70% beginning with resuscitation in the emergency department. A similar pediatric study from Brazil also reported marked improvement in survival with the same strategy. While these results have led to a recommendation for central venous pressure oxygen saturation measurements as an endpoint to guide titration of fluid therapy, the practicalities of reliably and rapidly establishing central venous access in most pediatric emergency departments have limited the application of this approach. Once central venous access is available, however, a $ScvO_2 > 70\%$ should be one goal of therapy. Other possible target physiologic endpoints (in addition to heart rate and skin perfusion) include invasive or noninvasive cardiac output measurements and blood lactate levels. The choice of fluid between crystalloid and colloid products is probably not important but pediatric sepsis guidelines state a preference for 5% albumin if available for initial resuscitation based on several small studies showing improved outcomes with albumin use.

If markers of perfusion have not improved with fluid administration within the first 30 to 60 minutes of care, the patient is considered to have fluid-resistant septic shock and ***vasopressors*** should be initiated. Current pediatric sepsis guidelines still suggest dopamine as the first-line agent for pediatric sepsis, though adult sepsis guidelines give equal first-line status to norepinephrine. Generally, dopamine and/or epinephrine are preferred for cold shock; norepinephrine is preferred for warm shock states. For cold shock, published guidelines suggest adding epinephrine relatively quickly if dopamine is ineffective at doses of up to 10 mcg/kg/min. In addition, clinicians should remember that sepsis is a dynamic process and the appropriate pressor may change as the clinical situation evolves. Since hypotension can develop rapidly in septic patients, an arterial catheter should be placed as soon as is practical for any patient requiring pressors for sepsis. Vasopressin infusions are sometimes used as a rescue therapy for patients failing catecholamine infusions but vasopressin has not been clearly shown to improve outcomes from severe sepsis.

If perfusion is still inadequate despite aggressive fluid and pressor support, the patient can be considered to have ***catecholamine-resistant septic shock***. This condition may be related to critical illness-related corticosteroid insufficiency (CIRCI), which is a condition of impaired adrenal responsiveness and low circulating cortisol levels that may occur in as many as 30% of critically ill patients. Several studies have suggested that low-dose hydrocortisone administration can speed the reversal of shock in patients with septic shock. Whether testing of adrenal responsiveness with an ACTH stimulation test improves identification of septic patients likely to respond to steroids is still controversial. Despite the uncertainties in this area, most published guidelines recommend hydrocortisone administration at a dose of 1 mg/kg every 6 hours up to 200 mg/day for patients with septic shock refractory to fluids and pressors.

Another essential element of treating sepsis is ***control of the source of infection***. Empiric broad-spectrum antibiotics should be administered within one hour of recognizing sepsis and should not be delayed while obtaining cultures. Drainage of abscesses or other infected spaces can be life-saving in patients with severe sepsis. In addition, because failure of one or more organs can develop rapidly, they should be anticipated and provisions made for intubation and mechanical ventilation, renal replacement therapy, or even ECMO for hemodynamic support as the situation progresses.

Brierley J et al: Clinical practice parameters for hemodynamic support of pediatric and neonatal septic shock: 2007 update. Crit Care Med 2009;37:666–688.

Cinel I, Opal SM: Molecular biology of inflammation and sepsis: A primer. Crit Care Med 2009;37(1):291–304.

Dellinger RP et al: Surviving Sepsis Campaign: International guidelines for management of severe sepsis and septic shock: 2008. Crit Care Med 2008;36:296–327.

Menon K et al: A prospective multicenter study of adrenal function in critically ill children. Am J Resp Crit Care Med 2010;182(2):246–251 [PMID: 20299532].

Surviving Sepsis Campaign website (a good source for information on sepsis including protocols and order bundles for the care of patients with sepsis). Available at: http://www.survivingsepsis.org/Pages/default.aspx

TRAUMATIC BRAIN INJURY & INTRACRANIAL HYPERTENSION

ESSENTIALS OF DIAGNOSIS & TYPICAL FEATURES

- Hypotension, hypoxia, hypoglycemia, and hyperthermia are harmful to the injured brain and can exacerbate brain damage. Timely identification and correction of these factors is essential.
- Early signs and symptoms of intracranial hypertension tend to be nonspecific. The classic Cushing triad of bradycardia, hypertension, and apnea occurs late and is often incomplete.

Traumatic Brain Injury

Trauma is the leading killer of children in the United States. Fifty percent of trauma-related deaths are due to traumatic brain injury, and many survivors endure lifelong disabilities. Prevention is the only true "therapy" for traumatic brain injury, and injury prevention strategies have helped reduce the incidence of this problem.

Traumatic brain injuries can be conceptualized as occurring in two phases. ***Primary injury*** occurs at the moment injury disrupts bone, blood vessels, and brain tissue. ***Secondary injury*** is the indirect result of the primary injury and develops within minutes to days after the initiating injury.

Secondary injuries are potentially reversible and include: (1) processes triggered by the primary injury, such as excitotoxicity (neuronal damage due to excitatory neurotransmitter release), oxidative stress, inflammation, and delayed neuronal death; and (2) additional insults to the vulnerable injured brain, including hypoxia, hypotension, hyperthermia, and hypoglycemia. Management of the head-injured child is directed at preventing and/or modifying the events contributing to secondary injury.

Intracranial Hypertension

One of the key elements of managing children with traumatic brain injuries is the management of intracranial hypertension, in large part because intracranial hypertension can promote and worsen secondary brain injury. ***Intracranial pressure (ICP)*** is the pressure inside the skull, and is generally less than 15 mm Hg in healthy children. Prolonged periods of intracranial hypertension (defined as ICP greater than 20 mm Hg) are associated with increased morbidity and mortality. Table 14–13 lists common causes of intracranial hypertension in children. The skull, containing the brain, CSF, and cerebral blood, contains a fixed volume. Under normal circumstances, these three components are in balance, such that an increase in the volume of one component is offset by a decrease in one of the other components, maintaining a constant intracranial pressure (Monroe-Kellie doctrine). As a result of a traumatic brain injury, the volume of any or all of these components may increase, resulting in increased intracranial pressure (ICP). The factors contributing to intracranial hypertension can be understood by considering each of these three components.

Table 14–13. Pediatric illnesses commonly associated with intracranial hypertension.

Diffuse processes
Trauma
Hypoxic-ischemic
Near-drowning
Cardiorespiratory arrest
Infectious
Encephalitis
Meningitis
Metabolic
Reye syndrome
Liver failure
Inborn errors of metabolism
Toxic
Lead intoxication
Vitamin A overdose
Focal processes
Trauma
Hypoxic-ischemic
Trauma
Stroke
Infectious
Abscess
Mass lesions
Tumors
Hematomas

The brain occupies about 80% of the volume within the skull. Apart from solid tumors, increases in the brain compartment are generally a result of cerebral edema. Cerebral edema can be divided into several forms: vasogenic, hydrostatic, interstitial, and cytotoxic. ***Vasogenic edema*** is frequently associated with trauma, tumors, abscesses, and infarct, and is due to breakdown of the tight endothelial junctions that make up the blood-brain barrier (BBB). As plasma constituents cross the BBB, extracellular water moves along fiber tracts into the brain parenchyma. This form of edema is thought to be at least partially responsive to corticosteroid therapy. ***Hydrostatic edema*** is due to transudation of fluid from the capillaries into the parenchyma as a result of elevated cerebral vascular pressures. This form of edema is frequently associated with acute, malignant hypertension, and is treated by judicious reduction of cerebral vascular pressures. ***Interstitial edema*** occurs primarily in lesions resulting in obstructed CSF flow and appears in a typical periventricular distribution; it is best treated by CSF drainage. ***Cytotoxic edema*** is the most common form of edema seen in the PICU and is the least easily treated. Cytotoxic edema occurs as a result of direct injury to brain cells, often leading to irreversible cell swelling and death. This form of cerebral edema is typical of traumatic brain injuries as well as hypoxic-ischemic injuries and metabolic disease.

CSF occupies an estimated 10% of the intracranial space. Intracranial hypertension due primarily to obstructed CSF flow or increased CSF volume (eg, hydrocephalus, primary or secondary) is generally easily diagnosed by CT scan and treated with appropriate drainage and shunting. CSF drainage can be of benefit in managing intracranial hypertension, however, even in the absence of overt hydrocephalus.

Cerebral blood volume comprises the final 10% of the intracranial space. Changes in cerebral blood volume generally result from alterations in vascular diameter in response to local metabolic demands or to local vascular pressures, responses termed autoregulation. Several factors interact to control cerebral blood volume via the autoregulatory responses of the cerebral vasculature. ***Metabolic autoregulation*** matches cerebral blood flow to tissue demands. High metabolic rates, such as those induced by fever or seizure activity, increase cerebral blood flow by causing vasodilation, which in turn increases cerebral blood volume; lower metabolic rates allow the vessels to constrict, reducing cerebral blood volume. Partial pressure of carbon dioxide is another important determinant, as elevations in blood PCO_2 lead to cerebral vasodilation and decreases in PCO_2 lead to vasoconstriction. ***Pressure autoregulation*** links cerebral blood volume to cerebral blood flow. This response attempts to maintain a constant cerebral blood flow rate over a range of systemic blood pressures. Within the autoregulatory range of blood pressure, the cerebral vessels dilate or constrict as appropriate to maintain constant cerebral blood flow. Once the cerebral vessels are maximally constricted, continued increases in systemic pressure may further increase cerebral blood flow and volume; conversely, once the vessels are maximally dilated, flow will fall as perfusing pressure falls. It is not unusual to see partial or complete loss of cerebral blood flow autoregulation in the event of injury. Cerebral blood flow then becomes dependent on systemic blood pressure (traditionally termed "pressure passive" blood flow).

Clinical Findings

Initial examination of the patient with traumatic brain injury should include assessment of airway patency, breathing, and cardiovascular function. In addition, mental status should be evaluated, and the Glasgow Coma Scale (GCS) score calculated. Once stabilized from a cardiac and respiratory standpoint, a more detailed neurological examination including cranial nerves, spontaneous movement of extremities, strength, sensory perception, and presence or absence of deep tendon reflexes should be performed. Cervical spine injury and immobilization should also be considered. Similar considerations apply in patients with suspected intracranial hypertension but no clinical history of trauma. In either setting, repeated neurologic examinations are needed to monitor the progression of intracranial hypertension.

The clinical presentation of intracranial hypertension is dependent on the nature, location and size of the lesions in the brain, as well as the amount of edema and infringement of CSF pathways (Table 14–14). Early signs and symptoms are nonspecific, particularly in young children. Inborn errors of metabolism need to be considered in cases where the etiology of coma is not apparent by history, physical examination, and neuroimaging. Head CT or magnetic resonance imaging (MRI) is generally needed to identify intracranial injuries, to determine the need for surgical intervention, to monitor the progression of injuries and cerebral edema, and to monitor for the development of complications.

Table 14–14. Signs and symptoms of intracranial hypertension in children.

Early
Poor feeding, vomiting
Irritability, lethargy
Seizures
Hypertension
Late
Coma
Decerebrate responses
Cranial nerve palsies
Abnormal respirations
Bradycardia
Hypertension
Apnea

Treatment

Continuous monitoring and correction of hemodynamic and respiratory abnormalities are essential for maintaining proper nutrient and oxygen supply to the brain after injury. Hypoxic episodes (PaO_2 less than 60 mm Hg) after TBI are associated with increased morbidity and mortality, and current treatment guidelines recommend early endotracheal intubation and initiation of mechanical ventilation. Episodes of agitation and/or pain can induce elevated ICP, and thus adequate sedation, either via intermittent dosing or continuous infusion, is also important. Several modalities may be used to monitor ICP, including placement of an external ventricular drain (EVD) in the lateral ventricle, and/or an intraparenchymal pressure monitor. Current treatment guidelines for children with severe TBI recommend ICP monitoring for all patients with GCS $\leq$ 8. Little evidence exists to support the utility of ICP measurement and ICP-directed therapies in conditions associated with global CNS injuries (eg, anoxic brain injuries).

Mechanical Therapies

Midline positioning and head elevation to 30° can aid in cerebral venous drainage of blood from the head, thereby reducing cerebral blood volume and ICP. In addition, cervical spine precautions must be maintained until a spinal cord injury has been ruled out. Timely surgical evacuation of hematomas and other pathologic masses remains a mainstay of TBI treatment, and decompressive craniectomy (removal of a portion of the skull and opening of the dura) can be of benefit in the treatment of refractory intracranial hypertension secondary to focal or diffuse injury. CSF drainage reduces ICP by reducing CSF volume, and can be accomplished by placement of an EVD in the lateral ventricles of the brain.

Medical Therapies

Treatment strategies for TBI in children are based, in part, on reducing ICP to normal levels. Studies in adult patients have demonstrated that more frequent and higher elevations in ICP predict worse outcomes, particularly when ICP rises over 20 mm Hg. As a result, treatment should be directed at reducing ICP to less than 20 mm Hg and preventing frequent spikes to higher levels. Another important concept for the treatment of intracranial hypertension is that of ***cerebral perfusion pressure (CPP),*** which is the driving pressure across the cerebral circulation and is defined as mean arterial pressure minus central venous pressure (CVP) or ICP, whichever is higher. Maintenance of CPP remains a second tier goal in most published guidelines for management of TBI and the appropriate target value is not clear in children, though most practitioners use 50–60 mm Hg. A suggested treatment algorithm for patients with documented intracranial hypertension based on best available evidence is presented in Figure 14–1. The information is largely drawn

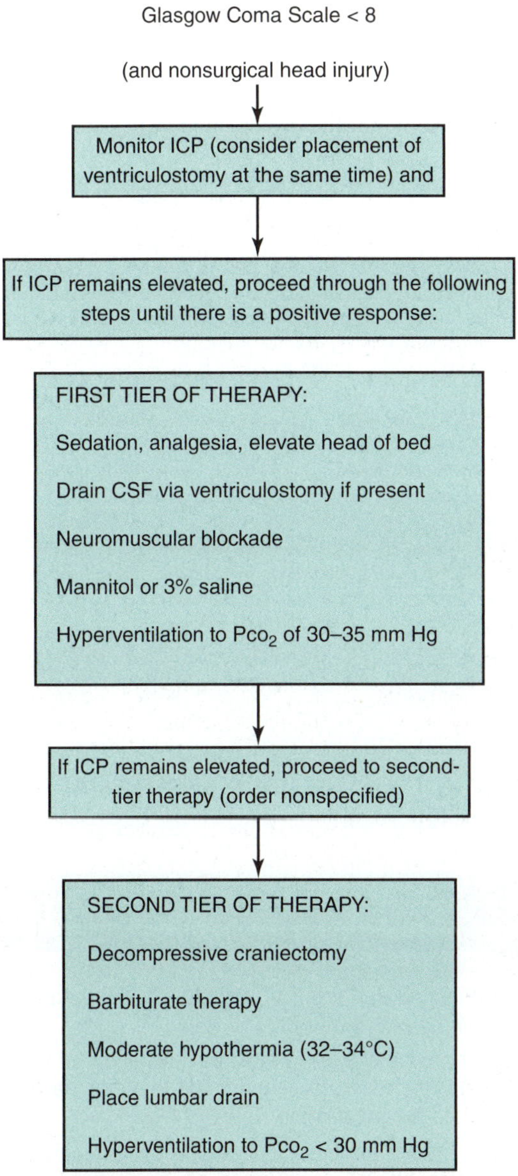

▲ **Figure 14–1.** Proposed treatment algorithm for intracranial hypertension in head injury. CSF, cerebrospinal fluid; ICP, intracranial pressure; Pco_2, partial pressure of arterial CO_2.

from experience with traumatic brain injuries, and the direct applicability of these concepts to other illnesses associated with intracranial hypertension remains unclear.

Osmotic therapies such as mannitol and hypertonic (3% or greater) saline can be effective treatments for elevated ICP regardless of etiology. These agents exert a rheologic effect, decreasing blood viscosity, which allows for increased blood flow and subsequent autoregulatory vasoconstriction. Cerebral vasoconstriction reduces cerebral blood volume, and therefore ICP. Osmotic agents also increase serum osmolarity and enhance movement of excess water out of brain cells and interstitium into blood vessels for removal by the kidney, an effect which enhances and prolongs the initial rheologic effects on ICP. Mannitol in doses of 0.25–1 g/kg can be used for intracranial hypertension unresponsive to sedation. Treatment with mannitol may result in a brisk diuresis, leading to hypovolemia and hypotension that exacerbate secondary injuries, and should be promptly treated with fluid resuscitation and/or vasopressors. Renal failure due to intravascular volume depletion and acute tubular necrosis is a rare side effect and is associated with serum osmolarity greater than 320 mOsm/L. Continuous infusion of 3% saline at 0.1–1 mL/kg/h can alternatively be used to increase osmolarity, using the minimum dose to achieve ICP of less than 20 mm Hg. Serum sodium and osmolarity should be followed to avoid a sodium level greater than 160 mEq/L or serum osmolarity greater than 320 mOsm/L.

Controlled ventilation is an important element of treating intracranial hypertension. Hyperventilation to PCO_2 levels less than 30 mm Hg—in the past a mainstay in the treatment of intracranial hypertension—is controversial and should only be used in emergent situations involving patients with acute ICP elevations unresponsive to other measures, such as sedation, paralysis, ventricular drainage, and osmotic diuretics. Although acutely effective in causing cerebral vasoconstriction, hyperventilation leads to much larger decreases in blood flow than in blood volume, such that hyperventilation necessary to control ICP may actually compromise CNS perfusion to uninjured brain and exacerbate secondary injury. This concept was confirmed by studies showing worse outcomes in head-injured patients consistently hyperventilated to a PCO_2 of 25 mm Hg or less. Mild hyperventilation, to maintain PCO_2 between 30–35 mm Hg, may be useful for managing intracranial hypertension in patients with severe brain injury. Due to the risks of worsening CNS ischemia, monitoring cerebral perfusion by blood flow studies or jugular bulb saturation is recommended for patients treated with extreme hyperventilation.

Current guidelines suggest the use of ***barbiturates*** for treating intracranial hypertension refractory to other measures. Barbiturates suppress cerebral metabolism and, through metabolic autoregulatory effects, reduce cerebral blood volume and ICP. Although effective in many instances for ICP elevations, these agents are potent cardiac depressants, and their use often leads to hypotension, necessitating the use of a pressor to maintain adequate cerebral and systemic perfusion pressures. In addition, plasma barbiturate levels correlate poorly with effect on ICP, and monitoring of CNS electrical activity by EEG is necessary to accurately titrate their use.

Temperature regulation and in particular maintenance of normothermia is essential. Hyperthermia increases cerebral metabolic demand and worsens outcome, and should be promptly recognized and treated with antipyretics and/or surface cooling devices. Induced hypothermia lowers cerebral metabolism, cerebral blood flow, and cerebral blood volume, but has not been shown to improve overall outcome.

Hemodynamic support is also crucial in managing patients with traumatic brain injuries. Fluid resuscitation with isotonic solutions is used to increase preload and cardiac performance. Vasopressors and inotropes increase contractility and afterload, thereby improving cardiac performance, mean arterial pressure, and CPP. Maintenance of adequate cardiac output and oxygen delivery to the CNS is critical in treating patients with intracranial hypertension. Studies in both adult and pediatric head injury patients show that even a single episode of hypotension is associated with a marked increase in mortality rates. Although age-appropriate thresholds for blood pressure in the context of severe TBI have not been delineated, a rational starting point for therapy would be maintenance of an adequate circulating blood volume, and a blood pressure at least well within the normal range for age.

Corticosteroids may be of use in reducing vasogenic cerebral edema surrounding tumors and other inflammatory CNS lesions but in general they have no role in the treatment of traumatic brain injuries or diffuse cerebral edema due to traumatic, ischemic, or metabolic injuries.

Complications

Complications are frequent in patients with traumatic brain injuries and should be anticipated. Seizures occur in approximately 30% of patients with severe head injury. Single early seizures do not require long-term treatment. Continuous electroencephalography (EEG) should be considered to determine if clinically unrecognized seizures or nonconvulsive status is present in patients with persistent altered mental status or in those requiring heavy sedation. Cerebral herniation presenting with Cushing triad of bradycardia, hypertension, and altered respirations is a medical emergency requiring intubation, infusion of mannitol, and brief period of hyperventilation while more definitive therapies are implemented. Cerebral infarctions may occur as a result of ischemia, thrombosis, and progressive edema compromising blood supply.

Prognosis

Many factors will affect prognosis of traumatic brain injury patients, especially the inciting event/severity of injury. Global hypoxic-ischemic events and inflicted brain injury have a worse outcome than uncomplicated, accidental traumatic brain injuries. Lack of improvement in neurological examination at 24–72 hours is associated with poor outcome. Follow-up studies have also demonstrated that "recovery" occurs over time, months to even years.

Quality Improvement

Early recognition of factors contributing to the development of secondary injury (including hypotension, hyperthermia, hypoglycemia, and hypoxia) and their timely treatment after brain injury are important considerations for improving outcome. Development of monitoring and treatment algorithms for brain-injured patients may reduce morbidity and mortality, although there is a paucity of data regarding effective monitoring and treatment in these patients.

Hutchison JS et al: Hypothermia therapy after traumatic brain injury in children. N Engl J Med 2008;358:2447–2456 [PMID: 18525042].

Jagannathan J et al: Long-term outcomes and prognostic factors in pediatric patients with severe traumatic injury and elevated intracranial pressure. J Neurosurg Pediatrics 2008;2:240–259 [PMID: 18831656].

Kochanek PM, Tasker RC: Pediatric Neurointensive Care: 2008 update for the *Rogers' Textbook of Pediatric Intensive Care.* Ped Crit Care Med 2009;10:517–523 [PMID: 19584637].

Mehta A et al: Relationship of intracranial pressure and cerebral perfusion pressure with outcome in young children after severe traumatic brain injury. Dev Neurosci 2010;32:413–419 [PMID: 20805152].

Vespa PM et al: Non-convulsive electrographic seizures after traumatic brain injury result in a delayed, prolonged increase in intracranial pressure and metabolic crisis. Crit Care Med 2007;35:2830–2836 [PMID: 18074483].

Zebrack M et al: Early resuscitation of children with moderate-to-severe traumatic brain injury. Pediatrics 2009;124:56–64 [PMID: 19703674].

SEDATION, ANALGESIA, & ANESTHESIA IN THE ICU

ESSENTIALS OF DIAGNOSIS & TYPICAL FEATURES

- Pain control and relief of anxiety are standard of care for all patients in the PICU.
- Sedation and analgesia must be individualized for each patient and reassessed frequently to avoid inadequate or excessive medication.
- Every medication has a unique set of physiologic effects and side effects, and should never be used without adequate monitoring and support to address potential adverse events.

Anxiety control and pain relief are important responsibilities of the critical care physician. It is well recognized that infants and children experience pain and that outcomes are improved in children receiving appropriate pain control. A child's anxiety in the PICU may heighten perception of pain to a level that causes deterioration of his or her condition. It is important to distinguish between anxiety and pain, because pharmacologic therapy may be directed at one or both of these symptoms (Table 14–15). Additionally, before

Table 14–15. Pain and anxiety control.

Drug	Dose and Method of Administration[a]	Advantages	Disadvantages	Usual Duration of Effect
Morphine	IV, 0.1 mg/kg; continuous infusion, 0.01–0.05 mg/kg/h	Excellent pain relief, reversible	Respiratory depression, hypotension, nausea, suppression of intestinal motility, histamine release	2–4 h
Meperidine	IV, 1 mg/kg	Good pain relief, reversible	Respiratory depression, histamine release, nausea, suppression of intestinal motility	2–4 h
Fentanyl	IV, 1–2 mcg/kg; continuous infusion, 0.5–2 mcg/kg/h	Excellent pain relief, reversible, short half-life	Respiratory depression, chest wall rigidity, severe nausea and vomiting	30 min
Diazepam	IV, 0.1 mg/kg	Sedation and seizure control	Respiratory depression, jaundice, phlebitis	1–3 h
Lorazepam	IV, 0.1 mg/kg	Longer half-life, sedation and seizure control	Nausea and vomiting, respiratory depression, phlebitis	2–4 h
Midazolam	IV, 0.1 mg/kg	Short half-life, only benzodiazepine given as continuous infusion	Respiratory depression	20–40 min

[a]Intravenous (IV) administration is most common in the ICU. The effects of morphine, meperidine, and fentanyl are reversible by administration of naloxone (opioid antagonist).

initiating or increasing sedative drugs, it is important to exclude or address physiologic causes of agitation, such as hypoxemia, hypercapnia, and cerebral hypoperfusion caused by low cardiac output.

Sedation

Sedative (anxiolytic) drugs are used to induce calmness without producing sleep—although at high doses, all anxiolytics will cause drowsiness and sleep. The five indications for the use of sedative drugs are to: (1) allay fear and anxiety, (2) manage acute confusional states, (3) facilitate treatment or diagnostic procedures, (4) facilitate mechanical ventilation, and (5) diminish physiologic responses to stress, such as tachycardia, hypertension, or increased ICP. Parenteral administration (bolus or infusion) allows titration of response. Sedatives fall into several classes, with the opioid and benzodiazepine classes serving as the mainstay of anxiety treatment in the PICU.

A. Benzodiazepines

Benzodiazepines possess anxiolytic, hypnotic, anticonvulsant, and skeletal muscle relaxant properties. Although their exact mode of action is unknown, it appears to be within the limbic system and to involve the neuroinhibitory transmitter γ-aminobutyric acid. Most benzodiazepines are metabolized in the liver, with their metabolites subsequently excreted in the urine; thus, patients in liver failure are likely to have long elimination times. Benzodiazepines can cause respiratory depression if given rapidly in high doses, and they potentiate the analgesic and respiratory depressive effects of opioids and barbiturates. Therefore, it is important to monitor cardiorespiratory status and have resuscitation equipment available. Three benzodiazepines with differing half-lives are presently used in the PICU.

Midazolam has the shortest half-life (1.5–3.5 hours) and is the only benzodiazepine that should be administered as a continuous IV infusion. It produces excellent retrograde amnesia lasting for 20–40 minutes after a single IV dose. Therefore, it can be used either for short-term sedation or for "awake" procedures, such as endoscopy, or as a continuous infusion in the anxious, restless patient. The single IV dose is 0.05–0.1 mg/kg, whereas a continuous infusion should be started at a rate of 0.1 mg/kg/h after an initial loading dose of 0.1 mg/kg. The midazolam infusion dosage must be titrated upward to achieve the desired effect. Midazolam is not an analgesic; therefore, small doses of an analgesic, such as morphine or fentanyl, may be needed.

Diazepam has a longer half-life than midazolam and can be given orally (PO) as well as by the IV route. Its disadvantage in the PICU is that its intermediary metabolite, nordazepam, has a very long half-life and may accumulate, prolonging sedation. It produces excellent anxiolysis and amnesia, and is also used to treat acute status epilepticus. The IV dose is 0.1 mg/kg, which can be repeated every 15 minutes to achieve the desired effect or until undesirable side effects (somnolence and respiratory depression) occur.

Lorazepam possesses the longest half-life of the three benzodiazepines discussed here and can be used to achieve sedation for as long as 6–8 hours. It has less effect on the cardiovascular and respiratory systems than other benzodiazepines and can be given PO, IV, or intramuscularly (IM). The IV route is most commonly used (0.1 mg/kg). Lorazepam can also be used to treat acute status epilepticus. Infusions of lorazepam should be avoided because its preservative, polyethylene glycol, can accumulate in patients with renal insufficiency and produce a metabolic acidosis.

B. Other sedatives

Chloral hydrate is an orally administered sedative and hypnotic agent frequently used in children. After administration, it is rapidly metabolized by the liver to its active form, trichloroethanol, which has an 8-hour half-life. A sedative dose is 6–20 mg/kg, usually given every 6–8 hours, whereas the hypnotic dose is up to 50 mg/kg up to a maximum of 1 g. The hypnotic dose is frequently used to sedate young children for prolonged outpatient radiologic procedures. Therapeutic doses of chloral hydrate have little effect on respiration or blood pressure. The drug is irritating to mucous membranes, however, and may cause gastric upset if administered on an empty stomach.

Ketamine is a phencyclidine derivative that produces a trance-like state of immobility and amnesia known as dissociative anesthesia. After IM or IV administration, it causes central sympathetic nervous system stimulation with resultant increases in heart rate, blood pressure, and cardiac output. Respiration is not depressed at therapeutic doses. Because salivary and tracheobronchial mucous gland secretions are increased, atropine may be administered 20 minutes prior to administering ketamine. A disadvantage of ketamine is the occurrence of unpleasant dreams or hallucinations, which occur less often in children, and can be reduced by the concurrent administration of a benzodiazepine. Ketamine is a negative inotrope but this effect is usually outweighed by its effect of increasing endogenous catecholamine release. As a result, it can be useful for the sedation of hemodynamically unstable patients. Additionally, its bronchodilator effects make it the induction agent of choice for patients with status asthmaticus requiring intubation. It is given as an IV injection of 1–2 mg/kg over 60 seconds, with supplementary doses of 0.5 mg/kg being required every 10–30 minutes to maintain an adequate level of sedation. Alternatively, it can be administered as an IM injection of 3–7 mg/kg, which usually produces the desired level of sedation within 3–4 minutes. If prolonged sedation is required, ketamine can be administered by IV infusion at doses of 3–20 mg/kg/h.

The ***antihistamines***, diphenhydramine and hydroxyzine, can be used as sedatives, but are not as effective as the benzodiazepines. Diphenhydramine produces sedation in only 50% of patients. It can be given IV, IM, or PO at a dose of 1 mg/kg. Hydroxyzine can be given either IM or PO. It is frequently used concurrently with morphine or meperidine, adding anxiolysis and potentiating their effects. The sedative effects of both drugs can last from 4 to 6 hours following a single dose.

Propofol is an anesthetic induction agent which can be used for procedural sedation in children. Its main advantages are a rapid recovery time and no cumulative effects resulting from its rapid hepatic metabolism. It has no analgesic properties and frequently causes pain on injection. Dose-related hypotension and metabolic acidosis have been reported in pediatric patients; the FDA recommends against the use of propofol in pediatric patients outside the controlled environment of the operating room.

Barbiturates (phenobarbital and thiopental) can cause direct myocardial and respiratory depression and are, in general, poor choices for sedation of seriously ill patients. Phenobarbital has a very long half-life (up to 4 days), and recovery from thiopental, although it is a short-acting barbiturate, can be prolonged because remobilization from tissue stores occurs.

Dexmedetomidine is an α_2-adrenoreceptor agonist with sedative, analgesic, and anxiolytic effects. It produces rapid sedation while maintaining a high degree of patient rousability. Dexmedetomidine has few side effects, but it can produce a dose-dependent bradycardia which can limit its use. Pediatric studies are ongoing to determine its role in the PICU. It may be useful as an adjunct therapy to limit benzodiazapine and opioid use and minimize withdrawal symptoms from these agents.

Analgesia

Opioid analgesics (morphine, fentanyl, codeine, and meperidine) are the mainstays of therapy for most forms of acute severe pain and for chronic cancer pain management. They possess both analgesic and dose-related sedative effects, although a range of plasma concentrations produce analgesia without sedation. In addition, opioids can cause respiratory depression, nausea, pruritus, slowed intestinal motility, meiosis, urinary retention, cough suppression, biliary spasm, and vasodilation. The dose of opioid required to produce adequate analgesia varies greatly between patients. Therefore, in the intensive care setting, a continuous infusion of morphine or fentanyl allows dosages to be easily titrated to achieve the desired effect.

In general, infants younger than age 3 months are more susceptible than older children to the respiratory depressant effects of opioids. Starting dosages for these patients should be about one-third to one-half the usual pediatric dose. Most opioids (except meperidine) have minimal cardiac depressive effects, and critically ill patients generally tolerate them well. Fentanyl does not cause the histamine release that morphine does, and thus produces less vasodilation and a less pronounced drop in systemic blood pressure. Opioids are metabolized in the liver, with metabolites excreted in the urine. Thus, patients with hepatic or renal impairment may have a prolonged response to their administration.

Long-term (> 7 days) administration and high doses (> 1.5–2.5 mg/kg cumulative fentanyl dose) of continuous infusions of opioids or benzodiazepines can lead to tolerance and physical dependence with the development of withdrawal symptoms (agitation, tachypnea, tachycardia, sweating, and diarrhea) upon acute termination of these drugs. In these patients, gradual tapering of the opioid dosage over a 5- to 10-day period may prevent withdrawal symptoms. The mechanism of opioid tolerance is related to conformational changes in the drug-receptor interaction, and the use of continuous infusions and synthetic opioids (in particular fentanyl) is associated with the faster development of tolerance.

Nonopioid analgesics used in the treatment of mild to moderate pain include acetaminophen, aspirin, and other nonsteroidal anti-inflammatory drugs (NSAIDs). ***Acetaminophen*** is the most commonly used analgesic in pediatrics in the United States and is the drug of choice for mild to moderate pain because of its low toxicity and lack of effect on bleeding time. It is metabolized by the liver. Suggested doses are 10–15 mg/kg PO or approximately 10–20 mg/kg per rectum every 4 hours. ***Aspirin*** is also an effective analgesic for mild to moderate pain at doses of 10–15 mg/kg PO every 4 hours. However, its prolongation of bleeding time, association with Reye syndrome, and propensity to cause gastric irritation limit its usefulness in pediatric practice. Aspirin and other NSAIDs are still useful, especially for pain of inflammatory origin, bone pain, and pain associated with rheumatic conditions. ***Ibuprofen*** and ***naproxen*** use remain limited in the pediatric intensive care setting given their deleterious effects on platelet function and propensity to cause gastritis. Naproxen is FDA-approved for children aged 2–12 years (5–7 mg/kg PO every 8–12 hours). Ibuprofen requires more frequent dosing intervals (4–10 mg/kg PO every 6–8 hours). All of the NSAIDs have a therapeutic ceiling after which no increase occurs in analgesic potency. They all can cause gastritis and should be given with antacids or with meals. These medications should be used with caution in people at risk for renal compromise or bleeding. The analgesic effects of acetaminophen, aspirin, and other NSAIDs are additive to those of opioids. Thus, if additional analgesia is required, their use should be continued and an appropriate oral opioid (codeine or morphine) or parenteral opioid (morphine or fentanyl) begun.

Additional Considerations

With any potent sedative or analgesic used in the PICU setting, appropriate patient monitoring (pulse oximetry, cardiorespiratory monitoring, and blood pressure monitoring) should be used during the period of administration, and equipment should be available to support prompt intervention if undesired side effects occur. In addition, the PICU regimen for sedation and analgesia must be carefully modified when the patient is transferred to the ward or a lower vigilance area. Patients with baseline respiratory, hepatic, or renal insufficiency are most predisposed to respiratory insufficiency from sedatives or opioid analgesics.

PICU patients will often respond best to continuous infusions of analgesics and sedatives. Advantages of continuous infusions of sedatives include a more constant level of sedation and increased patient comfort. Recently, however, there has been an increasing appreciation for the disadvantages of sedative agents, including both short- and long-term cognitive deficits and an increased risk for delirium. Daily interruption of all continuous sedation with titrated reintroduction as necessary has been shown in adult ICU patients to dramatically reduce the duration of mechanical ventilation and length of stay in the ICU. Currently, similar data are not available for pediatric patients but the untoward effects of ICU sedation in critically ill children remain a concern.

Patient-controlled analgesia is done via a computer-governed infusion pump for constant infusion or patient-regulated bolus infusion of opioid analgesics. The basal infusion mode is intended to provide a constant serum level of analgesic. The bolus mode allows the patient, by pushing a button, to self-administer additional doses for breakthrough pain. The patient is usually permitted six boluses an hour, with 10-minute lockouts. If the patient is using allotted hourly boluses, this usually means that the basal infusion rate is too low. The patient must understand the concept of patient-controlled analgesia in order to be a candidate for its use. In some circumstances in pediatrics, it is more appropriate for the nurse or parent to administer the bolus dose.

Naloxone reverses the analgesic, sedative, and respiratory depressive effects of opioid agonists. Its administration should be titrated to achieve the desired effect (eg, reversal of respiratory depression) because full reversal using 1–10 mcg/kg may cause acute anxiety, dysphoria, nausea, and vomiting. Furthermore, because the duration of effect of naloxone is shorter (30 minutes) than that of most opioids, the patient must be observed carefully for reappearance of the undesired effect.

Procedural sedation

Frequently pediatric patients will require relatively deep levels of sedation while undergoing a procedure (eg, vascular line placement or radiographic studies). Often these patients are not intubated and are not expected to require intubation and ventilator support. This technique is termed "moderate sedation/analgesia" and a systematic approach to it should include the following:

1. Pertinent history to elicit underlying illnesses
2. Physical examination focusing on the anatomy and adequacy of the child's airway (ie, large tonsils or facial deformity)
3. Informed consent
4. Appropriate patient fasting time from solids (6 hours) and liquids (2 hours)

5. Age- and size-appropriate equipment
6. Drug dosages calculated on a milligram-per-kilogram basis
7. Monitoring and documentation of vital signs (including continuous pulse oximetry, respiratory rate and pattern, and level of arousability)
8. Separate observers from the person performing the procedure to monitor deeply sedated patients
9. Presence of a practitioner capable of intubating and treating patients who enter a deeper state of sedation than initially anticipated

Short-acting agents are preferred for procedural sedation. Agents typically used include an opioid (usually fentanyl or morphine) and a benzodiazepine (most often midazolam). Another option is ketamine together with midazolam. It is important to select and become comfortable with a specific combination, and to learn its indications and potential complications. Using familiar agents and following the systematic approach outlined earlier have reduced anesthetic complications in these patients.

American Academy of Pediatrics; American Academy of Pediatric Dentistry, Cote CJ, Wilson S; Work Group on Sedation: Guidelines for monitoring and management of pediatric patients during and after sedation for diagnostic and therapeutic procedures. Pediatr 2006;118:2587 [PMID: 17142550].

Su F, Hammer GB: Dexmedetomidine: Pediatric pharmacology, clinical uses and safety. Expert Opin Drug Saf 2011 Jan;10(1):55–66 [Epub 2010 Aug 18] [PMID: 20718689].

Anand KJ et al: Tolerance and withdrawal from prolonged opioid use in critically ill children. Eunice Kennedy Shriver National Institute of Child Health and Human Development Collaborative Pediatric Critical Care Research Network. Pediatrics 2010 May;125(5):e1208–e1225 [PMID: 20403936].

Hartman ME, McCrory DC, Schulman SR: Efficacy of sedation regimens to facilitate mechanical ventilation in the pediatric intensive care unit: A systematic review. Pediatr Crit Care Med 2009 Mar;10(2):246–255 [Review] [PMID: 19188867].

Doyle L, Colletti JE: Pediatric procedural sedation and analgesia. Pediatr Clin North Am 2006;53:279 [PMID: 16574526].

NUTRITIONAL SUPPORT OF THE CRITICALLY ILL CHILD

ESSENTIALS OF DIAGNOSIS & TYPICAL FEATURES

- Critically ill children are more susceptible to metabolic stress than adults due to lower muscle and fat mass and higher resting energy requirements.
- Children with preexisting malnutrition are more likely to develop multiorgan system failure.
- Obese children are more likely to develop complications including sepsis, wound infection, and increased length of stay in the PICU.
- Changes in nutritional status can persist for 6 months after discharge in infants following prolonged PICU stay.
- Early enteral and parenteral feeding can improve nutrition deficits and may influence morbidity and mortality in critically ill infants and children.
- Acute protein energy malnutrition is associated with physiological instability and increased morbidity/mortality in the PICU.

When severely ill pediatric patients are admitted to the PICU, initial therapy is directed at the primary or underlying problem and at providing cardiorespiratory and hemodynamic support. Provision of adequate nutritional support is often overlooked early in the course of therapy. Malnutrition is, however, a major problem in hospitalized patients, leading to higher rates of infectious and noninfectious complications as well as longer hospital stays and increased hospital costs. In the pediatric ICU, it is estimated that as many as 20% of patients experience either acute or chronic malnutrition, a rate that is largely unchanged over the past 30 years. The etiology of malnutrition in PICU patients is typically multifactorial, related to increased demands due to the physiologic and metabolic stresses associated with critical illness (Table 14–16), to inaccurate assessments of caloric needs, and to inadequate delivery of nutrition at the bedside.

Nutritional Assessment

Pediatric Registered Dietitians (RDs) are integral members of the PICU team. Early assessment by a pediatric RD can be helpful to establish nutritional requirements and goals and to identify factors impeding adequate nutrition intake and tolerance. The caloric needs of the critically ill child can be estimated beginning with calculations of the basal metabolic rate (BMR) or the resting energy expenditure (REE). BMR represents the energy requirements of a healthy, fasting person who recently awoke from sleep, with normal temperature, and no stress, while REE represents the energy requirements of a healthy person at rest, with normal temperature and not fasting (Table 14–17). These closely related parameters are for practical purposes used interchangeably, though the REE tends to be approximately 10% above the BMR. The estimated basal metabolic need (BMR or REE) can then be multiplied by a stress factor related to the severity of the patient's illness to more accurately estimate overall energy requirements. Unfortunately, because these calculations are based on studies of healthy adults and children, they can be very inaccurate for use in critically ill children and lead to underfeeding or overfeeding. Indirect calorimetry (IC) is a more accurate means of directly measuring

Table 14–16. Physiologic and metabolic responses to severe illness.

Physiologic		
	Cardiovascular	
		Increased cardiac output
		Peripheral vasodilatation and capillary leak
		Expansion of vascular compartment
	Pulmonary	
		Increased minute ventilation
		Ventilation-perfusion mismatch
		Inefficient gas exchange
		Increased CO_2 responsiveness
	Skeletal muscle	
		Easier fatigability
		Slower relaxation
		Altered force-frequency pattern
	Renal	
		Salt and water retention
		Impaired concentrating ability
Metabolic		
	Hormone and biological response modifier levels	
		Increased insulin
		Increased glucocorticoids
		Increased catecholamines
		Increased interleukin-1
		Increased tumor necrosis factor
	Carbohydrate metabolism	
		Increased blood glucose
		Increased gluconeogenesis
		Increased glucose turnover
		Glucose intolerance
	Fat metabolism	
		Increased lipid turnover and utilization
		Insuppressible lipolysis
		Decreased ketogenesis
	Protein metabolism	
		Increased muscle protein catabolism
		Increased muscle branched-chain amino acid oxidation
		Increased serum amino acids
		Increased nitrogen losses

energy expenditure and determining caloric needs, though it is more difficult and expensive to perform and as a result is not always readily available. Identification of patients at highest risk for malnutrition (Table 14–17) for targeted use of IC assessment has been suggested as one strategy for optimizing the cost-benefit ratio of IC. This technique also requires collection of exhaled gases from the patient and can be inaccurate if a significant endotracheal tube leak is present, if the FIO_2 is > 60%, and during hemodialysis or continuous renal replacement. Either method or a combination of methods can be used to determine nutritional requirements based on patient's age and condition. Nutrition therapy is then gradually advanced to target, while the response is monitored and adjustments made as needed.

Table 14–17. Markers of high risk of malnutrition suggested as indications for targeted indirect calorimetry assessment of REE.

- Underweight (< fifth percentile for age) or overweight (> eighty-fifth percentile for age)
- > 10% weight gain or loss during ICU stay
- Failure to consistently meet prescribed caloric goals
- Failure to wean from respiratory support
- Need for muscle relaxants for > 7 days
- Neurologic injury with evidence of dysautonomia
- Oncologic diagnoses
- Burns
- Requiring mechanical ventilation for > 7 days
- Suspected hypermetabolic state (eg, status epilepticus, SIRS) or hypometabolic state (eg, hypothermia, induced coma)
- ICU length of stay > 4 weeks

Delivery of Nutrition

In adult ICU patients, ***enteral nutrition*** is associated with fewer infectious complications than parenteral nutrition. No such trials in pediatric patients exist, but it is generally accepted that enteral nutrition is preferred in critically ill children as well. Enteral nutrition is generally well tolerated, even in patients on vasoactive medications. Diarrhea, constipation, and abdominal distention are common in critically ill children, but may also reflect feeding intolerance. Use of an enteral feeding protocol and early transpyloric feeding may improve tolerance. The goal for protein intake should be 2–3 g/kg/d, but this may be difficult to achieve with pediatric formulas due to potential volume overload and adult formulas may be useful. Complications of enteral feeding include GI intolerance (vomiting, bleeding, diarrhea, and necrotizing enterocolitis), aspiration events/pneumonia, and mechanical issues (occlusion of tube, errors in tube placement). Meningitis, bacteremia, and death have been reported in neonates fed contaminated reconstituted powdered infant formulas.

Parenteral nutrition should be considered in critically ill children when enteral nutrition cannot be delivered or tolerated within 3–5 days. Although it is common practice to gradually increase the amino acid dose, evidence from preterm neonates shows that it is safe and efficacious to start parenteral amino acids at the target dose. Lipids should be included to decrease carbon dioxide production, minute ventilation, and fat storage, enhance lipid oxidation, augment protein retention, and prevent essential fatty acid deficiency. Hyperglycemia, hypertriglyceridemia, infection, and hepatobiliary abnormalities are all potential complications of parenteral nutrition. Metabolic evaluation (electrolytes, glucose, lipase, and liver function tests) should be followed regularly and the components of parenteral nutrition adjusted as needed.

Regardless of route of nutrition, ***monitoring*** should include routine physical examination, serial measures of growth (weight, skinfold thickness), serial monitoring of serum electrolyte and mineral concentrations, and repeated measurements of REE when available. Measurements of serum albumin provide limited information about nutritional status given the multiple other influences on albumin concentrations. Prealbumin and CRP measurements may be helpful, however. Prealbumin levels are a good marker of nutritional protein status; they drop during acute illness and return to normal during recovery. CRP levels are a marker of the acute phase response to illness and injury; they rise during acute illness and drop with recovery, typically in association with a return to anabolic metabolism and before increases in prealbumin.

Supplementation in Critical Illness

Pharmaconutrition is an area of ongoing research interest, though little prospective data is available to guide the use of supplements in critically ill children. ***Glutamine*** levels decrease during critical illness. Glutamine supplementation may improve GI, metabolic, antioxidant, and immune functions in a stressed state. Critically ill adults have improved outcomes with glutamine supplementation, but studies in critically ill infants and children have been conflicting. Glutamine supplementation in children with burns, trauma, and critical illness should be considered, since it may produce the same benefits as in adults. ***Arginine*** is important for immune function, protein synthesis, and tissue repair. Arginine supplementation may improve nitrogen intake and immune function in children with traumatic injuries, including burns.

Hulst JM et al: Causes and consequences of inadequate substrate supply to pediatric ICU patients. Curr Opin Clin Nutr Metab Care 2006;9:297 [PMID: 16607132].

Skillman HE, Wischmeyer PE: Nutrition therapy in critically ill infants and children. J Parent Enteral Nutr 2008;32:520–534 [PMID: 18753390].

Mehta NM, Duggan CP: Nutritional deficiencies during critical illness. Pediatr Clin North Am 2009 Oct; 56(5):1143–1160 [PMID: 19931068].

Mehta NM et al: A.S.P.E.N. clinical guidelines: Nutrition support of the critically ill child. J Parent Enteral Nutr 2009;33(3):260–276.

END-OF-LIFE CARE AND DEATH IN THE PICU

ESSENTIALS OF DIAGNOSIS & TYPICAL FEATURES

- End-of-life discussions in the PICU should include the patient, if possible, and family members as well as the medical team.
- PICU providers may assist in defining the limits of care provided, facilitating withdrawal of life support, and providing compassionate palliative care.
- The palliative care and ethics teams, if available, may facilitate end-of-life discussions in the PICU.
- Withdrawal of life-sustaining therapies should include a plan to treat any pain and discomfort in the patient.
- Brain death determination requires a systematic and age-appropriate evaluation consistent with institutional policies.
- Tissue and organ donation must be considered with every death.
- Grief/bereavement support for the family as well as medical team members should be provided following every death in the PICU.

Death in the PICU

In-hospital pediatric deaths occur infrequently. A large proportion of pediatric deaths occur in the PICU, however, and the PICU provider may be called upon to help define the limits to care provided, assist in the withdrawal of life-sustaining medical therapies (LSMT), and provide compassionate palliative care. End-of-life discussions may have occurred prior to PICU admission for some children with congenital or chronic diseases. For other children, their PICU stay may be the first time a child or family discusses end-of-life decisions. Regardless of the individual patient's situation, the medical team has a responsibility to facilitate discussions regarding the goals of care in an honest and sensitive manner.

Deaths without any limitations on patient care comprise a small minority (10%–12%) of pediatric ICU deaths. In these circumstances, most recent studies have found greater family satisfaction with the care provided if family members are allowed to witness ongoing resuscitative efforts. The remainder of pediatric deaths is divided between brain death declarations (23%) and decisions to limit or withdraw medical care (65%).

Brain Death

Severe neurologic injury can result in the irreversible loss of all brain functioning, or brain death. The concept of brain death arose when advances in ICU technologies allowed heart and lung function to be supported even in the absence of any brain activity. Brain death is diagnosed by a clinical exam (see Table 14–18) and is based on published guidelines. The general approach in the diagnosis of brain death is similar in most medical centers, but there can be subtle institutional variations. Therefore, it is imperative for PICU providers performing the brain death exam to be familiar with their own institutional policies on brain death declaration. A patient declared brain dead is legally dead and further

Table 14–18. Brain death examination.

- Normal blood pressure and temperature and no sedation medications or muscle relaxants.
- Flaccid coma with no evidence of cortical function.
- Absence of brain stem reflexes:
  - Apnea ("apnea test": no respirations seen with $PCO_2 > 60$ mm Hg and a change in $PCO_2 > 20$ mm Hg).
  - Fixed dilated pupils with no response to light.
  - Absence of corneal reflexes.
  - Absence of eye movements including spontaneous, oculocephalic (doll's eye), or oculovestibular (cold caloric). Do not perform oculocephalic maneuver if there is potential for cervical spine injury.
  - Absence of gag and cough reflex.
- Examination consistent throughout observation period as documented by two separate clinical exams by qualified physicians
- Recommended observation periods for the following ages:
  - Seven days to 2 mo old—Two examinations over 48 h with an ancillary study.[a]
  - Two months to 1 y—Two examinations over 24 h and consider ancillary study.[a]
  - Over 1 y—Two examinations over 12-24 h.
  - Teenage to adult—Two examinations over 6-12 h.

[a] Cerebral angiography, radionuclide scanning, electroencephalography, or transcranial Doppler ultrasonography.

medical support is no longer indicated, though the timing of discontinuation of medical support should be discussed and agreed upon with the patient's family.

Brain death is determined through a complete clinical assessment of the patient. First and foremost, the provider must be confident that the patient's condition is irreversible and must exclude any potentially reversible conditions that may produce signs similar to brain death. These may include hypotension, hypothermia, or the presence of excessive doses of sedating medications. The brain death exam is a formal clinical exam directed at demonstrating the absence of cortical function (flaccid coma without evidence of response to stimuli) and brainstem function (cranial nerve testing). In order to meet the definition of brain death, guidelines require that qualified physicians document two separate clinical exams consistent with brain death (ie, no evidence of brain function) separated by a period of observation. If a patient cannot tolerate some portion of the clinical exam (typically apnea testing) or is very young (especially < 1 year of age), an ancillary test such as electroencephalography or cerebral perfusion scan may provide supporting evidence of brain death. Once a child has been declared brain dead, their time of death is noted as occurring at the completion of the second exam even if they are still receiving cardiopulmonary support.

Limitation or Withdrawal of Medical Care

Most patients who die in the pediatric ICU will do so following a decision to limit or withdraw medical support rather than via a brain death declaration. The discussions leading to these decisions should include the patient (to the extent possible given their medical condition and developmental age), family members and members of the medical team. The primary goals of these discussions should be (1) to communicate information regarding the patient's medical status and anticipated prognosis, and (2) to clarify the goals of ongoing medical care both in regard to the patient's current status and in the event of an acute decompensation. If the opinion of the medical team is that the patient's condition is likely irreversible, the options for care include:

1. Continuing current support with escalation as deemed medically reasonable by the health care team
2. Continuing current support but not adding any new therapies
3. Withdrawal of life sustaining therapies such as mechanical ventilation and hemodynamic support

The first two options may include a decision to withhold cardiopulmonary resuscitation in the event of a respiratory or cardiac arrest (Do Not Attempt Resuscitation or DNAR). The third option presumes a DNAR but this must be explicitly written in the medical record and communicated to team members.

Discussions with patients and families regarding the decision to limit resuscitation or to withdraw LSMT should respect the following basic principles:

- Discussions should be conducted by experienced personnel with the ability to communicate in a clear and compassionate manner and should occur at an appropriate time and place.
- Cultural needs should be considered prior to major discussions and may include the need for a translator or spiritual guidance.
- Deliberations should begin with a clear statement that the goal is to make decisions in the best interest of the patient, and that the health care team can support the patient and family in making reasonable decisions based on that goal.
- Potential options regarding limitations of care or withdrawal of care should be clearly elucidated for the decision-makers.
- Withdrawal of LSMT can be considered when the pain and suffering inflicted by prolonging and supporting life outweighs the potential benefit for the individual. If there is no reasonable chance of recovery, the patient has the right to a natural death in a dignified and pain-free manner.
- The health care team should emphasize that decisions are not irrevocable; if at any time the family or health care providers wish to reconsider the decision, full medical therapy can be reinstituted until the situation is clarified.

Prior to the withdrawal of LSMT, the patient's family and care team should be prepared for the physiologic process of dying that the child will undergo. Key facets of the process to discuss include the possibility of agonal respirations, which can be disturbing to witness for family members and care providers, as well as the unpredictable length of time that the process may require. Additionally, the fact that patient will ultimately have a cardiopulmonary arrest and a member of the medical team will declare the time of death should be discussed. The family should also be reassured that the patient will be given appropriate doses of medications to treat signs and symptoms of pain or discomfort and that neither they nor the patient will be abandoned by the medical team during this process.

Palliative Care & Bioethics Consultation

Palliative care teams and ethics consultation services are essential resources to help the health care team and families address difficult end-of-life decision-making. For families of children with congenital or chronic diseases, the palliative care team may have established relationships with the patient and family during prior medical episodes. For patients with new conditions or whose prognosis has changed, the palliative care team may be newly introduced in the PICU. In either case, the palliative care team can bring invaluable support and resources for families during end-of-life discussions. If conflict arises surrounding decisions about limiting medical care, an ethics consultation in the ICU setting can aid the process by helping to identify, analyze, and resolve ethical problems. Ethics consultation can independently clarify views and allow the health care team, patient, and family to make decisions that respect patient autonomy and promote maximum benefit and minimal harm to the patient.

A more comprehensive discussion of palliative care can be found elsewhere in this book. Briefly, palliative care medicine has developed as a specialized field of practice to address the needs of dying children or children with a shortened lifespan. Many centers have developed palliative care teams that include medical personnel, social workers, and spiritual leaders to help families navigate the difficult process of dying and end-of-life decision-making, including withdrawal of support. Once the decision is made to limit or withdraw LSMT, a palliative care plan should be agreed on by all decision-makers, clarified to other health care providers and instituted with the primary goal of optimizing the patient's and family's experience prior to and following death. The plan, at minimum, should address the following issues:

1. Adequate pain control and sedation
2. Provision of warmth and cleanliness
3. Ongoing patient and family support and dignity

Tissue & Organ Donation

Organ transplantation is standard therapy for many pediatric conditions and many children die while awaiting a transplant due to short supply of organs. The gift of organ donation can be one positive outcome for a family from an otherwise tragic loss of their child's life. In fact, the 1986 U.S. Federal Required Request Law mandates that all donor-eligible families be approached about potential organ donation. The decision to donate must be made free of coercion, with informed consent, and without financial incentive. The state organ-procurement agencies provide support and education to care providers and families to make informed decisions.

To be a solid organ donor, the patient must be declared dead and have no conditions contraindicating donation. The most frequent type of solid organ donor in the PICU is a brain dead donor. However, the need for new donor organs has led to the emergence of protocols for procuring solid organs from non–heart beating donors. Although this practice has been described by many terms including Donation after Cardiac Death, the most recent nomenclature is Donation after Circulatory Determination of Death (DCDD). In these cases, the patient does not meet brain death criteria but has an irreversible disease process, and the family or patient has decided to withdraw life-sustaining therapy and consented to attempted organ donation. In the DCDD process, LSMT is withdrawn and comfort measures are provided as per usual care. The withdrawal of care may take place in the PICU or the operating room without any surgical staff present, depending upon institutional policy. Once the declaring physician has determined cessation of cardiac function, the patient is observed for an additional short time period for auto-resuscitation (the re-initiation of cardiac activity without medical intervention). After this waiting period, the patient is declared dead and the organs are harvested for donation. If the patient does not die within a predetermined time limit after discontinuation of LSMT, comfort measures continue but solid organ donation is abandoned due to unacceptably long ischemic times.

Tissue (heart valves, corneas, skin, and bone) can be donated following a "traditional" cardiac death (no pulse or respirations), brain death or DCDD.

Bereavement and Grief Support

After any pediatric death, bereavement and grief support for families and health care providers are essential components of comprehensive end-of-life care. Families may need information about care of the body after the death, funeral arrangements, and autopsy decisions as well as about educational, spiritual, and other supportive resources available. Members of the medical team may feel their own grief and sense of loss with the death of a patient. These emotions, if not appropriately addressed, can negatively affect their personal and professional lives. Therefore, similar supportive services should be available to health care workers caring for dying children.

Lee KJ et al: Alterations in end-of-life support in the pediatric intensive care unit. Pediatrics 2010;126(4):e859–e864.

Kolovos NS et al: Donation after cardiac death in pediatric critical care. Pediatr Crit Care Med 2007;8(1):47–49 [PMID: 17251881].

Meert KL et al: Exploring parents' environmental needs at the time of a child's death in the pediatric intensive care unit. Pediatr Crit Care Med 2008;9(6):623–628 [PMID: 18838930].

Shemie SD et al: Diagnosis of brain death in children. Lancet Neurol 2007;6:87 [PMID: 17166805].

Truog RD et al: Recommendations for end-of-life care in the intensive care unit: A consensus statement by the American College [corrected] of Critical Care Medicine. Crit Care Med 2008;36(3):953–963 [PMID: 18431285].

Truog RD et al: Toward interventions to improve end of life care in the pediatric intensive care unit. Crit Care Med 2006;34(11Suppl):S373–S379 [PMID: 17057601].

QUALITY IMPROVEMENT INITIATIVES IN THE PICU

Both adult and pediatric intensive care units have been areas of intense interest in quality improvement initiatives in recent years given the frequency and high cost of ICU-related complications. National collaboratives have identified six areas of focus for pediatric ICU quality and safety improvement efforts: risk adjustment (severity-adjusted mortality rates and length of stay measures), central venous catheter infection, mechanical ventilation, unplanned readmissions to the PICU, pain assessment, and medication safety. The two most widely applied quality initiatives in pediatric intensive care have been efforts to reduce central venous catheter-related infections and to reduce the incidence of ventilator-associated pneumonia. Efforts to reduce catheter-related infections have largely focused on implementation of procedure checklists to ensure adherence to strict sterile procedure during catheter insertion including hand hygiene, barrier precautions and site preparation, as well as sterile practice when accessing the catheter during care. Efforts to reduce ventilator-associated pneumonias include defined order sets ("order bundles") for mechanically ventilated patients specifying patient positioning, oral care, feeding, and endotracheal tube suctioning practices in an effort to reduce contamination of the airway and ETT with bacterial pathogens from either the patient's GI tract or from caregivers. Most of the data supporting these interventions have been derived from adult ICU populations and to date few large scale studies have been published documenting the efficacy of these measures in the pediatric ICU population. Those data that are available suggest that these initiatives are beneficial, though additional studies will likely be needed to refine and optimize these approaches in the pediatric ICU setting.

15 Skin

Joseph G. Morelli, MD
Lori D. Prok, MD

GENERAL PRINCIPLES

DIAGNOSIS OF SKIN DISORDERS

Examination of the skin requires that the entire surface of the body be palpated and inspected in good light. The onset and duration of each symptom should be recorded, together with a description of the primary lesion and any secondary changes, using the terminology in Table 15–1. In practice, characteristics of skin lesions are described in an order opposite to that shown in the table. Begin with distribution, then configuration, color, secondary changes, and primary changes. For example, guttate psoriasis could be described as generalized, discrete, red, or scaly papules.

TREATMENT OF SKIN DISORDERS

Topical Therapy

Treatment should be simple and aimed at preserving normal skin physiology. Topical therapy is often preferred because medication can be delivered in optimal concentrations to the desired site.

Water is an important therapeutic agent, and optimally hydrated skin is soft and smooth. This occurs at approximately 60% environmental humidity. Because water evaporates readily from the cutaneous surface, skin hydration (stratum corneum of the epidermis) is dependent on the water concentration in the air, and sweating contributes little. However, if sweat is prevented from evaporating (eg, in the axilla, groin), local humidity and hydration of the skin are increased. As humidity falls below 15%–20%, the stratum corneum shrinks and cracks; the epidermal barrier is lost and allows irritants to enter the skin and induce an inflammatory response. Decrease of transepidermal water loss will correct this condition. Therefore, dry and scaly skin is treated by using barriers to prevent evaporation (Table 15–2). Oils and ointments prevent evaporation for 8–12 hours, so they must be applied once or twice a day. In areas already occluded (axilla, diaper area), creams or lotions are preferred, but more frequent application may be necessary.

Overhydration (maceration) can also occur. As environmental humidity increases to 90%–100%, the number of water molecules absorbed by the stratum corneum increases and the tight lipid junctions between the cells of the stratum corneum are gradually replaced by weak hydrogen bonds; the cells eventually become widely separated, and the epidermal barrier falls apart. This occurs in immersion foot, diaper areas, axillae, and the like. It is desirable to enhance evaporation of water in these areas by air drying.

Wet Dressings

By placing the skin in an environment where the humidity is 100% and allowing the moisture to evaporate to 60%, pruritus is relieved. Evaporation of water stimulates cold-dependent nerve fibers in the skin, and this may prevent the transmission of the itching sensation via pain fibers to the central nervous system. It also is vasoconstrictive, thereby helping to reduce the erythema and also decreasing the inflammatory cellular response.

The simplest form of wet dressing consists of one set of wet underwear (eg, long johns) worn under dry pajamas. Cotton socks are also useful for hand or foot treatment. The underwear should be soaked in warm (not hot) water and wrung out until no more water can be expressed. Dressings can be worn overnight for a few days up to 1 week. When the condition improves, wet dressings are discontinued.

Topical Glucocorticoids

Twice-daily application of topical corticosteroids is the mainstay of treatment for all forms of dermatitis (Table 15–3). Topical steroids can also be used under wet dressings. After wet dressings are discontinued, topical steroids should be applied only to areas of active disease. They should never be applied to normal skin to prevent recurrence. Only low-potency steroids (see Table 15–3) are applied to the face or intertriginous areas.

Table 15–1. Examination of the skin.

Clinical Appearance	Description and Examples
Primary lesions (first to appear)	
Macule	Any circumscribed color change in the skin that is flat. Examples: white (vitiligo), brown (café au lait spot), purple (petechia).
Papule	A solid, elevated area < 1 cm in diameter whose top may be pointed, rounded, or flat. Examples: acne, warts, small lesions of psoriasis.
Plaque	A solid, circumscribed area > 1 cm in diameter, usually flat-topped. Example: psoriasis.
Vesicle	A circumscribed, elevated lesion < 1 cm in diameter and containing clear serous fluid. Example: blisters of herpes simplex.
Bulla	A circumscribed, elevated lesion > 1 cm in diameter and containing clear serous fluid. Example: bullous impetigo.
Pustule	A vesicle containing a purulent exudate. Examples: acne, folliculitis.
Nodule	A deep-seated mass with indistinct borders that elevates the overlying epidermis. Examples: tumors, granuloma annulare. If it moves with the skin on palpation, it is intradermal; if the skin moves over the nodule, it is subcutaneous.
Wheal	A circumscribed, flat-topped, firm elevation of skin resulting from tense edema of the papillary dermis. Example: urticaria.
Secondary changes	
Scales	Dry, thin plates of keratinized epidermal cells (stratum corneum). Examples: psoriasis, ichthyosis.
Lichenification	Induration of skin with exaggerated skin lines and a shiny surface resulting from chronic rubbing of the skin. Example: atopic dermatitis.
Erosion and oozing	A moist, circumscribed, slightly depressed area representing a blister base with the roof of the blister removed. Examples: burns, impetigo. Most oral blisters present as erosions.
Crusts	Dried exudate of plasma on the surface of the skin following disruption of the stratum corneum. Examples: impetigo, contact dermatitis.
Fissures	A linear split in the skin extending through the epidermis into the dermis. Example: angular cheilitis.
Scars	A flat, raised, or depressed area of fibrotic replacement of dermis or subcutaneous tissue. Examples: acne scar, burn scar.
Atrophy	Depression of the skin surface caused by thinning of one or more layers of skin. Example: lichen sclerosis.
Color	
	The lesion should be described as white, red, yellow, brown, tan, or blue. Particular attention should be given to the blanching of red lesions. Failure to blanch suggests bleeding into the dermis (petechiae).
Configuration of lesions	
Annular (circular)	Annular nodules represent granuloma annulare; annular scaly papules are more apt to be caused by dermatophyte infections.
Linear (straight lines)	Linear papules represent lichen striatus; linear vesicles, incontinentia pigmenti; linear papules with burrows, scabies.
Grouped	Grouped vesicles occur in herpes simplex or zoster.
Discrete	Discrete lesions are independent of each other.
Distribution	
	Note whether the eruption is generalized, acral (hands, feet, buttocks, face), or localized to a specific skin region.

Bewley A; Dermatology Working Group: Expert consensus: Time for a change in the way we advise our patient to use topical corticosteroids. Br J Dermatol 2008;158:917 [PMID: 18294314].

Chiang C, Eichenfield LC: Quantitative assessment of combination bathing and moisturizing regimens on skin hydration in atopic dermatitis. Pediatr Dermatol 2009;26:273 [PMID: 19706087].

Devillers AC, Oranje AP: Efficacy and safety of "wet wrap" dressings as an intervention treatment in children with severe and/or refractory atopic dermatitis: A critical review of the literature. Br J Dermatol 2006;154:579 [PMID: 16536797].

Table 15–2. Bases used for topical preparations.

Base	Combined with	Uses
Foam		Cosmetically elegant; increasing number of products available
Liquids		Wet dressings: relieve pruritus, vasoconstrict
	Powder	Shake lotions, drying pastes: relieve pruritus, vasoconstrict
	Grease and emulsifier; oil in water	Cream: penetrates quickly (10–15 min) and thus allows evaporation
	Excess grease and emulsifier; water in oil	Emollient cream: penetrates more slowly and thus retains moisture on skin
Grease		Ointments: occlusive (hold material on skin for prolonged time) and prevent evaporation of water
Gel		Transparent, colorless, semisolid emulsion: nongreasy, more drying and irritating than cream
Powder		Enhances evaporation

Characteristics of bases for topical preparations:

1. Thermolabile, low-residue foam vehicle is more cosmetically acceptable and uses novel permeability pathway for delivery.
2. Most greases are triglycerides (eg, Aquaphor, petrolatum, Eucerin).
3. Oils are fluid fats (eg, Alpha Keri, olive oil, mineral oil).
4. True fats (eg, lard, animal fats) contain free fatty acids that cause irritation.
5. Ointments (eg, Aquaphor, petrolatum) should not be used in intertriginous areas such as the axillae, between the toes, and in the perineum, because they increase maceration. Lotions or creams are preferred in these areas.
6. Oils and ointments hold medication on the skin for long periods and are therefore ideal for barriers or prophylaxis and for dried areas of skin. Medication gets into the skin more slowly from ointments.
7. Creams carry medication into skin and are preferable for intertriginous dermatitis.
8. Foams, solutions, gels, or lotions should be used for scalp treatments.

Table 15–3. Topical glucocorticoids.

Glucocorticoid	Concentrations
Low potency[a] = 1–9	
Hydrocortisone	0.5%, 1%, 2.5%
Desonide	0.05%
Moderate potency = 10–99	
Mometasone furoate	0.1%
Hydrocortisone valerate	0.2%
Fluocinolone acetonide	0.025%
Triamcinolone acetonide	0.01%
Amcinonide	0.1%
High potency = 100–499	
Desoximetasone	0.25%
Fluocinonide	0.05%
Halcinonide	0.1%
Super potency = 500–7500	
Betamethasone dipropionate	0.05%
Clobetasol propionate	0.05%

[a]1% hydrocortisone is defined as having a potency of 1.

DISORDERS OF THE SKIN IN NEWBORNS

TRANSIENT DISEASES IN NEWBORNS

1. Milia

Milia are tiny epidermal cysts filled with keratinous material. These 1- to 2-mm white papules occur predominantly on the face in 40% of newborns. Their intraoral counterparts are called Epstein pearls and occur in up to 60%–85% of neonates. These cystic structures spontaneously rupture and exfoliate their contents.

2. Sebaceous Gland Hyperplasia

Prominent white to yellow papules at the opening of pilosebaceous follicles without surrounding erythema—especially over the nose—represent overgrowth of sebaceous glands in response to maternal androgens. They occur in more than half of newborns and spontaneously regress in the first few months of life.

3. Neonatal Acne

Inflammatory papules and pustules with occasional comedones predominantly on the face occur in as many as 20% of newborns. Although neonatal acne can be present at birth, it most often occurs between 2 and 4 weeks of age. Spontaneous resolution occurs over a period of 6 months to 1 year. A rare entity that is often confused with neonatal acne is **neonatal cephalic pustulosis**. This is a more monomorphic eruption with red papules and pustules on the head and neck that appears in the first month of life. There is associated neutrophilic inflammation and yeasts of the genus *Malassezia*. This eruption will resolve spontaneously, but responds to topical antiyeast preparations.

4. Harlequin Color Change

A cutaneous vascular phenomenon unique to neonates in the first week of life occurs when the infant (particularly one of low birth weight) is placed on one side. The dependent half develops an erythematous flush with a sharp demarcation at the midline, and the upper half of the body becomes pale. The color change usually subsides within a few seconds after the infant is placed supine but may persist for as long as 20 minutes.

5. Mottling

A lacelike pattern of bluish, reticular discoloration representing dilated cutaneous vessels appears over the extremities and often the trunk of neonates exposed to lowered room temperature. This feature is transient and usually disappears completely on rewarming.

6. Erythema Toxicum

Up to 50% of full-term infants develop erythema toxicum. At 24–48 hours of age, blotchy erythematous macules 2–3 cm in diameter appear, most prominently on the chest but also on the back, face, and extremities. These are occasionally present at birth. Onset after 4–5 days of life is rare. The lesions vary in number from a few up to as many as 100. Incidence is much higher in full-term versus premature infants. The macular erythema may fade within 24–48 hours or may progress to formation of urticarial wheals in the center of the macules or, in 10% of cases, pustules. Examination of a Wright-stained smear of the lesion reveals numerous eosinophils. No organisms are seen on Gram stain. These findings may be accompanied by peripheral blood eosinophilia of up to 20%. The lesions fade and disappear within 5–7 days. Transient neonatal pustular melanosis is a pustular eruption in newborns of African-American descent. The pustules rupture leaving a collarette of scale surrounding a macular hyperpigmentation. Unlike erythema toxicum, the pustules contain mostly neutrophils and often involve the palms and soles.

7. Sucking Blisters

Bullae, either intact or as erosions (representing the blister base) without inflammatory borders, may occur over the forearms, wrists, thumbs, or upper lip. These presumably result from vigorous sucking in utero. They resolve without complications.

8. Miliaria

Obstruction of the eccrine sweat ducts occurs often in neonates and produces one of two clinical scenarios. Superficial obstruction in the stratum corneum causes miliaria crystallina, characterized by tiny (1- to 2-mm), superficial grouped vesicles without erythema over intertriginous areas and adjacent skin (eg, neck, upper chest). More commonly, obstruction of the eccrine duct deeper in the epidermis results in erythematous grouped papules in the same areas and is called miliaria rubra. Rarely, these may progress to pustules. Heat and high humidity predispose the patient to eccrine duct pore closure. Removal to a cooler environment is the treatment of choice.

9. Subcutaneous Fat Necrosis

This entity presents in the first 7 days of life as reddish or purple, sharply circumscribed, firm nodules occurring over the cheeks, buttocks, arms, and thighs. Cold injury is thought to play an important role. These lesions resolve spontaneously over a period of weeks, although in some instances they may calcify. Affected infants should be screened for hypocalcemia.

O'Connor NR et al: Newborn skin: Part I. Common rashes. Am Fam Physician 2008 Jan 1;77(1):47–52 [PMID: 18236822].

PIGMENT CELL BIRTHMARKS, NEVI, & MELANOMA

Birthmarks may involve an overgrowth of one or more of any of the normal components of skin (eg, pigment cells, blood vessels, lymph vessels). A nevus is a hamartoma of highly differentiated cells that retain their normal function.

1. Mongolian Spot

A blue-black macule found over the lumbosacral area in 90% of infants of Native-American, African-American, and Asian descent is called a mongolian spot. These spots are occasionally noted over the shoulders and back and may extend over the buttocks. Histologically, they consist of spindle-shaped pigment cells located deep in the dermis. The lesions fade somewhat with time as a result of darkening of the overlying skin, but some traces may persist into adult life.

2. Café au Lait Macule

A café au lait macule is a light brown, oval macule (dark brown on brown or black skin) that may be found anywhere on the body. Café au lait spots over 1.5 cm in greatest diameter are found in 10% of white and 22% of black children. These lesions persist throughout life and may increase in number with age. The presence of six or more such lesions over 1.5 cm in greatest diameter is a major diagnostic criterion for neurofibromatosis type 1 (NF-1). Patients with McCune-Albright syndrome (see Chapter 34) have a large, unilateral café au lait macule.

3. Spitz Nevus

A spitz nevus presents as a reddish-brown smooth solitary papule appearing on the face or extremities. Histologically, it consists of epithelioid and spindle shaped nevomelanocytes that may demonstrate nuclear pleomorphism. Although these lesions can look concerning histologically, they follow a benign clinical course in most cases.

ACQUIRED MELANOCYTIC NEVI

1. Common Moles

Well-demarcated, brown to brown-black macules represent junctional nevi. They can appear in the first years of life and increase with age. Histologically, single and nested melanocytes are present at the junction of the epidermis and dermis. Approximately 20% may progress to compound nevi—papular lesions with melanocytes both in junctional and intradermal locations. Intradermal nevi are often lighter in color and can be fleshy and pedunculated. Melanocytes in these lesions are located purely within the dermis. Nevi look dark blue (blue nevi) when they contain more deeply situated spindle-shaped melanocytes in the dermis.

2. Melanoma

Melanoma in prepubertal children is very rare. Pigmented lesions with variegated colors (red, white, blue), notched borders, asymmetrical shape, and very irregular or ulcerated surfaces should prompt suspicion of melanoma. Ulceration and bleeding are advanced signs of melanoma. If melanoma is suspected, wide local excision and pathologic examination should be performed.

3. Congenital Melanocytic Nevi

One in 100 infants is born with a congenital nevus. Congenital nevi tend to be larger and darker brown than acquired nevi and may have many terminal hairs. If the pigmented plaque covers more than 5% of the body surface area, it is considered a giant or large congenital nevus; these large nevi occur in 1 in 20,000 infants. Other classification systems characterize lesions over 20 centimeters as large. Often the lesions are so large they cover the entire trunk (bathing trunk nevi). Histologically, they are compound nevi with melanocytes often tracking around hair follicles and other adnexal structures deep in the dermis. The risk of malignant melanoma in small congenital nevi is controversial in the literature, but most likely very low, and similar to that of acquired nevi. Transformation to malignant melanoma in giant congenital nevi has been estimated between 1% and 5%. Of note, these melanomas often develop early in life (before puberty) and in a dermal location. Two-thirds of melanomas in children with giant congenital nevi develop in areas other than the skin.

Krengel S et al: Melanoma risk in congenital melanocytic naevi: A systematic review. Br J Dermatol 2006;155:1 [PMID: 16792745].

LaVigne EA et al: Clinical and dermascopic changes in common melanocytic nevi in school children: The Framingham school nevus study. Dermatology 2005;211:234 [PMID: 16205068].

Tannous ZS et al: Congenital melanocytic nevi: Clinical and histopathologic features, risk of melanoma, and clinical management. J Am Acad Dermatol 2005 Feb;52(2):197–203.

VASCULAR BIRTHMARKS

1. Capillary Malformations

Clinical Findings

Capillary malformations are an excess of capillaries in localized areas of skin. The degree of excess is variable. The color of these lesions ranges from light red-pink to dark red. Light red macules are found over the nape of the neck, upper eyelids, and glabella of newborns. Fifty percent of infants have such lesions over their necks. Eyelid and glabellar lesions usually fade completely within the first year of life. Lesions that occupy the total central forehead area usually do not fade. Those on the neck persist into adult life.

Port-wine stains are dark red macules appearing anywhere on the body. A bilateral facial port-wine stain or one covering the entire half of the face may be a clue to Sturge-Weber syndrome, which is characterized by seizures, mental retardation, glaucoma, and hemiplegia. (See Chapter 25.) Most infants with smaller, unilateral facial port-wine stains do not have Sturge-Weber syndrome. Similarly, a port-wine stain over an extremity may be associated with hypertrophy of the soft tissue and bone of that extremity (Klippel-Trénaunay syndrome).

Treatment

The pulsed dye laser is the treatment of choice for infants and children with port-wine stains.

Cordisco MR: An update on lasers in children. Curr Opin Pediatr 2009 Aug;21(4):499–504.

2. Hemangioma

Clinical Findings

A red, rubbery vascular plaque or nodule with a characteristic growth pattern is a hemangioma. The lesion is often not present at birth but is represented by a permanent blanched area on the skin that is supplanted at age 2–4 weeks by red papules. Hemangiomas then undergo a rapid growth or "proliferative" phase, where growth of the lesion is out of proportion to growth of the child. At 9–12 months, growth stabilizes, and the lesion slowly involutes over the next several years. Histologically, hemangiomas are benign tumors of capillary endothelial cells. They may be superficial, deep, or mixed. The terms *strawberry* and *cavernous* are misleading and should not be used. The biologic behavior of a hemangioma is the same despite its location. Fifty percent reach maximal regression by age 5 years, 70% by age 7 years, and 90% by age 9 years, leaving redundant skin, hypopigmentation, and telangiectasia. Local complications include superficial ulceration and secondary pyoderma. Rare complications include obstruction of vital structures such as the orbit or airway.

▶ Treatment

Complications that require immediate treatment are (1) visual obstruction (with resulting amblyopia), (2) airway obstruction (hemangiomas of the head and neck ["beard hemangiomas"] may be associated with subglottic hemangiomas), and (3) cardiac decompensation (high-output failure). Historically, the preferred treatment for complicated hemangiomas has been prednisolone, 2–3 mg/kg orally daily for 6–12 weeks. More recently, oral propranolol (2 mg/kg/day divided BID) has replaced systemic steroids as the treatment of choice at most institutions. Reported side effects are sleep disturbance, hypoglycemia, and bradycardia. Recommendations on pretreatment cardiac evaluation vary between institutions. Interferon α_{2a} has also been used to treat serious hemangiomas. However, 10% of patients with hemangiomas treated with interferon α_{2a} have developed spastic diplegia, and its use is very limited. If the lesion is ulcerated or bleeding, pulsed dye laser treatment is indicated to initiate ulcer healing and immediately control pain. The Kasabach-Merritt syndrome, characterized by platelet trapping with consumption coagulopathy, does not occur with solitary cutaneous hemangiomas. It is seen only with internal hemangiomas or the rare vascular tumors such as kaposiform hemangioendotheliomas and tufted angiomas.

Bagazgoitia et al: Propranolol for infantile hemangiomas. Pediatr Dermatol 2011 Mar-Apr;28(2):108–114.

MacFie et al: Diagnosis of vascular skin lesions in children: An audit and review. Pediatr Dermatol 2008 Jan-Feb;25(1):7–12 [Review].

3. Lymphatic Malformations

Lymphatic malformations may be superficial or deep. Superficial lymphatic malformations present as fluid-filled vesicles often described as resembling "frog spawn." Deep lymphatic malformations are rubbery, skin-colored nodules occurring most commonly in the parotid area (cystic hygromas) or on the tongue. They often result in grotesque enlargement of soft tissues. Histologically, they can be either macrocystic or microcystic.

▶ Treatment

Therapy includes sclerotherapy with injection of bleomycin, picibanil, or doxycycline, radiotherapy, or surgical excision.

Niti K et al: Microcystic lymphatic malformation (lymphangioma circumscriptum) treated using a minimally invasive technique of radiofrequency ablation and sclerotherapy. Dermatol Surg 2010 Nov;36(11):1711–1717.

EPIDERMAL BIRTHMARKS

1. Epidermal Nevus

▶ Clinical Findings

The majority of these birthmarks present in the first year of life; however, they can first be noted in adulthood. They are hamartomas of the epidermis that are warty to papillomatous plaques, often in a linear array. They range in color from skin-colored to dirty yellow to brown. Histologically they show a thickened epidermis with hyperkeratosis. The condition of widespread epidermal nevi associated with other developmental anomalies (central nervous system, eye, and skeletal) is called the epidermal nevus syndrome.

▶ Treatment

Treatment once or twice daily with topical calcipotriene may flatten some lesions. The only definitive cure is surgical excision.

Vujevich J, Mancini A: The epidermal nevus syndromes: Multisystem disorders. J Am Acad Dermatol 2004;50:957 [PMID: 15153903].

2. Nevus Sebaceus

▶ Clinical Findings

This is a hamartoma of sebaceous glands and underlying apocrine glands that is diagnosed by the appearance at birth of a yellowish, hairless plaque in the scalp or on the face. The lesions can be contiguous with an epidermal nevus on the face, and widespread lesions can constitute part of the epidermal nevus syndrome.

Histologically, nevus sebaceus represents an overabundance of sebaceous glands without hair follicles. At puberty, with androgenic stimulation, the sebaceous cells in the nevus divide, expand their cellular volume, and synthesize sebum, resulting in a warty mass.

▶ Treatment

Because it has been estimated that approximately 15% of these lesions will develop secondary epithelial tumors, including basal cell carcinomas (BCC), trichoblastomas, and other benign tumors, surgical excision at puberty is recommended. The majority of the tumors develop in adulthood, although BCCs have been reported in childhood and adolescence.

Rosen H et al: Management of nevus sebaceous and the risk of basal cell carcinoma: An 18-year review. Pediatr Dermatol 2009;26:676 [PMID: 19686305].

CONNECTIVE TISSUE BIRTHMARKS (JUVENILE ELASTOMA, COLLAGENOMA)

Clinical Findings

Connective tissue nevi are smooth, skin-colored papules 1–10 mm in diameter that are grouped on the trunk. A solitary, larger (5–10 cm) nodule is called a shagreen patch and is histologically indistinguishable from other connective tissue nevi that show thickened, abundant collagen bundles with or without associated increases of elastic tissue. Although the shagreen patch is a cutaneous clue to tuberous sclerosis (see Chapter 25), the other connective tissue nevi occur as isolated events.

Treatment

These nevi remain throughout life and need no treatment.

HEREDITARY SKIN DISORDERS

1. Ichthyosis

Ichthyosis is a term applied to several diseases characterized by the presence of excessive scales on the skin. These disorders represent a large and heterogeneous group of genetic and acquired defects of cornification of the skin. Classification of these diseases is clinically based, although the underlying genetic causes and pathophysiologic mechanisms responsible continue to be elucidated.

Disorders of keratinization are characterized as syndromic when the phenotype is expressed in the skin and other organs, or nonsyndromic when only the skin is affected. Ichthyoses may be inherited or acquired. Inherited disorders are identified by their underlying gene defect if known. Acquired ichthyosis may be associated with malignancy and medications, or a variety of autoimmune, inflammatory, nutritional, metabolic, infectious, and neurologic diseases. These disorders are diagnosed by clinical examination, with supportive findings on skin biopsy (including electron microscopy) and mutation analysis if available.

Treatment

Treatment consists of controlling scaling with lactic acid as ammonium hydroxide (Lac-Hydrin or AmLactin) 12% or urea cream 10%–40% applied once daily. Daily lubrication and a good dry skin care regimen are essential.

Oji V et al: Revised nomenclature and classification of inherited ichthyoses: Results of the First Ichthyosis Consensus Conference in Sorèze 2009. J Am Acad Dermatol 2010 Oct;63(4):607–641.

2. Epidermolysis Bullosa

This is a group of heritable disorders characterized by skin fragility with blistering. Four major subtypes are recognized, based on the ultrastructural level of skin cleavage (Table 15–4).

For the severely affected, much of the surface area of the skin may have blisters and erosions, requiring daily wound care and dressings. These children are prone to frequent skin infections, anemia, growth problems, mouth erosions and esophageal strictures, and chronic pain issues. They are also at increased risk of squamous cell carcinoma, a common cause of death in affected patients.

Table 15–4. Major epidermolysis bullosa subtypes.

Cleavage Level	Common Name	Targeted Protein(s)	Inheritance Pattern	Characteristic Clinical Features
Suprabasilar	Epidermolysis Bullosa Superficialis	Unknown	Autosomal dominant	Superficial erosions at birth; rare to no blistering
Suprabasilar	Plakophilin-deficient EB, Lethal acantholytic EB	Plakophilin, Desmoplakin	Autosomal recessive	Similar to above
Basilar	Epidermolysis bullosa simplex	Keratin 5 and 14	Autosomal dominant	Palm and sole blistering presents in early childhood with trauma
Basilar	EB simplex with muscular dystrophy	Plectin	Autosomal recessive	Blisters, muscular dystrophy
Basilar	EB with pyloric atresia	α-6 β-4 integrin	Autosomal recessive	Blisters, pyloric atresia
Junctional (within the basement membrane zone)	Junctional EB – Herlitz or non-Herlitz	Laminin 5, α-6 β-4 integrin, type XVII collagen	Autosomal recessive	Severe generalized blistering, oral involvement
Sub-basilar	Dystrophic EB or "dermolytic" EB	Type VII collagen	Autosomal dominant or recessive	Severe blisters and scarring

Treatment

Treatment consists of protection of the skin with topical emollients as well as nonstick dressings. The other medical needs and potential complications of the severe forms of epidermolysis bullosa require a multidisciplinary approach. For the less severe types, protecting areas of greatest trauma with padding and dressings as well as intermittent topical or oral antibiotics for superinfection are appropriate treatments. If hands and feet are involved, reducing skin friction with 5% glutaraldehyde every 3 days is helpful.

Fine JD et al: The classification of inherited epidermolysis bullosa (EB): Report of the Third International Consensus Meeting on Diagnosis and Classification of EB. J Am Acad Dermatol 2008 Jun;58(6):931–950 [Epub 2008 Apr 18].

COMMON SKIN DISEASES IN INFANTS, CHILDREN, & ADOLESCENTS

ACNE

Acne affects 85% of adolescents. The onset of adolescent acne is between ages 8 and 10 years in 40% of children. The early lesions are usually limited to the face and are primarily closed comedones (whiteheads; see following discussion).

Pathogenesis

The primary event in acne formation is obstruction of the sebaceous follicle and subsequent formation of the microcomedo (not evident clinically). This is the precursor to all future acne lesions. This phenomenon is androgen-dependent in adolescent acne. The four primary factors in the pathogenesis of acne are (1) plugging of the sebaceus follicle; (2) increased sebum production; (3) proliferation of *Propionibacterium acnes* in the obstructed follicle, and (4) inflammation. Many of these factors are influenced by androgens.

Drug-induced acne should be suspected in teenagers if all lesions are in the same stage at the same time and if involvement extends to the lower abdomen, lower back, arms, and legs. Drugs responsible for acne include corticotropin (ACTH), glucocorticoids, androgens, hydantoins, and isoniazid, each of which increases plasma testosterone.

Clinical Findings

Open comedones are the predominant clinical lesion in early adolescent acne. The black color is caused by oxidized melanin within the stratum corneum cellular plug. Open comedones do not progress to inflammatory lesions. Closed comedones, or whiteheads, are caused by obstruction just beneath the follicular opening in the neck of the sebaceous follicle, which produces a cystic swelling of the follicular duct directly beneath the epidermis. Most authorities believe that closed comedones are precursors of inflammatory acne lesions (red papules, pustules, nodules, and cysts). In typical adolescent acne, several different types of lesions are present simultaneously. Severe, chronic, inflammatory lesions may rarely occur as interconnecting, draining sinus tracts. Adolescents with cystic acne require prompt medical attention, because ruptured cysts and sinus tracts result in severe scar formation.

Differential Diagnosis

Consider rosacea, nevus comedonicus, flat warts, miliaria, molluscum contagiosum, and the angiofibromas of tuberous sclerosis.

Treatment

Different treatment options are listed in Table 15–5. Recent data have indicated that combination therapy that targets multiple pathogenic factors increases the efficacy of treatment and rate of improvement.

A. Topical Keratolytic Agents

Topical keratolytic agents address the plugging of the follicular opening with keratinocytes and include retinoids, benzoyl peroxide, and azelaic acid. The first-line treatment for both comedonal and inflammatory acne is a topical retinoid (tretinoin [retinoic acid], adapalene, and tazarotene). These are the most effective keratolytic agents and have been shown to prevent the microcomedone. These topical agents may be used once daily, or the combination of a retinoid applied to acne-bearing areas of the skin in the evening and a benzoyl peroxide gel or azelaic acid applied in the morning may be used. This regimen will control 80%–85% of cases of adolescent acne.

Table 15–5. Acne treatment.

Type of Lesion	Treatment
Comedonal acne	One of the following:
	Retinoic acid, 0.025, 0.05, or 0.1% cream; 0.01 or 0.025% gel; or 0.4% or 0.1% micro-gel Adapalene, 0.3% gel, 0.1% gel or solution; 0.05% cream
Papular inflammatory acne	One from first grouping, plus one of the following:
	Benzoyl peroxide, 2.5, 4, 5, 8, or 10% gel or lotion; 4 or 8% wash Azelaic acid, 15% or 20% cream Clindamycin, 1% lotion, solution, or gel
Pustular inflammatory acne	One from first grouping, plus one of the following oral antibiotics:
	Tetracycline, 250–500 mg, bid Minocycline or doxycycline, 50–100 mg, bid
Nodulocystic acne	Accutane, 1 mg/kg/d

B. Topical Antibiotics

Topical antibiotics are less effective than systemic antibiotics and at best are equivalent in potency to 250 mg of tetracycline orally once a day. One percent clindamycin phosphate solution is the most efficacious topical antibiotic. Most *P acnes* strains are now resistant to topical erythromycin solutions. Topical antibiotic therapy alone should never be used. Multiple studies have shown a combination of benzoyl peroxide or a retinoid and a topical antibiotic are more effective than the antibiotic alone. Benzoyl peroxide has been shown to help minimize the development of bacterial resistance at sites of application. The duration of application of topical antimicrobials should be limited unless benzoyl peroxide is used. Several combination products (benzoyl peroxide and clindamycin, tretinoin and clindamycin, adapalene and benzoyl peroxide) are available which may simplify the treatment regimen and increase patient compliance.

C. Systemic Antibiotics

Antibiotics that are concentrated in sebum, such as tetracycline, minocycline, and doxycycline, should be reserved for moderate to severe inflammatory acne. The usual dose of tetracycline is 0.5–1.0 g divided twice a day on an empty stomach; minocycline and doxycycline 50–100 mg taken once or twice daily can be taken with food. Monotherapy with oral antibiotics should never be used. Recent recommendations are that oral antibiotics should be used for a finite time period, and then discontinued as soon as there is improvement in the inflammatory lesions. The tetracycline antibiotics should not be given to children younger than 8 years of age due to the effect on dentition (staining of teeth). Doxycycline may induce significant photosensitivity, and minocycline can cause blueish-gray dyspigmentation of the skin, vertigo, headaches, and drug-induced lupus. These antibiotics have anti-inflammatory effects in addition to decreasing *P acnes* in the follicle.

D. Oral Retinoids

An oral retinoid, 13-*cis*-retinoic acid (isotretinoin; Accutane), is the most effective treatment for severe cystic acne. The precise mechanism of its action is unknown, but apoptosis of sebocytes, decreased sebaceous gland size, decreased sebum production, decreased follicular obstruction, decreased skin bacteria, and general anti-inflammatory activities have been described. The initial dosage is 0.5–1 mg/kg/day. This therapy is reserved for severe nodulocystic acne, or acne recalcitrant to aggressive standard therapy. Side effects include dryness and scaling of the skin, dry lips, and, occasionally, dry eyes and dry nose. Fifteen percent of patients may experience some mild achiness with athletic activities. Up to 10% of patients experience mild, reversible hair loss. Elevated liver enzymes and blood lipids have rarely been described. Acute depression may occur. Isotretinoin is teratogenic in young women of childbearing age. Because of this and the other side effects, it is not recommended unless strict adherence to the Food and Drug Administration (FDA) guidelines is ensured. The FDA has implemented a strict registration program (iPLEDGE) that must be used to obtain isotretinoin.

E. Other Acne Treatments

Hormonal therapy (oral contraceptives) is often an effective option for girls who have perimenstrual flares of acne or have not responded adequately to conventional therapy. Adolescents with endocrine disorders such as polycystic ovary syndrome also see improvement of their acne with hormonal therapy. Oral contraceptives can be added to a conventional therapeutic regimen and should always be used in female patients who are prescribed oral isotretinoin unless absolute contraindications exist. There is growing data regarding the use of light, laser, and photodynamic therapy in acne. However, existing studies are of variable quality, and although there is evidence to suggest that these therapies offer benefit in acne, the evidence is not sufficient to recommend any device as monotherapy in acne.

F. Patient Education and Follow-Up Visits

The multifactorial pathogenesis of acne and its role in the treatment plan must be explained to adolescent patients. Good general skin care includes washing the face consistently and using only oil-free, noncomedogenic cosmetics, face creams, and hair sprays. Acne therapy takes 8–12 weeks to produce improvement, and this delay must be stressed to the patient. Realistic expectations should be encouraged in the adolescent patient because no therapy will eradicate all future acne lesions. A written education sheet is useful. Follow-up visits should be made every 12–16 weeks. An objective method to chart improvement should be documented by the provider, because patients' assessment of improvement tends to be inaccurate.

Strauss JS et al: Guidelines of care for acne vulgaris management. J Am Acad Dermatol 2007;56:651 [PMID: 17276540].

Thiboutot D et al: New insights into the management of acne: An update from the Global Alliance to Improve Outcomes in Acne Group. J Am Acad Dermatol 2009;60:S1– S50 [PMID: 19376456].

BACTERIAL INFECTIONS OF THE SKIN

1. Impetigo

Erosions covered by honey-colored crusts are diagnostic of impetigo. Staphylococci and group A streptococci are important pathogens in this disease, which histologically consists of superficial invasion of bacteria into the upper epidermis, forming a subcorneal pustule.

Treatment

Impetigo should be treated with an antimicrobial agent effective against *Staphylococcus aureus* (β-lactamase–resistant penicillins or cephalosporins, clindamycin, amoxicillin–clavulanate) for 7–10 days. Topical mupirocin and fusidic acid (three times daily) are also effective.

2. Bullous Impetigo

All impetigo is bullous, with the blister forming just beneath the stratum corneum, but in "bullous impetigo" there is, in addition to the usual erosion covered by a honey-colored crust, a border filled with clear fluid. Staphylococci may be isolated from these lesions, and systemic signs of circulating exfoliatin are absent. Bullous impetigo lesions can be found anywhere on the skin, but a common location is the diaper area.

Treatment

Treatment with oral antistaphylococcal drugs for 7–10 days is effective. Application of cool compresses to debride crusts is a helpful symptomatic measure.

3. Ecthyma

Ecthyma is a firm, dry crust, surrounded by erythema that exudes purulent material. It represents invasion by group A β-hemolytic streptococci through the epidermis to the superficial dermis. This should not be confused with ecthyma gangrenosum. Lesions of ecthyma gangrenosum may be similar in appearance, but they are seen in a severely ill or immunocompromised patient and are due to systemic dissemination of bacteria, usually *Pseudomonas aeruginosa*, through the bloodstream.

Treatment

Treatment is with systemic penicillin.

4. Cellulitis

Cellulitis is characterized by erythematous, hot, tender, ill-defined, edematous plaques accompanied by regional lymphadenopathy. Histologically, this disorder represents invasion of microorganisms into the lower dermis and sometimes beyond, with obstruction of local lymphatics. Group A β-hemolytic streptococci and coagulase-positive staphylococci are the most common causes; pneumococci and *Haemophilus influenzae* are rare causes. Staphylococcal infections are usually more localized and more likely to have a purulent center; streptococcal infections spread more rapidly, but these characteristics cannot be used to specify the infecting agent. An entry site of prior trauma or infection (eg, varicella) is often present. Septicemia is a potential complication.

Treatment

Treatment is with an appropriate systemic antibiotic.

5. Folliculitis

A pustule at a follicular opening represents folliculitis. Deeper follicular infections are called furuncles (single follicle) and carbuncles (multiple follicles). Staphylococci and streptococci are the most frequent pathogens. Lesions are painless and tend to occur in crops, usually on the buttocks and extremities in children. Methicillin-resistant *Staphylococci aureus* (MRSA) is now an increasing cause of folliculitis and skin abscesses. Cultures of persistent or recurrent folliculitis for MRSA is advisable.

Treatment

Treatment consists of measures to remove follicular obstruction—either cool, wet compresses for 24 hours or keratolytics such as those used for acne. Topical or oral antistaphylococcal antibiotics may be required.

6. Abscess

An abscess occurs deep in the skin, at the bottom of a follicle or an apocrine gland, and is diagnosed as an erythematous, firm, acutely tender nodule with ill-defined borders. Staphylococci are the most common organisms.

Treatment

Treatment consists of incision and drainage and may require adjuvant systemic antibiotics. Recent studies have suggested that incision and drainage alone may be adequate for uncomplicated MRSA skin abscesses in otherwise healthy patients.

7. Scalded Skin Syndrome

This entity consists of the sudden onset of bright red, acutely painful skin, most obvious periorally, periorbitally, and in the flexural areas of the neck, the axillae, the popliteal and antecubital areas, and the groin. The slightest pressure on the skin results in severe pain and separation of the epidermis, leaving a glistening layer (the stratum granulosum of the epidermis) beneath. The disease is caused by a circulating toxin (exfoliatin) elaborated by phage group II staphylococci. Exfoliatin binds to desmoglein-1 resulting in a separation of cells in the granular layer. The causative staphylococci may be isolated not from the skin but rather from the nasopharynx, an abscess, sinus, blood culture, joint fluid, or other focus of infection.

Treatment

Treatment is with systemic antistaphylococcal drugs.

Odell CA: Community-associated methicillin-resistant Staphylococcus aureus (CA-MRSA) skin infections. Curr Opin Pediatr 2010 Jun;22(3):273–277 [Review].

Duong M et al: Randomized, controlled trial of antibiotics in the management of community-acquired skin abscesses in the pediatric patient. Ann Emerg Med 2009 Apr 29 [Epub ahead of print] [PMID: 19409657].

FUNGAL INFECTIONS OF THE SKIN

1. Dermatophyte Infections

Dermatophytes become attached to the superficial layer of the epidermis, nails, and hair, where they proliferate. Fungal infection should be suspected with any red and scaly lesion.

Classification & Clinical Findings

A. Tinea Capitis

Thickened, broken-off hairs with erythema and scaling of underlying scalp are the distinguishing features (Table 15–6). In endemic ringworm, hairs are broken off at the surface of the scalp, leaving a "black dot" appearance. Pustule formation and a boggy, fluctuant mass on the scalp occur in *Microsporum canis* and *Trichophyton tonsurans* infections. This mass, called a kerion, represents an exaggerated host response to the organism. Diffuse scaling of the scalp and pustules may also be seen. Fungal culture should be performed in all cases of suspected tinea capitis.

B. Tinea Corporis

Tinea corporis presents either as annular marginated plaques with a thin scale and clear center or as an annular confluent dermatitis. The most common organisms are *Trichophyton mentagrophytes*, *Trichophyton rubrum*, and *M canis*. The diagnosis is made by scraping thin scales from the border of the lesion, dissolving them in 20% potassium hydroxide (KOH), and examining for hyphae.

Table 15–6. Clinical features of tinea capitis.

Most Common Organisms	Clinical Appearance	Microscopic Appearance in KOH
Trichophyton tonsurans (90%)	Hairs broken off 2-3 mm from follicle; "black dot"; diffuse pustule; seborrheic dermatitis-like; no fluorescence	Hyphae and spores within hair
Microsporum canis (10%)	Thickened broken-off hairs that fluoresce yellow-green with Wood lamp	Small spores outside of hair; hyphae within hair

C. Tinea Cruris

Symmetrical, sharply marginated lesions in inguinal areas occur with tinea cruris. The most common organisms are *T rubrum*, *T mentagrophytes*, and *Epidermophyton floccosum*.

D. Tinea Pedis

The diagnosis of tinea pedis is becoming more common in the prepubertal child, although it is still most commonly seen in postpubertal males. Presentation is with red scaly soles, blisters on the instep of the foot, or fissuring between the toes.

E. Tinea Unguium (Onychomycosis)

Loosening of the nail plate from the nail bed (onycholysis), giving a yellow discoloration, is the first sign of fungal invasion of the nails. Thickening of the distal nail plate then occurs, followed by scaling and a crumbly appearance of the entire nail plate surface. *T rubrum* is the most common cause. The diagnosis is confirmed by KOH examination and fungal culture. Usually only one or two nails are involved. If every nail is involved, psoriasis, lichen planus, or idiopathic trachyonychia is a more likely diagnosis than fungal infection.

Treatment

The treatment of dermatophytosis is quite simple: If hair is involved, systemic therapy is necessary. For many providers, griseofulvin remains the treatment of choice. Topical antifungal agents do not enter hair or nails in sufficient concentration to clear the infection. The absorption of griseofulvin from the gastrointestinal tract is enhanced by a fatty meal; thus, whole milk or ice cream taken with the medication increases absorption. The dosage of griseofulvin is 20 mg/kg/d (maximum 500 mg/dose). With hair infections, cultures should be done every 4 weeks, and treatment should be continued for 4 weeks following a negative culture result. The side effects are few, and the drug has been used successfully in the newborn period. Terbinafine (62.5 mg/day, < 20 kg–125 mg/day, 20–40 kg–250 mg/day, > 40 kg) is also used. For nails, daily administration of topical ciclopirox 8% (Penlac nail lacquer) can be considered, as can terbenafine for 6–12 weeks or pulsed-dose itraconazole (50 mg/twice a day < 20 kg–100 mg/twice a day, 20–40 kg–200 mg/twice a day, > 40 kg) given in three 1-week pulses separated by 3 weeks.

Tinea corporis, tinea pedis, and tinea cruris can be treated effectively with topical medication after careful inspection to make certain that the hair and nails are not involved. Treatment with any of the imidazoles, allylamines, benzylamines, or ciclopirox applied twice daily for 3–4 weeks is recommended.

Andrews RM, McCarthy J, Carapetis JR et al: Skin disorders, including pyoderma, scabies, and tinea infections. Pediatr Clin N Am 2009;56:1421 [PMID: 19962029].

2. Tinea Versicolor

Tinea versicolor is a superficial infection caused by *Malassezia globosa*, a yeastlike fungus. It characteristically causes polycyclic connected hypopigmented macules and very fine scales in areas of sun-induced pigmentation. In winter, the polycyclic macules appear reddish brown.

Treatment

Treatment consists of application of selenium sulfide (Selsun), 2.5% suspension, zinc pyrithione shampoo, or topical antifungals. Selenium sulfide and zinc pyrithione shampoo should be applied to the whole body and left on overnight. Treatment can be repeated again in 1 week and then monthly thereafter. It tends to be somewhat irritating, and the patient should be warned about this difficulty. Topical antifungals are applied twice a day for 1–2 weeks.

3. Candida albicans Infections (See also Chapter 43)

Clinical Findings

In addition to being a frequent invader in diaper dermatitis, *Candida albicans* also infects the oral mucosa, where it appears as thick white patches with an erythematous base (thrush); the angles of the mouth, where it causes fissures and white exudate (perlêche); and the cuticular region of the fingers, where thickening of the cuticle, dull red erythema, and distortion of growth of the nail plate suggest the diagnosis of candidal paronychia. *Candida* dermatitis is characterized by sharply defined erythematous patches, sometimes with eroded areas. Pustules, vesicles, or papules may be present as satellite lesions. Similar infections may be found in other moist areas, such as the axillae and neck folds. This infection is more common in children who have recently received antibiotics.

Treatment

A topical imidazole cream is the drug of first choice for *C albicans* infections. In diaper dermatitis, the cream form can be applied twice a day. In oral thrush, nystatin suspension should be applied directly to the mucosa with the parent's finger or a cotton-tipped applicator, because it is not absorbed and acts topically. In candidal paronychia, the antifungal agent is applied over the area, covered with occlusive plastic wrapping, and left on overnight after the application is made airtight. Refractory candidiasis will respond to a brief course of oral fluconazole.

VIRAL INFECTIONS OF THE SKIN (SEE ALSO CHAPTER 40)

1. Herpes Simplex Infection

Clinical Findings

Painful, grouped vesicles or erosions on a red base suggest herpes simplex. Rapid immunofluorescent tests for herpes simplex virus (HSV) and varicella-zoster virus (VZV) are available. A Tzanck smear is done by scraping a vesicle base with a No. 15 blade, smearing on a glass slide, and staining the epithelial cells with Wright stain. The smear is positive if epidermal multinucleated giant cells are visualized. A positive Tzanck smear indicates herpesvirus infection (HSV or VZV). In infants and children, lesions resulting from herpes simplex type 1 are seen most commonly on the gingiva, lips, and face. Involvement of a digit (herpes whitlow) will occur if the child sucks the thumb or fingers. Herpes simplex type 2 lesions are seen on the genitalia and in the mouth in adolescents. Cutaneous dissemination of herpes simplex occurs in patients with atopic dermatitis (eczema herpeticum) and appears clinically as very tender, punched-out erosions among the eczematous skin changes.

Treatment

The treatment of HSV infections is discussed in Chapter 40.

2. Varicella-Zoster Infection

Clinical Findings

Grouped vesicles in a dermatome, usually on the trunk or face, suggest varicella-zoster reactivation. Zoster in children may not be painful and usually has a mild course. In patients with compromised host resistance, the appearance of an erythematous border around the vesicles is a good prognostic sign. Conversely, large bullae without a tendency to crusting and systemic illness imply a poor host response to the virus. Varicella-zoster and herpes simplex lesions undergo the same series of changes: papule, vesicle, pustule, crust, slightly depressed scar. Lesions of primary varicella appear in crops, and many different stages of lesions are present at the same time (eg, papules), eccentrically placed vesicles on an erythematous base ("dew drop" on a rose petal), erosions, and crusts.

Treatment

Antihistamines may be used for pruritus; cool baths or drying lotions such as calamine lotion are usually sufficient to relieve symptoms. In immunosuppressed children, intravenous or oral acyclovir should be used.

3. Human Immunodeficiency Virus Infection (See also Chapter 41)

Clinical Findings

The average time of onset of skin lesions after perinatally acquired HIV infection is 4 months; after transfusion-acquired infection, it is 11 months. Persistent oral candidiasis and recalcitrant candidal diaper rash are the most frequent cutaneous features of infantile HIV infection. Severe or recurrent herpetic gingivostomatitis, varicella-zoster infection, and molluscum contagiosum infection occur. Recurrent staphylococcal pyodermas, tinea of the face, and onychomycosis are also observed. A generalized dermatitis with features of seborrhea (severe cradle cap) is extremely common. In general, persistent, recurrent, or extensive skin infections should make one suspicious of HIV infection.

Treatment

The treatment of HIV infections is discussed in Chapter 41.

VIRUS-INDUCED TUMORS

1. Molluscum Contagiosum

Molluscum contagiosum is a poxvirus that induces the epidermis to proliferate, forming a pale papule. Molluscum contagiosum consists of umbilicated, flesh-colored papules in groups anywhere on the body. They are common in infants and preschool children, as well as sexually active adolescents.

Treatment

Treatment for molluscum is either immunological (topical imiquimod, oral cimetidine, intralesional candida antigen injection) or cytodestructive (topical cantharidin, cryotherapy with liquid nitrogen, and curettage). Left untreated, the lesions resolve over months to years.

2. Warts

Warts are skin-colored papules with rough (verrucous) surfaces. They are intraepidermal tumors caused by infection with human papillomavirus (HPV). There are over 100 types of this DNA virus, which induces the epidermal cells to proliferate, thus resulting in the warty growth. Flat warts are smoother and smaller than common warts and are often seen on the face. Certain types of HPV are associated with certain types of warts (eg, flat warts) or location of warts (eg, genital warts).

Treatment

No therapy for warts is ideal, and 30% of warts will clear in 6 months irrespective of the therapy chosen. As with molluscum, the treatment of warts is also immunological (topical imiquimod, oral cimetidine, intralesional candida antigen injection, and squaric acid contact therapy) or cytodestructive. Liquid nitrogen is painful, user dependent, and can lead to blistering and scarring. Topical salicylic acid may also be used. Large mosaic plantar warts are treated most effectively by applying 40% salicylic acid plaster cut with a scissors to fit the lesion. The adhesive side of the plaster is placed against the lesion and taped securely in place with duct or athletic tape. The plaster and tape should be placed on Monday and removed on Friday. Over the weekend, the patient should soak the skin in warm water for 30 minutes to soften it. Then the white, macerated tissue should be pared with a pumice stone, cuticle scissors, or a nail file. This procedure is repeated every week, and the patient is seen every 4 weeks. Most plantar warts resolve in 6–8 weeks when treated in this way. Vascular pulsed dye lasers are a useful adjunct therapy for the treatment of plantar warts.

For flat warts, a good response to 0.025% tretinoin gel or topical imiquimod (Aldara) cream, applied once daily for 3–4 weeks, has been reported.

Surgical excision, electrosurgery, and nonspecific burning laser surgery should be avoided; these modalities do not have higher cure rates and result in scarring. Cantharidin may cause small warts to become large warts and should not be used.

Venereal warts (condylomata acuminata) (see Chapter 44) may be treated with imiquimod, 25% podophyllum resin (podophyllin) in alcohol, or podofilox, a lower concentration of purified podophyllin, which is applied at home. Podophyllin should be painted on the lesions in the practitioner's office and then washed off after 4 hours. Re-treatment in 2–3 weeks may be necessary. Podofilox is applied by the patient once daily, Monday through Thursday, whereas imiquimod is used three times a week on alternating days. Lesions not on the vulvar mucous membrane but on the adjacent skin should be treated as a common wart and frozen.

No wart therapy is immediately and definitively successful. Realistic expectations should be set and appropriate follow-up treatments scheduled.

INSECT INFESTATIONS

1. Scabies

Clinical Findings

Scabies is suggested by linear burrows about the wrists, ankles, finger webs, areolas, anterior axillary folds, genitalia, or face (in infants). Often there are excoriations, honey-colored crusts, and pustules from secondary infection. Identification of the female mite or her eggs and feces is necessary to confirm the diagnosis. Scrape an unscratched papule or burrow with a No. 15 blade and examine microscopically in immersion oil to confirm the diagnosis. In a child who is often scratching, scrape under the fingernails. Examine the parents for unscratched burrows.

Treatment

Permethrin 5% is now the treatment of choice for scabies. It should be applied as a single overnight application. The need for re-treatment is rare. Oral ivermection 200 microgram/dose × 1 and repeated in 10 days may be used in resistant cases.

2. Pediculoses (Louse Infestations)

Clinical Findings

The presence of excoriated papules and pustules and a history of severe itching at night suggest infestation with the human body louse. This louse may be discovered in the seams of underwear but not on the body. In the scalp hair, the gelatinous nits of the head louse adhere tightly to the hair shaft. The pubic louse may be found crawling among pubic hairs, or blue-black macules may be found dispersed through the pubic region (maculae cerulea). The pubic louse is often seen on the eyelashes of newborns.

Treatment

Initial treatment of head lice is often instituted by parents with an over-the-counter pyrethrin or permethrin product. If head lice are not eradicated after two applications 7 days apart with these products, malathion 0.5% is highly effective but is toxic if ingested, and flammable. A second application 7–9 days after initial treatment may be necessary. Treatment of pubic lice is similar. Treatment of body lice is clean clothing and washing the infested clothing at high temperature.

Diamantis SA, Morrell DS, Burkhart CN: Pediatric infestations. Paediatr Ann 2009;38:326 [PMID: 19588676].

3. Papular Urticaria

Clinical Findings

Papular urticaria is characterized by grouped erythematous papules surrounded by an urticarial flare and distributed over the shoulders, upper arms, legs, and buttocks in infants. Although not a true infestation, these lesions represent delayed hypersensitivity reactions to stinging or biting insects. Fleas from dogs and cats are the usual offenders. Less commonly, mosquitoes, lice, scabies, and bird and grass mites are involved. The sensitivity is transient, lasting 4–6 months. Usually no other family members are affected. It is often difficult for the parents to understand why no one else is affected.

Treatment

The logical therapy is to remove the offending insect, although in most cases it is very difficult to identify the exact cause. Topical corticosteroids and oral antihistamines will control symptoms.

DERMATITIS (ECZEMA)

The terms *dermatitis* and *eczema* are currently used interchangeably in dermatology, although the term *eczema* truly denotes an acute weeping dermatosis. All forms of dermatitis, regardless of cause, may present with acute edema, erythema, and oozing with crusting, mild erythema alone, or lichenification. Lichenification is diagnosed by thickening of the skin with a shiny surface and exaggerated, deepened skin markings. It is the response of the skin to chronic rubbing or scratching.

Although the lesions of the various dermatoses are histologically indistinguishable, clinicians have nonetheless divided the disease group called dermatitis into several categories based on known causes in some cases and differing natural histories in others.

1. Atopic Dermatitis

Pathogenesis & Clinical Findings

Atopic dermatitis is a hereditary disorder characterized by dry skin, the presence of eczema, and onset before age 2 years. Many (not all) patients go through three clinical phases. In the first, infantile eczema, the dermatitis begins on the cheeks and scalp and frequently expresses itself as oval patches on the trunk, later involving the extensor surfaces of the extremities. The usual age at onset is 2–3 months, and this phase ends at age 18 months to 2 years. Only one-third of all infants with infantile eczema progress to phase 2 childhood or flexural eczema in which the predominant involvement is in the antecubital and popliteal fossae, the neck, the wrists, and sometimes the hands or feet. This phase lasts from age 2 years to adolescence. Only one-third of children with typical flexural eczema progress to adolescent eczema, which is usually manifested by the continuation of chronic flexural eczema along with hand and/or foot dermatitis. Atopic dermatitis is quite unusual after age 30 years.

Atopic dermatitis is a polygenic disease with positive and negative modifiers. Atopic dermatitis results from an interaction among susceptibility genes, the host environment, skin barrier defects, pharmacologic abnormalities, and immunologic response. The case for food and inhalant allergens as specific causes of atopic dermatitis is not strong. There is significant evidence that a primary defect in atopic dermatitis is an abnormality in the skin barrier formation due to defects in the filaggrin gene. Not all people with filaggrin abnormalities have atopic dermatitis and not all people with atopic dermatitis have filaggrin abnormalities.

A few patients with atopic dermatitis have immunodeficiency with recurrent pyodermas, unusual susceptibility to herpes simplex viruses, hyperimmunoglobulinemia E, defective neutrophil and monocyte chemotaxis, and impaired T-lymphocyte function. (See Chapter 33.)

A faulty epidermal barrier predisposes the patient with atopic dermatitis to dry, itchy skin. Inability to hold water within the stratum corneum results in rapid evaporation of water, shrinking of the stratum corneum, and cracks in the epidermal barrier. Such skin forms an ineffective barrier to the entry of various irritants. Chronic atopic dermatitis is frequently infected secondarily with *S aureus* or *Streptococcus pyogenes*. Patients with atopic dermatitis have a deficiency of antimicrobial peptides in their skin, which may account for the susceptibility to recurrent skin infection.

Treatment

A. Acute Stages

Application of wet dressings and medium-potency topical corticosteroids is the treatment of choice for acute, weeping atopic eczema. The use of wet dressings is outlined at the beginning of this chapter. Superinfection with *S aureus* and/or *Streptococcus pyogenes* may occur, and appropriate systemic antibiotics may be necessary. If the expected improvement is not seen, bacterial cultures should be obtained to identify the possibility of an organism resistant to standard therapy.

B. Chronic Stages

Treatment is aimed at avoiding irritants and restoring water to the skin. No soaps or harsh shampoos should be used, and the patient should avoid woolen or any rough clothing. Bathing is minimized to every second or third day. Twice daily lubrication of the skin is very important.

Nonperfumed creams or lotions are suitable lubricants. Plain petrolatum is an acceptable lubricant, but some people find it too greasy and during hot weather it may also cause considerable sweat retention. Liberal use of Cetaphil lotion four or five times daily as a substitute for soap is also satisfactory as a means of lubrication. A bedroom humidifier is often helpful. Topical corticosteroids should be limited to medium strength (see Table 15–3). There is seldom a reason to use super- or high-potency corticosteroids in atopic dermatitis. In superinfected atopic dermatitis, systemic antibiotics for 10–14 days are necessary.

Tacrolimus and pimecrolimus ointments are topical immunosuppressive agents that are effective in atopic dermatitis. Because of concerns about the development of malignancies, tacrolimus and pimecrolimus should be reserved for children older than 2 years of age with atopic dermatitis unresponsive to medium-potency topical steroids. It has been argued that an increased risk of malignancy has not been seen in immunologically normal individuals using these products. Recommendations for usage likely will change with time. Treatment failures in chronic atopic dermatitis are most often the result of noncompliance. This is a frustrating disease for parent and child. Return to a normal lifestyle for the parent and child is the ultimate goal of therapy.

Cork MJ et al: Epidermal barrier dysfunction in atopic dermatitis. J Invest Dermatol 2009;129:1892 [PMID: 19494826].

Batchelor JM, Grindlay DJ, Williams HC: What's new in atopic eczema? An analysis of systematic reviews published in 2008 and 2009. Clin Exp Dermatol 2010;35:823 [PMID: 20649899].

2. Nummular Eczema

Nummular eczema is characterized by numerous symmetrically distributed coin-shaped patches of dermatitis, principally on the extremities. These may be acute, oozing, and crusted or dry and scaling. The differential diagnosis should include tinea corporis, impetigo, and atopic dermatitis.

Treatment

The same topical measures should be used as for atopic dermatitis, although more potent topical steroids may be necessary.

3. Primary Irritant Contact Dermatitis (Diaper Dermatitis)

Contact dermatitis is of two types: primary irritant and allergic eczematous. Primary irritant dermatitis develops within a few hours, reaches peak severity at 24 hours, and then disappears. Allergic eczematous contact dermatitis (described in the next section) has a delayed onset of 18 hours, peaks at 48–72 hours, and often lasts as long as 2–3 weeks even if exposure to the offending antigen is discontinued.

Diaper dermatitis, the most common form of primary irritant contact dermatitis seen in pediatric practice, is caused by prolonged contact of the skin with urine and feces, which contain irritating chemicals such as urea and intestinal enzymes.

Clinical Findings

The diagnosis of diaper dermatitis is based on the picture of erythema and scaling of the skin in the perineal area and the history of prolonged skin contact with urine or feces. This is frequently seen in the "good baby" who sleeps many hours through the night without waking. In 80% of cases of diaper dermatitis lasting more than 3 days, the affected area is colonized with *C albicans* even before appearance of the classic signs of a beefy red, sharply marginated dermatitis with satellite lesions. Streptococcal perianal cellulitis and infantile psoriasis should be included in the differential diagnosis.

Treatment

Treatment consists of changing diapers frequently. The area should only be washed following a bowel movement. Washing should be done with a wash cloth and warm water only. Because rubber or plastic pants prevent evaporation of the contactant and enhance its penetration into the skin, they should be avoided as much as possible. Air drying is useful. Treatment of long-standing diaper dermatitis should include application of a barrier cream such as zinc oxide with each diaper change and an imidazole cream twice a day.

4. Allergic Eczematous Contact Dermatitis (Poison Ivy Dermatitis)

Clinical Findings

Plants such as poison ivy, poison sumac, and poison oak cause most cases of allergic contact dermatitis in children. Allergic contact dermatitis has all the features of delayed type (T-lymphocyte–mediated) hypersensitivity. Many substances may cause such a reaction; other than plants, nickel sulfate, potassium dichromate, and neomycin are the most common causes. Nickel is found to some degree in all metals. Nickel allergy is commonly seen on the ears secondary to the wearing of earrings, and near the umbilicus from pants snaps and belt buckles. The true incidence of allergic contact dermatitis in children is unknown. Children often present with acute dermatitis with blister formation, oozing, and crusting. Blisters are often linear and of acute onset.

Treatment

Treatment of contact dermatitis in localized areas is with potent topical corticosteroids. In severe generalized involvement, prednisone, 1–2 mg/kg/d orally for 10–14 days, can be used.

Bonitisis NG et al: Allergens responsible for allergic contact dermatitis among children: A systematic review and meta-analysis. Contact Dermatitis 2011;64:245 [PMID: 21480911].

Lee PW, Elsaie ML, Jacob SE: Allergic contact dermatitis in children: Common allergens and treatment: A review. Curr Opin Pediatr 2009;21:491 [PMID: 19584724].

5. Seborrheic Dermatitis

Clinical Findings

Seborrheic dermatitis is an erythematous scaly dermatitis accompanied by overproduction of sebum occurring in areas rich in sebaceous glands (ie, the face, scalp, and perineum). This common condition occurs predominantly in the newborn and at puberty, the ages at which hormonal stimulation of sebum production is maximal. Although it is tempting to speculate that overproduction of sebum causes the dermatitis, the exact relationship is unclear.

Seborrheic dermatitis on the scalp in infancy is clinically similar to atopic dermatitis, and the distinction may become clear only after other areas are involved. Psoriasis also occurs in seborrheic areas in older children and should be considered in the differential diagnosis.

Treatment

Seborrheic dermatitis responds well to low-potency topical corticosteroids.

Poindexter GB, Burkhart CN, Morrell DS: Therapies for pediatric seborrheic dermatitis. Pediatr Ann 2009;38:333 [PMID: 19588677].

6. Dandruff

Dandruff is physiologic scaling or mild seborrhea, in the form of greasy scalp scales. The cause is unknown. Treatment is with medicated dandruff shampoos.

7. Dry Skin Dermatitis (Asteatotic Eczema, Xerosis)

Children who live in arid climates are susceptible to dry skin, characterized by large cracked scales with erythematous borders. The stratum corneum is dependent on environmental humidity for its water, and below 30% environmental humidity the stratum corneum loses water, shrinks, and cracks. These cracks in the epidermal barrier allow irritating substances to enter the skin, predisposing the patient to dermatitis.

Treatment

Treatment consists of increasing the water content of the skin in the immediate external environment. House humidifiers are very useful. Minimize bathing to every second or third day.

Frequent soaping of the skin impairs its water-holding capacity and serves as an irritating alkali, and all soaps should therefore be avoided. Frequent use of emollients (eg, Cetaphil, Eucerin, Lubriderm) should be a major part of therapy.

8. Keratosis Pilaris

Follicular papules containing a white inspissated scale characterize keratosis pilaris. Individual lesions are discrete and may be red. They are prominent on the extensor surfaces of the upper arms and thighs and on the buttocks and cheeks. In severe cases, the lesions may be generalized.

Treatment

Treatment is with keratolytics such as urea cream or lactic acid, followed by skin hydration.

9. Pityriasis Alba

White, scaly macular areas with indistinct borders are seen over extensor surfaces of extremities and on the cheeks in children with pityriasis alba. Suntanning exaggerates these lesions. Histologic examination reveals a mild dermatitis. These lesions may be confused with tinea versicolor.

Treatment

Low-potency topical corticosteroids may help decrease any inflammatory component and may lead to faster return of normal pigmentation.

In SI et al: Clinical and histopathological characteristics of pityria sis alba. Clin Exp Dermatol 2009;34:591 [PMID: 19094127].

COMMON SKIN TUMORS

If the skin moves with the nodule on lateral palpation, the tumor is located within the dermis; if the skin moves over the nodule, it is subcutaneous. Seventy-five percent of lumps in childhood will be either epidermoid cysts (60%) or pilomatricomas (15%).

1. Epidermoid Cysts

Clinical Findings

Epidermoid cysts are the most common type of cutaneous cyst. Other names for epidermoid cysts are epidermal cysts, epidermal inclusion cysts, and "sebaceous" cysts. This last term is a misnomer since they contain neither sebum nor sebaceous glands. Epidermoid cysts can occur anywhere, but are most common on the face and upper trunk. They usually arise from and are lined by the stratified squamous epithelium of the follicular infundibulum. Clinically, epidermoid cysts are dermal nodules with a central punctum, representing the follicle associated with the cyst. They can reach several centimeters in diameter. **Dermoid cysts** are areas of sequestration of skin along embryonic fusion lines. They are present at birth and occur most commonly on the lateral eyebrow.

Treatment

Epidermoid cysts can rupture, causing a foreign-body inflammatory reaction, or become infected. Infectious complications should be treated with antibiotics. Definitive treatment of epidermoid and dermoid cysts is surgical excision.

2. Pilomatricomas

These are benign tumors of the hair matrix. They are most commonly seen on the face and upper trunk. They are firm and may be irregular. Their color varies, flesh colored or blue. The firmness is secondary to calcification of the tumor.

Treatment

Treatment is by surgical excision.

3. Granuloma Annulare

Violaceous circles or semicircles of nontender intradermal nodules found over the lower legs and ankles, the dorsum of the hands and wrists, and the trunk, in that order of frequency, suggest granuloma annulare. Histologically, the disease appears as a central area of tissue death (necrobiosis) surrounded by macrophages and lymphocytes.

Treatment

No treatment is necessary. Lesions resolve spontaneously within 1–2 years in most children.

4. Pyogenic Granuloma

These lesions appear over 1–2 weeks at times following skin trauma as a dark red papule with an ulcerated and crusted surface that may bleed easily with minor trauma. Histologically, this represents excessive new vessel formation with or without inflammation (granulation tissue). It should be regarded as an abnormal healing response.

Treatment

Pulsed dye laser for very small lesions or curettage followed by electrocautery are the treatments of choice.

5. Keloids

Keloids are scars of delayed onset that continue for up to several years to progress beyond the initial wound margins. The tendency to develop keloids is inherited. They are often found on the face, earlobes, neck, chest, and back.

Treatment

Treatment includes intralesional injection with triamcinolone acetonide, 20 mg/mL, or excision and injection with corticosteroids. For larger keloids, excision followed by postoperative radiotherapy may be indicated.

PAPULOSQUAMOUS ERUPTIONS

Papulosquamous eruptions (Table 15–7) comprise papules or plaques with varying degrees of scale.

1. Pityriasis Rosea

Pathogenesis & Clinical Findings

Pink to red, oval plaques with fine scales that tend to align with their long axis parallel to skin tension lines (eg, "Christmas tree pattern" on the back) are characteristic lesions of pityriasis rosea. In 20%–80% of cases, the generalized eruption is

Table 15–7. Papulosquamous eruptions in children.

Psoriasis
Pityriasis rosea
Tinea corporis
Lichen planus
Pityriasis lichenoides (acute or chronic)
Dermatomyositis
Lupus erythematosus
Pityriasis rubra pilaris
Secondary syphilis

preceded for up to 30 days by a solitary, larger, scaling plaque with central clearing and a scaly border (the herald patch). The herald patch is clinically similar to ringworm and can be confused. In whites, the lesions are primarily on the trunk; in blacks, lesions are primarily on the extremities and may be accentuated in the axillary and inguinal areas (inverse pityriasis rosea).

This disease is common in school-aged children and adolescents and is presumed to be viral in origin. The role of human herpesvirus 7 in the pathogenesis of pityriasis rosea is debated. The condition lasts 6–12 weeks and may be pruritic.

Differential Diagnosis

The major differential diagnosis is secondary syphilis, and a VDRL (Venereal Disease Research Laboratories) test should be done if syphilis is suspected, especially in high-risk patients with palm or sole involvement. Fever and widespread lymphadenopathy is often found in secondary syphilis. "Pityriasis rosea" lasting more than 12 weeks is likely to be pityriasis lichenoides.

Treatment

Exposure to natural sunlight may help hasten the resolution of lesions. Oral antihistamines and topical steroids can be used for pruritus. Often, no treatment is necessary. Pityriasis rosea that lasts more than 12 weeks should be referred to a dermatologist for evaluation.

Browning JC: An update on pityriasis rosea and other similar childhood exanthems. Curr Opin Pediatr 2009;21:481 [PMID: 19502983].

2. Psoriasis

Pathogenesis & Clinical Findings

Psoriasis is characterized by erythematous papules covered by thick white scales. Guttate (droplike) psoriasis is a common form in children that often follows an episode of streptococcal pharyngitis by 2–3 weeks. The sudden onset of small papules (3–8 mm), seen predominantly over the trunk and quickly covered with thick white scales, is characteristic of guttate psoriasis. Chronic psoriasis is marked by thick, large scaly plaques (5–10 cm) over the elbows, knees, scalp, and other sites of trauma. Pinpoint pits in the nail plate are seen, as well as yellow discoloration of the nail plate resulting from onycholysis. Psoriasis occurs frequently on the scalp, elbows, knees, periumbilical area, ears, sacral area, and genitalia. It should always be included in the differential diagnosis of "dermatitis" on the scalp or genitalia of children.

The pathogenesis of psoriasis is complex and incompletely understood. It has immune-mediated inflammation, is a familial condition, and multiple psoriasis susceptibility genes have been identified. There is increased epidermal turnover; psoriatic epidermis has a turnover time of 3–4 days versus 28 days for normal skin. These rapidly proliferating epidermal cells produce excessive stratum corneum, giving rise to thick, opaque scales.

Differential Diagnosis

Papulosquamous eruptions that present problems of differential diagnosis are listed in Table 15–7.

Treatment

Topical corticosteroids are the initial treatment of choice. Penetration of topical steroids through the enlarged epidermal barrier in psoriasis requires that more potent preparations be used, for example, fluocinonide 0.05% (Lidex) or clobetasol 0.05% (Temovate) ointment twice daily.

The second line of therapy is topical vitamin D3 medications such as calcipotriene (Dovonex) or the newer ointment, calcitriol (Vectical), applied twice daily or the combination of a superpotent topical steroid twice daily on weekends and calcipotriene twice daily on weekdays.

Topical retinoids such as tazarotene (0.1%, 0.5% cream, gel) can be used in combination with topical corticosteroids to help restore normal epidermal differentiation and turnover time. However, these treatments can cause skin to become dry.

Anthralin therapy is also useful. Anthralin is applied to the skin for a short contact time (eg, 20 minutes once daily) and then washed off with a neutral soap (eg, Dove). This can be used in combination with topical corticosteroids.

Crude coal tar therapy is messy and stains bedclothes. The newer tar gels (Estar, PsoriGel) and one foam product (Scytera) cause less staining and are most efficacious. They are applied twice daily. These preparations are sold over the counter and are not usually covered by insurance plans.

Scalp care using a tar shampoo requires leaving the shampoo on for 5 minutes, washing it off, and then shampooing with commercial shampoo to remove scales. It may be necessary to shampoo daily until scaling is reduced.

More severe cases of psoriasis are best treated by a dermatologist. Narrow band UVB phototherapy and multiple systemic medications and new biologic agents (antibodies, fusion proteins, and recombinant cytokines) are effective in more widespread, severe cases.

De Jager ME et al: Efficacy and safety of treatments for childhood psoriasis: A systematic literature review. J Am Acad Dermatol 2010;62:1013 [PMID: 19900732].

HAIR LOSS (ALOPECIA)

Hair loss in children (Table 15–8) imposes great emotional stress on the patient and the parent. A 60% hair loss in a single area is necessary before hair loss can be detected clinically. Examination should begin with the scalp to determine whether inflammation, scale, or infiltrative changes are present. The hair should be gently pulled to see if it is easily removable. Hairs should be examined microscopically for breaking and structural defects and to see whether growing or resting hairs are being shed. Placing removed hairs in mounting fluid (Permount) on a glass microscope slide makes them easy to examine.

Three diseases account for most cases of hair loss in children: alopecia areata, tinea capitis (described earlier in this chapter), and hair pulling.

1. Alopecia Areata

Clinical Findings

Complete hair loss in a localized area is called alopecia areata. This is the most common cause of hair loss in children. An immunologic pathogenic mechanism is suspected because dense infiltration of lymphocytes precedes hair loss. Fifty percent of children with alopecia areata completely regrow their hair within 12 months, although as many may have a relapse in the future.

A rare and unusual form of alopecia areata begins at the occiput and proceeds along the hair margins to the frontal scalp. This variety, called ophiasis, often eventuates in total scalp hair loss (alopecia totalis). The prognosis for regrowth in ophiasis is poor.

Treatment

Treatment of alopecia areata is difficult. Systemic corticosteroids given to suppress the inflammatory response will result in hair growth, but the hair may fall out again when the drug is discontinued. Systemic corticosteroids should never be used for a prolonged time period. Superpotent topical steroids, minoxidil (Rogaine), contact therapy, and anthralin are treatment options. In children with alopecia totalis, a wig is most helpful.

Alkhalifah A et al: Alopecia areata update. Part I. clinical picture, histopathology and pathogenesis. J Am Acad Dermatol 2010;62:177 [PMID: 21015945].

Alkhalifah A et al: Alopecia areata update. Part II. Treatment. J Am Acad Dermatol 2010;62:191 [PMID: 21015946].

2. Hair Pulling

Clinical Findings

Traumatic hair pulling causes the hair shafts to be broken off at different lengths, with an ill-defined area of hair loss, petechiae around follicular openings, and a wrinkled hair shaft on microscopic examination. This behavior may be merely habit, an acute reaction to severe stress, trichotillomania, or a sign of another psychiatric disorder. Eyelashes and eyebrows rather than scalp hair may be pulled out.

Treatment

If the behavior has a long history, psychiatric evaluation may be helpful. Cutting or oiling the hair to make it slippery is an aid to behavior modification.

Witkowskis AM, Schwartz RA, Janniger CK: Trichotillomania: An important psychocutaneous disorder. Cutis 2010;86:12 [PMID: 21049760].

REACTIVE ERYTHEMAS

1. Erythema Multiforme

Clinical Findings

Erythema multiforme begins with papules that later develop a dark center and then evolve into lesions with central bluish discoloration or blisters and the characteristic target lesions (iris lesions) that have three concentric circles of color change. Erythema multiforme has sometimes been diagnosed in patients with severe mucous membrane involvement, but Stevens-Johnson syndrome is the usual diagnosis when severe involvement of conjunctiva, oral cavity, and genital mucosa also occur.

Table 15–8. Other causes of hair loss in children.

Hair loss with scalp changes
Atrophy:
Lichen planus
Lupus erythematosus
Birthmarks:
Epidermal nevus
Nevus sebaceous
Aplasia cutis congenita
Hair loss with hair shaft defects (hair fails to grow out enough to require haircuts)
Monilethrix—alternating bands of thin and thick areas
Pili annulati—alternating bands of light and dark pigmentation
Pili torti—hair twisted 180 degrees, brittle
Trichorrhexis invaginata (bamboo hair)—intussusception of one hair into another
Trichorrhexis nodosa—nodules with fragmented hair

Many causes are suspected, particularly concomitant herpes simplex virus; drugs, especially sulfonamides; and *Mycoplasma* infections. Recurrent erythema multiforme is usually associated with reactivation of herpes simplex virus. In erythema multiforme, spontaneous healing occurs in 10–14 days, but Stevens-Johnson syndrome may last 6–8 weeks.

▶ Treatment

Treatment is symptomatic in uncomplicated erythema multiforme. Removal of offending drugs is an obvious measure. Oral antihistamines such as hydroxyzine, 2 mg/kg/d orally, are useful. Cool compresses and wet dressings will relieve pruritus. Steroids have not been demonstrated to be effective. Chronic acyclovir therapy has been successful in decreasing attacks in patients with herpes-associated recurrent erythema multiforme.

Wetter DA, Davis MD: Recurrent erythema multiforme: Clinical characteristics, etiologic associations, and treatment in a series of 48 patients at Mayo Clinic, 2000 to 2007. J Am Acad Dermatol 2010;62:45 [PMID: 19665257].

2. Drug Eruptions

Drugs may produce urticarial, morbilliform, scarlatiniform, pustular, bullous, or fixed skin eruptions. Urticaria may appear within minutes after drug administration, but most reactions begin 7–14 days after the drug is first administered. These eruptions may occur in patients who have received these drugs for long periods, and eruptions continue for days after the drug has been discontinued. Drug eruptions with fever, eosinophilia, and systemic symptoms (DRESS syndrome) is most commonly seen with anticonvulsants, but may be seen with other drugs. Drugs commonly implicated in skin reactions are listed in Table 15–9.

Newell BD, Horii KA: Cutaneous drug reactions in children. Pediatr Ann 2010;39:618 [PMID: 20954608].

Table 15–9. Common drug reactions.

Urticaria
Barbiturates
Opioids
Penicillins
Sulfonamides
Morbilliform eruption
Anticonvulsants
Cephalosporins
Penicillins
Sulfonamides
Fixed drug eruption, erythema multiforme, toxic epidermal necrolysis, Stevens-Johnson syndrome
Anticonvulsants
Nonsteroidal anti-inflammatory drugs
Sulfonamides
DRESS syndrome
Anticonvulsants
Photodermatitis
Psoralens
Sulfonamides
Tetracyclines
Thiazides

DRESS syndrome = drug eruptions with fever, eosinophilia, and systemic symptoms.

MISCELLANEOUS SKIN DISORDERS SEEN IN PEDIATRIC PRACTICE

1. Aphthous Stomatitis

Recurrent erosions on the gums, lips, tongue, palate, and buccal mucosa are often confused with herpes simplex. A smear of the base of such a lesion stained with Wright stain will aid in ruling out herpes simplex by the absence of epithelial multinucleate giant cells. A culture for herpes simplex is also useful in differential diagnostics. The cause remains unknown, but T-cell–mediated cytotoxicity to various viral antigens has been postulated.

▶ Treatment

There is no specific therapy for this condition. Rinsing the mouth with liquid antacids provides relief in most patients. Topical corticosteroids in a gel base may provide some relief. In severe cases that interfere with eating, prednisone, 1 mg/kg/d orally for 3–5 days, will suffice to abort an episode. Colchicine, 0.2–0.5 mg/d, sometimes reduces the frequency of attacks.

Chattopadhay A, Shetty KV: Recurrent aphthous stomatitis. Otolaryngol Clin North Am 2011;44:79 [PMID: 21093624].

2. Vitiligo

Vitiligo is characterized clinically by the development of areas of depigmentation. These are often symmetrical and occur mainly on extensor surfaces. The depigmentation results from a destruction of melanocytes. The basis for this destruction is unknown, but immunologically mediated damage is likely and vitiligo sometimes occurs in individuals with autoimmune endocrinopathies.

▶ Treatment

Treatment is with potent topical steroids or tacrolimus. Topical calcipotriene has also been used. Narrow-band ultraviolet B radiation (UVB 311 nm) may be used in severe cases. Response to treatment is slow often requiring many months to years.

Tamesis ME, Morellij JG: Vitiligo in childhood: A state of the art review. Pediatr Dermatol 2010;27:437 [PMID: 20553403].

16 Eye

Rebecca Sands Braverman, MD

Normal vision is a sense that develops during infancy and childhood. Pediatric ophthalmology emphasizes early diagnosis and treatment of pediatric eye diseases in order to obtain the best possible visual outcome. Eye disease in children is not always limited to the ocular system and may be a sign of systemic disease.

COMMON NONSPECIFIC SIGNS & SYMPTOMS

Nonspecific signs and symptoms commonly occur as the chief complaint or as an element of the history of a child with eye disease. Five of these findings are described here, along with a sixth—leukocoria—which is less common, but often has serious implications. Do not hesitate to seek the help of a pediatric ophthalmologist when you believe the diagnosis and treatment of these signs and symptoms requires in-depth clinical experience.

RED EYE

Redness (injection) of the bulbar conjunctiva or deeper vessels is a common presenting complaint. It may be mild and localized or diffuse and bilateral. Causes include superficial or penetrating foreign bodies, infection, allergy, and conjunctivitis associated with systemic entities such as Stevens-Johnson syndrome or Kawasaki disease. Irritating noxious agents also cause injection. Subconjunctival hemorrhage may be traumatic or spontaneous or may be associated with hematopoietic disease, vascular anomalies, or inflammatory processes. Uncommonly, an injected eye can be due to an intraocular or orbital tumor.

TEARING

Tearing in infants is usually due to nasolacrimal obstruction but may also be associated with congenital glaucoma, in which case photophobia and blepharospasm may also be present. Inflammation, allergic and viral diseases, or conjunctival and corneal irritation can also cause tearing.

DISCHARGE

Purulent discharge is usually associated with bacterial conjunctivitis. In infants and toddlers with nasolacrimal obstruction, a mucopurulent discharge may be present with low-grade, chronic dacryocystitis. Watery discharge occurs with viral infection, iritis, superficial foreign bodies, and nasolacrimal obstruction. Mucoid discharge may be a sign of allergic conjunctivitis or nasolacrimal obstruction. A mucoid discharge due to allergy typically contains eosinophils; a purulent bacterial discharge contains polymorphonuclear leukocytes.

PAIN & FOREIGN BODY SENSATION

Pain in or around the eye may be due to foreign bodies, corneal abrasions, lacerations, acute infections of the globe or ocular adnexa, iritis, and angle-closure glaucoma. Large refractive errors or poor accommodative ability may manifest as headaches. Trichiasis (inturned lashes) and contact lens problems also cause ocular discomfort.

PHOTOPHOBIA

Acute aversion to light may occur with corneal abrasions, foreign bodies, and iritis. Squinting of one eye in bright light is a common sign of intermittent exotropia. Photophobia is present in infants with glaucoma, albinism, aniridia, and retinal dystrophies such as achromatopsia. Photophobia is common after ocular surgery and after dilation of the pupil with mydriatic and cycloplegic agents. Photophobia in individuals with no ocular pathology may be due to migraine headache, meningitis, and retrobulbar optic neuritis.

LEUKOCORIA

Although not a common sign or complaint, leukocoria (a white pupil) is associated with serious diseases and requires prompt ophthalmologic consultation. Causes of leukocoria include retinoblastoma, retinopathy of prematurity, pupillary

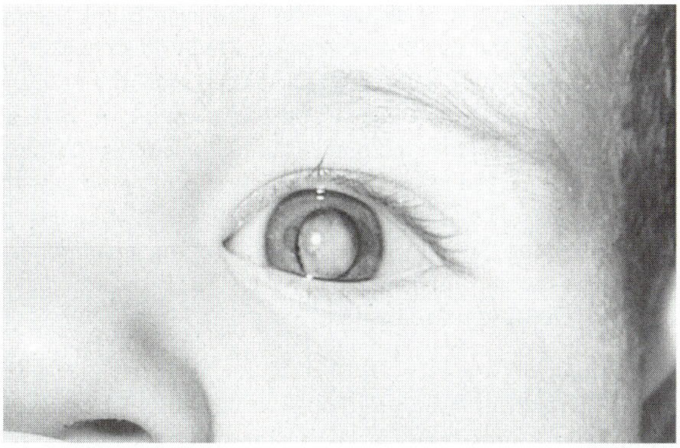

▲ **Figure 16–1.** Leukocoria of the left eye caused by retrolental membrane (persistent hyperplastic primary vitreous or persistent fetal vasculature).

membrane, cataract, vitreous opacities, retinal detachment, *Toxocara* infection, and retinal dysplasia (Figure 16–1).

REFRACTIVE ERRORS

ESSENTIALS OF DIAGNOSIS & TYPICAL FEATURES

- Significant refractive errors (myopia, hyperopia, astigmatism, or anisometropia) may cause decreased visual acuity, amblyopia, and strabismus.
- Symptoms and signs of uncorrected refractive error include blurred vision, squinting, headaches, fatigue with visual tasks, and failure of visual acuity screening.

Pathogenesis

Refractive error refers to the optical state of the eye (Figure 16–2). The shape of the cornea and, to a lesser extent, the shape of the lens and length of the eye play a role in the refractive state of the eye. Children at particular risk for refractive errors requiring correction with spectacles (glasses) include those who were born prematurely, those with Down syndrome, those who are offspring of parents with refractive errors, and those who have certain systemic conditions such as Stickler, Marfan, or Ehlers-Danlos syndrome.

Diagnosis

There are three common refractive errors: myopia, hyperopia, and astigmatism. Inequality of the refractive state between the two eyes (anisometropia) can cause amblyopia.

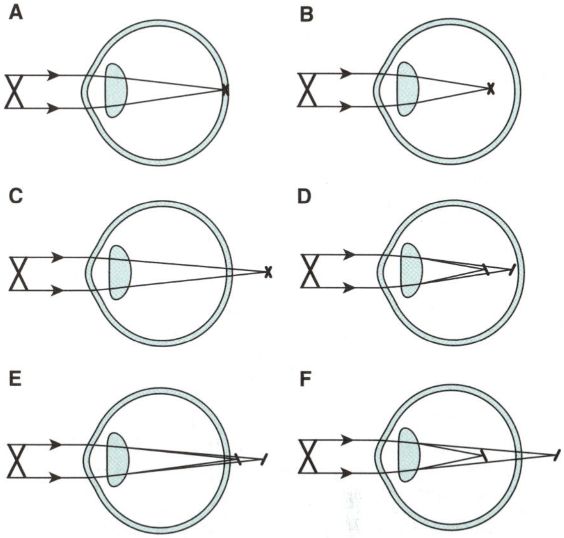

▲ **Figure 16–2.** Different refractive states of the eye. **A:** Emmetropia. Image plane from parallel rays of light falls on retina. **B:** Myopia. Image plane focuses anterior to retina. **C:** Hyperopia. Image plane focuses posterior to retina. **D:** Astigmatism, myopic type. Images in horizontal and vertical planes focus anterior to retina. **E:** Astigmatism, hyperopic type. Images in horizontal and vertical planes focus posterior to retina. **F:** Astigmatism, mixed type. Images in horizontal and vertical planes focus on either side of retina.

The refractive state is determined by an eye care professional via a procedure called refraction. The determination of the refractive state in a preverbal child often proves challenging. If there is concern that there may be a significant problem with a preverbal child's vision, they should be referred to an eye care professional specially trained for treating children.

Treatment

Not all refractive errors require correction, but severe errors can cause amblyopia (reduced vision with or without an organic lesion). Refractive errors in children are most commonly treated with glasses. Less often, contact lenses are required, usually for very high or asymmetrical refractive errors, or for adolescents who do not want to wear spectacles. Laser refractive surgery is not indicated for most children.

MYOPIA (NEARSIGHTEDNESS)

For the myopic or nearsighted individual, objects nearby are in focus; those at a distance are blurred. This is because the plane of focus is anterior to the retina. The onset is typically at about age 8 years and may progress throughout adolescence and young adulthood. A myopic person may squint to produce a pinhole effect, which improves distance vision. Divergent lenses provide clear distance vision. Many studies have attempted to slow or stop myopic progression. Atropine eye drops have shown some effect, but produce many side effects. A newer drug, pirenzepine, has shown promise in animal studies, but human studies have not shown a significant decrease in the magnitude of myopic progression.

HYPEROPIA (FARSIGHTEDNESS)

Saying that the hyperopic child is sighted for far (not near) vision is somewhat misleading, because the child can focus on near objects if the hyperopia is not excessive. Large amounts of uncorrected hyperopia can cause esotropia (inward deviation, or crossing, of the eyes) and amblyopia (see later sections on Amblyopia and Strabismus). Most infants have a hyperopic refraction that begins to diminish during the toddler years and does not require correction.

ASTIGMATISM

When either the cornea or the crystalline lens is not perfectly spherical, an image will not be sharply focused in one plane. Schematically, there will be two planes of focus. Both of the planes can be either in front of or behind the retina, or one of the planes can be in front of the retina and the other behind it. This refractive state is described as astigmatism. Large amounts of astigmatism not corrected at an early age can cause decreased vision from amblyopia, but proper refractive correction can prevent this.

OPHTHALMIC EXAMINATION

A history suggesting poor vision or misalignment of the eyes, visual acuity that falls outside the expected level for a specific age, eyelid malposition, abnormal pupil reactivity or shape, and presence of an asymmetric/abnormal red reflex requires referral to an ophthalmologist.

The American Academy of Pediatrics (AAP), American Association for Pediatric Ophthalmology and Strabismus (AAPOS), and the American Academy of Ophthalmology (AAO) policy statements for red reflex testing can be accessed at http://aappolicy.aappublications.org/.

Prompt detection and treatment of ocular conditions can prevent a lifetime of visual disability. The ophthalmic examination should be a part of every well-child assessment.

It is crucial to check newborn infants for vision or life threatening conditions that present with an abnormal red reflex that may be caused by cataracts or intraocular tumors. Eyelid ptosis (droopy eyelid) that obstructs the visual axis can cause permanent visual acuity loss from deprivation amblyopia and/or induced astigmatism, and requires urgent consultation with an ophthalmologist.

From birth to 3 years of age, the ophthalmic examination should include taking a history for ocular problems, vision assessment, inspection of the eyelids and eyes, pupil examination, ocular motility assessment, and red reflex check.

The ophthalmic examination of children older than 3 years should include taking a history for ocular problems, inspection of the eyelids and eyes, pupil examination, ocular motility assessment, and red reflex check and visual acuity testing with Allen, Lea, HOTV, Tumbling E, or Snellen symbols. Direct ophthalmoscopy should be attempted. Testing of binocular status can be accomplished by various tests, including the Random Dot E stereoacuity test.

HISTORY

Evaluation begins by ascertaining the chief complaint and taking a history of the present illness. Elements of the ocular history include onset of the complaint, its duration, whether it is monocular or binocular, treatment received thus far, and associated systemic symptoms. If an infectious disease is suspected, ask about possible contact with others having similar findings. The history should include prior ocular disease, perinatal and developmental history, any history of allergy, history of familial ocular disorders.

VISUAL ACUITY

Visual acuity testing is the most important test of visual function and should be part of every general physical examination (http://one.aao.org/Flash/VisionScreening/PediatricVisionScreening.html). Acuity should be tested in each eye individually, using an adhesive eye patch to prevent peeking. Glasses that were previously prescribed should be worn during vision screening. In older children who can cooperate, use of a pinhole will improve vision in children not wearing the appropriate spectacle prescription.

Vision Screening

Vision screening in the pediatric age group is a challenge, especially in younger and developmentally delayed children. Accuracy of the screening test being administered to a particular population and expense in terms of time, equipment, and personnel are some factors that must be considered in choosing a screening test. Vision screening should be done at well child visits. Further information on vision screening can be found at the AAP website (http://www.aap.org). Risk factors that should be screened for because they interfere with normal visual development and are amblyogenic include media opacities (such as cataracts), strabismus, and refractive errors that are different in the two eyes (anisometropia) or of large magnitude in both eyes.

In the sleeping newborn, the presence of a blepharospastic response to bright light is an adequate response. At age 6 weeks, eye-to-eye contact with slow, following movements is usually present. By age 3 months, the infant should demonstrate fixing and following ocular movements for objects at a distance of 2–3 ft. At age 6 months, interest in movement across the room is the norm. Vision can be recorded for the presence or absence of fixing and following behavior, and whether vision is steady (unsteady when nystagmus is present) and maintained.

In the verbal child, the use of familiar icons will allow for a quantitative test. Allen or Lea symbols with familiar pictures can be used to test children 2–3 years of age. When it is not possible to measure visual acuity or assess alignment in the preschool-aged child, random dot stereopsis testing (for depth perception) is effective in screening for manifest strabismus and amblyopia, but this test may miss some cases of anisometropic (unequal refractive error) amblyopia and small-angle strabismus, and is not designed to detect refractive errors.

Four-year-old children are often ready to play the tumbling E game (in which the child identifies the orientation of the letter E, which is turned in one of four directions) or the HOTV letters game (in which these four letters are shown individually at a distance and matched on a board that the child is holding). Literate children are tested with Snellen letters. Typical acuity levels in developmentally appropriate children are approximately 20/60 or better in children younger than 2–3 years, 20/40–20/30 in 3-year-old children, 20/30–20/25 in 4-year-old children, and 20/20 in literate children 5–6 years old. Referral criteria for children 3–5 years of age include visual acuity of less than 20/40 or 10/20 in either eye or a two-line difference between the eyes. Children 6 years or older should be referred if their visual acuity is less than 20/30 or 20/15 in either eye or a two-line difference is noted between the eyes.

The practitioner should be aware of two situations in which vision screening is complicated by nystagmus. Children who require a face turn or torticollis (in which the head is tilted to the right or left) to quiet the nystagmus will have poor visual acuity results when tested in the absence of the compensatory head posture. When latent nystagmus is present, acuity testing is particularly challenging (see later section on Nystagmus). Nystagmus appears or worsens when an eye is occluded, degrading central vision. To minimize the nystagmus, the occluder should be held about 12 inches in front of the eye not being tested. Testing both eyes simultaneously without occlusion often gives a better visual acuity measurement than when either eye is tested individually.

Traditional vision screening methods using eye charts in children aged 3–5 years require the child's cooperation as well as proficiency in testing by the examiner. Additional screening modalities including photoscreening and autorefractors have been used by various volunteer programs in schools, day care facilities, as well as physician offices. Photoscreening does not screen directly for amblyopia but for amblyogenic factors, which include strabismus, media opacities, eyelid ptosis, and refractive errors. Autorefractors can determine if there is a significant refractive error present in either eye or if there is a significant difference between the two eyes. Some autorefractors can also detect strabismus and eyelid ptosis. If the screening results suggest an amblyogenic factor, children are referred to an eye care professional for a complete eye examination. Problems exist with sensitivity and specificity of the instruments and poor follow-up for referrals made to eye care professionals. The cost-effectiveness of various vision screening modalities remains an area of continued research.

Davidson S, Quinn GE: The impact of pediatric vision disorders in adulthood. Pediatrics 2011 Feb;127(2):334–339 [Epub 2011 Jan 3] [Review] [PMID: 21199855].

Chou R, Dana T, Bougatsos C: Screening for visual impairment in children ages 1-5 years: Update for the USPSTF. Pediatrics 2011 Feb;127(2):e442–e479 [Epub 2011 Jan 31] [Review] [PMID: 21282269].

EXTERNAL EXAMINATION

Inspection of the anterior segment of the globe and its adnexa requires adequate illumination and often magnification. A penlight provides good illumination and should be used in both straight-ahead and oblique illumination. A Wood lamp or a blue filter cap placed over a penlight is needed for evaluation after applying a fluorescein. Immobilization of the child may be necessary. A drop of topical anesthetic may facilitate the examination.

In cases of suspected foreign body, pulling down on the lower lid provides excellent visualization of the inferior cul-de-sac (palpebral conjunctiva). Visualizing the upper cul-de-sac and superior bulbar conjunctiva is possible by having the patient look inferiorly while the upper lid is pulled away from the globe and the examiner peers into the upper recess. Illumination with a penlight is necessary. The upper lid should be everted to evaluate the superior tarsal conjunctiva (Figure 16–3).

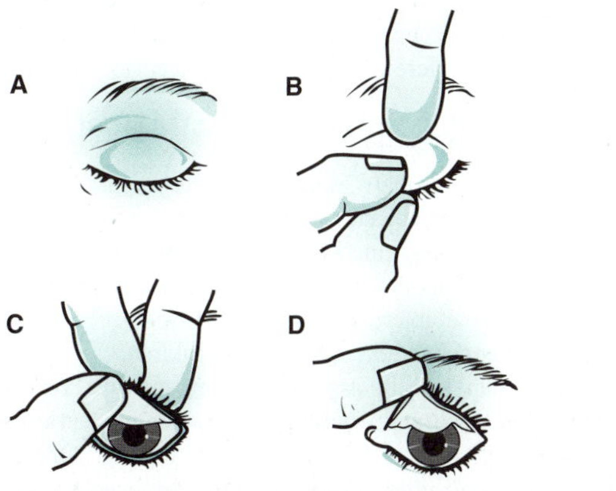

▲ **Figure 16–3.** Eversion of the upper lid. **A:** The patient looks downward. **B:** The fingers pull the lid down, and an index finger or cotton tip is placed on the upper tarsal border. **C:** The lid is pulled up over the finger. **D:** The lid is everted.

When indicated for further evaluation of the cornea, a small amount of fluorescein solution should be instilled into the lower cul-de-sac. Blue light will stain defects yellow-green. Disease-specific staining patterns may be observed. For example, herpes simplex lesions of the corneal epithelium produce a dendrite or branchlike pattern. A foreign body lodged beneath the upper lid shows one or more vertical lines of stain on the cornea due to the constant movement of the foreign body over the cornea. Contact lens overwear produces a central staining pattern. A fine, scattered punctate pattern may be a sign of viral keratitis or medication toxicity. Punctate erosions of the inferior third of the cornea can be seen with staphylococcal blepharitis or exposure keratitis secondary to incomplete lid closure.

PUPILS

The pupils should be evaluated for reaction to light, regularity of shape, and equality of size as well as for the presence of afferent pupillary defect. This defect, which occurs in optic nerve disease, is evaluated by the swinging flashlight test (see later section on Diseases of the Optic Nerve). Irregular pupils are associated with iritis, trauma, pupillary membranes, and structural defects such as iris coloboma (see later section on Iris Coloboma).

Pupils vary in size due to lighting conditions and age. In general, infants have miotic (constricted) pupils. Children have larger pupils than either infants or adults, whereas the elderly have miotic pupils.

Anisocoria, a size difference between the two pupils, may be physiologic if the size difference is within 1 mm and is the same in light and dark. Anisocoria occurs with Horner syndrome, third nerve palsy, Adie tonic pupil, iritis, and trauma. Medication could also cause abnormal pupil size or reactivity. For example, contact with atropine-like substances (belladonna alkaloids) will cause pupillary dilation and limit pupillary reaction. Systemic antihistamines and scopolamine patches, among other medicines, can dilate the pupils and interfere with accommodation (focusing).

ALIGNMENT & MOTILITY EVALUATION

Alignment and motility should be tested because amblyopia is associated with strabismus, a misalignment of the visual axes of the eyes. Besides alignment, ocular rotations should be evaluated in the six cardinal positions of gaze (Table 16–1; Figure 16–4). A small toy is an interesting target for testing ocular rotations in infants; a penlight works well in older children.

Alignment can be assessed in several ways. In order of increasing accuracy, these methods are observation, the corneal light reflex test, and cover testing. Observation is an educated guess about whether the eyes are properly aligned. Corneal light reflex evaluation (Hirschberg test) is performed by shining a light beam at the patient's eyes, observing the reflections off each cornea, and estimating whether these "reflexes" appear to be positioned properly. If the reflection of light is noted temporally on the cornea, esotropia is suspected (Figure 16–5). Nasal reflection of the light suggests exotropia (outward deviation). Accuracy of these tests increases with increasing angles of misalignment.

Another way of evaluating alignment is with the cover test, in which the patient fixes on a target while one eye is covered. If an esotropia or an exotropia is present, the deviated

Table 16–1. Function and innervation of each of the extraocular muscles.

Muscle	Function	Innervation
Medial rectus	Adductor	Oculomotor (third)
Lateral rectus	Abductor	Abducens (sixth)
Inferior rectus	Depressor, adductor, extorter	Oculomotor
Superior rectus	Elevator, adductor, intorter	Oculomotor
Inferior oblique	Elevator, abductor, extorter	Oculomotor
Superior oblique	Depressor, abductor, intorter	Trochlear (fourth)

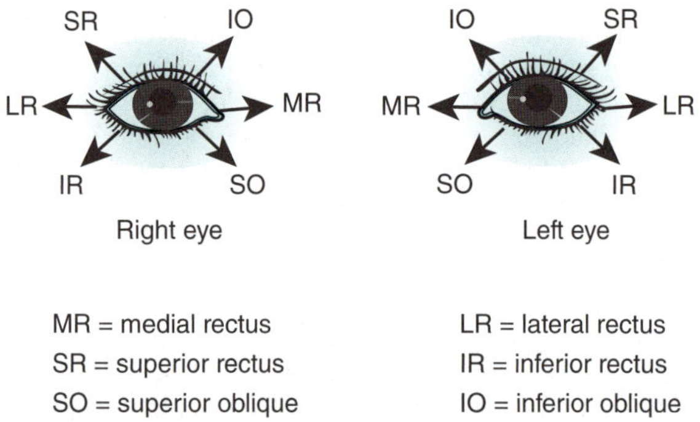

▲ **Figure 16–4.** Cardinal positions of gaze and muscles primarily tested in those fields of gaze. Arrow indicates position in which each muscle is tested.

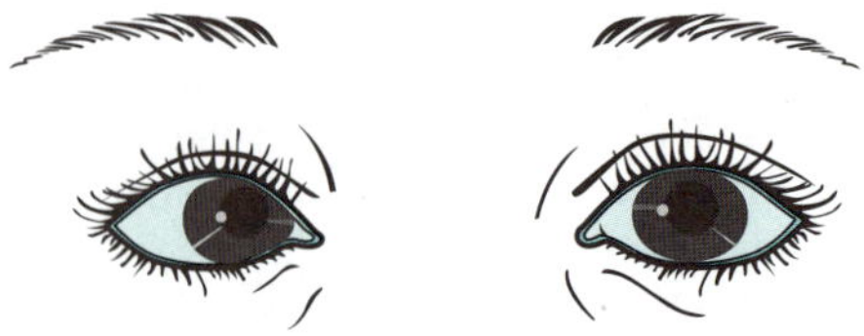

▲ **Figure 16–5.** Temporal displacement of light reflection showing esotropia (inward deviation) of the right eye. Nasal displacement of the reflection would show exotropia (outward deviation) of the left eye.

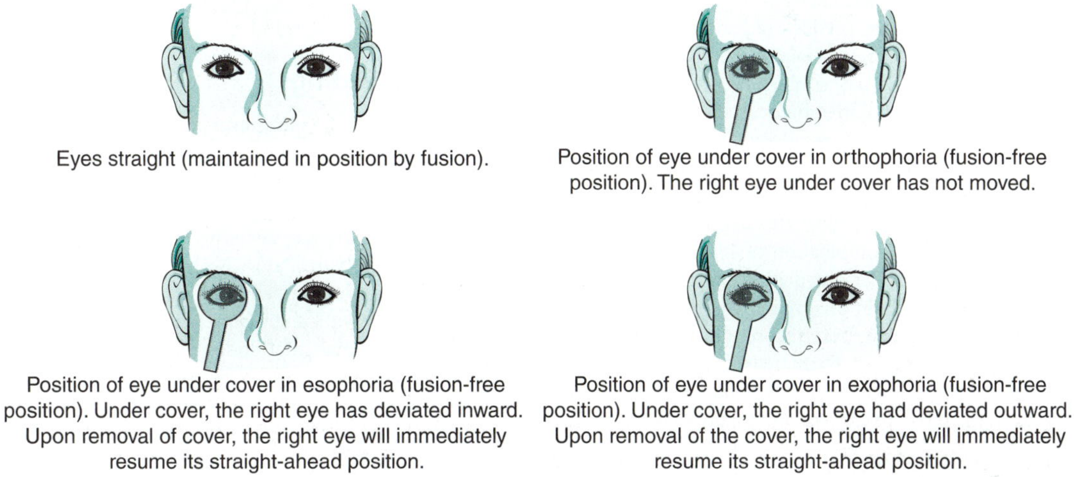

▲ **Figure 16–6.** Cover testing. The patient is instructed to look at a target at eye level 20 ft away. Note that in the presence of constant strabismus (ie, a tropia rather than a phoria), the deviation will remain when the cover is removed. (Reprinted, with permission, from Riordan-Eva P, Whitcher J: *Vaughan & Asbury's General Ophthalmology*, 17th ed. McGraw-Hill, 2008.)

eye will make a corrective movement to fixate on the target when the previously fixating eye is occluded. The other eye is tested similarly. When the occluder is removed from the eye just uncovered, a refixation movement of that eye indicates a phoria, or latent deviation, if alignment is reestablished. If the uncovered eye picks up fixation and strabismus is still present, then that eye can be presumed to be dominant and the nonpreferred eye possibly amblyopic. If the eye remains deviated after the occluder is removed, a tropia is noted to be present (Figure 16–6). A deviated eye that is blind or has very poor vision will not fixate on a target. Consequently, spurious results to cover testing may occur, as can happen with disinterest on the part of the patient, small-angle strabismus, and inexperience in administering cover tests.

Red Reflex Test

ESSENTIALS OF DIAGNOSIS & TYPICAL FEATURES

- The handheld ophthalmoscope is the tool necessary to check the red reflex of the eye.
- Simultaneous examination of both pupils at the same time is called the Brückner test.

▶ Clinical Findings

The examiner should see a round, red light in both eyes. The red reflex of each eye can be compared simultaneously when the observer is approximately 4 ft away from the patient. The largest diameter of light is shown through the ophthalmoscope, and no correction (zero setting) is dialed in the ophthalmoscope unless it is to compensate for the examiner's uncorrected refractive error. A red reflex chart is available through the AAP policy statement on red reflex testing on pediatric patients at http://aappolicy.aappublications.org/.

▶ Differential Diagnosis

The red reflex test (Brückner test) is useful for identifying disorders such as media opacities (eg, cataracts), large refractive errors, tumors such as retinoblastoma, and strabismus.

▶ Treatment

A difference in quality of the red reflexes between the two eyes constitutes a positive Brückner test and requires referral to an ophthalmologist.

American Academy of Pediatrics; Section on Ophthalmology; American Association for Pediatric Ophthalmology and Strabismus; American Academy of Ophthalmology; American Association of Certified Orthoptists: Red reflex examination in neonates, infants, and children. Pediatrics 2008 Dec;122(6):1401–1404 [Review]. Erratum in: Pediatrics 2009;123(4):1254 [PMID: 19047263].

OPHTHALMOSCOPIC EXAMINATION

A handheld direct ophthalmoscope allows visualization of the ocular fundus. As the patient's pupil becomes more constricted, viewing the fundus becomes more difficult. Although it is taught that pupillary dilation can precipitate an attack of closed-angle glaucoma in the predisposed adult, children are very rarely predisposed to angle closure. Exceptions include those with a dislocated lens, past surgery, or an eye previously compromised by a retrolental membrane, such as in retinopathy of prematurity. Therefore, if an adequate view of the fundus is precluded by a miotic pupil, use of a dilating agent (eg, one drop in each eye of 2.5% phenylephrine or 0.5% or 1% tropicamide) should provide adequate mydriasis (dilation). In infants, one drop of a combination of 1% phenylephrine with 0.2% cyclopentolate (Cyclomydril) is safer. Structures to be observed during ophthalmoscopy include the optic disk, blood vessels, the macular reflex, and retina, as well as the clarity of the vitreous media. By increasing the amount of plus lens dialed into the instrument, the point of focus moves anteriorly from the retina to the lens and finally to the cornea.

OCULAR TRAUMA

ESSENTIALS OF DIAGNOSIS & TYPICAL FEATURES

- A careful history of the events that lead to the ocular injury is crucial in the diagnosis and treatment of ocular trauma.
- The examination of the traumatized eye may be difficult in the child due to poor cooperation and significant discomfort.
- If the extent of the eye injury is difficult to determine or if it is sight threatening, urgent referral to an ophthalmologist is necessary.

OCULAR FOREIGN BODIES

ESSENTIALS OF DIAGNOSIS & TYPICAL FEATURES

- A foreign body of the eye/globe or adnexa may be difficult to visualize due to its small size or location.
- The clinician should always maintain a high index of suspicion for an occult or intraocular foreign body if the history suggests this, and ophthalmologic referral needs to be considered.

Prevention

Protective goggles or prescription glasses can help prevent ocular injuries and should be encouraged while participating in activities at risk for eye injuries, such as grinding metal, hammering, or sawing wood.

Clinical Findings

Foreign bodies on the globe and palpebral conjunctiva usually cause discomfort and red eye. The history may suggest the origin of the foreign body, such as being around a metal grinder or being outside on a windy day when a sudden foreign body sensation was encountered associated with tearing, redness, and pain. Pain with blinking suggests that the foreign body may be trapped between the eyelid and the eye.

Magnification with a slit lamp may be needed for inspection. Foreign bodies that lodge on the upper palpebral conjunctiva are best viewed by everting the lid on itself and removing the foreign body with a cotton applicator. The conjunctival surface (palpebral conjunctiva) of the lower lid presents no problem with visualization. After simple removal of a foreign body that is thought not to be contaminated, no other treatment is needed if no corneal abrasion has occurred.

Differential Diagnosis

Corneal abrasion, corneal ulcer, globe rupture/laceration.

Complications

Pain, infection, and potential vision loss from scarring.

Treatment

When foreign bodies are noted on the bulbar conjunctiva or cornea (Figure 16–7), removal is facilitated by using a topical anesthetic. If the foreign body is not too adherent, it can be dislodged with a stream of irrigating solution (Dacriose or saline) or with a cotton applicator after instillation of a topical anesthetic. Otherwise, a foreign body spud or needle is used to undermine the foreign body. This must be done with adequate magnification and illumination. An antibiotic ointment is then instilled. Ferrous corneal bodies often have an associated rust ring, which may be removed under slit-lamp visualization in cooperative children or under anesthesia if necessary.

Prognosis

Usually excellent if treatment is obtained shortly after injury.

CORNEAL ABRASION

ESSENTIALS OF DIAGNOSIS & TYPICAL FEATURES

- A corneal abrasion results in loss of the most superficial layer of corneal cells and causes severe ocular pain, tearing, and blepharospasm.
- An inciting event is usually identifiable as the cause of a corneal abrasion.

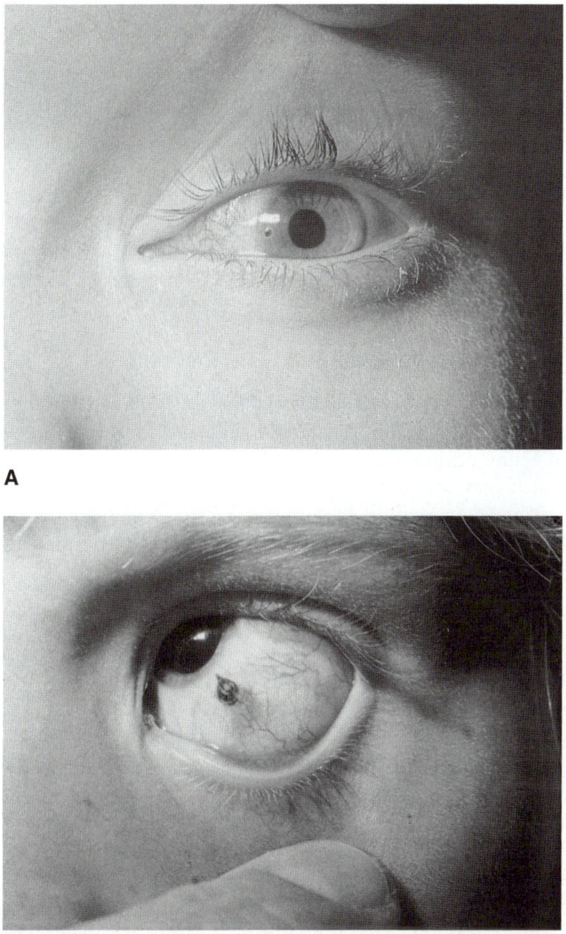

A

B

▲ **Figure 16–7.** **A:** Corneal foreign body at the nasal edge of the cornea. **B:** Subconjunctival foreign body of graphite.

Pathogenesis

Children often suffer corneal abrasions accidentally while playing with siblings or pets as well as participating in sports. Contact lens users frequently develop abrasions due to poorly fitting lenses, overnight wear, and use of torn or damaged lenses.

Prevention

Proper contact lens care and parental supervision can prevent activities that can lead to a corneal abrasion.

Clinical Findings

Symptom of a corneal abrasion is sudden and severe eye pain, usually after an inciting event such as an accidental finger poke to the eye. Decreased vision secondary to pain and tearing are common complaints. Eyelid edema, tearing, injection of the conjunctiva, and poor cooperation with the ocular examination due to pain are common signs of a corneal abrasion. Fluorescein dye is instilled into the eye and a cobalt blue or Wood lamp is used to illuminate the affected eye. The area with the abrasion will stain bright yellow.

Differential Diagnosis

Ocular or adnexal foreign bodies, corneal ulcer, corneal laceration.

Complications

Possible vision loss from corneal infection and scarring.

Treatment

Ophthalmic ointment, such as erythromycin ointment, lubricates the surface of the cornea and also helps prevent infections. Patching the affected eye when a large abrasion is present may provide comfort but is not advised for corneal abrasions caused by contact lens wear or other potentially contaminated sources. Large corneal abrasions result in referred pain to the ipsilateral brow. If a brow ache is present, it may be treated by the use of a topical cycloplegic agent such as 1% cyclopentolate. Daily follow-up is required until healing is complete.

Prognosis

Excellent if corneal infection and scarring do not occur.

INTRAOCULAR FOREIGN BODIES & PERFORATING OCULAR INJURIES

ESSENTIALS OF DIAGNOSIS & TYPICAL FEATURES

- Severe trauma may result in penetration of the eye by foreign bodies or retained foreign bodies, and is an ocular emergency.

Pathogenesis

Intraocular foreign bodies and penetrating injuries are most often caused by being in close proximity to high-velocity projectiles such as windshield glass broken during a motor vehicle accident, metal ground without use of protective safety goggles, and improperly detonated fireworks.

Prevention

Use protective eyewear when engaging in activities at risk for ocular injury.

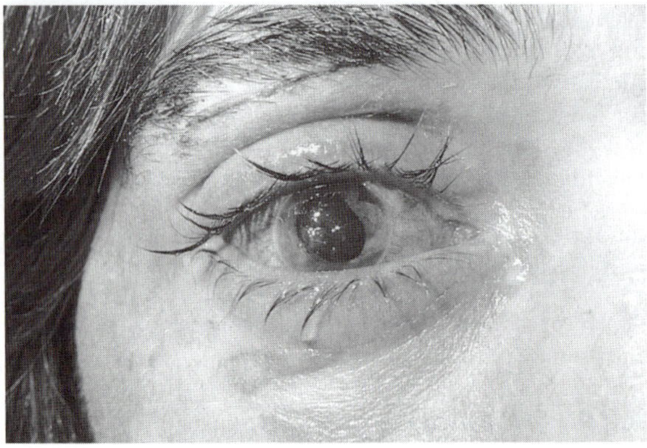

▲ **Figure 16–8.** Corneal laceration with irregular pupil and vitreous loss.

Clinical Findings

Sudden ocular pain occurs; vision loss, as well as multiple organ trauma, may be present.

Intraocular foreign bodies and corneal and scleral lacerations (ruptured globe) require emergency referral to an ophthalmologist. The diagnosis may be difficult if the obvious signs of corneal perforation (shallow anterior chamber with hyphema, traumatic cataract, and irregular pupil) are not present (Figure 16–8). Furthermore, nonradiopaque materials such as glass will not be seen on x-ray film.

Computed tomographic (CT) scan may be useful in evaluating ocular trauma, including bony injury and intraocular foreign bodies. Magnetic resonance imaging (MRI) must be avoided if a magnetic foreign body is suspected.

Differential Diagnosis

Corneal abrasion, superficial foreign body of the eye or eyelids.

Complications

Vision loss, intraocular infection, loss of the eye.

Treatment

In cases of suspected intraocular foreign body or perforation of the globe, it may be best to keep the child at rest, gently shield the eye with a metal shield or cut-down paper cup, and keep the extent of examination to a minimum to prevent expulsion of intraocular contents. In this setting, the child should be given nothing by mouth in case eye examination under anesthesia or surgical repair is required.

Prognosis

Depends on the extent of the trauma.

BLUNT ORBITAL TRAUMA

ESSENTIALS OF DIAGNOSIS & TYPICAL FEATURES

- Blunt orbital and soft tissue trauma may produce so-called black eye or ecchymosis (blue or purplish hemorrhagic areas) of the eyelids.

Pathogenesis

Trauma to the orbit from a closed fist, collision with another player during team sports, and falls are common causes of blunt orbital injuries. Orbital compartment syndrome, which may result from severe orbital trauma, is caused by hemorrhaging within the orbit or severe orbital edema (or both). This is an emergency which may lead to permanent vision loss if not treated urgently.

Prevention

Protective eyewear during athletic activities and adequate supervision of children at home and school.

Clinical Findings

Blunt trauma to the orbit may result in orbit fractures. The orbital floor is a common location for a fracture (called a blowout fracture). A specific fracture that occurs mainly in children after blunt orbit trauma is called the white-eyed blowout fracture. This results from a greenstick fracture of the orbit with entrapment of extraocular muscles. It is called "white-eyed" because the external orbital soft tissue injury may appear to be minimal, but the patient will have severe pain with eye movement, as well as nausea, vomiting, and restriction of eye movements.

A blowout fracture must be suspected in a patient with symptoms of double vision, pain with eye movements, and restriction of extraocular muscle movements after blunt orbital trauma. CT images of an orbital floor fracture often reveal herniation of orbital fat or the inferior rectus muscle into the maxillary sinus. Assessment of ocular motility, globe integrity, and intraocular pressure will determine the extent of the blunt orbital injury. Consultation with an ophthalmologist is necessary to determine the full spectrum of the patient's injuries.

Orbital compartment syndrome is an emergency requiring immediate treatment. Patients present with severe edema or ecchymosis of the eyelids (which makes it very difficult to open the eyelids), proptosis, and possibly an acute traumatic optic neuropathy resulting in decreased vision or an afferent pupillary defect. Neuroimaging may reveal a retrobulbar hemorrhage and proptosis.

Differential Diagnosis

Orbit fracture with or without muscle entrapment, globe rupture, orbital compartment syndrome, traumatic or ischemic optic neuropathy.

Treatment

Orbital compartment syndrome requires emergent lateral eyelid canthotomy and cantholysis to decompress the orbit. Treatment should not be delayed in order to image the orbits. Prompt treatment can prevent permanent vision loss.

Patients with clinical signs of muscle entrapment require urgent surgical repair to avoid permanent ischemic injury to the involved extraocular muscle. Large fractures may need repair to prevent enophthalmos, a sunken appearance to the orbit. This can usually be performed on a nonemergent basis.

Cold compresses or ice packs for brief periods (eg, 10 minutes at a time) are recommended in older children in the first 24 hours after injury to reduce hemorrhage and swelling.

Prognosis

The prognosis depends on the severity of the blunt trauma, associated ocular injuries, and extent of the orbit fractures.

Carroll SC, Ng SG: Outcomes of orbital blowout fracture surgery in children and adolescents. Br J Ophthalmol 2010 Jun;94(6):736–739 [PMID: 20508048].

LACERATIONS

ESSENTIALS OF DIAGNOSIS & TYPICAL FEATURES

- Inspection of the eyelids reveals the extent and severity of the traumatic laceration.
- Lacerations of the nasal third of the eyelid and involving the eyelid margin are at risk for lacrimal system injury and subsequent chronic tearing.

Pathogenesis

Lacerations of the eyelids and lacrimal system often result from dog bites, car accidents, falls, and fights.

Prevention

Supervision of children at home and while at school.

Clinical Findings

Eyelid lacerations may be partial or full thickness in depth depending on the extent of the injury. Foreign bodies such as glass or gravel may be present depending on the mechanism of the injury.

Differential Diagnosis

Lacerations involving the eyelid may or may not involve the nasolacrimal duct system or eyelid margin. Globe injury may be associated with eyelid lacerations as well.

Complications

Poor surgical repair of lacerations of the eyelid margin can result in eyelid malposition, which causes chronic ocular surface irritation and possible corneal scarring.

Treatment

Except for superficial lacerations away from the globe, repair in children is best performed in the operating room under general anesthesia. Special consideration must be given to lacerations involving the lid margin, significant tissue loss, full-thickness lacerations, lacerations that may involve the levator muscle in the upper lid, and to those that may involve the canaliculus (Figure 16–9). These injuries are best repaired by an ophthalmologist and may require intubation of the nasolacrimal system with silicone tubes.

Prognosis

It depends on severity of the injury, tissue loss, and adequacy of surgical repair.

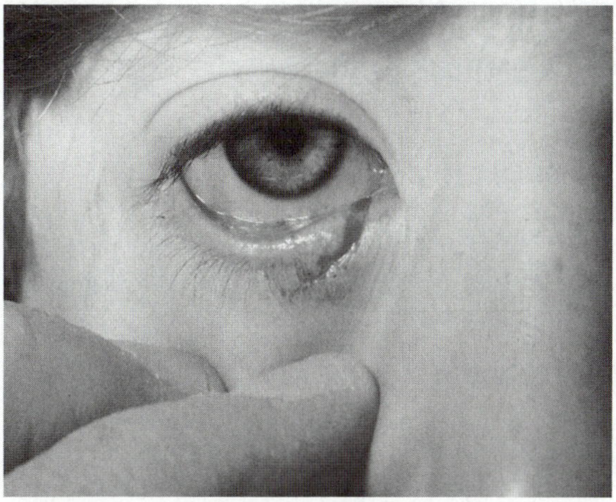

▲ **Figure 16–9.** Laceration involving right lower lid and canaliculus.

BURNS

ESSENTIALS OF DIAGNOSIS & TYPICAL FEATURES

- Severe thermal or chemical burns can result in permanent vision loss, ectropion or entropion of the lid, and scarring of the conjunctiva and cul-de-sac.

Pathogenesis

Chemical burns with strong acidic and alkaline agents can be blinding and constitute a true ocular emergency. Examples are burns caused by exploding batteries, spilled drain cleaner, and bleach. Eyelid burns can occur in toddlers from contact with a lighted cigarette. The cornea is often involved as well. Curling irons can cause similar burns. Burns of the conjunctiva and cornea may be thermal, radiant, or chemical. Radiant energy causes ultraviolet keratitis. Typical examples are welder's burn and burns associated with skiing without goggles in bright sunlight.

Prevention

Protective eyewear when engaging in activities that pose a potential risk for exposure to hazardous chemicals, radiant energy, or when explosive conditions are possible.

Clinical Findings

Superficial thermal burns cause pain, tearing, and injection. Corneal epithelial defects can be diagnosed using fluorescein dye, which will stain areas of the cornea bright yellow where the epithelium is absent. The fluorescein dye pattern will show a uniformly stippled appearance of the corneal epithelium in ultraviolet keratitis.

Differential Diagnosis

Corneal abrasion, iritis.

Complications

Significant corneal injury, especially if associated with an alkali burn, may lead to scarring and vision loss. Eyelid scarring can result in chronic exposure, dry eye, irritation, and entropion or ectropion.

Treatment

Alkalis tend to penetrate deeper than acids into ocular tissue and often causes severe injury. Damage to the conjunctival vessels gives the eye a white or blanched appearance, resulting in ocular ischemia. Immediate treatment consists of copious irrigation and removal of precipitates as soon as possible after the injury. Initial stabilization of the injury is initiated by using topical antibiotics and patching the injured eye closed. A cycloplegic agent such as cyclopentolate 1% may be added if corneal involvement is present. This reduces the pain from ciliary spasm and iritis that may accompany the injury. The patient should be referred to an ophthalmologist after immediate first aid has been given.

Prognosis

Depends on the severity of the injury.

HYPHEMA

ESSENTIALS OF DIAGNOSIS & TYPICAL FEATURES

- Slit-lamp examination or penlight examination may reveal a layer of blood within the anterior chamber. Other injuries to the globe and orbit are often present.
- A hyphema may be microscopic or may fill the entire anterior chamber (Figure 16–10).

Pathogenesis

Blunt trauma to the globe may cause a hyphema, or bleeding within the anterior chamber, from a ruptured vessel located near the root of the iris or in the anterior chamber angle.

Prevention

Protective eyewear and appropriate supervision at home and at school.

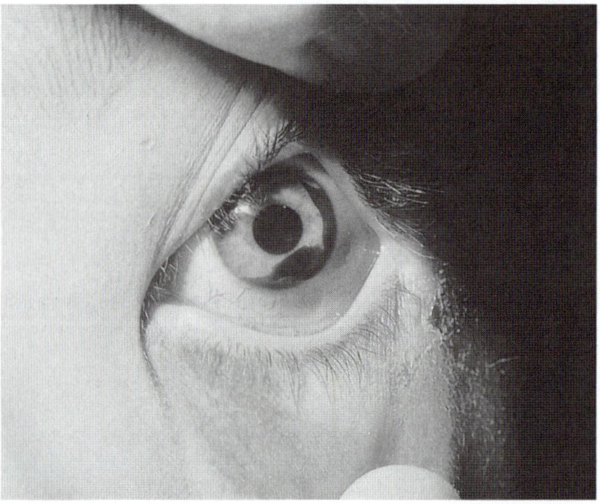

▲ **Figure 16–10.** Hyphema filling approximately 20% of the anterior chamber.

Clinical Findings

Blunt trauma severe enough to cause a hyphema may be associated with additional ocular injury, including iritis, lens subluxation, retinal edema or detachment, and glaucoma. In patients with sickle cell anemia or trait, even moderate elevations of intraocular pressure may quickly lead to optic atrophy and permanent vision loss. Therefore, all African Americans whose sickle cell status is unknown should be tested if hyphema is observed. These patients require extra vigilance in diagnosing and treating hyphema.

Differential Diagnosis

Nontraumatic causes of hyphema include juvenile xanthogranuloma and blood dyscrasias. Rarely, hyphema is noted in the newborn after a stressful birth.

Complications

Increased intraocular pressure, glaucoma, permanent corneal staining, and vision loss.

Treatment

A shield should be placed over the eye, the head elevated, and arrangements made for ophthalmologic referral.

Prognosis

The prognosis is worse if intraocular pressure is elevated, the patient has sickle cell disease, or if other associated ocular injuries are present.

ABUSIVE HEAD TRAUMA & NONACCIDENTAL TRAUMA

ESSENTIALS OF DIAGNOSIS & TYPICAL FEATURES

- Traumatic head trauma, commonly known as *shaken baby syndrome*, is a form of nonaccidental trauma characterized by a constellation of examination findings, including traumatic brain injury, retinal hemorrhages, and fractures of long bones or ribs.
- The history leading to the diagnosis of shaken baby syndrome is often vague and poorly correlated with the extent of injury.

Pathogenesis

The mechanism of injury has been ascribed to a rapid back and forth shaking of young children that results in brain and ocular injuries. It is now believed that injuries may also be the result of blunt impact. Additional injury may result from spinal cord injuries and hypoxia.

Clinical Findings

Victims often have multiple organ system involvement that includes, but is not limited to, traumatic brain injury, bone fractures, and retinal hemorrhages. The presentation can vary from irritability to emesis, change in mental status, or cardiopulmonary arrest.

Neuroimaging of the brain and a skeletal survey are used to diagnose shaken baby syndrome. Ophthalmic consultation and a dilated retinal examination are necessary to document retinal hemorrhages. Hemorrhages may be unilateral or bilateral and may be located in the posterior pole or periphery. Whereas retinal hemorrhages tend to resolve fairly quickly, those in the vitreous do not. If a blood clot lies over the macula, deprivation amblyopia may occur and may require intraocular surgery by a retinal specialist. Other ocular findings associated with nonaccidental trauma include lid ecchymosis, subconjunctival hemorrhage, hyphema, retinal folds, retinoschisis (traumatic separation of the retinal layers), and optic nerve edema. Acute-onset esotropia can also occur.

Differential Diagnosis

The differential diagnosis of retinal hemorrhages includes those secondary to a fall, seizures, chest compressions during cardiopulmonary resuscitation, blood dyscrasias, and Terson syndrome, among others. A team effort between the primary treating physician, neurosurgery, orthopedics, ophthalmology, and social services is often needed to determine the true cause of a patient's injuries.

Complications

The severity of injuries dictates the long-term outcome. Severely diffuse retinal hemorrhages, associated traumatic optic neuropathy, and cortical injury all adversely affect the potential for normal vision.

Treatment

Management of any systemic injuries is required. Observation by an ophthalmologist for resolution of retinal hemorrhages is the usual management. Vitreous hemorrhages or large preretinal hemorrhages that do not resolve within several weeks may need surgical treatment by a retinal specialist.

Prognosis

Depends on the severity of ocular and brain injuries.

Levin AV: Retinal hemorrhage in abusive head trauma. Pediatrics 2010 Nov;126(5):961–970 [Epub 2010 Oct 4] [Review] [PMID: 20921069].

PREVENTION OF OCULAR INJURIES

Air rifles, paintballs, and fireworks are responsible for many serious eye injuries in children. Golf injuries can be very severe. Bungee cords have been associated with multiple types of severe ocular trauma, including corneal abrasion, iris tears, hyphema, vitreous hemorrhage, retinal detachment, and blindness. Use of these items and associated activities should be avoided or very closely supervised. Safety goggles should be used in laboratories and industrial arts classes and when operating snow blowers, power lawn mowers, and power tools, or when using hammers and nails.

Sports-related eye injuries can be prevented with protective eyewear. Sports goggles and visors of polycarbonate plastic will prevent injuries in games using fast projectiles such as tennis or racquet balls, or where opponents may swing elbows or poke at the eye.

The one-eyed individual should be specifically advised to always wear polycarbonate eyeglasses and goggles for all sports. High-risk activities such as boxing and the martial arts should be avoided by one-eyed children.

DISORDERS OF THE OCULAR STRUCTURES

DISEASES OF THE EYELIDS

The eyelids can be affected by various dermatologic and infectious conditions.

Blepharitis

ESSENTIALS OF DIAGNOSIS & TYPICAL FEATURES

- Blepharitis is inflammation of the lid margin characterized by crusty debris at the base of the lashes, erythema of eyelid margins, and ocular irritation.

Pathogenesis

Blepharitis is caused by inflammation of the eyelid margin, meibomian gland obstruction, bacterial overgrowth, and tear film imbalance.

Prevention

Eyelid hygiene is essential to prevent or control blepharitis. Eyelid scrubs help to decrease the bacterial load on the eyelid margins and lashes. Warm compresses help to loosen the secretions of the meibomian glands.

Clinical Findings

Patients may present with dry eye symptoms, red and irritated eyelid margins, conjunctivitis, and decreased vision from corneal erosions or vascularization. When conjunctival injection accompanies blepharitis, the condition is known as blepharoconjunctivitis. *Staphylococcus* is the most common bacterial cause.

Differential Diagnosis

Chalazion, hordeolum, and rosacea blepharitis.

Complications

Permanent corneal and eyelid margin scarring in severe cases.

Treatment

Treatment includes lid scrubs with a nonburning baby shampoo several times a week, warm compresses to the eyelids, and application of a topical antibiotic ointment such as erythromycin or bacitracin at bedtime.

Prognosis

Generally good.

Chalazion

ESSENTIALS OF DIAGNOSIS & TYPICAL FEATURES

- A chalazion is an inflammation of the meibomian glands, which may produce a tender nodule over the tarsus of the upper or lower lid.
- Chalazion tends to be recurrent if eyelid hygiene is poor.

Pathogenesis

Obstruction of the eyelid margin meibomian glands with resultant inflammation, fibrosis, and granuloma formation.

Prevention

See earlier section on Blepharitis.

Clinical Findings

Eyelid nodule of variable size and localized erythema of the corresponding palpebral conjunctiva that may be associated with a yellow lipogranuloma (Figure 16–11).

Differential Diagnosis

Hordeolum, blepharitis.

Treatment

See earlier section on Blepharitis. Oral flax seed oil may also decrease the risk of recurrent chalazion. If incision and curettage are needed because the lesion is slow to resolve, the child will require a general anesthetic. Topical azithromycin (ophthalmic solution 1%) may also help decrease recurrence of chalazion, but is still under investigation.

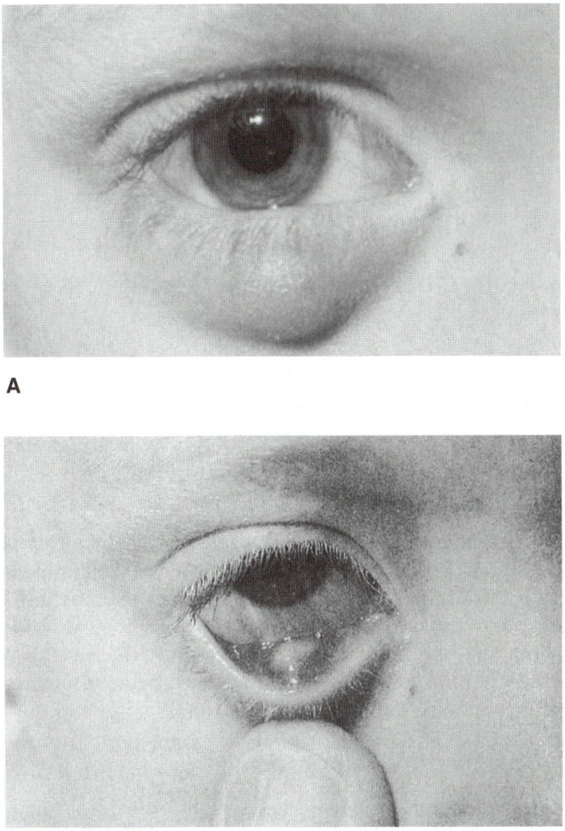

A

B

▲ **Figure 16–11.** Chalazion. **A:** Right lower lid, external view. **B:** Right lower lid conjunctival surface.

Prognosis

Generally good.

VIRAL EYELID DISEASE

ESSENTIALS OF DIAGNOSIS & TYPICAL FEATURES

- Viral infections of the eyelids can result in eyelid vesicles or papules.

Pathogenesis

Herpes simplex virus may involve the conjunctiva and lids at the time of primary herpes simplex infection resulting in blepharoconjunctivitis. Vesicular lesions with an erythematous base occur. Herpes zoster causes vesicular disease in association with a skin eruption in the dermatome of the ophthalmic branch of the trigeminal nerve. Molluscum contagiosum lesions are typically umbilicated papules. If near the lid margin, the lesions may cause conjunctivitis.

Prevention

Avoid contact with individuals with active viral infections.

Clinical Findings

A vesicular rash is the most common sign of herpes viral eyelid infection. Fluorescein dye should be administered topically to both eyes followed by examination with a cobalt blue light to determine if corneal or conjunctival involvement is present. Herpes simplex or herpes zoster can be diagnosed by rapid viral culture (24–48 hours) or detection of antigen in skin lesions (3 hours).

Differential Diagnosis

Impetigo.

Complications

Conjunctivitis, keratitis (corneal infection).

Treatment

Primary herpes simplex blepharoconjunctivitis should be treated with systemic acyclovir (a liquid formulation is available), valacyclovir, or famciclovir. When either the conjunctiva or the cornea is involved, treatment should include topical 1% trifluridine or 3% vidarabine.

Treatment of ophthalmic herpes zoster with nucleoside analogues within 5 days after onset may reduce the morbidity. When vesicles are present on the tip of the nose with herpes zoster (Hutchinson sign), ocular involvement, including iritis, is more likely.

Molluscum contagiosum lesions may be treated with cautery or excision.

Prognosis

Generally good unless corneal involvement is present.

MISCELLANEOUS EYELID INFECTIONS

Pediculosis

Pediculosis of the lids (phthiriasis palpebrarum) is caused by *Phthirus pubis*. Nits and adult lice can be seen on the eyelashes when viewed with appropriate magnification. Mechanical removal and application to the lid margins of phospholine iodide or 1% mercuric oxide ointment can be effective. Other bodily areas of involvement must also be treated if involved. Family members and contacts may also be infected (see Chapter 15).

Papillomavirus

Papillomavirus may infect the lid and conjunctiva. Warts may be recurrent, multiple, and difficult to treat. Treatment modalities include cryotherapy, cautery, carbon dioxide laser, and surgery.

Staphylococcal Infection

Localized staphylococcal infections of the glands of Zeis within the lid cause a sty (hordeolum) (Figure 16–12). When the infection coalesces and points internally or externally, it may discharge itself or require incision. The lesion is tender and red. Warm compresses help to shorten the acute process. Some practitioners prescribe a topical antibiotic ointment. Any coexisting blepharitis should be treated.

EYELID PTOSIS

ESSENTIALS OF DIAGNOSIS & TYPICAL FEATURES

- Eyelid ptosis results in a droopy eyelid that may be unilateral or bilateral. If the pupil is obstructed, deprivation amblyopia may result.

Pathogenesis

Ptosis—a droopy upper lid (Figure 16–13)—may be congenital or acquired but is usually congenital in children owing to a defective levator muscle. Other causes of ptosis are myasthenia gravis, lid injuries, third nerve palsy, and Horner syndrome (see next section). Ptosis may be associated with astigmatism and amblyopia.

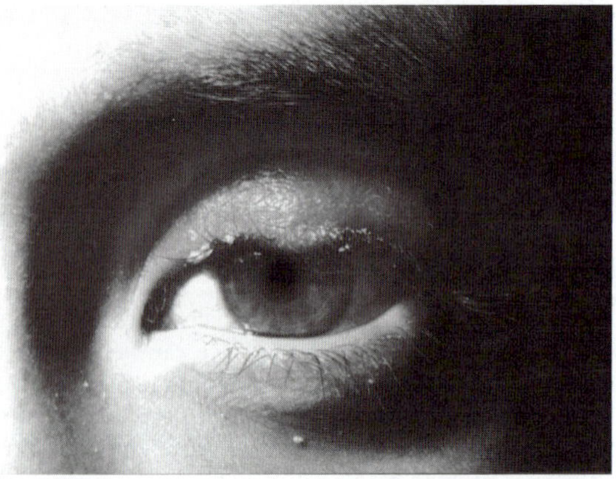

▲ **Figure 16–12.** Hordeolum and blepharitis, left upper lid.

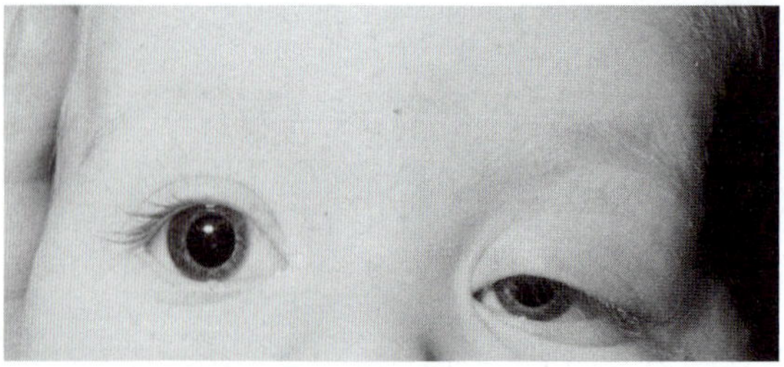

▲ **Figure 16–13.** Congenital ptosis of severe degree, left upper lid.

Prevention

Injury prevention.

Clinical Findings

An association sometimes seen with congenital ptosis is the Marcus Gunn jaw-winking phenomenon. Intermittent reduction of the ptosis occurs during mastication or sucking, due to a synkinesis or simultaneous firing of the external or internal pterygoid muscle (innervated by the trigeminal nerve) and the levator muscle (innervated by the oculomotor nerve).

Differential Diagnosis

Congenital ptosis, traumatic ptosis, neurogenic ptosis (oculomotor nerve palsy), Horner syndrome.

Complications

Deprivation amblyopia and induced astigmatism.

Treatment

Surgical correction is indicated for moderate to severe ptosis. Mild cases less often require operative management. Cosmesis may be better if surgery is delayed until most of the facial growth has occurred, usually around age 5 years.

Prognosis

The prognosis depends on the presence of amblyopia and whether it is adequately treated.

HORNER SYNDROME

ESSENTIALS OF DIAGNOSIS & TYPICAL FEATURES

- Horner syndrome, which may be congenital or acquired, presents with signs of unequal pupils (anisocoria), eyelid ptosis, iris heterochromia, and anhidrosis.

Pathogenesis

The syndrome is caused by an abnormality or lesion to the sympathetic chain. The congenital variety is most commonly the result of birth trauma. Acquired cases may occur in children who have had cardiothoracic surgery, trauma, or brainstem vascular malformation. Most worrisome is a Horner syndrome caused by neuroblastoma of the sympathetic chain in the apical lung region.

Prevention

Sympathetic chain injury avoidance during cardiothoracic surgery and delivery.

Clinical Findings

Parents may notice unequal pupils or different colored eyes. Penlight examination of the eyes may reveal unequal pupils (anisocoria), iris heterochromia, and eyelid ptosis of the affected eye.

The ptosis is usually mild with a well-defined upper lid crease. This differentiates it from congenital ptosis, which typically has a poorly defined lid crease. Another key finding of congenital Horner syndrome is heterochromia of the two irides, with the lighter colored iris occurring on the same side as the lesion (Figure 16–14). Anhidrosis can occur in congenital and acquired cases. Of note, not all of the three signs must be present to make the diagnosis.

Pharmacologic assessment of the pupils with topical cocaine and hydroxyamphetamine or epinephrine will help determine whether the Horner syndrome is due to a preganglionic or postganglionic lesion of the sympathetic chain. Preliminary studies suggest that topical apraclonidine may be useful in the diagnosis of Horner syndrome. Physical examination, including palpation of the neck and abdomen for masses, and MRI of structures in the head, neck, chest, and abdomen should be considered. An excellent screening test for neuroblastoma is the spot urine vanillylmandelic acid/creatinine ratio.

Differential Diagnosis

Congenital or neurogenic ptosis, physiologic anisocoria.

Complications

Depend on the etiology. Ptosis associated with Horner syndrome is usually mild and rarely results in amblyopia.

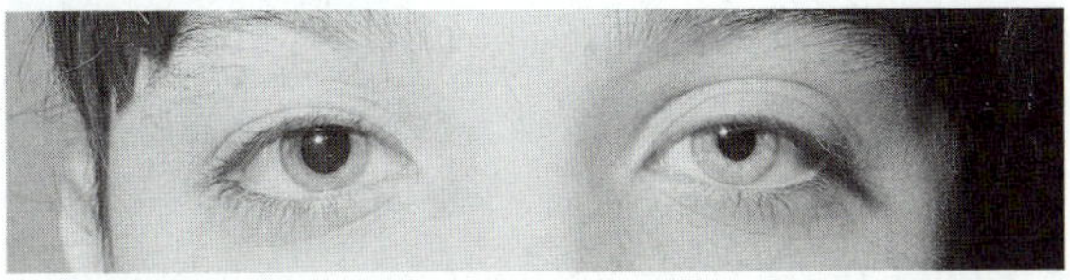

▲ **Figure 16–14.** Congenital Horner syndrome. Ptosis, miosis, and heterochromia. Lighter colored iris is on the affected left side.

Treatment

Management of any underlying disease is required. The ptosis and vision should be monitored by an ophthalmologist.

Prognosis

Depends on the etiology. The vision is usually normal.

EYELID TICS

Eyelid tics may occur as a transient phenomenon lasting several days to months. Although a tic may be an isolated finding in an otherwise healthy child, it may also occur in children with multiple tics, attention-deficit/hyperactivity disorder, or Tourette syndrome. Caffeine consumption may cause or exacerbate eyelid tics. If the disorder is a short-lived annoyance, no treatment is needed.

DISORDERS OF THE NASOLACRIMAL SYSTEM

NASOLACRIMAL DUCT OBSTRUCTION

ESSENTIALS OF DIAGNOSIS & TYPICAL FEATURES

- Nasolacrimal obstruction occurs in up to 6% of infants.
- Most cases clear spontaneously during the first year.

Pathogenesis

Obstruction in any part of the drainage system may result from incomplete canalization of the duct or membranous obstructions. Nasolacrimal obstruction may also occur in individuals with craniofacial abnormalities or Down syndrome.

Prevention

Not applicable.

Clinical Findings

Nasolacrimal duct obstruction presents with tearing and mucoid discharge from the affected eye. Signs and symptoms include tearing (epiphora), mucoid discharge especially in the morning, erythema of one or both lids, and conjunctivitis (Figure 16–15). Light sensitivity and blepharospasm suggest possible congenital glaucoma and warrant an urgent ophthalmic referral.

Differential Diagnosis

The differential diagnosis of tearing includes nasolacrimal duct obstruction, congenital glaucoma, foreign bodies, nasal disorders, and, in older children, allergies.

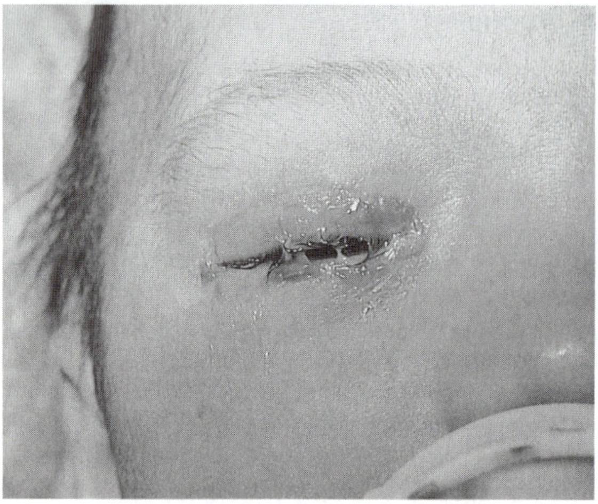

▲ **Figure 16–15.** Nasolacrimal obstruction, right eye. Mattering on upper and lower lids.

Complications

Dacryocystitis, preseptal cellulitis, orbital cellulitis.

Treatment

Massage over the nasolacrimal sac may empty debris from the nasolacrimal sac and clear the obstruction, although the efficacy of massage in clearing nasolacrimal obstruction is debated. Superinfection may occur, and treatment with topical antibiotics may help decrease the discharge.

The mainstay of surgical treatment is probing, which is successful 80% or more of the time, but the success rate may decrease after the infant reaches 1 year of age. Other surgical procedures, including infraction of the inferior nasal turbinate, balloon dilation, and silicone tube intubation, may be necessary if probing fails. Much less often, dacryocystorhinostomy is required.

Prognosis

Generally good with surgical treatment.

CONGENITAL DACRYOCYSTOCELE

ESSENTIALS OF DIAGNOSIS & TYPICAL FEATURES

- Presence of a nodular enlargement which may be blue in color, occurring shortly after birth over the nasolacrimal sac/medial eyelids.
- Dacryocystitis often occurs due to bacterial superinfection.

Pathogenesis

Congenital dacryocystocele is thought to result from obstructions proximal and distal to the nasolacrimal sac.

Prevention

Early intervention with nasolacrimal duct probing may prevent dacryocystitis.

Clinical Findings

At birth, the nasolacrimal sac is distended and has a bluish hue that often leads to an erroneous diagnosis of hemangioma. The tense and swollen sac displaces the medial canthus superiorly (Figure 16–16). Digital pressure over the nodule may result in reflux of tears, mucus, or purulent discharge from the inferior eyelid punctum. An intranasal duct cyst may be present beneath the inferior turbinate at the valve of Hasner. These cysts may be associated with respiratory distress.

Differential Diagnosis

Eyelid hemangioma, basal encephalocele.

Complications

Dacryocystitis, orbital cellulitis, sepsis, respiratory distress.

Treatment

Massage and warm compresses are rarely effective. Nasolacrimal duct probing and endoscopic marsupialization of the intranasal cyst under general anesthesia may be required. Hospital admission and systemic antibiotics are indicated if dacryocystitis is present. Consultation with an ear, nose, and throat specialist is recommended to aid in the diagnosis and treatment of an associated intranasal cyst.

Prognosis

Generally good.

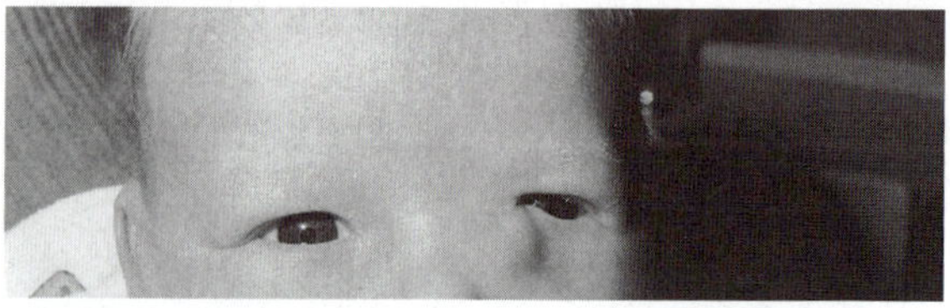

▲ **Figure 16–16.** Congenital dacryocystocele on the left side. Raised, bluish discolored mass of enlarged nasolacrimal sac. Note superiorly displaced medial canthus.

DACRYOCYSTITIS

ESSENTIALS OF DIAGNOSIS & TYPICAL FEATURES

- Dacryocystitis is an infection of the nasolacrimal sac that causes erythema and edema over the nasolacrimal sac.

Pathogenesis

Acute and chronic dacryocystitis are typically caused by bacteria that colonize the upper respiratory tract, such as *Staphylococcus aureus*, *Streptococcus pneumoniae*, *Streptococcus pyogenes*, *Streptococcus viridans*, *Moraxella catarrhalis*, and *Haemophilus* species.

Prevention

Treatment of nasolacrimal duct obstruction.

Clinical Findings

Acute dacryocystitis presents with inflammation, swelling, tenderness, and pain over the lacrimal sac (located inferior to the medial canthal tendon). Fever may be present. The infection may point externally (Figure 16–17). A purulent discharge and tearing can be expected, because the cause of infection is almost always nasolacrimal obstruction.

Signs of chronic dacryocystitis are mucopurulent debris on the lids and lashes, tearing, injection of the palpebral conjunctiva, and reflux of pus at the puncta when pressure is applied over the sac. Chronic dacryocystitis and recurrent episodes of low-grade dacryocystitis are caused by nasolacrimal obstruction.

Differential Diagnosis

Dacryocystocele, preseptal cellulitis.

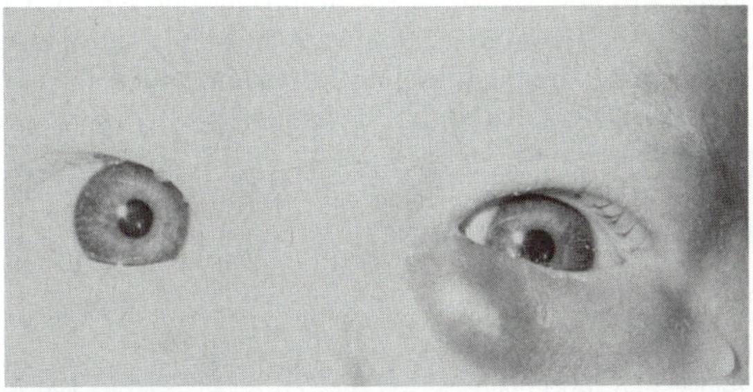

▲ **Figure 16–17.** Acute dacryocystitis in an 11-week-old infant.

Complications

Preseptal cellulitis, orbital cellulitis, sepsis.

Treatment

Severe acute dacryocystitis is treated with intravenous antibiotics after attempts at identifying the offending organism by culture and staining. Oral antibiotics can be tried in milder cases. Topical antibiotic administration is adjunctive and is also used with recurrent chronic infections. Warm compresses are beneficial. After the acute episode subsides—and in chronic cases—the nasolacrimal obstruction must be relieved surgically. If it cannot be drained via the intranasal portion of the nasolacrimal duct, external drainage may be necessary. This should be done as a last resort since a fistula may develop.

Prognosis

Generally good.

DISEASES OF THE CONJUNCTIVA

Conjunctivitis may be infectious, allergic, or associated with systemic disease. Trauma, irritation of the conjunctiva, and intraocular inflammation can cause injection of conjunctival vessels that can be confused with conjunctivitis.

OPHTHALMIA NEONATORUM

ESSENTIALS OF DIAGNOSIS & TYPICAL FEATURES

- Ophthalmia neonatorum (conjunctivitis in the newborn) occurs during the first month of life.

Pathogenesis

It may be due to inflammation resulting from silver nitrate prophylaxis given at birth, bacterial infection (gonococcal, staphylococcal, pneumococcal, or chlamydial), or viral infection. In developed countries, *Chlamydia* is the most common cause. Neonatal conjunctivitis may threaten vision if caused by *Neisseria gonorrhoeae*. Herpes simplex is a rare but serious cause of neonatal conjunctivitis, since it may indicate systemic herpes simplex infection.

Prevention

Treatment of maternal infections prior to delivery can prevent ophthalmia neonatorum. Although no single prophylactic medication can eliminate all cases of neonatal conjunctivitis, povidone-iodine may provide broader coverage against the organisms causing this disease than silver nitrate

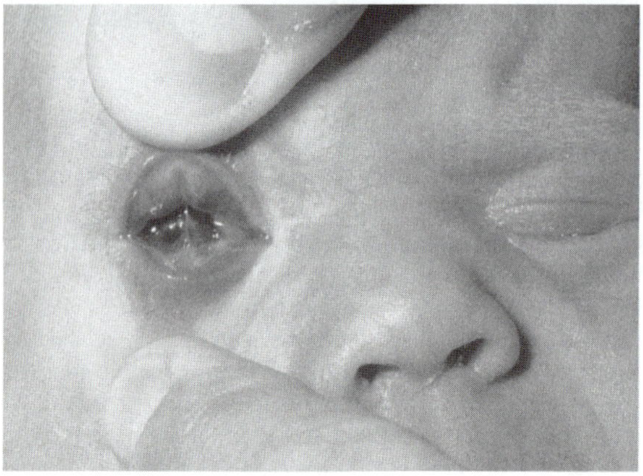

▲ **Figure 16–18.** Ophthalmia neonatorum due to *Chlamydia trachomatis* infection in a 2-week-old infant. Note marked lid and conjunctival inflammation.

or erythromycin ointment. Silver nitrate is not effective against *Chlamydia*. The choice of prophylactic agent is often dictated by local epidemiology and cost considerations, but erythromycin ophthalmic ointment is most often routinely administered immediately after birth to help prevent ophthalmia neonatorum.

▶ Clinical Findings

Ophthalmia neonatorum is characterized by redness and swelling of the lids and conjunctiva and by discharge (Figure 16–18). Gram staining, polymerase chain reaction amplification for *Chlamydia* and herpes simplex virus, and bacterial and viral cultures aid in making an etiologic diagnosis.

▶ Differential Diagnosis

Chemical/toxic conjunctivitis, viral conjunctivitis, bacterial conjunctivitis, chlamydial conjunctivitis.

▶ Complications

Chlamydia can cause a delayed-onset pneumonitis. Gonococcal infections can cause blindness through endophthalmitis as well as sepsis.

▶ Treatment

Treatment of these infections requires specific systemic antibiotics because they can cause serious infections in other organs. Parents should be examined and receive treatment when a sexually associated pathogen is present.

▶ Prognosis

Depends on the infectious agent as well as the rapidity of treatment.

BACTERIAL CONJUNCTIVITIS

ESSENTIALS OF DIAGNOSIS & TYPICAL FEATURES

- In general, bacterial conjunctivitis is accompanied by a purulent discharge.

▶ Pathogenesis

Common bacterial causes of conjunctivitis in older children include *Haemophilus* species, *S pneumoniae*, *M catarrhalis*, and *S aureus*.

▶ Prevention

Hand-washing and contact precautions.

▶ Clinical findings

Purulent discharge and conjunctival injection of one or both eyes. These symptoms may be associated with an upper respiratory infection. Regional lymphadenopathy is not a common finding in bacterial conjunctivitis except in cases of oculoglandular syndrome due to *S aureus*, group A β-hemolytic streptococci, *Mycobacterium tuberculosis* or atypical mycobacteria, *Francisella tularensis* (the agent of tularemia), and *Bartonella henselae* (the agent of cat-scratch disease).

▶ Differential Diagnosis

Viral, allergic, traumatic, or chemical/toxic conjunctivitis.

▶ Complications

Bacterial conjunctivitis is usually self-limited unless caused by *Chlamydia trachomatis*, *N gonorrhoeae*, and *Neisseria meningitidis* which may have systemic manifestations.

▶ Treatment

If conjunctivitis is not associated with systemic illness, topical antibiotics such as erythromycin, polymyxin-bacitracin, sulfacetamide, tobramycin, and fluoroquinolones are adequate. Systemic therapy is recommended for conjunctivitis associated with *C trachomatis*, *N gonorrhoeae*, and *N meningitidis*.

▶ Prognosis

Generally good.

Gold RS: Treatment of bacterial conjunctivitis in children. Pediatr Ann 2011 Feb;40(2):95–105 doi:10.3928/00904481-20110117-09 [PMID: 21323206].

VIRAL CONJUNCTIVITIS

ESSENTIALS OF DIAGNOSIS & TYPICAL FEATURES

- Children with viral conjunctivitis usually present with injection of the conjunctiva of one or both eyes and watery ocular discharge.

Pathogenesis

Adenovirus infection is often associated with pharyngitis, a follicular reaction and injection of the palpebral conjunctiva, and preauricular adenopathy (pharyngoconjunctival fever). Epidemics of adenoviral keratoconjunctivitis occur. Conjunctivitis may also be due to enterovirus and can occur as part of an acute measles illness. Herpes simplex virus may cause conjunctivitis or blepharoconjunctivitis.

Prevention

Hand-washing and contact precautions.

Clinical Findings

Watery discharge associated with conjunctival injection of one or both eyes. A vesicular rash involving the eyelids or face suggests herpes simplex virus.

Differential Diagnosis

Bacterial, allergic, traumatic, or chemical/toxic conjunctivitis.

Complications

Generally, viral conjunctivitis is self-limited. Herpes conjunctivitis may result in keratitis, which can affect visual acuity. This should be treated with antiviral therapy and the patient should be referred to an ophthalmologist.

Treatment

Treatment of adenovirus conjunctivitis is supportive. Children with presumed adenoviral keratoconjunctivitis are considered contagious 10–14 days from the day of onset. They should stay out of school and group activities as long as their eyes are red and tearing. Strict hand-washing precautions are recommended.

Herpes conjunctivitis can be treated with topical trifluridine 1% drops or 3% vidarabine ointment. Oral acyclovir may be used for treatment of the primary infection to decrease the duration and severity of the infection and as prophylaxis to reduce recurrence of herpes simplex ocular disease.

Prognosis

Generally good.

ALLERGIC CONJUNCTIVITIS

ESSENTIALS OF DIAGNOSIS & TYPICAL FEATURES

- A history of itchy, watery, red eyes, often associated with other allergy symptoms such as sneezing and rhinitis.

Prevention

Decrease exposure to allergens. This may be done by hand washing after handling dogs/cats, washing clothing, and bathing after being outdoors when pollen counts are elevated.

Clinical Findings

The history of itchy, watery, and red eyes is essential in making the diagnosis of allergic conjunctivitis. Redness of the conjunctiva, tearing, and discharge may be part of the history but need not be present on examination to make the diagnosis. Vernal conjunctivitis is a more severe form of allergic conjunctivitis occurring mostly in the spring and summer that is associated with intense tearing, itching, and a stringy discharge. Vernal allergic conjunctivitis is more common in males. Vernal conjunctivitis may present with giant cobblestone papillae (Figure 16–19) on the eyelid conjunctiva, nodules around the corneal limbus, and even sterile corneal ulcers. Contact lens wear may induce a conjunctivitis that appears similar to the palpebral form of vernal conjunctivitis.

Treatment

Topical ophthalmic solutions that combine both an antihistamine and mast cell stabilizers, including olopatadine 0.1%,

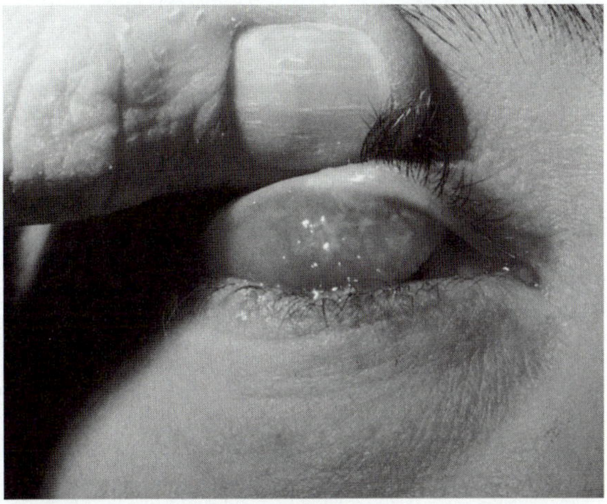

▲ **Figure 16–19.** Vernal conjunctivitis. Cobblestone papillae in superior tarsal conjunctiva.

epinastine HCl 0.05%, and ketotifen fumarate 0.025%, are very effective at treating allergic conjunctivitis. Other agents available include a combination topical vasoconstrictor plus an antihistamine (naphazoline antazoline), a nonsteroidal anti-inflammatory drug such as ketorolac tromethamine 0.5%, a mast cell stabilizer such as lodoxamide tromethamine 0.1%, or a corticosteroid such as prednisolone 0.125% (Table 16–2). Corticosteroids should be used with caution because their extended use causes glaucoma or cataracts in some patients. Systemic antihistamines and limitation of exposure to allergens may help reduce symptoms as well.

Prognosis

Generally good.

MUCOCUTANEOUS DISEASES

ESSENTIALS OF DIAGNOSIS & TYPICAL FEATURES

- Erythema multiforme, Stevens-Johnson syndrome, and toxic epidermal necrolysis are systemic conditions that often affect the eyes, as well as the skin, oral, and genitourinary mucosa.
- Ocular involvement may result in permanent conjunctival scarring, eyelid malposition, severe dry eye syndrome, and permanent vision loss.

Clinical Findings

Erythema multiforme, Stevens-Johnson syndrome, and toxic epidermal necrolysis may be caused by medications including: phenytoin, sulfonamides, NSAIDS and barbiturates or infections such as HSV or *Mycoplasma pneumonia*. With Stevens-Johnson syndrome, conjunctival changes include erythema and vesicular lesions that frequently rupture. Staining of the conjunctiva and/or cornea with fluorescein suggests severe ocular involvement and high risk for permanent ocular sequela, including symblepharon (adhesions) between the raw edges of the bulbar (eye) and palpebral (lid) conjunctivae.

Differential Diagnosis

Viral or bacterial conjunctivitis if the patient presents prior to cutaneous or mucosal eruptions.

Complications

Severe ocular involvement can result in permanent scarring of the conjunctiva leading to eyelid malposition, trichiasis

Table 16–2. Common ocular allergy medications.

Generic Name	Brand Name	Mechanism of Action	Side Effects	Dosage	Indications
Lodoxamide tromethamine 0.1%	Alomide	Mast cell stabilizer	Transient burning or stinging	1 drop 4 times daily—taper	Vernal kerato-conjunctivitis
Cromolyn Na 4%	Crolom, Opticrom	Mast cell stabilizer	Transient burning or stinging	1 drop 4–6 times daily	Vernal kerato-conjunctivitis
Olopatadine	Patanol	Mast cell stabilizer, H_1-receptor antagonist	Headache, burning or stinging	Twice daily (interval 6–8 h)	Itching due to allergic conjunctivitis
Ketorolac tromethamine 0.5%	Acular	Nonsteroidal anti-inflammatory	Transient burning or stinging	1 drop 4 times daily	Itching due to seasonal allergic conjunctivitis
Levocabastine HCl 0.05%	Livostin	H_1-receptor antagonist	Transient burning or stinging, headache	1 drop 4 times daily	Relief of symptoms of seasonal allergic conjunctivitis
Naphazoline HCl 0.1%	AK-Con, Naphcon, Opcon, Vasocon	Ocular decongestant, vasoconstrictor	Mydriasis, increased redness, irritation, discomfort, punctate keratitis, increased intraocular pressure, dizziness, headache, nausea, nervousness, hypertension, weakness, cardiac effects, hyperglycemia	Varies by preparation	Temporary relief of redness due to minor eye irritants
Pheniramine maleate	Component in AKCon A, Opcon-A, Naphcon-A	Antihistamine		1 drop every 3–4 h, as needed	Relief of symptoms of seasonal allergic conjunctivitis

(eyelashes touching the surface of the eye), and vision loss from chronic ocular irritation and extreme tear film deficiency.

Treatment

Treatment of the underlying disease, including discontinuation of offending medications and use of appropriate antimicrobials is necessary. Management of conjunctivitis associated with mucocutaneous disease depends on its severity. Artificial tears and ointment provide comfort and a topical corticosteroid may help prevent adhesions and dry eye in mild to moderate cases. Lysis of adhesions or use of a scleral ring by an ophthalmologist may be required. Surgical treatment of severe cases with amniotic membrane grafts may prevent visual disability by decreasing the risk of dry eye from tear-producing glands/goblet cell destruction, symblepharon, and trichiasis. Topical cyclosporine may help decrease the inflammatory reaction that leads to the destruction of tear-producing glands/goblet cells and subsequent dry eye syndrome.

Prognosis

It depends on the severity of the underlying condition. Guarded visual prognosis is made in severe cases.

Gregory DG: Treatment of acute Stevens-Johnson syndrome and toxic epidermal necrolysis using amniotic membrane: A review of 10 consecutive cases. Ophthalmology 2011 May;118(5):908–914 [Epub 2011 Mar 26] [PMID: 21440941].

DISORDERS OF THE IRIS

IRIS COLOBOMA

ESSENTIALS OF DIAGNOSIS & TYPICAL FEATURES

- Iris coloboma is a developmental defect due to incomplete closure of the anterior embryonal fissure.
- Iris coloboma may occur as an isolated defect or in association with various chromosomal abnormalities and syndromes.

Clinical Findings

Penlight examination of the pupils reveals a keyhole shape to the pupil rather than the normal round configuration (Figure 16–20). A dilated examination by an ophthalmologist is necessary to determine if the coloboma involves additional structures of the eye including the retina. If the retina is involved, vision may be poor. A genetic evaluation is usually recommended due to the high rate of associated genetic syndromes.

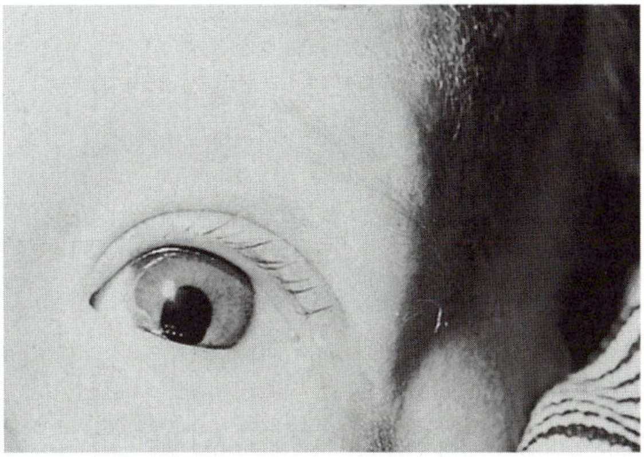

▲ **Figure 16–20.** Iris coloboma located inferiorly.

Differential Diagnosis

Microphthalmia, aniridia, previous iris trauma.

Complications

Low vision and rarely a secondary retinal detachment may need surgical intervention.

Treatment

Patients with coloboma should be monitored by an ophthalmologist for signs of amblyopia, significant refractive errors, and strabismus.

Prognosis

The prognosis depends on whether there are other ocular structures involved. Visual acuity is guarded if a large retinal coloboma is present.

ANIRIDIA

ESSENTIALS OF DIAGNOSIS & TYPICAL FEATURES

- Aniridia is a bilateral disorder that results in the absence of the majority of the iris (Figure 16–21).

Pathogenesis

Aniridia may occur as an autosomal dominant disease or in a sporadic form associated with Wilms tumor. The aniridia gene is located within the 11p13 chromosome region.

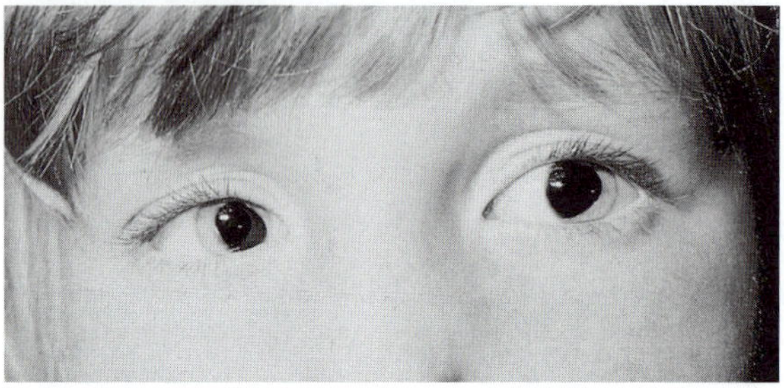

▲ **Figure 16–21.** Bilateral aniridia. Iris remnants present temporally in each eye.

Aniridia, genitourinary abnormalities, and developmental delay have been linked to an 11p deletion.

Clinical Findings

Slit-lamp or penlight examinations reveal little to no visible iris. Photophobia, nystagmus, and poor vision are present in aniridia. Abdominal ultrasonography is indicated in the sporadic form of aniridia to diagnose Wilms tumor. Genetic evaluation is indicated, as well. Cataract, corneal changes, macular hypoplasia, and glaucoma are often seen.

Differential Diagnosis

Microphthalmia, iris coloboma, previous iris trauma.

Complications

Low vision, cataracts, and glaucoma.

Treatment

An ophthalmologist should determine if cataracts or glaucoma are present in patients with aniridia. Surgical treatment of cataracts and glaucoma is often indicated. If Wilms tumor is present, treatment by an oncologist is necessary.

Prognosis

Patients tend to have low vision.

ALBINISM

ESSENTIALS OF DIAGNOSIS & TYPICAL FEATURES

- Albinism is caused by defective melanogenesis, usually as an autosomal recessive disease, but an X-linked form does occur.

Pathogenesis

Tyrosinase is an essential enzyme in the production of melanin. Many cases of complete albinism are caused by mutations of the tyrosinase gene. Albinism with some pigment production, especially in people of African descent, is more commonly caused by mutations of the *p* gene.

Clinical Findings

Affected individuals are usually legally blind and have nystagmus (see later section on Nystagmus). Iris, skin, and hair color vary with the type and severity of albinism as well as the individual's race. Iris transillumination is abnormal transmission of light through an iris with decreased pigment which can aid in the diagnosis of albinism. This may be obvious or may require slit-lamp examination with retroillumination to detect focal areas of transillumination. Other ocular abnormalities include foveal hypoplasia, abnormal optic pathway projections, strabismus, and poor stereoacuity.

Differential Diagnosis

Albinism may be associated with other systemic manifestations. Bleeding problems occur in individuals with Hermansky-Pudlak syndrome (chromosome 10q23 or 5q13), in which oculocutaneous albinism is associated with a platelet abnormality. Chédiak-Higashi syndrome (chromosome 1q42–44) is characterized by neutrophil defects, recurrent infections, and oculocutaneous albinism. Other conditions associated with albinism are Waardenburg, Prader-Willi, and Angelman syndromes.

Complications

Low vision, strabismus, high refractive errors, and visual field abnormalities.

Treatment

Children with albinism should be evaluated by a pediatric ophthalmologist in order to optimize their visual function. Low-vision aids such as telescopes, stand magnifiers, and large-print books are often required. Vision teachers in schools and ophthalmic specialists trained in treating low-vision patients can improve the patient's ability to perform activities of daily living and function within society. Affected individuals should use sunscreen and protective clothing to prevent skin cancer.

Prognosis

Vision is subnormal in most individuals.

MISCELLANEOUS IRIS CONDITIONS

Heterochromia, or a difference in iris color, can occur in congenital Horner syndrome, after iritis, or with tumors and nevi of the iris and use of topical prostaglandins. Malignant melanoma of the iris may also cause iris heterochromia. Acquired iris nodules (Lisch nodules), which occur in type 1 neurofibromatosis, usually become apparent by age 8 years. When seen on slit-lamp examination, Lisch nodules are 1–2 mm in diameter. They are often beige in color, although their appearance can vary. Iris xanthogranuloma occurring with juvenile xanthogranuloma can cause hyphema and glaucoma. Patients with juvenile xanthogranuloma should be evaluated by an ophthalmologist for ocular involvement.

GLAUCOMA

ESSENTIALS OF DIAGNOSIS & TYPICAL FEATURES

- Glaucoma is caused by increased intraocular pressure and results in vision loss due to optic nerve injury, corneal scarring, and amblyopia.
- Pediatric glaucoma can be congenital or acquired, pupillary block or angle closure, and unilateral or bilateral.
- Glaucoma can be classified on an anatomic basis into two types: open-angle and closed-angle.

Clinical Findings

Signs of glaucoma presenting within the first year of life include enlargement of the globe due to low scleral rigidity in the infant eye (buphthalmos), as well as tearing, photophobia, blepharospasm, corneal clouding due to edema, and optic nerve cupping. After age 3 years, usually only optic nerve changes occur. Findings may be unilateral or bilateral. In general, a red, inflamed eye is not typical of congenital or infantile glaucoma.

Sudden eye pain, redness, corneal clouding, and vision loss suggests possible pupillary block or angle-closure glaucoma. Urgent referral to an ophthalmologist is indicated. Genetic evaluation should be completed if other systemic abnormalities are noted.

Glaucoma also occurs with ocular and systemic syndromes such as aniridia, anterior segment dysgenesis, Sturge-Weber syndrome, the oculocerebrorenal syndrome of Lowe, and the Pierre Robin syndrome. Glaucoma can also occur with a traumatic hyphema, iritis, lens dislocation, intraocular tumor, and retinopathy of prematurity.

Differential Diagnosis

Buphthalmos is glaucoma until proven otherwise. The signs and symptoms of glaucoma are quite variable and should be urgently evaluated by an ophthalmologist.

Treatment

Treatment depends on the cause, but surgery is often indicated. Topical medications, which are available to decrease the intraocular pressure, have limited success in pediatric glaucoma.

Prognosis

Generally poor prognosis for glaucoma associated with congenital buphthalmos. In general, the prognosis is guarded.

Beck AD, Lynn MJ, Crandall J, Mobin-Uddin O: Surgical outcomes with 360-degree suture trabeculotomy in poor-prognosis primary congenital glaucoma and glaucoma associated with congenital anomalies or cataract surgery. J AAPOS 2011 Feb;15(1):54–58 [PubMed] [PMID: 21397807]; [PubMed Central] [PMCID: PMC3073639].

Mandal AK, Chakrabarti D: Update on congenital glaucoma. Indian J Ophthalmol 2011 Jan;59(Suppl):S148–S157 [PubMed] [PMID: 21150027]; [PubMed Central] [PMCID:PMC3038500].

UVEITIS

Inflammation of the uveal tract can be subdivided according to the uveal tissue primarily involved (iris, choroid, or retina) or by location (anterior, intermediate, or posterior uveitis). Perhaps the most commonly diagnosed form of uveitis in childhood is traumatic iridocyclitis or iritis.

ANTERIOR UVEITIS/IRIDOCYCLITIS/IRITIS

ESSENTIALS OF DIAGNOSIS & TYPICAL FEATURES

- Iridocyclitis associated with juvenile idiopathic arthritis may be asymptomatic despite severe ocular inflammation.

Pathogenesis

Iridocyclitis associated with juvenile idiopathic arthritis occurs most often in girls with pauciarticular arthritis and a positive antinuclear antibody test. Inflammatory bowel disease is also associated with iritis—perhaps more commonly with Crohn disease than with ulcerative colitis. Other causes of anterior uveitis in children include syphilis, tuberculosis, sarcoidosis, relapsing fever (borreliosis), and Lyme disease, all but the last also causing posterior uveitis. Juvenile spondyloarthropathies, including ankylosing spondylitis, Reiter syndrome, and psoriatic arthritis, are associated with anterior uveitis. A substantial percentage of cases are of unknown origin.

Clinical Findings

Injection, photophobia, pain, and blurred vision usually accompany iritis (anterior uveitis or iridocyclitis). An exception to this is iritis associated with juvenile idiopathic arthritis (see Chapter 29). The eye in such cases is quiet and asymptomatic, but slit-lamp examination reveals anterior chamber inflammation with inflammatory cells and protein flare. Children with juvenile idiopathic arthritis should be screened according to a schedule recommended by the AAP (http://www.aap.org). Children with Crohn disease or ulcerative colitis should have routine periodic ophthalmologic examinations to detect ocular inflammation, which may be asymptomatic, and cataracts if they have been receiving long-term systemic corticosteroids.

Other ocular findings of the anterior segment include conjunctivitis, episcleritis, and sterile corneal infiltrates. Posterior segment findings may include central serous retinochoroidopathy, panuveitis (inflammation of all uveal tissue), choroiditis, ischemic optic neuropathy, retinal vasculitis, neuroretinitis, and intermediate uveitis (see later section on Intermediate Uveitis).

Posterior subcapsular cataracts can develop in patients with or without ocular inflammation. Most, if not all, of these patients have been taking corticosteroids as part of the long-term treatment of their autoimmune disease.

Differential Diagnosis

Iridocyclitis due to autoimmune disorder, trauma, infection, malignancy, or idiopathic etiology.

Complications

Permanent decreased vision due to cataracts, secondary glaucoma, and band keratopathy.

Treatment

Treatment with a topical corticosteroid and a cycloplegic agent is aimed at quieting the inflammation and preventing or delaying the onset of cataract and glaucoma. Methotrexate and other systemic immunosuppressive agents can be used in refractory cases. Systemic antitumor necrosis factor agents such as etanercept, infliximab, and adalimumab show promise in treating refractory cases of uveitis.

Prognosis

It depends on the severity of ocular inflammation, development of cataracts, and secondary glaucoma.

POSTERIOR UVEITIS

ESSENTIALS OF DIAGNOSIS & TYPICAL FEATURES

- The terms *choroiditis, retinitis,* and *retinochoroiditis* denote the tissue layers primarily involved in posterior uveitis. Infectious agents are the most common cause of posterior uveitis in the pediatric population.

Clinical Findings

Children with posterior uveitis often present with systemic manifestations of a congenital infection. Examples include deafness, developmental delay, cataracts, "salt and pepper" retinopathy, and hearing and cardiac disorders seen in congenital rubella.

Serologic analysis and retinal examination by an ophthalmologist are used to identify the cause of posterior uveitis. Active toxoplasmosis (see Chapter 43) produces a white lesion appearing as a "headlight in the fog" owing to the overlying vitreitis. Inactive lesions have a hyperpigmented border. Contiguous white satellite lesions suggest reactivation of disease.

A granular "salt and pepper" retinopathy is characteristic of congenital rubella. In infants, the TORCH complex (toxoplasmosis, other infections, rubella, cytomegalovirus [CMV], and herpes simplex virus) and syphilis are congenital infections that cause chorioretinitis.

Congenital lymphocytic choriomeningitis is diagnosed by immunofluorescent antibody or enzyme-linked immunosorbent assay (ELISA) serologic testing. Congenital lymphocytic choriomeningitis virus may also present with chorioretinitis. The virus is transmitted to humans by consumption of food contaminated with rodent urine or feces. It most closely resembles congenital toxoplasmosis in presentation. Pregnant women should avoid exposure to rodents.

Ocular candidiasis occurs typically in an immunocompromised host or a premature infant in the intensive care nursery receiving hyperalimentation. Candidal chorioretinitis appears as multifocal, whitish yellow, fluffy retinal lesions that may spread into the vitreous and produce a so-called cotton or fungus ball vitritis.

Acute retinal necrosis syndrome is caused most often by varicella-zoster virus and occasionally by herpes simplex virus. Patients may present with vision loss and a red and painful eye. Ophthalmoscopy may show unilateral or bilateral patchy white areas of retina, arterial sheathing, vitreous haze, atrophic retinal scars, retinal detachment, and optic nerve involvement.

CMV infection is the most common cause of retinitis in immunocompromised children, especially those with human immunodeficiency virus (HIV) infection. CMV retinitis appears as a white retinal lesion, typically but not always associated with hemorrhage, or as a granular, indolent-appearing lesion with hemorrhage and a white periphery. Cotton-wool spots (nerve fiber layer infarcts) also commonly occur in HIV-positive patients.

In toddlers and older youngsters, *Toxocara canis* or *Toxocara cati* infections (ocular larva migrans; see Chapter 41) occur from ingesting soil contaminated with parasite eggs. The disease is usually unilateral. Common signs and symptoms include a red injected eye, leukocoria, and decreased vision. Funduscopic examination may show endophthalmitis (vitreous abscess) or localized granuloma. Diagnosis is based on the appearance of the lesion and serologic testing using ELISA for *T canis* and *T cati*.

Differential Diagnosis

Posterior uveitis due to autoimmune disorder, trauma, infection, malignancy, or idiopathic etiology.

Complications

Permanent vision loss due to retinal scarring and detachment.

Treatment

Congenital toxoplasmosis infections must be treated with systemic antimicrobials (see Chapter 43). Studies have shown improved ophthalmic and neurologic outcomes with prolonged treatment. Other infectious agents such as *Candida*, varicella, and CMV require systemic and/or intraocular injections of antimicrobial agents, and may require retinal surgery. Treatment of toxocariasis includes periocular corticosteroid injections and vitrectomy.

Prognosis

The prognosis for vision depends on the severity of retinal and systemic involvement.

INTERMEDIATE UVEITIS

ESSENTIALS OF DIAGNOSIS & TYPICAL FEATURES

- Intermediate uveitis or pars planitis is described as inflammation located in the far anterior periphery of the retina and vitreous base.

Clinical Findings

Patients with pars planitis often complain of decreased vision and floaters. They may also have a history of a red eye and ocular discomfort. Patients with intermediate uveitis often have decreased vision. A prolonged duration of the disease can lead to deprivation amblyopia and strabismus.

A dilated examination is required for observation of inflammation of the pars plana and vitritis. Slit-lamp and dilated funduscopic examinations by an ophthalmologist often reveal chronic signs of inflammation associated with intermediate uveitis, including macular edema, cataracts, increased intraocular pressure, irregular pupil, iris adhesion to the lens, and band keratopathy.

Differential Diagnosis

Intermediate uveitis is often idiopathic although there are several known etiologies. *Toxocara* infections with peripheral granuloma can be associated with intermediate uveitis, as can inflammatory bowel disease, multiple sclerosis, and sarcoidosis. Retinoblastoma and other neoplasms can imitate uveitis, causing a so-called masquerade syndrome.

Complications

Decreased vision due to macular edema, vitreous floaters, cataracts, and glaucoma.

Treatment

The most common treatment regimen for intermediate uveitis includes subtenon steroid injections, vitrectomy by a retinal surgeon, and systemic immunosuppression. Secondary glaucoma often requires tube shunt surgery.

Prognosis

The prognosis depends on the severity of the disease and associated secondary complications such as glaucoma and cataracts.

Sauberan DP: Pediatric uveitis. Int Ophthalmol Clin 2010 Fall;50(4):73–85 [Review] [PubMed] [PMID: 20930582].

OCULAR MANIFESTATIONS OF ACQUIRED IMMUNODEFICIENCY SYNDROME

ESSENTIALS OF DIAGNOSIS & TYPICAL FEATURES

- The advent of highly active antiretroviral therapy (HAART) has significantly reduced the incidence of CMV retinitis.
- Ocular infections are important manifestations of AIDS (see Chapter 39).
- As CD4 T-lymphocyte counts fall below 200/μL, opportunistic ocular infections increase in these patients.

Pathogenesis

Pathogens commonly causing eye infection include CMV and varicella-zoster virus. Acute retinal necrosis syndrome (see earlier section on Posterior Uveitis) is a severe necrotizing retinitis that often results in blindness in patients with AIDS. Most cases are thought to be caused by varicella-zoster virus. Other implicated agents are herpes simplex types 1 and 2.

Patients with CD4 counts below 50/μL are at high risk for CMV retinitis and should have a complete ocular evaluation by an ophthalmologist. Various retinal abnormalities may be present which include cotton-wool spots, retinal hemorrhages, microaneurysms, perivasculitis, and decreased visual acuity from ischemic maculopathy.

Immune recovery uveitis associated with HAART may result in decreased vision and may require treatment.

Differential Diagnosis

Decreased vision due to immune recovery uveitis, CMV retinitis, or acute retinal necrosis syndrome.

Complications

Retinal scarring, retinal detachment, and blindness.

Treatment

If immune recovery is sufficient with HAART, the patient may be able to discontinue anti-CMV therapy. However, active viral retinitis must be treated with antiviral agents. CMV retinitis is treated with intravenous ganciclovir but foscarnet may be required if resistance develops. Intravitreal ganciclovir or ganciclovir implants in conjunction with oral valganciclovir may be required in severe cases or in individuals intolerant to intravenous therapy. Acute retinal necrosis due to HSV or VZV must be treated with intravenous acyclovir, systemic steroids and intraocular surgery.

Prognosis

Viral retinitis generally has a poor prognosis.

Jabs DA, Ahuja A, Van Natta M, Lyon A, Srivastava S, Gangaputra S: Studies of the Ocular Complications of AIDS Research Group. Course of cytomegalovirus retinitis in the era of highly active antiretroviral therapy: Five-year outcomes. Ophthalmology 2010 Nov;117(11):2152–2161 e1-2 [Epub 2010 Jul 29] [PubMed] [PMID: 20673591]; [PubMed Central] [PMCID: PMC2963687].

Jabs DA: Cytomegalovirus retinitis and the acquired immunodeficiency syndrome—bench to bedside: LXVII Edward Jackson Memorial Lecture. Am J Ophthalmol 2011 Feb;151(2):198–216 e1 [Epub 2010 Dec 18] [PubMed] [PMID: 21168815]; [PubMed Central] [PMCID: PMC3057105].

DISORDERS OF THE CORNEA

CLOUDY CORNEA

ESSENTIALS OF DIAGNOSIS & TYPICAL FEATURES

- Corneal clouding can be caused by developmental abnormalities, metabolic disorders, trauma, and infection.

Clinical Findings

The cornea may have a white, hazy appearance on penlight examination. The red reflex may be decreased or absent.

Differential Diagnosis

Corneal clouding, tearing, blepharospasm, and photophobia in a newborn are signs of congenital glaucoma until proven otherwise. Peter anomaly and sclerocornea are congenital malformations of the anterior segment of the eye that are the most common causes of a cloudy cornea at birth. Direct trauma to the cornea during a forceps delivery can result in corneal haze and significant amblyopia. Systemic abnormalities such as developmental delay and liver or kidney failure suggest metabolic disorders such as mucopolysaccharidoses, Wilson disease, and cystinosis. Corneal infiltrates occur with viral infections, staphylococcal lid disease, corneal dystrophies, and interstitial keratitis due to congenital syphilis.

A complete ocular evaluation by an ophthalmologist is required and should be completed urgently when congenital glaucoma is suspected.

Complications

Vision loss is likely due to deprivation amblyopia.

Treatment

Treatment depends on the underlying condition. Surgical treatment of glaucoma and possible corneal transplantation or keratoprosthesis may be required.

Prognosis

Depends on the amount of corneal involvement and response to surgical treatment. Corneal transplants have a very high frequency of rejection and subsequently a poor prognosis in children.

Lowe MT, Keane MC, Coster DJ, Williams KA: The outcome of corneal transplantation in infants, children, and adolescents. Ophthalmology 2011 Mar;118(3):492–497 [Epub 2010 Oct 8] [PubMed] [PMID: 20932584].

Nallasamy S, Colby K: Keratoprosthesis: Procedure of choice for corneal opacities in children? Semin Ophthalmol 2010 Sep-Nov;25(5-6):244–248 [Review] [PubMed] [PMID: 21091007].

VIRAL KERATITIS

ESSENTIALS OF DIAGNOSIS & TYPICAL FEATURES

- Herpes simplex, herpes zoster, and adenovirus can all infect the cornea.

- When the corneal epithelium is involved, a dendritic or amoeboid pattern can be seen with fluorescein staining.

CLINICAL FINDINGS

Patients commonly present with a painful, red eye. Photophobia and decreased vision are also common complaints. Fever, malaise, and symptoms of upper respiratory tract infection may be present.

Fluorescein administration to the involved cornea will reveal areas of staining when viewed with a blue light if the corneal epithelium is involved. The pattern of epithelium staining may be dendritic (branch like) or irregular and round if a geographic ulcer is present. Slit-lamp examination may reveal white infiltrates beneath the corneal epithelium as a result of corneal stromal scarring or edema from viral infection of the corneal stromal tissue. Decreased visual acuity, photophobia, and conjunctivitis may also be noted.

Differential Diagnosis

Corneal abrasion, bacterial corneal ulcer, iritis.

Treatment

Topical antivirals such as trifluridine and vidarabine are indicated when herpes simplex infection is limited to the corneal epithelium, although additional systemic therapy is required in newborns. Topical corticosteroids may be a useful addition to antiviral therapy when stromal disease is present. The use of corticosteroids in the presence of herpetic disease should be undertaken only by an ophthalmologist because of the danger of worsening the disease. Oral acyclovir started in the early phase (first 5 days) may be helpful in treating herpes zoster eye disease. Acyclovir prophylaxis is helpful in preventing recurrent herpetic epithelial keratitis (see earlier section on Viral Conjunctivitis) and stromal keratitis caused by herpes simplex.

Adenovirus conjunctivitis may progress to keratitis 1–2 weeks after onset. Vision may be decreased. In most cases, no treatment is necessary because adenovirus keratitis is most often self-limiting. However, adenovirus is highly contagious and easily spread (see section on Viral Conjunctivitis).

Prognosis

Corneal involvement with herpes simplex can be recurrent and lead to blindness.

CORNEAL ULCERS

ESSENTIALS OF DIAGNOSIS & TYPICAL FEATURES

- Decreased vision, pain, injection, a white corneal infiltrate or ulcer (Figure 16–22), and hypopyon (pus in the anterior chamber) may all be present.

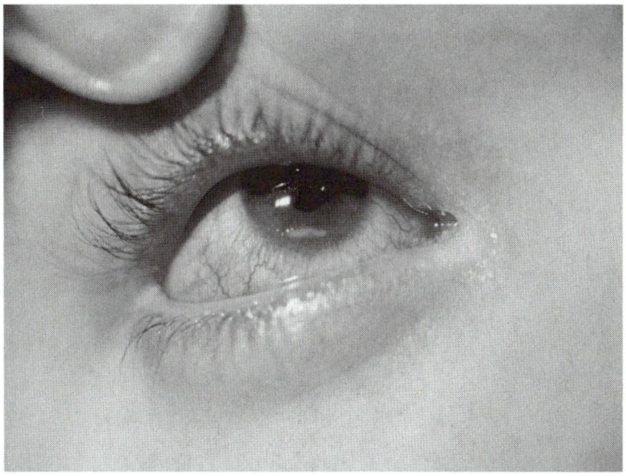

▲ **Figure 16–22.** Corneal ulcer. Note white infiltrate located on inferior cornea.

- Bacterial corneal ulcers in healthy children who are not contact lens wearers are usually secondary to corneal trauma from corneal abrasion or a penetrating foreign body.

Clinical findings

A corneal ulcer appears as a white spot on the surface of the cornea that stains with fluorescein. Associated symptoms include pain and decreased vision. Signs often include conjunctival injection, photophobia, tearing, and purulent discharge.

Differential Diagnosis

Viral keratitis, corneal abrasion, penetrating foreign body.

Complications

Permanent vision loss may result from corneal scarring. Corneal transplantation may be required.

Treatment

Prompt referral to an ophthalmologist is necessary for evaluation and management.

Prognosis

Depends on how large the ulcer is and whether the central cornea is involved.

DISORDERS OF THE LENS

Lens disorders involve abnormality of clarity or position. Lens opacification (cataract) can affect vision depending on its density, size, and position. Visual potential is also influenced by age at onset and the success of amblyopia treatment.

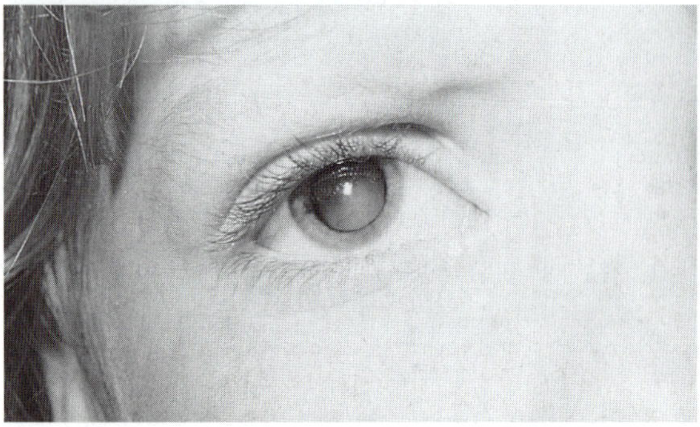

▲ **Figure 16–23.** Cataract causing leukocoria.

CATARACTS

ESSENTIALS OF DIAGNOSIS & TYPICAL FEATURES

- Cataracts in children may be unilateral or bilateral, may exist as isolated defects, or may be accompanied by other ocular disorders or systemic disease (Figure 16–23).

Clinical Findings

Leukocoria, poor fixation, and strabismus or nystagmus (or both) may be the presenting complaints. Absence of a red reflex in the newborn may be due to a cataract which requires an urgent referral to an ophthalmologist.

Laboratory investigation for infectious and metabolic causes of congenital cataracts is often indicated. Such investigation would include cultures or serologic tests for toxoplasmosis, rubella, CMV, herpes simplex virus, and syphilis, as well as evaluation for inborn metabolic errors, such as galactosemia or Lowe syndrome.

Differential Diagnosis

Cloudy cornea, intraocular tumor, retinal detachment.

Complications

Pediatric cataracts are frequently associated with severe deprivation amblyopia.

Treatment

Early diagnosis and treatment are necessary to prevent deprivation amblyopia in children younger than age 9 years, because they are visually immature. Cataracts that are visually significant require removal. Visually significant cataracts in infants are usually removed prior to 6 weeks of age to prevent deprivation amblyopia. Rehabilitation of the vision will require the correction of refractive errors and amblyopia treatment. Contact lenses, glasses, and artificial intraocular lenses are used to correct refractive errors after cataract extraction. Treatment of underlying concomitant congenital infections or systemic diseases must be instituted as appropriate.

Prognosis

The ultimate visual acuity depends on when the cataract was diagnosed and treated as well as compliance with amblyopia treatment. Glaucoma is often associated with pediatric cataracts and may result in a poor prognosis if not controlled.

DISLOCATED LENSES/ECTOPIA LENTIS

ESSENTIALS OF DIAGNOSIS & TYPICAL FEATURES

- Nontraumatic lens dislocation is usually bilateral.
- Subluxation causes refractive errors of large magnitude that are difficult to correct.

Pathogenesis

Systemic diseases, including Marfan syndrome, homocystinuria, Weill-Marchesani syndrome, sulfite oxidase deficiency, hyperlysinemia, syphilis, and Ehlers-Danlos syndrome, are often associated with dislocated lenses.

Clinical Findings

Slit-lamp examination reveals malposition of the intraocular lens. Refraction often reveals significant astigmatism. A complete ophthalmic evaluation, as well as genetic and metabolic evaluation, may be warranted.

Differential Diagnosis

Ectopia lentis due to systemic disease versus trauma.

Complications

Ectopia lentis can cause decreased vision and amblyopia due to induced refractive errors. Another ophthalmologic concern is pupillary block glaucoma, in which a malpositioned unstable lens interferes with the normal flow of aqueous humor from the ciliary body (posterior to the pupil), where it is produced, into the trabecular meshwork (anterior to the pupillary plane).

Treatment

Surgical lensectomy may be required if the visual acuity is not improved significantly with glasses or contact lenses.

Underlying metabolic and/or genetic disorders require a multidisciplinary approach.

Prognosis

Depends on the severity of the lens dislocation and need for lensectomy.

DISORDERS OF THE RETINA

RETINAL HEMORRHAGES IN THE NEWBORN

ESSENTIALS OF DIAGNOSIS & TYPICAL FEATURES

- Retinal hemorrhages are commonly seen in the otherwise healthy newborn.
- Retinal hemorrhages occur most often after vaginal delivery but can also be present after suction delivery or cesarean section.

Clinical Findings

A dilated retinal examination reveals unilateral or bilateral hemorrhages that can be located anywhere in the retina. They may appear as dot, blot, subretinal, or preretinal hemorrhages. They may also break into the vitreous. Examination of the retina of an otherwise healthy newborn infant is not indicated.

Differential Diagnosis

See earlier section on Abusive Head Trauma & Nonaccidental Trauma.

Treatment

Observation is indicated since retinal hemorrhages of the newborn usually disappear within the first month of life.

Prognosis

Excellent.

RETINOPATHY OF PREMATURITY

ESSENTIALS OF DIAGNOSIS & TYPICAL FEATURES

- Infants with a birth weight of less than 1500 g or gestational age of 32 weeks or less require retinal screening examinations for retinopathy of prematurity (ROP) by an ophthalmologist.
- Cost analysis studies have determined that screening and laser photoablation of ROP continue to be cost-effective medical interventions.
- The joint policy statement from the AAP, AAO, and AAPOS on screening examinations of premature infants for retinopathy of prematurity is available at http://www.pediatrics.org/cgi/content/full/117/2/572.

Pathogenesis

Premature infants with incomplete retinal vascularization are at risk for developing abnormal peripheral retinal vascularization, which may lead to retinal detachment and blindness. The cause of this disorder—including the role of supplemental oxygen in the neonatal period—is still not fully understood. Recent studies suggest that vascular endothelial growth factor may play a key role in ROP development. Other risk factors for severe ROP are bronchopulmonary dysplasia, intraventricular hemorrhage, sepsis, apnea and bradycardia, and mutations of the Norrie disease gene. White males, infants with zone 1 disease, and infants with very low birth weight and gestational age have a higher risk of developing severe ROP that requires treatment.

Prevention

The risk of vision loss from ROP can be reduced by timely screening of premature infants by an ophthalmologist.

Clinical Findings

The Cryotherapy for Retinopathy of Prematurity (CRYOROP) study outlined a standard nomenclature to describe the progression and severity of ROP (Table 16–3). Since retinal blood vessels emanate from the optic nerve and do not fully cover the developing retina until term, the optic nerve is used as the central landmark. The most immature zone of retina, zone 1, is the most posterior concentric

Table 16–3. Stages of retinopathy of prematurity.

Stage I	Demarcation line or border dividing the vascular from the avascular retina.
Stage II	Ridge. Line of stage I acquires volume and rises above the surface retina to become a ridge.
Stage III	Ridge with extraretinal fibrovascular proliferation.
Stage IV	Subtotal retinal detachment.
Stage V	Total retinal detachment.

imaginary circle around the optic nerve. Further out is zone 2, and beyond that is zone 3. Zone 1 disease is by definition more high-risk than disease in more anterior zones. Similarly, the stages of the abnormal vessels are numbered from zero (simply incomplete vascularization) through stages I–V.

Recommendations for initiating eye examination are outlined in the joint policy statement issued by the AAP, AAO, and AAPOS and are based on the gestational age at birth (http://www.pediatrics.org/cgi/content/full/117/2/572). The frequency of follow-up examinations depends on the findings and the risk factors for developing the disease. Most infants are evaluated every 1–2 weeks. ROP often resolves when the infant reaches 40 weeks' estimated gestational age. Examinations can be discontinued when the retinas are fully vascularized, or when the infant is 45 weeks' gestational age and has never had prethreshold disease or worse, or is vascularized out to zone 3 and never had zone 1 or 2 disease.

Complications

Low vision, retinal detachment.

Treatment

Surgical treatment of ROP is indicated when there is zone 1 ROP with any stage and plus disease, zone 1 ROP stage III without plus disease, zone 2 ROP with stage II or III and plus disease. The treatment of ROP within 72 hours can reduce the occurrence of bad visual outcomes by 50%. Diode laser treatment has largely replaced cryotherapy because it provides better access for treating zone 1 disease and causes less inflammation. However, some patients still progress to a retinal detachment, which can have a very poor prognosis for vision. Surgical treatment for a retinal detachment involves scleral buckling or a lens-sparing vitrectomy by an ophthalmologist specializing in vitreoretinal surgery. Intraocular injections of anti-vascular endothelial growth factor (anti-VEGF) agents such as bevacizumab and ranibizumab have been used in certain severe cases of ROP but long-term effects are still under investigation.

Prognosis

Most cases of ROP do not progress to retinal detachment and require no treatment. However, ROP remains a leading cause of blindness in children. Those with a history of ROP are at a much higher risk of developing strabismus, amblyopia, myopia, and glaucoma than the average child.

Faia LJ, Trese MT: Retinopathy of prematurity care: Screening to vitrectomy. Int Ophthalmol Clin 2011 Winter;51(1):1–16 [Review] [PubMed] [PMID: 21139474].

RETINOBLASTOMA

ESSENTIALS OF DIAGNOSIS & TYPICAL FEATURES

- Retinoblastoma is the most common primary intraocular malignancy of childhood, with an incidence estimated between 1:17,000 and 1:34,000 live births (see Chapter 29).
- Most patients present before age 3 years.

Pathogenesis

Inherited forms of retinoblastoma are autosomal dominant with high penetrance. The disease may consist of a solitary mass or multiple tumors in one or both eyes. All bilateral cases and some unilateral cases are caused by germinal mutations; however, most unilateral cases are caused by a somatic retinal mutation. In both situations, the mutation occurs in the retinoblastoma gene (*Rb*) at chromosome 13q14. This is a tumor suppressor gene. One mutated copy may be inherited in an autosomal dominant fashion (germline mutation). If a second mutation spontaneously occurs in any cell, tumorigenesis is likely. Individuals with a germinal mutation are at risk for the development of tumors other than retinoblastoma (pineal tumors, osteosarcoma, and other soft tissue sarcomas). All children with unilateral or bilateral retinoblastoma must be presumed to have the germline form, and followed expectantly for other tumors in the remaining eye and at extraocular sites. Approximately 15% of patients with unilateral disease have germline mutations.

Clinical Findings

The most common presenting sign in a child with previously undiagnosed retinoblastoma is leukocoria (see Figure 16–1). Evaluation of the pupillary red reflex is important, although a normal red reflex does not rule out retinoblastoma. Examination requires indirect ophthalmoscopy with scleral depression and pupillary dilation, performed by an ophthalmologist. Other presentations include strabismus, red eye, glaucoma, or pseudo-hypopyon (appearance of puslike material in the anterior chamber).

Genetic testing is available for patients with retinoblastoma. Once the causative mutation is found in an affected individual, unaffected members of the family should be tested to determine their personal and reproductive risk.

Differential Diagnosis

Retinal vasculature abnormalities seen in diseases such as Coats disease, uveitis, endophthalmitis.

Complications

Death if not adequately treated.

Treatment

The goal of treatment is to preserve the eye and as much useful vision as possible. Chemoreduction is used to reduce initial tumor volume. Local treatment with laser photocoagulation, cryotherapy, plaque radiotherapy, or thermotherapy can often preserve vision and spare the patient enucleation and radiation.

Prognosis

Generally good except in developing countries where children often succumb to their disease due to lack of treatment.

Shields CL, Shields JA: Retinoblastoma management: Advances in enucleation, intravenous chemoreduction, and intra-arterial chemotherapy. Curr Opin Ophthalmol 2010 May;21(3):203–212 [Review] [PubMed] [PMID: 20224400].

RETINAL DETACHMENT

ESSENTIALS OF DIAGNOSIS & TYPICAL FEATURES

- A retinal detachment may present as an abnormal or absent red reflex.
- Older children may complain of decreased vision, flashes, floaters, or visual field defects.

Pathogenesis

Common causes are trauma and high myopia. Other causes are ROP, Marfan syndrome, and Stickler syndrome.

Clinical Findings

Symptoms of detachment are floaters, flashing lights, and loss of visual field; however, children often cannot appreciate or verbalize their symptoms. A detachment may not be discovered until the child is referred after failing a vision screening examination, strabismus supervenes, or leukocoria is noted.

Differential Diagnosis

Intraocular tumor.

Complications

Vision loss, glaucoma, strabismus.

Treatment

Treatment of retinal detachment is surgical. For children with conditions predisposing to retinal detachment, or a strong family history, examinations under anesthesia by an ophthalmologist, with prophylactic laser treatment, may be recommended.

Prognosis

It depends on the location and duration of the detachment.

DIABETIC RETINOPATHY

ESSENTIALS OF DIAGNOSIS & TYPICAL FEATURES

- Diabetic retinopathy is a specific vascular complication of diabetes mellitus. Patients with type 1, or insulin-dependent, diabetes are at higher risk of developing severe proliferative retinopathy leading to visual loss than are those with type 2, or non–insulin-dependent, diabetes.
- The cost-effectiveness of screening examinations for diabetic retinopathy in children requires further evaluation.

Prevention

Control of diabetes is the best way to prevent ocular complications.

Clinical Findings

Acute onset of diabetes may be accompanied by sudden blurred vision due to myopia and cataracts.

In children older than age 9 years, referral to an ophthalmologist for screening of retinopathy should occur within 3–5 years after the onset of diabetes. Both conditions may be reversible with good glucose control. Young children with type 1 diabetes should be followed for the Wolfram, or DIDMOD, syndrome, in which diabetes mellitus occurs in conjunction with diabetes insipidus, optic atrophy, and deafness.

Complications

Vision loss due to vitreous hemorrhage, macular edema, neovascular glaucoma, cataracts, or retinal detachment.

Treatment

Severe proliferative diabetic retinopathy requires panretinal laser photocoagulation or vitreoretinal surgery (or both). Cataracts often require surgical removal and intraocular lens placement. Intraocular steroid injections have been used to treat macular edema in adults, but their role in children is not well established.

Prognosis

Depends on the severity of the retinopathy and associated complications.

DISEASES OF THE OPTIC NERVE

OPTIC NEUROPATHY

ESSENTIALS OF DIAGNOSIS & TYPICAL FEATURES

- Optic nerve function is evaluated by checking visual acuity, color vision, pupillary response, and visual fields.

Clinical Findings

Poor optic nerve function results in decreased central or peripheral vision, decreased color vision, strabismus, and nystagmus. Optic nerve disorders can be due to congenital malformation, malignancy, inflammation, infection, metabolic disorders, and trauma.

The swinging flashlight test is used to assess function of each optic nerve. It is performed by shining a light alternately in front of each pupil to check for an afferent pupillary defect or Marcus Gunn pupillary defect. An abnormal response in the affected eye is pupillary dilation when the light is directed into that eye after having been shown in the other eye with its healthy optic nerve. This results from poorer conduction along the optic nerve of the affected eye, which in turn results in less pupillary constriction of both eyes than occurs when the light is shined into the noninvolved eye. Hippus—rhythmic dilating and constricting movements of the pupil—can be confused with an afferent pupillary defect.

The optic nerve is evaluated as to size, shape, color, and vascularity. Occasionally, myelinization past the entrance of the optic nerve head occurs. It appears white, with a feathered edge (Figure 16–24). Myelinization onto the retina can be associated with myopia and amblyopia. Anatomic defects of the optic nerve include colobomatous defects and pits.

Treatment

Management of the underlying condition resulting in the optic neuropathy is necessary.

Prognosis

Depends on the severity of optic neuropathy and the underlying disease.

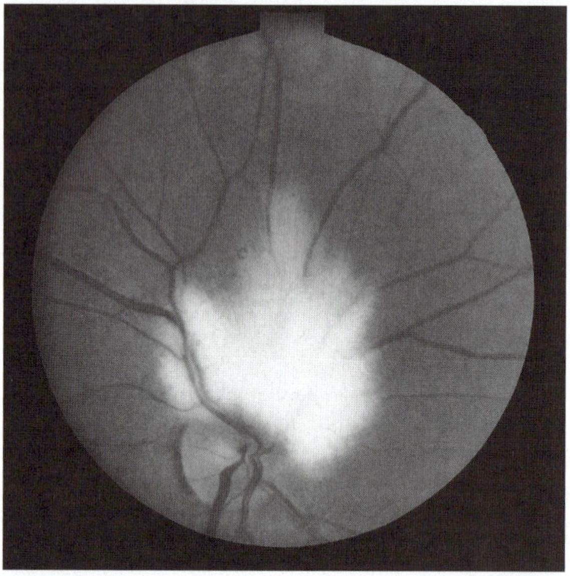

▲ **Figure 16–24.** Myelinization extending from optic nerve superiorly onto the retina.

OPTIC NERVE HYPOPLASIA

ESSENTIALS OF DIAGNOSIS & TYPICAL FEATURES

- Optic nerve hypoplasia may be associated with absence of the septum pellucidum and hypothalamic-pituitary dysfunction, which is known as septo-optic dysplasia, or de Morsier syndrome.
- Children with septo-optic dysplasia and hypocortisolism are at risk for sudden death during febrile illness from thermoregulatory disturbance and dehydration from diabetes insipidus.

Pathogenesis

Optic nerve hypoplasia may occur in infants of diabetic mothers and has also been associated with alcohol use or ingestion of quinine or phenytoin during pregnancy. Anatomically, the optic nerve may range from absent (aplasia) to almost full size, with a segmental defect.

Clinical Findings

Visual function with optic nerve hypoplasia ranges from mildly decreased to absent light perception. If only one eye is involved, the child usually presents with strabismus. If both eyes are affected, nystagmus is usually the presenting sign. Ophthalmoscopy is performed to directly visualize the optic nerves and to determine the severity of the hypoplasia. Neuroimaging of the brain and endocrine consultation should be performed in all patients with bilateral optic nerve hypoplasia.

Treatment

Sensory amblyopia and significant refractive errors should be treated by an ophthalmologist. Strabismus surgery may be necessary in certain patients. Endocrine abnormalities should be managed as necessary.

Prognosis

Severe bilateral optic nerve hypoplasia results in blindness.

PAPILLEDEMA

ESSENTIALS OF DIAGNOSIS & TYPICAL FEATURES

- Papilledema (optic nerve edema or choked disk) is associated with increased intracranial pressure due to any cause, such as tumor, craniosynostosis, or intracranial infection.

Pathogenesis

Hydrocephalus and intracranial tumors are common causes of papilledema. In pseudotumor cerebri (idiopathic intracranial hypertension), neuroimaging is normal but papilledema, headaches, and pulsating tinnitus may be present. Papilledema occurs almost equally in boys and girls and sometimes is associated with obesity or upper respiratory tract infection. Other associated causes are viral infections, corticosteroid use and withdrawal, sinus infection, trauma, tetracycline use, growth hormone, and venous sinus thrombosis (see Chapter 25, Neurologic & Muscular Disorders). Early in the illness the patient may not notice a change in vision, although the blind spot may be enlarged. Transient obscuration of vision (amaurosis fugax) may occur as the process becomes more long-standing. Further effects on vision will occur as the papilledema becomes chronic and ultimately leads to optic atrophy. Workup and treatment are directed toward finding the underlying systemic or central nervous system (CNS) cause.

Clinical Findings

Direct visualization of the optic nerve by ophthalmoscopy reveals an elevated disk with indistinct margins, increased vessel diameter, and hyperemia. Hemorrhages and exudates are present in more severe cases. Observed changes may be subtle to striking. Optic nerve head changes are bilateral and generally symmetrical.

Differential diagnosis

Pseudopapilledema (next section), optic nerve drusen.

Treatment

Treatment of idiopathic intracranial hypertension may be pharmacologic—for example, using acetazolamide, a carbonic anhydrase inhibitor, or a corticosteroid. Diagnostic lumbar puncture may also be curative. Optic nerve sheath fenestration and ventriculoperitoneal shunt are surgical interventions used when conservative measures fail.

Complications

Optic atrophy and vision loss.

Prognosis

Depends on the underlying etiology, duration, and control of the increased intracranial pressure.

PAPILLITIS

ESSENTIALS OF DIAGNOSIS & TYPICAL FEATURES

- Papillitis is a form of optic neuritis seen on ophthalmoscopic examination as an inflamed optic nerve head.
- Optic neuritis in the pediatric age group may be idiopathic or associated with multiple sclerosis, acute disseminated encephalomyelitis, Devic disease, or cat-scratch disease.

Clinical Findings

Papillitis may have the same appearance as papilledema. However, papillitis may be unilateral, whereas papilledema is almost always bilateral. Papillitis can be differentiated from papilledema by an afferent pupillary defect (Marcus Gunn pupil), by its greater effect in decreasing visual acuity and color vision, and by the presence of a central scotoma. Papilledema that is not yet chronic will not have as dramatic an effect on vision. Because increased intracranial pressure can cause both papilledema and a sixth (abducens) nerve palsy, papilledema can be differentiated from papillitis if esotropia and loss of abduction are also present. However, esotropia may also develop secondarily in an eye that has lost vision from papillitis. Retrobulbar neuritis, an inflamed optic nerve, but with a normal-appearing nerve head, is associated with pain and the other findings of papillitis. Pseudopapilledema is a normal variant of the optic disk, in which the disk appears elevated, with indistinct margins and a normal vascular pattern. Pseudopapilledema sometimes occurs in hyperopic individuals.

Workup of the patient with papillitis includes lumbar puncture and cerebrospinal fluid analysis. *B henselae* infection can be detected by serology. MRI is the preferred imaging study. An abnormal MRI is associated with a worse visual outcome.

Differential Diagnosis

Neoplastic optic nerve infiltration.

Complications

Decreased visual acuity, color vision, peripheral vision, and contrast sensitivity.

Treatment

Treatment of the underlying disease and use of systemic corticosteroids are necessary.

Prognosis

Depends on the underlying disease process.

OPTIC ATROPHY

ESSENTIALS OF DIAGNOSIS & TYPICAL FEATURES

- Optic atrophy is pallor of the optic nerve noted on ophthalmoscopy.

Clinical Findings

Optic atrophy is found in children most frequently after neurologic compromise during the perinatal period. An example would be a premature infant who develops an intraventricular hemorrhage. Hydrocephalus, glioma of the optic nerve, craniosynostosis, certain neurologic diseases, and toxins such as methyl alcohol can cause optic atrophy, as can certain inborn errors of metabolism, long-standing papilledema, or papillitis.

Direct examination of the optic nerve by ophthalmoscopy reveals an optic nerve head with a cream or white color and possibly cupping. Neuroimaging is necessary to delineate CNS abnormalities.

Complications

Vision loss, decreased peripheral vision, and contrast sensitivity.

Treatment

Treatment of the underlying condition is indicated.

Prognosis

Depends on the severity of the optic nerve atrophy and associated neurologic deficits.

DISEASES OF THE ORBIT

PERIORBITAL & ORBITAL CELLULITIS

ESSENTIALS OF DIAGNOSIS & TYPICAL FEATURES

- The fascia of the eyelids joins with the fibrous orbital septum to isolate the orbit from the lids.
- The orbital septum helps to decrease the risk of an eyelid infection from extending into the orbit.
- Infections arising anterior to the orbital septum are termed preseptal.
- Orbital cellulitis denotes infection posterior to the orbital septum and may cause serious complications, such as an acute ischemic optic neuropathy or cerebral abscess.

Pathogenesis

Preseptal (periorbital) cellulitis usually arises from a local exogenous source such as an abrasion of the eyelid, from other infections (hordeolum, dacryocystitis, or chalazion), or from infected varicella or insect bite lesions. *S aureus* and *S pyogenes* are the most common pathogens cultured from these sources. Preseptal infections in children younger than age 3 years also occur from bacteremia, although this is much less common since *Haemophilus influenzae* and *S pneumoniae* immunization are routinely administered. Bacteremia is still an occasional cause of this infection. Children with periorbital cellulitis from presumed bacteremia must be examined for additional foci of infection.

Orbital cellulitis almost always arises from contiguous sinus infection, because the walls of three sinuses make up portions of the orbital walls and infection can breach these walls or extend by way of a richly anastomosing venous system. The orbital contents can develop a phlegmon (orbital cellulitis), or frank pus can develop in the orbit (orbital abscess). The pathogenic agents are those of acute or chronic sinusitis—respiratory flora and anaerobes. *S aureus* is also frequently implicated.

The frequency of methicillin-resistant *S aureus* preseptal and orbital cellulitis has increased over the past several years.

Clinical Findings

Children with preseptal cellulitis present with erythematous and edematous eyelids, pain, and mild fever. The vision, eye movements, and eye itself are normal. Decreased vision, restricted eye movements, and an afferent pupillary defect suggest orbital cellulitis.

Orbital cellulitis presents with signs of periorbital disease as well as proptosis (a protruding eye), restricted eye movement, and pain with eye movement. Fever is usually high. CT scanning or MRI is required to establish the extent of the infection within the orbit and sinuses.

Differential diagnosis

Primary or metastatic neoplasm of the orbit, orbital pseudotumor (idiopathic orbital inflammation), orbital foreign body with secondary infection.

Complications

Preseptal cellulitis can progress to orbital cellulitis. Orbital cellulitis can result in permanent vision loss due to compressive optic neuropathy. Proptosis can cause corneal exposure, dryness, and scarring. Cavernous sinus thrombosis, intracranial extension, blindness, and death can result from severe orbital cellulitis.

Treatment

Therapy for preseptal and orbital cellulitis infection is with systemic antibiotics. Treatment of orbital infections may require surgical drainage for subperiosteal abscess in conjunction with intravenous antibiotics. Drainage of infected sinuses is often part of the therapy.

Prognosis

Most patients do well with timely treatment.

Seltz LB, Smith J, Durairaj VD, Enzenauer R, Todd J: Microbiology and antibiotic management of orbital cellulitis. Pediatrics 2011 Mar;127(3):e566–e572 [Epub 2011 Feb 14] [PubMed] [PMID: 21321025].

CRANIOFACIAL ANOMALIES

ESSENTIALS OF DIAGNOSIS & TYPICAL FEATURES

- Craniofacial anomalies can affect the orbit and visual system.
- Craniofacial anomalies occur with craniosynostoses and midface syndromes such as Treacher Collins and Pierre Robin syndromes.
- Fetal alcohol syndrome is associated with similar changes of the ocular adnexa.

Clinical Findings

Ocular abnormalities associated with craniofacial disease involving the orbits include visual impairment, proptosis, corneal exposure, hypertelorism (widely spaced orbits), strabismus, amblyopia, lid coloboma, papilledema, refractive errors, and optic atrophy.

Treatment

Orbital and ocular abnormalities associated with craniofacial anomalies often require a multispecialty approach. Management may require orbital and strabismus surgery. Ophthalmologists also treat amblyopia, refractive errors, and corneal exposure if present.

Taub PJ, Lampert JA: Pediatric Craniofacial Surgery: A Review for the Multidisciplinary Team. Cleft Palate Craniofac J 2011 Jul 8 [Epub ahead of print] [PubMed] [PMID: 21740182].

ORBITAL TUMORS

ESSENTIALS OF DIAGNOSIS & TYPICAL FEATURES

- Both benign and malignant orbital lesions occur in children.
- The most common benign tumor is capillary heman gioma (Figure 16–25).
- The most common primary malignant tumor of the orbit is rhabdomyosarcoma.

Clinical Findings

Capillary hemangiomas may be located superficially in the lid or deep in the orbit and can cause ptosis, refractive errors, and amblyopia. Deeper lesions may cause proptosis. Capillary hemangiomas in infants initially increase in size before involuting at about age 2–4 years.

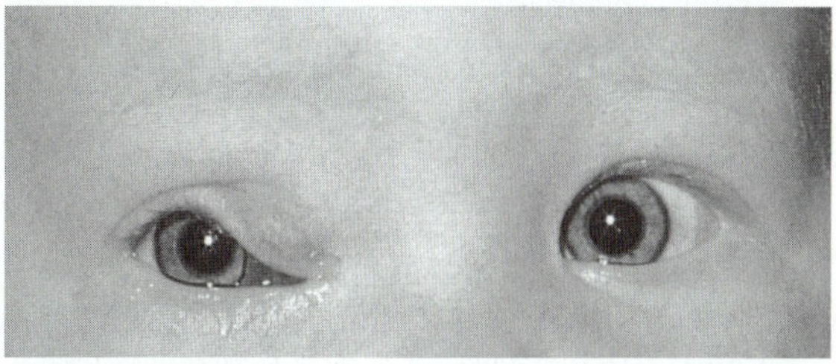

▲ **Figure 16–25.** Right upper lid hemangioma causing ptosis.

Orbital dermoid cysts vary in size and are usually found temporally at the brow and orbital rim or supranasally. These lesions are firm, well encapsulated, and mobile. Rupture of the cyst causes a severe inflammatory reaction.

Lymphangioma occurring in the orbit is typically poorly encapsulated, increases in size with upper respiratory infection, and is susceptible to hemorrhage. Other benign tumors of the orbit are orbital pseudotumor, neurofibroma, teratoma, and tumors arising from bone, connective tissue, and neural tissue.

Orbital rhabdomyosarcoma (see Chapter 31) grows rapidly and displaces the globe. The average age at onset is 6–7 years. The tumor is often initially mistaken for orbital swelling due to insignificant trauma.

Tumors metastatic to the orbit also occur; neuroblastoma is most common. The patient may exhibit proptosis, orbital ecchymosis (raccoon eyes), Horner syndrome, or opsoclonus (dancing eyes). Ewing sarcoma, leukemia, Burkitt lymphoma, and Langerhans cell histiocytosis may involve the orbit.

Examination of vision, eye movements, eyelids, and orbits often reveals amblyopia, eyelid malposition, strabismus, and proptosis. Neuroimaging with CT or MRI is required to delineate the location and size of orbital tumors.

Differential Diagnosis

Orbital pseudotumor (idiopathic orbital inflammation), orbital cellulitis.

Treatment

Therapy for capillary hemangiomas includes observation and intralesional or systemic corticosteroids. Recently, systemic beta blockers have shown success in treating capillary hemangiomas. Treatment is indicated if the lesion is large enough to cause amblyopia. Induced astigmatism or amblyopia (or both) are treated with glasses and patching, respectively. Treatment of orbital dermoids is by excision.

Rhabdomyosarcoma is treated with radiation and chemotherapy after biopsy confirms the diagnosis. With expeditious diagnosis and proper treatment, the survival rate of patients with orbital rhabdomyosarcoma confined to the orbit approaches 90%.

Treatment of metastatic disease requires management by an oncologist and may require chemotherapy and radiation therapy.

Prognosis

Depends on the underlying disease.

Moretti G, Guimarães R, Oliveira KM, Sanjar F, Voegels RL: Rhabdomyosarcoma of the head and neck: 24 cases and literature review. Braz J Otorhinolaryngol 2010 Aug;76(4):533–537 [Review English, Portuguese] [PubMed] [PMID: 20835543].

NYSTAGMUS

ESSENTIALS OF DIAGNOSIS & TYPICAL FEATURES

- Nystagmus is a rhythmic oscillation or jiggling of the eyes. It may be unilateral or bilateral, more pronounced in one eye, or gaze-dependent.

Pathogenesis

Nystagmus may be associated with esotropia or may occur with ocular lesions that cause deprivation amblyopia (eg, cataract and eyelid ptosis) or conditions in which the visual pathways are hypoplastic, sometimes referred to as "sensory nystagmus." Nystagmus is seen with optic nerve hypoplasia, macular hypoplasia, aniridia, and albinism. Nystagmus can also occur with normal ocular structures and seemingly normal CNS development, sometimes referred to as "motor nystagmus." In the latter instance, the nystagmus may be blocked in certain positions of gaze, in which case a face turn or torticollis may develop. Latent nystagmus occurs when one eye is occluded. This type of nystagmus occurs in patients with congenital esotropia. An associated amblyopia may be present.

Most nystagmus occurring in childhood is of ocular origin, but CNS disease and, less frequently, inner ear disease are other causes. A CNS cause is likely when the nystagmus is acquired. Patients should be referred to an ophthalmologist for evaluation.

Clinical Findings

Evaluation for iris transillumination defects caused by albinism should be performed since albinism is a common cause of nystagmus.

Spasmus nutans, in which a rapid, shimmering, disconjugate nystagmus occurs with head bobbing and torticollis. Glioma of the hypothalamus can mimic spasmus nutans. Neuroimaging may be necessary to determine if the cause of the nystagmus is due to a CNS disease. An electroretinogram may be required to rule out retinal pathology as the cause of nystagmus if neuroimaging is normal.

Differential Diagnosis

Opsoclonus.

Treatment

Therapy is directed at managing the underlying ocular or CNS disease. An ophthalmologist can optimize vision by correcting significant refractive errors and strabismus. The range of vision varies depending on the cause of the nystagmus. Some patients may benefit from extraocular muscle surgery and contact lenses.

Prognosis

Most affected individuals have subnormal vision but spasmus nutans usually improves with time.

AMBLYOPIA

ESSENTIALS OF DIAGNOSIS & TYPICAL FEATURES

- Amblyopia is a unilateral or bilateral reduction in vision due to strabismus, refractive errors, and/or visual deprivation.
- Amblyopia can occur only during the critical period of visual development in the first decade of life when the visual nervous system is plastic.
- Approximately 3% of the population is amblyopic.

Pathogenesis

Amblyopia is classified according to its cause. Strabismic amblyopia can occur in the nondominant eye of a strabismic child. Refractive amblyopia can occur in both eyes if significant refractive errors are untreated (ametropic or refractive amblyopia). Another type of refractive amblyopia can occur in the eye with the worse refractive error when imbalance is present between the eyes (anisometropic amblyopia). Deprivation amblyopia occurs when dense cataracts or complete ptosis prevents formation of a formed retinal image. Of the three types of amblyopia, the deprivation form of amblyopia results in the worst vision.

Prevention

Vision screening and referral to an eye care professional if amblyopia is suspected.

Clinical Findings

Screening for amblyopia should be a component of periodic well-child examinations. The single best screening technique to discover amblyopia is obtaining visual acuity in each eye. In preverbal children unable to respond to visual acuity assessment, amblyogenic factors are sought, including strabismus, media opacities, unequal Brückner reflexes (pupillary red reflexes), and a family history suggestive of strabismus, amblyopia, or ocular disease occurring in childhood (see earlier section on Ophthalmic Examination).

Treatment

The earlier treatment is begun, the better will be the chance of improving visual acuity. Treatment is usually discontinued after age 9 years. Amblyogenic factors such as refractive errors are addressed. Because of the extreme sensitivity of the visual nervous system in infants, congenital cataracts and media opacities must be diagnosed and treated within the first few weeks of life. Visual rehabilitation and amblyopia treatment must then be started to foster visual development.

After eradicating amblyogenic factors, the mainstay of treatment is patching the sound eye, which causes the visual nervous system to process input from the amblyopic eye and in that way permits the development of useful vision. Other treatment modalities include "fogging" the sound eye with cycloplegic drops (atropine), lenses, and filters.

Prognosis

Depends on the compliance with treatment but usually good.

STRABISMUS

ESSENTIALS OF DIAGNOSIS & TYPICAL FEATURES

- Strabismus is misalignment of the eyes.
- Its prevalence in childhood is about 2%–3%.
- Strabismus is categorized by the direction of the deviation (esotropia, exotropia, hypertropia, hypotropia) and its frequency (constant or intermittent).
- Strabismus may cause or be due to amblyopia.

Esotropia (Crossed Eyes)

ESSENTIALS OF DIAGNOSIS & TYPICAL FEATURES

- Pseudoesotropia can result from prominent epicanthal folds that give the appearance of crossed eyes when they are actually straight.
- Esotropia is deviation of the eyes toward the nose and may involve one or both eyes.

Pathogenesis

Congenital esotropia (infantile esotropia) has its onset in the first year of life in healthy infants. The deviation is large and obvious. Esotropia beginning in the first year also occurs in premature infants or children with a complicated perinatal history associated with CNS problems such as intracranial hemorrhage and periventricular leukomalacia. The most frequent type of acquired esotropia is the accommodative type

(Figure 16–26). Onset is usually between ages 2 and 5 years. The deviation is variable in magnitude and constancy and is often accompanied by amblyopia. One type of accommodative esotropia is associated with a high hyperopic refraction. In another type, the deviation is worse with near than with distant vision. This type of esodeviation is usually associated with lower refractive errors.

Esotropia is associated with certain syndromes. In Möbius syndrome (congenital facial diplegia), a sixth nerve palsy causing esotropia is associated with palsies of the 7th and 12th cranial nerves and limb deformities. Duane syndrome can affect the medial or lateral rectus muscles (or both). It may be an isolated defect or may be associated with a multitude of systemic defects (eg, Goldenhar syndrome). Duane syndrome is often misdiagnosed as a sixth (abducens) nerve palsy. The left eye is involved more commonly, but both eyes can be involved. Girls are affected more frequently. Children with unilateral paretic or restrictive causes of esotropia may develop face turns toward the affected eye to maintain binocularity.

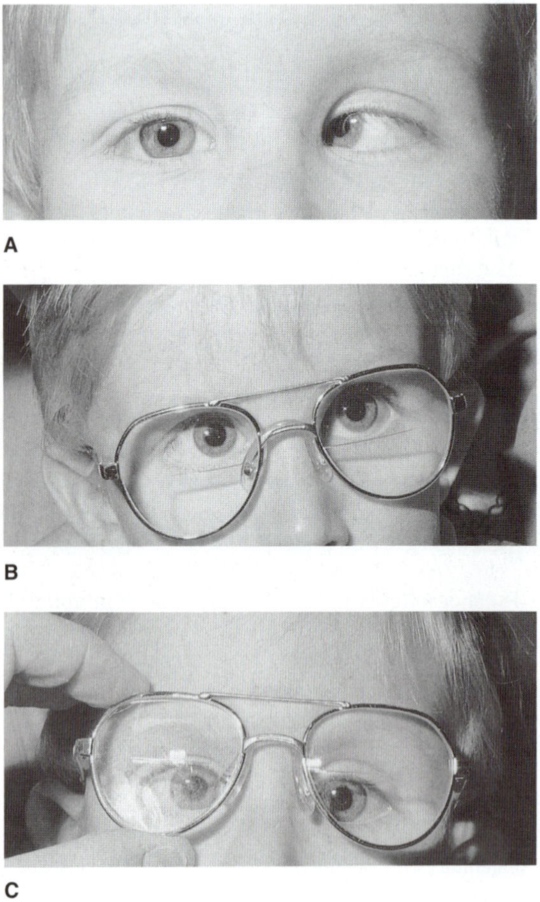

▲ **Figure 16–26.** Accommodative esotropia. **A:** Without glasses, esotropic; **B:** with glasses, well-aligned at distance; **C:** at near with bifocal correction.

After age 5 years, any esotropia of recent onset should arouse suspicion of CNS disease. Infratentorial masses, hydrocephalus, demyelinating diseases, and idiopathic intracranial hypertension are causes of abducens palsy, which appears as an esotropia, lateral rectus paralysis, and face turn. The face turn is an attempt to maintain binocularity away from the field of action of the paretic muscle. Papilledema is often, but not invariably, present with increased intracranial pressure.

Besides the vulnerability of the abducens nerve to increased intracranial pressure, it is susceptible to infection and inflammation. Otitis media and Gradenigo syndrome (inflammatory disease of the petrous bone) can cause sixth nerve palsy. Less commonly, migraine and diabetes mellitus are considerations in children with sixth nerve palsy.

Clinical Findings

Observation of the reflection of a penlight on the cornea, the corneal light reflex, is an accurate means of determining if the eyes are straight. If strabismus is present, the corneal light reflex will not be centered in both eyes. Observation of eye movements may reveal restriction of eye movements in certain positions of gaze. Alternate cover testing of the eyes while the child is fixating on a near and/or distant target will reveal refixation movements if the eyes are crossed.

Complications

Amblyopia and poor stereoacuity/depth perception.

Treatment

Motility, cycloplegic refraction, and a dilated funduscopic examination by an ophthalmologist are necessary to determine the etiology of esotropia. Some children require imaging studies and neurologic consultation.

Surgery is the mainstay of treatment for congenital esotropia. Controversy exists as to how young the child should be when surgery is performed so that the child can obtain an optimal binocular result. The age range is from younger than 6 months to 2 years.

Management of accommodative esotropia includes glasses with or without bifocals, amblyopia treatment, and in some cases surgery.

Underlying neurologic disease should be referred to the appropriate specialists for further management.

Prognosis

Usually good.

Exotropia (Wall-Eyed)

ESSENTIALS OF DIAGNOSIS & TYPICAL FEATURES

- Exotropia is a type of strabismus in which the eyes are divergent/wall-eyed (Figure 16–27).
- Exotropia may be intermittent or constant and involve one or both eyes.

Clinical Findings

The deviation most often begins intermittently and occurs after age 2 years. Congenital (infantile) exotropia is extremely rare in an otherwise healthy infant. Early-onset exotropia may occur in infants and children with severe neurologic problems.

Evaluation of the corneal light reflex reveals the penlight's reflection in the deviated eye is displaced nasally. All children with constant, congenital exotropia require CNS neuroimaging. Referral to an ophthalmologist is indicated.

Complications

Amblyopia and poor stereoacuity/depth perception.

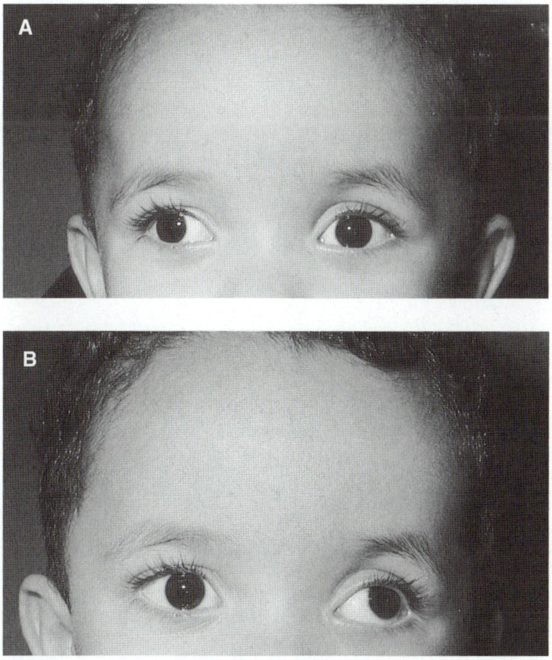

▲ **Figure 16–27.** Exotropia. **A:** Fixation with left eye. **B:** Fixation with right eye.

Treatment

Treatment of exotropia is with surgery, orthoptic exercises, patching, and occasionally glasses.

Prognosis

Generally good.

Granet DB, Khayali S: Amblyopia and strabismus. Pediatr Ann 2011 Feb;40(2):89–94 doi: 10.3928/00904481-20110117-08 [Review] [PubMed] [PMID: 21323205].

UNEXPLAINED DECREASED VISION IN INFANTS & CHILDREN

ESSENTIALS OF DIAGNOSIS & TYPICAL FEATURES

- Blindness in infants and children is commonly caused by retinal dystrophies, optic nerve disorders or cortical visual impairment due to significant central nervous system disease.

Pathogenesis

Occult causes of poor vision and blindness in children may be due to hereditary retinal dystrophies such as Leber congenital amaurosis and optic nerve abnormalities, including optic nerve hypoplasia and atrophy.

Cerebral visual impairment, also known as cortical blindness, is manifested as decreased visual attentiveness of varying degree. Cerebral visual impairment can be congenital or acquired. Insults to the optic pathways and higher cortical visual centers are responsible. Asphyxia, trauma, intracranial hemorrhage, and periventricular leukomalacia are some of the causes of cortical visual impairment.

Clinical Findings

Affected infants will have poor eye contact, fail to fixate and follow a visual target, and be unresponsive to visual threat. Wandering or roving eye movements and nystagmus are common. Eye poking is seen in some infants with low vision.

Referral to an ophthalmologist is indicated to determine the etiology of the low vision. Diagnostic tests such as an electroretinogram and visual evoked response may be required. Imaging studies of the brain, genetics, and neurology consultations may be useful.

Differential Diagnosis

Delayed visual maturation, vision loss due to an ocular versus neurologic disease.

Treatment

Low-vision aids enhance remaining vision. Devices used include magnifiers for both distance and near vision, closed-circuit television, and large-print reading materials. Vision rehabilitation specialists and support groups can help teach the affected child and their family how to best use these devices. Clinical trials are underway for treatment of Leber congenital amaurosis with gene therapy.

Prognosis

Generally poor for vision.

Brémond-Gignac D, Copin H, Lapillonne A, Milazzo S; European Network of Study and Research in Eye Development: Visual development in infants: physiological and pathological mechanisms. Curr Opin Ophthalmol 2011 Apr;22(Suppl):S1–S8 [Review] [PubMed] [PMID: 21478704].

LEARNING DISABILITIES & DYSLEXIA

ESSENTIALS OF DIAGNOSIS & TYPICAL FEATURES

- Learning disabilities and dyslexia result in poor reading comprehension and writing.
- Children often have vague complaints of ocular fatigue, headaches, and difficulty reading.

Clinical Findings

Evaluation of the child with learning disabilities and dyslexia should include ophthalmologic examination to identify any ocular disorders that could cause or contribute to poor school performance. Most children with learning difficulties have no demonstrable problems on ophthalmic examination.

Treatment

A multidisciplinary approach as suggested by the AAP, the AAPOS, and the AAO is recommended in evaluating children with learning disabilities. Although many therapies directed at "training the eyes" exist, scientific support for such approaches is weak.

Prognosis

Generally good.

Web Resources

American Academy of Ophthalmology: www.aao.org

American Association of Pediatric Ophthalmology and Strabismus: www.aapos.org

Oral Medicine & Dentistry

17

Ulrich Klein, DMD, DDS, MS

ISSUES IN PEDIATRIC ORAL HEALTH

Concept of the Dental Home

Analogous to the American Academy of Pediatrics' (AAP) concept of a "medical home," the American Academy of Pediatric Dentistry (AAPD) has promoted the concept of a "dental home." A dental home is best established by referring a child for oral health examination to a dentist who provides care for infants and young children (ie, pediatric dentist) 6 months after the first tooth erupts or by 12 months of age. The primary goal of the dental home is to encourage good oral health care habits that will allow the child to grow up free from dental disease. In partnership with the caregivers, the pediatric dentist develops a comprehensive, personalized preventive health care program based on an accurate risk assessment for dental disease. The pediatric dentist provides education on age-appropriate oral hygiene techniques and a tooth-friendly diet. Other functions of the dental home include provision of anticipatory guidance on growth and development, provision of comprehensive routine and emergency dental care, and referral to other dental specialists as needed. The dental home has the benefit of promoting continuity of care in a family-centered and culturally appropriate environment, and is associated with fewer emergency visits and reduced treatment costs. A child is less likely to develop dental anxiety if a number of positive experiences precede a less pleasant appointment.

Hale KJ: Oral health risk assessment timing and establishment of the dental home. Pediatrics 2003 May;111(5 Pt 1):1113–1116 [PMID: 12728101].

Perinatal Factors and Oral Health

The perinatal period offers a unique opportunity for oral health counseling from various health care providers aimed at women's self-care as well as future child care. They may be unaware of the consequences of their own poor oral health on that of their children. The vertical transmission of cariogenic bacteria from mother to child by licking a pacifier or sharing eating utensils is well documented. Colonization of the infant with Mutans streptococci (MS) is more likely when maternal salivary MS levels are high. The mother's oral hygiene, snacking habits, and socioeconomic status all have an influence on the infant's colonization with MS. Anticipatory guidance and dental treatment of the expectant mother can significantly reduce the child's risk of acquiring MS. Prenatal dental counseling should include education on the importance of regular dental visits and the role of fluoride in maternal and childhood oral health, counseling on appropriate maternal diet, and advice on reduction of MS colonization. Maternal MS levels and the risk of transmission to infants can be reduced by twice-daily use by the mother of chlorhexidine digluconate 0.12% for 2 weeks followed by chewing 100% xylitol gum for 5 minutes 3–5 times/d (total dose of xylitol 6–10 g/d).

Delayed dental development is characteristic of preterm infants and is also seen in infants with global developmental delay. Postnatal environmental tobacco smoke exposure increases susceptibility to childhood caries, an association that is independent of age, family income, geographic region, and frequency of dental visits. It is important to advise expectant mothers about this risk. The risk of oral anomalies is higher in preterm and low-birth-weight infants than in full-term infants. These anomalies may include a narrow palate caused by traumatic laryngoscopy or prolonged endotracheal intubation, hypoplasia of the enamel of primary dentition, and crown dilaceration of the permanent maxillary incisors. The role of palatal protection plates to prevent palatal "grooving" is not clear.

American Academy of Pediatric Dentistry: Guideline on Perinatal Oral Health Care. Pediatr Dent 2010;32(special issue):109–113.

Infant Oral Health Care

Infant oral health care is the foundation on which preventive dental care is built. Ideally, infant oral health care begins before caries develops so preventive measures can be implemented. The primary goals for an infant oral health program are (1) to establish with parents the goals of oral health, (2) to inform parents of their role in reaching these goals, (3) to motivate parents to learn and practice good preventive dental care, and (4) to initiate a long-term dental care relationship with parents. These goals can be achieved through oral examination of the child, risk assessment for oral disease, anticipatory parental guidance, and regular dental health supervision. This approach advances dental care beyond tooth monitoring toward true health promotion. Because pediatricians encounter new mothers and infants earlier than dentists, it is essential that they be aware of the infectious pathophysiology and risk factors for early childhood caries (ECC).

Pediatricians should incorporate oral health into anticipatory guidance by providing information on oral health in their offices and by referring children with special health care needs to a pediatric dentist as early as 6 months of age. Referral of healthy infants to establish a dental home should occur no later than 6 months after the first tooth erupts or 12 months of age (whichever comes first).

American Academy of Pediatric Dentistry: Guideline on Infant Oral Health Care. Pediatr Dent 2010;32(special issue):114–118.

Caries-risk Assessment

Caries-risk assessment is determining the likelihood of developing carious lesions based on biological and protective factors as well as clinical findings. By 6 months of age, every child should have a caries-risk assessment performed by a pediatric health care provider. The Caries Risk Assessment Form (Table 17–1) details risk indicators for the age group 0–3 years old that directly or indirectly influence development of dental caries. Caries management by risk assessment (CAMBRA) is another protocol for a comprehensive evaluation of the child and his/her family and integrates the many factors that contribute to the development of ECC into a practical and individualized strategy for caries control. Although the best predictor of future caries is the incidence of previous caries, this finding is not a practical preventative tool. Additional risk factors include the level of parental education and age of colonization with MS and lactobacilli. The earlier the colonization occurs, the greater the risk of severe decay.

The ultimate purpose of this assessment is the development of a caries management protocol. Based on a child's risk category and whether or not parents are engaged, interventions include diagnostics (regular recalls and determination of MS levels in saliva), optimization of the protective factors listed above, dietary counseling, and restorative measures as needed. More detailed information is available online at http://www.aapd.org/media/policies.asp.

Table 17–1. Caries-risk assessment for 0–3 year olds (modified from AAPD guideline on caries-risk assessment).

		High Risk	Moderate Risk	Protective
Biological Factors	Mother/primary caregiver has active caries	Yes		
	Parent/primary caregiver has low socioeconomic status	Yes		
	Child has >3 between meal sugar-containing snacks or beverages per day	Yes		
	Child is put to bed with a bottle containing natural or added sugar	Yes		
	Child has special health care needs		Yes	
	Child is a recent immigrant		Yes	
Protective Factors	Child receives optimally fluoridated drinking water and fluoride supplements			Yes
	Child has teeth brushed daily with fluoridated toothpaste			Yes
	Child receives topical fluoride from health professional			Yes
	Child has dental home/regular dental care			Yes
Clinical Findings	Child has white spot lesions or enamel defects	Yes		
	Child has visible cavities of fillings	Yes		
	Child is a recent immigrant		Yes	

American Academy of Pediatric Dentistry: Guideline on Caries-risk Assessment and Management for Infants, Children, and Adolescents. Pediatr Dent 2010;32(special issue):101–108.

Ramos-Gomez FJ et al: Caries risk assessment appropriate for the age 1 visit (infants and toddlers). J Calif Dent Assoc 2007 Oct;35(10): 687–702 [PMID: 18044377].

DENTAL CARIES

Dental caries is the most common chronic disease of childhood and the most prevalent unmet health need of U.S. children. Dental caries is largely a disease of poverty. Children and adolescents in low-income families account for 80% of patients with tooth decay.

Pathogenesis

Development of caries requires the interaction of four factors: (1) a host (tooth in the oral environment), (2) a suitable dietary substrate (fermentable carbohydrates), (3) cariogenic microorganisms that adhere to the tooth, and (4) time, measured as the frequency of exposure to fermentable carbohydrates and the duration of acid exposure. The main organisms implicated in the initiation of caries are *Streptococcus mutans* (MS) and *Streptococcus sobrinus. Lactobacillus acidophilus* and *Lactobacillus casei* are linked to the progression of caries. MS organisms are most commonly passed vertically from mother to child. A "window of infectivity" between ages 19 and 33 months has been described, but colonization can occur as early as 3 months of age. Earlier colonization increases the risk of caries. Dental plaque is an adherent biofilm on the tooth surface that harbors acidogenic bacteria in close proximity to the enamel. As bacteria metabolize sucrose, they produce lactic acid that solubilizes calcium phosphate in tooth enamel and dentin. Demineralization of the dental enamel occurs below pH 5.5 and is the first step in cariogenesis. The flow rate of saliva and its buffering capacity are important modifiers of demineralization. Demineralization of enamel and dentin can be halted or even reversed by redeposition of calcium, phosphate, and fluoride from saliva. If not halted, the carious process penetrates the enamel, advancing through the dentin toward the pulp of the tooth. In response, blood vessels in the pulp dilate and inflammatory cells begin to infiltrate (pulpitis). If the carious lesion is untreated, pulp exposure will occur, triggering invasion of more inflammatory cells and the eventual formation of a small pulp abscess. If this abscess can drain into the oral cavity, the apical tooth tissue may remain vital. However, if the radical pulp becomes necrotic, a periapical abscess develops (Figure 17–1). Although this process may be asymptomatic, it usually causes severe pain, fever, and swelling.

Clinical Findings & Treatment

The diagnosis of caries is usually made by visual and tactile oral examination. Radiographs are used to visualize caries on the surfaces between teeth. The initial defect observed on enamel beneath the dental plaque is the so-called "white-spot lesion," a white, chalky, decalcified area along the gingival margin or on approximated tooth surfaces. Frank carious lesions are light- to dark-brown spots or cavities of varying size on the tooth. A light shade of brown indicates more rampant decay. Arrested caries are almost black in color. In the early stages of decay, the tooth may be sensitive to temperature changes or sweets. Removing the carious tooth structure and filling the early defect with a restorative material can repair the tooth. As decay progresses deeper into the pulp, inflammation and pain increase. Eventually, the entire pulp becomes necrotic, and a choice must be made between root canal therapy (pulpectomy) or removal of the tooth. In the presence of cellulitis or facial space abscess, extraction and antibiotic therapy are the treatments of choice.

Cavitation is the late phase of disease. Filling cavities does not address the underlying pathologic process responsible for tooth decay. Unlike other infections, dental caries cannot be treated by a course of antibiotics. However, a daily dose of chlorhexidine gluconate rinse 0.12% for 2 weeks can significantly reduce the number of cariogenic bacteria in the mouth and delay recolonization for 3–6 weeks. Such treatment is recommended at 3-month intervals for patients with high levels of bacteria. Improvement in risk of dental caries can only be achieved by a sustained reduction in the number of cariogenic oral bacteria and by the creation of a favorable oral environment. Additionally, all active cavities must be restored to eliminate sources of reinfection. A patient and his/her family must be encouraged to change

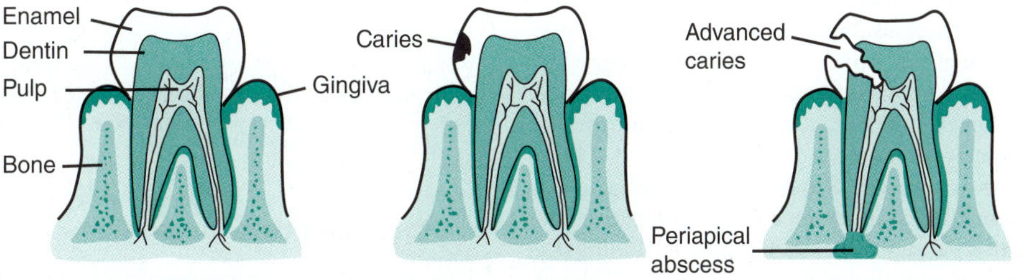

▲ **Figure 17–1.** Tooth anatomy and progression of caries.

diet and habits of oral hygiene in an effort to prevent further infection. Motivational interviewing has been shown to be more successful in setting these self-management goals than simple or stern recommendations. Regular dental visits, the periodicity of which should be determined by the risk level for developing carious lesions, must be maintained to monitor and reinforce these goals. The concept of prevention through timely and regular parent education, early diagnosis, and prompt intervention offers greater efficiency, better health outcomes, and lower costs than repeated restoration of diseased teeth.

Caries Prevention

Prevention of dental caries necessitates restoring the delicate balance between pathologic and protective factors. The former include cariogenic bacteria and fermentable carbohydrates. The latter consist of protective factors in saliva, and fluoride in food, beverages, drinking water, and oral care products. Saliva provides calcium, phosphate, proteins, antibacterial substances, and buffers to neutralize acid produced by bacteria in plaque.

A. Changes in Lifestyle

Oral hygiene practices should start soon after birth. The infant's gums should be cleaned daily using a moist, soft cloth. Once the teeth erupt, oral hygiene must be practiced in earnest, particularly in high-risk children. A small amount of fluoridated toothpaste ("smear layer") should be used on a small, soft toothbrush designed for infants. Because of a lack of manual dexterity in children younger than 8 years of age, parents need to brush for them twice daily and assist with flossing. Another important parental task is reducing the amount of substrate available to the bacteria by limiting the consumption of sugar-containing infant formulas, beverages, and snacks. Each such exposure produces an acidic oral environment for up to 30 minutes. The primary care physician and his/her team play an invaluable role in disseminating this information during early well-baby visits.

B. Fluorides

Fluorides are safe and effective in caries prevention through three topical mechanisms of action: inhibition of bacterial metabolism by interfering with enzyme activity; inhibition of demineralization; and enhancing remineralization. Fluoride can be applied professionally or by the patient under parental supervision. Although more than half the U.S. population has access to fluoridated community water, an increasing number of families consume processed water with unknown fluoride content. Fluorides affect the dentin and enamel of both erupted and unerupted teeth. Systemic effects are achieved by oral ingestion from sources such as fluoridated drinking water or fluoride supplements. Fluoridated toothpaste and mouth rinses deliver topical benefits. Table 17–2 shows the current ADA recommendations for dietary fluoride supplementation for children at high caries risk. They should be taken daily to maximize the caries risk prevention benefit. For children at low caries risk, dietary fluoride supplements are not recommended. The child's true exposure to fluoride must be evaluated before supplements are prescribed to avoid the mottled enamel (dental fluorosis) produced by excessive fluoride. Because children younger than 6 years of age cannot expectorate reliably, parents must monitor the use of fluoridated toothpaste, ensuring that only a "pea-sized" amount of the product is used at each brushing. Several factors are associated with a high risk for caries—orthodontic appliances, decreased salivary function, gastroesophageal reflux disease, cariogenic diet, physical inability to properly clean the teeth, mother or siblings with caries, personal history of caries. Individuals with these risk factors should be considered for additional topical fluoride therapy to supplement oral hygiene measures.

Table 17–2. Dietary fluoride supplementation schedule for children at high caries risk

Age	Concentration of Fluoride in Water		
	< 0.3 ppm F	0.3–0.6 ppm F	> 0.6 ppm F
Birth–6 mo	None	None	None
6 mo–3 y	0.25 mg	None	None
3–6 y	0.50 mg	0.25 mg	None
6–at least 16 y	1.00 mg	0.50 mg	None

Adapted from evidence-based clinical recommendations on the prescription of dietary fluoride supplements for caries prevention: A report of the American Dental Association Council on Scientific Affairs. Rozier RG et al; J Am Dent Assoc 2010 Dec;141(12):1480–1489 [PMID: 21158195].

Infants who consume concentrate infant formulas as the main source of nutrition may incur an increased risk for enamel fluorosis in the permanent dentition if those formulas are reconstituted with optimally fluoridated drinking water. It is important that practitioners evaluate all sources of fluoride intake when advising parents about the use of fluoridated toothpastes or prescribing fluoride supplements.

Berg J et al: Evidence-based clinical recommendations regarding fluoride intake from reconstituted infant formula and enamel fluorosis: A report of the American Dental Association Council on Scientific Affairs. J Am Dent Assoc 2011 Jan;142(1):79–87 [PMID: 21243832].

C. Other Adjunctive Measures

Consumption of beverages sweetened with artificial sweeteners instead of sugar can help reduce the intake of fermentable carbohydrates. While chewing gum helps to clean food debris from teeth and increases salivary flow, these beneficial effects are lost when sugar-containing gum is used. The AAP considers chewing gum a choking risk in smaller children. A significant reduction of salivary MS by the polyol sweetener xylitol has been described, but a dose of at least 5–10 g/d for adults and 5–7.5 g/d for toddlers aged 6–36 months with exposure times lasting several minutes three times daily are required to produce this effect. Topical application of 8 g/d xylitol syrup in 9–15 months old children twice per day for 12 months during primary tooth eruption could prevent up to 70% of dental caries. However, unclear labeling of the ingredients in xylitol-containing products makes the exact determination of the dose difficult and the high cost of foods containing xylitol limits its widespread use.

American Academy of Pediatric Dentistry: Policy on the Use of Xylitol in Caries Prevention. Pediatr Dent 2010;32(special issue):36–38.

Featherstone JD: The science and practice of caries prevention. J Am Dent Assoc 2000 Jul;131(7):887–899 [PMID: 10916327].

Early Childhood Caries

Formerly termed "baby bottle tooth decay" or "nursing bottle caries," early childhood caries (ECC) is a particularly virulent and rapidly progressive form of caries that begins on the smooth surfaces of the teeth soon after eruption. Lack of adequate preventive care as well as poor feeding habits such as the frequent consumption of liquids containing fermentable carbohydrates from a nursing bottle, frequent sipping from a no-spill sippy cup, taking a bottle to bed, and breastfeeding in combination with other carbohydrates place children at high risk for ECC. ECC typically involves the maxillary incisors but any other teeth may be affected.

ECC is defined as one or more decayed (d), missing (m), or filled (f) tooth surfaces (s) in any primary tooth in a child younger than 71 months of age. Any sign of smooth-surface caries in a child younger than 3 years is termed severe ECC (S-ECC). From 3–5 years, one or more decayed, missing, or filled smooth surfaces in maxillary front teeth or a total dmfs score of 4 or higher must be present to make a diagnosis of S-ECC. By age 5 years, a dmfs score of 6 or higher must be present to constitute S-ECC. Children with S-ECC are at higher risk for new carious lesions, more frequent hospitalizations, and emergency department visits. They are absent more often from school, may have below-normal height and weight gain, and have a diminished oral health-related quality of life. Although S-ECC can affect all children, it is 32 times more likely in children who consume sugary foods and whose mothers are of low socioeconomic status and education level.

Parents should be counseled to eliminate saliva-sharing activities and not to put infants to sleep with a bottle containing fermentable carbohydrates. After eruption of the first tooth, ad libitum breast-feeding should be discontinued and regular oral hygiene measures such as twice-daily use of fluoridated toothpaste, both in optimally fluoridated and fluoride-deficient communities, should be implemented. Infants should be weaned from the bottle at about 1 year of age and encouraged to drink from a noncovered cup mainly as part of a snack or meal. Frequent consumption of cariogenic liquids from a bottle or no-spill training cup should be avoided. The AAP recommends limiting juice to 4–6 oz/day for children 1–6 years of age.

Preventive strategies focused on the pregnant woman should start in the prenatal and perinatal periods. Maternal malnutrition during the third trimester, low birthweight, and systemic illness in the neonatal period can lead to tooth hypoplasia, which makes teeth more susceptible to caries. Later, motivational interviewing may help parents to reduce deleterious feeding habits and to adopt lifestyle changes within their family that address the multifactorial etiologies of early childhood caries.

American Academy of Pediatric Dentistry: Policy on Early Childhood Caries (ECC): Classifications, Con-sequences, and Preventive Strategies. Pediatr Dent 2010;32 (special issue):41–44.

Policy on Early Childhood Caries (ECC): Unique Challenges and Treatment Options. Pediatr Dent 2010;32(special issue):45–47.

Preventive Dental Treatment (Fluoride Varnish) by Physicians for High-Risk Populations

Since parents are more likely to take their very young child to a physician for well-child visits than to a dentist for oral health counseling, some states have established formal programs to entice medical offices to provide preventive dental services. These include dental screening, risk assessment, and referrals to dentists as needed, parent counseling about their child's oral health, and applications of fluoride varnish (ICD-9-CM Diagnosis Code V07.31: Need for Prophylactic Fluoride Administration). The latter consists of a resin base in which fluoride (5% NaF) is suspended. Its sticky nature allows for extended contact time of the fluoride with the tooth surface. Many studies have demonstrated the safety and efficacy of fluoride varnishes and have described a significant reduction in the decay rate of smooth surfaces as well as pits and fissures. A report on the effectiveness of a medical office-based preventive dental program in North Carolina found that it was successful in reducing caries-related treatments for children up to 6 years of age by 17%. Multiple fluoride varnish applications at the time of tooth emergence seemed to be most beneficial.

The varnish in single-dose packages (0.3–0.5 mL) should be stirred vigorously before application and the contents of larger tubes (5 mL) massaged to redissolve any precipitated fluoride. The former are preferable because consistent availability of fluoride cannot be guaranteed with multidose packages. The average amount of varnish needed depends on the number of teeth present and ranges from 0.1 mL for infants to 0.3 mL for preschool children. Teeth should be dried with gauze before application of the varnish with a small brush. It will set quickly to a dull yellow film upon contact with saliva. Caregivers should be instructed not to brush or floss and to give their child only soft foods until the next morning affording the fluoride enough time for absorption into enamel.

Miller EK, Vann WF Jr: The use of fluoride varnish in children: A critical review with treatment recommendations. J Clin Pediatr Dent 2008 Summer;32(4):259–264 [PMID: 18767454].

Pahel BT, Rozier RG, Stearns SC, Quiñonez RB: Effectiveness of preventive dental treatments by physicians for young Medicaid enrollees. Pediatrics 2011 Mar;127(3):e682–e689 [PMID: 21357343].

ORAL EXAMINATION OF THE NEWBORN & INFANT

The sagittal and vertical maxillomandibular relationships are different at birth. An anterior open bite is considered physiologic before the onset of tooth eruption. The infant's mouth is more triangularly shaped and its oral cavity is small and totally filled by the tongue due to a small and slightly retrognathic lower jaw. This newborn's pseudo micrognathia is due to ventral positioning of the fetus and will generally correct after birth by physiologic suckling.

Sucking Pads

Frequent breast-feeding can lead in some babies to formation of a lip callus ("sucking pad") at the midline of the upper lip. Since it does not bother the mother or the child, it should not be removed. It will generally go away within the baby's first year.

Newborns have a markedly larger corpus adiposum buccae on the outer side of the buccinator muscle called "sucking pads," which are supposed to strengthen and support the cheek during the act of sucking.

The mouth of the normal newborn is lined with an intact, smooth, moist, shiny mucosa (Figure 17–2). The alveolar ridges are continuous and relatively smooth. Within the alveolar bone are numerous tooth buds, which at birth are mostly primary teeth.

Teeth

Hard tissue formation of primary teeth begins at approximately 4 months' gestation. At birth, all 20 primary teeth are calcified. The central maxillary incisors are almost completely calcified while only the cusp tips of the maxillary and

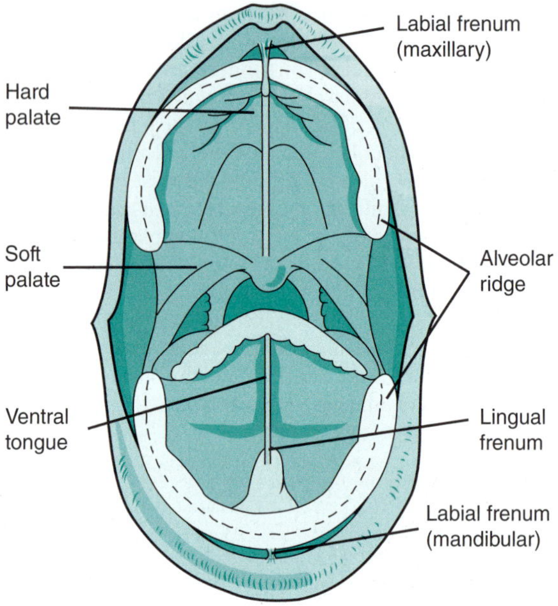

▲ **Figure 17–2.** Normal anatomy of the newborn mouth.

mandibular second molars are calcified. There is a trace of enamel on the first four permanent molars at birth.

The primary teeth usually begin to erupt at 6–7 months of age. On rare occasions (1:3000), natal teeth are present at birth or neonatal teeth erupt within the first month. These are most commonly (85%) mandibular primary incisors. They can be "real" primary teeth (90%) or supernumerary teeth (10%) and should be differentiated radiographically. Although the preferred approach is to leave the tooth in place, supernumerary and hypermobile immature primary teeth should be extracted. On occasion, such teeth must be smoothed or removed if their sharp incisal edge causes laceration of the tongue (Riga-Fede disease). If such teeth cause difficulties with breast feeding, pumping and bottling the milk is initially recommended while the infant is conditioned not to "bite" during suckling.

Frena

Noticeable but small maxillary and mandibular labial frena should be present (Figure 17–3). The "persisting tectolabial frenum" that is observed in 25% of all children tends to diminish in size with normal development. Its physiological purpose is to provide greater support to the upper lip during breastfeeding. Several small accessory frena may also be present farther posteriorly. In rare cases, as in oral-facial-digital syndrome, there are multiple thick tightly bound frena. Decisions about surgical correction should be based on the ability to maintain the child's gingival health and are best left until the late preteen years. Many thick frena do not require correction.

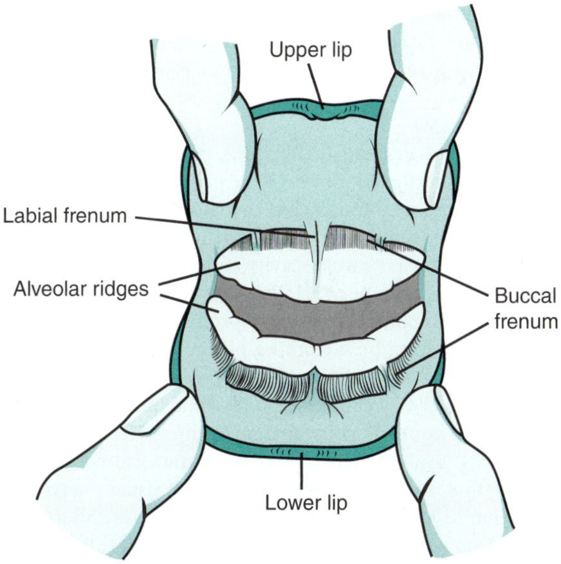

▲ **Figure 17–3.** The frena.

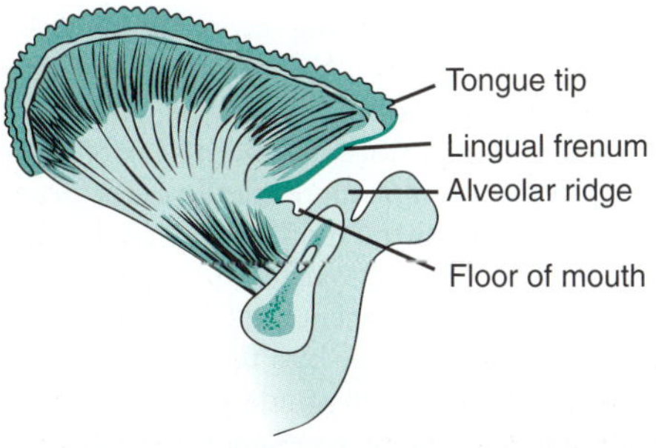

▲ **Figure 17–4.** Normal position of lingual frenum.

The tongue is connected to the floor of the mouth by the lingual frenum (Figures 17–3 and 17–4). This connection should not impede the free movement of the tongue. If the attachment is tight and high up on the alveolar ridge (Figure 17–5), it may restrict movement and interfere with the child's ability to produce "t," "d," and "l" sounds. This condition is called ankyloglossia (tongue-tie). Surgical correction may be indicated if the tongue cannot touch the maxillary incisors or the roof of the mouth. Earlier intervention (at age 3–4 years) is better than later, but there is usually no urgency for surgery in the neonatal period unless the child has difficulties to latch on properly to the mother's nipple and causes her pain during nursing.

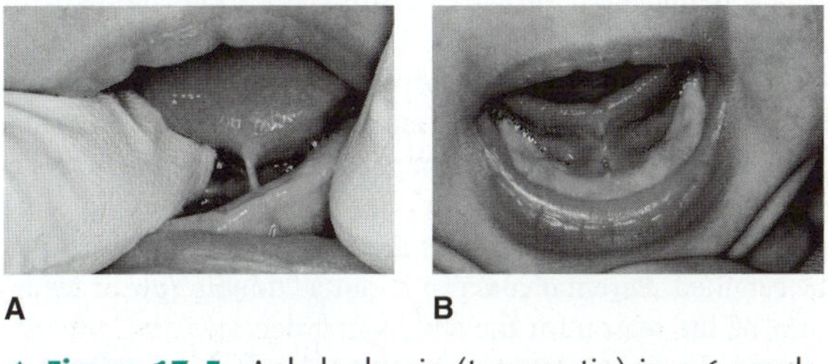

▲ **Figure 17–5.** Ankyloglossia (tongue-tie) in a 6-week old, before (A) and after (B) the release surgery.

Cleft Lip & Palate

The palate of the newborn should be intact and continuous from the alveolar ridge anteriorly to the uvula (see Figure 17–2). Cleft lip and palate are common defects with an incidence of 0.28–3.74 in 1000 live births globally. Incidence varies widely among races and ranges from 1 in 500 among Navaho Native Americans and Japanese to more than 1 in 800 in Caucasians and 1 in 2000 in African Americans. The cleft of the palate can be unilateral or bilateral (Figure 17–6). It can involve only the alveolar ridge, or the ridge and entire palate. Cleft palate may also present as an isolated submucous cleft or as bifid uvula. Although clefts present superficially as a cosmetic problem, they cause complex functional problems such as oro-antral communication and disruption of the maxillary alveolar ridge with significant associated dental problems such as irregularities in tooth numbers, delayed eruption, and malocclusion. They disturb the muscle arrangement of the perioral and the soft palate muscles by interrupting their continuity across the

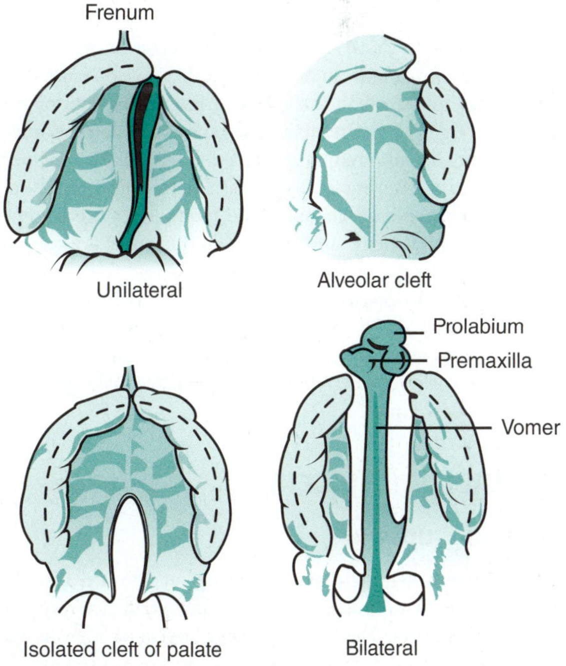

▲ **Figure 17–6.** Types of clefts.

midline. As a result, feeding, swallowing, speech, and ventilation of the middle ear are negatively affected.

Children with cleft lip and palate should be referred as soon as possible to a multidisciplinary cleft palate team for comprehensive assessment of their medical status, feeding problems, general development, dental development, hearing, facial esthetics, and overall functioning. Dental involvement in children with cleft palate is extensive, and treatment may begin immediately after birth with fabrication of a palatal obturator as a feeding aid. Nasoalveolar molding should be performed to lengthen the columella and to guide the protruding greater segment (in unilateral clefts) or the premaxilla (in bilateral clefts) back into the oral cavity, thus making surgical lip closure easier when it is performed usually after 10 weeks of age. Palate closure to approximate the muscles of the soft palate intended to restore its proper function and to facilitate the acquisition of normal speech without nasality follows at 12–18 months of age. The associated scar formation causes significant dentofacial growth disturbance. Orthodontic treatment aims to address the sagittal and transverse maxillary growth deficits as well as the frequent irregularities in tooth eruption and position. Between 8 and 10 years of age, an alveolar bone graft is indicated to add bony support to the incisor adjacent to the cleft and to enable eruption of the lateral incisor and canine on the cleft side. In some patients, orthognathic surgery to reposition the maxilla anteriorly and mandible posteriorly is needed in late adolescence after cessation of growth to complete their successful rehabilitation.

Other Soft Tissue Variations

Minor oral soft tissue variations can occur in newborns. Small, 1–2 mm round, smooth, white, or grayish lesions are sometimes noted on the buccal and lingual aspects of the alveolar ridges or the midpalatine raphe. The latter, called Epstein pearls, are remnants of epithelial tissue trapped along the raphe during fetal growth. The former, Bohn nodules, are remnants of mucous gland tissue. Both are benign, require no treatment, and usually disappear a few weeks after birth.

Some newborns may have small intraoral lymphangiomas on the alveolar ridge or the floor of the mouth. A dentist familiar with neonates should evaluate these and any other soft tissue variations that are more noticeable or larger than those just described.

ERUPTION OF THE TEETH

Normal Eruption

Primary teeth generally begin to erupt at about 6 months of age. The mandibular incisors usually erupt before the maxillary incisors. The first teeth may appear as early as age 3–4 months or as late as age 12–16 months. Many symptoms are ascribed to teething, but any association with fever, upper respiratory infection, or systemic illness is probably coincidental rather than related to the eruption process. Attributing fever to teething without thorough diagnostic evaluation for other sources has resulted in missing serious organic disease.

Common treatment for teething pain is the application of topical anesthetics or teething gels, available over the counter. Most of these agents contain benzocaine or, less commonly, lidocaine. If improperly used, they can cause numbness of the entire oral cavity and pharynx. Suppression of the gag reflex can be a serious side effect. Systemic analgesics such as acetaminophen or ibuprofen are safer and more effective. Chewing on a teething object can be beneficial, if only for distraction purposes.

Occasionally, swelling of the alveolar mucosa overlying an erupting tooth is seen during teething. This condition appears as localized red to purple, round, raised, smooth lesions that may be symptomatic but usually are not. Treatment is rarely needed, as these so-called eruption cysts or eruption hematomas resolve with tooth eruption.

Delayed Eruption

Premature loss of a primary tooth can either accelerate or delay eruption of the underlying secondary tooth. Typically, early eruption occurs when the permanent tooth is in its active eruption stage and the overlying primary tooth is removed within 6–9 months of its normal exfoliation. If loss of the primary tooth occurs more than 1 year before expected exfoliation, the permanent tooth will likely be delayed in eruption owing to healing that results in filling in of bone and gingiva over the permanent tooth. The loss of a primary tooth may cause adjacent teeth to tip or drift into the space and lead to space loss for the underlying permanent tooth. Placement of a space maintainer can prevent this.

Other local factors delaying or preventing tooth eruption include supernumerary teeth, cysts, tumors, overretained primary teeth, ankylosed primary teeth, and impaction. A generalized delay in eruption may be associated with global developmental delays, endocrinopathies (hypothyroidism or hypopituitarism), or other systemic conditions (cleidocranial dysplasia, rickets, or trisomy 21).

Ectopic Eruption

If the dental arch provides insufficient room, permanent teeth may erupt ectopically and cause a usually painless partial or complete root resorption in the adjacent primary tooth. This phenomenon is more common in the maxilla, with ectopic eruption of the maxillary first permanent molar being the most frequent. In the mandible, lower incisors may erupt lingually and thus the primary predecessor may be retained. Parental concern about a "double row of teeth" may be the reason for the child's first dental visit. If the primary teeth are not loose, the dentist should remove them to allow their successors to drift into proper position.

Impaction

Impaction occurs when a permanent tooth is prevented from erupting. Although crowding is the most frequent reason, over-retained primary or supernumerary teeth is another cause. The teeth most often affected in the developing dentition are the maxillary canines. Generally, they are brought into correct alignment through surgical exposure and orthodontic treatment.

Variations in Tooth Number

Failure of teeth to develop—a condition called hypodontia—is rare in the primary dentition, but occurs with an incidence of 5:100 in the permanent dentition. The most frequently missing teeth are the third molars followed by the lateral maxillary incisors and mandibular second premolars. Oligodontia, a condition in which only a few teeth develop, occurs in patients with ectodermal dysplasias.

Occasionally, supernumerary teeth are present, most typically in the maxillary incisor area, distal to the maxillary molars, or in the mandibular bicuspid region. Mesiodentes are peg-shaped supernumerary teeth situated at the maxillary midline that occur in about 5% of individuals. If they hinder eruption of adjacent permanent incisors, their timely removal is recommended.

Dean JA, Avery DR, McDonald RE: *McDonald and Avery Dentistry for the Child and Adolescent* 9th ed. Maryland Heights (MO): Mosby Elsevier.

PERIODONTAL DISEASE

Periodontal disease involves a tooth's supporting structures: bone, gingiva, and periodontal ligaments (Figure 17–7). It begins as inflammation of the gingival tissue adjacent to a tooth. Bacterial accumulation in the gingival sulcus causes irritation and inflammation. This initial phase, called dental plaque-induced disease, is found almost universally in children and adolescents. Systemic conditions, alterations in hormone levels (insulin, gonadotropin), medications, and malnutrition can intensify the inflammatory response to plaque. Generally, this condition responds well to removal of bacterial deposits and improved oral hygiene.

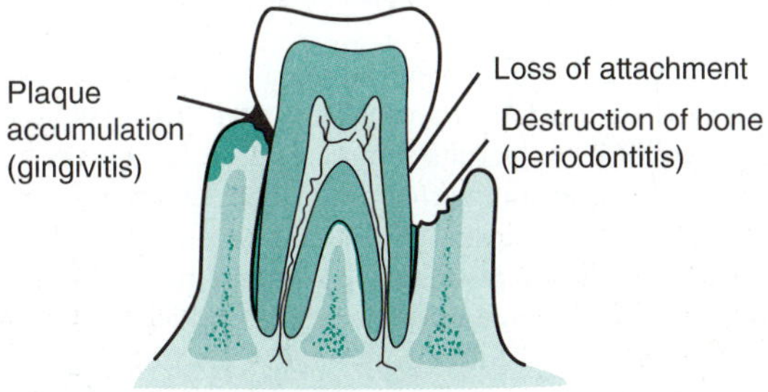

▲ **Figure 17–7.** Periodontal disease.

Periodontitis is characterized by loss of attachment and destruction of bone. Patients with localized aggressive periodontitis typically have severe alveolar bone loss around permanent first molars and incisors, whereas the generalized form involves other teeth as well. The prevalence is 0.2% in Caucasians, but higher (2.5%) in African Americans. Familial aggregation and functional defects such as anomalies of neutrophil chemotaxis, phagocytosis, and bacterial activity increase the risk of periodontitis. *Actinobacillus actinomycetemcomitans* in combination with *Bacteroides*-like species are implicated in this disease. Treatment consists of combined surgical and nonsurgical root debridement plus antibiotic therapy.

Periodontitis as a manifestation of systemic diseases can be associated with hematological (acquired neutropenia, leukemias) or genetic disorders such as Down-, PapillonLefèvre-, Chediak-Higashi-, hypophosphatasia-, and leukocyte adhesion deficiency syndromes. The incidence of necrotizing periodontal diseases is lower (1%) in North America than in developing countries (2%–5%). Necrotizing periodontal disease is characterized by interproximal ulceration and necrosis of the dental papillae, rapid onset of dental pain, and often fever. Predisposing factors include viral infections (including human immunodeficiency virus [HIV]), malnutrition, emotional stress, and systemic disease. The condition usually responds rapidly to treatment consisting of mechanical debridement with ultrasonic scalers, improved oral hygiene, and metronidazole and penicillin for febrile patients.

Armitage GC: Development of a classification system for periodontal diseases and conditions. Ann Periodontol 1999 Dec;4(1):1–6 [PMID: 10863370].

DENTAL EMERGENCIES

Orofacial Trauma

Orofacial trauma often consists only of abrasions or lacerations of the lips, gingiva, tongue, or oral mucosa (including the frena), without damage to the teeth. Lacerations should be cleansed, inspected for foreign bodies, and sutured if necessary. Occasionally, radiographs of the tongue, lips, or cheeks are needed to detect tooth fragments or other foreign bodies. All patients with facial trauma should be evaluated for jaw fractures. Blows to the chin are among the most common childhood orofacial traumas. They are also a leading cause of condylar fracture in the pediatric population. Condylar fracture should be suspected if pain or deviation occurs when the jaw is opened.

Tooth-related trauma affects any or all of the dental hard tissues and the pulp, the alveolar process, and the periodontal tissues. The range of luxation injuries includes concussion; subluxation; intrusive, extrusive, and lateral luxation; and avulsion. Figure 17–8 demonstrates the different luxation

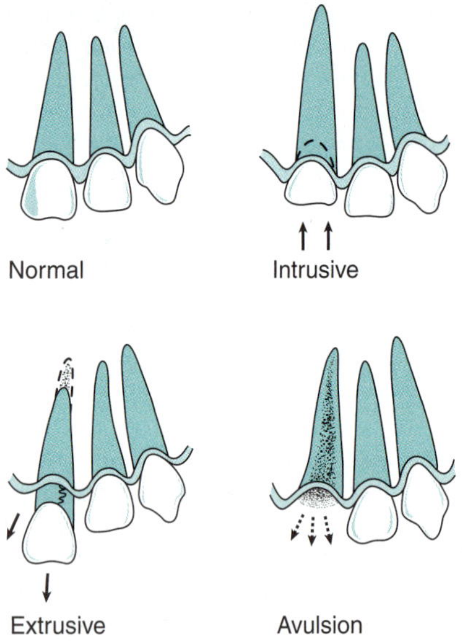

▲ **Figure 17–8.** Patterns of luxation injuries.

injuries, and Figure 17–9 shows the different degrees of tooth fractures.

The least problematic luxation injuries are concussion (no mobility) and subluxation (mobility without displacement). Unless mobility is extensive, this condition can be followed without active intervention, but pulp vitality should be periodically assessed.

Primary Teeth

The peak age for injuries to primary teeth is toddlerhood. Any treatment must include measures to ensure the integrity of the permanent teeth. Parents should be advised of any permanent tooth complications such as enamel hypocalcification or crown-root dilaceration caused by intrusion injuries of primary maxillary front teeth. An intrusive luxation is usually observed for a period of time to discern whether the tooth will spontaneously re-erupt (see Figure 17–8). Severe luxations in any direction are treated with extraction. Avulsed primary teeth are not replanted. In a root fracture, the crown and apical fragment are generally extracted. The latter should be left for physiologic resorption if its retrieval would result in potential damage to the permanent tooth.

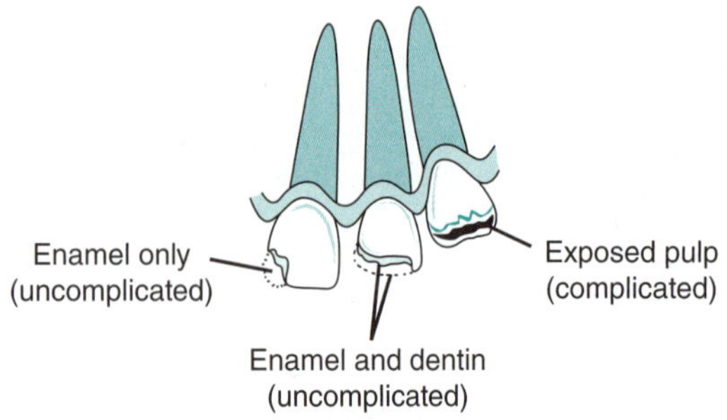

▲ **Figure 17–9.** Patterns of crown fractures.

Permanent Teeth

Because the prognosis for viability worsens rapidly as time outside the mouth increases, avulsed permanent teeth should be replanted at or near the site of injury following gentle rinsing with clean water. The patient should seek emergency dental care immediately thereafter. Hank's balanced salt solution is the best storage and transport medium for avulsed teeth that are to be replanted. The next best storage media in decreasing order are milk, saline, saliva (buccal vestibule), or water. The commercially available FDA-approved Save-a-Tooth kit should be part of first-aid kits in schools and sports facilities.

Intrusions of permanent teeth are corrected with surgical or orthodontic repositioning. Lateral and extrusive luxations are generally repositioned and splinted for up to 3 weeks. Root canal treatment is necessary in the majority of injuries. Factors to consider during treatment planning are root development (open or closed apex) and the extent of the luxation. Pulp necrosis; surface, inflammatory, and replacement resorption; or ankylosis may occur at any time during the healing process and determine the long-term outcome. All luxated and replanted teeth need to be followed regularly by a dentist.

Andreasen JO: *Traumatic Dental Injuries: A Manual.* 2nd ed. Wiley-Blackwell, 2003.

American Academy of Endodontists: Guidelines for the Treatment of Traumatic Dental Injuries 2004; Tooth Saving Tips. http://www.aae.org/guidelines/ Accessed July 2011.

Save-a-Tooth Emergency Tooth Preserving System. http://www.save-a-tooth.com/ Accessed July 2011.

Other Dental Emergencies

Dental emergencies other than trauma are usually associated with pain or swelling due to infection resulting from advanced caries. Odontogenic pain usually responds to acetaminophen or ibuprofen. Topical medications are of limited value.

A localized small swelling confined to the gingival tissue associated with a tooth is usually not an urgent situation. This "gumboil" or parulis represents an infection that has spread outward from the root of the tooth through the bone and periosteum. Usually it will drain and leave a fistulous tract. Facial cellulitis results if the infection invades the facial spaces. Elevated temperature (> 38.8°C), difficulty swallowing, and difficulty breathing are signs of more serious infection. Swelling of the midface—especially the bridge of the nose and the lower eyelid—should be urgently evaluated as a potential dental infection. Extraction of teeth or root canal therapy combined with antibiotics is the usual treatment. Hospitalization is a prudent choice for younger children with severe facial cellulitis especially if other risk factors are present—dehydration, airway compromise, or possible noncompliance. Inpatient treatment consists of intravenous antibiotics such as clindamycin or ampicillin-sulbactam (Unasyn) with incision, drainage, and removal of the source of infection.

ANTIBIOTICS IN PEDIATRIC DENTISTRY

The antibiotics of choice for odontogenic infection are penicillin and clindamycin.

Several patient groups require prophylactic antibiotic coverage prior to invasive dental manipulation. These include children with artificial heart valves, previous infectious endocarditis, certain congenital heart conditions, immunodeficiency, or central venous catheters. The American Heart Association published revised guidelines for infective endocarditis prophylaxis in April 2007.

Wilson W et al: Prevention of infective endocarditis: Guidelines from the American Heart Association: A guideline from the American Heart Association Rheumatic Fever, Endocarditis and Kawasaki Disease Committee, Council on Cardiovascular Disease in the Young, and the Council on Clinical Cardiology, Council on Cardiovascular Surgery and Anesthesia, and the Quality of Care and Outcomes Research Interdisciplinary Working Group. J Am Dent Assoc 2008 Jan;139(Suppl):3S–24S [PMID: 18167394].

SPECIAL PATIENT POPULATIONS

Children with Cancer

The most common source of systemic sepsis in the immunosuppressed patient with cancer is the oral cavity. Therefore, a dentist knowledgeable about pediatric oncology should evaluate children with cancer soon after diagnosis. The aim is to educate the patient and caregivers about the importance of good oral hygiene and to remove all existing and potential sources of infection such as abscessed teeth, extensive caries, teeth that will soon exfoliate, ragged or broken teeth, uneven fillings, and orthodontic appliances before the child becomes neutropenic as a consequence of chemotherapy. Younger patients have more oral problems than adults. After an initial evaluation and before the initiation of cancer therapy, a dental treatment plan should be developed in discussion with the medical team. Preventive strategies include reduction of refined sugars, fluoride therapy, lip care, and patient education. Chemotherapeutic drugs and local irradiation are cytotoxic to the oral mucosa, which becomes atrophic and develops mucositis. Oral pain may be severe and often leads to inadequate food and fluid intake, infections in the oral cavity, and an increased risk of septicemia. Meticulous oral hygiene reduces the risk of severe mucositis.

The pediatric oncology patient should be monitored throughout therapy to screen for infection, manage oral bleeding, and control oral pain. These patients can experience spontaneous oral hemorrhage, especially when the platelet count is less than 20,000/mL. Poor oral hygiene or areas of irritation can increase the chances of bleeding. Children receiving radiation therapy to the head and neck may develop xerostomia if salivary glands are in the path of the beam of radiation. Customized fluoride applicators and artificial saliva in combination with close follow-up are used to manage xerostomia aggressively to avoid rapid and extensive destruction of the teeth. Children receiving hematopoietic stem cell transplantation may require longer periods of immunosuppression. During the neutropenic phase of pretransplant conditioning, mucositis, xerostomia, oral pain, oral bleeding, and opportunistic infections may occur. Oral graft-versus-host disease as well as oral fungal and herpes simplex virus infections can be seen during the subsequent initial engraftment and hematopoietic reconstitution period. Long-term dental follow-up includes management of salivary dysfunction and craniofacial growth abnormalities from total body radiation and treatment of oral graft-versus-host disease.

Pediatric oncology patients need regular care by a dentist familiar with young children and their growth and development. Oral and maxillofacial growth disturbances can occur after therapy. Late effects of therapy include such morphologic changes as microdontia, hypocalcification, short and blunted roots, delayed eruption, and alterations in facial bone growth.

da Fonseca MA: Dental care of the pediatric cancer patient. Pediatr Dent 2004 Jan–Feb;26(1):53–57 [PMID: 15080359].

Children with Bleeding Disorders

Children with some genetic or acquired disorders of coagulation may require clotting factors before and after invasive dental procedures, including local block anesthesia. Oral surgical procedures on any child with a bleeding disorder should be planned in concert with the child's hematologist. Patients with hemophilia A and factor VIII antibodies (inhibitors) requiring surgery should be admitted to a hospital. Some patients with very mild factor VIII deficiency or von Willebrand disease type 1 may respond to DDAVP (1-deamino-8-D-arginine vasopressin), whereas von Willebrand types 2 and 3 require cryoprecipitate. Antifibrinolytic medications such as ε-aminocaproic and tranexamic acid are used successfully after dental treatment. Topical medications such as Gelfoam and thrombin can be used to control postoperative bleeding. Patients receiving anticoagulant therapy should generally not undergo dosage adjustment before surgical dental treatment because the risk of embolic complications is much higher than bleeding complications in those whose anticoagulant therapy is continued. However, the dentist is advised to consult with the hematologist to obtain the most recent INR (international normalized ratio) results and to discuss the most appropriate level of anticoagulation.

Children with Type 1 Diabetes

The incidence of caries is not increased in diabetic children if metabolic control is good. However, they are at higher risk for periodontal disease that usually starts at puberty with mild gingivitis, gum bleeding, and gingival recession. Care must be taken not to disturb the regular cycle of eating and insulin dosage. Anxiety associated with dental appointments can cause a major upset in the diabetic child's glycemic control. Postoperative pain or pain from dental abscess can disrupt their routine oral intake, necessitating adjustment of insulin doses.

ORTHODONTIC REFERRAL

A child's dentist usually initiates the referral to an orthodontist. For any child with a cleft palate or other craniofacial growth disorder, referral is indicated when maxillary permanent incisors are starting to erupt. Other localized problems such as anterior and/or posterior crossbites and disturbances associated with the eruption of maxillary and mandibular front teeth should be addressed early when they occur to restore proper function and normal craniofacial growth. Significant arch length deficiency resulting in severe crowding requires early decisions on how to guide the developing dentition through extractions of multiple primary and permanent teeth (ie, serial extraction sequence). Likewise, pronounced discrepancies in anterior-posterior skeletal jaw relationships warrant early evaluation by an orthodontist.

Ear, Nose, & Throat

18

Patricia J. Yoon, MD, FACS
Peggy E. Kelley, MD
Norman R. Friedman, MD

THE EAR

INFECTIONS OF THE EAR

The spectrum of infectious ear diseases includes the structures of the outer ear (otitis externa), the middle ear (otitis media), the mastoid bone (mastoiditis), and the inner ear (labyrinthitis).

1. Otitis Externa

ESSENTIALS OF DIAGNOSIS

- Infection of the ear canal skin.
- External auditory canal edema and minimal, thick drainage.
- Severe pain, worsened by manipulation of pinna.

Pathogenesis

Otitis externa is inflammation of the skin lining the ear canal and surrounding soft tissue. The most common cause is loss of the protective function of cerumen, leading to maceration of the underlying skin, such as occurs with swimming. Other causes include trauma to the ear canal as from using cotton swabs for cleaning or poorly fitted ear plugs while swimming; contact dermatitis; secondary infection of the canal from otitis media with a patent tympanostomy tube; and chronic drainage from a perforated tympanic membrane (TM). Infections due to *Staphylococcus aureus* or *Pseudomonas aeruginosa* are the most common.

Clinical Findings

A. Symptoms and Signs

Symptoms include pain and itching in the ear, especially with chewing or pressure on the tragus. Movement of the pinna or tragus causes considerable pain. Drainage may be minimal unless the otitis externa is from a draining tympanostomy tube or TM perforation. The ear canal is typically grossly swollen, and the patient may resist any attempt to insert an ear speculum. Debris is noticeable in the canal. It is often impossible to visualize the TM. Hearing is normal unless complete occlusion has occurred.

Differential Diagnosis

It can sometimes be difficult to distinguish this infection from a perforation of the TM with drainage or mastoiditis.

Complications

If untreated, facial cellulitis may result. Immunocompromised individuals can develop malignant otitis externa, which is a spread of the infection to the skull base with resultant osteomyelitis.

Treatment

Topical treatment usually suffices. Fluoroquinolone otic drops are recommended. In the absence of systemic symptoms, children with otitis externa secondary to draining tubes or perforations should be treated with topical therapy only. The topical therapy chosen must be safe for the inner ear (nonototoxic) because a perforation or patent tube allows the drops access to the middle and inner ear. If the TM cannot be seen, then a perforation should be presumed to exist. If the ear canal is patent, ototopical antibiotics are prescribed for 5–7 days as indicated. If the canal is too edematous to allow entry of the eardrops, a Pope ear wick (expandable sponge) is needed to assure antibiotic delivery. Oral antibiotics are indicated for any signs of invasive infection, such as fever, cellulitis of the face or auricle, or tender postauricular lymph nodes. In such cases, cultures of the ear canal discharge should be sent, and an antistaphylococcal antibiotic prescribed while awaiting culture results. Systemic antibiotics alone without local topical treatment will not successfully treat otitis externa. Narcotic analgesics may be required until the infection begins to resolve.

During the acute phase, the patient should keep the ear dry. The patient should be followed up in 1 week to document an intact TM. Children with intact TMs who are predisposed to external otitis should receive 2 or 3 drops of a 1:1 solution of white vinegar and 70% ethyl alcohol into the ears before and after swimming.

Kaushik V, Malik T, Saeed SR: Interventions for acute otitis externa. Cochrane Database of Systematic Reviews (1) CD004740 2010 [PMID: 20091565].

Roland PS et al: Consensus panel on role of potentially ototoxic antibiotics for topical middle ear use: Introduction, methodology, and recommendations. Otolaryngol Head Neck Surg 2004;130:S51 [PMID: 15543836].

2. Acute Otitis Media

ESSENTIALS OF DIAGNOSIS

- Acute onset of symptoms which may include fever, pain, decreased sleep, decreased appetite.
- Effusion (fluid in the middle ear).
- Inflammation.
- All of the above are needed to make diagnosis.

Pathogenesis

Otitis media is an infection associated with middle ear effusion (MEE) or with otorrhea (ear drainage) if a patent tympanostomy tube or perforation is present. Otitis media can be further classified by its associated clinical symptoms, otoscopic findings, duration, frequency, and complications. These more specific classifications are acute otitis media (AOM), otitis media with effusion (OME), and chronic suppurative otitis media.

Clinical Findings

A. Symptoms and Signs

In 2004, the American Academy of Pediatrics and of the American Academy of Family Physicians specified three criteria which must be present in order to make a diagnosis of acute otitis media (Table 18–1). These include acute onset of symptoms, presence of fluid in the middle ear, and signs and symptoms of inflammation.

The presence of an ear effusion is best determined by exam and either pneumatic otoscopy or tympanometry (Figure 18–1). To distinguish AOM from OME, signs and symptoms of middle-ear inflammation and acute infection must be present. Otoscopic findings specific for AOM include a bulging TM, impaired visibility of ossicular landmarks, yellow or white effusion (pus), opacified and inflamed eardrum, and sometimes squamous exudate or bullae on the eardrum. On the other hand, OME is associated with a retracted or neutral TM with decreased mobility. It may be opacified or have whitish or amber discoloration. Children with OME can develop superimposed AOM.

Table 18–1. Definition of acute otitis media (AOM).

A diagnosis of AOM requires (1) a history of acute onset of signs and symptoms, (2) the presence of MEE, and (3) signs and symptoms of middle-ear inflammation.

Elements of the definition of AOM are all of the following:

1. Recent, usually abrupt, onset of signs and symptoms of middle-ear inflammation and MEE
2. The presence of MEE that is indicated by any of the following:
   a. Bulging of the tympanic membrane
   b. Limited or absent mobility of the tympanic membrane
   c. Air-fluid level behind the tympanic membrane
   d. Otorrhea
3. Signs or symptoms of middle-ear inflammation as indicated by either
   a. Distinct erythema of the tympanic membrane or
   b. Distinct otalgia (discomfort clearly referable to the ear[s]) that results in interference with or precludes normal activity or sleep

B. Predisposing Factors

Otitis media is much more common in infants and young children due to the immature anatomy of the Eustachian tube and a multitude of other factors.

1. Eustachian tube dysfunction—The Eustachian tube regulates middle ear pressure and allows for drainage of middle ear. When obstructed, a vacuum develops in the middle ear, which can pull nasopharyngeal secretions and pathogens and serous fluid from the middle ear lining cells into the middle ear. This fluid is then prone to infection. The Eustachian tube of infants and small children is shorter, wider, and lies at a more horizontal angle than in adults; this is thought to contribute to the dysfunction. Infants with craniofacial disorders, such as Down syndrome or a cleft palate, may be particularly susceptible to AOM and OME.

2. Bacterial colonization—Nasopharyngeal colonization with *Streptococcus pneumoniae*, *Haemophilus influenzae*, or *Moraxella catarrhalis* increases the risk of otitis media, whereas colonization with normal flora such as viridans streptococci may prevent otitis by inhibiting growth of these pathogens. Colonization usually occurs sequentially with different pathogen serotypes sequentially, and there is risk of AOM with each new serotype acquired. Infants in day care acquire these at a younger age than those in home care. The increased number of children in day care over the past three decades has undoubtedly played a major role in the increase in AOM in the United States.

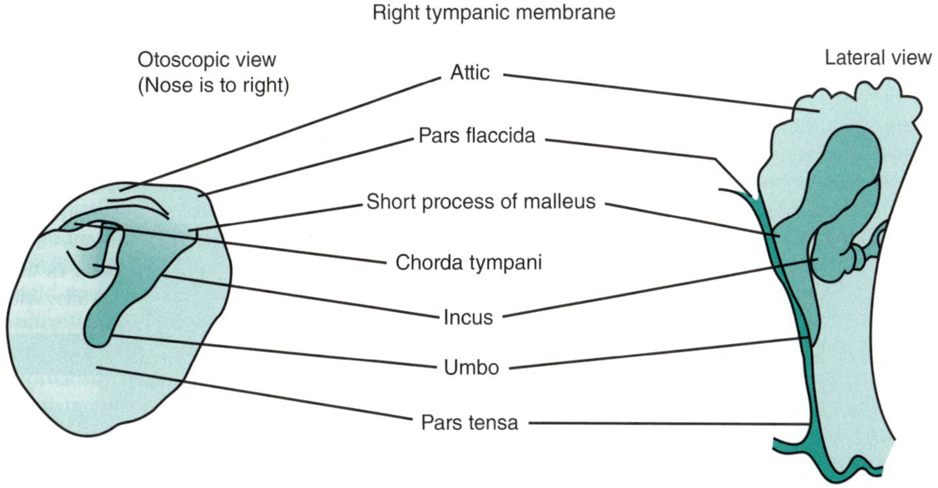

▲ **Figure 18–1.** Tympanic membrane.

3. Viral upper respiratory infections (URI)—Viral URIs increase the colonization of the nasopharynx with otitis pathogens. They also impair Eustachian tube function by causing both adenoidal swelling and edema of the Eustachian tube itself.

4. Smoke exposure—Passive smoking increases the risk of persistent MEE by enhancing colonization, prolonging the inflammatory response, and impeding drainage of the middle ear through the Eustachian tube. For infants aged 12–18 months, exposure to cigarettes at home is associated with an 11% per pack increase in the duration of MEE.

5. Impaired host immune defenses—Immunocompromised children such as those with selective IgA deficiency usually experience recurrent AOM, rhinosinusitis, and pneumonia. However, most children who experience recurrent or persistent otitis only have selective impairments of immune defenses against specific otitis pathogens. For example, a recent study showed some children have low-to-absent IgG_2 or IgA pneumococcal polysaccharide antibody responses (or both) after vaccination, despite normal serum levels of total IgG_2 and IgA. Also otitis media-prone children have a lower IgG response to an episode of acute otitis media than other children.

6. Bottle feeding—Breast feeding reduces the incidence of acute respiratory infections, provides IgA antibodies that reduce colonization with otitis pathogens, and decreases the aspiration of contaminated secretions into the middle ear space which can occur when a bottle is propped in the crib.

7. Genetic susceptibility—Although AOM is known to be multifactorial, and no gene for susceptibility has yet been identified, recent studies of twins and triplets suggest that as much as 70% of the risk is genetically determined.

C. Microbiology of Acute Otitis Media

The role of viral URI in precipitating otitis media is unquestionable, yet fewer than 12% of effusions culture positive for viruses. The URI usually precedes bacterial otitis media by 3–14 days and presumably sets the stage for bacterial infection by causing adenoid hypertrophy and eustachian tube dysfunction. The two viruses most clearly shown to precipitate otitis media are respiratory syncytial virus and influenza, accounting for the annual surge in otitis media cases from January to May in temperate climates.

There is some geographic variation in the pathogens causing AOM (Table 18–2). The microbiology of AOM has been changing. With widespread use of the pneumococcal conjugate vaccine, the incidence of *H influenza* is rising

Table 18–2. Bacteriology of acute otitis media.

	Denver (Author)	Kentucky[a] Pre-PCV7 (Prevnar)	Kentucky[a] Post-PCV7
Streptococcus pneumoniae	32	48	31
Haemophilus influenzae	50	41	56
Moraxella catarrhalis	8	9	11
Streptococcus pyogenes	4	2	2

[a]Data from Block SL et al: Community-wide vaccination with the heptavalent pneumococcal conjugate significantly alters the microbiology of acute otitis media. Pediatr Infect Dis J 2004;23:829.

while that of the *S pneumoniae* vaccine serotypes is declining (Table 18–2). There has also been an increase in disease caused by the penicillin-resistant *S pneumonia* serotypes not covered by the vaccine. These shifts in pneumococcal serotypes continue to influence treatment strategies and emphasize the need for continued surveillance. The third most common pathogen in some studies is *M catarrhalis,* which causes up to 25% of AOM cases in the United States. The fourth organism found is *Streptococcus pyogenes,* which is more common in school-aged children than in infants. This organism and *S pneumoniae* are the predominant causes of mastoiditis.

Drug-resistant *S pneumoniae* is a common pathogen in AOM and strains may be resistant to only one drug class (eg, penicillins or macrolides) or to multiple classes. Children with resistant strains tend to be younger and to have had more unresponsive infections. Antibiotic treatment in the preceding 3 months also increases the risk of harboring resistant pathogens. The prevalence of resistant strains no longer varies significantly among geographic areas within the United States, but it does vary worldwide. Lower incidences are found in countries using fewer courses of antibiotic per person. Nationwide resistance rates include 63% for trimethoprim–sulfamethoxazole, 32% for macrolides, and 2% for amoxicillin (dosed at 90 mg/kg/d). Oral cephalosporins vary widely in efficacy, with the highest resistance rates for cefixime and cefaclor and lowest rates (about 35%) for cefuroxime, cefprozil, cefpodoxime, and cefdinir. Over 90% of highly penicillin-resistant strains are still susceptible to clindamycin, rifampin, and fluoroquinolones. Fluoroquinolones are not yet approved for children younger than 16 years; however, studies are under way to assess their safety and efficacy in this age group.

D. Examination Techniques and Procedures

1. Pneumatic otoscopy—AOM is overdiagnosed. Contributing to errors in diagnosis are the temptation to accept the diagnosis without removing enough cerumen to adequately visualize the eardrum, and the mistaken belief that a red eardrum establishes the diagnosis. Redness of the eardrum is often a vascular flush caused by fever, crying, or even efforts to remove cerumen.

A pneumatic otoscope with a rubber suction bulb and tube is used to assess mobility of the TM. The speculum inserted into the patient's ear canal must be large enough to provide an airtight seal. The largest possible speculum (usually 3 or 4 mm) should be used to maximize the field of view. When the rubber bulb is squeezed, the TM should move freely with a snapping motion; if fluid is present in the middle ear space, the mobility of the TM will be absent or resemble a fluid wave. The ability to assess mobility is compromised by failure to achieve an adequate seal with the otoscope, poor visualization due to low light intensity, and mistaking the ear canal wall for the membrane.

2. Cerumen removal—Cerumen (ear wax) removal is an essential skill for anyone who cares for children. Impacted cerumen pushed against the TM can cause itching, otalgia, or hearing loss. Parents should be advised that ear wax protects the ear (cerumen contains lysozymes and immunoglobulins that inhibit infection) and usually comes out by itself; therefore, parents should never put anything solid into the ear canal to remove wax.

Cerumen may be safely removed under direct visualization through the operating head of an otoscope, provided two adults are present to hold the child. A size 0 plastic disposable ear curette may be used. Irrigation can also be used to remove hard or flaky cerumen. Asian children tend to have an ear wax variant that is dry and flaky. Wax can be softened with 1% sodium docusate solution, carbamyl peroxide solutions, mineral oil, or a few drops of detergent before irrigation is attempted. Irrigation with a soft bulb syringe is performed with water warmed to 35–38°C to prevent vertigo. A commercial jet tooth cleanser (eg, Water Pik) can be used, but it is important to set it at low power (2 or less) to prevent damage to the TM. A perforated TM or patent tympanostomy tube is a contraindication to any form of irrigation.

A home remedy for recurrent cerumen impaction is a few drops of oil such as mineral or olive oil a couple of times a week, warmed to body temperature to prevent dizziness.

3. Tympanometry—Tympanometry can be helpful in assessing middle ear status, particularly when pneumatic otoscopy is inconclusive or difficult to perform. Tympanometry cannot differentiate between AOM and OME, as it can only reveal the presence or absence of a MEE. It does not provide information as to whether the fluid is infected or whether the ear is inflamed. Tympanometry measures TM compliance and displays it in graphic form.

Tympanograms can be classified into four major patterns, as shown in Figure 18–2. The pattern shown in Figure 18–2A, characterized by maximum compliance at normal atmospheric pressure, indicates a normal TM, good Eustachian tube function, and absence of effusion. The pattern shown in Figure 18–2B identifies a nonmobile TM, which indicates MEE. The pattern shown in Figure 18–2C indicates an intact mobile TM with poor eustachian tube function and excessive negative pressure (worse than −300 mm H_2O air pressure) in the middle ear. Figure 18–2D shows a flat tracing with a large middle ear volume, indicating a patent tube or TM perforation.

4. Acoustic reflectometry—Acoustic reflectometry measures the spectral gradient of the TM using a handheld instrument, without requiring an airtight seal. Second generation models are more accurate than the original instruments and are available directly to consumers for home monitoring of middle ear effusions or for office use as an alternative to tympanometry.

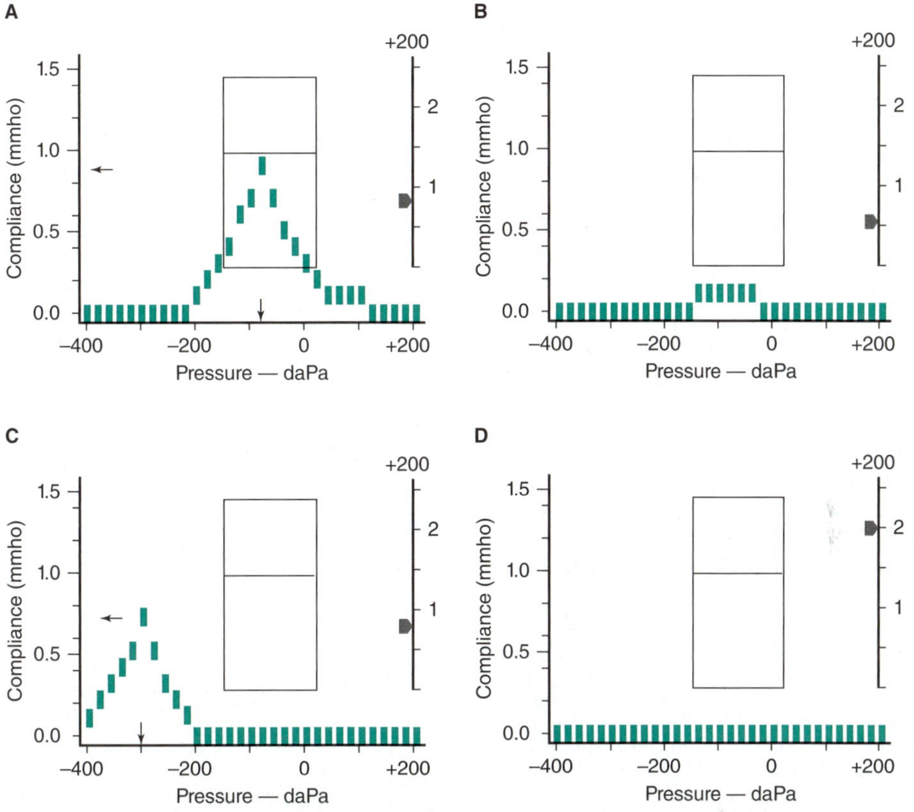

▲ **Figure 18–2.** Four types of tympanograms obtained with Welch-Allyn MicroTymp 2. **A:** Normal middle ear. **B:** Otitis media with effusion or acute otitis media. **C:** Negative middle ear pressure due to eustachian tube dysfunction. **D:** Patent tympanostomy tube or perforation in the tympanic membrane. Same as B except for a very large middle ear volume.

Differential Diagnosis

Chronic otitis media with effusion is sometimes mistaken for acute otitis media.

Complications

Complications of otitis media may involve damage to the middle ear structures, such as tympanosclerosis, retraction pockets, adhesions, ossicular erosion, cholesteatoma, perforations, and intratemporal and intracranial spread.

A. Tympanosclerosis, Retraction Pockets, Adhesive Otitis

White plaque-like patches on the TM are caused by chronic inflammation or trauma that produces granulation tissue and hyalinization.

The appearance of a small defect or invagination of the posterosuperior area of the pars tensa or in the pars flaccida suggests a retraction pocket. Retraction pockets occur when chronic inflammation and negative pressure in the middle ear space produce atrophy and atelectasis of the TM.

Continued inflammation can cause adhesions to form between the retracted TM and the ossicles. This condition, referred to as adhesive otitis, predisposes one to formation of a cholesteatoma or fixation and erosion of the ossicles.

B. Cholesteatoma

A greasy-looking mass or pearly white mass seen in a retraction pocket or perforation suggests a cholesteatoma. (See Figure 18–3.) If infection is superimposed, serous or purulent drainage will be seen, and the middle ear cavity may contain granulation tissue or even polyps. Persistent, recurrent, or

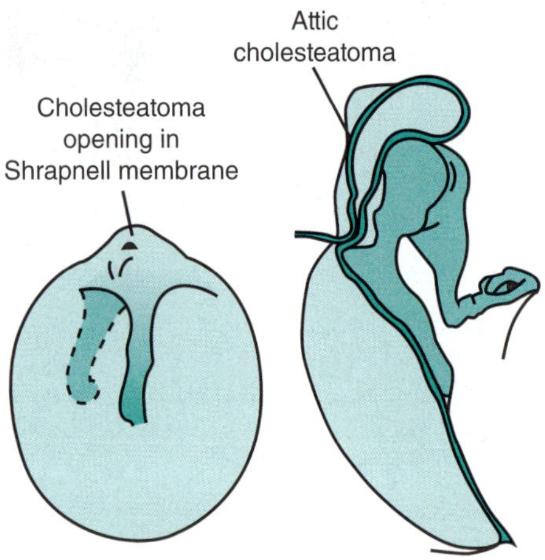

▲ **Figure 18–3.** Attic cholesteatoma, formed from an in-drawing of an attic retraction pocket.

foul smelling otorrhea following appropriate medical management should make one suspect a cholesteatoma.

C. Tympanic Membrane Perforation

Occasionally, an episode of AOM may result in rupture of the TM. Discharge from the ear is seen, and often there is rapid relief of pain. Perforations due to AOM usually heal spontaneously within a couple of weeks.

With TM perforation, a conductive hearing loss may or may not be present, depending on the size and location of the perforation.

When perforations fail to heal after 3–6 months, surgical repair may be needed. TM repair is generally delayed until the child is older and Eustachian tube function has improved. Procedures include paper patch myringoplasty, fat myringoplasty, and tympanoplasty. Tympanoplasty is generally deferred until around 7 years of age, which is approximately when the Eustachian tube reaches adult orientation. In otherwise healthy children, some surgeons will repair the perforated TM earlier if the contralateral nonperforated ear remains free of infection and effusion for 1 year.

In the presence of a perforation, water activities should be limited to surface swimming, preferably with the use of an ear mold.

D. Facial Nerve Paralysis

The facial nerve traverses the middle ear as it courses through the temporal bone to its exit at the stylomastoid foramen. Normally, the facial nerve is completely encased in bone, but occasionally bony dehiscence in the middle ear present, exposing the nerve to infection and making it susceptible to inflammation during an episode of AOM. The acute onset of a facial nerve paralysis should not be deemed idiopathic Bell's palsy until all other causes have been excluded. If middle ear fluid is present, prompt myringotomy and tube placement is indicated. CT is indicated if a cholesteatoma or mastoiditis is suspected.

E. Chronic Suppurative Otitis Media

Chronic suppurative otitis media is present when persistent otorrhea occurs in a child with tympanostomy tubes or TM perforations. Occasionally, it is a sign of cholesteatoma. Visualization of the TM, meticulous cleaning with culture of the drainage, and appropriate antimicrobial therapy are keys to management of cases not related to cholesteatoma. Successful treatment usually requires therapy with an antibiotic that covers *Pseudomonas* and anaerobes. Oral quinolone antibiotics are not yet approved for use in growing children, but studies suggest that topical quinolones for 14 days may be effective. It is very important to clean the ear canal by suction to allow delivery of the drops.

When chronic otorrhea is due to a cholesteatoma, medical therapy is not effective. If the discharge does not respond to 2 weeks of aggressive therapy, cholesteatoma, tuberculosis, or a fungal infection should be suspected. Serious central nervous system (CNS) complications such as extradural abscess, subdural abscess, brain abscess, meningitis, labyrinthitis, or lateral sinus thrombophlebitis can occur with extension of this process. Therefore, patients with facial palsy, vertigo, or other CNS signs should be referred immediately to an otolaryngologist.

▶ Treatment

A. Pain Management

Children with pain related to AOM may obtain relief from acetaminophen or ibuprofen, accompanied by a topical anesthetic drop (benzocaine and antipyrine) if the TM is not perforated.

B. The Observation Option (Watchful Waiting)

Doctors must often balance the desire of parents for treatment of AOM against the risk of increasing drug resistance due to overuse of antibiotics. Overdiagnosis of AOM is one of the most common reasons for antibiotic overuse. The natural history of untreated AOM is usually to improve through host defenses or by perforation of the TM; but mastoiditis was not an infrequent complication before the use of antibiotics.

In 2004, clinical practice guidelines were issued that suggested nontreatment of limited groups of children with AOM (Table 18–3). Key points are that children older than age 2 years with nonsevere disease were recommended for nontreatment for the first 48–72 hours after onset of symptoms. Those younger than age 2 years and older children with severe pain or fever were always recommended to receive immediate antibiotics. Children failing observation were to begin antibiotics after 48–72 hours. An option for the practitioner is to provide a prescription at the first visit,

Table 18–3. Criteria for initial antibiotic treatment in children with acute otitis media.

Age	Certain Diagnosis	Uncertain Diagnosis
< 6 mo	Antibacterial therapy	Antibacterial therapy
6 mo–2 y	Antibacterial therapy	Antibacterial therapy if severe illness; observation option[a] if nonsevere illness
≥ 2 y	Antibacterial therapy if severe illness; observation option[a] if nonsevere illness	Observation option[a]

[a]Nonsevere illness is mild otalgia and fever < 39°C in the past 24 h.

Table 18–4. Treatment of acute otitis media in an era of drug resistance.

First-line therapy
1. Amoxicillin, 90 mg/kg/d, up to 4 g/d. For children over age 2 y, give for 5 d; under age 2 y, for 10 d.
2. If amoxicillin has caused a rash, give cefuroxime (Ceftin), cefdinir (Omnicef), or cefpodoxime (Vantin).
3. If urticaria or other IgE-mediated events have occurred, give trimethoprim-sulfamethoxazole or azithromycin (Zithromax).
4. If child is unable to take oral medication, give single IM dose of ceftriaxone (Rocephin).

Second-line therapy[a]
1. Amoxicillin-clavulanate (Augmentin ES-600), given so that patient receives amoxicillin at 90 mg/kg/d.
2. If amoxicillin has caused allergic symptoms, see recommendations above.

Third-line therapy
1. Tympanocentesis is recommended to determine the cause.
2. Ceftriaxone (Rocephin), two doses given IM, 48 h apart, with option of a third dose.

Recurrences > 4 wk after first episode
1. A new pathogen is likely, so restart first-line therapy.
2. Be sure diagnosis is not OME, which may be observed for 3–6 mo without treatment.

[a]For clinical failure after 48–72 h of treatment, or for recurrences within 4 wk.
IM, intramuscular; OME, otitis media with effusion.

with instructions to fill only if no improvement is seen after the specified observation period. For infants younger than age 6 months, antibiotics are always recommended on the first visit, regardless of diagnostic certainty.

Recommendations differ for "certain" versus "uncertain" diagnosis, but clinicians should be able to make a correct diagnosis if they can master cerumen removal and pneumatic otoscopy. The guidelines emphasize the importance of establishing the presence of effusion, and differentiating between OME and AOM (see Table 18–3). Everyone agrees that overtreatment of OME by well-meaning providers has led to overuse of antibiotics for no discernible benefit.

C. Antibiotic Therapy

Amoxicillin remains the first-line antibiotic for treating otitis media, even with a high prevalence of drug-resistant *S pneumoniae,* because resistance to β-lactam antibiotics, such as amoxicillin, develops as a stepwise process over many years. A bacterial strain resistant to low levels of amoxicillin usually is eradicated by a higher dosage. Amoxicillin dosage may be raised considerably without toxicity; for example, a dosage of 200 mg/kg/d has been used to treat meningitis in children, and a maximum daily dose of 4 g has been used in adults. Studies have shown that increasing the dosage from 40 mg/kg to 90 mg/kg yields a drug concentration in middle ear fluid that surpasses the minimal level needed to inhibit 98% of all pneumococcal otitis media. A second advantage is that dosing amoxicillin at these higher levels may help delay stepwise emergence of resistance. High-dose amoxicillin will usually eradicate the most invasive pathogen, *S pneumoniae,* and if no improvement occurs, a second-line antibiotic may be chosen to cover *M catarrhalis* and β-lactamase–producing *H influenzae.*

Amoxicillin–clavulanate enhanced-strength (ES), with 90 mg/kg/d of amoxicillin dosing (14:1 ratio of amoxicillin to clavulanate), is an appropriate choice when a child is clinically failing after 48–72 hours on amoxicillin (Table 18–4). In this situation, the most likely pathogen is *H influenzae,* and the addition of clavulanate to amoxicillin will broaden the coverage while retaining efficacy against *S pneumoniae.* The regular strength formulations of amoxicillin–clavulanate (7:1 ratio) should not be doubled in dosage to achieve 90 mg/kg/d of amoxicillin, because the increased amount of clavulanate will cause diarrhea.

Three oral cephalosporins (cefuroxime, cefpodoxime, and cefdinir) are more β-lactamase–stable and are alternative choices for antibiotic therapy in children who develop papular rashes with amoxicillin (see Table 18–4). Unfortunately, the coverage of highly penicillin-resistant pneumococci with these agents is poor and only the intermediate-resistance classes are covered. Of these drugs, cefdinir suspension is most palatable; the other two have a bitter after-taste which is difficult to conceal. Newer flavoring agents may be helpful here. A second-line antibiotic is indicated when a child experiences symptomatic infection within 1 month of stopping amoxicillin; however, repeat use of high-dose amoxicillin is indicated if more than 4 weeks have passed without symptoms, because a new pathogen is usually present. Macrolides such as azithromycin and clarithromycin are not recommended as second-line agents because (1) *S pneumoniae* is resistant to macrolides is approximately 30% in respiratory isolates, and (2) because virtually all strains of *H influenzae* have an intrinsic macrolide efflux pump, which pumps antibiotic out of the bacterial cell. In a recent double tympanocentesis study, the on-therapy eradication rate of all pathogens was 94.2% for high-dose amoxicillin–clavulanate and 70.3% for azithromycin ($P < .001$).

If a child remains symptomatic for longer than 3 days while taking a second-line agent, a tympanocentesis is useful to identify the causative pathogen. Reasons for failure to eradicate a sensitive pathogen may be drug noncompliance, poor drug absorption, or vomiting of drug. If a highly resistant pneumococcus is found or if tympanocentesis is not feasible, intramuscular ceftriaxone at 50 mg/kg/d for 3 consecutive days is recommended. If a child has experienced anaphylaxis to amoxicillin, cephalosporins should not be substituted. However, the maculopapular rash frequently seen with amoxicillin is not IgE-mediated, so cephalosporins may be safely used.

Two new classes of antibiotics have been in active clinical trials for AOM: fluoroquinolones and ketolides. Ketolides, however, were recently removed from the market. Fluoroquinolones are divided into two classes; the older class includes ciprofloxacin, ofloxacin, and levofloxacin. The newer class includes gatifloxacin and moxifloxacin. Pneumococcal resistance has been seen in countries where fluoroquinolones were widely used in adults. The newer drugs have a lower tendency to select resistant *S pneumoniae,* because two mutations are required. In a double tympanocentesis study of high-risk children, gatifloxacin was shown to eradicate 96% of pathogens.

Figure 18–4 shows the recommended follow-up of AOM that resolves with a residual effusion at 3–4 weeks. Children, particularly those young enough to still be developing language skills, should be seen monthly for otoscopic examinations to determine if the effusion is persistent. Antibiotics and corticosteroids are no longer recommended for OME. An audiology evaluation should be performed after approximately 3 months of continuous bilateral effusion in children younger than 3 years and those at risk of language delay due to socioeconomic circumstances, craniofacial anomalies, or other risk factors. Children with hearing loss or speech delay should be referred to an otolaryngologist for possible ventilation tube placement. (See later section on Management of Otitis Media with Residual and Persistent Effusions.)

D. Duration of Therapy

The duration of antibiotic treatment is controversial. Only three recent trials have used stringent entry and outcome criteria. Success rates were higher following 10 days of therapy than shorter treatment courses in all three studies.

E. Tympanocentesis

Tympanocentesis is performed by placing a needle through the TM and aspirating the middle ear fluid. Indications for tympanocentesis are (1) AOM in an immunocompromised patient, (2) research studies, (3) evaluation for presumed sepsis or meningitis, such as in a neonate, (4) unresponsive otitis media despite courses of two appropriate antibiotics, and (5) acute mastoiditis or other suppurative complications. Tympanocentesis is performed with an open-headed operating otoscope and either a spinal needle and 3 mL syringe, or if available, an Alden-Senturia trap (Storz Instrument Co., St. Louis, MO) or the Tymp-Tap aspirator (Xomed Surgical Products, Jackson, FL) (Figure 18–5). The fluid is sent for culture and sensitivity.

F. Prevention of Acute Otitis Media

1. Antibiotic prophylaxis—Prolonged use of low doses of antibiotics, for periods of 6–12 months, has been the primary method of prophylaxis. However, due to concerns about resistant organisms, this method should be reserved for unusual situations. A situation in which prophylaxis might still be recommended is a child being considered for tympanostomy tube placement for recurrent infections who presents in late spring. A 1–2 month course of amoxicillin might prevent infection until the low-risk summer season when AOM is uncommon. Another situation would be in the child with patent tympanostomy tubes who experiences recurrent AOM and has been found to have an immune deficiency on more than one occasion. Antibiotic prophylaxis is not recommended for children with OME, despite earlier guidelines that made such a recommendation.

2. Lifestyle modifications—Parental education plays a major role in decreasing AOM. The following are some items to consider in children with frequent recurrences:

- Smoking is a risk factor both for upper respiratory infection and for AOM, and primary care physicians can provide literature on smoking cessation programs and on nicotine-containing gums or patches.
- Breast feeding protects children from AOM, but the mechanism is unknown. Also, propping a bottle of milk in the crib increases AOM risk.
- Removing pacifiers from infants was shown in Finland to reduce episodes of AOM by about one-third compared with a control group. The mechanism is uncertain but is likely to be related to effects on the eustachian tube.
- Day care is clearly a risk factor for AOM, but working parents may have few alternatives. Possible alternatives include care by relatives or care of the child in a home care setting with fewer children.

3. Surgery—Tympanostomy tubes are effective in the treatment of recurrent otitis media as well as OME, which will be discussed in the next section.

4. Immunologic evaluation and allergy testing—Parents often ask if an immune deficiency may be causing their child's frequent otitis episodes. While it is known that immunoglobulin subclass deficiencies are more common in immune-deficient children, the relationship is not straightforward. Furthermore, there is no practical immune therapy.

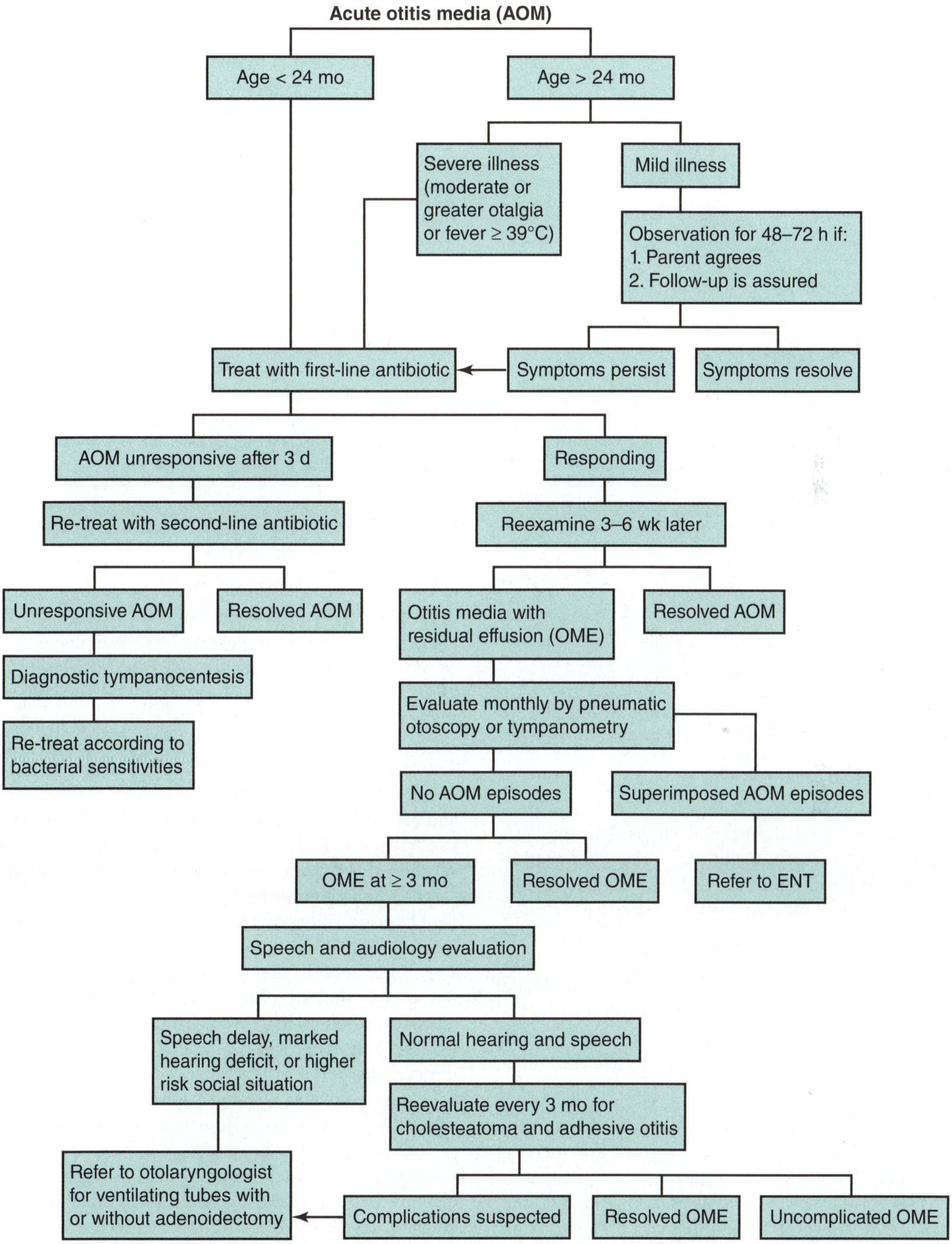

▲ **Figure 18–4.** Algorithm for acute otitis media. ENT, ear, nose, and throat consult.

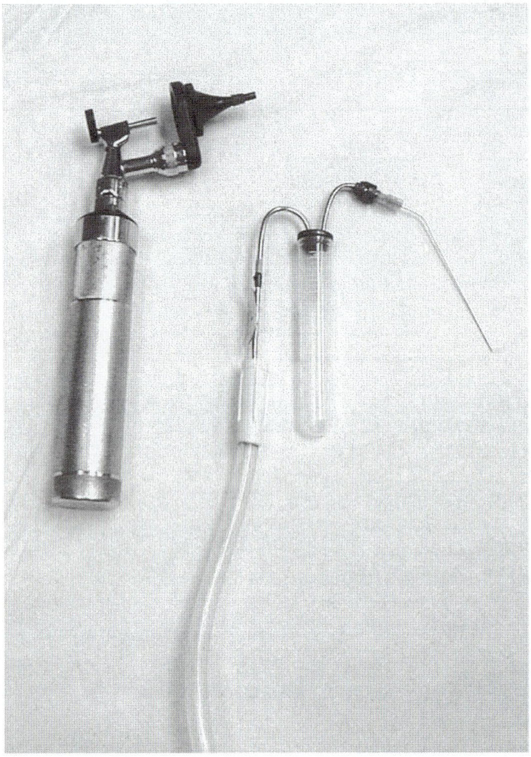

▲ **Figure 18–5.** Operating head and Alden-Senturia trap for tympanocentesis. 18-gauge spinal needle is attached and bent.

More serious immunodeficiencies such as selective IgA deficiency should be sought in children with a combination of recurrent AOM, rhinosinusitis, and pneumonia. Parents may also inquire about the role of allergy, since a generation ago many children with recurrent AOM were placed on milk elimination diets. No benefits were seen in the large group, but for certain individuals, eliminating all milk and milk-containing foods can eliminate ear infections. In the school-aged child or preschooler with an atopic background, skin testing may be beneficial in identifying allergens that can predispose to AOM.

5. Vaccines—With the increasing problems associated with antibiotic therapy and prophylaxis, vaccines are increasingly important. The seven-valent pneumococcal conjugate vaccine (PCV7) was designed to prevent meningitis and sepsis, not AOM. However, it did produce a 55% reduction in AOM resulting from the seven serotypes found in the vaccine; these strains include the serotypes most likely to be penicillin- and macrolide-resistant. Overall, PCV7 reduced AOM by 6% in a group of children in California, compared with a control group. More impressively, it reduced pressure equalization tube placements by 20% and greatly reduced AOM incidence in children having six or more episodes per year. Furthermore, studies are showing a herd immunity effect on the older siblings of vaccinated children, which may further reduce drug-resistant serotype circulation. PCV7 has recently been replaced by the newer PCV13.

In recent studies, intranasal influenza vaccine reduced the number of influenza-associated cases of AOM by 92%. For children older than 6 months with recurrent AOM, it seems prudent to recommend yearly influenza vaccine, although this is not yet an official recommendation.

Vaccines currently being studied in animals that hold promise for AOM prevention include a respiratory syncytial virus vaccine and a nontypeable *H influenzae* vaccine. Studies of pregnant women in the third trimester have shown that their pneumococcal antibody levels are raised by a heptavalent pneumococcal vaccine, which may also raise antibody levels in the offspring. A recent study showed that low cord blood pneumococcal antibody is a risk factor for AOM and OME, so passive transfer from the mother is a logical next step to study.

G. Management of Otitis Media with Residual and Persistent Effusions

Otitis media with effusion (OME) is treated to avoid the consequences of prolonged negative pressure on the TM and chronic conductive hearing loss. Available data show a causal relationship between conductive hearing loss due to OME and language delay. A significant relationship between fluctuating hearing loss from otitis media and speech perception abilities was found in a prospective Dutch study. The management options for otitis media with residual effusion at 6 weeks to 4 months include observation. Nasal and oral corticosteroids have not been found in large studies to decrease MEE over several months but may be helpful in certain patients with nasal obstruction from adenoid hypertrophy or allergic rhinitis.

The association of biofilm formation and otitis media with effusion has been found to explain the "sterile" effusion sometimes present when culturing middle ear fluid. Electron microscopy shows biofilm covering the middle ear mucosa and adenoids in patients with chronic otitis media. Currently work is being done to find ways to disrupt biofilms, including physical disruption, reduction, and eradication. Macrolides have been found to effectively disrupt biofilms in patients with otitis media, chronic sinusitis, and adenoiditis.

The guideline recommendation developed by the Agency for Healthcare Research and Quality for the management of OME is that ventilating tubes should be placed after an effusion has persisted for 4 months and is accompanied by a bilateral hearing impairment of 20 dB or greater. Earlier placement of ventilating tubes should depend on the child's developmental and behavioral status as well as on parental preference and tympanic membrane status. The value of ventilating tubes for treating unilateral effusions in otherwise healthy children is focused on preventing middle ear sequelae often such as a retracted or atelectatic drum.

Children who have otitis media and persistent effusion have an increased incidence of cholesteatoma, adhesive otitis, retraction pockets, membrane atrophy, and persistent membrane perforation. If a patient clears a persistent MEE, the physician should follow the patient monthly. As there is no way to identify the small proportion of candidate children for whom insertion of ventilating tubes will prevent damage, close follow-up of children with abnormal ears may be best accomplished by an otolaryngologist.

Prognosis

Prognosis is variable based on age of presentation, with a younger child at first otitis media episode being more likely to need surgical intervention. Other factors include genetics, socioeconomic factors, time of year born, and so on.

Hoberman A, Paradise J et al: Treatment of acute otitis media in children under 2 years of age. New England Journal of Medicine 2011 Jan 13;364(2):105–115 [PMID: 21226576].

Kaur R, Casey JR, Pichichero ME: Serum antibody response to three non-typeable Haemophilus influenzae outer membrane proteins during acute otitis media and nasopharyngeal colonization in otitis prone and non-otitis prone children. Vaccine 2011 Jan 29;29(5):1023–1028 [PMID: 21129398].

Ruohola A et al: Antibiotic treatment of acute otorrhea through tympanostomy tube: Randomized double-blind placebo-controlled study with daily follow-up. Pediatrics 2003;111:1061 [PMID: 12728089].

Saylam G et al: Association of adenoid surface biofilm formation and chronic otitis media with effusion. Arch Otolaryngol Head Neck Surg 2010 Jun;136(6):550–555 [PMID: 20566904].

Smith A, Buchinsky FJ, Post JC: Eradicating chronic ear, nose, and throat infections: A systematically conducted literature review of advances in biofilm treatment. [Review]. Otolaryngology—Head & Neck Surgery 2011 Mar;144(3):338–347 [PMID: 21493193].

Subcommittee on Management of Acute Otitis Media: Diagnosis and management of acute otitis media. Pediatrics 2004;113:1451 [PMID: 15121972].

Zumach A et al: Speech perception after early-life otitis media with fluctuating hearing loss. Audiology & Neuro-Otology 2011;16(5):304–314 [PMID: 21160177].

Web Resources

American Academy of Otolaryngology, Head and Neck Surgery (http://www.entnet.org): Information on diagnosis and treatment of acute and chronic ear disease, written by the Otolaryngology Academy. Information is presented for parents and treating providers.

American Academy of Pediatrics (http://www.aap.org/otitismedia/www/): Information on diagnosis and treatment of AOM, written for the American Academy of Pediatrics. Features video clips of TMs being insufflated, to help clinicians learn normal landmarks and pathologic states. Requires Apple QuickTime to run.

Centers for Disease Control and Prevention: Appropriate Antibiotic Use (http://www.cdc.gov/drugresistance): Offers excellent advice for clinicians on (1) distinguishing OME from AOM, (2) careful antibiotic use for respiratory infections, and (3) patient education material on these two topics.

The Ear Treatment Group at the University of Texas Medical Branch (http://www.atc.utmb.edu/aom/home.htm): An interactive site for medical students, residents, and physicians to learn about otitis media and to test their knowledge. Contains links to other otitis media–related resources as well as parent educational material.

3. Mastoiditis

ESSENTIALS OF DIAGNOSIS

- Complication of otitis media.
- Sixty percent younger than age 2 years.
- Often no prior history of recurrent otitis media.
- Postauricular pain, ear protrusion.

Pathogenesis

Mastoiditis occurs when infection spreads from the middle ear space to the mastoid portion of the temporal bone, which lies just behind the ear. It is filled with air-filled spaces. Mastoiditis can range in severity from inflammation of the mastoid periosteum to bony destruction of the mastoid air cells (coalescent mastoiditis) and abscess development. Mastoiditis can occur in any age group, but more than 60% of the patients are younger than age 2 years. Many children do not have a prior history of recurrent AOM.

Clinical Findings

A. Symptoms and Signs

Patients with mastoiditis usually have postauricular pain, fever, and an outwardly displaced pinna. On examination, the mastoid area often appears swollen and red. With disease progression it may become fluctuant. The earliest finding is severe tenderness on mastoid palpation. AOM is almost always present. Late findings are a pinna that is pushed forward by postauricular swelling and an ear canal that is narrowed due to pressure on the posterosuperior wall from the mastoid abscess. In infants younger than age 1 year, the swelling occurs superior to the ear and pushes the pinna downward rather than outward.

Meningitis can be a complication of acute mastoiditis and should be suspected when a child has associated high fever, stiff neck, severe headache, or other meningeal signs. Lumbar puncture should be performed for diagnosis. Brain abscess occurs in 2% of mastoiditis patients and may be associated with persistent headaches, recurring fever, or changes in sensorium. Facial palsy, cavernous sinus thrombosis, and thrombophlebitis may also be encountered.

B. Imaging Studies

The best way to determine the extent of disease is by computed tomography (CT) scan. In the acute phase, diffuse inflammatory clouding of the mastoid cells occurs, as is also seen in uncomplicated AOM. In more severe cases, bony destruction and resorption of the mastoid air cells may occur.

C. Microbiology

The most common pathogens are *S pneumoniae* and *S pyogenes,* with *S aureus* and *H influenzae* occasionally seen. Rarely gram-negative bacilli and anaerobes are isolated. Antibiotics may decrease the incidence and morbidity of acute mastoiditis. However, acute mastoiditis does still occur in children who are treated with antibiotics for an acute ear infection. In the Netherlands, where only 31% of AOM patients receive antibiotics, the incidence of acute mastoiditis is 4.2 per 100,000 person-years. In the United States, where more than 96% of patients with AOM receive antibiotics, the incidence of acute mastoiditis is 2 per 100,000 person-years. Moreover, despite the routine use of antibiotics, the incidence of acute mastoiditis has been rising in some cities. The pattern change may be secondary to the emergence of resistant *S pneumoniae.*

Differential Diagnosis

While the hallmark of mastoiditis is postauricular tenderness and ear protrusion, significant external otitis may also present with these signs.

Complications

Mastoiditis can progress to sigmoid sinus thrombosis, epidural abscess, or intraparenchymal brain abscess.

Treatment

1. Myringotomy with or without tube for mastoiditis without a subperiosteal abscess, followed by intravenous antibiotic therapy plus ofloxacin or ciprofloxacin ear drops
   (a) Ceftriaxone plus nafcillin or clindamycin until culture results return.
   (b) Culture directed antibiotic therapy for 2–3 weeks.
2. Surgical drainage of mastoid if no clinical improvement in 24–48 hours or if any signs or symptoms of intracranial complications arise. If the child has an isolated subperiosteal abscess and not coalescent mastoiditis, either needle aspiration or incision and drainage with an associated myringotomy has produced good clinical outcomes.
3. Cortical mastoidectomy is usual primary management for coalescent mastoiditis (with abscess formation and breakdown of the mastoid air cells). A recent review from the University of Texas–Southwestern reported that 39% of patients with mastoiditis required a mastoidectomy.
5. After significant clinical improvement is achieved with parenteral therapy, oral antibiotics are begun and should be continued for 3 weeks.

Prognosis

Prognosis for full recovery is good. Children for whom acute mastoiditis with abscess is their first ear infection are not necessarily prone to recurrent otitis media.

Bakhos D et al: Conservative management of acute mastoiditis in children. Archives of Otolaryngology—Head & Neck Surgery 2011 Apr;137(4):346–350 [PMID: 21502472].

Rosenfeld RM et al: Implications of the AHRQ evidence report on acute otitis media. Otolaryngol Head Neck Surg 2001;125:440 [PMID: 11700439].

ACUTE TRAUMA TO THE MIDDLE EAR

Head injuries, a blow to the ear canal, sudden impact with water, blast injuries, or the insertion of pointed instruments into the ear canal can lead to perforation of the TM, ossicular damage, and hematoma of the middle ear. One study reported that 50% of serious penetrating wounds of the TM were due to parental use of a cotton-tipped swab.

Treatment of middle ear hematomas consists mainly of watchful waiting. Antibiotics are not necessary unless signs of infection appear. The prognosis for unimpaired hearing depends on whether the ossicles have been dislocated or fractured. The patient needs to be followed with audiometry or by an otolaryngologist until hearing has returned to normal, which is expected within 6–8 weeks.

Traumatic perforations of the TM often do not heal spontaneously, in which case the patient should be referred to an otolaryngologist. Spontaneous healing may occur within 6 months of the perforation. If the perforation is clean and dry and there is no hearing change, then there is no urgency for specialty evaluation. Perforations caused by a foreign body should be attended to more urgently, especially if accompanied by vertigo.

EAR CANAL FOREIGN BODY

Numerous objects can be inserted into the ear canal by a child. If the object is large, wedged into place, or difficult to remove with available instruments, the patient should be referred to an otolaryngologist early rather than risk traumatizing the child or the ear canal or causing edema that will necessitate removal under anesthesia. An emergency condition exists if the foreign body is a disk-type battery, such as those used in clocks, watches, and hearing aids. An electric current is generated in the moist canal, and a severe burn with resultant scarring can occur in less than 4 hours.

Lin VY et al: Button batteries in the ear, nose and upper aerodigestive tract. Int J Pediatr Otorhinolaryngol 2004;68:473 [PMID: 15013616].

HEMATOMA OF THE PINNA

Trauma to the ear can result in a hematoma between the perichondrium and cartilage. This is different from a bruise, which does not change the ear shape, and where the blood is in the soft tissue outside of the perichondrial layer. A hematoma appears as a boggy purple swelling of the upper half of the ear. The cartilage folds are obscured. If untreated, pressure necrosis of the underlying cartilage may occur, resulting in "cauliflower ear." To prevent this cosmetic deformity, physicians should urgently refer patients to an otolaryngologist for drainage and application of a carefully molded pressure dressing.

CONGENITAL EAR MALFORMATIONS

Agenesis, known as atresia, of the external ear canal results in conductive hearing loss that requires evaluation in the first 3 months of life by hearing specialists and otolaryngologists.

Microtia is the term used for an external ear that is small, collapsed or only has an earlobe present. Incidence is highest in Native American and Latino populations and lowest in African populations. Reconstruction is begun in girls around age 6 and in boys around age 8–10 years. Often there is associated aural atresia as above.

"Lop ears," folded down or protruding ears (so-called Dumbo ears), are a source of much teasing and ridicule. In the past, surgical correction at age 5 or 6 years was offered. Taping the ears into correct anatomic position is very effective if performed in the first 72–96 hours of life. Tape is applied over a molding of wax and continued for 2 weeks. Another alternative for the ear that can be molded solely by finger pressure into a normal configuration is an incisionless otoplasty, which can be performed at a much earlier age than 5–6 years and is associated with little postoperative morbidity. Because no cartilage destruction is associated with this technique, future growth is unaffected.

An ear is low-set if the upper pole is below eyebrow level. This condition is often associated with renal malformations (eg, Potter syndrome), and renal ultrasound examination is suggested.

Preauricular tags, ectopic cartilage, fistulas, sinuses, and cysts require surgical correction, mainly for cosmetic reasons. Children exhibiting any of these findings should have their hearing tested. Renal ultrasound should be considered, as external ear anomalies may be associated with renal anomalies, as both form during the same period of embryogenesis. Most preauricular pits cause no symptoms. If one should become infected, the patient should receive antibiotic therapy and be referred to an otolaryngologist for eventual excision.

Brent B: Microtia repair with rib cartilage grafts: A review of personal experience with 1000 cases. Clin Plast Surg 2002;29:257 [PMID: 12120682].

Fritsch MH: Incisionless otoplasty. Otolaryngologic Clinics of North America 42(6):1199–1208 [PMID: 19962016].

Yotsuyanagi T et al: Nonsurgical treatment of various auricular deformities. Clin Plast Surg 2002;29:327 [PMID: 12120687].

IDENTIFICATION & MANAGEMENT OF HEARING LOSS

Hearing loss is classified as being conductive, sensorineural, or mixed in nature. Conductive hearing loss occurs when there is a blockage of sound transmission between the opening of the external ear and the cochlear receptor cells. The most common cause of conductive hearing loss in children is fluid in the middle ear. Sensorineural hearing loss is due to a defect in the neural transmission of sound, arising from a defect in the cochlear hair cells or the auditory nerve. Mixed hearing loss is characterized by elements of both conductive and sensorineural loss.

Hearing is measured in decibels (dB). The threshold, or 0 dB, refers to the level at which a sound is perceived in normal subjects 50% of the time. Hearing is considered normal if an individual's thresholds are within 15 dB of normal. In children, severity of hearing loss is commonly graded as follows: 16–30 dB mild, 31–60 dB moderate, 61–90 dB severe, and more than 91 dB profound.

Hearing loss can significantly impair a child's ability to communicate, and hinder academic, social, and emotional development. Studies suggest that periods of auditory deprivation may have enduring effects on auditory processing, even after normal hearing is restored. Even a unilateral loss may be associated with difficulties in school and behavioral issues. Early identification and management of any hearing impairment is therefore critical.

Conductive Hearing Loss

The most common cause of childhood conductive hearing loss is otitis media and related conditions such as middle ear effusion (MEE) and eustachian tube dysfunction. Other causes of conductive hearing loss may include external auditory canal atresia or stenosis, tympanic membrane perforation, cerumen impaction, cholesteatoma, and middle ear abnormalities, such as ossicular fixation or discontinuity. Often, a conductive loss may be corrected with surgery.

MEE may be serous, mucoid, or purulent, as in acute otitis media. Effusions are generally associated with a mild conductive hearing loss that normalizes once the effusion is gone. The American Academy of Pediatrics recommends that hearing and language skills be assessed in children who have recurrent acute otitis media or MEE lasting longer than 3 months.

Sensorineural Hearing Loss

Sensorineural hearing loss (SNHL) arises due to a defect in the cochlear receptor cells or the auditory nerve (cranial nerve VIII). The loss may be congenital (present at birth) or acquired. In both the congenital and acquired categories, the hearing loss may be either hereditary (due to a genetic mutation) or nonhereditary. It is estimated that SNHL affects 2–3 out of every 1000 live births, making this the most common congenital sensory impairment. The incidence is thought to be considerably higher among the neonatal intensive care unit population. Well-recognized risk factors for SNHL in neonates include positive family history of childhood SNHL, birthweight less than 1500 g, low Apgar scores (0–4 at 1 minute or 0–6 at 5 minutes), craniofacial anomalies, hypoxia, in-utero infections (eg, TORCH syndrome), hyperbilirubinemia requiring exchange transfusion, and mechanical ventilation for more than 5 days.

A. Congenital Hearing Loss

Nonhereditary causes account for approximately 50% of congenital hearing loss. These include prenatal infections, teratogenic drugs, and perinatal injuries. The other 50% is attributed to genetic factors. Among children with hereditary hearing loss, approximately one-third of cases are thought to be due to a known syndrome, while the other two-thirds are considered nonsyndromic.

Syndromic hearing impairment is associated with malformations of the external ear or other organs, or with medical problems involving other organ systems. Over 400 genetic syndromes that include hearing loss have been described. All patients being evaluated for hearing loss should also be evaluated for features commonly associated with these syndromes. These include branchial cleft cysts or sinuses, preauricular pits, ocular abnormalities, white forelock, café au lait spots, and craniofacial anomalies. Some of the more frequently mentioned syndromes associated with congenital hearing loss include the following: Waardenburg, branchio-oto-renal, Usher, Pendred, Jervell and Lange-Nielsen, and Alport.

Over 70% of hereditary hearing loss is nonsyndromic (ie, there are no associated visible abnormalities or related medical problems). The most common known mutation associated with nonsyndromic hearing loss is in the *GJB2* gene, which encodes the protein Connexin 26. The *GJB2* mutation has a carrier rate of about 3% in the general population. Most nonsyndromic hearing loss, including that due to the *GJB2* mutation, is autosomal recessive.

B. Acquired Hearing Loss

Hereditary hearing loss may be delayed in onset, as in Alport syndrome and most types of autosomal dominant nonsyndromic hearing loss. Vulnerability to aminoglycoside-induced hearing loss has also been linked to a mitochondrial gene defect.

Nongenetic etiologies for delayed-onset SNHL include exposure to ototoxic medications, meningitis, autoimmune or neoplastic conditions, noise exposure, and trauma. Infections such as syphilis or Lyme disease have been associated with hearing impairment. Hearing loss associated with congenital cytomegalovirus (CMV) infection may be present at birth, or may have a delayed onset. The loss is progressive in approximately half of all patients with congenital CMV-associated hearing loss. Other risk factors for delayed-onset, progressive loss include a history of persistent pulmonary hypertension and extracorporeal membrane oxygenation therapy.

Identification of Hearing Loss

A. Newborn Hearing Screening

Prior to the institution of universal newborn screening programs, the average age at identification of hearing loss was 30 months. Recognizing the importance of early detection, in 1993, a National Institutes of Health Consensus Panel recommended that all newborns be screened for hearing impairment prior to hospital discharge. Today, universal newborn hearing screening is mandated in almost all states, with a goal of hearing loss identification by 3 months of age, and appropriate intervention by the age of 6 months. Subjective testing is not reliable in infants, and therefore objective, physiologic methods are used for screening. Auditory brainstem response and otoacoustic emission testing are the two commonly employed screening modalities.

B. Office Clinical Assessment

A parent's report of his or her infant's behavior cannot be relied upon for identification of hearing loss. A deaf infant's behavior can appear normal and mislead parents as well as professionals. The following are some office screening techniques, but these may identify only gross hearing losses, and may not detect milder losses. If there is suspicion of hearing loss, it is important to refer the patient for formal audiometric testing by an audiologist who is experienced in testing the pediatric population.

1. Birth to 4 months—In response to a sudden loud sound (≥70 dB), an infant should show a startle reflex or blink the eyes.

2. Four months to 2 years—While an infant is distracted with a toy or bright object, a noisemaker is sounded softly outside the field of vision at the child's waist level. Normal responses are as follows: at 4 months, there is widening of the eyes, interruption of other activity, and perhaps a slight turning of the head in the direction of the sound; at 6 months, the head turns toward the sound; at 9 months or older, the child is usually able to locate a sound originating from below as well as turn to the appropriate side; after 1 year, the child is able to locate sound whether it comes from below or above.

After responses to soft sounds are noted, a loud horn or clacker should be used to produce an eye blink or startle reflex. This latter maneuver is necessary because deaf children are often visually alert and able to scan the environment so actively that their scanning can be mistaken for an appropriate response to the softer noise test. A deaf child will not blink in response to the loud sound. Consonant sounds such as "mama," "dada," and "baba" should be present in speech by age 11 months.

C. Audiologic Evaluation of Infants and Children

Audiometry subjectively evaluates hearing. There are several different methods used, based on patient age:

- Behavioral observational audiometry (birth to 6 months): Sounds are presented at various intensity levels, and the audiologist watches closely for a reaction, such as change in respiratory rate, starting or stopping of activity, startle, head turn, or muscle tensing. This method is highly tester-dependent and error-prone.
- Visual reinforcement audiometry (6 months to 2.5 years): Auditory stimulus is paired with positive reinforcement. For example, when a child reacts appropriately by turning toward a sound source, the behavior is rewarded by activation of a toy that lights up. After a brief conditioning period, the child localizes toward the tone, if audible, in anticipation of the lighted toy.
- Conditioned play audiometry (2.5–5 years): The child responds to sound stimulus by performing an activity, such as putting a peg into a board.
- Conventional audiometry (5 years and up): The child indicates when he or she hears a sound.

Objective methods such as auditory brainstem response and otoacoustic emission testing may be used if a child cannot be reliably tested using the above methods.

Referral

A child who fails newborn hearing screening or has a suspected hearing loss should be referred for further audiologic evaluation, and any child with hearing loss should be referred to an otolaryngologist for further workup and treatment. In addition to the infants who fall into the high-risk categories for SNHL as outlined earlier, hearing should be tested in children with a history of developmental delay, bacterial meningitis, ototoxic medication exposure, neurodegenerative disorders, or a history of infection such as mumps or measles. Children with bacterial meningitis should be referred immediately to an otolaryngologist, as cochlear ossification can occur, necessitating urgent cochlear implantation. Even if a newborn screening was passed, all infants who fall into a high-risk category for progressive or delayed-onset hearing loss should receive ongoing audiologic monitoring for 3 years and at appropriate intervals thereafter to avoid a missed diagnosis.

Prevention

Appropriate care may treat or prevent conditions causing hearing deficits. Aminoglycosides and diuretics, particularly in combination, are potentially ototoxic and should be used judiciously and monitored carefully. Given the association of a certain mitochondrial gene defect and aminoglycoside ototoxicity, use should be avoided, if possible, in patients with a family history of aminoglycoside-related hearing loss. Reduction of repeated exposure to loud noises may prevent high-frequency hearing loss associated with acoustic trauma. Any patient with sudden-onset SNHL should be seen by an otolaryngologist immediately, as in some cases, steroid therapy may reverse the loss if initiated right away.

Management of Hearing Loss

The importance of early intervention for receptive and expressive development is well established. The management of hearing loss depends on the type and severity of impairment. Conductive hearing loss is typically correctable by addressing the point in sound transmission at which efficiency is compromised. For example, hearing loss due to chronic effusions usually normalizes once the fluid has cleared, whether by natural means or by the placement of tympanostomy tubes. As of yet, SNHL is not reversible, although cochlear hair cell regeneration is an area of active research. Most sensorineural loss is managed with amplification. Cochlear implantation is an option for some children with severe-profound loss, and at the time of this writing, is FDA approved down to the age of 12 months. Unlike hearing aids, the cochlear implant does not amplify sound, but directly stimulates the cochlea with electrical impulses. Children with hearing loss should receive ongoing audiologic monitoring.

Choo D, Meinzen-Derr J: Universal newborn hearing screening in 2010. Curr Opin Otolaryngol Head Neck Surg 2010;18(5): 399–404 [PMID: 20808221].

Web Resources:

Smith RJH, Hildebrand MS, Van Camp G: Deafness and hereditary hearing loss overview. Last update Oct 14, 2010. Available at: http://www.ncbi.nlm.nih.gov/books/NBK1434/ Accessed Dec 5, 2011.

THE NOSE & PARANASAL SINUSES

ACUTE VIRAL RHINITIS (COMMON COLD; SEE ALSO CHAPTER 40)

The common cold (viral upper respiratory infection) is the most common pediatric infectious disease, and the incidence is higher in early childhood than in any other period of life. Children younger than 5 years typically have 6–12 colds per year. Approximately 30%–40% of these are caused by rhinoviruses. Other culprits include adenoviruses, coronaviruses, enteroviruses, influenza and parainfluenza viruses, and respiratory syncytial virus.

ESSENTIALS OF DIAGNOSIS

- Clear or mucoid rhinorrhea, nasal congestion, sore throat.
- Possible fever, particularly in younger children (under 5–6 years).
- Symptoms resolve by 7–10 days.

Clinical Findings

The patient usually experiences a sudden onset of clear or mucoid rhinorrhea, nasal congestion, sneezing, and sore throat. Cough or fever may develop. Although fever is usually not a prominent feature in older children and adults, in the first 5 or 6 years of life it can be as high as 40.6°C without superinfection. The nose, throat, and tympanic membranes may appear red and inflamed. The average duration of symptoms is about 1 week. Nasal secretions tend to become thicker and more purulent after day 2 of infection due to shedding of epithelial cells and influx of neutrophils. This discoloration should not be assumed to be a sign of bacterial rhinosinusitis, unless it persists beyond 10–14 days, by which time the patient should be experiencing significant symptomatic improvement.

Treatment

Treatment for the common cold is symptomatic (Figure 18–6). Acetaminophen or ibuprofen can be helpful for fever and pain. Humidification may provide relief for congestion and cough. Nasal saline drops and bulb suctioning may be used for an infant or child unable to blow his or her nose. A topical decongestant such as oxymetazoline may provide some relief, but should be discontinued within 3 days to prevent severe rebound nasal congestion or chemical rhinitis.

Available scientific data suggest that over-the-counter cold and cough medications are generally not effective in

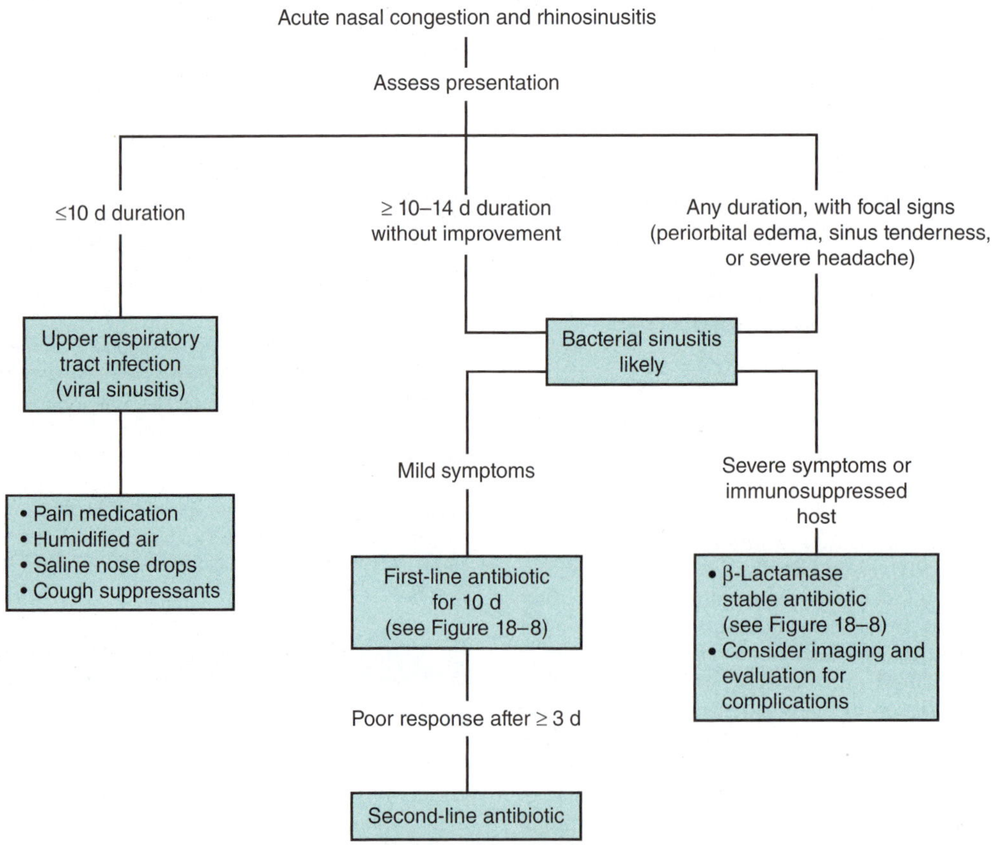

▲ **Figure 18–6.** Algorithm for acute nasal congestion and rhinosinusitis.

children. These medications may be associated with serious adverse effects, and it is recommended that they not be used in children under the age of 4 years. Antihistamines have not proven effective in relieving cold symptoms; in rhinoviral colds, increased levels of histamine are not observed. There is insufficient evidence of benefit to warrant the use of antibiotics for common cold symptoms. Oral decongestants have been found to provide some symptomatic relief in adults but have not been well studied in children. Cough suppression at night is the number one goal of many parents; however, studies have shown that antitussives, antihistamines, antihistamine-decongestant combinations and antitussive-bronchodilator combinations are no more effective than placebo. Use of narcotic antitussives is discouraged, as these have been associated with severe respiratory depression.

Education and reassurance may be the most important "therapy" for the common cold. Parents should be informed about the expected nature and duration of symptoms, efficacy and potential side effects of medications, and the signs and symptoms of complications of the common cold, such as bacterial rhinosinusitis, bronchiolitis, or pneumonia.

Arroll B, Kenealy T: Are antibiotics effective for acute purulent rhinitis? Systematic review and meta-analylsis of placebo controlled randomized trials. BMJ 2006;333(7562):279 [Epub 2006 July 21] [PMID: 16861253].

Smith SM, Schroeder K, Fahey T: Over-the-counter medications for acute cough in children and adults in ambulatory settings. Cochrane Database Syst Rev 2008;(1):CD001831 [PMID: 18253996].

Taverner D, Latte J: Nasal decongestants for the common cold. Cochrane Database Syst Rev 2007;(1):CD001953 [PMID: 17253470].

Web Resources:

U.S. Food and Drug Administration: Using over-the-counter cough and cold products in children. Posted Oct 22, 2008. Available at: http://www.fda.gov/ForConsumers/ConsumerUpdates/ucm048515.htm Accessed Dec 5, 2011.

RHINOSINUSITIS

The use of the term *rhinosinusitis* has replaced sinusitis. Rhinosinusitis acknowledges that the nasal *and* sinus mucosa are involved in similar and concurrent inflammatory processes.

1. Acute Bacterial Rhinosinusitis

Acute bacterial rhinosinusitis (ABRS) is a bacterial infection of the paranasal sinuses, which lasts less than 30 days and in which the symptoms resolve completely. It is almost always preceded by a viral upper respiratory infection (cold). Other predisposing conditions include allergies and trauma. The diagnosis of ABRS is made when a child with a cold does not improve by 10–14 days or worsens after 5–7 days. The maxillary and ethmoid sinuses are most commonly involved. These sinuses are present at birth. The sphenoid sinuses typically form by the age of 5 years, and the frontal sinuses by age 7–8 years. Frontal sinusitis is unusual before age 10 years.

ESSENTIALS OF DIAGNOSIS

- Upper respiratory infection symptoms are present 10 or more days beyond onset, or symptoms worsen within 10 days after an initial period of improvement.
- Symptoms may include nasal congestion, nasal drainage, postnasal drainage, facial pain, headache, and fever.
- Symptoms resolve completely within 30 days.

Pathogenesis

Situations that lead to inflammation of sinonasal mucosa and obstruction of sinus drainage pathways underlie the development of rhinosinusitis. A combination of anatomic, mucosal, microbial, and immune pathogenic factors is believed to be involved. Both viral and bacterial infections play integral roles in the pathogenesis. Viral upper respiratory infections may cause sinus mucosal injury and swelling, resulting in osteomeatal obstruction, loss of ciliary activity, and mucus hypersecretion. The bacterial pathogens that commonly cause acute rhinosinusitis are *S pneumoniae, H influenzae* (nontypeable), *M catarrhalis,* and β-hemolytic streptococci.

Clinical Findings

The onset of symptoms in ABRS may be gradual or sudden, and may commonly include nasal drainage, nasal congestion, facial pressure or pain, postnasal drainage, hyposmia or anosmia, fever, cough, fatigue, maxillary dental pain, and ear pressure or fullness. The physical examination is rarely helpful in making the diagnosis, as the findings are essentially the same as those in a child with an uncomplicated cold. Occasionally, sinuses may be tender to percussion, but this is typically seen only in older children and is of questionable reliability. Transillumination of the sinuses is difficult to perform and not very helpful unless the sinuses are grossly asymmetrical.

In complicated or immunocompromised patients, sinus aspiration and culture by an otolaryngologist should be considered for diagnostic purposes and to facilitate culture-directed antibiotic therapy. Gram stain or culture of nasal discharge does not necessarily correlate with cultures of sinus aspirates. If the patient is hospitalized because of rhinosinusitis-related complications, blood cultures should also be obtained.

Imaging of the sinuses during acute illness is not indicated except when evaluating for possible complications, or for patients with persistent symptoms which do not respond to medical therapy. As with the physical examination, the radiographic findings of ABRS, such as sinus opacification, fluid, and mucosal thickening, are also seen in viral upper respiratory infections.

Complications

Complications of ABRS occur when infection spreads to adjacent structures—the overlying tissues, the eye, or the brain. Streptococcus anginosus (milleri) is a particularly virulent organism commonly implicated in acute rhinosinusitis with complications.

Orbital complications are the most common, arising from the ethmoid sinuses. These complications usually begin as a preseptal cellulitis, but can progress to postseptal cellulitis, subperiosteal abscess, orbital abscess, and cavernous sinus thrombosis. Associated signs and symptoms include eyelid edema, restricted extraocular movements, proptosis, chemosis, and altered visual acuity (see Chapter 16).

The most common complication of frontal sinusitis is osteitis of the frontal bone, also known as Pott's puffy tumor. Intracranial extension of infection can lead to meningitis and to epidural, subdural, and brain abscesses. Frequently, children with complicated rhinosinusitis have no prior history of sinus infection.

Treatment

For children who are not improving by 10 days, or who have more severe symptoms, with fever of at least 39°C and purulent nasal drainage for at least 3–4 consecutive days, antibiotic therapy is recommended. Although some discrepancy exists, antibiotics are generally thought to decrease duration and severity of symptoms.

To minimize the number of children who receive antimicrobial therapy for uncomplicated viral upper respiratory infections, and to help combat antibiotic resistance, the American Academy of Pediatrics in 2001 issued guidelines for treatment. This algorithm is presented in Figure 18–7. Key decision points include severity of disease and risk factors for resistant organisms

For patients with mild-to-moderate symptoms, who are not in day care, and have not been on recent antibiotic therapy, high-dose amoxicillin is considered first-line therapy. For those with severe symptoms, in day care, or who were on antibiotics within the past 1–3 months, high-dose amoxicillin–clavulanate is recommended as first-line therapy. Cefuroxime, cefpodoxime, and cefdinir are recommended for patients with a non-type I hypersensitivity to penicillin. Macrolides should be reserved for patients with an anaphylactic reaction to penicillin. Other options for these patients include clindamycin or trimethoprim–sulfamethoxazole. However, it should be remembered that clindamycin is not effective against gram-negative organisms such as *H influenzae*.

Failure to improve after 48–72 hours suggests a resistant organism or potential complication. Second-line therapies should be initiated at this point, or, if the patient is already on amoxicillin–clavulanate or cephalosporin, intravenous antibiotic therapy should be considered. Imaging and referral for sinus aspiration should be strongly considered as well.

Patients who are toxic, or who have evidence of invasive infection or CNS complications, should be hospitalized immediately. Intravenous therapy with nafcillin or clindamycin plus a third-generation cephalosporin such as cefotaxime should be initiated until culture results become available.

Topical decongestants and oral combinations are frequently used in acute rhinosinusitis to promote drainage. Their effectiveness has not been proven, and concern has been raised about potential adverse effects related to impaired ciliary function, decreased blood flow to the mucosa, and reduced diffusion of antibiotic into the sinuses. Topical nasal decongestants should not be used for more than 3 days due to risk of rebound edema. Patients with underlying allergic rhinitis may benefit from intranasal cromolyn or corticosteroid nasal spray.

Esposito S, Bosis S, Bellasio M et al: From clinical practice to guidelines: how to recognize rhinosinusitis in children. Pediatr Allergy Immunol 2007;18(Suppl 18):53–55 [PMID: 17767610].

Principi N, Esposito S: New insights into pediatric rhinosinusitis. Pediatr Allergy Immunol 2007;18(Suppl 18):7–9 [PMID: 17767598].

2. Recurrent or Chronic Rhinosinusitis

Recurrent rhinosinusitis occurs when episodes of ABRS clear with antibiotic therapy but recur with each or most upper respiratory infections. Chronic rhinosinusitis is diagnosed when the child has not cleared the infection in the expected time but has not developed acute complications. Both symptoms and physical findings are required to support the diagnosis, and CT scan may be a useful adjuvant in making the diagnosis. Although recent meta-analysis evaluations have resulted in recommendations for ABRS, there is a paucity of data for the treatment of recurrent or chronic rhinosinusitis. Important factors to consider include allergies, anatomic variations, and disorders in host immunity. Mucosal inflammation leading to obstruction is most commonly caused by allergic rhinitis and occasionally by nonallergic rhinitis. Gastroesophageal reflux has also been implicated in chronic rhinosinusitis. Less commonly, chronic rhinosinusitis is caused by anatomic variations, such as septal deviation, polyp, or foreign body. Allergic polyps are unusual in children younger than age 10 years and should prompt a workup for cystic fibrosis. In cases of chronic or recurrent pyogenic pansinusitis, poor host resistance (eg, an immune defect, primary ciliary dyskinesia, or cystic fibrosis)—though rare—must be ruled out by immunoglobulin studies, electron microscopy studies of respiratory cilia, nasal nitric oxide measurements if available, a sweat chloride test, and genetic testing (see Chapters 19 and 37). Anaerobic and staphylococcal organisms are

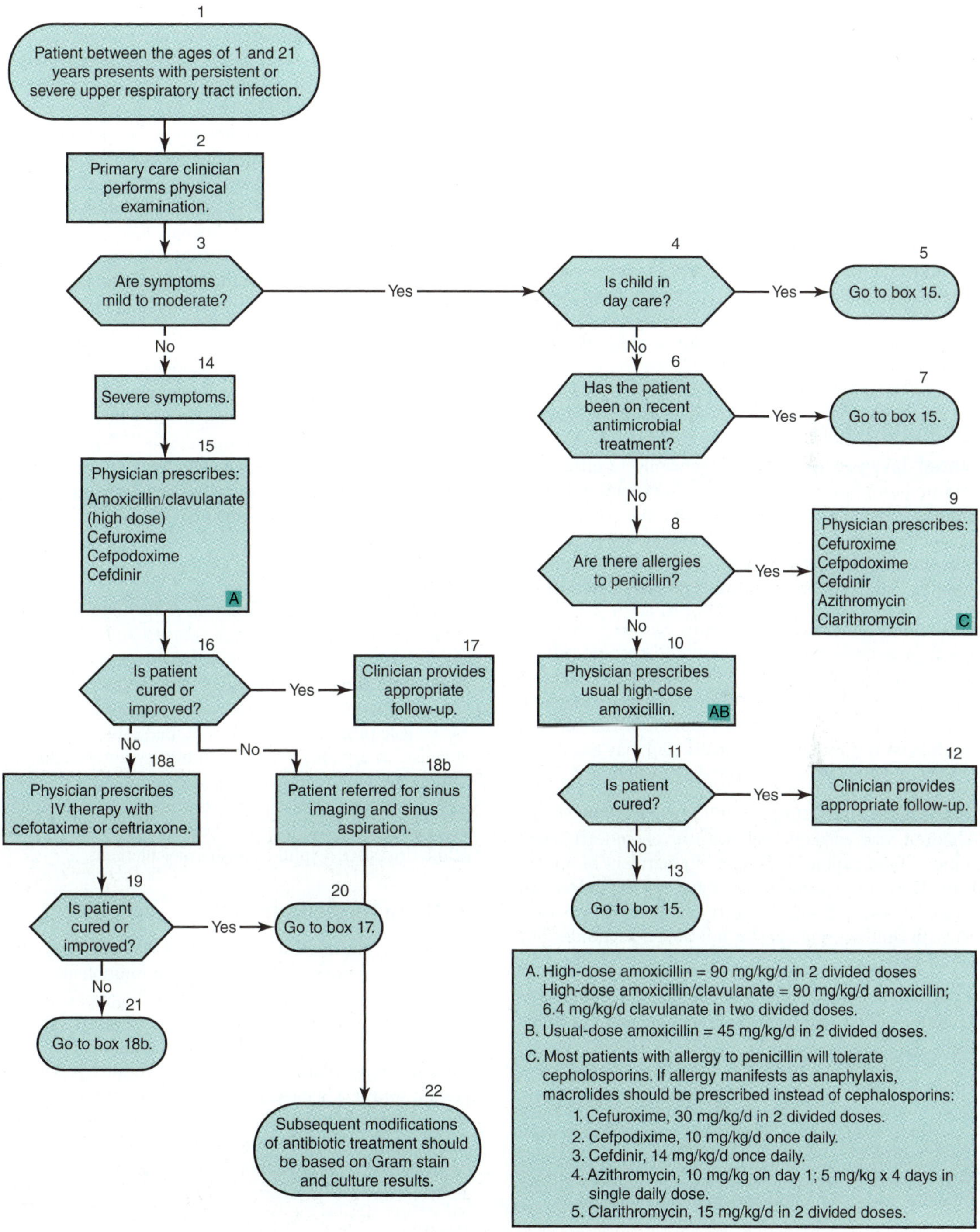

▲ **Figure 18–7.** Management of children with uncomplicated acute bacterial rhinosinusitis (ABRS). (Reproduced, with permission, from the American Academy of Pediatrics: Clinical practice guidelines: Management of sinusitis. Pediatrics 2001;108:798.)

often responsible for chronic rhinosinusitis. Evaluation by an allergist and an otolaryngologist may be useful in determining the underlying causes.

Treatment

A. Medical Therapy

Antibiotic therapy is similar to that used for ABRS, but the duration is longer, typically 3–4 weeks. Antimicrobial choice should include drugs effective against staphylococcal organisms. Adjuvant therapies such as saline nasal irrigation, decongestants, antihistamines, or topical intranasal steroids may be helpful depending on the underlying cause. A small percentage of children do not respond to medical therapy and will require surgery.

B. Surgical Therapy

1. Antral lavage—Antral lavage, generally regarded as a diagnostic procedure, may have some therapeutic value. An aspirate or a sample from the maxillary sinus is retrieved under anesthesia, either with a spinal needle or with a curved-tip instrument. The maxillary sinus is then irrigated. In the very young child, this may be the only procedure performed.

2. Adenoidectomy—Adenoidectomy has been shown to be effective in 60%–75% of children with chronic rhinosinusitis. The adenoids may serve as a reservoir of pathogenic bacteria and may also interfere with mucociliary clearance and drainage. Biofilms have been reported in the adenoids of children with chronic rhinosinusitis, and may explain the resistance of these infections to standard antibiotic therapy.

3. Endoscopic sinus surgery—Endoscopic sinus surgery in children was controversial because of concern about alteration of developing sinuses and impairment of midface growth. However, recent studies have not supported this concern. Endoscopic sinus surgery has been shown to be effective in children, and may be indicated if adenoidectomy is not effective.

4. External drainage—External drainage procedures are reserved for complications arising from ethmoid and frontal sinusitis.

Brietzke SE, Brigger MT: Adenoidectomy outcomes in pediatric rhinosinusitis: A meta-analysis. Int J Pedatr Otorhinolaryngol 2008;72(10):1541–1545 [PMID: 18723228].

Lusk R: Pediatric chronic rhinosinusitis. Curr Opin Otolaryngol Head Neck Surg 2006;14(6):393–396 [PMID: 17099346].

CHOANAL ATRESIA

Choanal atresia occurs in approximately 1 in 7000 live births. The female-male ratio is 2:1, as is the unilateral-bilateral ratio. Bilateral atresia results in severe respiratory distress at birth and requires immediate placement of an oral airway or intubation, and otolaryngology consultation for surgical treatment. Unilateral atresia usually appears later as a unilateral chronic nasal discharge that may be mistaken for chronic rhinosinusitis. Diagnosis may be suspected if a 6F catheter cannot be passed through the nose and is confirmed by axial CT scan. Approximately 50% of patients with bilateral choanal atresia have CHARGE association (**C**oloboma, **H**eart disease, **A**tresia of the choanae, **R**etarded growth and retarded development or CNS anomalies, **G**enital hypoplasia, and **E**ar anomalies or deafness) (see Chapter 37) or other congenital anomalies.

RECURRENT RHINITIS

Recurrent rhinitis is frequently seen in the office practice of pediatrics. The child is brought in with the chief complaint of having "one cold after another," "constant colds," or "always being sick." Approximately two-thirds of these children have recurrent colds; the rest have either allergic rhinitis or recurrent rhinosinusitis.

1. Allergic Rhinitis

Allergic rhinitis has significant morbidity and may contribute to the development of rhinosinusitis and asthma exacerbations. Symptoms may include nasal congestion, sneezing, rhinorrhea, and itchy nose, palate, throat, and eyes. On physical examination the nasal turbinates are swollen and may be red or pale pink. Several classes of medications have proven effective in treating allergic rhinitis symptoms, including intranasal corticosteroids, oral and intranasal antihistamines, leukotriene antagonists, and decongestants. Ipratropium nasal spray may also be used as an adjunctive therapy. Nasal saline rinses are helpful to wash away allergens.

2. Nonallergic Rhinitis

Nonallergic rhinitis also causes rhinorrhea and nasal congestion, but does not seem to involve an immunologic reaction. Its mechanism is not well understood. Triggers can include sudden changes in environmental temperature, air pollution, and other irritants such as tobacco smoke. Medications can also be associated with nonallergic rhinitis. Nasal decongestant sprays, when used for long periods of time, can cause *rhinitis medicamentosa*, which is a rebound nasal congestion which can be very difficult to treat. Oral decongestants, nasal corticosteroids, antihistamines, and ipratropium spray have all been shown to offer symptomatic relief.

Bachert C: A review of the efficacy of desloratadine, fexofenadine, and levocetirizine in the treatment of nasal congestion in patients with allergic rhinitis. Clin Ther 2009;31(5):921–944 [PMID: 19539095].

Web Resources:

American Academy of Allergy, Asthma, and Immunology: Rhinitis (Hay Fever): Tips to remember. Available at: http://www.aaaai.org/patients/publicedmat/tips/rhinitis.stm. Accessed Dec 5, 2011.

EPISTAXIS

The nose is an extremely vascular structure. In most cases, epistaxis (nosebleed) arises from the anterior portion of the nasal septum (Kiesselbach area). It is often due to dryness, vigorous nose rubbing, nose blowing, or nose picking. Examination of the anterior septum usually reveals a red, raw surface with fresh clots or old crusts. Presence of telangiectasias, hemangiomas, or varicosities should also be noted. If a patient has been using a nasal corticosteroid spray, check the patient's technique to make sure he or she is not directing the spray toward the septum. If proper technique does not reduce the nosebleeds, the spray should be discontinued.

In fewer than 5% of cases, epistaxis is caused by a bleeding disorder such as von Willebrand disease. A hematologic workup is warranted if any of the following is present: family history of a bleeding disorder; medical history of easy bleeding, particularly with circumcision or dental extraction; spontaneous bleeding at any site; bleeding that lasts for more than 30 minutes or blood that will not clot with direct pressure by the physician; onset before age 2 years; or a drop in hematocrit due to epistaxis. High blood pressure may rarely predispose to prolonged nosebleeds in children.

A nasopharyngeal angiofibroma may manifest as recurrent epistaxis. Adolescent boys are affected almost exclusively. CT scan with contrast of the nasal cavity and nasopharynx is diagnostic.

Treatment

The patient should sit up and lean forward so as not to swallow the blood. Swallowed blood may cause nausea and hematemesis. The nasal cavity should be cleared of clots by gentle blowing. The soft part of the nose below the nasal bones is pinched and held firmly enough to prevent arterial blood flow, with pressure over the bleeding site (anterior septum) being maintained for 5 minutes by the clock. For persistent bleeding, a one-time only application of oxymetazoline into the nasal cavity may be helpful. If bleeding continues, the bleeding site needs to be visualized. A small piece of gelatin sponge (Gelfoam) or collagen sponge (Surgicel) can be inserted over the bleeding site and held in place.

Friability of the nasal vessels is often due to dryness and can be decreased by increasing nasal moisture. This can be accomplished by daily application of a water-based ointment to the nose. A pea-sized amount of ointment is placed just inside the nose and spread by gently squeezing the nostrils. Twice-daily nasal saline irrigation and humidifier use may also be helpful. Aspirin and ibuprofen should be avoided, as should nose picking and vigorous nose blowing. Otolaryngology referral is indicated for refractory cases. Cautery of the nasal vessels is reserved for treatment failures.

NASAL INFECTION

A nasal furuncle is an infection of a hair follicle in the anterior nares. Hair plucking or nose picking can provide a route of entry. The most common organism is *S aureus*. A furuncle presents as an exquisitely tender, firm, red lump in the anterior nares. Treatment includes dicloxacillin or cephalexin orally for 5 days to prevent spread. The lesion should be gently incised and drained as soon as it points with a sterile needle. Topical bacitracin ointment may be of additional value. Because this lesion is in the drainage area of the cavernous sinus, the patient should be followed closely until healing is complete. Parents should be advised never to pick or squeeze a furuncle in this location—and neither should the physician. Associated cellulitis or spread requires hospitalization for administration of intravenous antibiotics.

A nasal septal abscess usually follows nasal trauma or a nasal furuncle. Examination reveals fluctuant gray septal swelling, which is usually bilateral. The possible complications are the same as for nasal septal hematoma (see following discussion). In addition, spread of the infection to the CNS is possible. Treatment consists of immediate hospitalization and incision and drainage by an otolaryngologist.

NASAL TRAUMA

Newborn infants rarely present with subluxation of the quadrangular cartilage of the septum. In this disorder, the top of the nose deviates to one side, the inferior septal border deviates to the other side, the columella leans, and the nasal tip is unstable. This disorder must be distinguished from the more common transient flattening of the nose caused by the birth process. In the past, physicians were encouraged to reduce all subluxations in the nursery. Otolaryngologists are more likely to perform the reduction under anesthesia for more difficult cases.

After nasal trauma, it is essential to examine the inside of the nose with a nasal speculum. Hematoma of the nasal septum must be ruled out as it poses a considerable risk of septal necrosis, leading to permanent nasal deformity. This diagnosis is confirmed by the abrupt onset of nasal obstruction following trauma and the presence of a boggy, widened nasal septum. The normal nasal septum is only 2–4 mm thick. A cotton swab can be used to palpate the septum. Treatment consists of immediate referral to an otolaryngologist for evacuation of the hematoma and packing of the nose.

Most blows to the nose result in epistaxis without fracture. A persistent nosebleed after trauma, crepitus, instability of the nasal bones, and external deformity of the nose indicate fracture. Septal injury cannot be ruled out by radiography, and can only be ruled out by careful intranasal examination. Patients with suspected nasal fractures should be referred to an otolaryngologist for definitive therapy. Since the nasal bones begin healing within 7 days, the child must ideally be seen by an otolaryngologist within 48–72 hours of the injury to allow time for fracture reduction before the bones become immobile.

FOREIGN BODIES IN THE NOSE

If this diagnosis is delayed, unilateral foul-smelling rhinorrhea, halitosis, bleeding, or nasal obstruction often result.

There are many ways to remove nasal foreign bodies. The obvious first maneuver is vigorous nose blowing if the child is old enough. The next step in removal requires nasal decongestion, good lighting, correct instrumentation, and physical restraint. Topical tetracaine or lidocaine may be used for anesthesia in young children. Nasal decongestion can be achieved by topical phenylephrine or oxymetazoline. When the child is properly restrained, most nasal foreign bodies can be removed using a pair of alligator forceps or right-angle instrument through an operating head otoscope. If the object seems unlikely to be removed on the first attempt, is wedged in, or is quite large, the patient should be referred to an otolaryngologist rather than worsening the situation through futile attempts at removal.

Because the nose is a moist cavity, the electrical current generated by disk-type batteries—such as those used in clocks, watches, and hearing aids—can cause necrosis of mucosa and cartilage destruction in less than 4 hours. Batteries constitute a true foreign body emergency.

THE THROAT & ORAL CAVITY

ACUTE STOMATITIS

1. Recurrent Aphthous Stomatitis

Aphthous ulcers, also known as canker sores, are small ulcers (3–10 mm) usually found on the inner aspect of the lips or on the tongue; rarely they may appear on the tonsils or palate. There is usually no associated fever and no cervical adenopathy. They are painful and last 1–2 weeks. They may recur numerous times throughout life. The cause is unknown, although an allergic or autoimmune basis is suspected.

Treatment consists of coating the lesions with a corticosteroid ointment, such as triamcinolone dental paste, twice daily. Pain can also be reduced by eating a bland diet, avoiding salty or acidic foods and juices, and giving acetaminophen or ibuprofen.

Other less common causes of recurrent oral ulcers include Behçet disease, familial Mediterranean fever, and PFAPA syndrome (**P**eriodic **F**ever, **A**phthous stomatitis, **P**haryngitis, and cervical **A**denopathy). PFAPA syndrome was first described in 1987, and its cause is unknown, although an immune etiology is suspected. It usually begins before the age of 5 years, continues through adolescence, and then resolves. The fever and other symptoms recur at regular intervals. Episodes may be dramatically improved with prednisone bursts, but recurrences typically continue. Episodes last approximately 5 days and are not associated with other URI symptoms or illnesses. PFAPA may resolve with prolonged cimetidine treatment or tonsillectomy (see following section on tonsillectomy). Otolaryngology referral is appropriate.

A diagnosis of Behçet disease requires two of the following: genital ulcers, uveitis, and erythema nodosum–like lesions. Patients with Mediterranean fever usually have a positive family history, serosal involvement, and recurrent fever.

Garavello W, Romagnoli M, Gaini RM: Effectiveness of adenotonsillectomy in PFAPA syndrome: A randomized study. J Pediatr 2009 Aug;155(2):250–253 [Epub 2009 May 21][PMID: 19464029].

Pignataro L et al: Outcome of tonsillectomy in selected patients with PFAPA syndrome. Arch Otolaryngol Head Neck Surg 2009 Jun;135(6):548–553 [PMID: 19528401].

2. Herpes Simplex Gingivostomatitis (See also Chapter 40)

In an initial infection with the herpes simplex virus, children usually develop 10 or more small ulcers (1–3 mm) of the buccal mucosa, anterior tonsillar pillars, inner lips, tongue, and gingival; the posterior pharynx is typically spared. The lesions are often associated with fever, tender cervical adenopathy, and generalized oral inflammation which precedes the development of the ulcers. Exposure to the virus occurs 3–50 days prior to the onset of symptoms. Affected children are commonly younger than 3 years of age. This gingivostomatitis lasts 7–10 days. Treatment is symptomatic, as described earlier for recurrent aphthous stomatitis, with the exception that corticosteroids are contraindicated. If the child is seen early in the course, he or she may be treated with a course of acyclovir. Due to pain, dehydration occasionally develops, requiring hospitalization. Herpetic laryngotracheitis is a rare complication.

3. Thrush (See also Chapter 43)

Oral candidiasis mainly affects infants and occasionally older children in a debilitated state. *Candida albicans* is a saprophyte that normally is not invasive unless the mouth is abraded or the patient is immunocompromised. The use of broad-spectrum antibiotics and systemic or inhaled corticosteroids may be contributing factors. Symptoms include oral pain and refusal of feedings. Lesions consist of white curdlike plaques, predominantly on the buccal mucosa, which cannot be washed away after a feeding. Another less common variation of oral candidal infection is erythematous candidiasis, which produces erythematous patches on the palate and dorsum of the tongue. This condition is associated primarily with patients who are taking broad-spectrum antibiotics or corticosteroids, or are HIV-positive.

Treatment consists of nystatin oral suspension. Large plaques may be removed with a moistened cotton-tipped applicator, and the nystatin may also be rubbed on the lesions with an applicator. Patients who do not respond to oral therapy or who are immunocompromised may require systemic antifungal agents. Parents should be advised to replace any items, such as a pacifier, that may have become contaminated with *Candida.*

4. Traumatic Oral Ulcers

Mechanical trauma most commonly occurs on the buccal mucosa secondary to biting by the molars. Thermal trauma, from very hot foods, can also cause ulcerative lesions. Chemical ulcers can be produced by mucosal contact with aspirin or other caustic agents. Oral ulcers can also occur with leukemia or on a recurrent basis with cyclic neutropenia.

PHARYNGITIS

Figure 18–8 is an algorithm for the management of a sore throat.

1. Acute Viral Pharyngitis & Tonsillitis

Over 90% of sore throats and fever in children are due to viral infections. The findings seldom point toward any particular viral agent, but four types of viral pharyngitis are sufficiently distinctive to warrant discussion below.

Clinical Findings

A. Infectious Mononucleosis

Findings include exudative tonsillitis, generalized cervical adenitis, and fever, usually in patients older than 5 years of age. A palpable spleen or axillary adenopathy increases the likelihood of the diagnosis. The presence of more than 10% atypical lymphocytes on a peripheral blood smear or a positive mononucleosis spot test supports the diagnosis, although these tests are often falsely negative in children younger than age 5 years. Epstein-Barr virus serology showing an elevated IgM-capsid antibody is definitive. Amoxicillin is contraindicated in patients suspected of having mononucleosis because the drug often precipitates a rash.

B. Herpangina

Herpangina ulcers are classically 3 mm in size, surrounded by a halo, and are found on the anterior tonsillar pillars, soft palate, and uvula; the anterior mouth and tonsils are spared. Herpangina is caused by the coxsackie A group of viruses, and a patient may have several bouts of the ulcers. Enteroviral polymerase chain reaction testing is widely available, but not typically indicated, as herpangina is a self-limiting illness.

C. Hand, Foot, and Mouth Disease

This entity is caused by several enteroviruses, only one of which (enterovirus 71) can rarely cause encephalitis. Ulcers occur anywhere in the mouth. Vesicles, pustules, or papules may be found on the palms, soles, interdigital areas, and buttocks. In younger children lesions may be seen on the distal extremities and even the face.

D. Pharyngoconjunctival Fever

This disorder is caused by an adenovirus and often is epidemic. Exudative tonsillitis, conjunctivitis, lymphadenopathy, and fever are the main findings. Treatment is symptomatic.

2. Acute Bacterial Pharyngitis

ESSENTIALS OF DIAGNOSIS

- Sore throat
- At least one of the following
  - i. Cervical lymphadenopathy (lymph nodes tender or >2 cm)
  - ii. Tonsillar exudates
  - iii. Positive culture for group A β-hemolytic streptococcus
  - iv. Fever greater than 38.3

Approximately 10% of children with sore throat and fever have a group A streptococcal infection. Less common causes of bacterial pharyngitis are *Mycoplasma pneumoniae, Chlamydia pneumoniae,* groups C and G streptococci, and *Arcanobacterium hemolyticum*. Of the five, *M pneumoniae* is by far the most common and may cause over one third of all pharyngitis cases in adolescents and adults.

Clinical Findings

Untreated streptococcal pharyngitis can result in acute rheumatic fever, glomerulonephritis, and suppurative complications (eg, cervical adenitis, peritonsillar abscess, otitis media, cellulitis, and septicemia). Sudden onset of sore throat, odynophagia, fever, headache, anterior cervical nodes, palatal petechiae, a beefy-red uvula, and a tonsillar exudate suggest streptococcal infection; however, the only way to make a definitive diagnosis is by throat culture or rapid antigen test. Rapid antigen tests are very specific, but have a sensitivity of only 85%–95%. Therefore, a positive test indicates *S pyogenes* infection, but a negative result requires confirmation by performing a culture. The presence of conjunctivitis,

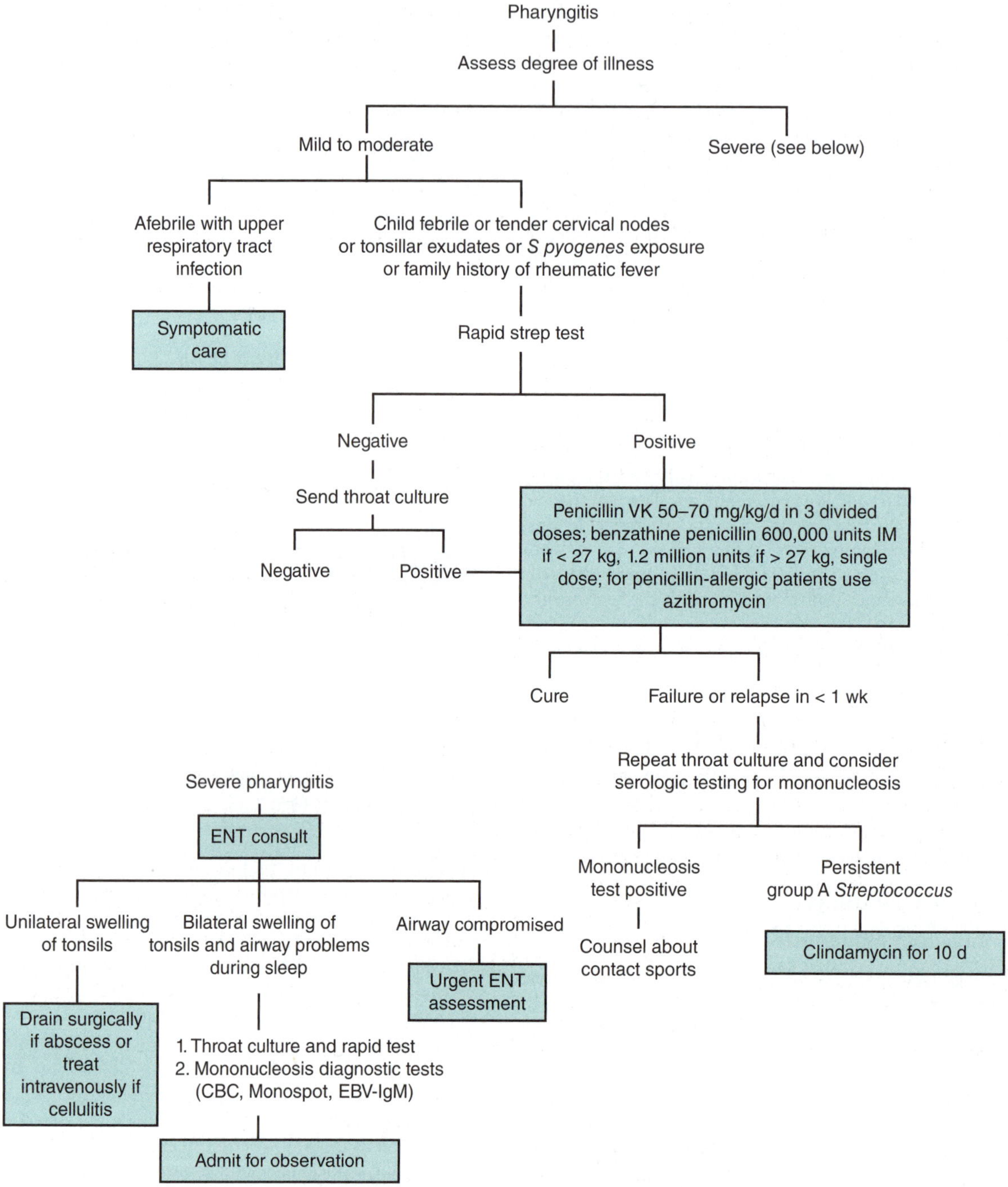

▲ **Figure 18–8.** Algorithm for pharyngitis. CBC, complete blood count; EBV, Epstein-Barr virus; ENT, ear, nose, and throat.

cough, hoarseness, symptoms of upper respiratory infection, anterior stomatitis, discrete ulcerative lesions, viral rash, and diarrhea should raise suspicion of a viral cause.

Occasionally, a child with group A streptococcal infection develops scarlet fever within 24–48 hours after the onset of symptoms. Scarlet fever is a diffuse, finely papular, erythematous eruption producing a bright red discoloration of the skin, which blanches on pressure. The rash is more intense in the skin creases. The tongue has a strawberry appearance.

A controversial but possible complication of streptococcal infections is childhood obsessive-compulsive disorder and/or tics. Pediatric Autoimmune Neuropsychiatric Disorders Associated with Streptococcus (PANDAS) is a yet unproven hypothesis.

Treatment

Suspected or proven group A streptococcal infection should be treated with a 10-day course of oral penicillin V potassium, a cephalosporin, or intramuscularly injected penicillin G benzathine LA (Table 18–5). Penicillin VK is equally effective if given in two or three divided doses in school-aged children. However, in adolescents, three doses are recommended. The American Heart Association endorses erythromycin as an alternative for penicillin-allergic patients.

The reported treatment failure rate after 10 days of penicillin VK administered three times daily varies from 6%–23%. However, over 50 years of treatment with penicillin, no group A streptococcal species have developed resistance to either penicillin or cephalosporins, so the cause of failure lies elsewhere. Patient compliance with 20 doses of medication is a large factor in failures, and intramuscular benzathine penicillin should be considered strongly in children who fail during or immediately after treatment. It has been suggested that the presence of β-lactamase–producing organisms in the pharynx may inactivate penicillin, but this has not been proven.

Children who fail to respond to treatment may be given amoxicillin–clavulanate or azithromycin. Approximately 5% of *S pyogenes* organisms are resistant to erythromycin, and trimethoprim–sulfamethoxazole is ineffective against group A streptococci. Further, because trimethoprim–sulfamethoxazole is ineffective in the eradication of pharyngeal organisms and is ineffective in the prevention of acute rheumatic fever when used as therapy for acute pharyngeal infections, it is not recommended.

Routine culturing after treatment is not recommended and is indicated only for those who remain symptomatic, have a recurrence of symptoms, or have had rheumatic fever. Of note, children who have had rheumatic fever are at a high risk of recurrence, so it is recommended that they receive long-term continuous antimicrobial prophylaxis.

In general, the carrier state is harmless, self-limited (2–6 months), and not contagious. There is little risk for the development of rheumatic fever. An attempt to eradicate the carrier state is warranted only if the patient or another family member has frequent streptococcal infections or when a family member or patient has a history of rheumatic fever or glomerulonephritis. If eradication is chosen, a course of clindamycin for 10 days or rifampin for 5 days should be used.

Table 18–5. Treatment of group A streptococcal pharyngitis.

Drug	Duration of Therapy	Dose	Clinical Cure Rate
Treatment of acute pharyngitis			
Penicillin	10 d	Penicillin V 50–75 mg/kg/d in 3 divided doses Benzathine penicillin 600,000 units IM if < 27 kg, 1.2 million units if > 27 kg, single dose	63%–64%
Amoxicillin	10 d	50 mg/kg/d once daily	86%
Azithromycin	5 d	12 mg/kg once daily	82%
Cephalexin	10 d	25–50 mg/kg/d in divided doses	94%
Eradication of carrier state			
Clindamycin	10 d	20 mg/kg/d in 3 divided doses	92% for carrier state
Penicillin + rifampin	10 d (rifampin final 4 d)	Penicillin V 50–75 mg/kg/d in 3 divided doses Benzathine penicillin 600,000 units IM if < 27 kg, 1.2 million units if > 27 kg, single dose Rifampin 20 mg/kg/d twice daily for 4 d	55%

Reproduced, and adapted, courtesy of Children's Hospital Colorado, from Suchitra R, Todd J: Commonly asked questions about group A streptococcal pharyngitis. Contagious Comments 2007;XXII(4).

In the past, daily penicillin prophylaxis was occasionally recommended; however, due to concerns about the development of drug resistance, tonsillectomy is now preferred.

Baugh RF et al; American Academy of Otolaryngology-Head and Neck Surgery Foundation. Clinical practice guideline: tonsillectomy in children. Otolaryngol Head Neck Surg 2011 Jan;144 (1 Suppl):S1–S30 [PMID: 21493257].

Gerber MA, Baltimore RS, Eaton CB, Gewitz M, Rowley AH, Shulman ST, Taubert KA: Prevention of rheumatic fever and diagnosis and treatment of acute Streptococcal pharyngitis: a scientific statement from the American Heart Association Rheumatic Fever, Endocarditis, and Kawasaki Disease Committee of the Council on Cardiovascular Disease in the Young, the Interdisciplinary Council on Functional Genomics and Translational Biology, and the Interdisciplinary Council on Quality of Care and Outcomes Research: endorsed by the American Academy of Pediatrics. Circulation 2009 Mar 24;119(11):1541–1551 [Epub 2009 Feb 26] [PMID: 19246689].

Shulman ST, Gerber MA: So what's wrong with penicillin for strep throat? Pediatrics 2004;113:1816 [PMID: 15173515].

PERITONSILLAR CELLULITIS OR ABSCESS (QUINSY)

ESSENTIALS OF DIAGNOSIS

- Severe sore throat
- Unilateral tonsillar swelling
- Deviation of the uvula
- Limited mouth opening (trismus)

Tonsillar infection occasionally penetrates the tonsillar capsule, spreading to the surrounding tissues, causing peritonsillar cellulitis. If untreated, necrosis occurs and a peritonsillar abscess forms. The most common pathogen is β-hemolytic streptococcus, but others include group D streptococcus, *S pneumoniae,* and anaerobes.

The patient complains of a severe sore throat even before the physical findings become marked. A high fever is usually present, and the process is almost always unilateral. The tonsil bulges medially, and the anterior tonsillar pillar is prominent. The soft palate and uvula on the involved side are edematous and displaced toward the uninvolved side. As the infection progresses, trismus, ear pain, dysphagia, and drooling may occur. The most serious complication of untreated peritonsillar abscess is a lateral pharyngeal abscess.

It is often difficult to differentiate peritonsillar cellulitis from abscess. In some children, it is possible to aspirate the peritonsillar space to diagnose and treat an abscess. However, it is reasonable to admit a child for 12–24 hours of intravenous antimicrobial therapy, because aggressive treatment of cellulitis can usually prevent suppuration. Therapy with penicillin or clindamycin is appropriate. Failure to respond to therapy during the first 12–24 hours indicates a high probability of abscess formation. An otolaryngologist should be consulted for incision and drainage or for aspiration under local or general anesthesia.

Recurrent peritonsillar abscesses are so uncommon (7%) that routine tonsillectomy for a single incident is not indicated unless other tonsillectomy indications exist. Hospitalized patients can be discharged on oral antibiotics when fever has resolved for 24 hours and dysphagia has improved.

RETROPHARYNGEAL ABSCESS

Retropharyngeal nodes drain the adenoids, nasopharynx, and paranasal sinuses and can become infected. The most common causes are β-hemolytic streptococci and *S aureus*. If this pyogenic adenitis goes untreated, a retropharyngeal abscess forms. The process occurs most commonly during the first 2 years of life. Beyond this age, retropharyngeal abscess usually results from superinfection of a penetrating injury of the posterior wall of the oropharynx.

The diagnosis of retropharyngeal abscess should be strongly suspected in an infant with fever, respiratory symptoms, and neck hyperextension. Dysphagia, drooling, dyspnea, and gurgling respirations are also found and are due to impingement by the abscess. Prominent swelling on one side of the posterior pharyngeal wall confirms the diagnosis. Swelling usually stops at the midline because a medial raphe divides the prevertebral space. Lateral neck soft tissue films show the retropharyngeal space to be wider than the C4 vertebral body.

Although retropharyngeal abscess is a surgical emergency, frequently it cannot be distinguished from retropharyngeal adenitis. Immediate hospitalization and intravenous antimicrobial therapy with a semisynthetic penicillin or clindamycin is the first step for most cases. Immediate surgical drainage is required when a definite abscess is seen radiographically or when the airway is compromised markedly. In most instances, a period of 12–24 hours of antimicrobial therapy will help to differentiate the two entities. In the child with adenitis, fever will decrease and oral intake will increase. A child with retropharyngeal abscess will continue to deteriorate. A surgeon should incise and drain the abscess under general anesthesia to prevent its extension.

LUDWIG ANGINA

Ludwig angina is a rapidly progressive cellulitis of the submandibular space that can cause airway obstruction and death. The submandibular space extends from the mucous membrane of the floor of the mouth to the muscular and fascial attachments of the hyoid bone. This infection is encountered infrequently in infants and children. The initiating factor in over 50% of cases is dental disease, including abscesses and extraction. Some patients have a history of lacerations and injuries to the floor of the mouth. Group A streptococci are the most common organism identified.

Symptoms include fever and tender swelling of the floor of the mouth. The tongue can become enlarged as well as tender and erythematous. Upward displacement of the tongue may cause dysphagia, drooling, and airway obstruction.

Treatment consists of high-dose intravenous clindamycin or ampicillin plus nafcillin until the culture results and sensitivities are available. Because the most common cause of death in Ludwig angina is sudden airway obstruction, the patient must be monitored closely in the intensive care unit and intubation provided for progressive respiratory distress. An otolaryngologist should be consulted to identify and perform a drainage procedure.

ACUTE CERVICAL ADENITIS

Local infections of the ear, nose, and throat can involve a regional lymph node and cause abscess formation. The typical case involves a unilateral, solitary, anterior cervical node. About 70% of these cases are due to β-hemolytic streptococcal infection, 20% to staphylococci, and the remainder to viruses, atypical mycobacteria, and *Bartonella henselae*. Methicillin-resistant *S aureus* (MRSA) must also be considered.

The initial evaluation of cervical adenitis should generally include a rapid group A streptococcal test, a complete blood count with differential looking for atypical lymphocytes, and a purified protein derivative skin test, looking for nontuberculous mycobacteria. If multiple enlarged nodes are found in addition to the sentinel node, a rapid mononucleosis test is useful. Early treatment with antibiotics prevents many cases of adenitis from progressing to suppuration. However, once fluctuation occurs, antibiotic therapy alone is often insufficient and needle aspiration may promote resolution. Depending on abscess size, an incision and drainage procedure may be necessary. Because of the increase in community acquired MRSA, it is a prudent to send a specimen for culture and sensitivity.

Cat-scratch disease is caused by *B henselae* causes indolent ("cold") adenopathy. The diagnosis is aided by the finding of a primary papule at the scratch site on the face. In over 90% of patients, there is a history of contact with kittens. The node is usually only mildly tender but may, over a month or more, suppurate and drain. About one-third of children have fever and malaise, and rarely neurologic sequelae and prolonged fever occur. Cat-scratch disease can be diagnosed by serologic testing, but testing is not always confirmatory. Blood should be drawn 2–8 weeks after onset of symptoms. Because most enlarged lymph nodes infected with *B henselae* spontaneously regress within 1–3 months, the benefit of antibiotics is controversial. In a placebo-controlled trial, azithromycin for 5 days caused a more rapid decrease in node size. Other drugs likely to be effective include rifampin, trimethoprim–sulfamethoxazole, erythromycin, clarithromycin, doxycycline, ciprofloxacin, and gentamicin.

Cervical lymphadenitis can be caused by nontuberculous mycobacterial species or *Mycobacterium avium* complex. Mycobacterial disease is unilateral and may involve several matted nodes. A characteristic violaceous appearance may develop over a prolonged period of time without systemic signs or much local pain. Atypical mycobacterial infections are often associated with positive purified protein derivative skin test reactions less than 10 mm in diameter, and a second-strength (250-test-unit) purified protein derivative skin test is virtually always positive.

Inman JC, Rowe M, Ghostine M, Fleck T: Pediatric neck abscesses: Changing organisms and empiric therapies. Laryngoscope 2008 Dec;118(12):2111–2114 [PMID: 18948832].

Wynne DM, Borg HK, Botma M, MacGregor F: Acute paediatric neck abscesses. Scott Med J 2008 Aug;53(3):17–20 [PMID: 18780520].

Differential Diagnosis

A. Neoplasms and Cervical Nodes

Malignant tumors usually are not suspected until adenopathy persists despite antibiotic treatment. Classically, malignant lymph nodes are painless, nontender, and firm to hard in consistency. They may be fixed to underlying tissues. They may occur as a single node, as unilateral nodes in a chain, bilateral cervical nodes, or as generalized adenopathy. Common malignancies that may manifest in the neck include Hodgkin disease, non-Hodgkin lymphoma, rhabdomyosarcoma, and thyroid carcinoma.

B. Imitators of Adenitis

Several structures in the neck can become infected and resemble a node. The first three masses are of congenital origin.

1. Thyroglossal duct cyst—These are in the midline, located between the hyoid bone and suprasternal notch. Thyroglossal duct cysts move upward when the tongue is protruded or with swallowing. Occasionally, a thyroglossal duct cyst may have a sinus tract with an opening just lateral to the midline. When infected, these can become acutely swollen and inflamed.

2. Branchial cleft cyst—These masses are found along the anterior border of the sternocleidomastoid muscle and are smooth and fluctuant. Occasionally a branchial cleft cyst may be attached to the overlying skin by a small dimple or a draining sinus tract. When infected, they can become a tender mass 3–5 cm in diameter.

3. Lymphatic malformation—Most of these lymphatic cysts are located in the posterior triangle just above the clavicle. These are soft and compressible and can be transilluminated. Over 60% of lymphatic malformations are noted at birth; the remaining malformations are usually seen by the time the child is age 2 years. If cysts become large enough, they can compromise the patient's ability to swallow and breathe.

4. Parotitis—The most common pitfall is mistaking parotitis for cervical adenitis. The parotid salivary gland crosses the angle of the jaw. Parotitis may be bacterial or viral and may occur unilaterally or bilaterally. Mumps was once the most common cause of viral parotitis, but due to routine vaccinations, parainfluenza is the primary viral cause in the United States. An amylase level will be elevated in parotitis.

5. Ranula—A ranula is a cyst in the floor of the mouth caused by obstruction of the ducts of the sublingual salivary gland. A "plunging" ranula extends below the mylohyoid muscle and can present as a neck mass.

6. Sternocleidomastoid muscle hematoma—These are noted at age 2–4 weeks. On close examination, the mass is found to be part of the muscle body and not movable. An associated torticollis usually confirms the diagnosis.

SNORING, MOUTH BREATHING, & UPPER AIRWAY OBSTRUCTION

In April 2002, the American Academy of Pediatrics (AAP) published a clinical practice guideline for the diagnosis and management of uncomplicated childhood obstructive sleep apnea syndrome (OSA). Currently, OSA is considered just one component of a broader spectrum of disease known as sleep-disordered breathing (SDB) which ranges from primary snoring (isolated snoring without apnea, arousals, or gas-exchange abnormalities) to upper airway resistance syndrome (UARS) to OSA. Historically, primary snoring (PS) has not been considered to be pathologic. The guideline emphasizes that pediatricians should screen all children for snoring and that complex high-risk patients should be referred to a specialist. The AAP is currently revising these guidelines but as of this writing they have not yet been published. At times, the terminology for SDB in the literature can be confusing since there SDB and OSA overlap. To simplify matters, the American Academy of Otolaryngology-Head and Neck Surgery (AAO-HNS) defines SDB as "an abnormal respiratory pattern during sleep and includes snoring, mouth breathing, and pauses in breathing. SDB encompasses a spectrum of disorders that increase in severity from snoring to obstructive sleep apnea." SDB is a presumptive diagnosis. OSA is diagnosed only by polysomnogram (PSG).

Polysomnography

The gold standard for diagnosis of OSA is a polysomnogram. A patient's history and clinical examination cannot predict the presence or severity of OSA. Similarly, an overnight oximetry study is a poor screening test for OSA; it may detect patients with severe disease but miss those with milder forms, such as upper airway resistance syndrome. Patients with this syndrome have an otherwise normal polysomnogram with the only evidence of obstruction being increased respiratory effort.

The criteria for diagnosing OSA differ between children and adults. An obstructive event occurs when airflow stops despite persistence of respiratory effort. A hypopnea episode is counted when airflow and respiratory effort decrease with an associated oxygen desaturation or arousal. Normative values for children are just being established. The American Academy of Sleep Medicine (AASM) states that for children, the occurrence of more than one apneic or hypopneic event per hour with duration of at least two respiratory cycles is abnormal. However, the AASM qualified its recommendation, stating that the criteria may be modified once more comprehensive data become available. One study of children between age 6 and 11 years found that a respiratory disturbance index of at least one event per hour, when associated with a 3% oxygen desaturation, was associated with daytime sleepiness and learning problems. If oxygen desaturations were absent, a respiratory disturbance index of five events per hour was associated with clinical symptoms.

Although an obstructive apnea index of greater than one event may be statistically significant, whether it is clinically relevant remains unclear. Any child with an apnea-plus-hypopnea index of greater than five events per hour appears to have clinically significant SDB. The dilemma is how to manage children with an apnea-plus-hypopnea index of more than one but fewer than five events per hour, as some of these children experience neurocognitive symptoms. Of note, many research studies have shown little correlation between the severity of OSA by PSG and neuropsychological morbidity.

Clinical Evaluation & Management

The AAO-HNS has developed clinical guidelines for otolaryngologists to facilitate their decision on whether to proceed with surgical treatment (usually adenotonsillectomy) or request a polysomnogram. A polysomnogram is generally recommended for children with SDB if they have any of the following comorbid conditions: obesity, Down syndrome, craniofacial abnormalities, neuromuscular disorders, sickle cell disease, or mucopolysaccharidoses. PSG is also recommended for children with SDB without the above comorbidities if the need for surgery is uncertain, or if there is discordance between tonsillar size on physical examination and the reported severity of SDB.

Most pediatric otolaryngologists perform adenotonsillectomy in healthy patients with SDB without obtaining a PSG. An adenotonsillectomy without PSG is usually recommended in a healthy child if the following are present:

1. Nighttime symptoms: habitual snoring along with gasping, pauses, or labored breathing. Other symptoms related to SDB may include night terrors, sleep walking, and secondary enuresis.
2. Daytime symptoms: unrefreshed sleep, attention deficit, hyperactivity, emotional lability, temperamental behavior,

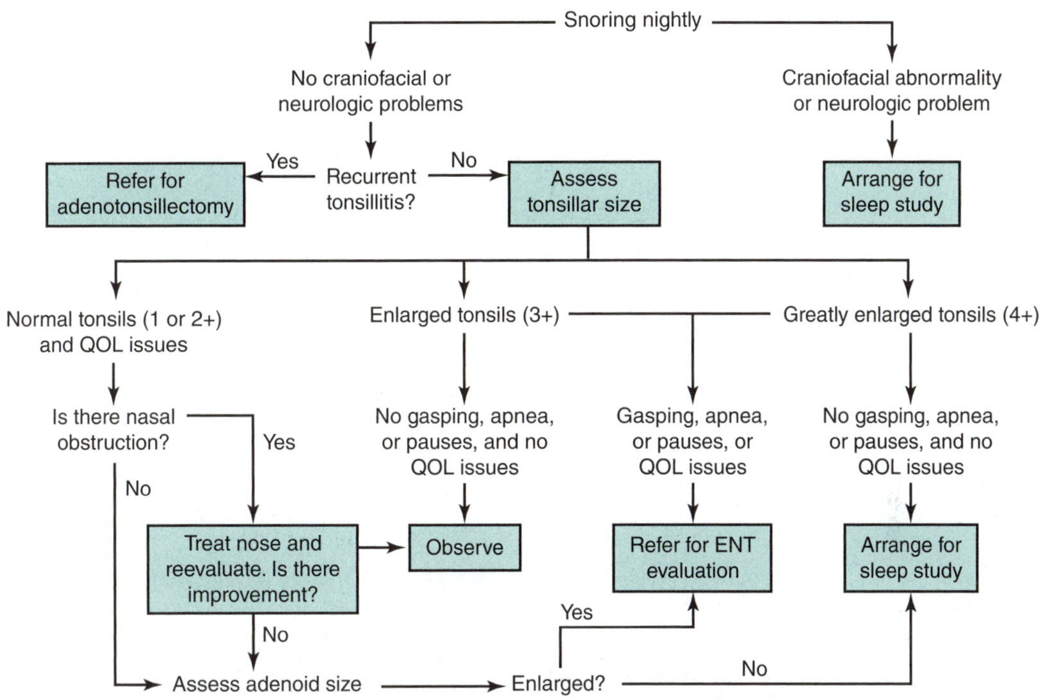

▲ **Figure 18–9.** Algorithm for snoring. ENT, ear, nose, and throat; QOL, quality of life.

poor weight gain, and daytime fatigue. Other signs include daytime mouth breathing or dysphagia.

3. Enlarged tonsils.

If the three findings cannot be confirmed, but the child has other indications for an adenotonsillectomy—ie, recurrent tonsillitis or markedly enlarged (4+) tonsils with dysphagia—surgery is also warranted.

Figure 18–9 is an algorithm for management of SDB complaints. The pathway relies on clinical symptoms and tonsil size. Of note, tonsil size alone does not predict the presence of significant SDB. Children without significant tonsil hypertrophy may still have SDB. Low muscle tone also contributes to an individual's propensity to experience SDB. However, measurement of muscle tone is not straightforward. Although the pathway states that an asymptomatic child with markedly enlarged tonsils (4+) should undergo an overnight polysomnographic study, a period of observation is reasonable. One's clinical suspicion of SDB should be heightened in the presence of enlarged tonsils, especially if the parents cannot provide a reliable history. If the child has no clinical symptoms and the tonsils are only moderately enlarged (3+), observation is appropriate. Educating the parents about the risks of SDB and what to look for is paramount.

A polysomnographic study is recommended for a child who has no adenotonsillar hypertrophy or nasal obstruction, but has significant symptoms of SDB. Other conditions, especially a periodic limb movement disorder, may mimic the daytime symptoms of SDB. If a polysomnogram indicates OSA in a child without adenotonsillar hypertrophy, a complete evaluation of the upper airway by awake flexible laryngoscopy should be performed to look for other possible sites of obstruction: nose, nasopharynx, hypopharynx (base of tongue or lingual tonsils), and larynx. The adenoids can also be assessed with a lateral neck x-ray. Alternative methods to evaluate a child for anatomical sites of obstruction include sedated ciné MRI of the upper airway or sleep endoscopy.

Allergic rhinitis is a common cause of nasal obstruction. If allergy is the suspected cause of SDB, a trial of intranasal corticosteroid spray is indicated. If enlarged tonsils (Figure 18–10) or adenoids are present, a referral to an otolaryngologist or a pediatric sleep laboratory is in order.

Complications & Sequelae

The importance of diagnosing SDB in children cannot be underestimated. SDB has been associated with problems in a multitude of realms, including social, behavioral, and neurocognitive. It has been shown to have significant impact on quality of life, and has been associated with

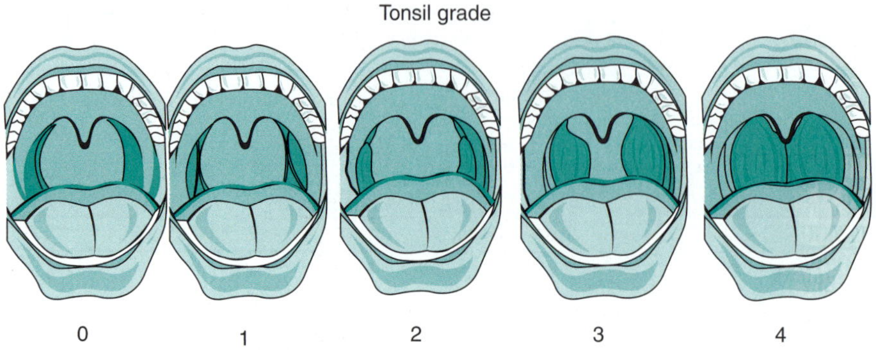

▲ **Figure 18–10.** A grading scale for tonsil size that ranges from 0 to 4. With grade 0 the tonsils are small and contained within the tonsillar fossa; in grade 4 the tonsils are so large they almost touch ("kissing"). (Reprinted, with permission, from Brodksy L: Modern assessment of tonsils and adenoids. Pediatr Clin North Am 1989;36:1551.)

growth impairment, and cardiovascular complications. Recent studies also suggest that SDB is associated with systemic inflammation.

Beebe DW: Neurobehavioral morbidity associated with disordered breathing during sleep in children: A comprehensive review. Sleep 2006;29:1115 [PMID: 17040000].

Gozal D, Kheirandish-Gozal L: The multiple challenges of obstructive sleep apnea in children: Morbidity and treatment. Curr Opin Pediatr 2008 Dec;20(6):654–658 [Review] [PMID: 19005334].

Loghmanee DA, Sheldon SH: Pediatric obstructive sleep apnea: An update. Pediatr Ann 2010 Dec;39(12):784–789; doi: 10.3928/00904481-20101116-09 [Review] [PMID: 21162487].

Mahmoud M, Gunter J, Sadhasivam S: Ciné MRI airway studies in children with sleep apnea: Optimal images and anesthetic challenges. Pediatr Radio 2009 Aug 11; [Epub ahead of print] [PMID: 19669745].

Nolan J, Brietzke SE: Systematic review of pediatric tonsil size and polysomnogram-measured obstructive sleep apnea severity. Otolaryngol Head Neck Surg 2011 Jun;144(6):844–850 [Epub 2011 Mar 11] [Review] [PMID: 21493309].

Roland PS et al; American Academy of Otolaryngology—Head and Neck Surgery Foundation. Clinical practice guideline: Polysomnography for sleep-disordered breathing prior to tonsillectomy in children. Otolaryngol Head Neck Surg 2011 Jul;145(1 Suppl):S1–S15 [Epub 2011 Jun 15] [PMID: 21676944].

Schechter MS: Technical report: Diagnosis and management of childhood obstructive sleep apnea syndrome. Pediatrics 2002;109:e69 [PMID: 11927742].

Web Resources

American Academy of Sleep Medicine educational site: http://www.sleepeducation.com

Child-friendly web site: http://www.sleepforkids.org/

National Sleep Foundation: http://www.sleepfoundation.org/

TONSILLECTOMY & ADENOIDECTOMY

Tonsillectomy

A tonsillectomy with or without adenoidectomy is typically performed for either hypertrophy or recurrent infections. Nowadays, the most common indication for an adenotonsillectomy is adenotonsillar hypertrophy that is associated with an obstructed breathing pattern at night (see earlier discussion of OSA and SDB). Besides producing airway obstruction, adenotonsillar hypertrophy may produce dysphagia or dental malocclusion. Rarely, hypertrophied tonsils may produce pulmonary hypertension or cor pulmonale.

Recurrent tonsillitis is a common reason for tonsillectomy. Tonsillitis is considered "recurrent" when a child has seven or more documented infections in 1 year, five per year for 2 years, or three per year for 3 years. For an infection to be considered clinically significant, there must be a sore throat and at least one of the following clinical features: cervical lymphadenopathy (tender lymph nodes or > 2 cm), OR tonsillar exudate, OR positive culture for group A β-hemolytic streptococcus, OR temperature greater than 38.3°C.

A tonsillectomy is reasonable if fewer infections are present but the child has missed multiple school days or has a complicated course. Other indications include recurrent peritonsillar abscess, persistent streptococcal carrier state, and multiple antibiotic allergies. Unless there a neoplasm is suspected, unilateral tonsillar hypertrophy is not an indication.

A new indication for tonsillectomy is PFAPA syndrome (see section on Recurrent Aphthous Stomatitis, earlier), in which fever recurs predictably, typically every 4–8 weeks. Tonsillectomy has been shown to eradicate or reduce symptoms recent studies.

Garavello W, Romagnoli M, Gaini RM: Effectiveness of adenotonsillectomy in PFAPA syndrome: A randomized study. J Pediatr 2009 Aug;155(2):250–253 [Epub 2009 May 21] [PMID: 19464029].

Gerber MA, Baltimore RS, Eaton CB, Gewitz M, Rowley AH, Shulman ST, Taubert KA: Prevention of rheumatic fever and diagnosis and treatment of acute Streptococcal pharyngitis: A scientific statement from the American Heart Association Rheumatic Fever, Endocarditis, and Kawasaki Disease Committee of the Council on Cardiovascular Disease in the Young, the Interdisciplinary Council on Functional Genomics and Translational Biology, and the Interdisciplinary Council on Quality of Care and Outcomes Research: endorsed by the American Academy of Pediatrics. Circulation 2009 Mar 24;119(11):1541–1551 [Epub 2009 Feb 26] [PMID: 19246689].

Pignataro L et al: Outcome of tonsillectomy in selected patients with PFAPA syndrome. Arch Otolaryngol Head Neck Surg 2009 Jun;135(6):548–553 [PMID: 19528401].

Web Resources

American Academy of Otolaryngology/Head and Neck Surgery–sponsored site dedicated to children: http://www.entnet.org/kidsent/

Adenoidectomy

The adenoids, composed of lymphoid tissue in the nasopharynx, are a component of the Waldeyer ring of lymphoid tissue, which also includes the palatine tonsils and lingual tonsils. Enlargement of the adenoids, with or without infection, can obstruct the upper airway, alter normal orofacial growth, and interfere with speech, swallowing, or Eustachian tube function. Children who are persistent mouthbreathers can develop dental malocclusion and "adenoid facies," where the face is pinched and the maxilla narrowed because the molding pressures of the orbicularis oris and buccinator muscles are unopposed by the tongue. The adenoids can also harbor biofilms, which have been associated with chronic rhinosinusitis and otitis media.

Indications for adenoidectomy with or without tonsillectomy include upper airway obstruction, orofacial conditions such as mandibular growth abnormalities and dental malocclusion, speech abnormalities, persistent middle ear effusion, recurrent otitis media, and chronic rhinosinusitis.

Complications of Tonsillectomy & Adenoidectomy

The mortality rate associated with tonsillectomy and adenoidectomy is reported to approximate that of general anesthesia alone. The rate of hemorrhage varies between 0.1% and 8.1%, depending on the definition of hemorrhage; the rate of postoperative transfusion is 0.04%. Other complications include permanently hypernasal speech (< 0.01%) and, more rarely, nasopharyngeal stenosis, atlantoaxial subluxation, mandibular condyle fracture, and psychological trauma.

Contraindications to Tonsillectomy & Adenoidectomy

A. Palatal Abnormalities

Adenoids should not be removed completely in a child with a cleft palate or submucous cleft palate because of the risk of velopharyngeal incompetence which may cause hypernasal speech and nasal regurgitation. If needed, a superior or partial adenoidectomy can be performed in a child with a palatal abnormality. A bifid uvula can be a sign of a palatal abnormality.

B. Bleeding Disorder

When suspected, bleeding disorders must be diagnosed and treated before tonsillectomy and adenoidectomy.

C. Acute Tonsillitis

An elective tonsillectomy and adenoidectomy can often be postponed until acute tonsillitis is resolved. Urgent tonsillectomy may be required for tonsillitis unresponsive to medical therapy.

DISORDERS OF THE LIPS

1. Labial Sucking Tubercle

A young infant may present with a small callus in the midupper lip. It usually is asymptomatic and disappears after cup feeding is initiated.

2. Cheilitis

Dry, cracked, scaling lips are usually caused by sun or wind exposure. Contact dermatitis from mouthpieces or various woodwind or brass instruments has also been reported. Licking the lips exacerbates cheilitis. Liberal use of lip balm gives excellent results.

3. Inclusion Cyst

Inclusion (retention) cysts are due to the obstruction of mucous glands or other mucous membrane structures. In the newborn, they occur on the hard palate or gums and are called Epstein pearls. These resolve spontaneously in 1–2 months. In older children, inclusion cysts usually occur on the palate, uvula, or tonsillar pillars. They appear as taut yellow sacs varying in size from 2 to 10 mm. Inclusion cysts that do not resolve spontaneously may undergo incision and drainage. Occasionally a mucous cyst on the lower lip (mucocele) requires excision for cosmetic reasons. Mucoceles pathologically are a blocked minor salivary gland.

DISORDERS OF THE TONGUE

1. Geographic Tongue (Benign Migratory Glossitis)

This condition of unknown etiology occurs in 1%–2% of the population with no age, sex, or racial predilection. It is characterized by irregularly shaped patches on the tongue that are devoid of papillae and surrounded by parakeratotic reddish borders. The pattern changes as alternating regeneration and desquamation occurs. The lesions are generally asymptomatic and require no treatment.

2. Fissured Tongue (Scrotal Tongue)

This condition is marked by numerous irregular fissures on the dorsum of the tongue. It occurs in approximately 1% of the population and is usually a dominant trait. It is also frequently seen in children with trisomy 21.

3. Coated Tongue (Furry Tongue)

The tongue normally becomes coated if mastication is impaired and the patient is taking a liquid or soft diet. Mouth breathing, fever, or dehydration can accentuate the process.

4. Macroglossia

Tongue hypertrophy and protrusion may be due to trisomy 21, Beckwith-Wiedemann syndrome, glycogen storage disease, cretinism, mucopolysaccharide storage disease, lymphangioma, or hemangioma. Tongue reduction procedures should be considered in otherwise healthy subjects when macroglossia affects airway patency.

HALITOSIS

Bad breath is usually due to acute stomatitis, pharyngitis, rhinosinusitis, nasal foreign body, or dental hygiene problems. In older children and adolescents, halitosis can be a manifestation of chronic rhinosinusitis, gastric bezoar, bronchiectasis, or lung abscess. The presence of orthodontic devices or dentures can cause halitosis if good dental hygiene is not maintained. Halitosis can also be caused by decaying food particles embedded in cryptic tonsils. In adolescents, tobacco use is a common cause. Mouthwashes and chewable breath fresheners give limited improvement. Treatment of the underlying cause is indicated, and a dental referral may be in order.

SALIVARY GLAND DISORDERS

1. Parotitis

A first episode of parotitis may safely be considered to be of viral origin, unless fluctuance is present. The leading cause was mumps until adoption of vaccination; now the leading viruses are parainfluenza and Epstein-Barr virus. HIV infection should be considered if the child is known to be at risk.

2. Suppurative Parotitis

Suppurative parotitis occurs chiefly in newborns and debilitated elderly patients. The parotid gland is swollen, tender, and often erythematous, usually unilaterally. The diagnosis is made by expression of purulent material from Stensen's duct. The material should be cultured. Fever and leukocytosis may be present. Treatment includes hospitalization and intravenous antibiotic therapy; the most common causative organism is *S aureus*.

3. Juvenile Recurrent Parotitis

Some children experience recurrent nonsuppurative parotid inflammation with swelling or pain and fever. Juvenile recurrent parotitis (JRP) is most prevalent between the ages of 3 and 6 years, and generally decreases by adolescence. The cause is unknown, but possible etiologic factors have been proposed, including ductal anomaly, autoimmune, allergy, and genetic. It usually occurs unilaterally. Treatment includes analgesics and some recommend an antistaphylococcal antibiotic for prophylaxis of bacterial infection and quicker resolution. Recently, endoscopy of Stensen's duct has been investigated not only to confirm the diagnosis but also to provide treatment.

Leerdam CM, Martin HC, Isaacs D: Recurrent parotitis of childhood. J Paediatr Child Health 2005 Dec;41(12):631–634 [PMID: 16398865].

Quenin S, Plouin-Gaudon I, Marchal F, Froehlich P, Disant F, Faure F: Juvenile recurrent parotitis: Sialendoscopic approach. Arch Otolaryngol Head Neck Surg 2008 Jul;134(7):715–719 [PMID: 18645120].

4. Tumors of the Parotid Gland

Mixed tumors, hemangiomas, sarcoidosis, and leukemia can manifest in the parotid gland as a hard or persistent mass. A cystic mass or multiple cystic masses may represent an HIV infection. Workup may require consultation with oncology, infectious disease, hematology, and otolaryngology.

5. Ranula

A ranula is a retention cyst of a sublingual salivary gland. It occurs on the floor of the mouth to one side of the lingual frenulum. It is thin-walled and contains a clear bluish fluid. Referral to an otolaryngologist for surgical management is the treatment of choice.

CONGENITAL ORAL MALFORMATIONS

1. Tongue-Tie (Ankyloglossia)

A short lingual frenulum can hinder both protrusion and elevation of the tongue. Puckering of the midline of the tongue with tongue movement is noted on physical examination. Ankyloglossia can cause feeding difficulties in the neonate, speech problems, and dental problems. When mild, treatment consists of reassurance. If the tongue cannot protrude past the teeth or alveolar ridge or move between the gums and cheek, referral to an otolaryngologist is indicated. A frenulectomy should be performed in the neonatal period if the infant is having difficulty latching onto the breast. In our practice, neonatal frenulectomy is performed in clinic. Early treatment is favored, as when an infant is even several months old, general anesthesia is required for the procedure to be performed safely.

Buryk M et al: Efficacy of neonatal release of ankyloglossia: A randomized trial. Pediatrics 2011 Aug;128(2):280–288 [PMID: 21768318].

2. Torus Palatini

Hard midline masses on the palate are called torus palatini. These are bony protrusions that form at suture lines of bone. Usually they are asymptomatic and require no therapy. They can be surgically reduced if necessary.

3. Cleft Lip & Cleft Palate (See Chapter 37)

A. Submucous Cleft Palate

A bifid uvula is present in 3% of healthy children. However, a close association exists between bifid uvula and submucous cleft palate. A submucous cleft can be diagnosed by noting a translucent zone in the middle of the soft palate (zona pellucida). Palpation of the hard palate reveals absence of the posterior bony protrusion. Affected children have a 40% risk of developing persistent middle ear effusion. They are at risk for velopharyngeal incompetence, or an inability to close the palate against the posterior pharyngeal wall, resulting in hypernasal speech. During feeding, some of these infants experience nasal regurgitation of food. Children with submucous cleft palate causing abnormal speech or significant nasal regurgitation of food should be referred for possible surgical repair.

B. High-Arched Palate

A high-arched palate is usually a genetic trait of no consequence. It also occurs in children who are chronic mouth breathers and in premature infants who undergo prolonged oral intubation. Some rare causes of high-arched palate are congenital disorders such as Marfan syndrome, Treacher Collins syndrome, and Ehlers-Danlos syndrome.

C. Pierre Robin Sequence

This group of congenital malformations is characterized by the triad of micrognathia, cleft palate, and glossoptosis. Affected children present as emergencies in the newborn period because of infringement on the airway by the tongue. The main objective of treatment is to prevent asphyxia until the mandible becomes large enough to accommodate the tongue. In some cases, this objective can be achieved by leaving the child in a prone position when unattended. Other airway manipulations such as a nasal trumpet may be necessary. Recently, distraction osteogenesis has been used to avoid tracheostomy. In severe cases, a tracheostomy is required. The child requires close observation and careful feeding until the problem is outgrown.

Mackay DR: Controversies in the diagnosis and management of the Robin sequence. Journal of Craniofacial Surgery 2011 Mar;22(2):415–420 [PMID: 21403570].

19 Respiratory Tract & Mediastinum

Monica J. Federico, MD
Paul Stillwell, MD
Robin R. Deterding, MD
Christopher D. Baker, MD
Vivek Balasubramaniam, MD
Edith T. Zemanick, MD
Scott D. Sagel, MD
Ann Halbower, MD
Casey J. Burg, MD
Gwendolyn S. Kerby, MD

RESPIRATORY TRACT

Pediatric pulmonary diseases account for almost 50% of deaths in children younger than age 1 year and about 20% of all hospitalizations of children younger than age 15 years. Approximately 7% of children have a chronic disorder of the lower respiratory system. Understanding the pathophysiology of many pediatric pulmonary diseases requires an appreciation of the normal growth and development of the lung.

GROWTH & DEVELOPMENT

The lung has its origins from an outpouching of the foregut during the fourth week of gestation. The development of the lung is divided into five overlapping stages.

1. *Embryonic stage* (3–7 weeks' gestation): During this stage, the primitive lung bud undergoes asymmetrical branching and then subsequent dichotomous branching, leading to the development of the conducting airways. This stage of lung development is dependent on a complex interaction of various growth factors originating in both the pulmonary epithelium and the splanchnic mesenchyme. It also sees the development of the large pulmonary arteries from the sixth aortic arch and the pulmonary veins as outgrowths of the left atrium. Abnormalities during this stage result in congenital abnormalities such as lung aplasia, tracheoesophageal fistula, and congenital pulmonary cysts.
2. *Pseudoglandular stage* (5–17 weeks' gestation): During this stage, which overlaps with the embryonic stage, the lung has a glandular appearance. The conducting airways (bronchi and bronchioles) form over these 12 weeks. The respiratory epithelium of these airways begins to differentiate, and the presence of cartilage, smooth muscle cells, and mucus glands are first seen. In addition, the pleuroperitoneal cavity divides into two distinct compartments. Abnormalities during this stage lead to pulmonary sequestration, congenital pulmonary airway malformation and congenital diaphragmatic hernia.
3. *Canalicular stage* (16–26 weeks' gestation): This stage witnesses the delineation of the pulmonary acinus. The alveolar type II cells differentiate into type I cells, the pulmonary capillary network develops, and the alveolar type I cells closely approximate with the developing capillary network. Abnormalities of development during this stage include neonatal respiratory distress syndrome and lung hypoplasia.
4. *Saccular stage* (26–36 weeks' gestation): During this stage further branching of the terminal saccules takes place as well as a thinning of the interstitium and fusion of the type I cell and capillary basement membrane in preparation for the lungs' function as a gas-exchange organ. This stage sees the beginning of an exponential increase in the epithelial surface area for gas exchange. During this stage of lung development the lung is able to fulfill its function, in terms of a gas-exchange organ.
5. *Alveolar stage* (36 weeks' gestation to 3–8 years of age): Controversy surrounds the length of this stage of lung development. During this stage, secondary alveolar septa form to increase the surface area for gas exchange, the capillary network has a rapid phase of growth, and true alveoli develop. Abnormalities during this stage lead to lung hypoplasia and can result in the development of bronchopulmonary dysplasia (BPD).

At birth, the lung assumes the gas-exchanging function served by the placenta in utero, placing immediate stress on all components of the respiratory system. Any abnormality in the lung, respiratory muscles, chest wall, airway, central respiratory control, or pulmonary circulation may therefore lead to problems at birth. For example, infants who are homozygous for an abnormality in the surfactant protein B gene will develop lethal pulmonary disease. Persistent pulmonary hypertension of the newborn due to a failure of the normal transition to a low-resistance pulmonary circulation at birth can complicate neonatal respiratory diseases. There is also mounting evidence that abnormalities during fetal and neonatal growth and development of the lung have long-standing effects into adulthood, such as reduced gas exchange, exercise intolerance, asthma, and an increased risk of chronic obstructive pulmonary disease.

Barker DJ: The intrauterine origins of cardiovascular and obstructive lung disease in adult life: The Marc Daniels Lecture 1990. J R Coll Physicians Lond 1991;25:129 [PMID: 2066923].

Bogue CW: Genetic and molecular basis of airway and lung development. In Haddad GG et al (editors): *Basic Mechanisms of Pediatric Respiratory Disease.* BC Decker, 2002.

Burri P: Structural aspects of prenatal and postnatal development and growth of the lung. In McDonald JA (editor): *Lung Growth and Development.* BC Decker, 1997.

Wharburton D et al: Molecular mechanisms of early lung specification and branching morphogenesis. Pediatr Res 2005;57(5 Pt 2) 26R [PMID: 15817505].

DIAGNOSTIC AIDS

PHYSICAL EXAMINATION OF THE RESPIRATORY TRACT

The four components of a complete pulmonary examination include inspection, palpation, auscultation, and percussion. *Inspection* of respiratory rate, depth, ease, symmetry, and rhythm of respiration is critical to the detection of pulmonary disease. In young children, an elevated respiratory rate may be an initial indicator of pneumonia or hypoxemia. In a study of children with respiratory illnesses, abnormalities of attentiveness, inconsolability, respiratory effort, color, and movement had good diagnostic accuracy in detecting hypoxemia. *Palpation* of tracheal position, symmetry of chest wall movement, and vibration with vocalization can help identify intrathoracic abnormalities. For example, a shift in tracheal position can suggest pneumothorax or significant atelectasis. Tactile fremitus may change with consolidation or air in the pleural space. *Auscultation* should assess the quality of breath sounds and detect the presence of abnormal sounds such as fine or coarse crackles, wheezing, or rhonchi. Wheezing or prolonged expiratory time compared to inspiratory time suggests intrathoracic airways obstruction. Tachypnea with an equal inspiratory and expiratory time suggests decreased lung compliance. Transmitted voice sounds in egophony and whispered pectoriloquy change with lung consolidation. It is important to know the lung anatomy in order to identify the location of abnormal findings (Figure 19–1). In older patients, unilateral crackles are the most valuable examination finding in pneumonia. *Percussion* may identify tympanic or dull sounds that can help define an intrathoracic process. (This component of the examination can prove challenging in young children, who may not cooperate.) Although chest radiography has replaced the utility of these tests, they can be helpful when imaging is not available.

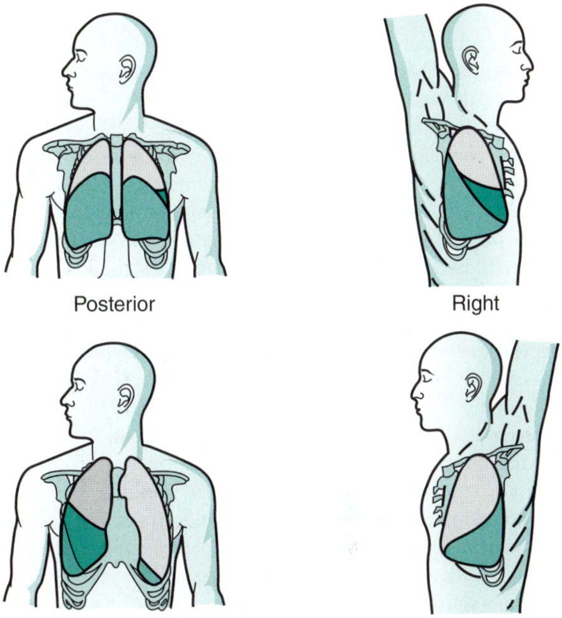

▲ **Figure 19–1.** Projections of the pulmonary lobes on the chest surface. The upper lobes are white, the right-middle lobe is the darker color, and the lower lobes are the lighter color.

Extrapulmonary manifestations of pulmonary disease include acute findings such as cyanosis and altered mental status and signs of chronic respiratory insufficiency such as growth failure, clubbing, and osteoarthropathy. Evidence of cor pulmonale (loud pulmonic component of the second heart sound, hepatomegaly, elevated neck veins, and rarely, peripheral edema) signifies pulmonary hypertension and may accompany advanced lung disease.

Respiratory disorders can be secondary to disease in other systems. It is therefore important to look for other conditions such as congenital heart disease, neuromuscular disease, immunodeficiency, autoimmune disease, and occult malignancy (arthritis or hepatosplenomegaly).

Palafox M et al: Diagnostic value of tachypnea in pneumonia defined radiologically. Arch Dis Child 2000;82:41 [PMID: 10630911].

Wipf JE et al: Diagnosing pneumonia by physical examination: Relevant or relic? Arch Intern Med 1999;159:1082 [PMID: 10335685].

PULMONARY FUNCTION TESTS

Pulmonary function tests are objective measures of lung and airway physiology that can help differentiate obstructive from restrictive lung diseases, measure disease severity, measure disease progression or improvement, and evaluate response to therapy. Because the range of normal values for a test may be wide, and because the predicted normal range changes dramatically with growth, serial determinations of lung function are often more informative than a single determination. Patient cooperation and reasonable effort is essential for almost all standard physiologic assessments. With a well-trained technician in a comfortable environment aided by visual incentives, and interactive computer-animated systems, most children age 4 years and older can produce satisfactory results. Lung function measurements in infants and toddlers are available at centers with specialized equipment and expertise. Tests of lung function are particularly valuable in the care of children with chronic respiratory disease. Children with cystic fibrosis (CF) perform pulmonary function testing as early as they can cooperate. The Expert Panel Report (3) for the diagnosis and management of asthma recommends pulmonary function testing be performed routinely for evaluation and management of asthmatic children age 5 and older.

Current spirometers use a pneumotachograph to record flow over the time of the test and to produce a volume-time tracing (spirogram) or a flow-volume curve. The patient inhales maximally, holds his or her breath for a short period, and then exhales as fast and hard as possible until they reach residual volume or for at least 3 seconds. The report values include forced vital capacity (FVC), which is the total volume of air that is exhaled, the forced expiratory volume in the first second of the exhalation (FEV_1), the ratio of the FEV_1/FVC, the forced expiratory flow at the middle of the vital capacity (FEF25-75), and the peak expiratory flow rate (PEFR). A suggested potential range of normal for these measurements is included in Table 19–1 and examples are shown in the figures included on the CD. Examples of obstructive processes include asthma, bronchopulmonary dysplasia, and cystic fibrosis (CF). Examples of restrictive problems include scoliosis, chest wall deformities that limit lung expansion, muscle weakness, and interstitial lung diseases such as collagen-vascular diseases, hypersensitivity pneumonitis, and interstitial fibrosis. Confirmation of restrictive lung or chest wall physiology requires lung volume measurements (eg, total lung capacity, residual volume, and functional residual capacity) that are usually only available at specialized centers.

The peak expiratory flow rate (PEFR), the maximal flow recorded during an FVC maneuver, can be assessed by handheld devices. These devices are not as well calibrated as spirometers and the PEFR measurement can vary greatly with patient effort, so they are not good substitutes for spirometry. However, peak flow monitoring can be helpful in following the course of a patient with asthma who is difficult to control or for patients with poor perception of their airflow obstruction.

Couriel JM, Child F: Applied physiology: Lung function tests in children. Curr Paediatrics 2006;16:413–419.

Galant SP, Nickerson B: Lung function measurement in the assessment of childhood asthma: Recent important developments. Curr Opin Allergy Clin Immunol 2010;10:149–154.

ASSESSMENT OF OXYGENATION & VENTILATION

Arterial blood gas measurements define the acid-base balance between respiration at the tissue level and in the lungs. Blood gas measurement is essential in critically ill children to evaluate hypoxemia, acidosis, and hypercarbia. Data from blood gas measurements can also be used to categorize acid-base disturbances as respiratory, metabolic, or mixed. Blood gas measurements are affected by abnormalities of respiratory control, gas exchange, respiratory mechanics, and the circulation. In pediatrics, hypoxemia (low partial pressure of arterial oxygen [PaO_2]) most commonly results from ventilation (V′) and perfusion (Q′) mismatch. Common pediatric diseases that may be associated with hypoxemia due to V′/Q′ mismatch include acute asthma, cystic fibrosis, pneumonia, bronchiolitis, and bronchopulmonary dysplasia (BPD). Other causes of hypoxemia include hypoventilation, shunts, and diffusion barrier for oxygen. Hypercapnia (elevated partial pressure of arterial carbon dioxide [$PaCO_2$]) results from inadequate alveolar ventilation (ie, inability to clear the CO_2 produced). This is termed *hypoventilation*. Causes include decreased central respiratory

Table 19–1. Classification of lung function abnormalities.

		Type of Lung Disease	
	Range of Normal	Obstructive[a]	Restrictive[b]
FVC (L)	80% to 120 % predicted	Normal or decreased	Decreased
FEV_1 (L)	80% to 120% predicted	Decreased	Decreased
FEV_1:FVC ratio	Greater than 82; less than 95	Decreased	Normal or increased
$FEF_{25\text{-}75}$ (L/sec)	60% to 140% predicted	Decreased	Normal, increased, or decreased

FEF_{25-75}, forced expiratory flow at 25%–75% of FVC; FEV_1, forced expiratory volume in the first second of exhalation; FVC, forced vital capacity.

Table 19–2. Normal arterial blood gas values on room air.

	pH	PaO_2 (mm Hg)	$PaCO_2$ (mm Hg)
Sea level	7.38–7.42	85–95	36–42
5000 ft	7.36–7.40	65–75	35–40

$PaCO_2$, partial pressure of arterial carbon dioxide; PaO_2, partial pressure of arterial oxygen; SaO_2, percent hemoglobin saturation.

drive, paralysis of respiratory muscles, and low-tidal-volume breathing as seen in restrictive lung diseases, severe scoliosis, or chest wall trauma. Hypercapnea can also occur when severe V′/Q′ mismatch is present such as may be present in CF or BPD. Table 19–2 gives normal values for arterial pH, PaO_2, and $PaCO_2$ at sea level and at 5000 ft.

Venous blood gas analysis or capillary blood gas analysis can be useful for the assessment of PCO_2 and pH, but not PaO_2 or saturation. Noninvasive assessment of oxygenation can be achieved with pulse oximetry (measuring light absorption by transilluminating the skin). Oxygenated hemoglobin absorbs red light at certain wavelengths. Measurement during a systolic pulse allows estimation of arterial oxygen saturation as the machine corrects for the light absorbed at the tissue level between pulses. No heating of the skin is necessary. Values of oxygen saturation are reliable as low as 80%. The pulse oximeter has reduced reliability during conditions causing reduced arterial pulsation such as hypothermia, hypotension, or infusion of vasoconstrictor drugs. Carbon monoxide bound by hemoglobin results in falsely high oxygen saturation readings. Transcutaneous assessment of PaO_2 is not commonly utilized because of the multiple factors that can interfere with accurate measurements.

Exhaled or end-tidal CO_2 monitoring can be used to noninvasively estimate arterial CO_2 content. It is used to monitor alveolar ventilation and is most accurate in patients without significant lung disease, particularly those with a good match of ventilation and perfusion and without airway obstruction. Monitoring of exhaled or end-tidal CO_2 is commonly used by anesthesia. Transcutaneous PCO_2 monitoring is even less reliable than transcutaneous PaO2 monitoring and should be used with caution if at all.

Ralston M et al (editors): *Pediatric Advanced Life Support Provider Manual.* American Heart Association and American Academy of Pediatrics, 2006.

Salyer JW: Neonatal and pediatric pulse oximetry. Respir Care 2003 Apr;48(4):386–396 [PMID: 12667266].

Soubani AO: Noninvasive monitoring of oxygen and carbon dioxide. Am J Emerg Med 2001;19:141 [PMID: 11239260].

Sullivan KJ, Kissoon N, Goodwin SR: End-tidal carbon dioxide monitoring in pediatric emergencies. Pediatr Emerg Care 2005 May;21(5):327–332 [PMID: 15874818].

Tobias JD: Transcutaneous carbon dioxide monitoring in infants and children. Paediatr Anaesth 2009 May;19(5):434–444 [PMID: 19236597].

CULTURE OF MATERIAL FROM THE RESPIRATORY TRACT

Sources of respiratory tract secretions for culture include expectorated and induced sputum, oropharyngeal swabs, tracheal aspirates, and bronchoalveolar lavage fluid. Spontaneously expectorated sputum is the least invasive way to collect a sample for culture though it is rarely available from patients younger than age 6 years. Oropharyngeal swabs are widely used as a surrogate for lower airway cultures in nonexpectorating patients, particularly children with CF. Sputum induction, performed by inhaling aerosolized hypertonic saline, is a relatively safe, noninvasive means of obtaining lower airway secretions. Sputum induction has been used in patients with CF and may be useful in patients with suspected *Mycobacterium tuberculosis, Pneumocystis jiroveci* pneumonia, or complicated community acquired pneumonia. Cultures from the lower respiratory tract can be obtained invasively by tracheal aspiration through an endotracheal tube or rigid bronchoscope, or by performing a bronchoalveolar lavage through a flexible bronchoscope. Other less commonly employed means of obtaining lung specimens include computed tomography (CT)–guided needle aspiration and lung biopsy, either open or thoracoscopic. Thoracentesis should be considered when pleural fluid is present.

Hatherill M et al: Induced sputum or gastric lavage for community-based diagnosis of childhood pulmonary tuberculosis? Arch Dis Child 2009;94:195–201.

Lahti E et al: Induced sputum in the diagnosis of childhood community-acquired pneumonia. Thorax 2009;64:252–257.

IMAGING OF THE RESPIRATORY TRACT

The plain chest radiograph remains the foundation for investigating the pediatric thorax. Both frontal (posterior-anterior) and lateral views should be obtained if feasible. The radiograph is useful for evaluating chest wall abnormalities, heart size and shape, mediastinum, diaphragm, and lung parenchyma. When pleural fluid is suspected, lateral decubitus radiographs may be helpful in determining the extent and mobility of the fluid. When a foreign body is suspected, forced expiratory radiographs may show focal air trapping and shift of the mediastinum to the contralateral side. Lateral neck radiographs can be useful in assessing the size of adenoids and tonsils and also in differentiating croup from epiglottitis, the latter being associated with the "thumbprint" sign.

Barium swallow is indicated for detection of swallowing dysfunction in patients with suspected aspiration, tracheoesophageal fistula, gastroesophageal reflux, vascular rings and slings, and achalasia. Airway fluoroscopy assesses both fixed airway obstruction (eg, tracheal stenosis, masses, or tracheal compression) and dynamic airway obstruction (eg, tracheomalacia). Fluoroscopy or ultrasound of the diaphragm can detect paralysis by demonstrating paradoxic movement of the involved hemidiaphragm.

Chest CT is useful in evaluation of congenital lung lesions, pleural disease (eg, effusion or recurrent pneumothorax), mediastinum (eg, lymphadenopathy), pulmonary nodules or masses. High-resolution CT is best for evaluating interstitial lung disease (ILD) or bronchiectasis while decreasing radiation exposure compared to a standard CT. Magnetic resonance imaging (MRI) is useful for defining vascular or bronchial anatomical abnormalities. Ventilation-perfusion scans can provide information about regional ventilation and perfusion and can help detect vascular malformations and pulmonary emboli. Pulmonary angiography is occasionally necessary to define the pulmonary vascular bed more precisely.

Schneebaum et al: Use and yield of chest computed tomography in the diagnostic evaluation of pediatric lung disease. Pediatrics 2009;124:472–479.

LARYNGOSCOPY & BRONCHOSCOPY

Direct visualization of the airways may be necessary to establish the etiology of a respiratory problem despite an extensive history and physical and sophisticated imaging. This can be achieved with rigid or flexible instrumentation. The indications for laryngoscopy include hoarseness, stridor, symptoms of obstructive sleep apnea, and laryngeal wheezing consistent with a diagnosis of vocal cord dysfunction; indications for bronchoscopy include wheezing, suspected foreign body, pneumonia, atelectasis, chronic cough, and hemoptysis. A flexible bronchoscope can also be used to assess placement and patency of an endotracheal tube. In general, the more specific the indication, the higher the diagnostic yield. Each method, rigid or flexible, has advantages. For some patients, both should be employed sequentially under the same anesthesia.

The rigid, open tube instruments have the best optics and allow surgical intervention to be easily achieved such as removal of a foreign body. Rigid bronchoscopy is done with general anesthesia. Flexible laryngoscopy may be done with topical anesthesia or light sedation and flexible bronchoscopy can be done with either conscious sedation or general anesthesia. The flexible bronchscopy is of a smaller caliber and allows more distal examination of the airways. Because it is smaller, the flexible bronchoscope does not stent the airway open during the procedure and often dynamic airway collapse is more easily documented by the flexible procedure. Bronchoalveolar lavage is often useful to sample the alveolar space for infection, inflammation, hemorrhage, or aspiration. Although removal of foreign bodies has been achieved with the flexible bronchoscope in larger children, the standard of care in most institutions is to remove foreign bodies via the rigid bronchoscope.

Transbronchial biopsy in children is limited to evaluation for infection and rejection in transplant patients due to poor diagnostic yield in most conditions. Transbronchial biopsy may have a role in diagnosing diffuse lung diseases such as sarcoidosis. Video-assisted thoracoscopic lung biopsy (VATS) provides a more substantial specimen for pathologic assessment.

Nicholai T: The role of rigid and flexible bronchoscopy in children. Paediatr Respir Rev 2011;12:190–195.

GENERAL THERAPY OF PEDIATRIC LUNG DISEASES

OXYGEN THERAPY

The primary goal of therapy with supplemental oxygen (O_2) is to relieve hypoxemia. In children with respiratory disease, oxygen can reduce the work of breathing, resulting in fewer respiratory symptoms; relax the pulmonary vasculature, lessening the potential for pulmonary hypertension and congestive heart failure; and improve feeding. Patients breathing spontaneously can be treated by nasal cannula, head hood, or mask (including simple, rebreathing, nonrebreathing, or Venturi masks). The general goal of oxygen therapy is to achieve an arterial oxygen tension of 65–90 mm Hg or an oxygen saturation above 92%, although lower PaO_2 or SpO_2 levels may be acceptable in certain situations. The actual oxygen concentration achieved by nasal cannula or mask depends on the flow rate, the type of mask used, and the patient's age. Small changes in flow rate during oxygen administration by nasal cannula can lead to substantial changes in inspired oxygen concentration in young infants. The amount of oxygen required to correct hypoxemia may vary according to the child's activity. It is not unusual, for example, for an infant with chronic lung disease to require 0.75 L/min while awake but 1 L/min while asleep or feeding.

Although the head hood is an efficient device for delivery of oxygen in young infants, the nasal cannula is used more often because it allows the infant greater mobility. The cannula has nasal prongs that are inserted in the nares. Flow through the nasal cannula should generally not exceed 3 L/min to avoid excessive drying of the mucosa. Even at high flow rates, oxygen by nasal cannula rarely delivers inspired oxygen concentrations greater than 40%–45%. In contrast, partial rebreathing and nonrebreathing masks or head hoods achieve inspired oxygen concentrations as high as 90%–100%.

Because the physical findings of hypoxemia are subtle, the adequacy of oxygenation should be measured by the arterial oxygen tension, or oxygen saturation. The advantages of the latter noninvasive method include the ability to obtain continuous measurements during various normal activities and to avoid artifacts caused by crying or breath-holding during attempts at arterial puncture. For children with chronic cardiopulmonary disorders that require supplemental oxygen therapy (eg, bronchopulmonary dysplasia or cystic fibrosis), frequent noninvasive assessments are essential to ensure the safety and adequacy of treatment.

AARC Clinical Practice Guidelines: Selection of an oxygen delivery device for neonatal and pediatric patients—2002 revision and update. Respir Care 2002;47:707–716.

Ralston M et al (editors): *Pediatric Advanced Life Support Provider Manual.* American Heart Association and American Academy of Pediatrics, 2006.

INHALATION OF MEDICATIONS

Inhalation of medications is a mainstay of therapy for pediatric respiratory conditions and are routinely used in patients with chronic diseases such as cystic fibrosis (CF), bronchopulmonary dysplasia (BPD), and asthma, as well as in acute illnesses such as infectious laryngotracheobronchitis and bronchiolitis. Short acting β agonists and anticholinergics provide acute bronchodilitation (relievers), whereas inhaled corticosteroids and cromones provide anti-inflammatory effects (controllers). Nebulised antibiotics have documented benefit in CF and nebulized mucolytic medications are used in CF and other conditions with impaired secretion control such as non-CF bronchiectasis. (See Table 19–3.)

The medications can be delivered by pressurized metered dose inhaler (pMDI), dry powder inhaler (DPI), or compressed air-driven wet nebulization (see Table 19–3) for currently available formulations. Careful attention to delivery technique is critical to optimize medication delivery to the airways. A valved holding chamber or similar spacer should be used with pMDI use, and this technique has been shown to be effective in infants as young as 4 months of age. A face-mask interface is recommended for both pMDI and wet nebulization in infants and toddlers; a simple mouth piece suffices for older children who can form a seal around the mouth piece. Delivery technique should be assessed and reviewed at each clinical visit.

Ahrens RC, Hess DR, Anderson P, Dhand R, Rau JL et al: Device selection and outcomes of aerosol therapy: Evidence-based guidelines. Chest 2005;127:335–371.

Janssens HM, Tiddens HA: Aerosol therapy: The special needs of young children. Paediatr Respir Rev 2006;7(Suppl 1).

AIRWAY CLEARANCE THERAPY

Chest physical therapy, with postural drainage, percussion, and forced expiratory maneuvers, has been widely used to improve the clearance of lower airway secretions in children with CF, bronchiectasis, and neuromuscular disorders. Currently available airway clearance techniques include: chest physiotherapy, autogenic drainage, blowing therapies (bubbles, pinwheels), active coughing, positive expiratory pressure (PEP) with handheld devices, intrapulmonary percussive ventilation, or high-frequency chest compression. The decision about which technique to use should be based on the patient's age and preference after trying different approaches. Daily exercise is an important adjunctive therapy for airway clearance and overall lung health. Cough-assist devices (eg, mechanical insufflator-exsufflators) are useful for children with a weak cough. For example, they are useful for children with neuromuscular disorders such as muscular dystrophy and spinal muscular atrophy. Bronchodilators or mucolytic medications may be given prior to or during airway clearance therapy. Inhaled corticosteroids and inhaled antibiotics should be given after airway clearance therapy so that the airways are first cleared of secretions, allowing the medications to maximally penetrate into the lung. Airway clearance has not been shown to be beneficial for patients with acute respiratory illnesses such as pneumonia, bronchiolitis, and asthma.

Table 19-3. Common uses for inhaled medications in pediatric respiratory illness.

Disease Process	Short Acting Bronchodilator	Anticholinergic Bronchodilator	Inhaled Steroid	Other
Asthma	Acute relief prior to exercise	Acute relief	Chronic use for control	Inhaled corticosteroid + long-acting bronchodilator for control
Bronchopulmonary dysplasia	Acute relief	Acute relief	Control if bronchial reactivity is present	
Cystic fibrosis	Prior to airway clearance	Limited data	Control if bronchial reactivity is present	Mucolytics and inhaled antibiotics
Infectious laryngotracheobronchitis (croup)	Acute relief (racemic epinephrine)		Acute relief (nebulized steroid)	
Bronchiolitis (acute infectious)	Acute relief (may have limited benefit)			Recent interest in inhaled epinephrine and hypertonic saline

De Boeck K et al: Airway clearance techniques to treat acute respiratory disorders in previously healthy children: Where is the evidence? Eur J Pediatr 2008;167;607–612.

Kravitz RM: Airway clearance in Duchenne muscular dystrophy. Pediatrics 2009;123:S231–S235.

Lester MK et al: Airway-Clearance therapy guidelines and implementation. Resp Care 2009;54(6):733–750.

AVOIDANCE OF ENVIRONMENTAL HAZARDS

There is increasing evidence that environmental insults can aggravate existing lung diseases and impair pulmonary function, but it remains unclear whether these insults actually cause lung disease in children. Outdoor air pollution (ozone and particulates), indoor pollution, diesel exhaust, and household fungi are examples. Environmental tobacco poisoning, either second or third hand, dramatically increases pulmonary morbidity. Many adolescents personally abuse tobacco and become addicted. Public health policies that limit smoke exposure and reduce advertising to children have had a positive impact. Smoking family members should be advised to quit smoking and do everything possible to minimize environmental smoke exposure to the children around them. Homes with mold should have remediation, particularly if children with lung disease are in residence. Ozone exposure can be limited by avoiding outdoor activities during the height of daily ozone levels, but additional public policy changes will be required to further reduce ozone pollutants in the air.

For children with asthma, family pets may be a significant trigger as can household cockroach infestation. Families should also be counseled about risks of foreign body aspiration in curious toddlers.

Anderson ME, Bogdan GM: Environments, indoor air quality, and children. Pediatr Clin N Am 2007;54:295–307.

Committee on Environmental Health: Spectrum of noninfectious health effects from molds. Pediatrics 2006;118:2582.

Tzivian L: Outdoor air pollution and asthma in children. J Asthma 2011;48:470.

DISORDERS OF THE CONDUCTING AIRWAYS

The conducting airways (the nose, mouth, pharynx, larynx, trachea, bronchi, and bronchioles) direct inspired air to the gas-exchange units of the lung; they do not participate in gas exchange themselves. Airflow obstruction in the conducting airways can occur at extrathoracic sites (eg, above the thoracic inlet) or at intrathoracic sites (eg, below the thoracic inlet). Extrathoracic or upper airway obstruction disrupts the inspiratory phase of respiration and is often manifest by stridor or "noisy breathing." Intrathoracic obstruction disrupts the expiratory phase of respiration and is often manifest by wheezing and prolongation of the expiratory phase. After assessing whether the obstruction is extrathoracic or intrathoracic the next challenge is to determine if the obstruction is fixed or variable (Table 19–4). Fixed obstructions disrupt each breath and the abnormal sounds are consistently heard. Fixed obstructions are often associated with anatomic abnormalities that may be amenable to surgical correction. With variable obstruction the abnormal breathing pattern is interspersed with normal quiet breathing. Variable obstructions are often due to dynamic changes in airway caliber that occurs with laryngomalacia, tracheomalacia, or bronchomalacia. The onset and progression of the obstruction can provide important clues to the etiology and can help determine the urgency of evaluation and management. Obstructions due to dynamic airway collapse often improve with age, whereas fixed obstructions typically progress or fail to improve with age. Acute onset extrathoracic obstruction is often infectious. Clinical indications that the obstruction is severe include high-pitched stridor or wheezing, bi-phasic stridor or wheezing, poor intensity breath sounds, severe retractions, and poor color or cyanosis.

Helpful diagnostic studies in the evaluation of extrathoracic obstruction include chest and lateral neck radiographs, airway

Table 19–4. Classification and causes of upper airway obstruction.

Fixed, Extrathoracic, Not Acute	Fixed, Extrathoracic, Acute	Fixed Intrathoracic, Intrinsic	Fixed, Intrathoracic, Extrinsic
Vocal cord paralysis	Infectious laryngotracheobronchitis	Tracheal stenosis	Tumor (compressing the airways)
Laryngeal atresia/web	Epiglottitis	Complete tracheal rings	Vascular ring or sling
Laryngocele/cyst	Bacterial tracheitis	Foreign body aspiration	Bronchogenic cyst
Laryngeal papillomas	Anaphylaxis	Endobronchial tumor	Congenital pulmonary adenomatoid malformation
Subglottic hemangioma	Angioneurotic edema		Esophageal duplication
Tracheal web	Foreign body aspiration		Congenital lobar overdistention
Peritonsillar abscess			
Choanal atresia			
Retropharyngeal abscess			

fluoroscopy, and barium swallow. In patients who have symptoms of severe chronic obstruction, an electrocardiogram and/or echocardiogram should be obtained to evaluate for right ventricular hypertrophy and pulmonary hypertension. Patients with obstructive sleep apnea should have polysomnography (see section on sleep abnormalities). In older children, pulmonary function tests can differentiate fixed from variable airflow obstruction and identify the site of variable obstruction. Treatment should be directed at relieving airway obstruction and correcting the underlying condition if possible.

Helpful diagnostic studies for intrathoracic obstruction include two-view chest radiographs, a sweat test, and pulmonary function tests in older children. Other diagnostic studies are dictated by the history and physical findings. Treatment should be directed toward the primary cause of the obstruction, but generally includes a trial of bronchodilators. If noninvasive studies are unable to establish the cause of airway obstruction, laryngoscopy and bronchoscopy remain the procedures of choice to establish the precise diagnosis.

LARYNGOMALACIA AND CONGENITAL DISORDERS OF THE EXTRATHORACIC AIRWAY

ESSENTIALS OF DIAGNOSIS & TYPICAL FEATURES

- Presentation from birth or within the first few months of life.
- Inspiratory sounds usually of a high-pitched ("croup") nature but can be variable.
- Moderate to severe symptoms require visualization of the airway.

LARYNGOMALACIA

Laryngomalacia is a benign congenital disorder in which the cartilaginous support for the supraglottic structures is underdeveloped. It is the most common cause of variable extrathoracic airway obstruction. Laryngomalacia usually presents in the first 6 weeks of life as **persistent stridor**. Stridor has been reported to be worse in the supine position, with increased activity, with upper respiratory infections, and during feeding; however, the clinical presentation can be variable. Patients may have oxygen desaturation during sleep. Gastroesophageal reflux may also be associated with laryngomalacia requiring treatment. The condition usually improves with age and resolves by the time the child is 2–3 years old. The diagnosis is established by direct laryngoscopy, which shows inspiratory collapse of an omega-shaped epiglottis (with or without long, redundant arytenoids). In mildly affected patients with a typical presentation (those without stridor at rest or retractions), treatment is not usually needed. However, in patients with severe symptoms of airway obstruction associated with feeding difficulties, failure to thrive, obstructive sleep apnea, respiratory insufficiency, or severe dyspnea, surgical epiglottoplasty may be beneficial.

Meier, Jeremy D et al: Improved growth curve measurements after supraglottoplasty. The Laryngoscope 2011:121(7):1574 [PMID: 21647914].

Thompson, Dana M et al: Laryngomalacia: Factors that influence disease severity and outcomes of management. Current Opinion in Otolaryngology & Head and Neck Surgery 2010:18(6):564 [PMID: 20962644].

OTHER CAUSES OF CONGENITAL EXTRATHORACIC OBSTRUCTION

Other rare congenital lesions of the larynx (laryngeal atresia, laryngeal web, laryngocele and cyst of the larynx, subglottic hemangioma, and laryngeal cleft) usually present as fixed extrathoracic obstruction. Fixed extrathoracic obstructions are best evaluated by direct laryngoscopy. Laryngeal atresia presents immediately after birth with severe respiratory distress and is usually fatal. Laryngeal web, representing fusion of the anterior portion of the true vocal cords, is associated with hoarseness, aphonia, and stridor. Surgical correction is usually necessary depending on the degree of airway obstruction.

Congenital cysts and laryngoceles are believed to have similar origin. Cysts are more superficial, whereas laryngoceles communicate with the interior of the larynx. Cysts are generally fluid-filled, whereas laryngoceles may be either air or fluid-filled. Airway obstruction is usually prominent and requires surgery or laser therapy.

Subglottic hemangiomas are seen in infancy with progressive signs of upper airway obstruction and can be associated with similar lesions of the skin (but not always). Although these lesions tend to regress spontaneously, medical management with Propranolol to speed regression has successfully changed the management paradigm in this area. In severe airway obstruction, surgical treatment or even tracheostomy may be required.

Laryngeal cleft is an uncommon condition resulting from failure of posterior cricoid fusion. Patients with this condition may have stridor or silent aspiration. Recent reports have shown that a type 1 laryngeal cleft (above the vocal cords) may not always show aspiration on a modified barium swallow while more severe type 2 and 3 laryngeal clefts almost always do. All types of clefts may result in recurrent or chronic pneumonia and failure to thrive. Laryngeal clefts can be diagnosed using direct laryngoscopy with attention to spreading and assessing the degree of tissue above the vocal folds. The decision to correct type 1 clefts should be made after multidisciplinary consideration of the pulmonary complications and other comorbidities. Repair may be addressed surgically or with an injection laryngoplasty. More severe clefts require surgical repair and may require tracheostomy. The return of normal swallow function without aspiration may take months to occur even after repair.

Ahmad SM, Soliman AM: Congenital anomalies of the larynx. Otolaryngol Clin North Am 2007 Feb;40(1):177–191 [PMID: 17346567].

Cohen, Michael et al: Injection laryngoplasty for type 1 laryngeal cleft in children. Otolaryngology—Head and Neck Surgery 2011;144(5):789 [PMID: 21493369].

Kieran SM et al: The lipid laden macrophage index as a marker of aspiration in patients with type I and II laryngeal clefts. Int J Pediatr Otorhinolaryngol 2010;74(7):743–746 [PMID: 20394993].

Starkey, E et al: Propranolol for infantile haemangiomas: A review. Archives of Disease in Childhood 2011;96(9):890 [PMID: 21622997].

Steehler, Matthew K et al: Management of subglottic cysts with Mitomycin-C-A case series and literature review. International Journal of Pediatric Otorhinolaryngology 2011;75(3):360 [PMID: 21239066].

ACQUIRED DISORDERS OF THE EXTRATHORACIC AIRWAY

ESSENTIALS OF DIAGNOSIS & TYPICAL FEATURES

- Presentation may be acute or subacute depending on diagnosis.
- Inspiratory sounds consistent with stridor. Pitch can be variable depending on diagnosis.
- Life-threatening condition can occur, requiring careful patient assessment.

FOREIGN BODY ASPIRATION

ESSENTIALS OF DIAGNOSIS & TYPICAL FEATURES

- Sudden onset of coughing or respiratory distress.
- Difficulty vocalizing.

Aspiration of a foreign body into the respiratory tract is rarely observed. Onset is generally sudden, with a history of the child running with food in the mouth or playing with seeds, small coins, or toys. Symptoms at the time of the ingestion are often abrupt and include cough, choking, or wheezing.

The foreign body can lodge itself anywhere along the respiratory tract. Often it is trapped in the supraglottic airway, triggering protective reflexes that result in laryngospasm. Small objects such as coins may pass through the glottis and obstruct the trachea. Foreign bodies that lodge in the esophagus may compress the airway and cause dysphagia and respiratory distress.

Objects most commonly seen in foreign body aspiration include peanuts, hot dogs, popcorn, small coins, hard candy, and small toys. Children aged 6 months to 4 years are at highest risk, and many deaths are caused by foreign body aspiration and airway obstruction each year.

Clinical Findings

The diagnosis is established by acute onset of choking along with *inability* to vocalize or cough and cyanosis with marked distress (complete obstruction), or with drooling, stridor, and *ability* to vocalize (partial obstruction). More typically, the foreign body lodges in the supraglottic airway, triggering protective reflexes that result in laryngospasm. Without treatment, progressive cyanosis, loss of consciousness, seizures, bradycardia, and cardiopulmonary arrest can follow.

Treatment

The emergency treatment of upper airway obstruction due to foreign body aspiration is somewhat controversial. If *complete* obstruction is present, then one must intervene immediately. If partial obstruction is present, then the choking subject should be allowed to use his or her own cough reflex to remove the foreign body. If after a brief observation period the obstruction increases or the airway becomes completely obstructed, acute intervention is required. The American Academy of Pediatrics and the American Heart Association distinguish between children younger than and older than age 1 year. A choking infant younger than age 1 year should be placed face down over the rescuer's arm, with the head positioned below the trunk. Five measured back blows are delivered rapidly between the infant's scapulas with the heel of the rescuer's hand. If obstruction persists, the infant should be rolled over and five rapid chest compressions performed (similar to cardiopulmonary resuscitation). This sequence is repeated until the obstruction is relieved. In a choking child older than age 1 year, abdominal thrusts (Heimlich maneuver) may be performed, with special care in younger children because of concern about possible intra-abdominal organ injury.

Blind finger sweeps should *not* be performed in infants or children because the finger may actually push the foreign body further into the airway causing further obstruction. The airway may be opened by jaw thrust, and if the foreign body can be directly visualized, careful removal with the fingers or instruments (Magill forceps) can be attempted. Patients with persistent apnea and inability to achieve adequate ventilation may require emergency intubation, tracheotomy, or needle cricothyrotomy, depending on the setting and the rescuer's skills.

Ralston M et al (editors): *Pediatric Advanced Life Support Provider Manual.* American Heart Association and American Academy of Pediatrics, 2006.

CROUP SYNDROME

Croup describes acute inflammatory diseases of the larynx, including viral croup (laryngotracheobronchitis), epiglottitis (supraglottitis), and bacterial tracheitis. These are the main entities in the differential diagnosis for patients presenting with acute stridor, although spasmodic croup, angioneurotic edema, laryngeal or esophageal foreign body, and retropharyngeal abscess should be considered as well.

1. Viral Croup

Viral croup generally affects younger children in the fall and early winter months and is most often caused by parainfluenza virus serotypes. Other organisms causing croup include respiratory syncytial virus (RSV), human coronavirus NL63, rhinovirus, human metapneumovirus, influenza virus, rubeola virus, adenovirus, and *Mycoplasma pneumoniae.* Although inflammation of the entire airway is usually present, edema formation in the subglottic space accounts for the predominant signs of upper airway obstruction.

Clinical Findings

A. Symptoms and Signs

Usually a prodrome of upper respiratory tract symptoms is followed by a barking cough and stridor. Fever is usually absent or low grade but may on occasion be high grade. Patients with mild disease may have stridor when agitated. As obstruction worsens, stridor occurs at rest, accompanied in severe cases by retractions, air hunger, and cyanosis. On examination, the presence of cough and the absence of drooling favor the diagnosis of viral croup over epiglottitis.

B. Imaging

Lateral neck radiographs in patients with classic presentations are not required but can be diagnostically supportive if the x-ray shows subglottic narrowing without the irregularities seen in tracheitis and a normal epiglottis. However, a severely ill patient should never be left unattended in the imaging suite.

Treatment

Treatment of viral croup is based on the symptoms. Mild croup, signified by a barking cough and no stridor at rest, requires supportive therapy with oral hydration and minimal handling. Mist therapy has historically been used but clinical studies do not demonstrate effectiveness. Conversely, patients with stridor at rest require active intervention. Oxygen should be administered to patients with oxygen desaturation. Nebulized racemic epinephrine (2.25% solution; 0.05 mL/kg to a maximum of 1.5 mL diluted in sterile saline) is commonly used because it has a rapid onset of action within 10–30 minutes. Both racemic epinephrine and epinephrine hydrochloride (L-epinephrine, an isomer) are effective in alleviating symptoms and decreasing the need for intubation.

The efficacy of glucocorticoids in croup is now firmly established. Dexamethasone, 0.6 mg/kg intramuscularly as one dose, improves symptoms, reduces the duration of hospitalizations and frequency of intubations, and permits earlier discharge from the emergency department. Oral dexamethasone (0.15 mg/kg) may be equally effective. Inhaled budesonide (2–4 mg) also improves symptoms and decreases hospital stay. Onset of action occurs within 2 hours, and this agent may be as effective as dexamethasone. Dexamethasone has also been shown to be more effective than prednisolone in equivalent doses.

If symptoms resolve within 3 hours of glucocorticoids and nebulized epinephrine, patients can safely be discharged without fear of a sudden rebound in symptoms. If, however, recurrent nebulized epinephrine treatments are required or if respiratory distress persists, patients require hospitalization for close observation, supportive care, and nebulization treatments as needed. Hospitalized patients with persistent symptoms over 3–4 days despite treatment should initiate consideration of another underlying cause.

Patients with impending respiratory failure require an artificial airway. Intubation with an endotracheal tube of slightly smaller diameter than would ordinarily be used is reasonably safe. Extubation should be accomplished within 2–3 days to minimize the risk of laryngeal injury. If the patient fails extubation, tracheostomy may be required.

Prognosis

Most children with viral croup have an uneventful course and improve within a few days. Some evidence suggests that patients with a history of croup associated with wheezing may have airway hyperreactivity. It is not always clear if the hyperreactivity was present prior to the croup episode or if the viral infection causing croup altered airway function.

2. Epiglottitis

With the introduction of the *Haemophilus influenzae* conjugate vaccine, the incidence of epiglottitis has dramatically decreased and epiglottitis is rare in countries with immunization programs. If disease occurs, it is likely to be associated with *H influenzae* in unimmunized children, or another organism such as nontypeable *H influenzae, Neisseria meningitides,* or *Streptococcus* species in immunized populations.

Clinical Findings

A. Symptoms and Signs

The classic presentation is a sudden onset of high fever, dysphagia, drooling, muffled voice, inspiratory retractions, cyanosis, and soft stridor. Patients often sit in the so-called sniffing dog position, which gives them the best airway possible under the circumstances. Progression to total airway obstruction may occur and result in respiratory arrest. The definitive diagnosis is made by direct inspection of the epiglottis, a procedure that should be done by an experienced airway specialist under controlled conditions (usually in the operating room). The typical findings are a cherry-red and swollen epiglottis and swollen arytenoids.

B. Imaging

Diagnostically, lateral neck radiographs may be helpful in demonstrating a classic "thumbprint" sign. Obtaining radiographs, however, may delay important airway intervention.

Treatment

Once the diagnosis of epiglottitis is made, endotracheal intubation must be performed immediately in children but not necessarily in adult populations. Most anesthesiologists prefer general anesthesia (but not muscle relaxants) to facilitate intubation. After an airway is established, cultures of the blood and epiglottis should be obtained and the patient should be started on appropriate intravenous antibiotics to cover H influenzae and Streptococcus species (ceftriaxone sodium or an equivalent cephalosporin). Extubation can usually be accomplished in 24–48 hours, when direct inspection shows significant reduction in the size of the epiglottis. Intravenous antibiotics should be continued for 2–3 days, followed by oral antibiotics to complete a 10-day course.

Prognosis

Prompt recognition and appropriate treatment usually results in rapid resolution of swelling and inflammation. Recurrence is unusual.

Guardiani, Elizabeth et al: Supraglottitis in the era following widespread immunization against Haemophilus influenzae type B: Evolving principles in diagnosis and management. The Laryngoscope 2010;120(11):2183 [PMID: 20925091].

Tibballs, James et al: Symptoms and signs differentiating croup and epiglottitis. Journal of Paediatrics and Child Health 2011;47(3):77 [PMID: 21091577].

3. Bacterial Tracheitis

Bacterial tracheitis (pseudomembranous croup) is a severe, life-threatening form of laryngotracheobronchitis. As the management of severe viral croup has been improved with the use of dexamethasone and vaccination has decreased the incidence of epiglottitis, tracheitis is a more common cause of a pediatric airway emergency requiring admission to the pediatric intensive care unit. This diagnosis must be high in the differential when a patient presents with severe upper airway obstruction and fever. The organism most often isolated is *Staphylococcus aureus,* but organisms such as *H influenzae,* group A *Streptococcus pyogenes, Neisseria* species, *Moraxella catarrhalis,* and others have been reported. A viral prodrome is common. Viral coinfections are described and should be treated especially Influenza A and H1N1. The disease probably represents localized mucosal invasion of bacteria in patients with primary viral croup, resulting in inflammatory edema, purulent secretions, and pseudomembranes. Although cultures of the tracheal secretions are frequently positive, blood cultures are almost always negative.

Clinical Findings

A. Symptoms and Signs

The early clinical picture is similar to that of viral croup. However, instead of gradual improvement, patients develop higher fever, toxicity, and progressive or intermittent severe upper airway obstruction that is unresponsive to standard croup therapy. The incidence of sudden respiratory arrest or progressive respiratory failure is high; in such instances, airway intervention is required. Findings of toxic shock and the acute respiratory distress syndrome may also be seen. Recently, subsets of patients with tracheal membranes have been reported with a less severe initial clinical presentation. Nevertheless, these patients are still at risk for life-threatening airway obstruction. Aggressive medical treatment and debridement still must occur in these patients.

B. Laboratory Findings and Imaging

The white cell count is usually elevated with a left shift. Cultures of tracheal secretions usually demonstrate one of the causative organisms. Lateral neck radiographs show a normal epiglottis but severe subglottic and tracheal narrowing. Irregularity of the contour of the proximal tracheal mucosa can frequently be seen radiographically and should elicit concern for tracheitis. Bronchoscopy showing a normal epiglottis and the presence of copious purulent tracheal secretions and membranes confirms the diagnosis.

Treatment

Patients with suspected bacterial tracheitis will require direct visualization of the airway in a controlled environment and debridement of the airway. Most patients will be intubated because the incidence of respiratory arrest or progressive respiratory failure is high. Patients may also require further debridement, humidification, frequent suctioning, and intensive care monitoring to prevent endotracheal tube obstruction by purulent tracheal secretions. Intravenous antibiotics to cover *S aureus, H influenzae,* and the other organisms are indicated. Thick secretions persist for several days, usually resulting in longer periods of intubation for bacterial tracheitis than for epiglottitis or croup. Despite the severity of this illness, the reported mortality rate is very low if it is recognized and treated promptly.

Hopkins, Brandon S et al: H1N1 influenza A presenting as bacterial tracheitis. Otolaryngology—Head and Neck Surgery 2010;142(4):612 [PMID: 20304287].

Tebruegge M et al: Bacterial tracheitis: A multi-centre perspective. Scand J Infect Dis 2009:1–10 [PMID: 19401934].

VOCAL CORD PARALYSIS

Unilateral or bilateral vocal cord paralysis may be congenital, or more commonly may result from injury to the recurrent laryngeal nerves. Risk factors for acquired paralysis include difficult delivery (especially face presentation), neck and thoracic surgery (eg, ductal ligation or repair of tracheo-esophageal fistula), trauma, mediastinal masses, and central nervous system disease (eg, Arnold-Chiari malformation). Patients usually present with varying degrees of hoarseness, aspiration, or high-pitched stridor. Unilateral cord paralysis is more likely to occur on the left because of the longer course of the left recurrent laryngeal nerve and its proximity to major thoracic structures. Patients with unilateral paralysis are usually hoarse but rarely have stridor. With bilateral cord paralysis, the closer to midline the cords are positioned, the greater the airway obstruction; the more lateral the cords are positioned, the greater the tendency to aspirate and experience hoarseness or aphonia. If partial function is preserved (paresis), the adductor muscles tend to operate better than the abductors, with a resultant high-pitched inspiratory stridor and normal voice.

Airway intervention (tracheostomy) is rarely indicated in unilateral paralysis but is often necessary for bilateral paralysis. Clinically, paralysis can be assessed by direct visualization of vocal cord function with laryngoscopy or more invasively by recording the electrical activity of the muscles (electromyography). Electromyogram recordings can differentiate vocal fold paralysis from arytenoid dislocation, which has prognostic value. Recovery is related to the severity of nerve injury and the potential for healing.

SUBGLOTTIC STENOSIS

Subglottic stenosis may be congenital, or more commonly may result from endotracheal intubation. Neonates and infants are particularly vulnerable to subglottic injury from intubation. The subglottis is the narrowest part of an infant's airway, and the cricoid cartilage, which supports the subglottis, is the only cartilage that completely encircles the airway. The clinical presentation may vary from totally asymptomatic to the typical picture of severe upper airway obstruction. Patients with signs of stridor who repeatedly fail extubation are likely to have subglottic stenosis. Subglottic stenosis should also be suspected in children with multiple, prolonged, or severe episodes of croup. Diagnosis is made by direct visualization of the subglottic space with bronchoscopy and maneuvers to size the airway. Tracheostomy is often required when airway compromise is severe. Surgical intervention is ultimately required to correct the stenosis. Laryngotracheal reconstruction in which a cartilage graft from another source (eg, rib) is used to expand the airway has become the standard procedure for symptomatic subglottic stenosis in children.

Khariwala SS et al: Laryngotracheal consequences of pediatric cardiac surgery. Arch Otolaryngol Head Neck Surg 2005;131:336 [PMID: 15837903].

O'Connor, Tony E et al: Laryngotracheoplasty to avoid tracheostomy in neonatal and infant subglottic stenosis. Otolaryngology—Head and Neck Surgery 2011;144(3):435 [PMID: 21493209].

Quesnel, Alicia M et al: Minimally invasive endoscopic management of subglottic stenosis in children: Success and failure. International Journal of Pediatric Otorhinolaryngology 2011;75(5):652 [PMID: 21377219].

Schroeder JW et al: Congenital laryngeal stenosis. Otolaryngol Clin North Am 2008;41(5):865–875, viii [PMID: 18775338].

RECURRENT RESPIRATORY PAPILLOMATOSIS

Papillomas of the larynx are benign, warty growths that are difficult to treat and are the most common laryngeal neoplasm in children. Human papillomaviruses (HPV) 6, 11, and 16 have been implicated as causative agents. A substantial percentage of mothers of patients with laryngeal papillomas have a history of genital condylomas at the time of delivery, so the virus may be acquired during passage through an infected birth canal.

The age at onset is usually 2–4 years, but juvenile-onset recurrent respiratory papillomatosis is well documented. A younger age of onset may be a worse prognostic indicator. Patients usually develop hoarseness, voice changes, croupy cough, or stridor that can lead to life-threatening airway obstruction. Diagnosis is by direct laryngoscopy. The larynx was involved at the time of diagnosis in more than 95% of patients, most of whom had only one site involved.

Prevention with a newly developed human papillomavirus vaccine for woman may be the most effect strategy. However, once disease has occurred treatment is directed toward relieving airway obstruction, usually by surgical removal of the lesions. Tracheostomy is necessary when life-threatening obstruction or respiratory arrest occurs. Various surgical procedures (laser, cup forceps, or cryosurgery) have been used to remove papillomas, but recurrences are the rule, and frequent reoperation may be needed. The lesions occasionally spread down the trachea and bronchi, making surgical removal more difficult. Treatment also includes intralesional cidofovir. Interferon therapy remains controversial. Fortunately, spontaneous remissions do occur, usually by puberty, so that the goal of therapy is to maintain an adequate airway until remission occurs.

CONGENITAL CAUSES OF INTRATHORACIC AIRWAY OBSTRUCTION

MALACIA OF AIRWAYS

ESSENTIALS OF DIAGNOSIS & TYPICAL FEATURES

- Chronic monophonic wheeze with or without a barking cough.
- Respiratory symptoms do not respond to bronchodilators.

General Considerations

Tracheomalacia or bronchomalacia exists when the cartilaginous framework of the airway is inadequate to maintain airway patency. Because the cartilage of the infant airway is normally soft, all infants may have some degree of dynamic collapse of the central airway when pressure outside the airway exceeds intraluminal pressure. In tracheomalacia, whether congenital or acquired, dynamic collapse leads to airway obstruction. Congenital tracheomalacia and bronchomalacia may also be associated with developmental abnormalities such as tracheoesophageal fistula, vascular ring, or cardiac anomalies causing extrinsic airway compression during development. Tracheomalacia is also associated with various syndromes. Congenital tracheomalacia may be localized to part of the trachea, but can also involve the entire trachea as well as the remainder of the conducting airways. In severe cases, cartilage in the involved area may be missing or underdeveloped. Acquired tracheomalacia has been associated with long-term ventilation of premature newborns, tracheoesophageal fistula, severe tracheobronchitis, and airway compression due to anomalies of the great vessels and congenital heart disease, tumors, abscess or infection, and cysts.

Clinical Findings

Coarse wheezing, cough, stridor, recurrent illnesses, recurrent wheezing that does not respond to bronchodilators, or radiographic changes are common findings. Symptoms classically present insidiously over the first few months of life and can increase with agitation, excitement, activity, or upper respiratory tract infections. Diagnosis can be made by airway fluoroscopy or bronchoscopy. Barium swallow may be indicated to rule out coexisting conditions such as vascular compression.

Treatment

Conservative treatment is usually indicated for the isolated condition, which generally improves over time with growth. Coexisting lesions such as tracheoesophageal fistulas and vascular rings need primary repair. In severe cases of tracheomalacia, intubation or tracheostomy may be necessary. Unfortunately, tracheostomy alone is seldom satisfactory because airway collapse continues to exist below the tip of the artificial airway. Positive pressure ventilation may be required to stent the collapsing airway. Surgical approaches to the problem (tracheopexy or aortopexy) may be considered as alternatives prior to or in an effort to wean off of ventilatory support.

Carden KA et al: Tracheomalacia and tracheobronchomalacia in children and adults: An in-depth review. Chest 2005;127:984 [PMID: 15764786].

Masters IB, Chang AB: Interventions for primary (intrinsic) tracheomalacia in children. Cochrane Database Syst Rev 2005;(4):CD005304 [PMID: 16235399].

VASCULAR RINGS & SLINGS

General Considerations

The most common vascular anomaly to compress the trachea or esophagus is a vascular ring. A vascular ring can be formed by a double aortic arch or a right aortic arch with left ligamentum arteriosum or a patent ductus arteriosus. The pulmonary sling is created when the left pulmonary artery branches off the right pulmonary artery. Other common vascular anomalies include an anomalous innominate artery, a left carotid artery, and an aberrant right subclavian artery. All but the right subclavian artery can cause tracheal compression. The pulmonary sling may compress the trachea but can also compress the right upper lobe bronchus or the right mainstem takeoff. Of note, a pulmonary sling is associated with long segment tracheal stenosis 50% of the time.

Laboratory Findings and Imaging Studies

Symptoms of chronic airway obstruction (stridor, coarse wheezing, and croupy cough) are often worse in the supine position. Respiratory compromise is most severe with double aortic arch and may lead to apnea, respiratory arrest, or even death. Esophageal compression, present in all but anomalous innominate or carotid artery, may result in feeding difficulties, including dysphagia and vomiting. Barium swallow showing esophageal compression is the mainstay of diagnosis. Chest radiographs and echocardiograms may miss abnormalities. Anatomy can be further defined by angiography, chest CT with contrast, MRI or magnetic resonance angiography, or bronchoscopy.

Treatment

Patients with significant symptoms require surgical correction, especially those with double aortic arch. Patients usually improve following correction but may have persistent but milder symptoms of airway obstruction due to associated tracheomalacia.

Humphrey C et al: Decade of experience with vascular rings at a single institution. Pediatrics 2006;117:e903 [PMID: 16585275].
McLaren CA, Elliott MJ, Roebuck DJ: Vascular compression of the airway in children. Paediatr Respir Rev 2008;9(2):85–94 [PMID: 18513668].

BRONCHOGENIC CYSTS

General Considerations

Bronchogenic cysts generally occur in the middle mediastinum (see later section on Mediastinal Masses) near the carina and adjacent to the major bronchi but can be found elsewhere in the lung. They range in size from 2 to 10 cm. Cyst walls are thin and may contain air, pus, mucus, or blood. Cysts develop from abnormal lung budding of the primitive foregut. They can be seen in conjunction with other congenital pulmonary malformations such as pulmonary sequestration or lobar emphysema.

Clinical Findings

Bronchogenic cysts can present acutely with respiratory distress in early childhood due to airway compression or with symptoms of infection. Other patients present with chronic symptoms such as chronic wheezing, cough, intermittent tachypnea, recurrent pneumonia, or recurrent stridor, depending on the location and size of the cysts and the degree of airway compression. Still other patients remain asymptomatic until adulthood. However, all asymptomatic cysts will eventually become symptomatic with chest pain being the most common presenting complaint. The physical examination is often normal. Positive examination findings might include tracheal deviation from the midline and decreased breath sounds; percussion over involved lobes may be hyperresonant due to air trapping.

The choice of diagnostic studies for bronchogenic cysts is controversial. Chest radiographs can show air trapping and hyperinflation of the affected lobes or may show a spherical lesion with or without an air-fluid level. However, smaller lesions may not be seen on chest radiographs. CT scan is the preferred imaging study and can differentiate solid versus cystic mediastinal masses and define the cyst's relationship to the airways and the rest of the lung. A barium swallow can help determine whether the lesion communicates with the gastrointestinal tract. MRI and ultrasound are other imaging modalities used.

Treatment

Treatment is surgical resection. Postoperatively, vigorous pulmonary physiotherapy is required to prevent complications (atelectasis or infection of the lung distal to the site of resection of the cyst).

Eber E: Antenatal diagnosis of congenital thoracic malformations: Early surgery, late surgery, or no surgery? Semin Respir Crit Care Med 2007;28(3)355–366.
McAdams HP et al: Bronchogenic cyst: Imaging features with clinical and histopathologic correlation. Radiology 2000;217:441 [PMID: 11058643].

ACQUIRED CAUSES OF INTRATHORACIC AIRWAY OBSTRUCTION

FOREIGN BODY ASPIRATION

ESSENTIALS OF DIAGNOSIS & TYPICAL FEATURES

- Sudden onset of coughing, wheezing, or respiratory distress.
- Asymmetrical physical findings of decreased breath sounds or localized wheezing.
- Asymmetrical radiographic findings, especially with forced expiratory view.

Clinical Findings

A. Symptoms and Signs

Respiratory symptoms and signs vary depending on the site of obstruction and the duration following the acute episode. For example, a large or central airway obstruction may cause marked distress. The acute cough or wheezing caused by a foreign body in the lower respiratory tract may diminish over time only to recur later as chronic cough or persistent wheezing, monophonic wheezing, asymmetrical breath sounds on chest examination, or recurrent pneumonia in one location. Foreign body aspiration should be suspected in children with chronic cough, persistent wheezing, or recurrent pneumonia. Long-standing foreign bodies may lead to bronchiectasis or lung abscess. Hearing asymmetrical breath sounds or localized wheezing also suggests a foreign body.

B. Laboratory Findings and Imaging Studies

Inspiratory and forced expiratory (obtained by manually compressing the abdomen during expiration) chest radiographs should be obtained if foreign body aspiration is suspected. Chest radiographs may be normal up to 25% of the time. If abnormal, the initial inspiratory view may show localized hyperinflation due to the ball-valve effect of the foreign body, causing distal air trapping or aeration within an area of atelectasis. A positive forced expiratory study shows a mediastinal shift away from the affected side. If airway obstruction is complete, atelectasis and related volume loss will be the major radiologic findings. Lateral decubitus views may be helpful if the child is too young to cooperate. Chest fluoroscopy is an alternative approach for detecting air trapping and mediastinal shift.

Treatment

When a foreign body is highly suspected, a normal chest radiograph should not rule out the possibility of an airway foreign body. If clinical suspicion persists based on two of three findings—history of possible aspiration, focal abnormal lung examination, or an abnormal chest radiograph—then a bronchoscopy is indicated. Rigid bronchoscopy under general anesthesia is recommended. Flexible bronchoscopy may be helpful for follow-up evaluations (after the foreign object has been removed).

Children with suspected acute foreign body aspiration should be admitted to the hospital for evaluation and treatment. Chest postural drainage is no longer recommended because the foreign body may become dislodged and obstruct a major central airway. Bronchoscopy should not be delayed in children with respiratory distress but should be performed as soon as the diagnosis is made—even in children with more chronic symptoms. Following the removal of the foreign body, β-adrenergic nebulization treatments followed by chest physiotherapy are recommended to help clear related mucus or treat bronchospasm. Failure to identify a foreign body in the lower respiratory tract can result in bronchiectasis or lung abscess. This risk justifies an aggressive approach to suspected foreign bodies in suspicious cases.

Chiu CY et al: Factors predicting early diagnosis of foreign body aspiration in children. Pediatr Emerg Care 2005;21:161 [PMID: 15744193].

Cohen S, Avital A, Godfrey S, Gross M, Kerem E, Springer C: Suspected foreign body inhalation in children: What are the indications for bronchoscopy? J Pediatr 2009 Aug;155(2):276–280 [Epub 2009 May 15] [PMID: 19446848].

DISORDERS OF MUCOCILIARY CLEARANCE

Mucociliary clearance is the primary defense mechanism for the lung. Inhaled particles including microbial pathogens are also entrapped in mucus on the airway surface, then cleared by the coordinated action of cilia. The volume and composition of airway surface liquid influence the efficiency of ciliary function and mucus clearance. Mucous that cannot be cleared normally can obstruct the airways. If mucociliary clearance is not normal, bacteria that are not cleared can lead to a vicious cycle of infection and inflammation and increased mucous production. The two main genetic diseases of mucociliary clearance involve disorders of ion transport (cystic fibrosis, CF) and disorders in ciliary function (primary ciliary dyskinesia, PCD).

CYSTIC FIBROSIS

ESSENTIALS OF DIAGNOSIS & TYPICAL FEATURES

- Greasy, bulky, malodorous stools; failure to thrive.
- Recurrent respiratory infections.
- Digital clubbing on examination.
- Bronchiectasis on chest imaging.
- Sweat chloride > 60 mmol/L.

General Considerations

CF, an autosomal recessive disease, results in a syndrome of chronic sinopulmonary infections, malabsorption, and nutritional abnormalities. It is one of the most common lethal genetic diseases in the United States, with an incidence of approximately 1:3000 among Caucasians and 1:9200 in the U.S. Hispanic population. Although abnormalities occur in the hepatic, gastrointestinal, and male reproductive systems, lung disease is the major cause of morbidity and mortality. Most individuals with CF develop obstructive lung disease associated with chronic infection that leads to progressive loss of pulmonary function.

The cause of CF is a defect in a single gene on chromosome 7 that encodes an epithelial chloride channel called the CF transmembrane conductance regulator (CFTR) protein. The most common mutation is ΔF508, although approximately 1500 other disease-causing mutations in the CF gene have been identified. Gene mutations lead to defects or deficiencies in CFTR, causing problems in salt and water movement across cell membranes, resulting in abnormally thick secretions in various organ systems and critically altering host defense in the lung.

Clinical Findings

A. Symptoms and Signs

All states in the US and many other countries now perform newborn screening for CF by measuring immunoreactive trypsin (IRT), a pancreatic enzyme, in blood with or without concurrent DNA testing. Most infants with CF have elevated IRT in the newborn period, although false negative results are possible. In newborns with positive newborn screen, the diagnosis of CF must be confirmed by sweat testing, mutation analysis, or both (http://www.cff.org/AboutCF/Testing/NewbornScreening/).

Approximately 15% of newborns with CF present at birth with meconium ileus, a severe intestinal obstruction resulting from inspissation of tenacious meconium in the terminal ileum. Meconium ileus is virtually diagnostic of CF, so the infant should be treated presumptively as having CF until a sweat test or genotyping can be obtained.

During infancy and beyond, a common presentation of CF is failure to thrive due to malabsorption from exocrine pancreatic insufficiency. These children fail to gain weight despite good appetite and typically have frequent, bulky, foul-smelling, oily stools. These symptoms are the result of severe exocrine pancreatic insufficiency, the failure of the pancreas to produce sufficient digestive enzymes to allow breakdown and absorption of fats and protein. Pancreatic insufficiency occurs in more than 85% of persons with CF. (Chapter 22 describes gastrointestinal and hepatobiliary manifestations of CF; see also Table 22–9 there.) Infants with undiagnosed CF may also present with hypoproteinemia with or without edema, anemia, and deficiency of the fat-soluble vitamins A, D, E, and K, because of ongoing steatorrhea.

From a respiratory standpoint, clinical manifestations include productive cough, wheezing, recurrent pneumonias, progressive obstructive airways disease, exercise intolerance, dyspnea, and hemoptysis. Chronic airway infection with bacteria, including *S aureus* and *H influenzae,* often begins in the first few months of life, even in asymptomatic infants. Eventually, *Pseudomonas aeruginosa* becomes the predominant pathogen. Chronic infection with the mucoid phenotype of *P aeruginosa* is associated with a more rapid decline in pulmonary function. Chronic infection leads to airflow obstruction and progressive airway and lung destruction resulting in bronchiectasis. Methicillin-resistant *S aureus* is increasingly prevalent in CF and may worsen lung disease.

An acute change in respiratory signs and symptoms from the subject's baseline is generically termed a pulmonary exacerbation. Clinically, an exacerbation is typically manifested by increased cough and sputum production, decreased exercise tolerance, malaise, and anorexia. These symptoms are usually associated with decreased measures of lung function. Treatment for pulmonary exacerbations generally consists of antibiotics and augmented airway clearance.

CF should also be considered in infants and children who present with severe dehydration and hypochloremic alkalosis. Other findings that should prompt a diagnostic evaluation for CF include unexplained bronchiectasis, rectal prolapse, nasal polyps, chronic sinusitis, and unexplained pancreatitis or cirrhosis.

B. Laboratory Findings and Imaging Studies

The diagnosis of CF is made by a sweat chloride concentration greater than 60 mmol/L in the presence of one or more typical clinical features (chronic sinopulmonary disease, pancreatic insufficiency, salt loss syndromes) or an appropriate family history (sibling or first cousin who has CF). Sweat tests should be performed at a CF Foundation–accredited laboratory. A diagnosis can also be confirmed by genotyping that reveals two disease-causing mutations. Intermediate sweat chloride values of 30–60 may be associated with either mild CFTR mutations or CFTR-related metabolic syndrome (CFRM). Patients with mild CFTR mutations typically have adequate pancreatic exocrine function, but are still at risk for severe lung disease. CFRM patients appear to have even milder disease phenotypes, but the natural history of this condition is still being defined.

Treatment

It is strongly recommended that individuals with CF be followed at a CF Foundation–accredited CF care center (http://www.cff.org).

The cornerstone of gastrointestinal treatment is pancreatic enzyme supplementation combined with a high calorie, high protein, and high fat diet. Persons with CF are required to take pancreatic enzyme capsules immediately prior to each meal and with snacks. Individuals should also take daily multivitamins that contain vitamins A, D, E, and K. Caloric supplements are often added to the patient's diet to optimize growth. Daily salt supplementation also is recommended to prevent hyponatremia, especially during hot weather.

Airway clearance therapy and aggressive antibiotic use form the mainstays of treatment for CF lung disease. Antibiotic therapy appears to be one of the primary reasons for the increased life expectancy of persons with CF. Respiratory treatments typically include recombinant human DNAse (Pulmozyme), inhaled hypertonic saline, and for those with chronic *Pseudomonas* infection, inhaled tobramycin (TOBI) or inhaled aztreonam, and chronic oral azithromycin. These therapies have been shown to maintain lung function and reduce the need for hospitalizations and intravenous antibiotics. Early detection of *P aeruginosa* and treatment with inhaled tobramycin can often eradicate the bacteria and delay chronic infection. Bronchodilators and anti-inflammatory therapies are also frequently used. Recent clinical trials using protein-rescue therapies to improve CFTR function have shown encouraging results, and may lead to novel pharmaceutical approaches to treatment.

Prognosis

A few decades ago, CF was fatal in early childhood. Now the median life expectancy is around 35 years of age. The rate of lung disease progression usually determines survival. Lung transplantation may be performed in those with end-stage lung disease. In addition, new treatments, including gene therapy trials and agents that modulate CFTR protein function, are being developed based on improved understanding of the disease at the cellular and molecular levels.

Cohen-Cymberknow M et al: Managing cystic fibrosis: Strategies that increase life expectancy and improve quality of life. Am J Respir Crit Care Med 2011;183(11):1463–1471.

Farrell PM et al: Guidelines for diagnosis of cystic fibrosis in newborns through older adults: Cystic Fibrosis Foundation consensus report. J Pediatr 2008;153:S4–S14.

Mogayzel PJ Jr et al: Update in cystic fibrosis 2010. Am J Respir Crit Care Med 2011;183(12):1620–1624.

PRIMARY CILIARY DYSKINESIA

ESSENTIALS OF DIAGNOSIS & TYPICAL FEATURES

- Chronic bronchitis, sinusitis, and otitis.
- Situs inversus in approximately 50% of cases.
- Unexplained respiratory distress in the newborn period.
- Consistent ultrastructural defect of cilia demonstrated by electron microscopy.

General Considerations

Primary ciliary dyskinesia (PCD), also known as immotile cilia syndrome, is a rare, inherited, usually autosomal recessive disorder with impaired ciliary function leading to progressive sinopulmonary disease. It is believed to occur in approximately 1 in 15,000 births. Half of the patients with PCD have their internal organs reversed (situs abnormalities), and men are usually infertile. The triad of situs inversus totalis, bronchiectasis, and chronic sinusitis is known as Kartagener syndrome.

Clinical Findings

A. Symptoms and Signs

Upper and lower respiratory tract manifestations are cardinal features of PCD. The majority of children with PCD present in the immediate newborn period with respiratory distress (commonly diagnosed as neonatal pneumonia or transient tachypnea of the newborn), suggesting cilia are critical for effective clearance of fetal lung fluid. Upper respiratory tract problems include chronic year-around nasal drainage that may begin in the first weeks of life, chronic sinusitis, and chronic serous otitis media. If myrinotomy tubes are placed, chronic otorrhea often ensues. These children commonly have associated conductive hearing loss with chronic middle ear effusion. Lower respiratory tract features include chronic productive cough, chronic and recurrent bronchitis, and recurrent pneumonia. They are at risk to develop bronchiectasis. Situs inversus totalis, a unique feature in Kartagener triad, occurs in approximately 50% of patients with PCD.

B. Laboratory Findings and Imaging Studies

The diagnosis of PCD currently requires a compatible clinical phenotype and identification of ultrastructural and/or functional defects of the cilia. Examination of ciliary ultrastructure by transmission electron microscopy remains the cornerstone test for PCD. Cilia samples may be obtained from either the upper airways (nasal passage) or lower airways (trachea). Semen collection from older male patients can also be obtained to analyze sperm tails, which have the same ultrastructure as cilia. Several ciliary ultrastructural defects have been described, but the classic primary (genetic) abnormalities are absence or shortening of outer or inner dynein arms, absence of radial spokes, or loss of the central pair of microtubules with transposition of a peripheral doublet to the center. Significant expertise is required to produce high-quality transmission electron micrographs of cilia, and to distinguish primary (genetic) defects from secondary (acquired) defects in ciliary ultrastructure. Measurement of nasal nitric oxide has proven to be a useful screening and adjunctive diagnostic test for PCD in children ages 5 and older based on very low levels in PCD. Genetic testing is emerging for PCD and demonstrates extensive genetic heterogeneity. Some genes and gene mutations involved in PCD have been defined. Approximately one-third of PCD cases have identifiable gene mutations in one of six different genes.

Treatment

At present, no specific therapies are available to correct the ciliary dysfunction in PCD. Treatment is not evidence based and recommendations are largely extrapolated from CF and other suppurative lung diseases. Respiratory management includes routine pulmonary monitoring (lung function testing, respiratory cultures, chest imaging), airway clearance by combinations of physiotherapy and physical exercise, and aggressive treatment of upper and lower airways infections.

Prognosis

The progression of lung disease in PCD is quite variable and for most affected individuals is less severe than in CF. Importantly, though, persons with PCD are at risk for chronic lung disease with bronchiectasis. With monitoring and aggressive treatment during times of illness, most individuals with PCD should experience a normal or near-normal life span.

A national consortium, the "Genetic Disorders of Mucociliary Clearance Consortium," a member of the Rare Disease Clinical Research Network (http://rarediseasesnetwork.epi.usf.edu/gdmcc/index.htm), has been established to improve diagnosis and treatment of children with suspected or confirmed PCD.

Barbato A et al: Primary ciliary dyskinesia: A consensus statement of diagnostic and treatment approaches in children. Eur Respir J 2009;34:1264–1276 [PMID: 19948909].

Leigh MW, Zariwala MA, Knowles MR: Primary ciliary dyskinesia: Improving the diagnostic approach. Curr Opin Pediatr 2009;21:320–325 [PMID: 19300264].

BRONCHIOLITIS OBLITERANS

Bronchiolitis obliterans is a rare chronic obstructive lung disease characterized by complete obliteration of the small airways following a severe insult. The most common form in children is postinfectious, following a lower airway tract infection with adenovirus, although influenza, rubeola, *Bordetella,* and *Mycoplasma* are also implicated. Other causes include connective tissue diseases, chronic aspiration, Stevens-Johnson syndrome, posttransplantation (lung or bone marrow) and inhalational injury. Many cases of bronchiolitis obliterans are idiopathic. Adenovirus-induced bronchiolitis obliterans occurs more frequently in the Native American population. Mechanical ventilation for severe adenoviral respiratory infection is a strong risk factor for development of bronchiolitis obliterans.

Clinical Findings

A. Symptoms and Signs

Persons with bronchiolitis obliterans usually experience dyspnea, coughing, and exercise intolerance. This diagnosis should be considered in children with persistent cough, wheezing, crackles, or hypoxemia persisting longer than 60 days following a lower respiratory tract infection.

B. Laboratory Findings and Imaging Studies

Chest radiograph abnormalities include evidence of heterogeneous air trapping and airway wall thickening. Traction bronchiectasis can occur as the disease progresses. Ventilation-perfusion scans show a pattern of ventilation and perfusion mismatch. Pulmonary angiograms reveal decreased vasculature in involved lung, and bronchograms show marked pruning of the bronchial tree. Classic findings on chest high-resolution CT include a mosaic perfusion pattern, vascular attenuation, and central bronchiectasis. This finding along with pulmonary function testing showing airway obstruction unresponsive to bronchodilators may be diagnostic in some patients with the appropriate clinical history.

Differential Diagnosis

Poorly treated asthma, CF, and BPD must be considered in children with persistent airway obstruction. A trial of medications (including bronchodilators and corticosteroids) may help to determine the reversibility of the process when the primary differential is between asthma and bronchiolitis obliterans. Others without classic findings on CT scan and lung function testing may require a lung biopsy.

Complications

Sequelae of bronchiolitis obliterans include persistent airway obstruction, recurrent wheezing, bronchiectasis, chronic atelectasis, recurrent pneumonia, and unilateral hyperlucent lung syndrome.

Treatment

Supportive care including supplemental oxygen for hypoxemia, routine vaccination, avoidance of environmental irritant exposure, exercise, and nutritional support should be provided. Ongoing airway damage due to problems such as aspiration should be prevented. Inhaled bronchodilators may reverse airway obstruction if the disease has a reactive component. Corticosteroids (inhaled, daily, or pulse dosing) may help reverse the obstruction or prevent ongoing damage. Antibiotics should be used as indicated for pneumonia. Azithromycin has been shown to have therapeutic properties for airway injury in CF, diffuse panbronchiolitis, and in bronchiolitis obliterans syndrome (BOS) after lung transplantation, providing some rationale for a trial of this medication for bronchiolitis obliterans. Lung transplant may be an option for patients with severe, progressive disease.

Prognosis

Prognosis depends in part on the underlying cause as well as the age of onset. Postinfectious bronchiolitis obliterans tends to be nonprogressive with low mortality and the possibility of slow improvement with time. Conversely, posttransplantation or Stevens-Johnson syndrome–related bronchiolitis obliterans may have a rapidly progressive course leading to death or need for lung transplantation.

Fischer, GB et al: Post infectious bronchiolitis obliterans in children. Paediatric Respiratory Reviews 2010;11:233–239.

Moonnumakal SP et al: Bronchiolitis obliterans in children. Curr Opin Pediatr 2008;20(3):272–278 [PMID: 18475095].

CONGENITAL MALFORMATIONS OF THE LUNG PARENCHYMA

What follows is a brief description of selected congenital pulmonary malformations.

PULMONARY AGENESIS & HYPOPLASIA

In unilateral pulmonary agenesis (complete absence of one lung), the trachea continues into a main bronchus and often has complete tracheal rings. The left lung is affected more often than the right. With compensatory postnatal growth, the remaining lung often herniates into the contralateral chest. Chest radiographs show a mediastinal shift toward the affected side, and vertebral abnormalities may be present. Absent or incomplete lung development may be associated with other congenital abnormalities, such as absence of one or both kidneys or fusion of ribs, and the outcome is primarily related to the severity of associated lesions. About 50% of patients survive; the mortality rate is higher with agenesis of the right lung than of the left lung. This difference is probably not related to the higher incidence of associated anomalies but rather to a greater shift in the mediastinum that leads to tracheal compression and distortion of vascular structures.

Pulmonary hypoplasia is incomplete development of one or both lungs, characterized by a reduction in alveolar number and a reduction in airway branches. Pulmonary hypoplasia is present in up to 10%–15% of perinatal autopsies. The hypoplasia can be a result of an intrathoracic mass, resulting in lack of space for the lungs to grow; decreased size of the thorax; decreased fetal breathing movements; decreased blood flow to the lungs; or possibly a primary mesodermal defect affecting multiple organ systems. Congenital diaphragmatic hernia is the most common cause, with an incidence of 1:2200 births. Other causes include extralobar sequestration, diaphragmatic eventration or hypoplasia, thoracic neuroblastoma, fetal hydrops, and fetal hydrochylothorax. Chest cage abnormalities, diaphragmatic elevation, oligohydramnios, chromosomal abnormalities, severe musculoskeletal disorders, and cardiac lesions may also result in hypoplastic lungs. Postnatal factors may play important roles. For example, infants with advanced BPD can have pulmonary hypoplasia.

Clinical Findings

A. Symptoms and Signs

The clinical presentation is highly variable and is related to the severity of hypoplasia as well as associated abnormalities. Lung hypoplasia is often associated with pneumothorax in newborns. Some newborns present with perinatal stress, severe acute respiratory distress, and persistent pulmonary hypertension of the newborn secondary to primary pulmonary hypoplasia (without associated anomalies). Children with lesser degrees of hypoplasia may present with chronic cough, tachypnea, wheezing, and recurrent pneumonia.

B. Laboratory Findings and Imaging Studies

Chest radiographic findings include variable degrees of volume loss in a small hemithorax with mediastinal shift. Pulmonary agenesis should be suspected if tracheal deviation is evident on the chest radiograph. The chest CT scan is the optimal diagnostic imaging procedure if the chest radiograph is not definitive. Ventilation-perfusion scans, angiography, and bronchoscopy are often helpful in the evaluation, demonstrating decreased pulmonary vascularity or premature blunting of airways associated with the maldeveloped lung tissue. The degree of respiratory impairment is defined by analysis of arterial blood gases.

Treatment & Prognosis

Treatment is supportive. The outcome is determined by the severity of underlying medical problems, the extent of the hypoplasia, and the degree of pulmonary hypertension.

Berrocal T et al: Congenital anomalies of the tracheobronchial tree, lung and mediastinum: Embryology, radiology, and pathology. Radiographics 2004:24(1):e17 [PMID: 14610245].

Chinoy MR: Pulmonary hypoplasia and congenital diaphragmatic hernia: Advances in the pathogenetics and regulation of lung development. J Surg Res 2002;106:209 [PMID: 12127828].

Laudy JA, Wladimiroff JW: The fetal lung 2: Pulmonary hypoplasia. Ultrasound Obstet Gynecol 2000;16:482 [PMID: 11169336].

Winn HN et al: Neonatal pulmonary hypoplasia and perinatal mortality in patients with midtrimester rupture of amniotic membranes—A critical analysis. Am J Obstet Gynecol 2000;182:1638 [PMID: 10871491].

PULMONARY SEQUESTRATION

Pulmonary sequestration is nonfunctional pulmonary tissue that does not communicate with the tracheobronchial tree and receives its blood supply from one or more anomalous systemic arteries. This abnormality originates during the embryonic period of lung development. It is classified as either extralobar or intralobar. Extralobar sequestration is a mass of pulmonary parenchyma anatomically separate from the normal lung, with a distinct pleural investment. Its blood supply derives from the systemic circulation (more typical), from pulmonary vessels, or from both. Rarely, it communicates with the esophagus or stomach. Pathologically, extralobar sequestration appears as a solitary thoracic lesion near the diaphragm. Abdominal sites are rare. Size varies from 0.5 to 12 cm. The left side is involved in more than 90% of cases. In contrast to intralobar sequestrations, venous drainage is usually through the systemic or portal venous system.

Histologic findings include uniformly dilated bronchioles, alveolar ducts, and alveoli. Occasionally the bronchial structure appears normal; however, often the cartilage in the wall is deficient, or no cartilage-containing structures can be found. Lymphangiectasia is sometimes found within the lesion. Extralobar sequestration can be associated with other anomalies, including bronchogenic cysts, heart defects, and diaphragmatic hernia, the latter occurring in over half of cases.

Intralobar sequestration is an isolated segment of lung within the normal pleural investment that often receives blood from one or more arteries arising from the aorta or its branches. Intralobar sequestration is usually found within the lower lobes (98%), two-thirds are found on the left side, and it is rarely associated with other congenital anomalies (< 2% vs 50% with extralobar sequestration). It rarely presents in the newborn period (unlike extralobar sequestration). Some researchers have hypothesized that intralobar sequestration is an acquired lesion secondary to chronic infection. Clinical presentation includes chronic cough, wheezing, or recurrent pneumonias. Rarely, patients with intralobar sequestration can present with hemoptysis. Diagnosis is often made by angiography, which shows large systemic arteries perfusing the lesion. Recently spiral CT scans with contrast or magnetic resonance angiography have proved useful in identifying anomalous systemic arterial supply to the lung. Treatment is usually by surgical resection.

Alton H: Pulmonary vascular imaging. Paediatr Respir Rev 2001;2:227 [PMID: 12052324].

Conran RM, Stocker JT: Extralobar sequestration with frequently associated congenital cystic adenomatoid malformation, type 2: Report of 50 cases. Pediatr Dev Pathol 1999;2:454 [PMID: 10441623].

Eber E: Antenatal diagnosis of congenital thoracic malformations: Early surgery, late surgery, or no surgery? Semin Respir Crit Care Med 2007;28:355 [PMID: 17562505].

Halkic N et al: Pulmonary sequestration: A review of 26 cases. Eur J Cardiothorac Surg 1998;14:127 [PMID: 9754996].

Salmons S: Pulmonary sequestration. Neonatal Netw 2000;19:27 [PMID: 11949021].

Zylak CJ et al: Developmental lung anomalies in the adult: Radiologic-pathologic correlation. Radiographics 2002;22(Spec No):S25 [PMID: 12376599].

CONGENITAL LOBAR EMPHYSEMA

Patients with congenital lobar emphysema—also known as infantile lobar emphysema, congenital localized emphysema, unilobar obstructive emphysema, congenital hypertrophic lobar emphysema, or congenital lobar overinflation—present most commonly with severe neonatal respiratory distress or progressive respiratory impairment during the first year of life. Rarely the mild or intermittent nature of the symptoms in older children or young adults results in delayed diagnosis. Most patients are white males. Although the cause of congenital lobar emphysema is not well understood, some lesions show bronchial cartilaginous dysplasia due to abnormal orientation or distribution of the bronchial cartilage. This leads to expiratory collapse, producing obstruction and the symptoms outlined in the following discussion.

Clinical Findings

A. Symptoms and Signs

Clinical features include respiratory distress, tachypnea, cyanosis, wheezing, retractions, and cough. Breath sounds are reduced on the affected side, perhaps with hyperresonance to percussion, mediastinal displacement, and bulging of the chest wall on the affected side.

B. Imaging Studies

Radiologic findings include overdistention of the affected lobe (usually an upper or middle lobe; > 99%), with wide separation of bronchovascular markings, collapse of adjacent lung, shift of the mediastinum away from the affected side, and a depressed diaphragm on the affected side. The radiographic diagnosis may be confusing in the newborn because of retention of alveolar fluid in the affected lobe causing the appearance of a homogeneous density. Other diagnostic studies include chest radiograph with fluoroscopy, ventilation-perfusion study, and chest CT scan followed by bronchoscopy, angiography, and exploratory thoracotomy.

Differential Diagnosis

The differential diagnosis of congenital lobar emphysema includes pneumothorax, pneumatocele, atelectasis with compensatory hyperinflation, diaphragmatic hernia, and congenital cystic adenomatoid malformation. The most common site of involvement is the left upper lobe (42%) or right middle lobe (35%). Evaluation must differentiate regional obstructive emphysema from lobar hyperinflation secondary to an uncomplicated ball-valve mechanism due to extrinsic compression from a mass (ie, bronchogenic cyst, tumor, lymphadenopathy, foreign body, pseudotumor or plasma cell granuloma, or vascular compression) or intrinsic obstruction from a mucus plug due to infection and inflammation from various causes.

Treatment

When respiratory distress is marked, a segmental or complete lobectomy is usually required. Less symptomatic older children may do equally well with or without lobectomy.

Babu R et al: Prenatal sonographic features of congenital lobar emphysema. Fetal Diagn Ther 2001;16:200 [PMID: 11399878].

Horak E et al: Congenital cystic lung disease: Diagnostic and therapeutic considerations. Clin Pediatr 2003;42:251 [PMID: 12739924].

Mandelbaum I et al: Congenital lobar obstructive emphysema: Report of eight cases and literature review. Ann Surg 1965;162:1075 [PMID: 5845589].

CONGENITAL PULMONARY AIRWAY (CYSTIC ADENOMATOID) MALFORMATION

Patients with congenital pulmonary airway malformation CPAM (previously known as congenital cystic adenomatoid malformations), which are unilateral, hamartomatous lesions, generally present with marked respiratory distress within the first days of life. This disorder accounts for 95% of cases of congenital cystic lung disease.

Right and left lungs are involved with equal frequency. These lesions originate during the first 4–6 weeks of gestation during the embryonic period of lung development. They appear as glandlike, space-occupying masses or have an increase in terminal respiratory structures, forming intercommunicating cysts of various sizes, lined by cuboidal or ciliated pseudostratified columnar epithelium. The lesions may have polypoid formations of mucosa, with focally increased elastic tissue in the cyst wall beneath the bronchial type of epithelium. Air passages appear malformed and tend to lack cartilage.

There are five types of such malformations.

Type 0, also known as acinar dysplasia or agenesis istracheal or bronchial in origin, is rare and incompatible with life. The lungs are small, firm and microscopically are made up entirely of irregular bronchial type structures.

Type 1, a large cyst lesion (bronchial or bronchiolar origin), is most common (50%–65%) and consists of single or multiple large cysts (> 2 cm in diameter) with features of mature lung tissue, including a pseudostratified epithelium. Type 1 is amenable to surgical resection. A mediastinal shift is evident on examination or chest radiograph in 80% of patients and can mimic infantile lobar emphysema. Approximately 75% of type 1 lesions are on the right side. A survival rate of 90% is generally reported. There are some reports of bronchioloalveolar carcinoma in patients with type 1 CPAM although this does not necessitate urgent resection.

Type 2 lesions, small cyst lesions (bronchiolar origin) and (10%–40% of cases), consist of multiple small cysts (< 2 cm) resembling dilated simple bronchioles and are often (60%) associated with other anomalies, especially renal agenesis or dysgenesis, cardiac malformations, extralobar sequestration and intestinal atresia. Approximately 60% of type 2 lesions are on the left side. Mediastinal shift is evident less often (10%) than in type 1, and the survival rate is worse (40%). Microscopically the lesion is composed of dilated bronchioles lined by cuboidal to low columnar epithelium and separated by alveolar duct-like structures.

Type 3 lesions, adenomatoid lesion (bronchiolar/alveolar duct origin) and (5%–10% of cases), consist of small cysts (< 0.5 cm). These are the "classic" CPAM (or CCAM). They appear as bulky, firm masses with mediastinal shift and carry the risk of hydrops from mass shift resulting in caval obstruction and cardiac compression (80% of cases). The lesion will often involve the entire lobe and microscopically random bronchiolar/alveolar duct-like structures are seen. There is a striking absence of any small, medium, or large pulmonary arteries within the lesion. Often the adjacent or uninvolved lung is hypoplastic. The reported survival rate is 50%.

Type 4 lesions, "unlined" cyst (distal acinar origin) and (10%–15% of cases), appear to be a hamartomatous malformation of the distal acinus. The cysts are large thin walled and found at the periphery of the lung. The cysts are lined by flattened epithelial (type I) cells.

Clinical Findings

A. Symptoms and Signs

Clinically, respiratory distress is noted soon after birth. Expansion of the cysts occurs with the onset of breathing and produces compression of normal lung areas with mediastinal herniation. Breath sounds are decreased. With type 3 lesions, dullness to percussion may be present. Older patients can present with a spontaneous pneumothorax or with pneumonia-like symptoms. Recently more patients are diagnosed with these lesions on prenatal ultrasound.

B. Laboratory Findings and Imaging Studies

With type 1 lesions, chest radiographs show an intrapulmonary mass of soft tissue density with scattered radiolucent areas of varying sizes and shapes, usually with a mediastinal shift and pulmonary herniation. Placement of a radiopaque feeding tube into the stomach helps in the differentiation from diaphragmatic hernia. Type 2 lesions appear similar except that the cysts are smaller. Type 3 lesions may appear as a solid homogeneous mass filling the hemithorax and causing a marked mediastinal shift. Type 4 lesions are large air-filled cysts localized to one lobe. Differentiation from sequestration is not difficult because congenital CPAM have no systemic blood supply.

Treatment

In cases of prenatal diagnosis, the treatment of these lesions is variable and does not need antenatal intervention. Up to 6%–10% of these have regressed spontaneously and thus they need to be followed serially, prenatally. Attention must be paid to the development of hydrops as a complication of these lesions. Postnatal treatment of types 1 and 3 lesions involves surgical removal of the affected lobe. Resection is often indicated because of the risk of infection and air trapping, since the malformation communicates with the tracheobronchial tree but mucous clearance is compromised. Because type 2 lesions are often associated with other severe anomalies, management may be more complex. Segmental resection is not feasible because smaller cysts may expand after removal of the more obviously affected area. CPAM have been reported to have malignant potential; therefore, expectant management with observation alone should proceed with caution. Recent development of intrauterine surgery for congenital malformations has led to promising results.

Biyyam DR et al: Congenital lung abnormalities: Embryologic features, prenatal diagnosis, and postnatal radiologic-pathologic correlation. Radiographics: A Review Publication of the Radiological Society of North America, Inc. 2010;30(6):1721–1738 [PMID: 21071385].

Calvert JK et al: Outcome of antenatally suspected congenital cystic adenomatoid malformation of the lung: 10 years' experience 1991–2001. Arch Dis Child Fetal Neonatal Ed 2006;91:F26 [PMID: 16131533].

MacSweeney F et al: An assessment of the expanded classification of congenital cystic adenomatoid malformations and their relationship to malignant transformation. Am J Surg Pathol 2003;27:1139 [PMID: 12883247].

Stocker JT: Congenital pulmonary airway malformation: A new name for and an expanded classification of congenital cystic adenomatoid malformation of the lung. Symposium 24: non-neoplastic lung disease. Histopathology 2002;41(Suppl 2):424–430.

Wilson RD et al: Cystic adenomatoid malformation of the lung: Review of genetics, prenatal diagnosis, and in utero treatment. Am J Med Genet A 2006;140:151 [PMID: 16353256].

ACQUIRED ABNORMALITIES OF THE LUNG PARENCHYMA

BRONCHOPULMONARY DYSPLASIA

ESSENTIALS OF DIAGNOSIS & TYPICAL FEATURES

- Acute respiratory distress in the first week of life.
- Required oxygen therapy or mechanical ventilation, with persistent oxygen requirement at 36 weeks' gestational age or 28 days of life.
- Persistent respiratory abnormalities, including physical signs and radiographic findings.

General Considerations

Broncopulmonary Dysplasia (BPD) remains one of the most significant sequelae of acute respiratory distress in the neonatal intensive care unit, with an incidence of about 30% for infants with a birth weight of less than 1000 g. This disease was first characterized in 1967 when Northway first reported the clinical, radiologic, and pathologic findings in a group of preterm newborns that required prolonged mechanical ventilation and oxygen therapy to treat hyaline membrane disease (HMD). The progression from acute HMD to chronic lung disease was divided into four stages: acute respiratory distress shortly after birth (stage I); clinical and radiographic worsening of the acute lung disease, often due to increased pulmonary blood flow secondary to a patent ductus arteriosus (stage II); and progressive signs of chronic lung disease (stages III and IV).

The pathologic findings and clinical course of BPD in recent years have changed due to a combination of new therapies (artificial surfactants, prenatal glucocorticoids, and protective ventilatory strategies) and increased survival of infants born at earlier gestational ages. Although the incidence of BPD has not changed, the severity of the lung disease has decreased. Pathologically this "new" BPD is a developmental disorder of the lung characterized by decreased surface area for gas exchange, reduced inflammation, and a dysmorphic vascular structure.

Pathogenesis

The precise mechanism that results in the development of BPD is unclear. Current studies indicate that these babies have abnormal lung mechanics due to structural immaturity of the alveolar-capillary network, surfactant deficiency, atelectasis, and pulmonary edema. Furthermore, mechanical ventilation causes barotrauma and supplemental oxygen may lead to toxic oxygen metabolites in a child whose antioxidant defense mechanisms are not sufficiently mature. These ongoing injuries to the lungs lead to a vicious cycle of ventilator and oxygen requirement which results in progressive lung injury. As a result, the lungs of extremely preterm newborns with BPD show simplified histology with fewer alveoli, early inflammation, and hypercellularity followed by healing with fibrosis. Excessive fluid administration, patent ductus arteriosus, pulmonary interstitial emphysema, pneumothorax, infection, pulmonary hypertension, and inflammatory stimuli secondary to lung injury or infection also play important roles in the pathogenesis of the disease.

Clinical Findings

A recent summary of a National Institutes of Health workshop on BPD proposed a definition of the disease that includes oxygen requirement for more than 28 days, a history of positive pressure ventilation or continuous positive airway pressure, and gestational age. The new definition accommodates several key observations regarding the disease, as follows: (1) although most of these children were born preterm and had hyaline membrane disease, full-term newborns with such disorders as meconium aspiration, diaphragmatic hernia, or persistent pulmonary hypertension also can develop BPD; (2) some extremely preterm newborns require minimal ventilator support yet subsequently develop a prolonged oxygen requirement despite the absence of severe acute manifestations of respiratory failure; (3) newborns dying within the first weeks of life can already have the aggressive, fibroproliferative pathologic lesions that resemble BPD; and (4) physiologic abnormalities (increased airway resistance) and biochemical markers of lung injury (altered protease-antiprotease ratios and increased inflammatory cells and mediators), which may be predictive of BPD, are already present in the first week of life.

The clinical course of infants with BPD ranges from a mild increased oxygen requirement that gradually evolves over a few months to more severe disease requiring chronic tracheostomy and mechanical ventilation, often for as long as the first 2 years of life. In general, patients show slow, steady improvements in oxygen or ventilator requirements but can have respiratory exacerbations leading to frequent and prolonged hospitalizations. Clinical management generally includes careful attention to growth, nutrition (the caloric requirements of infants with oxygen dependence and respiratory distress are quite high), metabolic status, developmental and neurologic status, and related problems, along with the various cardiopulmonary abnormalities.

Treatment

A. Medical Therapy

Early use of surfactant therapy with adequate lung recruitment increases the chance for survival without BPD and can decrease the overall mortality and reduce the need for ventilation. Short courses of postnatal glucocorticoid therapy have been helpful in increasing the success of weaning from the ventilator. Longer courses of postnatal glucocorticoids have been linked to an increased incidence of cerebral palsy. Inhaled corticosteroids together with occasional use of β-adrenergic agonists are commonly part of the treatment plan but the overall effect on the course of BPD is not clear.

Salt and water retention secondary to chronic hypoxemia, hypercapnia, or other stimuli may be present. Chronic or intermittent diuretic therapy is commonly used if rales or signs of persistent pulmonary edema are present; clinical studies show acute improvement in lung function with this therapy. Unfortunately, diuretics often have adverse effects, including severe volume contraction, hypokalemia, alkalosis, hyponatremia, and nephrocalcinosis. Potassium and arginine chloride supplements are commonly required.

B. Airway Evaluation

Children with significant stridor, sleep apnea, chronic wheezing, or excessive respiratory distress need diagnostic bronchoscopy to evaluate for structural lesions (eg, subglottic stenosis, vocal cord paralysis, tracheal stenosis, tracheobronchomalacia, bronchial stenosis, or airway granulomas). In addition, the contribution of gastroesophageal reflux and aspiration should be considered in the face of worsening chronic lung disease.

C. Management of Pulmonary Hypertension

Infants with BPD are at risk of developing pulmonary hypertension, and in many of these children even mild hypoxemia can cause significant elevations of pulmonary arterial pressure. To minimize the harmful effects of hypoxemia, the arterial oxygen saturation should be kept above 93% in children with pulmonary hypertension, with care to avoid hyperoxia during retinal vascular development. Electrocardiographic and echocardiographic studies should be performed to monitor for the development of right ventricular hypertrophy. Management of neonatal pulmonary hypertension should involve expert consultation with a pulmonary hypertension specialist. If right ventricular hypertrophy persists or if it develops when it was not previously present, intermittent hypoxemia should be considered and further assessments of oxygenation pursued, especially while the infant sleeps. Cardiac catheterization may be necessary to diagnose unsuspected cardiac or pulmonary lesions and to measure the response of the pulmonary vascular vasodilators such as nitric oxide before chronic therapy is initiated. Infants with a history of intubation can develop obstructive sleep apnea secondary to a high-arched palate or subglottic narrowing. Barium esophagram, esophageal pH probe studies, and bronchoscopy can be used to diagnose gastroesophageal reflux, aspiration, and airway abnormalities that contribute to the underlying pathophysiology. Long-term care should include monitoring for systemic hypertension and the development of left ventricular hypertrophy.

D. Nutrition and Immunizations

Nutritional problems in infants with BPD may be due to increased oxygen consumption, feeding difficulties, gastroesophageal reflux, and chronic hypoxemia. Hypercaloric formulas and gastrostomy tubes are often required to ensure adequate intake while avoiding overhydration. Routine vaccinations including the influenza vaccine are recommended. With the onset of acute wheezing secondary to suspected viral infection, rapid diagnostic testing for RSV infection may facilitate early treatment. Immune prophylaxis of RSV reduces the morbidity of bronchiolitis in infants with BPD.

E. Ventilation

For children with BPD who remain ventilator-dependent, attempts should be made to maintain $PaCO_2$ below 60 mm Hg—even when pH is normal—because of the potential adverse effects of hypercapnia on salt and water retention, cardiac function, and perhaps pulmonary vascular tone. Changes in ventilator settings in children with severe lung disease should be slow, because the effects of many of the changes may not be apparent for days.

Differential Diagnosis

The differential diagnosis of BPD includes meconium aspiration syndrome, congenital infection (eg, with cytomegalovirus or *Ureaplasma*), cystic adenomatoid malformation, recurrent aspiration, pulmonary lymphangiectasia, total anomalous pulmonary venous return, overhydration, and idiopathic pulmonary fibrosis.

Prognosis

Surfactant replacement therapy has had a significantly and markedly beneficial effect on reducing morbidity and mortality from BPD. Infants of younger gestational age are surviving in greater numbers. Surprisingly, the effect of neonatal care has not significantly decreased the incidence of BPD. The disorder typically develops in the most immature infants. The long-term outlook for most survivors is favorable. Follow-up studies suggest that lung function may be altered for life. Hyperinflation and damage to small airways has been reported in children 10 years after the first signs of BPD. In addition, these infants are at a higher risk for developing such sequelae as persistent hypoxemia, airway hyperreactivity, exercise intolerance, pulmonary hypertension, chronic obstructive pulmonary disease, and abnormal lung growth. As smaller, more immature infants survive, abnormal neurodevelopmental outcomes become more likely. The incidence of cerebral palsy, hearing loss, vision abnormalities, spastic diplegia, and developmental delays is increased. Feeding abnormalities, behavior difficulties, and increased irritability have also been reported. A focus on good nutrition and prophylaxis against respiratory pathogens and airway hyperreactivity provide the best outcomes. Patience, continued family support, attention to developmental issues and school performance, and speech and physical therapy help to improve the long-term outlook.

Baraldi E, Filippone M: Chronic lung disease after premature birth. N Engl J Med 2007;357:1946 [PMID: 17989387].

Chess PR et al: Pathogenesis of bronchopulmonary dysplasia. Semin Perinatol 2006;30:171 [PMID: 16860156].

Higgins RD et al: Executive summary of the workshop on oxygen in neonatal therapies: Controversies and opportunities for research. Pediatrics 2007;119:790 [PMID: 17403851].

Northway WH et al: Pulmonary disease following respiratory therapy of hyaline membrane disease: Bronchopulmonary dysplasia. N Engl J Med 1967;276:357 [PMID: 5334613].

Stocks J, Coates A, Bush A: Lung function in infants and young children with chronic lung disease of infancy: The next steps? Pediatr Pulmonol 2007;42:3 [PMID: 17123320].

Thébaud B, Abman SH: Bronchopulmonary dysplasia: Where have all the vessels gone? Roles of angiogenic growth factors in chronic lung disease. Am J Respir Crit Care Med 2007 May 15;175:978–985 [PMID: 17272782].

COMMUNITY AQUIRED BACTERIAL PNEUMONIA

ESSENTIALS OF DIAGNOSIS & TYPICAL FEATURES

- Fever, cough, dyspnea.
- Abnormal chest examination (crackles or decreased breath sounds).
- Abnormal chest radiograph (infiltrates, hilar adenopathy, pleural effusion).

General Considerations

Lower respiratory tract infections (LRTI) are a major cause of childhood mortality in disadvantaged areas of the world. The infectious etiologies vary widely by geographic region and by the age of the child. In developed countries, the majority of pneumonias are caused by viral agents and bacterial pneumonia is a less common cause. Discrimination between viral and bacterial pneumonia is challenging as neither the white blood cell count nor differential nor the chest radiograph are strong predictors. In areas where the technology is readily available, chest radiography is recommended to establish with certainty the presence of pneumonia. The most common cause of bacterial pneumonia in children of all ages is *S pneumoniae*. Bacterial pneumonia usually follows a viral lower respiratory tract infection. Children at high risk for bacterial pneumonia are those with compromised pulmonary defense systems. For example, children with abnormal mucociliary clearance, immunocompromised children, children who aspirate their own secretions or who aspirate while eating, and malnourished children are at increased risk for bacterial pneumonia.

Clinical Findings

A. Symptoms and Signs

The pathogen, severity of the infection, and age of the patient may cause substantial variations in the presentation of community-acquired pneumonia (CAP). Infants may have few or nonspecific findings on history and physical examination. Immunocompetent older patients may not appear to be seriously ill. Fevers (over 39°C), tachypnea, and cough are hallmarks of CAP. Chest auscultation may reveal crackles or decreased breath sounds in the setting of consolidation or an associated pleural effusion. Some patients may have additional extrapulmonary findings, such as meningismus or abdominal pain, due to pneumonia itself. Others may have evidence of infection at other sites due to the same organism causing their pneumonia: meningitis, otitis media, sinusitis, pericarditis, epiglottitis, or abscesses.

B. Laboratory Findings and Imaging Studies

An elevated peripheral white blood cell count with a left shift may be a marker of bacterial pneumonia. A low white blood count (< 5000/μL) can be an ominous finding in this disease. Blood cultures should be obtained in children admitted to the hospital with pneumonia, although approximately 10% or less will be positive, even with known bacterial pneumonia. Air space or consolidation in a lobar distribution on chest x-ray suggests bacterial pneumonia; interstitial or peribronchial infiltrates suggest a viral infection. If a pleural effusion is suspected, radiographs should be taken in the lateral decubitus position. Severity of the infection may not correlate with radiographic findings and clinical improvement precedes radiographic resolution. A diagnostic (and possibly therapeutic) thoracocentesis should be performed in a child with a pleural effusion. Sputum cultures may be helpful in older children capable of providing a satisfactory sample. Bacterial antigen detection may be nonspecific for pneumonia. Procalcitonin and C-reative protein markers are not specific for bacterial or viral pneumonia. The spectrum of potential pathogens to be considered includes aerobic, anaerobic, and acid-fast bacteria as well as *Chlamydia trachomatis, Chlamydia pneumoniae, C psittaci, Coxiella burnetii* (Q fever), *P jiroveci, B pertussis, M pneumoniae, Legionella pneumophila,* and respiratory viruses. *S pneumoniae* is the most prevalent bacterial pathogen.

Invasive diagnostic procedures (bronchial brushing or washing, lung puncture, or open or thoracoscopic lung biopsy) should be undertaken in critically ill patients when other means do not adequately identify the cause (see earlier section on Culture of Material from the Respiratory Tract).

Differential Diagnosis

Noninfectious pulmonary disease (including gastric aspiration, foreign body aspiration, atelectasis, congenital malformations, congestive heart failure, malignancy, tumors such as plasma cell granuloma, chronic ILD, and pulmonary hemosiderosis) should be considered in the differential diagnosis of localized or diffuse infiltrates. When effusions are present, additional noninfectious disorders such as collagen diseases, neoplasm, and pulmonary infarction should also be considered.

Complications

Empyema can occur frequently with staphylococcal, pneumococcal, and group A β-hemolytic streptococcal pneumonia. Distal sites of infection—meningitis, otitis media, sinusitis (especially of the ethmoids), and septicemia—may be present, particularly with disease due to *S pneumoniae* or *H influenzae*. Certain immunocompromised patients, such as those who have undergone splenectomy or who have hemoglobin SS or SC disease or thalassemia, are especially prone to overwhelming sepsis with these organisms.

Treatment

If a bacterial pneumonia is suspected, empiric antibiotic therapy should be considered. In children less than 5 years old with an abnormal chest x-ray or suggestive clinical findings, the most likely bacterial pathogen is *S pneumoniae* and the antibiotic of choice is amoxicillin for outpatient management. The suggested dose is 80–100 mg/kg/d. Second-generation cephalosporins are recommended for children allergic to penicillin, or a macrolide can be effective. Children older than 5 years are more likely to have atypical pneumonia (eg, *Mycoplasma*) and a macrolide might be the best empiric antibiotic choice. When possible, therapy can be guided by the antibiotic sensitivity pattern of the organisms isolated. (For further discussion, see Chapter 39.) An appropriate antiviral (eg, amantadine, rimantidine, osetamivir, zanamivir) should be considered for the child with pneumonia due to influenza. Whether a child should be hospitalized depends on his or her age, the severity of illness, the suspected organism, and the anticipated reliability of adherence to the treatment regimen at home. All children younger than 3 months of age are generally admitted to the hospital for treatment of bacterial pneumonia. Children older than 3 months of age with febrile pneumonias, infants generally—and toddlers often—require admission. Moderate to severe respiratory distress, apnea, hypoxemia, poor feeding, clinical deterioration on treatment, or associated complications (large effusions, empyema, or abscess) indicate the need for immediate hospitalization. Careful outpatient follow-up within 12 hours to 5 days is often indicated in those not admitted.

Additional therapeutic considerations include oxygen, humidification of inspired gases, hydration and electrolyte supplementation, and nutrition. Removal of pleural fluid for diagnostic purposes is indicated initially to guide antimicrobial therapy. Removal of pleural fluid for therapeutic purposes may also be indicated.

Prognosis

In developed countries, for the immunocompetent host in whom bacterial pneumonia is adequately recognized and treated, the survival rate is high. For example, the mortality rate from uncomplicated pneumococcal pneumonia is less than 1%. If the patient survives the initial illness, persistently abnormal pulmonary function following empyema is surprisingly uncommon, even when treatment has been delayed or inappropriate.

Durbin WJ, Stille C: Pneumonia. Pediatr Rev 2008;29(5):147–158 [PMID: 18450836].

Stein RT, Marostica PJ: Community-acquired pneumonia: A review and recent advances. Pediatr Pulmonol 2007;42(12):1095–1103.

PARAPNEUMONIC EFFUSION & EMPYEMA

ESSENTIALS OF DIAGNOSIS & TYPICAL FEATURES

- Respiratory distress and chest pain.
- Fever.
- Chest x-ray showing a meniscus or layering fluid on a lateral decubitus film.

General Considerations

Bacterial pneumonia is often accompanied by pleural effusion. Some of these effusions harbor infection, and others are inflammatory reactions to pneumonia. The nomenclature in this area is somewhat confusing. Some authors use the term *empyema* for grossly purulent fluid and *parapneumonic effusion* for nonpurulent fluid. It is clear, however, that some nonpurulent effusions will also contain organisms and represent either partially treated or early empyema. It is probably best to refer to all effusions associated with pneumonia as parapneumonic effusions, some of which are infected and some not.

The most common organism associated with empyema is *S pneumoniae*. Other common organisms include *H influenzae* and *S aureus*. Less common causes are group A streptococci, gram-negative organisms, anaerobic organisms, and *M pneumoniae*. Effusions associated with tuberculosis are almost always sterile and constitute an inflammatory reaction.

Clinical Findings

A. Symptoms and Signs

Patients usually present with typical signs of pneumonia, including fever, tachypnea, and cough. They may have chest pain, decreased breath sounds, and dullness to percussion on the affected side and may prefer to lie on the affected side. With large effusions, there may be tracheal deviation to the contralateral side.

B. Diagnostic Studies

The white blood cell count is often elevated, with left shift. Blood cultures are sometimes positive. The tuberculin skin test is positive in most cases of tuberculosis. Thoracentesis reveals findings consistent with an exudate. Cells in the pleural fluid are usually neutrophils in bacterial disease and lymphocytes in tuberculous effusions. In bacterial disease, pleural fluid pH and glucose are often low. A pH less than 7.2 suggests active bacterial infection. The pH of the specimen should be determined in a blood gas syringe sent to the laboratory on ice. Extra heparin should not be used in the syringe as it can falsely lower the pH. Although in adults the presence of low pH and glucose indicates the need for aggressive and thorough drainage procedures, the prognostic significance of these findings in children is unknown. Gram stain, cultures, and counterimmunoelectrophoresis are often positive for the offending organism.

The presence of pleural fluid is suggested by a homogeneous density that obscures the underlying lung on chest radiograph. Large effusions may cause a shift of the mediastinum to the contralateral side. Small effusions may only blunt the costophrenic angle. Lateral decubitus radiographs may help to detect freely movable fluid by demonstrating a layering-out effect. If the fluid is loculated, no such effect is perceived. Ultrasonography can be extremely valuable in localizing the fluid and detecting loculations, especially when thoracentesis is contemplated, but availability may be limited. Chest CT scan can help determine whether the fluid is intraparenchymal or extraparenchymal and can direct further care of complicated pneumonias.

Treatment

After initial thoracentesis and identification of the organism, appropriate intravenous antibiotics and adequate drainage of the fluid remain the mainstay of therapy, but the approach is debated. Although there is a trend toward managing smaller pneumococcal empyemas without a chest tube, larger effusions require chest tube drainage. Often the empyema has been present for more than 7 days, increasing the chance for loculation of fluid. Evidence of early interventions using thoracoscopic techniques such as VATS may reduce morbidity and has been shown to shorten length of hospital stay when done by an experienced surgeon. While there is growing use of VATS as first-line therapy, it is not standard of care. Studies in adults show that aggressive management with drainage of pleural cavity fluid and release of adhesions with fibrinolytics is cost effective and also decreases the length of stay. There are limited studies of fibrinolytics in children. The therapeutic choice will vary depending on the resources available and the preferences of the clinician.

Prognosis

The prognosis is related to the severity of disease but is generally excellent, with complete or nearly complete recovery expected in most instances.

Gates RL et al: Drainage, fibrinolytics, or surgery: A comparison of treatment options in pediatric empyema. J Pediatr Surg 2004;39:1638 [PMID: 15547825].

Jaffe A, Balfour-Lynn IM: Management of empyema in children. Pediatr Pulmonol 2005;40:148–156 [PMID: 15965900].

ATYPICAL PNEUMONIAS: VIRAL PNEUMONIA

ESSENTIALS OF DIAGNOSIS & TYPICAL FEATURES

- Upper respiratory infection prodrome (fever, coryza, cough, hoarseness).
- Wheezing or rales.
- Myalgia, malaise, headache (older children).

General Considerations

Most pneumonias in children are caused by viruses. RSV, parainfluenza (1, 2, and 3) viruses, influenza (A and B) viruses, and human metapneumovirus are responsible for the large majority of cases. Severity of disease, severity of fever, radiographic findings, and the characteristics of cough or lung sounds do not reliably differentiate viral from bacterial pneumonias. Furthermore, such infections may coexist. However, substantial pleural effusions, pneumatoceles, abscesses, lobar consolidation with lobar volume expansion, and "round" pneumonias are generally inconsistent with viral disease.

Clinical Findings

A. Symptoms and Signs

An upper respiratory infection frequently precedes the onset of lower respiratory disease due to viruses. Although wheezing or stridor may be prominent in viral disease, cough, signs of respiratory distress (tachypnea, retractions, grunting, and nasal flaring), and physical findings (rales and decreased breath sounds) may not be distinguishable from those in bacterial pneumonia.

B. Laboratory Findings

The peripheral white blood cell count can be normal or slightly elevated and is not useful in distinguishing viral from bacterial disease.

Rapid viral diagnostic methods—such as fluorescent antibody tests or enzyme-linked immunosorbent assay and/or polymerase chain reaction (PCR)—should be performed on nasopharyngeal secretions to confirm this diagnosis in high-risk patients and for epidemiology or infection control. Rapid diagnosis of RSV infection does not preclude the possibility of concomitant infection with other pathogens.

C. Imaging Studies

Chest radiographs frequently show perihilar streaking, increased interstitial markings, peribronchial cuffing, or patchy bronchopneumonia. Lobar consolidation or atelectasis may occur, however. Hyperinflation of the lungs may occur when involvement of the small airways is prominent.

Differential Diagnosis—The differential diagnosis of viral pneumonia is the same as for bacterial pneumonia. Patients with prominent wheezing may have asthma, airway obstruction caused by foreign body aspiration, acute bacterial or viral tracheitis, or parasitic disease.

Complications

Viral pneumonia or laryngotracheobronchitis may predispose the patient to subsequent bacterial tracheitis or pneumonia as immediate sequelae. Bronchiolitis obliterans or severe chronic respiratory failure may follow adenovirus pneumonia. The results of studies evaluating the development of asthma after a viral pneumonia are variable. Bronchiectasis, chronic ILD, and unilateral hyperlucent lung (Sawyer-James syndrome) may follow measles, adenovirus, and influenza pneumonias.

Treatment

General supportive care for viral pneumonia does not differ from that for bacterial pneumonia. Patients can be quite ill and should be hospitalized according to the level of their illness. Because bacterial disease often cannot be definitively excluded, antibiotics may be indicated.

Patients at risk for life-threatening RSV infections (eg, those with BPD or other severe pulmonary conditions, congenital heart disease, or significant immunocompromise) should be hospitalized and ribavirin should be considered. Rapid viral diagnostic tests may be a useful guide for such therapy (see the following section regarding prevention). These high-risk patients and all children 6 months to 5 years of age should be immunized annually against influenza A and B viruses. Despite immunization, however, influenza infection can still occur. When available epidemiologic data indicate an active influenza A infection in the community, rimantadine, amantadine hydrochloride, or oseltamivir phosphate should be considered early for high-risk infants and children who appear to be infected. Children with suspected viral pneumonia should be placed in respiratory isolation.

Prognosis

Although most children with viral pneumonia recover uneventfully, worsening asthma, abnormal pulmonary function or chest radiographs, persistent respiratory insufficiency, and even death may occur in high-risk patients such as newborns or those with underlying lung, cardiac, or immunodeficiency disease. Patients with adenovirus infection or those concomitantly infected with RSV and second pathogens such as influenza, adenovirus, cytomegalovirus, or *P jiroveci* also have a worse prognosis.

Don M, Caniani M, Korppi M: Community-acquired pneumonia in children: What's old? What's new? Acta Paediatrica 2010;99:1602–1608.

Durbin WJ, Stille C: Pneumonia. Pediatr Rev 2008;29:147–160 [PMID: 18450836].

Ruuskanen O, Lahti E, Jennings LC, Murdoch DR: Viral pneumonia. Lancet 2011;377:1364–1375.

BRONCHIOLITIS

ESSENTIALS OF DIAGNOSIS & TYPICAL FEATURES

- Clinical syndrome characterized by one or more of the following findings: coughing, tachypnea, labored breathing, and hypoxia.
- Irritability, poor feeding, vomiting.
- Wheezing and crackles on chest auscultation.

Bronchiolitis is the most common serious acute respiratory illness in infants and young children. The diagnosis of bronchiolitis is based upon clinical findings including an upper respiratory infection that has progressed to cough, tachypnea, respiratory distress, and crackles or wheeze by physical examination. In most literature from the United States, this definition of bronchiolitis specifically applies to children younger than 2 years old. One to 3% of infants with bronchiolitis will require hospitalization, especially during the winter months. RSV is by far the most common viral cause of acute bronchiolitis. Parainfluenza, human metapneumovirus, influenza, adenovirus, *Mycoplasma, Chlamydia, Ureaplasma, Bocavirus,* and *Pneumocystis* are less common causes of bronchiolitis during early infancy.

Clinical Findings

A. Symptoms and Signs

The usual course of RSV bronchiolitis is 1–2 days of fever, rhinorrhea, and cough, followed by wheezing, tachypnea, and respiratory distress. Typically the breathing pattern is shallow, with rapid respirations. Nasal flaring, cyanosis, retractions, and rales may be present, along with prolongation of the expiratory phase and wheezing, depending on the severity of illness. Some young infants present with apnea and few findings on auscultation but may subsequently develop rales, rhonchi, and expiratory wheezing.

B. Laboratory Findings and Imaging Studies

A viral nasal wash may be performed to identify the causative pathogen but is not necessary to make the diagnosis of bronchiolitis. The peripheral white blood cell count may be normal or may show a mild lymphocytosis. Chest radiographs are not indicated in children who have bilateral, symmetrical findings on examination, who are not in significant respiratory distress, and who do not have elevated temperature for the child's age. If obtained, chest radiograph findings are generally nonspecific and typically include hyperinflation, peribronchial cuffing, increased interstitial markings, and subsegmental atelectasis.

Complications

The most common complication of bronchiolitis is superinfection with a bacterial pathogen such as *Streptococcus pneumoniae* leading to pneumonia. The results of studies investigating the risk for the subsequent development of chronic airway hyperreactivity (asthma) are variable. Bronchiolitis due to RSV infection contributes substantially to morbidity and mortality in children with underlying medical disorders, including chronic lung disease of prematurity, CF, congenital heart disease, and immunodeficiency.

Prevention & Treatment

The most effective preventions against RSV infection are proper handwashing techniques and reducing exposure to potential environmental risk factors. Major challenges have impeded the development of an RSV vaccine, but a licensed product may be expected in the near future. Prophylaxis with a monoclonal antibody (palivizumab) has proven effective in reducing the rate of hospitalization and associated morbidities in high-risk premature infants and those with chronic cardiopulmonary conditions.

Although most children with RSV bronchiolitis are readily treated as outpatients, hospitalization is required in infected children with hypoxemia on room air, a history of apnea, moderate tachypnea with feeding difficulties, and marked respiratory distress with retractions. Children at high risk for hospitalization include infants younger than 6 months of age, especially with any history of prematurity, and those with underlying chronic cardiopulmonary disorders. While in the hospital, treatment should include supportive strategies such as frequent suctioning and providing adequate fluids to maintain hydration. If hypoxemia is present, supplemental oxygen should be administered. There is no evidence to support the use of antibiotics in children with bronchiolitis unless there is evidence of an associated bacterial pneumonia. Bronchodilators and corticosteroids have not been shown to change the severity or the length of the illness in bronchiolitis and therefore are not recommended. Studies evaluating the effectiveness of hypertonic saline and the combination of oral dexamethasone and inhaled epinephrine in children with bronchiolitis seen in the emergency department and inpatient setting are ongoing.

Patients at risk for life-threatening RSV infections (eg, children under 24 months of age whose gestational age is less than 35 weeks, children under 24 months of age with other severe pulmonary conditions, congenital heart disease, neuromuscular disease, or significant immunocompromise) should be considered for RSV prophylaxis therapy. For more detail, refer to the American Academy of Pediatrics 2009 guidelines. High-risk patients with RSV bronchiolitis may need to be hospitalized and treated with ribavirin.

Prognosis

The prognosis for the majority of infants with acute bronchiolitis is very good. With improved supportive care and prophylaxis with palivizumab, the mortality rate among high-risk infants has decreased substantially.

American Academy of Pediatrics Subcommittee on Diagnosis and Management of Bronchiolitis: Diagnosis and management of bronchiolitis. Pediatrics 2006;118:1774 [PMID: 17015575].

Committee in Infectious Disease: From the American Academy of Pediatrics: policy statements—Modified recommendations for the use of palivizumab for prevention of respiratory syncitial virus infections. Pediatrics 2009;124(6):1694–1701 [PMID: 19736258].

Guilbert TW, Bacharier LB: Controversies in the treatment of the acutely wheezing infant. AJRCCM 2011;183(10):1284–1285 [PMID: 21596826].

Simoes EA: Maternal smoking, asthma, and bronchiolitis: Clear cut association or equivocal evidence? Pediatrics 2007;119:1210 [PMID: 17545392].

CHLAMYDIAL PNEUMONIAS (SEE ALSO CHAPTER 40)

ESSENTIALS OF DIAGNOSIS & TYPICAL FEATURES

- Cough, pharyngitis, tachypnea, rales, few wheezes, fever.
- Inclusion conjunctivitis, eosinophilia, and elevated immunoglobulins in some cases.

General Considerations

In children, *C pneumoniae* is a common respiratory pathogen and may cause 5%–20% of all community-acquired pneumonias. Often these lower respiratory tract illnesses are mild or asymptomatic, although this can occasionally be a serious pathogen.

Pulmonary disease due to *C trachomatis* usually evolves gradually as the infection descends the respiratory tract. Infants may appear quite well despite the presence of significant pulmonary illness. Infant infections are now at epidemic proportions in urban environments worldwide. *C pneumoniae* is now recognized as a common cause of respiratory infections in adults and children.

Clinical Findings

A. Symptoms and Signs

Cough is usually present. It can have a staccato character and resemble the cough of pertussis. The infant is usually tachypneic. Scattered inspiratory rales are commonly heard; wheezes are rarely heard. Significant fever suggests a different or additional diagnosis. About 50% of infants with *C trachomatis* pneumonia have active inclusion conjunctivitis or a history of it. Rhinopharyngitis with nasal discharge or otitis media may have occurred or may be currently present. Female patients may have vulvovaginitis.

B. Laboratory Findings and Imaging Studies

Although patients may frequently be hypoxemic, carbon dioxide retention is not common. Peripheral blood eosinophilia (400 cells/mL) has been observed.

C trachomatis can be identified in nasopharyngeal washings using fluorescent antibody or culture techniques. *C pneumoniae* isolation can be difficult and the diagnosis is often made by serologic testing. These tests can be performed to confirm this diagnosis in difficult to diagnose or high-risk patients and for epidemiology or infection control.

Chest radiographs may reveal diffuse interstitial and patchy alveolar infiltrates, peribronchial thickening, or focal consolidation. A small pleural reaction can be present. Despite the usual absence of wheezes, hyperexpansion is commonly present.

Differential Diagnosis

Bacterial, viral, and fungal (*P jiroveci*) pneumonias should be considered in the differential diagnosis. Premature infants and those with BPD may also have chlamydial pneumonia. *C pneumoniae* is often accompanied by coinfection with other pathogens, particularly *S pneumoniae* and *M pneumoniae*.

Treatment

A macrolide or sulfisoxazole therapy should be administered. Hospitalization may be required for children with significant respiratory distress, coughing paroxysms, or posttussive apnea. Oxygen therapy may be required for prolonged periods in some patients.

Prognosis

An increased incidence of obstructive airway disease and abnormal pulmonary function tests may occur for at least 7–8 years following infection.

Brunetti L et al: The role of pulmonary infection in pediatric asthma. Allergy Asthma Proc 2007;28:190 [PMID: 17479603].

Don M, Canciani M, Korppi M: Community acquired pneumonia in children: What's old? What's new? Acta Paediatr 2010;99(11):1602–1608 [PMID: 20573146].

MYCOPLASMAL PNEUMONIA (SEE ALSO CHAPTER 42)

ESSENTIALS OF DIAGNOSIS & TYPICAL FEATURES

- Fever.
- Cough.
- Most common in children older than age 5 years.

General Considerations

M pneumoniae is a common cause of symptomatic pneumonia in older children although it may be seen in children younger than 5 years of age. Endemic and epidemic infection can occur. The incubation period is long (2–3 weeks), and the onset of symptoms is slow. Although the lung is the primary infection site, extrapulmonary complications sometimes occur.

Clinical Findings

A. Symptoms and Signs

Fever, cough, headache, and malaise are common symptoms as the illness evolves. Although cough is usually dry at the onset, sputum production may develop as the illness progresses. Sore throat, otitis media, otitis externa, and bullous myringitis may occur. Rales are frequently present on chest examination; decreased breath sounds or dullness to percussion over the involved area may be present.

B. Laboratory Findings and Imaging Studies

The total and differential white blood cell counts are usually normal. Enzyme immunoassay (EIA) and complement fixation are sensitive and specific for *M pneumoniae.* The cold hemagglutinin titer may be elevated during the acute presentation. A titer of 1:64 or higher supports the diagnosis. Acute and convalescent titers for *M pneumoniae* demonstrating a fourfold or greater rise in specific antibodies confirm the diagnosis. Diagnosis of mycoplasmal pneumonia by polymerase chain reaction is also available.

Chest radiographs usually demonstrate interstitial or bronchopneumonic infiltrates, frequently in the middle or lower lobes. Pleural effusions are extremely uncommon.

Complications

Extrapulmonary involvement of the blood, central nervous system, skin, heart, or joints can occur. Direct Coombs–positive autoimmune hemolytic anemia, occasionally a life-threatening disorder, is the most common hematologic abnormality that can accompany *M pneumoniae* infection. Coagulation defects and thrombocytopenia can also occur. Cerebral infarction, meningoencephalitis, Guillain-Barré syndrome, cranial nerve involvement, and psychosis all have been described. A wide variety of skin rashes, including erythema multiforme and Stevens-Johnson syndrome, can occur. Myocarditis, pericarditis, and a rheumatic fever–like illness can also occur.

Treatment

Antibiotic therapy with a macrolide for 7–10 days usually shortens the course of illness. Ciprofloxacin is a possible alternative. Supportive measures, including hydration, antipyretics, and bed rest, are helpful.

Prognosis

In the absence of the less common extrapulmonary complications, the outlook for recovery is excellent. The extent to which *M pneumoniae* can initiate or exacerbate chronic lung disease is not well understood.

Brunetti L et al: The role of pulmonary infection in pediatric asthma. Allergy Asthma Proc 2007;28:190 [PMID: 17479603].

Don M, Canciani M, Korppi M: Community acquired pneumonia in children: What's old? What's new? Acta Paediatr 2010;99(11):1602–1608 [PMID: 20573146].

Waites KB: New concepts of *Mycoplasma pneumoniae* infections in children. Pediatr Pulmonol 2003;36:267 [PMID: 12950038].

TUBERCULOSIS (SEE ALSO CHAPTER 42)

ESSENTIALS OF DIAGNOSIS & TYPICAL FEATURES

- Positive tuberculin skin test or anergic host.
- Positive culture for *M tuberculosis*.
- Symptoms of active disease (if present): chronic cough, anorexia, weight loss or poor weight gain, fever, night sweats.

General Considerations

Tuberculosis is a widespread and deadly disease resulting from infection with *M tuberculosis*. The clinical spectrum of disease includes asymptomatic primary infection, calcified nodules, pleural effusions, progressive primary cavitating lesions, contiguous spread into adjacent thoracic structures, acute miliary tuberculosis, and acute respiratory distress syndrome, overwhelming reactivation infection in the immunocompromised host, occult lymphohematogenous spread, and metastatic extrapulmonary involvement at almost any site. Because transmission is usually through respiratory droplets, isolated pulmonary parenchymal tuberculosis constitutes more than 85% of presenting cases. Pulmonary tuberculosis is the focus of discussion here; additional manifestations of tuberculosis are discussed in Chapter 42.

Following a resurgence in the 1980s and early 1990s, tuberculosis has declined among all age groups in the United States, including children. This trend has continued through 2006, the most recent year for which data are available. However, the disease remains a significant cause of morbidity and mortality worldwide.

Clinical Findings

A. Symptoms and Signs

Most children with tuberculosis are asymptomatic and present with a positive tuberculin skin test. Symptoms of active disease, if present, might include chronic cough, anorexia, weight loss or poor weight gain, fever, and night sweats. Children can also present with symptoms of airway obstruction with secondary bacterial pneumonia or airway collapse resulting from hilar adenopathy.

Because most children infected with tuberculosis are asymptomatic, a clue to infection may be contact with an individual with tuberculosis—often an elderly relative, a caregiver, or a person previously residing in a region where tuberculosis is endemic—or a history of travel to or residence in such an area. Homeless and extremely impoverished children are also at high risk, as are those in contact with high-risk adults (patients with AIDS, residents or employees of correctional institutions or nursing homes, drug users, and health care workers). Once exposed, pediatric patients at risk for developing active disease include infants and those with malnutrition, AIDS, diabetes mellitus, or immunosuppression (cancer chemotherapy or corticosteroids).

The symptoms of active disease listed previously most often occur during the first year of infection. Thereafter, infection remains quiescent until adolescence, when reactivation of pulmonary tuberculosis is common. At any stage, chronic cough, anorexia, weight loss or poor weight gain, and fever are useful clinical signs of reactivation. Of note, except in patients with complications or advanced disease, physical findings are few.

B. Laboratory Findings and Imaging Studies

A positive tuberculin skin test is defined by the size of induration as measured by a medical provider 48–72 hours after intradermal injection of 5 tuberculin units of purified protein derivative (PPD). A positive test is defined as an induration greater than or equal to 5 mm in patients who are at high risk for developing active disease (ie, immunocompromised, those with a history of a positive test or radiograph, children younger than 4 years, and those known to have close contact with someone with active disease); greater than 10 mm in patients from or exposed to high-risk populations (ie, born in countries with a high prevalence, users of injected drugs, having poor access to health care, or living in facilities such as jails, homeless shelters, or nursing homes); and greater than 15 mm in those who are at low risk. Tine tests should not be used. Appropriate control skin tests, such as those for hypersensitivity to diphtheria-tetanus, mumps, or *Candida albicans,* should be applied in patients with suspected or proven immunosuppression or in those with possible severe disseminated disease. If the patient fails to respond to PPD, the possibility of tuberculosis is not excluded. In suspected cases, the patient, immediate family, and suspected carriers should also be tuberculin-tested. Because healing—rather than progression—is the usual course in the uncompromised host, a positive tuberculin test may be the only manifestation. The primary focus (usually single) and associated nodal involvement may not be seen radiographically. For patients born outside the United States or those who have received a previous bacillus Calmette-Guérin immunization, induration greater than 5 mm should be considered positive and further evaluated.

There are new serum immunological tests that are currently being studied in adults and children, for example, T-spot. TB (Oxford Immunotec, U.K.) and Quantiferon-TB Gold (Cellestis, Australia) are now being used in adults. Guidelines for interpretation of the tests in pediatrics are not available. In addition, it is not clear how to distinguish new infection from latent infections using these immunological assays.

C. Imaging Studies

Anteroposterior and lateral chest radiographs should be obtained in all suspected cases. Culture for *M tuberculosis* is critical for proving the diagnosis and for defining drug susceptibility. Early morning gastric lavage following an overnight fast should be performed on three occasions in infants and children with suspected active pulmonary tuberculosis before treatment is started, when the severity of illness allows. Although stains for acid-fast bacilli on this material are of little value, this is the ideal culture site. Despite the increasing importance of isolating organisms because of multiple drug resistance, only 40% of children will yield positive cultures.

D. Special Tests

Sputum cultures from older children and adolescents can also be useful. Stains and cultures of bronchial secretions can be obtained using bronchoscopy. When pleural effusions are present, pleural biopsy for cultures and histopathologic examination for granulomas or organisms provide diagnostic information. Meningeal involvement is also possible in young children, and lumbar puncture should be considered in their initial evaluation.

Differential Diagnosis

Fungal diseases that affect mainly the lungs, such as histoplasmosis, coccidioidomycosis, cryptococcosis, and North American blastomycosis, may resemble tuberculosis and in cases where the diagnosis is unclear, should be excluded by biopsy or appropriate serologic studies. Atypical tuberculous organisms may involve the lungs, especially in the immunocompromised patient. Depending on the presentation, diagnoses such as lymphoreticular and other malignancies, collagen-vascular disorders, or other pulmonary infections may be considered.

Complications

In addition to those complications listed in the sections on general considerations and clinical findings, lymphadenitis, meningitis, osteomyelitis, arthritis, enteritis, peritonitis, and renal, ocular, middle ear, and cutaneous disease may occur. Infants born to parents infected with *M tuberculosis* are at great risk for developing illness. The possibility of life-threatening airway compromise must always be considered in patients with large mediastinal or hilar lesions.

Treatment

Because the risk of hepatitis due to isoniazid is extremely low in children, this drug is indicated in those with a positive tuberculin skin test. This greatly reduces the risk of subsequent active disease and complications with minimal morbidity. Isoniazid plus rifampin treatment for 6 months, plus pyrazinamide during the first 2 months, is indicated when the chest radiograph is abnormal or when extrapulmonary disease is present. Without pyrazinamide, isoniazid plus rifampin must be given for 9 months. In general, the more severe tuberculous complications are treated with a larger number of drugs (see Chapter 42). Enforced, directly observed therapy (twice or three times weekly) is indicated when nonadherence is suspected. Recommendations for antituberculosis chemotherapy based on disease stage are continuously being updated. The most current edition of the American Academy of Pediatrics *Red Book* is a reliable source for these protocols.

Corticosteroids are used to control inflammation in selected patients with potentially life-threatening airway compression by lymph nodes, acute pericardial effusion, massive pleural effusion with mediastinal shift, or miliary tuberculosis with respiratory failure.

Prognosis

In patients with an intact immune system, modern antituberculous therapy offers good potential for recovery. The outlook for patients with immunodeficiencies, organisms resistant to multiple drugs, poor drug adherence, or advanced complications is guarded. Organisms resistant to multiple drugs are increasingly common. Resistance emerges either because the physician prescribes an inadequate regimen or because the patient discontinues medications. When resistance to or intolerance of isoniazid and rifampin prevents their use, cure rates are 50% or less.

Newton S et al: Paediatric tuberculosis. Lancet Infect Dis 2008;8:498–510 [PMID: 18652996].

Powell DA, Hunt WG: Tuberculosis in children: An update. Adv Pediatr 2006;53:279 [PMID: 17089872].

ASPIRATION PNEUMONIA

ESSENTIALS OF DIAGNOSIS & TYPICAL FEATURES

- History of recurrent aspiration or an aspiration event.
- New onset respiratory distress, oxygen requirement, or in some children, fever, after the aspiration or in a child with known aspiration.
- Focal findings on physical examination (usually in the side).

Patients whose anatomic defense mechanisms are impaired are at risk of aspiration pneumonia (Table 19–5). Acute disease is commonly caused by bacteria present in the mouth (especially gram-negative anaerobes). Chronic aspiration often causes recurrent bouts of acute febrile pneumonia. It may also lead to chronic focal infiltrates, atelectasis, an illness resembling asthma or ILD, bronchiectasis, or failure to thrive.

Table 19–5. Risk factors for aspiration pneumonia.

Seizures
Depressed sensorium
Recurrent gastroesophageal reflux, emesis, or gastrointestinal obstruction
Neuromuscular disorders with suck-swallow dysfunction
Anatomic abnormalities (laryngeal cleft, tracheoesophageal fistula, vocal cord paralysis)
Debilitating illnesses
Occult brainstem lesions
Near-drowning
Nasogastric, endotracheal, or tracheostomy tubes
Severe periodontal disease

Clinical Findings

A. Symptoms and Signs

Acute onset of fever, cough, respiratory distress, or hypoxemia in a patient at risk suggests aspiration pneumonia. Chest physical findings, such as rales, rhonchi, or decreased breath sounds, may initially be limited to the lung region into which aspiration occurred. Although any region may be affected, the right side—especially the right upper lobe in the supine patient—is commonly affected. In patients with chronic aspiration, diffuse wheezing may occur. Generalized rales may also be present. Such patients may not develop acute febrile pneumonias.

B. Laboratory Findings and Imaging Studies

Chest radiographs may reveal lobar consolidation or atelectasis and focal or generalized alveolar or interstitial infiltrates. In some patients with chronic aspiration, perihilar infiltrates with or without bilateral air trapping may be seen.

In severely ill patients with acute febrile illnesses, and especially when the pneumonia is complicated by a pleural effusion, a bacteriologic diagnosis should be made. In addition to blood cultures and cultures of the pleural fluid, cultures of tracheobronchial secretions and bronchoalveolar lavage specimens may be considered (see earlier section on Culture of Material from the Respiratory Tract).

In patients with chronic aspiration pneumonitis, documentation of aspiration as the cause of illness may be elusive. Barium contrast studies using liquids of increasing consistency may provide evidence of suck-swallow dysfunction or laryngeal cleft. Bolus barium swallow studies with good distention of the esophagus may help to identify an occult tracheoesophageal fistula. Gastroesophageal reflux may be a risk factor for aspiration while the child is sleeping, and an overnight or 24-hour esophageal pH probe studies may also help establish the diagnosis of gastroesophageal reflux. Although radionuclide scans are commonly used, the yield from such studies is disappointingly low. Rigid bronchoscopy in infants or flexible bronchoscopy in older children can be used to identify anatomic abnormalities such as tracheal cleft and tracheoesophageal fistula. Flexible bronchoscopy and bronchoalveolar lavage specimens to search for lipid-laden macrophages can also suggest chronic aspiration.

Differential Diagnosis

In the acutely ill patient, bacterial and viral pneumonias should be considered. In the chronically ill patient, the differential diagnosis may include disorders causing recurrent pneumonia (eg, immunodeficiencies, ciliary dysfunction, or foreign body), chronic wheezing, or interstitial lung disorders (see next section), depending on the presentation.

Complications

Empyema or lung abscess may complicate acute aspiration pneumonia. Chronic aspiration may also result in bronchiectasis.

Treatment

Aspiration pneumonia leads to a chemical pneumonitis and, in some cases, supportive treatment is the only recommended therapy. Antimicrobial therapy for patients who are acutely ill from aspiration pneumonia includes coverage for gram-negative anaerobic organisms. In general, clindamycin is appropriate initial coverage. However, in some hospital-acquired infections, additional coverage for multiple resistant *P aeruginosa,* streptococci, and other organisms may be required.

Treatment of recurrent and chronic aspiration pneumonia may include the following: surgical correction of anatomic abnormalities; improved oral hygiene; improved hydration; and inhaled bronchodilators, chest physical therapy, and suctioning. In patients with compromise of the central nervous system, exclusive feeding by gastrostomy and (in some) tracheostomy may be required to control airway secretions. Gastroesophageal reflux, if present in these patients, also often requires surgical correction.

Prognosis

The outlook is directly related to the disorder causing aspiration.

Boesch RP et al: Advances in the diagnosis and management of chronic pulmonary aspiration in children. Eur Respir J 2006;28(4):847–861 [PMID: 17012631].

Brook I: Anaerobic pulmonary infections in children. Pediatr Emerg Care 2004;20:636 [PMID: 15599270].

Methany NA et al: Tracheobronchial aspiration of gastric contents in critically ill tube-fed patients: Frequency, outcomes, and risk factors. Crit Care Med 2006;34:687 [PMID: 16484901].

CHILDREN'S INTERSTITIAL LUNG DISEASE SYNDROME

ESSENTIALS OF DIAGNOSIS & TYPICAL FEATURES

- Occurs acutely in the neonatal period or subacutely in infancy or childhood.
- Infants and young children have different diagnoses than adolescents and adults.
- Presence of three to five of the following criteria in the absence of any identified primary etiology is suggestive of an interstitial lung disease (ILD) syndrome:
  - Symptoms of impaired respiratory function (cough, tachypnea, retractions, exercise intolerance).
  - Evidence of impaired gas exchange (resting hypoxemia or hypercarbia, desaturation with exercise).
  - Diffuse infiltrates on imaging.
  - Presence of adventitious sounds (crackles, wheezing).
  - Abnormal spirometry, lung volumes, or carbon monoxide diffusing capacity.
- History of exposure (eg, birds, organic dusts, drug therapy, hot tubs, molds), previous lung disease, immunosuppression, symptoms of connective tissue disease; family history of familial lung disease (especially ILD) or early infant death from lung disease.

General Considerations

Children's **I**nterstitial **L**ung **D**isease (chILD) syndrome is a constellation of signs and symptoms and not a specific diagnosis. Once recognized, chILD syndrome should elicit a search for a more specific rare ILD. Other disorders can present as chILD syndrome and must be excluded as the primary cause of symptoms. These disorders include CF, cardiac disease, asthma, acute infection, immunodeficiency, neuromuscular disease, scoliosis, thoracic cage abnormality, typical BPD or premature respiratory distress syndrome, and confirmed significant aspiration on a swallow study. However, if patients present with symptoms out of proportion to the diagnosis, consideration should be given to ILD disorders.

Clinical Findings

A. Symptoms and Signs

chILD syndrome may present acutely in the newborn period with respiratory failure or gradually over time with a chronic dry cough or a history of dyspnea on exertion. The child with more advanced disease may have increased dyspnea, tachypnea, retractions, cyanosis, clubbing, failure to thrive, or weight loss.

B. Laboratory Findings

Once chILD syndrome is recognized, initial evaluations should be directed at ruling out known conditions. The initial evaluations should include the following diagnostic studies depending upon the age and presentation of the child: radiographs, modified barium swallow, pulmonary function tests, and skin tests (see earlier section on Tuberculosis); complete blood count and erythrocyte sedimentation rate; sweat chloride test for CF; electrocardiogram or echocardiogram; serum immunoglobulins and other immunologic evaluations; sputum studies (see later section on Pneumonia in the Immunocompromised Host); and possibly studies for Epstein-Barr virus, cytomegalovirus, *M pneumoniae, Chlamydia, Pneumocystis,* and *Ureaplasma urealyticum.*

C. Imaging Studies

Chest radiographs are normal in up to 10%–15% of patients. Frequently, specific chILD disorders can be suspected by findings on controlled volume inspiratory and expiratory high-resolution CT, which should be considered early in the course of evaluation. Diagnoses of bronchiolitis obliterans (BO) and neuroendocrine cell hyperplasia of infancy (NEHI) can be made using CT findings in the right clinical context. Infants and children younger than age 5 years require sedation, which allows either infant pulmonary function testing or bronchoscopy evaluations to be completed at the same time. The lowest possible dose of radiation should always be used and this point should be emphasized at centers not specialized in pediatric care.

D. Special Tests

On pulmonary function testing, multiple patterns can be seen depending on the specific ILD condition such as (1) a restrictive pattern of decreased lung volumes, compliance, and carbon monoxide diffusing capacity, (2) an obstructive pattern with hyperinflation, or (3) a mixed obstructive-restrictive pattern. Infant pulmonary function testing can provide insight into pulmonary mechanics and different chILD disorders, especially NEHI. Exercise-induced or nocturnal hypoxemia is often the earliest detectable abnormality of lung function in children.

During the second evaluation phase, bronchoscopy is performed to exclude anatomic abnormalities, obtain multiple nasal brushings to examine cilia if primary ciliary dyskinesia (PCD) is considered a possibility, and obtain bronchoalveolar lavage for microbiologic and cytologic testing.

In patients with static or slowly progressing disease, one can then await results of bronchoscopic studies. In patients with acute, rapidly progressive disease, this stage should be combined with video-assisted thoracoscopic biopsy. Lung biopsy is the most reliable method for definitive diagnosis when analyzed by pathologists experienced in chILD disorders. A new chILD histology classification has been proposed to improve diagnostic yields. Tissue should be processed in a standard manner for special stains and cultures, electron microscopy, and immunofluorescence for immune complexes if indicated. Although transbronchial biopsy may be useful in diagnosing a few diffuse disorders and graft rejection in transplantation (eg, sarcoidosis), its overall usefulness in chILD is limited at this time.

E. Genetic Testing

Genomic mutational analysis of tissue or blood for surfactant proteins B and C (SP-B, SP-C) and *ABCA3* is now offered in clinical laboratories and should be considered in most patients with diffuse lung disease or a strong family history of ILD. Recently other genetic mutations have been reported for rare chILD that offer diagnostic information. A newly recognized disorder associated with the thyroid transcription factor–1 protein (*NKX2.1* gene) can result in variable phenotypes of Brain, Thyroid, Lung Syndrome. Children with unexplained lung disease and hypotonia or developmental delays with or without hypothyroidism and newborns with severe RDS and congenital hypothyroidism should be screened for this disorder. Other genetic disorders that cause ILD include alveolar capillary dysplasia (FOXF1 found in 30% of patients), pulmonary alveolar microlithiasis (SLC34A2), and lysinuric protein intolerance (SLC7A7).

Differential Diagnosis

chILD syndrome is composed of a group of diverse conditions that can differ from adult ILD conditions. Common adult causes of ILD such as UIP (usual interstitial pneumonitis, also known as idiopathic pulmonary fibrosis), which is associated with a high mortality rate, and respiratory bronchiolitis, associated with smoking, have not been found in children. Conversely, newly identified conditions unique to infancy, such as neuroendocrine cell hyperplasia of infancy (NEHI) or pulmonary interstitial glycogenosis (PIG), have not been described in adults. Other chILD conditions include the genetically recognized surfactant dysfunction mutations SP-B, SP-C, *ABCA3* and *NKX2.1*; developmental abnormalities; and growth disorders, especially in younger children. Older children are more likely to have SP-C or *ABCA3* surfactant mutations, hypersensitivity pneumonitis, or collagen-vascular disease. Other known conditions must also be ruled out.

Complications

Respiratory failure or pulmonary hypertension may occur. Somatic growth deficiencies often require nutritional supplementation. Mortality and morbidity can be significant in some chILD disorders.

Treatment

Therapy for known causes of ILD such as infection, aspiration, or cardiac disorders should be directed toward the primary disorder. It must be recognized that treatment for chILD conditions is anecdotal and based on case reports and small case series. In noninflammatory chILD syndrome conditions such as neuroendocrine cell hyperplasia of infancy or developmental or growth abnormalities, treatment is supportive and may not require corticosteroids. For chILD conditions such as surfactant dysfunction mutations, pulmonary interstitial glycogenosis, hypersensitivity pneumonitis, and systemic collagen-vascular disease, patients are frequently treated initially with glucocorticoids. Treat of pulmonary interstitial glycogenosis requires careful considerations of the risk and benefits of treatment. Other conditions may require oral (2 mg/kg/d for 6 weeks) or monthly pulse glucocorticoids (IV doses of 10–30 mg/kg for 1–3 days). Many patients require even more protracted therapy with alternate-day prednisone. Chloroquine (5–10 mg/kg/d) may be useful in selected disorders such as desquamative interstitial pneumonitis, surfactant dysfunction mutations, or refractory disease. In refractory cases, azathioprine and cyclophosphamide may be tried. Cyclophosphamide is needed in severe cases of diffuse alveolar hemorrhage associated with pulmonary capillaritis. Finally, some patients with severe disease may require long-term mechanical ventilation or lung transplantation for survival. chILD disorders should be evaluated and cared for by a multidisciplinary team experienced in chILD. The chILD Family Foundation can provide further supportive resources for families (http://www.childfoundation.us).

Prognosis

The prognosis is guarded in children with ILD due to collagen-vascular disease, surfactant dysfunction mutations, and developmental disorders (eg, alveolar-capillary dysplasia). Other conditions such as neuroendocrine cell hyperplasia of infancy and pulmonary interstitial glycogenosis have not had deaths reported.

HYPERSENSITIVITY PNEUMONITIS

General Considerations

Hypersensitivity pneumonitis, or extrinsic allergic alveolitis, is a T-cell–mediated disease involving the peripheral airways, interstitium, and alveoli and presents as a distinct form of chILD. Both acute and chronic forms may occur. In children, the most common forms are brought on by exposure to domestic and occasionally wild birds or bird droppings (eg, pigeons, parakeets, parrots, or doves) also known as bird fanciers lung. Intensity, duration, and genetic predisposition are all important factors. However, inhalation of almost any organic dust (moldy hay, compost, logs or tree bark, sawdust, or aerosols from humidifiers or hot tubs) can cause disease. Methotrexate-induced hypersensitivity has also been described in a child with juvenile rheumatoid arthritis. Hot tub lung can be caused by exposure to aerosolized *Mycobacterium avium* complex. A high level of suspicion and a thorough history are required for diagnosis.

Clinical Findings

A. Symptoms and Signs

Episodic cough and fever can occur with acute exposures. Chronic exposure results in weight loss, fatigue, dyspnea, cyanosis, and ultimately, respiratory failure.

B. Laboratory Findings

Acute exposure may be followed by polymorphonuclear leukocytosis with eosinophilia and evidence of airway obstruction on pulmonary function testing. Chronic disease results in a restrictive picture on lung function tests.

The serologic key to diagnosis is the finding of precipitins (precipitating IgG antibodies) to the organic materials that contain avian proteins or fungal or bacterial antigens. Ideally, to identify avian proteins, the patient's sera should be tested with antigens from droppings of the suspected species of bird. However, exposure may invoke precipitins without causing disease.

Bronchoscopy with bronchoalveolar lavage findings of lymphocytosis or *M avium* complex may be suggestive. Normal cell counts may help rule out acute hypersensitivity pneumonitis.

Differential Diagnosis

Patients with mainly acute symptoms must be differentiated from those with atopic asthma. Patients with chronic symptoms must be distinguished from those with collagen-vascular, immunologic, or primary interstitial pulmonary disorders.

Complications

Prolonged exposure to offending antigens may result in pulmonary hypertension due to chronic hypoxemia, irreversible restrictive lung disease due to pulmonary fibrosis, or respiratory failure.

Treatment & Prognosis

Complete elimination of exposure to the offending antigens is required. If drug-induced hypersensitivity pneumonitis is suspected, discontinuation is required. Corticosteroids may hasten recovery. With appropriate early diagnosis and identification and avoidance of offending antigens, the prognosis is excellent.

EOSINOPHILIC PNEUMONIA

General Considerations

Eosinophilic pneumonia is another rare condition that can be considered under the heading of chILD syndrome. A spectrum of diseases should be considered under this heading: (1) allergic bronchopulmonary helminthiasis (ABPH), (2) pulmonary eosinophilia with asthma (allergic bronchopulmonary aspergillosis and related disorders), (3) hypereosinophilic mucoid impaction, (4) bronchocentric granulomatosis, and (5) collagen-vascular disorders. The former term, *Löffler syndrome* (transient migratory pulmonary infiltrates and eosinophilia), is no longer used because most patients had undiagnosed ABPH, medication reactions (see http://www.pneumotox.com), or allergic bronchopulmonary aspergillosis. Many of these disorders occur in children with personal or family histories of allergies or asthma. ABPH may be related to hypersensitivity to migratory parasitic nematodes (*Ascaris, Strongyloides, Ancylostoma, Toxocara,* or *Trichuris*) and larval forms of filariae (*Wuchereria bancrofti*).

Allergic bronchopulmonary aspergillosis is related to hypersensitivity to the fungus *Aspergillus*. Hypersensitivity to other fungi has also been documented. Eosinophilic pneumonias are rare but can be associated with drug hypersensitivity, sarcoidosis, Hodgkin disease or other lymphomas, and bacterial infections, including brucellosis and those caused by *M tuberculosis* and atypical mycobacteria.

Clinical Findings

A. Symptoms and Signs

Cough, wheezing, and dyspnea are common presenting complaints. In allergic bronchopulmonary helminthiasis, fever, malaise, sputum production, and rarely hemoptysis may be present. In allergic bronchopulmonary aspergillosis, patients may present with all of these findings and occasionally produce brown mucus plugs. Anorexia, weight loss, night sweats, and clubbing can also occur.

B. Laboratory Findings and Imaging Studies

Elevated absolute peripheral blood eosinophil counts (3000/μL and often exceeding 50% of leukocytes) are present in ABPH and allergic bronchopulmonary aspergillosis. Serum IgE levels as high as 1000–10,000 IU/mL are common. In allergic bronchopulmonary aspergillosis, the serum IgE concentration appears to correlate with activity of the disease. Stools should be examined for ova and parasites—often several times—to clarify the diagnosis. Isohemagglutinin titers are often markedly elevated in ABPH.

In allergic bronchopulmonary aspergillosis and related disorders, patients may show central bronchiectasis on chest radiograph (so-called tramlines) or CT scan. Saccular proximal bronchiectasis of the upper lobes is pathognomonic. Although the chest radiograph may be normal, peribronchial haziness, focal or platelike atelectasis, or patchy to massive consolidation can occur. Positive immediate skin tests, serum IgG precipitating antibodies, or IgE specific for the offending fungus is present.

Differential Diagnosis

These disorders must be differentiated from exacerbations of asthma, CF, or other underlying lung disorders that cause infiltrates to appear on chest radiographs. Allergic bronchopulmonary aspergillosis can occur in patients with CF.

Complications

Delayed recognition and treatment of allergic bronchopulmonary aspergillosis may cause progressive lung damage and bronchiectasis. Lesions of the conducting airways in bronchocentric granulomatosis can extend into adjacent lung parenchyma and pulmonary arteries, resulting in secondary vasculitis.

Treatment

Therapy for the specific parasite causing ABPH should be given, and corticosteroids may be required when illness is severe. Treatment of disease due to microfilariae is both diagnostic and therapeutic. Allergic bronchopulmonary aspergillosis and related disorders are treated with prolonged courses of oral corticosteroids, bronchodilators, and chest physical therapy. In patients with CF, itraconazole may decrease corticosteroid doses for those with allergic bronchopulmonary aspergillosis. Pulmonary vasculitis associated with collagen-vascular disease is usually treated with high-dose steroids or cytotoxic agents.

Jeong YJ et al: Eosinophilic lung diseases: A clinical, radiologic, and pathologic overview. Radiographics 2007;27:617 [PMID: 17495282].

Nathan N et al: Chronic eosinophilic pneumonia in a 13-year-old child. Eur J Pediatr 2008;167(10):1203–1207 [PMID: 18202853].

PNEUMONIA IN THE IMMUNOCOMPROMISED HOST

General Considerations

Immunocompromised children can present with focal pneumonia or ILD. Pneumonia in an immunocompromised host may be due to any common bacteria (streptococci, staphylococci, or *M pneumoniae*) or less common pathogens such as *Toxoplasma gondii, P jiroveci, Aspergillus* species, *Mucor* species, *Candida* species, *Cryptococcus neoformans,* gram-negative enteric and anaerobic bacteria, *Nocardia* species, *L pneumophila,* mycobacteria, and viruses (cytomegalovirus, varicella-zoster, herpes simplex, influenza virus, RSV, human metapneumovirus, or adenovirus). Multiple organisms are commonly present. The underlying cause of the immunocompromised state often determines the spectrum of infectious agents responsible for disease (see also Chapter 33 on Immunodeficiency).

Clinical Findings

A. Symptoms and Signs

Patients often present with subtle signs such as mild cough, tachypnea, or low-grade fever that can rapidly progress to high fever, respiratory distress, and hypoxemia or chILD syndrome. An obvious portal of infection, such as an intravascular catheter, may predispose to bacterial or fungal infection.

B. Laboratory Findings and Imaging Studies

Fungal, parasitic, or bacterial infection, especially with antibiotic-resistant bacteria, should be suspected in the neutropenic child. Cultures of peripheral blood, sputum, tracheobronchial secretions, urine, nasopharynx or sinuses, bone marrow, pleural fluid, biopsied lymph nodes, or skin lesions or cultures through intravascular catheters should be obtained as soon as infection is suspected. Currently, serum and bronchoalveolar lavage (BAL) galactomannan (GM) assays for invasive pulmonary aspergillosis are being used in some centers to help guide therapy.

Invasive methods are commonly required to make a diagnosis. Appropriate samples should be obtained soon after a patient with pneumonia fails to respond to initial treatment. The results of these procedures usually lead to important changes in empiric preoperative therapy. Sputum is often unavailable. Bronchoalveolar lavage frequently provides the diagnosis of one or more organisms and should be done early in evaluation. The combined use of a wash, brushing, and lavage has a high yield. In patients with rapidly advancing disease, lung biopsy becomes more urgent. The morbidity and mortality of this procedure can be reduced by a surgeon skilled in video-assisted thoracoscopic surgical (VATS) techniques. Because of the multiplicity of organisms that may cause disease, a comprehensive set of studies should be done on lavage and biopsy material. These consist of rapid diagnostic studies, including fluorescent antibody studies for *Legionella*; rapid culture and antigen detection for viruses; Gram, acid-fast, and fungal stains; cytologic examination for viral inclusions; cultures for viruses, anaerobic and aerobic bacteria, fungi, mycobacteria, and *Legionella*; and rapid immunofluorescent studies for *P jiroveci*.

Chest radiographs and increasingly high-resolution CT scans may be useful in identifying the pattern and extent of disease. In *P jiroveci* pneumonia, dyspnea and hypoxemia may be marked despite minimal radiographic abnormalities.

Differential Diagnosis

The organisms causing disease vary with the type of immunocompromise present. For example, the splenectomized patient may be overwhelmed by infection with *S pneumoniae* or *H influenzae*. The child receiving immunosuppressant therapy or chemotherapy is more likely to have *P jiroveci* infection. The febrile neutropenic child who has been receiving adequate doses of intravenous broad-spectrum antibiotics may have fungal disease. The key to diagnosis is to consider all possibilities of infection.

Depending on the form of immunocompromise, perhaps only half to two-thirds of new pulmonary infiltrates in such patients represents infection. The remainder are caused by pulmonary toxicity of radiation, chemotherapy, or other drugs; pulmonary disorders, including hemorrhage, embolism, atelectasis, or aspiration; idiopathic pneumonia syndrome or acute respiratory distress syndrome in bone marrow transplant patients; recurrence or extension of primary malignant growths or immunologic disorders; transfusion reactions, leukostasis, or tumor cell lysis; or ILD, such as lymphocytic interstitial pneumonitis with HIV infection.

Complications

Progressive respiratory failure, shock, multiple organ damage, disseminated infection, and death commonly occur in the infected immunocompromised host if the primary etiology is not treated effectively.

Treatment

Broad-spectrum intravenous antibiotics are indicated early in febrile, neutropenic, or immunocompromised children. Trimethoprim–sulfamethoxazole (for *Pneumocystis*) and macrolides (for *Legionella*) are also indicated early in the treatment of immunocompromised children before an organism is identified. Further therapy should be based on studies of specimens obtained from bronchoalveolar lavage or lung biopsy. Recent data suggest that use of noninvasive ventilation strategies early in the course of pulmonary insufficiency or respiratory failure may decrease mortality.

Prognosis

Prognosis is based on the severity of the underlying immunocompromise, appropriate early diagnosis and treatment, and the infecting organisms. Intubation and mechanical ventilation have been associated with high mortality rates, especially in hematopoietic stem cell transplant patients.

Collaco, J Michael et al: Pulmonary dysfunction in pediatric hematopoietic stem cell transplant patients: Overview, diagnostic considerations, and infectious complications. Pediatric Blood & Cancer 2007;49(2):117 [PMID: 17029246].

Nouér, Simone A et al: Earlier response assessment in invasive aspergillosis based on the kinetics of serum Aspergillus galactomannan: Proposal for a new definition. Clinical Infectious Diseases 2011;53(7):671 [PMID: 21846834].

LUNG ABSCESS

General Considerations

Lung abscesses are most likely to occur in immunocompromised patients; in those with severe infections elsewhere (embolic spread); or in those with recurrent aspiration, malnutrition, or blunt chest trauma. Although organisms such as *S aureus, H influenzae, S pneumoniae,* and viridans streptococci more commonly affect the previously normal host, anaerobic and gram-negative organisms as well as *Nocardia, Legionella* species, and fungi (*Candida* and *Aspergillus*) should also be considered in the immunocompromised host.

Clinical Findings

A. Symptoms and Signs

High fever, malaise, and weight loss are often present. Symptoms and signs referable to the chest may or may not be present. In infants, evidence of respiratory distress can be present.

B. Laboratory Findings and Imaging Studies

Elevated peripheral white blood cell count with a neutrophil predominance or an elevated erythrocyte sedimentation rate may be present. Blood cultures are rarely positive except in the overwhelmed host.

Chest radiographs usually reveal single or multiple thick-walled lung cavities. Air-fluid levels can be present. Local compressive atelectasis, pleural thickening, or adenopathy may also occur. Chest CT scan may provide better localization and understanding of the lesions.

In patients producing sputum, stains and cultures may provide the diagnosis. Direct percutaneous aspiration of material for stains and cultures guided by fluoroscopy or ultrasonography or CT imaging should be considered in the severely compromised or ill.

Differential Diagnosis

Loculated pyopneumothorax, an *Echinococcus* cyst, neoplasms, plasma cell granuloma, and infected congenital cysts and sequestrations should be considered. Pneumatoceles, non–fluid-filled cysts, are common in children with empyema and usually resolve over time.

Complications

Although complications due to abscesses are now rare, mediastinal shift, tension pneumothorax, and spontaneous rupture can occur. Diagnostic maneuvers such as radiology-guided lung puncture to drain and culture the abscess may also cause a pneumothorax or a bronchopulmonary fistula.

Treatment

Because of the risks of lung puncture, uncomplicated abscesses are frequently conservatively treated in the uncompromised host with appropriate broad-spectrum antibiotics directed at *S aureus, H influenzae,* and streptococci. Additional coverage for anaerobic and gram-negative organisms should be provided for others. Prolonged therapy (3 weeks or more) may be required. Attempts to drain abscesses via bronchoscopy have caused life-threatening airway compromise. Surgical drainage or lobectomy is occasionally required, primarily in immunocompromised patients. However, such procedures may themselves cause life-threatening complications.

Prognosis

Although radiographic resolution may be very slow, resolution occurs in most patients without risk factors for lower respiratory tract infections or loss of pulmonary function. In the immunocompromised host, the outlook depends on the underlying disorder.

Chan PC et al: Clinical management and outcome of childhood lung abscess: A 16-year experience. J Microbiol Immunol Infect 2005;38:183 [PMID: 15986068].

BRONCHIECTASIS

ESSENTIALS OF DIAGNOSIS & TYPICAL FEATURES

- Chronic cough with sputum production.
- Rhonchi or wheezes (or both) on chest auscultation.
- Diagnosis is confirmed by high-resolution CT scan.

General Considerations

Bronchiectasis is the permanent dilation of bronchi resulting from airway obstruction by retained mucus secretions or inflammation in response to chronic or repeated infection. It occurs either as a consequence of a preceding illness (severe pneumonia or foreign body aspiration) or as a manifestation of an underlying systemic disorder (CF, PCD, chronic aspiration or immunodeficiency).

Clinical Findings

A. Symptoms and Signs

Persons with bronchiectasis will typically have chronic cough, purulent sputum, fever, and weight loss. Recurrent respiratory infections and dyspnea on exertion are also common. Hemoptysis occurs less frequently in children than in adults with bronchiectasis. On physical examination, finger clubbing may be seen. Rales, rhonchi, and decreased air entry are often noted over the bronchiectatic areas.

B. Laboratory Findings and Imaging Studies

The most common bacteria detected in cultures from the lower respiratory tract include *Streptococcus pneumoniae, S aureus,* nontypeable *H influenza,* and *Pseudomonas aeruginosa.* Nontuberculous mycobacterial species may also be detected in patients with bronchiectasis.

Chest radiographs may be mildly abnormal with slightly increased bronchovascular markings or areas of atelectasis, or they may demonstrate cystic changes in one or more areas of the lung. The extent of bronchiectasis is best defined by high-resolution CT scan of the lung, which often reveals far wider involvement of lung than expected from the chest radiograph. Airflow obstruction and air trapping often is seen on pulmonary function testing. Evaluation of lung function after use of a bronchodilator is helpful in assessing the benefit a patient may have from bronchodilators. Serial assessments of lung function help define the progression or resolution of the disease.

Differential Diagnosis

Bronchiectasis has numerous causes. It can occur following severe respiratory tract infections by bacteria (*Staph aureus,*

Bordetella pertussis), viruses (adenovirus), or other organisms (*M tuberculosis*). Bronchiectasis can also be due to persistent inflammation and is commonly seen in persons with recurrent aspiration pneumonia, CF, PCD, immunodeficiency, and collagen-vascular conditions. Other diagnostic considerations include foreign body aspiration and allergic bronchopulmonary aspergillosis.

Treatment

Aggressive antibiotic therapy during pulmonary exacerbations and routine airway clearance are mainstays of treatment. Inhaled hyperosmolar agents (hypertonic saline) were shown in small clinical trials to improve lung function and secretion clearance in non-CF bronchiectasis. Chronic antibiotic use, inhaled mucolytics (DNAse), anti-inflammatory therapy, and bronchodilators have not been proven effective in non-CF bronchiectasis, although individual patients may benefit.

Surgical removal of an area of lung affected with severe bronchiectasis is considered when the response to medical therapy is poor. Other indications for operation include severe localized disease, repeated hemoptysis, and recurrent pneumonia in one area of lung. If bronchiectasis is widespread, surgical resection offers little advantage.

Prognosis

The prognosis depends on the underlying cause and severity of bronchiectasis, the extent of lung involvement, and the response to medical management. Good pulmonary hygiene and avoidance of infectious complications in the involved areas of lung may reverse cylindric bronchiectasis.

Bilton D: Update on non-cystic fibrosis bronchiectasis. Curr Opin Pulm Med 2008;14:595–599.

Redding GJ: Bronchiectasis in children. Pediatr Clin North Am 2009;56:157–171, xi.

DISEASES OF THE PULMONARY CIRCULATION

PULMONARY HEMORRHAGE

General Considerations

Pulmonary hemorrhage can be caused by a spectrum of disorders affecting the large and small airways and alveoli. It can occur as an acute or chronic process. If pulmonary hemorrhage is subacute or chronic, hemosiderin-laden macrophages can be found in the sputum and tracheal or gastric aspirate as soon as 72 hours after the bleeding begins. Many cases are secondary to infection (bacterial, mycobacterial, parasitic, viral, or fungal), lung abscess, bronchiectasis (CF or other causes), foreign body, coagulopathy (often with overwhelming sepsis), or elevated pulmonary venous pressure (secondary to congestive heart failure or anatomic heart lesions). Other causes include lung contusion from trauma, pulmonary embolus with infarction, arteriovenous fistula or telangiectasias, autoimmune vasculitis, pulmonary sequestration, agenesis of a single pulmonary artery, and esophageal duplication or bronchogenic cyst. In children, pulmonary hemorrhage due to airway tumors (eg, bronchial adenoma or left atrial myxoma) is quite rare.

Hemorrhage involving the alveoli is termed diffuse alveolar hemorrhage. Diffuse alveolar hemorrhage may be idiopathic or drug-related or may occur in Goodpasture syndrome, rapidly progressive glomerulonephritis, and systemic vasculitides (often associated with such collagen-vascular diseases as systemic lupus erythematosus, rheumatoid arthritis, Wegener granulomatosis, polyarteritis nodosa, Henoch-Schönlein purpura, and Behçet disease). Idiopathic pulmonary hemosiderosis refers to the accumulation of hemosiderin in the lung, especially the alveolar macrophage, as a result of chronic or recurrent hemorrhage (usually from pulmonary capillaries) that is not associated with the previously listed causes. Children and young adults are mainly affected, with the age at onset ranging from 6 months to 20 years.

Pulmonary hemorrhage and pulmonary hemosiderosis have been reported in infants who were exposed to a toxigenic mold, *Stachybotrys chartarum,* as well as other fungi found in older homes with recent water damage. Environmental tobacco smoke was also frequently present in the environment. Other forms of hypersensitivity pneumonitis have also been reported to cause pulmonary bleeding.

Clinical Findings

A. Symptoms and Signs

Pulmonary hemorrhage has as many symptoms as it has causes. Large airway hemorrhage presents with hemoptysis and symptoms of the underlying cause, such as infection, foreign body, or bronchiectasis in CF. Hemoptysis from larger airways is often bright red or contains clots. Some children or young adults with diffuse alveolar hemorrhage present with massive hemoptysis, marked respiratory distress, stridor, or a pneumonia-like syndrome. However, most patients with diffuse alveolar hemorrhage and idiopathic pulmonary hemosiderosis present with nonspecific respiratory symptoms (cough, tachypnea, and retractions) with or without hemoptysis, poor growth, and fatigue that waxes and wanes. Fever, abdominal pain, digital clubbing, and chest pain may also be reported. Jaundice and hepatosplenomegaly may be present with chronic bleeding. Physical examination often reveals decreased breath sounds, rales, rhonchi, or wheezing.

B. Laboratory Findings and Imaging Studies

Laboratory studies vary depending on the cause of hemorrhage. When gross hemoptysis is present, large airway bronchiectasis, epistaxis, foreign body, and arteriovenous or pulmonary malformations should be ruled out. Flexible bronchoscopy and imaging (MRI or CT-assisted angiography) can be used to localize the site of bleeding. Alveolar bleeding with hemoptysis is often frothy and pink. The differential diagnosis includes the disorders causing diffuse alveolar hemorrhage. Following long-standing idiopathic pulmonary hemorrhage, iron deficiency anemia and heme-positive sputum are present. Nonspecific findings may include lymphocytosis and an elevated erythrocyte sedimentation rate. Peripheral eosinophilia is present in up to 25% of patients. Chest radiographs demonstrate a range of findings, from transient perihilar infiltrates to large, fluffy alveolar infiltrates with or without atelectasis and mediastinal adenopathy. Pulmonary function testing generally reveals restrictive impairment, with low lung volumes, poor compliance, and an increased diffusion capacity. Hemosiderin-laden macrophages are found in bronchial or gastric aspirates. The diagnostic usefulness of lung biopsy is controversial.

Patients with diffuse alveolar hemorrhage with an underlying systemic disease may need a lung biopsy. In patients with systemic lupus erythematosus, Wegener granulomatosis, and occasionally Goodpasture syndrome diffuse alveolar hemorrhage can occur with the histologic entity known as necrotizing pulmonary capillaritis. On lung biopsy, the alveolar septa are infiltrated with neutrophils, and alveolar hemorrhage is acute or chronic. The septa can fill with edema or fibrinoid necrosis. In idiopathic pulmonary hemosiderosis, you can see a mild form of capillaritis associated with alveolar hemorrhage that may be focal or diffuse. An immune-mediated process may cause idiopathic pulmonary hemosiderosis and capillaritis by biopsy, although no serologic marker has yet been identified. Although capillaritis has been described without evidence of underlying systemic disease, the search for collagen-vascular disease, vasculitis, or pulmonary fibrosis should be exhaustive.

The investigation should include serologic studies such as circulating antineutrophilic cytoplasmic autoantibodies for Wegener granulomatosis, perinuclear antineutrophilic cytoplasmic autoantibodies for microscopic polyangiitis, antinuclear antibodies for systemic lupus erythematosus, and anti–basement membrane antibodies for Goodpasture syndrome. α_1-Antitrypsin deficiency has been associated with vasculitides and should be considered.

Suspected cases of cow's milk–induced pulmonary hemosiderosis (Heiner syndrome) can be confirmed by laboratory findings that include high titers of serum precipitins to multiple constituents of cow's milk and positive intradermal skin tests to various cow's milk proteins. Improvement after an empiric trial of a diet free of cow's milk also supports the diagnosis.

Differential Diagnosis

Bleeding from the nose or mouth can present as hemoptysis. Therefore, a complete examination of the nose and mouth is required before confirming the diagnosis of intrapulmonary bleeding. Hematemesis can also be confused with hemoptysis; confirming that the blood was produced after coughing and not with emesis should, therefore, also be part of the initial evaluations. A complete past medical history including underlying systemic illness and cardiac or vascular anomalies may direct the search for the site of respiratory bleeding.

Treatment

Therapy should be aimed at direct treatment of the underlying disease. In severe bleeding, intubation with application of positive pressure during mechanical ventilation may help attenuate bleeding. Patients with cystic fibrosis or bronchiectasis from other causes who develop massive (> 240 ml) or recurrent hemoptysis, bronchial artery embolization may be necessary. An interventional radiologist with experience with this procedure should be consulted immediately. Although its use requires anticoagulation, extracorporal life support has resulted in the survival of children with severe pulmonary hemorrhage. For more chronic bleeding, supportive measures, including iron therapy, supplemental oxygen, and blood transfusions, may be needed. A diet free of cow's milk should be tried in infants. Systemic corticosteroids have been used for various causes of diffuse alveolar hemorrhage and have been particularly successful in those secondary to collagen-vascular disorders and vasculitis. Case reports have been published describing the variable effectiveness of steroids, chloroquine, cyclophosphamide, and azathioprine for idiopathic pulmonary hemosiderosis.

Prognosis

The outcome of pulmonary hemorrhage depends on the cause of the bleeding and how much blood has been lost. The course of idiopathic pulmonary hemosiderosis is variable, characterized by a waxing and waning course of intermittent intrapulmonary bleeds and the gradual development of pulmonary fibrosis over time. The severity of the underlying renal disease contributes to the mortality rates associated with Goodpasture syndrome and Wegener granulomatosis. Diffuse alveolar hemorrhage is considered a lethal pulmonary complication of systemic lupus erythematosus.

Bull TM et al: Pulmonary vascular manifestations of mixed connective tissue disease. Rheum Dis Clin North Am 2005;31:451 [PMID: 16084318].

Flume PA et al: Cystic fibrosis pulmonary guidelines–pulmonary complications: Hemoptysis and pneumothorax. Am J Respir Crit Care Med 2010;182(3):298 [PMID: 20675678].

Godfrey S: Pulmonary hemorrhage/hemoptysis in children. Pediatr Pulmonol 2004;37:476 [PMID: 15114547].

Ioachimescu OC et al: Idiopathic pulmonary haemosiderosis revisited. Eur Respir J 2004;24:162 [PMID: 15293620].

Sherman J et al: Time course of hemosiderin production and clearance by human pulmonary macrophages. Chest 1984;86:409 [PMID: 6468000].

PULMONARY EMBOLISM

General Considerations

Although pulmonary embolism is rarely diagnosed in children, the incidence is probably underestimated because it is often not considered in the differential diagnosis of respiratory distress. It occurs most commonly in children with: sickle cell anemia as part of the acute chest syndrome, malignancy, rheumatic fever, infective endocarditis, schistosomiasis, bone fracture, dehydration, polycythemia, nephrotic syndrome, atrial fibrillation, and other conditions. A recent report suggests that a majority of children with pulmonary emboli referred for hematology evaluation have coagulation regulatory protein abnormalities and antiphospholipid antibodies. Emboli may be single or multiple, large or small, with clinical signs and symptoms dependent on the severity of pulmonary vascular obstruction. In children, tumor emboli are a more common cause of massive pulmonary embolism than embolization from a lower extremity deep venous thrombosis.

Clinical Findings

A. Symptoms and Signs

Pulmonary embolism usually presents clinically as an acute onset of dyspnea and tachypnea. Heart palpitations or a sense of impending doom may be reported.

Pleuritic chest pain and hemoptysis may be present (not common), along with splinting, cyanosis, and tachycardia. Massive emboli may be present with syncope and cardiac arrhythmias. Physical examination is usually normal (except for tachycardia and tachypnea) unless the embolism is associated with an underlying disorder. Mild hypoxemia, rales, focal wheezing, or a pleural friction rub may be found.

B. Laboratory Findings and Imaging Studies

Radiographic findings may be normal, but a peripheral infiltrate, small pleural effusion, or elevated hemidiaphragm can be present. If the emboli are massive, differential blood flow and pulmonary artery enlargement may be appreciated. The electrocardiogram is usually normal unless the pulmonary embolus is massive. Echocardiography is useful in detecting the presence of a large proximal embolus. A negative D-dimer has a more than 95% negative predictive value for an embolus. Ventilation-perfusion scans show localized areas of ventilation without perfusion.

Spiral CT with contrast may be helpful, but pulmonary angiography is the gold standard. A recent case series suggests that bedside chest ultrasound may aid in diagnosing pulmonary emboli, particularly in critically ill children. Further evaluation may include Doppler ultrasound studies of the legs to search for deep venous thrombosis. Coagulation studies, including assessments of antithrombin III, fibrinogen, antiphospholipid antibodies, homocystine, coagulation regulatory proteins (proteins C and S, and factor V Leiden), and the prothrombin G20210A mutation should be obtained. Abnormalities have been demonstrated in 70% of the hematology referrals in one pediatric institution.

Treatment

Acute treatment includes supplemental oxygen, sedation, and anticoagulation. Current recommendations include heparin administration to maintain an activated partial thromboplastin time that is 1.5 or more times the control value for the first 24 hours. Urokinase or tissue plasminogen activator can be used to help dissolve the embolus. These therapies should be followed by warfarin therapy for at least 6 weeks with an international normalized ratio (INR) greater than 2. In patients with identifiable deep venous thrombosis of the lower extremities and significant pulmonary emboli (with hemodynamic compromise despite anticoagulation), inferior vena caval interruption may be necessary. However, long-term prospective data regarding this latter therapy are lacking.

Baird JS et al: Massive pulmonary embolism in children. J Pediatr 2010;156:148 [PMID: 20006766].

Bounameaux H: Review: ELISA D-dimer is sensitive but not specific in diagnosing pulmonary embolism in an ambulatory clinical setting. ACP J Club 2003;138:24 [PMID: 12511136].

Konstantinides S et al: Heparin plus alteplase compared with heparin alone in patients with submassive pulmonary embolism. N Engl J Med 2002;347:1143 [PMID: 12374874].

Kosiak M et al: Is chest sonography a breakthrough in diagnosis of pulmonary thromboembolism in children? Pediatr Pulmonol 2008;43:1183 [PMID: 19009615].

Rahimtoola A et al: Acute pulmonary embolism: An update on diagnosis and management. Curr Probl Cardiology 2005;30:61 [PMID: 15650680].

PULMONARY EDEMA

General Considerations

Pulmonary edema is excessive accumulation of extravascular fluid in the lung. This occurs when fluid is filtered into the lungs faster than it can be removed, leading to changes in lung mechanics such as decreased lung compliance, worsening hypoxemia from ventilation-perfusion mismatch, bronchial compression, and if advanced, decreased surfactant function. There are two basic types of pulmonary edema: increased pressure (cardiogenic or hydrostatic) and increased permeability (noncardiogenic or primary). Hydrostatic pulmonary edema is usually due to excessive increases in pulmonary venous pressure, which is most commonly due to congestive heart failure from multiple causes. Postobstructive pulmonary edema occurs when airway occlusion (or its sudden relief) causes a sudden drop in airway pressure which leads to increased venous return and decreased left heart blood flow. These changes result in elevated hydrostatic pressures and transudation of fluid from the pulmonary capillaries to the alveolar space.

In contrast, many lung diseases, especially acute respiratory distress syndrome, are characterized by the development of pulmonary edema secondary to changes in permeability due to injury to the alveolocapillary barrier. In these settings, pulmonary edema occurs independently of the elevations of pulmonary venous pressure.

Clinical Findings

A. Symptoms and Signs

Cyanosis, tachypnea, tachycardia, and respiratory distress are commonly present. Physical findings include rales, diminished breath sounds, and (in young infants) expiratory wheezing. More severe disease is characterized by progressive respiratory distress with marked retractions, dyspnea, and severe hypoxemia.

B. Imaging Studies

Chest radiographic findings depend on the cause of the edema. Pulmonary vessels are prominent, often with diffuse interstitial or alveolar infiltrates. Heart size is usually normal in permeability edema but enlarged in hydrostatic edema.

Treatment

Although specific therapy depends on the underlying cause, supplemental oxygen therapy, and ventilator support may be indicated. Diuretics, digoxin, and vasodilators may be indicated for congestive heart failure along with restriction of salt and water. Loop diuretics, such as furosemide, are primarily beneficial because they increase systemic venous capacitance, not because they induce diuresis. Improvement can even be seen in anuric patients. Recommended interventions for permeability edema are reduction of vascular volume and maintenance of the lowest central venous or pulmonary arterial wedge pressure possible without sacrificing cardiac output or causing hypotension (see following discussion). β-Adrenergic agonists such as terbutaline have been shown to increase alveolar clearance of lung water, perhaps through the action of a sodium-potassium channel pump. Maintaining normal albumin levels and a hematocrit concentration above 30 maintains the filtration of lung liquid toward the capillaries, avoiding low oncotic pressure.

High altitude pulmonary edema (HAPE) occurs when susceptible individuals develop noncardiogenic edema after rapid ascent to altitudes above 3000 m. Children may develop HAPE with variation in severity. Oxygen therapy and prompt descent are the cornerstones of therapy for this illness.

Bartsch P et al: Physiologic aspects of high-altitude pulmonary edema. J Appl Physiol 2005;98:1101.

O'Brodovich H: Pulmonary edema in infants and children. Curr Opin Pediatr 2005;17:381 [PMID: 15891430].

Redding GJ: Current concepts in adult respiratory distress syndrome in children. Curr Opin Pediatr 2001;13:261 [PMID: 11389362].

Udeshi A et al: Postobstructive pulmonary edema. Journal of Critical Care 2010;25:508 [PMID: 20413250].

CONGENITAL PULMONARY LYMPHANGIECTASIA

General Considerations

Structurally, congenital pulmonary lymphangiectasia appears as dilated subpleural and interlobular lymphatic channels and may present as part of a generalized lymphangiectasis (in association with obstructive cardiovascular lesions—especially total anomalous pulmonary venous return) or as an isolated idiopathic lesion. Pathologically, the lung appears firm, bulky, and noncompressible, with prominent cystic lymphatics visible beneath the pleura. On cut section, dilated lymphatics are present near the hilum, along interlobular septa, around bronchovascular bundles, and beneath the pleura. Histologically, dilated lymphatics have a thin endothelial cell lining overlying a delicate network of elastin and collagen.

Clinical Findings

Congenital pulmonary lymphangiectasia is a rare, usually fatal disease that generally presents as acute or persistent respiratory distress at birth. Although most patients do not survive the newborn period, some survive longer, and there are case reports of its diagnosis later in childhood. Congenital pulmonary lymphangiectasia may be associated with features of Noonan syndrome, asplenia, total anomalous pulmonary venous return, septal defects, atrioventricular canal, hypoplastic left heart, aortic arch malformations, and renal malformations. Chylothorax has been reported. Chest radiographic findings include a ground-glass appearance, prominent interstitial markings suggesting lymphatic distention, diffuse hyperlucency of the pulmonary parenchyma, and hyperinflation with depression of the diaphragm.

Prognosis

Although the onset of symptoms may be delayed for as long as the first few months of life, prolonged survival is rare. Most deaths occur within weeks after birth. However, more recent studies have shown that respiratory symptoms do improve after the first year of life suggesting that maximal medical treatment remains warranted. In those with the most severe disease, rapid diagnosis is essential in order to expedite the option of lung transplantation.

Barker PM et al: Primary pulmonary lymphangiectasia in infancy and childhood. Eur Respir J 2004;24(3):413 [PMID: 15358700].

Esther CR et al: Pulmonary lymphangiectasia: Diagnosis and clinical course. Pediatr Pulmonol 2004;38:308 [PMID: 15334508].

Huber A et al: Congenital pulmonary lymphangiectasia. Pediatr Pulmonol 1991;10:310 [PMID: 1896243].

Mettauer N et al: Outcome of children with pulmonary lymphangiectasis. Pediatr Pulmonol 2009;44:351 [PMID: 19330773].

DISORDERS OF THE CHEST WALL AND DIAPHRAGM

SCOLIOSIS

Scoliosis is defined as lateral curvature of the spine and is commonly categorized as idiopathic, congenital, or neuromuscular. No pulmonary impairment is typically seen with a Cobb angle showing thoracic curvature of less than 35 degrees. Most cases of idiopathic scoliosis occur in adolescent girls and are corrected before significant pulmonary impairment occurs. Congenital scoliosis of severe degree or with other major abnormalities carries a more guarded prognosis. Patients with progressive neuromuscular disease, such as Duchenne muscular dystrophy, can be at risk for respiratory failure due to severe scoliosis. Severe scoliosis can also lead to impaired lung function and possible death from cor pulmonale if uncorrected. (See also Chapter 26.)

Greiner KA: Adolescent idiopathic scoliosis: Radiologic decision-making. Am Fam Physician 2002;65:1817 [PMID: 12018804].

Kearon C et al: Factors determining pulmonary function in adolescent idiopathic thoracic scoliosis. Am Rev Respir Dis 1993;148:288 [PMID: 8342890].

PECTUS CARINATUM

Pectus carinatum is a protrusion of the upper or lower (more common) portion of the sternum, more commonly seen in males. Again, although the disorder may have a psychological impact, impedance of cardiopulmonary function is debated. The decision to repair this deformity is often based upon cosmetic concerns, but research has shown that those with reduced endurance or dyspnea with mild exercise experienced marked improvement within 6 months following repair, suggesting possible physiologic indications. Pectus carinatum may be associated with systemic diseases such as the mucopolysaccharidoses and congenital heart disease.

Borowitz D et al: Pulmonary function and exercise response in patients with pectus excavatum after Nuss repair. J Pediatr Surg 2003;38:544 [PMID: 12677562].

Lawson ML et al: Impact of pectus excavatum on pulmonary function before and after repair with the Nuss procedure. J Pediatr Surg 2005;40:174 [PMID: 15868581].

Malek MH et al: Ventilatory and cardiovascular responses to exercise in patients with pectus excavatum. Chest 2003;124:870 [PMID: 12970011].

PECTUS EXCAVATUM

Pectus excavatum is anterior depression of the chest wall that may be symmetrical or asymmetrical with respect to the midline. Its presence can be psychologically difficult for the patient. Whether or not it is cause for cardiopulmonary limitations is controversial. While subjective exertional dyspnea can be reported and may improve with repair, objective cardiopulmonary function may not change postoperatively. Therefore, the decision to repair the deformity may be based on cosmetic or physiologic considerations. Surgical literature provides more information regarding long-term outcomes following repair. Timing of repair is critical in light of growth plate maturation. Pectus excavatum may be associated with congenital heart disease.

Fonkalsrud EW, Anselmo DM: Less extensive techniques for repair of pectus carinatum: The undertreated chest deformity. J Am Coll Surg 2004;198:898 [PMID: 15194071].

Williams AM, Crabbe DC: Pectus deformities of the anterior chest wall. Paediatr Respir Rev 2003;4:237 [PMID: 12880759].

NEUROMUSCULAR DISORDERS

Neuromuscular disorders are discussed in detail in Chapter 25. Weakness of the respiratory and pharyngeal muscles leads to chronic or recurrent pneumonia secondary to weak cough and poor mucous clearance, aspiration and infection, persistent atelectasis, hypoventilation, and respiratory failure in severe cases. Scoliosis, which frequently accompanies longstanding neuromuscular disorders, may further compromise respiratory function. Children born with significant neuromuscular weakness may present with signs and symptoms of respiratory compromise early in life. The time to presentation for children with progressive or acquired neuromuscular disease will depend upon the progression of their disease. Typical examination findings in children at increased risk for pulmonary disease are a weak cough, decreased air exchange, crackles, wheezing, and dullness to percussion. The child also may have symptoms of obstructive sleep apnea and decreased lung function by spirometry and/or lung volume analysis. Signs of cor pulmonale (loud pulmonary component to the second heart sound, hepatomegaly, and elevated neck veins) may be evident in advanced cases. Chest radiographs generally show small lung volumes. If chronic aspiration is present, increased interstitial infiltrates and areas of atelectasis or consolidation may be present. Arterial blood gases demonstrate hypoxemia in the early stages and compensated respiratory acidosis in the late stages. Typical pulmonary function abnormalities include low lung volumes and decreased inspiratory force generated against an occluded airway.

Treatment is supportive and includes vigorous pulmonary toilet, antibiotics with infection, and oxygen to correct hypoxemia. Consideration of bilevel positive airway pressure and mechanical airway clearance support, like mechanical inexsufflation, should be introduced before respiratory failure is present. Unfortunately, despite aggressive medical therapy, many neuromuscular conditions progress to respiratory failure and death. The decision to intubate and ventilate is a difficult one; it should be made only when there is real hope that deterioration, though acute, is potentially reversible or when chronic ventilation is wanted. Chronic mechanical ventilation using either noninvasive or invasive techniques is being used more frequently in patients with chronic respiratory insufficiency.

Finder JD et al: Respiratory care of the patient with Duchenne muscular dystrophy: ATS consensus statement. Am J Respir Crit Care Med 2004;170:456 [PMID: 15302625].

Miske LJ et al: Use of the mechanical in-exsufflator in pediatric patients with neuromuscular disease and impaired cough. Chest 2004;125:1406 [PMID: 15078753].

Panitch HB: The pathophysiology of respiratory impairment in pediatric neuromuscular diseases. Pediatric 2009;123(Suppl 4): S215–S218 [PMID: 19420146].

EVENTRATION OF THE DIAPHRAGM

ESSENTIALS OF DIAGNOSIS & TYPICAL FEATURES

- Respiratory distress in a newborn.
- Recurrent pneumonia.
- Persistent elevation of the diaphragm by chest x-ray.

General Considerations

Eventration of the diaphragm occurs when striated muscle is replaced with connective tissue and is demonstrated on radiograph by elevation of a part or whole of the diaphragm. There are two types: congenital and acquired. The congenital type is thought to represent incomplete formation of the diaphragm in utero. The acquired type is related to atrophy of diaphragm muscles secondary to prenatal or postnatal phrenic nerve injury. The differential diagnosis of eventration includes phrenic nerve injury and partial diaphragmatic hernia.

Clinical Findings

A. Symptoms and Signs

The degree of respiratory distress depends on the amount of paradoxical motion of the diaphragm. When the diaphragm moves upward during inspiration, instability of the inferior border of the chest wall increases the work of breathing and can lead to respiratory muscle fatigue and potential failure when stressed. Symptoms include persistent increased work of breathing, particularly with feeding or failure to extubate.

B. Laboratory Findings and Imaging Studies

Small eventrations may be an incidental finding on a chest radiograph, commonly seen on the right side. Ultrasound provides useful information to further define a suspected eventration. When defects are small, there is no paradoxical movement of the diaphragm and little symptomatology. When defects are large, paradoxical movement of the diaphragm may be present.

Treatment

Treatment is based on severity of symptoms. If symptoms persist for 2–4 weeks, the diaphragm is surgically plicated, which stabilizes it. Function returns to the diaphragm in about 50% of cases of phrenic nerve injury whether or not plication was performed. Recovery periods of up to 100 days have been reported in these cases.

Clements BS: Congenital malformations of the lungs and airways. In Taussig LM, Landau LI (editors): *Pediatric Respiratory Medicine*. Mosby, 1999.

Eren S et al: Congenital diaphragmatic eventration as a cause of anterior mediastinal mass in children: Imaging modalities and literature review. Eur J Radiol 2004;51:85 [PMID: 15186890].

DISORDERS OF THE PLEURA & PLEURAL CAVITY

The *parietal* pleura covers the inner surface of the chest wall. The *visceral* pleura covers the outer surface of the lungs. Disease processes can lead to accumulation of air or fluid or both in the pleural space. Pleural effusions are classified as transudates or exudates. Transudates occur when there is imbalance between hydrostatic and oncotic pressure, so that fluid filtration exceeds reabsorption (eg, congestive heart failure). Exudates form as a result of inflammation of the pleural surface leading to increased capillary permeability (eg, parapneumonic effusions). Other pleural effusions include chylothorax and hemothorax.

Thoracentesis is helpful in characterizing the fluid and providing definitive diagnosis. Recovered fluid is considered an exudate (as opposed to a transudate) if any of the following are found: a pleural fluid–serum protein ratio greater than 0.5, a pleural fluid–serum lactate dehydrogenase ratio greater than 0.6, or a pleural fluid lactate dehydrogenase level greater than 200 U/L. Important additional studies on pleural fluid include cell count; pH and glucose; Gram stain, acid-fast and fungal stains; aerobic and anaerobic cultures; counterimmunoelectrophoresis for specific organisms; and occasionally, amylase concentration. Cytologic examination of pleural fluid should be performed to rule out leukemia or other neoplasm.

Hilliard TN et al: Management of parapneumonic effusion and empyema. Arch Dis Child 2003;88:915 [PMID: 14500314].

HEMOTHORAX

Accumulation of blood in the pleural space can be caused by surgical or accidental trauma, coagulation defects, and pleural or pulmonary tumors. A parapneumonic effusion is defined as a hemothorax when the hematocrit of the fluid is more than 50% of the peripheral blood. With blunt trauma, hemopneumothorax may be present. Symptoms are related to blood loss and compression of underlying lung parenchyma. There is some risk of secondary infection, resulting in empyema.

Treatment

Drainage of a hemothorax is required when significant compromise of pulmonary function is present, as with hemopneumothorax. In uncomplicated cases, observation is indicated because blood is readily absorbed spontaneously from the pleural space.

VATS has been used successfully in the management of hemothorax. Chest CT scan is helpful to select patients who may require surgery, as identification of blood and the volume of blood may be more predictive by this method than by chest radiograph.

Bliss D, Silen M: Pediatric thoracic trauma. Crit Care Med 2002; 30(Suppl):S409 [PMID: 12528782].

Muzumdar H, Arens R: Pleural fluid. Pediatr Rev 2007;28(12): 462–464 [PMID: 18055645].

CHYLOTHORAX

The accumulation of chyle, fluid of intestinal origin containing fat digestion products mostly lipids), in the pleural space usually results from accidental or surgical trauma to the thoracic duct. The most common cause of a pleural effusion in the first few days of life is a chylothorax. In a newborn, chylothorax can be due to congenital abnormalities of the lymph vessels or secondary to birth trauma. In an older child, chylothoracies can be due to: laceration or obstruction of the thoracic duct due to trauma or any surgery involving the chest wall (cardiac surgery, scoliosis repair etc); obstruction of the vessels due to a benign or malignant mass or lymphadenopathy; or increased venous pressure due to obstruction or left ventricular failure. Symptoms of chylothorax are related to the amount of fluid accumulation and the degree of compromise of underlying pulmonary parenchyma. Thoracentesis reveals typical milky fluid (unless the patient has been fasting) containing chiefly T lymphocytes.

Treatment

Treatment should be conservative because many chylothoraces resolve spontaneously. Oral feedings with medium-chain triglycerides reduce lymphatic flow through the thoracic duct. Recent literature has shown somatostatin and octreotide as viable therapeutic options. Drainage of chylous effusions should be performed only for respiratory compromised because the fluid often rapidly reaccumulates. Repeated or continuous drainage may lead to protein malnutrition and T-cell depletion, rendering the patient relatively immunocompromised. If reaccumulation of fluid persists, surgical ligation of the thoracic duct or sclerosis of the pleural space can be attempted, although the results may be less than satisfactory.

Helin RD, Angeles ST, Bhat R: Octreotide therapy for chylothorax in infants and children: A brief review. Pediatr Crit Care Med 2006 Nov;7(6):576–579 [PMID: 16878051].

Soto-Martinez M, Massie J: Chylothorax: Diagnosis and management in children. Paediatr Respir Rev 2009;10(4):199–207 [PMID: 19879510].

PNEUMOTHORAX & RELATED AIR LEAK SYNDROMES

ESSENTIALS OF DIAGNOSIS & TYPICAL FEATURES

- Sudden onset shortness of breath.
- Focal area of absent breath sounds on chest auscultation.
- Shift of the trachea away from the area with absent breath sounds.

Pneumothorax can occur spontaneously in newborns and in older children, or more commonly, as a result of birth trauma, positive pressure ventilation, underlying obstructive or restrictive lung disease, or rupture of a congenital or acquired lung cyst. Pneumothorax can also occur as an acute complication of tracheostomy. Air usually dissects from the alveolar spaces into the interstitial spaces of the lung. Migration to the visceral pleura ultimately leads to rupture into the pleural space. Associated conditions include pneumomediastinum, pneumopericardium, pneumoperitoneum, and subcutaneous emphysema. These conditions are more commonly associated with dissection of air into the interstitial spaces of the lung with retrograde dissection along the bronchovascular bundles toward the hilum.

Clinical Findings

A. Symptoms and Signs

The clinical spectrum can vary from asymptomatic to severe respiratory distress. Associated symptoms include cyanosis, chest pain, and dyspnea. Physical examination may reveal decreased breath sounds and hyperresonance to percussion on the affected side with tracheal deviation to the opposite side. When pneumothorax is under tension, cardiac function may be compromised, resulting in hypotension or narrowing of the pulse pressure. Pneumopericardium is a life-threatening condition that presents with muffled heart tones and shock. Pneumomediastinum rarely causes other than chest pain symptoms by itself.

B. Diagnostic Studies

Chest radiographs usually demonstrate the presence of free air in the pleural space. If the pneumothorax is large and under tension, compressive atelectasis of the underlying lung and shift of the mediastinum to the opposite side may be demonstrated. Cross-table lateral and lateral decubitus radiographs can aid in the diagnosis of free air. Pneumopericardium is identified by the presence of air completely surrounding the heart, whereas in patients with pneumomediastinum, the heart and mediastinal structures may be outlined with air, but the air does not involve the diaphragmatic cardiac border. Chest CT scan may be helpful with recurrent spontaneous pneumothoraces to look for subtle pulmonary disease not seen on chest radiograph, but this is debated.

Differential Diagnosis

Acute deterioration of a patient on a ventilator can be caused by tension pneumothorax, obstruction or dislodgment of the endotracheal tube, or ventilator failure. Radiographically, pneumothorax must be distinguished from diaphragmatic hernia, lung cysts, congenital lobar emphysema, and cystic adenomatoid malformation, but this task is usually not difficult.

Treatment

Small (<15%) or asymptomatic pneumothoraces usually do not require treatment and can be managed with close observation. Larger or symptomatic pneumothoraces require drainage, although inhalation of 100% oxygen to wash out blood nitrogen can be tried. Needle aspiration should be used to relieve tension acutely, followed by chest tube or pigtail catheter placement. Pneumopericardium requires immediate identification, and if clinically symptomatic, needle aspiration to prevent death, followed by pericardial tube placement.

Prognosis

In older patients with spontaneous pneumothorax, recurrences are common; sclerosing and surgical procedures are often required.

Baumann MH et al: Management of spontaneous pneumothorax: An American College of Chest Physicians Delphi Consensus Statement. ACCP Pneumothorax Consensus Group. Chest 2001;119:590 [PMID: 11171742].

Johnson NN, Toledo A, Endom EE: Pnuemothorax, pneumomediastinum, and pulmonary embolism. Pediatri Clin North Am 2010;57(6):1357–1383 [PMID: 21111122].

MEDIASTINUM

MEDIASTINAL MASSES

General Considerations

Children with mediastinal masses may present because of symptoms produced by pressure on the esophagus, airways, nerves, or vessels within the mediastinum, or the masses may be discovered on a routine chest radiograph. Once the mass is identified, localization to one of four mediastinal compartments aids in the differential diagnosis. The superior mediastinum is the area above the pericardium that is bordered inferiorly by an imaginary line from the manubrium to the fourth thoracic vertebra. The anterior mediastinum is bordered by the sternum anteriorly and the pericardium posteriorly, and the posterior mediastinum is defined by the pericardium and diaphragm anteriorly and the lower eight thoracic vertebrae posteriorly. The middle mediastinum is surrounded by these three compartments.

Clinical Findings

A. Symptoms and Signs

Respiratory symptoms, when present, are due to pressure on an airway (cough or wheezing) or an infection (unresolving pneumonia in one area of lung). Hemoptysis can also occur but is an unusual presenting symptom. Dysphagia may occur secondary to compression of the esophagus. Pressure on the recurrent laryngeal nerve can cause hoarseness due to paralysis of the left vocal cord. Superior vena caval syndrome presents with dilation of neck vessels and other signs and symptoms of venous obstruction from the head and neck: superior mediastinal syndrome presents similarly but includes tracheal compression.

B. Laboratory Findings and Imaging

The mass is initially defined by frontal and lateral chest radiographs together with thoracic CT scans or MRI. A barium esophagram may also help define the extent of a mass. Other studies that may be required include angiography (to define the blood supply to large tumors), electrocardiography, echocardiography, ultrasound of the thorax, fungal and mycobacterial skin tests, and urinary catecholamine assays. MRI or myelography may be necessary in children suspected of having a neurogenic tumor in the posterior mediastinum. Mediastinal masses, particularly anterior masses, can cause life-threatening airway compromise during sedation even in patients with mild symptoms; thus, any sedation or anesthesia should be avoided if possible and performed cautiously if absolutely necessary.

Differential Diagnosis

The differential diagnosis of mediastinal masses is determined by their location. Within the superior mediastinum, one may find cystic hygromas, vascular or neurogenic tumors, thymic masses, teratomas, intrathoracic thyroid tissue, mediastinal abscess, and esophageal lesions. Within the anterior mediastinum, thymic tissue (thymomas, hyperplasia, cysts and intrathoracic thyroid) and teratomas, vascular tumors, and lymphatic tissue (lymphomas, leukemia, or reactive lymphadenopathy) give rise to masses. Within the middle mediastinum one may again find lymphomas and hypertrophic lymph nodes, granulomas, bronchogenic or enterogenous cysts, metastases, and pericardial cysts. Abnormalities of the great vessels and aortic aneurysms may also present as masses in this compartment. Within the posterior mediastinum, neurogenic tumors, enterogenous cysts, thoracic meningoceles, or aortic aneurysms may be present.

In some series, more than 50% of mediastinal tumors occur in the posterior mediastinum and are mainly neurogenic tumors or enterogenous cysts. Most neurogenic tumors in children younger than age 4 years are malignant (neuroblastoma or neuroganglioblastoma), whereas a benign ganglioneuroma is the most common histologic type in older children. In the middle and anterior mediastinum, lymphoma and leukemia are the primary concern. Definitive diagnosis in most instances relies on surgery to obtain the mass or a part of the mass for histologic examination.

Treatment & Prognosis

The appropriate therapy and the response to therapy depend on the cause of the mediastinal mass.

Franco A et al: Imaging evaluation of pediatric mediastinal masses. Radiol Clin North Am 2005;43:325 [PMID: 15737372].

Garey CL et al: Management of anterior mediastinal masses in children. Eur J Pediatr Surg 2011;July 12 e-published.

SLEEP-DISORDERED BREATHING

General Considerations

Sleep apnea is recognized as a major public health problem in adults, with the risk of excessive daytime sleepiness, driving accidents, poor work performance, and effects on mental health. Pediatric sleep disorders are less commonly recognized because of a lack of training in sleep problem recognition and the presentation, risks, and outcome all differ from those in adults. The spectrum of sleep-disordered breathing includes obstructive sleep apnea, upper airway resistance disorder, and primary snoring. Sleep apnea is defined as cessation of breathing and can be classified as obstructive (the attempt to breathe through an obstructed airway) or central (the lack of effort to breathe). Snoring, mouth breathing, and upper airway obstruction are discussed in Chapter 18.

Clinical Findings & Differential Diagnosis

A. Obstructive Sleep Apnea

Obstructive sleep apnea occurs in normal children with an incidence of about 2%, increasing in children with craniofacial abnormalities, neuropathies, or other medical problems. The incidence also increases when children are medicated with hypnotics, sedatives, or anticonvulsants. While not all children who snore have sleep apnea, there is evidence that snoring without gas-exchange abnormalities has neurobehavioral consequences. Obstructive sleep apnea should be suspected whenever a child presents with frequent or habitual snoring, witnessed apnea, labored breathing, frequent nighttime arousals, failure to thrive, oxygen desaturations, life-threatening events, behavior abnormalities, obesity, or craniofacial abnormalities. Upper airway resistance syndrome is characterized by daytime fatigue or sleepiness in the presence of a snoring without gas-exchange abnormalities on the polysomnogram. Symptoms are similar to obstructive sleep apnea, including snoring, change in appetite, poor performance in school, and problems with behavior. This chronic flow limitation often improves with treatment. In children, airway obstruction is often associated with adenotonsillar hypertrophy. Tonsillar hypertrophy is most common between the ages of two and seven years. Obesity is widely recognized as an etiologic component in adult OSA and has been similarly cited in children. In children, consequences of sleep apnea include failure to thrive, pulmonary hypertension, deficits of cognition, poor school performance, and psychiatric or behavioral problems.

B. Central Sleep Apnea

Central apneas are seen in infants and children. These are pauses in breathing without concomitant effort. Clinical significance is uncertain, but they may be relevant if they occur frequently or gas-exchange problems or sleep fragmentation occurs. Healthy children have been shown to have central apneas lasting 25 seconds without clear consequences. In comparison, central hypoventilation syndrome patients have intact voluntary control of ventilation, but lack automatic control. During sleep, they will hypoventilate to the point at which they need ventilatory support that may require treatment with positive airway pressure and a rated tidal volume via a noninvasive mask or tracheostomy. Central hypoventilation may occur with low tidal volume breathing and not discreet central apneas, and requires treatment of gas-exchange problems.

C. Diagnostic Studies

Several studies have shown that clinical history and physical exam alone are not enough to identify children with

OSA and that polysomnography should be performed in all suspected cases. This test measures sleep state with electroencephalogram leads and electromyography, airflow at the nose, chest and abdominal muscle movement, heart rate and rhythm, gas exchange (CO_2 and oxygenation), and leg movements, along with other potential data including body position, vibrations representing snoring, and esophageal pH/impedence. Polysomnography allows diagnosis of various forms of apnea, sleep fragmentation, periodic limb movement disorder, or other sleep disorders of children. Overnight oximetry is not an ideal study to diagnose obstructive sleep apnea. While it may identify subjects with severe obstructive sleep apnea, its sensitivity is low. Literature has shown normal oximetry studies in half a population of subjects with polysomnographically confirmed obstructive sleep apnea.

Treatment

First-line therapy for obstructive sleep apnea in children is adenotonsillectomy, which improves the clinical status for most children with normal craniofacial structure. Even children with craniofacial anomalies or neuromuscular disorders may benefit, although additional treatment with continuous positive airway pressure may be indicated (Roland et al: S1–S15). Down syndrome presents unique challenges: up to half of these children can still have obstructive sleep apnea despite adenotonsillectomy. Treatment of young or developmentally delayed children with apnea also presents several challenges. (See Chapter 18 for additional discussion.) Other therapies, such as, nasal steroids, leukotriene modifiers (Goldbart et al: 364–370), oral appliances, rapid maxillary expanders, and weight loss have their roles in select patient populations.

Because the presentation of sleep apnea is quite varied among children, pediatric sleep disorder centers are the referral of choice for testing and initiation of therapy.

Aurora RN et al: American Academy of Sleep Medicine. Practice parameters for the respiratory indications for polysomnography in children. Sleep 2011 Mar 1;34(3):379–388 [PMID: 21359087].

Capdevila OS et al: Pediatric obstructive sleep apnea: Complications, management, and long-term outcomes. Proc Am Thorac Soc 2008;5(2):274–282.

Marcus CL: Sleep-disordered breathing in children. Am J Respir Crit Care Med 2001;164:16 [PMID: 11435234].

Owens JA: Neurocognitive and behavioral impact of sleep disordered breathing in children. Pediatr Pulmonol 2009 May;44(5):417–422 [PMID: 19382210].

Sateia MJ (editor): *The International Classification of Sleep Disorders,* 2nd ed. American Academy of Sleep Medicine, 2005.

Section on Pediatric Pulmonology, Subcommittee on Obstructive Sleep Apnea Syndrome, American Academy of Pediatrics: Clinical practice guideline: Diagnosis and management of childhood obstructive sleep apnea syndrome. Pediatrics 2002;109:704 [PMID: 11927718].

APPARENT LIFE-THREATENING EVENTS IN INFANCY

General Considerations

Apparent life-threatening events (ALTEs) are characterized as being frightening to the observer and commonly include some combination of apnea, color change (usually cyanosis or pallor), a marked change in muscle tone (usually extreme limpness), choking, or gagging. The observer sometimes fears the infant has died. The most frequent problems associated with an ALTE are gastrointestinal (~50%), neurologic (30%), respiratory (20%), cardiovascular (5%), metabolic and endocrine (< 5%), or diverse other problems, including child abuse. Up to 50% of ALTEs remain unexplained and are referred to as apnea of infancy. The relationship between ALTE and future risk of sudden infant death syndrome (SIDS) is not clear, as ALTE infants tend to be slightly younger and found more often while the caretaker is awake. The term *apparent life-threatening event* replaced "near-miss SIDS" in order to distance the event from a direct association with SIDS. Literature has reported an increased risk when extreme cardiopulmonary events were present at the time of the ALTE. About 12%–15% of both SIDS victims and infants dying unexpectedly of a known cause (SUDI) have had a prior history of ALTE, but most do not.

The mechanism for ALTEs is unknown, but because they do not occur after infancy, immaturity is felt to play a major role. Classic studies on the nervous system, reflexes, or responses to apnea or gastroesophageal reflux during sleep in infants and immature animals show profound cardiovascular changes during stimulation of the vagus nerve where adults would not be affected. More recently, an association of endogenous opioids and opioid-induced respiratory depression has been implicated as an association with ALTE in infants, and is an area of exciting research. The following section describes an approach to the patient who has undergone an ALTE, taking note of the very broad differential diagnosis and uncertainties in both evaluation and treatment.

Clinical Findings & Differential Diagnosis

A. History and Physical Examination

Table 19–6 classifies disorders associated with ALTEs. As seen from the outset, the causes of ALTEs are multifactorial, but it is the response to the trigger that creates a symptom cluster unique to infants. A careful history is often the most helpful part of the evaluation. In a large epidemiological study of infants who later died of SIDS or SUDI, a careful history using a "baby check" score was useful in identifying infants who were seriously ill. It is useful to determine whether the infant has been ill or essentially well. A history of several days of poor feeding, temperature instability, or respiratory or gastrointestinal symptoms suggests an infectious process. Reports of "struggling to breathe" or "trying to breathe" imply airway

Table 19–6. Potential causes of apparent life-threatening events.

Infectious	Viral: respiratory syncytial virus and other respiratory *viruses* Bacterial: sepsis, pertussis, Chlamydia
Gastrointestinal	Gastroesophageal reflux with or without obstructive apnea
Respiratory	Airway abnormality; vascular rings, pulmonary slings, tracheomalacia Pneumonia
Neurologic	Seizure disorder Central nervous system infection: meningitis, encephalitis Vasovagal response Leigh encephalopathy Brain tumor
Cardiovascular	Congenital malformation Dysrhythmias Cardiomyopathy
Nonaccidental trauma	Battering Drug overdose Munchausen syndrome by proxy
No definable cause	Apnea of infancy

obstruction. Association of the episodes with feeding implies discoordinated swallowing, gastroesophageal reflux, or delayed gastric emptying, or may imply an airway abnormality, but these awake episodes may lead to very different diagnoses than those episodes occurring during sleep. Episodes that typically follow crying may be related to breath-holding. Association of episodes with sleeping may also suggest seizure, gastroesophageal reflux, apnea of infancy, or sleep-disordered breathing. Attempts should be made to determine the duration of the episode, but this is often difficult. It is helpful to role-play the episode with the family. Details regarding the measures taken to resuscitate the infant and the infant's recovery from the episode may be useful in determining severity.

The physical examination provides further direction in pursuing the diagnosis. Fever or hypothermia suggests infection. An altered state of consciousness implies a postictal state or drug overdose. Respiratory distress implies cardiac or pulmonary lesions.

Apneic episodes have been linked to child abuse in several ways. Head injury following nonaccidental trauma may be first brought to medical attention because of apnea. Other signs of abuse are usually immediately apparent in such cases. Drug overdose, either accidental or intentional, may also present with apnea. Several series document that apneic episodes may be falsely reported by parents seeking attention (ie, Munchausen syndrome by proxy). Parents may physically interfere with a child's respiratory efforts, in which case pinch marks on the nares are sometimes found.

B. Laboratory Findings

Most patients are hospitalized for observation in order to reduce stress on the family and allow prompt completion of the evaluation. Laboratory evaluation includes a complete blood count for evidence of infection. Diagnostic testing should be based very heavily on the history and physical exam. Laboratory evaluation might include a complete blood count, blood culture with urinalysis and urine culture for evidence of infection, especially in the face of fever, hypothermia, or an abnormal physical exam. Serum electrolytes might be considered as elevations in serum bicarbonate suggest chronic hypoventilation, whereas decreases suggest acute acidosis, perhaps due to hypoxia during the episode. Chronic acidosis suggests an inherited metabolic disorder. Arterial blood gas studies provide an initial assessment of oxygenation and acid-base status, and low PaO_2 or elevated $PaCO_2$ (or both) implies cardiorespiratory disease. A significant base deficit suggests that the episode was accompanied by hypoxia or circulatory impairment. Oxygen saturation measurements in the hospital assess oxygenation status during different activities and are more comprehensive than a single blood gas sample. Because apnea has been associated with respiratory infections, diagnostic studies for RSV and other viruses, pertussis, and *Chlamydia* may help with diagnosis. Apnea occurring with infection often precedes other physical findings.

C. Imaging

The chest radiograph is examined for infiltrates suggesting acute infection or chronic aspiration and for cardiac size as a clue to intrinsic cardiac disease. If the episode might have involved airway obstruction, the airway should be examined either directly, by fiberoptic bronchoscopy, or radiographically, by CT or barium swallow. Barium swallow is a useful tool to rule out the possibility of anatomic abnormalities such as vascular ring and tracheoesophageal fistula. Esophageal pH monitoring is only helpful if the infant has sufficiently acidified the stomach, and can underestimate the degree of reflux for nonacid events. Impedence monitors improve this interpretation. Gastroesophageal reflux is one of the most common findings in infants with ALTE; however, it may be a marker of autonomic immaturity as opposed to a diagnosis for the event. Most infants with reflux and apnea can be given medical antireflux treatment. Infants with reflux and repeated episodes of apnea may benefit from a surgical antireflux procedure.

D. Polysomnography and Other Studies

ALTEs occur in the same age group as infants who die of sudden death (2–4 months is the peak age). Sleep-disordered breathing has been implicated as a possible cause of ALTEs and perhaps sudden death. Depending on the discretion of the clinician in appropriate scenarios, polysomnograms can be useful to determine abnormalities of cardiorespiratory function, sleep state, oxygen saturation, CO_2 retention, and seizure activity. They can be used in conjunction with pH monitoring to determine the contribution of reflux to apnea. Esophageal pressure manometry can be useful to detect subtle changes in respiratory effort related to partial obstructive breathing (hypopnea). Infants may be at more risk of adverse events from sleep-disordered breathing due to their immature nervous system.

There are several neurologic causes of ALTEs, and seizure disorder has been found to be a cause of ALTE in a significant number of cases. Apnea as the sole manifestation of a seizure disorder is unusual but may occur. In cases of repeated episodes, 24-hour electroencephalographic monitoring may be helpful in detecting a seizure disorder.

Treatment

Therapy is directed at the underlying cause if one is found. After blood cultures are taken, antibiotics should be given to infants who appear toxic. Seizure disorders are treated with anticonvulsants. Gastroesophageal reflux should be treated, but may not prevent future episodes of ALTE. Vascular rings and pulmonary slings must be corrected surgically because of severe morbidity and high mortality rates when untreated.

The approach to care of infants with ALTEs where no definable cause can be ascertained is controversial. Home monitoring has been used in the past as treatment, but the efficacy of monitoring has not been demonstrated in controlled trials. With more than 30 years of home monitoring, the sudden infant death rate did not change due to this intervention. Although monitors can detect central apnea or bradycardia, they do not predict which children will have future ALTEs, and they do not detect obstructive forms of breathing a common form of apnea in infants. Apnea monitors are prone to frequent false alarms, and it must be noted that many parents cannot handle the stress associated with having a monitor in the home. Parents should be taught cardiopulmonary resuscitation prior to discharge and should prevent modifiable risk factors for infant death discussed below. The decision to monitor these infants involves the participation of the family. Infants with severe initial episodes or repeated severe episodes are now thought to be at significantly increased risk. A monitor with an oxygen saturation detection capability may identify episodes earlier. The caregiver responsible for prescribing a monitor should have a plan for the data acquisition, and the discontinuation of the monitor so that the parents can be prepared. Oxygen has been used as therapy for ALTEs for several reasons. Oxygen reduces periodic breathing of infancy, an immature pattern of breathing that can cause some degree of oxygen desaturation. Second, infants have small chest capacities with increased chest wall compliance that reduces lung volume. Oxygen can increase the baseline saturation, reducing the severity of desaturation with short apneas. Respiratory stimulants such as caffeine and aminophylline have been used in specific cases of central apnea or periodic breathing.

Any infant seen by a caregiver under one year of age should be evaluated for the presence of modifiable SIDS risk factors. Parents should be educated on how to avoid these risk factors, especially in infants at increased risk such as former preterm infants, children exposed to cigarette smoke environmentally or prior to birth, African American or Native American infants, and infants in poor socioeconomic areas. Updates on recommendations for the prevention of unexpected death in infants was recently published by the American Academy of Pediatrics (SIDS and Other Sleep-Related Infant Deaths: Expansion of Recommendations for a Safe Infant Sleeping Environment 1030–1039) and especially applies to infants after an ALTE. The reference should be read in full, but new recommendations include:

- Always place a baby on its back to sleep (this includes a baby with reflux).
- A baby should always sleep in its own space such as a crib, bassinette, or pack & play. A baby should not sleep on an adult bed, couch, armchair, futon, or other soft surface. Use a firm mattress designed for the crib, bassinet, or pack & play with a tight fitting sheet. The mattress should be flat, not elevated and with no soft bedding underneath or on top.
- Share a room, but not a bed, with a baby.
- There should be nothing in a baby's sleep space, other than the baby. Avoid overheating, overwrapping, and covering the face and head; use appropriate baby sleep clothing or sleep sack.
- Breastfeeding a baby is recommended.
- Consider offering a pacifier to a baby at nap and sleep time.
- Avoid or limit a baby's exposure to cigarette smoke.
- Car seats, swings, and baby slings should NOT be used for sleep.
- Avoid the use of adult beds, bed rails, and in-bed co-sleepers, which increase the risk of suffocation and entrapment.

SUDDEN INFANT DEATH SYNDROME

General Considerations

SIDS is defined as the sudden death of an infant younger than age 1 year that remains unexplained after a thorough case investigation, including performance of a complete autopsy, examination of the death scene, and review of the clinical history. The postmortem examination is an important feature of the definition because approximately 20% of cases of sudden death can be explained by autopsy findings. The incidence of SIDS in the United States has declined to less than 1 in 1000 live births over the last 15 years; however, it has leveled off. Reduction of prone sleeping after the "Back to Sleep" campaign was in large part responsible for the reduction of SIDS from a high of 2 infants per 1000 births, but new evidence shows the increase of sudden unexpected deaths of infants (SUDI) due to accidental suffocation and unsafe sleep surfaces.

Epidemiology & Pathogenesis

Epidemiologic and pathologic data constitute most of what is known about SIDS. The number of deaths peaks between ages 2 and 4 months. Most deaths occur between midnight and 8 AM, while the infant and often the caregiver are sleeping. In fact, the only unifying features of all SIDS cases are age and sleep. SIDS is more common among ethnic and racial minorities and socioeconomically disadvantaged populations. Racial disparity in the prevalence of prone positioning or especially in co-sleeping (Fu, Moon, and Hauck: 376–382) may also be contributing to the continued disparity in SIDS rates between black and white infants. There is a 3:2 male predominance in most series. Other risk factors include low birth weight, teenage or drug-addicted mothers, multiparity, crowded living conditions, maternal smoking, and a family history of SIDS. Most of these risk factors are associated with a two- to threefold elevation of incidence but are not specific enough to be useful in predicting which infants will die unexpectedly. Recent immunization is not a risk factor.

The most consistent pathologic findings are intrathoracic petechiae and mild inflammation and congestion of the respiratory tract. More subtle pathologic findings include brainstem gliosis, extramedullary hematopoiesis, and increases in periadrenal brown fat. These latter findings suggest that infants who succumb to SIDS have had intermittent or chronic hypoxia before death.

The mechanism or mechanisms of death in SIDS are unknown. For example, it is unknown whether the initiating event at the time of death is cessation of breathing, cardiac arrhythmia, or asystole. Hypotheses have included upper airway obstruction, catecholamine excess, and increased fetal hemoglobin. However, maldevelopment or delay in maturation of the brainstem, which is responsible for arousal, remains the predominant theory. A history of mild symptoms of upper respiratory infection before death is not uncommon, and SIDS victims are sometimes seen by physicians a day or so before death. The postmortem examination is essential for the diagnosis of SIDS and may help the family by excluding other possible causes of death. A death scene investigation is also important in determining the cause of sudden unexpected deaths in infancy.

Families must be supported following the death of an infant. The National SIDS Resource Center (http://www.sidscenter.org) provides information about psychosocial support groups and counseling for families of SIDS victims.

Prevention

Since 1990, SIDS rates have declined more than 60% worldwide. Population studies in New Zealand and Europe identified risk factors, which when changed had a major effect on the incidence of SIDS. Since 1994, the American Academy of Pediatrics' "Back-to-Sleep" campaign has promoted education about SIDS risk factors in the United States. The new updated recommendations are printed above and are available on line (SIDS and Other Sleep-Related Infant Deaths: Expansion of Recommendations for a Safe Infant Sleeping Environment 1030–1039). Modifiable risk factors include sleeping position, bottle feeding, maternal smoking, and infant overheating. The prone sleep position could contribute to SIDS through decreased arousal or rebreathing of exhaled gases. The side position, often used in hospitals and then mimicked at home, increases risk of SIDS compared with the supine position. Maternal smoking, especially prenatal maternal smoking, increases the risk of SIDS. Investigations of tobacco effects on the autonomic nervous system of the developing fetus, pulmonary growth and function of the newborn, or its combination with viral infection all point to differences in SIDS compared with control subjects. New data demonstrates decreased risk of SIDS with the use of pacifiers and breast feeding.

Table 19–7. American Academy of Pediatrics recommendations regarding sudden infant death syndrome (SIDS) risk reduction.

"Back-to-sleep" (supine sleeping position)
Firm sleep surface designed for infant sleep
Pillows/loose bedding, loose blankets should be out of the crib
Share a room, not a bed with the infant
Do not smoke during pregnancy, and smoke-free environment after birth
Consider offering a pacifier at nap and bed time
Avoid overheating, overwrapping, and head covering
Avoid commercial devices marketed to reduce the risk of SIDS
Do not use home monitors as a strategy to reduce the risk of SIDS
Encourage tummy time while awake

The health care provider is instrumental in parental education regarding the modifiable risk factors for SIDS (Table 19–7). The health care provider should screen all infants for SIDS risk factors, and include awareness of the child care setting, as many parents rely on others to watch their children, where the importance of risk factors may not be recognized. Hospitals should set an example by placing infants in the supine position with no blankets in the bed prior to discharge. At present, the data shows that the environment is key to the safety of the infant, and unsafe sleep environments are responsible for the recent increase in accidental suffocation, asphyxia and entrapment.

Aurora RN et al: Practice parameters for the respiratory indications for polysomnography in children. Sleep 34.3 2011;379–388.

Platt MW et al: A clinical comparison of SIDS and explained sudden infant deaths: how healthy and how normal? CESDI SUDI Research Group. Confidential Inquiry into Stillbirths and Deaths in Infancy study. Arch Dis Child 82.2 2000;98–106.

SIDS and Other Sleep-Related Infant Deaths: Expansion of Recommendations for a Safe Infant Sleeping Environment. Pediatrics 128.5 2011;1030–1039.

Cardiovascular Diseases

20

Jeffrey R. Darst, MD
Kathryn K. Collins, MD
Shelley D. Miyamoto, MD

Eight in 1000 infants are born with a congenital heart defect. Advances in medical and surgical care allow more than 90% of such children to enter adulthood. It is important that pediatric cardiac care include not only the diagnosis and treatment of congenital heart disease but also the prevention of risk factors for adult cardiovascular disease—obesity, smoking, and hyperlipidemia. Acquired and familial heart diseases such as Kawasaki disease, viral myocarditis, cardiomyopathies, and rheumatic heart disease are also a significant cause of morbidity and mortality in children.

DIAGNOSTIC EVALUATION

HISTORY

Most congenital defects lead either to decreased pulmonary blood flow or to increased pulmonary blood flow with associated pulmonary congestion. Symptoms vary according to the alteration in pulmonary blood flow (Table 20–1). The presence of other cardiovascular symptoms such as palpitations and chest pain should be determined by history in the older child, paying particular attention to the timing (at rest or activity-related), onset, and termination (gradual vs sudden), as well as precipitating and relieving factors.

PHYSICAL EXAMINATION

General

The examination begins with a visual assessment of mental status, signs of distress, perfusion, and skin color. Documentation of heart rate, respiratory rate, blood pressure (in all four extremities), and oxygen saturation is essential. Many congenital cardiac defects occur as part of a genetic syndrome (Table 20–2), and complete assessment includes evaluation of dysmorphic features that may be clues to the associated cardiac defect.

Cardiovascular Examination

A. Inspection and Palpation

Chest conformation should be noted in the supine position. A precordial bulge indicates cardiomegaly. Palpation may reveal increased precordial activity, right ventricular lift, or left-sided heave; a diffuse point of maximal impulse; or a precordial thrill caused by a grade IV/VI or greater murmur. The thrill of aortic stenosis is found in the suprasternal notch. In patients with severe pulmonary hypertension, a palpable pulmonary closure (P_2) is frequently noted at the upper left sternal border.

B. Auscultation

1. Heart sounds—The first heart sound (S_1) is the sound of atrioventricular (AV) valve closure. It is best heard at the lower left sternal border and is usually medium-pitched. Although S_1 has multiple components, only one of these (M_1—closure of the mitral valve) is usually audible.

The second heart sound (S_2) is the sound of semilunar valve closure. It is best heard at the upper left sternal border. S_2 has two component sounds, A_2 and P_2 (aortic and pulmonic valve closure). Splitting of S_2 varies with respiration, widening with inspiration and narrowing with expiration. Abnormal splitting of S_2 may be an indication of cardiac disease (Table 20–3). A prominent or loud P_2 is associated with pulmonary hypertension.

The third heart sound (S_3) is the sound of rapid left ventricular filling. It occurs in early diastole, after S_2, and is medium- to low-pitched. In healthy children, S_3 diminishes or disappears when going from supine to sitting or standing. A pathologic S_3 is often heard in the presence of poor cardiac function or a large left-to-right shunt. The fourth heart sound (S_4) is associated with atrial contraction and increased atrial pressure and has a low pitch similar to that of S_3. It occurs just prior to S_1 and is not normally audible. It is heard in the presence of atrial contraction into a noncompliant

Table 20–1. Symptoms of increased and decreased pulmonary blood flow.

Decreased Pulmonary Blood Flow	Increased Pulmonary Blood Flow
Infant/toddler	
Cyanosis	Tachypnea with activity/feeds
Squatting	Diaphoresis
Loss of consciousness	Poor weight gain
Older child	
Dizziness	Exercise intolerance
Syncope	Dyspnea on exertion, diaphoresis

Table 20–2. Cardiac defects in common syndromes.

Genetic Syndrome	Commonly Associated Cardiac Defect
Down syndrome	AVSD
Turner syndrome	Bicuspid aortic valve, coarctation, dilated aortic root, hypertension
Noonan syndrome	Dysplastic pulmonic valve, HCM
Williams-Beuren syndrome	Supravalvular aortic stenosis, PPS
Marfan syndrome	MVP, MR, dilated aortic root
Fetal alcohol syndrome	VSD, ASD
Maternal rubella	PDA, PPS

ASD, atrial septal defect; AVSD, atrioventricular septal defect; HCM, hypertrophic cardiomyopathy; MR, mitral regurgitation; MVP, mitral valve prolapse; PDA, patent ductus arteriosus; PPS, peripheral pulmonary stenosis; VSD, ventricular septal defect.

Table 20–3. Abnormal splitting of S_2.

Causes of wide split S_2
RV volume overload: ASD, anomalous pulmonary venous return, PI
RV pressure overload: Pulmonary valve stenosis
Delayed RV conduction: RBBB
Causes of narrow split S_2
Pulmonary hypertension
Single semilunar valve (aortic atresia, pulmonary atresia, truncus arteriosus)

ASD, atrial septal defect; PI, pulmonic insufficiency; RBBB, right bundle branch block; RV, right ventricle.

ventricle as in hypertrophic or restrictive cardiomyopathy or from other causes of diastolic dysfunction.

Ejection clicks are usually related to dilated great vessels or valve abnormalities. They are heard during ventricular systole and are classified as early, mid, or late. Early ejection clicks at the mid left sternal border are from the pulmonic valve. Aortic clicks are typically best heard at the apex. In contrast to aortic clicks, pulmonic clicks vary with respiration, becoming louder during inspiration. A mid to late ejection click at the apex is most typically caused by mitral valve prolapse.

2. Murmurs—A heart murmur is the most common cardiovascular finding leading to a cardiology referral. Innocent or functional heart murmurs are common, and 40%–45% of children have an innocent murmur at some time during childhood.

A. Characteristics—All murmurs should be described based on the following characteristics:

(1) Location and radiation—Where the murmur is best heard and where the sound extends.

(2) Relationship to cardiac cycle and duration—Systolic ejection (immediately following S_1 with a crescendo/decrescendo change in intensity), pansystolic (occurring throughout most of systole and of constant intensity), diastolic, or continuous. The timing of the murmur provides valuable clues as to underlying pathology (Table 20–4).

(3) Intensity—Grade I describes a soft murmur heard with difficulty; grade II, soft but easily heard; grade III, loud but without a thrill; grade IV, loud and associated with a precordial thrill; grade V, loud, with a thrill, and audible with the edge of the stethoscope; grade VI, very loud and audible with the stethoscope off the chest.

(4) Quality—Harsh, musical, or rough; high, medium, or low in pitch.

(5) Variation with position—Audible changes in murmur when the patient is supine, sitting, standing, or squatting.

B. Innocent murmurs—The six most common innocent murmurs of childhood are

(1) Newborn murmur—Heard in the first few days of life, this murmur is at the lower left sternal border, without significant radiation. It has a soft, short, vibratory grade I–II/VI quality that often subsides when mild pressure is applied to the abdomen. It usually disappears by age 2–3 weeks.

(2) Peripheral pulmonary artery stenosis (PPS)—This murmur, often heard in newborns, is caused by the normal branching of the pulmonary artery. It is heard with equal intensity at the upper left sternal border, at the back, and in one or both axilla. It is a soft, short, high-pitched, grade I–II/VI systolic ejection murmur and usually disappears by age 2. This murmur must be differentiated from true peripheral pulmonary stenosis (Williams syndrome, Alagille syndrome, or rubella syndrome), coarctation of the thoracic aorta, and valvular pulmonary stenosis. Characteristic facial features, extracardiac physical exam findings, history, and laboratory abnormalities suggestive of the syndromes listed above are the best way to differentiate true peripheral pulmonary stenosis from benign PPS of infancy as the murmurs can be similar.

Table 20–4. Pathologic murmurs.

Systolic Ejection	Pansystolic	Diastolic	Continuous
Semilunar valve stenosis (AS/PS/truncal stenosis)	VSD	Semilunar valve regurgitation	Runoff lesions
ASD	AVVR (MR/TR)	AI/PI/truncal insufficiency	PDA/AVM/aortopulmonary collaterals
Coarctation		AV valve stenosis (MS/TS)	

AI/PI, aortic insufficiency/pulmonic insufficiency; AS/PS, aortic stenosis/pulmonic stenosis; ASD, atrial septal defect; AV, atrioventricular; MS/TS, mitral stenosis/tricuspid stenosis; AVVR, atrioventricular valve regurgitation; MR/TR, mitral regurgitation/tricuspid regurgitation; PDA/AVM, patent ductus arteriosus/arteriovenous malformation; VSD, ventricular septal defect.

(3) Still murmur—This is the most common innocent murmur of early childhood. It is typically heard between 2 and 7 years of age. It is the loudest midway between the apex and the lower left sternal border. Still murmur is a musical or vibratory, short, high-pitched, grade I–III early systolic murmur. It is loudest when the patient is supine. It diminishes or disappears with inspiration or when the patient is sitting. The Still murmur is louder in patients with fever, anemia, or sinus tachycardia from any reason.

(4) Pulmonary ejection murmur—This is the most common innocent murmur in older children and adults. It is heard from age 3 years onward. It is usually a soft systolic ejection murmur, grade I–II in intensity at the upper left sternal border. The murmur is louder when the patient is supine or when cardiac output is increased. The pulmonary ejection murmur must be differentiated from murmurs of pulmonary stenosis, coarctation of the aorta, atrial septal defect (ASD), and peripheral pulmonary artery stenosis.

(5) Venous hum—A venous hum is usually heard after age 2 years. It is located in the infraclavicular area on the right. It is a continuous musical hum of grade I–III intensity and may be accentuated in diastole and with inspiration. It is best heard in the sitting position. Turning the child's neck, placing the child supine, and compressing the jugular vein obliterates the venous hum. Venous hum is caused by turbulence at the confluence of the subclavian and jugular veins.

(6) Innominate or carotid bruit—This murmur is more common in the older child and adolescents. It is heard in the right supraclavicular area. It is a long systolic ejection murmur, somewhat harsh and of grade II–III intensity. The bruit can be accentuated by light pressure on the carotid artery and must be differentiated from all types of aortic stenosis. The characteristic findings of aortic stenosis are outlined in more detail later in this chapter.

When functional murmurs are found in a child, the physician should assure the parents that these are normal heart sounds of the developing child and that they do not represent heart disease.

Extracardiac Examination

A. Arterial Pulse Rate and Rhythm

Cardiac rate and rhythm vary greatly during infancy and childhood, so multiple determinations should be made. This is particularly important for infants (Table 20–5) whose heart rates vary with activity. The rhythm may be regular or there may be a normal phasic variation with respiration (sinus arrhythmia).

B. Arterial Pulse Quality and Amplitude

A bounding pulse is characteristic of run-off lesions, including patent ductus arteriosus (PDA), aortic regurgitation, arteriovenous malformation, or any condition with a low diastolic pressure (fever, anemia, or septic shock). Narrow or thready pulses occur in patients with conditions reducing cardiac output such as cardiomyopathy, myocarditis, pericardial tamponade, or severe aortic stenosis. A reduction in pulse amplitude or blood pressure (> 10 mm Hg) with inspiration is referred to as pulsus paradoxus and is a telltale sign of pericardial tamponade. The pulses of the upper and lower extremities should be compared. The femoral pulse should be palpable and equal in amplitude and simultaneous with the brachial pulse. A femoral pulse that is absent or weak, or that is delayed in comparison with the brachial pulse, suggests coarctation of the aorta.

Table 20–5. Resting heart rates.

Age	Low	High
< 1 mo	80	160
1–3 mo	80	200
2–24 mo	70	120
2–10 y	60	90
11–18 y	40	90

C. Arterial Blood Pressure

Blood pressures should be obtained in the upper and lower extremities. Systolic pressure in the lower extremities should be greater than or equal to that in the upper extremities. The cuff must cover the same relative area of the arm and leg. Measurements should be repeated several times. A lower blood pressure in the lower extremities suggests coarctation of the aorta.

D. Cyanosis of the Extremities

Cyanosis results from an increased concentration (> 4–5 g/dL) of reduced hemoglobin in the blood. Bluish skin color is usually, but not always, a sign. Visible cyanosis also accompanies low cardiac output, hypothermia, and systemic venous congestion, even in the presence of adequate oxygenation. Cyanosis should be judged only by the color of the mucous membranes (lips). Bluish discoloration around the mouth (acrocyanosis) is a feature of skin that has not been exposed to sun, and it does not correlate with cyanosis.

E. Clubbing of the Fingers and Toes

Clubbing is often associated with severe cyanotic congenital heart disease. It usually appears after age 1 year. Hypoxemia with cyanosis is the most common cause, but clubbing also occurs in patients with endocarditis, chronic liver disease, inflammatory bowel diseases, chronic pulmonary disease, and lung abscess. Digital clubbing may be a benign genetic variant.

F. Edema

Edema of dependent areas (lower extremities in the older child and the face and sacrum in the younger child) is characteristic of elevated right heart pressure, which may be seen with tricuspid valve pathology or right ventricular (RV) dysfunction (right heart failure) from a variety of causes including left ventricular (LV) dysfunction.

G. Abdomen

Hepatomegaly is the cardinal sign of right heart failure in the infant and child. Left heart failure can ultimately lead to right heart failure and therefore, hepatomegaly may also be seen in the child with pulmonary edema from lesions causing left-to-right shunting (pulmonary overcirculation) or left ventricular failure. Splenomegaly may be present in patients with long-standing heart failure (HF), and is characteristic of infective endocarditis. Ascites is also a feature of chronic right heart failure. Examination of the abdomen may reveal shifting dullness or a fluid wave.

Finley JP et al: Assessing children's heart sounds at a distance with digital recordings. Pediatrics 2006;118:2322–2325 [PMID: 17142514].

Mahnke CB et al: Utility of store-and-forward pediatric telecardiology evaluation in distinguishing normal from pathologic pediatric heart sounds. Clin Pediatr (Phila) 2008;47:919–925 [PMID: 18626106].

Markel H: The stethoscope and the art of listening. N Engl J Med 2006;354:551–553 [PMID: 16467541].

ELECTROCARDIOGRAPHY

The electrocardiogram (ECG) is essential in the evaluation of the cardiovascular system. The heart rate should first be determined, then the cardiac rhythm (Is the patient in a normal sinus rhythm or other rhythm as evidenced by a P wave with a consistent PR interval before every QRS complex?), and then the axis (Are the P and QRS axes normal for patient age?). Once the initial assessment of rate, rhythm, and axis is performed, attention can be directed toward assessment of chamber enlargement and finally to assessment of cardiac intervals and ST segments.

Age-Related Variations

The ECG evolves with age. The rate decreases and intervals increase with age. RV dominance in the newborn changes to LV dominance in the older infant, child, and adult. The normal ECG of the 1-week-old infant is abnormal for a 1-year-old child, and the ECG of a 5-year-old child is abnormal for an adult.

Electrocardiographic Interpretation

Figure 20–1 defines the events recorded by the ECG.

A. Rate

The heart rate varies markedly with age, activity, and state of emotional and physical well-being. In most infants and younger children, the heart rate ranges from 70 to 200 beats/min depending on the above.

B. Rhythm

Sinus rhythm should always be present in healthy children. Extra heart beats representing premature atrial and ventricular contractions are common during childhood, with atrial ectopy predominating in infants and ventricular ectopy during adolescence. Isolated premature beats in patients with normal heart structure and function are usually benign.

C. Axis

1. P wave axis—The P wave is generated from atrial contraction beginning in the high right atrium at the site of the sinus node. The impulse proceeds leftward and inferiorly, thus leading to a positive deflection in all left-sided and inferior leads (II, III, and aVF) and negative in lead aVR.

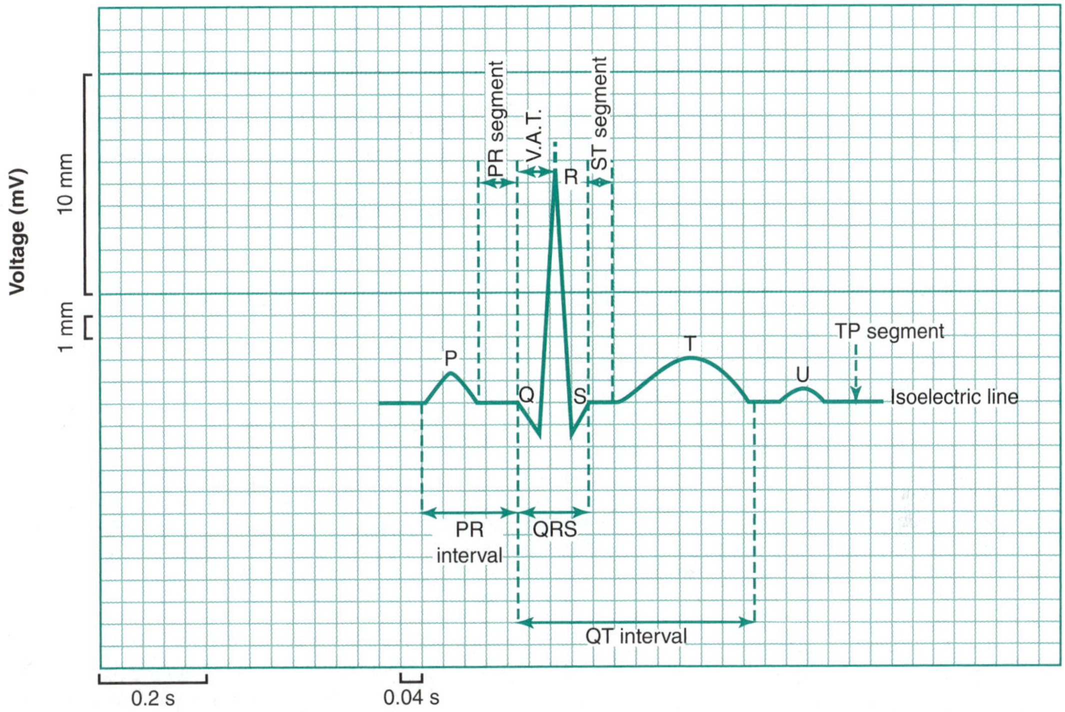

▲ **Figure 20–1.** Complexes and intervals of the electrocardiogram.

2. QRS axis—The net voltage should be positive in leads I and aVF in children with a normal axis. In infants and young children, RV dominance may persist, leading to a negative deflection in lead I. Several congenital cardiac lesions are associated with alterations in the normal QRS axis (Table 20–6).

D. P Wave

In the pediatric patient, the amplitude of the P wave is normally no greater than 3 mm and the duration no more than 0.08 second. The P wave is best seen in leads II and V_1.

Table 20–6. QRS axis deviation.

Right Axis Deviation	Left Axis Deviation
Tetralogy of Fallot Transposition of the great arteries Total anomalous pulmonary venous return Atrial septal defect	Atrioventricular septal defect Pulmonary atresia with intact ventricular septum Tricuspid atresia

E. PR Interval

The PR is measured from the beginning of the P wave to the beginning of the QRS complex. It increases with age and with slower rates. The PR interval ranges from a minimum of 0.10 second in infants to a maximum of 0.18 second in older children with slow rates. The PR interval is commonly prolonged in patients who have rheumatic heart disease and those receiving digitalis.

F. QRS Complex

This represents ventricular depolarization, and its amplitude and direction of force (axis) reveal the relative size of the ventricular mass in hypertrophy, hypoplasia, and infarction. Abnormal ventricular conduction (eg, right or left bundle-branch block) is also revealed.

G. QT Interval

This interval is measured from the beginning of the QRS complex to the end of the T wave. The QT duration may be prolonged as a primary condition or secondarily due to drugs or electrolyte imbalances (Table 20–7). The normal

Table 20–7. Causes of QT prolongation.[a]

Cardiac medications
Antiarrhythmics: IA (quinidine, procainamide, disopyramide) class III (amiodarone, sotalol)
Inotropic agents: dobutamine, dopamine, epinephrine, isoproterenol
Noncardiac medications
Antibiotics/antivirals: azithromycin, clarithromycin, levofloxacin, amantadine
Antipsychotics: risperidol, thioridazine, lithium, haloperidol
Sedatives: chloral hydrate, methadone
Other: albuterol, levalbuterol, ondansetron, phenytoin, pseudoephedrine
Electrolyte disturbances: hypokalemia, hypomagnesemia, hypocalcemia

[a]Partial list only.

QT duration is rate-related and must be corrected using the Bazett formula:

$$QTc = \frac{\text{QT intervals (s)}}{\sqrt{\text{R-R intervals (s)}}}$$

The normal QTc is less than or equal to 0.44 second.

H. ST Segment

This segment, lying between the end of the QRS complex and the beginning of the T wave, is affected by drugs, electrolyte imbalances, or myocardial injury.

I. T Wave

The T wave represents myocardial repolarization and is altered by electrolytes, myocardial hypertrophy, and ischemia.

J. Impression

The ultimate impression of the ECG is derived from a systematic analysis of all the features above as compared with expected normal values for the child's age.

O'Connor M, McDaniel N, Brady WJ: The pediatric electrocardiogram: part I: Age-related interpretation. Am J Emerg Med 2008 May:26(4):506–512 [PMID: 18416018].

CHEST RADIOGRAPH

Evaluation of the chest radiograph for cardiac disease should focus on (1) position of the heart, (2) position of the abdominal viscera, (3) cardiac size, (4) cardiac configuration, and (5) character of the pulmonary vasculature. The standard posteroanterior and left lateral chest radiographs are used (Figure 20–2).

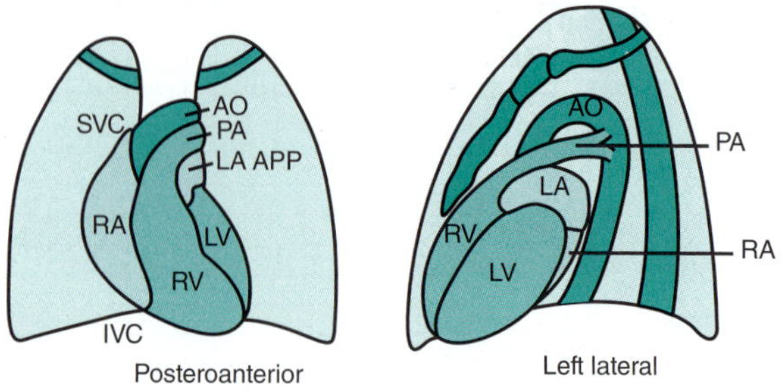

▲ **Figure 20–2.** Position of cardiovascular structures in principal radiograph views. AO, aorta; IVC, inferior vena cava; LA, left atrium; LA APP, left atrial appendage; LV, left ventricle; PA, pulmonary artery; RA, right atrium; RV, right ventricle; SVC, superior vena cava.

Cardiac position is either levocardia (heart predominantly in the left chest), dextrocardia (heart predominantly in the right chest), or mesocardia (midline heart). The position of the liver and stomach bubble is either in the normal position (abdominal situs solitus), inverted with the stomach bubble on the right (abdominal situs inversus), or variable with midline liver (abdominal situs ambiguous). The heart appears relatively large in normal newborns at least in part due to a prominent thymic shadow. The heart size should be less than 50% of the chest diameter in children older than age 1 year. The cardiac configuration on chest radiograph may provide useful diagnostic information (Table 20–8). Some congenital cardiac lesions have a characteristic radiographic appearance that suggests the diagnosis but should not be viewed as conclusive (Table 20–9). The pulmonary vasculature should be assessed. The presence of increased or decreased pulmonary blood flow suggests a possible congenital cardiac diagnosis, particularly in the cyanotic infant (Table 20–10).

Laya BF et al: The accuracy of chest radiographs in the detection of congenital heart disease and in the diagnosis of specific congenital cardiac lesions. Pediatr Radiol 2006;36:677–681 [PMID: 16547698].

Table 20–8. Radiographic changes with cardiac chamber enlargement.

Chamber Enlarged	Change in Cardiac Silhouette on Anteroposterior Film
Right ventricle	Apex of the heart is tipped upward
Left ventricle	Apex of the heart is tipped downward
Left atrium	Double shadow behind cardiac silhouette Increase in subcarinal angle
Right atrium	Prominence of right atrial border of the heart

Table 20–9. Lesion-specific chest radiographic findings.

Diagnosis	Chest Radiograph Appearance
D-transposition of the great arteries	Egg on a string
Tetralogy of Fallot	Boot-shaped heart
Unobstructed total anomalous pulmonary venous drainage	Snowman
Obstructed total anomalous pulmonary venous drainage	Small heart with congested lungs
Coarctation	Figure 3 sign + rib notching

Table 20–10. Alterations in pulmonary blood flow in cyanotic cardiac lesions.

Increased Pulmonary Blood Flow	Decreased Pulmonary Blood Flow
Total anomalous pulmonary venous return	Pulmonic stenosis
Tricuspid atresia with large ventricular septal defect	Tricuspid atresia/restrictive ventricular septal defect
Transposition of the great arteries	Tetralogy of Fallot
Truncus arteriosus	Pulmonary atresia with intact ventricular septum

Dextrocardia

Dextrocardia is a radiographic term used when the heart is on the right side of the chest. When dextrocardia occurs with reversal of position of the other important organs of the chest and abdomen (eg, liver, lungs, and spleen), the condition is called situs inversus totalis, and the heart is usually normal. When dextrocardia occurs with the other organs normally located (situs solitus), the heart usually has severe defects.

Other situs abnormalities include situs ambiguous with the liver central and anterior in the upper abdomen and the stomach pushed posteriorly; bilateral right-sidedness (asplenia syndrome); and bilateral left-sidedness (polysplenia syndrome). In virtually all cases of situs ambiguous, congenital heart disease is present.

ECHOCARDIOGRAPHY

Echocardiography is a fundamental tool of pediatric cardiology. Using multiple ultrasound modalities (two-dimensional imaging, Doppler, and M-mode), cardiac anatomy, blood flow, intracardiac pressures, and ventricular function can be assessed. Echocardiography is based on the physical principles of sound waves. The ultrasound frequencies utilized in cardiac imaging range from 2 to 10 million cycles/s.

M-mode echocardiography uses short bursts of ultrasound sent from a transducer. At acoustic interfaces, sound waves are reflected back to the transducer. The time it takes for the sound wave to return to the transducer is measured and the distance to the interface is calculated. That calculated distance is displayed against time, and a one-dimensional image is constructed that demonstrates cardiac motion. **Two-dimensional imaging** extends this technique by sending a rapid series of ultrasound bursts across a 90-degree sector, which allows construction of a two-dimensional image of the heart. **Doppler ultrasound** measures blood flow. The ultrasound transducer sends out a known frequency of sound which reflects off moving red blood cells. The transducer receives the reflected frequency and compares it with the transmitted frequency. The blood flow velocity can be calculated from the measured frequency shift. This information is used to estimate pressure gradients by the simplified Bernouli equation, in which the pressure gradient is equal to four times the calculated velocity (Pressure gradient = $4(V^2)$).

A transthoracic echocardiogram is obtained by placing the transducer on areas of the chest where there is minimal lung interference. At each transducer position, the beam is swept through the heart and, while a two-dimensional image appears on the screen, a three-dimensional image of the heart is constructed in the interpreter's mind. Complex intracardiac anatomy and spatial relationships can be described, making possible the accurate diagnosis of simple and complex congenital heart disease. In addition to structural details, Doppler gives information about intracardiac blood flow and pressure gradients. Commonly used Doppler techniques include color flow imaging, pulsed-wave, and continuous-wave Doppler. Color flow imaging gives general information on the direction and velocity of flow. Pulsed- and continuous-wave Doppler imagings give more precise measurements of blood velocity. The role of M-mode in the ultrasound examination has decreased as other ultrasound modalities have been developed. M-mode is still used to measure LV end-diastolic and end-systolic dimensions and permits calculation of the LV-shortening fraction, a standard estimate of LV function (SF = LV end-diastolic volume – LV systolic volume/LV end-diastolic volume).

A typical transthoracic echocardiogram performed by a skilled sonographer takes about 30 minutes, and patients must be still for the examination. Frequently infants and children cannot cooperate for the examination and sedation is required. Transesophageal echocardiography requires general anesthesia in infants and children and is primarily used to guide interventional procedures and surgical repair of congenital heart disease. In cases of difficult imaging windows due to patient size, air interference or when looking for evidence of vegetations on cardiac valves, transesophageal echocardiography may be necessary.

Although echocardiography is an excellent tool for cardiac examination, there are limitations to the technique.

Two-dimensional imaging can accurately diagnose intracardiac anatomy, but some extracardiac structures such as the distal pulmonary arteries are more difficult to assess. Doppler imaging estimates pressure gradients accurately and assessment of diastolic function by echocardiography is improving. However, exact hemodynamic data is still best determined by cardiac catheterization.

It is important to note that fetal echocardiography plays an important role in the prenatal diagnosis of complex congenital heart disease. A fetal echocardiogram is recommended if the fetus is considered high risk for the development of congenital heart disease or if there is suspicion for structural heart disease or fetal arrhythmias based on the obstetric fetal ultrasound. In utero management of fetal arrhythmias and post-delivery planning for the fetus with complex heart disease has resulted in improved outcomes for this challenging group of patients.

Ayres NA et al: Indications and guidelines for performance of transesophageal echocardiography in the patient with pediatric acquired or congenital heart disease: Report from the task force of the Pediatric Council of the American Society of Echocardiography. J Am Soc Echocardiogr 2005;18:91–98 [PMID: 15637497].

Cheitlin MD et al: ACC/AHA/ASE 2003 guideline update for the clinical application of echocardiography: Summary article: A report of the American College of Cardiology/American Heart Association Task Force on Practice Guidelines (ACC/AHA/ASE Committee to Update the 1997 Guidelines for the Clinical Application of Echocardiography). Circulation 2003;108:1146–1162 [PMID: 12952829].

NUCLEAR CARDIOLOGY

Nuclear imaging is not commonly used in pediatric cardiology, but can be a useful adjunct to cardiopulmonary exercise testing in assessing both fixed and reversible areas of myocardial ischemia. It is valuable in evaluating myocardial perfusion in patients with Kawasaki disease, repaired anomalous left coronary artery or other coronary anomalies, myocardial bridging in the setting of hypertrophic cardiomyopathy (HCM), or chest pain in association with ECG changes with exercise.

MAGNETIC RESONANCE IMAGING

Magnetic resonance imaging (MRI) of the heart is valuable for evaluation and noninvasive follow-up of many congenital heart defects. It is particularly useful in imaging the thoracic vessels, which are difficult to image by transthoracic echocardiogram. Cardiac gated imaging allows dynamic evaluation of structure and blood flow of the heart and great vessels. Cardiac MRI provides unique and precise imaging in patients with newly diagnosed or repaired aortic coarctation and defines the aortic dilation in Marfan, Turner, and Loeys-Dietz syndromes. Cardiac MRI can quantify regurgitant lesions such as pulmonary insufficiency (PI) after repair of tetralogy of Fallot (ToF) and can define ventricular function, chamber size, and wall thickness in patients with inadequate echocardiographic images or cardiomyopathies. MRI is especially useful to characterize right ventricular size and function as this chamber is often difficult to image comprehensively by echocardiogram. Because it allows computer manipulation of images of the heart and great vessels, three-dimensional MRI is an ideal noninvasive way of obtaining accurate reconstructions of the heart. General anesthesia is often required to facilitate cardiac MRI performance in children < 8 years.

Woodard PK et al: Cardiac MRI in the management of congenital heart disease in children, adolescents, and young adults. Curr Treat Options Cardiovasc Med 2008;10:419–424 [PMID: 18814831].

CARDIOPULMONARY STRESS TESTING

Most children with heart disease are capable of normal activity. Data on cardiac function after exercise are essential to prevent unnecessary restriction of activities. The response to exercise is helpful in determining the need for and the timing of cardiovascular surgery and is a useful objective outcome measure of the results of medical and surgical interventions.

Bicycle ergometers or treadmills can be used in children as young as age 5 years. The addition of a metabolic cart enables one to assess whether exercise impairment is secondary to cardiac limitation, pulmonary limitation, deconditioning, or lack of effort. Exercise variables include the ECG, blood pressure response to exercise, oxygen saturation, ventilation, maximal oxygen consumption, and peak workload attained. Cardiopulmonary stress testing is routine in children with congenital cardiac lesions to ascertain limitations, develop exercise programs, assess the effect of therapies, and decide on the need for cardiac transplantation. Stress testing is also employed in children with structurally normal hearts with complaints of exercise-induced symptoms in order to rule out cardiac or pulmonary pathology. Significant stress ischemia or dysrhythmias warrant physical restrictions or appropriate therapy. Children with poor performance due to suboptimal conditioning benefit from a planned exercise program.

Arvidsson D, Slinde F, Hulthén L, Sunnegårdh J: Physical activity, sports participation and aerobic fitness in children who have undergone surgery for congenital heart defects.Acta Paediatr 2009 Sep;98(9):1475–1482 [PMID: 19489769].

ARTERIAL BLOOD GASES

Quantitating the partial oxygen pressure (Po_2) or o_2 saturation during the administration of 100% oxygen is the most useful method of distinguishing cyanosis produced primarily by heart disease or by lung disease in sick infants. In cyanotic heart disease, the partial arterial oxygen pressure (Pao_2) increases very little when 100% oxygen is administered over the values obtained while breathing room air.

Table 20–11. Examples of responses to 10 minutes of 100% oxygen in lung disease and heart disease.

	Lung Disease		Heart Disease	
	Room Air	100% O_2	Room Air	100% O_2
Color	Blue → Pink		Blue → Blue	
Oximetry	60% → 99%		60% → 62%	
Pao_2 (mm Hg)	35 → 120		35 → 38	

Pao_2, partial arterial oxygen pressure.
Data from Mahle WT et al: Role of pulse oximetry in examining newborns for congenital heart disease: A scientific statement from the AHA and AAP. Pediatrics 2009;124:823–836 [PMID: 19581259].

However, Pao_2 usually increases significantly when oxygen is administered to a patient with lung disease. Table 20–11 illustrates the responses seen in patients with heart or lung disease during the hyperoxic test. Larger studies are needed to determine if pulse oximetry should be used routinely in the newborn evaluation to screen for major cardiac defects.

CARDIAC CATHETERIZATION & ANGIOCARDIOGRAPHY

Cardiac catheterization is an invasive method to evaluate anatomic and physiologic conditions in congenital or acquired heart disease. Management decisions may be made based on hemodynamic, oximetric, or angiographic data obtained through a catheterization. In an increasing number of cases, intervention may be performed during a catheterization that may palliate, or even cure, a congenital heart defect without open heart surgery.

Interventional Cardiac Catheterization

Cardiac catheterization can be performed to evaluate the effects of pharmaceutical therapy. An example of this use of catheterization is monitoring changes in pulmonary vascular resistance during the administration of nitric oxide or prostacyclin in a child with primary pulmonary hypertension. Electrophysiologic evaluation and ablation of abnormal electrical pathways in children can be performed by qualified personnel in the pediatric catheterization laboratory.

Various procedures are commonly performed in the catheterization laboratory that can improve or cure congenital malformations. Lesions that result in abnormal flow near or within the heart can be occluded, such as a patent ductus arteriosus, atrial septal defect, or ventricular septal defect. Obstruction of heart valves can be addressed through balloon valvuloplasty. Intervention may also be performed on vascular obstruction through angioplasty or stent placement in pulmonary arteries or the aorta. Systemic and pulmonary veins can be modified in a similar fashion, unfortunately sometimes with variable success. More recently, newer devices are now available to allow patients to undergo replacement of failing heart valves without open heart surgery.

Although the risks of cardiac catheterization are very low for elective studies in older children (< 0.1%), the risk of major complications in distressed infants is about 2%. Interventional procedures, particularly in unstable babies and children, increase these risks further.

Cardiac Catheterization Data

Figure 20–3 shows oxygen saturation (in percent) and pressure (in millimeters of mercury) values obtained at cardiac catheterization from the chambers and great arteries of the heart. These values represent the normal range for a child.

A. Oxygen Content and Saturation; Pulmonary (Q_p) and Systemic (Q_s) Blood Flow (Cardiac Output)

In most catheterization laboratories, left-to-right shunting is determined by changes of blood oxygen content through saturation sampling in the right side of the heart. Oxygenated blood that mixes with nonoxygenated blood

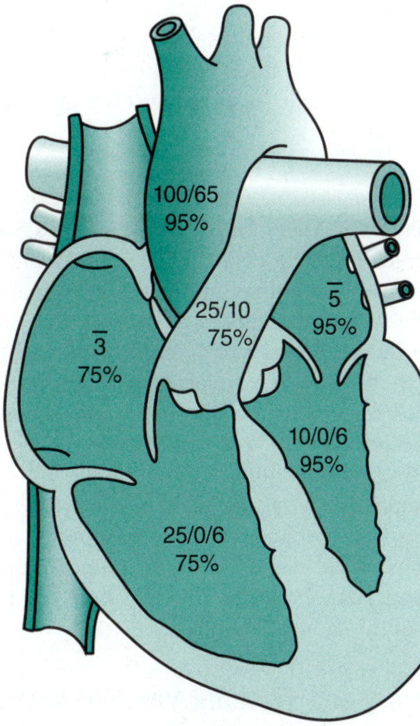

▲ **Figure 20–3.** Pressures (in millimeters of mercury) and oxygen saturation (in percent) obtained by cardiac catheterization in a healthy child. 3, mean pressure of 3 mm Hg in the right atrium; 5, mean pressure of 5 mm Hg in the left atrium.

will result in an increase in saturation of the mixed blood compared to "plain" venous blood. A significant increase in oxygen saturation between two locations in the right side of the heart indicates the presence of a left-to-right shunt at the site of the increase. Subnormal saturation suggests the presence of a right-to-left shunt or an abnormal pulmonary process.

The Fick principle allows for calculation of cardiac output. Systemic cardiac output, often referred to as Qs, represents blood flow from the heart to the body. Pulmonary blood flow, known as Qp, is blood flow from the heart to the lungs. These can be calculated during a catheterization, with similar equations. The equations, shown below, account for changes in the patient's heart rate and size through the inclusion of oxygen consumption. Hemoglobin (Hb) and oxygen saturations within the heart also affect the result (13.6 is a constant based on the milliliters of oxygen carried by one gram of hemoglobin).

$$\text{Systemic cardiac output (L/min)} = \frac{\text{Oxygen consumption (mL/min)}}{(\text{Hb})(13.6)(\text{aortic sat} - \text{mixed venous sat})}$$

$$\text{Pulmonary blood flow (L/min)} = \frac{\text{Oxygen consumption (mL/min)}}{(\text{Hb})(13.6)(\text{pulmonary vein sat} - \text{pulmonary artery sat})}$$

In a normal heart, systemic cardiac output and pulmonary blood flow are equal. If there is a difference, a left-to-right shunt (Qp > Qs) or right-to-left shunt (Qs > Qp) is present.

B. Pressures

Pressures should be determined in all chambers and major vessels entered. Systolic pressure in the right ventricle should be equal to the systolic pressure in the pulmonary artery. Likewise, the systolic pressure in the left ventricle should be equal to the systolic pressure of the aorta. The mean pressure in the atria should be nearly equal to the diastolic pressure of the ventricles. If a gradient in pressure exists, an obstruction is present, and the severity of the gradient is one criterion for the necessity of intervention.

For example, an RV systolic pressure of 100 mm Hg and a pulmonary artery systolic pressure of 20 mm Hg, a gradient of 80 mm Hg, would classify as severe pulmonary valve stenosis. Balloon pulmonary valvuloplasty would be indicated at the time of the catheterization.

C. Pulmonary and Systemic Vascular Resistance

The vascular resistance is calculated from the following formula and reported in units or in dynes × cm^{-5}/m^2:

$$\text{Resistance} = \frac{\text{Pressure}}{\text{Flow}}$$

The pressure drop used to determine pulmonary vascular resistance is calculated by subtracting the left atrial pressure (or pulmonary artery wedge pressure) from the mean pulmonary artery pressure. This pressure drop is divided by pulmonary blood flow (via the Fick principle, see above). Similarly, systemic vascular resistance is determined by subtracting the mean central venous pressure from the mean systemic arterial pressure and dividing this pressure drop by systemic blood flow.

Normal pulmonary vascular resistance is less than 3 U/m^2, or 240 dynes × cm^{-5}/m^2. Systemic vascular resistance normally covers a wider range, from 15 to 30 U/m^2, or from 1200 to 2400 dynes × cm^{-5}/m^2. The ratio of pulmonary to systemic vascular resistance is usually less than 0.3.

High pulmonary resistance or a high ratio of resistance denotes abnormal pulmonary vasculature. It often represents increased risk in patients with congenital heart disease or pulmonary hypertension and results in higher risk of death in severely affected patients.

Hill KD, Lim DS, Everett AD, Ivy DD, Moore JD: Assessment of pulmonary hypertension in the pediatric catheterization laboratory: Current insights from the Magic registry. Catheter Cardiovasc Interv 2010 Nov 15;76(6):865–873.

McElhinney DB, Hellenbrand WE, Zahn EM, Jones TK, Cheatham JP, Lock JE, Vincent JA: Short- and medium-term outcomes after transcatheter pulmonary valve placement in the expanded multicenter US melody valve trial. Circulation. 2010 Aug 3;122(5):507–516.

PERINATAL & NEONATAL CIRCULATION

At birth, two events affect the cardiovascular and pulmonary system: (1) the umbilical cord is clamped, removing the placenta from the maternal circulation; and (2) breathing commences. As a result, marked changes in the circulation occur. During fetal life, the placenta offers low resistance to blood flow. In contrast, the pulmonary arterioles are markedly constricted and there is high resistance to blood flow in the lungs. Therefore, the majority of blood entering the right side of the heart travels from the right atrium into the left atrium across the foramen ovale (right-to-left shunt). In addition, most of the blood that makes its way into the right ventricle and then pulmonary arteries will flow from the pulmonary artery into the aorta through the ductus arteriosus (right-to-left shunt). Subsequently, pulmonary blood flow accounts for only 7%–10% of the combined in utero ventricular output. At birth, pulmonary blood flow dramatically increases with the fall in pulmonary vascular resistance and pressure. The causes of prolonged high pulmonary vascular resistance include physical factors (lack of an adequate air-liquid interface or ventilation), low oxygen tension, and vasoactive mediators such as elevated endothelin peptide levels or leukotrienes. Clamping the umbilical cord produces an immediate increase in resistance to flow in the systemic circuit.

As breathing commences, the Po_2 of the small pulmonary arterioles increases, resulting in a decrease in pulmonary vascular resistance. Increased oxygen tension, rhythmic lung distention, and production of nitric oxide as well as prostacyclin play major roles in the fall in pulmonary vascular resistance at birth. The pulmonary vascular resistance falls below that of the systemic circuit, resulting in a reversal in direction of blood flow across the ductus arteriosus and marked increase in pulmonary blood flow.

Functional closure of the ductus arteriosus begins shortly after birth. The ductus arteriosus usually remains patent for 1–5 days. During the first hour after birth, a small right-to-left shunt is present (as in the fetus). However, after 1 hour, bidirectional shunting occurs, with the left-to-right direction predominating. In most cases, right-to-left shunting disappears completely by 8 hours. In patients with severe hypoxia (eg, in the syndrome of persistent pulmonary hypertension of the newborn), pulmonary vascular resistance remains high, resulting in a continued right-to-left shunt. Increased Po_2 of the arterial blood causes spasm of the ductus. Although flow through the ductus arteriosus usually is gone by 5 days of life, the vessel does not close anatomically for 7–14 days.

In fetal life, the foramen ovale serves as a one-way valve shunting blood from the inferior vena cava through the right atrium into the left atrium. At birth, because of the changes in the pulmonary and systemic vascular resistance and the increase in the quantity of blood returning from the pulmonary veins to the left atrium, the left atrial pressure rises above that of the right atrium. This functionally closes the flap of the foramen ovale, preventing flow of blood across the septum. The foramen ovale remains probe patent in 10%–15% of adults.

Persistent pulmonary hypertension is a clinical syndrome of full-term infants. The neonate develops tachypnea, cyanosis, and pulmonary hypertension during the first 8 hours after delivery. These infants have massive right-to-left ductal and/or foramen shunting for 3–7 days because of high pulmonary vascular resistance. Progressive hypoxia and acidosis will cause early death unless the pulmonary resistance can be lowered. Postmortem findings include increased thickness of the pulmonary arteriolar media. Increased alveolar Po_2 with hyperventilation, alkalosis, paralysis, surfactant administration, high-frequency ventilation, and cardiac inotropes can usually reverse this process. Inhaled nitric oxide selectively dilates pulmonary vasculature, produces a sustained improvement in oxygenation, and has resulted in improved outcomes.

In the normal newborn, pulmonary vascular resistance and pulmonary arterial pressure continue to fall during the first weeks of life as a result of demuscularization of the pulmonary arterioles. Adult levels of pulmonary resistance and pressure are normally achieved by 4–6 weeks of age. It is at this time typically that signs of pulmonary overcirculation associated with left-to-right shunt lesions (VSD or atrioventricular septal defect [AVSD]) appear.

Konduri GG, Kim UO: Advances in the diagnosis and management of persistent pulmonary hypertension of the newborn. Pediatr Clin North Am 2009;56:579–600, Table of Contents [PMID: 19501693].

Rudolph AM: The fetal circulation and congenital heart disease. Arch Dis Child Fetal Neonatal Ed 2010;95(2):F132–F136 [PMID: 19321508].

HEART FAILURE

Heart failure (HF) is the clinical condition in which the heart fails to meet the circulatory and metabolic needs of the body. The term *congestive heart failure* is not always accurate, as some patients with significant cardiac dysfunction have symptoms of exercise intolerance and fatigue without evidence of congestion. Right and left heart failure can result from volume or pressure overload of the respective ventricle or an intrinsic abnormality of the ventricular myocardium. Causes of right ventricular volume overload include an ASD, pulmonary insufficiency, or anomalous pulmonary venous return. Left ventricular volume overload occurs with any left-to-right shunting lesion (eg, VSD, PDA), aortic insufficiency, or a systemic arteriovenous malformation. Causes of right ventricular failure as a result of pressure overload include pulmonary hypertension, valvar pulmonary stenosis, or severe branch pulmonary artery stenosis. Left ventricular pressure overload results from left heart obstructive lesions such as aortic stenosis (sub-valvar, valvar, or supra-valvar) or coarctation of the aorta. Abnormalities of the right ventricular myocardium that can result in right heart failure include Ebstein's anomaly (atrialization of the right ventricle) and arrhythmogenic right ventricular dysplasia (a genetic disorder where the right ventricular myocardium is replaced by fat). Abnormalities of the left ventricular myocardium are more common and include dilated cardiomyopathy, myocarditis, or hypertrophic cardiomyopathy. As a result of elevated left atrial pressure and impaired relaxation of the left ventricle, left heart failure can lead to right heart failure. Other causes of HF in infants include AV septal defect, coronary artery anomalies, and chronic atrial tachyarrhythmias. Metabolic, mitochondrial, and neuromuscular disorders with associated cardiomyopathy present at various ages depending on the etiology. HF due to acquired conditions such as myocarditis can occur at any age. Children with HF may present with irritability, diaphoresis with feeds, fatigue, exercise intolerance, or evidence of pulmonary congestion (see Table 20–1).

Treatment of Heart Failure

The therapy of HF should be directed toward the underlying cause as well as the symptoms. Regardless of the etiology, neurohormonal activation occurs early when ventricular systolic dysfunction is present. Plasma catecholamine levels (eg, norepinephrine) increase causing tachycardia, diaphoresis, and, by activating the renin-angiotensin system, peripheral vasoconstriction and salt and water retention. There is no gold standard diagnostic or therapeutic approach to HF in children. Treatment must be individualized and therapies should be aimed at improving cardiac performance by targeting the three determinants of cardiac performance: (1) preload, (2) afterload, and (3) contractility.

Inpatient Management of Heart Failure

Patients with cardiac decompensation may require hospitalization for initiation or augmentation of HF therapy. Table 20–12 demonstrates intravenous inotropic agents used to augment cardiac output and their relative effect on heart rate, systemic vascular resistance, and cardiac index. The drug used will depend in part on the cause of the HF.

A. Inotropic and Mechanical Support

1. Afterload reduction

A. Milrinone—This selective phosphodiesterase inhibitor increases cyclic adenosine monophosphate, thereby improving the inotropic state of the heart. In addition to a dose-dependent increase in cardiac contractility, milrinone is a systemic and pulmonary vasodilator and thus an effective agent in both right and left ventricular systolic dysfunction. Milrinone reduces the incidence of low cardiac output syndrome following open-heart surgery. The usual dosage range is 0.25–0.75 mcg/kg/min.

B. Nitroglycerin—Nitroglycerin functions primarily as a dilator of venous capacitance vessels and causes a reduction of right and left atrial pressure. Systemic blood pressure may also fall, and reflex tachycardia may occur. Nitroglycerin is used to improve coronary blood flow and may be especially useful when cardiac output is reduced because of coronary under-perfusion following congenital heart surgery. The usual intravenous dosage range is 1–3 mcg/kg/min.

2. Enhancement of contractility

A. Dopamine—This naturally occurring catecholamine increases myocardial contractility primarily via cardiac β-adrenergic activation. Dopamine also directly acts on renal dopamine receptors to improve renal perfusion. The usual dose range for HF is 3–10 mcg/kg/min.

B. Dobutamine—This synthetic catecholamine increases myocardial contractility secondary to cardiospecific β-adrenergic activation and produces little peripheral vasoconstriction. Dobutamine does not usually cause marked tachycardia, which is a distinct advantage. However, the drug does not selectively improve renal perfusion as does dopamine. The usual dose range is essentially the same as for dopamine.

3. Mechanical circulatory support—Mechanical support is indicated in children with severe, refractory myocardial failure secondary to cardiomyopathy, myocarditis, or following cardiac surgery. Mechanical support is used for a limited time while cardiac function improves or as a bridge to cardiac transplantation.

A. Extracorporeal membrane oxygenation (ECMO)—ECMO is a temporary means of providing oxygenation, carbon dioxide removal, and hemodynamic support to patients with cardiac or pulmonary failure refractory to conventional therapy. The blood removed from the patient via a catheter positioned in the venous system (eg, superior vena cava or right atrium) passes through a membrane oxygenator and then is delivered back to the patient through a catheter in the arterial system (eg, aorta or common carotid artery). Flow rates are adjusted to maintain adequate systemic perfusion, as judged by mean arterial blood pressure, acid-base status, end-organ function, and mixed venous oxygen saturation. The patient is monitored closely for improvement in cardiac contractility. Risks are significant and include severe

Table 20–12. Intravenous inotropic agents.

Drug	Dose	Renal Perfusion	Heart Rate	Cardiac Index	SVR
Dopamine	2-5 mcg/kg/min	↑ via vasodilation	0	0	0
	5-10	↑/↓-depending on balance of ↑ cardiac index and ↑SVR	↑	↑	↑↓
	> 10	↓	↑	↑	↑
Dobutamine	2.5-10 mcg/kg/min	↑ via ↑ cardiac index	↑	↑	↑↓
Epinephrine	0.2-2.0 mcg/kg/min	↓	↑	↑	↓
Norepinephrine	0.05-0.1 mcg/kg/min	↓	0	↑	↑↑
Isoproterenol	0.05-2.0 mcg/kg/min	0	↑↑	↑	↓↓

SVR, systemic vascular resistance.

internal and external bleeding, infection, thrombosis, and pump failure.

B. Ventricular assist devices—Use of ventricular assist devices is limited in children by patient size, availability, and institutional expertise. These devices allow for less invasive hemodynamic support than ECMO. A cannula is usually positioned in the apex of the ventricle and removes blood from the ventricle using a battery-operated pump. Blood is then returned to the patient through a separate cannula positioned in the aorta or pulmonary artery, depending on the ventricle being supported. Biventricular support can be done if necessary. Ventricular assist carries lower risk of pump failure than ECMO, but the risk of infection, thrombosis and bleeding complications remains.

Outpatient Management of Heart Failure

A. Medications

1. Afterload-reducing agents—Oral afterload-reducing agents improve cardiac output by decreasing systemic vascular resistance. Angiotensin-converting enzyme (ACE) inhibitors (captopril, enalapril, and lisinopril) are first-line therapy in children with HF requiring long-term treatment. These agents block angiotensin II–mediated systemic vasoconstriction and are particularly useful in children with structurally normal hearts but reduced LV myocardial function (eg, myocarditis or dilated cardiomyopathies [DCMs]). They are also useful in ameliorating mitral and aortic insufficiency and have a role in controlling refractory HF in patients with large left-to-right shunts in whom systemic vascular resistance is elevated.

2. β-Blockade—Although clearly beneficial in adults with HF, a randomized, controlled study of the use of a β-blocker (carvedilol) in children with HF did not demonstrate any significant improvement compared to placebo. However, β-blockers may still be useful adjunctive therapy in some children with refractory HF already taking ACE inhibitors. In the setting of HF, excessive circulating catecholamines are present due to activation of the sympathetic nervous system. Although beneficial acutely, this compensatory response over time produces myocardial fibrosis, myocyte hypertrophy, and myocyte apoptosis that contribute to the progression of HF. β-Blockers (eg, carvedilol and metoprolol) antagonize this sympathetic activation and may offset these deleterious effects. Side effects of β-blockers are significant and include bradycardia, hypotension, and worsening HF in some patients.

3. Diuretics—Diuretic therapy may be necessary in HF to maintain the euvolemic state and control symptoms related to pulmonary or hepatic congestion.

A. Furosemide—This rapid-acting loop diuretic may be given intravenously or orally. It removes large amounts of potassium and chloride from the body, producing hypochloremic metabolic alkalosis when used chronically. Electrolytes should be monitored during long-term therapy.

B. Thiazides—Thiazides are distal tubular diuretics used to complement furosemide in severe cases of HF.

C. Spironolactone—Spironolactone is a potassium-sparing aldosterone inhibitor. It is used frequently in conjunction with furosemide or thiazides for its enhanced diuretic function. Because it spares potassium, supplemental potassium may be avoided. Spironolactone has benefit in adults with HF regardless of its diuretic effect as aldosterone is associated with the development of fibrosis, sodium retention, and vascular dysfunction. This effect has not been proven in children.

4. Digitalis—Digitalis is a cardiac glycoside with a positive inotropic effect on the heart and an associated decrease in systemic vascular resistance. The preparation of digitalis used in clinical practice is digoxin. Large studies in adult patients with HF have not demonstrated decreased mortality of HF with digoxin use, but treatment is associated with reduced hospitalization rates for HF exacerbations. There are no controlled studies in children.

A. Digitalis toxicity—Any dysrhythmia that occurs during digoxin therapy should be attributed to the drug until proven otherwise. Ventricular bigeminy and first-, second-, or third-degree AV block are characteristic of digoxin toxicity. A trough level should be obtained if digoxin toxicity is suspected.

B. Digitalis poisoning—This acute emergency must be treated without delay. Digoxin poisoning most commonly occurs in toddlers who have taken their parents' or grandparents' medications. The child's stomach should be emptied immediately by gastric lavage even if several hours have passed since ingestion. Patients who have ingested massive amounts of digoxin should receive large doses of activated charcoal. In advanced heart block, atropine or temporary ventricular pacing may be needed. Digoxin immune Fab can be used to reverse potentially life-threatening intoxication. Antiarrhythmic agents may be useful.

5. Fluid restriction—Fluid restriction is rarely necessary in children with HF due to the effectiveness of diuretics and the tendency of infants and children with HF to self-regulate intake. Ensuring adequate caloric intake to promote growth is a more important goal in children with HF.

Morales DL, Zafar F, Rossano JW et al: Use of ventricular assist devices in children across the United States: analysis of 7.5 million pediatric hospitalizations. Ann Thorac Surg 2010 Oct;90(4):1313–1318, discussion 1318–1319 [PMID: 20868835].

Rosenthal D et al: International Society for Heart and Lung Transplantation: Practice guidelines for management of heart failure in children. J Heart Lung Transplant 2004;23:1313 [PMID: 15607659].

GENETIC BASIS OF CONGENITAL HEART DISEASE

Environmental factors such as maternal diabetes, alcohol consumption, progesterone use, viral infection, and other maternal teratogen exposure are associated with an increased incidence of cardiac malformations. However, the importance of genetics as a cause of congenital heart disease is becoming more evident as advances in the field occur. Microdeletion in the long arm of chromosome 22 (22q11) is associated with DiGeorge syndrome. These children often have conotruncal abnormalities such as truncus arteriosus, tetralogy of Fallot, double-outlet RV, or interrupted aortic arch. Alagille, Noonan, Holt-Oram, and Williams syndromes and the Trisomies 13, 18, and 21 are all commonly associated with congenital heart lesions. Understanding these associations as well as further targeted study investigating the genetic basis of other cardiac lesions will offer opportunities for early diagnosis, gene therapy, and recurrence risk counseling for families.

Pierpont ME et al: Genetic basis for congenital heart defects: Current knowledge: A scientific statement from the American Heart Association Congenital Cardiac Defects Committee, Council on Cardiovascular Disease in the Young: Endorsed by the American Academy of Pediatrics. Circulation 2007;115:3015–3038 [PMID: 17519398].

ACYANOTIC CONGENITAL HEART DISEASE

DEFECTS IN SEPTATION

1. Atrial Septal Defect

ESSENTIALS OF DIAGNOSIS & TYPICAL FEATURES

- Fixed, widely split S_2, RV heave.
- Grade I–III/VI systolic ejection murmur at the pulmonary area.
- Large shunts cause a diastolic flow murmur at the lower left sternal border (increased flow across the tricuspid valve).
- ECG shows rsR′ in lead V_1.
- Frequently asymptomatic.

General Considerations

Atrial septal defect (ASD) is an opening in the atrial septum permitting the shunting of blood between the atria. There are three major types: ostium secundum, ostium primum, and sinus venosus. Ostium secundum is the most common type and represents an embryologic deficiency in the septum secundum or too large of a central hole in the septum primum. Ostium primum defect is associated with atrioventricular septal defects. The sinus venosus defect is frequently associated with abnormal pulmonary venous return, as the location of the sinus venosus is intimately related to the right upper pulmonary vein.

Ostium secundum ASD occurs in 10% of patients with congenital heart disease and is two times more common in females than in males. The defect is most often sporadic but may be familial or have a genetic basis (Holt-Oram syndrome). After the third decade, atrial arrhythmias or pulmonary vascular disease may develop. Irreversible pulmonary hypertension resulting in cyanosis as atrial level shunting becomes right-to-left and ultimately right heart failure can occur and is a life-limiting process (Eisenmenger syndrome).

Clinical Findings

A. Symptoms and Signs

Most infants and children with an ASD have no cardiovascular symptoms. Older children and adults can present with exercise intolerance, easy fatigability, or, rarely, heart failure. The direction of flow across the ASD is determined by the compliance of the ventricles. Because the right ventricle is normally more compliant, shunting across the ASD is left-to-right as blood follows the path of least resistance. Therefore, cyanosis does not occur unless RV dysfunction occurs, usually as a result of pulmonary hypertension, leading to reversal of the shunt across the defect.

Peripheral pulses are normal and equal. The heart is usually hyperactive, with an RV heave felt best at the mid to lower left sternal border. S_2 at the pulmonary area is widely split and often fixed. In the absence of associated pulmonary hypertension, the pulmonary component is normal in intensity. A grade I–III/VI ejection-type systolic murmur is heard best at the left sternal border in the second intercostal space. This murmur is caused by increased flow across the pulmonic valve, not flow across the ASD. A mid-diastolic murmur is often heard in the fourth intercostal space at the left sternal border. This murmur is caused by increased flow across the tricuspid valve during diastole. The presence of this murmur suggests high flow with a pulmonary-to-systemic blood flow ratio greater than 2:1.

B. Imaging

Radiographs may show cardiac enlargement. The main pulmonary artery may be dilated and pulmonary vascular markings increased in large defects owing to the increased pulmonary blood flow.

C. Electrocardiography

The usual ECG shows right axis deviation. In the right precordial leads, an rsR′ pattern is usually present. A mutation in the cardiac homeobox gene (*NKX2-5*) is associated with an ASD, and AV block would be seen on the ECG.

D. Echocardiography

Echocardiography shows a dilated right atrium and RV. Direct visualization of the exact anatomic location of the ASD by two-dimensional echocardiography, and demonstration of a left-to-right shunt through the defect by color-flow Doppler, confirms the diagnosis and has eliminated the need for cardiac catheterization prior to surgical or catheter closure of the defect. Assessment of all pulmonary veins should be made to rule out associated anomalous pulmonary venous return.

E. Cardiac Catheterization

Although cardiac catheterization is rarely needed for diagnostic purposes, transcatheter closure of an ostium secundum ASD is now the preferred method of treatment.

If a catheterization is performed, oximetry shows a significant step-up in oxygen saturation from the superior vena cava to the right atrium. The pulmonary artery pressure and pulmonary vascular resistance are usually normal. The Qp: Qs may vary from 1.5:1 to 4:1.

▶ Treatment

Surgical or catheterization closure is generally recommended for symptomatic children with a large atrial level defect and associated right heart dilation. In the asymptomatic child with a large hemodynamically significant defect, closure is performed electively at age 1–3 years. Most defects are amenable to nonoperative device closure during cardiac catheterization, but the defect must have adequate tissue rims on all sides on which to anchor the device. The mortality for surgical closure is less than 1%. When closure is performed by age 3 years, late complications of RV dysfunction and dysrhythmias are avoided.

▶ Course & Prognosis

Patients usually tolerate an ASD well in the first two decades of life, and the defect often goes unnoticed until middle or late adulthood. Pulmonary hypertension and reversal of the shunt are rare late complications. Infective endocarditis (IE) is uncommon. Spontaneous closure occurs, most frequently in children with a defect less than 4 mm in diameter, therefore outpatient follow-up is recommended. Exercise tolerance and oxygen consumption in surgically corrected children are generally normal, and restriction of physical activity is unnecessary.

Arrington CB et al: An assessment of the electrocardiogram as a screening test for large atrial septal defects in children. J Electrocardiol 2007;40:484–488 [PMID: 17673249].

Butera G et al: Treatment of isolated secundum atrial septal defects: Impact of age and defect morphology in 1,013 consecutive patients. Am Heart J 2008;156:706–712 [PMID: 18926151].

2. Ventricular Septal Defect

ESSENTIALS OF DIAGNOSIS & TYPICAL FEATURES

- Holosystolic murmur at lower left sternal border with RV heave.
- Presentation and course depend on size of defect and the pulmonary vascular resistance.
- Clinical features are failure to thrive, tachypnea, and diaphoresis with feeds.
- Left-to-right shunt with normal pulmonary vascular resistance.
- Large defects may cause Eisenmenger syndrome if not repaired early.

▶ General Considerations

Ventricular septal defect (VSD) is the most common congenital heart malformation, accounting for about 30% of all congenital heart disease. Defects in the ventricular septum occur both in the membranous portion of the septum (most common) and the muscular portion. VSDs follow one of four courses:

A. Small, Hemodynamically Insignificant Ventricular Septal Defects

Between 80% and 85% of VSDs are small (< 3 mm in diameter) at birth and will close spontaneously. In general, small defects in the muscular interventricular septum will close sooner than those in the membranous septum. In most cases, a small VSD never requires surgical closure. Fifty percent of small VSDs will close by age 2 years, and 90% by age 6 years, with most of the remaining closing during the school years. Parents should be told at the time of diagnosis that nearly all small VSDs will eventually close.

B. Moderate-Sized Ventricular Septal Defects

Asymptomatic patients with moderate-sized VSDs (3–5 mm in diameter) account for 3%–5% of children with VSDs. In general, these children do not have clear indicators for surgical closure. Historically, in those who had cardiac catheterization, the ratio of pulmonary to systemic blood flow is usually less than 2:1, and serial cardiac catheterizations demonstrate that the shunts get progressively smaller. If the patient is asymptomatic and without evidence of pulmonary hypertension, these defects can be followed serially as some close spontaneously over time.

C. Large Ventricular Septal Defects with Normal Pulmonary Vascular Resistance

These defects are usually 6–10 mm in diameter. Unless they become markedly smaller within a few months after birth, they often require surgery. The timing of surgery depends on the clinical situation. Many infants with large VSDs and normal pulmonary vascular resistance develop symptoms of failure to thrive, tachypnea, diaphoresis with feeds by age 3–6 months, and require correction at that time. Surgery before age 2 years in patients with large VSDs essentially eliminates the risk of pulmonary vascular disease.

D. Large Ventricular Septal Defects with Pulmonary Vascular Obstructive Disease

The direction of flow across a VSD is determined by the resistance in the systemic and pulmonary vasculature, explaining why flow is usually left-to-right. In large VSDs, ventricular pressures are equalized, resulting in increased pulmonary artery pressure. In addition, shear stress caused by increased volume in the pulmonary circuit causes increased resistance over time. The vast majority of patients with inoperable pulmonary hypertension develop the condition progressively. The combined data of the multicenter National History Study indicate that almost all cases of irreversible pulmonary hypertension can be prevented by surgical repair of a large VSD before age 2 years.

Clinical Findings

A. Symptoms and Signs

Patients with small or moderate left-to-right shunts usually have no cardiovascular symptoms. Patients with large left-to-right shunts are usually ill early in infancy. These infants have frequent respiratory infections and gain weight slowly. Dyspnea, diaphoresis, and fatigue are common. These symptoms can develop as early as 1–6 months of age. After the first year, symptoms usually improve, although easy fatigability may persist. Older children may experience exercise intolerance. Over time, in children and adolescents with persistent large left-to-right shunt, the pulmonary vascular bed undergoes structural changes, leading to increased pulmonary vascular resistance and reversal of the shunt from left-to-right to right-to-left (Eisenmenger syndrome). Cyanosis will then be present.

1. Small left-to-right shunt—No lifts, heaves, or thrills are present. The first sound at the apex is normal, and the second sound at the pulmonary area is split physiologically. A grade II–IV/VI, medium- to high-pitched, harsh pansystolic murmur is heard best at the left sternal border in the third and fourth intercostal spaces. The murmur radiates over the entire precordium. No diastolic murmurs are heard.

2. Moderate left-to-right shunt—Slight prominence of the precordium with moderate LV heave is evident. A systolic thrill may be palpable at the lower left sternal border between the third and fourth intercostal spaces. The second sound at the pulmonary area is most often split but may be single. A grade III–IV/VI, harsh pansystolic murmur is heard best at the lower left sternal border in the fourth intercostal space. A mitral diastolic flow murmur indicates that pulmonary blood flow and subsequently the pulmonary venous return are significantly increased by the large shunt.

3. Large ventricular septal defects with pulmonary hypertension—The precordium is prominent, and the sternum bulges. Both LV and RV heaves are palpable. S_2 is palpable in the pulmonary area. A thrill may be present at the lower left sternal border. S_2 is usually single or narrowly split, with accentuation of the pulmonary component. The murmur ranges from grade I to IV/VI and is usually harsh and pansystolic. Occasionally, when the defect is large or ventricular pressures approach equivalency, a murmur is difficult to hear. A diastolic flow murmur may be heard, depending on the size of the shunt.

B. Imaging

In patients with small shunts, the chest radiograph may be normal. Patients with large shunts have significant cardiac enlargement involving both the left and right ventricles and the left atrium. The main pulmonary artery segment may be dilated. The pulmonary vascular markings are increased.

C. Electrocardiography

The ECG is normal in small left-to-right shunts. Left ventricular hypertrophy (LVH) usually occurs in patients with large left-to-right shunts and normal pulmonary vascular resistance. Combined ventricular enlargement occurs in patients with pulmonary hypertension caused by increased flow, increased resistance, or both. Pure RV hypertrophy occurs in patients with pulmonary hypertension secondary to pulmonary vascular obstruction induced by long-standing left-to-right shunt (Eisenmenger syndrome).

D. Echocardiography

Two-dimensional echocardiography can reveal the size of a VSD and identify its anatomic location. Multiple defects can be detected by combining two-dimensional and color-flow imaging. Doppler can further evaluate the VSD by estimating the pressure difference between the left and right ventricles. A pressure difference greater than 50 mm Hg in the left ventricle compared to the right ventricle confirms the absence of severe pulmonary hypertension.

E. Cardiac Catheterization and Angiocardiography

The ability to describe the VSD anatomy and estimate the pulmonary artery pressures on the basis of the gradient across the VSD allows for the vast majority of isolated defects to be repaired without cardiac catheterization and angiocardiography. Catheterization is indicated in those patients with increased pulmonary vascular resistance. The pulmonary artery pressure may vary from normal to systemic (equal to the aortic pressure). Pulmonary artery wedge pressure (a surrogate for direct left atrial pressure) may be normal to increased. Pulmonary vascular resistance varies from normal to markedly increased. Angiocardiographic examination defines the number, size, and location of the defects.

Treatment

A. Medical Management

Patients who develop symptoms should receive anticongestive treatment (see section on Heart Failure, earlier), particularly diuretics and systemic afterload reduction. If the patient does not respond to anticongestive measures, or if he or she shows progressive pulmonary hypertension, surgery is indicated without delay.

B. Surgical Treatment

Patients with cardiomegaly, poor growth, poor exercise tolerance, or other clinical abnormalities who have a significant shunt (> 2:1) without significant pulmonary hypertension typically undergo surgical repair at age 3–6 months. A synthetic or pericardial patch is used for primary closure. The age of elective surgery has decreased and most defects are now closed in infancy. Patients with pulmonary artery pressures equal to systemic pressure undergo surgical repair well before age 2 years to avoid pulmonary vascular disease. In most centers, these children have surgery before age 1 year. As a result, Eisenmenger syndrome has been virtually eliminated. The surgical mortality rate for VSD closure is below 2%.

Transcatheter closure of muscular VSDs is now becoming common. Perimembranous VSDs have also been closed in children during catheterization, but a high incidence of complete heart block after placement of the occluding device has slowed the acceptance of this approach.

Course & Prognosis

Significant late dysrhythmias are uncommon. Functional exercise capacity and oxygen consumption are usually normal, and physical restrictions are unnecessary. Adults with corrected defects have normal quality of life. After surgical VSD closure, antibiotic prophylaxis for bacterial endocarditis can be discontinued 6 months after surgery.

Butera G et al: Transcatheter closure of perimembranous ventricular septal defects: Early and long-term results. J Am Coll Cardiol 2007;50:1189–1195 [PMID: 17868812].

Sondheimer HM, Rahimi-Alangi K: Current management of ventricular septal defect. Cardiol Young 2006;16(Suppl 3):131–135 [PMID: 17378052].

3. Atrioventricular Septal Defect

ESSENTIALS OF DIAGNOSIS & TYPICAL FEATURES

- Murmur often inaudible in neonates.
- Loud pulmonary component of S_2.
- Common in infants with Down syndrome.
- ECG with extreme left axis deviation.

General Considerations

Atrioventricular septal defect (AVSD) results from incomplete fusion of the embryonic endocardial cushions. The endocardial cushions help to form the "crux" of the heart, which includes the lower portion of the atrial septum, the membranous portion of the ventricular septum, and the septal leaflets of the tricuspid and mitral valves. AVSD accounts for about 4% of all congenital heart disease. Sixty percent of children with Down syndrome have congenital heart disease, and of these, 35%–40% have an AVSD.

AVSDs are defined as partial or complete. The physiology of the defect is determined by the location of the AV valves. If the valves are located in the midportion of the defect (complete AVSD), both atrial and ventricular components of the septal defect are present and the left- and right-sided AV valves share a common ring or orifice. In the partial form, there is a low insertion of the AV valves, resulting in a primum ASD without a ventricular defect component. In partial AVSD, there are two separate AV valve orifices and usually a cleft in the left-sided valve.

Partial AVSD behaves like an isolated ASD with variable amounts of regurgitation through the cleft in the left AV valve. The complete form causes large left-to-right shunts at both the ventricular and atrial levels with variable degrees of AV valve regurgitation. If there is increased pulmonary vascular resistance, the shunts may be bidirectional. Bidirectional shunting is more common in Down syndrome or in older children who have not undergone repair.

Clinical Findings

A. Symptoms and Signs

The partial form may produce symptoms similar to ostium secundum ASD. Patients with complete AVSD usually are severely affected. HF manifesting as failure to thrive, tachypnea, and diaphoresis with feeding often develops in infancy, and recurrent bouts of pneumonia are common.

In the neonate with the complete form, the murmur may be inaudible due to relatively equal systemic and pulmonary vascular resistance (PVR). After 4–6 weeks, as PVR drops, a nonspecific systolic murmur develops. The murmur is usually not as harsh as that of an isolated VSD. There is both right- and left-sided cardiac enlargement. S_2 is loud, and a pronounced diastolic flow murmur may be heard at the apex and the lower left sternal border.

If severe pulmonary vascular obstructive disease is present, there is usually dominant RV enlargement. S_2 is palpable at the pulmonary area and no thrill is felt. A nonspecific short systolic murmur is heard at the lower left sternal border. No diastolic flow murmurs are heard. If a right-to-left shunt is present, cyanosis will be evident.

B. Imaging

Cardiac enlargement is always present. In the complete form, all four chambers are enlarged. Pulmonary vascular markings are increased. In patients with pulmonary vascular obstructive disease, only the main pulmonary artery segment and its branches are prominent and the peripheral pulmonary vascular markings are usually decreased.

C. Electrocardiography

In all forms of AVSD, there is extreme left axis deviation with a counterclockwise loop in the frontal plane. The ECG is an important diagnostic tool. Only 5% of isolated VSDs have this ECG abnormality. First-degree heart block occurs in over 50% of patients. Right, left, or combined ventricular hypertrophy is present depending on the particular defect and the presence or absence of pulmonary hypertension.

D. Echocardiography

Echocardiography is the diagnostic test of choice. The anatomy can be well visualized by two-dimensional echocardiography. Both AV valves are at the same level, compared with the normal heart in which the tricuspid valve is more apically positioned. The size of the atrial and ventricular components of the defect can be measured. AV valve regurgitation can be detected. The LV outflow tract is elongated (gooseneck appearance), which produces systemic outflow obstruction in some patients.

E. Cardiac Catheterization and Angiocardiography

Cardiac catheterization is not routinely used to evaluate AVSD but may be used to assess pulmonary artery pressures and resistance in the older infant with Down syndrome, as this patient group is predisposed to early-onset pulmonary hypertension. Increased oxygen saturation in the RV or the right atrium identifies the level of the shunt. Angiocardiography reveals the characteristic gooseneck deformity of the LV outflow tract in the complete form.

Treatment

Spontaneous closure of this type of defect does not occur and therefore surgery is required. In the partial form, surgery carries a low mortality rate (1%–2%), but patients require follow-up because of late-occurring LV outflow tract obstruction and mitral valve dysfunction. The complete form carries a higher mortality rate. Complete correction in the first year of life, prior to the onset of irreversible pulmonary hypertension, is obligatory. If possible, primary correction should be performed when the child is well and weighs more than 5 kg. During surgery, transesophageal echocardiography is used to assess the adequacy of repair before discontinuing cardiopulmonary bypass.

Craig B: Atrioventricular septal defect: From fetus to adult. Heart 2006;92:1879–1885 [PMID: 17105897].

Kobayashi M, Takahashi Y, Ando M: Ideal timing of surgical repair of isolated complete atrioventricular septal defect. Interact Cardiovasc Thorac Surg 2007;6:24–26 [PMID: 17669760].

PATENT (PERSISTENT) DUCTUS ARTERIOSUS

ESSENTIALS OF DIAGNOSIS & TYPICAL FEATURES

- Continuous machinery type murmur.
- Bounding peripheral pulses if large ductus present.
- Presentation and course depends on size of the ductus and the pulmonary vascular resistance.
- Clinical features of a large ductus are failure to thrive, tachypnea, and diaphoresis with feeds.
- Left-to-right shunt with normal pulmonary vascular resistance.

General Considerations

PDA is the persistence of the normal fetal vessel joining the pulmonary artery to the aorta. It closes spontaneously in normal-term infants at 1–5 days of age. PDA accounts for 10% of all congenital heart disease. The incidence of PDA is higher in infants born at altitudes over 10,000 ft. It is twice as common in females as in males. The frequency of PDA in preterm infants weighing less than 1500 g ranges from 20% to 60%. The defect may occur as an isolated abnormality or with associated lesions, commonly coarctation of the aorta and VSD. Patency of the ductus arteriosus may be necessary in some patients with complex forms of congenital heart disease (eg, hypoplastic left heart syndrome [HLHS], pulmonary atresia). Prostaglandin E_2 (PGE_2) is a product of arachidonic acid metabolism and continuous intravenous infusion maintains ductal patency.

Clinical Findings

A. Symptoms and Signs

The clinical findings and course depend on the size of the shunt and the degree of pulmonary hypertension.

1. Moderate to large patent ductus arteriosus—Pulses are bounding, and pulse pressure is widened due to diastolic runoff through the ductus. S_1 is normal and S_2 is usually narrowly split. In large shunts, S_2 may have a paradoxical split (eg, S_2 narrows on inspiration and widens on expiration). Paradoxical splitting is caused by volume overload of the LV and prolonged ejection of blood from this chamber.

The murmur is characteristic. It is a rough machinery murmur maximal at the second left intercostal space. It begins shortly after S_1, rises to a peak at S_2, and passes through the S_2 into diastole, where it becomes a decrescendo murmur and fades before the S_1. The murmur tends to radiate well to the anterior lung fields but relatively poorly to the posterior lung fields. A diastolic flow murmur is often heard at the apex.

2. Patent ductus arteriosus with increased pulmonary vascular resistance—Flow across the ductus is diminished. S_2 is single and accentuated, and no significant heart murmur is present. The pulses are normal rather than bounding.

B. Imaging

In an isolated PDA, the appearance of the chest radiograph depends on the size of the shunt. If the shunt is small, the heart is not enlarged. If the shunt is large, both left atrial and LV enlargement may be seen. The aorta and the main pulmonary artery segment may also be prominent.

C. Electrocardiography

The ECG may be normal or may show LVH, depending on the size of the shunt. In patients with pulmonary hypertension caused by increased blood flow, biventricular hypertrophy usually occurs. In pulmonary vascular obstructive disease, pure right ventricular hypertrophy (RVH) occurs.

D. Echocardiography

Echocardiography provides direct visualization of the ductus and confirms the direction and degree of shunting. High-velocity left-to-right flow argues against abnormally elevated pulmonary vascular resistance, and as pulmonary vascular resistance drops during the neonatal period, higher velocity left-to-right shunting is usually seen. If suprasystemic pulmonary vascular resistance is present, flow across the ductus will be seen from right to left. Associated cardiac lesions and ductal-dependent pulmonary or systemic blood flow must be recognized by echocardiography, as closure of a PDA in this setting would be contraindicated.

E. Cardiac Catheterization and Angiocardiography

Children with an isolated PDA no longer require a cardiac catheterization for diagnostic purposes. However, children weighing more than 5 kg with a PDA routinely undergo PDA closure in the catheterization laboratory with a vascular plug or coils.

Treatment

Surgical closure is indicated when the PDA is large and the patient is small. Caution must be given to closing a PDA in patients with pulmonary vascular obstructive disease and right-to-left shunting across the ductus as this could result in RV failure. Patients with large left-to-right shunts require repair by age 1 year to prevent the development of progressive pulmonary vascular obstructive disease. Symptomatic PDA with normal pulmonary artery pressure can be safely coil or device-occluded in the catheterization laboratory after the child has reached 5 kg.

Patients with nonreactive pulmonary vascular obstruction, pulmonary vascular resistance greater than 10 Wood units (normal, < 3), and a ratio of pulmonary to systemic resistance greater than 0.7 (normal, < 0.3) despite vasodilator therapy (eg, nitric oxide) should not undergo PDA closure. These patients are made worse by PDA closure because the flow through the ductus allows preserved RV function and maintains cardiac output to the systemic circulation. These patients can be managed with pulmonary vasodilator therapy, but eventually may require heart-lung transplant in severe cases.

Presence of a symptomatic PDA is common in preterm infants. Indomethacin, a prostaglandin synthesis inhibitor, is often used to close the PDA in premature infants. Indomethacin does not close the PDA of full-term infants or children. The success of indomethacin therapy is as high as 80%–90% in premature infants with a birth weight greater than 1200 g, but it is less successful in smaller infants. Indomethacin (0.1–0.3 mg/kg orally every 8–24 hours or 0.1–0.3 mg/kg parenterally every 12 hours) can be used if there is adequate renal, hematologic, and hepatic function. Because indomethacin may impair renal function, urine output, BUN, and creatinine should be monitored during therapy. If indomethacin is not effective and the ductus remains hemodynamically significant, surgical ligation should be performed. If the ductus partially closes so that the shunt is no longer hemodynamically significant, surgery is not needed, and a second course of indomethacin may be used. Recent studies from Europe indicate that ibuprofen may be as effective as indomethacin for medical closure of preterm PDA.

Course & Prognosis

Patients with an isolated PDA and small-to-moderate shunts usually do well without surgery. However, in the third or fourth decade of life, symptoms of easy fatigability, dyspnea on exertion, and exercise intolerance appear in those patients who develop pulmonary hypertension and/or HF. Percutaneous closure can be done later in life if there has not been development of severe pulmonary vascular disease.

Spontaneous closure of a PDA may occur up to age 1 year, especially in preterm infants. After age 1 year, spontaneous closure is rare. Because IE is a potential complication, some cardiologists recommend closure if the defect persists beyond age 1 year, even if it is small. Most of these patients undergo percutaneous occlusion as opposed to surgical ligation.

The prognosis for patients with large shunts or pulmonary hypertension is not as good. Poor growth and development, frequent pneumonias, and HF occur in these children. Patients beyond the newborn period with a hemodynamically significant PDA should have transcatheter device closure of their PDA.

Cherif A, Jabnoun S, Khrouf N: Oral ibuprofen in early curative closure of patent ductus arteriosus in very premature infants. Am J Perinatol 2007;24:339–345 [PMID: 17564958].

Takata H, Higaki T, Sugiyama H et al: Long-term outcome of coil occlusion in patients with patent ductus arteriosus. Circ J 2011 Feb;75(2):407–412 [PMID: 21173496].

RIGHT-SIDED OBSTRUCTIVE LESIONS

1. Pulmonary Valve Stenosis

ESSENTIALS OF DIAGNOSIS & TYPICAL FEATURES

- No symptoms in mild or moderate stenosis.
- Cyanosis and a high incidence of right-sided HF in ductal-dependent lesions.
- RV lift with systolic ejection click heard at the third left intercostal space.
- S_2 widely split with soft to inaudible P_2; grade I–VI/VI systolic ejection murmur, maximal at the pulmonary area.
- Dilated pulmonary artery on chest radiograph.

General Considerations

Pulmonic valve stenosis accounts for 10% of all congenital heart disease. In the usual case, the cusps of the pulmonary valve are fused to form a membrane or diaphragm with a hole in the middle from 2 to 10 mm in diameter. Occasionally, only two cusps are fused, producing a bicuspid pulmonary valve. In more severe cases, secondary infundibular (subvalvular) stenosis occurs. The pulmonary valve annulus is usually small with moderate to marked poststenotic dilation of the main pulmonary artery. Patients with Noonan syndrome frequently have pulmonary stenosis and hypertrophic cardiomyopathy (HCM).

Obstruction to blood flow across the pulmonary valve causes an increase in RV pressure. Pressures greater than systemic are potentially life-threatening and are associated with critical obstruction. Because of the increased RV strain, severe right ventricular hypertrophy (RVH) and eventual RV failure can occur.

When obstruction is severe and the ventricular septum is intact, a right-to-left shunt will often occur at the atrial level through a patent foramen ovale (PFO). In neonates with severe obstruction and minimal antegrade pulmonary blood flow (critical PS), left-to-right flow through the ductus is essential, making prostaglandin a necessary intervention at the time of birth. These infants are cyanotic at presentation.

Clinical Findings

A. Symptoms and Signs

Patients with mild or even moderate valvular pulmonary stenosis are acyanotic and asymptomatic. Patients with severe valvular obstruction may develop cyanosis early. Patients with mild to moderate obstruction are usually well developed and well nourished. They are not prone to pulmonary infections. The pulses are normal. The precordium may be prominent, often with palpable RV heave. A systolic thrill is often present in the pulmonary area. In patients with mild to moderate stenosis, a prominent ejection click of pulmonary origin is heard at the third left intercostal space. The click varies with respiration, being more prominent during expiration than inspiration. In severe stenosis, the click tends to merge with S_1. S_2 varies with the degree of stenosis. In mild pulmonic stenosis, S_2 is normal. In moderate pulmonic stenosis, S_2 is more widely split and the pulmonary component is softer. In severe pulmonary stenosis, S_2 is single because the pulmonary component cannot be heard. A rough systolic ejection murmur is best heard at the second left interspace. It radiates well to the back. With severe pulmonary valve obstruction, the murmur is usually short. No diastolic murmurs are audible.

B. Imaging

The heart size is normal. Poststenotic dilation of the main pulmonary artery and the left pulmonary artery often occurs.

C. Electrocardiography

The ECG is usually normal with mild obstruction. RVH is present with moderate to severe pulmonic stenosis. In severe obstruction, RV hypertrophy with an RV strain pattern (deep inversion of the T wave) occurs in the right precordial leads (V_{3R}, V_1, V_2). Right atrial enlargement may be present. Right axis deviation occurs in moderate to severe stenosis.

D. Echocardiography

The diagnosis often is made by physical examination, but the echocardiogram confirms the diagnosis, defines the anatomy, and can identify any associated lesions. The pulmonary valve has thickened leaflets with reduced valve leaflet excursion. The transvalvular pressure gradient can be estimated accurately by Doppler, which provides an estimate of RV pressure and can assist in determining the appropriate time to intervene.

E. Cardiac Catheterization and Angiocardiography

Pulmonic stenosis is easily diagnosed by physical examination, ECG, and echocardiography. Catheterization is reserved for therapeutic balloon valvuloplasty. In severe cases with associated RV dysfunction, a right-to-left shunt at the atrial level is indicated by a lower left atrial saturation than pulmonary vein saturation. Pulmonary artery pressure is normal. The gradient across the pulmonary valve varies from 10 to 200 mm Hg. In severe cases, the right atrial pressure is elevated, with a predominant "a" wave. Angiocardiography in the RV shows a thick pulmonary valve with a narrow opening producing a jet of contrast into the pulmonary artery. Infundibular (RV outflow tract) hypertrophy may be present and may contribute to obstruction to pulmonary blood flow.

Treatment

Treatment of pulmonic stenosis is recommended for children with RV systolic pressure greater than two-thirds of systemic pressure. Immediate correction is indicated for patients with systemic or suprasystemic RV pressure. Percutaneous balloon valvuloplasty is the procedure of choice. It is as effective as surgery in relieving obstruction and causes less valve insufficiency. Surgery is needed to treat pulmonic valve stenosis when balloon pulmonic valvuloplasty is unsuccessful.

Course & Prognosis

Patients with mild pulmonary stenosis live normal lives. Even those with moderate stenosis are rarely symptomatic. Those with severe valvular obstruction may develop cyanosis in infancy as described above.

After balloon pulmonary valvuloplasty or surgery, most patients have good maximum exercise capacity unless they have significant pulmonary insufficiency (PI). Limitation of physical activity is unwarranted. The quality of life of adults with successfully treated pulmonary stenosis and minimal PI is normal. Patients with PI, a frequent side effect of intervention, may be significantly limited in exercise performance. Severe PI leads to progressive RV dilation and dysfunction, which may precipitate ventricular arrhythmias or right heart failure in adulthood. Patients with severe PI may benefit from replacement of the pulmonic valve.

Drossner DM, Mahle WT: A management strategy for mild valvar pulmonary stenosis. Pediatr Cardiol 2008;29:649–652 [PMID: 18193316].

Harrild DM, Powell AJ, Tran TX et al: Long-term pulmonary regurgitation following balloon valvuloplasty for pulmonary stenosis risk factors and relationship to exercise capacity and ventricular volume and function. J Am Coll Cardiol 2010 Mar 9;55(10):1041–1047 [PMID: 20202522].

2. Subvalvular Pulmonary Stenosis

Isolated infundibular (subvalvular) pulmonary stenosis is rare. More commonly it is found in combination with other lesions, such as in tetralogy of Fallot. Infundibular hypertrophy that is associated with a small perimembranous VSD may lead to a "double-chambered RV" characterized by obstruction between the inflow and outflow portion of the RV. One should suspect such an abnormality if there is a prominent precordial thrill, no audible pulmonary ejection click, and a murmur maximal in the third and fourth intercostal spaces rather than in the second intercostal space. The clinical picture is otherwise identical to that of pulmonic valve stenosis. Intervention, if indicated, is always surgical because this condition does not improve with balloon catheter dilation.

3. Supravalvular Pulmonary Stenosis

Supravalvular pulmonary stenosis is a relatively rare condition defined by narrowing of the main pulmonary artery. The clinical picture may be identical to valvular pulmonary stenosis, although the murmur is maximal in the first intercostal space at the left sternal border and in the suprasternal notch. No ejection click is audible, as the valve itself is not involved. The murmur radiates toward the neck and over the lung fields. Children with William syndrome can have supravalvular and peripheral pulmonary stenosis as well as supravalvular aortic stenosis.

4. Peripheral (Branch) Pulmonary Artery Stenosis

In peripheral pulmonary stenosis, there are multiple narrowings of the branches of the pulmonary arteries, sometimes extending into the vessels in the periphery of the lungs. Systolic murmurs may be heard over both lung fields, anteriorly and posteriorly, radiating to the axilla. Mild, nonpathologic pulmonary branch stenosis produces a murmur in infancy that resolves by 6 months of age. William syndrome, Alagille syndrome, and congenital rubella are commonly associated with severe forms of peripheral pulmonary artery stenosis. Surgery is often unsuccessful, as areas of stenoses near and beyond the hilum of the lungs are not accessible to the surgeons. Transcatheter balloon angioplasty and even stent placement are used to treat this condition, with moderate success. In some instances, the stenoses improve spontaneously with age.

5. Ebstein Malformation of the Tricuspid Valve

In Ebstein malformation of the tricuspid valve, the septal leaflet of the tricuspid valve is displaced toward the apex of the heart and is attached to the endocardium of the RV rather than at the tricuspid annulus. As a result, a large portion of the RV functions physiologically as part of the right atrium. This "atrialized" portion of the RV is thin-walled and does not contribute to RV output. The portion of the ventricle below the displaced tricuspid valve is diminished in volume and represents the functioning RV.

Clinical Findings

A. Symptoms and Signs

The clinical picture of Ebstein malformation varies with the degree of displacement of the tricuspid valve. In the most extreme form, the septal leaflet is markedly displaced into the RV outflow tract, causing obstruction of antegrade flow into the pulmonary artery and there is very little functioning RV as the majority of the ventricle is "atrialized." The degree of tricuspid insufficiency may be so severe that forward (antegrade) flow out the RV outflow tract is further diminished leading to a right-to-left atrial level shunt and cyanosis. At the opposite extreme when antegrade pulmonary blood flow is adequate, symptoms may not develop until adulthood when tachyarrhythmias associated with right atrial dilation or reentrant electrical pathways occur. These older patients typically have less displacement of the septal leaflet of the tricuspid valve and therefore more functional RV tissue.

B. Imaging

The chest radiograph usually shows cardiomegaly with prominence of the right heart border. The extent of cardiomegaly depends on the degree of tricuspid valve insufficiency and the presence and size of the atrial level shunt. Massive cardiomegaly with a "wall-to-wall heart" (the heart shadow extends across the entire chest cavity from right-to-left) occurs with severe tricuspid valve displacement and/or a restrictive atrial level defect.

C. Electrocardiography

ECG may be normal but usually shows right atrial enlargement and right bundle-branch block (RBBB). There is an association between Ebstein anomaly and Wolff-Parkinson-White (WPW) syndrome, in which case a delta wave is present (short PR with a slurred upstroke of the QRS).

D. Echocardiography

Echocardiography is necessary to confirm the diagnosis and may aid in predicting outcome. Degree of tricuspid valve displacement, size of the right atrium, and presence of associated atrial level shunt all affect outcome. The size of the atrialized portion of the RV is determined by echocardiography, and, in severe cases, the atrialized RV can become so enlarged that it encroaches on the LV, impeding LV filling and function.

Course & Prognosis

In cyanotic neonates, PGE_2 is used to maintain pulmonary blood flow via the ductus arteriosus until pulmonary vascular resistance decreases, facilitating antegrade pulmonary artery flow. If the neonate remains significantly cyanotic, surgical intervention is required, but the outcome is poor.

The type of surgical repair varies and depends on the severity of the disease. For example, in order to decrease the amount of tricuspid regurgitation surgery may involve atrial plication and tricuspid valve repair. The success of the procedure is highly variable. Late arrhythmias are common due to the preexisting atrial dilation. If a significant Ebstein malformation is not treated, atrial tachyarrhythmias frequently begin during adolescence. Postoperative exercise tolerance improves but remains lower than age-related norms.

6. Other Rare Right-Sided Malformations

A. Absence of a Pulmonary Artery

Absence of a pulmonary artery (left or right) may be an isolated malformation or may occur in association with other congenital heart lesions. It occurs occasionally in patients with tetralogy of Fallot.

B. Absence of the Pulmonary Valve

Absence of the pulmonary valve is rare and usually associated with a VSD. In about 50% of cases, infundibular pulmonary stenosis is also present (ToF with absent pulmonary valve).

Alsoufi B et al: Surgical outcomes in the treatment of patients with tetralogy of Fallot and absent pulmonary valve. Eur J Cardiothorac Surg 2007;31:354–359; discussion 359 [PMID: 17215132].

Knott-Craig CJ et al: Repair of neonates and young infants with Ebstein's anomaly and related disorders. Ann Thorac Surg 2007;84:587–592; discussion 592–593 [PMID: 17643640].

LEFT-SIDED LESIONS

1. Coarctation of the Aorta

ESSENTIALS OF DIAGNOSIS & TYPICAL FEATURES

- Absent or diminished femoral pulses.
- Upper to lower extremity systolic blood pressure gradient of > 20 mm Hg.
- Blowing systolic murmur in the back or left axilla.

General Considerations

Coarctation of the aorta is a narrowing in the aortic arch that usually occurs in the proximal descending aorta near the takeoff of the left subclavian artery near the ductus arteriosus. The abdominal aorta is rarely involved. Coarctation accounts for about 6% of all congenital heart disease. Three times as many males as females are affected. Many affected females have Turner syndrome (45, XO). The incidence of associated bicuspid aortic valve with coarctation is 80%–85%.

Clinical Findings

A. Symptoms and Signs

The cardinal physical finding is decreased or absent femoral pulses. Infants with severe coarctation have equal upper and lower extremity pulses from birth until the ductus arteriosus closes (ductal patency ensures flow to the descending aorta distal to the level of obstruction). Approximately 40% of children with coarctation will present as young infants. Coarctation alone, or in combination with VSD, ASD, or other congenital cardiac anomalies, is the leading cause of HF in the first month of life.

Coarctation presents insidiously in the 60% of children with no symptoms in infancy. Coarctation is usually diagnosed by a pulse discrepancy between the arms and legs on physical examination or by right arm hypertension on blood pressure measurement. The pulses in the legs are diminished or absent. The left subclavian artery is occasionally involved in the coarctation, in which case the left brachial pulse is also weak. The pathognomonic murmur of coarctation is heard in the left axilla and the left back. The murmur is usually systolic but may spill into diastole, as forward flow continues across the narrow coarctation site throughout the cardiac cycle. A systolic ejection murmur is often heard at the aortic area and the lower left sternal border along with an apical ejection click if there is an associated bicuspid aortic valve.

B. Imaging

In the older child, radiographs may show a normal-sized heart, or more often some degree of LV enlargement. The aorta proximal to the coarctation is prominent. The aortic outline may indent at the level of the coarctation. The poststenotic segment is often dilated. This combination of abnormalities results in the "figure 3" sign on chest radiograph. Notching of the ribs caused by marked enlargement of the intercostal collaterals can be seen. In patients with severe coarctation and associated HF, marked cardiac enlargement and pulmonary venous congestion occur.

C. Electrocardiography

ECGs in older children may be normal or may show LVH. ECG usually shows RVH in infants with severe coarctation because the RV serves as the systemic ventricle during fetal life.

D. Echocardiography

Two-dimensional echocardiography and color-flow Doppler are used to visualize the coarctation directly, and continuous-wave Doppler estimates the degree of obstruction. Diastolic runoff flow is detected by continuous-wave Doppler if the obstruction is significant. In neonates with a PDA, a coarctation cannot be ruled out, as stenosis of the arch may evolve as the PDA closes. Identification of lesions such as a bicuspid aortic valve or mitral abnormalities may suggest the presence of a coarctation. In the face of poor LV systolic function, the gradient across the coarctation will be low, as the failing LV is unable to generate very much pressure proximal to the narrowing.

E. Cardiac Catheterization and Angiocardiography

Cardiac catheterization and angiocardiography are rarely performed for diagnosis in infants or children with coarctation, but are used if transcatheter intervention is planned. If completed, these studies demonstrate the anatomy and severity of the coarctation and assess the adequacy of collateral circulation.

Treatment

Infants with coarctation of the aorta and HF may present in extremis secondary to LV dysfunction and low cardiac output. Resuscitative measures include PGE_2 infusion (0.05–0.1 mcg/kg/min) to reopen the ductus arteriosus. End-organ damage distal to the coarctation is not uncommon, and inotropic support is frequently needed. Once stabilized, the infant should undergo corrective repair. In patients with poor LV function, balloon angioplasty of the coarctation is sometimes performed as a palliative measure. Recent data suggest that balloon angioplasty of the aorta can be the definitive procedure in many patients with good LV function. Surgery also has a high success rate. The main complication of both surgery and balloon angioplasty is recurrent coarctation. Fortunately, this complication is treatable in the catheterization laboratory. In older patients, particularly those of adult size, transcatheter stent placement is effective for recurrent coarctation.

Course & Prognosis

Children who survive the neonatal period without developing HF do well through childhood and adolescence. Fatal complications (eg, hypertensive encephalopathy or intracranial bleeding) are uncommon in childhood. Infective endarteritis is rare before adolescence, but can occur in both repaired and unrepaired coarctation. Children with coarctation corrected after age 5 years are at increased risk for systemic hypertension and myocardial dysfunction even with successful surgery. Exercise testing is mandatory for these children prior to their participation in athletic activities.

Golden AB, Hellenbrand WE: Coarctation of the aorta: Stenting in children and adults. Catheter Cardiovasc Interv 2007;69:289–299 [PMID: 17191237].

Rodes-Cabau J et al: Comparison of surgical and transcatheter treatment for native coarctation of the aorta in patients > or = 1 year old. The Quebec Native Coarctation of the Aorta study. Am Heart J 2007;154:186–192 [PMID: 17584575].

2. Aortic Stenosis

ESSENTIALS OF DIAGNOSIS & TYPICAL FEATURES

- Harsh systolic ejection murmur at the upper right sternal border with radiation to the neck.
- Thrill in the carotid arteries.
- Systolic click at the apex.
- Dilation of the ascending aorta on chest radiograph.

General Considerations

Aortic stenosis is defined as obstruction to outflow from the LV at or near the aortic valve producing a systolic pressure gradient of more than 10 mm Hg between the LV and the aorta. Aortic stenosis accounts for approximately 7% of congenital heart disease. There are three anatomic types of congenital aortic stenosis.

A. Valvular Aortic Stenosis (75%)

In critical aortic stenosis presenting in infancy, the aortic valve is usually a unicuspid diaphragm-like structure without well-defined commissures. A bicuspid aortic valve or a trileaflet valve with partially fused leaflets is another anatomic possibility that can be associated with aortic stenosis. Aortic stenosis is more common in males than in females.

B. Subvalvular Aortic Stenosis (23%)

In this type, a membranous or fibrous ring occurs just below the aortic valve that causes obstruction to LV outflow. The aortic valve itself and the anterior leaflet of the mitral valve are often malformed.

C. Supravalvular Aortic Stenosis (2%)

In this type, constriction of the ascending aorta occurs just above the coronary arteries. The condition is often familial, and two different genetic patterns are found, one with abnormal facies and mental retardation (William syndrome) and one with normal facies and no developmental delay.

Clinical Findings

A. Symptoms and Signs

Although isolated valvular aortic stenosis seldom causes symptoms in infancy, severe HF occasionally occurs when critical obstruction is present at birth. Response to medical therapy is poor; therefore, an aggressive approach using interventional catheterization or surgery is required. The physical findings vary depending on the anatomic type of lesion:

1. Valvular aortic stenosis—If the stenosis is severe with a gradient greater than 80 mm Hg, pulses are diminished with a slow upstroke; otherwise, pulses are usually normal. Cardiac examination reveals an LV thrust at the apex. A systolic thrill at the right base, the suprasternal notch, and over both carotid arteries may accompany moderate disease.

A prominent aortic ejection click is best heard at the apex. The click corresponds to the opening of the aortic valve. It is separated from S_1 by a short but appreciable interval. It does not vary with respiration. S_2 at the pulmonary area is normal. A loud, rough, medium- to high-pitched ejection-type systolic murmur is evident. It is loudest at the first and second intercostal spaces, radiating well into the suprasternal notch and along the carotids. The grade of the murmur correlates well with the severity of the stenosis.

2. Discrete membranous subvalvular aortic stenosis—The findings are the same as those of valvular aortic stenosis except for the absence of a click. The murmur and thrill are usually somewhat more intense at the left sternal border in the third and fourth intercostal spaces. In the setting of aortic insufficiency, a diastolic murmur is commonly heard.

3. Supravalvular aortic stenosis—The thrill and murmur are best heard in the suprasternal notch and along the carotids but are well transmitted over the aortic area and near the mid left sternal border. There may be a difference in pulses and blood pressure between the right and left arms if the narrowing is just distal to the takeoff of the innominate artery, with more prominent pulse and pressure in the right arm (the Coanda effect).

Of those not presenting in infancy, most patients with aortic stenosis have no cardiovascular symptoms. Except in the most severe cases, patients do well until the third to fifth decades of life. Some patients have mild exercise intolerance and fatigability. In a small percentage of patients, significant symptoms (eg, chest pain with exercise, dizziness, and syncope) manifest in the first decade. Sudden death is uncommon but may occur in all forms of aortic stenosis with the greatest risk in patients with subvalvular obstruction.

B. Imaging

In most cases the heart is not enlarged. The LV, however, may be slightly prominent. In valvular aortic stenosis, dilation of the ascending aorta is frequently seen.

C. Electrocardiography

Patients with mild aortic stenosis have normal ECGs. Some patients with severe obstruction have LVH and LV strain but even in severe cases, 25% of ECGs are normal. Progressive LVH on serial ECGs indicates a significant obstruction. LV strain is one indication for surgery.

D. Echocardiography

This is a reliable noninvasive technique for the evaluation of all forms of aortic stenosis. Doppler accurately estimates the transvalvular gradient, and the level of obstruction can be confirmed by both two-dimensional echocardiographic images and by the level of flow disturbance revealed by color Doppler.

E. Cardiac Catheterization and Angiocardiography

Left heart catheterization demonstrates the pressure differential between the LV and the aorta and the anatomic level at which the gradient exists. Echocardiography is the standard method for following the severity of aortic valve stenosis, and catheterization is reserved for patients whose resting gradient has reached 60–80 mm Hg and in whom intervention is planned. For those with valvular aortic stenosis, balloon valvuloplasty is usually the first option. In subvalvular or supravalvular aortic stenosis, interventional catheterization is not effective and surgery is required.

▶ Treatment

Percutaneous balloon valvuloplasty is now standard initial treatment for patients with valvular aortic stenosis. Surgery should be considered in symptomatic patients with a high resting gradient (60–80 mm Hg) despite balloon angioplasty, or coexisting aortic insufficiency. In many cases, the gradient cannot be significantly diminished by valvuloplasty without producing aortic insufficiency. Patients who develop significant aortic insufficiency require surgical intervention to repair or replace the valve. The Ross procedure is an alternative to mechanical valve placement in infants and children. In this procedure, the patient's own pulmonic valve is moved to the aortic position, and an RV-to-pulmonary artery conduit is used to replace the pulmonic valve. Discrete subvalvular aortic stenosis is usually surgically repaired at a lesser gradient because continued trauma to the aortic valve by the subvalvular jet may damage the valve and produce aortic insufficiency. Unfortunately, simple resection is followed by recurrence in more than 25% of patients with subvalvular aortic stenosis. Supravalvar aortic stenosis may also require surgical repair and is commonly associated with William syndrome.

▶ Course & Prognosis

All forms of LV outflow tract obstruction tend to be progressive. Pediatric patients with LV outflow tract obstruction—with the exception of those with critical aortic stenosis of infancy—are usually asymptomatic. Symptoms accompanying severe unoperated obstruction (angina, syncope, or HF) are rare but imply serious disease. Children whose obstruction is mild to moderate have normal oxygen consumption and maximum voluntary working capacity. Children in this category with normal resting and exercising (stress) ECGs may safely participate in vigorous physical activity, including nonisometric competitive sports. Children with severe aortic stenosis are predisposed to ventricular dysrhythmias and should refrain from vigorous activity and avoid all isometric exercise.

Mavroudis C, Backer CL, Kaushal S: Aortic stenosis and aortic insufficiency in children: Impact of valvuloplasty and modified Ross-Konno procedure. Semin Thorac Cardiovasc Surg Pediatr Card Surg Annu 2009;76–86 [PMID: 19349019].

McLean KM, Lorts A, Pearl JM: Current treatments for congenital aortic stenosis. Curr Opin Cardiol 2006;21:200–204 [PMID: 16601457].

3. Mitral Valve Prolapse

ESSENTIALS OF DIAGNOSIS & TYPICAL FEATURES

- Midsystolic click.
- Late systolic "whooping" or "honking" murmur.
- Typical symptoms include chest pain, palpitations, and dizziness.
- Often overdiagnosed on routine cardiac ultrasound.

▶ General Considerations

In this condition as the mitral valve closes during systole, it moves posteriorly or superiorly (prolapses) into the left atrium. Mitral valve prolapse (MVP) occurs in about 2% of thin female adolescents, a minority of whom have concomitant mitral insufficiency. Although MVP is usually an isolated lesion, it can occur in association with connective tissue disorders such as Marfan, Loeys-Dietz, and Ehlers-Danlos syndromes. These coexisting conditions should be ruled out by clinical examination.

▶ Clinical Findings

A. Symptoms and Signs

Most patients with MVP are asymptomatic. Chest pain, palpitations, and dizziness may be reported, but it is unclear whether these symptoms are more common in affected patients than in the normal population. Chest pain on exertion is rare and should be assessed with cardiopulmonary stress testing. Significant dysrhythmias have been reported, including increased ventricular ectopy and nonsustained ventricular tachycardia. If significant mitral regurgitation is present, atrial arrhythmias may also occur. Standard auscultation technique must be modified to diagnose MVP. A midsystolic click (with or without a systolic murmur) is elicited best in the standing position and is the hallmark of this entity. Conversely, maneuvers that increase LV volume, such as squatting or handgrip exercise, will cause delay or obliteration of the click-murmur complex. The systolic click usually is heard at the apex but may be audible at the left sternal border. A late, short systolic murmur after the click implies mitral insufficiency and is much less common than isolated prolapse. The murmur is not holosystolic, in contrast to rheumatic mitral insufficiency.

B. Imaging

Most chest radiographs are normal and are not usually indicated in this condition. In the rare case of significant mitral valve insufficiency, the left atrium may be enlarged.

C. Electrocardiography

The ECG may be normal. Diffuse flattening or inversion of T waves may occur in the precordial leads. U waves are sometimes prominent.

D. Echocardiography

Significant posterior systolic movement of the mitral valve leaflets to the atrial side of the mitral annulus is diagnostic. Echocardiography assesses the degree of myxomatous change of the mitral valve and the degree of mitral insufficiency.

E. Other Testing

Invasive procedures are rarely indicated. Holter monitoring or event recorders may be useful in establishing the presence of ventricular dysrhythmias in patients with palpitations.

Treatment & Prognosis

Propranolol may be effective in treatment of coexisting arrhythmias. Prophylaxis for infectious endocarditis is no longer indicated, based on 2007 AHA guidelines.

The natural course of this condition is not well defined. Twenty years of observation indicate that isolated MVP in childhood is usually a benign entity. Surgery for mitral insufficiency is rarely needed.

Knackstedt C et al: Ventricular fibrillation due to severe mitral valve prolapse. Int J Cardiol 2007;116:e101–e102 [PMID: 17137658].

Mechleb BK et al: Mitral valve prolapse: Relationship of echocardiography characteristics to natural history. Echocardiography 2006;23:434–437 [PMID: 16686634].

4. Other Congenital Left Heart Valvular Lesions

A. Congenital Mitral Stenosis

Congenital mitral stenosis is a rare disorder in which the valve leaflets are thickened and/or fused, producing a diaphragm- or funnel-like structure with a central opening. In many cases the subvalve apparatus (papillary muscles and chordae) is also abnormal. When mitral stenosis occurs with other left-sided obstructive lesions, such as subaortic stenosis and coarctation of the aorta, the complex is called Shone syndrome. Most patients develop symptoms early in life with tachypnea, dyspnea, and failure to thrive. Physical examination reveals an accentuated S_1 and a loud pulmonary closure sound. No opening snap is heard. In most cases, a presystolic crescendo murmur is heard at the apex. Occasionally, only a mid-diastolic murmur can be heard. ECG shows right axis deviation, biatrial enlargement, and RVH. Chest radiograph reveals left atrial enlargement and frequent pulmonary venous congestion. Echocardiography shows abnormal mitral valve structures with reduced leaflet excursion and left atrial enlargement. Cardiac catheterization reveals an elevated pulmonary capillary wedge pressure and pulmonary hypertension, owing to the elevated left atrial pressure.

Mitral valve repair or mitral valve replacement with a prosthetic mitral valve may be performed, even in young infants, but it is a technically difficult procedure. Mitral valve repair is the preferred surgical option, as valve replacement has a poor outcome in infants and very young children.

B. Cor Triatriatum

Cor triatriatum is a rare abnormality in which the pulmonary veins join in a confluence that is not completely incorporated into the left atrium. The pulmonary vein confluence communicates with the left atrium through an opening of variable size, and may be obstructed. Patients may present in a similar way as those with mitral stenosis. Clinical findings depend on the degree of obstruction of pulmonary venous flow into the left atrium. If the communication between the confluence and the left atrium is small and restrictive to flow, symptoms develop early in life. Echocardiography reveals a linear density in the left atrium with a pressure gradient present between the pulmonary venous chamber and the true left atrium. Cardiac catheterization may be needed if the diagnosis is in doubt. High pulmonary wedge pressure and low left atrial pressure (with the catheter passed through the foramen ovale into the true left atrium) support the diagnosis. Angiocardiography identifies the pulmonary vein confluence and the anatomic left atria. Surgical repair is always required in the presence of an obstructive membrane, and long-term results are good. Coexisting mitral valve abnormalities may be noted, including a supravalvular mitral ring or a dysplastic mitral valve.

C. Congenital Mitral Regurgitation

Congenital mitral regurgitation is a rare abnormality usually associated with other congenital heart lesions, such as congenitally corrected transposition of the great arteries (ccTGA), AV septal defect, and coronary artery anomalies (anomalous left coronary artery from the pulmonary artery). Isolated congenital mitral regurgitation is very rare. It is sometimes present in patients with connective tissue disorders (Marfan or Loeys-Dietz syndrome), usually related to a myxomatous prolapsing mitral valve.

D. Congenital Aortic Regurgitation

Congenital aortic regurgitation is rare. The most common associations are bicuspid aortic valve, with or without coarctation of the aorta; VSD with aortic cusp prolapse; and fenestration of the aortic valve cusp (one or more holes in the cusp).

Beierlein W et al: Long-term follow-up after mitral valve replacement in childhood: Poor event-free survival in the young child. Eur J Cardiothorac Surg 2007;31:860–865 [PMID: 17383889].

DISEASES OF THE AORTA

Although more common in mid to late adulthood, aortic dilation and dissection may occur in children. Although the aorta may not be dilated at birth, the structural abnormality that predisposes to dilation is presumed to be congenital. Patients at risk for progressive aortic dilation and dissection include those with isolated bicuspid aortic valve, Marfan syndrome, Loeys-Dietz syndrome, Turner syndrome, and type IV Ehlers-Danlos syndrome.

1. Bicuspid Aortic Valve

Patients with bicuspid aortic valves have an increased incidence of aortic dilation and dissection, regardless of the presence of aortic stenosis. Histologic examination demonstrates cystic medial degeneration of the aortic wall, similar to that seen in patients with Marfan syndrome. Patients with an isolated bicuspid aortic valve require regular follow-up even in the absence of aortic insufficiency or aortic stenosis. Significant aortic root dilation requiring surgical intervention typically does not occur until adulthood.

2. Marfan and Loeys-Dietz Syndromes

Marfan syndrome is an autosomal dominant disorder of connective tissue caused by a mutation in the fibrillin-1 gene. Spontaneous mutations account for 25%–30% of cases, and thus family history is not always helpful. Patients are diagnosed by the Ghent criteria and must have at a minimum, major involvement of two body systems plus involvement of a third body system or a positive family history. Body systems involved include cardiovascular, ocular, musculoskeletal, pulmonary, and integumentary. Cardiac manifestations include aortic root dilation and MVP, which may be present at birth. Patients are at risk for aortic dilation and dissection and are restricted from competitive athletics, contact sports, and isometric activities. β-Blockers or ACE inhibitors are used to lower blood pressure and slow the rate of aortic dilation. More recently, studies are ongoing to evaluate the effectiveness of angiotensin receptor blockers (losartan). Elective surgical intervention is performed in patients of adult size when the aortic root dimension reaches 50 mm or if there is an increase of greater than 1 cm in root dimension in 1 year. The ratio of actual to expected aortic root dimension is used to determine the need for surgery in the young child. Surgical options include replacement of the dilated aortic root with a composite valve graft (Bentall technique) or a David procedure in which the patient's own aortic valve is spared and a Dacron tube graft is used to replace the dilated ascending aorta. Young age at diagnosis was previously thought to confer a poor prognosis; however, early diagnosis with close follow-up and early medical therapy has more recently been associated with more favorable outcome. Ventricular dysrhythmias may contribute to the mortality in Marfan syndrome.

Loeys-Dietz syndrome is a connective tissue disorder first described in 2005. Many patients with Loeys-Dietz were thought to have Marfan syndrome in the past. Loeys-Dietz is a result of a mutation in the transforming growth factor β (TGFβ) receptor and is associated with musculoskeletal, skin, and cardiovascular abnormalities. Cardiovascular involvement includes mitral and tricuspid valve prolapse, aneurysms of the PDA, and aortic and pulmonary artery dilation. Dissection and aneurysm formation of arteries throughout the body can occur including in the head and neck vessels.

3. Turner Syndrome

Cardiovascular abnormalities are common in Turner syndrome. Patients are at risk for aortic dissection, typically during adulthood. Risk factors include hypertension regardless of cause, aortic dilation, bicuspid aortic valve, and coarctation of the aorta. There are rare reports of aortic dissection in adult Turner syndrome patients in the absence of any risk factors suggesting that there is a vasculopathic component to this syndrome. Patients with Turner syndrome require routine follow-up from adolescence onward to monitor for this potentially lethal complication.

Beroukhim RS, Roosevelt G, Yetman AT: Comparison of the pattern of aortic dilation in children with the Marfan's syndrome versus children with a bicuspid aortic valve. Am J Cardiol 2006;98:1094–1095 [PMID: 17027578].

Brooke BS, Habashi JP, Judge DP et al: Angiotensin II blockade and aortic-root dilation in Marfan's syndrome. N Engl J Med 2008 Jun 26;358(26):2787–2795 [PMID: 18579813].

Dulac Y et al: Cardiovascular abnormalities in Turner's syndrome: What prevention? Arch Cardiovasc Dis 2008;101:485–490 [PMID: 18848691].

Everitt MD et al: Cardiovascular surgery in children with Marfan syndrome or Loeys-Dietz syndrome. J Thorac Cardiovasc Surg 2009;137:1327–1332; discussion 1332–1333 [PMID: 19464442].

CORONARY ARTERY ABNORMALITIES

Several anomalies involve the origin, course, and distribution of the coronary arteries. Abnormal origin or course of the coronary arteries are often asymptomatic and can go undetected. However, in some instances these children are at risk for sudden death. The most common congenital coronary artery abnormality in infants is anomalous origin of the left coronary artery from the pulmonary artery (ALCAPA) and is discussed in more detail here.

Anomalous Origin of the Left Coronary Artery from the Pulmonary Artery

In this condition, the left coronary artery arises from the pulmonary artery rather than the aorta. In neonates, whose pulmonary artery pressure is high, perfusion of the left coronary artery may be adequate and the infant may be asymptomatic. By age 2 months the pulmonary arterial pressure falls, causing a progressive decrease in myocardial perfusion provided by the anomalous left coronary artery. Ischemia and infarction of the LV is the result. Immediate surgery is indicated to reimplant the left coronary artery and restore myocardial perfusion.

Clinical Findings

A. Symptoms and Signs

Neonates appear healthy and growth and development are relatively normal until pulmonary artery pressure decreases. Detailed questioning may disclose a history of intermittent abdominal pain (fussiness or irritability), pallor, wheezing, and sweating, especially during or after feeding. Presentation may be subtle, with nonspecific complaints of "fussiness" or intermittent "colic." The colic and fussiness are probably attacks of true angina. Presentation may be fulminant at age 2–4 months with sudden, severe HF due to LV dysfunction and mitral insufficiency. On physical examination, the infants are usually well developed and well nourished. The pulses are typically weak but equal. A prominent left precordial bulge is present. A gallop and/or holosystolic murmur of mitral regurgitation is sometimes present, though frequently auscultation alone reveals no obvious abnormalities.

B. Imaging

Chest radiographs show cardiac enlargement, left atrial enlargement, and may show pulmonary venous congestion if left ventricular function has been compromised.

C. Electrocardiography

On the ECG, there is T-wave inversion in leads I and aVL. The precordial leads also show T-wave inversion from V_4–V_7. Deep and wide Q waves are present in leads I, aVL, and sometimes in V_4–V_6. These findings of myocardial infarction are similar to those in adults.

D. Echocardiography

The diagnosis can be made with two-dimensional echo techniques by visualizing a single large right coronary artery arising from the aorta and visualization of the anomalous left coronary artery arising from the main pulmonary artery. Flow reversal in the left coronary (heading *toward* the pulmonary artery, rather than away from the aorta) confirms the diagnosis. LV dysfunction, echo-bright (ischemic) papillary muscles, and mitral regurgitation are commonly seen.

E. Cardiac Catheterization and Angiocardiography

Angiogram of the aorta fails to show the origin of the left coronary artery. A large right coronary artery fills directly from the aorta, and contrast flows from the right coronary system via collaterals into the left coronary artery and finally into the pulmonary artery. Angiogram of the RV or main pulmonary artery may show the origin of the anomalous vessel. Rarely, a left-to-right shunt may be detected as oxygenated blood passes through the collateral system without delivering oxygen to the myocardium, and passes into the pulmonary artery.

Treatment & Prognosis

The prognosis of ALCAPA is guarded and depends in part on the clinical appearance of the patient at presentation. Medical management with diuretics and afterload reduction can help stabilize a critically ill patient, but surgical intervention should not be delayed. Surgery involves reimplantation of the anomalous coronary button onto the aorta. The mitral valve may have to be replaced, depending on the degree of injury to the papillary muscles and associated mitral insufficiency. Although a life-threatening problem, cardiac function nearly always recovers if the infant survives the surgery and postoperative period.

Lange R et al: Long-term results of repair of anomalous origin of the left coronary artery from the pulmonary artery. Ann Thorac Surg 2007;83:1463–1471 [PMID: 17383358].

CYANOTIC CONGENITAL HEART DISEASE

TETRALOGY OF FALLOT

ESSENTIALS OF DIAGNOSIS & TYPICAL FEATURES

- Hypoxemic spells during infancy.
- Right-sided aortic arch in 25% of patients.
- Systolic ejection murmur at the upper left sternal border.

General Considerations

In tetralogy of Fallot (ToF), a single embryologic abnormality causes multiple morphologic problems. Anterior deviation of the infundibular (pulmonary outflow) septum causes narrowing of the right ventricular outflow tract. This deviation also results in a VSD and the aorta then overrides the crest of the ventricular septum. The RV hypertrophies, not because of pulmonary stenosis, but because it is pumping against systemic resistance across a (usually) large VSD. ToF is the most common cyanotic cardiac lesion and accounts for 10% of all congenital heart disease. A right-sided aortic arch is present in 25% of cases, and ASD occurs in 15%.

Obstruction to RV outflow with a large VSD causes a right-to-left shunt at the ventricular level with arterial desaturation. The greater the obstruction and the lower the systemic vascular resistance, the greater is the right-to-left shunt. ToF is associated with deletions in the long arm of chromosome 22 (22q11, DiGeorge syndrome) in as many as 15% of affected children. This is especially common in those with an associated right aortic arch.

Clinical Findings

A. Symptoms and Signs

Clinical findings vary with the degree of RV outflow obstruction. Patients with mild obstruction are minimally cyanotic or acyanotic. Those with severe obstruction are deeply cyanotic from birth. Few children are asymptomatic. In those with significant RV outflow obstruction, many have cyanosis at birth, and nearly all have cyanosis by age 4 months. The cyanosis usually is progressive, as subvalvular obstruction increases. Growth and development are not typically delayed, but easy fatigability and dyspnea on exertion are common. The fingers and toes show variable clubbing depending on age and severity of cyanosis. Historically, older children with ToF would frequently squat to increase systemic vascular resistance. This decreased the amount of right-to-left shunt, forcing blood through the pulmonary circuit, and would help ward off cyanotic spells. Squatting is rarely seen as the diagnosis is now made in infancy.

Hypoxemic spells, also called cyanotic or "Tet spells," are one of the hallmarks of severe ToF. These spells can occur spontaneously and at any time, but in infants occur most commonly with crying or feeding, while in older children they can occur with exercise. They are characterized by (1) sudden onset of cyanosis or deepening of cyanosis; (2) dyspnea; (3) alterations in consciousness, from irritability to syncope; and (4) decrease or disappearance of the systolic murmur (as RV the outflow tract becomes completely obstructed). These episodes most commonly start at age 4–6 months. Cyanotic spells are treated acutely by administration of oxygen and placing the patient in the knee-chest position (to increase systemic vascular resistance). Intravenous morphine should be administered cautiously, but is helpful for its sedative effect. Propranolol produces β-blockade and may reduce the obstruction across the RV outflow tract through its negative inotropic action. Acidosis, if present, should be corrected with intravenous sodium bicarbonate. Chronic oral prophylaxis of cyanotic spells with propranolol may be useful to delay surgery, but the onset of Tet spells usually prompts surgical intervention. In fact, in the current era, elective surgical repair generally occurs around the age of 3 months so as to avoid the development of Tet spells.

On examination, an RV lift is palpable. S_2 is predominantly aortic and single. A grade II–IV/VI, rough, systolic ejection murmur is present at the left sternal border in the third intercostal space and radiates well to the back.

B. Laboratory Findings

Hemoglobin, hematocrit, and red blood cell count are usually elevated in older infants or children secondary to chronic arterial desaturation.

C. Imaging

Chest radiographs show a normal-size heart. The RV is hypertrophied, often shown by an upturning of the apex (boot-shaped heart). The main pulmonary artery segment is usually concave and, if there is a right aortic arch, the aortic knob is to the right of the trachea. The pulmonary vascular markings are usually decreased.

D. Electrocardiography

The QRS axis is rightward, ranging from +90 to +180 degrees. The P waves are usually normal. RVH is always present, but RV strain patterns are rare.

E. Echocardiography

Two-dimensional imaging is diagnostic, revealing thickening of the RV wall, overriding of the aorta, and a large subaortic VSD. Obstruction at the level of the infundibulum and pulmonary valve can be identified, and the size of the proximal pulmonary arteries can be measured. The anatomy of the coronary arteries should be visualized, as abnormal branches crossing the RV outflow tract are at risk for transection during surgical enlargement of the area.

F. Cardiac Catheterization and Angiocardiography

Cardiac catheterization is generally done mainly in those patients with hypoplastic pulmonary arteries. If a catheterization is done, it reveals a right-to-left shunt at the ventricular level in most cases. Arterial desaturation of varying degrees is present. The RV pressure is at systemic levels and the pressure tracing in the RV is identical to that in the LV if the VSD is large. The pulmonary artery pressure is invariably low. Pressure gradients may be noted at the pulmonary valvular level, the infundibular level, or both. RV angiography reveals RV outflow obstruction and a right-to-left shunt at the ventricular level. The major indications for cardiac catheterization are to establish coronary artery and distal pulmonary artery anatomy if not able to be clearly defined by echocardiography.

Treatment

A. Palliative Treatment

Most centers currently advocate complete repair of ToF during the neonatal or infant period regardless of patient size. However, some centers prefer palliative treatment for small neonates in whom complete correction is deemed risky. Some patients may be palliated by balloon dilation or even stent placement in the RV outflow tract during infancy.

Neonates with very little antegrade pulmonary blood flow due to severe RV outflow tract obstruction may be dependent on their ductus arteriosus. In these patients, the pulmonary arteries are often severely hypoplastic and the most common surgical palliation is the insertion of a GoreTex shunt from the subclavian artery to the ipsilateral pulmonary artery (modified Blalock-Taussig shunt) to replace the ductus arteriosus (which is ligated and divided). This secures a source of pulmonary blood flow regardless of the level of infundibular or valvular obstruction, and some believe, allows for growth of the patient's pulmonary arteries (which are usually small) prior to complete surgical correction.

B. Total Correction

Open-heart surgery for repair of ToF is performed at ages ranging from birth to 2 years, depending on the patient's anatomy and the experience of the surgical center. The current surgical trend is toward earlier repair for symptomatic infants. The major limiting anatomic feature of total correction is the size of the pulmonary arteries. During surgery, the VSD is closed and the obstruction to RV outflow removed. Although a valve sparing procedure is preferred, in many cases a transannular patch is placed across the RV outflow tract as the pulmonary valve is contributing to the obstruction. When a transannular patch repair is done, the patient has pulmonary insufficiency that is usually well tolerated for years. However, pulmonary valve replacement is eventually necessary once symptoms (usually exercise intolerance) and right ventricular dilation occur. Surgical mortality is low.

Course & Prognosis

Infants with severe ToF are usually deeply cyanotic at birth. These children require early surgery, either a Blalock-Taussig shunt or complete repair. All children with ToF eventually require open-heart surgery. Complete repair before age 2 years usually produces a good result, and patients are currently living well into adulthood. Depending on the extent of the repair required, patients frequently require additional surgery 10–15 years after their initial repair for replacement of the pulmonary valve. Transcatheter pulmonary valves are now performed in some adolescents and young adults with a history of ToF, avoiding the need for open heart surgery. Patients with ToF are at risk for sudden death due to ventricular dysrhythmias. A competent pulmonary valve without a dilated RV appears to diminish arrhythmias and enhance exercise performance.

Harrild DM et al: Pulmonary valve replacement in tetralogy of Fallot: Impact on survival and ventricular tachycardia. Circulation 2009;119:445–451 [PMID: 19139389].

Lurz P et al: Percutaneous pulmonary valve implantation. Semin Thorac Cardiovasc Surg Pediatr Card Surg Annu 2009;112–117 [PMID: 19349024].

PULMONARY ATRESIA WITH VENTRICULAR SEPTAL DEFECT

ESSENTIALS OF DIAGNOSIS & TYPICAL FEATURES

- Symptoms depend on degree of pulmonary blood flow.
- Pulmonary blood flow via PDA and/or aortopulmonary collaterals.

This condition, complete atresia of the pulmonary valve in association with a VSD, is essentially an extreme form of ToF. Because there is no antegrade flow from the RV to the pulmonary artery, pulmonary blood flow must be derived from a PDA or from multiple aortopulmonary collateral arteries (MAPCAs). Symptoms depend on the amount of pulmonary blood flow. If flow is adequate, patients may be stable. If pulmonary flow is inadequate, severe hypoxemia occurs and immediate palliation is required. Newborns are stabilized with intravenous prostaglandin E_1 (PGE_1) to maintain the PDA while being prepared for surgery. Rarely, if the ductus does not contribute significantly to pulmonary blood flow (eg, the MAPCAs alone are sufficient), PGE_1 may be discontinued. Once stabilized, a palliative aortopulmonary shunt (synthetic shunt from the innominate artery to the pulmonary artery, also known as a Blalock-Taussig shunt) or complete repair is undertaken. The decision to perform palliation or complete repair in a newborn with this diagnosis is dependent on surgical expertise and preference in combination with pulmonary artery anatomy. In many centers, a palliative shunt is performed in newborns with severely hypoplastic pulmonary arteries or in those with only MAPCAs as a source of pulmonary blood flow. The goal of the shunt is to augment pulmonary blood flow and encourage vascular growth, and open-heart surgical correction is planned several months later. In children with MAPCAs, relocation of the MAPCAs is performed so that they are connected to the pulmonary artery (unifocalization) to complete the repair.

Echocardiography is usually diagnostic. Cardiac catheterization and angiocardiography are usually required to confirm the source(s) of pulmonary blood flow and document size of the distal pulmonary arteries. Cardiac MRI can also be a useful imaging modality for this diagnosis.

Pulmonary vascular disease is common in pulmonary atresia with VSD, due both to intrinsic abnormalities of the pulmonary vasculature and to abnormal amounts of pulmonary blood flow. Even patients who have undergone surgical correction as infants are at risk. Pulmonary vascular disease is a common cause of death as early as the third decade of life.

Ishibashi N et al: Clinical results of staged repair with complete unifocalization for pulmonary atresia with ventricular septal defect and major aortopulmonary collateral arteries. Eur J Cardiothorac Surg 2007;32:202–208 [PMID: 17512210].

PULMONARY ATRESIA WITH INTACT VENTRICULAR SEPTUM

ESSENTIALS OF DIAGNOSIS & TYPICAL FEATURES

- Completely different lesion from pulmonary atresia with VSD.
- Cyanosis at birth.
- Pulmonary blood flow is always ductal dependent with rare aortopulmonary collateral arteries being present.
- RV-dependent coronary arteries sometimes are present.

General Considerations

Although pulmonary atresia with intact ventricular septum (PA/IVS) sounds as if it might be related to pulmonary atresia with VSD, it is a distinct cardiac condition. As the name suggests, the pulmonary valve is atretic. The pulmonic annulus usually has a small diaphragm consisting of the fused valve cusps. The ventricular septum is intact. The main pulmonary artery segment is usually present and closely approximated to the atretic valve, but is somewhat hypoplastic. Although the RV is always reduced in size, the degree of reduction is variable. The size of the RV is critical to the success of surgical repair. In some children with PA/IVS, the RV is adequate for an ultimate two-ventricular repair. A normal RV has three component parts (inlet, trabecular or body, and outlet). The absence of any one of the components makes adequate RV function unlikely and a single ventricle palliative approach is necessary. Even with all three components, some RVs are inadequate.

After birth, the pulmonary flow is provided by the ductus arteriosus. MAPCAs are usually *not* present in this disease, in contrast to pulmonary atresia with VSD. A continuous infusion of PGE_1 must be started as soon as possible after birth to maintain ductal patency.

Clinical Findings

A. Symptoms and Signs

Neonates are usually cyanotic and become more so as the ductus arteriosus closes. A blowing systolic murmur resulting from the associated PDA may be heard at the pulmonary area. A holosystolic murmur is often heard at the lower left sternal border, as many children develop tricuspid insufficiency if the RV is of good size and egress from that ventricle is only through the tricuspid valve. A PFO or ASD is essential for decompression of the right side of the heart.

B. Imaging

The heart size varies from small to markedly enlarged depending on the degree of tricuspid insufficiency. With severe tricuspid insufficiency, right atrial enlargement may be massive and the cardiac silhouette may fill the chest on radiograph. In patients with an associated hypoplastic tricuspid valve and or RV, most of the systemic venous return travels right-to-left across the ASD and so the heart size can be normal.

C. Electrocardiography

ECG reveals a left axis for age (45–90 degrees) in the frontal plane. Left ventricular forces dominate the ECG, and there is a paucity of RV forces, particularly with a hypoplastic RV. Findings of right atrial enlargement are usually striking.

D. Echocardiography

Echocardiography shows atresia of the pulmonary valve with varying degrees of RV cavity and tricuspid annulus hypoplasia. Patency of an intra-atrial communication is verified by echocardiography.

E. Cardiac Catheterization and Angiocardiography

RV pressure is often suprasystemic. Angiogram of the RV reveals no filling of the pulmonary artery. It also demonstrates the size of the RV chamber, relative hypoplasia of the three components of the RV, and the presence or absence of tricuspid regurgitation. Some children with pulmonary atresia and an intact ventricular septum have sinusoids between the RV and the coronary arteries. The presence of sinusoids indicates that the coronary circulation may depend on high right ventricular pressure. Any attempt to decompress the RV in patients with RV-dependent coronary circulation causes myocardial infarction and death because of the precipitous decrease in coronary perfusion.

Treatment & Prognosis

As in all ductal-dependent lesions, PGE_1 is used to stabilize the patient and maintain patency of the ductus until surgery can be performed. Surgery is usually undertaken in the first week of life. Unrestricted flow through the ASD is a necessity, since egress of blood from the right heart can only occur across the atrial defect and into the left atrium. A Rashkind balloon atrial septostomy may be required to open a communication across the atrial septum. If the RV is tripartite and an eventual two-chamber repair is planned, the pulmonary valve plate may be perforated and dilated during cardiac catheterization in the newborn to allow antegrade flow from the RV to the pulmonary artery and thus encourage RV cavity growth. If the RV is inadequate, if significant sinusoids are present, if there is RV-dependent coronary circulation (lack of antegrade filling of the coronaries from the aorta), or if the pulmonic valve cannot be opened successfully during cardiac catheterization, a Blalock-Taussig shunt is performed to establish pulmonary blood flow. Later in infancy, a communication between the RV and pulmonary artery can be created to stimulate RV cavity growth. If either RV dimension or function is inadequate for two-ventricular repair, an approach similar to that taken for a single ventricle pathway best serves these children (see section on Hypoplastic Left Heart Syndrome). Children with significant sinusoids or coronary artery abnormalities are considered for cardiac transplantation because they are at risk for coronary insufficiency and sudden death.

The prognosis in this condition is guarded. Ultimate plans for two-ventricular repair, Fontan procedure, or cardiac transplantation depend on the patient's anatomy.

Alwi M: Management algorithm in pulmonary atresia with intact ventricular septum. Catheter Cardiovasc Interv 2006 May;67(5):679–686 [Review] [PMID: 16572430].

Tuo G, Volpe P, Bondanza S et al: Impact of prenatal diagnosis on outcome of pulmonary atresia and intact ventricular septum. J Matern Fetal Neonatal Med 2011 Jun 24 [PMID: 21699439].

TRICUSPID ATRESIA

ESSENTIALS OF DIAGNOSIS & TYPICAL FEATURES

- Marked cyanosis present from birth.
- ECG with left axis deviation, right atrial enlargement, and LVH.

General Considerations

In tricuspid atresia, there is complete atresia of the tricuspid valve with no direct communication between the right atrium and the RV. There are two types of tricuspid atresia based on the relationship of the great arteries (normally related or transposed great arteries). The entire systemic venous return must flow through the atrial septum (either ASD or PFO) to reach the left atrium. The left atrium thus receives both the systemic venous return and the pulmonary venous return. Complete mixing occurs in the left atrium, resulting in variable degrees of arterial desaturation.

Because there is no flow to the RV, development of the RV depends on the presence of a ventricular left-to-right shunt. Severe hypoplasia of the RV occurs when there is no VSD or when the VSD is small.

Clinical Findings

A. Symptoms and Signs

Symptoms usually develop in early infancy with cyanosis present at birth in most infants. Growth and development are poor, and the infant usually exhibits exhaustion during feedings, tachypnea, and dyspnea. Patients with increased pulmonary blood flow may develop HF with less prominent cyanosis. The degree of pulmonary blood flow is most dependent on pulmonary vascular resistance. Those patients with low pulmonary vascular resistance will have increased pulmonary blood flow. A murmur from the VSD is usually present and heard best at the lower left sternal border. Digital clubbing is present in older children with long-standing cyanosis.

B. Imaging

The heart is slightly to markedly enlarged. The main pulmonary artery segment is usually small or absent. The size of the right atrium is moderately to massively enlarged, depending on the size of the communication at the atrial level. The pulmonary vascular markings are usually decreased. Pulmonary vascular markings may be increased if pulmonary blood flow is not restricted by the VSD or pulmonary stenosis.

C. Electrocardiography

The ECG shows marked left axis deviation. The P waves are tall and peaked, indicative of right atrial hypertrophy. LVH or LV dominance is found in almost all cases. RV forces on the ECG are usually low or absent.

D. Echocardiography

Two-dimensional methods are diagnostic and show absence of the tricuspid valve, the relationship between the great arteries, the anatomy of the VSD, presence of an ASD or PFO, and the size of the pulmonary arteries. Color-flow Doppler imaging can help identify atrial level shunting and levels of restriction of pulmonary blood flow, either at the VSD or in the RV outflow tract.

E. Cardiac Catheterization and Angiocardiography

Catheterization reveals a right-to-left shunt at the atrial level. Because of mixing in the left atrium, oxygen saturations in the LV, RV, pulmonary artery, and aorta are identical to those in the left atrium. Right atrial pressure is increased if the ASD is restrictive. LV and systemic pressures are normal. The catheter cannot be passed through the tricuspid valve from the right atrium to the RV. A balloon atrial septostomy is performed if a restrictive PFO or ASD is present.

Treatment & Prognosis

In infants with unrestricted pulmonary blood flow, conventional anticongestive therapy with diuretics and afterload reduction should be given until the infant begins to outgrow the VSD. Sometimes, a pulmonary artery band is needed to protect the pulmonary bed from excessive flow and development of pulmonary vascular disease.

Staged palliation of tricuspid atresia is the usual surgical approach. In infants with diminished pulmonary blood flow, PGE_1 is given until an aortopulmonary shunt (Blalock-Taussig or BT shunt) can be performed. A Glenn procedure (superior vena cava to pulmonary artery anastomosis) is done with takedown of the aortopulmonary/BT shunt at 4–6 months when saturations begin to fall, and completion of the Fontan procedure (redirection of inferior vena cava and superior vena cava to pulmonary artery) is performed when the child reaches around 15 kg.

The prognosis for patients with tricuspid atresia depends on achieving a pulmonary blood flow that permits adequate oxygenation of the tissues without producing HF. The long-term prognosis for children treated by the Fontan procedure is unknown, although patients now are living into their late 20s and early 30s. In the short term, the best results for the Fontan procedure occur in children with low pulmonary artery pressures prior to open-heart surgery.

Wald RM et al: Outcome after prenatal diagnosis of tricuspid atresia: A multicenter experience. Am Heart J 2007;153:772–778 [PMID: 17452152].

HYPOPLASTIC LEFT HEART SYNDROME

ESSENTIALS OF DIAGNOSIS & TYPICAL FEATURES

- Mild cyanosis at birth.
- Minimal auscultatory findings.
- Rapid onset of shock with ductal closure.

General Considerations

Hypoplastic left heart syndrome (HLHS) includes several conditions in which obstructive lesions of the left heart are associated with hypoplasia of the LV. The syndrome occurs in 1.4%–3.8% of infants with congenital heart disease.

Stenosis or atresia of the mitral and aortic valves is the rule. In the neonate, survival depends on a PDA because ante-grade flow into the systemic circulation is inadequate or nonexistent. The PDA provides the only flow to the aorta and coronary arteries. Children with HLHS are usually stable at birth, but they deteriorate rapidly as the ductus closes in the first week of life. Untreated, the average age at death is the first week of life. Rarely, the ductus remains patent and infants may survive for weeks to months without PGE_1 therapy.

The diagnosis is often made prepartum by fetal echocardiography. Prepartum diagnosis aids in counseling for the expectant parents and planning for the delivery of the infant at or near a center with experience in treating HLHS.

Clinical Findings

A. Symptoms and Signs

Neonates with HLHS appear stable at birth because the ductus is patent. They deteriorate rapidly as the ductus closes, with shock and acidosis secondary to inadequate systemic perfusion. Oxygen saturation may actually increase for a period of time as the ductus closes due to increased blood flowing to the lungs.

B. Imaging

Chest radiograph in the first day of life may be relatively unremarkable, with the exception of a small cardiac silhouette. Later, chest radiographs demonstrate cardiac enlargement with severe pulmonary venous congestion if the PDA has begun closing or if the baby has been placed on supplemental oxygen increasing pulmonary blood flow.

C. Electrocardiography

The ECG shows right axis deviation, right atrial enlargement, and RVH with a relative paucity of LV forces. The small Q wave in lead V_6 may be absent, and a qR pattern is often seen in lead V_1.

D. Echocardiography

Echocardiography is diagnostic. A hypoplastic aorta and LV with atretic or severely stenotic mitral and aortic valves are diagnostic. The systemic circulation is dependent on the PDA. Color-flow Doppler imaging shows retrograde flow in the ascending aorta, as the coronary arteries must be supplied by the ductus via the small native aorta.

▶ Treatment & Prognosis

Initiation of PGE_1 is essential and lifesaving, as systemic circulation depends on a patent ductus arteriosus. Later management depends on balancing pulmonary and systemic blood flow both of which depend on the RV. At a few days of age the pulmonary resistance falls, favoring pulmonary over-circulation and systemic underperfusion. Therapy is then directed at encouraging systemic blood flow. Despite hypoxia and cyanosis, supplemental oxygen is avoided as this will decrease pulmonary resistance and lead to further increases in pulmonary blood flow. In some centers, nitrogen is used to decrease inspired oxygen to as low as 17%. This therapy must be carefully monitored, but results in increased pulmonary arterial resistance, which encourages systemic blood flow and improves systemic perfusion. Systemic afterload reduction will also increase systemic perfusion. Adequate perfusion can usually be obtained by keeping systemic O_2 saturation between 65% and 80%, or more accurately a PO_2 of 40 mm Hg.

A choice must be made shortly after birth among several treatment options. In the Norwood procedure, the relatively normal main pulmonary artery is transected and connected to the small ascending aorta. The entire aortic arch must be reconstructed due to its small size. Then, either a Blalock-Taussig shunt (from the subclavian artery to the pulmonary artery) or a Sano shunt (from the RV to the pulmonary artery) must be created to restore pulmonary blood flow. Children who have a Norwood procedure will later require a Glenn anastomosis (superior vena cava to pulmonary artery with takedown of the systemic-pulmonary shunt) and then a Fontan (inferior vena cava to pulmonary artery, completing the systemic venous bypass of the heart) at ages 6 months and 2–3 years, respectively. Although this is a major improvement over nonsurgical intervention, HLHS remains one of the most challenging lesions in pediatric cardiology, as survival is 70%–90% after stage I of the Norwood and 60%–70% at 5 years.

Orthotopic heart transplantation is also a treatment option for newborns with HLHS, but in the current era is typically only performed in infants who are considered poor Norwood candidates. Survival after transplantation is better than that after the Norwood operation, but death while awaiting transplantation increases overall mortality to the same level as the Norwood with 72% survival at 5 years. Heart transplantation is more commonly utilized in the event of a failed surgical palliation or if the systemic RV fails (often in adolescence or young adulthood).

Recently, some centers offer a "hybrid" approach to HLHS as a result of collaboration between surgeons and interventional cardiologists. In the hybrid procedure, the chest is opened surgically and the branch pulmonary arteries are banded, to limit pulmonary blood flow. Then, also through the open chest, a PDA stent is placed by the interventionalist to maintain systemic output. The second stage is considered a "comprehensive Glenn," in which the pulmonary artery bands and ductal stent are taken down, and the superior vena cava is surgically connected to the pulmonary arteries. Aortic arch reconstruction is done during the second stage, in contrast to the Norwood operation. Survival after the first-stage "hybrid" is greater than 90% at the most experienced centers. Long-term follow-up data are not yet available.

Alsoufi B: New developments in the treatment of hypoplastic left heart syndrome. Pediatrics 2007;119:109–117 [PMID: 17200277].

Atz AM, Travison TG, Williams IA et al: Prenatal diagnosis and risk factors for preoperative death in neonates with single right ventricle and systemic outflow obstruction: screening data from the Pediatric Heart Network Single Ventricle Reconstruction Trial(*). J Thorac Cardiovasc Surg 2010 Dec;140(6):1245–1250 [Epub 2010 Jun 18] [PMID: 20561642].

TRANSPOSITION OF THE GREAT ARTERIES

ESSENTIALS OF DIAGNOSIS & TYPICAL FEATURES

- Cyanotic newborn without respiratory distress.
- More common in males.

General Considerations

Transposition of the great arteries (TGA) is the second most common cyanotic congenital heart disease, accounting for 5% of all cases of congenital heart disease. The male-to-female ratio is 3:1. It is caused by an embryologic abnormality in the spiral division of the truncus arteriosus in which the aorta arises from the RV and the pulmonary artery from the LV. This is referred to as "ventriculoarterial discordance." Patients may have a VSD, or the ventricular septum may be intact. Left unrepaired, transposition is associated with a high incidence of early pulmonary vascular obstructive disease. Because pulmonary and systemic circulations are in parallel, survival is impossible without mixing between the two circuits. Specifically an interatrial communication (PFO or ASD) is critically important. The majority of mixing occurs at the atrial level (some mixing can occur at the level of the ductus as well), so even in the presence of a VSD an adequate interatrial communication is needed. If the atrial communication is inadequate at birth, the patient is severely cyanotic.

Clinical Findings

A. Symptoms and Signs

Many neonates are large (up to 4 kg) and profoundly cyanotic without respiratory distress or a significant murmur. Infants with a large VSD may be less cyanotic and they usually have a prominent murmur. The findings on cardiovascular examination depend on the intracardiac defects. Obstruction to outflow from either ventricle is possible, and coarctation must be ruled out.

B. Imaging

The chest radiograph in transposition is usually nondiagnostic. Sometimes there is an "egg on a string" appearance because the aorta is directly anterior to the main pulmonary artery, giving the image of a narrow mediastinum.

C. Electrocardiography

Because the newborn ECG normally has RV predominance, the ECG in transposition is of little help, as it will frequently look normal.

D. Echocardiography

Two-dimensional imaging and Doppler evaluation demonstrate the anatomy and physiology well. The aorta arises from the RV and the pulmonary artery arises from the LV. Associated defects, such as a VSD, RV or LV outflow tract obstruction, or coarctation, must be evaluated. The atrial septum should be closely examined, as any restriction could prove detrimental as the child awaits repair. The coronary anatomy is variable and must be defined prior to surgery.

E. Cardiac Catheterization and Angiocardiography

A Rashkind balloon atrial septostomy is frequently performed in complete transposition if the interatrial communication is restrictive. This procedure can be done at the bedside with echocardiographic guidance in many cases. The coronary anatomy can be delineated by ascending aortography if not well seen by echocardiography.

Treatment

Early corrective surgery is recommended. The arterial switch operation (ASO) has replaced the previously performed atrial switch procedures (Mustard and Senning operations). The ASO is performed at age 4–7 days. The arteries are transected above the level of the valves and switched, while the coronaries are separately reimplanted. Small associated VSDs may be left to close on their own, but large VSDs are repaired. The ASD is also closed. Early surgical repair (< 14 days of age) is vital for patients with TGA and an intact ventricular septum to avoid potential deconditioning of the LV as it pumps to the low-resistance pulmonary circulation. If a large, unrestrictive VSD is present, LV pressure is maintained at systemic levels, the LV does not become deconditioned, and corrective surgery can be delayed for a few months. Surgery should be performed by age 3–4 months in those with TGA and a VSD because of the high risk of early pulmonary vascular disease associated with this defect.

Survival after the ASO is greater than 95% in major centers. The main advantage of the *arterial* switch procedure in comparison to the *atrial* switch procedures (Mustard and Senning operations) is that the systemic ventricle is the LV. Patients who have undergone an *atrial* switch have an RV as their systemic ventricle, leaving them with significant late risk of RV failure and need for heart transplantation.

Lalezari S, Bruggemans EF, Blom NA, Hazekamp MG: Thirty-year experience with the arterial switch operation. Ann Thorac Surg 2011 Sep;92(3):973–979 [PMID: 21871285].

Warnes CA: Transposition of the great arteries. Circulation 2006; 114:2699–2709 [PMID: 17159076].

1. Congenitally Corrected Transposition of the Great Arteries

Congenitally corrected transposition of the great arteries (ccTGA) is a relatively uncommon congenital heart disease. Patients may present with cyanosis, heart failure, or be asymptomatic, depending on the associated lesions. In ccTGA, both atrioventricular and ventriculoarterial discordance occurs so that the right atrium connects to a morphologic LV, which supports the pulmonary artery. Conversely, the left atrium empties via a tricuspid valve into a morphologic RV, which supports the aorta. Common associated lesions are VSD and pulmonary stenosis. A dysplastic left-sided tricuspid valve is almost always present. In the absence of associated lesions, patients with ccTGA are often undiagnosed until adulthood when they present with left-sided AV valve insufficiency or arrhythmias.

Previously, surgical repair was directed at VSD closure and relief of pulmonary outflow tract obstruction—a technique that maintained the RV as the systemic ventricle with outflow to the aorta. It is now recognized that these patients have a reduced life span due to systemic RV failure; thus other surgical techniques have been advocated. The double-switch procedure is one such technique. An atrial level switch (Mustard or Senning technique) is performed, in which pulmonary and systemic venous blood are baffled such that they drain into the contralateral ventricle (systemic venous return drains into the RV and pulmonary venous return drains into the LV). An ASO then restores the morphologic LV to its position as systemic ventricle.

Patients with ccTGA have an increased incidence of complete heart block with an estimated risk of 1% per year and an overall frequency of 50%.

Malhotra SP, Reddy VM, Qiu M et al: The hemi-Mustard/bidirectional Glenn atrial switch procedure in the double-switch operation for congenitally corrected transposition of the great arteries: Rationale and midterm results. J Thorac Cardiovasc Surg 2011 Jan;141(1):162–170 [Epub 2010 Nov 5] [PMID: 21055773].

2. Double-Outlet Right Ventricle

In this uncommon malformation, both great arteries arise from the RV. There is always a VSD that allows blood to exit the LV. Presenting symptoms depend on the relationship of the VSD to the semilunar valves. The VSD can be in variable positions, and the great arteries could be normally related or malposed. In the absence of outflow obstruction, a large left-to-right shunt exists and the clinical picture resembles that of a large VSD. Pulmonary stenosis may be present, particularly if the VSD is remote from the pulmonary artery. This physiology is similar to ToF. Alternatively, if the VSD is nearer the pulmonary artery, aortic outflow may be obstructed (called the Taussig-Bing malformation). Early primary correction is the goal. LV flow is directed to the aorta across the VSD (closing the VSD), and an RV to pulmonary artery conduit is placed to maintain unobstructed flow through the pulmonary circulation. If the aorta is far from the VSD, an arterial switch may be necessary. Echocardiography is usually sufficient to make the diagnosis and determine the orientation of the great vessels and their relationship to the VSD.

Mahle WT et al: Anatomy, echocardiography, and surgical approach to double outlet right ventricle. Cardiol Young 2008;18(Suppl 3): 39–51 [PMID: 19094378].

TOTAL ANOMALOUS PULMONARY VENOUS RETURN

ESSENTIALS OF DIAGNOSIS & TYPICAL FEATURES

- Abnormal pulmonary venous connection *leading to* cyanosis.
- Occurs with or without a murmur and may have accentuated P_2.
- Right atrial enlargement and RVH.

General Considerations

This malformation accounts for 2% of all congenital heart lesions. Instead of the pulmonary veins draining into the left atrium, the veins empty into a confluence that usually is located behind the left atrium. However, the confluence is not connected to the left atrium and instead the pulmonary venous blood drains into the systemic venous system. Therefore, there is complete mixing of the systemic and pulmonary venous blood at the level of the right atrium. The presentation of a patient with total anomalous pulmonary venous return (TAPVR) depends on the route of drainage into the systemic circulation and whether or not this drainage route is obstructed.

The malformation is classified as either intra-, supra-, or infracardiac. Intracardiac TAPVR occurs when the pulmonary venous confluence drains directly into the heart, usually via the coronary sinus into the right atrium (rarely direct drainage into the right atrium). Supracardiac (or supradiaphragmatic) return is defined as a confluence that drains into the right superior vena cava, innominate vein, or persistent left superior vena cava. In infracardiac (or infradiaphragmatic) return, the confluence drains below the diaphragm usually into the portal venous system which empties into the inferior vena cava. Infracardiac pulmonary venous return is very frequently obstructed. This obstruction to pulmonary venous drainage makes this lesion a potential surgical emergency. Supracardiac veins may also be obstructed, though less commonly. Rarely, the pulmonary venous confluence drains to more than one location, called mixed TAPVR.

Because the entire venous drainage from the body returns to the right atrium, a right-to-left shunt must be present at the atrial level, either as an ASD or a PFO. Occasionally, the atrial septum is restrictive and balloon septostomy is needed at birth to allow filling of the left heart.

Clinical Findings

A. Unobstructed Pulmonary Venous Return

Patients with unobstructed TAPVR and a large atrial communication tend to have high pulmonary blood flow and typically present with cardiomegaly and HF rather than cyanosis. Oxygen saturations in the high 80s or low 90s are common. Most patients in this group have mild to moderate elevation of pulmonary artery pressure owing to elevated pulmonary blood flow. In most instances, pulmonary artery pressure does not reach systemic levels.

1. Symptoms and signs—Patients may have mild cyanosis in the neonatal period and early infancy. Thereafter, they do relatively well except for frequent respiratory infections. They are usually small and thin, resembling patients with other large left-to-right shunts. Examination discloses dusky nail beds and mucous membranes, but overt cyanosis and digital clubbing are usually absent. The arterial pulses are normal. An RV heave is palpable, and P_2 is increased. A systolic and diastolic murmur may be heard as a result of increased flow across the pulmonary and tricuspid valves, respectively.

2. Imaging—Chest radiography reveals cardiomegaly involving the right heart and pulmonary artery. Pulmonary vascular markings are increased. The characteristic cardiac contour, called a "snowman" or "figure 8," is often seen when the anomalous veins drain via a persistent left superior vena cava to the innominate vein and then the right superior vena cava, but this is not apparent until about 3 months of age when the vertical and innominate veins have dilated.

3. Electrocardiography—ECG shows right axis deviation and varying degrees of right atrial enlargement and right ventricular hypertrophy. A qR pattern is often seen over the right precordial leads.

4. Echocardiography—Demonstration by echocardiography of a discrete chamber posterior to the left atrium is strongly suggestive of the diagnosis. The availability of two-dimensional echocardiography plus color-flow Doppler has increased diagnostic accuracy such that diagnostic cardiac catheterization is rarely required.

B. With Obstructed Pulmonary Venous Return

This group includes essentially all patients with infracardiac TAPVR and a few of the patients in whom venous drainage is into a systemic vein above the diaphragm. The pulmonary venous return is usually obstructed at the level of the ascending or descending vein that connects the confluence to the systemic veins to which it is draining. Obstruction can be caused from extravascular structures (such as the diaphragm), or by inherent stenosis within the ascending or descending vein.

1. Symptoms and signs—Infants usually present shortly after birth with severe cyanosis and respiratory distress and require early corrective surgery. Cardiac examination discloses a striking RV impulse. S_2 is markedly accentuated and single. Although there is often no murmur, sometimes, a systolic murmur is heard over the pulmonary area with radiation over the lung fields. Diastolic murmurs are uncommon.

2. Imaging—The heart is usually small and pulmonary venous congestion severe with associated air bronchograms. The chest radiographic appearance may lead to an erroneous diagnosis of severe lung disease. In less severe cases, the heart size may be normal or slightly enlarged with mild pulmonary venous congestion.

3. Electrocardiography—The ECG shows right axis deviation, right atrial enlargement, and RVH.

4. Echocardiography—Echocardiography shows a small left atrium and LV, a dilated right heart with high RV pressure. For infracardiac TAPVR, appearance of a vessel lying parallel and anterior to the descending aorta and to the left of the inferior vena cava may represent the vein draining the confluence caudally toward the diaphragm. Color-flow Doppler echocardiography may reveal flow disturbance, commonly near the confluence or in the liver, where flow is obstructed.

5. Cardiac catheterization and angiocardiography—If echocardiography does not confirm the anatomy, cardiac catheterization and angiography demonstrate the site of entry of the anomalous veins. Catheterization can also assist in calculating the ratio of pulmonary to systemic blood flow and the degree of pulmonary hypertension and pulmonary vascular resistance.

Treatment

Surgery is always required for TAPVR. If pulmonary venous return is obstructed, surgery must be performed immediately (obstructed TAPVR represents one of the few surgical emergencies in congenital heart disease). In unobstructed TAPVR, surgery may be delayed for weeks to months. The timing of surgery is determined by the child's weight gain and the risk of pulmonary infection. If early surgery is not required and the atrial septum is restrictive, a balloon atrial septostomy can be performed in newborns.

Course & Prognosis

Most children with TAPVR do well after surgery. However, some surgical survivors develop late stenosis of the pulmonary veins. Pulmonary vein stenosis is an intractable condition that is difficult to treat either with interventional catheterization or surgery and has a poor prognosis and mortality is high in this subgroup of patients. A heart-lung transplant may be the only remaining option available to those with severe pulmonary vein stenosis. By avoiding direct suturing at the pulmonary venous ostia, the chance of recurrent stenosis at the anastomotic site is lessened. Unfortunately, any manipulation of the pulmonary veins increases the risk of stenosis.

Seale AN, Uemura H, Webber SA et al: Total anomalous pulmonary venous connection: Morphology and outcome from an international population-based study. Circulation 2010 Dec 21;122(25):2718–2726 [Epub 2010 Dec 6] [PMID: 21135364].

TRUNCUS ARTERIOSUS

ESSENTIALS OF DIAGNOSIS & TYPICAL FEATURES

- Early HF with or without cyanosis.
- Systolic ejection click.

General Considerations

Truncus arteriosus accounts for less than 1% of congenital heart malformations. A single great artery arises from the heart, giving rise to the systemic, pulmonary, and coronary circulations. Truncus develops embryologically as a result of failure of the division of the common truncus arteriosus into the aorta and the pulmonary artery. A VSD is always present. The number of truncal valve leaflets varies from two to six, and the valve may be insufficient or stenotic.

Truncus arteriosus is divided into subtypes by the anatomy of the pulmonary circulation. A single main pulmonary artery may arise from the base of the trunk and gives rise to branch pulmonary arteries (type 1). Alternatively, the pulmonary arteries may arise separately from the common trunk, either in close association with one another (type 2) or widely separated (type 3). This lesion can occur in association with an interrupted aortic arch.

In patients with truncus, blood from both ventricles leaves the heart through a single exit. Thus, oxygen saturation in the pulmonary artery is equal to that in the systemic arteries. The degree of systemic arterial oxygen saturation depends on the ratio of pulmonary to systemic blood flow. If pulmonary vascular resistance is normal, the pulmonary blood flow is greater than the systemic blood flow and the saturation is relatively high. If pulmonary vascular resistance is elevated because of pulmonary vascular obstructive disease or small pulmonary arteries, pulmonary blood flow is reduced and oxygen saturation is low. The systolic pressures are systemic in both ventricles.

Clinical Findings

A. Symptoms and Signs

High pulmonary blood flow characterizes most patients with truncus arteriosus. These patients are usually minimally cyanotic and present in HF. Examination of the heart reveals a hyperactive precordium. A systolic thrill is common at the lower left sternal border. A loud early systolic ejection click is commonly heard. S_2 is single and accentuated. A loud holosystolic murmur is audible at the left lower sternal border. A diastolic flow murmur can often be heard at the apex due to increased pulmonary venous return crossing the mitral valve. An additional diastolic murmur of truncal insufficiency may be present.

Patients with decreased pulmonary blood flow are more profoundly cyanotic early. The most common manifestations are growth retardation, easy fatigability, and HF. The heart is not hyperactive. S_1 and S_2 are single and loud. A systolic murmur is heard at the lower left sternal border. No mitral flow murmur is heard, as pulmonary venous return is decreased. A loud systolic ejection click is commonly heard. In the current era, this lesion is often diagnosed by prenatal screening echocardiography.

B. Imaging

The common radiographic findings are a boot-shaped heart, absence of the main pulmonary artery segment, and a large aorta that has a right arch 30% of the time. The pulmonary vascular markings vary with the degree of pulmonary blood flow.

C. Electrocardiography

The axis is usually normal. RVH or combined ventricular hypertrophy is commonly present.

D. Echocardiography

Images generally show override of a single great artery (similar to ToF, but no second great artery arises directly from the heart). The origin of the pulmonary arteries and the degree of truncal valve abnormality can be defined. Color-flow Doppler can aid in the description of pulmonary flow and the function of the truncal valve, both of which are critical to management. Echocardiography is critical in identifying associated lesions which will impact surgical planning, such as the presence of an interrupted aortic arch.

E. Angiocardiography

Cardiac catheterization is not routinely performed but may be of value in older infants in whom pulmonary vascular disease must be ruled out. The single most important angiogram would be from the truncal root, as both the origin of the pulmonary arteries and the amount of truncal insufficiency would be seen from one injection.

Treatment

Anticongestive measures are needed for patients with high pulmonary blood flow and congestive failure. Surgery is always required in this condition. Because of HF and the risk of development of pulmonary vascular disease, surgery is usually performed in the neonatal period or early infancy. The VSD is closed to allow LV egress to the truncal valve. The pulmonary artery (type 1) or arteries (types 2–3) are separated from the truncus as a block, and a valved conduit is fashioned from the RV to the pulmonary circulation.

Course & Prognosis

Children with a good surgical result generally do well. Outcome is also dependent to some degree on anatomy and integrity of the truncal valve, which becomes the "neoaortic" valve. Patients with a dysplastic valve may eventually require surgical repair or replacement of this valve. In addition, similar to patients with ToF, they eventually outgrow the RV-to-pulmonary artery conduit placed in infancy and require revision of the conduit in later childhood. The risk of early pulmonary vascular obstructive disease is high in the unrepaired patient and a decision to delay open-heart surgery beyond age 4–6 months is not wise even in stable patients.

Henaine R, Azarnoush K, Belli E et al: Fate of the truncal valve in truncus arteriosus. Ann Thorac Surg 2008 Jan;85(1):172–178 [PMID: 18154803].

Konstantinov IE, Karamlou T, Blackstone EH et al: Truncus arteriosus associated with interrupted aortic arch in 50 neonates: A Congenital Heart Surgeons Society study. Ann Thorac Surg 2006 Jan;81(1):214–222 [PMID: 16368368].

QUALITY IMPROVEMENT IN CONGENITAL HEART DISEASE

The National Pediatric Cardiology-Quality Improvement Collaborative (NPC-QIC) was formed in response to the Joint Council on Congenital Heart Disease (JCCHD) initiative to improve outcomes of children with heart disease. The mission of the NPC-QIC is to build a collaborative network of pediatric cardiologists and an associated database to serve as the foundation for improvement projects. The inaugural project of the NPC-QIC was an improvement project aimed at improving survival and quality of life of infants with HLHS between stages 1 (Norwood) and 2 (bidirectional Glenn) of their palliative surgery.

As outcomes improve and even those with complex congenital heart disease are surviving into adulthood, the care of adults with congenital heart disease is an expanding area of need within pediatric cardiology. Subspecialty clinics addressing the needs of adults with repaired or palliated congenital heart disease are needed to assess and advise patients regarding such adult issues as the impact of pregnancy, the risks of anticoagulation during pregnancy, and appropriate adult career choices.

Baker-Smith CM, Neish SR, Klitzner TS et al: Variation in postoperative care following stage I palliation for single-ventricle patients: A report from the Joint Council on Congenital Heart Disease National Quality Improvement Collaborative. Congenit Heart Dis 2011 Mar-Apr;6(2):116–127 [PMID: 21426525].

NPC-QIC website: http://jcchdqi.org/

ACQUIRED HEART DISEASE

RHEUMATIC FEVER

Rheumatic fever remains a major cause of morbidity and mortality in developing countries that suffer from poverty, overcrowding, and poor access to health care. Even in developed countries, rheumatic fever has not been entirely eradicated. The overall incidence in the United States is less than 1 per 100,000. There have been regional resurgences, such as in Utah in the 1980s, with an incidence of nearly 12 per 100,000 children between the ages of 3 and 17 years.

Group A β-hemolytic streptococcal infection of the upper respiratory tract is the essential trigger in predisposed individuals. Only certain serotypes of group A Streptococcus cause rheumatic fever. The latest attempts to define host susceptibility implicate immune response genes that are present in approximately 15% of the population. The immune response triggered by infection of the pharynx with group A streptococci consists of (1) sensitization of B lymphocytes by streptococcal antigens, (2) formation of anti-streptococcal antibody, (3) formation of immune complexes that cross-react with cardiac sarcolemma antigens, and (4) myocardial and valvular inflammatory response.

The peak age of risk in the United States is 5–15 years. The disease is slightly more common in girls and in African Americans. The annual death rate from rheumatic heart disease in school-aged children (whites and nonwhites) recorded in the 1980s was less than 1 per 100,000.

Clinical Findings

Two major or one major and two minor manifestations (plus supporting evidence of streptococcal infection) based on the modified Jones criteria are needed for the diagnosis of acute rheumatic fever (Table 20–13). Except in cases of rheumatic fever manifesting solely as Sydenham chorea or long-standing carditis, there should be clear evidence of a streptococcal infection such as scarlet fever, a positive throat culture for group A β-hemolytic Streptococcus, and

Table 20–13. Jones criteria (modified) for diagnosis of rheumatic fever.

Major manifestations
Carditis
Polyarthritis
Sydenham chorea
Erythema marginatum
Subcutaneous nodules
Minor manifestations
Clinical
Previous rheumatic fever or rheumatic heart disease
Polyarthralgia
Fever
Laboratory
Acute phase reaction: elevated erythrocyte sedimentation rate, C-reactive protein, leukocytosis
Prolonged PR interval
Plus
Supporting evidence of preceding streptococcal infection, ie, increased titers of antistreptolysin O or other streptococcal antibodies, positive throat culture for group A Streptococcus

increased antistreptolysin O or other streptococcal antibody titers. The antistreptolysin O titer is significantly higher in rheumatic fever than in uncomplicated streptococcal infections.

A. Carditis

Carditis is the most serious consequence of rheumatic fever and varies from minimal to life-threatening HF. The term *carditis* implies pancardiac inflammation, but it may be limited to valves, myocardium, or pericardium. Valvulitis is frequently seen, with the mitral valve most commonly affected. Mitral insufficiency is the most common valvular residua of acute rheumatic carditis. Mitral stenosis after acute rheumatic fever is rarely encountered until 5–10 years after the first episode. Thus, mitral stenosis is much more commonly seen in adults than in children.

An early decrescendo diastolic murmur consistent with aortic insufficiency is occasionally encountered as the sole valvular manifestation of rheumatic carditis. The aortic valve is the second most common valve affected in polyvalvular as well as in single-valve disease. The aortic valve is involved more often in males and in African Americans. Dominant aortic stenosis of rheumatic origin does not occur in pediatric patients. In one large study, the shortest length of time observed for a patient to develop dominant aortic stenosis secondary to rheumatic heart disease was 20 years.

B. Polyarthritis

The large joints (knees, hips, wrists, elbows, and shoulders) are most commonly involved and the arthritis is typically migratory. Joint swelling and associated limitation of movement should be present. This is one of the more common major criteria, occurring in 80% of patients. Arthralgia alone is not a major criterion.

C. Sydenham Chorea

Sydenham chorea is characterized by involuntary and purposeless movements and is often associated with emotional lability. These symptoms become progressively worse and may be accompanied by ataxia and slurring of speech. Muscular weakness becomes apparent following the onset of the involuntary movements. Chorea is self-limiting, although it may last up to 3 months. Chorea may not be apparent for months to years after the acute episode of rheumatic fever.

D. Erythema Marginatum

A macular, serpiginous, erythematous rash with a sharply demarcated border appears primarily on the trunk and the extremities. The face is usually spared.

E. Subcutaneous Nodules

These usually occur only in severe cases, and then most commonly over the joints, scalp, and spinal column. The nodules vary from a few millimeters to 2 cm in diameter and are nontender and freely movable under the skin.

Treatment & Prophylaxis

A. Treatment of the Acute Episode

1. Anti-infective therapy—Eradication of the streptococcal infection is essential. Long-acting benzathine penicillin is the drug of choice. Depending on the age and weight of the patient, a single intramuscular injection of 0.6–1.2 million units is effective; alternatively, give penicillin V, 250–500 mg orally 2–3 times a day for 10 days, or amoxicillin, 50 mg/kg (maximum 1 g) once daily for 10 days. Narrow-spectrum cephalosporins, clindamycin, azithromycin, or clarithromycin are used in those allergic to penicillin.

2. Anti-inflammatory agents

A. ASPIRIN—Aspirin, 30–60 mg/kg/d, is given in four divided doses. This dose is usually sufficient to effect dramatic relief of arthritis and fever. Higher dosages carry a greater risk of side effects and there are no proven short- or long-term benefits of high doses that produce salicylate blood levels of 20–30 mg/dL. The duration of therapy is tailored to meet the needs of the patient, but 2–6 weeks of therapy with reduction in dose toward the end of the course is usually sufficient. Other nonsteroidal anti-inflammatory agents used because of concerns about Reye syndrome are less effective than aspirin.

B. CORTICOSTEROIDS—Corticosteroids are seldom indicated except in the rare patient with severe carditis and HF, in whom they may be lifesaving. Steroids are given as follows: prednisone, 2 mg/kg/d orally for 2 weeks; reduce prednisone to 1 mg/kg/d during the third week, and begin aspirin, 50 mg/kg/d; stop prednisone at the end of 3 weeks, and continue aspirin for 8 weeks or until the C-reactive protein is negative and the sedimentation rate is falling.

3. Therapy in heart failure—Treatment for HF is based on symptoms and severity of valve involvement and cardiac dysfunction (see section on Heart Failure, earlier).

4. Bed rest and ambulation—Bed rest is not required in most cases. Activity level should be commensurate with symptoms and children should be allowed to self-limit their activity level while affected. Most acute episodes of rheumatic fever are managed on an outpatient basis.

B. Treatment After the Acute Episode

1. Prevention—Prevention is critical, as patients who have had rheumatic fever are at greater risk of recurrence if future group A β-hemolytic streptococcal infections are inadequately treated. Follow-up visits are essential to reinforce the necessity for prophylaxis, with regular intramuscular long-acting benzathine penicillin injections preferred to oral medication due to better adherence. Long-term (possibly lifelong) prophylaxis is recommended for patients with residual rheumatic heart disease. More commonly, with no or transient cardiac involvement, 5–10 years of therapy or discontinuance in early adulthood (age 21) (whichever is longer) is an effective approach.

The following preventive regimens are in current use:

A. **Penicillin G benzathine**—600,000 units for less than 27 kg, 1.2 million units for more than 27 kg intramuscularly every 4 weeks is the drug of choice.

B. **Penicillin V**—250 mg orally twice daily is much less effective than intramuscular penicillin benzathine G (5.5 vs 0.4 streptococcal infections per 100 patient-years).

C. **Sulfadiazine**—500 mg for less than 27 kg and 1 g for more than 27 kg, once daily. Blood dyscrasias and lesser effectiveness in reducing streptococcal infections make this drug less satisfactory than penicillin benzathine G. This is the recommended regimen for penicillin-allergic patients.

D. **Erythromycin**—250 mg orally twice a day may be given to patients who are allergic to both penicillin and sulfonamides. Azithromycin or clarithromycin may also be used.

2. Residual valvular damage—As described above, the mitral and aortic valves are most commonly affected by rheumatic fever and the severity of carditis is quite variable. In the most severe cases, cardiac failure or the need for a valve replacement can occur in the acute setting. In less severe cases, valve abnormalities can persist, requiring lifelong medical management and eventual valve replacement. Other patients fully recover without residual cardiac sequelae.

Although antibiotic prophylaxis to protect against endocarditis used to be recommended for those with residual valvular abnormalities, the criteria for prevention of IE were revised in 2007 and routine prophylaxis is recommended only if a prosthetic valve is in place.

Gerber MA et al: Prevention of rheumatic fever and diagnosis and treatment of acute Streptococcal pharyngitis: A scientific statement from the American Heart Association Rheumatic Fever, Endocarditis, and Kawasaki Disease Committee of the Council on Cardiovascular Disease in the Young, the Interdisciplinary Council on Functional Genomics and Translational Biology, and the Interdisciplinary Council on Quality of Care and Outcomes Research: Endorsed by the American Academy of Pediatrics. Circulation 2009;119:1541–1551 [PMID: 19246689].

KAWASAKI DISEASE

Kawasaki disease was first described in Japan in 1967 and was initially called mucocutaneous lymph node syndrome. The cause is unclear and there is no specific diagnostic test. Kawasaki disease is the leading cause of acquired heart disease in children in the United States. Eighty percent of patients are younger than 5 years old (median age at diagnosis is 2 years), and the male-to-female ratio is 1.5:1. Diagnostic criteria are fever for more than 5 days and at least four of the following features: (1) bilateral, painless, nonexudative conjunctivitis; (2) lip or oral cavity changes (eg, lip cracking and fissuring, strawberry tongue, and inflammation of the oral mucosa); (3) cervical lymphadenopathy greater than or equal to 1.5 cm in diameter and usually unilateral; (4) polymorphous exanthema; and (5) extremity changes (redness and swelling of the hands and feet with subsequent desquamation). Clinical features not part of the diagnostic criteria, but frequently associated with Kawasaki disease, are shown in Table 20–14.

The potential for cardiovascular complications is the most serious aspect of Kawasaki disease. Complications during the acute illness include myocarditis, pericarditis, valvular heart disease (usually mitral or aortic regurgitation), and coronary arteritis. Patients with fever for at least 5 days but fewer than four of the diagnostic features can be diagnosed with incomplete Kawasaki disease, especially if they have coronary artery abnormalities detected by echocardiography. Comprehensive recommendations regarding the evaluation for children with suspected incomplete Kawasaki disease were outlined in a 2004 Statement by the American Heart Association (see references at the end of this section).

Coronary artery lesions range from mild transient dilation of a coronary artery to large aneurysms. Aneurysms rarely form before day 10 of illness. Untreated patients have a 15%–25% risk of developing coronary aneurysms. Those at greatest risk for aneurysm formation are males, young infants (< 6 months), and those not treated with intravenous immunoglobulin (IVIG). Most coronary artery aneurysms resolve within 5 years of diagnosis; however, as aneurysms

Table 20–14. Noncardiac manifestations of Kawasaki disease.

System	Associated Signs and Symptoms
Gastrointestinal	Vomiting, diarrhea, gallbladder hydrops, elevated transaminases
Blood	Elevated ESR or CRP, leukocytosis, hypoalbuminemia, mild anemia in acute phase and thrombocytosis in subacute phase (usually second to third week of illness)
Renal	Sterile pyuria, proteinuria
Respiratory	Cough, hoarseness, infiltrate on chest radiograph
Joint	Arthralgia and arthritis
Neurologic	Mononuclear pleocytosis of cerebrospinal fluid, irritability, facial palsy

CRP, C-reactive protein; ESR, erythrocyte sedimentation rate.

resolve, associated obstruction or stenosis (19% of all aneurysms) may develop, which may result in coronary ischemia. Giant aneurysms (> 8 mm) are less likely to resolve, and nearly 50% eventually become stenotic. Of additional concern, acute thrombosis of an aneurysm can occur, resulting in myocardial infarction that is fatal in approximately 20% of cases.

Treatment

Immediate management of Kawasaki disease includes IVIG and high-dose aspirin. This therapy is effective in decreasing the incidence of coronary artery dilation and aneurysm formation. The currently recommended regimen is 2 g/kg of IVIG administered over 10–12 hours and 80–100 mg/kg/d of aspirin in four divided doses. The duration of high-dose aspirin is institution-dependent: many centers reduce the dose once the patient is afebrile for 48–72 hours; others continue through 5 afebrile days or day 14 of the illness. Once high-dose aspirin is discontinued, low-dose aspirin (3–5 mg/kg/d) is given through the subacute phase of the illness (6–8 weeks) or until coronary artery abnormalities resolve. If fever recurs within 48–72 hours of the initial treatment course and no other source of the fever is detected, a second dose of IVIG is often recommended; however, the effectiveness of this approach has not been clearly demonstrated. A recent multicenter, randomized, double-blind, placebo-controlled study (Newburger et al) demonstrated no beneficial effect of pulsed corticosteroids on the development of coronary abnormalities in patients responsive to IVIG. However, corticosteroids or other anti-inflammatory therapy (eg, infliximab) should be considered for patients with persistent fever despite one or two infusions of IVIG.

Follow-up of patients with treated Kawasaki disease depends on the degree of coronary involvement. In those with no or minimal coronary disease at the time of diagnosis, an echocardiogram 2 weeks and again 6–8 weeks after diagnosis is sufficient. Repeat echocardiography more than 8 weeks after diagnosis in those with no coronary abnormalities is optional. In 2004, the AHA published updated guidelines for the long-term management of Kawasaki disease based on the risk level of the patient. The risk stratification and recommended follow-up is reviewed in Table 20–15.

McCrindle BW et al: Coronary artery involvement in children with Kawasaki disease: Risk factors from analysis of serial normalized measurements. Circulation 2007 Jul 10;116(2):174–179.

Newburger JW et al: Diagnosis, treatment, and long-term management of Kawasaki disease: A statement for health professionals from the Committee on Rheumatic Fever, Endocarditis and Kawasaki Disease, Council on Cardiovascular Disease in the Young, American Heart Association. Circulation 2004 Oct 26;110(17):2747–2771.

Table 20–15. Long-term management in Kawasaki disease.

Risk Level	Definition	Management Guidelines
I	No coronary artery changes at any stage of the illness	No ASA is needed beyond the subacute phase (6–8 wk). No follow-up beyond the first year.
II	Transient ectasia of coronary arteries during the acute phase	Same as above, or clinical follow-up ± ECG every 3–5 y.
III	Single small to medium coronary aneurysm	ASA until abnormality resolves. Annual follow-up with ECG and echo if < 10 y and every other-year stress testing if > 10 y.
IV	Giant aneurysm or multiple small to medium aneurysms without obstruction	Long-term ASA ± warfarin. Annual follow-up with ECG, echo, and stress testing.
V	Coronary artery obstruction	Long-term ASA ± warfarin ± calcium channel blocker to reduce myocardial oxygen consumption. Echo and ECG every 6 mo. Stress testing and Holter examination annually.

ASA, acetyl salicylic acid; ECG, electrocardiogram; echo, echocardiogram.

Newburger JW et al: Randomized trial of pulsed corticosteroid therapy for primary treatment of Kawasaki disease. N Engl J Med 2007 Feb 15;356(7):663–675.

INFECTIVE ENDOCARDITIS

ESSENTIALS OF DIAGNOSIS & TYPICAL FEATURES

- Positive blood culture.
- Intracardiac oscillating mass, abscess, or new valve regurgitation on echocardiogram.
- Fever.
- Elevated erythrocyte sedimentation rate or C-reactive protein.

General Considerations

Bacterial or fungal infection of the endocardium of the heart is rare and usually occurs in the setting of a preexisting abnormality of the heart or great arteries. It may occur in a normal heart during septicemia or as a consequence of infected indwelling central catheters.

The frequency of infective endocarditis (IE) appears to be increasing for several reasons: (1) increased survival in children with congenital heart disease, (2) greater use of central venous catheters, and (3) increased use of prosthetic material and valves. Pediatric patients without preexisting heart disease are also at increased risk for IE because of (1) increased survival rates for children with immune deficiencies, (2) long-term use of indwelling lines in ill newborns and patients with chronic diseases, and (3) increased intravenous drug abuse.

Patients at greatest risk are children with unrepaired or palliated cyanotic heart disease (especially in the presence of an aorta to pulmonary shunt), those with implanted prosthetic material, and patients who have had a prior episode of IE. Common organisms causing IE are viridans streptococci (30%–40% of cases), *Staphylococcus aureus* (25%–30%), and fungal agents (about 5%).

Clinical Findings

A. History

The majority of patients with IE have a history of heart disease. There may or may not be an antecedent infection or surgical procedure (cardiac surgery, tooth extraction, tonsillectomy). Transient bacteremia occurs frequently during normal daily activities such as flossing or brushing teeth, using a toothpick and even when chewing food. Although dental and nonsterile surgical procedures also can result in transient bacteremias, these episodes are much less frequent for a given individual. This may be why a clear inciting event is often not identified in association with IE and also underlies the recent changes in guidelines for antibiotic prophylaxis to prevent IE (for details, see Wilson et al reference).

B. Symptoms, Signs, and Laboratory Findings

Although IE can present in a fulminant fashion with cardiovascular collapse, often it presents in an indolent manner with fever, malaise, and weight loss. Joint pain and vomiting are less common. On physical examination, there may be a new or changing murmur, splenomegaly, and hepatomegaly. Classic findings of Osler nodes (tender nodules, usually on the pulp of the fingers), Janeway lesions (nontender hemorrhagic macules on palms and soles), splinter hemorrhages, and Roth spots (retinal hemorrhage) are uncommonly noted in children. Laboratory findings include multiple positive blood cultures, elevated erythrocyte sedimentation rate or C-reactive protein, and hematuria. Transthoracic echocardiography can identify large vegetations in some patients, but transesophageal imaging has better sensitivity and may be necessary if the diagnosis remains in question.

Table 20–16. Conditions requiring antibiotic prophylaxis for the prevention of infective endocarditis (IE).

Prosthetic cardiac valves
Prior episode of IE
Congenital heart disease (CHD)
Palliated cyanotic CHD
For 6 months postprocedure if CHD repair involves implanted prosthetic material
Repair of CHD with residual defect bordered by prosthetic material
Cardiac transplant with valvulopathy

Prevention

In 2007, the AHA revised criteria for patients requiring prophylaxis for IE (Table 20–16). Only the high-risk patients listed require antibiotics before dental work (tooth extraction or cleaning) and procedures involving the respiratory tract or infected skin or musculoskeletal structures. IE prophylaxis is *not* recommended for gastrointestinal or genitourinary procedures, body piercing, or tattooing.

Recommended propylaxis is under 40 kg, 50 mg/kg of oral amoxicillin for patients <40 kg and 2000 mg for those >40 kg. This dose is to be given 1 hour prior to procedure. If the patient is allergic to amoxicillin, alternative prophylactic antibiotics are recommended in the AHA guidelines.

Treatment

In general, appropriate antibiotic therapy should be initiated as soon as IE is suspected and several large volume blood cultures have been obtained via separate venipunctures. Therapy can be tailored once the pathogen and sensitivities are defined. Vancomycin or a β-lactam antibiotic, with or without gentamicin, for a 6-week course is the most common regimen. If HF occurs and progresses in the face of adequate antibiotic therapy, surgical excision of the infected area and prosthetic valve replacement must be considered.

Course & Prognosis

Factors associated with a poor outcome are delayed diagnosis, presence of prosthetic material, perioperative associated IE, and *S aureus* infection. Mortality for bacterial endocarditis in children ranges from 10% to 25%, with fungal infections having a much greater mortality (50% or more).

Wilson W et al: Prevention of infective endocarditis: Guidelines from the American Heart Association: A guideline from the American Heart Association Rheumatic Fever, Endocarditis, and Kawasaki Disease Committee, Council on Cardiovascular Disease in the Young, and the Council on Clinical Cardiology, Council on Cardiovascular Surgery and Anesthesia, and the Quality of Care and Outcomes Research Interdisciplinary Working Group. Circulation 2007;116:1736–1754 [PMID: 17446442].

PERICARDITIS

ESSENTIALS OF DIAGNOSIS & TYPICAL FEATURES

- Chest pain made worse by deep inspiration and decreased by leaning forward.
- Fever and tachycardia.
- Shortness of breath.
- Pericardial friction rub.
- ECG with elevated ST segments.

General Considerations

Pericarditis is an inflammation of the pericardium and is commonly related to an infectious process. The most common cause of pericarditis in children is viral infection (eg, coxsackievirus, mumps, Epstein-Barr, adenovirus, influenza, and human immunodeficiency virus [HIV]). Purulent pericarditis results from bacterial infection (eg, pneumococci, streptococci, staphylococci, and *Haemophilus influenzae*) and is less common but potentially life-threatening.

In some cases, pericardial disease occurs in association with a generalized process. Associations include rheumatic fever, rheumatoid arthritis, uremia, systemic lupus erythematosus, malignancy, and tuberculosis. Pericarditis after cardiac surgery (postpericardiotomy syndrome) is most commonly seen after surgical closure of an ASD. Postpericardiotomy syndrome appears to be autoimmune in nature with high titers of antiheart antibody and evidence of acute or reactivated viral illness. The syndrome is often self-limited and responds well to short courses of aspirin or corticosteroids.

Clinical Findings

A. Symptoms and Signs

Childhood pericarditis usually presents with sharp stabbing mid chest, shoulder, and neck pain made worse by deep inspiration or coughing, and decreased by sitting up and leaning forward. Shortness of breath and grunting respirations are common. Physical findings depend on the presence of fluid accumulation in the pericardial space (effusion). In the absence of significant accumulation, a characteristic scratchy, high-pitched friction rub may be heard. If the effusion is large, heart sounds are distant and muffled and a friction rub may not be present. In the absence of cardiac tamponade, the peripheral, venous, and arterial pulses are normal.

Cardiac tamponade occurs in association with a large effusion, or one that has rapidly accumulated. Tamponade is characterized by jugular venous distention, tachycardia, hepatomegaly, peripheral edema, and pulsus paradoxus, in which systolic blood pressure drops more than 10 mm Hg during inspiration. Decreased cardiac filling and subsequent decrease in cardiac output result in signs of right heart failure and the potential for cardiovascular collapse.

B. Imaging

In pericarditis with a significant pericardial effusion, the cardiac silhouette is enlarged. The cardiac silhouette can appear normal if the effusion has developed over an extremely short period of time.

C. Electrocardiography

The ST segments are commonly elevated in acute pericarditis. Low voltages or electrical alternans (alteration in QRS amplitude between beats) can be seen with large pericardial effusions.

D. Echocardiography

Echocardiography is essential in diagnosis and management of pericarditis. Serial studies allow direct, noninvasive estimate of the volume of fluid and its change over time. Echocardiography also demonstrates cardiac tamponade if there is compression of the atria or respiratory alteration of ventricular inflow.

Treatment

Treatment depends on the cause of pericarditis and the size of the associated effusion. Viral pericarditis is usually self-limited and symptoms can be improved with nonsteroidal anti-inflammatory therapy. Purulent pericarditis requires immediate evacuation of the fluid and appropriate antibiotic therapy. Cardiac tamponade from any cause must be treated by immediate removal of the fluid, usually via pericardiocentesis. Pericardiocentesis should also be considered if the underlying cause is unclear or identification of the pathogen is necessary for targeted therapy. In the setting of recurrent or persistent effusions, a surgical pericardiectomy or pericardial window may be necessary. Diuretics should be avoided in the patient with cardiac tamponade because they reduce ventricular preload and can exacerbate the degree of cardiac decompensation.

Prognosis

Prognosis depends to a great extent on the cause of pericardial disease. Constrictive pericarditis can develop following infectious pericarditis (especially if bacterial or tuberculous) and can be a difficult problem to manage. Cardiac tamponade will result in death unless the fluid is evacuated.

Ratnapalan S, Brown K, Benson L: Children presenting with acute pericarditis to the emergency department. Pediatr Emerg Care 2011 Jul;27(7):581–585 [PMID: 21712753].

CARDIOMYOPATHY

There are five classified forms of cardiomyopathy in children: (1) dilated, (2) hypertrophic, (3) restrictive, (4) arrhythmogenic right ventricular dysplasia (ARVD), and (5) left ventricular noncompaction. Discussion will be limited to the first three forms, which are the most common.

1. Dilated Cardiomyopathy

This most frequent of the childhood cardiomyopathies occurs with an annual incidence of 4–8 cases per 100,000 population in the United States and Europe. Although usually idiopathic, identifiable causes of dilated cardiomyopathy (DCM) include viral myocarditis, untreated tachyarrhythmias, left heart obstructive lesions, congenital abnormalities of the coronary arteries, medication toxicity (eg, anthracycline), and genetic (eg, dystrophin gene defects, sarcomeric mutations) and metabolic diseases (inborn errors of fatty acid oxidation and mitochondrial oxidative phosphorylation defects). Genetic causes are being discovered at an increasing rate with commercial testing now available for some of the more common genes.

Clinical Findings

A. Signs and Symptoms

As myocardial function fails and the heart dilates, cardiac output falls, and affected children develop decreased exercise tolerance, failure to thrive, diaphoresis, and tachypnea. As the heart continues to deteriorate, congestive signs such as hepatomegaly and rales develop, and a prominent gallop can be appreciated on examination. The initial diagnosis in a previously healthy child can be difficult, as presenting symptoms can resemble a viral respiratory infection, pneumonia, or asthma.

B. Imaging

Chest radiograph shows generalized cardiomegaly with or without pulmonary venous congestion.

C. Electrocardiography

Sinus tachycardia with ST-T segment changes is commonly seen on ECG. The criteria for right and left ventricular hypertrophy may also be met and the QT interval may be prolonged. Evaluation for the presence of supraventricular arrhythmias on ECG is critical, as this is one of the few treatable and reversible causes of DCM in children.

D. Echocardiography

The echocardiogram shows LV and left atrial enlargement with decreased LV-shortening fraction and ejection fraction. The calculated end-diastolic and end-systolic dimensions are increased and mitral insufficiency is commonly seen. A careful evaluation for evidence of structural abnormalities (especially coronary artery anomalies or left heart obstructive lesions) must be performed in infant patients.

E. Other Testing

Cardiac catheterization is useful to evaluate hemodynamic status and coronary artery anatomy. Endomyocardial biopsies can aid in diagnosis. Biopsy specimens may show inflammation consistent with acute myocarditis, abnormal myocyte architecture, and myocardial fibrosis. Electron micrographs may reveal evidence of mitochondrial or other metabolic disorders. Polymerase chain reaction (PCR) testing may be performed on biopsied specimens to detect viral genome products in infectious myocarditis. Skeletal muscle biopsy may be helpful in patients with evidence of skeletal muscle involvement. Cardiopulmonary stress testing is useful for measuring response to medical therapy and as an objective assessment of the cardiac limitations on exercise.

Treatment & Prognosis

Outpatient management of pediatric DCM usually entails combinations of afterload-reducing agents and diuretics (see section on Heart Failure, earlier). In 2007, Shaddy et al published the results of a multicenter, placebo-controlled, double-blind trial of carvedilol in children with HF. Children did not receive the same beneficial effects of β-blocker therapy as adults with HF, possibly due to the heterogenous nature of HF in children, but perhaps there are inherent differences in pediatric and adult HF. Aspirin or warfarin may be used to prevent thrombus formation in the dilated and poorly contractile cardiac chambers. Arrhythmias are more common in dilated hearts. Antiarrhythmic agents that do not suppress myocardial contractility, such as amiodarone, are used. Despite widespread use of internal defibrillators in the adult population, the technical difficulty of implanting internal defibrillators and the risk of adverse events (eg, high frequency of inappropriate discharge, vascular obstruction) in children limit their use.

Therapy of the underlying cause of cardiomyopathy is always indicated if possible. Unfortunately despite complete evaluation, a diagnosis is discovered in less than 30% of patients with DCM. If medical management is unsuccessful, cardiac transplantation is considered.

2. Hypertrophic Cardiomyopathy

The most common cause of hypertrophic cardiomyopathy (HCM) is familial hypertrophic cardiomyopathy, which is found in 1 in 500 individuals. HCM is the leading cause of sudden cardiac death in young persons. The most common presentation is in an older child, adolescent, or adult, although it may occur in neonates. Causes of nonfamilial HCM in neonates and young children include glycogen storage disease, Noonan syndrome (including related syndromes such as LEOPARD and Costello syndrome), Friedreich ataxia, maternal gestational diabetes, mitochondrial disorders, and other metabolic disorders.

A. Familial Hypertrophic Cardiomyopathy

In the familial form, HCM is most commonly caused by a mutation in one of the several genes that encode proteins of the cardiac sarcomere (β-myosin heavy chain, cardiac troponin T or I, α-tropomyosin, and myosin-binding protein C).

1. Clinical findings—Patients may be asymptomatic despite having significant hypertrophy, or may present with symptoms of inadequate coronary perfusion or HF such as angina, syncope, palpitations, or exercise intolerance. Patients may experience sudden cardiac death as their initial presentation, often precipitated by sporting activities. Although the cardiac examination may be normal on presentation, some patients develop a left precordial bulge with a diffuse point of maximal impulse. An LV heave or an S_4 gallop may be present. If outflow tract obstruction exists, a systolic ejection murmur will be audible. A murmur may not be audible at rest but may be provoked with exercise or positional maneuvers that decrease left ventricular volume (standing), thereby increasing the outflow tract obstruction.

A. ECHOCARDIOGRAPHY—The diagnosis of HCM is usually made by echocardiography and in most familial cases demonstrates asymmetrical septal hypertrophy. Young patients with metabolic or other nonfamilial causes are more likely to have concentric hypertrophy. Systolic anterior motion of the mitral valve leaflet may occur and contribute to LV outflow tract obstruction. The mitral valve leaflet may become distorted and result in mitral insufficiency. LV outflow tract obstruction may be present at rest or provoked with either amyl nitrate or monitored exercise. Systolic function is most often hypercontractile in young children but may deteriorate over time, resulting in poor contractility and LV dilation. Diastolic function is almost always abnormal.

B. ELECTROCARDIOGRAPHY—The ECG may be normal, but more typically demonstrates deep Q waves in the inferolateral leads (II, III, aVF, V_5, and V_6) secondary to the increased mass of the hypertrophied septum. ST-segment abnormalities may be seen in the same leads. Age-dependent criteria for LVH are often present as are criteria for left atrial enlargement.

C. OTHER TESTING—Cardiopulmonary stress testing is valuable to evaluate for provocable LV outflow tract obstruction, ischemia, and arrhythmias, and to determine prognosis. Extreme LVH and a blunted blood pressure response to exercise have both been associated with increased mortality in children. Cardiac MRI is useful for defining areas of myocardial fibrosis or scarring. Patients are at risk for myocardial ischemia, possibly as a result of systolic compression of the intramyocardial septal perforators, myocardial bridging of epicardial coronary arteries, or an imbalance of coronary artery supply and demand due to the presence of massive myocardial hypertrophy.

D. CARDIAC CATHETERIZATION—Cardiac catheterization is often performed in patients with HCM who have angina, syncope, resuscitated sudden death, or a worrisome stress test. Hemodynamic findings include elevated left atrial pressure secondary to impaired diastolic filling. If midcavitary LV outflow tract obstruction is present, an associated pressure gradient will be evident. Provocation of LV outflow tract obstruction with either rapid atrial pacing or isoproterenol may be sought, but this is not commonly done in children. Angiography demonstrates a "ballerina slipper" configuration of the LV secondary to the midcavitary LV obliteration during systole. The myocardial biopsy specimen demonstrates myofiber disarray.

2. Treatment and prognosis—Treatment varies depending on symptoms and phenotype. Affected patients are restricted from competitive athletics and isometric exercise due to associated risk of sudden cardiac death. Patients with resting or latent LV outflow tract obstruction may be treated with β-blockers, verapamil, or disopyramide with variable success in alleviating obstruction. Patients with severe symptoms despite medical therapy and an LV outflow tract gradient may require additional intervention. Surgical myectomy with resection of part of the hypertrophied septum has been used in symptomatic patients with good results. At the time of myectomy, the mitral valve may require repair or replacement in patients with a long history of systolic anterior motion of the mitral valve. Ethanol ablation is used in adults with HCM and LV outflow tract obstruction. This procedure involves selective infiltration of ethanol in a coronary septal artery branch to induce a small targeted myocardial infarction. This leads to a reduction in septal size and improvement of obstruction. The long-term effects of this procedure are unknown and it is not currently employed in children. Although dual-chamber pacing has been used in children with good relief of obstruction, larger series demonstrate no significant improvement in obstruction. Risk stratification with respect to sudden death is important in HCM. Consideration for placement of internal defibrillators in adult patients are based on the known risk factors for sudden cardiac death: severe hypertrophy (>3 cm septal thickness in adults), documented ventricular arrhythmias, syncope, abnormal blood pressure response to exercise, resuscitated sudden death, or a strong family history of HCM with associated sudden death. The criteria for defibrillator placement in children are not as well defined.

B. Glycogen Storage Disease of the Heart

There are at least 10 types of glycogen storage disease. The type that primarily involves the heart is Pompe disease (GSD IIa) in which acid maltase, necessary for hydrolysis of the outer branches of glycogen, is absent. There is marked deposition of glycogen within the myocardium. Affected infants are well at birth, but symptoms of growth and developmental delay, feeding problems, and cardiac failure occur by the sixth month of life. Physical examination reveals generalized muscular weakness, a large tongue, and cardiomegaly without significant heart murmurs. Chest radiographs reveal cardiomegaly with or without pulmonary venous congestion. The ECG shows a short PR interval and LVH with ST depression and T-wave inversion over the left precordial leads. Echocardiography shows severe concentric LVH. Children with Pompe disease usually die before age 1 year. Death may be sudden or result from progressive HF. Recent enzyme replacement clinical trials have shown some promise in reversing hypertrophy and preserving cardiac function.

3. Restrictive Cardiomyopathy

Restrictive cardiomyopathy is a rare entity in the pediatric population, accounting for less than 5% of all cases of cardiomyopathy. The cause is usually idiopathic but can be familial or secondary to an infiltrative process (eg, amyloidosis).

Clinical Findings

Patients present with signs of congestive HF as a consequence of diastolic dysfunction in the setting of preserved systolic function. The left ventricle is more severely affected than the right ventricle in restrictive cardiomyopathy, but the right ventricle is also affected in most cases resulting in signs and symptoms consistent with biventricular congestion. Patients often present with exercise intolerance, fatigue, chest pain and orthopnea. Physical examination is remarkable for a prominent S_4 and jugular venous distention.

A. Electrocardiography

ECG demonstrates marked right and left atrial enlargement with normal ventricular voltages. ST-T–wave abnormalities including a prolonged QTc interval may be present.

B. Echocardiography

The diagnosis is confirmed echocardiographically by the presence of normal-sized ventricles with normal systolic function and massively dilated atria. Cardiac MRI is useful in ruling out pericardial abnormalities (restrictive or constrictive pericarditis) and infiltrative disorders.

Treatment & Prognosis

Anticongestive therapy is used for symptomatic relief. The high risk of sudden death in restrictive cardiomyopathy and the propensity for rapid progression of irreversible pulmonary hypertension warrant close follow-up with early consideration of cardiac transplantation.

Chen LR et al: Reversal of cardiac dysfunction after enzyme replacement in patients with infantile-onset Pompe disease. J Pediatr 2009 Aug;155(2):271–275, e272.

Colan SD et al: Epidemiology and cause-specific outcome of hypertrophic cardiomyopathy in children: Findings from the Pediatric Cardiomyopathy Registry. Circulation 2007 Feb 13; 115(6):773–781.

Decker JA et al: Risk factors and mode of death in isolated hypertrophic cardiomyopathy in children. J Am Coll Cardiol 2009 Jul 14;54(3):250–254.

Shaddy RE et al: Carvedilol for children and adolescents with heart failure: A randomized controlled trial. JAMA 2007 Sep 12; 298(10):1171–1179.

Towbin JA et al: Incidence, causes, and outcomes of dilated cardiomyopathy in children. JAMA 2006 Oct 18;296(15):1867–1876.

MYOCARDITIS

The most common causes of viral myocarditis are adenoviruses, coxsackie A and B viruses, echoviruses, parvovirus, cytomegalovirus, and influenza A virus. HIV can also cause myocarditis. The ability to identify the pathogen has been enhanced by PCR technology, which replicates identifiable segments of the viral genome from the myocardium of affected children.

Clinical Findings

A. Symptoms and Signs

There are two major clinical patterns. In the first, sudden-onset HF occurs in an infant or child who was relatively healthy in the hours to days previously. This malignant form of the disease is usually secondary to overwhelming viremia with tissue invasion in multiple organ systems including the heart. In the second pattern, the onset of cardiac symptoms is gradual and there is often a history of upper respiratory tract infection or gastroenteritis in the previous month. This more insidious form may have a late postinfectious or autoimmune component. Acute and chronic presentations occur at any age and with all types of myocarditis.

The signs of HF are variable, but in a decompensated patient with fulminant myocarditis include pale gray skin; rapid, weak, and thready pulses; and breathlessness. In those with a more subacute presentation signs include increased work of breathing such as orthopnea, difficulty with feeding in infants, exercise intolerance and edema of the face and extremities. The patient is usually tachycardic and heart sounds may be muffled and distant; an S_3 or S_4 gallop (or both) are common. Murmurs are usually absent, although a murmur of tricuspid or mitral insufficiency may be heard. Moist rales are usually present at both lung bases. The liver is enlarged and frequently tender.

B. Imaging

Generalized cardiomegaly is seen on radiographs along with moderate to marked pulmonary venous congestion.

C. Electrocardiography

The ECG is variable. Classically, there is low-voltage QRS in all frontal and precordial leads with ST-segment depression and inversion of T waves in leads I, III, and aVF (and in the left precordial leads during the acute stage). Dysrhythmias are common, and AV and intraventricular conduction disturbances may be present.

D. Echocardiography

Echocardiography demonstrates four-chamber dilation with poor ventricular function and AV valve regurgitation. A pericardial effusion may be present. Patients with a more acute presentation may have less ventricular dilation than those with a longer history of HF-related symptoms.

E. Myocardial Biopsy

An endomyocardial biopsy may be helpful in the diagnosis of viral myocarditis. An inflammatory infiltrate with myocyte damage can be seen by hematoxylin and eosin staining. Viral PCR testing of the biopsy specimen may yield a positive result in 30%–40% of patients suspected to have myocarditis. However, myocarditis is thought to be a "patchy" process, so it is possible that biopsy results are falsely negative if the area of active myocarditis was missed.

F. Cardiac MRI

Cardiac MRI is increasing in use as a potential diagnostic modality for myocarditis. Abnormalities in T2-weighted imaging (consistent with myocardial edema, inflammation) and global relative enhancement (evidence of capillary leak) are evident in patients with acute myocarditis. This imaging method requires general anesthesia in infants and young children, which is associated with significant risk in those with HF and must be a consideration when ordering this test.

Treatment

The inpatient cardiac support measures outlined previously in the section on heart failure are used in the treatment of these patients. The use of digitalis in a rapidly deteriorating child with myocarditis is dangerous and should be undertaken with great caution, as it may cause ventricular dysrhythmias.

Administration of immunomodulating medications such as corticosteroids for myocarditis is controversial. If the patient's condition deteriorates despite anticongestive measures, corticosteroids are commonly used, although conclusive data supporting their effectiveness are lacking. Subsequent to the successful use of IVIG in children with Kawasaki disease, there have been several trials of IVIG in presumed viral myocarditis. The therapeutic value of IVIG remains unconfirmed. Initiation of mechanical circulatory support in those with fulminant or severe myocarditis is another therapeutic option as a bridge to transplantation or recovery.

Prognosis

The prognosis of myocarditis is determined by the age at onset and the response to therapy. Children presenting with fulminant myocarditis and severe hemodynamic compromise have a 75% early mortality. Those at highest risk for a poor outcome are those presenting in the first year of life. Although complete recovery is possible, many patients recover clinically but have persistent LV dysfunction and a need for ongoing medical therapy for HF. It is possible that subclinical myocarditis in childhood is the pathophysiologic basis for some of the "idiopathic" DCMs later in life. Children with myocarditis whose ventricular function fails to return to normal may be candidates for cardiac transplantation if they remain symptomatic or suffer growth failure despite maximal medical management.

May LJ, Patton DJ, Fruitman DS: The evolving approach to paediatric myocarditis: A review of the current literature. Cardiol Young 2011 Jun;21(3):241–251 [Epub 2011 Jan 28] [PMID: 21272427].

PREVENTIVE CARDIOLOGY

HYPERTENSION

Blood pressure should be determined at every pediatric visit beginning at 3 years. Because blood pressure is being more carefully monitored, systemic hypertension has become more widely recognized as a pediatric problem. Pediatric standards for blood pressure have been published. Blood pressures in children must be obtained when the child is relaxed and an appropriate-size cuff must always be used. The widest cuff that fits between the axilla and the antecubital fossa should be used (covers 60%–75% of the upper arm). Most children aged 10–11 years need a standard adult cuff (bladder width of 12 cm), and many high school students need a large adult cuff (width of 16 cm) or leg cuff (width of 18 cm). The pressure coinciding with the onset (K_1) and the loss (K_5) of the Korotkoff sounds determines the systolic and diastolic blood pressure, respectively. The 95th percentile value for blood pressure (Table 20–17) is similar for both sexes and all three major ethnic groups. If a properly measured blood pressure exceeds the 95th percentile, the measurement should be repeated several times over a 2- to 4-week interval. If it is elevated persistently, a search for the cause should be undertaken. Although most hypertension in children is essential, the incidence of treatable causes is higher in children than in adults; these include conditions such as coarctation of the aorta, renal artery stenosis, chronic renal disease, and pheochromocytoma, as well as medication side effects (eg, steroids). If no cause is identified, and hypertension is deemed essential, antihypertensive therapy should be initiated and nutritional and exercise counseling given. β-Blockers or ACE inhibitors are the usual first-line medical therapies for essential hypertension in children.

Falkner B: Hypertension in children and adolescents: Epidemiology and natural history. Pediatr Nephrol 2009 [PMID: 19421783].

ATHEROSCLEROSIS & DYSLIPIDEMIAS

Awareness of coronary artery risk factors in general, and atherosclerosis in particular, has risen dramatically in the general population since the mid-1970s. Although coronary artery disease is still the leading cause of death in the United States, the age-adjusted incidence of death from ischemic heart disease has been decreasing as a result of improved diet, decreased smoking, awareness and treatment of hypertension, and an increase in physical activity. The level of serum lipids in childhood usually remains constant through adolescence. Biochemical abnormalities in the lipid profile appearing early in childhood correlate with higher risk for coronary artery disease in adulthood. Low-density lipoprotein (LDL) is atherogenic, while its counterpart, high-density lipoprotein (HDL) has been identified as an anti-atherogenic factor.

Table 20–17. The 95th percentile value for blood pressure (mm Hg) taken in the sitting position.[a]

	Sea Level			10,000 ft		
Age (y)	S	Dm	Dd	S	Dm	Dd
5				92	72	62
6	106	64	60	96	74	66
7	108	72	66	98	76	70
8	110	76	70	104	80	70
9	114	80	76	106	80	70
10	118	82	76	108	80	70
11	124	82	78	108	80	72
12	128	84	78	108	80	72
13	132	84	80	116	84	76
14	136	86	80	120	84	76
15	140	88	80	120	84	80
16	140	90	80	120	84	80
17	140	92	80	122	84	80
18	140	92	80	130	84	80

[a]Blood pressures: S, systolic (Korotkoff sound 1; onset of tapping); Dm, diastolic muffling (Korotkoff sound 4); Dd, diastolic disappearance (Korotkoff sound 5).

Routine lipid screening of children at age 3 years remains controversial. The National Cholesterol Education Program recommends selective screening in children with high-risk family members, defined as a parent with total cholesterol greater than 240 mg/dL or a parent or grandparent with early-onset cardiovascular disease. When children have LDL levels greater than 130 mg/dL on two successive tests, dietary lifestyle counseling is appropriate. Dietary modification may decrease cholesterol levels by 5%–20%. If the patient is unresponsive to diet change and at extreme risk (eg, LDL > 160 mg/dL, HDL < 35 mg/dL, and a history of cardiovascular disease in a first-degree relative at an age < 40 years), drug therapy may be indicated. Cholestyramine, a bile acid–binding resin, is rarely used today due to poor adherence. The 3-hydroxy-3-methylglutaryl coenzyme A (HMG-CoA) reductase inhibitors (statins) are more commonly used in the pediatric population. Niacin is useful for treatment of hypertriglyceridemia.

Gidding SS et al: Dietary recommendations for children and adolescents: A guide for practitioners: Consensus statement from the American Heart Association. Circulation 2005 Sep 27;112(13):2061–2075.

McCrindle BW et al: Drug therapy of high-risk lipid abnormalities in children and adolescents: A scientific statement from the American Heart Association Atherosclerosis, Hypertension, and Obesity in Youth Committee, Council of Cardiovascular Disease in the Young, with the Council on Cardiovascular Nursing. Circulation 2007 Apr 10;115(14):1948–1967.

CHEST PAIN

Overview

Chest pain is a common pediatric complaint, accounting for 6 in 1000 visits to urban emergency departments and urgent care clinics. Although children with chest pain are commonly referred for cardiac evaluation, chest pain in children is rarely cardiac in origin. Other more likely causes of chest pain in children include reactive airways disease, musculoskeletal pain, esophagitis, gastritis, and functional pain.

Detailed history and physical examination should guide the pediatrician to the appropriate workup of chest pain. Rarely is there a need for laboratory tests or evaluation by a specialist. The duration, location, intensity, frequency, and radiation of the pain should be documented, and possible triggering events preceding the pain should be explored. For instance, chest pain following exertion may lead to a more elaborate evaluation for a cardiac disorder. The timing of the pain in relation to meals may suggest a gastrointestinal cause. The patient should also be asked about how pain relief is achieved. A social history to reveal psychosocial stressors and cigarette smoke exposure may be revealing. On physical examination, attention must be placed on the vital signs; general appearance of the child; the chest wall musculature; cardiac, pulmonary, and abdominal examination findings; and quality of peripheral pulses. If the pain can be reproduced through direct palpation of the chest wall, it is almost always musculoskeletal in origin.

Etiology

Cardiac disease is a rare cause of chest pain, but, if misdiagnosed, it may be life-threatening. Although myocardial infarction rarely occurs in healthy children, patients with diabetes mellitus, chronic anemia, abnormal coronary artery anatomy, or HCM may be at increased risk for ischemia. A history of Kawasaki disease with coronary involvement is a risk for myocardial infarction secondary to thrombosis of coronary aneurysms. More than 50% of children and adolescents who exhibit sequelae from Kawasaki disease arrive at the emergency department with chest pain.

Young children may mistake palpitations for chest pain. Supraventricular tachycardia (SVT), atrial flutter, premature ventricular contractions (PVCs), or ventricular tachycardia may be described as chest pain in children. Structural lesions that can cause chest pain include aortic stenosis, pulmonary stenosis, and mitral valve prolapse. Structural cardiac lesions are usually accompanied by significant findings on cardiac examination. Of children with mitral valve prolapse, 30% will complain of chest pain presumably caused by papillary muscle ischemia. Other cardiac lesions causing chest pain include DCM, myocarditis, pericarditis, rheumatic carditis, and aortic dissection.

Noncardiac chest pain may be due to a respiratory illness, reactive airway disease, pneumonia, pneumothorax, or pulmonary embolism. Gastrointestinal causes of chest pain include reflux, esophagitis, and foreign body ingestion. The most common cause of chest pain (30% of children) is inflammation of musculoskeletal structures of the chest wall. Costochondritis is caused by inflammation of the costochondral joints and is usually unilateral and reproducible on examination.

In most cases sophisticated testing is not required. However, if a cardiac origin is suspected, a pediatric cardiologist should be consulted. Evaluation in these instances may include an ECG, chest radiograph, echocardiogram, Holter monitor, or serum troponin levels if there are known risk factors for ischemia.

Hanson CL, Hokanson JS: Etiology of chest pain in children and adolescents referred to cardiology clinic. WMJ 2011 Apr;110(2):58–62 [PMID: 21560558].

CARDIAC TRANSPLANTATION

Cardiac transplantation is an effective therapeutic modality for infants and children with end-stage cardiac disease. Indications for transplantation include (1) progressive HF despite maximal medical therapy, (2) complex congenital heart diseases that are not amenable to surgical repair or palliation, or in instances in which the surgical palliative approach has an equal or higher risk of mortality compared with transplantation, and (3) malignant arrhythmias unresponsive to medical therapy, catheter ablation, or automatic implantable cardiodefibrillator. Approximately 300–400 pediatric cardiac transplant procedures are performed annually in the United States. Infant (< 1 year of age) transplants account for 30% of pediatric cardiac transplants. The current estimated graft half-life for children undergoing cardiac transplantation in infancy is over 18 years, while overall pediatric heart transplant graft half-life is approximately 14 years. This is a rapidly evolving field, and the most recent data indicate an optimistic future for the transplant recipient.

Careful evaluation of the recipient and the donor is performed prior to cardiac transplantation. Assessment of the recipient's pulmonary vascular resistance is critical, as irreversible and severe pulmonary hypertension is a risk factor for post-transplant right heart failure and early death. End-organ function of the recipient may also influence post-transplant outcome and should be evaluated closely. Donor-related factors that can have an impact on outcome include cardiac function, amount of inotropic support needed, active infection (HIV and hepatitis B and C are contraindications to donation), donor size, and ischemic time to transplantation.

Immunosuppression

The ideal post-transplant immunosuppressive regimen allows the immune system to continue to recognize and respond to foreign antigens in a productive manner while avoiding graft rejection. Although there are many different regimens, calcineurin inhibitors (eg, cyclosporine and tacrolimus) remain the mainstay of maintenance immunosuppression in pediatric heart transplantation. Calcineurin inhibitors may be used in isolation in children considered to be at low risk for graft rejection. Double-drug therapy includes the addition of antimetabolite or antiproliferative medications such as azathioprine, mycophenolate mofetil, or sirolimus. Because of the significant adverse side effects of corticosteroids in children, many centers attempt to avoid chronic steroid use. Growth retardation, susceptibility to infection, impaired wound healing, hypertension, diabetes, osteoporosis, and a cushingoid appearance are some of the consequences of long-term steroid use.

Graft Rejection

Despite advances in immunosuppression, graft rejection remains the leading cause of death in the first 3 years after transplantation. The pathophysiologic mechanisms of rejection are not entirely known. T cells are required for rejection, but multiple cell lines and mechanisms are likely involved. Because graft rejection can present in the absence of clinical symptomatology, monitoring for and diagnosing rejection in a timely fashion can be difficult. Screening regimens include serial physical examinations, electrocardiography, echocardiography, and cardiac catheterization with endomyocardial biopsy.

Rejection Surveillance

A. Symptoms and Signs

Acute graft rejection may not cause symptoms in the early stages. With progression patients may develop tachycardia, tachypnea, rales, a gallop rhythm, or hepatosplenomegaly. Infants and young children may present with irritability, poor feeding, vomiting, or lethargy. The goal is to detect rejection prior to the development of hemodynamic compromise, as there is 50% mortality in the year following an episode of rejection, resulting in cardiovascular compromise.

B. Imaging

In an actively rejecting patient, chest radiographs may show cardiomegaly, pulmonary edema, or pleural effusions.

C. Electrocardiography

Abnormalities in conduction can be present, although the most typical finding is reduced QRS voltages. Both atrial and ventricular arrhythmias can occur in rejection.

D. Echocardiography

Echocardiography is a noninvasive rejection surveillance tool that is especially useful in infant recipients, but helpful in all ages. Changes in ventricular compliance and function may initially be subtle, but are progressive with increasing duration of the rejection episode. A new pericardial effusion or worsening valvular insufficiency may also indicate rejection.

E. Cardiac Catheterization and Endomyocardial Biopsy

Hemodynamic assessment including ventricular filling pressures, cardiac output, and oxygen consumption can be obtained via cardiac catheterization. The endomyocardial biopsy is useful in diagnosing acute graft rejection. However, because not all episodes of symptomatic rejection result in a positive biopsy result, this tool is not universally reliable. The appearance of infiltrating lymphocytes with myocellular damage on the biopsy is the hallmark of cell-mediated graft rejection and is helpful if present.

Treatment of Graft Rejection

The goal of graft rejection treatment is to reverse the immunologic inflammatory cascade. High-dose corticosteroids are the first line of treatment. Frequently additional therapy with antithymocyte biologic preparations such as antithymocyte globulin (a rabbit based polyclonal antibody) is needed to reverse rejection. Most rejection episodes can be treated effectively if diagnosed promptly. Usually graft function returns to its baseline state, although severe rejection episodes can result in chronic graft failure, graft loss, and patient death even with optimal therapy. Antibody mediated rejection is another form of acute rejection that is treated in a similar fashion as T-cell mediated rejection, but the addition of plasmapheresis and IVIG to the treatment regimen may improve outcomes. The diagnosis of antibody mediated rejection varies across centers, but can be a combination of clinical findings consistent with rejection in the absence of evidence of cell-mediated rejection, evidence of complement deposition on endomyocardial biopsy and new or increasing antibody production (typically anti-human lymphocyte antigen [HLA] antibodies) in the circulation.

Course & Prognosis

The quality of life of pediatric heart transplant recipients is usually quite good. The risk of infection is low after the immediate post-transplant period in spite of chronic immunosuppression. Cytomegalovirus is the most common pathogen responsible for infection-related morbidity and mortality in heart transplant recipients. Most children tolerate environmental pathogens well. Nonadherence with lifetime immunosuppression is of great concern especially in adolescent patients. Several recent studies have identified nonadherence as the leading cause of late death. Post-transplant lymphoproliferative disorder, a syndrome related to Epstein-Barr virus infection, can result in a Burkitt-like lymphoma that usually responds to a reduction in immunosuppression, but occasionally must be treated with chemotherapy and can be fatal. The overwhelming majority of children are not physically limited and do not require restrictions related to the cardiovascular system.

The greatest long-term concern after heart transplantation is related to cardiac allograft vasculopathy (transplant coronary artery disease). Cardiac allograft vasculopathy results from intimal proliferation within the lumen of the coronary arteries that can ultimately result in complete luminal occlusion. These lesions are diffuse and often involve distal vessels and thus are usually not amenable to bypass grafting, angioplasty, or stent placement. The etiology of these lesions has an immune basis, but the specifics are not known making targeted therapy challenging. Overall, despite the concerns of immunosuppression, the risk of late rejection, and coronary disease, the majority of pediatric patients enjoy a good quality of life with survival rates that are improving. Currently, 10-year survival is around 60% overall for pediatric recipients. Newer, more specific, and more effective immunosuppressive agents are currently being tried in clinical studies or are being evaluated in preclinical studies, making the future promising for children after cardiac transplantation. Donor availability remains a major limitation to the expansion of indications for cardiac transplantation.

QUALITY IMPROVEMENT FOR PEDIATRIC HEART TRANSPLANTATION

The Pediatric Heart Transplant Study (PHTS) group is a consortium of over 40 pediatric heart transplant centers in North America and Europe that maintains an event-driven database that is used to support research aimed at improving treatment options and outcomes for children in need of a heart transplant or who have had a transplant. This group was established in 1993 and has published over 40 manuscripts in peer-reviewed journals. Each participating center receives an annual report that details center-specific outcomes compared to the collaborative group as a whole. This report is utilized for internal quality assurance purposes and as a performance benchmark.

Canter CE et al: Indications for heart transplantation in pediatric heart disease: A scientific statement from the American Heart Association Council on Cardiovascular Disease in the Young; the Councils on Clinical Cardiology, Cardiovascular Nursing, and Cardiovascular Surgery and Anesthesia; and the Quality of Care and Outcomes Research Interdisciplinary Working Group. Circulation 2007 Feb 6;115(5):658–676.

Kirk R, Edwards LB, Kucheryavaya AY et al: The Registry of the International Society for Heart and Lung Transplantation: Thirteenth official pediatric heart transplantation report—2010. J Heart Lung Transplant. 2010 Oct;29(10):1119–1128 No abstract available [PMID: 20870166].

PHTS website: http://www.uab.edu/ctsresearch/phts/index.html

PRIMARY PULMONARY HYPERTENSION

ESSENTIALS OF DIAGNOSIS & TYPICAL FEATURES

- Often subtle with symptoms of dyspnea, fatigue, chest pain, and syncope.
- Loud pulmonary component of S_2; ECG with RVH.
- Implies exclusion of secondary causes of pulmonary hypertension.
- Rare, progressive, and often fatal disease without treatment.

General Considerations

Unexplained or primary pulmonary hypertension (PPH) in children is a rare disease with an estimated overall incidence of 1–2 persons per million worldwide. Pulmonary hypertension is defined as a mean pulmonary pressure greater than 25 mm Hg at rest or greater than 30 mm Hg during exercise. PPH is a diagnosis made after exclusion of all other causes of pulmonary hypertension. Secondary pulmonary hypertension is most commonly associated with congenital heart disease, pulmonary parenchymal disease, causes of chronic hypoxia (upper airway obstruction), thrombosis, liver disease, hemoglobinopathies, and collagen vascular disease. PPH is difficult to diagnose in the early stages because of its subtle manifestations. Most patients with PPH are young adult women, although the gender incidence is equal in children. Historically, the diagnosis of PPH in individuals younger than 16 years of age carried a median survival of only 10 months. Fortunately, survival is improving with the advent of new therapies. Familial PPH occurs in 6%–12% of affected individuals. When a clear familial association is known, the disease shows evidence of genetic anticipation, presenting at younger ages in subsequent generations.

Clinical Findings

A. Symptoms and Signs

The clinical picture varies with the severity of pulmonary hypertension, and usually early symptoms are subtle, delaying the diagnosis. Initial symptoms may be dyspnea, palpitations, or chest pain, often brought on by strenuous exercise or competitive sports. Syncope may be the first symptom, which usually implies severe disease. As the disease progresses, patients have signs of low cardiac output and right heart failure. Right heart failure may be manifested by hepatomegaly, peripheral edema, and an S_3 gallop on examination. Murmurs of pulmonary regurgitation and tricuspid regurgitation may be present, and the pulmonary component of S_2 is usually pronounced.

B. Imaging

The chest radiograph most often reveals a prominent main pulmonary artery, and the RV may be enlarged. The peripheral pulmonary vascular markings may be normal or diminished. However, in 6% of patients with confirmed PPH, the chest radiograph is normal.

C. Electrocardiography

The ECG usually shows RVH with an upright T wave in V_1 (when it should be negative in young children) or a qR complex in lead V_1 or V_{3R}. Also present may be evidence of right axis deviation and right atrial enlargement.

D. Echocardiography

The echocardiogram is an essential tool for excluding congenital heart disease as a cause of pulmonary hypertension. It frequently shows RVH and dilation. In the absence of other structural disease, any tricuspid and PI jets can be used to estimate pulmonary artery systolic and diastolic pressures, respectively. Other echocardiographic modalities such as myocardial performance index and input vascular impedance are in the early stages of use in evaluation of pulmonary hypertension.

E. Cardiac Catheterization and Angiocardiography

Cardiac catheterization is the best method for diagnosing PPH and determining the severity of disease. As an invasive test, it carries with it associated risks and should be performed with caution. The procedure is performed to rule out cardiac (eg, restrictive cardiomyopathy) or vascular (eg, pulmonary vein stenosis) causes of pulmonary hypertension, determine the severity of disease, and define treatment strategies. The reactivity of the pulmonary vascular bed to short-acting vasodilator agents (oxygen, nitric oxide, or prostacyclin) can be assessed and used to determine treatment options. Angiography may show a decrease in the number of small pulmonary arteries with tortuous vessels.

F. Other Evaluation Modalities

Cardiac MRI is used in some patients to evaluate right ventricular function, pulmonary artery anatomy, and hemo-dynamics, as well as thromboembolic phenomena. Cardiopulmonary exercise testing using cycle ergometry correlates with disease severity. More simply, a 6-minute walk test, in which distance walked and perceived level of exertion are measured, has a strong independent association with mortality in late disease.

Treatment

The goal of therapy is to reduce pulmonary artery pressure, increase cardiac output, and improve quality of life. Cardiac catheterization data are used to determine the proper treatment. Patients responsive to pulmonary vasodilators are given calcium channel blockers such as nifedipine or diltiazem. Patients unresponsive to vasodilators initially receive one of three classes of drugs: prostanoids (such as epoprostenol), endothelin receptor antagonists (such as bosentan), or phosphodiesterase inhibitors (such as sildenafil). All of these agents have distinct mechanisms of action that can reduce pulmonary vascular resistance. Warfarin is commonly used for anticoagulation to prevent thromboembolic events, usually with a goal to maintain the INR between 1.5 and 2.0.

Atrial septostomy is indicated in some patients with refractory pulmonary hypertension and symptoms. Cardiac output falls as pulmonary vascular resistance rises, so an interatrial shunt can preserve left heart output, albeit with deoxygenated blood. Lung transplantation should be considered in patients with intractable pulmonary hypertension and in those with associated anatomic lesions that contribute to high pulmonary arterial pressure, like pulmonary vein stenosis. Heart-lung transplant procedures appear to have survival benefits over isolated lung transplantation in patients with pulmonary hypertension. Recurrence of pulmonary hypertension is rare after heart-lung transplant.

Although survival is less than 10 months in children with untreated pulmonary hypertension, recent studies have showed improved survival rates of more than 95% at 5 years with calcium channel blockade, and more than 80% at 5 years in children requiring epoprostenol.

Abman SH, Ivy DD: Recent progress in understanding pediatric pulmonary hypertension. Curr Opin Pediatr 2011 Jun;23(3):298–304 [PMID: 21572384].

Lammers AE, Adatia I, Cerro MJ et al: Functional classification of pulmonary hypertension in children: Report from the PVRI pediatric taskforce, Panama 2011. Pulm Circ 2011 Aug 2;1(2):280–285 [PMID: 21874157].

DISORDERS OF RATE & RHYTHM

Cardiac rhythm abnormalities occur in two different patient populations: children with congenital heart disease or children who are otherwise healthy with a normal heart structure. Children with congenital heart are at risk for a cardiac rhythm abnormalities based on the underlying heart defect itself, the changes in cardiac muscle cells associated with a chronic state of altered cardiac hemodynamics, and any operative procedures with surgical suture lines/scars which place the patient at higher risk for certain types of arrhythmias. Children with a normal heart structure have an intrinsic abnormality of the electrical conduction system within the heart.

The evaluation and treatment of cardiac rhythm disorders have advanced significantly over the last several decades. Arguably, the most significant advancements in the last few years have continued in the area of the genetic basis of rhythm disorders such as long QT syndrome which will be discussed at the end of the chapter. Treatment for cardiac rhythm abnormalities includes clinical monitoring with no intervention, antiarrhythmic medications, invasive electrophysiology study and ablation procedures, pacemakers, and internal cardioverter/defibrillators.

Deal BJ et al: Arrhythmic complications associated with the treatment of patients with congenital cardiac disease: Consensus definitions from the Multi-Societal Database Committee for Pediatric and Congenital Heart Disease. Cardiol Young 2008 Dec;18(Suppl 2):202–205.

DISORDERS OF THE SINUS NODE

SINUS ARRHYTHMIA

Phasic variation in the heart rate (sinus arrhythmia) is normal. Typically, the sinus rate varies with the respiratory cycle (heart rate increases with inspiration and decreases with expiration), whereas P-QRS-T intervals remain stable. Sinus arrhythmia may occur in association with respiratory distress or increased intracranial pressure, or it may be present in normal children. In isolation, it never requires treatment; however, it may be associated with sinus node dysfunction or autonomic nervous system dysfunction.

SINUS BRADYCARDIA

Sinus bradycardia is defined as a heart rate below the normal limit for age (neonates to 6 years, 60 beats/min; 7–11 years, 45 beats/min; > 12 years, 40 beats/min). Sinus bradycardia is often seen in athletic children. In critically ill patients, causes of sinus bradycardia include hypoxia, central nervous system damage, eating disorders, and medication side effects. Only symptomatic bradycardia (syncope, low cardiac output, or exercise intolerance) requires treatment (atropine, isoproterenol, or cardiac pacing).

SINUS TACHYCARDIA

The heart rate normally accelerates in response to stress (eg, exercise, anxiety, fever, hypovolemia, anemia, or HF). Although sinus tachycardia in the normal heart is well tolerated, symptomatic tachycardia with decreased cardiac output warrants evaluation for structural heart disease, cardiomyopathy or true tachyarrhythmias. The first evaluation should be made with a 12-lead ECG to determine the precise mechanism of the rapid rate. Treatment may be indicated for correction of the underlying cause of sinus tachycardia (eg, transfusion for anemia or correction of hypovolemia or fever).

SINUS NODE DYSFUNCTION

Sinus node dysfunction is a clinical syndrome of inappropriate sinus nodal function and rate. The abnormality may be a true anatomic defect of the sinus node or its surrounding tissue, or it may be an abnormality of autonomic input. It is defined as one or more of the following: severe sinus bradycardia, marked sinus arrhythmia, sinus pause or arrest, chronotropic incompetence (inability of the heart rate to increase with activity or other demands), or combined bradyarrhythmias and tachyarrhythmias. It is usually associated with postoperative repair of congenital heart disease (most commonly the Mustard or Senning repair for complete TGA or the Fontan procedure), but it is also seen in normal hearts, in unoperated congenital heart disease, and in acquired heart diseases. Symptoms usually manifest between ages 2 and 17 years and consist of episodes of presyncope, syncope, palpitations, pallor, or exercise intolerance.

The evaluation of sinus node dysfunction may involve the following: baseline ECG, 24-hour ambulatory ECG monitoring, exercise stress test, and transient event monitoring. Treatment for sinus node dysfunction is indicated only in symptomatic patients. Bradyarrhythmias are treated with vagolytic (atropine) or adrenergic (aminophylline) agents or permanent cardiac pacemakers.

PREMATURE BEATS

Atrial Premature Beats

Atrial premature beats are triggered by an ectopic focus in the atrium. They are one of the most common premature beats occurring in pediatric patients, particularly during the fetal and newborn periods. The premature beat may be conducted (followed by a QRS) or nonconducted (not followed by a QRS, as the beat has occurred so early that the AV node is still refractory) (Figure 20–4). A brief pause usually occurs until the next normal sinus beat occurs. As an isolated finding, atrial premature beats are benign and require no treatment.

Junctional Premature Beats

Junctional premature beats arise in the atrioventricular node or the bundle of His. They induce a normal QRS complex with no preceding P wave. Junctional premature beats are usually benign and require no specific therapy.

Ventricular Premature Beats

Ventricular premature beats are sometimes referred to as premature ventricular contractions (PVC) or as ventricular ectopy. They are relatively common, occurring in 1%–2% of patients with normal hearts. They are characterized by an early beat with a wide QRS complex, without a preceding P wave, and with a full compensatory pause following this early beat (Figure 20–5). Ventricular premature beats originating from a single ectopic focus all have the same configuration; those of multifocal origin show varying configurations. The consecutive occurrence of two ventricular premature beats is referred to as a ventricular couplet and of three or more as ventricular tachycardia. Most ventricular premature beats in otherwise normal patients are usually benign. However, most patients are evaluated further with tests such as a 24-hour ambulatory ECG or with exercise testing to rule out concerning arrhythmias. An echocardiogram may be performed to evaluate ventricular function. The significance of ventricular premature beats can be confirmed by having the patient exercise. As the heart rate increases, benign ventricular premature beats usually disappear. If exercise results in an increase or coupling of contractions, underlying disease may be present. Multifocal ventricular premature beats are always abnormal and may be more dangerous. They may be associated with drug overdose (tricyclic antidepressants or digoxin toxicity), electrolyte imbalance, myocarditis, or hypoxia. Treatment is directed at correcting the underlying disorder.

SUPRAVENTRICULAR TACHYCARDIA

Supraventricular tachycardia (SVT) is a term used to describe any rapid rhythm originating from the atrium, the atrioventricular node, or an accessory pathway. These tachycardias

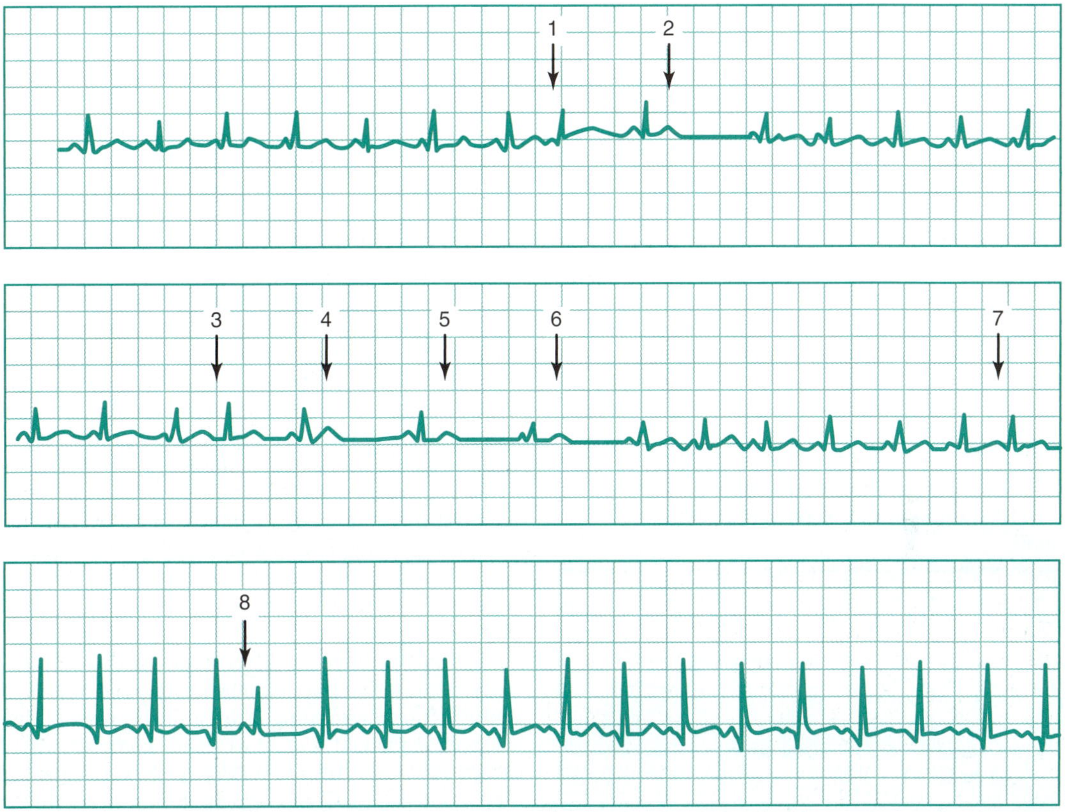

▲ **Figure 20–4.** Lead II rhythm strip with premature atrial contractions. Beats 1, 3, 7, and 8 are conducted to the ventricles, whereas beats 2, 4, 5, and 6 are not.

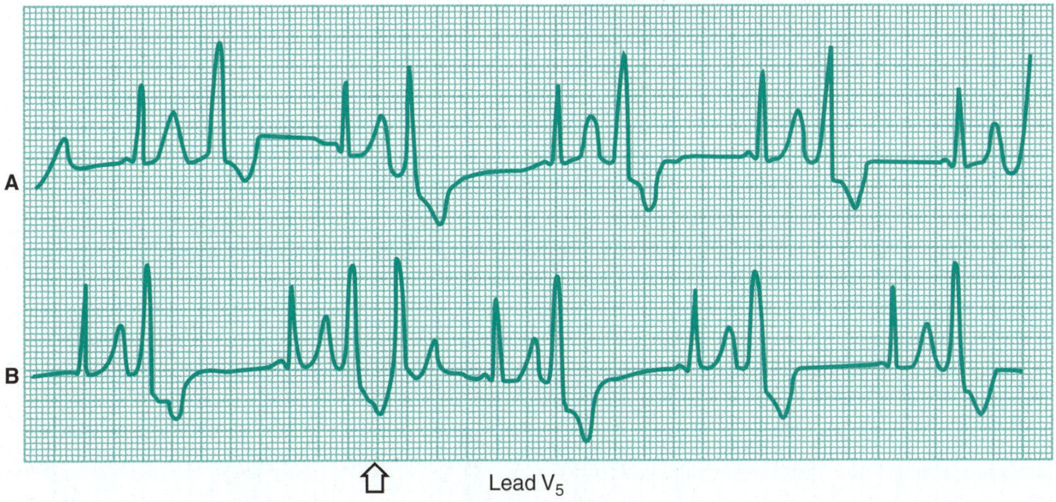

▲ **Figure 20–5.** Lead V_5 rhythm strip with unifocal premature ventricular contractions in a bigeminy pattern. The arrow shows a ventricular couplet.

are rapid, narrow complex tachycardias. The mode of presentation depends on the heart rate, the presence of underlying cardiac structural or functional abnormalities, coexisting illness, and patient age. An otherwise healthy child with SVT may complain of intermittent periods of rapid heartbeats. An infant with SVT may have poor feeding and increased fatigue (manifesting as less awake time). Incessant tachycardia, even if fairly slow (120–150 beats/min), may cause myocardial dysfunction and HF if left untreated. In children with preexisting HF or an underlying systemic disease such as anemia or sepsis, SVT may result in decreased heart function and further signs of hemodynamic instability.

The mechanisms of tachycardia are generally divided into reentrant and automatic mechanisms and can be described by the location of tachycardia origination (Table 20–18).

Table 20–18. Mechanism of supraventricular tachycardia.

Site of Origination	Automatic Mechanisms	Reentrant Mechanisms
Sinus node	Sinus tachycardia	Sinoatrial node reentry
Atrium	Ectopic atrial tachycardia Multifocal atrial tachycardia	Atrial flutter Intra-atrial reentrant tachycardia Atrial fibrillation
Atrioventricular node	Junctional ectopic tachycardia	Atrioventricular nodal reentrant tachycardia (AVNRT)
Accessory pathways		Concealed accessory pathways Wolff-Parkinson-White (WPW) syndrome Permanent form of junctional reciprocating tachycardia (PJRT) Mahaim fiber tachycardia

Reentrant tachycardias represent approximately 80% of pediatric arrhythmias. Reentrant tachycardias have the following characteristics: they initiate abruptly, they have a fixed rate, they have little variation with fever or internal catecholamines, and they terminate abruptly. They can be terminated to sinus rhythm with maneuvers such as vagal maneuvers, administration of adenosine, pacing maneuvers, or DC cardioversion. (For vagal maneuvers or adenosine, the atrioventricular node must be part of the reentrant circuit.) Reentrant tachycardia mechanisms involve two connections where electrical conduction travels down one of the pathways and then backs up the other, creating a sustained repetitive circular loop. The circuit can be confined to the atrium (*atrial flutter* in a normal heart or *intra-atrial reentrant tachycardia* in a patient with congenital heart disease) (Figure 20–6). It may be confined within the AV node (*AV nodal reentrant tachycardia*), or it may encompass an accessory connection between atria and ventricle (*accessory pathway–mediated tachycardia*). If, during tachycardia, the electrical impulse travels antegrade (from atria to ventricles) through the AV node and retrograde (from ventricle to atria) back up the accessory pathway, orthodromic reciprocating tachycardia is present. If, instead, the impulse travels antegrade through the accessory pathway and retrograde up through the AV node, antidromic reciprocating tachycardia is present. This latter tachycardia would present as a wide complex tachycardia. *Wolff-Parkinson-White* (WPW) *syndrome* is a subclass of reentrant tachycardia in which, during sinus rhythm, the impulse travels antegrade down the accessory connection, bypassing the AV node and creating ventricular preexcitation (early eccentric activation of the ventricle with a short PR interval and slurred upstroke of the QRS, a delta wave) (Figure 20–7). Most patients with WPW have otherwise structurally normal hearts. However, WPW has been noted to occur with increased frequency in association with the following congenital cardiac lesions: tricuspid atresia,

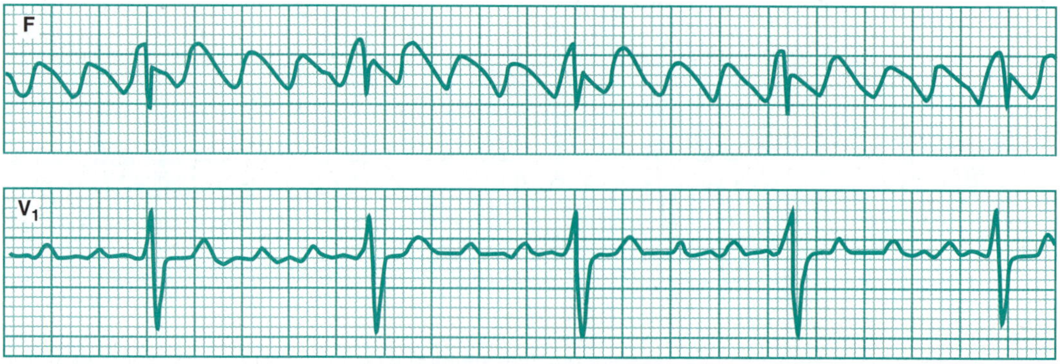

▲ **Figure 20–6.** Leads aVF (F) and V_1, showing atrial flutter with "sawtooth" atrial flutter waves.

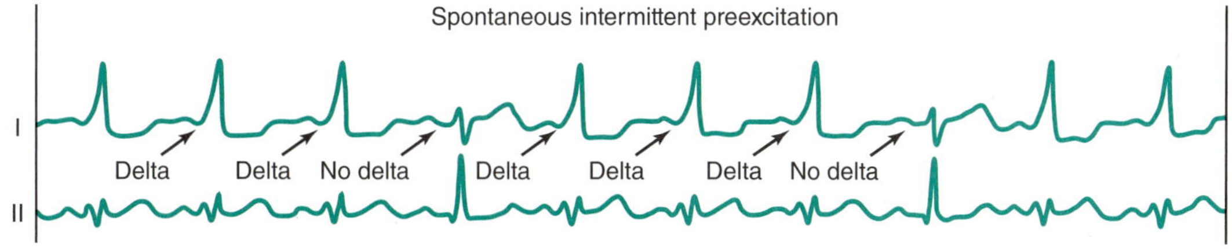

▲ **Figure 20–7.** Leads I and II with spontaneous intermittent ventricular preexcitation (Wolff-Parkinson-White syndrome).

Ebstein anomaly of the tricuspid valve, HCM, and ccTGA. Different than other causes of tachycardias described above where the arrhythmia is not life threatening, there have been rare cases of sudden collapse from WPW syndrome. The mechanism of this sudden event is the development of atrial fibrillation, conducting down a rapid accessory pathway to the ventricle leading to ventricular fibrillation and sudden death. For this reason, most centers recommend that even asymptomatic patients undergo an invasive procedure to assess the conduction properties of the WPW accessory pathway (described under treatment for tachyarrhythmias).

Improved surgical survival for patients with congenital heart disease has created a new, increasingly prevalent, chronic arrhythmia which is similar to atrial flutter in a normal heart structure. These arrhythmias have been referred to by many names: intra-atrial reentrant tachycardia, incisional tachycardia, macroreentry, or postoperative atrial flutter. In this tachycardia, electrically isolated corridors of atrial myocardium (eg, the tricuspid valve–inferior vena cava isthmus, or the region between an atrial incision and the crista terminalis) act as pathways for sustained reentrant circuits of electrical activity. These tachycardias are chronic, medically refractory, and clinically incapacitating.

The automatic tachycardias represent approximately 20% of childhood arrhythmias. The characteristics of these types of arrhythmias include gradual onset, rate variability, variations in rate with fever or increasing internal catecholamines, and gradual offset. Maneuvers such as vagal maneuvers, adenosine, and attempt pacing can alter the rhythm temporarily but they do not result in termination of the rhythm to sinus rhythm as would be seen in the reentrant tachycardias. Automatic tachycardias can be episodic or incessant. They are usually under autonomic influence. When they are incessant, they are usually associated with HF and a clinical picture of DCM. Automatic tachycardias are created when a focus of cardiac tissue develops an abnormally fast spontaneous rate of depolarization. For ectopic atrial tachycardia, the ECG demonstrates a normal QRS complex preceded by an abnormal P wave (Figure 20–8). Junctional ectopic tachycardia does not have a P wave preceding the QRS waves and may be associated with AV dissociation or 1:1 retrograde conduction.

Doniger SJ, Sharieff GQ: Pediatric dysrhythmias. Pediatr Clin North Am 2006 Feb;53(1):85–105, vi.

Schlechte EA, Boramanand N, Funk M: Supraventricular tachycardia in the pediatric primary care setting: Age-related presentation, diagnosis, and management. J Pediatr Health Care 2008 Sep–Oct;22(5):289–299.

Clinical Findings

A. Symptoms and Signs

Presentation varies with age. Infants tend to turn pale and mottled with onset of tachycardia and may become irritable. With long duration of tachycardia, symptoms of HF develop. Older children complain of dizziness, palpitations, fatigue, and chest pain. Heart rates range from 240–300 beats/min in the younger child to 150–180 beats/min in the teenager. HF is less common in children than in infants. Tachycardia may be associated with either congenital heart defects or acquired conditions such as cardiomyopathies and myocarditis.

B. Imaging

Chest radiographs are normal during the early course of tachycardia and therefore are usually not obtained. If HF is present, the heart is enlarged and pulmonary venous congestion is evident.

C. Electrocardiography

ECG is the most important tool in the diagnosis of SVT and to define the precise tachycardia mechanism. Findings include a heart rate that is rapid and out of proportion to the patient's physical status (eg, a rate of 140 beats/min with an abnormal P wave while quiet and asleep). For reentrant mechanisms, the rhythm would be extremely regular with little variability. For automatic mechanisms, the rhythm would be irregular with a gradual increasing and decreasing of the rate. The QRS complex is usually the same as during normal sinus rhythm. However, the QRS complex is occasionally widened (SVT with aberrant ventricular conduction), in which case the condition may be difficult to differentiate from ventricular tachycardia. The presence of

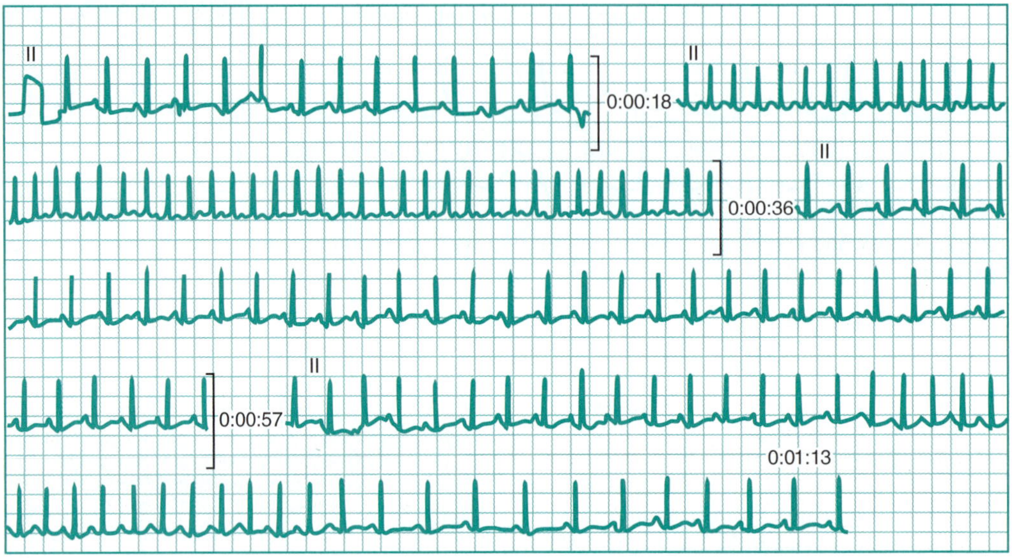

▲ **Figure 20–8.** Lead II rhythm strip of ectopic atrial tachycardia. The tracing demonstrates a variable rate with a maximum of 260 beats/min, an abnormal P wave, and a gradual termination.

P waves and their association with the QRS are important in determining tachycardia mechanism. With automatic tachycardias, there is often a 1:1 or 2:1 A: V relationship with P waves preceding the QRS. With reentrant tachycardias, such as accessory pathway–mediated tachycardias, a small retrograde P wave can often be seen just after the QRS. With atrioventricular nodal reentrant tachycardia, P waves cannot be identified as they are occurring at the same time as the QRS.

Treatment

A. Acute Treatment

During the initial episodes of SVT, patients require close monitoring. Correction of acidosis and electrolyte abnormalities is also indicated. The following acute treatments are effective in terminating tachycardia only for patients with reentrant SVT. Acute treatment for automatic SVT is aimed at rate control, usually with a β-blocker.

1. Vagal maneuvers—The "diving reflex" produced by placing an ice bag on the nasal bridge for 20 seconds (for infants) or by immersing the face in ice water (for children or adolescents) will increase parasympathetic tone and terminate some tachycardias. The Valsalva maneuver, which can be performed by older compliant children, may also terminate reentrant tachycardias.

2. Adenosine—Adenosine transiently blocks AV conduction and terminates tachycardias that incorporate the AV node or may aid in the diagnosis of arrhythmias confined to the atrium by causing a pause in ventricular conduction, so one can identify the presence of multiple P waves. The dose is 100–250 mcg/kg by rapid intravenous bolus. It is antagonized by aminophylline and should be used with caution in patients with sinus node dysfunction or asthma.

3. Transesophageal atrial pacing—Atrial overdrive pacing and termination can be performed from a bipolar electrode-tipped catheter positioned in the esophagus adjacent to the left atrium. Overdrive pacing at rates approximately 30% faster than the tachycardia rate will interrupt a reentrant tachycardia circuit and restore sinus rhythm.

4. Direct current cardioversion—Direct current cardioversion (0.5–2 synchronized J/kg) should be used immediately when a patient presents in cardiovascular collapse. This will convert a reentrant mechanism to sinus. Automatic tachycardia will not respond to cardioversion.

B. Chronic Treatment

Once the patient has been diagnosed with SVT and the mechanism has been evaluated, then long-term treatment options can be considered. Options include monitoring clinically for tachycardia recurrences, medical management with antiarrhythmic medications, or an invasive electrophysiology study and ablation procedure. In infancy and early childhood, antiarrhythmic medications are the mainstay of therapy. Medications such as digoxin and β-blockers are the first-line therapies. Other antiarrhythmic medications (eg, verapamil, flecainide, propafenone, sotalol, and amiodarone) have increased pharmacologic actions and are extremely effective. However, these medications also have serious side effects, including proarrhythmia (production of arrhythmias) and sudden death, and should be used only under the direction of a pediatric cardiologist.

Tachycardias, both automatic and reentrant, can be more definitively addressed with an invasive electrophysiology study and ablation procedure. This is a nonsurgical transvascular catheter technique that desiccates an arrhythmia focus or accessory pathway and permanently cures an arrhythmia. The ablation catheters can utilize either a heat source (radiofrequency) or a cool source (cryoablation). The latter has been reported to be safer around the normal conduction pathway and thus decreases the risk of inadvertent atrioventricular block. The success rate from an ablation procedure in a patient with a normal heart structure is > 90%, with a recurrence risk of < 10%. The procedure can be performed in infants or adults. In children younger than age 4 years, the risks of procedural complications or failed ablation are potentially higher, and the procedure should be reserved for those whose arrhythmias are refractory to medical management. The high success rate, low complication and low recurrence rates, in addition to the elimination of the need for chronic antiarrhythmic medications have made ablation procedures the primary treatment option in most pediatric cardiovascular centers. In patients with congenital heart disease, electrophysiology study and ablation procedures are also utilized to address arrhythmia substrates. The success rate of these procedures is lower than in patients with a normal heart structure, often reported in the 75%–80% range.

Prognosis

SVT in infants and children generally carries an excellent prognosis. It can be treated with medical management or with the potentially curative ablation procedures. There are, however, rare cases of incessant SVT leading to HF and there is reported sudden collapse from atrial fibrillation in the presence of WPW. All patients with complaints of rapid heartbeats or other symptoms where there is a concern for tachyarrhythmia should be referred for evaluation.

Harahsheh A et al: Risk factors for atrioventricular tachycardia degenerating to atrial flutter/fibrillation in the young with Wolff-Parkinson-White. Pacing Clin Electrophysiol 2008 Oct;31(10):1307–1312.

Lee PC et al: The results of radiofrequency catheter ablation of supraventricular tachycardia in children. Pacing Clin Electrophysiol 2007 May;30(5):655–661.

VENTRICULAR TACHYCARDIA

Ventricular tachycardia is uncommon in childhood (Figure 20–9). It is usually associated with underlying abnormalities of the myocardium (myocarditis, cardiomyopathy, myocardial tumors, or postoperative congenital heart disease) or toxicity (hypoxia, electrolyte imbalance, or drug toxicity). On occasion, it can be secondary to a primary electrical abnormality in an otherwise normal heart. Sustained ventricular tachycardia can be an unstable situation, and, if left untreated, it could degenerate into ventricular fibrillation and sudden collapse.

Ventricular tachycardia needs to be differentiated from accelerated idioventricular rhythm. The latter is a sustained ventricular tachycardia occurring in neonates with normal hearts, with a ventricular tachycardia rate within 10% of the preceding sinus rate. This is a self-limiting arrhythmia that requires no treatment.

Acute termination of ventricular tachycardia involves restoration of the normal myocardium when possible (correction of electrolyte imbalance, drug toxicity, etc) and direct current cardioversion (1–4 J/kg), cardioversion with

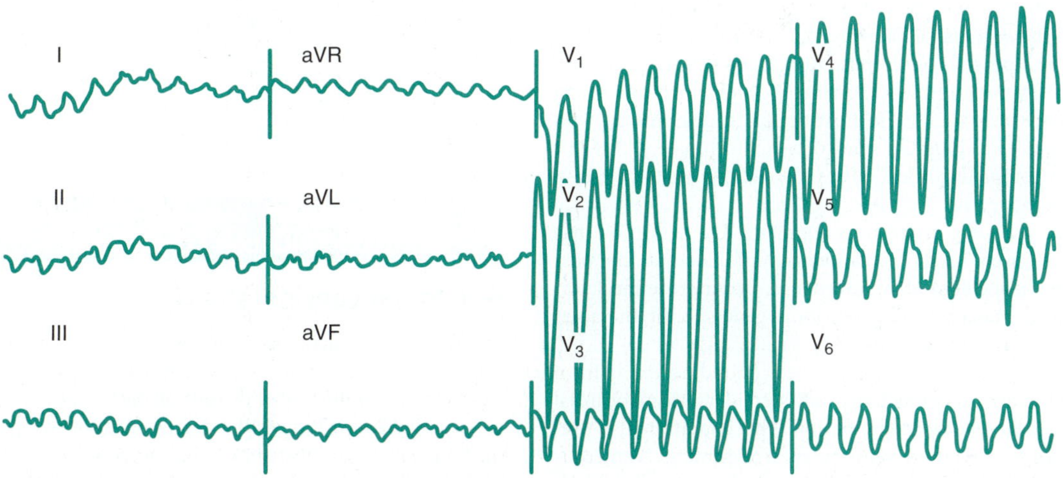

▲ **Figure 20–9.** Twelve-lead ECG from a child with imipramine toxicity and ventricular tachycardia.

lidocaine (1 mg/kg), or with amiodarone (5 mg/kg load). Chronic suppression of ventricular arrhythmias with antiarrhythmic drugs has many side effects (including proarrhythmia and death), and it must be initiated in the hospital under the direction of a pediatric cardiologist. If the etiology of the tachycardia is a primary electrical abnormality, then catheter ablation procedures can be offered in select patients as a potentially curative treatment option. Ablation for ventricular tachycardia in the pediatric population is much less commonly performed compared to ablation for SVT.

Batra A, Silka MJ: Ventricular arrhythmias. Prog Pediatr Cardiol 2000 May 1;11(1):39–45.

Hayashi M et al: Incidence and risk factors of arrhythmic events in catecholaminergic polymorphic ventricular tachycardia. Circulation 2009 May 12;119(18):2426–2434.

LONG QT SYNDROME

Long QT syndrome is a malignant disorder of cardiac conduction where cardiac repolarization is prolonged (QTc measurement on ECG) and this predisposes the patient to sudden episodes of syncope, seizures, or sudden death (5% per year if untreated). The mechanism is a pause-dependent initiation of torsades de pointes, a multifocal ventricular tachycardia. It can be congenital or acquired. Congenital long QT syndrome is inherited in an autosomal dominant (more common) or recessive pattern or it may occur spontaneously (less likely). The recessive inheritance pattern is associated with congenital deafness and the Jervell and Lange-Nielsen syndrome. Congenital long QT syndrome is caused by a defect in one of several genes that code for ion channels in cardiac myocytes. As many as 10 genes have been identified and these defects explain 75% of the patient population with symptoms and signs consistent with long QT. The diagnosis of long QT syndrome is suspected in a patient or a family with a history of sudden syncope, seizures, documented dysrrhythmia, or cardiac arrest. Evaluation includes an ECG which shows a long QTc measurement, 24-hour ambulatory ECG, and possibly an exercise test. There is a commercially available genetic test for the primary genes which cause long QT syndrome. This test is most helpful in determining who in a family has long QT syndrome. Unfortunately, this test cannot completely rule it out as there continues to be a 25% false negative rate.

The mainstay of treatment for long QT syndrome has been exercise restriction, treatment with β-blockade, and possibly the placement of an internal cardioverter/defibrillator. Within the next several years, more gene-specific therapies are anticipated to be developed.

Long QT syndrome can also be acquired, resulting from altered ventricular repolarization secondary to myocardial toxins, ischemia, or inflammation. This condition also predisposes a patient to ventricular arrhythmias. Numerous medications can also cause QT prolongation.

Collins KK, Van Hare GF: Advances in congenital long QT syndrome. Curr Opin Pediatr 2006 Oct;18(5):497–502.

Kapoor JR: Long-QT syndrome. N Engl J Med 2008 May 1;358(18):1967–1968; author reply 1968.

Vetter VL et al: Cardiovascular monitoring of children and adolescents with heart disease receiving medications for attention deficit/hyperactivity disorder [corrected]: A scientific statement from the American Heart Association Council on Cardiovascular Disease in the Young Congenital Cardiac Defects Committee and the Council on Cardiovascular Nursing. Circulation 2008 May 6;117(18):2407–2423.

SUDDEN DEATH

Everyone in a family, school, community, are affected when an otherwise healthy child dies suddenly and unexpectedly. There are several cardiac causes of sudden death. Long QT syndrome and HCM are two of the most common cause of sudden death in young athletes. Other causes include dilated or restrictive cardiomyopathies, arrhythmogenic RV dysplasia, congenital structural anomalies of the coronary arteries, and primary arrhythmias such as catecholamine sensitive ventricular tachycardia or Brugada syndrome. Many of these causes are genetic and thus family members of the patient may also be unknowingly affected. Arrhythmias in patients with postoperative congenital heart disease are important causes of morbidity and mortality and may present as sudden death events.

Because of the genetic nature of some of the causes of sudden death, it is necessary to conduct a detailed family history looking for seizures, syncope, or early sudden death. Family members should be examined with an arrhythmia screen consisting of a physical examination, ECG, and echocardiography to detect arrhythmias or cardiomyopathies.

Bar-Cohen Y, Silka MJ: Sudden cardiac death in pediatrics. Curr Opin Pediatr 2008 Oct;20(5):517–521.

DeMaso DR, Neto LB, Hirshberg J: Psychological and quality-of-life issues in the young patient with an implantable cardioverter-defibrillator. Heart Rhythm 2009 Jan;6(1):130–132.

Denjoy I et al: Arrhythmic sudden death in children. Arch Cardiovasc Dis 2008 Feb;101(2):121–125.

Wren C: Screening children with a family history of sudden cardiac death. Heart 2006 Jul;92(7):1001–1006.

DISORDERS OF ATRIOVENTRICULAR CONDUCTION

General Considerations

The atrioventricular node is the electrical connection between the atrium and the ventricles. Atrioventricular blocks involve a slowing or disruption of this connection and are described according to the degree of this slowing or disruption. The term 'heart block' has been utilized, although 'atrioventricular block' is more precise.

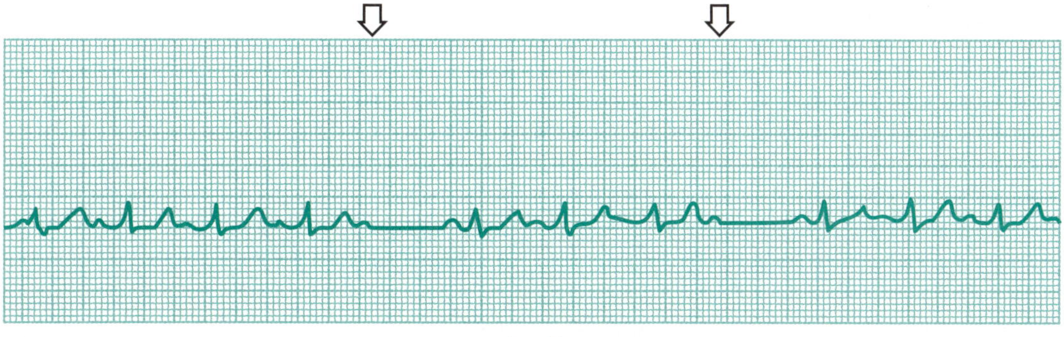

▲ **Figure 20–10.** Lead I rhythm strip with Mobitz type I (Wenckebach) second-degree heart block. There is progressive lengthening of the PR interval prior to the nonconducted P wave (*arrows*).

First-Degree Atrioventricular Block

First-degree atrioventricular block is an ECG diagnosis of prolongation of the PR interval. The block does not in itself cause problems. It may be associated with structural congenital heart defects, namely AV septal defects and ccTGA, and with diseases such as rheumatic carditis. The PR interval is prolonged in patients receiving digoxin therapy.

Second-Degree Atrioventricular Block

Mobitz type I (Wenckebach) atrioventricular block is recognized by progressive prolongation of the PR interval until there is no QRS following a P wave (Figure 20–10). Mobitz type I block occurs in normal hearts at rest and is usually benign. In Mobitz type II block, there is no progressive lengthening of the PR interval before the dropped beat (Figure 20–11). Mobitz type II block is frequently associated with organic heart disease, and a complete evaluation is necessary.

Complete Atrioventricular Block

In complete atrioventricular block, the atria and ventricles beat independently. Ventricular rates can range from 40 to 80 beats/min, whereas atrial rates are faster (Figure 20–12). The most common form of complete atrioventricular block is congenital complete atrioventricular block which occurs in a fetus or infant with an otherwise normal heart. There is a very high association with maternal systemic lupus erythematosus antibodies and therefore it is recommended to screen the mother of an affected infant even if the mother has no symptoms of collagen vascular disease. Congenital complete atrioventricular block is also associated with some forms of congenital heart disease (congenitally corrected transposition of the great vessels and AV septal defect). Acquired complete atrioventricular block may be secondary to acute myocarditis, drug toxicity, electrolyte imbalance, hypoxia, and cardiac surgery.

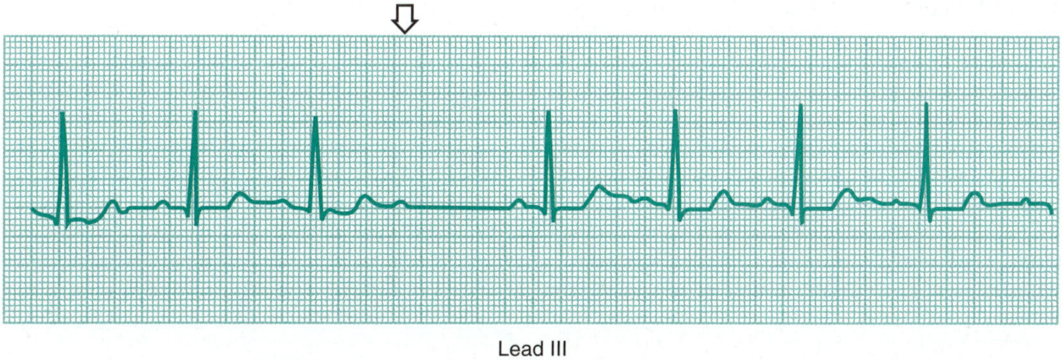

▲ **Figure 20–11.** Lead III rhythm strip with Mobitz type II second-degree heart block. There is a consistent PR interval with occasional loss of AV conduction (*arrow*).

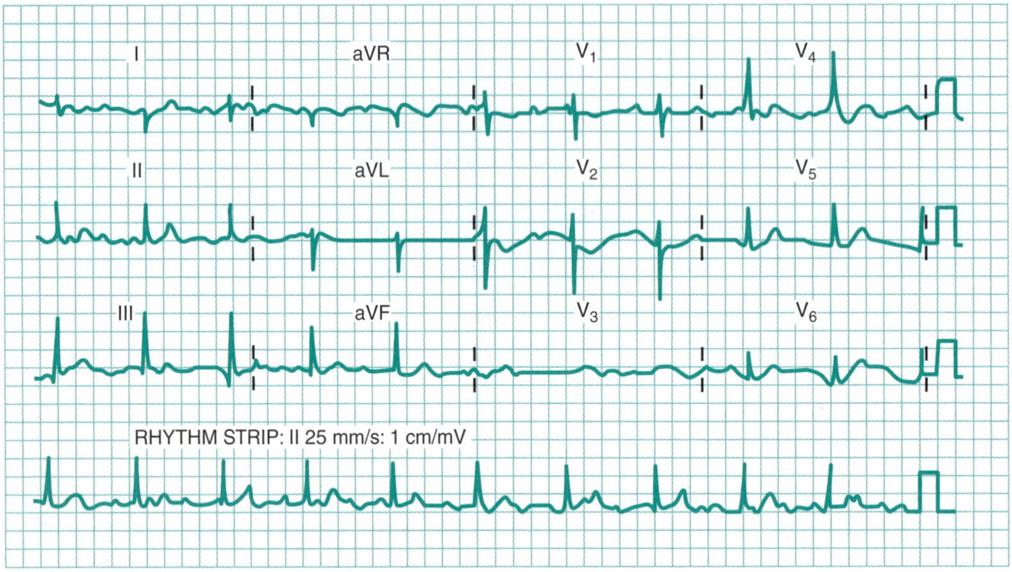

▲ **Figure 20–12.** Twelve-lead ECG and lead II rhythm strip of complete heart block. The atrial rate is 150 beats/min, and the ventricular rate is 60 beats/min.

Clinical Findings

The primary finding in infants and children with complete atrioventricular block is a significantly low heart rate for age. The diagnosis is often made prenatally when fetal bradycardia is documented. An ultrasound is then conducted as well as a fetal echocardiogram of the heart. With the fetal echocardiogram, atrial and ventricular contractions can be distinguished and the atrial rate is documented as being higher than the ventricular rate with no relationship to each other. If the heart rates are sufficiently low, then there will be low cardiac output, decreased cardiac function, and the development of hydrops fetalis. Postnatal adaptation largely depends on the heart rate; infants with heart rates less than 55 beats/min are at significantly greater risk for low cardiac output, HF, and death. Wide QRS complexes and a rapid atrial rate are also poor prognostic signs. Most patients have an innocent flow murmur from increased stroke volume. In symptomatic patients, the heart can be quite enlarged, and pulmonary edema may be present.

Complete atrioventricular block can also occur in older patients. Patients may be asymptomatic or may present with presyncope, syncope, or fatigue. Complete cardiac evaluation, including ECG, echocardiography, and Holter monitoring, is necessary to assess the patient for ventricular dysfunction and to relate any symptoms to concurrent arrhythmias.

Treatment

When diagnosis of complete atrioventricular block is made in a fetus, the treatment depends on gestational age, ventricular rate, and the presence or absence of hydrops. Some centers have advocated the administration of steroids, intravenous immune globulin (IVIG) and/or β-adrenergic stimulation treatment of the mother in some instances (fetuses that have associated heart failure). Emergent delivery is sometimes warranted. Postnatal treatment for neonates or older patients who present with significant symptoms and require immediate intervention includes temporary support by the infusions of isoproterenol, temporary transvenous pacing wires, or by temporary transcutaneous pacemakers if needed. The relationship of complete congenital atrioventricular block to auto-antibody production and cardiomyopathy is the basis for the consideration of immune modulation with steroids and IVIG in neonates in addition to their mothers. Long-term treatment involves the placement of a permanent pacemaker.

Jayaprasad N, Johnson F, Venugopal K: Congenital complete heart block and maternal connective tissue disease. Int J Cardiol 2006 Sep 20;112(2):153–158.

Villain E: Indications for pacing in patients with congenital heart disease. Pacing Clin Electrophysiol 2008 Feb;31(Suppl 1):S17–S20.

Trucco SM et al: Use of intravenous gamma globulin and corticosteroids in the treatment of maternal autoantibody-mediated cardiomyopathy. J Am Coll Cardiol. 2011 Feb8:57(6):715–723 [PMID: 21292131].

SYNCOPE (FAINTING)

Syncope is a sudden transient loss of consciousness that resolves spontaneously. The common form of syncope (simple fainting) occurs in 15% of children and is a disorder of control of heart rate and blood pressure by the autonomic nervous system that causes hypotension or bradycardia. It is often associated with rapid rising and postural hypotension, prolonged standing, or hypovolemia. Patients exhibit vagal symptoms such as pallor, nausea, or diaphoresis. Syncope, also known as autonomic dysfunction, can be evaluated with head-up tilt table testing. The patient is placed supine on a tilt table, and then—under constant heart rate and blood pressure monitoring—is tilted to the upright position. If symptoms develop, they can be classified as vasodepressor (hypotension), cardioinhibitory (bradycardia), or mixed.

Syncope is usually self-limited (can recur over approximately 6 months to 2 years) and can be controlled with dietary salt and volume loading to prevent hypovolemia. In refractory cases, medications to manipulate the autonomic nervous system have been useful. Fludrocortisone (0.1 mg/kg/d) is a mineralocorticoid that causes renal salt resorption and thus increases intravascular volume. Although β-blockers have been used for treatment of syncope, there is a paucity of data regarding their effectiveness. Vagolytic agents (disopyramide, 2.5 mg/kg four times daily) help control hypervagotonia, and the selective serotonin reuptake inhibitors have also been effective in alleviating symptoms. Syncope that occurs during exercise or stress or is associated with a positive family history is a warning sign that a serious underlying dysrhythmia may be present, calling for further investigation.

Johnsrude CL: Current approach to pediatric syncope. Pediatr Cardiol 2000 Nov–Dec;21(6):522–531.

21 Gastrointestinal Tract

Shikha S. Sundaram, MD, MSCI
Edward J. Hoffenberg, MD
Robert E. Kramer, MD
Judith M. Sondheimer, MD
Glenn T. Furuta, MD

DISORDERS OF THE ESOPHAGUS

GASTROESOPHAGEAL REFLUX AND GERD

ESSENTIALS OF DIAGNOSIS & TYPICAL FEATURES

- Recurrent postprandial spitting and vomiting in healthy infants that resolves spontaneously is uncomplicated gastroesophageal reflux.
- Heartburn and regurgitation in older children characterizes gastroesophageal reflux disease (GERD).
- Chronic complications of GERD include esophagitis, stricture, anemia, and Barrett esophagus.
- Diagnosis is clinical in infancy with upper gastrointestinal (GI) radiograph to rule out other anatomical GI diseases.

Clinical Findings

A. Infants with Gastroesophageal Reflux

Gastroesophageal (GE) reflux is common in young infants and a physiological event. Frequent postprandial regurgitation, ranging from effortless to forceful, is the most common infant symptom. Infant GE is usually benign and is common in neurologically impaired infants.

Reflux of gastric contents into the esophagus occurs during spontaneous relaxations of the lower esophageal sphincter that are unaccompanied by swallowing. Low pressures in the lower esophageal sphincter or developmental immaturity of the sphincter are not causes of GE reflux in infants. Normal factors promoting reflux in infants are their small stomach capacity, frequent large-volume feedings, short esophageal length, supine positioning, and slow swallowing response to the flow of refluxed material up the esophagus. Infants' individual responses to the stimulus of reflux, particularly the maturity of their self-settling skills, are important factors determining the severity of reflux-related symptoms.

An important differential point in evaluating infants with GE reflux is whether the vomited material contains bile. Bile-stained emesis in an infant requires immediate evaluation as it may be a symptom of intestinal obstruction (malrotation with volvulus, intussusception). When, in rare cases, it causes failure to thrive, food refusal, colic, rumination, and neck contortions (Sandifer syndrome), it is termed GERD. Apneic spells in young infants, especially occurring with position change after feeding, may be caused by GERD.

B. Older Children with Reflux

GE reflux disease (GERD) is diagnosed when reflux causes persistent symptoms with or without inflammation of the esophagus. Older children with GERD complain of adult-type symptoms of regurgitation into the mouth, heartburn, and dysphagia. Esophagitis can occur as a complication of GERD and requires endoscopy with biopsy for diagnostic confirmation. Children with asthma, cystic fibrosis, developmental handicaps, hiatal hernia, and repaired tracheoesophageal fistula are at increased risk of GERD and esophagitis.

C. Diagnostic Studies

In thriving infants, GE reflux is a clinical diagnosis. An upper GI series rules out anatomic causes of vomiting but is not a test for GERD.

In older children with heartburn, a trial of acid-suppressing medication may be both diagnostic and therapeutic. Persistent symptoms should be investigated by upper GI series and endoscopy to rule out other organic causes. pH or impedance esophageal monitoring studies may be helpful to recognize associations between episodic or unusual symptoms and reflux events. pH studies quantify the number and duration of acid reflux events. Esophageal intraluminal impedance monitoring is a pH-independent method of detecting fluid movements in the esophagus. These studies have shown that episodes of nonacid reflux occur as frequently as acid reflux episodes and that treatment with acid-suppressing medications changes the proportions of acid versus nonacid events, not the total number of events. Esophagoscopy with biopsy is not diagnostic of GERD, but esophagitis can be identified.

Treatment & Prognosis

Reflux resolves spontaneously in 85% of affected infants by 12 months of age, coincident with assumption of erect posture and initiation of solid feedings. Until then, regurgitation volume may be reduced by offering small feedings at frequent intervals and by thickening feedings with rice cereal (2–3 tsp/oz of formula). Prethickened "antireflux" formulas are available. Histamine-2 (H2)–receptor antagonists (ranitidine, 5 mg/kg/d in two doses) or proton pump inhibitors (omeprazole, lansoprazole, pantopraole, 0.5–1.0 mg/kg/d in one dose) do not reduce the frequency of reflux but may reduce pain. Prokinetic agents such as metoclopramide hasten gastric emptying and improve esophageal motor function, but studies have not shown efficacy in controlling symptoms. A two week trial of protein hydrolysate formula (hypoallergenic) sometimes controls emesis and pain behavior in infants with protein sensitivity. Special formulas and acid suppression agents are costly and should be discontinued if there is no improvement in 2 weeks.

Spontaneous resolution is less likely in older children with GERD. Episodic heartburn pain may be controlled with intermittent use of acid blockers. Patients with more severe heartburn or esophagitis require chronic acid suppression. Untreated GERD esophagitis may cause feeding dysfunction, esophageal stricture, and anemia. Barrett esophagus, a precancerous condition, is rare in childhood but can occur in patients with very long-standing esophagitis.

Antireflux surgery (fundoplication) is indicated when GERD is unresponsive to medications thus leading to severe symptoms that include: (1) persistent vomiting with failure to thrive, (2) esophagitis or esophageal stricture, (see Figure 21–1), (3) life-threatening apneic spells, or (4) chronic pulmonary disease unresponsive. Fundoplication also may be considered early in patients whose response to medication is likely to be poor—those with large hiatal hernia, neurologic handicap, previous tracheoesophageal (TE) fistula surgery, or severe esophagitis. Prior to performing a fundoplication, all other causes of esophagitis should be ruled out, ie, eosinophilic esophagitis.

Rudolph CD et al: Guidelines for evaluation and treatment of gastroesophageal reflux in infants and children: Recommendations of the North American Society for Pediatric Gastroenterology and Nutrition. J Pediatr Gastroenterol Nutr 2001;23(Suppl):1 [PMID: 11525610].

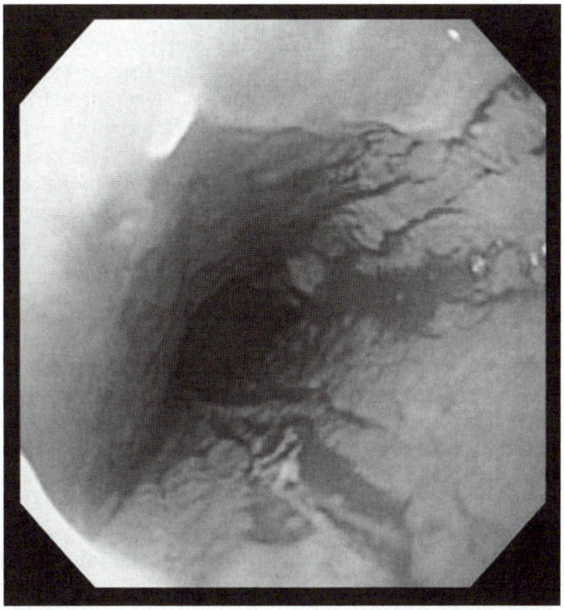

▲ **Figure 21–1.** Esophagitis associated with gastroesophageal reflux disease. Mucosa is erythematous with loss of vascular pattern.

Sherman PM et al: A global, evidence-based consensus on the definition of gastroesophageal reflux disease in the pediatric population. Am J Gastroenterol 2009 May;104(5):1278–1295 [PMID: 19352345].

EOSINOPHILIC ESOPHAGITIS-(EoE)

ESSENTIALS OF DIAGNOSIS & TYPICAL FEATURES

- Feeding dysfunction, dysphagia, esophageal food impaction, and heartburn.
- Must rule out other causes for esophageal eosinophilia before assigning diagnosis of EoE.
- Esophagoscopy may reveal white eosinophilic exudates, ringlike esophageal folds, and esophageal stricture. Esophageal mucosal biopsy shows dense eosinophilic infiltrate of the epithelium.

Clinical Findings

A. Symptoms and Signs

This recently recognized entity occurs in all ages and most frequently affects boys. Common initial presentations in young children include feeding dysfunction and vague nonspecific symptoms of GERD such as abdominal pain, vomiting, and regurgitation. If a history of careful and lengthy chewing, long mealtimes, washing food down with liquid, or avoiding highly textured foods is encountered, one may suspect EoE. In adolescents, symptoms of solid food dysphagia, heartburn, and acute and recurrent food impactions predominate. If a child's symptoms are unresponsive to medical and/or surgical management of GERD, EoE should be strongly considered as a diagnostic possibility. A family or personal history of atopy, asthma, and dysphagia is not uncommon.

B. Laboratory Findings

The esophageal mucosa usually appears abnormal with features of thickening, longitudinal mucosal fissures, and circumferential mucosal rings. The esophagus is often sprinkled with pinpoint white exudates that superficially resemble Candida. On microscopic examination, the white spots are composed of eosinophils (see Figure 21–2). Basal cell layers of the esophageal mucosa are hypertrophied and infiltrated by eosinophils (usually more than 15 per 40 × light microscopic field). A lengthy stricture may be seen which can split merely with the passage of an endoscope. Serum IgE may be elevated but this is not a diagnostic finding. Specific allergens can often be identified by skin testing and patient can sometimes identify foods that precipitate pain and dysphagia.

Differential Diagnosis

The most common differential conditions are peptic esophagitis and Candidal esophagitis. EoE may be part of a generalized eosinophilic gastroenteropathy, a very rare, steroid-responsive entity. Patients with eosinophilic gastroenteropathy can also present with gastric outlet obstruction or intestinal caused by large local infiltrates of eosinophils in the antrum, duodenum, and cecum.

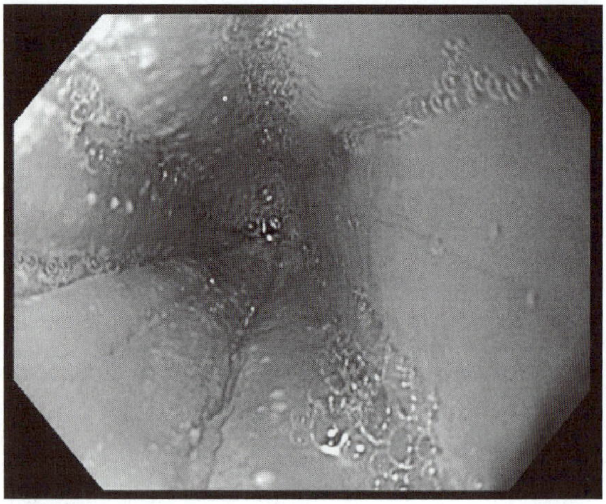

▲ **Figure 21–2.** Esophagitis associated with eosinophilic esophagitis. Mucosa contains linear folds, white exudate, and has loss of vascular pattern.

Diagnosis

The diagnosis of EoE is based on clinical and histopathological features. Symptoms referable to esophageal dysfunction as listed before must be seen in association with esophageal eosinophilia and normal gastric and duodenal mucosa. Other causes for esophageal eosinophilia, in particular, GERD, must be ruled out.

Treatment

Nutritional exclusion of offending allergens (elemental diet, removal of allergenic foods) is effective treatment. Such diets are useful in young children, but adherence in older children can be difficult. Topical corticosteroids also offer an effective treatment choice. Steroids are puffed in the mouth and swallowed from a metered dose pulmonary inhaler. Two puffs of fluticasone from an inhaler twice daily using an age-appropriate metered dose is a common recommendation. Patients should not rinse their mouth or eat for 30 minutes to maximize the effectiveness. Systemic corticosteroids benefit most patients with more acute or severe symptoms. Esophageal dilation may be required to treat strictures. The association of EoE and esophageal malignancy has not been identified. Parent and family support is available at American Partnership for Eosinophilic Disorders APFED.org.

Liacouras CA et al: Eosinophilic esophagitis: Updated consensus recommendations for children and adults. J Allergy Clin Immunol 2011;128:3–20.

ACHALASIA OF THE ESOPHAGUS

ESSENTIALS OF DIAGNOSIS & TYPICAL FEATURES

- Gradual onset of distal esophageal obstruction.
- Dysphagia, esophageal food impaction, chronic pulmonary aspiration.
- Failure of lower esophageal relaxation during swallowing with abnormalities of esophageal peristalsis.
- High or low resting pressure of the lower esophageal sphincter.

Clinical Findings

A. Symptoms and Signs

Achalasia most commonly occurs in children who are greater than 5 years of age but cases during infancy have been reported. The most common presenting symptoms are dysphagia, postprandial vomiting, retrosternal pain, early satiety, weight loss, and solid food impaction. Patients may eat slowly and often require large amounts of fluid when ingesting solid food. Dysphagia is relieved by repeated forceful swallowing or vomiting. Familial cases occur in Allgrove syndrome (alacrima, adrenal insufficiency, and achalasia, associated with a defect in the AAAS gene on 12q13, encoding the ALADIN protein) and familial dysautonomia. A recent study of achalasia patients revealed electron micrographic evidence of mast cells in close proximity to nerve fibers, suggesting a role in the pathogenesis of achalasia. Chronic cough, wheezing, recurrent aspiration pneumonitis, anemia, and poor weight gain are common.

B. Imaging and Manometry

Barium esophagram shows a dilated esophagus with a tapered "beak" at the gastroesophageal junction. Esophageal dilation may not be present in infants because of the short duration of distal obstruction. Fluoroscopy shows irregular tertiary contractions of the esophageal wall, indicative of disordered esophageal peristalsis. Esophageal manometry may show high resting pressure of the lower esophageal sphincter, failure of sphincter relaxation after swallowing, and abnormal esophageal peristalsis. Adult studies, using high resolution manometry, suggest varying subtypes of achalasia, which may predict likelihood of response to different therapies.

C. Differential Diagnosis

Congenital or peptic esophageal stricture, esophageal webs, and esophageal masses may mimic achalasia. Eosinophilic esophagitis commonly presents with symptoms of dysphagia and food impaction, similar to achalasia. Cricopharyngeal achalasia or spasm is a rare cause of dysphagia in children, but shares some clinical features of primary achalasia involving the lower esophageal sphincter. Intestinal pseudo-obstruction, multiple endocrine neoplasia type 2b, systemic amyloidosis, and postvagotomy syndrome cause esophageal dysmotility and symptoms similar to achalasia. Teenage girls may be suspected of having an eating disorder. In Chagas disease, caused by the parasite *Trypanosoma cruzi*, nNOS and ganglion cells are diminished or absent in the muscular layers of the lower esophageal sphincter causing an acquired achalasia.

Treatment & Prognosis

Endoscopic injection of botulinum toxin paralyzes the lower esophageal sphincter and temporarily relieves obstruction, but has relapse rates of greater than 50%. Pneumatic dilation of the lower esophageal sphincter produces temporary relief of obstruction that may last weeks to years. Due to concerns that dilation may increase inflammation between the esophageal mucosal and muscular layers, some have advocated surgical myotomy as the best initial treatment. While long-lasting functional relief is achieved by surgically dividing the lower esophageal sphincter (Heller myotomy), recurrence risk of obstructive symptoms following myotomy in children has been reported to be as high as 27%. Postoperative gastroesophageal reflux disease is common leading some to perform a fundoplication at the same time as myotomy. In a large retrospective pediatric study, general response rates of pneumatic dilation compared to Heller myotomy were not significantly different, though recent studies suggest that children over six may have better outcomes with pneumatic dilation. Self-expanding metal stents have been used with success in adults with achalasia, but have not been studied in children.

Because of the shorter duration of esophageal obstruction in children, there is less secondary dilation of the esophagus. Thus, the prognosis for return or retention of some normal esophageal motor function after surgery is better than in adults.

Pastor AC et al: A single center 26-year experience with treatment of esophageal achalasia: Is there an optimal method? J Pediatr Surg 2009; 44(7):1349 [PMID: 19573660].

CAUSTIC BURNS OF THE ESOPHAGUS

ESSENTIALS OF DIAGNOSIS & TYPICAL FEATURES

- Reported history of ingestion, with or without evidence of oropharyngeal injury.
- Odynophagia, drooling, and food refusal typical of esophageal injury.
- Endoscopic evaluation of severity and extent of injury at 24–48 hours postingestion.
- Significant risk for development of esophageal strictures, especially in second and third degree lesions.

Clinical Findings

A. Symptoms and Signs

Ingestion of caustic solids or liquids ($pH < 2$ or $pH > 12$) produces esophageal lesions ranging from superficial inflammation to deep necrosis with ulceration, perforation, mediastinitis, or peritonitis. Acidic substances typically lead to limited injury because of the small volume ingested due to the sour taste. In addition, acid ingestions often lead to superficial coagulative necrosis with eschar formation. Conversely, the more benign taste of alkali ingestions may allow for larger volume ingestions, subsequent liquifactive necrosis that can lead to deeper mucosal penetration.

Beyond the pH, factors which determine the severity of injury from a caustic ingestion include the amount ingested, the physical state of the agent, and the duration of mucosal exposure time. For these reasons, powdered or gel formulations of dishwashing detergent are especially dangerous, due to their innocuous taste, high pH, and tendency to stick to the mucosa. Symptoms of hoarseness, stridor, and dyspnea suggest associated airway injury, while odynophagia, drooling, and food refusal are typical with more severe esophageal injury. The lips, mouth, and airway should be examined in suspected caustic ingestion, although up to 12% of children without oral lesions can have significant esophageal injury.

B. Imaging Studies

Esophagoscopy is often a routine part of the evaluation in caustic ingestions to determine the severity and extent of the esophageal injury. Timing of endoscopy is important, however, as endoscopy may not indicate the true severity of injury if it is performed too early (less than 24–48 hours) and may increase the risk of perforation if it is performed too late (> 72 hours) due to formation of granulation tissue. Grading of esophageal lesions into first degree (superficial injury, erythema only), second degree (transmucosal with erythema, ulceration, and sloughing), and third degree (transmural with circumferential sloughing and deep mucosal ulceration) can help predict prognosis. Circumferential lesions should be particularly noted, since they carry the highest risk of stricture formation. Endoscopic esophageal dilation may eventually be necessary but should not be performed in the acute phase of injury. Elevation of white blood cell count was found in a recent pediatric study to be a sensitive, but not specific, indicator of high grade injury. Plain radiographs of the chest and abdomen may be performed if there is clinical suspicion of perforation. Contrast studies of the esophagus should be performed when endoscopic evaluation is not available, as they are unlikely to detect grade 1 and grade 2 lesions. Some centers have advocated conservative management with upper GI series within 3 weeks of injury, reserving endoscopic evaluation for those with evidence of stricture.

Treatment & Prognosis

Clinical observation is always prudent, as it is often difficult to predict the severity of esophageal injury at presentation. Vomiting should not be induced and administration of buffering agents should be avoided to prevent an exothermic reaction in the stomach. Intravenous corticosteroids (eg, methylprednisolone, 1–2 mg/kg/d) are given immediately to reduce oral swelling and laryngeal edema. Many centers advocate continued corticosteroids for the first week to decrease the risk of stricture formation; however, meta-analysis has not been able to show a clinical benefit from this practice. Intravenous fluids are necessary if dysphagia prevents oral intake. Treatment may be stopped if there are only first-degree burns at endoscopy. Broad spectrum antibiotic coverage with third generation cephalosporins has been postulated to decrease stricture formation by preventing bacterial colonization into necrotic tissue. When radiographs show erosion into the mediastinum or peritoneum, antibiotics are mandatory. Use of acid-blockade to decrease additional injury from acid reflux is often employed.

Esophageal strictures develop in areas of anatomic narrowing (thoracic inlet, GE junction, or point of compression where the left bronchus crosses the esophagus), where contact with the caustic agent is more prolonged. Strictures may develop quickly or gradually over several months. Strictures occur only with full-thickness esophageal necrosis and prevalence of stricture formation varies from 10% to 50%. Shortening of the esophagus is a late complication that may cause hiatal hernia. Repeated esophageal dilations may be necessary as a stricture develops and esophageal stenting may be beneficial during early management. Newer, fully covered, self-expanding, removable esophageal stents, now available in pediatric sizes, may offer additional options for recurrent caustic strictures. In a recent multicenter analysis, endoscopic administration of topical mitomycin-C was effective in treatment of refractory caustic strictures of the esophagus. Surgical replacement of the esophagus by colonic interposition or gastric tube may be needed for long strictures resistant to dilation.

Riffat F, Cheng A: Pediatric caustic ingestion: 50 consecutive cases and a review of the literature. Dis Esophagus 2009;22:89–94 [PMID: 18847446].

Bicakci U, Tander B, Deveci G, Rizalar R, Ariturk E, Bernay F: Minimally invasive management of children with caustic ingestion: Less pain for patients. Pediatr Surg Int 2010;26(3):251–255 [PMID: 19936762].

Betalli P et al: Update on management of caustic and foreign body ingestion in children. Diagn Ther Endosc 2009 [Epub 2009 Nov 8] [PMID: 19902009].

FOREIGN BODIES IN THE ALIMENTARY TRACT

In the pediatric population, ingestion of nonfood items is a common occurrence and accounts for 80% of documented foreign body ingestions. Fortunately 80%–90% of foreign bodies pass spontaneously with only 10%–20% requiring endoscopic or surgical management. At presentation, the most common symptoms are dysphagia, odynophagia, drooling, regurgitation, and abdominal pain. A high index of suspicion should be maintained for toddlers presenting with these symptoms, even without a witnessed ingestion. If the ingestion is witnessed, the timing of the event is important to note as it will have implications for the timing of any necessary endoscopic procedures for removal. Contrast studies should be avoided, as they may interfere with endoscopy and some hypertonic contrast materials may cause pulmonary edema if aspirated in the case of an obstructed esophagus.

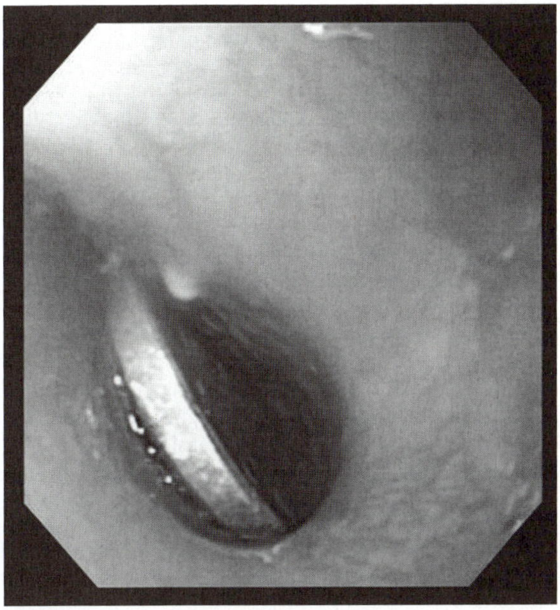

▲ **Figure 21–3.** Foreign body in esophagus. Coin is lodged in the esophageal lumen.

The most common foreign bodies ingested by children are coins (see Figure 21–3). Ingested foreign bodies tend to lodge in narrowed areas—valleculae, thoracic inlet, GE junction, pylorus, ligament of Treitz, and ileocecal junction, congenital or acquired intestinal stenoses. Esophageal foreign bodies should be removed within 24 hours to avoid ulceration, which can lead to serious complications such as erosion into a vessel or stricture formation. Disk-shaped batteries lodged in the esophagus are especially concerning and should be removed immediately. They may cause an electrical thermal injury in as little as two hours and have resulted in death from subsequent aorto-enteric fistula formation, even weeks after removal as described in a recent report. Disk-shaped batteries in the stomach will generally pass uneventfully, but should be monitored closely to ensure prompt passage. Rates of significant injury and death have increased in recent years with the transition to higher voltage lithium batteries. Impaction of a foreign body or food bolus in the esophagus should also raise suspicion for a possible underlying esophageal stricture, from eosinophilic esophagitis, peptic disease, or congenital anomaly. The use of glucagon for esophageal food impaction is controversial, but use of meat tenderizer should definitely be avoided due to mortality risk from perforation.

Smooth foreign bodies in the stomach, such as buttons or coins, may be monitored without attempting removal for up to several months if the child is free of symptoms. Straight pins, screws, and nails, with a blunt end that is heavier than the sharp end, generally pass without incident. Wooden toothpicks should be removed as they carry mouth flora which may cause abscess formation if the toothpick becomes imbedded in the bowel wall. They have also been known to migrate through the intestine into the pericardium, liver, and inferior vena cava. Large, open safety pins should be removed from the stomach because they may not pass the pyloric sphincter and may cause perforation. Objects longer than 5 cm, however, may be unable to pass the ligament of Treitz and should be removed. Magnets require consideration for removal only if there has been more than one ingested, due to the risk of fistula or erosion of mucosal tissue trapped between two adherent magnets. The use of balanced electrolyte lavage solutions containing polyethylene glycol may help the passage of small, smooth foreign bodies lodged in the stomach or intestine. Lavage is especially useful in hastening the passage of disk-shaped batteries or ingested tablets that may be toxic. Failure of a smooth foreign body to exit the stomach after several days suggests the possibility of gastric outlet obstruction.

Most foreign bodies can be removed from the esophagus or stomach by a skilled endoscopist. In some circumstances an alternative technique can be used. An experienced radiologist using fluoroscopy can utilize a Foley catheter with balloon inflated below the foreign body to extract smooth, round esophageal foreign bodies in the upper esophagus while the patient is placed in the Trendelenberg position. Contraindications include precarious airway, history that foreign body has been present for several days and previous esophageal surgery.

Adu-Frimpong J, Sorrell J: Magnetic toys: The emerging problem in pediatric ingestions. Pediatr Emerg Care 2009;25:42–43 [PMID: 19148014].

Brumbaugh DE, Colson SB, Sandoval JA, Karrer FM, Bealer JF, Litovitz T, Kramer RE: Management of button battery-induced hemorrhage in children. J Pediatr Gastroenterol Nutr 2011;52(5):585–589 [PMID: 21502830].

Litovitz T, Whitaker N, Clark L, White NC, Marsolec M: Emerging battery-ingestion hazard: Clinical implications. Pediatrics 2010;125(6):1168–1177.

Wong KK, Fang CX, Tam PK: Selective upper endoscopy for foreign body ingestion in children: An evaluation of management protocol after 282 cases. J Pediatr Surg 2006;41:2016–2018 [PMID: 17161195].

DISORDERS OF THE STOMACH AND DUODENUM

HIATAL HERNIA

In paraesophageal hiatal hernias, the esophagus and gastroesophageal (GE) junction are in their normal anatomic position, but the gastric cardia is herniated through the diaphragmatic hiatus alongside the GE junction. In sliding hiatal hernias, the GE junction and a portion of the proximal stomach are displaced above the diaphragmatic hiatus. Sliding hiatal hernias are common. Congenital paraesophageal hernias are rare in childhood; patients may present with recurrent pulmonary infections, vomiting, anemia, failure to thrive or dysphagia. The most common cause of paraesophageal hernia is previous fundoplication surgery. Radiographic studies typically reveal a cystic mass in the posterior mediastinum or a dilated esophagus. The diagnosis is typically made with an upper GI series or a CT scan of the chest and abdomen. Controversy exists about using biosynthetic mesh in the repair of these iatrogenic hernias, as its use definitely decreases the risk of recurrent hernia but has also been associated with esophageal erosion in children. GE reflux may accompany sliding hiatal hernias, although most produce no symptoms. Fundoplication is indicated if paraesophageal or sliding hiatal hernias produce persistent symptoms, though the presence of a preoperative hiatal hernia has been found to triple the risk of recurrent GERD following fundoplication.

Karpelowsky JS, Wieselthaler N, Rode H: Primary paraesophageal hernia in children. J Pediatr Surg 2006;41:1588–1593 [PMID: 16952596].

Ngerncham M, Barnhart DC, Haricharan RN, Roseman JM, Georgeson KE, Harmon CM: Risk factors for recurrent gastroesophageal reflux disease after fundoplication in pediatric patients: A case-control study. J Pediatr Surg 2007;42(9):1778–1785 [PMID: 17848234].

St Pete SD, Ostlie DJ, Holcomb GW III: The use of biosynthetic mesh to enhance hiatal repair at the time of redo Nissen fundoplication. J Pediatr Surg 2007;42:1298–1301 [PMID: 17618902].

PYLORIC STENOSIS

ESSENTIALS OF DIAGNOSIS & TYPICAL FEATURES

- Postnatal muscular hypertrophy of the pylorus.
- Progressive gastric outlet obstruction, nonbilious vomiting, dehydration, and alkalosis in infants younger than 12 weeks.
- Upper GI contrast radiographs or abdominal ultrasound are diagnostic.

The cause of postnatal pyloric muscular hypertrophy with gastric outlet obstruction is unknown. The incidence is 1–8 per 1000 births, with a 4:1 male predominance. A positive family history is present in 13% of patients. Recent studies suggest that erythromycin in the neonatal period is associated with a higher incidence of pyloric stenosis in infants younger than 30 days, though the mean age at diagnosis in a large population-based study was 43.1 days. Studies investigating the risk of pyloric stenosis with macrolide antibiotic exposure via breastmilk have shown conflicting results.

Clinical Findings

A. Symptoms and Signs

Projectile postprandial vomiting usually begins between 2 and 4 weeks of age but may start as late as 12 weeks. Vomiting starts at birth in about 10% of cases and onset of symptoms may be delayed in preterm infants. Vomitus is rarely bilious but may be blood-streaked. Infants are usually hungry and nurse avidly. Constipation, weight loss, fretfulness, dehydration, and finally apathy occur. The upper abdomen may be distended after feeding, and prominent gastric peristaltic waves from left to right may be seen. An oval mass, 5–15 mm in longest dimension can be felt on deep palpation in the right upper abdomen, especially after vomiting. This palpable "olive", however, was only present in 13.6% of patients studied.

B. Laboratory Findings

Hypochloremic alkalosis with potassium depletion are the classic metabolic findings, though low chloride may be seen in as few as 23% and alkalosis in 14.4%. Dehydration causes elevated hemoglobin and hematocrit. Mild unconjugated bilirubinemia occurs in 2%–5% of cases.

C. Imaging

A barium upper GI series reveals retention of contrast in the stomach and a long narrow pyloric channel with a double track of barium. The hypertrophied muscle mass produces typical semilunar filling defects in the antrum. Isolated pylorospasm is common in young infants, and by itself is insufficient to make a diagnosis of pyloric stenosis. Ultrasonography shows a hypoechoic muscle ring greater than 4-mm thick with a hyperdense center and a pyloric channel length greater than 15 mm. Infants presenting younger than 21 days may not fulfill these classic ultrasonographic criteria and may require clinical judgement to interpret "borderline" measures of pyloric muscle thickness.

Treatment & Prognosis

Ramstedt pyloromyotomy is the treatment of choice and consists of incision down to the mucosa along the pyloric length. The procedure can be performed laparoscopically, with similar efficacy and improved cosmetic results compared to open procedures. An alternative, double Y, form of pyloromyotomy has been investigated and early results suggest more rapid resolution of vomiting and increased weight gain in the first postoperative week compared to the traditional Ramstedt procedure. Treatment of dehydration and electrolyte imbalance is mandatory before surgical treatment, even if it takes 24–48 hours. Use of IV cimetidine and other acid-blocking agents has been shown in small studies to rapidly correct metabolic alkalosis, allowing more rapid progression to surgery and resolution of symptoms. Patients often vomit postoperatively as a consequence of gastritis, esophagitis, or associated GE reflux. The outlook after surgery is excellent, though patients may show as much as a four times greater risk for development of chronic abdominal pain of childhood. The postoperative barium radiograph remains abnormal for many months despite relief of symptoms.

Alalayet YF, Miserez M, Mansoor K, Khan AM: Double-Y pylo-romyotomy: A new technique for the surgical management of infantile hypertrophic pyloric stenosis. Eur J Pediatr Surg 2009;19:17–20 [PMID: 19221947].

Goldstein LH et al: The safety of macrolides during lactation. Breastfeed Med 2009 [PMID: 19366316].

Leong MM et al: Epidemiological features of infantile hypertrophic pyloric stenosis in Taiwanese children: A Nation-Wide Analysis of Cases during 1997–2007. PLoS One 2011;6(5):e19404 [PMID: 21559291].

GASTRIC & DUODENAL ULCER

ESSENTIALS OF DIAGNOSIS & TYPICAL FEATURES

- Localized erosions of gastric or duodenal mucosa.
- Pain and bleeding are the most common symptoms.
- Underlying severe illness, *Helicobacter pylori* infection, and nonsteroidal anti-inflammatory drugs (NSAIDs) are the most common causes.
- Diagnosis by endoscopy.

General Considerations

Gastric and duodenal ulcers occur at any age. Boys are affected more frequently than girls. In the United States, most childhood gastric and duodenal ulcers are associated with underlying illness, toxins, or drugs that cause breakdown in mucosal defenses.

Worldwide, the most common cause of gastric and duodenal ulcer is infection of the gastric mucosa with *Helicobacter pylori*. Infection causes nodular gastritis and duodenal or gastric ulcer. Long-standing infection is associated with gastric lymphoid tumors and adenocarcinoma. Between 10% and 20% of North American children have antibodies against *H pylori*. Antibody prevalence increases with age, poor sanitation, crowded living conditions, and family exposure. In some developing countries, over 90% of schoolchildren have serologic evidence of past or present infection. In contrast to ulcers secondary to *H pylori*, non-*H pylori* ulcers tend to occur as frequently in girls as boys, present at a younger age, and are more likely to recur. In a large study of over 1000 children undergoing endoscopy, 5.4% had ulcers, with 47% of these due to *H pylori*, 16.5% related to NSAID's and 35.8% unrelated to either *H pylori* or NASID's. Recent evidence suggests that the prevalence of non-*H pylori* peptic ulcers is increasing.

Illnesses predisposing to secondary ulcers include central nervous system disease, burns, sepsis, multiorgan system failure, chronic lung disease, Crohn disease, cirrhosis, and rheumatoid arthritis. The most common drugs causing secondary ulcers are aspirin, alcohol, and NSAIDs. NSAID use causes ulcers throughout the upper GI tract but most often in the stomach and duodenum. Severe ulcerative lesions in full-term neonates have been found to be associated with maternal antacid use in the last month of pregnancy.

Clinical Findings

A. Symptoms and Signs

In children younger than 6 years, vomiting and upper GI bleeding are the most common symptoms of gastric and duodenal ulcer. Older children are more likely to complain of abdominal pain. The first attack of acute *H pylori* gastritis may be accompanied by vomiting and hematemesis. Ulcers in the pyloric channel may cause gastric outlet obstruction. Chronic blood loss may cause iron-deficiency anemia. Deep penetration of the ulcer may erode into a mucosal arteriole and cause acute hemorrhage. Penetrating duodenal ulcers (especially common during cancer chemotherapy, immunosuppression, and in the intensive care setting) may perforate the duodenal wall resulting in peritonitis or abscess.

B. Diagnostic Studies

Upper GI endoscopy is the most accurate diagnostic examination. It also allows for identification of other causes of peptic symptoms such as esophagitis, eosinophilic enteropathy, and celiac disease. Upper GI barium radiographs may show an ulcer crater. Soft signs suggestive of peptic disease in adults (duodenal spasticity and thick irregular folds) are not reliable indicators in children. Assessment for *H pylori* may be performed either by urease activity on gastric biopsies, or by evaluation of breath after administration of radiolabeled urea by mouth. Both methods have shown sensitivity and specificity of greater than 95% in children as young as two. *H pylori* antigens can be measured in stool and may be an effective, noninvasive test for infection. Serum antibodies against *H pylori* have poor sensitivity and specificity and do not prove that there is active infection or that treatment is needed. If endoscopy is not available, the *H pylori* IgG is more reliable than the IgA or IgM in identifying active infection. Endoscopic appearances demonstrate a white exudative base with erythematous margins (see Figure 21–4). For severe or recurrent ulcerations not caused by *H pylori*, stress or medications, a serum gastrin level

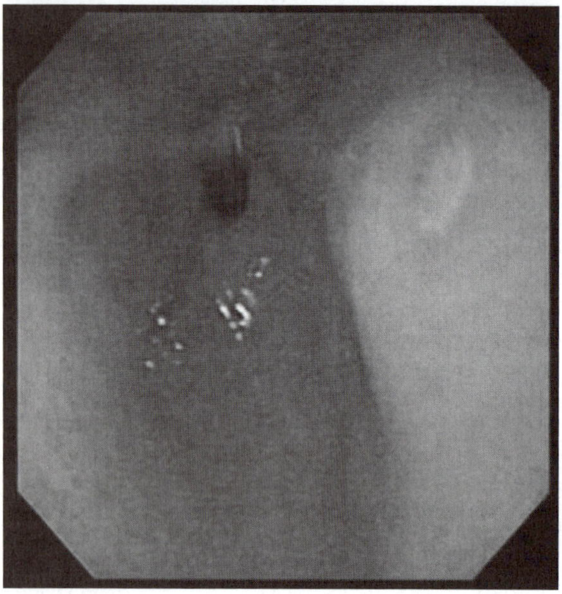

▲ **Figure 21–4.** Gastric ulcer. White exudate coats the ulcer bed of antral ulcer that is surrounded by an erythematous margin.

may be considered to evaluate for a gastrin-secreting tumor (Zollinger-Ellison syndrome), though mild to moderate elevation in gastrin levels can be seen with use of proton pump inhibitor drugs.

Treatment

Acid suppression or neutralization is the mainstay of ulcer therapy. Liquid antacids in the volumes needed to neutralize gastric acid are usually unacceptable to children. H2-receptor antagonists and proton pump inhibitors are more effective and usually produce endoscopic healing in 4–8 weeks.

Alternatively, 7–14 day courses of sucralfate may be helpful as a mucosal protective agent to speed healing and decrease symptoms. Bland "ulcer diets" do not speed healing, but foods causing pain should be avoided. Caffeine should be avoided because it increases gastric acid secretion. Aspirin, alcohol, NSAIDs, and other gastric irritants should be avoided as well.

Treatment of *H pylori* infection requires eradication of the organism. Spontaneous clearance of infection may occur. The optimal medical regimen is still undetermined. Combinations of amoxicillin, metronidazole, clarithromycin, and bismuth subsalicylate for 10–14 days, or amoxicillin for 14 days with omeprazole for 6 weeks are both effective. Clarithromycin for 7 days with a proton pump inhibitor for 6 weeks also is also effective. Resistance to antibiotics is common. An unresolved clinical question is whether recurrent courses of antibiotics should be used to eradicate resistant *H pylori* infection. Some epidemiologic data suggest that the incidence of GERD and Barrett esophagus is increasing in white males as a consequence of aggressive eradication of *H pylori*.

Endoscopic therapy of bleeding ulcers may be considered for severe or refractory lesions posing a risk for significant morbidity or mortality. Therapeutic options include injection therapy, application of monopolar or bipolar electrocoagulation, placement of clipping devices, or use of argon plasma coagulation.

Huang SC, Sheu BS, Lee SC, Yang HB, Yang YJ: Etiology and treatment of childhood peptic ulcer disease in Taiwan: A single center 9-year experience. J Formos Med Assoc 2010;109(1):75–81 [PMID: 20123589].

Tam YH, Lee KH, To KF et al: Helicobacter pylori-positive versus Helicobacter pylori-negative idiopathic peptic ulcers in children with their long-term outcomes. J Pediatr Gastroenterol Nutr 2009;48(3):299–305 [PMID: 1927478].

CONGENITAL DIAPHRAGMATIC HERNIA

Herniation of abdominal contents through the diaphragm usually occurs through a posteriolateral defect in the diaphragm (foramen of Bochdalek). In about 5% of cases, the diaphragmatic defect is retrosternal (foramen of Morgagni). Hernias result from failure of the diaphragmatic anlagen to fuse and divide the thoracic and abdominal cavities at 8–10 weeks' gestation. All degrees of protrusion of abdominal viscera through the diaphragmatic opening may occur. Eighty percent of posteriolateral defects involve the left diaphragm. In eventration of the diaphragm, a leaf of the diaphragm with hypoplastic muscular elements balloons into the chest and leads to similar but milder symptoms. With the advent of inhaled nitric oxide, high-frequency oscillatory ventilation and extracorporeal membrane oxygenation, recent one-year survival rates in neonates with CDH are as high as 82%. Fetal surgery with tracheal occlusion has been advocated for severely affected fetuses with low lung-to-head ratio. Otherwise, operative repair is usually performed in the newborn period, with increasing utilization of lapascopic and thoracoscopic minimally invasive approaches to decrease complications. A recent review, however, has shown these minimally invasive surgeries to have a higher risk of short-term recurrent hernia. Occasionally, diaphragmatic hernia is first identified in an older infant or child during incidental radiograph or routine physical examination. These children usually have a much more favorable prognosis than neonates. Congenital diaphragmatic hernia (CDH) survivors are often found to have a dilated esophagus and significant GE reflux, which may be related to findings of abnormal intrinsic innervation of the lower esophagus.

Mettauer NL, Pierce CM, Cassidy JV, Kiely EM, Petros AJ: One-year survival in congenital diaphragmatic hernia, 1995–2006. Arch Dis Child 2009;94:407 [PMID: 19383869].

Sinha CK et al: Congenital diaphragmatic hernia: Prognostic indices in the fetal endoluminal tracheal occlusion era. J Pediatr Surg 2009;44:312–316 [PMID: 1923152].

Tsao K, Lally PA, Lally KP: Congenital Diaphragmatic Hernia Study Group. Minimally invasive repair of congenital diaphragmatic hernia. J Pediatr Surg 2011;46(6):1158–1164 [PMID: 21683215].

CONGENITAL DUODENAL OBSTRUCTION

General Considerations

Obstruction is generally classified into intrinsic and extrinsic causes, although rare cases of simultaneous intrinsic and extrinsic anomalies have been reported. Extrinsic duodenal obstruction is usually due to congenital peritoneal bands associated with intestinal malrotation, annular pancreas, or duodenal duplication. In rare cases, a preduodenal portal vein has been associated with extrinsic obstruction as well. Intrinsic obstruction is caused by stenosis, mucosal diaphragm (so-called wind sock deformity), or duodenal atresia. In atresia, the duodenal lumen may be obliterated by a membrane or completely interrupted with a fibrous cord between the two segments. Atresia is more often distal to the ampulla of Vater than proximal. In about two-thirds of patients with congenital duodenal obstruction there are other associated anomalies.

Imaging Studies

Diagnosis of congenital duodenal obstructions is often made prenatally by ultrasound. Prenatal diagnosis predicts complete obstruction in 77% of cases and is associated with polyhydramnios, prematurity, and higher risk of maternal-fetal complications. Presence of a "double bubble" on ultrasound, in association with an echogenic band in the second portion of the duodenum, was found to be 100% sensitive and specific for an annular pancreas. Postnatal abdominal plain radiographs show gaseous distention of the stomach and proximal duodenum (the "double-bubble" radiologic sign). With protracted vomiting, there is less air in the stomach and less abdominal distention. Absence of distal intestinal gas suggests atresia or severe extrinsic obstruction, whereas a pattern of intestinal air scattered over the lower abdomen may indicate partial duodenal obstruction. Barium enema may be helpful in determining the presence of malrotation or atresia in the lower GI tract.

Clinical Findings

A. Duodenal Atresia

Maternal polyhydramnios is common and often leads to prenatal diagnosis by ultrasonography. Vomiting (usually bile-stained) and epigastric distention begin within a few hours of birth. Meconium may be passed normally. Duodenal atresia is often associated with other congenital anomalies (30%), including esophageal atresia, intestinal atresias, and cardiac and renal anomalies. Prematurity (25%–50%) and Down syndrome (20%–30%) are also associated.

B. Duodenal Stenosis

In this condition, duodenal obstruction is not complete. Onset of obvious obstructive symptoms may be delayed for weeks or years. Although the stenotic area is usually distal to the ampulla of Vater, the vomitus does not always contain bile. Duodenal stenosis or atresia is the most common GI tract malformation in children with Down syndrome, occurring in 3.9%.

C. Annular Pancreas

Annular pancreas is a rotational defect in which normal fusion of the dorsal and ventral pancreatic anlagen does not occur, and a ring of pancreatic tissue encircles the duodenum. The presenting symptom is duodenal obstruction. Down syndrome and congenital anomalies of the GI tract occur frequently. Polyhydramnios is common. Symptoms may develop late in childhood or even in adulthood if the obstruction is not complete in infancy. Treatment consists of duodenoduodenostomy or duodenojejunostomy without operative dissection or division of the pancreatic annulus.

Treatment & Prognosis

Generally speaking, duodenoduodenostomy is performed to bypass the area of stenosis or atresia. For duodenal stenoses, however, there have been isolated reports of successful endoscopic treatment with balloon dilation. Thorough surgical exploration is typically done to ensure that no lower GI tract anomalies are present. More recent reports document the safety and utility of a laparoscopic approach. The mortality rate is increased in infants with prematurity, Down syndrome, and associated congenital anomalies. Duodenal dilation and hypomotility from antenatal obstruction may cause duodenal dysmotility with obstructive symptoms even after surgical treatment. Placement of transanastomotic feeding tubes at the time of the initial repair has been found to result in more rapid progression to full enteral feeds and decreased need for parenteral nutrition. The overall prognosis for these patients is good, with the majority of their mortality risk due to associated anomalies other than duodenal obstruction.

Calisti A et al: Prenatal diagnosis of duodenal obstruction selects cases with a higher risk of maternal-foetal complications and demands in utero transfer to a tertiary centre. Fetal Diagn Ther 2008;24:478–482 [PMID: 19047796].

Freeman SB et al: Congenital gastrointestinal defects in Down syndrome: A report from the Atlanta and National Down Syndrome Projects. Clin Genet 2009;75:180–184 [PMID: 19021635].

Hall NJ, Drewett M, Wheeler RA, Griffiths DM, Kitteringham LJ, Burge DM: Trans-anastomotic tubes reduce the need for central venous access and parenteral nutrition in infants with congenital duodenal obstruction. Pediatr Surg Int 2011 Apr 8 [Epub ahead of print] [PMID: 21476073].

Mustafawi AR, Hassan ME: Congenital duodenal obstruction in children: A decade's experience. Eur J Pediatr Surg 2008;18:93–97 [PMID: 18437652].

DISORDERS OF THE SMALL INTESTINE

INTESTINAL ATRESIA & STENOSIS

Excluding anal anomalies, intestinal atresia, or stenosis accounts for one-third of all cases of neonatal intestinal obstruction (see Chapter 2). Antenatal ultrasound can identify intestinal atresia in utero; polyhydramnios occurs in most affected pregnancies. Sensitivity of antenatal ultrasound is greater in more proximal atresias. Other congenital anomalies may be present in up to 54% of cases and 52% are delivered preterm. In apparently isolated atresia cases, occult congenital cardiac anomalies have been reported in as many as 30%. In one large population-based study, the prevalence was 2.9 per 10,000 births, although there is some evidence that the prevalence may be increasing. The localization and relative incidence of atresias and stenoses are listed in Table 21–1. Although jejunal and ileal atresias are often grouped together, there is data to suggest that jejunal atresias are associated with increased morbidity and mortality compared to ileal atresia. These differences may be related to increased compliance of the jejunal wall, resulting in more proximal dilation and subsequent loss in peristaltic activity.

Bile-stained vomiting and abdominal distention begin in the first 48 hours of life. Multiple sites in the intestine may be affected and the overall length of the small intestine may be significantly shortened. Radiographic features include dilated loops of small bowel and absence of colonic gas. Barium enema reveals narrow-caliber microcolon because of lack of intestinal flow distal to the atresia. In over 10% of patients with intestinal atresia the mesentery is absent, and the superior mesenteric artery cannot be identified beyond the origin of the right colic and ileocolic arteries. The ileum coils around one of these two arteries, giving rise to the so-called Christmas tree deformity on contrast radiographs. The tenuous blood supply often compromises surgical anastomoses. The differential diagnosis of intestinal atresia includes Hirschsprung disease, paralytic ileus secondary to sepsis, midgut volvulus, and meconium ileus. Surgery is mandatory. Postoperative complications include short bowel syndrome in 15% and small bowel hypomotility secondary to antenatal obstruction. Overall mortality has been reported at 8%, with increased risk in low birth weight and premature infants.

Burjonrappa S, Crete E, Bouchard S: Comparative outcomes in intestinal atresia: A clinical outcome and pathophysiology analysis. Pediatr Surg Int 2011;27(4):437–442 [PMID: 20820789].

Olgun H, Karacan M, Caner I, Oral A, Ceviz N: Congenital cardiac malformations in neonates with apparently isolated gastrointestinal malformations. Pediatr Int 2009;51:260–262 [PMID: 19405929].

Stollman TH et al: Decreased mortality but increased morbidity in neonates with jejunoileal atresia: A study of 114 cases over a 34-year period. J Pediatr Surg 2009;44:217–221 [PMID: 19159746].

Walker K et al: A population-based study of the outcome after small bowel atresia/stenosis in New South Wales and the Australian Capital Territory, Australia, 1992–2003. J Pediatr Surg 2008;43:484–488 [PMID: 18358286].

INTESTINAL MALROTATION

General Considerations

The midgut extends from the duodenojejunal junction to the mid transverse colon. It is supplied by the superior mesenteric artery, which runs in the root of the mesentery. During gestation, the midgut elongates into the umbilical sac, returning to an intra-abdominal position during the 10th week of gestation. The root of the mesentery rotates in a counterclockwise direction during retraction causing the colon to cross the abdominal cavity ventrally. The cecum moves from the left to the right lower quadrant, and the duodenum crosses dorsally becoming partly retroperitoneal. When rotation is incomplete, the dorsal fixation of the mesentery is defective and shortened, so that the bowel from the ligament of Treitz to the mid transverse colon may rotate around its narrow mesenteric root and occlude the superior

Table 21–1. Localization and relative frequency of congenital gastrointestinal atresias and stenoses.

	Area Involved	Type of Lesion	Relative Frequency
Pylorus		Atresia; web or diaphragm	1%
Duodenum	80% are distal to the ampulla of Vater	Atresia, stenosis; web or diaphragm	45%
Jejunoileal	Proximal jejunum and distal ileum	Atresia (multiple in 6%–29%); stenosis	50%
Colon	Left colon and rectum	Atresia (usually associated with atresias of the small bowel)	5%–9%

mesenteric artery (volvulus). From autopsy studies it is estimated that up to 1% of the general population may have intestinal malrotation, which is diagnosed in the first year of life in 70%–90% of patients.

Clinical Findings

A. Symptoms and Signs

Malrotation with volvulus accounts for 10% of neonatal intestinal obstructions. Most infants present in the first 3 weeks of life with bile-stained vomiting or with overt small bowel obstruction. Intrauterine volvulus may cause intestinal obstruction or perforation at birth. The neonate may present with ascites or meconium peritonitis. Later presenting signs include intermittent intestinal obstruction, malabsorption, protein-losing enteropathy, or diarrhea. Associated congenital anomalies, especially cardiac, occur in over 25% of symptomatic patients. Many of these may be found in a subgroup of malrotation patients with heterotaxy syndromes, with associated asplenia or polysplenia. Older children and adults with undiagnosed malrotation typically present with chronic GI symptoms of nausea, vomiting, diarrhea, abdominal pain, dyspepsia, bloating, and early satiety.

B. Imaging

An upper GI series is considered the gold standard for diagnosis, with a reported sensitivity of 96%, and classically shows the duodenojejunal junction and the jejunum on the right side of the spine. The diagnosis of malrotation can be further confirmed by barium enema, which may demonstrate a mobile cecum located in the midline, right upper quadrant, or left abdomen. Plain films of the abdomen in the newborn period may show a "double bubble" sign, resulting in a misdiagnosis of duodenal atresia. CT scan and ultrasound of the abdomen may be used to make the diagnosis as well, and are characterized by the "whirlpool sign" denoting midgut volvulus. Reversal of the normal position of the SMA and SMV may be seen in malrotation, though normal position may be found in up to 29% of patients. Identification of the third portion of the duodenum within the retroperitoneum makes malrotation very unlikely.

Treatment & Prognosis

Surgical treatment of malrotation is the Ladd procedure. In young infants, the Ladd procedure should be performed even if volvulus has not occurred. The duodenum is mobilized, the short mesenteric root is extended, and the bowel is then fixed in a more normal distribution. Treatment of malrotation discovered in children older than age 12 months is uncertain. Because volvulus can occur at any age, surgical repair is usually recommended, even in asymptomatic children. Laparoscopic repair of malrotation is possible but is technically difficult and is never performed in the presence of volvulus.

Midgut volvulus is a surgical emergency. Bowel necrosis results from occlusion of the superior mesenteric artery. When necrosis is extensive, it is recommended that a first operation include only reduction of the volvulus with lysis of mesenteric bands. Resection of necrotic bowel should be delayed if possible until a second-look operation 24–48 hours later can be undertaken in the hope that more bowel can be salvaged. The prognosis is guarded if perforation, peritonitis, or extensive intestinal necrosis is present. Midgut volvulus is one of the most common indications for small bowel transplant in children, responsible for 10% of cases in a recent series.

Lampl B, Levin TL, Berdon WE, Cowles RA: Malrotation and midgut volvulus: A historical review and current controversies in diagnosis and management. Pediatr Radiol 2009;39:359–366 [PMID: 19241073].

Sizemore AW, Rabbani KZ, Ladd A, Applegate KE: Diagnostic performance of the upper gastrointestinal series in the evaluation of children with clinically suspected malrotation. Pediatr Radiol 2008;38:518–528 [PMID: 18265969].

Taylor GA: CT appearance of the duodenum and mesenteric vessels in children with normal and abnormal bowel rotation. Pediatr Radiol 2011 [Epub ahead of print] [PMID: 21594544].

SHORT BOWEL SYNDROME

General Considerations

The most common cause of short bowel syndrome in children is neonatal intestinal resection. Necrotizing enterocolitis is the most common reason for resection (45%). Other causes include intestinal atresias (23%), gastroschisis (15%), volvulus (15%), and, less commonly, congenital short bowel, long-segment Hirschsprung disease, and ischemic bowel. If bowel resection is extensive, the infant may be left with an intestine of insufficient length to support normal absorption and growth. Estimates of the small bowel length of a newborn range from 150 to 300 cm. Neonatal short bowel syndrome is defined as removal of more than 50% of the small intestinal length. In patients with 50% resection, it is almost certain that intravenous nutrition will be required for months to years to support growth. The use of serum citrulline levels as an indirect measure of bowel length has been proposed and shows promise in predicting patients' ability to be weaned off of parenteral nutrition.

The intestine remaining after resection does not undergo compensatory increase in length. However, if nutrition can be maintained, enterocytes will proliferate, villi will lengthen, and the intestine will elongate in proportion to the child's increasing height. These adaptations may eventually be sufficient for the patient's nutritional needs. Achieving independence from intravenous nutrition is less likely when less than 30 cm of small intestine remain after surgery. An intact colon and intact ileocecal sphincter are factors improving prognosis in short bowel syndrome.

Symptoms and Signs

Generally, patients present with feeding intolerance and failure to thrive. Often due to prematurity, severity of illness, and subsequent oral aversion, these patients take little or no enteral nutrition orally in the initial period of their illness. Enteral nutrition, primarily delivered via a feeding device, is often limited by symptoms of diarrhea, abdominal distention, vomiting, or fluid and electrolyte disturbances. The inability to provide and/or absorb adequate nutrition enterally results in growth failure, unless supplementation is given parenterally.

Treatment & Prognosis

The use of multidisciplinary intestinal rehabilitation programs improves morbidity and mortality through the use of combined medical, nutritional, and surgical therapies. Emerging medical therapy with glucagon-like peptide 2 analogues shows promise in increasing absorption and bowel adaptation in early trials. Surgical bowel-lengthening procedures, such as the Bianchi and the serial transverse enteroplasty (STEP) procedures, have been successful in allowing weaning from TPN in up to 50% of patients in reported series. The STEP procedure offers the advantage of being less technically demanding and potentially repeatable, if the bowel dilates sufficiently after the initial procedure. Intestinal transplantation is an option for children with very short residual intestinal segments, with recently reported one-year and three-year survival rates of 83% and 60% respectively.

Five-year survival for infants with greater than 50% bowel resection or requiring TPN for more than 2 months due to short bowel syndrome has been reported at 73%. Liver failure (a consequence of intravenous nutrition, recurrent infection, and other injuries) is the most common cause of death in patients with short bowel syndrome. Recent research on TPN-associated liver disease has focused on altering the ratio of omega-3 and omega-6 lipids to decrease liver injury. Additional attention has been given to reducing the incidence of sepsis through the use of ethanol and antibiotic locks in central venous catheters.

Diamond IR, Pencharz PB, Wales PW: What is the current role for parenteral lipid emulsions containing omega-3 fatty acids in infants with short bowel syndrome? Minerva Pediatr 2009;61:263–272 [PMID: 19461570].

Fitzgibbons S et al: Relationship between serum citrulline levels and progression to parenteral nutrition independence in children with short bowel syndrome. J Pediatr Surg 2009;44:928–932 [PMID: 19433172].

Kato T et al: Intestinal and multivisceral transplantation in children. Ann Surg 2006;243:756–764 [PMID: 16772779].

Sudan D: Advances in the nontransplant medical and surgical management of intestinal failure. Curr Opin Organ Transplant 2009;14:274–279 [PMID: 19373087].

Wallis K, Walters JR, Gabe S: Short bowel syndrome: The role of GLP-2 on improving outcome. Curr Opin Clin Nutr Metab Care 2009 [PMID: 19474717].

INTUSSUSCEPTION

Intussusception is the most frequent cause of intestinal obstruction in the first 2 years of life. It is three times more common in males than in females. In 85% of cases, the cause is not apparent. Small bowel polyp, Meckel diverticulum, omphalomesenteric remnant, duplication, Henoch-Schönlein purpura, lymphoma, lipoma, parasites, foreign bodies, and viral enteritis with hypertrophy of Peyer patches all have been implicated as causes. Rotavirus vaccines have been implicated as a potential risk factor for intussusception, but several studies investigating this association have not found any increased risk over placebo. Viral PCR studies have suggested that nonenteric adenovirus may be correlated with intussusception in children. Intussusception of the small intestine occurs in patients with celiac disease and cystic fibrosis related to the bulk of stool in the terminal ileum. In children older than 6 years, lymphoma is the most common cause. Intermittent small bowel intussusception is a rare cause of recurrent abdominal pain.

In its usual form, the intussusception starts just proximal to the ileocecal valve and extends for varying distances into the colon. The terminal ileum telescopes into the colon. Swelling, hemorrhage, incarceration, vascular compromise, and necrosis of the intussuscepted ileum may occur, as well as intestinal perforation and peritonitis.

Clinical Findings

Characteristically, a thriving infant 3–12 months of age develops recurring paroxysms of abdominal pain with screaming and drawing up of the knees. Vomiting and diarrhea occur soon afterward (90% of cases) and bloody bowel movements with mucus appear within the next 12 hours (50%). The child is characteristically lethargic between paroxysms and may be febrile. The abdomen is tender and often distended. A sausage-shaped mass may be palpated, usually in the upper mid abdomen. An intussusception can persist for several days if obstruction is not complete, and patients may present with intermittent attacks of enterocolitis. In older children, sudden attacks of abdominal pain may be related to chronic recurrent intussusception with spontaneous reduction.

Diagnosis and Treatment

The combination of abdominal pain, lethargy, vomiting, and a suspicious abdominal radiograph was found to have a sensitivity of 95% in identifying intussusceptions in children. Abdominal ultrasound has also been used as an initial screening study and has been found to be a cost-effective way of decreasing unnecessary radiation exposure from air and contrast enemas. Barium enema and air enema are both diagnostic and therapeutic. Reduction of the intussusception by barium enema should not be attempted if signs of strangulated bowel, perforation, or toxicity are present. Air insufflation of the colon under fluoroscopic guidance is a safe alternative to barium enema that has excellent diagnostic sensitivity and specificity without the risk of contaminating the abdominal cavity with barium. Care is required in performing either air or barium enema because ischemic damage to the colon secondary to vascular compromise increases the risk of perforation.

Surgery is required in extremely ill patients, in patients with evidence of bowel perforation, or in those in whom hydrostatic or pneumatic reduction has been unsuccessful (25%). Surgery has the advantage of identifying a lead point such as a Meckel diverticulum. Surgical reduction of intussusception is associated with a lower recurrence rate than pneumatic reduction.

Prognosis

The prognosis relates directly to the duration of the intussusception before reduction. Successful reduction by enema was decreased from 59% to 36% in a large cohort if symptom duration was greater than 24 hours. Similarly, of those requiring surgery the risk of subsequent bowel resection was increased from 17% to 39% in patients with symptoms greater than 24 hours. The mortality rate with treatment is 1%–2%. The patient should be observed carefully after hydrostatic or pneumatic reduction because intussusception recurs within 24 hours in 3%–4% of patients. Intussusception patients older than five years have a greater risk of persistent symptoms, having an underlying lead point and recurrence of intussusception.

Kaiser AD, Applegate KE, Ladd AP: Current success in the treatment of intussusception in children. Surgery 2007;142:469–475 [PMID: 17950338].

Prevention of rotavirus disease: Updated guidelines for use of rotavirus vaccine. Pediatrics 2009;123:1412–1420 [PMID: 19332437].

INGUINAL HERNIA

A peritoneal sac precedes the testicle as it descends from the genital ridge to the scrotum. The lower portion of this sac envelops the testis as the tunica vaginalis, and the remainder normally atrophies by the time of birth forming a cord (processus vaginalis). In some cases, peritoneal fluid may become trapped in the tunica vaginalis (noncommunicating hydrocele). If the processus vaginalis remains open, peritoneal fluid or an abdominal structure may be forced into it (indirect inguinal hernia).

Inguinal hernias are most often indirect and occur more frequently (9:1) in boys than in girls. Hernias may present at any age. The incidence in preterm male infants is close to 5% and is reported in 30% of male infants weighing 1000 g or less.

Clinical Findings

No symptoms are associated with an empty processus vaginalis. In most cases, a hernia is a painless inguinal swelling. The mother of the infant may be the only person to see the mass, as it may retract when the infant is active, cold, frightened, or agitated. A history of inguinal fullness associated with coughing or long periods of standing, or presence of a firm, globular, and tender swelling, sometimes associated with vomiting and abdominal distention are clinical clues. In some instances, a herniated loop of intestine may become partially obstructed leading to severe pain. Rarely, bowel becomes trapped in the hernia sac, and complete intestinal obstruction occurs. Gangrene of the hernia contents or testis may occur. In girls, the ovary may prolapse into the hernia sac presenting as a mass below the inguinal ligament. Suggestive histories are often the only criterion for diagnosis, along with the "silk glove" feel of the rubbing together of the two walls of the empty hernia sac.

Differential Diagnosis

Inguinal lymph nodes may be mistaken for a hernia. Nodes are usually multiple with more discrete borders. A hydrocele of the cord should transilluminate. An undescended testis is usually mobile in the canal and is associated with absence of the gonad in the scrotum.

Treatment

Incarceration of an inguinal hernia is more likely to occur in boys and in children younger than 10 months of age. Manual reduction of incarcerated inguinal hernias can be attempted after the sedated infant is placed in the Trendelenburg position with an ice bag on the affected side. Manual reduction is contraindicated if incarceration has been present for more than 12 hours or if bloody stools are noted. Surgery is indicated if a hernia has ever incarcerated. Hydroceles frequently resolve by age 2 years. Controversy remains about whether the side opposite a unilateral hernia should be surgically explored. Exploration of the unaffected groin can document an open processus vaginalis, but patency does not always guarantee that herniation will occur, especially in patients older than age 1 year, in whom the risk of contralateral hernia is about 10%.

Antonoff MB, Kreykes NS, Saltzman DA, Acton RD: American Academy of Pediatrics Section on Surgery hernia survey revisited. J Pediatr Surg 2005 Jun;40(6):1009–1014 [PMID: 15991187].

UMBILICAL HERNIA

Umbilical hernias are more common in full-term, African American infants. Small bowel may incarcerate in small-diameter umbilical hernias. Most umbilical hernias regress spontaneously if the fascial defect has a diameter of less than 1 cm. Hernias persisting after age 4 years should be treated surgically. Reducing the hernia and strapping the skin over the abdominal wall defect does not accelerate healing.

PATENT OMPHALOMESENTERIC DUCT

The omphalomesenteric duct is an embryonic remnant connecting the ileum to the undersurface of the umbilicus. It may be patent, completely occluded as a fibrous cord, or may have blind cystic areas. Fecal discharge from the umbilicus suggests a patent omphalomesenteric duct. A fibrous cord may become the focal point of an intestinal volvulus. Mucoid umbilical discharge may indicate a mucocele in the omphalomesenteric remnant with an opening at the umbilicus. A closed mucocele may protrude through the umbilicus and be mistaken for an umbilical granuloma because it is firm and bright red. Cauterization of a mucocele is not recommended. Surgical excision of omphalomesenteric remnants is indicated. Ultrasound examination or abdominal computed tomography (CT) can help confirm the diagnosis of omphalomesenteric duct remnant.

MECKEL DIVERTICULUM

Meckel diverticulum is the most common form of omphalomesenteric duct remnant and is usually located on the antimesenteric border of the mid to distal ileum. It occurs in 1.5% of the population and in the majority of cases causes no symptoms. Familial cases have been reported. If complications occur, they are three times more common in males than in females. More than 50% of complications occur in the first 2 years of life.

Clinical Findings

A. Symptoms and Signs

Forty to sixty percent of symptomatic patients have painless episodes of maroon or melanotic rectal bleeding. Bleeding is due to deep ileal ulcers adjacent to the diverticulum caused by acid secreted by heterotopic gastric tissue and may be voluminous enough to cause shock and anemia. Occult bleeding is less common. Intestinal obstruction occurs in 25% of symptomatic patients as a result of ileocolonic intussusception. Intestinal volvulus may occur around a fibrous remnant of the vitelline duct extending from the tip of the diverticulum to the abdominal wall. In some patients, entrapment of bowel under a band running between the diverticulum and the base of the mesentery occurs. Meckel diverticula may be trapped in an inguinal hernia (Littre hernia). Diverticulitis occurs in 10%–20% of symptomatic patients and is clinically indistinguishable from acute appendicitis. Perforation and peritonitis may occur.

B. Imaging

Diagnosis of Meckel diverticulum is made with a Meckel scan. Technetium-99 (^{99m}Tc)-pertechnetate is taken up by the heterotopic gastric mucosa in the diverticulum and outlines the diverticulum on a nuclear scan. Giving pentagastrin or cimetidine before administering the radionuclide increases ^{99m}Tc-pertechnetate uptake and retention by the heterotopic gastric mucosa and can increase the sensitivity of the test.

Treatment & Prognosis

Treatment is surgical. At laparoscopy or laparotomy, the ileum proximal and distal to the diverticulum may reveal ulcerations and heterotopic gastric tissue adjacent to the neck of the diverticulum. The prognosis for Meckel diverticulum is good.

ACUTE APPENDICITIS

General Considerations

Acute appendicitis is the most common indication for emergency abdominal surgery in childhood. The frequency increases with age and peaks between 15 and 30 years. Obstruction of the appendix by fecalith (25%) is a common predisposing factor. Parasites may rarely cause obstruction (especially ascarids) and most of the remaining cases are idiopathic.

The incidence of perforation is high in childhood (40%), especially in children younger than age 2 years, in whom pain is often poorly localized and symptoms nonspecific. To avoid delay in diagnosis, it is important to maintain close communication with parents and perform a thorough initial physical examination with sequential examinations at frequent intervals over several hours to correctly interpret the evolving symptoms and signs.

Clinical Findings

A. Symptoms and Signs

The typical patient has fever and periumbilical abdominal pain, which then localizes to the right lower quadrant with signs of peritoneal irritation. Anorexia, vomiting, constipation, and diarrhea also occur. Contrary to the vomiting of acute gastroenteritis which usually precedes abdominal pain, vomiting in appendicitis usually follows the onset of pain and is often bilious. The clinical picture is frequently atypical, especially in young children and infants. A rectal examination may clarify the site of tenderness or reveal a localized appendiceal mass. Serial examinations are critical in differentiating appendicitis from the many other conditions that transiently mimic its symptoms.

B. Laboratory Findings

The white blood cell count is seldom higher than 15,000/μL. Pyuria, fecal leukocytes, and guaiac-positive stool are sometimes present. The combination of elevated CRP and leukocytosis has been reported to have positive predictive value of 92% for acute appendicitis, although having normal values for both measures does not exclude the diagnosis. Levels of

IL-6 show promise as a potential biomarker for acute appendicitis, usually peaking within 24 hours of onset of pain.

C. Imaging

A radio-opaque fecalith reportedly is present in two-thirds of cases of ruptured appendix. In experienced hands, ultrasonography of the appendix shows a noncompressible, thickened appendix in 93% of cases. A localized fluid collection adjacent to or surrounding the appendix may also be seen. Abdominal CT after rectal instillation of contrast with thin cuts in the area of the appendix may be diagnostic. An otherwise normal abdominal CT scan with a nonvisualized appendix has still been reported to have a negative predictive value of 99%. Analysis of diagnostic strategies for pediatric patients with suspected appendicitis has shown abdominal ultrasound, followed by CT scan for negative studies, to be the most cost-effective compared to CT or ultrasound alone. Indium-labeled white blood cell scan may localize to an inflamed appendix. Enlarged mesenteric lymph nodes are a nondiagnostic finding.

Differential Diagnosis

The presence of pneumonia, pleural effusion, urinary tract infection, right-sided kidney stone, cholecystitis, perihepatitis, and pelvic inflammatory disease may mimic appendicitis. Acute gastroenteritis with Yersinia enterocolitica may present as pseudoappendicitis in 17% of cases. Other medical and surgical conditions causing acute abdomen should also be considered (see Table 21–7).

Treatment & Prognosis

Exploratory laparotomy or laparoscopy is indicated when the diagnosis of acute appendicitis cannot be ruled out after a period of close observation. Postoperative antibiotic therapy is reserved for patients with gangrenous or perforated appendix. A single intraoperative dose of cefoxitin or cefotetan is recommended for all patients to prevent postoperative infection. Nonoperative management of perforated appendicitis with antibiotic therapy and image-guided drainage of abdominal abscesses has become more commonplace. Failure of nonoperative management may occur in up to 38% of patients and is more commonly associated with bandemia on admission and persistent fever after the initial 24 hours of antibiotics. The mortality rate is less than 1% during childhood, despite the high incidence of perforation. In uncomplicated nonruptured appendicitis, a laparoscopic approach is associated with a shortened hospital stay.

Bundy DG et al: Does this child have appendicitis? JAMA 2007;298:438 [PMID: 17652298].

Garcia K et al: Suspected appendicitis in children: Diagnostic importance of normal abdominopelvic CT findings with nonvisualized appendix. Radiology 2009;250(2):531–537 [PMID: 19188320].

Kharbanda AB, Cosme Y, Liu K, Spitalnik SL, Dayan PS: Discriminative accuracy of novel and traditional biomarkers in children with suspected appendicitis adjusted for duration of abdominal pain. Acad Emerg Med 2011;18(6):567–574 [PMID: 21676053].

Wan MJ et al: Acute appendicitis in young children: Cost-effectiveness of US versus CT in diagnosis—a Markov decision analytic model. Radiology 2009;250(2):378–386 [PMID: 19098225].

Whyte C, Levin T, Harris BH: Early decisions in perforated appendicitis in children: Lessons from a study of nonoperative management. J Pediatr Surg 2008;43(8):1459–1463 [PMID: 18675635].

DUPLICATIONS OF THE GASTROINTESTINAL TRACT

Enteric duplications are congenital spherical or tubular structures found most commonly in the ileum. Other common locations of duplication are the duodenum, rectum, and esophagus. Duplications usually contain fluid and sometimes blood if necrosis has taken place. Most duplications are attached to the mesenteric side of the gut and generally do not communicate with the intestinal lumen. The epithelial lining of the duplication is usually of the same type as the bowel from which it originates. Some duplications (neuroenteric cysts) are attached to the spinal cord and are associated with hemivertebrae and anterior or posterior spina bifida.

Symptoms of vomiting, abdominal distention, colicky pain, rectal bleeding, partial or total intestinal obstruction, or an abdominal mass may start in infancy. Diarrhea and malabsorption may result from bacterial overgrowth in communicating duplications. Physical examination may reveal a rounded, smooth, movable mass, and barium radiograph or CT of the abdomen may show a noncalcified cystic mass displacing other organs. ^{99m}Tc-pertechnetate scan may help identify duplications containing gastric mucosa. Duplications of the ileum can give rise to an intussusception. Prompt surgical treatment is indicated.

DISORDERS OF THE COLON

CONGENITAL AGANGLIONIC MEGACOLON (HIRSCHSPRUNG DISEASE)

General Considerations

Hirschsprung disease results from an absence of ganglion cells in the mucosal and muscular layers of the colon. Neural crest cells fail to migrate into the mesodermal layers of the gut during gestation, possibly secondary to abnormal end-organ cell surface receptors or local deficiency of nitric oxide synthesis. The absence of ganglion cells results in failure of the colonic muscles to relax in front of an advancing bolus. The rectum (30%) or rectosigmoid (44%) is usually affected. The entire colon may be aganglionic (8%). Segmental aganglionosis is rare.

The aganglionic segment has normal or slightly narrowed caliber with dilation of the normal colon proximal to the obstructing aganglionic segment. The mucosa of the dilated colonic segment may become thin and inflamed, causing diarrhea, bleeding, and protein loss (enterocolitis).

A familial pattern has been described, particularly in total colonic aganglionosis. The disease is four times more common in boys than girls, and 10%–15% of patients have Down syndrome. Mutations in the ret proto-oncogene have been identified in about 15% of cases.

Clinical Findings

A. Symptoms and Signs

Failure of the newborn to pass meconium, followed by vomiting, abdominal distention, and reluctance to feed, suggests the diagnosis of Hirschsprung disease. Most children with Hirschsprung disease do not pass stool in the first 24 hours of their life. Enterocolitis manifested by fever, explosive diarrhea, and prostration is reported in approximately 50% of affected newborns. Enterocolitis may lead to inflammatory and ischemic changes in the colon, with perforation and sepsis. In some patients, especially those with short segments involved, symptoms are not obvious at birth. In later infancy, alternating obstipation and diarrhea predominate. The older child is more likely to have constipation alone. The stools are foul-smelling and ribbon-like. The abdomen is distended with prominent veins. Peristaltic waves are visible and fecal masses palpable. Intermittent bouts of intestinal obstruction, hypochromic anemia, hypoproteinemia, and failure to thrive are common. Encopresis is rare.

On digital rectal examination, the anal canal and rectum are devoid of fecal material despite obvious retained stool on abdominal examination or radiographs. If the aganglionic segment is short, there may be a gush of flatus and stool as the finger is withdrawn.

Infants of diabetic mothers may have similar symptoms and, in this setting, small left colon syndrome should be suspected. Meglumine diatrizoate (Gastrografin) enema is both diagnostic and therapeutic in small left colon syndrome as it reveals a meconium plug in the left colon, which is often passed during the diagnostic radiograph. The left colon is narrow but usually functional.

B. Laboratory Findings

Ganglion cells are absent in both the submucosal and muscular layers of involved bowel. Special stains may show nerve trunk hypertrophy and increased acetylcholinesterase activity. Ganglionated bowel above the aganglionic segment is sometimes found to contain more than normal numbers of ganglion cells in abnormal locations (neuronal dysplasia).

C. Imaging

Plain abdominal radiographs may reveal dilated proximal colon and absence of gas in the pelvic colon. Barium enema using a catheter without a balloon and with the tip inserted barely beyond the anal sphincter usually demonstrates a narrow distal segment with a sharp transition to the proximal dilated (normal) colon. Transition zones may not be seen in neonates since the normal proximal bowel has not had time to become dilated. Retention of barium for 24–48 hours is not diagnostic of Hirschsprung disease in older children as it typically occurs in retentive constipation as well.

D. Special Examinations

Rectal manometric testing reveals failure of reflex relaxation of the internal anal sphincter after distention of the rectum in all patients with Hirschsprung disease, regardless of the length of the aganglionic segment. In occasional patients, a nonrelaxing internal anal sphincter is the only abnormality. This condition is often called "ultrashort segment Hirschsprung disease."

Differential Diagnosis

Hirschsprung disease accounts for 15%–20% of cases of neonatal intestinal obstruction. It must be differentiated from the small left colon syndrome by biopsy. In childhood, Hirschsprung disease must be differentiated from retentive constipation. In older infants and children, it can also be confused with celiac disease because of the striking abdominal distention and failure to thrive.

Treatment & Prognosis

Treatment is surgical. Diverting colostomy (or ileostomy) is performed proximal to the aganglionic segment. In unstable infants, resection of the aganglionic segment may be postponed. At the time of definitive surgery, the transition zone between ganglionated and nonganglionated bowel is identified. Aganglionic bowel is resected, and a pull-through of ganglionated bowel to the preanal rectal remnant is made. Several surgical techniques, including laparoscopic pull-through, are in use. In children with ultrashort segment disease, an internal anal sphincter myotomy or botulinum toxin injection of the internal anal sphincter may control symptoms.

Complications after surgery include fecal retention, fecal incontinence, anastomotic breakdown, or anastomotic stricture. Postoperative obstruction may result from inadvertent retention of a distal aganglionic colon segment or postoperative destruction of ganglion cells secondary to vascular impairment. Neuronal dysplasia of the remaining bowel may produce a pseudo-obstruction syndrome. Enterocolitis occurs postoperatively in 15% of patients.

Gariepy CE: Developmental disorders of the enteric nervous system: Genetic and molecular bases. J Pediatr Gastroenterol Nutr 2004;39:5 [PMID: 15187773].

CONSTIPATION

Chronic constipation in childhood is defined as two or more of the following characteristics for 2 months: (1) less than 3 bowel movements per week; (2) more than 1 episode of encopresis per week; (3) impaction of the rectum with stool; (4) passage of stool so large it obstructs the toilet; (5) retentive posturing and fecal withholding; and (6) pain with defecation. Retention of feces in the rectum results in encopresis (involuntary fecal leakage) in 60% of children with constipation. Most constipation in childhood is a result of voluntary or involuntary retentive behavior (chronic retentive constipation). About 2% of healthy primary school children have chronic retentive constipation. The ratio of males to females may be as high as 4:1.

Clinical Findings

Infants younger than age 3 months often grunt, strain, and turn red in the face while passing normal stools. Failure to appreciate this normal developmental pattern may lead to the unwise use of laxatives or enemas. Infants and children may, however, develop the ability to ignore the sensation of rectal fullness and retain stool. Many factors reinforce this behavior, which results in impaction of the rectum and overflow incontinence or encopresis. Among these are painful defecation; skeletal muscle weakness; psychological issues, especially those relating to control and authority; modesty and distaste for school bathrooms; medications; and other factors listed in Table 21–2. The dilated rectum gradually becomes less sensitive to fullness, thus perpetuating the problem.

Differential Diagnosis

One must distinguish between chronic retentive constipation from Hirschsprung disease as summarized in Table 21–3.

Treatment

Increased intake of high-residue foods such as bran, whole wheat, fruits, and vegetables may be sufficient therapy in mild constipation. Increased water drinking is important for both dietary and medical approaches. If diet change alone is ineffective, medications may be required. Barley malt extract (Maltsupex), 1–2 tsp added to feedings two or three times daily, or polyethylene glycol solution (MiraLax), 0.8–1 g/kg/d, are safe stool softeners in infants and children. Stool softeners such as dioctyl sodium sulfosuccinate, 5–10 mg/kg/d, may be less effective in children with voluntary stool retention. Stimulant laxatives such as standardized extract of senna fruit (Senokot syrup, ExLax) can be used for short periods to relieve fecal impaction. If encopresis is present, treatment should start with relieving fecal impaction. Disimpaction can be achieved in several ways, including medications such as hypertonic phosphate or saline enemas, mineral oil

Table 21–2. Causes of constipation.

Functional or retentive causes	**Abnormalities of myenteric ganglion cells**
Dietary causes	Hirschsprung disease
Undernutrition, dehydration	Waardenburg syndrome
Excessive milk intake	Multiple endocrine neoplasia 2a
Lack of bulk	**Hypo- and hyperganglionosis**
Cathartic abuse	von Recklinghausen disease
Drugs	Multiple endocrine neoplasia 2b
Narcotics	Intestinal neuronal dysplasia
Antihistamines	Chronic intestinal pseudo-obstruction
Some antidepressants	**Spinal cord defects**
Vincristine	**Metabolic and endocrine disorders**
Structural defects of gastrointestinal tract	Hypothyroidism
Anus and rectum	Hyperparathyroidism
Fissure, hemorrhoids, abscess	Renal tubular acidosis
Anterior ectopic anus	Diabetes insipidus (dehydration)
Anal and rectal stenosis	Vitamin D intoxication (hypercalcemia)
Presacral teratoma	Idiopathic hypercalcemia
Small bowel and colon	**Skeletal muscle weakness or incoordination**
Tumor, stricture	Cerebral palsy
Chronic volvulus	Muscular dystrophy/myotonia
Intussusception	
Smooth muscle diseases	
Scleroderma and dermatomyositis	
Systemic lupus erythematosus	
Chronic intestinal pseudo-obstruction	

Modified and reproduced, with permission, from Silverman A, Roy CC: Pediatric Clinical Gastroenterology, 3rd ed. Mosby, 1983.

Table 21–3. Differentiation of retentive constipation and Hirschsprung disease.

	Retentive Constipation	Hirschsprung Disease
Onset	2–3 y	At birth
Abdominal distention	Rare	Present
Nutrition and growth	Normal	Poor
Soiling and retentive behavior	Intermittent or constant	Rare
Rectal examination	Ampulla full	Ampulla may be empty
Rectal biopsy	Ganglion cells present	Ganglion cells absent
Rectal manometry	Normal rectoanal reflex	Nonrelaxation of internal anal sphincter after rectal distention
Barium enema	Distended rectum	Narrow distal segment with proximal megacolon

(2–3 mL/kg/d), and nonabsorbable osmotic agents such as polyethylene glycol (MiraLax, 1 g/kg/d) and milk of magnesia (1–2 mL/kg/d). Effective stool softeners should thereafter be given regularly in doses sufficient to induce two or three loose bowel movements per day. After several weeks to months of regular loose stools, stool softeners can be tapered and stopped. Mineral oil should not be given to nonambulatory infants, physically handicapped or bed-bound children, or any child with GE reflux. Aspiration of mineral oil may cause lipid pneumonia. A multiple vitamin supplement is recommended while mineral oil is given. Recurrence of encopresis is common and should be treated promptly with a short course of stimulant laxatives or an enema. Psychiatric consultation may be indicated for patients with resistant symptoms or severe emotional disturbances.

Benninga M et al: The Paris Consensus on Childhood Constipation Terminology (PACCT) Group. J Pediatr Gastroenterol Nutr 2005;40:273 [PMID: 15735478].

Constipation Guidelines Committee of the North American Society for Pediatric Gastroenterology, Hepatology and Nutrition: Evaluation and treatment of constipation in infants and children: Recommendations of the North American Society for Pediatric Gastroenterology, Hepatology and Nutrition. J Pediatr Gastroenterol Nutr 2006;43:e1 [PMID: 16954945].

ANAL FISSURE

Anal fissure is a slitlike tear in the squamous epithelium of the anus, that usually occurs secondary to the passage of large, hard fecal masses. Anal stenosis, anal crypt abscess, and trauma can be contributory factors. Sexual abuse must be considered in children with large, irregular, or multiple anal fissures. Anal fissures may be the presenting sign of Crohn disease in older children.

The infant or child with anal fissure typically cries with defecation and will try to hold back stools. Sparse, bright red bleeding is seen on the outside of the stool or on the toilet tissue following defecation. The fissure can often be seen if the patient is examined in a knee-chest position with the buttocks spread apart. When a fissure cannot be identified, it is essential to rule out other causes of rectal bleeding such as juvenile polyp, perianal inflammation due to group A β-hemolytic streptococcus, or inflammatory bowel disease. Anal fissures should be treated promptly to break the constipation, fissure, pain, retention, constipation cycle. A stool softener should be given. Anal dilation relieves sphincter spasm. Warm sitz baths after defecation may be helpful. Rarely, silver nitrate cauterization or surgery is indicated. Anal surgery should be avoided in patients with Crohn disease because of the high risk of recurrence and progression after surgery.

CONGENITAL ANORECTAL ANOMALIES

1. Anterior Displacement of the Anus

Anterior displacement of the anus is a common anomaly of infant girls. Its usual presentation in infants is constipation and straining with stool. On physical examination, the anus looks normal but is ventrally displaced, located close to the vaginal fourchette (in females) or to the base of the scrotum (in males). The diagnosis is made in girls if the distance from the vaginal fourchette to the center of the anal opening is less than 25% of the total distance from fourchette to coccyx. In boys, the diagnosis is made if the distance from the base of the scrotum to the anal aperture is less than 33% of the total distance from scrotum to coccyx. In severe anterior displacement, when the anal opening is located less than 10% of the distance from the vaginal fourchette to the coccyx, the anal sphincter muscle may not completely encircle the anal opening and severe obstipation similar to that seen in imperforate anus may occur. Indeed, extreme anterior displacement of the anus may be a form of imperforate anus. Surgery is not needed in most cases. Stool softeners or occasional glycerin suppositories usually relieve straining. This problem improves significantly by age 3–4 years as normal toddler lordosis disappears.

2. Anal Stenosis

Anal stenosis usually presents in the newborn period. The anal aperture may be very small and filled with a dot of meconium. Defecation is difficult, with ribbon-like stools, blood and mucus per rectum, fecal impaction, and abdominal distention. This malformation accounts for about 10% of anorectal anomalies. Anal stenosis may not be apparent at birth because the anus looks normal. Rectal bleeding in a straining infant often leads to a rectal examination which reveals a tight ring in the anal canal. Dilation of the anal ring is usually curative but may have to be repeated daily for several weeks.

3. Imperforate Anus

Imperforate anus in its numerous forms accounts for 75% of all anorectal anomalies. These anomalies are often complicated by associated anomalies of the urinary and genital tract. They are more common in males than in females and require careful diagnostic evaluation immediately to assess the extent of bowel, urinary, genital, and other organ system anomalies, including spinal cord and heart.

Infants with low imperforate anus fail to pass meconium. There may be a greenish bulging membrane obstructing the anal aperture. Perforation of the anal membrane is a relatively simple surgical procedure. A skin tag shaped like a "bucket handle" is seen on the perineum of some males below which a stenotic aperture can be seen. The aperture is sometimes surrounded by normal anal musculature, but in many cases the aperture is a rectoperineal fistula and the anal musculature is displaced posteriorly or is absent. Eighty to ninety percent of patients with low imperforate anus are continent after surgery.

In high imperforate anus, physical examination usually shows no anal musculature. There may be a rectoperineal, rectovesicular, rectourethral, or rectovaginal fistula; hypoplastic buttocks; cloacal anomalies; and sometimes, evidence of distal neurologic deficit. It is critical in these cases to fully evaluate the complex anatomy and neurologic function before attempting corrective surgery. A diverting colostomy is usually performed to protect the urinary tract and relieve obstruction. After reparative surgery, only 30% of patients with high imperforate anus achieve fecal continence.

Levitt MA, Pena A: Outcomes from the correction of anorectal malformations. Curr Opin Pediatr 2005;17:394 [PMID: 15891433].

PSEUDOMEMBRANOUS ENTEROCOLITIS

Pseudomembranous enterocolitis occurs when previous antibiotic use allows overgrowth of *Clostridium difficile* and toxin secretion. *C difficile* infection may range in severity from mere antibiotic-associated diarrhea to pseudomembranous enterocolitis. The onset of colitis ranges from 1–14 days after initiation of antibiotic therapy to as many as 30 days after antibiotics have been discontinued. Clindamycin was one of the first antibiotics associated with pseudomembranous colitis. Almost all antibiotics are now recognized to be potential causes, although erythromycin seems less likely than most. In pediatric patients, amoxicillin and cephalosporins are commonly associated with pseudomembranous enterocolitis, probably because of their widespread use. Although antibiotic use is the most common antecedent of pseudomembranous colitis, previous GI surgery and antimetabolite therapy in cancer patients are also associated with its development.

C difficile secretes enterotoxins that cause necrotizing inflammation of the colon mucosa. The patient characteristically has fever, abdominal distention, tenesmus, diarrhea, and generalized abdominal tenderness. Chronic presentations with low-grade fever, diarrhea, and abdominal pain have been described. Diarrheal stools contain sheets of neutrophils and sometimes gross blood. Plain abdominal radiographs show a thickened colon wall and ileus. On colonoscopy, the colon is covered by small, raised white plaques (pseudomembranes) with areas of apparently normal bowel in between (see Figure 21–5). Biopsy specimens show "exploding crypts or volcano lesion"—an eruption of white cells that appears to be shooting out of affected crypts. Stool cultures often show overgrowth of *Staphylococcus aureus*, which is probably an opportunistic organism growing in the necrotic tissue. *C difficile* can be cultured in specialized laboratories. Identification of stool toxins is the usual method of diagnosis. Use of real time PCR has been replacing more traditional EIA methods of stool toxin detection, due to improved sensitivity. Infants up to 18–24 months of age may have toxins in the stool but generally do not develop disease or require therapy. *C difficile* may be a component of the normal flora in up to 50% of infants, who seem to not have sufficient receptors for the toxins to produce disease.

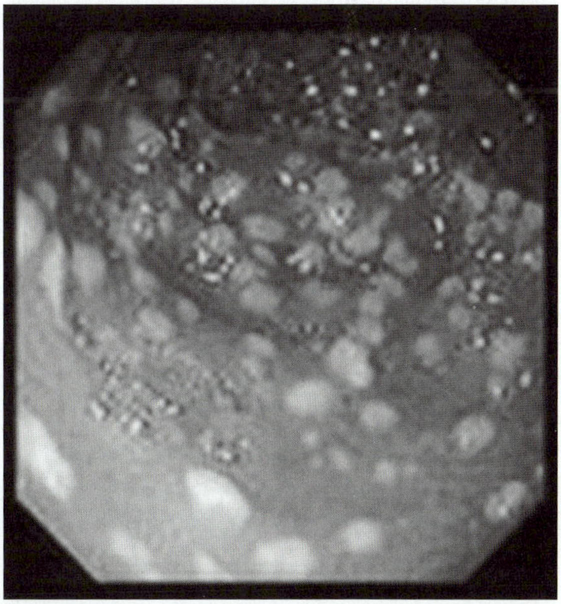

▲ **Figure 21–5.** Clostridium difficile associated pseudomembranes. Colonic mucosa is covered with plaques coated with white exudates.

In recent years, there has been an alarming increase in the incidence, morbidity, and mortality of *C difficile* reported in Europe, Canada, and the United States. At least a portion of this increase seems to be due to the expansion of a new strain of *C difficile*, identified as the North American Pulsed Field type 1 (NAP1) *C difficile*, which has been found to have increased toxin production, sporulation, and antibiotic resistance. Surveillance from children's hospitals seems to mirror the increase in incidence of *C difficile* in adults, but not necessarily the increase in morbidity and mortality. Pediatric hospitalizations in the United States due to *C difficile* have almost doubled between 1997 and 2006. The NAP1 strain was identified in 19% of *C difficile* isolates in a recent pediatric study.

Standard treatment of pseudomembranous colitis consists of stopping antibiotics and instituting therapy with oral vancomycin (30–50 mg/kg/d) or metronidazole (30 mg/kg/d). Vancomycin is many times more expensive than metronidazole and no more efficacious. Metronidazole can be given intravenously in patients with vomiting or ileus. With increasing virulence and antibiotic resistance being reported, alternative therapies, such as Rifaxamin and Nitazoxanide, are being used and show similar response rates as oral Vancomycin. Relapse occurs after treatment in 10%–50% of patients because of exsporulation of residual spores in the colon. Spores are very hardy and may remain viable on inanimate surfaces for up to 12 months. Retreatment with the same antibiotic regimen is usually effective, but multiple relapses are possible and may be a significant management problem. Adjunctive strategies such as *Sachromyces boulardii* probiotic therapy, cholestyramine as a toxin-binder, and pulsed courses of antibiotics have been used for refractory disease. Ulcerative colitis may be an underlying problem in cases of apparent recurrent *C difficile*.

Kim J et al: Epidemiological features of *Clostridium difficile*-associated disease among inpatients at children's hospitals in the United States, 2001–2006. Pediatrics 2008;122(6):1266–1270 [PMID: 19047244].

Toltzis P et al: Presence of the epidemic North American Pulsed Field type 1 *Clostridium difficile* strain in hospitalized children. J Pediatr 2009;154(4):607–608 [PMID: 19324222].

Zilberberg MD, Tillotson GS, McDonald C: *Clostridium difficile* infections among hospitalized children, United States, 1997–2006. 2010;16(4):604–609 [PMID: 20350373].

DISORDERS OF THE PERITONEAL CAVITY

PERITONITIS

Primary bacterial peritonitis accounts for less than 2% of childhood peritonitis. The most common causative organisms are *Escherichia coli*, other enteric organisms, hemolytic streptococci, and pneumococci. Primary peritonitis occurs in patients with splenectomy, splenic dysfunction, or ascites (nephrotic syndrome, advanced liver disease, kwashiorkor). It also occurs in infants with pyelonephritis or pneumonia.

Secondary peritonitis is much more common. It is associated with peritoneal dialysis, penetrating abdominal trauma, or ruptured viscus. The organisms associated with secondary peritonitis vary with the cause. Organisms not commonly pathogenic such as *Staphylococcus epidermidis* and *Candida* may cause secondary peritonitis in patients receiving peritoneal dialysis. Multiple enteric organisms may be isolated after penetrating abdominal injury, bowel perforation, or ruptured appendicitis. Intra-abdominal abscesses may form in pelvic, subhepatic, or subphrenic areas, but discrete localization of infection is less common in young infants than in adults.

Symptoms of peritonitis include abdominal pain, fever, nausea, vomiting, acidosis, and shock. Respirations are shallow. The abdomen is tender, rigid, and distended, with involuntary guarding. Bowel sounds may be absent. Diarrhea is fairly common in primary peritonitis and less so in secondary peritonitis. Most peritonitis is an acute medical emergency. In patients receiving peritoneal dialysis, peritonitis can be a chronic infection causing milder symptoms.

Leukocyte count is high initially (> 20,000/μL) with a predominance of immature forms, and later may fall to neutropenic levels, especially in primary peritonitis. Abdominal imaging can confirm the presence of ascites. Bacterial peritonitis should be suspected if paracentesis fluid contains more than 500 leukocytes/μL or more than 32 mg/dL of lactate; if it has a pH less than 7.34; or if the pH is over 0.1 pH unit less than arterial blood pH. Diagnosis is made by Gram stain and culture, preferably of 5–10 mL of fluid for optimal yield. The blood culture is often positive in primary peritonitis.

Antibiotic treatment and supportive therapy for dehydration, shock, and acidosis are indicated. Surgical treatment of the underlying cause of secondary peritonitis is critical. Removal of infected peritoneal dialysis catheters in patients with secondary peritonitis is sometimes necessary and almost always required if *Candida* infection is present.

European Association for the Study of the Liver: EASL clinical practice guidelines on the management of ascites, spontaneous bacterial peritonitis, and hepatorenal syndrome in cirrhosis. J Hepatol 2010 Sep;53(3):397–417.

Koulaouzidis A et al: Spontaneous bacterial peritonitis. World J Gastroenterol 2009 Mar 7;15(9):1042–1049.

CHYLOUS ASCITES

Neonatal chylous ascites may be due to congenital infection or developmental abnormality of the lymphatic system (intestinal lymphangiectasia). If the thoracic duct is involved, chylothorax may be present. Later in life, chylous ascites may result from congenital lymphangiectasia, retroperitoneal or lymphatic tumors, peritoneal bands, abdominal trauma, or infection, or it may occur after cardiac or abdominal surgery. It may be associated with intestinal malrotation.

Clinical Findings

A. Symptoms and Signs

Both congenital and acquired lymphatic obstruction cause chylous ascites, diarrhea, and failure to thrive. The abdomen is distended, with a fluid wave and shifting dullness. Unilateral or generalized peripheral edema may be present.

B. Laboratory Findings

Laboratory findings include hypoalbuminemia, hypogammaglobulinemia, and lymphopenia. Ascitic fluid contains lymphocytes and has the biochemical composition of chyle if the patient has just been fed; otherwise, it is indistinguishable from ascites secondary to cirrhosis.

Differential Diagnosis

Chylous ascites must be differentiated from ascites due to liver disease and in the older child, from constrictive pericarditis, chronically elevated right heart pressure, malignancy, infection, or inflammatory diseases causing lymphatic obstruction. In the newborn, urinary ascites from anatomic abnormalities of the kidney or collecting system must be considered. A simple test to diagnose urinary ascites is a urea nitrogen or creatinine concentration of abdominal fluid. Neither of these is present in chylous or hepatic ascites

Complications & Sequelae

Chylous ascites caused by intestinal lymphatic obstruction is associated with fat malabsorption and protein loss. Intestinal loss of albumin and γ-globulin may lead to edema and increase the risk of infection. Rapidly accumulating chylous ascites may cause respiratory complications. The primary infections and malignancies causing chylous ascites may be life-threatening.

Treatment & Prognosis

Little can be done to correct congenital abnormalities due to hypoplasia, aplasia, or ectasia of the lymphatics unless they are surgically resectable. More recently, somatostatin and fibrin glue have been tried with varying success. Treatment is supportive, consisting mainly of a very high-protein diet and careful attention to infections. Shunting of peritoneal fluid into the venous system is sometimes effective. A fat-free diet supplemented with medium-chain triglycerides decreases the formation of chylous ascites. Total parenteral nutrition may rarely be necessary. Infusions of albumin generally provide only temporary relief and are rarely used for chronic management. In the neonate, congenital chylous ascites may spontaneously disappear following one or more paracenteses and a medium-chain triglyceride diet.

Chye JK et al: Neonatal chylous ascites: Report of 3 cases and review of the literature. Pediatr Surg Int 1997;12:296 [PMID: 9099650].

Karagol BS et al: Acta Paediatr 2010 Sep;99:1307–1310.

GASTROINTESTINAL TUMORS & MALIGNANCIES

JUVENILE POLYPS

Juvenile polyps are usually pedunculated and solitary (see Figure 21–6). The head of the polyp is composed of hyperplastic glandular and vascular elements, often with cystic transformation. Juvenile polyps are benign, and 80% occur in the rectosigmoid. Their incidence is highest between ages 3 and 5 years. They are rare before age 1 year and usually autoamputate by age 15 years. They are more frequent in boys. The painless passage of small amounts of bright red blood on a normal or constipated stool is the most frequent manifestation. Abdominal pain is rare, but a juvenile polyp can be the lead point for an intussusception. Low-lying polyps may prolapse during defecation.

Rarely, many juvenile polyps may be present in the colon, causing anemia, diarrhea, and protein loss. A few cases of generalized juvenile polyposis involving the stomach, small bowel, and colon have been reported. These cases are associated with a slightly increased risk of cancer.

Colonoscopy is diagnostic and therapeutic when polyps are suspected. After removal of the polyp by electrocautery, nothing further should be done if histologic findings confirm the diagnosis. There is a slight risk of developing further juvenile polyps. Other polyposis syndromes are summarized in Table 21–4.

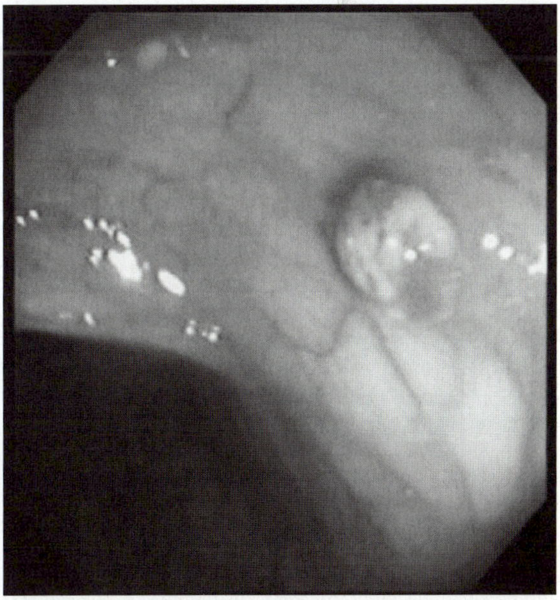

▲ **Figure 21–6.** Juvenile polyp. Solitary, smooth polyp coated with exudate and erythematous pattern that lies on the surface of a normal colonic mucosa.

Table 21–4. Gastrointestinal polyposis syndromes.

	Location	Number	Histology	Extraintestinal Findings	Malignant Potential	Recommended Therapy
Juvenile polyps	Colon	Single (70%) Several (30%)	Hyperplastic, hamartomatous	None	None	Remove polyp for continuous bleeding or prolapse.
Familial juvenile polyposis coli[a]	Colon	> 10	Hyperplastic with focal adenomatous change	None	10%–25%; higher if familial	Remove all polyps. Consider colectomy if very numerous or adenomatous.
Generalized juvenile polyposis[a]	Stomach, small bowel, colon	Multiple	Hyperplastic with focal adenomatous change	Hydrocephaly, cardiac lesions, mesenteric lymphangioma, malrotation	10%–25%	Colectomy and close surveillance.
Familial adenomatous polyposis[a]	Colon; less commonly, stomach and small bowel	Multiple	Adenomatous	None	95%–100%	Colectomy by age 18 years.
Peutz-Jeghers syndrome[a]	Small bowel, stomach, colon	Multiple	Hamartomatous	Pigmented cutaneous and oral macules; ovarian cysts and tumors; bony exostoses	2%–3%	Remove accessible polyps or those causing obstruction or bleeding.
Gardner syndrome	Colon; less commonly, stomach and small bowel	Multiple	Adenomatous	Cysts, tumors, and desmoids of skin and bone; ampullary tumors; other tumors, retinal pigmentations can be a screening tool in families	95%–100%	Colectomy by age 18 y. Upper tract surveillance.
Cronkhite-Canada syndrome	Stomach, colon; less commonly, esophagus and small bowel	Multiple	Hamartomatous	Alopecia; onychodystrophy; hyper-pigmentation	Rare	None.
Turcot syndrome[b]	Colon	Multiple	Adenomatous	Thyroid and brain tumors are the usual presentation	Possible	Central nervous system screening most important.

[a]Autosomal dominant.
[b]Autosomal recessive.

Barnard J: Screening and surveillance recommendations for pediatric gastrointestinal polyposis syndrome. J Pediatr Gastroenterol Nutr 2009 Apr;48(Suppl 2):575–578 [PMID: 19300132].

Beggs AD et al: Puetz-Jeghers Syndrome: A systematic review and recommendations for management. Gut 2010 Jul;59(7):975–986 [PMID: 20581245].

Hamartomatous Polyposis Syndromes: Nat Clin Pract Gastroenterol Hepatol. 2007 Sep;4(9):492–502.

CANCERS OF THE ESOPHAGUS, SMALL BOWEL, & COLON

Esophageal cancer is rare in childhood. Cysts, leiomyomas, and hamartomas predominate. Caustic injury of the esophagus increases the very long-term risk of squamous cell carcinoma. Chronic peptic esophagitis is associated with Barrett esophagus, a precancerous lesion. Simple GE reflux in infancy without esophagitis is not a risk for cancer of the esophagus.

The most common gastric or small bowel cancer in children is lymphoma or lymphosarcoma. Intermittent abdominal pain, abdominal mass, intussusception, or a celiac-like picture may be present. Carcinoid tumors are usually benign and most often an incidental finding in the appendix. Metastasis is rare. The carcinoid syndrome (flushing, sweating, hypertension, diarrhea, and vomiting), associated with serotonin secretion, only occurs with metastatic carcinoid tumors.

Adenocarcinoma of the colon is rare in childhood. The transverse colon and rectosigmoid are the two most commonly affected sites. The low 5-year survival rate relates to the nonspecificity of presenting complaints and the large percentage of undifferentiated types. Children with a family history of colon cancer, chronic ulcerative colitis, or familial polyposis syndromes are at greater risk.

MESENTERIC CYSTS

These rare tumors may be small or large, single or multiloculated. They are thin-walled and contain serous, chylous, or hemorrhagic fluid. They are commonly located in the small bowel mesentery but are also found in the mesocolon. Most mesenteric cysts cause no symptoms. Traction on the mesentery may lead to colicky abdominal pain, which can be mild and recurrent but may appear acutely with vomiting. Volvulus may occur around a cyst, and hemorrhage into a cyst may be mild or hemodynamically significant. A rounded mass can occasionally be palpated or seen on radiograph displacing adjacent intestine. Abdominal ultrasonography is usually diagnostic. Surgical removal is indicated.

Tan JJ: Mesenteric cysts: An institution experience over 14 years and review of the literature. Worl J Surg 2009 Sep;33(9):1961–1965 [PMID: 19609826].

INTESTINAL HEMANGIOMA

Hemangiomas of the bowel may cause acute or chronic blood loss. They may also cause intussusception, local stricture, or intramural hematoma. Thrombocytopenia and consumptive coagulopathy are occasional complications. Some lesions are telangiectasias (Rendu-Osler-Weber syndrome), and others are capillary hemangiomas. The largest group is cavernous hemangiomas, which are composed of large, thin-walled vessels arising from the submucosal vascular plexus. They may protrude into the lumen as polypoid lesions or may invade the intestine from mucosa to serosa.

MAJOR GASTROINTESTINAL SYMPTOMS & SIGNS

ACUTE DIARRHEA

Viruses are the most common cause of acute gastroenteritis in developing and developed countries. Bacterial and parasitic enteric infections are discussed in Chapters 42 and 43. Of the viral agents causing enteric infection, rotavirus, a 67-nm double-stranded RNA virus with at least eight serotypes, is the most common. As with most viral pathogens, rotavirus affects the small intestine, causing voluminous watery diarrhea without leukocytes or blood. In the United States, rotavirus primarily affects infants between 3 and 15 months of age. The peak incidence in the United States is in the winter with sporadic cases occurring at other times. The virus is transmitted via the fecal-oral route and survives for hours on hands and for days on environmental surfaces.

1. Rotavirus Infection

The incubation period for rotavirus is 1–3 days. Symptoms caused by rotavirus are similar to other viral pathogens. Vomiting is the first symptom in 80%–90% of patients, followed within 24 hours by low-grade fever and watery diarrhea. Diarrhea usually lasts 4–8 days but may last longer in young infants or immunocompromised patients. Rotavirus cannot be definitively diagnosed on clinical grounds alone. Rotavirus antigens can be identified in stool or virus can be seen by scanning electron microscopy. The specific identification of rotavirus is not required in every case, however, as treatment is nonspecific. Additionally laboratory testing is also generally unnecessary, but when obtained will usually show a normal white blood cell count. As patients become dehydrated due to unreplaced fecal water loss, they may become hypernatremic. Metabolic acidosis can occur from bicarbonate loss in the stool, ketosis from poor intake, and in severe cases, lactic acidemia occurs from hypotension and hypoperfusion. Stools do not contain blood or white blood cells.

Treatment is nonspecific and supportive, aimed at replacement of fluid and electrolyte deficits, along with ongoing losses, especially in small infants. (Oral and intravenous therapy are discussed in Chapter 45.) The use of oral rehydration solutions is appropriate in most cases. The use of clear liquids or hypocaloric (dilute formula) diets for more than 48 hours is not advisable. Early initiation of refeeding is recommended. Intestinal lactase levels are reduced during rotavirus infection. Therefore, the brief use of a lactose-free diet is associated with a shorter period of diarrhea but is not critical to successful recovery in healthy infants. Reduced fat intake during recovery may decrease nausea and vomiting.

Antidiarrheal medications are ineffective (kaolin-pectin combinations) and in some circumstances can be dangerous (loperamide, tincture of opium, diphenoxylate with atropine). Bismuth subsalicylate preparations may reduce stool volume but are not critical to recovery. Oral immunoglobulin or specific antiviral agents have occasionally been useful in limiting duration of disease in immunocompromised patients.

Most children are infected with rotavirus more than once, with the first infection being the most severe. Some protective immunity is imparted by the first infection. Prevention of infection occurs primarily by good hygiene and prevention of fecal-oral contamination. As treatment for rotavirus is nonspecific, prevention of illness is critical. The American Academy of Pediatrics issued guidelines in January 2007 recommending the routine use of bovine-based pentavalent rotavirus vaccine to be given orally to infants at 2, 4, and 6 months of age.

2. Other Viral Infections Causing Acute Diarrhea

Other viral pathogens causing diarrhea in children can be identified in stool by electron microscopy, viral culture, or enzyme-linked immunoassay. Depending on the geographic location, enteric adenoviruses (serotypes 40 and 41) or caliciviruses are the next most common viral pathogens in infants. The symptoms of enteric adenovirus infection are similar to those of rotavirus, but infection is not seasonal and the duration of illness may be longer. The Norwalk agent (now called norovirus), a calicivirus, is a small RNA virus that mainly causes vomiting but can also cause diarrhea in older children and adults, usually in common source outbreaks. The duration of symptoms is short, usually 24–48 hours. Other potentially pathogenic viruses include astroviruses, corona-like viruses, and other small round viruses.

Cytomegalovirus rarely causes diarrhea in immunocompetent children but may cause erosive colitis or enteritis in immunocompromised hosts. Cytomegalovirus enteritis is particularly common after solid organ and bone marrow transplantation and in the late stages of HIV infection. Probiotics are moderately effective in treating acute viral gastroenteritis in healthy children. Probiotics should be used with extreme caution, however, in immunocompromised, chronically debilitated, or seriously ill children.

American Academy of Pediatrics Committee on Infectious Diseases: Prevention of rotavirus disease: Guidelines for the use of rotavirus vaccine. Pediatrics 2007;119:171 [PMID: 17200286].

Bernstein DT: Rotavirus overview. Pediatric Infect Dis J 2009 March;28(Suppl 3):S50–S53 [PMID: 19252423].

DW Thomas et al: Probiotics and prebiotics in pediatrics. Pediatrics 2010 Dec;126(6):1217–1231.

O'Ryan M et al: An update on management of severe acute infectious gastroenteritis in children. Expert Rev Anti Infect Ther 2010 Jun; 8(6):671–682 [PMID: 20521895].

CHRONIC DIARRHEA

Bowel habits are variable, making the specific diagnosis of chronic diarrhea difficult. Some healthy infants may have 5–8 stools daily. A gradual or sudden increase in the number and volume of stools to more than 15 g/kg/d combined with an increase in fluidity should raise a suspicion that an organic cause of chronic diarrhea is present. Diarrhea may result from (1) interruption of normal cell transport processes for water, electrolytes, or nutrients; (2) decrease in surface area available for absorption secondary to shortened bowel or mucosal disease; (3) increase in intestinal motility; (4) increase in unabsorbable osmotically active molecules in the intestinal lumen; (5) increase in intestinal permeability, leading to increased loss of water and electrolytes; and (6) stimulation of enterocyte secretion by toxins or cytokines. The most common entities causing chronic diarrhea are listed below. Malabsorption syndromes, which also cause chronic or recurrent diarrhea, are considered separately.

1. Causes of Chronic Diarrhea

A. Antibiotic Therapy

Diarrhea is reported in up to 60% of children receiving antibiotics. Only a small fraction of these patients have *C difficile*–related pseudomembranous enterocolitis. Eradication of normal gut flora and overgrowth of other organisms may cause antibiotic associated diarrhea. Most antibiotic-associated diarrhea is watery, is not associated with systemic symptoms, and decreases when antibiotic therapy is stopped. Recent data suggests that the use of probiotics may decrease the incidence and severity of this diarrhea by helping to restore intestinal microbial balance.

B. Extraintestinal Infections

Infections of the urinary tract and upper respiratory tract (especially otitis media) are at times associated with diarrhea, though the mechanism is incompletely understood. Antibiotic treatment of the primary infection, toxins released by infecting organisms, and local irritation of the rectum (in patients with bladder infection) may play a role.

C. Malnutrition

Malnutrition is associated with an increased frequency of enteral infections. Decreased bile acid synthesis, decreased pancreatic enzyme output, decreased disaccharidase activity, altered motility, and changes in the intestinal flora all may contribute to diarrhea. In addition, severely malnourished children are at higher risk of enteric infections because of depressed immune functions, both cellular and humoral.

D. Diet and Medications

Overfeeding may cause diarrhea, especially in young infants. Relative deficiency of pancreatic amylase in young infants causes osmotic diarrhea after starchy foods. Fruit juices, especially those high in fructose or sorbitol, produce diarrhea because these osmotically active sugars are poorly absorbed. Intestinal irritants (spices and foods high in fiber) and histamine-containing or histamine-releasing foods (eg, citrus fruits, tomatoes, fermented cheeses, red wines, and scombroid fish) may also cause diarrhea.

Laxative abuse in association with eating disorders or Münchausen syndrome by proxy can cause unpredictable diarrhea. A high concentration of magnesium in the stool may indicate overuse of milk of magnesia or other magnesium-containing laxatives. Detection of other laxative preparations in the stool or circulation requires sophisticated analysis not available in most laboratories. A high index of suspicion and careful observation may be required to make this diagnosis.

E. Allergic Diarrhea

Diarrhea resulting from allergy to dietary proteins is a frequently entertained but rarely proven diagnosis. Gastrointestinal symptoms from cow's milk protein allergy are more common in infants younger than age 12 months. See Diarrhea section 7.

In contrast to the self limited cow's milk protein allergy of infancy, infants and older children may develop more severe diarrhea caused by a systemic allergic reaction. For instance, food protein induced enterocolitis syndrome (FPIES) is a life-threatening condition occurring during infancy manifested by large volume diarrhea, acidosis, and shock as a result of an allergic reaction to common food proteins such as milk and soy. Patients require hospitalization for volume resuscitation and strict avoidance of allergens. Reintroduction of allergens should be performed in a controlled setting by an experienced allergist.

Older children may develop a celiac-like syndrome secondary to milk protein resulting in flattening of small bowel villi, steatorrhea, hypoproteinemia, occult blood loss, and chronic diarrhea. Skin testing is not reliable since it detects circulating antibodies, not the T-cell–mediated responses that are probably responsible for food sensitivity reactions. Double-blind oral challenge with the suspected food under careful observation is often necessary to confirm this intestinal protein allergy. Small bowel biopsy findings are nonspecific. The diagnosis is often confirmed by either double-blind oral challenge with the suspected food or dietary elimination of the food followed by disappearance of occult blood in the stool and improvement in other symptoms. Consultation with an allergist is recommended for long-term management of patients with this disease.

Anaphylactic, IgE-mediated reactions to foods can occur in both young and older children. After ingestion, the patient quickly develops vomiting, then diarrhea, pallor, and hypotension. In these cases, RAST and skin testing is positive. Food challenges should be undertaken in a setting in which resuscitation can be performed as there is often a progressively more severe reaction with subsequent ingestions. The close association between ingestion and symptoms usually leaves little doubt about the diagnosis.

F. Chronic Nonspecific Diarrhea

Chronic nonspecific diarrhea, also called toddler's diarrhea, is the most common cause of loose stools in otherwise thriving children. The typical patient is a healthy, thriving child aged 6–20 months who has three to six loose stools per day during the waking hours. They do not have blood in their stools. They grow normally and may have a family history of functional bowel disease. No organic etiology is found for their diarrhea, with stool tests for blood, white blood cells, fat, parasites, and bacterial pathogens being negative. Diarrhea may worsen with a low-residue, low-fat, or high-carbohydrate diet and during periods of stress and infection. Excessive fruit juice ingestion seems to worsen symptoms. This syndrome resolves spontaneously usually by age 3½ years. Possible causes of this diarrhea include abnormalities of bile acid absorption in the terminal ileum, excess intake of osmotically active carbohydrates and abnormal motor function. A change in dietary fiber (either increasing fiber if deficient or decreasing fiber if excessive), a slight increase in dietary fat, and restriction of osmotically active carbohydrates like fruit juices will usually help control symptoms. If these measures fail, loperamide (0.1–0.2 mg/kg/d in two or three divided doses) can be used as needed for symptomatic relief.

G. Immunologic Causes of Chronic Diarrhea

Chronic diarrhea is common in immune deficiency states, especially IgA deficiency and T-cell abnormalities. The causes of the diarrhea include common bacterial, viral, fungal, or parasitic organisms usually considered nonpathogenic (rotavirus, *Blastocystis hominis, Candida*), or unusual organisms (cytomegalovirus, *Cryptosporidium, Isospora belli, Mycobacterium* spp, microsporidia).

Between 50% and 60% of patients with idiopathic acquired hypogammaglobulinemia have steatorrhea and intestinal villous atrophy. Lymphonodular hyperplasia of the small intestine is also prominent. Patients with congenital or Bruton-type agammaglobulinemia usually have diarrhea and abnormal intestinal morphology. Patients with isolated IgA deficiency have chronic diarrhea, a celiac disease like picture, lymphoid nodular hyperplasia, and are prone to giardiasis. Patients with isolated defects of cellular immunity, combined cellular and humoral immune incompetence, and HIV infection may have severe chronic diarrhea leading to malnutrition but often the cause cannot be identified. Chronic granulomatous disease may be associated with intestinal symptoms suggestive of chronic inflammatory bowel disease. Specific treatments are available for many of the unusual pathogens causing diarrhea in the immunocompromised host. Thus, a vigorous diagnostic search for specific pathogens is warranted in these individuals. In addition, treatment must be directed toward correcting the immunologic defect.

H. Other Causes of Chronic Diarrhea

Most infections of the GI tract are acute and resolve spontaneously or with specific antibiotic therapy. Organisms most prone to cause chronic or recurrent diarrhea in immunocompetent children are *Giardia lamblia, Entameba histolytica, Salmonella* species, and *Yersinia*. Infection with these organisms requires a small innoculum. Some patients may develop a postinfectious diarrhea, with persistent diarrhea present despite the eradication of the offending organism, either viral or bacterial. Bacterial overgrowth of the small bowel in patients with short bowel syndrome, those undergoing chemotherapy, or with anatomic abnormalities may experience chronic diarrhea.

Pancreatic insufficiency due to cystic fibrosis or Shwachman–Diamond Syndrome may result in chronic diarrhea, typically in conjunction with failure to thrive. Certain extremely rare malignancies of childhood (neuroblastoma, ganglioneuroma, metastatic carcinoid, pancreatic VIPoma, or gastrinoma) may secrete substances such as gastrin and vasoactive intestinal polypeptide (VIP) that promote small intestinal secretion of water and electrolytes. Children may present with large volume, chronic and intermittent watery diarrhea that does not cease when they discontinue oral feedings.

Dennehy PH: Acute diarrheal disease in children: Epidemiology, prevention, and treatment. Infect Dis Clin North Am 2005 Sept;19(3):585–602 [PMID: 16102650].

Grimwood K et al: Acute and persistent diarrhea. Pediatr Clin North Am 2009 Dec;56(6):1343–1361 [PMID: 19962025].

Ramaswamy K et al: Infectious diarrhea in children. Gastro Clin North America 2001 Sept;30(3):611–624 [PMID: 11586548].

GASTROINTESTINAL BLEEDING

Vomiting blood and passing blood per rectum are alarming symptoms. The history, physical examination, and initial evaluation are key to identifying the bleeding source. In large volume, acute gastrointestinal (GI) bleeding, the primary focus, however, should first center on stabilizing the patient to ensure adequate hemodynamic support.

History

The first goal of the history is to determine if GI bleeding is truly blood, and if the source is the GI tract. A number of substances simulate hematochezia or melena (Table 21–5). The presence of blood should be confirmed chemically with guiac testing. Coughing, tonsillitis, lost teeth, menarche, or epistaxis may cause what appears to be occult or overt GI bleeding. A careful history of the specifics surrounding the bleeding is critical. Is the blood in emesis, stool, or both? How much blood is there and what is its color and character? History of NSAID use and other medications should be ascertained. Inquiry about associated dysphagia, epigastric pain, or retrosternal pain should be made and, if present, suggest gastroesophageal reflux or a peptic cause of bleeding. Table 21-6 gives further cues in the presentation to help identify the source of bleeding.

Other important aspects of the history include foreign body/caustic ingestion, history of chronic illnesses (especially liver/biliary disease), personal or family history of food allergy/atopy, current and recent medications, associated symptoms (pain, vomiting, diarrhea, fever, weight loss), and family history of GI disorders (IBD, celiac disease, liver disease, bleeding/coagulation disorder). In addition to these historical features, the age of the patient offers additional clues to determine the likely etiology. Table 21–6 lists causes of gastrointestinal bleeding by age and presentation.

Table 21–5. Identification of sites of gastrointestinal bleeding.

Symptom or Sign	Location of Bleeding Lesion
Effortless bright red blood from the mouth	Nasopharyngeal or oral lesions; tonsillitis; esophageal varices; lacerations of esophageal or gastric mucosa (Mallory-Weiss syndrome)
Vomiting of bright red blood or of "coffee grounds"	Lesion proximal to ligament of Treitz
Melanotic stool	Lesion proximal to ligament of Treitz, upper small bowel. Blood loss in excess of 50–100 mL/24 h
Bright red or dark red blood in stools	Lesion in the ileum or colon. (Massive upper gastrointestinal bleeding may also be associated with bright red blood in stool.)
Streak of blood on outside of a stool	Lesion in the rectal ampulla or anal canal

Physical Examination

The most important aspect of the examination and initial assessment is to determine if the child is acutely or chronically ill and initiate supportive measures as rapidly as necessary. The physical examination should be thorough. Physical signs of portal hypertension, intestinal obstruction, or coagulopathy are particularly important. The nasal passages should be inspected for signs of recent epistaxis, the vagina for menstrual blood, and the anus for fissures and hemorrhoids. Skin exam should assess for hemangiomas, eczema, petechiae, or purpura.

A systolic blood pressure below 100 mm Hg and a pulse rate above 100 beats/min in an older child suggest at least a 20% reduction of blood volume. A pulse rate increase of 20 beats/min or a drop in systolic blood pressure greater than 10 mm Hg when the patient sits up is also a sensitive index of volume depletion. Tachycardia may be the initial indication of persistent bleeding.

Laboratory Findings

Initial laboratory investigations should include a CBC, PT, and PTT, at minimum. In specific cases it may be prudent to add a liver profile (with suspected variceal bleeding), ESR/CRP (with possible inflammatory bowel disease), BUN/Creatinine (for possible hemolytic uremic syndrome), stool culture/*C difficile* toxin assay (for acute bloody diarrhea suggestive of infectious colitis). Low MCV in association with anemia suggests chronic GI losses and may warrant addition of iron studies as well. Serial determination of vital signs and hematocrit are essential to assess ongoing bleeding. Detection of blood in the gastric aspirate confirms a bleeding site proximal to the ligament of Treitz. However, its absence does not rule out the duodenum as the source. Testing the stool for occult blood will help in monitoring ongoing loss of blood.

Imaging Studies

In infants with acute onset of bloody stools, multiple-view plain X-rays of the abdomen are helpful in assessing for

Table 21–6. Differential diagnosis of gastrointestinal bleeding in children by symptoms and age at presentation.

	Infant	Child (2–12 y)	Adolescent (> 12 y)
Hematemesis	Swallowed maternal blood Peptic esophagitis Mallory-Weiss tear Gastritis Gastric ulcer Duodenal ulcer	Epistaxis Peptic esophagitis Caustic ingestion Mallory-Weiss tear Esophageal varices Gastritis Gastric ulcer Duodenal ulcer Hereditary hemorrhagic telangiectasia Hemobilia Henoch-Schönlein purpura	Esophageal ulcer Peptic esophagitis Mallory-Weiss tear Esophageal varices Gastric ulcer Gastritis Duodenal ulcer Hereditary hemorrhagic telangiectasia Hemobilia Henoch-Schönlein purpura
Painless melena	Duodenal ulcer Duodenal duplication Ileal duplication Meckel diverticulum Gastric heterotopia[a]	Duodenal ulcer Duodenal duplication Ileal duplication Meckel diverticulum Gastric heterotopia[a]	Duodenal ulcer Leiomyoma (sarcoma)
Melena with pain, obstruction, peritonitis, perforation	Necrotizing enterocolitis Intussusception[b] Volvulus	Duodenal ulcer Hemobilia[c] Intussusception[b] Volvulus Ileal ulcer (isolated)	Duodenal ulcer Hemobilia[c] Crohn disease (ileal ulcer)
Hematochezia with diarrhea, crampy abdominal pain	Infectious colitis Pseudomembranous colitis Eosinophilic colitis Hirschsprung enterocolitis	Infectious colitis Pseudomembranous colitis Granulomatous (Crohn) colitis Hemolytic-uremic syndrome Henoch-Schönlein purpura Lymphonodular hyperplasia	Infectious colitis Pseudomembranous colitis Granulomatous (Crohn) colitis Hemolytic-uremic syndrome Henoch-Schönlein purpura
Hematochezia without diarrhea or abdominal pain	Anal fissure Eosinophilic colitis Rectal gastric mucosa heterotopia Colonic hemangiomas	Anal fissure Solitary rectal ulcer Juvenile polyp Lymphonodular hyperplasia	Anal fissure Hemorrhoid Solitary rectal ulcer Colonic arteriovenous malformation

[a]Ectopic gastric tissue in jejunum or ileum without Meckel diverticulum.
[b]Classically, "currant jelly" stool.
[c]Often accompanied by vomiting and right upper quadrant pain.
Reproduced, with permission, from Treem WR: Gastrointestinal bleeding in children. Gastrointest Endosc Clin North Am 1994;4:75.

pneumatosis intestinalis or signs of obstruction. Children less than two, with a history and examination suggestive of intussusception, should undergo air or water-soluble contrast enema. Painless, large volume bleeding may prompt performance of a ^{99}Tc-pertectnetate nuclear scan to assess for a Meckel diverticulum. Pretreatment with a histamine-2-receptor antagonist may be helpful in increasing the sensitivity of this study; however, a negative scan does not preclude the diagnosis. CT scan of the abdomen with oral and IV contrast may be indicated to look for structural and inflammatory causes of bleeding. Persistent bleeding without a clear source may prompt consideration of a radioisotope tagged RBC scan with technetium ^{99m}Tc -sulfur colloid, though the bleeding must be active at the time of the study, with a rate of at least 0.1 mL/min. Angiography is generally less sensitive, requiring 1–2 mL/min.

Treatment

In severe bleeding, the ABC's of resuscitation should be performed. Adequate IV access is critical in these cases to ensure fluid boluses and blood products are able to be delivered. If a hemorrhagic diathesis is detected, vitamin K should be given intravenously and additional blood products should be administered as needed to correct any underlying coagulopathy. In severe bleeding, the need for volume replacement is monitored by measurement of central venous pressure. In less severe cases, vital signs, serial hematocrits, and gastric aspirates are sufficient.

In suspected upper GI bleeding, gastric lavage with saline should be performed but there is no value of lavage in controlling bleeding. After stabilization, upper intestinal endoscopy may be considered to identify the bleeding site. Endoscopy is superior to barium contrast study for lesions such as esophageal varices, stress ulcers, and gastritis. Acid suppression with intravenous histamine-2-antagonists or, preferably proton pump inhibitors, may be helpful in suspected peptic causes of bleeding. Colonoscopy may identify the source of bright red rectal bleeding but should be performed as an emergency procedure only if the extent of bleeding warrants immediate investigation and if plain abdominal radiographs show no signs of intestinal obstruction. Colonoscopy on an unprepped colon is often inadequate for making a diagnosis. Capsule endoscopy may help identify the site of bleeding if colonoscopy and upper endoscopy findings are negative. Push or balloon enteroscopy may be helpful to perform therapeutic interventions, obtain biopsies or mark small bowel lesions (prior to laparotomy/laparoscopy) identified on capsule endoscopy.

Persistent vascular bleeding (varices [see Figure 21–7], vascular anomalies) may be relieved temporarily using intravenous octreotide, 1–4 μg/kg/h. Sustained infusion of octreotide may be used for up to 48 hours if needed with careful monitoring of glucose homeostasis. Bleeding from esophageal varices may be stopped by compression with a Sengstaken-Blakemore tube. Endoscopic sclerosis or banding of bleeding varices is effective treatment.

If gastric decompression, acid suppressive therapy, and transfusion are ineffective in stopping ulcer bleeding, endoscopic therapy with argon plasma coagulation, local injection of epinephrine, electrocautery, or application of hemostatic clips may be employed. If bleeding remains refractory to therapy, emergency surgery may be necessary.

Boyle JT: Gastrointestinal bleeding in infants and children. Pediatr Rev 2008;29(2):39–52 [PMID: 18245300].

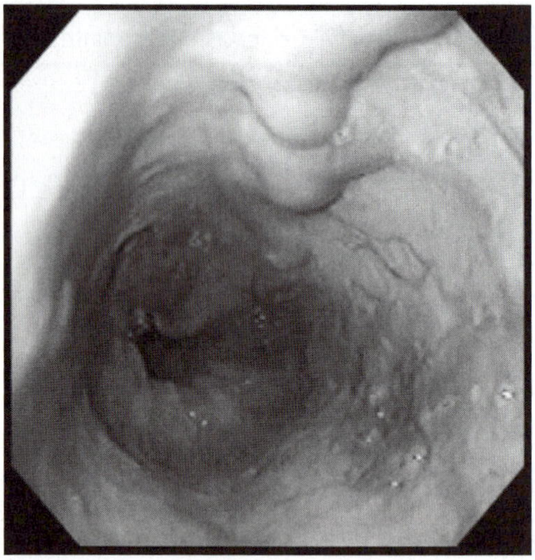

▲ **Figure 21–7.** Esophageal varices. Serpiginous esophageal varix extending to the esophageal lower esophageal sphincter.

VOMITING

Vomiting is an extremely complex activity. The centers controlling and coordinating vomiting are in the paraventricular nuclei of the brain. These nuclei receive afferent input from many sources, including drugs and neurotransmitters in cerebrospinal fluid, the chemoreceptor trigger zone (CTZ) near the distal fourth ventricle, the vestibular apparatus of the ear, the GI tract and other abdominal organs, and even from higher cortical areas. Vagal afferents from the gut to brain are stimulated by ingested drugs and toxins, mechanical stretch, inflammation, and local neurotransmitters. Additionally, local feedback loops in the gut also appear capable of initiating vomiting.

Vomiting is the presenting symptom of many pediatric conditions. It is the pediatrician's difficult job to find the underlying cause. The most common cause of vomiting in childhood is probably acute viral gastroenteritis. However, obstruction and acute or chronic inflammation of the GI tract and associated structures are also major causes. Central nervous system inflammation, pressure, or tumor may cause vomiting. Metabolic derangements associated with inborn errors of metabolism, sepsis, and drug intoxication can stimulate either the CTZ or the brain directly to promote vomiting. Regurgitation associated with GE reflux of infants should be distinguished from vomiting. In this instance, spontaneous relaxation of the lower esophageal sphincter creates a common cavity between the stomach and esophagus. Because the resting pressure of the thorax is negative, the mildly positive pressure of the abdominal cavity (~ 6 mm Hg) pushes gastric contents into the esophagus, causing an effortless flow into the mouth. Occasionally, regurgitated fluid stimulates the pharyngeal afferents and provokes gagging or even a complete vomiting complex.

Control of vomiting with medication is rarely necessary in acute gastroenteritis, but may relieve vomiting and decrease the need for intravenous fluids and/or hospitalization. Antihistamines and anticholinergics are appropriate for motion sickness because of their labyrinthine effects. 5-HT_3 receptor antagonists (ondansetron, granisetron) are useful for vomiting associated with surgery and chemotherapy. Benzodiazepines, corticosteroids, and substituted benzamides are also used in chemotherapy-induced vomiting. Butyrophenones (droperidol, haloperidone) are powerful drugs that block the D2 receptor in the CTZ and are used for intractable vomiting in acute gastritis, chemotherapy, and after surgery. Phenothiazines are helpful in chemotherapy, cyclic vomiting, and acute GI infection but are not recommended for outpatient use because of extrapyramidal side effects.

Levine DA: Anti-emetics for acute gastroenteritis in children. Curr Opin Pediatr 2009 Jun;21(3);294–298 [PMID: 19381093].

DeCamp LR et al: Use of anti-emetic agents in acute gastroenteritis: A systematic review and meta-analysis. Arch Pediatr Adolesc Med 2008 Sep;162(9):858–865 [PMID: 18762604].

1. Cyclic Vomiting Syndrome

Clinical Findings

Cyclic vomiting syndrome (CVS) is characterized by recurrent episodes of stereotypical vomiting in children usually older than 1 year of age. The emesis is forceful and frequent, occurring up to six times per hour for up to 72 hours or more. Episode frequency ranges from two to three per month to less than one per year. Nausea, retching, and small-volume bilious emesis continue even after the stomach is emptied. Hematemesis secondary to forceful vomiting may occur. Patients experience abdominal pain, anorexia, and rarely, diarrhea. Autonomic symptoms, such as pallor, sweating, temperature instability, and lethargy are common and give the patient a very ill appearance. The episodes end suddenly, often after a period of sleep. In some children, dehydration, electrolyte imbalance, and shock may occur. Between episodes, the child is completely healthy.

The cause of CVS is unknown; however, a relationship to migraine headaches has long been recognized. Family history is positive for migraine in 50%–70% of cases and many patients develop migraine headaches as adults. Research suggests that abnormalities of neurotransmitters and hormones provoke CVS. About one quarter of patients have typical migraine symptoms during episodes: premonitory sensation, headache, photophobia, and phonophobia. Identifiable triggers include infection, positive or negative emotional stress, diet (chocolate, cheese, monosodium glutamate), menses, or motion sickness.

Differential Diagnosis

Conditions that mimic CVS include drug toxicity, increased intracranial pressure, seizures, brain tumor, Chiari malformation, recurrent sinusitis, choledochal cyst, gallstones, recurrent small bowel obstruction, inflammatory bowel disease, familial pancreatitis, obstructive uropathy, recurrent urinary infection, diabetes, mitochondrial diseases, disorders of fatty and organic acid metabolism, adrenal insufficiency, and Münchausen syndrome by proxy. Although tests for GE reflux are often positive in these patients, it is unlikely that GE reflux and CVS are related.

Treatment

Avoidance of triggers prevents episodes in some patients. Sleep can also end an episode although some children awaken and resume vomiting. Diphenhydramine or lorazepam is used at the onset of spells in some children to reduce nausea and induce sleep. Early use of antimigraine medications (sumatriptan), antiemetics (ondansetron), or antihistamines can abort spells in some patients. Once a spell is well established, intravenous fluids are often required to end it. With careful supervision, some children with predictable spells can receive intravenous fluids at home. Several approaches usually are tried before an effective therapy is found. Preventing spells with prophylactic propranolol, amitriptyline, or antihistamines is effective in some patients with frequent or disabling spells. Some patients have been successfully treated with anticonvulsants.

Sudel B, Li BU: Treatment options for cyclic vomiting syndrome. Curr Treat Options Gastroenterol 2005;8:387 [PMID: 16162304].

RECURRENT ABDOMINAL PAIN

Approximately 2%–4% of all pediatric office visits occur because of unexplained, recurrent abdominal pain. In addition, up to 17% of adolescents have been reported to have recurrent abdominal pain. Based on the Rome III criteria, the descriptive term "recurrent abdominal pain" has been discarded for the more meaningful term "functional abdominal pain," which encompasses four entities: functional dyspepsia, irritable bowel syndrome, abdominal migraines, and functional abdominal pain not otherwise specified.

Clinical Findings

A. Symptoms and Signs

Children with functional abdominal pain experience recurrent attacks of abdominal pain or discomfort at least once per week for at least 2 months. Attacks of pain are of variable duration and intensity. Parents or patients commonly report that the pain is constant, all day, every day. The pain is usually localized to the periumbilical area, but may also be more generalized. The pain occurs primarily during the day, but may prevent children from falling to sleep at night. The pain may be associated with pallor, nausea, or vomiting. The pain may also be associated with dramatic reactions such as frantic crying, clutching the abdomen, and doubling over. Parents may become alarmed, and take their children into the emergency departments, where the evaluation is negative for an acute abdomen. School attendance may suffer, and enjoyable family events may be disrupted.

Alarm symptoms that would suggest a more severe organic etiology are absent. These include dysphagia, persistent vomiting, gastrointestinal blood loss, pain leading to night awakening, rashes or joint aches. In addition, these children do not have a history of unintentional weight loss or fevers.

Functional abdominal pain usually bears little relationship to bowel habits and physical activity. However, some patients have a symptom constellation suggestive of irritable bowel syndrome, including bloating, postprandial pain, lower abdominal discomfort, and erratic stool habits with a sensation of obstipation or incomplete evacuation of stool. A precipitating or stressful situation in the child's life at the time the pains began can sometimes be elicited. School phobia may be a precipitant. A history of functional GI complaints is often found in family members. A family history, however, of inflammatory bowel disease, peptic ulcer disease, and celiac disease is absent.

A thorough physical examination that includes a rectal examination is essential and usually normal. Complaints of abdominal tenderness elicited during palpation may be out of proportion to visible signs of distress.

B. Laboratory Findings

Complete blood count, sedimentation rate, and stool test for occult blood are usually a sufficient evaluation. Extraintestinal sources such as kidney, spleen, and genitourinary tract may require assessment. In the adolescent female patient, ultrasound of the abdomen and pelvis may be helpful to detect gallbladder or ovarian pathology. If the pain is atypical, further testing suggested by symptoms and family history should be done. This may include additional imaging studies or endoscopic analysis.

Differential Diagnosis

Abdominal pain secondary to disorders causing acute abdomen are listed in Table 21–7. Pinworms, mesenteric lymphadenitis, and chronic appendicitis are improbable causes of recurrent abdominal pain. *H pylori* infection does not cause recurrent abdominal pain. Lactose intolerance usually causes abdominal distention, gas, and diarrhea with milk ingestion. At times, however, abdominal discomfort may be the only symptom. Abdominal migraine and cyclic vomiting are rare conditions with an episodic character often associated with vomiting. The incidence of peptic gastritis, esophagitis, duodenitis, and ulcer disease is probably underappreciated.

Treatment & Prognosis

Treatment consists of reassurance based on a thorough history and physical examination and a sympathetic, age-appropriate explanation of the nature of functional pain. The concept of "visceral hyperalgesia" or increased pain signaling from physiologic stimuli such as gas, acid secretion, or stool is one that parents can understand and helps them to respond appropriately to the child's complaints. Reassurance without education is rarely helpful. Regular activity should be resumed, especially school attendance. Therapy for psychosocial stressors, including biofeedback therapy, may be necessary. In older patients, and in those with what appears to be visceral hyperalgesia, amitriptyline in low doses may occasionally be helpful. Antispasmodic medications are rarely helpful and should be reserved for patients with more typical irritable bowel complaints.

Table 21–7. Differential diagnosis of acute abdomen.

Gastrointestinal Causes	**Hepatobiliary Causes**
Appendicitis	Cholecystitis
Bowel Obstruction	Cholangitis
Perforated Ulcer	Hepatic Abscess
Ischemic Colitis	Splenic Rupture
Volvulus	Splenic Infarction
Intussusception	**Urologic/Gynecologic Causes**
Pancreatitis	Acute cystitis
Incarcerated Hernia	Nephrolithiasis
Toxic Megacolon	Ruptured Ectopic Pregnancy
Abdominal Vasculitis	Ovarian Torsion
Intra-abdominal Abscess	Testicular Torsion
Other Causes	Acute salpingitis
Diabetic Ketoacidosis	Pelvic Inflammatory Disease
Lead Poisoning	
Porphyria	
Abdominal Sickle Cell Crisis	

Chiou E et al: Management of functional abdominal pain and irritable bowel syndrome in children and adolescents. Expert Rev Gastroenterol Hepatol 2010 Jun; 4(3):293–304 [PMID; 20528117].

Drossman DA: The functional gastrointestinal disorders and the Rome III process. Gastroenterology 2006;130:1377–1390 [PMID: 16678553].

Grover M: Functional abdominal pain. Curr Gastroenterol Rep 2010 Oct;12(5):391–398 [PMID: 20694840].

Rasquin A et al: Childhood functional gastrointestinal disorders: Child/adolescent. Gastroenterology 2006;130:1527 [PMID: 16678566].

ACUTE ABDOMEN

An acute abdomen is a constellation of findings indicating an intra-abdominal process that may require surgery. A degree of urgency is implied when this diagnosis is suspected. The pain of an acute abdomen intensifies over time and is rarely relieved without definitive treatment. Pain is often accompanied by nausea, vomiting, diarrhea, fever, and anorexia. Pain may be localized or generalized. The abdomen may be distended and tense and bowel sounds reduced or obstructive. Patients appear ill and are reluctant to be examined or moved. The acute abdomen is usually a result of infection of the intra-abdominal or pelvic organs but also occurs with intestinal obstruction, intestinal perforation, inflammatory conditions, trauma, and some metabolic disorders. Some of the conditions causing acute abdomen are listed in Table 21–7. Reaching a timely and accurate diagnosis is critical and requires skill in physical diagnosis, recognition of the symptoms of a large number of conditions, and a judicious selection of laboratory and radiologic tests. (Acute appendicitis is discussed earlier in the section on Disorders of the Small Intestine.)

MALABSORPTION SYNDROMES

Malabsorption of ingested food has many causes (Table 21–8). Shortening of the small bowel (usually via surgical resection) and mucosal damage (celiac disease) both reduce surface area. Impaired motility interferes with normal propulsive

Table 21–8. Malabsorption syndromes.

Intraluminal abnormalities
- Acid hypersecretion (eg, Zollinger-Ellison syndrome)
- Exocrine pancreatic insufficiency:
  - Cystic fibrosis
  - Shwachman syndrome
  - Malnutrition
- Enzyme deficiency
  - Enterokinase deficiency
  - Trypsinogen deficiency
  - Co-lipase deficiency
- Decreased intraluminal bile acids
  - Chronic parenchymal liver disease
  - Biliary obstruction
  - Bile acid loss (short gut, ileal disease)
  - Bile acid deconjugation by bacterial overgrowth

Mucosal abnormalities
- Infection (eg, *Giardia*, *Cryptosporidium*)
- Graft versus host disease
- Mucosal injury:
  - Celiac disease
  - Allergic enteropathy
  - IBD
  - Radiation enteritis
- Enzyme deficiency:
  - Lactase deficiency
  - Sucrase-isomaltase deficiency
- Short bowel syndrome

Vascular abnormalities
- Ischemic bowel:
  - Vasculitis: lupus, mixed connective tissue disorder
  - Congestive heart failure
- Intestinal lymphangiectasia

Metabolic genetic disease
- Abetalipoproteinemia
- Congenital secretory diarrheas
- Lysinuric protein intolerance
- Cystinosis

movements and mixing of food with pancreatic and biliary secretions. Dysmotility also allows anaerobic bacteria proliferation with subsequent bacterial overgrowth and increased carbohydrate fermentation with resultant acidic diarrhea. Another problem of bacterial overgrowth occurs when bacterial deconjugation of bile acids leads to fat malabsorption as seen in intestinal pseudo-obstruction, postoperative blind loop syndrome. Impaired intestinal lymphatic (congenital lymphangiectasia) or venous drainage also causes malabsorption. Diseases reducing pancreatic exocrine function (cystic fibrosis, Shwachman syndrome) or the production and flow of biliary secretions cause nutrient malabsorption. Malabsorption of specific nutrients may be genetically determined (disaccharidase deficiency, glucose-galactose malabsorption, and abetalipoproteinemia).

▶ Clinical Findings

Diarrhea, vomiting, anorexia, abdominal pain, failure to thrive, and abdominal distention are common. Stools associated with fat malabsorption are characterized as bulky, foul, greasy and pale; in contrast, those seen with osmotic diarrhea are loose, watery, and acidic. Stool microscopic examination for neutral fat (pancreatic insufficiency as in cystic fibrosis) and fatty acids (as in mucosal injury, liver disease) may be useful.

Quantifying fat malabsorption requires timed stool collection comparing ingested to excreted fat volume. Stool loss of 10%–15% of ingested fat is normal in infancy, while loss of 5% of ingested fat is normal for 1–10 year olds. Fat soluble vitamin deficiency occurs with long standing fat malabsorption and is manifested by prolonged prothrombin time (vitamin K) and low levels of serum carotene (vitamin A), vitamin E, and vitamin D. Loss of serum proteins across the intestinal mucosa is suggested by elevated fecal α1-antitrypsin levels. Disaccharide or monosaccharide malabsorption manifests by stool pH < 5.5 due to lactic acid and presence of reducing substances in the stool. Specific enzyme deficiencies may be evaluated by breath hydrogen test after ingestion of various carbohydrates, or small intestinal biopsy showing normal histology and measurement of specific disaccharidase activity. Other screening tests suggesting a specific diagnosis include sweat chloride concentration (cystic fibrosis), intestinal mucosal biopsy (celiac disease, lymphangiectasia, inflammatory bowel disease), liver and gallbladder function tests, and pancreatic secretion after stimulation with secretin and cholecystokinin. Some of the most common disorders associated with malabsorption in pediatric patients are detailed below.

1. Protein-Losing Enteropathy

Loss of plasma proteins into the GI tract occurs in association with intestinal inflammation, intestinal graft-versus-host disease, acute and chronic intestinal infections, venous and lymphatic obstruction or malformations, and infiltration of the intestine or its lymphatics and vasculature by malignant cells. Chronic elevation of venous pressure in children with the Fontan procedure and elevated right sided heart pressures may produce protein-losing enteropathy.

▶ Clinical Findings

Signs and symptoms are mainly those caused by hypoproteinemia and in some instances by fat malabsorption: edema, ascites, poor weight gain, anemia, and specific vitamin (fat-soluble vitamins A, D, E, K) and mineral deficiencies. Serum albumin and globulins may be decreased. Fecal α1-antitrypsin is elevated (> 3 mg/g dry weight stool; slightly higher in breast-fed infants). Disorders associated with protein-losing enteropathy are listed in Table 21–9. In the presence of intestinal bleeding, fecal α1-antitrypsin measurements are falsely high.

▶ Differential Diagnosis

Hypoalbuminemia may be due to increased catabolism, poor protein intake, impaired hepatic protein synthesis, or congenital malformations of lymphatics outside the GI tract. Protein losses in the urine from nephritis and nephrotic syndrome may also cause hypoalbuminemia.

▶ Treatment

Albumin infusion, diuretics, and a high-protein, low-fat diet may control symptoms. Nutritional deficiencies should be addressed. Treatment must be directed toward identifying and treating the underlying cause.

Table 21–9. Disorders associated with protein-losing enteropathy.

Cardiac disease
Congestive heart failure
Constrictive pericarditis
Cardiomyopathy
Post-Fontan procedure with elevated right atrial pressure
Lymphatic disease
Primary congenital lymphangiectasia
Secondary lymphangiectasia
Malrotation
Malignancy: lymphoma, retroperitoneal tumor
Other: sarcoid, arsenic poisoning
Inflammation
Giant hypertrophic gastritis (Ménétrier disease), often secondary to cytomegalovirus infection or *Helicobacter pylori*
Infection: TB, C difficile, parasite (eg, Giardia), bacteria (eg, salmonella)
Allergic enteropathy
Celiac disease
Radiation enteritis
Graft-vs.-host disease
Inflammatory Bowel Disease
Hirschprung disease
Necrotizing enterocolitis
Vascular disorders
Systemic lupus erythematosis and mixed connective tissue disorder

2. Celiac Disease (Gluten Enteropathy)

ESSENTIALS OF DIAGNOSIS & TYPICAL FEATURES

- Clinical features suggestive of celiac disease include abdominal distention, diarrhea, fatty stools, failure to thrive, irritability, hypoproteinemia, and edema.
- Serum antibodies to tissue transglutaminase, endomysium, or deamidated gliadin peptides are present.
- Duodenal biopsy shows villous atrophy and increased intraepithelial lymphocytes.
- Clinical improvement on gluten-free diet.

Celiac disease (CD) is an immune-mediated enteropathy triggered by gluten, a protein in wheat, rye, barley, and (rarely) oats. CD presents anytime after gluten is introduced in the diet, with symptoms of abdominal pain, diarrhea, vomiting, distention, and sometimes constipation. Other manifestations include oral ulcers, a pruritic rash (dermatitis herpetiformis), growth and pubertal delay, iron-deficiency anemia, decreased bone mineralization, and arthritis. Disease frequency in Western populations approaches 1 in 100. Associated conditions include type 1 diabetes (4%–10%), Down syndrome (5%–12%), Turner syndrome (4%–8%), IgA deficiency (2%–8%), autoimmune thyroiditis (8%), and family history of CD (5%–10%). Almost all CD patients express HLA-DQ2 or DQ8 tissue antigens.

Clinical Findings

A. Symptoms and Signs

1. Gastrointestinal manifestations—The classic form of CD consists of GI symptoms with onset soon after gluten containing foods are introduced in the diet, usually between 6 and 24 months of age. Chronic diarrhea, abdominal distention, irritability, anorexia, vomiting, and poor weight gain are typical. Celiac crisis, with dehydration, hypotension, hypokalemia, and explosive diarrhea, is rare. Older children may have chronic abdominal pain, chronic constipation, bloating, and diarrhea that mimic symptoms of lactose intolerance, functional abdominal pain, or irritable bowel syndrome.

2. Nongastrointestinal manifestations—Adolescents may present with delayed puberty or short stature, and in females, delayed menarche. CD should be considered in children with unexplained iron-deficiency anemia, decreased bone mineral density, elevated liver function enzymes, arthritis, or epilepsy with cerebral calcifications. A number of asymptomatic children are identified only by screening because of a risk factor, such as having type 1 diabetes or a relative with diabetes or CD. The need for early screening and treatment in asymptomatic individuals is unclear.

B. Laboratory Findings

1. Serologic and genetic testing—Screening tests exist with excellent sensitivity and specificity. In IgA sufficient patients these are the IgA antitissue transglutaminase, IgA antiendomysial and IgA/IgG antideamidated gliadin peptide antibodies. In the presence of IgA deficiency, IgG-based anti-tissue transglutaminase and antiendomysium antibodies are available. Genetic testing for HLA-DQ2 and DQ8 has a high negative predictive value, and is useful in assessing risk for CD in family members, but not for screening for the presence of CD.

2. Stools—Stools may have increased levels of partially digested fat, and may be acidic from secondary lactose intolerance.

3. Hypoproteinemia—Hypoalbuminemia can be severe enough to lead to edema. There is evidence of increased protein loss in the gut lumen and poor hepatic synthesis secondary to malnutrition.

4. Anemia—Anemia with low MCV and evidence of iron deficiency is common.

C. Biopsy Findings

Endoscopic small intestinal biopsy is recommended for diagnosis of celiac disease. Patients should remain on a diet containing gluten until biopsy. Characteristic duodenal biopsy findings on light microscopy are villous atrophy and increased numbers of intraepithelial lymphocytes. The findings may be patchy so multiple biopsies should be obtained and reviewed by an experienced pathologist.

Differential Diagnosis

The differential diagnosis includes disorders causing malabsorption and villous atrophy. These include food allergies, Crohn disease, postinfectious diarrhea, immunodeficiencies, graft versus host disease, and hypergastrinemia (Zollinger-Ellison syndrome).

Treatment

A. Diet

Treatment is dietary gluten restriction for life. All sources of wheat, rye, and barley are eliminated. Most, but not all, patients tolerate oats. The intestinal mucosa should normalize by 6–12 months while lactose intolerance resolves often within a few weeks. Supplemental calories, vitamins, and minerals are indicated only in the acute phase. Celiac disease related antibody titers decrease on a gluten-free diet.

B. Corticosteroids

Corticosteroids are indicated only in patients with celiac crisis with profound anorexia, malnutrition, diarrhea, edema, abdominal distention, and hypokalemia.

Prognosis

Enteropathy-associated T-cell lymphoma of the small bowel occurs with increased frequency in adults with long-standing untreated disease. Individuals with poor adherence to gluten-free diet may be at increased risk for fractures, iron deficiency anemia, and infertility.

Catassi C, Fasano A: Celiac disease diagnosis: Simple rules are better than complicated algorithms. Am J Med 2010 Aug;123(8): 691–693 [PMID: 20670718].

Hill I et al: Guidelines for the diagnosis and treatment of celiac disease in children: Recommendations of the North American Society for Pediatric Gastroenterology, Hepatology and Nutrition. J Pediatr Gastroenterol Nutr 2005;40:1 [PMID: 15625418].

3. Disaccharidase Deficiency

Starches and the disaccharides sucrose and lactose are the most important dietary carbohydrates. Dietary disaccharides and the oligosaccharide products of pancreatic amylase action on starch require hydrolysis by intestinal brush border disaccharidases before absorption takes place. Disaccharidase levels are higher in the jejunum and proximal ileum than in the distal ileum and duodenum. Several features characterize primary disaccharidase deficiency, including the fact that a single enzyme is affected, disaccharide intolerance is permanent, intestinal histologic findings are normal, and a positive family history is common. Because disaccharidases are located on the luminal surface of intestinal enterocytes, they are susceptible to mucosal damage. Many conditions, especially viral enteritis, cause secondary disaccharidase deficiency and lactase is usually the most severely depressed.

A. Lactase Deficiency

Congenital lactase deficiency is extremely rare. All human ethnic groups are lactase-sufficient at birth. Genetic or familial lactase deficiency appears after 5 years of age. In Asians, Alaskan natives, and Native Americans, genetic lactase deficiency develops in virtually 100%. In Africans, the incidence in most tribes is over 80%. In African Americans, the incidence is about 70%, and among Caucasian Americans, the incidence is between 30% and 60%. Acquired or secondary lactase deficiency caused by intestinal injury due to viral infection, inflammatory disease, radiation, and drugs is very common, and may be self-limited resolving within a few weeks after resolution of the acute illness.

Lactose ingestion in deficient individuals causes variable degrees of diarrhea, abdominal distention, flatus, and abdominal pain depending on the residual enzyme activity and the dose of lactose. Stools are liquid or frothy with a pH < 5.5 owing to the presence of organic acids. Reducing substances are present in fresh stools. Diagnostic tests include genetic testing, lactose breath test with a rise in breath hydrogen content due to fermentation of undigested lactose by normal colonic flora, and a lactose load test in which blood glucose fails to rise more than 10 mg/dL after ingestion of 1 g/kg of lactose. Symptoms resolve when dietary lactose is restricted or lactase supplementation is added to milk products or taken with meals to enhance lactose hydrolysis.

B. Sucrase-Isomaltase Deficiency

This condition is inherited in an autosomal recessive fashion and is most common in Greenland, Iceland, and among Alaskan natives. The condition is rare in other groups. Abdominal distention, failure to thrive, and watery diarrhea are the presenting symptoms. Stools are usually watery and acidic. Because sucrose is not a reducing sugar, stool may test negative for reducing substances unless the sucrose is hydrolyzed by colon bacteria. Diagnosis is made by oral sucrose tolerance testing (1 g/kg) with elevated breath hydrogen content, or by testing a snap frozen intestinal biopsy for enzyme activity. There are partial enzyme deficiencies. Treatment is avoidance of sucrose and starches rich in amylopectin, or the use of sacrosidase enzyme supplement.

Treem WR et al: Saccharosidase therapy for congenital sucrase-isomaltase deficiency. J Pediatr Gastroenterol Nutr 1999;28:137 [PMID: 9932843].

www.csidinfo.com

www.ivpcare.com

4. Glucose-Galactose Malabsorption

Glucose-galactose malabsorption is a rare disorder in which the sodium-glucose transport protein is defective. Transport of glucose in the intestinal epithelium and renal tubule is impaired. Diarrhea begins with the first feedings, accompanied by reducing sugar in the stool and acidosis. Small bowel histologic findings are normal. Glycosuria and aminoaciduria may occur. The glucose tolerance test is flat. Fructose is well tolerated. Diarrhea subsides promptly on withdrawal of glucose and galactose from the diet. The acquired form of glucose-galactose malabsorption occurs mainly in infants younger than age 6 months, usually following acute viral or bacterial enteritis.

In the congenital disease, exclusion of glucose and galactose from the diet is mandatory. A satisfactory formula is one with a carbohydrate-free base plus added fructose. The prognosis is good if the disease is diagnosed early, because tolerance for glucose and galactose improves with age. In secondary monosaccharide intolerance, prolonged parenteral nutrition may be required until intestinal transport mechanisms for monosaccharides return.

El-Naggar W et al: Nephrocalcinosis in glucose-galactose malabsorption: Association with renal tubular acidosis. Pediatr Nephrol 2005;20:1336 [PMID: 16010597].

Wright EM et al: Molecular basis for glucose-galactose malabsorption. Cell Biochem Biophys 2002;36:115 [PMID: 12139397].

5. Dietary Fructose Intolerance

Fructose malabsorption occurs when fructose is in excess of glucose, often with consumption of high fructose corn syrup. Malabsorbed fructose is fermented by colonic bacteria and excess hydrogen and other gasses are produced. Symptoms include abdominal pain, bloating, flatulence, and diarrhea. These symptoms may lead to diagnosis of irritable bowel syndrome. The capacity for human fructose absorption has a wide range, and may be inducible by dietary consumption. Diagnosis is made with a fructose breath hydrogen test and is bolstered by the occurrence of symptoms during the test.

Kyaw MH, Mayberry JF: Fructose malabsorption: True condition or a variance from normality. J Clin Gastroenterol 2011 Jan;45(1):16–21 [PMID: 20818234].

6. Intestinal Lymphangiectasia

This form of protein-losing enteropathy results from a congenital ectasia of the bowel lymphatic system often associated with abnormalities of the lymphatics in the extremities. Obstruction of lymphatic drainage of the intestine leads to rupture of the intestinal lacteals with leakage of lymph into the lumen of the bowel. Fat loss in the stool may be significant. Chronic loss of lymphocytes and immunoglobulins increases the susceptibility to infections.

Clinical Findings

Peripheral edema, diarrhea, abdominal distention, chylous effusions, and repeated infections are common. Laboratory findings are reduced serum albumin, decreased immunoglobulin levels, lymphocytopenia, and anemia. Serum calcium and magnesium are frequently depressed as these cations are lost in complex with unabsorbed fatty acids. Lymphocytes may be seen on a stool smear. Fecal α1-antitrypsin is elevated. Radiographic studies reveal an edematous small bowel mucosal pattern, and biopsy findings reveal dilated lacteals in the villi and lamina propria. If only the lymphatics of the deeper layers of bowel or intestinal mesenteries are involved, laparotomy may be necessary to establish the diagnosis. Capsule (camera) endoscopy shows diagnostic brightness secondary to the fat-filled lacteals.

Differential Diagnosis

Other causes of protein-losing enteropathy must be considered, although an associated lymphedematous extremity strongly favors this diagnosis.

Treatment & Prognosis

A high-protein diet (6–7 g/kg/d may be needed) enriched with medium-chain triglycerides as a fat source usually allows for adequate nutrition and growth in patients with intestinal mucosal lymphangiectasia. The serum albumin may not normalize. Vitamin and calcium supplements should be given. Parenteral nutritional supplementation may be needed temporarily. Surgery may be curative if the lesion is localized to a small area of the bowel or in cases of constrictive pericarditis or obstructing tumors. IV albumin and immune globulin may also be used to control symptoms but are usually not needed chronically. The prognosis is not favorable, although remission may occur with age. Malignant degeneration of the abnormal lymphatics may occur, and intestinal lymphoma of the B-cell type may be a long-term complication.

7. Cow's Milk Protein Intolerance

Milk protein intolerance refers to a nonallergic food sensitivity and is more common in males than females and in young infants with a family history of atopy. The estimated prevalence is 0.5%–1.0%. Symptoms may occur while the infant is still exclusively breastfed. The most common form is a healthy infant with flecks of blood in the stool. Infants may present with loose mucoid stools that are blood streaked but otherwise appear well. These symptoms typically occur as a result of cow's milk protein that is either present in formula or breast milk. A family history of atopy is common in these infants. Skin testing is not reliable and not indicated. Treatment consists of eliminating the source of the protein; in the breast-fed infant, maternal avoidance of milk protein will usually reduce signs of colitis. Substituting a protein hydrolysate formula for cow's milk-based formula may reduce symptoms. Allergic colitis in young infants is self-limited, usually disappearing by 8–12 months of age. Since no long-term consequences of this problem have been identified, some suggest that if the symptoms are mild and the infant is thriving, no treatment may be indicated. Colonoscopy is not required for diagnosis, but rectal biopsies, if performed, show mild lymphonodular hyperplasia, mucosal edema, and eosinophilia.

In older children, milk protein sensitivity may induce eosinophilic gastroenteritis with protein-losing enteropathy, iron deficiency, hypoalbuminemia, and hypogammaglobulinemia. A celiac-like syndrome with villous atrophy, malabsorption, hypoalbuminemia, occult blood in the stool, and anemia can occur.

Kneepkens CM, Meijer Y: Clinical practice: Diagnosis and treatment of cow's milk allergy. Eur J Pediatr 2009 Aug;168(8):891–896 [PMID: 19271238].

Xanthakos SA et al: Prevalence and outcome of allergic colitis in healthy infants with rectal bleeding: A prospective cohort study. J Pediatr Gastroenterol Nutr 2005;41:16–22 [PMID: 15990624].

8. Pancreatic Insufficiency

The most common cause of pancreatic exocrine insufficiency in childhood is cystic fibrosis. Decreased secretion of pancreatic digestive enzymes is caused by obstruction of the exocrine ducts by thick secretions, which destroys pancreatic acinar cells. Destruction of acinar cells may occur before birth. Some genotypes of cystic fibrosis have partially or completely preserved pancreatic exocrine function. Other conditions associated with exocrine pancreatic insufficiency are discussed in Chapter 22.

9. Other Genetic Disorders Causing Malabsorption

A. Abetalipoproteinemia

Abetalipoproteinemia is an autosomal recessive condition in which the secretion of triglyceride-rich lipoproteins from the small intestine (chylomicrons) and liver (very low-density lipoproteins) is abnormal. Profound steatosis of the intestinal enterocytes (and hepatocytes) and severe fat malabsorption occur. Deficiencies of fat-soluble vitamins develop with neurologic complications of vitamin E deficiency and atypical retinitis pigmentosa. Serum cholesterol level is very low, and red cell membrane lipids are abnormal, causing acanthosis of red blood cells, which may be the key to diagnosis.

B. Acrodermatitis Enteropathica

Acrodermatitis enteropathica is an autosomal recessive condition in which the intestine has a selective inability to absorb zinc. The condition usually becomes obvious at the time of weaning from breast feeding and is characterized by rash on the extremities, rashes around the body orifices, eczema, profound failure to thrive, steatorrhea, diarrhea, and immune deficiency. Zinc supplementation by mouth results in rapid improvement.

INFLAMMATORY BOWEL DISEASE

General Considerations

Inflammatory bowel disease (IBD), a chronic relapsing inflammatory disease, is most commonly differentiated into Crohn disease (CrD) and ulcerative colitis (UC). The etiology is most likely multifactorial, involving a complex interaction of environmental and genetic factors leading to maladaptive immune responses to flora in the GI tract. The genetic association is clear, with 5%–30% of patients identifying a family member with IBD, and a 10–20 relative risk of a sibling developing IBD. The 15%–36% concordance rate for monozygotic twins indicates that genetics is important but not sufficient for development of IBD.

Clinical Findings

A. Symptoms and Signs

IBD may present in diverse ways depending on the site and type of involvement. Most commonly, inflammation causes abdominal pain, diarrhea, bloody stools, fever, anorexia, fatigue, and weight loss. CrD may also present as a stricturing process with abdominal pain and intestinal obstruction, or as a penetrating/fistulizing process with abscess, perianal disease, or acute symptoms suggestive of appendicitis. UC usually presents with crampy abdominal pain, diarrhea, and blood in the stool.

CrD can affect any part of the GI tract from the lips to the anus. In pediatrics, CrD most often affects the terminal ileum and colon although it may have a patchy distribution with skip areas of uninvolved bowel. UC is limited to the colon, and in children usually involves the entire colon (pancolitis) without skip areas. The younger the age of onset, the more likely the course will be severe.

Extraintestinal manifestations are common in both forms of IBD and may precede the intestinal complaints. These include uveitis, recurrent oral aphthous ulcers, arthritis, growth and pubertal delay, liver involvement (typically primary sclerosing cholangitis), rash (erythema nodosa and pyoderma gangrenosum), and iron-deficiency anemia.

B. Diagnostic Testing

Diagnosis is based on typical presentation, course, radiographic, endoscopic, and histologic findings, and exclusion of other disorders. No single test is diagnostic. Patients with IBD often have low hemoglobin, iron, and serum albumin levels, and elevated ESR and CRP and fecal calprotectin. IBD-related serum antibodies are present in most, with antibodies to *Saccharomyces cerevisiae* (ASCA) in 60% of patients with CrD, while serum perinuclear antineutrophil cytoplasmic antibodies (pANCA) are present in approximately 70% of UC patients. These, and other IBD-related antibodies, may be helpful in differentiating CrD from UC, but are neither sensitive nor specific enough to be diagnostic. Barium upper GI radiographs with small bowel follow-through may reveal small bowel disease, especially terminal ileal thickening with separation of bowel loops, and enteric fistulas. Abdominal imaging with US, CT, or magnetic resonance may show mucosal and mural edema and exclude other etiologies.

Upper endoscopy and ileocolonoscopy are the most useful diagnostic modalities, revealing severity and extent of upper intestinal, ileal, and colonic involvement. Granulomas are found in only 25%–50% of CrD cases. Deep linear ulcers, white exudate (see Figure 21–8), apthous lesions (see Figure 21–9), patchy involvement, and perianal disease suggest CrD. Superficial and continuous involvement of the colon sparing the upper GI tract are most consistent with UC. Both forms of IBD may have mild gastritis and/or duodenitis.

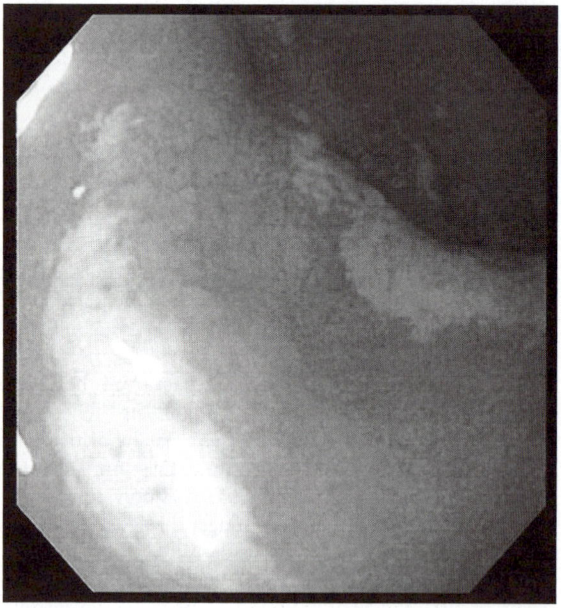

▲ **Figure 21–8.** Ulcerative colitis. White exudate is present overlying an abnormal colonic mucosa that has lost its typical vascular pattern.

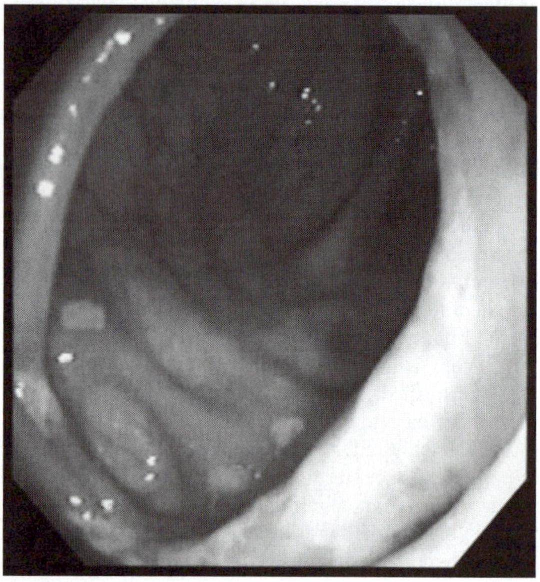

▲ **Figure 21–9.** Crohns colitis. Discrete apthous lesions are scattered across a thickened mucosa with some areas with normal vascular pattern.

Differential Diagnosis

When extraintestinal symptoms predominate, CrD can be mistaken for rheumatoid arthritis, systemic lupus erythematosus, celiac disease, or hypopituitarism. The acute onset of ileocolitis may be mistaken for intestinal obstruction, appendicitis, lymphoma, amebiasis, or tuberculosis. Malabsorption symptoms suggest celiac disease, peptic ulcer, *Giardia* infection, food protein allergy, anorexia nervosa, or growth failure from endocrine causes. Perianal disease may suggest child abuse. Crampy diarrhea and blood in the stool can also occur with infection such as *Shigella, Salmonella, Yersinia, Campylobacter, E histolytica*, enteroinvasive *E coli* (*E coli O157*), *Aeromonas hydrophila, Giardia*, and *C difficile*, and, if immunocompromised, CMV. Mild IBD mimics irritable bowel syndrome, or lactose intolerance. Eosinophilic gastroenteropathy and vasculitic lesions should also be considered. Behçet disease should be considered if there are deep intestinal ulcers, and is characterized by oral aphthous ulcerations along with at least two of the following: genital ulcers, synovitis, posterior uveitis, meningoencephalitis, and pustular vasculitis. Chronic granulomatous disease and sarcoidosis also cause granulomas.

Complications

A. Crohn Disease

Nutritional complications from chronic active disease, malabsorption, anorexia, protein losing enteropathy, bile salt malabsorption, or secondary lactose intolerance include failure to thrive, short stature, decreased bone mineralization, and specific nutrient deficiencies, including iron, calcium, zinc, and vitamin D. In addition, corticosteroid therapy may impact growth and bone mineral density. Induction of remission usually allows for improved nutrition and resumption of normal growth velocity. Most patients achieve reasonable final adult height. Intestinal obstruction, fistulae, abdominal abscess, perianal disease, pyoderma gangrenosum, arthritis, and amyloidosis occur. Crohn colitis carries a risk for adenocarcinoma of the colon.

B. Ulcerative Colitis

Even with the typical features and course of UC, up to 3%–5% of patients may have an ultimate diagnosis of CrD. Arthritis, uveitis, pyoderma gangrenosum, and malnutrition all occur. Growth failure and delayed puberty are less common than in CrD. Liver disease (chronic active hepatitis, sclerosing cholangitis) is more common. Adenocarcinoma of the colon occurs with an incidence of 1%–2% per year after the first 7–8 years of disease in patients with pan-colitis and is significantly higher in patients with both UC and sclerosing cholangitis Therefore, after 7–8 years of disease, cancer screening with routine colonoscopy and multiple biopsies is recommended. Persistent metaplasia, aneuploidy, or dysplasia indicates need for colectomy.

Treatment

A. Medical Treatment

Therapy for pediatric IBD involves induction of remission followed by a different approach for maintenance of remission. In addition, nutritional deficiencies need to be addressed to promote normal growth and development. Treatment includes anti-inflammatory, immunomodulatory, antidiarrheal, antibiotic, and biological options. No medical therapy is uniformly effective in all patients. In severe CrD, growth hormone may be needed to attain full height potential.

1. Diet—Ensuring adequate nutrition for normal growth as well as for puberty can be challenging. In addition to total calories, micronutrient, calcium, and vitamin deficiencies should be replenished. Restrictive or bland diets are counterproductive because they usually result in poor intake. A high-protein, high-carbohydrate diet with normal amounts of fat is recommended. A diet with decreased fiber may provoke symptoms during active colitis or partial intestinal obstruction; however, increased fiber may benefit mucosal health via bacterial production of fatty acids when disease is inactive. Low-lactose diet or lactase replacement may be needed temporarily for small bowel CrD. Ileal disease may require antibiotics to treat bacterial overgrowth, and extra fat-soluble vitamins due to increased losses. Supplemental calories in the form of liquid diets or enteral (NG tube supplements) are well tolerated and promote catch-up growth in severe CrD. Bowel rest with liquid or elemental diet or parenteral nutrition is a therapy for CrD relapses, and promotes linear growth and sexual development. Diet therapies are less effective in UC.

2. Aminosalicylates (ASA)—Multiple preparations of 5-ASA derivatives are available and are used to induce and maintain remission in mild CrD and UC. Common preparations including 5-ASA products such as sulfasalazine (50 mg/kg/d), or balsalazide (0.75–2.5 g PO tid) or mesalamine products, are available in tablets, granules, and delayed release formulations targeting specific locations in the GI tract (adult dose range 2.4–4.8 g/d). Side effects include skin rash, nausea, headache, and abdominal pain, hair loss, diarrhea, and rarely nephritis, pericarditis, serum sickness, hemolytic anemia, aplastic anemia, and pancreatitis. Sulfasalazine, in which sulfa delivers the 5-ASA, may cause sulfa-related side effects including photosensitivity and rash.

3. Corticosteroids—Patients with moderate to severe CrD and UC generally respond quickly to corticosteroids. Methylprednisolone (1 mg/kg/d) may be given intravenously when disease is severe. For moderate disease, prednisone (1 mg/kg/d, orally in one to two divided doses) is given until symptomatic response, followed by gradual tapering over 4–8 weeks. A flare is common during the taper, requiring reinduction and a slower taper course. Steroid dependence is an indication for use of an immunomodulator. Ileocecal CrD is effectively treated with budesonide (9 mg QAM) with several advantages over systemic steroids based on its property of undergoing "single-pass" clearance by the liver. Thus, this preparation limits systemic corticosteroid side effects of weight gain, mood swings, acne, striae, and bone demineralization. Corticosteroid enemas and foams are useful topical agents for distal proctitis or left-sided colitis and do not have the systemic side effects of oral or IV preparations. While on corticosteroids, consideration should be given to calcium and vitamin D supplementation as well as acid suppression to prevent gastritis,

Varicella immunity should be confirmed by history or antibody screen and parents counseled as to risks and therapy after varicella exposure.

4. Immunomodulators: azathioprine (AZA), 6-mercaptopurine (6MP), and methotrexate (MTX)—If IBD is moderate to severe, or the patient is steroid-dependent, immunomodulators are effective in maintaining remission and reducing the need for corticosteroids. AZA (2–3 mg/kg/d PO) or 6MP (1–2 mg/kg/d PO) provides effective maintenance therapy for moderate to severe CrD. The optimal dose of AZA or 6MP depends on the enzyme thiopurine methylene transferase (TPMT), which should be assessed before starting therapy to determine dosing. For individuals deficient in TPMT, MTX should be used; for intermediate enzyme activity, dose is reduced by 50%.

In cases where adherence may be an issue, or where dose adjustments may be necessary, AZA or 6MP metabolites may be measured in red blood cells by specialized testing. Maximum therapeutic efficacy may not be seen for 2–3 months after beginning treatment. Side effects include pancreatitis, hepatotoxicity, and bone marrow suppression.

MTX, effective in CrD but not UC, has a more rapid onset of action, usually 2–3 weeks, and is given in weekly doses, orally or intramuscularly. Most common side effect is nausea, while serious adverse events include bone marrow, liver, lung, and kidney toxicities. MTX is well known to cause fetal death and deformities.

5. Antibiotics—Metronidazole (15–30 mg/kg/d in three divided doses) and ciprofloxacin have been used to treat perianal CrD and bacterial overgrowth. Peripheral neuropathy may occur with prolonged use of metronidazole.

6. Biologicals—Infliximab, a chimeric monoclonal antibody against tumor necrosis factor-α (TNFα) is used for moderate to severe CrD and UC, and for fistulizing disease. Adalimumab and certolizumab are similar injectable agents expected to be approved for use in pediatrics. Most patients require repeated doses, and recurrence of disease often occurs within 12 months of stopping therapy. Use of biologics is associated with risk for infusion reactions, injection site reactions, and increased risk for opportunistic infections and for malignancy, especially hepatosplenic T-cell lymphoma.

7. Other agents—Cyclosporine or tacrolimus may be used instead of a biologic agent for severe, steroid-resistant IBD. Because of side effects and loss of response with time, these agents are more often used as a "bridge" to more definitive therapy (such as colectomy for UC). Thalidomide has been used, especially in patients with oral and vaginal ulcers secondary to CrD. Its mechanism of action may include prevention of TNF secretion or antiangiogenic activity. This medication must be used under strict supervision in postpubescent female patients because of the risk of teratogenesis. Probiotics and prebiotics are frequently used but with very limited data on efficacy.

B. Surgical Treatment

1. Crohn disease—Surgery is not curative for CrD. Indications for surgery in CrD include stricture, obstruction, uncontrollable bleeding, perforation, abscess, fistula, and failure of medical management. Up to 50% of patients with CrD eventually require a surgical procedure and repeated surgery is common. Surgery to correct growth retardation and promote attainment of height potential must be performed before the completion of puberty.

2. Ulcerative colitis—Surgery is curative and is recommended for patients with steroid dependence or steroid resistance, uncontrolled hemorrhage, toxic megacolon, high-grade dysplasia, or malignant tumors. Colectomy may also be performed for prevention of colorectal cancer after 7–8 years of disease. Colectomy usually requires a temporary ileostomy with J pouch formation. After ileostomy takedown, pouchitis develops in up to 25% of patients, manifested by diarrhea and cramping, but usually responds to ciprofloxacin. Liver disease associated with UC (sclerosing cholangitis) is not improved by colectomy.

REFERENCES

deRidder L et al: Infliximab use in children and adolescents with inflammatory bowel disease. J Pediatr Gastroenterol Nutr 2007;45:3 [PMID: 17592358].

Differentiating ulcerative colitis from Crohn disease in children and young adults: Report of the working group of the North American Society for Pediatric Gastroenterology, Hepatology and Nutrition and the Crohn and Colitis Foundation of America. J Pediatr Gastroenterol Nutr 2007;44:53 [PMID: 17460505].

Kotlyar DS et al: A systematic review of factors that contribute to hepatosplenic T-cell lymphoma in patients with inflammatory bowel disease. Clin Gastroenterol Hepatol 2011 Jan;9(1):36–41 [PMID: 20888436].

Mackey AC et al: Hepatosplenic T cell lymphoma associated with infliximab use in young patients treated for inflammatory bowel disease. J Pediatr Gastroenterol Nutr 2007;44:265–267 [PMID: 17255842].

Markowitz J: Current treatment of inflammatory bowel disease in children. Dig Liver Dis 2008;40:16–21 [PMID: 17988965].

Oliva-Hemker M et al: Relapsing inflammatory bowel disease working group. J Pediatr Gastroenterol Nutr 2008;47:266–272 [PMID: 18664886].

Thomas DW, Greer FR: Probiotics and prebiotics in pediatrics. Pediatrics 2010;126:1217–1231 [PMID: 21115585].

Web Resources

http://www.ccfa.org

http://www.naspghan.org/wmspage.cfm?parm1=354

http://health.nih.gov/topic/CrohnsDisease/DigestiveSystem

http://health.nih.gov/topic/UlcerativeColitis

http://www.ucandcrohns.org/

General References

Petar M, Markowitz JE, Baldassano RN: Pediatric Inflammatory Bowel Disease. Springer, 2008 [ISBN: 978-0-387-73480-4; e-ISBN 978-0-0387-73481-1].

Walker WA et al (editors): *Pediatric Gastrointestinal Disease*, 4th ed. BC Decker, 2004.

Wyllie R et al (editors): *Pediatric Gastrointestinal and Liver Disease*, 3rd ed. WB Saunders, 2006.

Liver & Pancreas

22

Ronald J. Sokol, MD
Michael R. Narkewicz, MD

LIVER DISORDERS

PROLONGED NEONATAL CHOLESTATIC JAUNDICE

Key clinical features of disorders causing prolonged neonatacholestasis are (1) jaundice with elevated serum conjugated (or direct) bilirubin fraction (> 2 mg/dL or > 20% of total bilirubin), (2) variably acholic stools, (3) dark urine, and (4) hepatomegaly.

Prolonged neonatal cholestasis (conditions with decreased bile flow) is caused by both intrahepatic and extrahepatic diseases. Specific clinical clues (Table 22–1) distinguish these two major categories of jaundice in 85% of cases. Histologic examination of percutaneous liver biopsy specimens increases the accuracy of differentiation to 95% (Table 22–2).

INTRAHEPATIC CHOLESTASIS

ESSENTIALS OF DIAGNOSIS & TYPICAL FEATURES

- Elevated total and conjugated bilirubin.
- Hepatomegaly and dark urine.
- Patency of extrahepatic biliary tree.

General Considerations

Intrahepatic cholestasis is characterized by impaired hepatocyte secretion of bile and patency of the extrahepatic biliary system. A specific cause can be identified in about 60% of cases. Patency of the extrahepatic biliary tract is suggested by pigmented stools and lack of bile duct proliferation on liver biopsy. It can be confirmed least invasively by hepatobiliary scintigraphy using technetium-99m (^{99m}Tc)-diethyliminodiacetic acid (diethyl-IDA [DIDA]). Radioactivity in the bowel within 4–24 hours is evidence of bile duct patency, as is finding bilirubin in duodenal aspirates. Patency can also be determined by cholangiography carried out either intraoperatively, percutaneously by transhepatic cholecystography, or by endoscopic retrograde cholangiopan-creatography (ERCP) using a pediatric-size side-viewing endoscope. Magnetic resonance cholangiopancreatography in infants is of limited use and highly dependent on the operator and equipment.

1. Perinatal or Neonatal Hepatitis Resulting from Infection

This diagnosis is considered in infants with jaundice, hepatomegaly, vomiting, lethargy, fever, and petechiae. It is important to identify perinatally acquired viral, bacterial, or protozoal infections (Table 22–3). Infection may occur transplacentally, by ascent through the cervix into amniotic fluid, from swallowed contaminated fluids (maternal blood, urine, vaginal secretions) during delivery, from blood transfusions administered in the early neonatal period, or from breast milk or environmental exposure. Infectious agents associated with neonatal intrahepatic cholestasis include herpes simplex virus, varicella virus, enteroviruses (coxsackievirus and echovirus), cytomegalovirus (CMV), rubella virus, adenovirus, parvovirus, human herpesvirus type 6 (HHV-6), hepatitis B virus (HBV), human immunodeficiency virus (HIV), *Treponema pallidum,* and *Toxoplasma gondii.* Although hepatitis C may be transmitted vertically, it rarely causes neonatal cholestasis. The degree of liver cell injury caused by these agents is variable, ranging from massive hepatic necrosis (herpes simplex, enteroviruses) to focal necrosis and mild inflammation (CMV, HBV). Serum bilirubin, bile acids, alanine aminotransferase (ALT), aspartate aminotransferase (AST), and alkaline phosphatase are elevated. The infant is jaundiced, may have petechiae or rash, and generally appears ill.

Table 22–1. Characteristic clinical features of intrahepatic and extrahepatic neonatal cholestasis.

Intrahepatic	Extrahepatic
Preterm infant, small for gestational age, appears ill	Full-term infant, seems well
Hepatosplenomegaly, other organ or system involvement	Hepatomegaly (firm to hard)
Stools with some pigment	Acholic stools
Associated cause identified (infections, metabolic, familial, etc)	Polysplenia or asplenia syndromes, midline liver

Table 22–2. Characteristic histologic features of intrahepatic and extrahepatic neonatal cholestasis.

	Intrahepatic	Extrahepatic
Giant cells	+++	+
Lobules	Disarray	Normal
Portal reaction	Inflammation, minimal fibrosis	Fibrosis, lymphocytic infiltrate
Neoductular proliferation	Rare	Marked
Other	Steatosis, extramedullary hematopoiesis	Portal bile duct plugging, bile lakes

Clinical Findings

A. Symptoms and Signs

Clinical symptoms typically present in the first 2 weeks of life, but may appear as late as age 2–3 months. Jaundice may be noted as early as the first 24 hours of life. Poor oral intake, poor sucking reflex, lethargy, and vomiting are frequent. Stools may be normal to pale in color, but are seldom acholic. Dark urine stains the diaper. Hepatomegaly is present, and the liver has a uniform firm consistency. Splenomegaly is variably present. Macular, papular, vesicular, or petechial rashes may occur. In less severe cases, failure to thrive may be the primary problem. Unusual presentations include neonatal

Table 22–3. Infectious causes of neonatal hepatitis.

Infectious Agent	Diagnostic Tests	Specimens	Treatment
Cytomegalovirus	Culture and PCR, liver histology, IgM/[a]IgG	Urine, blood, liver	Ganciclovir (Foscarnet)[b]
Herpes simplex	PCR and culture, liver histology, Ag (skin)	Liver, blood, eye, throat, rectal, CSF, skin	Acyclovir
Rubella	Culture, IgM/[a]IgG	Liver, blood, urine	Supportive
Varicella	Culture, PCR, Ag (skin)	Skin, blood, CSF, liver	Acyclovir (Foscarnet)[b]
Parvovirus	Serum IgM/[a]IgG, PCR	Blood	Supportive, IVIG
Enteroviruses	Culture and PCR	Blood, urine, CSF, throat, rectal, liver	IVIG
Adenovirus	Culture and PCR	Nasal/throat, rectal, blood, liver, urine	No established therapy, Cidofovir or IVIG may have value
Hepatitis B virus (HBV)	HBsAg, HBcAg IgM, HBV DNA	Serum	Supportive for acute infection
Hepatitis C virus (HCV)	HCV PCR, HCV IgG	Serum	Supportive for acute infection
Treponema pallidum	Serology; darkfield exam (skin)	Serum, CSF	Penicillin
Toxoplasma gondii	IgM/[a]IgG, PCR, culture	Serum, CSF, liver	Pyrimethamine and sulfadiazine with folinic acid for 6 mo
Mycobacterium tuberculosis	Chest radiograph, liver tissue histologic stains and culture, gastric aspirate stain and culture	Serum, liver, gastric aspirate	INH, pyrazinamide, rifampin (If multiply-drug resistant TB is present, consult a specialist)
Bacterial infection	Cultures or PCR testing	Blood, urine, other cultures	Appropriate antibiotics

[a]IgG = positive indicates maternal infection and transfer of antibody transplacentally; negative indicates unlikelihood of infection in mother and infant.
[b]Use foscarnet for resistant viruses. Treat only if symptomatic.
[c]Discontinue streptomycin as soon as possible.
Ag, viral antigen testing; CSF, cerebrospinal fluid; HBcAg, hepatitis B core antigen; HBsAg, hepatitis B surface antigen; INH, isoniazid; IVIG, intravenous gamma globulin; PCR, polymerase chain reaction test for viral DNA or RNA; PPD, purified protein derivative.

liver failure, hypoproteinemia, anasarca (nonhemolytic hydrops), and hemorrhagic disease of the newborn.

B. Diagnostic Studies

Neutropenia, thrombocytopenia, and signs of mild hemolysis are common. Mixed hyperbilirubinemia, elevated aminotransferases with near-normal alkaline phosphatase, prolongation of clotting studies, mild acidosis, and elevated cord serum IgM suggest congenital infection. Nasopharyngeal washings, urine, stool, serum, and cerebrospinal fluid (CSF) should be cultured for virus and tested for pathogen-specific nucleic acid. Specific IgM antibody may be useful, as are long-bone radiographs to determine the presence of "celery stalking" in the metaphyseal regions of the humeri, femurs, and tibias. When indicated, computed tomography (CT) scans can identify intracranial calcifications (especially with CMV and toxoplasmosis). Hepatobiliary scintigraphy shows decreased hepatic clearance of the circulating isotope with excretion into the gut. Careful ophthalmologic examination may be useful for diagnosis of herpes simplex virus, CMV, toxoplasmosis, and rubella.

A percutaneous liver biopsy is useful in distinguishing intrahepatic from extrahepatic cholestasis, but may not identify a specific infectious agent (see Table 22–2). Exceptions are the typical inclusions of CMV in hepatocytes or bile duct epithelial cells, the presence of intranuclear acidophilic inclusions of herpes simplex or varicella-zoster virus, the presence of adenovirus basophilic intranuclear inclusions, or positive immunohistochemical stains for several viruses. Variable degrees of lobular disarray characterized by focal necrosis, multinucleated giant-cell transformation, and ballooned pale hepatocytes with loss of cordlike arrangement of liver cells are usual. Intrahepatocytic and canalicular cholestasis may be prominent. Portal changes are not striking, but modest neoductular proliferation and mild fibrosis may occur. Viral cultures, immunohistochemical stains, or polymerase chain reaction (PCR) testing of biopsy material may be helpful.

Differential Diagnosis

Great care must be taken to distinguish infectious causes of intrahepatic cholestasis from genetic or metabolic disorders because the clinical presentations are similar. Galactosemia, congenital fructose intolerance, and tyrosinemia must be investigated promptly, because specific dietary or drug therapy is available. These infants may also have concomitant bacteremia. α_1-antitrypsin deficiency, cystic fibrosis, bile acid synthesis defects, progressive familial intrahepatic cholestasis, mitochondrial respiratory chain disorders, and neonatal iron storage disease must also be considered. Specific physical features may suggest Alagille, athrogryposis/renal dysfunction/cholestasis (ARC) or Zellweger syndrome. Idiopathic neonatal hepatitis can be indistinguishable from infectious causes.

Patients with intrahepatic cholestasis frequently appear ill, whereas infants with extrahepatic cholestasis do not typically appear ill, have stools that are usually completely acholic, and have an enlarged, firm liver. Histologic findings are described in Table 22–2.

Treatment

Most forms of viral neonatal hepatitis are treated symptomatically. However, infections with herpes simplex virus, varicella, CMV, parvovirus, and toxoplasmosis have specific treatments (see Table 22–3). Fluids and adequate calories are encouraged. Intravenous dextrose is needed if feedings are not well tolerated. The consequences of cholestasis are treated as indicated (Table 22–4). Vitamin K orally or by injection and vitamins D and E orally should be provided. Choleretics (ursodeoxycholic acid [UDCA] or cholestyramine) are used if cholestasis persists. Corticosteroids are contraindicated. Penicillin for suspected syphilis, specific antiviral therapy, or antibiotics for bacterial hepatitis need to be administered promptly.

Prognosis

Multiple organ involvement is commonly associated with neonatal infectious hepatitis and has a poor outcome. Hepatic or cardiac failure, intractable acidosis, or intracranial hemorrhage may be fatal in herpesvirus, adenovirus, or enterovirus infections, and occasionally in CMV or rubella infection. HBV rarely causes fulminant neonatal hepatitis; most infected infants are immunotolerant to hepatitis B. Although persistent liver disease with any virus can result in mild chronic hepatitis, portal fibrosis, or cirrhosis, the liver usually recovers without fibrosis after acute infections. Chronic cholestasis, although rare following infections, may lead to dental enamel hypoplasia, failure to thrive, biliary rickets, severe pruritus, and xanthoma.

2. Specific Infectious Agents

A. Neonatal Hepatitis B Virus Disease

Vertical transmission of HBV may occur at any time during perinatal life. Most cases of neonatal disease are acquired from mothers who are asymptomatic carriers of HBV. Although HBV has been found in most body fluids, including breast milk, neonatal transmission occurs primarily from exposure to maternal blood at delivery and only occasionally transplacentally. In chronic hepatitis B surface antigen (HBsAg)–carrier mothers, neonatal acquisition risk is greatest if the mother (1) is also hepatitis B "e" antigen (HBeAg)–positive and hepatitis B "e" antibody (HBeAb)–negative, (2) has high serum levels of hepatitis B core antibody (HBcAb), or (3) has high blood levels of HBV DNA, indicating circulating infectious virus.

Table 22–4. Treatment of complications of chronic cholestatic liver disease.

Indication	Treatment	Dose	Toxicity
Intrahepatic cholestasis	Phenobarbital	3–10 mg/kg/d	Drowsiness, irritability, interference with vitamin D metabolism
	Cholestyramine or colestipol hydrochloride	250–500 mg/kg/d	Constipation, acidosis, binding of drugs, increased steatorrhea
	Ursodeoxycholic acid	15–20 mg/kg/d	Transient increase in pruritus
Pruritus	Phenobarbital	3–10 mg/kg/d	Drowsiness, irritability, interference with vitamin D metabolism
	Cholestyramine or colestipol	250–500 mg/kg/d	Constipation, acidosis, binding of drugs, increased steatorrhea
	Antihistamines: diphenhydramine hydrochloride	5–10 mg/kg/d	Drowsiness
	Hydroxyzine	2–5 mg/kg/d	Drowsiness
	Ultraviolet light B	Exposure as needed	Skin burn
	Carbamazepine	20–40 mg/kg/d	Hepatotoxicity, marrow suppression, fluid retention
	Rifampin	10 mg/kg/d	Hepatotoxicity, marrow suppression
	Ursodeoxycholic acid	15–20 mg/kg/d	Transient increase in pruritus
	Naltrexone	1 mg/kg/day	Irritability, vomiting
Steatorrhea	Formula containing medium-chain triglycerides (eg, Pregestimil or Alimentum)	120–150 kcal/kg/d for infants	Expensive
	Oil supplement containing medium-chain triglycerides	1–2 mL/kg/d	Diarrhea, aspiration
Malabsorption of fat-soluble vitamins	Vitamin A	10,000–25,000 U/d	Hepatitis, pseudotumor cerebri, bone lesions
	Vitamin D	800–5000 U/d	Hypercalcemia, hypercalciuria
	25-Hydroxy-cholecalciferol (25-OH vitamin D)	3–5 mcg/kg/d	Hypercalcemia, hypercalciuria
	1,25-Dihydroxycholecalciferol (1,25 OH_2 vitamin D)	0.05–0.2 mcg/kg/d	Hypercalcemia, hypercalciuria
	Vitamin E (oral)	25–200 IU/kg/d	Potentiation of vitamin K deficiency
	Vitamin E (oral, TPGS[a])	15–25 IU/kg/d	Potentiation of vitamin K deficiency
	Vitamin E (intramuscular)	1–2 mg/kg/d	Muscle calcifications
	Vitamin K (oral)	2.5 mg twice per week to 5 mg/d	
	Vitamin K (intramuscular)	2–5 mg each 4 wk	
Malabsorption of other nutrients	Multiple vitamin	One to two times the standard dose	
	Calcium	25–100 mg/kg/d	Hypercalcemia, hypercalciuria
	Phosphorus	25–50 mg/kg/d	Gastrointestinal intolerance
	Zinc	1 mg/kg/d	Interference with copper and iron absorption

[a]D-α-Tocopheryl polyethylene glycol-1000 succinate.

Neonatal HBV liver disease is extremely variable. The infant has a 70%–90% chance of acquiring HBV at birth from an HBsAg/HBeAg-positive mother if the infant does not receive prophylaxis. Most infected infants develop a prolonged asymptomatic immunotolerant stage of HBV infection. Fulminant hepatic necrosis and liver failure rarely occurs in infants. Other patients develop chronic hepatitis with focal hepatocyte necrosis and a mild portal inflammatory response. Cholestasis is intracellular and canalicular. Chronic hepatitis may persist for many years, with serologic evidence of persisting antigenemia (HBsAg) and mildly elevated serum aminotransferases. Chronic hepatitis may rarely progress to cirrhosis within 1–2 years. Most infected infants have only mild evidence, if any, of liver injury.

To prevent perinatal transmission, all infants of mothers who are HBsAg-positive (regardless of HBeAg status) should receive hepatitis B immunoglobulin (HBIG) and hepatitis B vaccine within the first 24 hours after birth and vaccine again at ages 1 and 6 months. (See Chapter 10.) This prevents HBV infection in 85%–95% of infants. HBIG can provide some protection when given as late as 72 hours after birth. If not given at birth it can be administered as late as 7 days postpartum as long as the infant has received the vaccine. Universal HBV immunization at birth, with two follow-up doses, is recommended for all infants. Universal screening of pregnant women for HbsAg is conducted to determine which infants will need HBIG.

B. Neonatal Bacterial Hepatitis

Most bacterial liver infections in newborns are acquired by transplacental invasion from amnionitis with ascending spread from maternal vaginal or cervical infection. Onset is abrupt, usually within 48–72 hours after delivery, with signs of sepsis and often shock. Jaundice appears early with direct hyperbilirubinemia. The liver enlarges rapidly, and the histologic picture is that of diffuse hepatitis with or without microabscess. The most common organisms involved are *Escherichia coli, Listeria monocytogenes*, and group B streptococci. Neonatal liver abscesses caused by *E coli* or *Staphylococcus aureus* may result from omphalitis or umbilical vein catheterization. Bacterial hepatitis and neonatal liver abscesses require specific antibiotics in optimal doses and combinations and, rarely, surgical or radiologic interventional drainage. Deaths are common, but survivors show no long-term consequences of liver disease.

C. Neonatal Jaundice with Urinary Tract Infection

Urinary tract infections typically present with cholestasis between the second and fourth weeks of life. Lethargy, fever, poor appetite, jaundice, and hepatomegaly may be present. Except for mixed hyperbilirubinemia, other liver function tests (LFTs) are mildly abnormal. Leukocytosis is present, and infection is confirmed by urine culture. The liver impairment is caused by the action of endotoxin and cytokines on bile secretion.

Treatment of the infection leads to resolution of the cholestasis without hepatic sequelae. Metabolic liver diseases, such as galactosemia and tyrosinemia, may present with gram-negative bacterial urinary tract infection and must be excluded.

Berardi A, Lugli L, Rossi C, Maria CL, Guidotti I, Gallo C, Ferrari F: Neonatal herpes simplex virus. J Matern Fetal Neonatal Med 2011 Oct;24(Suppl 1):88–90 [PMID: 21942600].

Chang MH: Hepatitis B virus infection. Semin Fetal Neonatal Med 2007;12:160 [PMID: 17336170].

Lin K, Vickery J: Screening for hepatitis B virus infection in pregnant women: Evidence for the U.S. Preventive Services Task Force reaffirmation recommendation statement. Ann Intern Med 2009;150:874–876 [PMID: 19528566].

3. Intrahepatic Cholestasis Resulting from Inborn Errors of Metabolism, Familial, & "Toxic" Causes

These cholestatic syndromes caused by specific enzyme deficiencies, other genetic disorders, or certain toxins share findings of intrahepatic cholestasis (ie, jaundice, hepatomegaly, and normal to completely acholic stools). Specific clinical conditions have characteristic clinical signs.

A. Enzyme Deficiencies and Other Inherited Disorders

Establishing the specific diagnosis as early as possible is important because dietary or pharmacologic treatment may be available (Table 22–5). Reversal of liver disease and clinical symptoms is prompt and maintained in several disorders as long as the diet is maintained. As with other genetic disorders, parents of the affected infant should be offered genetic counseling. For some disorders, prenatal genetic diagnosis is available.

Cholestasis caused by metabolic diseases (eg, galactosemia, hereditary fructose intolerance, and tyrosinemia) is frequently accompanied by vomiting, lethargy, poor feeding, hypoglycemia, or irritability. The infants often appear septic; gram-negative bacteria can be cultured from blood in 25%–50% of symptomatic cases, especially in patients with galactosemia and cholestasis. Neonatal screening programs for galactosemia usually detect the disorder before cholestasis develops. Other metabolic and genetic causes of neonatal intrahepatic cholestasis are outlined in Table 22–5. Treatment of these disorders is discussed in Chapter 36.

B. "Toxic" Causes of Neonatal Cholestasis

1. Neonatal ischemic-hypoxic conditions—Perinatal events that result in hypoperfusion of the gastrointestinal system are sometimes followed within 1–2 weeks by cholestasis. This occurs in preterm infants with respiratory distress, severe hypoxia, hypoglycemia, shock, and acidosis.

Table 22–5. Metabolic and genetic causes of neonatal cholestasis.

Disease	Inborn Error	Hepatic Pathology	Diagnostic Studies
Galactosemia	Galactose-1-phosphate uridyltransferase	Cholestasis, steatosis, necrosis, pseudoacini, fibrosis	Galactose-1-phosphate uridylyltransferase assay of red blood cells
Fructose intolerance	Fructose-1-phosphate aldolase	Steatosis, necrosis, pseudoacini, fibrosis	Liver fructose-1-phosphate aldolase assay or genotyping[a]
Tyrosinemia	Fumarylacetoacetase	Necrosis, steatosis, pseudoacini, portal fibrosis	Urinary succinylacetone, fumarylacetoacetase assay of red blood cells
Cystic fibrosis	Cystic fibrosis transmembrane conductance regulator gene	Cholestasis, neoductular proliferation, excess bile duct mucus, portal fibrosis	Sweat test and genotyping[a]
Hypopituitarism	Deficient production of pituitary hormones	Cholestasis, giant cells	Thyroxine, TSH, cortisol levels
α_1-Antitrypsin deficiency	Abnormal α_1-antitrypsin molecule (PiZZ phenotype)	Giant cells, cholestasis, steatosis, neoductular proliferation, fibrosis, PAS-diastase–resistant cytoplasmic globules	Serum α_1-antitrypsin phenotype or genotype
Gaucher disease	β-Glucosidase	Cholestasis, cytoplasmic inclusions in Kupffer cells (foam cells)	β-Glucosidase assay in leukocytes
Niemann-Pick type C disease	Lysosomal sphingomyelinase	Cholestasis, cytoplasmic inclusions in Kupffer cells	Sphingomyelinase assay of leukocytes or liver or fibroblasts (type C); genotyping
Glycogen storage disease type IV	Branching enzyme	Fibrosis, cirrhosis, PAS-diastase–resistant cytoplasmic inclusions	Branching enzyme analysis of leukocytes or liver, genotyping
Neonatal hemochromatosis	Transplacental alloimmunization	Giant cells, portal fibrosis, hemosiderosis, cirrhosis	Histology, iron stains, lip biopsy, abdominal MRI
Peroxisomal disorders (eg, Zellweger syndrome)	Deficient peroxisomal enzymes or assembly	Cholestasis, necrosis, fibrosis, cirrhosis, hemosiderosis	Plasma very-long-chain fatty acids, qualitative bile acids, plasmalogen, pipecolic acid, liver electron microscopy, genotyping of leukocyte DNA
Abnormalities in bile acid metabolism	Several enzyme deficiencies defined	Cholestasis, necrosis, giant cells	Urine, serum, duodenal fluid analyzed for bile acids by fast atom bombardment–mass spectroscopy
Byler disease and syndrome (PFIC types I and II)	*FIC-1* and *BSEP* genes	Cholestasis, necrosis, giant cells, fibrosis	Histology, family history, normal cholesterol, low or normal γ-glutamyl transpeptidase, genotyping
Arthrygryposis/renal dysfunction/ cholestasis syndrome	*VPS33B* genes	Cholestasis, fibrosis	Genotyping
MDR3 deficiency (PFIC type III)	*MDR3* gene	Cholestasis, bile duct proliferation, portal fibrosis	Bile phospholipid level, genotyping
Alagille syndrome (syndromic paucity of interlobular bile ducts)	*JAGGED1* gene and *NOTCH2* mutations	Cholestasis, paucity of interlobular bile ducts, increased copper levels	Three or more clinical features, liver histology, genotyping of leukocyte DNA
Mitochondrial hepatopathies (respiratory chain diseases and mtDNA depletion)	*POLG, BCS1l, SCO1, DGUOK,* and *MPV17* gene mutations	Cholestasis, steatosis, portal fibrosis, abnormal mitochondria on electron microscopy	mtDNA depletion studies, respiratory chain studies on liver or muscle, genotyping

[a]Performed on leukocyte DNA

IV, intravenous; MDR3, multiple-drug resistance protein type 3; MRI, magnetic resonance imaging; mtDNA, mitochondrial DNA; PAS, periodic acid–Schiff; PFIC, progressive familial intrahepatic cholestasis; TSH, thyroid-stimulating hormone.

When these perinatal conditions develop in association with gastrointestinal lesions, such as ruptured omphalocele, gastroschisis, or necrotizing enterocolitis, a subsequent cholestatic picture is common (25%–50% of cases). Liver function studies reveal mixed hyperbilirubinemia, elevated alkaline phosphatase and γ-glutamyl transpeptidase (GGT) values, and variable elevation of the aminotransferases. Stools are seldom persistently acholic.

The mainstays of treatment are choleretics (Ursodiol), introduction of enteral feedings using special formulas as soon as possible, and nutrient supplementation until the cholestasis resolves (see Table 22–4). As long as no severe intestinal problem is present (eg, short gut syndrome or intestinal failure), resolution of the hepatic abnormalities is the rule.

2. Prolonged parenteral nutrition—Cholestasis may develop after 1–2 weeks in premature newborns receiving parenteral nutrition. Even full-term infants with significant intestinal atresia, resections, or dysmotility may develop parenteral nutrition–associated cholestasis. Contributing factors include toxicity of intravenous amino acids, diminished stimulation of bile flow from prolonged absence of feedings, frequent episodes of sepsis, small intestinal bacterial overgrowth with translocation of intestinal bacteria and their cell wall products, missing nutrients or antioxidants, photooxidation of amino acids, infusion of lipid hydroperoxides or plant sterols, and the "physiologic cholestatic" propensity of the premature infant. Histology of the liver may resemble that of biliary atresia. Early introduction of feedings has reduced the frequency of this disorder. The prognosis is generally good; however, occasional cases progress to cirrhosis, liver failure, and hepatoma, particularly in infants with intestinal failure. These infants may require liver and intestinal transplantation. Oral erythromycin as a pro-motility agent may reduce the incidence of cholestasis in very-low-birth-weight infants. Intravenous fish oil–based lipid emulsions or reduction in soy-oil based lipid emulsions may reverse features of cholestasis.

3. Inspissated bile syndrome—The syndrome is the result of accumulation of bile in canaliculi and in the small- and medium-sized bile ducts in hemolytic disease of the newborn (Rh, ABO) and in some infants receiving parenteral nutrition. The same mechanisms may cause intrinsic obstruction of the common bile duct. An ischemia-reperfusion injury may also contribute to cholestasis in Rh incompatibility. Stools may become acholic and levels of bilirubin, primarily conjugated, may reach 40 mg/dL. If inspissation of bile occurs within the extrahepatic biliary tree, differentiation from biliary atresia may be difficult. Although most cases improve slowly over 2–6 months, persistence of complete cholestasis for more than 1–2 weeks requires further studies (ultrasonography, DIDA scanning, liver biopsy) with possible cholangiography. Irrigation of the common bile duct is sometimes necessary to dislodge the obstructing inspissated biliary material.

Cober MP et al: Intravenous fat emulsions reduction for patients with parenteral nutrition-associated liver disease. J Pediatr 2011 Oct 6 [Epub ahead of print] [PMID: 21982303].

Dicken BJ et al: More evidence on the use of parenteral omega-3 lipids in pediatric intestinal failure. J Pediatr 2011 Jul;159(1): 170–171 [PMID: 21669322].

Morotti RA et al: Progressive familial intrahepatic cholestasis (PFIC) type 1, 2, and 3: A review of the liver pathology findings. Semin Liver Dis 2011 Feb;31(1):3–10 [PMID: 21344347].

Ng PC et al: High-dose oral erythromycin decreased the incidence of parenteral nutrition-associated cholestasis in preterm infants. Gastroenterology 2007;132:1726 [PMID: 17484870].

4. Idiopathic Neonatal Hepatitis (Giant-Cell Hepatitis)

This common type of cholestatic jaundice is of unknown cause and presents with features of cholestasis and a typical liver biopsy appearance; it accounts for 25%–40% of cases of neonatal intrahepatic cholestasis. The degree of cholestasis is variable, and the disorder may be indistinguishable from extrahepatic causes in 10% of cases. Many cases of this disorder have been shown in recent years to have specific etiologies. Viral infections, α_1-antitrypsin deficiency, Alagille syndrome, Niemann-Pick type C disease (NPC), progressive familial intrahepatic cholestasis (PFIC), and bile acid synthesis defects may present in a similar clinical and histologic manner. In idiopathic neonatal hepatitis, PFIC types I and II and ARC syndrome, and disease due to bile acid synthesis defects, the GGT levels are normal or low. Electron microscopy of the liver biopsy (and genotyping) may help distinguish NPC and PFIC.

Intrauterine growth retardation, prematurity, poor feeding, emesis, poor growth, and partially or intermittently acholic stools are characteristic of intrahepatic cholestasis. Patients with neonatal lupus erythematosus may present with giant-cell hepatitis; however, thrombocytopenia, rash, or congenital heart block is usually also present.

In cases of suspected idiopathic neonatal hepatitis (diagnosed in the absence of infectious, metabolic, and toxic causes), patency of the biliary tree should be verified to exclude extrahepatic surgical disorders. HIDA scanning and ultrasonography may be helpful in this regard if stools are acholic. Liver biopsy findings are usually diagnostic after age 6–8 weeks (see Table 22–2), but may be misleading before age 6 weeks. Failure to detect patency of the biliary tree, nondiagnostic liver biopsy findings, or persisting complete cholestasis (acholic stools) are indications for minilaparotomy and intraoperative cholangiography performed by an experienced surgeon, ERCP, percutaneous cholecystography, or magnetic resonance cholangiopancreatography (MRCP). Occasionally, a small but patent (hypoplastic) extrahepatic biliary tree is demonstrated (as in Alagille syndrome); it is probably the result, rather than the cause, of diminished bile flow. Surgical reconstruction of hypoplastic biliary trees should not be attempted.

Once a patent extrahepatic tree is confirmed, therapy should include choleretics, a special formula with medium-chain triglycerides (eg, Pregestimil, Alimentum) or breast milk (if growth is adequate), and supplemental fat-soluble vitamins in water-soluble form (see Table 22–4). This therapy is continued as long as significant cholestasis remains (conjugated bilirubin > 1 mg/dL). Fat-soluble vitamin serum levels should be monitored while supplements are given and repeated at least once after their discontinuation.

Eighty percent of patients recover without significant hepatic fibrosis. However, failure to resolve the cholestatic picture by age 6–12 months is associated with progressive liver disease and evolving cirrhosis. This may occur with either normal or diminished numbers of interlobular bile ducts (paucity of interlobular ducts). Liver transplantation has been successful when signs of hepatic decompensation are noted (rising bilirubin, coagulopathy, intractable ascites).

Torbenson M et al: Neonatal giant cell hepatitis: Histological and etiological findings. Am J Surg Pathol 2010 Oct;34(10):1498–1503 [PMID: 20871223].

Wang JS, Tan N, Dhawan A: Significance of low or normal serum gamma glutamyl transferase level in infants with idiopathic neonatal hepatitis. Eur J Pediatr 2006;165:795–801 [PMID: 16770572].

5. Paucity of Interlobular Bile Ducts

Forms of intrahepatic cholestasis caused by decreased numbers of interlobular bile ducts (< 0.5 bile ducts per portal tract) may be classified according to whether they are associated with other malformations. Alagille syndrome (syndromic paucity or arteriohepatic dysplasia) is caused by mutations in the gene *JAGGED1*, located on chromosome 20p, which codes for a ligand of the notch receptor, or more rarely in the gene *NOTCH2*. Alagille syndrome is recognized by the characteristic facies, which becomes more obvious with age. The forehead is prominent. The eyes are set deep and sometimes widely apart (hypertelorism). The chin is small and slightly pointed and projects forward. The ears are prominent. The stool color varies with the severity of cholestasis. Pruritus begins by age 3–6 months. Firm, smooth hepatomegaly may be present. Cardiac murmurs are present in 95% of patients, and butterfly vertebrae (incomplete fusion of the vertebral body or anterior arch) are present in 50%. Xanthomas develop as hypercholesterolemia becomes a problem. Occasionally, early cholestasis is mild and not recognized or the patient presents with complex congenital heart disease (eg, tetralogy of Fallot).

Conjugated hyperbilirubinemia may be mild to severe (2–15 mg/dL). Serum alkaline phosphatase, GGT, and cholesterol are markedly elevated, especially early in life. Serum bile acids are always elevated, aminotransferases are mildly increased, but clotting factors and other liver proteins are usually normal.

Cardiac involvement includes peripheral pulmonary artery, branch pulmonary artery, or pulmonary valvular stenoses, atrial septal defect, coarctation of the aorta, and tetralogy of Fallot. Up to 10%–15% of patients have intracranial vascular abnormalities or may develop intracranial hemorrhage or stroke early in childhood.

Eye abnormalities (posterior embryotoxon or a prominent Schwalbe line in 90%) and renal abnormalities (dysplastic kidneys, renal tubular ectasia, single kidney, hematuria) are also characteristic. Growth retardation with normal to increased levels of growth hormone (growth hormone resistance) is common. Some patients may rarely have pancreatic insufficiency that may contribute to the fat malabsorption. Although variable, the intelligence quotient is frequently low. Hypogonadism with micropenis may be present. A weak, high-pitched voice may develop. Neurologic disorders resulting from vitamin E deficiency (areflexia, ataxia, ophthalmoplegia) eventually develop in many unsupplemented children and may be profound.

In the nonsyndromic form, paucity of interlobular bile ducts occurs in the absence of the extrahepatic malformations. Paucity may also occur in α_1-antitrypsin deficiency, Zellweger syndrome, in association with lymphedema (Aagenaes syndrome), PFIC, cystic fibrosis, CMV or rubella infection, and inborn errors of bile acid metabolism.

High doses (250 mg/kg/d) of cholestyramine may control pruritus, lower cholesterol, and clear xanthomas. Ursodiol (15–25 mg/kg/d) appears to be more effective and causes fewer side effects than cholestyramine. Naltrexone (1 mg/kg/day) is occasionally required. Nutritional therapy to prevent wasting and deficiencies of fat-soluble vitamins is of particular importance because of the severity of cholestasis (see Table 22–4).

Prognosis is more favorable in the syndromic than in the nonsyndromic varieties. In the former, only 30%–40% of patients have severe complications of disease, whereas over 70% of patients with nonsyndromic varieties progress to cirrhosis. Many of this latter group may have forms of PFIC. In Alagille syndrome, cholestasis may improve by age 2–4 years, with minimal residual hepatic fibrosis. Survival into adulthood despite raised serum bile acids, aminotransferases, and alkaline phosphatase occurs in about 50% of cases. Several patients have developed hepatocellular carcinoma. Hypogonadism has been noted; however, fertility is not obviously affected in most cases. Cardiovascular anomalies may shorten life expectancy. Some patients have persistent, severe cholestasis, rendering their quality of life poor. Pruritus may respond to partial external biliary diversion or ileal exclusion. Recurrent bone fractures may result from metabolic bone disease. Liver transplantation has been successfully performed under these circumstances. Intracranial hemorrhage, moya moya disease, or stroke may occur in up to 10%–12% of affected children.

Kamath BM et al: Medical management of Alagille syndrome. J Pediatr Gastroenterol Nutr 2010 Jun;50(6):580–586 [PMID: 20479679].

Subramaniam P et al: Diagnosis of Alagille syndrome-25 years of experience at King's College Hospital. J Pediatr Gastroenterol Nutr 2011 Jan;52(1):84–89 [PMID: 21119543].

6. Progressive Familial Intrahepatic Cholestasis (PFIC; Byler Disease and Byler Syndrome)

PFIC is a group of disorders presenting as pruritus, diarrhea, jaundice, fat-soluble vitamin deficiencies, and failure to thrive in the first 6–12 months of life. PFIC type I (Byler disease), caused by mutations in the *FIC1* gene, is associated with low to normal serum levels of GGT and cholesterol and elevated levels of bilirubin, aminotransferases, and bile acids. Diarrhea and pruritus are common. Pancreatitis and hearing loss may develop. Liver biopsy demonstrates cellular cholestasis, sometimes with a paucity of interlobular bile ducts and centrolobular fibrosis that progresses to cirrhosis. Electron microscopy shows diagnostic granular "Byler bile" in canaliculi. Treatment includes administration of UDCA, partial biliary diversion or ileal exclusion if the condition is unresponsive to UDCA, and liver transplantation if unresponsive to these therapies. With partial biliary diversion or ileal exclusion surgery, many patients show improved growth and liver histology, reduction in symptoms and, thus, avoid liver transplantation.

PFIC type II is caused by mutations in the bile salt export pump (*BSEP*) gene, which codes for an adenosine triphosphate–dependent canalicular bile salt transport protein. These patients are clinically and biochemically similar to PFIC type I patients, but liver histology includes numerous "giant cells." There is an increased incidence of hepatocellular carcinoma in these patients. Treatment is similar to PFIC type I although close monitoring for hepatocellular carcinoma is essential.

PFIC type III is caused by mutations in the multiple drug resistance protein type 3 (*MDR3*) gene, which encodes a canalicular protein that pumps phospholipid into bile. Serum GGT and bile acid levels are both elevated, bile duct proliferation and portal tract fibrosis are seen in liver biopsies, and bile phospholipid levels are low. Treatment is similar to that for other forms of PFIC except that partial biliary diversion is not recommended. Bile acid synthesis defects are clinically similar to PFIC types I and II, with low serum levels of GGT and cholesterol; however, the serum level of total bile acids is inappropriately normal or low and urine bile acid analysis may identify a synthesis defect. Treatment of bile acid synthesis defects is with oral cholic acid and UDCA.

Arnell H et al: Follow-up in children with progressive familial intrahepatic cholestasis after partial external biliary diversion. J Pediatr Gastroenterol Nutr 2010 Oct;51(4):494–499 [PMID: 20683202].

Davit-Spraul A et al: Progressive familial intrahepatic cholestasis. Orphanet J Rare Dis 2009;4:1 [Review] [PMID: 19133130].

Knisely AS et al: Hepatocellular carcinoma in ten children under five years of age with bile salt export pump deficiency. Hepatology 2006;44:478 [PMID: 16871584].

EXTRAHEPATIC NEONATAL CHOLESTASIS

Extrahepatic neonatal cholestasis is characterized by complete and persistent cholestasis (acholic stools) in the first 3 months of life; lack of patency of the extrahepatic biliary tree proved by intraoperative, percutaneous, or endoscopic cholangiography; firm to hard hepatomegaly; and typical features on histologic examination of liver biopsy tissue (see Table 22–2). Causes include biliary atresia, choledochal cyst, spontaneous perforation of the extrahepatic ducts, and intrinsic or extrinsic obstruction of the common duct.

1. Biliary Atresia

General Considerations

Biliary atresia is the progressive fibroinflammatory obliteration of the lumen of all, or part of, the extrahepatic biliary tree presenting within the first 3 months of life. Biliary atresia occurs in 1:10,000–1:18,000 births, and the incidence in both sexes is equal, except in Asian Americans where the incidence is higher and the disorder is more common in girls. There are at least two types of biliary atresia: the perinatal form (80% of cases), in which a perinatal insult is believed to initiate inflammatory obstruction and fibrosis of the biliary tree, and the fetal-embryonic form (20% of cases), in which the extrahepatic biliary system did not develop normally. In the perinatal form, meconium and initial stools are usually normal in color, suggesting early patency of the ducts. Evidence obtained from surgically removed remnants of the extrahepatic biliary tree suggests an inflammatory sclerosing cholangiopathy. Recent research supports an autoimmune reaction that is responsible for intrahepatic bile duct injury and fibrosis. Although an infectious cause seems reasonable, no agent has been consistently found in such cases. A role for reovirus type 3, CMV and rotavirus group C has been suggested. In the fetal-embryonic type, the bile duct presumably did not develop normally and is associated with other nonhepatic congenital anomalies. The association of biliary atresia with the polysplenia syndrome (heterotaxia, preduodenal portal vein, interruption of the inferior vena cava, polysplenia, and midline liver) and asplenia syndrome supports an embryonic origin of biliary atresia in these cases.

Clinical Findings

A. Symptoms and Signs

Jaundice may be noted in the newborn period or develops about age 2–3 weeks. Urine stains the diaper; and stools are often pale yellow, buff-colored, gray, or acholic. Seepage of bilirubin products across the intestinal mucosa may give some yellow coloration to the stools. Hepatomegaly is common, and the liver may feel firm to hard; splenomegaly develops later. Pruritus, digital clubbing, xanthomas, and a rachitic rosary may be noted in older patients. By age 2–6 months, the growth curve reveals poor weight gain.

Ascites, failure to thrive, bone fractures, and bleeding complications occur later.

B. Laboratory Findings and Imaging

No single laboratory test will consistently differentiate biliary atresia from other causes of complete obstructive jaundice. A HIDA scan showing lack of intestinal excretion is always present in biliary atresia, but may be seen with intrahepatic cholestasis. MRCP may be of some value to define biliary atresia. Although biliary atresia is suggested by persistent elevation of serum GGT or alkaline phosphatase levels, high cholesterol levels, and prolonged prothrombin time (PT), these findings have also been reported in severe neonatal hepatitis, α_1-antitrypsin deficiency, and bile duct paucity. Furthermore, these tests will not differentiate the location of the obstruction within the extrahepatic system. Generally, the aminotransferases are elevated only modestly in biliary atresia. Serum proteins and blood clotting factors are not affected early in the disease. Routine chest radiograph may reveal abnormalities suggestive of polysplenia syndrome. Ultrasonography of the biliary system should be performed to exclude the presence of choledochal cyst and intra-abdominal anomalies; a triangular cord sign in the hepatic porta suggests biliary atresia. Liver biopsy specimens (particularly if obtained after age 6–8 weeks) can differentiate intrahepatic causes of cholestasis from biliary atresia in over 90% of cases (see Table 22–2).

Differential Diagnosis

The major diagnostic dilemma is distinguishing between this entity and neonatal hepatitis, bile duct paucity, metabolic liver disease (particularly α_1-antitrypsin deficiency), choledochal cyst, or intrinsic bile duct obstruction (stones, bile plugs). Although spontaneous perforation of extrahepatic bile ducts leads to jaundice and acholic stools, the infants in such cases are usually quite ill with chemical peritonitis from biliary ascites, and hepatomegaly is not found.

If the diagnosis of biliary atresia cannot be excluded by the diagnostic evaluation and percutaneous liver biopsy, surgical exploration should be performed as soon as possible. Laparotomy or laparoscopy must include liver biopsy and an operative cholangiogram if a gallbladder is present. The presence of yellow bile in the gallbladder implies patency of the proximal extrahepatic duct system. Radiographic visualization of cholangiographic contrast in the duodenum excludes obstruction to the distal extrahepatic ducts.

Treatment

In the absence of surgical correction or transplantation, biliary cirrhosis, hepatic failure, and death occur uniformly by age 18–24 months.

Except for the occasional example of correctable biliary atresia, in which choledochojejunostomy is feasible, the standard procedure is hepatoportoenterostomy (Kasai procedure). Occasionally, portocholecystostomy (gallbladder Kasai procedure) may be performed if the gallbladder is present and the passage from it to the duodenum is patent. These procedures are best done in specialized centers where experienced surgical, pediatric, and nursing personnel are available. Surgery should be performed as early as possible (ideally before 45 days of life); the Kasai procedure should generally not be undertaken in infants older than age 4 months, because the likelihood of bile drainage at this age is very low. Orthotopic liver transplantation is now indicated for patients who do not undergo the Kasai procedure, who fail to drain bile after the Kasai procedure, or who progress to end-stage biliary cirrhosis despite surgical treatment. The 3- to 5-year survival rate following liver transplantation for biliary atresia is at least 80%–90%. Biliary atresia is the leading indication for pediatric liver transplantation.

Whether or not the Kasai procedure is performed, supportive medical treatment consists of vitamin and caloric support (vitamins A, D, E, and K and formulas containing medium-chain triglycerides [Pregestimil or Alimentum]) (see Table 22–4). Monitoring of fat-soluble vitamin levels is essential to assure adequate supplementation. Suspected bacterial infections (eg, ascending cholangitis) should be treated promptly with broad-spectrum antibiotics, and any bleeding tendency should be corrected with intramuscular vitamin K. Ascites can be managed initially with reduced sodium intake and spironolactone. Choleretics and bile acid–binding products (cholestyramine, aluminum hydroxide gel) are of little use. The value of UDCA remains to be determined. Antibiotic prophylaxis reduces the rate of cholangitis. The role of post-Kasai corticosteroids is controversial.

Prognosis

When bile flow is sustained following portoenterostomy (serum total bilirubin < 2 mg/dL by 3 months of age), the 10-year survival rate without liver transplantation is up to 35%. Death is usually caused by liver failure, sepsis, acidosis, or respiratory failure secondary to intractable ascites. Esophageal variceal hemorrhage develops in 40% of patients, yet terminal hemorrhage is unusual. Occasional long-term survivors develop hepatopulmonary syndrome (intrapulmonary right to left shunting of blood resulting in hypoxia) or portopulmonary hypertension (pulmonary arterial hypertension in patients with portal hypertension). Liver transplantation has dramatically changed the outlook for these patients.

Davenport M et al: Randomized, double-blind, placebo-controlled trial of corticosteroids after Kasai portoenterostomy for biliary atresia. Hepatology 2007;46:1821–1827 [PMID: 17935230].

Serinet MO et al: Impact of age at Kasai operation on its results in late childhood and adolescence: A rational basis for biliary atresia screening. Pediatrics 2009;123:1280–1286 [PMID: 19403492].

Shneider BL et al: A multicenter study of the outcome of biliary atresia in the United States, 1997 to 2000. J Pediatr 2006;148:467 [PMID: 16647406].

Sokol RJ et al: Screening and outcomes in biliary atresia: Summary of a National Institutes of Health workshop. Hepatology 2007;46:566 [PMID: 17661405].

Superina R et al: The anatomic pattern of biliary atresia identified at time of Kasai hepatoportoenterostomy and early postoperative clearance of jaundice are significant predictors of transplant-free survival. Ann Surg 2011 Oct;254(4):577–585 [PMID: 21869674].

2. Choledochal Cyst

ESSENTIALS OF DIAGNOSIS

- Abnormal abdominal ultrasound with cyst of the biliary tree.

Clinical Features

A. Symptoms and Signs

In most cases, the clinical manifestations, basic laboratory findings, and histopathologic features on liver biopsy are indistinguishable from those associated with biliary atresia. In older children, choledochal cyst presents as recurrent episodes of right upper quadrant abdominal pain, vomiting, obstructive jaundice, pancreatitis, or as a right abdominal mass. Choledochal cysts cause only 2%–5% of cases of extrahepatic neonatal cholestasis; the incidence is higher in girls and patients of Asian descent. Neonatal symptomatic cysts are usually associated with atresia of the distal common duct—accounting for the diagnostic dilemma—and may simply be part of the spectrum of biliary atresia.

B. Imaging Studies

Ultrasonography or magnetic resonance imaging (MRI) reveals the presence of a cyst.

Treatment

Immediate surgery is indicated for neonates once abnormalities in clotting factors have been corrected and bacterial cholangitis, if present, has been treated with intravenous antibiotics. Excision of the cyst and choledocho-Roux-en-Y jejunal anastomosis are recommended. In some cases, because of technical problems, only the mucosa of the cyst can be removed with jejunal anastomosis to the proximal bile duct. Anastomosis of cyst to jejunum or duodenum is not recommended.

Prognosis

The prognosis depends on the presence or absence of associated evidence of atresia and the appearance of the intrahepatic ducts. If atresia is found, the prognosis is similar to that described in the preceding section. If an isolated extrahepatic cyst is encountered, the outcome is generally excellent, with resolution of the jaundice and return to normal liver architecture. However, bouts of ascending cholangitis may occur, particularly if intrahepatic cysts are present or stricture of the anastomotic site develops. The risk of bile duct carcinoma developing within the cyst is about 5%–15% in adulthood; therefore, cystectomy or excision of cyst mucosa should be undertaken whenever possible.

Hung MH et al: Choledochal cysts in infants and children: Experiences over a 20-year period at a single institution. Eur J Pediatr 2011 Sep;170(9):1179–1185 [PMID: 21350805].

Tsai MS et al: Clinicopathological feature and surgical outcome of choledochal cyst in different age groups: The implication of surgical timing. J Gastrointest Surg 2008;12:2191 [PMID: 18677540].

3. Spontaneous Perforation of the Extrahepatic Bile Ducts

The sudden appearance of obstructive jaundice, acholic stools, and abdominal enlargement with ascites in a sick newborn is suggestive of this condition. The liver is usually normal in size, and a yellow-green discoloration can often be discerned under the umbilicus or in the scrotum. In 24% of cases, stones or sludge obstructs the common bile duct. DIDA scan or ERCP shows leakage from the biliary tree, and ultrasonography confirms ascites or fluid around the bile duct.

Treatment is surgical. Simple drainage, without attempts at oversewing the perforation, is sufficient in primary perforations. A diversion anastomosis is constructed in cases associated with choledochal cyst or stenosis. The prognosis is generally good.

Evans K et al: Spontaneous perforation of the bile duct in infancy and childhood: A systematic review. J Pediatr Gastroenterol Nutr 2010 Jun;50(6):677–681 [PMID: 20400907].

Sahnoun L et al: Spontaneous perforation of the extrahepatic bile duct in infancy: Report of two cases and literature review. Eur J Pediatr Surg 2007;17:132 [PMID: 17503309].

OTHER NEONATAL HYPERBILIRUBINEMIC CONDITIONS (NONCHOLESTATIC NONHEMOLYTIC)

Two other groups of disorders are associated with hyperbilirubinemia: (1) unconjugated hyperbilirubinemia, present in breast milk jaundice, Lucey-Driscoll syndrome, congenital hypothyroidism, upper intestinal obstruction, Gilbert disease, Crigler-Najjar syndrome, and drug-induced hyperbilirubinemia; and (2) conjugated noncholestatic hyperbilirubinemia, present in the Dubin-Johnson syndrome and Rotor syndrome.

1. Unconjugated Hyperbilirubinemia

A. Breast Milk Jaundice

Persistent elevation of the indirect bilirubin fraction (> 80% of total bilirubin) may occur in up to 36% of breast-fed infants. Enhanced β-glucuronidase activity in breast milk is one factor that increases absorption of unconjugated bilirubin. Substances (eg, L-aspartic acid) in casein hydrolysate formulas inhibit this enzyme. The increased enterohepatic shunting of unconjugated bilirubin exceeds the normal conjugating capacity in the liver of these infants. The mutation for Gilbert syndrome (UDP-glucuronyltransferase 1A1 [*UGT1A1*]) predisposes to breast milk jaundice and to more prolonged jaundice. Neonates who carry the 211 and 388 variants in the *UGT1A1* and *OATP 2* genes, respectively, and feed with breast milk, are at high risk to develop severe hyperbilirubinemia. Low volumes of ingested breast milk may also contribute to jaundice in the first week of life.

Hyperbilirubinemia does not usually exceed 20 mg/dL, with most cases in the range of 10–15 mg/dL. Jaundice is noticeable by the fifth to seventh day of breast feeding. It may accentuate the underlying physiologic jaundice—especially early, when total fluid intake may be less than optimal. Except for jaundice, the physical examination is normal; urine does not stain the diaper, and the stools are golden yellow.

The jaundice peaks before the third week of life and clears before age 3 months in almost all infants, even when breast feeding is continued. All infants who remain jaundiced past age 2–3 weeks should have measurements of conjugated bilirubin to exclude cholestasis and hepatobiliary disease.

Kernicterus has rarely been reported in association with this condition. In special situations, breast feeding may be discontinued temporarily and replaced by formula feedings for 2–3 days until serum bilirubin decreases by 2–8 mg/dL. Cow's milk formulas inhibit the intestinal reabsorption of unconjugated bilirubin. When breast feeding is reinstituted, the serum bilirubin may increase slightly, but not to the previous level. Phototherapy is not indicated in the healthy full-term infant with this condition unless bilirubin levels meet high-risk levels as defined by the American Academy of Pediatrics.

Bhutani VK et al: Expert Committee for Severe Neonatal Hyperbilirubinemia; European Society for Pediatric Research; American Academy of Pediatrics: Management of jaundice and prevention of severe neonatal hyperbilirubinemia in infants ≥ 35 weeks gestation. Neonatology 2008;94(1):63–67 [Epub 2008 Jan 17] [PMID: 18204221].

Huang MJ et al: Risk factors for severe hyperbilirubinemia in neonates. Pediatr Res 2004;56:682–689 [Epub 2004 Aug 19] [PMID: 15319464].

Preer GL, Philipp BL: Understanding and managing breast milk jaundice. Arch Dis Child Fetal Neonatal Ed 2010 Aug 5 [Epub ahead of print] [PMID: 20688866].

B. Congenital Hypothyroidism

Although the differential diagnosis of indirect hyperbilirubinemia should always include congenital hypothyroidism, the diagnosis is usually suggested by clinical and physical clues or from the newborn screening results. The jaundice clears quickly with replacement thyroid hormone therapy, although the mechanism is unclear.

Tiker F: Congenital hypothyroidism and early severe hyperbilirubinemia. Clin Pediatr (Phila) 2003;42:365 [PMID: 12800733].

C. Upper Intestinal Obstruction

The association of indirect hyperbilirubinemia with high intestinal obstruction (eg, duodenal atresia, annular pancreas, pyloric stenosis) in the newborn has been observed repeatedly; the mechanism is unknown. Diminished levels of hepatic glucuronyl transferase are found on liver biopsy in pyloric stenosis, and genetic studies suggest that this indirect hyperbilirubinemia may be an early sign of Gilbert syndrome.

Treatment is that of the underlying obstructive condition (usually surgical). Jaundice disappears once adequate nutrition is achieved.

Hua L et al: The role of UGT1A1*28 mutation in jaundiced infants with hypertrophic pyloric stenosis. Pediatr Res 2005;58:881–884 [PMID: 16257926].

D. Gilbert Syndrome

Gilbert syndrome is a common form of familial hyperbilirubinemia present in 3%–7% of the population. It is associated with a partial reduction of hepatic bilirubin uridine diphosphate-glucuronyl transferase activity. Affected infants may have more rapid increase in jaundice in the newborn, accentuated breast milk jaundice, and jaundice with intestinal obstruction. During puberty and beyond, mild fluctuating jaundice, especially with illness and vague constitutional symptoms, is common. Shortened red blood cell survival in some patients is thought to be caused by reduced activity of enzymes involved in heme biosynthesis (protoporphyrinogen oxidase). Reduction of hyperbilirubinemia has been achieved in patients by administration of phenobarbital (5–8 mg/kg/d), although this therapy is not justified.

The disease is inherited as an abnormality of the promoter region of uridine diphosphate-glucuronyl transferase-1 (*UDGT1*); however, another factor appears to be necessary for disease expression. The homozygous (16%) and heterozygous states (40%) are common. Males are affected more often than females (4:1) for reasons that are not clear. Serum unconjugated bilirubin is generally less than 3–6 mg/dL, although unusual cases may exceed 8 mg/dL. The findings on liver biopsy and most other LFTs are normal. An increase of 1.4 mg/dL or more in the level of unconjugated bilirubin after a 2-day fast (300 kcal/d) is consistent with the diagnosis of Gilbert syndrome. Genetic testing is available but rarely needed. No treatment is necessary.

Claridge LC et al: Gilbert's syndrome. BMJ 2011 Apr 19;342:d2293 [PMID: 21508045].

Bartlett MG, Gourley GR: Assessment of UGT polymorphisms and neonatal jaundice. Semin Perinatol 2011 Jun;35(3):127–133 [PMID: 21641485].

E. Crigler-Najjar Syndrome

Infants with type 1 Crigler-Najjar syndrome usually develop rapid severe unconjugated hyperbilirubinemia (> 30–40 mg/dL) with neurologic consequences (kernicterus). Consanguinity is often present. Prompt recognition of this entity and treatment with exchange transfusions are required, followed by phototherapy. Some patients have no neurologic signs until adolescence or early adulthood, at which time deterioration may occur suddenly. For diagnosis of this condition, it is useful to obtain a duodenal bile specimen, which characteristically will be colorless and contain a predominance of unconjugated bilirubin, small amounts of monoconjugates, and only traces of diconjugated bilirubin. Phenobarbital administration does not significantly alter these findings, nor does it lower serum bilirubin levels. UGT genetic testing is available. The deficiency in UGT1 is inherited in an autosomal recessive pattern. A combination of aggressive phototherapy and cholestyramine may keep bilirubin levels below 25 mg/dL. The use of tin protoporphyrin or tin mesoporphyrin remains experimental. Orlistat therapy may decrease bilirubin in a subset of patients. Liver transplantation is curative and may prevent kernicterus if performed early. Auxiliary orthotopic transplantation also relieves the jaundice while the patient retains native liver. Hepatocyte transplantation is experimental and future gene therapy may be possible

A milder form (type 2) with both autosomal dominant and recessive inheritance is rarely associated with neurologic complications. Hyperbilirubinemia is less severe, and the bile is pigmented and contains small amounts of bilirubin monoglucuronide and diglucuronide. Patients with this form respond to phenobarbital (4 mg/kg/d in infants) with lowering of serum bilirubin levels. An increased proportion of monoconjugated and diconjugated bilirubin in the bile follows phenobarbital treatment. Liver biopsy findings and LFTs are consistently normal in both types.

Bartlett MG, Gourley GR: Assessment of UGT polymorphisms and neonatal jaundice. Semin Perinatol 2011 Jun;35(3):127–133 [PMID: 21641485].

Kohli S et al: Novel human pathological mutations. Gene symbol: UGT1A1 Disease: Crigler-Najjar syndrome 1. Hum Genet 2010 Apr;127(4):485 No abstract available [PMID: 21488310].

F. Drug-Induced Hyperbilirubinemia

Vitamin K_3 (menadiol) may elevate indirect bilirubin levels by causing hemolysis. Vitamin K_1 (phytonadione) can be used safely in neonates. Carbamazepine can cause conjugated hyperbilirubinemia in infancy. Rifampin and antiretroviral protease inhibitors may cause unconjugated hyperbilirubinemia. Other drugs (eg, ceftriaxone, sulfonamides) may displace bilirubin from albumin, potentially increasing the risk of kernicterus—especially in the sick premature infant.

2. Conjugated Noncholestatic Hyperbilirubinemia (Dubin-Johnson Syndrome & Rotor Syndrome)

These diagnoses are suspected when persistent or recurrent conjugated hyperbilirubinemia and jaundice occur and liver function tests are normal. The basic defect in Dubin-Johnson syndrome is in the multiple organic anion transport protein 2 (*MRP2*) of the bile canaliculus, causing impaired hepatocyte excretion of conjugated bilirubin into bile. A variable degree of impairment in uptake and conjugation complicates the clinical picture. Transmission is autosomal recessive, so a positive family history is occasionally obtained. In Rotor syndrome, the defect lies in hepatic uptake and storage of bilirubin. Bile acids are metabolized normally, so that cholestasis does not occur. Bilirubin values range from 2 to 5 mg/dL, and other LFTs are normal.

In Rotor syndrome, the liver is normal; in Dubin-Johnson syndrome, it is darkly pigmented on gross inspection and may be enlarged. Microscopic examination reveals numerous dark-brown pigment granules consisting of polymers of epinephrine metabolites, especially in the centrilobular regions. However, the amount of pigment varies within families, and some jaundiced family members may have no demonstrable pigmentation in the liver. Otherwise, the liver is histologically normal. Oral cholecystography fails to visualize the gall-bladder in Dubin-Johnson syndrome, but is normal in Rotor syndrome. Differences in the excretion patterns of bromosulfophthalein, in results of HIDA cholescintigraphy, in urinary coproporphyrin I and III levels, and in the serum pattern of monoglucuronide and diglucuronide conjugates of bilirubin can help distinguish between these two conditions. Genotyping of *MRP2* is available.

Choleretic agents (eg, UDCA) may help reduce the cholestasis in infants with Dubin-Johnson syndrome.

Rastogi A, Krishnani N, Pandey R: Dubin-Johnson syndrome—a clinicopathologic study of twenty cases. Indian J Pathol Microbiol 2006;49:500–504 [PMID: 17183837].

Strassburg CP: Hyperbilirubinemia syndromes (Gilbert-Meulengracht, Crigler-Najjar, Dubin-Johnson, and Rotor syndrome). Best Pract Res Clin Gastroenterol 2010 Oct;24(5): 555–571 [PMID: 20955959].

HEPATITIS A

ESSENTIALS OF DIAGNOSIS & TYPICAL FEATURES

- Gastrointestinal upset (anorexia, vomiting, diarrhea).
- Jaundice.

- Liver tenderness and enlargement.
- Abnormal LFTs.
- Local epidemic of hepatitis A infection.
- Positive anti-hepatitis A virus (HAV) IgM antibody.

Pathogenesis

Hepatitis A virus (HAV) infection occurs in both epidemic and sporadic fashion (Table 22–6). Fecal-oral route is the mode of transmission in epidemic outbreaks from contaminated food or water supplies, including by food handlers. HAV viral particles are found in stools during the acute phase of hepatitis A infection. Sporadic cases usually result from contact with an infected individual. Transmission through blood products obtained during the viremic phase is a rare event, although it has occurred in a newborn nursery.

Prevention

Isolation of the patient during initial phases of illness is indicated, although most patients with hepatitis A are noninfectious by the time the disease becomes overt. Stool, diapers, and other fecally stained clothing should be handled with care for 1 week after the appearance of jaundice.

Passive-active immunization of exposed susceptible persons can be achieved by giving standard immune globulin, 0.02–0.04 mL/kg intramuscularly. Illness is prevented in 80%–90% of individuals if immune globulin is given within 1–2 weeks of exposure. Alternatively, HAV vaccine can be given following exposure, with equal efficacy at preventing symptomatic HAV infection. Individuals traveling to endemic disease areas should receive HAV vaccine or

HEPATITIS VIRUS ABBREVIATIONS	
HAV	Hepatitis A virus
Anti-HAV IgM	IgM antibody to HAV
HBV	Hepatitis B virus
HBsAg	HBV surface antigen
HBcAg	HBV core antigen
HBeAg	HBV e antigen
Anti-HBs	Antibody to HBsAg
Anti-HBc	Antibody to HBcAg
Anti-HBc IgM	IgM antibody to HBcAg
Anti-HBe	Antibody to HBeAg
HCV	Hepatitis C virus
Anti-HCV	Antibody to HCV
HDV	Hepatitis D (delta) virus
Anti-HDV	Antibody to HDV
HEV	Hepatitis E virus
Anti-HEV	Antibody to HEV

Table 22–6. Hepatitis viruses.

	HAV	HBV	HCV	HDV	HEV
Type of virus	Enterovirus (RNA)	Hepadnavirus (DNA)	Flavivirus (RNA)	Deltavirus (RNA)	Hepevirus (family not assigned) (RNA)
Transmission routes	Fecal-oral	Parenteral, sexual, vertical	Parenteral, sexual, vertical	Parenteral, sexual	Fecal-oral
Incubation period (days)	15–40	45–160	30–150	20–90	14–65
Diagnostic test	Anti-HAV IgM	HBsAg, anti-HBc IgM, DNA PCR	Anti-HCV, RNA PCR	Anti-HDV antibody	Anti-HEV IgM
Mortality rate (acute)	0.1%–0.2%	0.5%–2%	1%–2%	2%–20%	1%–2% (10%–20% in pregnant women)
Carrier state	No	Yes	Yes	Yes	No
Vaccine available	Yes	Yes	No	Yes (HBV)	Yes (experimental)
Treatment	None	Interferon-α (pegylated interferon in adults), nucleoside analogues (lamivudine, tenofovir, adefovir; entecavir or telbivudine for children > 16 y old);	Pegylated interferon plus ribavirin	Treatment for HBV	None

HAV, hepatitis A virus; HBc, hepatitis B core; HBsAg, hepatitis B surface antigen; HBV, hepatitis B virus; HDV, hepatitis D (delta) virus; HEV, hepatitis E virus; PCR, polymerase chain reaction.

0.02–0.06 mL/kg of immune globulin as prophylaxis if there is insufficient time (< 2 weeks) for the initial dose of vaccine. All children older than 12 months with chronic liver disease should receive two doses of HAV vaccine 6 months apart. It is currently recommended that all children 12–23 months of age receive HAV vaccination in the United States. Lifelong immunity to HAV follows infection.

Antibody to HAV appears within 1–4 weeks of clinical symptoms. Although the great majority of children with infectious hepatitis are asymptomatic or have mild disease and recover completely, some will develop fulminant hepatitis leading to death or requiring liver transplantation.

Clinical Findings

A. History

Historical risk factors may include direct exposure to a previously jaundiced individual or recently arrived international adoptee from a high prevalence country, consumption of seafood, contaminated water or imported fruits or vegetables, attendance in a day care center, or recent travel to an area of endemic infection. Following an incubation period of 15–40 days, nonspecific symptoms usually precede the development of jaundice by 5–10 days. In developing countries, hepatitis A is common and most children are exposed to HAV by age 10 years, while only 20% are exposed by age 20 years in developed countries.

B. Symptoms and Signs

The overt form of the disease is easily recognized by the clinical manifestations. However, two-thirds of children are asymptomatic, and two-thirds of symptomatic children are anicteric. Therefore, the presenting symptoms in children with HAV resemble gastroenteritis. Fever, anorexia, vomiting, headache, and abdominal pain are typical and dark urine precedes jaundice, which peaks in 1–2 weeks and then begins to subside. The stools may become light- or clay-colored. Clinical improvement can occur as jaundice develops. Tender hepatomegaly and jaundice are typically present; splenomegaly is variable.

C. Laboratory Findings

Serum aminotransferases and conjugated and unconjugated bilirubin levels are elevated. Although unusual, hypoalbuminemia, hypoglycemia, and marked prolongation of PT (international normalized ratio [INR] > 2.0) are serious prognostic findings. Diagnosis is made by a positive anti-HAV IgM, whereas anti-HAV IgG persists after recovery.

Percutaneous liver biopsy is rarely indicated. "Balloon cells" and acidophilic bodies are characteristic histologic findings. Liver cell necrosis may be diffuse or focal, with accompanying infiltration of inflammatory cells containing polymorphonuclear leukocytes, lymphocytes, macrophages, and plasma cells, particularly in portal areas. Some bile duct proliferation may be seen in the perilobular portal areas alongside areas of bile stasis. Regenerative liver cells and proliferation of reticuloendothelial cells are present. Occasionally massive hepatocyte necrosis portends a poor prognosis.

Differential Diagnosis

Before jaundice appears, the symptoms are those of nonspecific viral enteritis. Other diseases with somewhat similar onset include pancreatitis, infectious mononucleosis, leptospirosis, drug-induced hepatitis, Wilson disease, autoimmune hepatitis (AIH), and other hepatitis viruses. Acquired CMV disease may also mimic HAV, although lymphadenopathy is usually present in the former.

Treatment

No specific treatment measures are required although bed rest is reasonable for the child who appears ill. Sedatives and corticosteroids should be avoided. During the icteric phase, lower-fat foods may diminish gastrointestinal symptoms, but do not affect overall outcome. Drugs and elective surgery should be avoided. Hospitalization is recommended for children with coagulopathy, encephalopathy, or severe vomiting.

Prognosis

Ninety-nine percent of children recover without sequelae. Persons with underlying chronic liver disease have an increased risk of death. In rare cases of fulminant HAV hepatitis, the patient may die within days to weeks and requires evaluation for liver transplantation. The prognosis is poor if hepatic coma or ascites develop; liver transplantation is indicated under these circumstances and is life-saving. Incomplete resolution can cause a prolonged hepatitis; however, resolution invariably occurs without long-term hepatic sequelae. Rare cases of aplastic anemia following acute infectious hepatitis have been reported. A benign relapse of symptoms may occur in 10%–15% of cases after 6–10 weeks of apparent resolution.

American Academy of Pediatrics Committee on Infectious Diseases: Hepatitis A vaccine recommendations. Pediatrics 2007;120:189 [PMID: 17606579].

Marshall H et al: Long-term (5 year) antibody persistence following two- and three-dose regimens of a combined hepatitis A and B vaccine in children aged 1–11 years. Vaccine 2010;17:4411 [PMID: 20434544].

Sweet K et al: Hepatitis A infection in recent international adoptees and their contacts in Minnesota, 2007–2009. Pediatrics 2011;128:e333 [PMID: 21727017].

Victor JC et al: Hepatitis A vaccine versus immune globulin for postexposure prophylaxis. N Engl J Med 2007;357:1685 [PMID: 17947390].

HEPATITIS B

ESSENTIALS OF DIAGNOSIS & TYPICAL FEATURES

- Gastrointestinal upset, anorexia, vomiting, diarrhea.
- Jaundice, tender hepatomegaly, abnormal LFTs.
- Serologic evidence of hepatitis B disease: HBsAg, HBeAg, anti-HBc IgM.
- History of parenteral, sexual, or household exposure or maternal HBsAg carriage.

General Considerations

In contrast to HAV, HBV infection has a longer incubation period of 45–160 days (see Table 22–6). HBV is a DNA virus that is usually acquired perinatally from a carrier mother, or later in life from exposure to contaminated blood through shared needles, needle sticks, skin piercing, tattoos, or sexual transmission. Transmission via blood products has been almost eliminated by donor-screening and donor blood testing protocols.

Pathophysiology

The HBV particle is composed of a core (28-nm particle) that is found in the nucleus of infected liver cells and a double outer shell (surface antigen). The surface antigen in blood is termed HBsAg, which elicits an antibody (anti-HBs). The core antigen is termed HBcAg and its antibody is anti-HBc. Anti-HBc IgM antibody indicates recent viral infection. Another important antigen-antibody system associated with HBV disease is the "e" (envelope) antigen system. HBeAg, a truncated soluble form of HBcAg, correlates with active virus replication. Persistence of HBeAg is a marker of infectivity, whereas the appearance of anti-HBe generally implies termination of viral replication. However, HBV mutant viruses (precore mutant) may replicate with negative HBeAg tests and positive tests for anti-HBe antibody and are associated with a more virulent form of the disease. Circulating HBV DNA (measured by PCR) also indicates viral replication.

Prevention

Hepatitis B vaccination is the preferred method for prevention. Universal immunization of all infants born in the United States and of adolescents is now recommended, as it is in most other countries. Other control methods include screening of blood donors and pregnant women, use of properly sterilized needles and surgical equipment, avoidance of sexual contact with carriers, general adoption of safe sex practices, and vaccination of household contacts, sexual partners, medical personnel, and those at high risk. For postexposure prophylaxis, use either the HBV vaccine alone (see Chapter 10) or together with administration of HBIG (0.06 mL/kg intramuscularly, given as soon as possible after exposure, up to 7 days). The risk of vertical transmission is dramatically reduced with the combination of newborn vaccination and HBIG administration.

Clinical Findings

A. Symptoms and Signs

Most infants and young children are completely asymptomatic, especially if the infection is acquired vertically. Symptoms of acute hepatitis B infection include slight fever (which may be absent), malaise, and mild gastrointestinal upset. Visible jaundice is usually the first significant finding and is accompanied by darkening of the urine and pale or clay-colored stools. Hepatomegaly is frequently present. Occasionally an antigen-antibody complex presentation antedates the appearance of icterus, and is characterized by macular rash, urticaria, and arthritis. HBV infection more rarely presents as a glomerulonephritis or nephrotic syndrome from immune complexes.

B. Laboratory Findings

The diagnosis of acute HBV infection is confirmed by the presence of HBsAg and anti-HBc IgM. Recovery from acute infection is accompanied by HBsAg clearance and appearance of anti-HBs and anti-HBc IgG. Individuals who are immune by vaccination are positive for anti-HBs, but negative for anti-HBc IgG. Chronic infection is defined as the presence of HBsAg for at least 6 months. Vertical transmission to newborns is documented by positive HBsAg. LFT results are similar to those discussed earlier for hepatitis A. Liver biopsy is most useful in chronic infection to determine the degree of fibrosis and inflammation. Hepatitis and a ground glass appearance of the hepatocytes may be present. Renal involvement may be suspected on the basis of urinary findings suggesting glomerulonephritis or nephrotic syndrome.

Differential Diagnosis

The differentiation between HAV and HBV disease is made easier by a history of parenteral exposure, an HBsAg-positive parent, or an unusually long period of incubation. HBV and hepatitis C virus (HCV) infection or Epstein-Barr virus (EBV) infection are differentiated serologically. The history may suggest a drug-induced hepatitis, especially if a serum sickness prodrome is reported. AIH, Wilson disease, hemochromatosis, nonalcoholic fatty liver disease (NAFLD), α_1-antitrypsin deficiency, and drug-induced hepatitis should also be considered.

Treatment

Supportive measures such as bed rest and a nutritious diet are used during the active symptomatic stage of acute HBV infection. Corticosteroids are contraindicated. No other treatment is needed for acute HBV infection. For acute infection complicated by acute liver failure, nucleoside or nucleotide therapy may be helpful. For patients with progressive disease (chronic hepatitis with fibrosis), there are currently two approved treatment options. Treatment with α-interferon (5–6 million U/m^2 of body surface area injected subcutaneously three times a week for 4–6 months) inhibits viral replication in 30%–40% of patients, normalizes the ALT level, and leads to the disappearance of HBeAg and the appearance of anti-HBe. Side effects are common. Younger children may respond better than older children. Orally administered nucleoside analog therapy (lamivudine 3 mg/kg/d up to 100 mg/d for children > 2 years old or adefovir 10 mg/d for children > 12 years old and entecavir [0.5 mg once daily] or telbivudine [600 mg once daily] for children > 16 years old) leads to a successful response in 25% of treated children, with minimal side effects, but may require long-term treatment. However, resistant organisms can emerge, more frequently with lamivudine. Pegylated interferon, several oral antiviral agents (with much lower rates of resistance), and combination therapy are promising options being tested in children. Asymptomatic HBsAg carriers (normal serum ALT, no hepatomegaly) do not respond to either therapy alone. Liver transplantation is successful in acute fulminant hepatitis B; however, reinfection is common following liver transplantation for chronic hepatitis B unless long-term HBIG or antivirals are used.

Prognosis

The prognosis for acute HBV infection is good in older children, although fulminant hepatitis (< 0.1%) or chronic hepatitis and cirrhosis (up to 10%) may supervene. The course of the acute disease is variable, but jaundice seldom persists for more than 2 weeks. HBsAg disappears in 95% of cases at the time of clinical recovery. Chronic infection may occur, particularly in children with vertical transmission, Down syndrome, or leukemia, and in those undergoing chronic hemodialysis. Persistence of neonatally acquired HBsAg occurs in 70%–90% of infants without immunoprophylaxis or vaccination. The presence of HBeAg in the HBsAg carrier indicates ongoing viral replication. However, 1%–2% of children infected at birth will show spontaneous seroconversion of HBeAg each year. If HBV infection is acquired later in childhood, HBV is cleared and recovery occurs in 90%–95% of patients. Chronic hepatitis B disease predisposes the patient to development of hepatocellular carcinoma. Once chronic HBV infection is established, surveillance for development of hepatocellular carcinoma with serum α-fetoprotein is performed biannually and ultrasonography yearly. Routine HBV vaccination of newborns in endemic countries has reduced the incidence of fulminant hepatic failure, chronic hepatitis, and hepatocellular carcinoma in children.

Haber BA et al: Recommendations for screening, monitoring, and referral of pediatric chronic hepatitis B. Pediatrics 2009;124:183 [PMID: 19805457].

Jonas MM et al: Treatment of children with chronic hepatitis B virus infection in the United States: Patient selection and therapeutic options. Hepatology 2010;52:2192 [PMID: 20890947].

Kansu A et al: Comparison of two different regimens of combined interferon-alpha2a and lamivudine therapy in children with chronic hepatitis B infection. Antivir Ther 2006;11:255 [PMID: 16640106].

Kurbegov AC, Sokol RJ: Hepatitis B therapy in children. Expert Rev Gastroenterol Hepatol 2009;3:39 [PMID: 19210112].

Ni YH: Natural history of hepatitis B virus infection: Pediatric perspective. J Gastroenterol 2011;46:1 [PMID: 20812021].

HEPATITIS C

General Considerations

Hepatitis C virus (HCV) is the most common cause of non-B chronic hepatitis (90% of posttransfusion hepatitis cases; see Table 22–6). Risk factors in adults and older children include illicit use of intravenous drugs (40%), occupational or sexual exposure (10%), and transfusions (10%); 30% of cases have no known risk factors. In children, most cases are now associated with transmission from an infected mother (vertical transmission) or other household transmission. In the past, children with hemophilia or on chronic hemodialysis were at significant risk. The risk from transfused blood products has diminished greatly (from 1–2:100 to < 1:100,000 units of blood) since the advent of blood testing for ALT and anti-HCV. HCV infection has also been caused by contaminated immune serum globulin preparations. Vertical transmission from HCV-infected mothers occurs more commonly with mothers who are HIV-positive (15%–20%) compared with those who are HIV-negative (5%–6%). About 0.4% of adolescents and 1.5% of adults in the United States have serologic evidence of infection. Vertically infected infants often have elevated ALT levels, but do not appear ill; long-term outcome is unknown; however, 20%–30% of infants clear the infection spontaneously by 2 years of age. Transmission of the virus from breast milk is very rare. HCV rarely causes fulminant hepatitis in children or adults in Western countries, but different serotypes do so in Asia.

HCV is a single-stranded RNA virus in the flavivirus family. At least seven genotypes of HCV exist. Several well-defined HCV antigens are the basis for serologic antibody tests. The third-generation enzyme-linked immunosorbent assay (ELISA) test for anti-HCV is highly accurate. Anti-HCV is generally present when symptoms occur; however, test results may be negative in the first few months of infection. The presence of HCV RNA in serum indicates active infection.

Prevention

At present, the only effective means of prevention is avoidance of exposure by eliminating risk-taking behaviors such as illicit use of intravenous drugs. There is no effective prevention for vertical transmission, but avoidance of fetal scalp monitoring in infant of mothers with HCV has been suggested. Elective cesarean delivery of HCV-infected pregnant women with a high titer of circulating virus may lessen the likelihood for vertical transmission. There is no vaccine, and no benefit from using immune globulin in infants born to infected mothers. Breast feeding is generally allowed unless there is bleeding into the milk.

Clinical Findings

A. Symptoms and Signs

Most childhood cases, especially those acquired vertically, are asymptomatic despite development of chronic hepatitis. The incubation period is 1–5 months, with insidious onset of symptoms. Flu-like prodromal symptoms and jaundice occur in less than 25% of cases. Hepatosplenomegaly may or may not be evident in chronic hepatitis. Ascites, clubbing, palmar erythema, or spider angiomas are rare and indicate progression to cirrhosis.

B. Laboratory Findings

Fluctuating mild to moderate elevations of aminotransferases over long periods are characteristic of chronic HCV infection; however, normal aminotransferases are common in children. Diagnosis is established by the presence of anti-HCV (third-generation ELISA) confirmed by the radioimmunoblot assay or detection of HCV RNA by PCR. Anti-HCV is acquired passively at birth from infected mothers and cannot be used to confirm disease in the neonate for the first 15 months. HCV RNA testing should be performed in suspected cases. Results of this test may be negative in the first month of life, but become positive by 4 months.

Percutaneous liver biopsy should be considered in chronic cases. Histologic examination shows portal triaditis with chronic inflammatory cells, occasional lymphocyte nodules in portal tracts, mild macrovesicular steatosis, and variable bridging necrosis, fibrosis, and cirrhosis; most children have only mild to moderate fibrosis on liver biopsy. Cirrhosis in adults generally requires 20–30 years of chronic HCV infection, but it has occasionally developed sooner in children.

Differential Diagnosis

HCV disease should be distinguished from HAV and HBV disease by serologic testing. Other causes of cirrhosis in children should be considered in cases of chronic illness, such as Wilson disease, α_1-antitrypsin deficiency, AIH, drug-induced hepatitis, or steatohepatitis.

Treatment

Treatment of acute HCV hepatitis with pegylated interferon has a high response rate in adults, but has not been studied in children. Indications for treatment of chronic infection in children are unclear, but generally include chronic hepatitis and fibrosis. Current treatment of children, consisting of pegylated interferon-α 2a or 2b (104 mcg/m^2 BSA weekly for 2a and 60 mcg/m^2 BSA weekly for 2b) and ribavirin (15 mg/kg/d), results in sustained response rates of 40%–50% in genotype 1. The response is up to 80% for genotypes 2 and 3. Protease inhibitors lead to improved response in adults with genotype 1 infection when combined with pegylated interferon and ribavirin, but have not been studied in children. End-stage liver disease secondary to HCV responds well to liver transplantation, although re-infection of the transplanted liver is very common and occasionally rapidly progressive. Pre- and posttransplant antiviral therapy may reduce the risk of reinfection.

Prognosis

Following an acute infection with HCV, 70%–80% of adults and older children develop a chronic infection. Approximately 5% of children at risk for vertical infection with HCV become infected and up to 30% spontaneously clear the infection by 2 years of age. Twenty percent of adults with chronic HCV develop cirrhosis by 30 years. The majority of children with chronic HCV have mild inflammation and fibrosis on liver biopsy, although cirrhosis may develop rapidly in rare cases or after decades. The longer-term outcome in children is less well defined. Limited 30-year follow-up of infants exposed to HCV by transfusion suggests a lower rate of progression to cirrhosis compared to adults. The prognosis for infants infected at birth with concomitant HIV infection is unknown, but the course appears benign for the first 10 years of life. In adults, chronic HCV infection has been associated with mixed cryoglobulinemia, polyarteritis nodosa, a siccalike syndrome, and membranoproliferative glomerulonephritis, as well as hepatocellular carcinoma.

Goodman GD et al: Pathology of chronic hepatitis C in children: Liver biopsy findings in the PEDS-C trial. Hepatology 2008;47:836 [PMID: 18167062].

Hu J et al: Treatment of hepatitis C in children: A systematic review. PLoS One 2010;5:e11542 [PMID: 20644626].

Schwarz KB et al: The combination of ribavirin and peginterferon is superior to peginterferon and placebo for children and adolescents with chronic hepatitis C. Gastroenterology 2011; 140:450 [PMID: 21036173].

Wirth S et al: High sustained virologic response rates in children with chronic hepatitis C receiving peginterferon alfa-2b plus ribavirin. J Hepatol 2010;52:501 [PMID: 20189674].

HEPATITIS D (DELTA AGENT)

The hepatitis D virus (HDV) is a 36-nm defective virus that requires the presence of HBsAg to be infectious (see Table 22–6). Thus, HDV infection can occur only in the presence of HBV infection. Transmission is by parenteral exposure or intimate contact. HDV is rare in North America. HDV can infect simultaneously with HBV, causing acute hepatitis, or can superinfect a patient with chronic HBV infection, predisposing the individual to chronic hepatitis or fulminant hepatitis. In children, the association between chronic HDV coinfection with HBV and chronic hepatitis and cirrhosis is strong. Vertical HDV transmission is rare. Patients should be screened for HDV by anti-HDV IgG, which indicates active or previous infection; active infection is confirmed by detecting HDV RNA by PCR or by detecting HDV IgM antibody. Treatment is directed at therapy for HBV infection or for fulminant hepatic failure.

Hughes SA et al: Hepatitis delta virus. Lancet 2011;378:73 [PMID: 21511329].

HEPATITIS E

Hepatitis E virus (HEV) infection is a cause of enterically transmitted, epidemic hepatitis (see Table 22–6). It is rare in the United States. HEV is a hepevirus that is transmitted via the fecal-oral route. It occurs predominantly in developing countries in association with water-borne epidemics, and has only a 3% secondary attack rate in household contacts. Areas reporting epidemics include Southeast Asia, China, the Indian subcontinent, the Middle East, northern and western Africa, Mexico, and Central America, with sporadic cases in the United States and Europe. Recent reports suggest zoonotic transmission can occur in low endemic regions. Its clinical manifestations resemble HAV infection except that symptomatic disease is rare in children, more common in adolescents and adults, and is associated with a high mortality (10%–20%) in pregnant women, particularly in the third trimester. HEV infection in individuals with chronic liver disease can cause acute deterioration. Zoonotic transmission from pigs, boars and deer can lead to chronic infection and cirrhosis in immunocompromised individuals. Outside of these settings chronic disease is not reported. Diagnosis is established by detecting anti-HEV IgM antibody or by HEV PCR. A recombinant vaccine is being tested. There is no effective treatment.

Aggarwal R: Hepatitis E: Historical, contemporary and future perspectives. J Gastroenterol Hepatol 2011;26 S1:72 [PMID: 21199517].

OTHER HEPATITIS VIRUSES

Other undiscovered viruses may be the cause of cases of acute liver failure (ALF)/severe hepatitis in children, in some cases in association with aplastic anemia. Aplastic anemia occurs in a small proportion of patients recovering from hepatitis and in 10%–20% of those undergoing liver transplantation for ALF of unknown etiology. Parvovirus has been associated with severe hepatitis; the prognosis is relatively good in children. Infectious mononucleosis (EBV) is commonly associated with acute hepatitis. CMV, adenovirus, herpes simplex virus, HHV-6, HIV, brucella, Q-fever, and leptospirosis are other infectious causes of acute hepatitis.

Aydim M et al: Detection of human parvovirus B19 in children with acute hepatitis. Ann Trop Paediatr 2006;26:25 [PMID: 16494701].

Cacheux W et al: HHV-6-related acute liver failure in two immunocompetent adults: Favourable outcome after liver transplantation and/or ganciclovir therapy. J Intern Med 2005;258:573 [PMID: 16313481].

ACUTE LIVER FAILURE

ESSENTIALS OF DIAGNOSIS & TYPICAL FEATURES

- Acute hepatitis with deepening jaundice.
- Extreme elevation of AST and ALT.
- Prolonged PT and INR.
- Encephalopathy and cerebral edema.
- Asterixis and fetor hepaticus.

General Considerations

Acute Liver Failure (ALF) is defined as acute liver dysfunction associated with significant hepatic synthetic dysfunction evidenced by a vitamin K-resistant coagulopathy (INR > 2.0) within 6 weeks after the onset of liver injury. This is often associated with encephalopathy, but in young children, encephalopathy may be difficult to detect or absent. Without liver transplantation, mortality is approximately 50% in children. An unusually virulent infectious agent or aggressive host immune response is postulated in many cases. A cause is not found in the majority of cases. The common identifiable causes of ALF are shown in Table 22–7. Patients with immunologic deficiency diseases and those receiving immunosuppressive drugs are vulnerable to herpes viruses. In children with HIV infection, nucleoside reverse transcriptase inhibitors have triggered lactic acidosis and liver failure. In patients with underlying respiratory chain defects, valproic acid may trigger ALF.

Clinical Findings

A. History

In some patients, the disease presents with the rapid development of deepening jaundice, bleeding, confusion, and

Table 22–7. Common identifiable causes[a] of ALF by age.

Neonates	Infections: herpesviruses and enteroviruses. Metabolic: neonatal iron storage disease, galactosemia, fructosemia, tyrosinemia, FAO, mitochondrial disorders. Ischemia: congenital heart disease.
Infants 1–24 mo	Infections: HAV, HBV. Metabolic: FAO, mitochondrial disorders, tyrosinemia. Drug: acetaminophen, valproate. Immune: AIH, HLH.
Children	Infections: EBV, HAV. Metabolic: FAO, Wilson disease. Drug: acetaminophen, valproate, others. Immune: AIH.
Adolescents	Infections: EBV, HAV. Metabolic: FAO, Wilson disease, fatty liver of pregnancy. Drug: acetaminophen, valproate, herbs, "ecstasy", others. Immune: AIH.

[a]Unknown cause of ALF remains the most common etiology.
ALF, acute liver failure; AIH, autoimmune hepatitis; EBV, Epstein-Barr virus; HAV, hepatitis A; HBV, hepatitis B; FAO, fatty acid oxidation defects; HLH, hemophagocytic lymphohistiocytosis.

progressive coma, while others are asymptomatic at the onset and then suddenly become severely ill during the second week of the disease. Jaundice, fever, anorexia, vomiting, and abdominal pain are the most common symptoms. A careful history of drug and toxin exposure is the key to determining a drug induced cause.

B. Symptoms and Signs

Deep jaundice with tender hepatomegaly is common early with a progressive shrinking of the liver, often with worsening hepatic function. Signs of chronic liver disease (splenomegaly, spider hemangiomata) should suggest an underlying chronic liver disease. Hyper-reflexia and positive extensor plantar responses are seen before encephalopathy. A characteristic breath odor (fetor hepaticus) is present. Impairment of renal function, manifested by either oliguria or anuria, is an ominous sign.

C. Laboratory Findings

Characteristic findings include elevated serum bilirubin levels (usually > 15–20 mg/dL), sustained very high AST and ALT (> 3000 U/L) that may decrease terminally, low serum albumin, hypoglycemia, and prolonged PT and INR. Blood ammonia levels become elevated, whereas blood urea nitrogen is often very low. Prolonged PT from disseminated intravascular coagulation (DIC) can be differentiated by determination of factor V (low in ALF and DIC) and VIII (normal to high in ALF and low in DIC). Terminally, AST and ALT, which were greatly elevated (2000–10,000 U/L), may improve as the liver gets smaller and undergoes massive necrosis and collapse. A high AST and ALT with normal bilirubin suggests acetaminophen or metabolic causes.

Differential Diagnosis

Severe hepatitis, with or without coagulopathy, due to infections, metabolic, autoimmune or drug can initially mimic ALF. Acute leukemia, cardiomyopathy, and Budd-Chiari syndrome can mimic severe hepatitis. Patients with Reye syndrome or urea cycle defects are typically anicteric.

Complications

The development of renal failure and depth of hepatic coma are major factors in the prognosis. Patients in stage 4 coma (unresponsiveness to verbal stimuli, decorticate or decerebrate posturing) rarely survive without liver transplantation and may have residual central nervous system deficits. Cerebral edema, which usually accompanies coma, is frequently the cause of death. Extreme prolongation of PT or INR greater than 3.5 predicts poor recovery except with acetaminophen overdose. Sepsis, hemorrhage, renal failure, or cardiorespiratory arrest is a common terminal event.

Treatment

The mainstay of therapy is excellent critical care while investigating for potentially treatable causes. Several therapies have failed to affect outcome, including exchange transfusion, plasmapheresis with plasma exchange, total body washout, charcoal hemoperfusion, and hemodialysis using a special high-permeability membrane. Hyperammonemia and bleeding should be controlled. Extracorporeal hepatic support devices are being developed to help bridge patients to liver transplantation or allow for liver regeneration. Orthotopic liver transplantation is successful with 60%–80% 1- to 3-year survival; however, up to 50% of patients spontaneously recover and will not need transplant and patients in grade 4 coma may not always recover cerebral function. Therefore, patients in ALF should be transferred prior to the development of hepatic coma to centers where liver transplantation can be performed. Criteria for deciding when to perform transplantation are not firmly established; however, serum bilirubin over 20 mg/dL, INR greater than 4, and factor V levels less than 20% indicate a poor prognosis. Living related donors may be required for transplantation in a timely fashion. The prognosis is better for acetaminophen ingestion, particularly when *N*-acetylcysteine treatment is given. Corticosteroids may be harmful, except in AIH for which steroids may reverse ALF. Acyclovir is essential in herpes simplex or varicella-zoster virus infection. For hyperammonemia, oral antibiotics such as metronidazole, neomycin, or gentamicin are used, as well as lactulose, 1–2 mL/kg three or four times daily, which reduces blood ammonia levels and traps ammonia in the colon.

Close monitoring of fluid and electrolytes is mandatory and requires a central venous line. Adequate dextrose should be infused (6–8 mg/kg/min) to maintain normal blood glucose and cellular metabolism. Diuretics, sedatives, and tranquilizers should be used sparingly. Early signs of cerebral edema are treated with infusions of mannitol (0.5–1.0 g/kg). Comatose patients should be intubated, given mechanical ventilatory support, and monitored for signs of infection. Coagulopathy is treated with fresh-frozen plasma, recombinant factor VIIa, other clotting factor concentrates, platelet infusions, or exchange transfusion for bleeding or procedures. Plasmapheresis and hemodialysis may help stabilize a patient while awaiting liver transplantation. Monitoring for increased intracranial pressure (hepatic coma stages 3 and 4) in patients awaiting liver transplantation is advocated by some. Continuous venous-venous dialysis may be helpful to maintain fluid balance.

Prognosis

The prognosis is primarily dependent on the etiology and depth of coma. Only 20%–30% of children with stage 3 or 4 hepatic encephalopathy will have a spontaneous recovery. Children with acute acetaminophen toxicity have a high rate of spontaneous survival, while 40% of children with indeterminate ALF (of unknown etiology) will have a spontaneous recovery. Data from a recent large study suggest that the spontaneous recovery rate is about 40%–50% when all causes of ALF are combined; 30% of patients will receive a liver transplant; and 20% will die without a transplant. Exchange transfusions or other modes of heroic therapy do not improve survival figures. Indeterminate ALF, nonacetaminophen drug induced ALF, and ALF in infants are associated with a poorer prognosis. Acetaminophen and AIH as a cause or rising levels of factors V and VII, coupled with rising levels of serum α-fetoprotein, may signify a more favorable prognosis. The 1-year survival rate in patients who undergo liver transplantation for ALF is 60%–85%.

Dhawan A: Etiology and prognosis of acute liver failure in children. Liver Transpl 2008;14:S80 [PMID: 18825678].

Miloh T et al: Improved outcomes in pediatric liver transplantation for acute liver failure. Pediatr Transplant 2010;14:863 [PMID: 20609170].

Narkewicz MR et al: Pattern of diagnostic evaluation for the causes of pediatric acute liver failure: An opportunity for quality improvement. J Pediatr 2009;155:801 [PMID: 1963443].

Squires RH: Acute liver failure in children. Semin Liver Dis 2008;28:153 [PMID: 18452115].

Sundaram SS et al: Characterization and outcomes of young infants with acute liver failure. J Pediatr 2011 [epub ahead of print] [PMID: 21621221].

AUTOIMMUNE HEPATITIS

ESSENTIALS OF DIAGNOSIS & TYPICAL FEATURES

- Acute or chronic hepatitis.
- Hypergammaglobulinemia.
- Positive antinuclear antibodies (ANA), anti-smooth muscle antibodies (ASMA), anti-liver-kidney microsomal (LKM) antibodies, or anti-soluble liver antigen antibodies (SLA).

Clinical Findings

A. History

Gradual onset of jaundice which may be asymptomatic or associated with fever, malaise, rash, arthritis, amenorrhea, gynecomastia, acne, pleurisy, pericarditis, or ulcerative colitis may be noted on history. A family history of autoimmune disease is often present and a high prevalence of seroimmunologic abnormalities has also been noted in relatives.

B. Symptoms and Signs

Asymptomatic hepatomegaly or splenomegaly may be found on examination. Occasionally patients present in ALF. Cutaneous signs of chronic liver disease may be noted (eg, spider angiomas, palmar erythema, and digital clubbing). Hepatosplenomegaly is frequently present. AIH can present as ALF, more commonly in those patients with AIH type 2 (anti-LKM-positive). Jaundice is not always present.

C. Laboratory Findings

LFTs reveal moderate elevations of serum bilirubin, AST, ALT, and serum alkaline phosphatase. Serum albumin may be low. Serum IgG levels are generally elevated (in the range of 2–6 g/dL). Low levels of C3 complement have been reported. Three subtypes of disease have been described based on autoantibodies present: type 1—ASMA (antiactin); type 2—anti-LKM (anti-cytochrome P-450); and type 3—anti-SLA. A genetic susceptibility to AIH is suggested by the increased incidence of the histocompatibility antigens HLA-A1 and HLA-B8. Liver biopsy shows loss of the lobular limiting plate, and interface hepatitis ("piecemeal" necrosis). Portal fibrosis, an inflammatory reaction of lymphocytes and plasma cells in the portal areas and perivascularly, and some bile duct and Kupffer cell proliferation and pseudolobule formation may be present. Cirrhosis may exist at diagnosis in up to 50% of patients.

Differential Diagnosis

Laboratory and histologic findings differentiate other types of chronic hepatitis (eg, HBV, HCV, and HDV infection; steatohepatitis; Wilson disease; α_1-antitrypsin deficiency; primary sclerosing cholangitis [PSC]). PSC occasionally presents in a manner similar to AIH, including the presence of autoantibodies. Ten to fifteen percent of pediatric patients have an "overlap syndrome" of AIH and PSC. Anti-HCV antibodies can be falsely positive and should be confirmed by HCV PCR. Drug-induced (minocycline, isoniazid, methyldopa, pemoline) chronic hepatitis should be ruled out.

Complications

Untreated disease that continues for months to years eventually results in cirrhosis, with complications of portal hypertension. Persistent malaise, fatigue, amenorrhea, and anorexia parallel disease activity. Bleeding from esophageal varices and development of ascites usually usher in hepatic failure.

Treatment

Corticosteroids (prednisone, 2 mg/kg/d maximum 60 mg) decrease the mortality rate during the early active phase of the disease. Recent data in adults suggests budesonide may be as efficacious as prednisone with less steroid side effects. Azathioprine or 6-mercaptopurine (6-MP), 1–2 mg/kg/d, is of value in decreasing the side effects of long-term corticosteroid therapy, but should not be used alone during the induction phase of treatment. Steroids are reduced over a 3- to 12-month period, and azathioprine is continued for at least 1–2 years if AST and ALT remain consistently normal. Whether a patient should be weaned completely off steroids is controversial. Liver biopsy is performed before stopping azathioprine or 6-MP therapy; if inflammation persists, then azathioprine or 6-MP is continued. Thiopurine methyltransferase activity in red blood cells should be assessed prior to starting azathioprine or 6-MP, to prevent extremely high blood levels and severe bone marrow toxicity. Relapses are treated similarly. Many patients require chronic azathioprine or 6-MP therapy. Cyclosporine, tacrolimus, or methotrexate may be helpful in poorly responsive cases. Mycophenolate mofetil can be substituted for azathioprine or 6-MP. Liver transplantation is indicated when disease progresses to decompensated cirrhosis despite therapy or in cases presenting in ALF that do not respond to therapy. Steroid therapy may be lifesaving in those presenting in ALF.

Prognosis

The overall prognosis for AIH is improved significantly with early therapy. Some studies report cures (normal histologic findings) in 15%–20% of patients. Relapses (seen clinically and histologically) occur in 40%–50% of patients after cessation of therapy; remissions follow repeat treatment. Survival for 10 years is common despite residual cirrhosis. Of children with AIH, 20%–50% eventually require liver transplantation. Complications of portal hypertension (bleeding varices, ascites, spontaneous bacterial peritonitis, and hepatopulmonary syndrome) require specific therapy. Liver transplantation is successful 70%–90% of the time. Disease recurs after transplantation 10%–50% of the time and is treated similarly to pretransplant disease.

Chai PF et al: Childhood autoimmune liver disease: Indications and outcome of liver transplantation. J Pediatr Gastroenterol Nutr 2010;50:295 [PMID: 20118802].

Greene MT, Whitington PF: Outcomes in pediatric autoimmune hepatitis. Curr Gastroenterol Rep 2009;11:248 [PMID: 19463226].

Mieli-Vergani G, Vergani D: Autoimmune hepatitis in children: What is different from adult AIH? Semin Liver Dis 2009;29:297 [PMID: 19676002].

NONALCOHOLIC FATTY LIVER DISEASE

ESSENTIALS OF DIAGNOSIS & TYPICAL FEATURES

- Hepatomegaly in patient with BMI > 95th percentile.
- Elevated ALT > AST.
- Detection of fatty infiltration of the liver on ultrasound.
- Histologic evidence of fat in the liver.
- Insulin resistance.

Nonalcoholic fatty liver disease (NAFLD) is now the most common form of chronic liver disease in children, affecting up to 10% of children in the United States. Most cases are associated with overweight state or type 2 diabetes mellitus. The prevalence of NAFLD is related to the prevalence of obesity in the population, which is estimated at 3%–9% for children and adolescents with significant racial and ethic variability. One to 3% of adolescents in the United States may have nonalcoholic steatohepatitis (NASH), based on the observation that 15%–25% of American adolescents are overweight or obese and that roughly 40% will have NAFLD and 10% will have NASH.

Prevention

The most effective therapy is prevention of excess weight gain.

Clinical Findings

A. History

Most patients with NAFLD are asymptomatic and discovered upon routine screening. Obesity and insulin resistance are known risk factors.

B. Symptoms and Signs

Patients with NAFLD present with asymptomatic soft hepatomegaly. Physical findings of insulin resistance (acanthosis nigrans) are frequently present.

C. Laboratory Findings

Many patients will have normal transaminases, but evidence for increased hepatic fat on ultrasound or liver biopsy. If NASH is present, mild to moderately elevated aminotransferases (2–10 times the upper limit of normal) are also present, but recent work suggests that the upper limit of ALT in children should be 25–30 independent of the local laboratory value. ALT is frequently higher than AST. Alkaline phosphatase and GGT may be mildly elevated, but bilirubin is normal. Elevated insulin levels are common. Liver biopsy shows micro- or macrovesicular steatosis in simple NAFLD; NASH also has portal tract inflammation, Mallory bodies, and variable degrees of portal fibrosis to cirrhosis. There are no established reliable biochemical predictors of the degree of hepatic fibrosis, but new biomarkers, like patatin-like phospholipase domain-containing 3 polymorphisms and hyaluronic acid, show promise.

D. Imaging

Ultrasonography or CT scanning indicates fat density in the liver. Transient elastography is a research tool that shows promise in estimating hepatic fibrosis.

Differential Diagnosis

Steatohepatitis is also associated with Wilson disease, hereditary fructose intolerance, tyrosinemia, HCV hepatitis, cystic fibrosis, fatty acid oxidation defects, kwashiorkor, Reye syndrome, respiratory chain defects, and toxic hepatopathy (ethanol and others).

Complications

Untreated, NAFLD with hepatic inflammation can progress to cirrhosis and portal hypertension. Dyslipidemia, hypertension, and insulin resistance are more common in children and adolescents with NAFLD.

Treatment

Treatment is weight reduction and exercise for obesity or treatment for the other causes. To date, no medications have affected NAFLD in controlled trials. In addition, improved control of insulin resistance with metformin or pioglitazone is also under study in NASH.

Prognosis

Although untreated, NAFLD can progress to cirrhosis and liver failure, there is a very high response rate to weight reduction. However, success in achieving long-term weight reduction is low in children and adults.

Lavine JE et al: Effect of vitamin E or metformin for treatment of nonalcoholic fatty liver disease in children and adolescents: The TONIC randomized controlled trial. JAMA 2011;27:1659 [PMID: 21521847].

Loomba R et al: Advances in pediatric nonalcoholic fatty liver disease. Hepatology 2009 [Epub] [PMID: 19637286].

Mencin AA, Lavine JE: Nonalcoholic fatty liver disease in children. Curr Opin Clini Nutr Metab Care 2011;14:151 [PMID: 21178608].

Schwimmer JB et al: SAFETY study: Alanine aminotransferase cutoff values are set too high for reliable detection of pediatric chronic liver disease. Gastroenterology 2010;138:1357 [PMID: 20064512].

α_1-ANTITRYPSIN DEFICIENCY LIVER DISEASE

ESSENTIALS OF DIAGNOSIS & TYPICAL FEATURES

- Serum α_1-antitrypsin level < 50–80 mg/dL.
- Identification of a specific protease inhibitor (Pi) phenotype (PiZZ, PiSZ) or genotype.
- Detection of diastase-resistant glycoprotein deposits in periportal hepatocytes.
- Histologic evidence of liver disease.
- Family history of early-onset pulmonary disease or liver disease.

General Considerations

The disease is caused by a deficiency in α_1-antitrypsin, a protease inhibitor (Pi) system, predisposing patients to chronic liver disease, and an early onset of pulmonary emphysema. It is most often associated with the Pi phenotypes ZZ and SZ. The accumulation of misfolded aggregates of α_1-antitrypsin protein in the liver causes the liver injury by unclear mechanisms.

Clinical Findings

A. Symptoms and Signs

α_1-Antitrypsin deficiency should be considered in all infants with neonatal cholestasis. About 10%–20% of affected individuals present with neonatal cholestasis. Serum GGT is usually, but not always, elevated. Jaundice, acholic stools, and malabsorption may also be present. Infants are often small for gestational age, and hepatosplenomegaly may be present. The family history may be positive for emphysema or cirrhosis.

The disease can also present in older children, where hepatomegaly or physical findings suggestive of cirrhosis and portal hypertension should always lead one to consider α_1-antitrypsin deficiency. Recurrent pulmonary disease (bronchitis, pneumonia) may be present in a few older children. However, very few children have significant pulmonary involvement. Most affected children are completely asymptomatic, with no laboratory or clinical evidence of liver or lung disease.

B. Laboratory Findings

Levels of the α_1-globulin fraction may be less than 0.2 gm/dL on serum protein electrophoresis. α_1-Antitrypsin level is low (< 50–80 mg/dL) in homozygotes (ZZ). Specific Pi phenotyping should be done to confirm the diagnosis. Genotyping is also available. LFTs often reflect underlying hepatic pathologic changes. Hyperbilirubinemia (mixed) and elevated aminotransferases, alkaline phosphatase, and GGT are present early. Hyperbilirubinemia generally resolves, while aminotransferase and GGT elevation may persist. Signs of cirrhosis and hypersplenism may develop even when LFTs are normal.

Liver biopsy findings after age 6 months show diastase-resistant, periodic acid–Schiff staining intracellular globules, particularly in periportal zones. These may be absent prior to age 6 months, but when present are characteristic of α_1-antitrypsin deficiency.

Differential Diagnosis

In newborns, other specific causes of neonatal cholestasis need to be considered, including biliary atresia. In older children, other causes of insidious cirrhosis (eg, HBV or HCV infection, AIH, Wilson disease, cystic fibrosis, and glycogen storage disease) should be considered.

Complications

Of all infants with PiZZ α_1-antitrypsin deficiency, only 15%–20% develop liver disease in childhood, and many have clinical recovery. Thus, other genetic or environmental modifiers must be involved. An associated abnormality in the microsomal disposal of accumulated aggregates may contribute to the liver disease phenotype. The complications of portal hypertension, cirrhosis, and chronic cholestasis predominate in affected children. Occasionally, children develop paucity of interlobular bile ducts.

Early-onset pulmonary emphysema occurs in young adults (age 30–40 years), particularly in smokers. An increased susceptibility to hepatocellular carcinoma has been noted in cirrhosis associated with α_1-antitrypsin deficiency.

Treatment

There is no specific treatment for the liver disease of this disorder. Replacement of the protein by transfusion therapy is used to prevent or treat pulmonary disease in affected adults. The neonatal cholestatic condition is treated with choleretics, medium-chain triglyceride–containing formula, and water-soluble preparations of fat-soluble vitamins (see Table 22–4). UCDA may reduce AST, ALT, and GGT, but its effect on outcome is unknown. Portal hypertension, esophageal bleeding, ascites, and other complications are treated as described elsewhere. Hepatitis A and B vaccines should be given to children with α_1-antitrypsin deficiency. Genetic counseling is indicated when the diagnosis is made. Diagnosis by prenatal screening is possible. Liver transplantation, performed for development of end-stage liver disease, cures the deficiency and prevents the development of pulmonary disease. Passive and active cigarette smoke exposure should be eliminated to help prevent pulmonary manifestations, and obesity should be avoided.

Prognosis

Of those patients presenting with neonatal cholestasis, approximately 10%–25% will need liver transplantation in the first 5 years of life, 15%–25% during childhood or adolescence, and 50%–75% will survive into adulthood with variable degrees of liver fibrosis. A correlation between histologic patterns and clinical course has been documented in the infantile form of the disease. Liver failure can be expected 5–15 years after development of cirrhosis. Recurrence or persistence of hyperbilirubinemia along with worsening coagulation studies indicates the need for evaluation for liver transplantation. Decompensated cirrhosis caused by this disease is an indication for liver transplantation; the survival rate should reach 80%–90%. Pulmonary involvement is prevented by liver transplantation. Heterozygotes may have a slightly higher incidence of liver disease. The exact relationship between low levels of serum α_1-antitrypsin and the development of liver disease is unclear. Emphysema develops because of a lack of inhibition of neutrophil elastase, which destroys pulmonary connective tissue.

Gotzsche PC, Johansen HK: Intravenous alpha-1 antitrypsin augmentation therapy for treating patients with alpha-1 antitrypsin deficiency and lung disease. Cochrane Database Syst Rev 2010: CD007851 [PMID: 20614465].

Lykavieris P et al: Liver disease associated with ZZ alpha1-antitrypsin deficiency and ursodeoxycholic acid therapy in children. J Pediatr Gastroenterol Nutr 2008;47:623 [PMID: 18955864].

Teckman JH: Alpha 1-antitrypsin deficiency in childhood. Semin Liv Dis 2007;27:274 [PMID: 17682974].

WILSON DISEASE (HEPATOLENTICULAR DEGENERATION)

ESSENTIALS OF DIAGNOSIS & TYPICAL FEATURES

- Acute or chronic liver disease.
- Deteriorating neurologic status.
- Kayser-Fleischer rings.
- Elevated liver copper.
- Abnormalities in levels of ceruloplasmin and serum and urine copper.

General Considerations

Wilson disease is caused by mutations in the gene *ATP7B* on chromosome 13 coding for a specific P-type adenosine triphosphatase involved in copper transport. This results in impaired bile excretion of copper and incorporation of copper into ceruloplasmin by the liver. The accumulated hepatic copper causes oxidant (free-radical) damage to the liver. Subsequently, copper accumulates in the basal ganglia and other tissues. The disease should be considered in all children older than age 2 years with evidence of liver disease (especially with hemolysis) or with suggestive neurologic signs. A family history is often present, and 25% of patients are identified by screening asymptomatic homozygous family members. The disease is autosomal recessive and occurs in 1:30,000 live births in all populations.

Clinical Findings

A. Symptoms and Signs

Hepatic involvement may present as ALF, acute hepatitis, chronic liver disease, cholelithiasis, or as cirrhosis with portal hypertension. Findings may include jaundice, hepatomegaly early in childhood, splenomegaly, and Kayser-Fleischer rings. The disease is considered after 3–4 years of age. The later onset of neurologic or psychiatric manifestations after age 10 years may include tremor, dysarthria, and drooling. Deterioration in school performance can be the earliest neurologic expression of disease. The Kayser-Fleischer ring is a brown band at the junction of the iris and cornea, generally requiring slit-lamp examination for detection. Absence of Kayser-Fleischer rings does not exclude this diagnosis.

B. Laboratory Findings

The laboratory diagnosis can be challenging. Serum ceruloplasmin levels (measured by the oxidase method) are usually less than 20 mg/dL. (Normal values are 23–43 mg/dL.) Low values, however, occur normally in infants younger than 3 months, and in at least 10%–20% of homozygotes the levels may be within the lower end of the normal range (20–30 mg/dL), particularly if immunoassays are used to measure ceruloplasmin. Rare patients with higher ceruloplasmin levels have been reported. Serum copper levels are low, but the overlap with normal is too great for satisfactory discrimination. In acute fulminant Wilson disease, serum copper levels are elevated markedly, owing to hepatic necrosis and release of copper. The presence of anemia, hemolysis, very high serum bilirubin levels (> 20–30 mg/dL), low alkaline phosphatase, and low uric acid are characteristic of acute Wilson disease. Urine copper excretion in children older than 3 years is normally less than 30 mcg/d; in Wilson disease, it is generally greater than 100 mcg/d although recent reports suggest it can be as low as > 40 mcg/d. Finally, the tissue content of copper from a liver biopsy, normally less than 40–50 mcg/g dry tissue, is greater than 250 mcg/g in most Wilson disease patients, but may be as low as > 75 mcg/d when characteristic liver histology is present.

Glycosuria and aminoaciduria have been reported. Hemolysis and gallstones may be present; bone lesions simulating those of osteochondritis dissecans have also been found.

The coarse nodular cirrhosis, macrovesicular steatosis, and glycogenated nuclei in hepatocytes seen on liver biopsy may distinguish Wilson disease from other types of cirrhosis. Early in the disease, vacuolation of liver cells, steatosis, and lipofuscin granules can be seen, as well as Mallory bodies. The presence of Mallory bodies in a child is strongly suggestive of Wilson disease. Stains for copper may sometimes be negative despite high copper content in the liver. Therefore, quantitative liver copper levels must be determined biochemically on biopsy specimens. Electron microscopy findings of abnormal mitochondria may be helpful.

Differential Diagnosis

During the icteric phase, acute or chronic viral hepatitis, α_1-antitrypsin deficiency, AIH, and drug-induced hepatitis are the usual diagnostic possibilities. NASH may have similar histology and be confused with Wilson disease in overweight patients. Later, other causes of cirrhosis and portal hypertension require consideration. Laboratory testing for serum ceruloplasmin, 24-hour urine copper excretion, liver copper concentration, and a slit-lamp examination of the cornea will differentiate Wilson disease from the others. Urinary copper excretion during penicillamine challenge (500 mg twice a day in the older child or adult) may also be helpful. Genetic testing of *ATP7B* is available and may be necessary in confusing cases. Other copper storage diseases that occur in early childhood include Indian childhood cirrhosis, Tyrolean childhood cirrhosis, and idiopathic copper toxicosis. However, ceruloplasmin concentrations are normal to elevated in these conditions.

Complications

Cirrhosis, hepatic coma, progressive neurologic degeneration, and death are the rule in the untreated patient. The complications of portal hypertension (variceal hemorrhage, ascites) may be present at diagnosis. Progressive central nervous system disease and terminal aspiration pneumonia were common in untreated older people. Acute hemolytic disease may result in acute renal failure and profound jaundice as part of the presentation of fulminant hepatitis.

Treatment

Copper chelation with D-penicillamine or trientine hydrochloride, 750–1500 mg/d orally, is the treatment of choice, whether or not the patient is symptomatic. The target dose for children is 20 mg/kg/d; begin with 250 mg/d and increase the dose weekly by 250 mg increments. Strict dietary restriction of copper intake is not practical. Supplementation with zinc acetate (25–50 mg orally, three times daily) may reduce copper absorption but must not be given at same time as copper chelators. Copper chelation or zinc therapy is continued for life, although doses of chelators may be reduced transiently at the time of surgery or early in pregnancy. Vitamin B_6 (25 mg) is given daily during therapy with penicillamine to prevent optic neuritis. In some countries, after a clinical response to penicillamine or trientine, zinc therapy is substituted and continued for life. Tetrathiomolybdate is being tested as an alternative therapy. Noncompliance with any of the drug regimens (including zinc therapy) can lead to sudden fulminant liver failure and death.

Liver transplantation is indicated for all cases of acute fulminant disease with hemolysis and renal failure, for progressive hepatic decompensation despite several months of therapy, and severe progressive hepatic insufficiency in patients who inadvisedly discontinue penicillamine, triene, or zinc therapy.

Prognosis

The prognosis of untreated Wilson disease is poor. The fulminant presentation is fatal without liver transplantation. Copper chelation reduces hepatic copper content, reverses many of the liver lesions, and can stabilize the clinical course of established cirrhosis. Neurologic symptoms generally respond to therapy. All siblings should be immediately screened and homozygotes given treatment with copper chelation or zinc acetate therapy, even if asymptomatic. Recent data suggest that zinc monotherapy may not be as effective for hepatic Wilson disease as copper chelation. Genetic testing (haplotype analysis or genotyping) is available clinically if there is any doubt about the diagnosis and for family members.

Arnon R et al: Wilson disease in children: Serum aminotransferases and urinary copper on triethylene tetramine dihydrochloride (trientine) treatment. J Pediatr Gastroenterol Nutr 2007;44:596 [PMID: 17460493].

Roberts EA, Schilsky ML: American Association for Study of Liver Diseases (AASLD): Diagnosis and treatment of Wilson disease: An update. Hepatology 2008;47:2089–2111 [PMID: 18506894].

Rosencrantz R, Schilsky M: Wilson disease: Pathogenesis and clinical considerations in diagnosis and treatment. Semin Liver Dis 2011 Aug;31(3):245–259 [PMID: 21901655].

Weiss KH et al: Zinc monotherapy is not as effective as chelating agents in treatment of Wilson disease. Gastroenterology 2011 Apr;140(4):1189–1198 [PMID: 21185835].

CIRRHOSIS

ESSENTIALS OF DIAGNOSIS & TYPICAL FEATURES

- Underlying liver disease.
- Nodular hard liver and splenomegaly.
- Nodular liver on abdominal imaging.
- Liver biopsy demonstrating cirrhosis.

General Considerations

Cirrhosis is a histologically defined condition of the liver characterized by diffuse hepatocyte injury and regeneration, an increase in connective tissue (bridging fibrosis), and disorganization of the lobular and vascular architecture (regenerative nodules). It may be micronodular or macronodular in appearance. It is the vasculature distortion that leads to increased resistance to blood flow, producing portal hypertension and its consequences.

Many liver diseases may progress to cirrhosis. In children, the two most common forms of cirrhosis are postnecrotic and biliary, each of which has different causes, symptoms, and treatments. Both forms can eventually lead to liver failure and death.

Clinical Findings

A. History

Many children with cirrhosis may be asymptomatic early in the course. Malaise, loss of appetite, failure to thrive, and nausea are frequent complaints, especially in anicteric varieties. Easy bruising may be reported. Jaundice may or may not be present.

B. Symptoms and Signs

The first indication of underlying liver disease may be splenomegaly, ascites, gastrointestinal hemorrhage, or hepatic encephalopathy. Variable hepatomegaly, spider angiomas, warm skin, palmar erythema, or digital clubbing may be present. A small, shrunken liver may present. Most often, the liver is enlarged slightly, especially in the subxiphoid region, where it has a firm to hard quality and an irregular edge. Splenomegaly generally precedes other complications of portal hypertension. Ascites may be detected as shifting dullness or a fluid wave. Gynecomastia may be noted in males. Digital clubbing occurs in 10%–15% of cases. Pretibial edema often occurs, reflecting underlying hypoproteinemia. In adolescent girls, irregularities of menstruation or/and amenorrhea may be early complaints.

In biliary cirrhosis, patients often have jaundice, dark urine, pruritus, hepatomegaly, and sometimes xanthomas in addition to the previously mentioned clinical findings. Malnutrition and failure to thrive due to steatorrhea may be more apparent in this form of cirrhosis.

C. Laboratory Findings

Mild abnormalities of AST and ALT are often present, with a decreased level of albumin and a variable increase in the level of γ-globulins. PT is prolonged and may be unresponsive to vitamin K administration. Burr and target red cells may be noted on the peripheral blood smear. Anemia, thrombocytopenia, and leukopenia are present if hypersplenism exists. However, blood tests may be normal in patients with cirrhosis.

In biliary cirrhosis, elevated conjugated bilirubin, bile acids, GGT, alkaline phosphatase, and cholesterol are common.

D. Imaging

Hepatic ultrasound, CT, or MRI examination may demonstrate abnormal hepatic texture and nodules. In biliary cirrhosis, abnormalities of the biliary tree may be apparent.

E. Pathologic Findings

Liver biopsy findings of regenerating nodules and surrounding fibrosis are hallmarks of cirrhosis. Pathologic features of biliary cirrhosis also include canalicular and hepatocyte cholestasis, as well as plugging of bile ducts. The interlobular bile ducts may be increased or decreased, depending on the cause and the stage of the disease process.

Differential Diagnosis

In the pediatric population, postnecrotic cirrhosis is often a result of acute or chronic liver disease (eg, viral hepatitis [HBV, HCV], autoimmune or drug-induced hepatitis, idiopathic neonatal giant-cell hepatitis); more recently, NAFLD; or certain inborn errors of metabolism (see Table 22–5). The evolution to cirrhosis may be insidious, with no recognized icteric phase, as in some cases of HBV or HCV infection, Wilson disease, hemochromatosis, or α_1-antitrypsin deficiency. At the time of diagnosis of cirrhosis, the underlying liver disease may be active, with abnormal LFTs; or it may be quiescent, with normal LFTs. Most cases of biliary cirrhosis result from congenital abnormalities of the bile ducts (biliary atresia, choledochal cyst), tumors of the bile duct, Caroli disease, PFIC, PSC, paucity of the intrahepatic bile ducts, and cystic fibrosis. Occasionally, cirrhosis may follow a hypersensitivity reaction to certain drugs such as phenytoin. Parasites (*Opisthorchis sinensis, Fasciola*, and *Ascaris*) may be causative in children living in endemic areas.

Complications

Major complications of cirrhosis in childhood include progressive nutritional disturbances, hormonal disturbances, and the evolution of portal hypertension and its complications. Hepatocellular carcinoma occurs with increased frequency in the cirrhotic liver, especially in patients with the chronic form of hereditary tyrosinemia or after long-standing HBV or HCV disease.

Treatment

At present, there is no proven medical treatment for cirrhosis, but whenever a treatable condition is identified (eg, Wilson disease, galactosemia, congenital fructose intolerance, AIH) or an offending agent eliminated (HBV, HCV, drugs, toxins), disease progression can be altered; occasionally regression of fibrosis has been noted. Recent evidence suggests that cirrhosis from HCV may be reversed by successful antiviral therapy. Children with cirrhosis should receive the hepatitis A and B vaccines, and they should be monitored for the development of hepatocellular carcinoma with serial serum α-fetoprotein determinations annually and abdominal ultrasound for hepatic nodules at least each 2–3 years. Liver transplantation may be appropriate in patients with: cirrhosis caused by a progressive disease; evidence of worsening hepatic synthetic function; or complications of cirrhosis that are no longer manageable.

Prognosis

Postnecrotic cirrhosis has an unpredictable course. Without transplantation, affected patients may die from liver failure within 10–15 years. Patients with a rising bilirubin, a vitamin K–resistant coagulopathy, or diuretic refractory ascites usually survive less than 1–2 years. The terminal event in some patients may be generalized hemorrhage, sepsis, or cardiorespiratory arrest. For patients with biliary cirrhosis, the prognosis is similar, except for those with surgically corrected lesions that result in regression or stabilization of the underlying liver condition. With liver transplantation, the long-term survival rate is 70%–90%.

Hardy SC, Kleinman RE: Cirrhosis and chronic liver failure. In Suchy FJ, Sokol RJ, Balistreri WF (editors): *Liver Disease in Children*, 3rd ed. Cambridge University Press, 2007:97–137.

Leonis MA, Balistreri WF: Evaluation and management of end-stage liver disease in children. Gastroenterology 2008;134:1741 [PMID: 18471551].

PORTAL HYPERTENSION

ESSENTIALS OF DIAGNOSIS & TYPICAL FEATURES

- Splenomegaly.
- Recurrent ascites.
- Variceal hemorrhage.
- Hypersplenism.

General Considerations

Portal hypertension is defined as an increase in the portal venous pressure to more than 5 mm Hg greater than the inferior vena caval pressure. Portal hypertension is most commonly a result of cirrhosis. Portal hypertension without cirrhosis may be divided into prehepatic, suprahepatic, and intrahepatic causes. Although the specific lesions vary somewhat in their clinical signs and symptoms, the consequences of portal hypertension are common to all.

A. Prehepatic Portal Hypertension

Prehepatic portal hypertension from acquired abnormalities of the portal and splenic veins accounts for 30%–50% of cases of variceal hemorrhage in children. A history of neonatal omphalitis, sepsis, dehydration, or umbilical vein catheterization may be present. Causes in older children include local trauma, peritonitis (pyelophlebitis), hypercoagulable states, and pancreatitis. Symptoms may occur before age 1 year, but in most cases the diagnosis is not made until age 3–5 years. Patients with a positive neonatal history tend to be symptomatic earlier.

A variety of portal or splenic vein malformations, some of which may be congenital, have been described, including defects in valves and atretic segments. Cavernous transformation is probably the result of attempted collateralization around the thrombosed portal vein rather than a congenital malformation. The site of the venous obstruction may be anywhere from the hilum of the liver to the hilum of the spleen.

B. Suprahepatic Vein Occlusion or Thrombosis (Budd-Chiari Syndrome)

No cause can be demonstrated in most instances in children, while tumor, medications, and hypercoagulable states are common causes in adults. The occasional association of hepatic vein thrombosis in inflammatory bowel disease favors the presence of endogenous toxins traversing the liver. Vasculitis leading to endophlebitis of the hepatic veins has been described. In addition, hepatic vein obstruction may be secondary to tumor, abdominal trauma, hyperthermia, or sepsis, or it may occur following the repair of an omphalocele or gastroschisis. Congenital vena caval bands, webs, a membrane, or stricture above the hepatic veins are sometimes causative. Hepatic vein thrombosis may be a complication of oral contraceptive medications. Underlying thrombotic conditions (deficiency of antithrombin III, protein C or S, or factor V Leiden; antiphospholipid antibodies; or mutations of the prothrombin gene) are common in adults.

C. Intrahepatic Portal Hypertension

1. Cirrhosis—See previous section.

2. Veno-occlusive disease (acute stage)—This entity now occurs most frequently in bone marrow transplant recipients. It may also develop after chemotherapy for acute leukemia, particularly with thioguanine. Additional causes include the ingestion of pyrrolizidine alkaloids ("bush tea") or other herbal teas, and a familial form of the disease occurring in congenital immunodeficiency states. The acute form of the disease generally occurs in the first month after bone marrow transplantation and is heralded by the triad of weight gain (ascites), tender hepatomegaly, and jaundice.

3. Congenital hepatic fibrosis—This is a rare autosomal recessive cause of intrahepatic presinusoidal portal hypertension (see Table 22–9). Liver biopsy is generally diagnostic, demonstrating Von Meyenburg complexes (abnormal clusters of ectatic bile ducts). On angiography, the intrahepatic branches of the portal vein may be duplicated. Autosomal recessive polycystic kidney disease is frequently associated with this disorder.

4. Other rare causes—Hepatoportal sclerosis (idiopathic portal hypertension, noncirrhotic portal fibrosis), focal nodular regeneration of the liver, and schistosomal hepatic fibrosis are also rare causes of intrahepatic presinusoidal portal hypertension.

Clinical Findings

A. Symptoms and Signs

For prehepatic portal hypertension, splenomegaly in an otherwise well child is the most constant physical sign. Recurrent episodes of abdominal distention resulting from ascites may be noted. The usual presenting symptoms are hematemesis and melena.

The presence of prehepatic portal hypertension is suggested by the following: (1) an episode of severe infection in the newborn period or early infancy—especially omphalitis, sepsis, gastroenteritis, severe dehydration, or prolonged or difficult umbilical vein catheterizations; (2) no previous evidence of liver disease; (3) a history of well-being prior to onset or recognition of symptoms; and (4) normal liver size and tests with splenomegaly.

Most patients with suprahepatic portal hypertension present with abdominal pain, tender hepatomegaly of acute onset, and abdominal enlargement caused by ascites. Jaundice is present in only 25% of patients. Vomiting, hematemesis, and diarrhea are less common. Cutaneous signs of chronic liver disease are often absent, as the obstruction is usually acute. Distended superficial veins on the back and the anterior abdomen, along with dependent edema, are seen when inferior vena cava obstruction affects hepatic vein outflow. Absence of hepatojugular reflux (jugular distention when pressure is applied to the liver) is a helpful clinical sign.

The symptoms and signs of intrahepatic portal hypertension are generally those of cirrhosis (see earlier section on Cirrhosis).

B. Laboratory Findings and Imaging

Most other common causes of splenomegaly or hepatosplenomegaly may be excluded by appropriate laboratory tests. Cultures, EBV titers, hepatitis serologies, blood smear examination, bone marrow studies, and LFTs may be necessary. In prehepatic portal hypertension, LFTs are generally normal. In Budd-Chiari syndrome and veno-occlusive disease, mild to moderate hyperbilirubinemia with modest elevations of aminotransferases and PT are often present. Significant early increases in fibrinolytic parameters (especially plasminogen activator inhibitor 1) have been reported in veno-occlusive disease. Hypersplenism with mild leucopenia and thrombocytopenia is often present. Upper endoscopy may reveal varices in symptomatic patients.

Doppler-assisted ultrasound scanning of the liver, portal vein, splenic vein, inferior vena cava, and hepatic veins may assist in defining the vascular anatomy. In prehepatic portal hypertension, abnormalities of the portal or splenic vein may be apparent, whereas the hepatic veins are normal. When noncirrhotic portal hypertension is suspected, angiography often is diagnostic. Selective arteriography of the superior mesenteric artery or MRI is recommended prior to surgical shunting to determine the patency of the superior mesenteric vein.

For suprahepatic portal hypertension, an inferior vena cavogram using catheters from above or below the suspected obstruction may reveal an intrinsic filling defect, an infiltrating tumor, or extrinsic compression of the inferior vena cava by an adjacent lesion. A large caudate lobe of the liver suggests Budd-Chiari syndrome. Care must be taken in interpreting extrinsic pressure defects of the subdiaphragmatic inferior vena cava if ascites is significant.

Simultaneous wedged hepatic vein pressure and hepatic venography are useful to demonstrate obstruction to major hepatic vein ostia and smaller vessels. In the absence of obstruction, reflux across the sinusoids into the portal vein branches can be accomplished. Pressures should also be taken from the right heart and supradiaphragmatic portion of the inferior vena cava to eliminate constrictive pericarditis and pulmonary hypertension from the differential diagnosis.

Differential Diagnosis

All causes of splenomegaly must be included in the differential diagnosis. The most common ones are infections, immune thrombocytopenic purpura, blood dyscrasias, lipidosis, reticuloendotheliosis, cirrhosis of the liver, and cysts or hemangiomas of the spleen. When hematemesis or melena occurs, other causes of gastrointestinal bleeding are possible, such as gastric or duodenal ulcers, tumors, duplications, and inflammatory bowel disease.

Because ascites is almost always present in suprahepatic portal hypertension, cirrhosis resulting from any cause must be excluded. Other suprahepatic (cardiac, pulmonary) causes of portal hypertension must also be ruled out. Although ascites may occur in prehepatic portal hypertension, it is uncommon.

Complications

The major manifestation and complication of portal hypertension is bleeding from esophageal varices. Fatal exsanguination is uncommon, but hypovolemic shock or resulting anemia may require prompt treatment. Hypersplenism with leukopenia and thrombocytopenia occurs, but seldom causes major symptoms. Rupture of the enlarged spleen secondary to trauma is always a threat. Retroperitoneal edema has been reported (Clatworthy sign).

Without treatment, complete and persistent hepatic vein obstruction in suprahepatic portal hypertension leads to liver failure, coma, and death. A nonportal type of cirrhosis may develop in the chronic form of hepatic veno-occlusive disease in which small- and medium-sized hepatic veins are affected. Death from renal failure may occur in rare cases of congenital hepatic fibrosis.

Treatment

Definitive treatment of noncirrhotic portal hypertension is generally lacking. Aggressive medical treatment of the complications of prehepatic portal hypertension is generally quite effective. Excellent results with either portosystemic shunt or the mesorex (mesenterico–left portal bypass) shunt. When possible, the mesorex shunt is the preferred technique. Veno-occlusive disease may be prevented somewhat by the prophylactic use of UCDA or defibrotide prior to conditioning for bone marrow transplantation. Treatment with defibrotide and withdrawal of the suspected offending agent, if possible, may increase the chance of recovery. Transjugular intrahepatic portosystemic shunts have been successful bridging to recovery in veno-occlusive disease. For suprahepatic portal hypertension, efforts should be directed at correcting the underlying cause, if possible. Either surgical or angiographic relief of obstruction should be attempted if a defined obstruction of the vessels is apparent. Liver transplantation, if not contraindicated, should be considered early if direct correction is not possible. In most cases, management of portal hypertension is directed at management of the complications (Table 22–8).

Prognosis

For prehepatic portal hypertension, the prognosis depends on the site of the block, the effectiveness of variceal eradication, the availability of suitable vessels for shunting procedures, and the experience of the surgeon. In patients treated by medical means, bleeding episodes seem to diminish with adolescence.

The prognosis in patients treated by medical and supportive therapy may be better than in the surgically treated group, especially when surgery is performed at an early age, although no comparative study has been done. Portacaval encephalopathy is unusual after shunting except when protein intake is excessive, but neurologic outcome may be better in patients who receive a mesorex shunt when compared with medical management alone.

The mortality rate of hepatic vein obstruction is very high (95%). In veno-occlusive disease, the prognosis is better, with complete recovery possible in 50% of acute forms and 5%–10% of subacute forms.

DeLeve LD et al: Vascular disorders of the liver. Hepatology 2009;49:1729 [PMID: 19399912].

Mileti E, Rosenthal P: Management of portal hypertension in children. Curr Gastroenterol Rep 2011;13:10 [PMID: 20927620].

Plessier A, Valla DC: Budd-Chiari syndrome. Semin Liver Dis 2008;28:259 [PMID: 18814079].

Goyet J: Mesoportal bypass for extrahepatic portal vein obstruction in children: Close to a cure for most! J Pediatr Surg 2010;45:272 [PMID: 20105620].

Table 22–8. Treatment of complications of portal hypertension.

Complication	Diagnosis	Treatment
Bleeding esophageal varices	Endoscopic verification of variceal bleeding.	Endosclerosis or variceal band ligation. Octreotide, 30 mcg/m^2 BSA/h intravenous. Pediatric Sengstaken-Blakemore tube. Surgical portosystemic shunt, TIPS, surgical variceal ligation, selective venous embolization, OLT. Propranolol may be useful to prevent recurrent bleeding.
Ascites	Clinical examination (fluid wave, shifting dullness), abdominal ultrasonography.	Sodium restriction (1–2 mEq/kg/d), spironolactone (3–5 mg/kg/d), furosemide (1–2 mg/kg/d), intravenous albumin (0.5–1 g/kg per dose), paracentesis, peritoneovenous (LeVeen) shunt, TIPS, surgical portosystemic shunt, OLT.[a]
Hepatic encephalopathy	Abnormal neurologic examination, elevated plasma ammonia.	Protein restriction (0.5–1 g/kg/d), intravenous glucose (6–8 mg/kg/min), neomycin (2–4 g/m^2 BSA PO in four doses), rifaximin (200 mg three times a day in children > 12 y), lactulose (1 mL/kg per dose [up to 30 mL] every 4–6 h PO), plasmapheresis, hemodialysis, OLT.[a]
Hypersplenism	Low WBC count, platelets, and/or hemoglobin. Splenomegaly.	No intervention, partial splenic embolization, surgical portosystemic shunt, TIPS, OLT. Splenectomy may worsen variceal bleeding.

[a]In order of sequential management.
BSA, body surface area; OLT, orthotopic liver transplantation; TIPS, transjugular intrahepatic portosystemic shunt; WBC, white blood cell.

BILIARY TRACT DISEASE

1. Cholelithiasis

ESSENTIALS OF DIAGNOSIS & TYPICAL FEATURES

- Episodic right upper quadrant abdominal pain.
- Elevated bilirubin, alkaline phosphatase, and GGT.
- Stones or sludge seen on abdominal ultrasound.

General Considerations

Gallstones may develop at all ages in the pediatric population and in utero. Gallstones may be divided into cholesterol stones (which contain more than 50% cholesterol) and pigment (black [sterile bile] and brown [infected bile]) stones. Pigment stones predominate in the first decade of life, while cholesterol stones account for up to 90% of gallstones in adolescence. For some patients, gallbladder dysfunction is associated with biliary sludge formation, which may evolve into "sludge balls" or tumefaction bile and then into gallstones. The process is reversible in many patients.

Clinical Findings

A. History

Most symptomatic gallstones are associated with acute or recurrent episodes of moderate to severe, sharp right upper quadrant or epigastric pain. The pain may radiate substernally or to the right shoulder. On rare occasions, the presentation may include a history of jaundice, back pain, or generalized abdominal discomfort, when it is associated with pancreatitis, suggesting stone impaction in the common duct or ampulla hepatopancreatica. Nausea and vomiting may occur during attacks. Pain episodes often occur postprandially, especially after ingestion of fatty foods. The groups at risk for gallstones include patients with known or suspected hemolytic disease; females; teenagers with prior pregnancy; obese individuals; individuals with rapid weight loss; children with portal vein thrombosis; certain racial or ethnic groups, particularly Native Americans (Pima Indians) and Hispanics; infants and children with ileal disease (Crohn disease) or prior ileal resection; patients with cystic fibrosis or Wilson disease; infants on prolonged parenteral hyperalimentation and those with bile acid transporter defects. Other, less certain risk factors include a positive family history, use of birth control pills, and diabetes mellitus.

B. Symptoms and Signs

During acute episodes of pain, tenderness is present in the right upper quadrant or epigastrium, with a positive inspiratory arrest (Murphy sign), usually without peritoneal signs. While rarely present, scleral icterus is helpful. Evidence of underlying hemolytic disease in addition to icterus may include pallor (anemia), splenomegaly, tachycardia, and high-output cardiac murmur. Fever is unusual in uncomplicated cases.

C. Laboratory Findings

Laboratory tests are usually normal unless calculi have lodged in the extrahepatic biliary system, in which case the serum bilirubin and GGT (or alkaline phosphatase) may be elevated. Amylase and lipase levels may be increased if stone obstruction occurs at the ampulla hepatopancreatica.

D. Imaging

Ultrasound evaluation is the best imaging technique, showing abnormal intraluminal contents (stones, sludge) as well as anatomic alterations of the gallbladder or dilation of the biliary ductal system. The presence of an anechoic acoustic shadow differentiates calculi from intraluminal sludge or sludge balls. Ceftriaxone may cause similar findings. Plain abdominal radiographs will show calculi with a high calcium content in the region of the gallbladder in up to 15% of patients. Lack of visualization of the gallbladder with hepatobiliary scintigraphy suggests chronic cholecystitis. In selected cases, ERCP, MRCP, or endoscopic ultrasound may be helpful in defining subtle abnormalities of the bile ducts and locating intraductal stones.

Differential Diagnosis

Other abnormal conditions of the biliary system with similar presentation are summarized in Table 22–9. Liver disease (hepatitis, abscess, or tumor) can cause similar symptoms or signs. Peptic disease, reflux esophagitis, paraesophageal hiatal hernia, cardiac disease, and pneumomediastinum must be considered when the pain is epigastric or substernal in location. Renal or pancreatic disease is a possible explanation if the pain is localized to the right flank or mid back. Subcapsular or supracapsular lesions of the liver (abscess, tumor, or hematoma) or right lower lobe infiltrate may also be a cause of nontraumatic right shoulder pain.

Complications

Major problems are related to stone impaction in either the cystic or common duct, which may lead to stricture formation or perforation. Acute distention and subsequent perforation of the gallbladder may occur when gallstones cause obstruction of the cystic duct. Stones impacted at the level of the ampulla hepatopancreatica often cause gallstone pancreatitis.

Treatment

Symptomatic cholelithiasis is treated by laparoscopic cholecystectomy or open cholecystectomy in selected cases. Intra-operative cholangiography via the cystic duct is recommended so that the physician can be certain the biliary system is free of retained stones. Calculi in the extrahepatic bile ducts may be removed at ERCP.

Gallstones developing in premature infants on parenteral nutrition can be followed by ultrasound examination. Most of the infants are asymptomatic, and the stones will resolve in 3–36 months. Gallstone dissolution using cholelitholytics (UCDA) or mechanical means (lithotripsy) has not been approved for children. Asymptomatic gallstones do not usually require treatment, as less than 20% will eventually cause problems.

Prognosis

The prognosis is excellent in uncomplicated cases that come to standard cholecystectomy.

Bogue CO et al: Risk factors, complications and outcomes of gallstones in children: A single center review. J Pediatr Gastroenterol Nutr 2010;50:303 [PMID: 20118803].

St Peter SD et al: Laparoscopic cholecystectomy in the pediatric population. J Laparoendosc Adv Surg Tech A 2008;18:127 [PMID: 18266591].

2. Primary Sclerosing Cholangitis

ESSENTIALS OF DIAGNOSIS & TYPICAL FEATURES

- Pruritus and jaundice.
- Elevated GGT.
- Associated with inflammatory bowel disease.
- Abnormal ERCP or MRCP.

General Considerations

PSC is a progressive liver disease of unknown cause, characterized by chronic inflammation and fibrosis of the intrahepatic or extrahepatic bile ducts (or both), with eventual obliteration of peripheral bile ducts, cholangiographic evidence of strictures, and dilation of all or parts of the biliary tree. PSC is more common in males with inflammatory bowel disease, particularly ulcerative colitis. It can also be seen with histiocytosis X, autoimmune hepatitis, IgG4 autoimmune pancreatitis, sicca syndromes, congenital and acquired immunodeficiency syndromes, and cystic fibrosis.

Clinical Findings

A. Symptoms and Signs

PSC often has an insidious onset. Clinical symptoms may include abdominal pain, fatigue, pruritus, and jaundice. Acholic stools and steatorrhea can occur. Physical findings include hepatomegaly, splenomegaly, and jaundice.

B. Laboratory Findings

The earliest finding may be asymptomatic elevation of the GGT. Subsequent laboratory abnormalities include elevated levels of alkaline phosphatase and bile acids. Later, cholestatic jaundice and elevated AST and ALT may occur. Patients with associated inflammatory bowel disease often test positive for perinuclear antineutrophil cytoplasmic antibodies. Other markers of autoimmune liver disease (ANA and ASMA) are often found, but are not specific for PSC. Sclerosing cholangitis due to cryptosporidia is common in immunodeficiency syndromes.

Table 22–9. Biliary tract diseases of childhood.

	Acute Hydrops Transient Dilation of Gallbladder[a,b]	Choledochal Cyst[c] (see Figure 22–1)	Acalculous Cholecystitis[d]	Caroli Disease[e] (Idiopathic Intrahepatic Bile Duct Dilation)	Congenital Hepatic Fibrosis[f]	Biliary Dyskinesia[g]
Predisposing or associated conditions	Premature infants with prolonged fasting or systemic illness. Hepatitis. Abnormalities of cystic duct. Kawasaki disease. Bacterial sepsis, EBV.	Congenital lesion. Female sex. Asians. Rarely with Caroli disease or congenital hepatic fibrosis.	Systemic illness, sepsis (*Streptococcus, Salmonella, Klebsiella*, etc), HIV infection. Gallbladder stasis, obstruction of cystic duct (stones, nodes, tumor).	Congenital lesion. Also found in congenital hepatic fibrosis or with choledochal cyst. Female sex. Autosomal recessive polycystic kidney disease.	Familial (autosomal recessive) 25% with autosomal recessive polycystic kidney disease (PKHD1 mutation). Choledochal cyst. Caroli disease. Meckel-Gruber, Ivemark, or Jeune syndrome.	Adolescents.
Symptoms	Absent in premature infants. Vomiting, abdominal pain in older children.	Abdominal pain, vomiting, jaundice.	Acute severe abdominal pain, vomiting, fever.	Recurrent abdominal pain, vomiting. Fever, jaundice when cholangitis occurs.	Hematemesis, melena from bleeding esophageal varices.	Intermittent RUQ pain.
Signs	RUQ abdominal mass. Tenderness in some.	Icterus, acholic stools, dark urine in neonatal period. RUQ abdominal mass or tenderness in older children.	Tenderness in mid and right upper abdomen. Occasional palpable mass in RUQ.	Icterus, hepatomegaly.	Hepatosplenomegaly.	Usually normal exam.
Laboratory abnormalities	Most are normal. Increased WBC count during sepsis (may be decreased in premature infants). Abnormal LFTs in hepatitis.	Conjugated hyperbilirubinemia, elevated GGT, slightly increased AST. Elevated pancreatic serum amylase common.	Elevated WBC count, normal or slight abnormality of LFTs.	Abnormal LFTs. Increased WBC count with cholangitis. Urine abnormalities if associated with congenital hepatic fibrosis.	Low platelet and WBC count (hypersplenism), slight elevation of AST, GGT. Inability to concentrate urine.	Usually normal.
Diagnostic studies most useful	Gallbladder US.	Gallbladder US, hepatobiliary scintigraphy, MRCP, or ERCP.	Scintigraphy to confirm nonfunction of gallbladder. US or abdominal CT scan to rule out other neighboring disease.	Transhepatic cholangiography, MRCP, ERCP, scintigraphy, US, intravenous pyelography.	Liver biopsy. US of liver and kidneys. Upper endoscopy.	Normal US, CCK stimulated hepatobiliary scintigraphy demonstrating a very reduced ejection fraction.
Treatment	Treatment of associated condition. Needle or tube cystostomy rarely required. Cholecystectomy seldom indicated.	Surgical resection and choledochojejunostomy.	Broad-spectrum antibiotic coverage, then cholecystectomy.	Antibiotics and surgical or endoscopic drainage for cholangitis. Liver transplantation for some. Lobectomy for localized disease.	Treatment of portal hypertension. Liver and kidney transplantation for some.	Cholecystectomy in well selected cases. Biliary sphincterotomy in rare cases.

Complications	Perforation with bile peritonitis rare.	Progressive biliary cirrhosis. Increased incidence of cholangiocarcinoma. Cholangitis in some.	Perforation and bile peritonitis, sepsis, abscess or fistula formation. Pancreatitis.	Sepsis with episodes of cholangitis, biliary cirrhosis, portal hypertension. Intraductal stones. Cholangiocarcinoma.	Bleeding from varices. Splenic rupture, severe thrombocytopenia. Progressive renal failure.	Continued pain after surgery.
Prognosis	Excellent with resolution of underlying condition. Consider cystic duct obstruction if disorder fails to resolve.	Depends on anatomic type of cyst, associated condition, and success of surgery. Liver transplantation required in some.	Good with early diagnosis and treatment.	Poor, with gradual deterioration of liver function. Multiple surgical drainage procedures expected. Liver transplantation should improve long-term prognosis.	Good in absence of serious renal involvement and with control of portal hypertension. Slightly increased risk of cholangiocarcinoma.	Good short-term outcome in well-selected patients.

[a]Crankson S et al: Acute hydrops of the gallbladder in childhood. Eur J Pediatr 1992;151:318 [PMID: 9788647].
[b]Zulian F et al: Acute surgical abdomen as presenting manifestation of Kawasaki disease. J Pediatr 2003;142:731 [PMID: 12838207].
[c]Edil BH et al: Choledochal cyst disease in children and adults: A 30-year single-institution experience. J Am Coll Surg 2008;206:1000 [PMID: 18471743].
[d]Imamoglu M et al: Acute acalculous cholecystitis in children: Diagnosis and treatment. J Pediatr Surg 2002;37:36 [PMID: 11781983].
[e]Yonem O, Bayraktar Y: Clinical characteristics of Caroli's syndrome. World J Gastroenterol 2007;13:1934 [PMID: 17461493].
[f]Veigel MC et al: Fibropolycystic liver disease in children. Pediatr Radiol 2009;39:317–327; quiz 420 [PMID: 19083218].
[g]Hofeldt M et al: Laparoscopic cholecystectomy for treatment of biliary dyskinesia is safe and effective in the pediatric population. Am Surg 2008;74:1069 [PMID: 19062663].
AST, aspartate aminotransferase; CCK, cholecystokinin; CT, computed tomography; EBV, Epstein-Barr virus; ERCP, endoscopic retrograde cholangiopancreatography; GGTx, Y-glutamyl transpeptidase; HIV, human immunodeficiency virus; LFT, liver function test; MRCP, magnetic resonance cholangiopancreatography; RUQ, right upper quadrant; US, ultrasound; WBC, white blood cell.

C. Imaging

Ultrasound may show dilated intrahepatic bile ducts behind strictures. MRCP is the diagnostic study of choice, demonstrating irregularities of the biliary tree. ERCP may be more sensitive for the diagnosis of irregularities of the intrahepatic biliary tree.

Differential Diagnosis

The differential diagnosis includes infectious hepatitis, secondary cholangitis, AIH, metabolic liver disease, cystic fibrosis, choledochal cyst, or other anomalies of the biliary tree, including Caroli disease, choledochal cyst, and congenital hepatic fibrosis (see Table 22–9).

Complications

Complications include secondary bacterial cholangitis, pancreatitis, biliary fibrosis, and cirrhosis. Progression to liver failure is common, and the risk of cholangiocarcinoma is higher in PSC.

Treatment

No completely effective treatment is available. Ursodeoxycholic acid use is controversial as in high doses it may worsen disease in adults. Oral vancomycin may improve outcome. Patients with autoimmune markers and autoimmune sclerosing cholangitis or IgG4 cholangitis may benefit from treatment with corticosteroids and azathioprine. Antibiotic treatment of cholangitis and dilation and stenting of dominant bile duct strictures can reduce symptoms. Liver transplantation is effective for patients with end-stage complications, but the disease may recur in up to 10%.

Prognosis

The majority of patients will eventually require liver transplantation, and PSC is the fifth leading indication for liver transplantation in the United States. The median duration from the time of diagnosis to end-stage liver disease is 12–15 years.

Kerkar N, Miloh T: Sclerosing cholangitis: Pediatric perspective. Curr Gastroenterol Rep 2010;12:195 [PMID: 20425475].

Mieli-Vergani G, Vergani D: Unique features of primary sclerosing cholangitis in children. Curr Opin Gastroenterol 2010;26:265 [PMID: 20393280].

Miloh T et al: A retrospective single-center review of primary sclerosing cholangitis in children. Clin Gastroenterol Hepatol 2009;7:239 [PMID: 19121649].

3. Other Biliary Tract Disorders

For a schematic representation of the various types of choledochal cysts, see Figure 22–1. For summary information on acute hydrops, choledochal cyst, acalculous cholecystitis, Caroli disease, biliary dyskinesia, and congenital hepatic fibrosis, see Table 22–9.

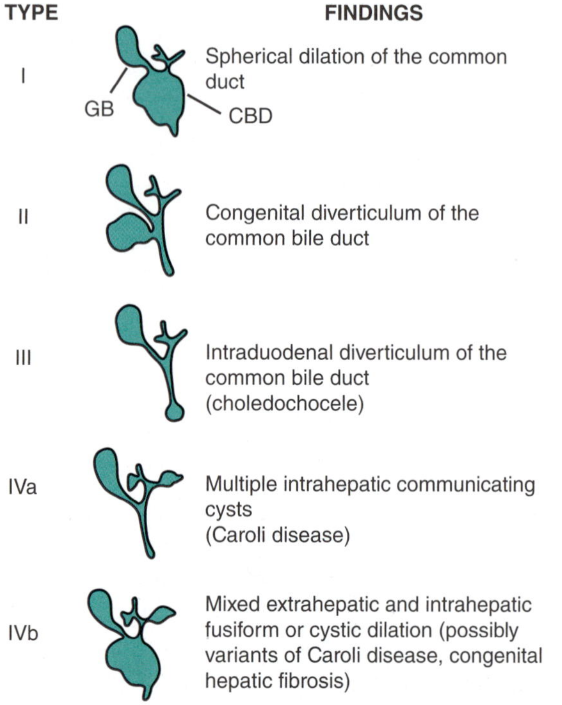

▲ **Figure 22–1.** Classification of cystic dilation of the bile ducts. Types I, II, and III are extrahepatic choledochal cysts. Type IVa is solely intrahepatic, and type IVb is both intrahepatic and extrahepatic.

PYOGENIC & AMEBIC LIVER ABSCESS

ESSENTIALS OF DIAGNOSIS & TYPICAL FEATURES

- Fever and painful enlarged liver.
- Ultrasound of liver demonstrating an abscess.
- Positive serum ameba antibody or positive bacterial culture of abscess fluid.

General Considerations

Pyogenic liver abscesses are rare in developed countries, but remain a significant issue in developing countries. The most common cause is *S aureus*, with enteric bacteria less common; fungal abscesses also occur. The resulting lesion tends to be solitary and located in the right hepatic lobe. Unusual causes include omphalitis, subacute infective endocarditis, pyelonephritis, Crohn disease, and perinephric abscess. In immunocompromised patients, *S aureus*, gram-negative organisms, and fungi may seed the liver from the arterial system. Multiple pyogenic liver abscesses are associated with severe sepsis. Children receiving anti-inflammatory and immunosuppressive agents and children with defects in white blood cell function (chronic granulomatous disease) are prone to pyogenic hepatic abscesses, especially those caused by *S aureus*.

Amebic liver abscess can occur when *Entamoeba histolytica* invasion occurs via the large bowel, although a history of diarrhea (colitis-like picture) is not always obtained.

Clinical Findings

A. History

With any liver abscess, nonspecific complaints of fever, chills, malaise, and abdominal pain are frequent. Amoebic liver abscess is rare in children. An increased risk is associated with travel in areas of endemic infection (Mexico, Southeast Asia) within 5 months of presentation.

B. Symptoms and Signs

Weight loss is very common, especially when diagnosis is delayed. A few patients have shaking chills and jaundice. The dominant complaint is a constant dull pain over an enlarged liver that is tender to palpation. An elevated hemidiaphragm with reduced or absent respiratory excursion may be demonstrated on physical examination and confirmed by fluoroscopy.

Fever and abdominal pain are the two most common symptoms of amebic liver abscess. Abdominal tenderness and hepatomegaly are present in over 50%. An occasional prodrome may include cough, dyspnea, and shoulder pain when rupture of the abscess into the right chest occurs.

C. Laboratory Findings

Laboratory studies show leukocytosis and, at times, anemia. LFTs may be normal or reveal mild elevation of transaminases and alkaline phosphatase. Early in the course, LFTs may suggest mild hepatitis. Blood cultures may be positive. The distinction between pyogenic and amebic abscesses is best made by indirect hemagglutination test for specific antibody (which is positive in more than 95% of patients with amebic liver disease) and the prompt clinical response of the latter to antiamebic therapy (metronidazole). Examination of material obtained by needle aspiration of the abscess using ultrasound guidance is often diagnostic.

D. Imaging

Ultrasound liver scan is the most useful diagnostic aid in evaluating pyogenic and amebic abscesses, detecting lesions as small as 1–2 cm. MRI, CT, or nuclear scanning with gallium or technetium sulfur colloid may be useful in differentiating tumor or hydatid cyst. Consolidation of the right lower lobe is common (10%–30% of patients) in amebic abscess.

Differential Diagnosis

Hepatitis, hepatoma, hydatid cyst, gallbladder disease, or biliary tract infections can mimic liver abscess. Subphrenic abscesses, empyema, and pneumonia may give a similar picture. Inflammatory disease of the intestines or of the biliary system may be complicated by liver abscess.

Complications

Spontaneous rupture of the abscess may occur with extension of infection into the subphrenic space, thorax, peritoneal cavity, and, occasionally, the pericardium. Bronchopleural fistula with large sputum production and hemoptysis can develop in severe cases. Simultaneously, the amebic liver abscess may be secondarily infected with bacteria (in 10%–20% of patients). Metastatic hematogenous spread to the lungs and the brain has been reported.

Treatment

Ultrasound- or CT-guided percutaneous needle aspiration for aerobic and anaerobic culture with simultaneous placement of a catheter for drainage, combined with appropriate antibiotic therapy, is the treatment of choice for solitary pyogenic liver abscess. Multiple liver abscesses may also be treated successfully by this method. Surgical intervention may be indicated if rupture occurs outside the capsule of the liver or if enterohepatic fistulae are suspected.

Amebic abscesses in uncomplicated cases should be treated promptly with oral metronidazole, 35–50 mg/kg/d, in three divided doses for 10 days. Intravenous metronidazole can be used for patients unable to take oral medication. Failure to improve after 72 hours of drug therapy suggests superimposed bacterial infection or an incorrect diagnosis. At this point, needle aspiration or surgical drainage is indicated. Once oral feedings can be tolerated, a luminal amebicide such as iodoquinol should be initiated. Resolution of the abscess cavity occurs over 3–6 months.

Prognosis

With drainage and antibiotics, the cure rate is about 90%. Mortality rates have improved, but remain at 15% for pyogenic liver abscess, especially with extrahepatic complications, and less than 1% for amebic abscess.

Mishra K et al: Liver abscess in children: An overview. World J Pediatr 2010;6:210 [PMID: 20706820].

Singh O et al: Comparative study of catheter drainage and needle aspiration in management of large liver abscesses. Indian J Gastroenterol 2009;28:88 [PMID: 19907956].

LIVER TUMORS

ESSENTIALS OF DIAGNOSIS & TYPICAL FEATURES

- Abdominal enlargement and pain, weight loss, anemia.
- Hepatomegaly with or without a definable mass.
- Mass lesion on imaging studies.
- Laparotomy and tissue biopsy.

General Considerations

Primary epithelial neoplasms of the liver represent 0.2%–5.8% of all malignant conditions in children. After Wilms tumor and neuroblastoma, hepatomas are the third most common intra-abdominal cancer. The incidence is higher in Southeast Asia, where childhood cirrhosis is more common. This trend is changing with improved prevention of chronic hepatitis B infections. There are two basic morphologic types with certain clinical and prognostic differences. Hepatoblastoma predominates in male infants and children and accounts for 79% of liver cancer in children, with most cases appearing before age 5 years. There is an increased risk of hepatoblastoma in Beckwith-Wiedemann syndrome, hemihypertrophy, familial adenomatosis polyposis coli, and in premature or low-birth-weight infants. Most lesions are found in the right lobe of the liver. Pathologic differentiation from hepatocellular carcinoma, the other major malignant tumor of the liver, may be difficult. Hepatocellular carcinoma occurs more frequently after age 3 years, carries a worse prognosis than hepatoblastoma, and causes more abdominal discomfort.

Patients with chronic HBV or HCV infection, cirrhosis, glycogen storage disease type I, tyrosinemia, or α_1-antitrypsin deficiency have an increased risk for hepatocellular carcinoma. The late development of hepatocellular carcinoma in patients receiving androgens for treatment of Fanconi syndrome and aplastic anemia must also be kept in mind. The use of anabolic steroids by body-conscious adolescents poses a risk of hepatic neoplasia.

An interesting aspect of primary epithelial neoplasms of the liver is the increased incidence of associated anomalies and endocrine abnormalities. Virilization has been reported as a consequence of gonadotropin activity of the tumor. Feminization with bilateral gynecomastia may occur in association with high estradiol levels in the blood, the latter a consequence of increased aromatization of circulating androgens by the liver. Leydig cell hyperplasia without spermatogenesis is found on testicular biopsy. Hemihypertrophy, congenital absence of the kidney, macroglossia, and Meckel diverticulum have been found in association with hepatocellular carcinoma.

Clinical Findings

A. History

A noticeable increase in abdominal girth with or without pain is the most constant feature of the history. A parent may note a bulge in the upper abdomen or report feeling a hard mass. Constitutional symptoms (eg, anorexia, fatigue, fever, and chills) may be present. Teenage boys may complain of gynecomastia.

B. Symptoms and Signs

Weight loss, pallor, and abdominal pain associated with a large abdomen are common. Physical examination reveals hepatomegaly with or without a definite tumor mass, usually to the right of the midline. In the absence of cirrhosis, signs of chronic liver disease are usually absent. However, evidence of virilization or feminization in prepubertal children may be noted.

C. Laboratory Findings

Normal LFTs are the rule. Anemia frequently occurs, especially in cases of hepatoblastoma. Cystathioninuria has been reported. α-Fetoprotein levels are often elevated, especially in hepatoblastoma. Estradiol levels are sometimes elevated. Tissue diagnosis is best obtained at laparotomy, although ultrasound- or CT-guided needle biopsy of the liver mass can be used.

D. Imaging

Ultrasonography, CT, and MRI are useful for diagnosis, staging, and following tumor response to therapy. A scintigraphic study of bone and chest CT are generally part of the preoperative workup to evaluate metastatic disease.

Differential Diagnosis

In the absence of a palpable mass, the differential diagnosis is that of hepatomegaly with or without anemia or jaundice. Hematologic and nutritional conditions should be ruled out, as well as HBV and HCV infection, α_1-antitrypsin deficiency disease, lipid storage diseases, histiocytosis X, glycogen storage disease, tyrosinemia, congenital hepatic fibrosis, cysts, adenoma, focal nodular hyperplasia, inflammatory pseudotumor, and hemangiomas. If fever is present, hepatic abscess (pyogenic or amebic) must be considered. Veno-occlusive disease and hepatic vein thrombosis are rare possibilities. Tumors in the left lobe may be mistaken for pancreatic pseudocysts.

Complications

Progressive enlargement of the tumor, abdominal discomfort, ascites, respiratory difficulty, and widespread metastases (especially to the lungs and the abdominal lymph nodes) are the rule. Rupture of the neoplastic liver and intraperitoneal hemorrhage have been reported. Progressive anemia and emaciation predispose the patient to an early septic death.

Treatment

For tumors that are resectable, an aggressive surgical approach with complete resection of the lesion offers the only chance for cure. It appears that every isolated lung metastasis should also be surgically resected. Radiotherapy and chemotherapy have been disappointing in the treatment of hepatocellular carcinoma, although hepatoblastomas are generally more responsive. Chemotherapy may be used for initial cytoreduction of tumors (especially hepatoblastoma) found to be unresectable at the time of primary surgery (see Chapter 31 for additional discussion). Second-look celiotomy has, in some cases, allowed resection of the tumor, resulting in a reduced mortality rate. Liver transplantation can be an option in hepatoblastoma with 85% 10-year survival in patients with unresectable disease limited to the liver. For hepatocellular carcinoma, the survival rate is poor due to the typically advanced stage at diagnosis. The survival rate may be better for those patients in whom the tumor is incidental to another disorder (tyrosinemia, biliary atresia, cirrhosis) or is less than a total of 7 cm diameter without vascular invasion. In HBV-endemic areas, childhood HBV vaccination has reduced the incidence of hepatocellular carcinoma.

Prognosis

If the tumor is completely removed, the survival rate is 90% for hepatoblastoma and 33% for hepatocellular carcinoma. If metastases are present, survival is reduced to 40% for hepatoblastoma. In well-selected candidates for liver transplantation for unresectable hepatoblastoma, survival approaches 65%.

Gupta AA et al: Critical review of controversial issues in the management of advanced pediatric liver tumors. Pediatr Blood Cancer 2011;56:1013 [PMID: 21488153].

Finegold MJ et al: Liver tumors: Pediatric population. Liver Transpl 2008;14:1545 [PMID: 18975283].

Kim T et al: Surgery for hepatoblastoma: From laparoscopic resection to liver transplantation. Hepatogastroenterology 2011;58:896 [PMID: 21830412].

Meyers RL: Tumors of the liver in children. Surg Oncol 2007;16:195 [PMID: 17714939].

Tajiri H et al: Reduction of hepatocellular carcinoma in childhood after introduction of selective vaccination against hepatitis B virus for infants born to HBV carrier mothers. Cancer Causes Control 2011;22:523 [PMID: 21191808].

LIVER TRANSPLANTATION

Orthotopic liver transplantation is indicated in children with end-stage liver disease, acute fulminant hepatic failure, or complications from metabolic liver disorders. Multiple options for immunosuppression (eg, cyclosporine, tacrolimus, monoclonal antibodies against T cells, and interleukin 2 [IL-2] receptor, mycophenolate mofetil, and sirolimus), individualization of immunosuppression, better candidate selection, improvements in surgical techniques, anticipatory monitoring for complications (eg, CMV and EBV infections, hypertension, renal dysfunction, and dyslipidemias) and experience in postoperative management have contributed to improved results. The major indications for childhood transplantation are shown in Table 22–10.

Children who are potential candidates for liver transplantation should be referred early for evaluation because the limiting factor for success is the small donor pool. In addition to full-sized cadaveric organs, children may also receive reduced segment or split cadaveric livers and live donor donation, all of which have expanded the donor pool. Ten percent of recipients require retransplantation. In general, 80%–90% of children survive at least 2–5 years after transplantation, with long-term survival expected to be comparable. Lifetime immunosuppression therapy, using combinations of tacrolimus, cyclosporine, prednisone, azathioprine, mycophenolate mofetil, or sirolimus, with its incumbent risks, is generally necessary to prevent rejection. Several studies have examined immunosuppression withdrawal, which can occasionally be performed successfully; however, criteria for which patients can survive off immunosuppression have not been determined. The minimal amount of immunosuppression that will prevent allograft rejection should be chosen. The overall quality of life for children with a transplanted liver appears to be excellent. There is an increased risk (up to 25%) of

Table 22–10. Indications for pediatric liver transplantation.

Indication	Percent of Pediatric Transplants
Biliary atresia (failed Kasai or decompensated cirrhosis)	39.6
Metabolic diseases (α_1-antitrypsin deficiency, urea cycle enzyme defects, Wilson disease, tyrosinemia)	14.6
Nonbiliary atresia cholestatic disorders (eg, Alagille syndrome, PFIC)	13.6
Acute liver failure	13.2
Cirrhosis (autoimmune hepatitis, hepatitis B and C)	8.0
Hepatic malignancies (unresectable hepatoblastoma, HCC, others)	5.8
Other	5.2

PFIC, progressive familial intrahepatic cholestasis.

renal dysfunction and low intelligence scores. The lifelong risk of EBV-induced lymphoproliferative disease, which is approximately 5%, is related to age and EBV exposure status at time of transplantation, and intensity of immunosuppression. Various protocols are being tested for prevention and treatment of lymphoproliferative disease.

Alonso EM, Sorensen LG: Cognitive development following pediatric solid organ transplantation. Curr Opin Organ Transplant 2009;14:522 [PMID: 19625964].

Anthony SJ et al: Quality of life after pediatric solid organ transplantation. Pediatr Clin North Am 2010;57:559 [PMID: 20371052].

Campbell KM et al: High prevalence of renal dysfunction in long-term survivors after pediatric liver transplantation. J Pediatr 2006;148:475 [PMID: 16647407].

Kamath BM, Olthoff KM: Liver transplantation in children: Update 2010. Pediatr Clin North Am 2010;57:401 [PMID: 20371044].

PANCREATIC DISORDERS

ACUTE PANCREATITIS

ESSENTIALS OF DIAGNOSIS & TYPICAL FEATURES

- Epigastric abdominal pain radiating to the back.
- Nausea and vomiting.
- Elevated serum amylase and lipase.
- Evidence of pancreatic inflammation by CT or ultrasound.

General Considerations

The rate of hospitalization for acute pancreatitis in children is 0.02–0.09/1000 U.S. population. The incidence of pediatric acute pancreatitis seems to be increasing. Most cases of acute pancreatitis are the result of drugs, viral infections, systemic diseases, abdominal trauma, or obstruction of pancreatic flow. More than 20% are idiopathic. Causes of pancreatic obstruction include stones, choledochal cyst, tumors of the duodenum, pancreas divisum, and ascariasis. Acute pancreatitis has been seen following treatment with sulfasalazine, thiazides, valproic acid, azathioprine, mercaptopurine, asparaginase, antiretroviral drugs (especially didanosine), high-dose corticosteroids, and other drugs. It may also occur in cystic fibrosis, systemic lupus erythematosus, α_1-antitrypsin deficiency, diabetes mellitus, Crohn disease, glycogen storage disease type I, hyperlipidemia types I and V, hyperparathyroidism, Henoch-Schönlein purpura, Reye syndrome, organic acidopathies, Kawasaki disease, or chronic renal failure; during rapid refeeding in cases of malnutrition; following spinal fusion surgery; and in families. Alcohol-induced pancreatitis should be considered in the teenage patient.

Clinical Findings

A. History

An acute onset of persistent (hours to days), moderate to severe upper abdominal and midabdominal pain occasionally referred to the back, frequently associated with vomiting, or nausea is the common presenting picture.

B. Symptoms and Signs

The abdomen is tender, but not rigid, and bowel sounds are diminished, suggesting peritoneal irritation. Abdominal distention is common in infants and younger children and classic symptoms of abdominal pain, tenderness and nausea are less common in this age group. Jaundice is unusual. Ascites may be noted, and a left-sided pleural effusion is present in some patients. Periumbilical and flank bruising indicate hemorrhagic pancreatitis.

C. Laboratory Findings

An elevated serum amylase or lipase (more than three times normal) is the key laboratory finding. The elevated serum lipase persists longer than serum amylase. Infants younger than 6 months may not have an elevated amylase or lipase. In this setting, an elevated immunoreactive trypsinogen may be more sensitive. Pancreatic lipase can help differentiate nonpancreatic causes (eg, salivary, intestinal, or tuboovarian) of serum amylase elevation. Leukocytosis, hyperglycemia (serum glucose > 300 mg/dL), hypocalcemia, falling hematocrit, rising blood urea nitrogen, hypoxemia, and acidosis may all occur in severe cases and imply a poor prognosis.

D. Imaging

Plain radiographic films of the abdomen may show a localized ileus (sentinel loop). Ultrasonography is primarily used to assess for biliary tract disease leading to pancreatitis, but can show decreased echodensity of the pancreas in comparison with the left lobe of the liver. The pancreas is often difficult to image with ultrasound due to overlying gas. CT scanning images the pancreas more consistently and is better for detecting pancreatic phlegmon, pseudocyst, necrosis, or abscess formation. ERCP or MRCP may be useful in confirming patency of the main pancreatic duct in cases of abdominal trauma; in recurrent acute pancreatitis; or in revealing stones, ductal strictures, and pancreas divisum.

Differential Diagnosis

Other causes of acute upper abdominal pain include gastritis; peptic ulcer disease; duodenal ulcer; hepatitis; liver abscess; cholelithiasis; cholecystitis; choledocholithiasis; acute gastroenteritis or atypical appendicitis; pneumonia; volvulus; intussusception; and nonaccidental trauma.

Complications

Early complications include shock, fluid and electrolyte disturbances, ileus, acute respiratory distress syndrome, and hypocalcemia. Hypervolemia due to renal insufficiency related to renal tubular necrosis may occur. The gastrointestinal, neurologic, musculoskeletal, hepatobiliary, dermatologic, and hematologic systems may also be involved. Early predictors of a more aggressive course include renal dysfunction, significant fluid requirements, and multisystem organ dysfunction. Five to 20% of patients can develop a pseudo-cyst 1–4 weeks later that may be asymptomatic or present with recurrence of abdominal pain and rise in the serum amylase. Up to 60%–70% of pseudocysts resolve spontaneously. Infection, hemorrhage, rupture, or fistulization may occur. Phlegmon formation is rare in children, but when present may extend from the gland into the retroperitoneum or into the lesser sac. Most regress, but some require drainage. Infection may occur in this inflammatory mass. Pancreatic abscess formation, which is rare (3%–5%), develops 2–3 weeks after the initial insult. Fever, leukocytosis, and pain suggest this complication; diagnosis is made by ultrasound or CT scanning. Chronic pancreatitis, exocrine or endocrine pancreatic insufficiency, and pancreatic lithiasis are rare sequelae of acute pancreatitis.

Treatment

Medical management includes careful attention to fluids, electrolytes, and respiratory status. Gastric decompression may be helpful if there is significant vomiting. Pain should be controlled with opioids. Acid suppression may be helpful. Nutrition is provided by the parenteral or enteral (jejunal or gastric) route. Broad-spectrum antibiotic coverage is useful only in necrotizing pancreatitis. Drugs known to produce acute pancreatitis should be discontinued. Surgical treatment is reserved for traumatic disruption of the gland, intraductal stone, other anatomic obstructive lesions, and unresolved or infected pseudocysts or abscesses. Early endoscopic decompression of the biliary system reduces the morbidity associated with pancreatitis caused by obstruction of the common bile duct.

Prognosis

In the pediatric age group, the prognosis is surprisingly good with conservative management.

Lowe ME, Greer JB: Pancreatitis in children and adolescents. Curr Gastroenterol Rep 2008;10:128 [PMID: 18342688].

Morinville VD et al: Increasing incidence of acute pancreatitis at an American pediatric tertiary care center: Is greater awareness among physicians responsible? Pancreas 2010;39:5 [PMID: 19752770].

CHRONIC PANCREATITIS

Chronic pancreatitis is differentiated from acute pancreatitis in that the pancreas remains structurally or functionally abnormal after an attack.

The causes are multiple and can be divided into toxic-metabolic (eg, alcohol, chronic renal failure, hypercalcemia), idiopathic, genetic (increasingly recognized in children and adolescents), autoimmune, recurrent and severe acute pancreatitis, and obstructive pancreatitis (eg, pancreas divisum, choledochal cyst).

Clinical Findings

A. History

The diagnosis often is delayed by the nonspecificity of symptoms and the lack of persistent laboratory abnormalities. There is usually a prolonged history of recurrent upper abdominal pain of variable severity. Radiation of the pain into the back is a frequent complaint.

B. Symptoms and Signs

Fever and vomiting are rare. Diarrhea, due to steatorrhea, and symptoms of diabetes may develop later in the course. Malnutrition due to acquired exocrine pancreatic insufficiency may also occur.

C. Laboratory Findings

Serum amylase and lipase levels are usually elevated during early acute attacks, but are often normal in the chronic phase. Pancreatic insufficiency may be diagnosed by demonstration of a low fecal pancreatic elastase 1. Mutations of the cationic trypsinogen gene, the pancreatic secretory trypsin inhibitor, and the cystic fibrosis transmembrane conductance regulator gene (*CFTR*) are associated with recurrent acute and chronic pancreatitis. Elevated blood glucose and glycohemoglobin levels and glycosuria frequently occur in protracted disease. Sweat chloride should be checked for cystic fibrosis, α_1-antitrypsin level or phenotype, and serum calcium for hyperparathyroidism.

D. Imaging

Radiographs of the abdomen may show pancreatic calcifications in up to 30% of patients. Ultrasound or CT examination demonstrates an abnormal gland (enlargement or atrophy), ductal dilation, and calculi in up to 80%. CT is the initial imaging procedure of choice. MRCP or ERCP can show ductal dilation, stones, strictures, or stenotic segments. Endoscopic ultrasound in the diagnosis and staging of chronic pancreatitis is being evaluated.

Differential Diagnosis

Other causes of recurrent abdominal pain must be considered. Specific causes of pancreatitis such as hyperparathyroidism;

systemic lupus erythematosus; infectious disease; α_1-antitrypsin deficiency; and ductal obstruction by tumors, stones, or helminths must be excluded by appropriate tests.

Complications

Disabling abdominal pain, steatorrhea, malnutrition, pancreatic pseudocysts, and diabetes are the most frequent long-term complications. Pancreatic carcinoma occurs more frequently in patients with chronic pancreatitis, and in up to 40% of patients with hereditary pancreatitis by age 70.

Treatment

Medical management of acute attacks is indicated (see section on Acute Pancreatitis, earlier). If ductal obstruction is strongly suspected, endoscopic therapy (balloon dilation, stenting, stone removal, or sphincterotomy) should be pursued. Relapses occur in most patients. Pancreatic enzyme therapy should be used in patients with pancreatic insufficiency. Antioxidant therapy is being investigated. Pseudocysts may be marsupialized to the surface or drained into the stomach or into a loop of jejunum if they fail to regress spontaneously. Lateral pancreaticojejunostomy or the Frey procedure can reduce pain in pediatric patients with a dilated pancreatic duct and may prevent or delay progression of functional pancreatic impairment. Pancreatectomy and islet cell autotransplantation has been used in selected cases of chronic pancreatitis.

Prognosis

In the absence of a correctable lesion, the prognosis is not good. Disabling episodes of pain, pancreatic insufficiency, diabetes, and pancreatic cancer may ensue. Narcotic addiction and suicide are risks in teenagers with disabling disease.

Bellin MD et al: Outcome after pancreatectomy and islet autotransplantation in a pediatric population. J Pediatr Gastroenterol Nutr 2008;47:37 [PMID: 18607267].

Lal A, Lal DR: Hereditary pancreatitis. Pediatr Surg Int 2010;26:1193 [PMID: 20697897].

Witt H: Gene mutations in children with chronic pancreatitis. Pancreatology 2001;1:432 [PMID: 12120220].

GASTROINTESTINAL & HEPATOBILIARY MANIFESTATIONS OF CYSTIC FIBROSIS

Cystic fibrosis is a disease with protean manifestations. Although pulmonary and pancreatic involvement dominate the clinical picture for most patients (see Chapter 19), various other organs can be involved. Table 22–11 lists the important gastrointestinal, pancreatic, and hepatobiliary conditions that may affect patients with cystic fibrosis along with their clinical findings, incidence, most useful diagnostic studies, and preferred treatment.

Bhardwaj S et al: Hepatobiliary abnormalities and disease in cystic fibrosis: Epidemiology and outcomes through adulthood. J Clin Gastroenterol 2009;43:858 [PMID: 19525864].

Borowitz D et al: Gastrointestinal outcomes and confounders in cystic fibrosis. J Pediatr Gastroenterol Nutr 2005;41:273 [PMID: 16131979].

Borowitz D et al: Use of fecal elastase-1 to classify pancreatic status in patients with cystic fibrosis. J Pediatr 2004;145:322 [PMID: 15343184].

Houwen RH et al: Defining DIOS and constipation in cystic fibrosis with a multicentre study on the incidence, characteristics, and treatment of DIOS. J Pediatr Gastroenterol Nutr 2010;50:38 [PMID: 19525866].

Littlewood JM et al: Diagnosis and treatment of intestinal malabsorption in cystic fibrosis. Pediatr Pulmonol 2006;41:35 [PMID: 16288483].

Munck A et al: Pancreatic enzyme replacement therapy for young cystic fibrosis patients. J Cyst Fibros 2009;8:14 [PMID: 18718819].

Rowland M et al: Outcome in cystic fibrosis liver disease. Am J Gastroenterol 2011;106:104 [PMID: 20736939].

SYNDROMES WITH PANCREATIC EXOCRINE INSUFFICIENCY

Several syndromes are associated with exocrine pancreatic insufficiency. Patients present with a history of failure to thrive, diarrhea, fatty stools, and an absence of respiratory symptoms. Laboratory findings include a normal sweat chloride; low fecal pancreatic elastase 1; and low to absent pancreatic lipase, amylase, and trypsin levels on duodenal intubation. Each disorder has several associated clinical features that aid in the differential diagnosis. In Shwachman-Diamond syndrome, pancreatic exocrine hypoplasia with widespread fatty replacement of the glandular acinar tissue is associated with neutropenia because of maturational arrest of the granulocyte series. Bone marrow failure is seen in one third. Metaphyseal dysostosis and an elevated fetal hemoglobin level are common; immunoglobulin deficiency and hepatic dysfunction are also reported. CT examination of the pancreas demonstrates the widespread fatty replacement. Serum immunoreactive trypsinogen levels are extremely low.

Other associations of exocrine pancreatic insufficiency include (1) aplastic alae, aplasia cutis, deafness (Johanson-Blizzard syndrome); (2) sideroblastic anemia, developmental delay, seizures, and liver dysfunction (Pearson bone marrow pancreas syndrome); (3) duodenal atresia or stenosis; (4) malnutrition; and (5) pancreatic hypoplasia or agenesis.

The complications and sequelae of exocrine pancreatic insufficiency are malnutrition, diarrhea, and growth failure. The degree of steatorrhea may lessen with age. Intragastric lipolysis by lingual lipase may compensate in patients with low or absent pancreatic function. In Shwachman syndrome, the major sequel is short stature. Increased numbers of infections may result from chronic neutropenia and the reduced neutrophil mobility that is present in many patients. An increased incidence of leukemia has been noted in these patients.

Table 22–11. Gastrointestinal and hepatobiliary manifestations of cystic fibrosis.

Organ	Condition	Symptoms	Age at Presentation	Incidence (%)	Diagnostic Evaluation	Management
Esophagus	Gastroesophageal reflux, esophagitis	Pyrosis, dysphagia, epigastric pain, hematemesis.	All ages.	10–20	Endoscopy and biopsy, overnight pH study.	H_2 blockers, PPIs, surgical antireflux procedure.
	Varices	Hematemesis, melena.	Childhood and adolescents.	3–5	Endoscopy.	Endosclerosis, band ligation, drugs (see text), TIPS, surgical shunt, liver transplantation (see Table 22–8).
Stomach	Gastritis	Upper abdominal pain, vomiting, hematemesis.	School age and older.	10–25	Endoscopy and biopsy.	H_2 blockers, PPIs.
	Hiatal hernia	Reflux symptoms (see above), epigastric pain.	School age and older.	3–5	UGI; endoscopy.	As above. Surgery in some.
Intestine	Meconium ileus	Abdominal distention, bilious emesis.	Neonate.	10–15	Radiologic studies, plain abdominal films; contrast enema shows microcolon.	Dislodgement of obstruction with Gastrografin enema. Surgery if unsuccessful or if case complicated by atresia, perforation, or volvulus.
	Distal intestinal obstruction syndrome	Abdominal pain, acute and recurrent; distention; occasional vomiting.	Any age, usually school age through adolescence.	5–10	Palpable mass in right lower quadrant, radiologic studies.	Gastrografin enema, intestinal lavage solution, diet, bulk laxatives, adjustment of pancreatic enzyme intake.
	Intussusception	Acute, intermittent abdominal pain; distention; emesis.	Infants through adolescence.	1–3	Radiographic studies, barium enema.	Reduction by barium or air enema or surgery if needed. Diet. Bulk laxatives. Adjustment of pancreatic enzyme intake.
	Rectal prolapse	Anal discomfort, rectal bleeding.	Infants and children to age 4–5 y.	15–25	Visual mass protruding from anus.	Manual reduction, adjustment of pancreatic enzyme dosage, reassurance as problem resolves by age 3–5 y.
	Carbohydrate intolerance	Abdominal pain, flatulence, continued diarrhea with adequate enzyme replacement therapy.	Any age.	10–25	Intestinal mucosal biopsy and disaccharidase analysis. Lactose breathe hydrogen test.	Reduce lactose intake; lactase; reduction of gastric hyperacidity if mucosa shows partial villous atrophy. Beware concurrent celiac disease or *Giardia* infection.
	Small bowel bacterial overgrowth	Abdominal pain, flatulence, continued diarrhea with adequate enzyme replacement therapy.	Any age: Higher risk with previous intestinal surgery.	Unknown	Culture of duodenal fluid, glucose breath hydrogen test.	Probiotic therapy, oral antibiotics (metronidazole, trimethoprim-sulfamethoxazole).

(*Continued*)

Table 22–11. Gastrointestinal and hepatobiliary manifestations of cystic fibrosis. (*Continued*)

Organ	Condition	Symptoms	Age at Presentation	Incidence (%)	Diagnostic Evaluation	Management
Pancreas	Total exocrine insufficiency	Diarrhea, steatorrhea, malnutrition, failure to thrive. Fat-soluble vitamin deficiency.	Neonate through infancy.	85–90	72-h fecal fat evaluation, fecal pancreatic elastase 1, direct pancreatic function tests.	Pancreatic enzyme replacement, may need elemental formula, fat-soluble vitamin supplements.
	Pancreatic sufficiency (partial exocrine insufficiency)	Occasional diarrhea, mild growth delay.	Any age.	10–15	72-h fecal fat evaluation, direct pancreatic function tests, fecal pancreatic elastase.	Pancreatic enzyme replacement in selected patients. Fat-soluble vitamin supplements as indicated by biochemical evaluation.
	Pancreatitis	Recurrent abdominal pain, vomiting.	Older children through adolescence. Primarily in patients with partial pancreatic sufficiency.	0.1	Increased serum lipase and amylase, CT, MRCP, ERCP.	Endoscopic removal of sludge or stones if present, endoscopic papillotomy.
	Diabetes	Weight loss, polyuria, polydipsia.	Older children through adolescence.	5–7	Glucose tolerance test and insulin levels.	Diet, insulin.
Liver	Steatosis	Hepatomegaly, often in setting of malnutrition, elevated ALT.	Neonates and infants, but can be seen at all ages.	20–60	US showing homogeneous increased echogenicity. Liver biopsy.	Improved nutrition, replacement of pancreatic enzymes, vitamins, and essential fatty acids.
	Hepatic fibrosis	Hepatomegaly, firm liver. May have abnormal AST, ALT.	Infants and older patients. Prevalence uncertain.	10–70	US showing heterogeneous echogenicity. Liver biopsy.	As above. Ursodeoxycholic acid.
	Cirrhosis	Hepatosplenomegaly, hematemesis from esophageal varices; hypersplenism, jaundice, ascites late in course.	Infants through adolescence.	5–10	US showing nodular liver, signs of portal hypertension. Liver biopsy, endoscopy.	Improved nutrition, ursodeoxycholic acid, endosclerosis or band ligation of varices, or partial splenic embolization, liver transplantation.
	Neonatal jaundice	Cholestatic jaundice hepatomegaly; often seen with meconium ileus.	Neonates.	0.1–1	Sweat chloride test, liver biopsy	Nutritional support, special formula with medium-chain triglyceride–containing oil, pancreatic enzyme replacement, vitamin supplements.
Gallbladder	Microgallbladder	None.	Congenital—present at any age.	30	US or hepatobiliary scintigraphy.	None needed.
	Cholelithiasis	Recurrent right upper quadrant abdominal pain, rarely jaundice.	School age through adolescence.	1–10	US.	Surgery if symptomatic and low-risk, trial of cholelitholytics in others.
Extrahepatic bile ducts	Intraluminal obstruction (sludge, stones, tumor)	Jaundice, hepatomegaly, abdominal pain.	Neonates, then older children through adolescence.	Rare in neonates (< 0.1)	US and hepatobiliary scintigraphy, MRCP.	Surgery in neonates; ERCP in older patients or surgery.
	Extraluminal obstruction (intrapancreatic compression, tumor)	As above.	Older children to adults.	Rare (< 1)	As above.	Surgical biliary drainage procedure or ERCP.

ALT, alanine aminotransferase; AST, aspartate aminotransferase; CT, computed tomography; ERCP, endoscopic retrograde cholangiopancreatography; MRCP, magnetic resonance cholangiopancreatography; PPI, proton pump inhibitor; TIPS, transjugular intrahepatic portosystemic shunt; UGI, upper gastrointestinal; US; abdominal ultrasound.

Pancreatic enzyme and fat-soluble vitamin replacement are required therapy in most patients. The prognosis appears to be good for those able to survive the increased number of bacterial infections early in life and lack severe associated defects.

Chen R et al: Neonatal and late-onset diabetes mellitus caused by failure of pancreatic development: Report of 4 more cases and a review of the literature. Pediatrics 2008;121:1541 [PMID: 18519458].

Dror Y: Shwachman-Diamond syndrome. Pediatr Blood Cancer 2005;45:892 [PMID: 16047374].

Durie PR: Pancreatic aspects of cystic fibrosis and other inherited causes of pancreatic dysfunction. Med Clin North Am 2000;84:609 [PMID: 10872418].

Rezaei N et al: Eponym Johanson-Blizzard syndrome. Eur J Pediatr 2011;170:179 [PMID: 20556422].

Seneca S et al: Pearson marrow pancreas syndrome: A molecular study and clinical management. Clin Genet 1997;51:338 [PMID: 9212183].

Toiviainen-Salo S et al: Magnetic resonance imaging findings of the pancreas in patients with Shwachman-Diamond syndrome and mutations in the SBDS gene. J Pediatr 2008;152(3):434 [PMID: 18280855].

ISOLATED EXOCRINE PANCREATIC ENZYME DEFECT

Normal premature infants and most newborns produce little, if any, pancreatic amylase following meals or exogenous hormonal stimulation. This temporary physiologic insufficiency may persist for the first 3–6 months of life and be responsible for diarrhea when complex carbohydrates (cereals) are introduced into the diet.

Congenital pancreatic lipase deficiency and congenital colipase deficiency are extremely rare disorders, causing diarrhea and variable malnutrition with malabsorption of dietary fat and fat-soluble vitamins. The sweat chloride level is normal and neutropenia is absent. Treatment is oral replacement of pancreatic enzymes and a low-fat diet or formula containing medium-chain triglycerides.

Exocrine pancreatic insufficiency of proteolytic enzymes (eg, trypsinogen, trypsin, chymotrypsin) is caused by enterokinase deficiency, a duodenal mucosal enzyme required for activation of the pancreatic proenzymes. These patients present with malnutrition associated with hypoproteinemia and edema, but do not have respiratory symptoms and have a normal sweat test. They respond to pancreatic enzyme replacement therapy and feeding formulas that contain a casein hydrolysate (eg, Nutramigen, Pregestimil).

Durie PR: Pancreatic aspects of cystic fibrosis and other inherited causes of pancreatic dysfunction. Med Clin North Am 2000;84:609 [PMID: 10872418].

McKenna LL: Pancreatic disorders in the newborn. Neonatal Netw 2000;19:13 [PMID: 11949098].

Stormon MO, Durie PR: Pathophysiologic basis of exocrine pancreatic dysfunction in childhood. J Pediatr Gastroenterol Nutr 2002;35:8 [PMID: 12142803].

Table 22–12. Pancreatic tumors.

	Age	Major Findings	Diagnosis	Treatment	Associated Conditions
Insulinoma	Any age	Hypoglycemia, seizures; high serum insulin; weight gain; abdominal pain and mass infrequent	CT scan, MRI, PET, EUS, SRS	Surgery, diazoxide, SSTA	MEN1
Adenocarcinoma	Any age	Epigastric pain, mass, weight loss, anemia, biliary obstruction	Ultrasound, CT scan, MRI, EUS	Surgery	Chronic pancreatitis
Gastrinoma	Older than age 5–8 y	Male sex, gastric hypersecretion, peptic symptoms, multiple ulcers, gastrointestinal bleeding, anemia, diarrhea	Elevated fasting gastrin and postsecretin suppression test (> 300 pg/mL), CT scan, MRI, EUS, SRS, laparotomy	PPI, surgical resection, total gastrectomy, SSTA	Zollinger-Ellison syndrome, MEN1, neurofibromatosis
VIPoma	Any age (more common 2–4 y old)	Secretory diarrhea, hypokalemia, hypochlorhydria, weight loss, flushing	Elevated VIP levels (> 75 pg/mL); sometimes, elevated serum gastrin and pancreatic polypeptide; CT, EUS, SRS	Surgery, SSTA, IV fluids	
Glucagonoma	Older patients	Diabetes, necrolytic migratory erythema, diarrhea, anemia, thrombotic events, depression	Elevated glucagon, hyperglycemia, gastrin, VIP, CT, MRI, EUS, SRS	Surgery, SSTA	

CT, computed tomography; EUS, endoscopic ultrasound; IV, intravenous; MEN1, multiple endocrine neoplasia syndrome type I; MRI, magnetic resonance imaging; PPI, proton pump inhibitor; PET, Positron emission tomography; SRS, somatostatin-receptor scintigraphy; SSTA, somatostatin analogue; VIP, vasoactive intestinal polypeptide.

PANCREATIC TUMORS

Pancreatic tumors, whether benign or malignant, are rare. They most often arise from ductal or acinar epithelium (malignant adenocarcinoma) or from islet (endocrine) components within the gland, such as the benign insulinoma (adenoma) derived from β cells. Other pancreatic tumors originate from these pluripotential endocrine cells (eg, gastrinoma, VIPoma, glucagonoma), and produce diverse symptoms, because they release biologically active polypeptides from this ectopic location. The clinical features of these tumors are summarized in Table 22–12. The differential diagnosis of pancreatic tumors includes Wilms tumor, neuroblastoma, and malignant lymphoma. In older children, endoscopic ultrasonography can aid in localizing these tumors.

Doherty GM: Rare endocrine tumours of the GI tract. Best Pract Res Clin Gastroenterol 2005;19:807 [PMID: 16253902].

Nissen NN et al: Pancreatic neuroendocrine tumors: Presentation, management, and outcomes. Am Surg 2009;75:1025 [PMID: 19886158].

Yu DC et al: Childhood pancreatic tumors: A single institution experience. J Pediatr Surg 2009;44:2267 [PMID: 20006007].

REFERENCES

Kleinman R et al (editors): *Walker's Pediatric Gastrointestinal Disease: Physiology, Diagnosis, Management,* 5th ed. BC Decker Inc, 2008.

Suchy FJ, Sokol RJ, Balistreri WF (editors): *Liver Disease in Children,* 3rd ed. Cambridge University Press, 2007.

Wyllie R, Hyams JS (editors): *Pediatric Gastrointestinal and Liver Disease,* 4th ed. Elsevier, 2011.

Fluid, Electrolyte, & Acid-Base Disorders & Therapy

23

Douglas M. Ford, MD

REGULATION OF BODY FLUIDS, ELECTROLYTES, & TONICITY

Total body water (TBW) constitutes 50%–75% of the total body mass, depending on age, sex, and fat content. After an initial postnatal diuresis, the TBW slowly decreases to the adult range near puberty (Figure 23–1). TBW is divided into the intracellular and extracellular spaces. Intracellular fluid (ICF) accounts for two-thirds of the TBW and extracellular fluid (ECF), for one-third. The ECF is further compartmentalized into plasma (intravascular) volume and interstitial fluid (ISF).

The principal constituents of plasma are sodium, chloride, bicarbonate, and protein (primarily albumin). The ISF is similar to plasma but lacks significant amounts of protein (Figure 23–2). Conversely, the ICF is rich in potassium, magnesium, phosphates, sulfates, and protein.

An understanding of osmotic shifts between the ECF and ICF is fundamental to understanding disorders of fluid balance. Iso-osmolality is generally maintained between fluid compartments. Because the cell membrane is water-permeable, abnormal fluid shifts occur if the concentration of solutes that cannot permeate the cell membrane in the ECF does not equal the concentration of such solutes in the ICF. Thus, NaCl, mannitol, and glucose (in the setting of hyperglycemia) remain restricted to the ECF space and contribute effective osmoles by obligating water to remain in the ECF compartment. In contrast, a freely permeable solute such as urea does not contribute effective osmoles because it is not restricted to the ECF and readily crosses cell membranes. Tonicity, or effective osmolality, differs from measured osmolality in that it accounts only for osmotically active impermeable solutes rather than all osmotically active solutes, including those that are permeable to cell membranes. Osmolality may be estimated by the following formula:

$$\text{mOsm/kg} = 2(\text{Na}^+,\ \text{mEq/L}) + \frac{\text{Glucose, mg/dL}}{18} + \frac{\text{BUN, mg/dL}}{2.8}$$

Although osmolality and osmolarity differ, the former being an expression of osmotic activity per weight (kg) and the latter per volume (L) of solution, for clinical purposes they are similar and occasionally used interchangeably. Oncotic pressure, or colloid osmotic pressure, represents the osmotic activity of macromolecular constituents such as albumin in the plasma and body fluids.

The principal mechanisms that regulate ECF volume and tonicity are antidiuretic hormone (ADH), thirst, aldosterone, and atrial natriuretic factor (ANF).

Antidiuretic Hormone

In the kidney, ADH increases water reabsorption in the cortical and medullary collecting ducts, leading to formation of concentrated urine. In the absence of ADH, dilute urine is produced. Under normal conditions, ADH secretion is regulated by the tonicity of body fluids rather than the fluid volume and becomes detectable at a plasma osmolality of 280 mOsm/kg or greater. However, tonicity may be sacrificed to preserve ECF volume, as in the case of hyponatremic dehydration, wherein ADH secretion and renal water retention are maximal.

Thirst

Water intake is commonly determined by cultural factors rather than by thirst. Thirst is not physiologically stimulated until plasma osmolality reaches 290 mOsm/kg, a level at which ADH levels are sufficient to induce maximal antidiuresis. Thirst provides control over a wide range of fluid volumes and can even be a response to an absence of or lack of responsiveness to ADH, which results in the production of copious, dilute urine, as in diabetes insipidus. One who cannot perceive thirst develops profound problems with fluid balance.

Aldosterone

Aldosterone is released from the adrenal cortex in response to decreased effective circulating volume and stimulation of the renin-angiotensin-aldosterone axis or in response to

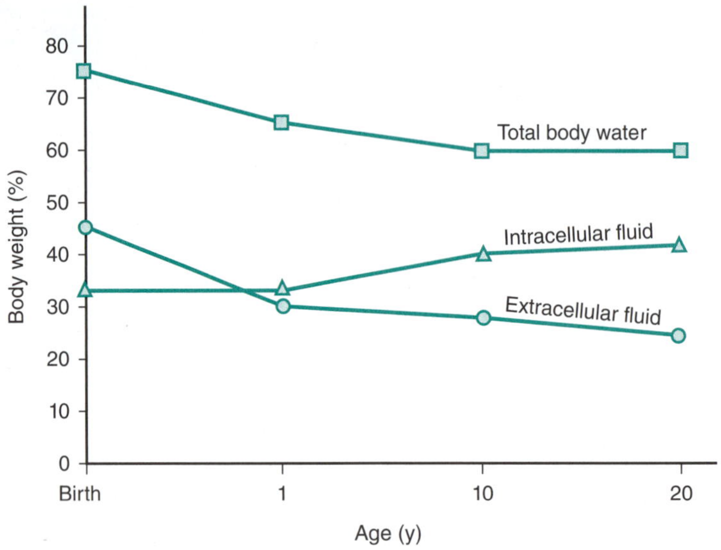

▲ **Figure 23–1. Body water compartments related to age.** (Modified, with permission, from Friis-Hansen B: Body water compartments in children: Changes during growth and related changes in body composition. Pediatrics 1961;28:169.)

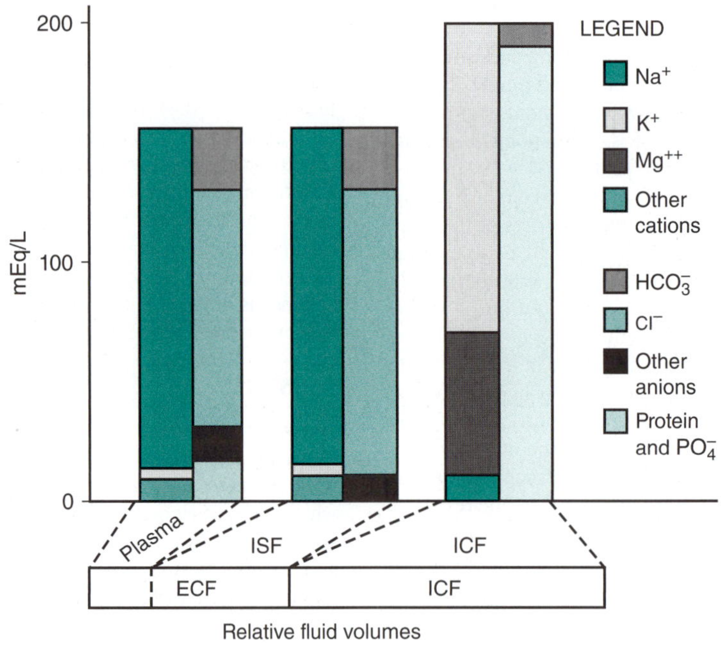

▲ **Figure 23–2. Composition of body fluids.** ECF, extracellular fluid; ICF, intracellular fluid; ISF, interstitial fluid.

increasing plasma K^+. Aldosterone enhances renal tubular reabsorption of Na^+ in exchange for K^+, and to a lesser degree H^+. At a constant osmolality, retention of Na^+ leads to expansion of ECF volume and suppression of aldosterone release.

Atrial Natriuretic Factor

ANF, a polypeptide hormone secreted principally by the cardiac atria in response to atrial dilation, plays an important role in regulation of blood volume and blood pressure. ANF inhibits renin secretion and aldosterone synthesis and causes an increase in glomerular filtration rate and renal sodium excretion. ANF also guards against excessive plasma volume expansion in the face of increased ECF volume by shifting fluid from the vascular to the interstitial compartment. ANF inhibits angiotensin II– and norepinephrine-induced vasoconstriction and acts in the brain to decrease the desire for salt and inhibit the release of ADH. Thus, the net effect of ANF is a decrease in blood volume and blood pressure associated with natriuresis and diuresis.

ACID-BASE BALANCE

The pH of arterial blood is maintained between 7.38 and 7.42 to ensure that pH-sensitive enzyme systems function normally. Acid-base balance is maintained by interaction of the lungs, kidneys, and systemic buffering systems. Over 50% of the blood's buffering capacity is provided by the carbonic acid–bicarbonate system, roughly 30% by hemoglobin, and the remainder by phosphates and ammonium. The carbonic acid–bicarbonate system, depicted chemically as

$$CO_2 + H_2O \leftrightarrow H_2CO_3 \leftrightarrow H^+ + HCO_3^-$$

interacts via the lungs and kidneys, and in conjunction with the nonbicarbonate systems, to stabilize systemic pH. The concentration of dissolved CO_2 in blood is established by the respiratory system and that of HCO_3^- by the kidneys. Disturbances in acid-base balance are initially stabilized by chemical buffering, compensated for by pulmonary or renal regulation of CO_2 or HCO_3^-, and ultimately corrected when the primary cause of the acid-base disturbance is eliminated.

Renal regulation of acid-base balance is accomplished by the reabsorption of filtered HCO_3^- primarily in the proximal tubule, and the excretion of H^+ or HCO_3^- in the distal nephron to match the net input of acid or base. When urine is alkalinized, HCO_3^- enters the kidney and is ultimately lost in the urine. Alkalinization of the urine may occur when an absolute or relative excess of bicarbonate exists. However, urinary alkalinization will not occur if there is a deficiency of Na^+ or K^+, because HCO_3^- must also be retained to maintain electroneutrality. In contrast, the urine may be acidified if an absolute or relative decrease occurs in systemic HCO_3^-. In this setting, proximal tubular HCO_3^- reabsorption and distal tubular H^+ excretion are maximal. A "paradoxical aciduria" with low urinary pH may be seen in the setting of

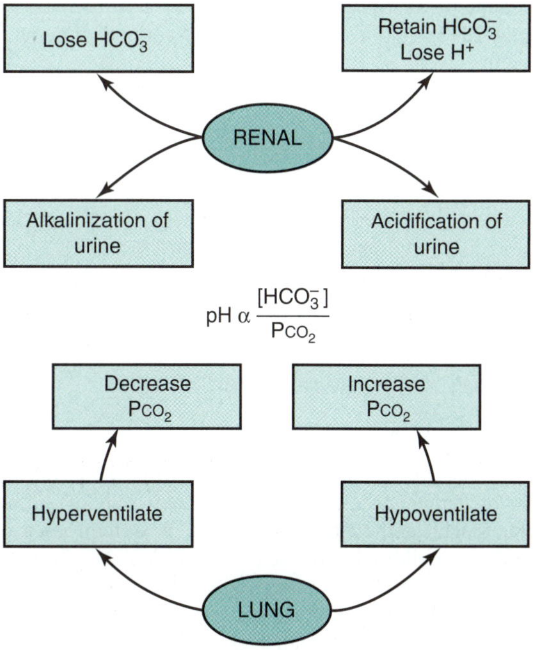

▲ **Figure 23–3.** Maintaining metabolic stability via compensatory mechanisms.

hypokalemic metabolic alkalosis and systemic K^+ depletion wherein H^+ is exchanged and excreted in preference to K^+ in response to mineralocorticoid. Some of the processes involved in acid-base regulation are shown in Figure 23–3.

FLUID & ELECTROLYTE MANAGEMENT

Therapy of fluid and electrolyte disorders is directed toward providing maintenance fluid and electrolyte requirements, replenishing prior losses, and replacing persistent abnormal losses. Therapy should be phased to (1) rapidly expand the ECF volume and restore tissue perfusion, (2) replenish fluid and electrolyte deficits while correcting attendant acid-base abnormalities, (3) meet the patient's nutritional needs, and (4) replace ongoing losses.

The cornerstone of therapy involves an understanding of maintenance fluid and electrolyte requirements. Maintenance requirements call for provision of enough water, glucose, and electrolytes to prevent deterioration of body stores for a euvolemic patient. During short-term parenteral therapy, sufficient glucose is provided to prevent ketosis and limit protein catabolism, although this is usually little more than 20% of the patient's true caloric needs. Prior to the administration of maintenance fluids, it is important to consider the patient's volume status and to determine whether intravenous fluids are truly needed.

Table 23–1. Caloric and water needs per unit of body weight.

Body Weight (kg)	kcal/kg	mL of Water/kg
3–10	100	100
11–20	1000 kcal + 50 kcal/kg for each kg > 10 kg	1000 mL + 50 mL/kg for each kg > 10 kg
> 20	1500 kcal + 20 kcal/kg for each kg > 20 kg	1500 mL + 20 mL/kg for each kg > 20 kg

Data from Holliday MA, Segar WE: The maintenance need for water in parenteral fluid therapy. Pediatrics 1957;19:823.

Various models have been devised to facilitate calculation of maintenance requirements based on body surface area, weight, and caloric expenditure. A system based on caloric expenditure is most helpful, because 1 mL of water is needed for each kilocalorie expended. The system presented in Table 23–1 is based on caloric needs and is applicable to children weighing more than 3 kg.

As depicted in Table 23–1, a child weighing 30 kg would need 1700 kcal or 1700 mL of water daily. If the child received parenteral fluids for 2 days, the fluid would usually contain 5% glucose, which would provide 340 kcal/d, or 20% of the maintenance caloric needs. Maintenance fluid requirements take into account normal insensible water losses and water lost in sweat, urine, and stool, and assume the patient to be afebrile, at their true dry weight and relatively inactive. Thus, if excessive losses occur, standard "maintenance fluids" will be inadequate. In contrast, if losses are reduced for any reason, standard "maintenance fluid" administration would be excessive. Maintenance requirements are greater for low-birth-weight and preterm infants. Table 23–2 lists other factors that commonly alter fluid and caloric needs.

Electrolyte losses occur primarily through the urinary tract and to a lesser degree via the skin and stool. Although maintenance electrolyte estimates vary, reasonable approximations for maintenance needs are 3–4 mEq Na^+/100 kcal and 2 mEq K^+/100 kcal or 30–40 mEq Na^+/L and 20 mEq K^+/L, respectively, of intravenous fluid. However, the observant clinician should be alert to the potential for hyponatremia to develop in hospitalized patients receiving hypotonic intravenous solutions. The clinical relevance of hospital acquired hyponatremia is a very important issue. It has been suggested that the judicious use of isotonic fluids, or at least 0.45 normal saline solution, rather than hypotonic fluids be considered to avoid hyponatremia with its attendant complications. In recent years, there also has been a trend for total parenteral nutrition, or hyperalimentation, solution sodium, and other electrolytes to be calculated and ordered on a milliequivalents-per-kilogram basis rather than the more classic milliequivalents-per-liter basis (eg, 0.2 or 0.45 normal). It is extremely important to understand that if the administered fluid volume is decreased in this setting, as the child is weaned from supplemental IV fluids to enteral intake, the sodium and other electrolytes will need to be reduced accordingly to avoid progressively increasing IV fluid tonicity that can result in hypernatremia or other electrolyte derangements.

It is helpful to monitor the patient's daily weight, urinary output, fluid input, and urine specific gravity. If fluid or electrolyte balance is abnormal, serial determination of electrolyte concentrations, blood urea nitrogen, and creatinine may be necessary. In patients with significant burns, anuria, oliguria, or persistent abnormal losses (eg, from a stoma, or polyuria secondary to a renal concentrating defect), it is important to measure output, and if needed its components, so appropriate replacement can be provided.

Table 23–2. Alterations of maintenance fluid requirements.

Factor	Altered Requirement
Fever	12% per degree C[a]
Hyperventilation	10–60 mL/100 kcal
Sweating	10–25 mL/100 kcal
Hyperthyroidism	Variable: 25%–50%
Gastrointestinal loss and renal disease	Monitor and analyze output. Adjust therapy accordingly.

[a]Do not correct for 38°C; correct 24% for 39°C.

DEHYDRATION

Depletion of body fluids is one of the most commonly encountered problems in clinical pediatrics. Children have a high incidence of gastrointestinal diseases, including gastroenteritis, and may demonstrate gastrointestinal symptoms in nongastrointestinal conditions, such as pneumonia or meningitis. Infants and young children often decrease their oral intake when ill, and their high ratio of surface area to weight promotes significant evaporative losses. Renal concentrating mechanisms do not maximally conserve water in early life, and fever may significantly increase fluid needs. Dehydration decreases ECF volume, leading to decreased tissue perfusion, progressive uremia and abnormal renal function studies, compensatory tachycardia, and lactic acidosis. The clinical effects of dehydration relate to the degree of dehydration and to the relative amounts of salt and water lost. Caregivers must be particularly aware of dehydration occurring in breast-fed newborn infants who go home soon after birth and whose mothers fail to produce enough milk. This problem is more common in the hot summer months and has been associated with severe dehydration, brain damage, and death.

The clinical evaluation of a child with dehydration should focus on the composition and volume of fluid intake; the frequency and amount of vomiting, diarrhea, and urine output; the degree and duration of fever; the nature of any administered medications; and the existence of underlying medical conditions. A recently recorded weight, if known, can be very helpful in calculating the magnitude of dehydration. Important clinical features in estimating the degree of dehydration include the capillary refill time, postural blood pressure, and heart rate changes; dryness of the lips and mucous membranes; lack of tears; lack of external jugular venous filling when supine; a sunken fontanelle in an infant; oliguria; and altered mental status (Table 23–3). Children generally respond to a decrease in circulating volume with a compensatory increase in pulse rate and may maintain their blood pressure in the face of severe dehydration. A low or falling blood pressure is, therefore, a late sign of shock in children, and when present should prompt emergent treatment. Salient laboratory parameters include a high urine specific gravity (in the absence of an underlying renal concentrating defect as seen in diabetes insipidus or chronic obstructive or reflux nephropathy), a relatively greater elevation in blood urea nitrogen than in serum creatinine, a low urinary [Na^+] excretion (< 20 mEq/L), and an elevated hematocrit or serum albumin level secondary to hemoconcentration.

Emergent intravenous therapy is indicated when there is evidence of compromised perfusion (inadequate capillary refill, tachycardia, poor color, oliguria, or hypotension). The initial goal is to rapidly expand the plasma volume and to prevent circulatory collapse. A 20-mL/kg bolus of isotonic fluid should be given intravenously as rapidly as possible. Either colloid (5% albumin) or crystalloid (normal saline or Ringer lactate) may be used. Colloid is particularly useful in hypernatremic patients in shock, in malnourished infants, and in neonates. If no intravenous site is available, fluid may be administered intraosseously through the marrow space of the tibia. If there is no response to the first fluid bolus, a second bolus may be given. When adequate tissue perfusion is demonstrated by improved capillary refill, decreased pulse rate and urine output, and improved mental status, deficit replacement may be instituted. If adequate perfusion is not restored after 40 mL/kg of isotonic fluids, other pathologic processes must be considered such as sepsis, occult hemorrhage, or cardiogenic shock. Isotonic dehydration may be treated by providing half of the remaining fluid deficit over 8 hours and the second half over the ensuing 16 hours in the form of 5% dextrose with 0.2%–0.45% saline containing 20 mEq/L of KCl. In the presence of metabolic acidosis, potassium acetate may be considered. Maintenance fluids and replacement of ongoing losses should also be provided. Typical electrolyte compositions of various body fluids are depicted in Table 23–4, although it may be necessary to measure the specific constituents of a patient's fluid losses to guide therapy. If the patient is unable to eat for a prolonged period, nutritional needs must be met through hyperalimentation or enteral tube feedings.

Oral rehydration may be provided to children with mild to moderate dehydration. Clear liquid beverages found in the home, such as broth, soda, juice, and tea are inappropriate for the treatment of dehydration. Commercially available solutions provide 45–75 mEq/L of Na^+, 20–25 mEq/L of K^+, 30–34 mEq/L of citrate or bicarbonate, and 2%–2.5% of

Table 23–3. Clinical manifestations of dehydration.

Clinical Signs	Degree of Dehydration: Mild	Moderate	Severe
Decrease in body weight	3-5%	6-10%	11-15%
Skin			
Turgor	Normal ±	Decreased	Markedly decreased
Color	Normal	Pale	Markedly decreased
Mucous membranes	Dry →	→	Mottled or gray; parched
Hemodynamic signs			
Pulse	Normal	Slight increase	Tachycardia
Capillary refill	2-3 s	3-4 s	> 4 s
Blood pressure	Normal →	→	Low
Perfusion	Normal →	→	Circulatory collapse
Fluid loss			
Urinary output	Mild oliguria	Oliguria	Anuria
Tears	Decreased		Absent
Urinary indices			
Specific gravity	> 1.020 →	→	Anuria
Urine [Na^+]	< 20 mEq/L →	→	Anuria

Table 23–4. Typical electrolyte compositions of various body fluids.

	Na^+ (mEq/L)	K^+ (mEq/L)	HCO_3^- (mEq/L)
Diarrhea	10–90	10–80	40
Gastric	20–80	5–20	0
Small intestine	100–140	5–15	40
Ileostomy	45–135	3–15	40

Data from Winters RW: *Principles of Pediatric Fluid Therapy.* Little, Brown, 1973.

Table 23–5. Estimated water and electrolyte deficits in dehydration (moderate to severe).

Type of Dehydration	H_2O (mL/kg)	Na^+ (mEq/kg)	K^+ (mEq/kg)	Cl^- and HCO_3^- (mEq/kg)
Isotonic	100–150	8–10	8–10	16–20
Hypotonic	50–100	10–14	10–14	20–28
Hypertonic	120–180	2–5	2–5	4–10

Adapted, with permission, from Winters RW: *Principles of Pediatric Fluid Therapy.* Little, Brown, 1982.

glucose. Frequent small aliquots (5–15 mL) should be given to provide approximately 50 mL/kg over 4 hours for mild dehydration and up to 100 mL/kg over 6 hours for moderate dehydration. Oral rehydration is contraindicated in children with altered levels of consciousness or respiratory distress who cannot drink freely; in children suspected of having an acute surgical abdomen; in infants with greater than 10% volume depletion; in children with hemodynamic instability; and in the setting of severe hyponatremia ($[Na^+]$ < 120 mEq/L) or hypernatremia ($[Na^+]$ > 160 mEq/L). Failure of oral rehydration due to persistent vomiting or inability to keep up with losses mandates intravenous therapy. Successful oral rehydration requires explicit instructions to caregivers and close clinical follow up of the child.

The type of dehydration is characterized by the serum $[Na^+]$. If relatively more solute is lost than water, the $[Na^+]$ falls, and hyponatremic dehydration ($[Na^+]$ < 130 mEq/L) ensues. This is important clinically because hypotonicity of the plasma contributes to further volume loss from the ECF into the intracellular space. Thus, tissue perfusion is more significantly impaired for a given degree of hyponatremic dehydration than for a comparable degree of isotonic or hypertonic dehydration. It is important to note, however, that significant solute losses also occur in hypernatremic dehydration. Furthermore, because plasma volume is somewhat protected in hypernatremic dehydration, it poses the risk of the clinician underestimating the severity of dehydration. Typical fluid and electrolyte losses associated with each form of dehydration are shown in Table 23–5.

HYPONATREMIA

Hyponatremia may be factitious in the presence of high plasma lipids or proteins, which decrease the percentage of plasma volume that is water. Hyponatremia in the absence of hypotonicity also occurs when an osmotically active solute, such as glucose or mannitol, is added to the ECF. Water drawn from the ICF dilutes the serum $[Na^+]$ despite isotonicity or hypertonicity.

Patients with hyponatremic dehydration generally demonstrate typical signs and symptoms of dehydration (see Table 23–3), because the vascular space is compromised as water leaves the ECF to maintain osmotic neutrality. The treatment of hyponatremic dehydration is fairly straightforward. The magnitude of the sodium deficit may be calculated by the following formula:

$$Na^+ \text{ deficit} = (Na^+\text{desired} - Na + \text{observed}) \times \text{Bodyweight (kg)} \times 0.6$$

Half of the deficit is replenished in the first 8 hours of therapy, and the remainder is given over the following 16 hours. Maintenance and replacement fluids should also be provided. The deficit plus maintenance calculations generally approximate 5% dextrose with 0.45% saline. The rise in serum $[Na^+]$ should not exceed 0.5–1.0 mEq/L/h or more than 20 mEq/L/24 h unless the patient demonstrates central nervous system (CNS) symptoms that warrant more rapid initial correction. The dangers of too rapid correction of hyponatremia include cerebral dehydration and injury due to fluid shifts from the ICF compartment.

Hypovolemic hyponatremia also occurs in cerebral salt wasting associated with CNS insults, a condition characterized by high urine output and elevated urinary $[Na^+]$ (> 80 mEq/L) due to an increase in ANF. This must be distinguished from the syndrome of inappropriate secretion of ADH (SIADH), which may also become manifest in CNS conditions and certain pulmonary disorders. In contrast to cerebral salt wasting, SIADH is characterized by euvolemia or mild volume expansion and relatively low urine output due to ADH-induced water retention. Urinary $[Na^+]$ is high in both conditions, though generally not as high as in SIADH. It is important to distinguish between these two conditions, because the treatment of the former involves replacement of urinary salt and water losses, whereas the treatment of SIADH involves water restriction.

In cases of severe hyponatremia (serum $[Na^+]$ < 120 mEq/L) with CNS symptoms, intravenous 3% NaCl may be given over 1 hour to raise the $[Na^+]$ to 120 mEq/L, to alleviate CNS manifestations and sequelae. In general, 6 mL/kg of 3% NaCl will raise the serum $[Na^+]$ by about 5 mEq/L. If 3% NaCl is administered, estimated Na^+ and fluid deficits should be adjusted accordingly. Further correction should proceed slowly, as outlined earlier.

Hypervolemic hyponatremia may occur in edematous disorders such as nephrotic syndrome, congestive heart failure, and cirrhosis, wherein water is retained in excess of salt. Treatment involves restriction of Na^+ and water and correction of the underlying disorder. Hypervolemic hyponatremia due to water intoxication is characterized by a maximally dilute urine (specific gravity < 1.003) and is also treated with water restriction.

HYPERNATREMIA

Although diarrhea is commonly associated with hyponatremic or isonatremic dehydration, hypernatremia may develop in the presence of persistent fever or decreased fluid intake or in response to improperly mixed rehydration solutions. Extreme care is required to treat hypernatremic dehydration appropriately. If the serum [Na^+] falls precipitously, the osmolality of the ECF drops more rapidly than that of the CNS. Water shifts from the ECF compartment into the CNS to maintain osmotic neutrality. If hypertonicity is corrected too rapidly (a drop in [Na^+] of greater than 0.5–1 mEq/L/h), cerebral edema, seizures, and CNS injury may occur. Thus, following the initial restoration of adequate tissue perfusion using isotonic fluids, a gradual decrease in serum [Na^+] is desired (10–15 mEq/L/d). This is commonly achieved using 5% dextrose with 0.2% saline to replace the calculated fluid deficit over 48 hours. Maintenance and replacement fluids should also be provided. If the serum [Na^+] is not correcting appropriately, the free water deficit may be estimated as 4 mL/kg of free water for each milliequivalent of serum [Na^+] above 145 mEq/L and provided as 5% dextrose over 48 hours. If metabolic acidosis is also present, it must be corrected slowly to avoid CNS irritability. Potassium is provided as indicated—as the acetate salt if necessary. Electrolyte concentrations should be assessed every 2 hours in order to control the decline in serum [Na^+]. Elevations of blood glucose and blood urea nitrogen may worsen the hyperosmolar state in hypernatremic dehydration and should also be monitored closely. Hyperglycemia is often associated with hypernatremic dehydration and may necessitate lower intravenous glucose concentrations (eg, 2.5%).

Patients with diabetes insipidus, whether nephrogenic or central in origin, are prone to develop profound hypernatremic dehydration as a result of unremitting urinary-free water losses (urine specific gravity < 1.010), particularly during superimposed gastrointestinal illnesses associated with vomiting or diarrhea. Treatment involves restoration of fluid and electrolyte deficits as described earlier as well as replacement of excessive water losses. Formal water deprivation testing to distinguish responsiveness to ADH should only be done during daylight hours after restoration of normal fluid volume status.

However, if a child presents with marked dehydration and a serum Na^+ greater than 150 mEq/L, it may prove helpful and timely to obtain a plasma vasopressin level at the time of their initial presentation. The evaluation and treatment of nephrogenic and central diabetes insipidus are discussed in detail in Chapters 24 and 34, respectively.

Hypervolemic hypernatremia (salt poisoning), associated with excess total body salt and water, may occur as a consequence of providing improperly mixed formula, excessive NaCl or $NaHCO_3$ administration, or as a feature of primary hyperaldosteronism. Treatment includes the use of diuretics, and potentially, concomitant water replacement or even dialysis.

POTASSIUM DISORDERS

The predominantly intracellular distribution of potassium is maintained by the actions of Na^+-K^+-ATPase in the cell membranes. Potassium is shifted into the ECF and plasma by acidemia and into the ICF in the setting of alkalosis, hypochloremia, or in conjunction with insulin-induced cellular glucose uptake. The ratio of intracellular to extracellular K^+ is the major determinant of the cellular resting membrane potential and contributes to the action potential in neural and muscular tissue. Abnormalities of K^+ balance are potentially life-threatening. In the kidney, K^+ is filtered at the glomerulus, reabsorbed in the proximal tubule, and excreted in the distal tubule. Distal tubular K^+ excretion is regulated primarily by aldosterone. Renal K^+ excretion continues for significant periods even after the intake of K^+ is decreased. Thus, by the time urinary [K^+] decreases, the systemic K^+ pool has been depleted significantly.

The causes of net K^+ loss are primarily renal in origin. Gastrointestinal losses through nasogastric suction or vomiting reduce total body K^+ to some degree. However, the resultant volume depletion results in an increase in plasma aldosterone, promoting renal excretion of K^+ in exchange for Na^+ reclamation to preserve circulatory volume. Diuretics (especially thiazides), mineralocorticoids, and intrinsic renal tubular diseases (eg, Bartter syndrome) enhance the renal excretion of K^+. Clinically, hypokalemia is associated with neuromuscular excitability, decreased peristalsis or ileus, hyporeflexia, paralysis, rhabdomyolysis, and arrhythmias. Electrocardiographic changes include flattened T waves, a shortened PR interval, and the appearance of U waves. Arrhythmias associated with hypokalemia include premature ventricular contractions; atrial, nodal, or ventricular tachycardia; and ventricular fibrillation. Hypokalemia increases responsiveness to digitalis and may precipitate overt digitalis toxicity. In the presence of arrhythmias, extreme muscle weakness, or respiratory compromise, intravenous K^+ should be given. If the patient is hypophosphatemic ([PO_4^{3-}] < 2 mg/dL), a phosphate salt may be used. The first priority in the treatment of hypokalemia is the restoration of an adequate serum [K^+]. Providing maintenance amounts of K^+ is usually sufficient; however, when the serum [K^+] is dangerously low and K^+ must be administered intravenously, it is imperative that the patient have a cardiac monitor. Intravenous K^+ should generally not be given faster than at a rate of 0.3 mEq/kg/h. Oral K^+ supplements may be needed for weeks to replenish depleted body stores.

Hyperkalemia—due to decreased renal K^+ excretion, mineralocorticoid deficiency or unresponsiveness, or K^+ release from the ICF compartment—is characterized by muscle weakness, paresthesias, and tetany; ascending paralysis; and arrhythmias. Electrocardiographic changes associated with hyperkalemia include peaked T waves, widening of the QRS complex, and arrhythmias such as sinus bradycardia or sinus arrest, atrioventricular block, nodal or idioventricular rhythms, and ventricular tachycardia or fibrillation. The severity of hyperkalemia depends on the electrocardiographic changes, the status of the other electrolytes, and the stability of the underlying disorder. A rhythm strip should be obtained when significant hyperkalemia is suspected. If the serum [K^+] is less than 6.5 mEq/L, discontinuing K^+ supplementation is usually sufficient. If the serum [K^+] is greater than 7 mEq/L or if potentiating factors such as hyponatremia, digitalis toxicity, and renal failure are present, more aggressive therapy is needed. If electrocardiographic changes or arrhythmias are present, treatment must be initiated promptly. Intravenous 10% calcium gluconate (0.2–0.5 mL/kg over 2–10 minutes) will rapidly ameliorate depolarization and may be repeated after 5 minutes if electrocardiographic changes persist. Calcium should be given only with a cardiac monitor in place and should be discontinued if bradycardia develops. The intravenous administration of a diuretic that acts in the loop of Henle, such as furosemide (1–2 mg/kg), will augment renal K^+ excretion and can be very helpful in lowering serum and total body [K^+]. Administering Na^+ and increasing systemic pH with bicarbonate therapy (1–2 mEq/kg) will shift K^+ from the ECF to the ICF compartment, as will therapy with a β-agonist such as albuterol. In nondiabetic patients, 0.5 g/kg of glucose over 1–2 hours will enhance endogenous insulin secretion, lowering serum [K^+] 1–2 mEq/L. Administration of intravenous glucose and insulin may be needed as a simultaneous drip (0.5–1 g/kg glucose and 0.3 units of regular insulin per gram of glucose) given over 2 hours with monitoring of the serum glucose level every 15 minutes.

The therapies outlined above provide transient benefits. Ultimately, K^+ must be reduced to normal levels by reestablishing adequate renal excretion using diuretics or optimizing urinary flow, using ion exchange resins such as sodium polystyrene sulfonate orally or as a retention enema (0.2–0.5 g/kg orally or 1 g/kg as an enema), or by dialysis.

ACID-BASE DISTURBANCES

When evaluating a disturbance in acid-base balance, the systemic pH, partial carbon dioxide pressure (Pco_2), serum [HCO_3^-], and anion gap must be considered. The anion gap, $Na^+ - (Cl^- + HCO_3^-)$, is an expression of the unmeasured anions in the plasma and is normally 12 ± 4 mEq/L. An increase above normal suggests the presence of an unmeasured anion, such as occurs in diabetic ketoacidosis, lactic acidosis, salicylate intoxication, and so on. Although the base excess (or deficit) is also used clinically, it is important to recall that this expression of acid-base balance is influenced by the renal response to respiratory disorders and cannot be interpreted independently (as in a compensated respiratory acidosis, wherein the base excess may be quite large). Recently, there has been greater interest in the Stewart approach to acid-base disturbances and the calculation of the "strong ion difference," which is beyond the scope of the present discussion. The interested reader is referred to the review by Gunnerson and Kellum listed in the references at the end of this chapter.

METABOLIC ACIDOSIS

Metabolic acidosis is characterized by a primary decrease in serum [HCO_3^-] and systemic pH due to the loss of HCO_3^- from the kidneys or gastrointestinal tract, the addition of an acid (from external sources or via altered metabolic processes), or the rapid dilution of the ECF with non-bicarbonate–containing solution (usually normal saline). When HCO_3^- is lost through the kidneys or gastrointestinal tract, Cl^- must be reabsorbed with Na^+ disproportionately, resulting in a hyperchloremic acidosis with a normal anion gap. Thus, a normal anion gap acidosis in the absence of diarrhea or other bicarbonate-rich gastrointestinal losses suggests the possibility of renal tubular acidosis and should be evaluated appropriately. (See Chapter 24.) In contrast, acidosis that results from addition of an unmeasured acid is associated with a widened anion gap. Examples are diabetic ketoacidosis, lactic acidosis, starvation, uremia, toxin ingestion (salicylates, ethylene glycol, or methanol), and certain inborn errors of organic or amino acid metabolism. Dehydration may also result in a widened anion gap acidosis as a result of inadequate tissue perfusion, decreased O_2 delivery, and subsequent lactic and keto acid production. Respiratory compensation is accomplished through an increase in minute ventilation and a decrease in Pco_2. The patient's history, physical findings, and laboratory features should lead to the appropriate diagnosis.

The ingestion of unknown toxins or the possibility of an inborn error of metabolism (see Chapter 36) must be considered in children without an obvious cause for a widened anion gap acidosis. Unfortunately, some hospital laboratories fail to include ethylene glycol or methanol in their standard toxicology screens, so assay of these toxins must be requested specifically. This is of critical importance when therapy with fomepizole (4-methylpyrazole) must be considered for either ingestion—and instituted promptly to obviate profound toxicity. Ethylene glycol (eg, antifreeze) is particularly worrisome because of its sweet taste and accounts for a significant number of toxin ingestions. Screening by fluorescence of urine under a Wood lamp is relatively simple but does not replace specific laboratory assessment. Salicylate intoxication has a stimulatory effect on the respiratory center of the CNS; thus, patients may initially present with respiratory alkalosis or mixed respiratory alkalosis and widened anion gap acidosis.

Most types of metabolic acidosis will resolve with correction of the underlying disorder, improved renal perfusion, and acid excretion. Intravenous $NaHCO_3$ administration may be considered in the setting of metabolic acidosis when the pH is less than 7.0 or the $[HCO_3^-]$ is less than 5 mEq/L, but only if adequate ventilation is ensured. The dose (in milliequivalents) of $NaHCO_3$ may be calculated as

$$\text{Weight (kg)} \times \text{Base deficit} \times 0.3$$

and given as a continuous infusion over 1 hour. The effect of $NaHCO_3$ in lowering serum potassium and ionized calcium concentrations must also be considered and monitored.

METABOLIC ALKALOSIS

Metabolic alkalosis is characterized by a primary increase in $[HCO_3^-]$ and pH resulting from a loss of strong acid or gain of buffer base. The most common cause for a metabolic alkalosis is the loss of gastric juice via nasogastric suction or vomiting. This results in a Cl^--responsive alkalosis, characterized by a low urinary $[Cl^-]$ (< 20 mEq/L) indicative of a volume-contracted state that will be responsive to the provision of adequate Cl^- salt (usually in the form of normal saline). Cystic fibrosis may also be associated with a Cl^--responsive alkalosis due to the high losses of NaCl through the sweat, whereas congenital Cl^--losing diarrhea is a rare cause of Cl^--responsive metabolic alkalosis. Chloride-resistant alkaloses are characterized by a urinary $[Cl^-]$ greater than 20 mEq/L and include Bartter syndrome, Cushing syndrome, and primary hyperaldosteronism, conditions associated with primary increases in urinary $[Cl^-]$, or volume-expanded states lacking stimuli for renal Cl^- reabsorption. Thus, the urinary $[Cl^-]$ is helpful in distinguishing the nature of a metabolic alkalosis, but must be specifically requested in many laboratories because it is not routinely included in urine electrolyte panels. The serum $[K^+]$ is also low in these settings (hypokalemic metabolic alkalosis) owing to a combination of increased mineralocorticoid activity associated with volume contraction, the shift of K^+ to the ICF compartment, preferential reabsorption of Na^+ rather than K^+ to preserve intravascular volume, or primary mineralocorticoid excess.

RESPIRATORY ACIDOSIS

Respiratory acidosis develops when alveolar ventilation is decreased, increasing P_{CO_2} and lowering systemic pH. The kidneys compensate for respiratory acidosis by increasing HCO_3^- reabsorption, a process that takes several days to fully manifest. Patients with acute respiratory acidoses frequently demonstrate air hunger with retractions and the use of accessory respiratory muscles. Respiratory acidoses occur in upper or lower airway obstruction, ventilation-perfusion disturbances, CNS depression, and neuromuscular defects. Hypercapnia is not as detrimental as the hypoxia that usually accompanies these disorders. The goal of therapy is to correct or compensate for the underlying pathologic process to improve alveolar ventilation. Bicarbonate therapy is not indicated in a pure respiratory acidosis, because it will worsen the acidosis by shifting the equilibrium of the carbonic acid–bicarbonate buffer system to increase P_{CO_2}.

RESPIRATORY ALKALOSIS

Respiratory alkalosis occurs when hyperventilation results in a decrease in P_{CO_2} and an increase in systemic pH. Depending on the acuity of the respiratory alkalosis, there may be an associated compensatory loss of bicarbonate by the kidneys manifested as a low serum bicarbonate level and a normal anion gap that may be misinterpreted as a normal anion gap acidosis if all acid-base parameters are not considered. Patients may experience tingling, paresthesias, dizziness, palpitations, syncope, or even tetany and seizures due to the associated decrease in ionized calcium. Causes of respiratory alkalosis include psychobehavioral disturbances, CNS irritation from meningitis or encephalitis, salicylate intoxication, and iatrogenic over ventilation in patients who are intubated and mechanically ventilated. Therapy is directed toward the causal process. Rebreathing into a paper bag will decrease the severity of symptoms in acute hyperventilation.

REFERENCES

Adrogue JA, Madias NE: Management of life-threatening acid-base disorders: Parts 1 and 2. N Engl J Med 1998;338:26, 107 [PMID: 9414329].

Avner ED: Clinical disorders of water metabolism: Hyponatremia and hypernatremia. Pediatr Ann 1995;24:23 [PMID: 7715960].

Choong K et al: Hypotonic versus isotonic maintenance fluids after surgery for children: A randomized controlled trial. Pediatrics 2011;128:980–983 [PMID: 22007013].

Fall PJ: A stepwise approach to acid-base disorders. Practical patient evaluation for metabolic acidosis and other conditions. Postgraduate Med 2000;107:249 [PMID: 10728149].

Finberg L et al: *Water and Electrolytes in Pediatrics: Physiology, Pathophysiology and Treatment*, 2nd ed. WB Saunders, 1993.

Friedman A: Fluid and electrolyte therapy: A primer. Pediatr Nephrol 2009;7:1189 [PMID: 19444484].

Gunnerson KJ, Kellum JA: Acid-base and electrolyte analysis in critically ill patients: Are we ready for the new millennium? Curr Opin Crit Care 2003;9:468 [PMID: 14639065].

Hellerstein S: Fluids and electrolytes: Physiology. Pediatr Rev 1993;14:70 [PMID: 8493184].

Jospe N, Forbes G: Fluids and electrolytes: Clinical aspects. Pediatr Rev 1996;17:395 [PMID: 8937172].

Kappy MS, Ganong CA: Cerebral salt wasting in children: The role of atrial natriuretic hormone. Adv Pediatr 1996;43:271 [PMID: 8794180].

Liebelt EL: Clinical and laboratory evaluation and management of children with vomiting, diarrhea, and dehydration. Curr Opin Pediatr 1998;10:461 [PMID: 9818241].

McDonald RA: Disorders of potassium balance. Pediatr Ann 1995;24:31 [PMID: 7715961].

Moritz AL, Ayus JC: Prevention of hospital-acquired hyponatremia: A case for using isotonic saline. Pediatrics 2003;111:227 [PMID: 12563043].

Moritz ML, Ayus JC: Prevention of hospital-acquired hyponatremia: Do we have the answers? Pediatrics 2011;128:980–983 [PMID: 22007008].

Roberts KB: Fluid and electrolytes: Parenteral fluid therapy. Pediatr Rev 2001;22:380 [PMID: 11691948].

Watkins SL: The basics of fluid and electrolyte therapy. Pediatr Ann 1995;24:16 [PMID: 7715959].

White ML, Liebelt: Update on antidotes for pediatric poisoning. Pediatr Emerg Care 2006;22:740 [PMID:17110870].

Kidney & Urinary Tract

24

Gary M. Lum, MD

EVALUATION OF THE KIDNEY & URINARY TRACT

HISTORY

When renal disease is suspected, the history should include

1. Family history of cystic disease, hereditary nephritis, deafness, dialysis, or renal transplantation
2. Preceding acute or chronic illnesses (eg, urinary tract infection, pharyngitis, impetigo, or endocarditis)
3. Rashes or joint pains
4. Growth delay or failure to thrive
5. Polyuria, polydipsia, enuresis, urinary frequency, or dysuria
6. Documentation of hematuria, proteinuria, or discolored urine
7. Pain (abdominal, costovertebral angle, or flank) or trauma
8. Sudden weight gain or edema
9. Drug or toxin exposure
10. Data pertaining to the newborn with suspected urinary tract disease: prenatal ultrasonographic studies, birth asphyxia, Apgar scores, oligohydramnios, dysmorphic features, abdominal masses, voiding patterns, anomalous development, and umbilical artery catheterization

PHYSICAL EXAMINATION

Important aspects of the physical examination include the height, weight, skin lesions (café au lait or ash leaf spots), pallor, edema, or skeletal deformities. Anomalies of the ears, eyes, or external genitalia may be associated with renal anomalies or disease. The blood pressure should be measured in a quiet setting. The cuff should cover two-thirds of the child's upper arm, and peripheral pulses should be noted. The abdomen should be palpated, with attention to the kidneys, abdominal masses, musculature, and the presence of ascites. An ultrasonic device is useful for measurements in infants.

LABORATORY EVALUATION OF RENAL FUNCTION

Serum Analysis

The standard indicators of renal function are serum levels of urea nitrogen and creatinine; their ratio is normally about 10:1. This ratio may increase when renal perfusion or urine flow is decreased, as in urinary tract obstruction or dehydration. Because serum urea nitrogen levels are more affected by these and other factors (eg, nitrogen intake, catabolism, use of corticosteroids) than are creatinine levels, the most reliable single indicator of glomerular function is the serum level of creatinine. For example, an increase in serum creatinine from 0.5 to 1.0 mg/dL represents a 50% decrease in glomerular filtration rate. The serum creatinine level of small children should be well under 0.8 mg/dL. Only larger adolescents should have levels exceeding 1 mg/dL. Less precise but nonetheless important indicators of possible renal disease are abnormalities of serum electrolytes, pH, calcium, phosphorus, magnesium, albumin, or complement.

Glomerular Filtration Rate

The endogenous creatinine clearance (C_{cr}) in milliliters per minute estimates the glomerular filtration rate (GFR). A 24-hour urine collection is usually obtained; however, in small children from whom collection is difficult, a 12-hour daytime specimen, collected when urine flow rate is greatest, is acceptable. The procedure for collecting a timed urine specimen should be explained carefully so that the parent or patient understands fully the rationale of (1) first emptying the bladder (discarding that urine) and noting the time; and (2) putting all urine subsequently voided into the collection receptacle, including the last void, 12 or 24 hours later. Reliability of the 24-hour collection can be checked by measuring the total 24-hour creatinine excretion in the specimen. Total daily creatinine excretion (creatinine index) should be 14–20 mg/kg. Creatinine indices on either side of this range suggest collections that were either inadequate or excessive. Calculation by the following formula requires measurements of plasma creatinine (P_{cr}) in mg/mL, urine creatinine (U_{cr}) in mg/mL, and urine volume (V) expressed as mL/min:

$$C_{cr} = \frac{U_{cr}V}{P_{cr}}$$

Creatinine is a reflection of body muscle mass. Because accepted ranges of normal C_{cr} are based on adult parameters, correction for size is needed to determine normal ranges in children. Clearance is corrected to a standard body surface area of 1.73 m^2 in the formula:

$$\text{"Corrected" } C = \frac{\text{Patient's } C_{cr} \times 1.73\ \text{m}^2}{\text{Patient's body surface area}}$$

Although 80–125 mL/min/1.73 m^2 is the normal range for C_{cr}, estimates at the lower end of this range may indicate problems.

A reliable formula for quick approximation of C_{cr} is based on plasma creatinine level and length in centimeters:

$$C_{cr}(\text{mL/min/1.73 m}^2) = \frac{0.55 \times \text{Height in cm}}{P_{cr} \text{ in mg/dL}}$$

Note: Because this formula takes into account the body surface area, further correction is not necessary. Use 0.45 × length in centimeters for newborns and for infants younger than age 1 year. This method of calculation does not replace creatinine clearance determinations, but is useful when a serum creatinine might be thought to be too high, but one is not sure.

Urine Concentrating Ability

Inability to concentrate urine causes polyuria, polydipsia, or enuresis and is often the first sign of chronic renal failure. The first morning void should be concentrated (specific gravity 1.020 or higher). Evaluation of other abnormalities of urinary concentration or dilution is discussed later in the sections on specific disease entities, such as diabetes insipidus.

Urinalysis

Commercially available dipsticks can be used to check the urine for red blood cells (RBCs), hemoglobin, leukocytes, nitrites, and protein and to approximate its pH. Positive results for blood should always be confirmed by microscopy, and is the only way to determine if there is significant crystalluria. Significant proteinuria (> 150 mg/dL) detected by dipstick should be confirmed by quantitation, either with a 24-hour collection or by the protein/creatinine ratio of a random specimen.

In children with asymptomatic hematuria or proteinuria, the search for renal origins will yield the most results. Isolated proteinuria may reflect urologic abnormalities, benign excretion, or glomerular alterations. RBC casts suggest glomerulonephritis (GN), but the absence of casts does not rule out this disease. Anatomic abnormalities such as cystic disease may also cause hematuria.

Benign hematuria, including benign familial hematuria, is diagnosed by exclusion. In this group are children whose hematuria is caused by asymptomatic hypercalciuria. Figure 24–1 suggests an approach to the renal workup of hematuria. GN is discussed in more detail later in this chapter.

Combined proteinuria and hematuria is characteristic of more significant glomerular disease. Quantitation of proteinuria is customarily accomplished by a timed collection (eg, over a 24-hour period). However, given the frequency of errors in collection in the pediatric population, the degree of proteinuria may be estimated by the ratio of protein mg/dL/creatinine mg/dL in a random urine sample. A protein-to-creatinine ratio above 0.2 is abnormal. If the laboratory reports this as mg protein/gram of creatinine, normal is 200 or less.

In the evaluation of asymptomatic proteinuria, orthostatic or postural proteinuria should be ruled out. The protein present in urine voided on arising in the morning is compared with that in urine formed in the upright position during the rest of the day. This can be accomplished simply by comparing the protein/creatinine ratios of the two urine samples. If the urine formed in the supine position (the first morning void having been accumulated in the bladder while sleeping) is normal and proteinuria is occurring only during upright posture, this demonstrates postural (benign) proteinuria. If both samples are abnormal, proteinuria would be considered "persistent."

An approach to the workup of isolated proteinuria is shown in Figure 24–2. Note that corticosteroid therapy is indicated in the algorithm because this may be initiated prior to referral. Other renal lesions with proteinuric manifestations are discussed later in this chapter.

Special Tests of Renal Function

Measurements of urinary sodium, creatinine, and osmolality are useful in differentiating prerenal from renal causes of renal insufficiency, such as acute tubular necrosis. Prolonged underperfusion causes varying increases in serum creatinine and blood urea nitrogen (BUN) concentrations, prompting the need to differentiate between this state and acute tubular necrosis (see section on Acute Renal Failure, later). The physiologic response to decreased renal perfusion is decreased urinary output, increased urine osmolality, increased urinary solutes (eg, creatinine), and decreased urinary sodium (usually < 20 mEq/L).

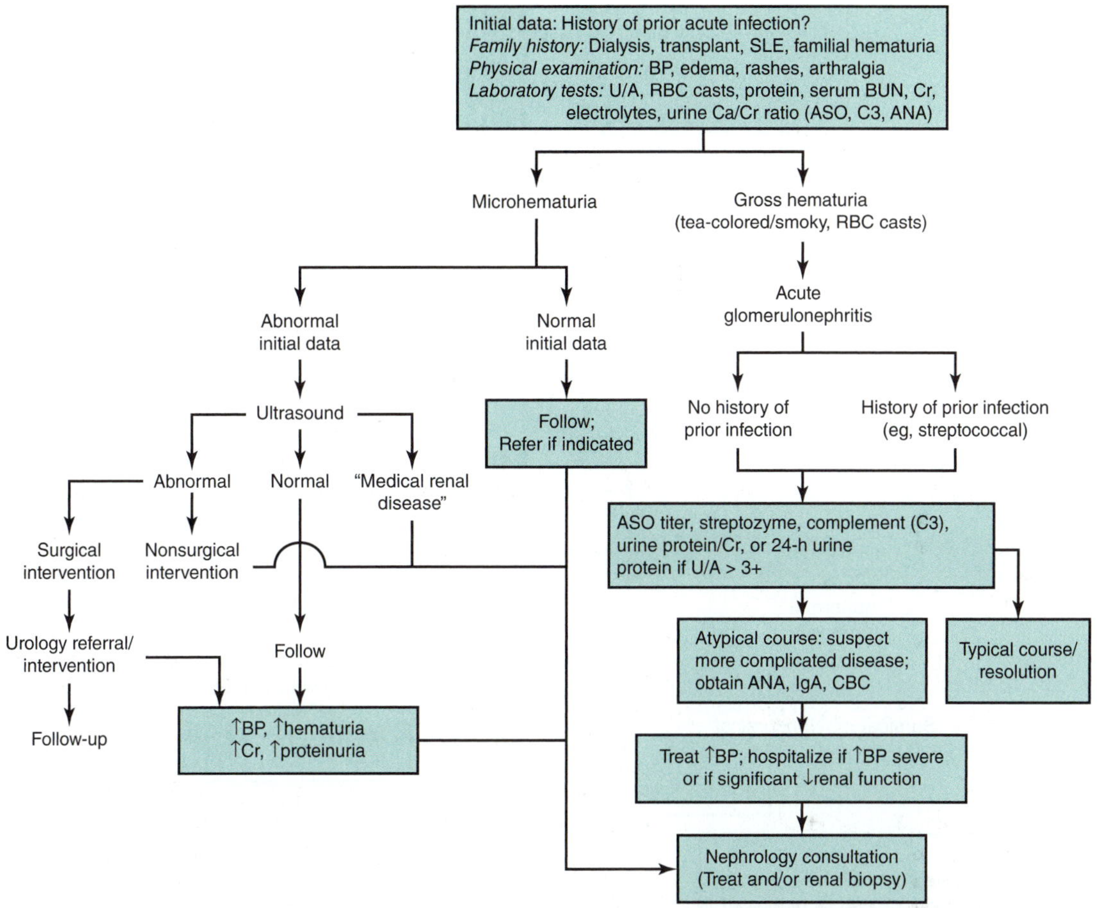

▲ **Figure 24–1.** Approach to the renal workup of hematuria. (Exclude UTI, lithiasis, trauma, bleeding disorders, sickle cell disease.) Complement is depressed in acute poststreptococcal type of glomerulonephritis (about 30 days), chronic glomerulonephritis (persistent), and lupus. ANA, antinuclear antibody; ASO, antistreptolysin antibody; BP, blood pressure; BUN, blood urea nitrogen; C3, complement; Ca, calcium; CBC, complete blood count; Cr, creatinine; IgA, immunoglobulin A; RBC, red blood cell; SLE, systemic lupus erythematosus; U/A, urinalysis.

The presence of certain substances in urine may suggest tubular dysfunction. For example, urine glucose should be less than 5 mg/dL. Hyperphosphaturia occurs with significant tubular abnormalities (eg, Fanconi syndrome). Measurement of the phosphate concentration of a 24-hour urine specimen and evaluation of tubular reabsorption of phosphorus (TRP) will help document renal tubular diseases as well as hyperparathyroid states. TRP (expressed as percentage of reabsorption) is calculated as follows:

$$\text{TRP} = 100\left[1 - \frac{S_{cr} \times \text{UPO}_4}{\text{SPO}_4 \times U_{cr}}\right]$$

where S_{cr} = serum creatinine; U_{cr} = urine creatinine; SPO_4 = serum phosphate; and UPO_4 = urine phosphate. All values for creatinine and phosphate are expressed in milligrams per deciliter for purposes of calculation. A TRP value of 80% or more is considered normal, although it depends somewhat on the value of SPO_4.

The urinary excretion of amino acids in generalized tubular disease reflects a quantitative increase rather than a qualitative change. Diseases affecting proximal tubular reabsorption of bicarbonate—including isolated renal tubular acidosis (RTA), Fanconi syndrome (which occurs in diseases such as cystinosis), and chronic renal failure—are discussed later in the chapter.

LABORATORY EVALUATION OF IMMUNOLOGIC FUNCTION

Many parenchymal renal diseases are thought to have immune causation, although the mechanisms are largely unknown. Examples include (1) deposition of circulating antigen-antibody complexes that are directly injurious or incite injurious

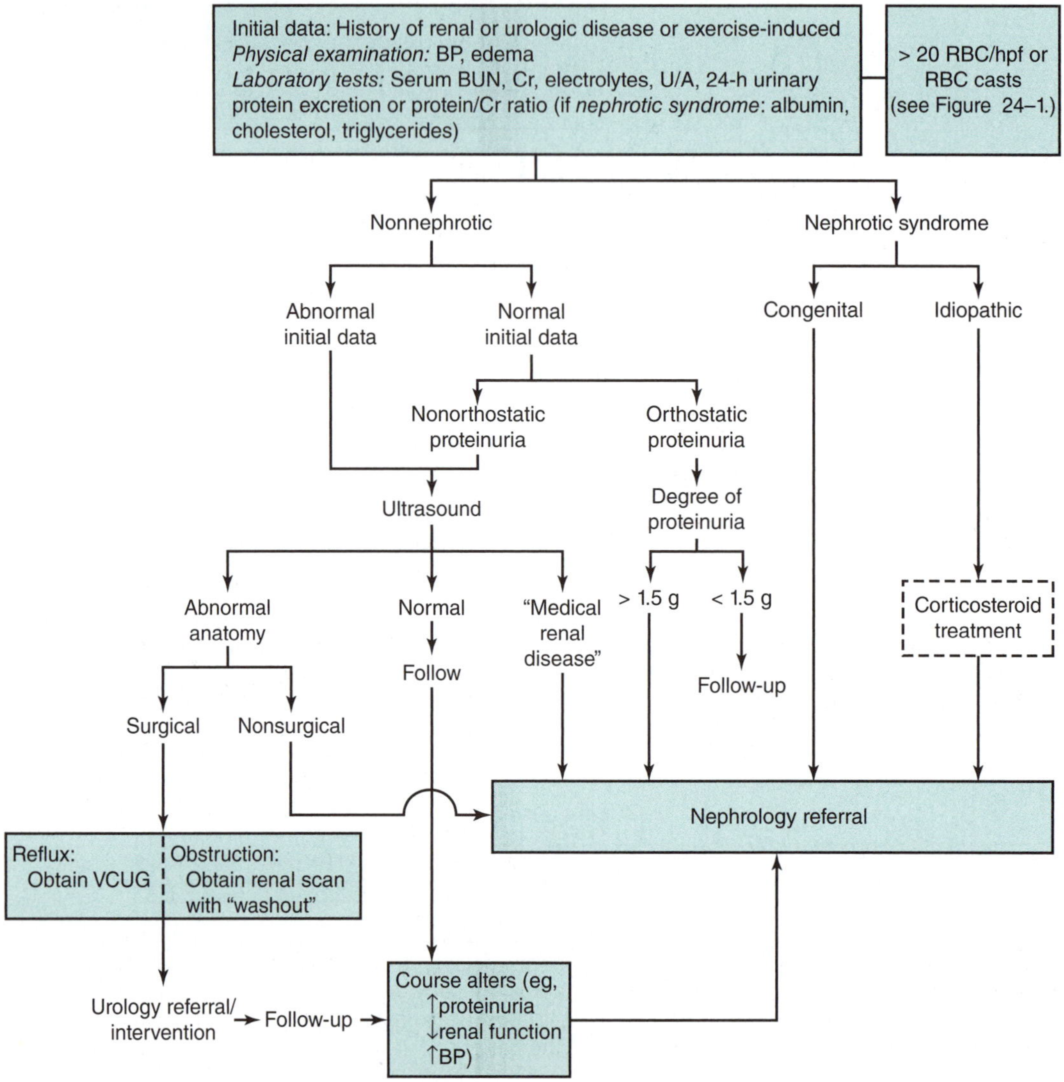

▲ **Figure 24–2.** Approach to the workup of isolated proteinuria. BP, blood pressure; Cr, creatinine; hpf, high-power field; RBC, red blood cell; U/A, urinalysis; VCUG, voiding cystourethrogram. Rules out benign postural proteinuria with urine protein/creatine ratio of first morning void (recumbent urine) versus day void (upright). Will normalize within a month in poststreptococcal glomerulonephritis.

responses and (2) formation of antibody directed against the glomerular basement membrane (rare in children).

C3 and C4 complement components should be measured when immune-mediated renal injury or chronic GN is suspected. Where clinically indicated, antinuclear antibodies, hepatitis B surface antigen, and rheumatoid factor should be obtained. In rare cases, coldprecipitable proteins (cryoglobulins), C3 "nephritic" factor, or antiglomerular basement membrane (anti-GBM) antibody measurements may help confirm a specific diagnosis. At some point in the workup, the diagnosis may be supported or confirmed by histologic examination of renal tissue.

RADIOGRAPHIC EVALUATION

Renal ultrasonography is a useful noninvasive tool for evaluating renal parenchymal disease, urinary tract abnormalities, or renal blood flow. Excretory urography is used to assess the anatomy and function of the kidneys, collecting system, and bladder. Radioisotope studies provide information about renal anatomy, blood flow, and integrity and function of the glomerular, tubular, and collecting systems. Renal stones are best seen by computed tomography.

Voiding cystourethrography or cystoscopy is indicated when vesicoureteral reflux (VUR) or bladder outlet obstruction is suspected. Cystoscopy is rarely useful in the evaluation of asymptomatic hematuria or proteinuria in children.

Renal arteriography or venography is indicated to define vascular abnormalities (eg, renal artery stenosis) prior to surgical intervention or transluminal angiography. Less invasive measures such as ultrasonography and Doppler studies can demonstrate renal blood flow or thromboses. More specific identification of stenoses of the renal artery is accomplished by magnetic resonance arteriography.

RENAL BIOPSY

Histologic information is valuable for diagnosis, to guide treatment, and to inform prognosis. Satisfactory evaluation of renal tissue requires examination by light, immunofluorescence, and electron microscopy.

When a biopsy is anticipated, a pediatric nephrologist should be consulted. In children, percutaneous renal biopsy with a biopsy needle is an acceptable low-risk procedure—avoiding the risks of general anesthesia—when performed by an experienced physician. A surgeon should perform the biopsy procedure if operative exposure of the kidney is necessary, if a risk factor (eg, bleeding disorder) is present, or if a "wedge" biopsy is preferred.

CONGENITAL ANOMALIES OF THE URINARY TRACT

RENAL PARENCHYMAL ANOMALIES

About 10% of children have congenital anomalies of the genitourinary tract, which range in severity from asymptomatic to lethal. Some asymptomatic abnormalities may have significant complications. For example, patients with "horseshoe" kidney (kidneys fused in their lower poles) have a higher incidence of renal calculi. Unilateral agenesis is usually accompanied by compensatory hypertrophy of the contralateral kidney and thus should be compatible with normal renal function. Supernumerary and ectopic kidneys are usually of no significance. Abnormal genitourinary development is associated with varying degrees of renal dysgenesis and dysfunction ranging from mild forms to complete renal agenesis. In neonates, bilateral renal agenesis is associated with severe oligohydramnios, pulmonary hypoplasia, abnormal (Potter) facies, and early death.

1. Renal Dysgenesis

Renal dysgenesis is a spectrum of anomalies. In simple hypoplasia, which may be unilateral or bilateral, the affected kidneys are smaller than normal. In some forms of dysgenesis, immature, undifferentiated renal tissue persists. In some situations, the number of normal nephrons is insufficient to sustain life once the child reaches a critical body size. The lack of renal tissue may not be readily discernible in the newborn period because the infant's urine production, though poor in concentration, may be adequate in volume. Often, the search for renal insufficiency is initiated only when growth fails or chronic renal failure develops.

Other forms of renal dysgenesis include oligomeganephronia (characterized by the presence of only a few large glomeruli) and the cystic dysplasias (characterized by the presence of renal cysts). This group includes microcystic disease (congenital nephrosis). A simple cyst within a kidney may be clinically unimportant because it does not predispose to progressive polycystic development. An entire kidney lost to multicystic development with concomitant hypertrophy and normal function of the contralateral side may also be of little clinical consequence. Nonetheless, even a simple cyst could pose problems if it becomes a site for stone formation, infection, or bleeding.

2. Polycystic Kidney Disease

Autosomal recessive polycystic kidney disease is increasingly diagnosed by prenatal ultrasound. In its most severe form, the cystic kidneys are nonfunctional in utero, and, therefore, newborns can have Potter facies and other complications of oligohydramnios. In infancy and childhood, kidney enlargement by cysts may initially be recognized by abdominal palpation of renal masses. Hypertension is an early problem. The rate of the progression of renal insufficiency varies, as does growth failure and other complications of chronic renal failure. Two genes (*ADPKD1* and *ADPKD2*) account for 80% and 10% of cases of autosomal dominant polycystic kidney disease, respectively. Susceptibility of family members is detected by gene linkage studies. Renal ultrasound identifies cysts in about 80% of affected children by age 5 years. Children with this diagnosis need close monitoring for the development and treatment of hypertension, and their families should be offered genetic counseling. Management of end-stage renal failure is by dialysis or renal transplantation.

3. Medullary Cystic Disease (Juvenile Nephronophthisis)

Medullary cystic disease is characterized by cysts of varying sizes in the renal medulla with tubular and interstitial nephritis. Children present with renal failure and signs of tubular dysfunction (decreased concentrating ability, Fanconi syndrome). This lesion should not be confused with medullary sponge kidney (renal tubular ectasia), a frequently asymptomatic disease occurring in adults.

DISTAL URINARY TRACT ANOMALIES

1. Obstructive Uropathy

Obstruction at the ureteropelvic junction may be the result of intrinsic muscle abnormalities, aberrant vessels, or fibrous bands. The lesion can cause hydronephrosis and usually presents as an abdominal mass in the newborn. Obstruction can occur in other parts of the ureter, especially at its entrance into the bladder, causing proximal hydroureter and hydronephrosis. Renal radionuclide scan with furosemide "wash-out" will reveal or rule out obstruction as the cause of the hydronephrosis. Whether intrinsic or extrinsic, urinary tract obstruction should be relieved surgically as soon as possible to minimize damage to the kidneys.

Severe bladder malformations such as exstrophy are clinically obvious and a surgical challenge. More subtle—but urgent in terms of diagnosis—is obstruction of urine flow from vestigial posterior urethral valves. This anomaly, which occurs almost exclusively in males, usually presents in newborns with anuria or a poor voiding stream secondary to severe obstruction of urine flow. The kidneys and bladder may be easily palpable. Leakage (ureteric perforation, although rare) proximal to the obstruction may produce urinary ascites. Surgical drainage of urine is urgently required to prevent irreversible damage.

Prune belly syndrome is an association of urinary tract anomalies with cryptorchidism and absent abdominal musculature. Although complex anomalies, especially renal dysplasia, usually cause early death or the need for dialysis or transplantation, some patients have lived into the third decade with varying degrees of renal insufficiency. Timely urinary diversion is essential to sustain renal function.

Other complex malformations and external genital anomalies such as hypospadias are beyond the scope of this text. The challenge presented by urologic abnormalities resulting in severe compromise and destruction of renal tissue is to preserve all remaining renal function and treat the complications of progressive chronic renal failure. Involvement of a specialist in pediatric urology in early management is essential.

2. Reflux Nephropathy

The retrograde flow of urine from the bladder into the ureter (vesicoureteral reflux) may cause renal scarring and subsequent renal insufficiency or hypertension, or both, especially in the presence of urinary tract infection. A finding of hydronephrosis on renal ultrasound is suggestive of vesicoureteral reflux. Its presence can be confirmed or eliminated by a voiding cystourethrogram, which would also be obtained to rule out reflux in the evaluation of urinary tract infection. Low-grade reflux may resolve in the absence of infection, in which case antibiotic prophylaxis (advised with any degree of reflux) is undertaken while awaiting signs of spontaneous resolution. Surgery may be required for chronic severe reflux.

HEMATURIA & GLOMERULAR DISEASE

MICROHEMATURIA

Children with painful hematuria should be investigated for urinary tract infection (UTI) or direct injury to the urinary tract. Dysuria is common in cystitis or urethritis; associated back pain suggests the possibility of pyelonephritis; colicky flank pain may indicate the passage of a stone. Bright red blood or clots in the urine are associated with bleeding disorders, trauma, and arteriovenous malformations. Abdominal masses suggest the presence of urinary tract obstruction, cystic disease, or tumors of the renal or perirenal structures.

Asymptomatic hematuria is a challenge because clinical and diagnostic data are required to decide whether to refer the child to a nephrologist. The diagnosis of hematuria should not rely solely on a urine "dipstick" evaluation, but should be verified by a microscopic RBC count. Ruling out hypercalciuria as a cause of hematuria by a random urine calcium/creatinine ratio is one of the initial steps in the evaluation of hematuria. A value above 0.2 requires verification with a 24-hour collection. Hypercalciuria is excretion of calcium in excess of 4 mg/kg/d. Figure 24–1 delineates the out-patient approach to renal hematuria. The concern regarding the differential diagnosis is the possible presence of glomerular disease.

GLOMERULONEPHRITIS

The various types of glomerulonephritis (GN) have similar manifestations. Table 24–1 lists the most commonly encountered disorders in the differential diagnosis of childhood GN, including their clinical and histopathologic abnormalities. Severe glomerular histopathologic and clinical entities, such as anti-GBM antibody disease (Goodpasture syndrome), Wegener granulomatosis, and idiopathic, rapidly progressive GN, may be considered in the differential diagnosis of acute GN, but these disorders are exceedingly rare in children.

1. Acute Poststreptococcal Glomerulonephritis

The diagnosis of acute poststreptoccocal glomerulonephritis is supported by a recent history (7–14 days previously) of group A β-hemolytic streptococcal infection, typically involving the pharynx or skin. If a positive culture is not available, recent infection may be supported by an elevated antistreptolysin O titer or by high titers of other antistreptococcal antibodies. Other infections can cause similar glomerular injury; thus, "postinfection" glomerulonephritis (GN) may be a better term for this type of acute glomerulonephritis (AGN). In most cases, recovery is expected and usually complete within weeks. If the diagnosis is in question, or if the renal function of a patient with postinfection GN progressively deteriorates, a renal biopsy should be performed and treatment with corticosteroids initiated.

Table 24–1. Glomerular diseases encountered in childhood.

Entity	Clinical Course	Prognosis
Postinfection glomerulonephritis (GN). Onset occurs 10–14 d after acute illness, commonly streptococcal. Characteristics include acute onset, tea-colored urine, mild to severe renal insufficiency, and edema.	Acute phase is usually over in 2 wk. Complete resolution occurs in 95% of cases. Severity of renal failure and hypertension varies. Microhematuria may persist to 18 mo. Hypocomplementemia resolves in 1–30 d.	Excellent. Chronic disease is rare. Severe proteinuria, atypical presentation or course, or persistent hypocomplementemia suggest another entity.
Membranoproliferative GN. Presentation ranges from mild microhematuria to acute GN syndrome. Diagnosis is made by renal biopsy. Etiology is unknown. Types I and II are most common. Lesion is chronic.	Course can be mild to severe (rapid deterioration in renal function); may mimic postinfection GN. Proteinuria can be severe. Complement depression is intermittent to persistent. Hypertension is usually significant.	Type I may respond to corticosteroids. Type II (dense deposit disease) is less responsive to treatment; function decrease varies from immediate to as long as 15 y in 30%–50% of untreated cases.
IgA nephropathy. Classic presentation is asymptomatic gross hematuria during acute unrelated illness, with microhematuria between episodes. Occasional instances of acute GN syndrome occur. Etiology is unknown. Diagnosis is made by biopsy.	90% of cases resolve in 1–5 y. Gross hematuric episodes resolve with recovery from acute illness. Severity of renal insufficiency and hypertension varies. Proteinuria occurs in more severe, atypical cases.	Generally good; a small percentage develops chronic renal failure. Proteinuria in the nephrotic range is a poor sign. There is no universally accepted medication. (Corticosteroids may be useful in severe cases.)
Henoch-Schönlein purpura GN. Degree of renal involvement varies. Asymptomatic microhematuria is most common, but GN syndrome can occur. Renal biopsy is recommended in severe cases; it can provide prognostic information.	Presentation varies with severity of renal lesion. In rare cases, may progress rapidly to serious renal failure. Hypertension varies. Proteinuria in the nephrotic range and severe decline in function can occur.	Overall, prognosis is good. Patients presenting with > 50% reduction in function or proteinuria exceeding 1 g/24 h may develop chronic renal failure. Severity of renal biopsy picture can best guide approach in such cases. There is no universally accepted medication therapy.
GN of systemic lupus erythematosus (SLE). Microhematuria and proteinuria are rarely first signs of this systemic disease. Renal involvement varies, but severe GN may ensue with remissions and exacerbations throughout the course.	Renal involvement is mild to severe. Clinical complexity depends on degree of renal insufficiency and other systems involved. Serum complement is depressed. Hypertension is significant. Manifestations of the severity of the renal lesion guide therapeutic intervention.	Renal involvement accounts for most significant morbidity in SLE. Control of hypertension affects renal prognosis. Medication is guided by symptoms, serology, and renal lesion. End-stage renal failure can occur.
Hereditary GN (eg, Alport syndrome). Transmission is autosomal-dominant/X-linked, with family history marked by end-stage renal failure, especially in young males. Deafness and eye abnormalities are associated.	There is no acute syndrome. Females are generally less affected but are carriers. Hypertension and increasing proteinuria occur with advancing renal failure. There is no known treatment.	Progressive proteinuria and hypertension occur early, with gradual decline in renal function in those most severely affected. Disease progresses to end-stage renal failure in most males.

The clinical presentation of GN is gross hematuria generally accompanied by varying degrees of increase in serum creatinine, edema, and hypertension. Urine may be coffee-colored or tea-colored. Microscopic examination of urine reveals RBCs too numerous to count. Microscopy may reveal RBC casts. If present, these are diagnostic of GN, but their absence does not exclude the diagnosis. Edema is often seen (periorbital, facial, extremities), caused by sodium and water retention resulting from alteration in glomerular function. Symptoms are usually nonspecific. In cases accompanied by hypertension (a common finding), headache may be present. Fever is uncommon. Severe glomerular injury (which usually occurs in severe, acute presentations of the more chronic or destructive forms of GN) may be accompanied by massive proteinuria (nephrotic syndrome), anasarca, ascites, and severe compromise of renal function.

Typical poststreptococcal GN has no specific treatment. Antibiotic therapy is indicated if an infection is still present. Disturbances in renal function and resulting hypertension may require close monitoring, reduction in salt intake, diuretics, or other antihypertensive drugs. In severe cases of renal failure, hemodialysis or peritoneal dialysis may be necessary. Corticosteroids may also be administered in an attempt to influence the course of the GN.

The acute abnormalities generally resolve in 2–3 weeks. Low levels of serum complement (C3) may normalize as early as 24 hours or as late as 30 days after onset. Other complement-consuming glomerulonephritides include membranoproliferative GN (chronic GN with persistent complement depression) and lupus GN. In poststreptococcal GN, although microscopic hematuria may persist for as long as a year, 85% of children recover completely. Persistent deterioration in renal function, urinary abnormalities beyond 18 months, persistent hypocomplementemia, and nephrotic syndrome are ominous signs. If any of these is present, a renal biopsy is indicated.

2. IgA Nephropathy

When asymptomatic gross hematuria appears to accompany a minor acute febrile illness or other stressful occurrence, the diagnosis of IgA nephropathy may be entertained. In contrast to postinfection GN, IgA nephropathy is not associated with prior streptococcal infection, complement is not depressed, and in 50% of cases, serum immunoglobin A is elevated. Often there are no associated symptoms or signs. Gross hematuria resolves within days, and there are no serious sequelae in 85% of cases. Treatment is not indicated, and the prognosis is good in most cases. Prognosis is guarded, however, if severe proteinuria, hypertension, or renal insufficiency is present or develops. In such instances, although no treatment is universally accepted, corticosteroids and other immunosuppressive drugs are used. Omega-3 fatty acids from fish oils are thought to be helpful.

3. Henoch-Schönlein Purpura

The diagnosis of Henoch-Schönlein purpura rests on the presence of a typical maculopapular and purpuric rash found primarily, but not exclusively, on the dorsal surfaces of the lower extremities and buttocks. Most children have abdominal pain, and bloody diarrhea may be present. Joint pain is common, and, depending on the extent of renal involvement, hypertension may be present. Joint and abdominal pain responds to treatment with corticosteroids. Renal involvement ranges from mild GN with microhematuria to severe GN and varying degrees of renal insufficiency. GN with massive proteinuria and renal insufficiency carries a poor prognosis. Twenty percent of such cases result in end-stage renal failure. There is no universally accepted treatment, but corticosteroids are often administered (see Chapter 30).

4. Membranoproliferative Glomerulonephritis

The most common "chronic" form of GN in childhood is membranoproliferative GN. The diagnosis is established from the histologic appearance of the glomeruli on biopsy tissue. There are two major histologic types of membranoproliferative GN. Clinically, type II carries the worse prognosis, as end-stage renal failure develops in most cases. Type I more often responds to treatment with corticosteroids. C3 is depressed (in both types) and may be useful as a marker of response to treatment.

5. Lupus Glomerulonephritis

The diagnosis of systemic lupus erythematosus (SLE) is based on its numerous clinical features and abnormal laboratory findings that include a positive antinuclear antibody test, depressed serum complement, and increased serum double-stranded DNA. Renal involvement is indicated by varying degrees of hematuria and proteinuria. More severe cases are accompanied by renal insufficiency and hypertension. Significant renal involvement requires treatment with immunosuppressive drugs and close monitoring. End-stage renal failure develops in 10%–15% of patients with childhood SLE.

6. Hereditary Glomerulonephritis

The most commonly encountered hereditary GN is Alport syndrome, characterized by hearing loss and GN, occurring predominantly in males. It is a chronic form of GN and thus does not present with the clinical features typically seen in patients with acute processes. A family history is generally present, but there is a spontaneous mutation rate of about 18%. In individuals with the progressive form of GN, end-stage renal failure occurs, usually in the second to third decade of life. Although currently there is no treatment for this disorder, careful management of associated hypertension may slow the process.

Ahn SY, Ingulli E: Acute poststreptococcal glomerulonephritis: An update. Curr Opin Pediatr 2008;20:157–162 [PMID: 18332711].

Sanders JT, Wyatt RJ: IgA nephropathy and Henoch-Schönlein purpura nephritis. Curr Opin Pediatr 2008;20:163–170 [PMID: 18332712].

ACUTE INTERSTITIAL NEPHRITIS

Acute interstitial nephritis is characterized by diffuse or focal inflammation and edema of the renal interstitium and secondary involvement of the tubules. The condition is most commonly drug related (eg, β-lactam–containing antibiotics, such as methicillin).

Fever, rigor, abdominal or flank pain, and rashes may occur in drug-associated cases. Urinalysis usually reveals leukocyturia and hematuria. Hansel staining of the urinary sediment often demonstrates eosinophils. The inflammation can cause significant deterioration of renal function. If the diagnosis is unclear because of the absence of a history of drug or toxin exposure or the absence of eosinophils in the urine, a renal biopsy may be performed to demonstrate the characteristic tubular and interstitial inflammation. Immediate identification and removal of the causative agent is imperative and may be all that is necessary. Treatment with corticosteroids is helpful in patients with progressive renal insufficiency or nephrotic syndrome. Severe renal failure requires supportive dialysis.

Gonzalez E et al: Early steroid treatment improves the recovery of renal function in patients with drug-induced acute interstitial nephritis. Kidney Int 2008;73:940–946 [PMID: 18185501].

PROTEINURIA & RENAL DISEASE

Urine is rarely completely protein-free, but the average excretion is well below 150 mg/24 h. Small increases in urinary protein can accompany febrile illnesses or exertion and in some cases occur while in the upright posture.

An algorithm for investigation of isolated proteinuria is presented in Figure 24–2. In idiopathic nephrotic syndrome without associated features of GN, treatment with corticosteroids may be initiated. Nephrologic advice or follow-up should be sought, especially in patients with difficult or frequently relapsing unexplained proteinuria.

CONGENITAL NEPHROSIS

Congenital nephrosis is a rare autosomal recessive disorder. The kidneys are pale and large and may show microcystic dilations (microcystic disease) of the proximal tubules and glomerular abnormalities, including proliferation, crescent formation, and thickening of capillary walls. The pathogenesis is not well understood.

Infants with congenital nephrosis commonly have low birth weight, a large placenta, wide cranial sutures, and delayed ossification. Mild edema may be seen after the first few weeks of life. Anasarca follows, and the abdomen can become greatly distended by ascites. Massive proteinuria associated with typical-appearing nephrotic syndrome and hyperlipidemia is the rule. Hematuria is common. If the patient lives long enough, progressive renal failure occurs. Most affected infants succumb to infections by a few months of life.

Treatment prior to dialysis and transplantation has little to offer other than nutritional support and management of the chronic renal failure.

IDIOPATHIC NEPHROTIC SYNDROME OF CHILDHOOD (MINIMAL CHANGE DISEASE)

Nephrotic syndrome is characterized by proteinuria, hypoproteinemia, edema, and hyperlipidemia. It may occur as a result of any form of glomerular disease and may rarely be associated with a several extrarenal conditions. In young children, the disease usually takes the form of idiopathic nephrotic syndrome of childhood (nil disease, lipoid nephrosis, minimal change disease), which has characteristic clinical and laboratory findings, but no well-understood cause.

Clinical Findings

Affected patients are generally younger than age 6 years at onset. Typically, periorbital swelling and oliguria are noted, often following an influenza-like syndrome. Within a few days, increasing edema—even anasarca—becomes evident. Most children have few complaints other than vague malaise or abdominal pain. With significant "third spacing" of plasma volume, however, some children may present with hypotension. With marked edema, dyspnea due to pleural effusions may also occur.

Despite heavy proteinuria, the urine sediment is usually normal, although microscopic hematuria may be present. Plasma albumin concentration is low, and lipid levels increased. When azotemia occurs, it is usually secondary to intravascular volume depletion.

Glomerular morphology is unremarkable except for fusion of foot processes of the glomerular basement membrane. This nonspecific finding is associated with many proteinuric states.

Complications

Infections (eg, peritonitis) sometimes occur, and *Streptococcus pneumoniae* is frequently the cause. Hypercoagulability may be present, and thromboembolic phenomena are commonly reported. Hypertension can be noted, and renal insufficiency can result from decreased renal perfusion.

Treatment & Prognosis

As soon as the diagnosis of idiopathic nephrotic syndrome is made, corticosteroid treatment should be started. Prednisone, 2 mg/kg/d (maximum, 60 mg/d), is given for 6 weeks as a single daily dose. The same dose is then administered on an alternate-day schedule for 6 weeks; thereafter, the dose is tapered gradually and discontinued over the ensuing 2 months. The goal of this regimen is the disappearance of proteinuria. If remission is not achieved during the initial phase of corticosteroid treatment, additional nephrologic consultation should be obtained. If remission is achieved, only to be followed by relapse, the treatment course may be repeated. A renal biopsy is often considered when there is little or no response to treatment. One should take into account that the histologic findings may not alter the treatment plan, which is designed to eliminate the nephrotic syndrome regardless of underlying renal histology.

Unless the edema causes symptoms such as respiratory compromise due to ascites, diuretics should be used with extreme care. Patients may have decreased circulating volume and are also at risk for venous thrombosis. Careful restoration of compromised circulating volume with intravenous albumin infusion and administration of diuretics is helpful in mobilizing edema. Infections such as peritonitis should be treated promptly to reduce morbidity. Immunization with pneumococcal vaccine is advised.

A favorable response of proteinuria to corticosteroids and subsequent favorable response during relapse suggests a good prognosis. Failure to respond or early relapse usually heralds a prolonged series of relapses. This not only may indicate the presence of more serious nephropathy, but presents a challenge in choosing future therapy. Chlorambucil or cyclophosphamide drug therapy is usually effective only in children who respond to corticosteroids. Patients who do not respond to corticosteroids or who relapse frequently should be referred to a pediatric nephrologist. Intravenous methylprednisolone may be helpful in more refractory cases. When the protracted use of corticosteroids raises concerns of toxicity, concomitant treatment with either cyclosporin A or tacrolimus appears to be helpful.

FOCAL GLOMERULAR SCLEROSIS

Focal glomerular sclerosis is one cause of corticosteroid-resistant or frequent relapsing nephrotic syndrome. The cause is unknown. The diagnosis is made by renal biopsy, which shows normal-appearing glomeruli as well as some partially or completely sclerosed glomeruli. The lesion has serious prognostic implications because as many as 15%–20% of cases can progress to end-stage renal failure. The response to corticosteroid treatment is variable. In difficult cases, cyclosporin A or tacrolimus have been used in addition to corticosteroids. There are increasing reports that poorly responsive cases may respond to rituximab, a monoclonal antibody against the B-cell surface antigen CD20. Recurrence of focal glomerular sclerosis resulting in nephrotic syndrome may occur after renal transplantation. The recurrence is usually treated with plasmapheresis or rituximab (this drug is finding encouraging utility in treating the nephrotic syndrome of membranous or mesangial nephropathy as well as minimal change disease).

MESANGIAL NEPHROPATHY (MESANGIAL GLOMERULONEPHRITIS)

Mesangial nephropathy is another form of corticosteroid-resistant nephrotic syndrome. The renal biopsy shows a distinct increase in the mesangial matrix of the glomeruli. Very often the expanded mesangium contains deposits of IgM demonstrable on immunofluorescent staining. The cause is unknown. Corticosteroid therapy may induce remission, but relapses are common. Choices for treating this type of nephrotic syndrome are the same as noted earlier.

MEMBRANOUS NEPHROPATHY (MEMBRANOUS GLOMERULONEPHRITIS)

Although largely idiopathic in nature, membranous nephropathy can be found in association with hepatitis B antigenemia, SLE, congenital and secondary syphilis, renal vein thrombosis; with immunologic disorders such as autoimmune thyroiditis; and with administration of drugs such as penicillamine. The pathogenesis is unknown, but the glomerular lesion is thought to be the result of prolonged deposition of circulating antigen-antibody complexes.

The onset of membranous nephropathy may be insidious or may resemble that of idiopathic nephrotic syndrome of childhood (see earlier section). It occurs more often in older children and adults. The proteinuria of membranous nephropathy responds poorly to corticosteroid therapy, although low-dose corticosteroid therapy may reduce or delay development of chronic renal insufficiency. The diagnosis is made by renal biopsy.

Fine RN: Recurrence of nephrotic syndrome/focal segmental glomerulosclerosis following renal transplantation in children. Pediatr Nephrol 2007;22:496 [PMID: 17186280].

Gipson DS et al: Management of childhood onset nephrotic syndrome. Pediatrics 2009;124:747–757 [PMID: 19651590].

DISEASES OF THE RENAL VESSELS

RENAL VEIN THROMBOSIS

In newborns, renal vein thrombosis may complicate sepsis or dehydration. It may be observed in infants of diabetic mothers, may be associated with umbilical vein catheterization, or may result from any condition that produces a hypercoagulable state (eg, clotting factor deficiency, SLE, or thrombocytosis). Renal vein thrombosis is less common in older children and adolescents. It may develop following trauma or without any apparent predisposing factors. Spontaneous renal vein thrombosis has been associated with membranous glomerulonephropathy. Nephrotic syndrome may either cause or result from renal vein thrombosis.

Clinical Findings

Renal vein thrombosis in newborns is generally characterized by the sudden development of an abdominal mass. If the thrombosis is bilateral, oliguria may be present; urine output may be normal with a unilateral thrombus. In older children, flank pain, sometimes with a palpable mass, is a common presentation.

No single laboratory test is diagnostic of renal vein thrombosis. Hematuria usually is present; proteinuria is less constant. In the newborn, thrombocytopenia may be found, but it is rare in older children. The diagnosis is made by ultrasonography and Doppler flow studies.

Treatment

Anticoagulation with heparin is the treatment of choice in newborns and older children. In the newborn, a course of heparin combined with treatment of the underlying problem is usually all that is required. Management in other cases is less straightforward. The tendency for recurrence and embolization has led some to recommend long-term anticoagulation. If an underlying membranous GN is suspected, biopsy should be performed.

Course & Prognosis

The mortality rate in newborns from renal vein thrombosis depends on the underlying cause. With unilateral renal venous thromboses at any age, the prognosis for adequate renal function is good. Renal vein thrombosis may rarely recur in the same kidney or occur in the other kidney years after the original episode of thrombus formation. Extension into the vena cava with pulmonary emboli is possible.

RENAL ARTERIAL DISEASE

Arterial disease (eg, fibromuscular hyperplasia, congenital stenosis) is a rare cause of hypertension in children. Although few clinical clues are specific to underlying arterial lesions, they should be suspected in children with severe hypertension, with onset at or before age 10 years, or with delayed visualization on nuclear scan of the kidneys. The diagnosis is established by renal arteriography with selective renal vein renin measurements. Some of these lesions may be approached by transluminal angioplasty or surgery (see section on Hypertension), but repair may be technically impossible in small children. Although thrombosis of renal arteries is rare, it should be considered in a patient with acute onset of hypertension and hematuria in an appropriate setting (eg, in association with hyperviscosity or umbilical artery catheterization). Early diagnosis and treatment provides the best chance of reestablishing renal blood flow.

Tullus K: Renovascular hypertension in children. Lancet 2008;371: 1453–1463 [PMID: 18440428].

HEMOLYTIC-UREMIC SYNDROME

Hemolytic-uremic syndrome is the most common glomerular vascular cause of acute renal failure in childhood. The diarrhea-associated form is usually the result of infection with Shiga toxin–producing (also called verotoxin-producing) strains of *Shigella* or *Escherichia coli*. Ingestion of undercooked ground beef or unpasteurized foods is a common source. There are many serotypes, but the most common pathogen in the United States is *E coli* O157:H7. Bloody diarrhea is the usual presenting complaint, followed by hemolysis and renal failure. Circulating verotoxin causes endothelial damage, which leads to platelet deposition, microvascular occlusion with subsequent hemolysis, and thrombocytopenia. Similar microvascular endothelial activation may also be triggered by drugs (eg, cyclosporin A); by viruses (human immunodeficiency virus [HIV]); and by pneumococcal infections, in which bacterial neuraminidase exposes the Thomsen-Friedenreich antigen on RBCs, platelets, and endothelial cells, thereby causing platelet aggregation, endothelial damage, and hemolysis. Rare cases are caused by genetic factors (eg, congenitally depressed C3 complement and factor H deficiency).

Clinical Findings

Hemolytic-uremic syndrome due to Shigella or *E coli* begins with a prodrome of abdominal pain, diarrhea, and vomiting. Oliguria, pallor, and bleeding manifestations, principally gastrointestinal, occur next. Hypertension and seizures develop in some children—especially those who develop severe renal failure and fluid overload. There may also be significant endothelial involvement in the central nervous system (CNS).

Anemia is profound, and RBC fragments are seen on blood smears. A high reticulocyte count confirms the hemolytic nature of the anemia, but may not be noted in the presence of renal failure. Thrombocytopenia is profound, but other coagulation abnormalities are less consistent. Serum fibrin split products are often present, but fulminant disseminated intravascular coagulation is rare. Hematuria and proteinuria are often present. The serum complement level is normal except in those cases related to congenital predisposition.

Complications

These usually result from renal failure. Neurologic problems, particularly seizures, may result from hyponatremia, hypertension, or CNS vascular disease. Severe bleeding, transfusion requirements, and hospital-acquired infections must be anticipated.

Treatment

Meticulous attention to fluid and electrolyte status is crucial. The use of antimotility agents and antibiotics for hemolytic-uremic syndrome caused by gastrointestinal infection is believed to worsen the disease. Antibiotics may upregulate and cause the release of large amounts of bacterial Shiga toxin. Timely dialysis improves the prognosis. Since prostacyclin-stimulating factor, a potent inhibitor of platelet aggregation, may be absent in some cases, plasma infusion or plasmapheresis has been advocated in severe cases (generally in those cases with severe CNS involvement). Platelet inhibitors have also been tried, but the results have not been impressive, especially late in the disease. Nonetheless, using a platelet inhibitor early in the disease in an attempt to halt platelet consumption and microvascular occlusion may obviate the need for platelet transfusions and reduce the progression of renal failure. RBC and platelet transfusions may be necessary. Although the risk of volume overload is significant, this can be minimized by dialysis. Erythropoietin (epoetin alfa) treatment may reduce RBC transfusion needs. Although no therapy is universally accepted, strict control of hypertension, adequate nutrition support, and the timely use of dialysis reduce morbidity and mortality. If renal failure is "nonoliguric," and if urine output is sufficient to ensure against fluid overload and electrolyte abnormalities, management of renal failure without dialysis is possible.

Course & Prognosis

Most commonly, children recover from the acute episode within 2–3 weeks. Some residual renal disease (including hypertension) occurs in about 30%, and end-stage renal failure occurs in about 15%. Thus, follow-up of children recovering from hemolytic-uremic syndrome should include serial determinations of renal function for 1–2 years and monitoring of blood pressure for 5 years. Mortality (about 3%–5%) is most likely in the early phase, primarily resulting from CNS or cardiac complications.

Copelovitch L, Kaplan BS: *Streptococcus pneumoniae*–associated hemolytic uremic syndrome. Pediatr Nephrol 2008;23:1951–1956 [PMID: 17564729].

Iijima K et al: Management of diarrhea-associated hemolytic uremic syndrome in children. Clin Exp Nephrol 2008;12:16–19 [PMID: 18175052].

RENAL FAILURE

ACUTE RENAL FAILURE

Acute renal failure is the sudden inability to excrete urine of sufficient quantity or composition to maintain body fluid home-ostasis. The most common cause in children is dehydration. However, encountering signs of acute renal insufficiency in a hospitalized patient raises many other possibilities: impaired renal perfusion or renal ischemia, acute renal disease, renal vascular compromise, acute tubular necrosis, or obstructive uropathy. Table 24–2 lists such prerenal, renal, and postrenal causes.

Clinical Findings

The hallmark of early renal failure is oliguria. Although an exact etiologic diagnosis may be unclear at the onset, classifying oliguria as outlined in Table 24–2 is helpful in determining if an immediately reversible cause is present.

If the cause of elevation in serum BUN and creatinine or oliguria is unclear, entities that can be quickly addressed and corrected (eg, volume depletion) should be considered first. Once normal renal perfusion is ensured and no clinical evidence for de novo renal disease is present, a diagnosis of acute tubular necrosis (vasomotor nephropathy, ischemic injury) may be entertained.

A. Prerenal Causes

The most common cause of decreased renal function in children is compromised renal perfusion. It is usually secondary to dehydration, although abnormalities of renal vasculature and poor cardiac performance may also be considered. Table 24–3 lists the urinary indices helpful in distinguishing these "prerenal" conditions from true renal parenchymal insult, such as in acute tubular necrosis.

B. Renal Causes

Causes of renal failure intrinsic to the kidneys include acute glomerulonephritides, hemolytic-uremic syndrome, acute interstitial nephritis, and nephrotoxic injury. The diagnosis of acute tubular necrosis (vasomotor nephropathy)—which is reserved for those cases in which renal ischemic insult is believed to be the likely cause—should be considered when correction of prerenal or postrenal problems does not improve renal function and there is no evidence of de novo renal disease.

C. Postrenal Causes

Postrenal failure, usually found in newborns with urologic anatomic abnormalities, is accompanied by varying degrees of renal insufficiency. The approach to the problem in the very young is addressed earlier in the chapter, but one should always keep in mind the possibility of acute urinary tract obstruction in acute renal failure, especially in the setting of anuria of acute onset.

Complications

The clinical severity of the complications depends on the degree of renal functional impairment and oliguria. Common complications include (1) fluid overload (hypertension, congestive heart failure, and pulmonary edema), (2) electrolyte disturbances (hyperkalemia), (3) metabolic acidosis, (4) hyperphosphatemia, and (5) uremia.

Table 24–2. Classification of renal failure.

Prerenal
- Dehydration due to gastroenteritis, malnutrition, or diarrhea
- Hemorrhage, aortic or renal vessel injury, trauma, cardiac disease or surgery, renal arterial thrombosis
- Diabetic acidosis
- Hypovolemia associated with capillary leak or nephrotic syndrome
- Shock
- Heart failure

Renal
- Hemolytic-uremic syndrome
- Acute glomerulonephritis
- Prolonged renal hypoperfusion
- Nephrotoxins
- Acute tubular necrosis or vasomotor nephropathy
- Renal (cortical) necrosis
- Intravascular coagulation: septic shock, hemorrhage
- Diseases of renal vessels
- Iatrogenic (eg, drug toxicity)
- Sepsis with shock
- Drowning, especially fresh water
- Crystalluria: sulfonamide or uric acid
- Hypercalcemia from cancer treatment
- Hepatic failure

Postrenal
- Obstruction due to tumor, hematoma, posterior urethral valves, ureteropelvic junction stricture, ureterovesical junction stricture, ureterocele
- Stones
- Trauma to a solitary kidney or collecting system
- Renal vein thrombosis

Table 24–3. Urine studies.

	Prerenal Failure	Acute Tubular Necrosis
Urine osmolality	50 mOsm/kg > plasma osmolality	≤ plasma osmolality
Urine sodium	< 10 mEq/L	> 20 mEq/L
Ratio of urine creatinine to plasma creatinine	> 40:1	< 40:1
Specific gravity	> 1.020	1.012–1.018

Treatment

An indwelling bladder catheter is inserted to ascertain urine output. If urine volume is insignificant and renal failure is established, the catheter should be removed to minimize infection risk. Prerenal or postrenal factors should be excluded or rectified, and normal circulating volume maintained with appropriate fluids. Strict measurement of input and output must be maintained, and input adjusted as reduction in output dictates. The patient's response is assessed by physical examination and urinary output. Measurement of central venous pressure may be indicated. Increasing urine output with diuretics, such as furosemide (1–5 mg/kg, per dose, intravenously, maximum of 200 mg), can be attempted. The effective dose will depend on the amount of functional compromise (if < 50% function, initiate attempt at diuresis with maximum dose). If a response does not occur within 1 hour and the urine output remains low (< 0.5 mL/kg/h), the furosemide dose, if not already maximized, should be increased up to 5 mg/kg. In some cases, the addition of a long-acting thiazide diuretic, such as metolazone, may improve the response. If no diuresis occurs with maximum dosing, further administration of diuretics should cease.

If these maneuvers stimulate some urine flow but biochemical evidence of acute renal failure persists, the resulting nonoliguric acute renal failure should be more manageable. Fluid overload and dialysis may be averted. However, if the medications and nutrients required exceed the renal capacity for excretion, and there is no increase in urine output with the use of maximum doses of diuretics (loop diuretic plus a thiazide diuretic) dialysis is indicated. Institution of dialysis before the early complications of acute renal failure develop is likely to improve clinical management and outcome. It is important to adjust medication dosage according to the degree of renal function.

A. Acute Dialysis: Indications

Immediate indications for dialysis are (1) severe hyperkalemia; (2) unrelenting metabolic acidosis (usually in a situation where fluid overload prevents sodium bicarbonate administration); (3) fluid overload with or without severe hypertension or congestive heart failure (a situation in which volume concerns would seriously compromise administration of adequate nutritional support or of necessary intravenous medications); and (4) symptoms of uremia, usually manifested in children by CNS depression.

B. Methods of Dialysis

Peritoneal dialysis is generally preferred in children because of the ease of performance and patient tolerance. Although peritoneal dialysis is technically less efficient than hemodialysis, hemodynamic stability and metabolic control can be better sustained because this technique can be applied on a relatively continuous basis. Hemodialysis should be considered (1) if rapid removal of toxins is desired, (2) if the size of the patient makes hemodialysis less technically cumbersome and hemodynamically well tolerated, or (3) if impediments to efficient peritoneal dialysis are present (eg, ileus, adhesions). Furthermore, if vascular access and usage of anticoagulation are not impediments, a slow, continuous hemodialytic process (continuous renal replacement treatment) may be applied.

C. Complications of Dialysis

Complications of peritoneal dialysis include peritonitis, volume depletion, and technical complications such as dialysate leakage and respiratory compromise from intra-abdominal dialysate fluid. Peritonitis can be avoided by strict aseptic technique. Peritoneal fluid cultures are obtained as clinically indicated. Leakage is reduced by good catheter placement technique and appropriate intra-abdominal dialysate volumes. Adjustment of the electrolyte concentration of dialysate is important to maintain electrolyte balance. Potassium (absent from standard dialysate solutions) can be added to the dialysate as required. Phosphate is also absent because hyperphosphatemia is an expected problem in renal failure. Nonetheless, if phosphate intake is inadequate, hypophosphatemia must be addressed. Correction of fluid overload is accomplished by using high osmolar dialysis fluids. Higher dextrose concentrations (maximum 4.25%) can correct fluid overload rapidly at the risk of causing hyperglycemia. Fluid removal may also be increased with more frequent exchanges of the dialysate, but rapid osmotic transfer of water may result in hypernatremia.

Even in small infants, hemodialysis can rapidly correct major metabolic and electrolyte disturbances, as well as volume overload. The process is highly efficient, but the speed of the changes can cause problems such as hemodynamic instability. Anticoagulation is usually required. Careful monitoring of the appropriate biochemical parameters is important. Note that during or immediately following the procedure, blood sampling will produce misleading results because equilibration between extravascular compartments and the blood will not have been achieved. Vascular access must be obtained and carefully monitored. Hemodialysis is generally intermittent and utilized as clinically indicated. If need be, continuous renal replacement therapy (CRRT) may be used to maintain more minute to minute, continuous metabolic and fluid control.

Course & Prognosis

The course and prognosis of acute renal failure vary with the etiology. If severe oliguria occurs in acute tubular necrosis, it usually lasts about 10 days. Anuria or oliguria lasting longer than 3 weeks makes the diagnosis of acute tubular necrosis unlikely and favors alternative diagnoses such as vascular injury, severe ischemia (cortical necrosis), GN, or obstruction. The diuretic phase begins with an increase in urinary output to large volumes of isosthenuric urine containing sodium levels of 80–150 mEq/L. During the recovery phase, signs and symptoms subside rapidly, although polyuria may persist for several days or weeks. Urinary abnormalities usually disappear completely within a few months. If renal recovery does not ensue, arrangements are made for chronic dialysis and eventual renal transplantation.

Andreoli SP: Acute kidney injury in children. Pediatr Nephrol 2009;24:253–263 [PMID: 19083019].

Walters S et al: Dialysis and pediatric acute kidney injury: Choice of renal support modality. Pediatr Nephrol 2009;24:37–48 [PMID: 18483748].

CHRONIC RENAL FAILURE

Chronic renal failure in children most commonly results from developmental abnormalities of the kidneys or urinary tract. Infants with renal agenesis are not expected to survive. Depending on the degree of dysgenesis (including multicystic development), the resulting renal function will determine outcome. Abnormal development of the urinary tract may not permit normal renal development. Obstructive uropathy or severe VUR nephropathy, without (or despite) surgical intervention, continues to cause a significant amount of progressive renal insufficiency in children. In older children, the chronic glomerulonephritides and nephropathies, irreversible nephrotoxic injury, or hemolytic-uremic syndrome may also cause chronic renal failure.

Chronic renal failure may follow acute GN or develop with chronic GN in the absence of an obvious acute episode. Growth failure depends on age at presentation and the rapidity of functional decline. Some of the chronic glomerulonephritides (eg, membranoproliferative GN) can progress unnoticed if subtle abnormalities of the urinary sediment are undetected or ignored. Any child with a history of chronic GN or significant renal injury needs close follow-up and monitoring of renal function and blood pressure.

Complications

Any remaining unaffected renal tissue can compensate for gradual loss of functioning nephrons in progressive chronic renal failure, but complications of renal insufficiency appear when compensatory ability is overwhelmed. In children who have developmentally reduced function and are unable to concentrate the urine, polyuria and dehydration are more likely to be problems than fluid overload. Output may be expected to gradually diminish as renal failure progresses to end stage; however, some children can continue to produce generous quantities of urine (but not of good quality) even though they require dialysis. A salt-wasting state can also occur. In contrast, children who develop chronic renal failure due to glomerular disease or renal injury will characteristically retain sodium and water and develop hypertension.

Metabolic acidosis and growth retardation occur early in chronic renal failure. Disturbances in calcium, phosphorus, and vitamin D metabolism leading to renal osteodystrophy and rickets require prompt attention. Although increased parathyroid hormone (in response to decrease serum calcium from lack of renal activated vitamin D, and/or rising serum phosphorus—as glomerular function decreases increase levels of PTH are needed to improve renal tubular excretion) can maintain a normal serum calcium and serum phosphate level early in the course, but at the expense of the skeleton. The increase in parathyroid hormone will also be reflected in an increase in alkaline phosphatase.

Uremic symptoms occur late in chronic renal failure, and include anorexia, nausea, and malaise. CNS features range from confusion, apathy, and lethargy to stupor and coma. Associated electrolyte abnormalities may precipitate seizures. More commonly, seizures are a result of untreated hypertension or hypocalcemia (especially with rapid correction of acidosis). Anemia (normochromic and normocytic from decreased renal erythropoietin synthesis) is common. Platelet dysfunction and other abnormalities of the coagulation system may be present. Bleeding—especially gastrointestinal bleeding—may be a problem. Uremic pericarditis, congestive heart failure, pulmonary edema, and hypertension may occur.

Treatment

A. Management of Complications

Treatment of chronic renal failure is primarily aimed at controlling the associated complications. Hypertension, hyperkalemia, hyperphosphatemia, acidosis, and anemia are among the early problems. Acidosis may be treated with sodium citrate solutions, as long as the added sodium will not aggravate hypertension. Sodium restriction is advisable when hypertension is present. Hyperphosphatemia is controlled by dietary restriction and dietary phosphate binders (eg, calcium carbonate). Vitamin D should be given to maintain normal serum calcium. When the BUN level exceeds approximately 50 mg/dL, or if the child is lethargic or anorexic, dietary protein should be restricted. Potassium restriction will be necessary as the GFR falls to a level where urinary output decreases sharply. Diet must be maintained to provide the child's daily requirements.

Renal function must be monitored regularly (creatinine and BUN), and serum electrolytes, calcium, phosphorus, alkaline phosphatase, and hemoglobin and hematocrit levels monitored to guide changes in fluid and dietary management as well as dosages of phosphate binder, citrate buffer, vitamin D, blood pressure medications, and epoetin alfa. Growth failure may be treated with human recombinant growth hormone. These treatments require careful monitoring to minimize symptoms while the need for chronic dialysis and transplantation continues to be assessed.

Care must be taken to avoid medications that aggravate hypertension; increase the body burden of sodium, potassium, or phosphate; or increase production of BUN. Successful management relies greatly on education of the patient and family.

Attention must also be directed toward the psychosocial needs of the patient and family as they adjust to chronic illness and the eventual need for dialysis and kidney transplantation.

B. Dialysis and Transplantation

Chronic peritoneal dialysis (home-based) and hemodialysis provide life-saving treatment for children prior to renal transplantation. The best measure of the success of chronic dialysis in children is the level of physical and psychosocial rehabilitation achieved, such as continued participation in day-to-day activities and school attendance. Although catch-up growth rarely occurs, patients can grow at an acceptable rate even though they may remain in the lower percentiles. Use of epoetin alfa, growth hormone, and better control of renal osteodystrophy contribute to improved outcome.

At present, the graft survival rate for living-related kidney transplants is 90% at 1 year, 85% at 2 years, and 75% at 5 years. With cadaveric transplantation, graft survivals are 76%, 71%, and 62%, respectively. Overall, the mortality rate is 4% for recipients of living-related donors and 6.8% for recipients of cadaver organs. These percentages are affected by the increased mortality, reported to be as high as 75%, in infants younger than age 1 year, primarily due to technical issues and complications of immunosuppression. A body weight of at least 15 kg is associated with a significantly improved survival rate. Adequate growth and well-being are directly related to acceptance of the graft, the degree of normal function, and the side effects of medications.

Carey WA et al: Outcomes of dialysis initiated during the neonatal period for treatment of end-stage renal disease: A North American Pediatric Renal Trials and Collaborative Studies special analysis. Pediatrics 2007;119:468 [PMID: 17224455].

Rees L: Long-term outcome after renal transplantation in childhood. Pediatr Nephrol 2009;24:475–484 [PMID: 17687572].

Shroff R, Ledermann S: Long-term outcome of chronic dialysis in children. Pediatr Nephrol 2009;24:463–474 [PMID: 18214549].

HYPERTENSION

Hypertension in children is commonly of renal origin. It is anticipated as a complication of known renal parenchymal disease, but it may be found on routine physical examination in an otherwise normal child. Increased understanding of the roles of water and salt retention and overactivity of the renin-angiotensin system has done much to guide therapy; nevertheless, not all forms of hypertension can be explained by these two mechanisms.

The causes of renal hypertension in the newborn period include (1) congenital anomalies of the kidneys or renal vasculature, (2) obstruction of the urinary tract, (3) thrombosis of renal vasculature or kidneys, and (4) volume overload. Some instances of apparent paradoxic elevations of blood pressure have been reported in clinical situations in which chronic diuretic therapy is used, such as in bronchopulmonary dysplasia. Hypertensive infants and older children should be examined for renal, vascular, or aortic abnormalities (eg, thrombosis, neurofibromatosis, coarctation) as well as some endocrine disorders, including pheochromocytoma, glucocorticoid-remedial aldosteronism, primary hyperaldosteronism, pseudoaldosteronism (Liddle syndrome) and pseudohypoaldosteroism (Gordon syndrome).

Clinical Findings

A child is normotensive if the average recorded systolic and diastolic blood pressures are lower than the 90th percentile for age and sex. The 90th percentile in the newborn period is approximately 85–90/55–65 mm Hg for both sexes. In the first year of life, the acceptable levels are 90–100/60–67 mm Hg. Incremental increases with growth occur, gradually approaching young adult ranges of 100–120/65–75 mm Hg in the late teens. Careful measurement of blood pressure requires correct cuff size and reliable equipment. The cuff should be wide enough to cover two-thirds of the upper arm and should encircle the arm completely without an overlap in the inflatable bladder. Although an anxious child may have an elevation in blood pressure, abnormal readings must not be too hastily attributed to this cause. Repeat measurement is helpful, especially after the child has been consoled.

Routine laboratory studies include serum BUN, creatinine and electrolytes, a complete blood count, urinalysis, and urine culture. Abnormal BUN and creatinine would support underlying renal disease as the cause and serum electrolytes demonstrating hypokalemic alkalosis may represent either hyperaldosteronism or pseudoaldosteronism in which case urine sodium and chloride should be measured. Renal ultrasonography with Doppler flow is helpful in determining the possible presence of renal scarring, urinary tract obstruction or renovascular flow disturbances as a cause of hypertension. A renal biopsy (which rarely reveals the cause of hypertension unless clinical evidence of renal disease is present) should be undertaken with special care in the hypertensive patient and preferably after pressures have been controlled by therapy. Figure 24–3 presents a suggested approach to the outpatient workup of hypertension.

Treatment

A. Acute Hypertensive Emergencies

A hypertensive emergency exists when CNS signs of hypertension appear, such as papilledema or encephalopathy. Retinal hemorrhages or exudates also indicate a need for prompt and effective control. In children, end-organ abnormalities secondary to hypertension commonly are not present. Treatment varies with the clinical presentation. The primary classes of useful antihypertensive drugs are (1) diuretics, (2) α- and β-adrenergic blockers, (3) angiotensin-converting enzyme inhibitors, (4) calcium channel blockers, and (5) vasodilators.

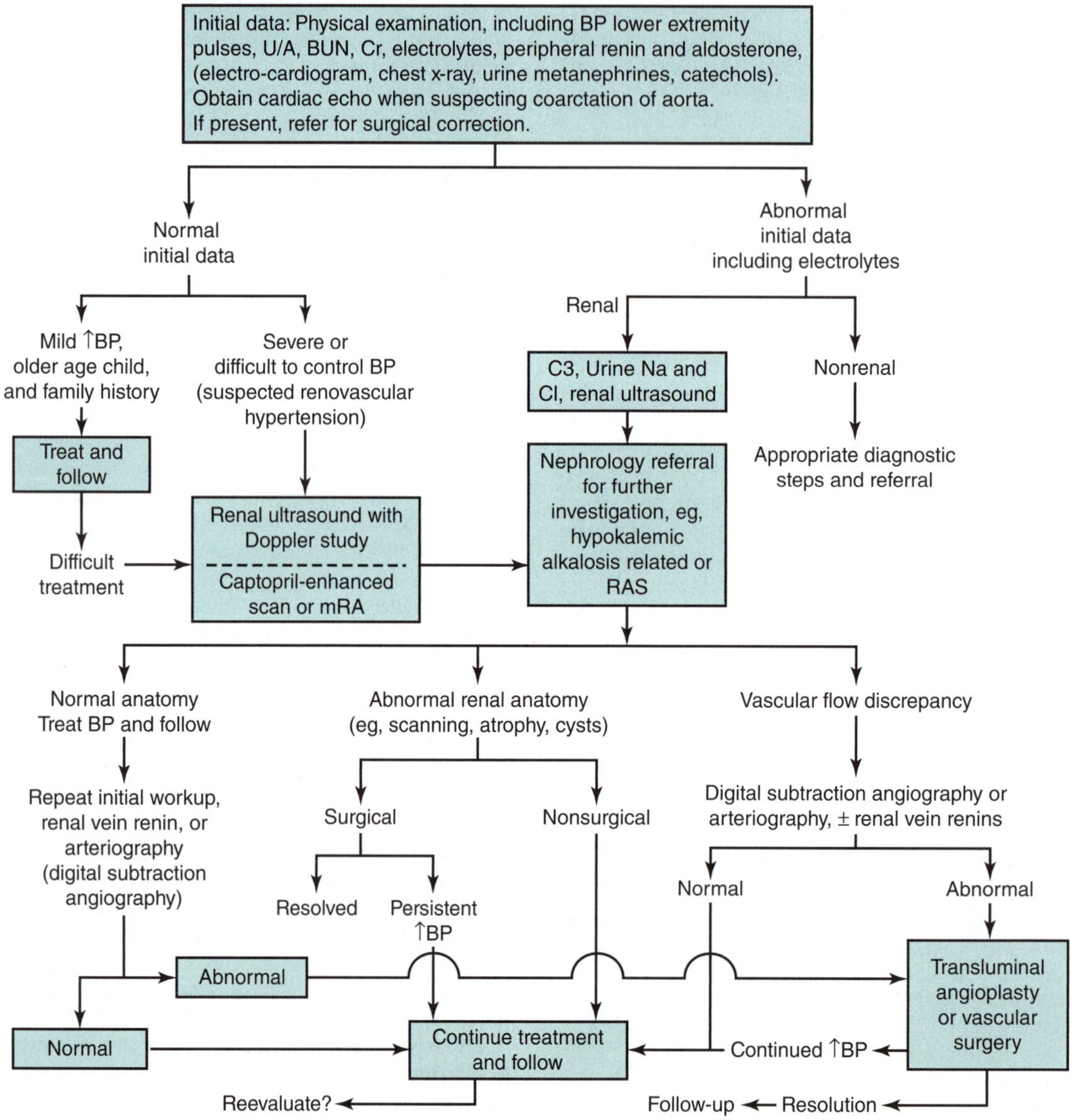

▲ **Figure 24–3.** Approach to the outpatient workup of hypertension. ANA, antinuclear antibody; BP, blood pressure; BUN, blood urea nitrogen; C3, complement; Cr, creatinine; mRA, magnetic resonance angiography; U/A, urinalysis.

Whatever method is used to control emergent hypertension, medications for sustained control should also be initiated so that normal blood pressure will be maintained when the emergent measures are discontinued (Table 24–4). Acute elevations of blood pressure not exceeding the 95th percentile for age may be treated with oral antihypertensives, aiming for progressive improvement and control within 48 hours.

1. Sublingual nifedipine—This calcium channel blocker is rapid acting, and, in appropriate doses, should not result in hypotensive blood pressure levels. The liquid from a 10-mg capsule can be drawn into a syringe and the dosage approximated. The exact dosage for children who weigh less than 10–30 kg is difficult to ascertain by this method, but 5 mg is a safe starting point. Because the treatment is given for rising blood pressure, it is unlikely that the effects will be greater than desired. Larger children with malignant hypertension require 10 mg. In such cases, the capsule may simply be pierced and the medication squeezed under the patient's tongue. In children who are able to swallow capsules, and are large enough for a 10-mg dose, the child may bite the capsule,

Table 24–4. Antihypertensive drugs for emergency treatment.

Drug	Oral Dose	Major Side Effects[a]
Nifedipine	0.25–0.5 mg/kg SL	Flushing, tachycardia
Labetalol	1–3 mg/kg/h IV	Secondary to β-blocking activity
Sodium nitroprusside	0.5–10 mg/kg/min IV drip	Cyanide toxicity, sodium and water retention
Furosemide	1–5 mg/kg IV	Secondary to severe volume contraction, hypokalemia
Esmolol hydrochloride	Load 500 mcg/kg/ over 1 minute followed by continuous 50–200 mcg/kg, titrate	Secondary to β blocking
Hydralazine	0.1–0.2 mg/kg IV	Sodium and water retention, tachycardia, flushing

[a]Many more side effects than those listed have been reported. IV, intravenous; SL, sublingual.

then swallow it for rapid onset of the drug. IV medication to achieve sustained control should be initiated as soon as possible.

2. Sodium nitroprusside—Sodium nitroprusside is considered one of the most rapidly effective IV medications to gain control of malignant hypertension but long-term usage is limited by fear of possible thiocyanate toxicity especially in renal failure. As with other vasodilators, it will result in reflex tachycardia requiring the addition of a β blocker, and fluid retention requiring addition of a diuretic.

3. Furosemide—Administered at 1–5 mg/kg intravenously, this diuretic reduces blood volume and enhances the effectiveness of antihypertensive drugs.

4. Labetalol or Esmolol—IV forms of β blockers can be very effective if there are no cardiac or respiratory contraindications to their use.

5. Intravenous hydralazine—This vasodilator is sometimes effective. Dosage varies according to the severity of the hypertension and should begin at about 0.15 mg/kg. Will cause physiologic responses requiring addition of β blocker and diuretic.

B. Sustained Hypertension

Several choices are available for treatment (Table 24–5). A single drug such as a β-blocker (unless contraindicated, eg, in reactive airway disease) may be adequate to treat mild hypertension. Diuretics are useful to treat renal insufficiency, but the disadvantages of possible electrolyte imbalance must be considered. Single-drug therapy with an angiotensin-converting enzyme inhibitor is useful, especially because most hypertension in children is renal in origin. Calcium channel blockers are increasingly useful, and appear well tolerated in children. The use of the vasodilator type of antihypertensive drug requires concomitant administration of a diuretic to counter the effect of vasodilation on increasing renal sodium and water retention and a β-blocker to counter reflex tachycardia. Minoxidil, considered the most powerful of the orally administered vasodilators, can be extremely efficacious in the treatment of severe, sustained hypertension, but its effect is greatly offset by these other effects. Hirsutism is also a significant side effect. Hydralazine hydrochloride may still be the most common vasodilator in pediatric use—but, again, the necessity of using two additional drugs for maximum benefit relegates use to severe situations calling for management with three or four drugs. The advice of a pediatric nephrologist should be sought.

Table 24–5. Antihypertensive drugs for ambulatory treatment.

Drug	Oral Dose	Major Side Effects[a]
Hydrochlorothiazide	2–4 mg/kg/24 h as single dose or in 2 divided doses	Potassium depletion, hyperuricemia
Furosemide	1–5 mg/kg per dose, 2–3 doses per day	Potassium and volume depletion
Hydralazine	0.75 mg/kg/24 h in 4–6 divided doses	Lupus erythematosus, tachycardia, headache
Amlodipine	0.2–0.5 mg/kg/d in 2 divided doses	Fatigue, headache, facial flushing
Propranolol	0.2–5 mg/kg per dose, 2–3 doses per day	Syncope, cardiac failure, hypoglycemia
Minoxidil	0.15 mg/kg per dose, 2–3 doses per day	Tachycardia, angina, fluid retention, hirsutism
Captopril	0.3–2 mg/kg per dose, 2–3 doses per day	Rash, hyperkalemia, glomerulopathy
Lisinopril	0.5–1 mg/kg/d in 2 divided doses	Hyperkalemia, cough
Nifedipine	0.5–1 mg/kg/d, 3 doses per day	Flushing, tachycardia

[a]Many more side effects than those listed have been reported.

Flynn JT: Hypertension in the young: Epidemiology, sequelae and therapy. Nephrol Dial Transplant 2009;24:370 [PMID: 18996836].

Hogg RJ et al: A multicenter study of the pharmacokinetics of lisinopril in pediatric patients with hypertension. Pediatr Nephrol 2007;22:695 [PMID: 17216247].

INHERITED OR DEVELOPMENTAL DEFECTS OF THE KIDNEYS

There are many developmental, hereditary, or metabolic defects of the kidneys and collecting system. The clinical consequences include metabolic abnormalities, failure to thrive, nephrolithiasis, renal glomerular or tubular dysfunction, and chronic renal failure. Table 24–6 lists some of the major entities.

DISORDERS OF THE RENAL TUBULES

Three subtypes of renal tubular acidosis (RTA) are recognized: (1) the classic form, called type I or distal RTA; (2) the bicarbonate-wasting form, called type II or proximal RTA; and (3) type IV, or hyperkalemic RTA (rare in children), which is associated with hyporeninemic hypoaldosteronism. Types I and II and their variants are encountered most frequently in children. Type III is a combination of types I and II.

Other primary tubular disorders in childhood, such as glycinuria, hypouricemia, or renal glycosuria, may result from a defect in a single tubular transport pathway (see Table 24–6).

1. Distal Renal Tubular Acidosis (Type I)

The most common form of distal RTA in childhood is the hereditary form. The clinical presentation is one of failure to thrive, anorexia, vomiting, and dehydration. Hyperchloremic metabolic acidosis, hypokalemia, and a urinary pH exceeding 6.5 are found. Acidosis is more severe in the presence of a bicarbonate "leak." This variant of distal RTA with bicarbonate wasting has been called type III but for clinical purposes need not be considered as a distinct entity. Concomitant hypercalciuria may lead to rickets, nephrocalcinosis, nephrolithiasis, and renal failure.

Other situations that may be responsible for distal RTA are found in some of the entities listed in Table 24–6.

Table 24–6. Inherited or developmental defects of the urinary tract.

Cystic diseases of genetic origin
- Polycystic disease
  - Autosomal recessive form (infantile)
  - Autosomal dominant form (adult)
  - Other syndromes that include either form
- Cortical cysts
  - Several syndromes are known to have various renal cystic manifestations, including "simple" cysts; may not have significant effect on renal functional status or be associated with progressive disease
- Medullary cysts
  - Medullary sponge kidney
  - Medullary cystic disease (nephronophthisis)
- Hereditary and familial cystic dysplasia
  - Congenital nephrosis
  - "Finnish" disease

Dysplastic renal diseases
- Renal aplasia (unilateral, bilateral)
- Renal hypoplasia (unilateral, bilateral, total, segmental)
- Multicystic renal dysplasia (unilateral, bilateral, multilocular, postobstructive)
- Familial and hereditary renal dysplasias
- Oligomeganephronia

Hereditary diseases associated with nephritis
- Hereditary nephritis with deafness and ocular defects (Alport syndrome)
- Nail-patella syndrome
- Familial hyperprolinemia
- Hereditary nephrotic syndrome
- Hereditary osteolysis with nephropathy
- Hereditary nephritis with thoracic asphyxiant dystrophy syndrome

Hereditary diseases associated with intrarenal deposition of metabolites
- Angiokeratoma corporis diffusum (Fabry disease)
- Heredopathia atactica polyneuritiformis (Refsum disease)
- Various storage diseases (eg, G_{M1} monosialogangliosidosis, Hurler syndrome, Niemann-Pick disease, familial metachromatic leukodystrophy, glycogenosis type I [von Gierke disease], glycogenosis type II [Pompe disease])
- Hereditary amyloidosis (familial Mediterranean fever, heredofamilial urticaria with deafness and neuropathy, primary familial amyloidosis with polyneuropathy)

Hereditary renal diseases associated with tubular transport defects
- Hartnup disease
- Fanconi anemia
- Oculocerebrorenal syndrome of Lowe
- Cystinosis (infantile, adolescent, adult types)
- Wilson disease
- Galactosemia
- Hereditary fructose intolerance
- Renal tubular acidosis (many types)
- Hereditary tyrosinemia
- Renal glycosuria
- Vitamin D–resistant rickets
- Pseudohypoparathyroidism
- Vasopressin-resistant diabetes insipidus
- Hypouricemia

Hereditary diseases associated with lithiasis
- Hyperoxaluria
- L-Glyceric aciduria
- Xanthinuria
- Lesch-Nyhan syndrome and variants, gout
- Nephropathy due to familial hyperparathyroidism
- Cystinuria (types I, II, III)
- Glycinuria

Miscellaneous
- Hereditary intestinal vitamin B_{12} malabsorption
- Total and partial lipodystrophy
- Sickle cell anemia
- Bartter syndrome

Distal RTA results from a defect in the distal nephron, in the tubular transport of hydrogen ion, or in the maintenance of a steep enough gradient for proper excretion of hydrogen ion. This defect can be accompanied by degrees of bicarbonate wasting.

The classic test for distal RTA is an acid load from NH_4Cl. The test is cumbersome and can produce severe acidosis. A clinical trial of alkali administration should be used to rule out proximal (type II) RTA. The dose of alkali required to achieve a normal plasma bicarbonate concentration in patients with distal RTA is low (seldom exceeding 2–3 mEq/kg/24 h)—in contrast to that required in proximal RTA (> 10 mEq/kg/24 h). Higher doses are needed, however, if distal RTA is accompanied by bicarbonate wasting. Correction of acidosis can result in reduced complications and improved growth.

Distal RTA is usually permanent, although it sometimes occurs as a secondary complication. If the defect is not caused by a significant tubular disorder and renal damage is prevented, the prognosis with treatment is good.

2. Proximal Renal Tubular Acidosis (Type II)

Proximal RTA, the most common form of RTA in childhood, is characterized by an alkaline urine pH, loss of bicarbonate in the urine, and mildly reduced serum bicarbonate concentration. This occurs as a result of a lower than normal bicarbonate threshold, above which bicarbonate appears in the urine. Thus, urinary acidification can occur when the concentration of serum bicarbonate drops below that threshold, and bicarbonate disappears from the urine; this ability to eventually acidify the urine thus reflects normal distal tubular function.

Proximal RTA is often an isolated defect, and in the newborn can be considered an aspect of renal immaturity. Onset in infants is accompanied by failure to thrive, hyperchloremic acidosis, hypokalemia, and, rarely, nephrocalcinosis. Secondary forms result from reflux or obstructive uropathy or occur in association with other tubular disorders (see Table 24–6). Proximal RTA requires more than 3 mEq/kg of alkali per day to correct the acidosis. Serum bicarbonate should be monitored weekly until a level of at least 20 mEq/L is attained.

Citrate solutions (eg, Bicitra, Polycitra) are somewhat more easily tolerated than sodium bicarbonate. Bicitra contains 1 mEq/mL of Na^+ and citrate. Polycitra contains 2 mEq/mL of citrate and 1 mEq each of Na^+ and K^+. The required daily dosage is divided into three doses. Potassium supplementation may be required, because the added sodium load presented to the distal tubule may exaggerate potassium losses.

The prognosis is excellent in cases of isolated defects, especially when the problem is related to renal immaturity. Alkali therapy can usually be discontinued after several months to 2 years. Growth should be normal, and the gradual increase in the serum bicarbonate level to greater than 22 mEq/L heralds the presence of a raised bicarbonate threshold in the tubules. If the defect is part of a more complex tubular abnormality (Fanconi syndrome with attendant phosphaturia, glycosuria, and amino aciduria), the prognosis depends on the underlying disorder or syndrome.

OCULOCEREBRORENAL SYNDROME (LOWE SYNDROME)

Lowe syndrome results from various mutations in the *ORCL1* gene, which codes for a Golgi apparatus phosphatase. Affected males have anomalies involving the eyes, brain, and kidneys. The physical stigmata and degree of mental retardation vary with the location of the mutation. In addition to congenital cataracts and buphthalmos, the typical facies includes prominent epicanthal folds, frontal prominence, and a tendency to scaphocephaly. Muscle hypotonia is a prominent finding. The renal abnormalities are of tubule function and include hypophosphatemic rickets with low serum phosphorus levels, low to normal serum calcium levels, elevated serum alkaline phosphatase levels, RTA, and aminoaciduria. Treatment includes alkali therapy, phosphate replacement, and vitamin D. Antenatal diagnosis is possible.

HYPOKALEMIC ALKALOSIS (BARTTER SYNDROME, GITELMAN SYNDROME, & LIDDLE SYNDROME)

Bartter syndrome is characterized by severe hypokalemic, hypochloremic metabolic alkalosis, extremely high levels of circulating renin and aldosterone, and a paradoxic absence of hypertension. On renal biopsy, a striking juxtaglomerular hyperplasia is seen.

A neonatal form of Bartter syndrome is thought to result from mutations in two genes affecting either Na^+–K^+ or K^+ transport. These patients have life-threatening episodes of fever and dehydration with hypercalciuria and early-onset nephrocalcinosis. Classic Bartter syndrome presenting in infancy with polyuria and growth retardation (but not nephrocalcinosis) is thought to result from mutations in a chloride channel gene. Gitelman syndrome occurs in older children and features episodes of muscle weakness, tetany, hypokalemia, and hypomagnesemia. These children have hypocalciuria. In Liddle syndrome, the presenting significant clinical abnormality may at first be hypertension, although hypokalemia may also be evident. Serum rennin and aldosterone are low and serum sodium is elevated.

Treatment with prostaglandin inhibitors and potassium-conserving diuretics (eg, amiloride combined with magnesium supplements) and potassium and magnesium where indicated is beneficial in Bartter syndrome and Gitelman syndrome. Although the prognosis is guarded, a few patients seem to have less severe forms of the disease that are compatible with long survival times. Treatment in Liddle syndrome is with a low sodium diet and potassium sparing diuretics, excluding spironolactone, since it acts by regulation of aldosterone.

CYSTINOSIS

There are three types of cystinosis: adult, adolescent, and infantile. The adolescent type is characterized by cystine deposition, which, if not treated with phosphocysteamine (Cystagon) which aids in the metabolic conversion of cystine (unable to exit cells) to cysteine (able to exit cells), is accompanied by the development of the renal Fanconi syndrome (renal tubular dysfunction) and varying degrees of renal failure. Growth is usually normal. The infantile type is the most common and the most severe. Characteristically, children present in the first or second year of life with Fanconi syndrome and, without the metabolic benefit of Cystagon treatment, progress to end-stage renal failure.

Cystinosis results from mutations in the *CTNS* gene, which codes for a cystine transporter. About 50% of patients share an identical deletion. Inheritance is autosomal recessive. Cystine is stored in cellular lysosomes in virtually all tissues. Eventually, cystine accumulation results in cell damage and cell death, particularly in the renal tubules. Renal failure between ages 6 and 12 years is common in the infantile form.

Whenever the diagnosis of cystinosis is suspected, slit-lamp examination of the corneas should be performed. Cystine crystal deposition causes an almost pathognomonic ground-glass "dazzle" appearance. Increased white cell cystine levels are diagnostic. Hypothyroidism is common.

Cystagon therapy is helpful in the treatment of cystinosis and can retard progression of renal failure and the accumulation of cystine in other organs. Depending on the progression of chronic renal failure, management is directed toward all side effects of renal failure, with particular attention paid to the control of renal osteodystrophy. Dialysis and transplantation may be needed.

Nesterova G, Gahl W: Nephropathic cystinosis: Late complications of a multisystem disease. Pediatr Nephrol 2008;32:863–878 [PMID: 18008091].

NEPHROGENIC DIABETES INSIPIDUS

The congenital X-linked recessive form of nephrogenic (no response to vasopressin) diabetes insipidus results from mutations in the vasopressin receptor, *AVPR2*. Autosomal (recessive and dominant) forms of nephrogenic diabetes insipidus are caused by mutations of the *AQP2* gene that codes for a water channel protein, aquaporin-2. Genetic counseling and mutation testing are available.

Urine concentrating ability is impaired in a number of other conditions—sickle cell anemia, pyelonephritis, potassium depletion, hypercalcemia, cystinosis and other renal tubular disorders, and obstructive uropathy—and as a result of nephrotoxic drugs. Children receiving lithium treatment should be monitored for the development of nephrogenic diabetes insipidus.

The symptoms of nephrogenic diabetes insipidus are polyuria, polydipsia, and failure to thrive. In some children, particularly if the solute intake is unrestricted, adjustment to an elevated serum osmolality may develop. These children are particularly susceptible to episodes of dehydration, fever, vomiting, and convulsions.

The diagnosis can be suspected on the basis of a history of polydipsia and polyuria insensitive to the administration of vasopressin, desmopressin acetate, or lypressin. The diagnosis is confirmed by performing a vasopressin test. Carefully monitored water restriction does not increase the tubular reabsorption of water (TcH_2O) to above 3 mL/min/m^2. Urine osmolality remains lower than 450 mOsm/kg, whereas serum osmolality rises and total body weight falls. Before weight reduction of more than 5% occurs or before serum osmolality exceeds 320 mOsm/kg, vasopressin should be administered.

In infants, it is usually best to allow water as demanded and to restrict salt. Serum sodium levels should be evaluated at intervals to avoid hyperosmolality from inadvertent water restriction. In later childhood, sodium intake should continue to be restricted to 2.0–2.5 mEq/kg/24 h.

Treatment with hydrochlorothiazide is helpful, and many patients show improvement with administration of prostaglandin inhibitors such as indomethacin or tolmetin.

Linshaw MA: Back to basics: Congenital nephrogenic diabetes insipidus. Pediatr Rev 2007;28:372–380 [PMID: 17908859].

NEPHROLITHIASIS

Renal calculi in children may result from inborn errors of metabolism, such as cystine in cystinuria, glycine in hyperglycinuria, urates in Lesch-Nyhan syndrome, and oxalates in oxalosis. Stones may occur secondary to hypercalciuria in distal tubular acidosis, and large stones are quite often seen in children with spina bifida who have paralyzed lower limbs or any situation where immobilization promotes calcium mobilization from bones. Treatment is limited to that of the primary condition, if possible. Surgical removal of stones or lithotrypsy should be considered only for obstruction, intractable severe pain, and chronic infection.

Tanaka ST, Pope JC 4th: Pediatric stone disease. Curr Urol Rev 2009;10:138–143 [PMID: 19239819].

1. Cystinuria

Cystinuria, like Hartnup disease and several other disorders, is primarily an abnormality of amino acid transport across both the enteric and proximal renal tubular epithelium. There are at least three biochemical types. In the first type, the bowel transport of basic amino acids and cystine is impaired, but transport of cysteine is not impaired. In the renal tubule, basic amino acids are again rejected by the tubule, but cystine absorption appears to be normal. The reason for cystinuria remains obscure. Heterozygous individuals have no aminoaciduria. The second type is similar to the first except that heterozygous individuals excrete excess cystine and lysine in the urine, and cystine transport in the bowel is normal. In the third type, only the nephron is involved. The only clinical manifestations are related to stone formation: ureteral colic, dysuria, hematuria, proteinuria, and secondary UTI. Urinary excretion of cystine, lysine, arginine, and ornithine is increased.

The most reliable way to prevent stone formation is to maintain a constantly high free-water clearance. This involves generous fluid intake. Alkalinization of the urine is helpful. If these measures do not prevent significant renal lithiasis, the use of tiopronin (Thiola) is recommended.

Ahmed K et al: Management of cystinuric patients: An observational, retrospective, single-centre analysis. Urol Int 2008;80P: 141–144 [PMID: 18362482].

2. Primary Hyperoxaluria

Oxalate in humans is derived from the oxidative deamination of glycine to glyoxylate, from the serine-glycolate pathway, and from ascorbic acid. At least two enzymatic blocks have been described. Type I is a deficiency of liver-specific peroxisomal alanine–glyoxylate aminotransferase. Type II is glyoxylate reductase deficiency.

Excess oxalate combines with calcium to form insoluble deposits in the kidneys, lungs, and other tissues, beginning during childhood. The joints are occasionally involved, but the main effect is on the kidneys, where progressive oxalate deposition leads to fibrosis and eventual renal failure.

Pyridoxine supplementation and a low-oxalate diet have been tried as therapy, but the overall prognosis is poor, and most patients succumb to uremia by early adulthood. Renal transplantation is not very successful because of destruction of the transplant kidney. However, encouraging results have been obtained with concomitant liver transplantation, correcting the metabolic defect.

Hyperoxaluria may also be a consequence of severe ileal disease or ileal resection.

URINARY TRACT INFECTIONS

It is estimated that 8% of girls and 2% of boys will acquire UTIs in childhood. Girls older than age 6 months have UTIs far more commonly than boys, whereas uncircumcised boys younger than 3 months of age have more UTIs than girls. Circumcision reduces the risk of UTI in boys. The density of distal urethral and periurethral bacterial colonization with uropathogenic bacteria correlates with the risk of UTI in children. Most UTIs are ascending infections. Specific adhesins present on the fimbria of uropathogenic bacteria allow colonization of the uroepithelium in the urethra and bladder and increase the likelihood of UTI. The organisms most commonly responsible for UTI are fecal flora, most commonly *E coli* (> 85%), *Klebsiella*, *Proteus*, other gram-negative bacteria, and, less frequently, *Enterococcus* or coagulase-negative staphylococci.

Pathogenesis

Dysfunctional voiding, which is uncoordinated relaxation of the urethral sphincter during voiding, leads to incomplete emptying of the bladder, increasing the risk of bacterial colonization. Similarly, any condition that interferes with complete emptying of the bladder, such as constipation or neurogenic bladder, increases the risk of UTI. Poor perineal hygiene, structural abnormalities of the urinary tract, catheterization, instrumentation of the urinary tract, and sexual activity increase the risk as well.

The inflammatory response to pyelonephritis may produce renal parenchymal scars. Such scars in infancy and childhood may contribute to hypertension, renal disease, and renal failure later in life.

Clinical Findings

A. Symptoms and Signs

Newborns and infants with UTI have nonspecific signs, including fever, hypothermia, jaundice, poor feeding, irritability, vomiting, failure to thrive, and sepsis. Strong, foul-smelling or cloudy urine may be noted. Preschool children may have abdominal or flank pain, vomiting, fever, urinary frequency, dysuria, urgency, or enuresis. School-aged children commonly have classic signs of cystitis (frequency, dysuria, and urgency) or pyelonephritis (fever, vomiting, and flank pain). Costovertebral tenderness is unusual in young children, but may be demonstrated by school-aged children. Physical examination should include attention to blood pressure determination, abdominal examination, and a genitourinary examination. Urethritis, poor perineal hygiene, herpes simplex virus, or other genitourinary infections may be apparent on examination.

B. Laboratory Findings

Screening urinalysis indicates pyuria (> 5 WBCs/high-power field) in most children with UTI, but many children with pyuria do not have UTI. White cells from the urethra or vagina may be present in urine or may be in the urine because of a systemic infection. The leukocyte esterase test correlates well with pyuria, but has a similar false-positive rate. The detection of urinary nitrite by dipstick is highly correlated with enteric organisms being cultured from urine. Most young children (70%) with UTI have negative nitrite tests. They empty their bladders frequently, and it requires several hours for bacteria to convert ingested nitrates to nitrite in the bladder. The sensitivity of nitrite detection is highest on a first morning void. Gram stain of unspun urine correlates well with culture recovery of 10^5 colony-forming units (cfu)/mL or more, but this test is frequently unavailable outside the hospital.

The gold standard for diagnosis remains the culture of a properly collected urine specimen. Collection of urine for urinalysis and culture is difficult in children due to frequent contamination of the sample. In toilet-trained, cooperative, older children, a midstream, clean-catch method is satisfactory. Although cleaning of the perineum does not improve specimen quality, straddling of the toilet to separate the labia in girls, retraction of the foreskin in boys, and collecting midstream urine significantly reduce contamination. In infants and young children, bladder catheterization or suprapubic collection is necessary in most cases to avoid contaminated samples. Bagged urine specimens are helpful only if negative. Specimens that are not immediately cultured should be refrigerated and kept cold during transport. Any growth is considered significant from a suprapubic culture. Quantitative recovery of 10^5 cfu/mL or more is considered significant on clean-catch specimens, and 10^4–10^5 is considered significant on catheterized specimens. Usually the recovery of multiple organisms indicates contamination, but some contaminated specimens yield only a single species.

Asymptomatic bacteriuria is detected in 0.5%–1.0% of children who are screened with urine culture. Asymptomatic bacteriuria is believed to represent colonization of the urinary tract with nonuropathogenic bacteria. Treatment may increase the risk of symptomatic UTI by eliminating nonpathogenic colonization. Screening urine cultures in nonsymptomatic children are, therefore, generally discouraged. Repeated urine cultures are often helpful in differentiating asymptomatic bacteriuria from contamination of the culture versus true UTI.

Urinary function during UTI should be assessed by measurement of BUN and serum creatinine concentration.

C. Imaging

Because congenital urologic abnormalities increase the risk of UTI, radiologic evaluation of first UTI has been routinely recommended. These recommendations usually include routine ultrasound of the kidneys and voiding cystourethrogram (VCUG). VUR is a congenital abnormality present in about 1% of the population beyond infancy that is detected by VCUG. VUR is graded using the international scale (I—reflux into ureter; II—reflux to the kidneys; III—reflux to kidneys with dilation of ureter only; IV—reflux with dilation of ureter and mild blunting of renal calyces; V—reflux with dilation of ureter and blunting of renal calyces). Reflux is detected in 30%–50% of children 1 year of age and younger. The natural history of reflux is to improve, and 80% of reflux of grades I, II, or III will resolve or significantly improve within 3 years following detection.

VCUG should be done selectively on children with a first UTI. Children with a suspected urologic abnormality due to weak stream, dribbling, or perineal abnormalities should be studied with VCUG. Boys with a first UTI should be studied to detect posterior urethral valves, an important congenital abnormality that requires surgery. Children older than 3 years of age who are otherwise healthy and growing well usually can be followed clinically and do not need VCUG for a first UTI. The yield in sexually active teenagers is also very low.

Ultrasonographic examination of kidneys should be done acutely in children with pyelonephritis who have not improved after 3–5 days of antimicrobial treatment adjusted for the susceptibility of the organism. The examination is done to detect renal or perirenal abscesses or obstruction of the kidneys.

Treatment

A. Antibiotic Therapy

Management of UTI is influenced by clinical assessment. Very young children (younger than 3 months) and children with dehydration, toxicity, or sepsis should be admitted to the hospital and treated with parenteral antimicrobials. Older infants and children who are not seriously ill can be treated as outpatients. Initial antimicrobial therapy is based on prior history of infection and antimicrobial use, as well as location of the infection in the urinary tract.

Uncomplicated cystitis can be treated with amoxicillin, trimethoprim–sulfamethoxazole, or a first-generation cephalosporin. These antimicrobials are concentrated in the lower urinary tract, and high cure rates are common. There are significant differences in the rates of antimicrobial resistance, so knowledge of the rates in the local community is important. More seriously ill children are initially treated parenterally with a third-generation cephalosporin or aminoglycoside. The initial antimicrobial choice is adjusted after culture and susceptibility are known. The recommended duration of antimicrobial therapy for uncomplicated cystitis is 7–10 days. For sexually mature teenagers with cystitis, fluoroquinolones such as ciprofloxacin and levofloxacin for 3 days are effective and cost-effective. Short-course therapy of cystitis is not recommended in children, because differentiating upper and lower tract disease may be difficult, and higher failure rates are reported in most studies of short-course therapy.

Acute pyelonephritis is usually treated for 10 days. In nontoxic children > 3 months of age who are not vomiting, oral treatment with an agent such as cefixime can be used. In sicker children, parenteral therapy may be required initially. Most of these children can complete therapy orally once symptomatic improvement has occurred. A repeat urine culture 24–48 hours after beginning therapy is not needed if the child is improving and doing well.

B. Follow-Up

Children with UTI should be followed with screening urinalysis 1 and 2 months after resolution of UTI. Dipstick nitrite determination can be used at home by parents on first morning voided urine in children with frequently recurring UTI.

C. Prophylactic Antimicrobials

Selected children with frequently recurring UTI may benefit from prophylactic antimicrobials. In children with high-grade

VUR, prophylactic antimicrobials may be beneficial in reducing UTI, as an alternative to surgical correction, or in the interval prior to surgical therapy. Many experts recommend surgical correction of higher-grade reflux, particularly grade V. Trimethoprim–sulfamethoxazole and nitrofurantoin are approved for prophylaxis. The use of broader-spectrum antimicrobials leads to colonization and infection with resistant strains.

Children with dysfunctional voiding generally do not benefit from prophylactic antimicrobials; rather, addressing the underlying dysfunctional voiding is most important.

DeMuri GP, Wald ER: Imaging and antimicrobial prophylaxis following the diagnosis of urinary tract infection in children. Pediatr Infect Dis J 2008;27:553–554 [PMID: 18520594].

Williams G, Craig JC: Prevention of recurrent urinary tract infection in children. Curr Opin Infect Dis 2009;22:72–76 [PMID: 19532083].

REFERENCE

Geary DF, Schaefer F: *Comprehensive Pediatric Nephrology*, 1st ed. Mosby, Inc, 2008.

25 Neurologic & Muscular Disorders

Timothy J. Bernard, MD
Kelly Knupp, MD
Michele L. Yang, MD
Sita Kedia, MD
Paul M. Levisohn, MD
Paul G. Moe, MD

NEUROLOGIC ASSESSMENT & NEURODIAGNOSTIC PROCEDURES

HISTORY & EXAMINATION

History

Even in an era of increasingly sophisticated neurodiagnostic testing, the assessment of the child with a possible neurologic disorder begins with history, general physical exam as well as detailed neurologic examination. The standard pediatric history and physical examination are presented in Chapter 9. A careful history will allow the clinician to establish the nature and course of the illness. The progression of the illness, that is, acute, chronic, progressive or static, episodic or continuous, will help to determine the approach to the evaluation. Insidious developmental delay or weakness might demand more detailed exploration of pregnancy, family, and social history as well as developmental landmarks. In situations that the developmental history may be vague, other resources such as extended family members and baby books may provide clarification of prior development. Episodic events such as headaches or seizures warrant more emphasis on precise details preceding and during these events. Often times spells can now be videotaped and this can provide important details that will assist in diagnosis.

Neurologic Examination

A general physical examination is an essential aspect of the assessment. Growth parameters and head circumference should be charted (see Chapter 3). A developmental assessment using an appropriate screening tool is part of every neurologic evaluation of the infant and young child and can be used to document a child's developmental status. Chapter 3 delineates age-appropriate developmental landmarks (see Tables 3–1 and 3–2). Multiple instruments are available for screening infants and children. Among these are the Denver Developmental Screening Test II (see Figure 3–12), which is particularly helpful in infants and is often used to document development as opposed to screening. The Ages & Stages Questionnaires®, Third Edition (ASQ-3) is a parent-completed screening tool, which is widely used when assessing infants and young children. The Modified Checklist for Autism in Toddlers (M-CHAT™) is a screening tool for assessing toddlers between 16 and 30 months of age for risk of autism spectrum disorders. The specifics of the neurologic examination are determined by the age of the child and the ability to cooperate in the examination. Expected newborn-infant reflexes and automations and other examination suggestions pertinent to that age group are included in Chapter 2. The hallmark of neurologic diagnosis is *location,* that is, where in the nervous system is the "lesion?" While not all childhood neurologic disorders are easily localized, the part of the nervous system involved, for example, central versus neuromuscular, can often be defined and will act as a guide for evaluation and diagnosis.

Table 25–1 outlines components of the neurologic examination. Much of the examination of the frightened infant or toddler is by necessity observational. An organized approach to the examination is thus imperative. Playing games will engage a toddler or preschooler: throwing and catching a ball, stacking blocks, hopping, jogging, counting, and drawing (circles, lines) can reduce anxiety and allow assessment of fine and gross motor coordination, balance, and handedness. In the older child, "casual" conversation can reveal both language and cognitive competence as will drawing, writing, calculating, and spelling.

DIAGNOSTIC TESTING

Electroencephalography

Electroencephalography (EEG) is a noninvasive method for recording cerebral activity. The background patterns of the EEG vary by both age and clinical state of the subject, for example, infant, toddler, adolescent; awake, drowsy, or asleep. Intermittent activity often reflects disordered central nervous system (CNS) function. The EEG has its greatest clinical applicability in the study of seizure disorders. An EEG may demonstrate "epileptiform activity," that is, patterns that indicate risk for seizures and epilepsy, though may not necessarily be diagnostic of such. At times, however, the findings on an EEG are diagnostic, as in the hypsarrhythmic pattern of infantile spasms (West syndrome) or generalized three-cycle-per-second spike-wave pattern of absence epilepsy. Availability of time-locked video recording with EEG has increased the utility of the test in assessing episodic disorders and has become almost routine in many EEG laboratories. In addition, EEG is used in the evaluation of altered mental status and of relatively static disorders, such as neurodegenerative diseases, tumors, cerebrovascular accidents, and other neurologic disorders causing brain dysfunction. EEG can now be performed for either short or long periods of time and in some institutions may also be available for longer durations as an outpatient study as an ambulatory EEG. The limitations and benefits of each type of study need to be understood to be used properly.

Routine EEG is the standard short duration, outpatient EEG. The limitations of routine EEG are not inconsiderable. In most cases, the duration of the actual tracing is less than 30 minutes. Therefore, events of interest are usually not recorded. Due to the short duration of recording, electrodes are placed using a temporary adhesive; therefore, if the child is unable to cooperate, the tracing may be uninterpretable. Medications used for sedation for an uncooperative child, especially barbiturates and benzodiazepines, may produce artifact in the tracing which can confuse interpretation and in addition may decrease the likelihood of recording abnormalities of interest such as epileptiform discharges. The EEG itself, in isolation, is rarely diagnostic but is one part of the child's clinical picture. Individuals without a history of epilepsy, especially children, may have an abnormal EEG. EEG findings such as those occasionally seen in migraine, learning

Table 25–1. Neurologic examination: toddler age and up.

Category	Operation	Assesses
Mental status	Level of consciousness; orientation, language, cortical function developmental screen (age specific questions); activity level; affect.	Both cortical and subcortical pathways
Cranial nerves	CN I: omit most of the time (smell). CN II: pupils (light reflex), vision (acuity), fields, fundi. CN III, IV, VI: extraocular movements, pupils, convergence, (strabismus?). CN V: facial sensation (upper, middle, lower; V_1, V_2, V_3); motor—move jaw laterally, open, close against resistance. CN VII: upper—eye closure, brow; lower—grimace, show teeth. CN VIII: whispered voice from 10–20 ft each ear. Tuning fork tests. CN IX, X: sensation? Movement of palate to "ahh" or tongue blade ("gagging"—often omit). CN XI: turning head right, left; flexing against resistance. CN XII: protrude tongue, push it out cheek. Push left, right against resistance (examiner's thumb).	
Motor	Tone: trunk (infant)—hold prone, supine; manipulate relaxed limbs; hold under arms. Strength: proximal/distal—shoulder abduction/grasp; get up from floor (hips); dorsiflexion of foot. 0 = no movement; 1 = trace; 3 = against gravity; 5 = normal (0–5 grading strength)	Brain: "suprasegmental" influence Cord: lower motor neuron-"segmental" component
Reflexes	Tendon reflexes: biceps, triceps, brachioradialis, knee, ankle. Cutaneous: abdominal (cremasteric).	Pyramidal tract Spinal cord: sensory/motor nerve arc
Station	Standing, eyes open, closed, hands out (Romberg test): truncal balance.	Cerebellum (vermis) Posterior columns
Gait	Walking (running in hall); heel-toe (tandem gait) forward, backward. Balance on each foot.	Cerebellum (vermis)
Coordination (truncal, limb)	Balance on each foot; hopping; finger-nose-finger pursuit. Stack blocks. Reach for a rattle. Rapid alternating movements.	Cerebellum: lateral lobes
Sensory	Light touch, sharp (pain), vibration (tuning fork-toe, finger, on bone), position (same). Cortical: 2 point, finger writing, object identification, position limb in space, barognosis (weight).	Peripheral nerve Posterior column Anterior/lateral column Parietal lobe

disabilities, or behavior disorders are often nonspecific and do not reflect structural brain damage. When questions arise regarding the clinical significance of EEG findings, referral to a pediatric EEG laboratory may be appropriate.

Outpatient ambulatory EEG recordings have become increasingly useful with the advent of digital technology, which allows the child to be recorded using a small instrument while at home or at school. Due to more prolonged recording, ambulatory EEG can be useful in assessing events of interest to ascertain if they are due to epileptic seizures. Likewise, recording the EEG during nocturnal polysomnographic studies can help differentiate between nonepileptic sleep-related events from nocturnal epileptic seizures arising from sleep.

Prolonged bedside EEG recordings are useful in the assessment of patients with altered mental status, suspected nonconvulsive status epilepticus, and drug-induced coma (for the treatment of increased intracranial pressure or status epilepticus), as well as infants with hypoxic ischemic encephalopathy. The EEG is now less commonly used for determining so-called brain death (electrocerebral inactivity).

Continuous video-EEG monitoring has allowed neurologists specializing in the care of the child with epilepsy to assess the patient with medically intractable epilepsy for surgical treatment. Correlating video with EEG has also proven useful in characterizing spells that may or may not be seizures. When children are admitted to the hospital, medications are often reduced or discontinued, increasing the likelihood of recording an event. The children are admitted to a specialized unit (epilepsy monitoring unit [EMU]) for up to a week or more. This may also be an option for children who are not able to tolerate brief recordings as the electrode application is placed with more permanent adhesive and once electrodes are placed removal is difficult allowing for less artifact while a child is moving. Computed tomography (CT) scans, evoked potentials, positron emission tomography (PET), regional cerebral blood flow studies, single-photon emission computed tomography (SPECT), and magnetic resonance imaging (MRI) supplement the EEG and neurologic exam as a diagnostic and prognostic tool.

Evoked Potentials

Cortical visual, auditory, or somatosensory evoked potentials (evoked responses) may be recorded from the scalp surface over the temporal, occipital, or frontoparietal cortex after repetitive stimulation of the retina by light flashes, the cochlea by sounds, or a nerve by galvanic stimuli of varying frequency and intensity, respectively. Computer averaging is used to recognize and enhance these responses while subtracting or suppressing the asynchronous background EEG activity. The presence or absence of evoked potential waves and their latencies (time from stimulus to wave peak or time between peaks) figures in the clinical interpretation. These studies are no longer routinely obtained in assessing the child with neurologic disorders, but at times can be helpful. Much of this testing requires cooperation, or in the young child, sedation.

Auditory evoked responses are now the standard for screening hearing in the neonate. An uncooperative patient can be assessed objectively, making the technique particularly useful in high-risk infants and in mentally retarded or autistic patients. Intraoperative somatosensory evoked potentials are used on a more routine basis during spine surgery to assist the surgeon during placement of instrumentation for early identification of potentially reversible spinal cord injury. Similar techniques are used in other surgeries that are at risk of nerve injury such as craniofacial surgeries.

Lumbar Puncture

Assessing cerebral spinal fluid is a necessity in some clinical situations. Spinal fluid is usually obtained by inserting a small-gauge needle (eg, No. 22) through the L3–L4 intervertebral space into the thecal sac while the patient is lying in a lateral recumbent position. After an opening pressure is measured, fluid is removed to examine for evidence of infection, inflammation, or evidence of metabolic disorders (Table 25–2). Fluid is often sent for red and white cell counts, for determination of the concentrations of protein and glucose, for viral polymerase chain reaction (PCR), and for viral and bacterial cultures. In some cases, additional information is obtained with special staining techniques for mycobacteria and fungus. Additional fluid may be sent for testing for specific viral agents, antibody titer determinations, cytopathologic study, lactate and pyruvate concentrations, and amino acid and neurotransmitter analysis. Lumbar puncture is imperative when bacterial meningitis is suspected. Caution must be exercised, however, when signs of increased intracranial pressure (eg, papilledema) or focal neurologic signs are present that might indicate a substantial risk of precipitating tentorial or tonsillar herniation.

PEDIATRIC NEURORADIOLOGIC PROCEDURES

Computed Tomography

CT scanning is a noninvasive technique which allows visualization of intracranial contents using x-ray to compute images. It consists of a series of cross-sectional (axial) roentgenograms. Radiation exposure is approximately the same as that from a skull radiographic series. CT images record very small variations in tissue density using thin x-ray beams which allow measurement of photon transmission through the head. Serial images are obtained which allow computation of x-ray absorption and computation of images which appear as serial slices. Because x-ray absorption is measured, bone interferes with the ability to view intracranial structures, a significant limitation. New scanning techniques allow rapid acquisition of data, often without sedation. CT scanning is of high sensitivity (88%–96% of lesions larger than 1–2 cm can be seen) but low specificity (tumor, infection, or infarct may look the same). It is particularly useful for assessment of trauma, allowing excellent visualization of

Table 25–2. Characteristics of cerebrospinal fluid in the normal child and in central nervous system infections and inflammatory conditions.

Condition	Initial Pressure (mm H_2O)	Appearance	Cells/μL	Protein (mg/dL)	Glucose (mg/dL)	Other Tests	Comments
Normal	< 160	Clear	0–5 lymphocytes; first 3 mo, 1–3 PMNs; neonates, up to 30 lymphocytes, rare RBCs	15–35 (lumbar), 5–15 (ventricular); up to 150 (lumbar) for short time after birth; to 6 mo up to 65	50–80 (two-thirds of blood glucose); may be increased after seizure	CSF-IgG index[a] < 0.7[a]; LDH 2–27 U/L	CSF protein in first month may be up to 170 mg/dL in small-for-date or premature infants; no increase in WBCs due to seizure
Bloody tap	Normal or low	Bloody (sometimes with clot)	One additional WBC/700 RBCs;[b] RBCs not crenated	One additional milligram per 800 RBCs[b]	Normal	RBC number should fall between first and third tubes; wait 5 min between tubes	Spin down fluid, supernatant will be clear and colorless[c]
Bacterial meningitis, acute	200–750+	Opalescent to purulent	Up to thousands, mostly PMNs; early, few cells	Up to hundreds	Decreased; may be none	Smear and culture mandatory; LDH > 24 U/L; lactate, IL-8, TNF elevated, correlate with prognosis	Very early, glucose may be normal; PCR meningococci and pneumococci in plasma, CSF may aid diagnosis
Bacterial meningitis, partially treated	Usually increased	Clear or opalescent	Usually increased; PMNs usually predominate	Elevated	Normal or decreased	LDH usually > 24 U/L; PCR may still be positive	Smear and culture may be negative if antibiotics have been in use
Tuberculous meningitis	150–750+	Opalescent; fibrin web or pellicle	250–500, mostly lymphocytes; early, more PMNs	45–500; parallels cell count; increases over time	Decreased; may be none	Smear for acid-fast organism: CSF culture and inoculation; PCR	Consider AIDS, a common comorbidity of tuberculosis
Fungal meningitis	Increased	Variable; often clear	10–500; early, more PMNs; then mostly lymphocytes	Elevated and increasing	Decreased	India ink preparations, cryptococcal antigen, PCR, culture, inoculations, immunofluorescence tests	Often superimposed in patients who are debilitated or on immunosuppressive therapy
Aseptic meningoencephalitis (viral meningitis, or parameningeal disease); encephalitis is similar	Normal or slightly increased	Clear unless cell count > 300/μL	None to a few hundred, mostly lymphocytes; PMNs predominate early	20–125	Normal; may be low in mumps, herpes, or other viral infections	CSF, stool, blood, throat washings for viral cultures; LDH < 28 U/L; PCR for HSV, CMV, EBV, enterovirus, etc	Acute and convalescent antibody titers for some viruses; in mumps, up to 1000 lymphocytes; serum amylase often elevated; up to 1000 cells present in enteroviral infection

(Continued)

Table 25–2. Characteristics of cerebrospinal fluid in the normal child and in central nervous system infections and inflammatory conditions. (*Continued*)

Condition	Initial Pressure (mm H_2O)	Appearance	Cells/µL	Protein (mg/dL)	Glucose (mg/dL)	Other Tests	Comments
Parainfectious encephalomyelitis (ADEM)	80–450, usually increased	Usually clear	0–50+, mostly lymphocytes; lower numbers, even 0, in MS	15–75	Normal	CSF-IgG index, oligoclonal bands variable; in MS, moderate increase	No organisms; fulminant cases resemble bacterial meningitis
Polyneuritis	Normal and occasionally increased	Early: normal; late: xanthochromic if protein high	Normal; occasionally slight increase	Early: normal; late: 45–1500	Normal	CSF-IgG index may be increased; oligoclonal bands variable	Try to find cause (viral infections, toxins, lupus, diabetes, etc)
Meningeal carcinomatosis	Often elevated	Clear to opalescent	Cytologic identification of tumor cells	Often mildly to moderately elevated	Often depressed	Cytology	Seen with leukemia, medulloblastoma, meningeal melanosis, histiocytosis X
Brain abscess	Normal or increased	Usually clear	5–500 in 80%; mostly PMNs	Usually slightly increased	Normal; occasionally decreased	Imaging study of brain (MRI)	Cell count related to proximity to meninges; findings as in purulent meningitis if abscess ruptures

[a]CSF-IgG index = (CSF IgG/serum IgG)/(CSF albumin/serum albumin).
[b]Many studies document pitfalls in using these ratios due to WBC lysis. Clinical judgment and repeat lumbar punctures may be necessary to rule out meningitis in this situation.
[c]CSF WBC (predicted) = CSF RBC × (blood WBC/blood RBC). O:P ratio = (observed CSF WBC)/(predicted CSF WBC). Also, do WBC:RBC ratio. If O:P ratio ≤ 0.01, and WBC:RBC ratio ≤ 1:100, meningitis is absent.

ADEM, acute disseminated encephalomyelitis; AIDS, acquired immunodeficiency syndrome; CMV, cytomegalovirus; CSF, cerebrospinal fluid; EBV, Epstein-Barr virus; HSV, herpes simplex virus; IL-8, interleukin 8; LDH, lactate dehydrogenase; MRI, magnetic resonance imaging; MS, multiple sclerosis; PCR, polymerase chain reaction; PMN, polymorphonuclear neutrophil; RBC, red blood cell; TNF, tumor necrosis factor; WBC, white blood cell.

intracranial blood. It also allows visualization of the ventricular system and is the method of choice for assessing hydrocephalus. It can also be particularly useful in determining presence of intracranial calcifications associated with intrauterine infections, slow growing tumors old injury, metabolic disease, and tubers in patients with tuberous sclerosis complex. Intravenous injection of iodized contrast media may aid in defining structures as well as vasculature and patency of sinuses (eg, evaluating sinus thrombosis) but is not routinely used. CT angiography (CTA) is possible using contrast and specialized techniques to visualize vascular anatomy. CT angiography can replace catheter angiography in evaluation of stroke allowing visualization of major arteries as well as the site of an acute thrombosis. Radiation exposure is a disadvantage of all CT scanning. Radiation exposure is generally decreased in children receiving CT compared to adults, decreasing some visualization of stuctures.

Magnetic Resonance Imaging

MRI is a noninvasive technique that provides high-resolution images of soft tissues. It is particularly useful in evaluating intracranial tissues and spinal cord. MRI uses the magnetic properties of certain nuclei to produce diagnostically useful signals (Table 25–3). The technique is based on detecting the response (resonance) of hydrogen proton nuclei to applied radiofrequency electromagnetic radiation. The strength of MRI signals varies with the relationship of water to protein and the amount of lipid in the tissue MRI can provide information about the histologic, physiologic, and biochemical status of tissues in addition to gross anatomic data. A recent advance has been the use of very powerful magnets (3 Tesla) which allow more detailed visualization, although the clinical utility of 3T MRI scans has not been fully defined. Sedation is often necessary for MRI scans in children who are unable to lie still for 45 minutes to avoid any movement artifact.

MRI delineates brain structure, brain tumors, edema, ischemic and hemorrhagic lesions, hydrocephalus, vascular disorders, inflammatory and infectious lesions, and degenerative processes. MRI can be used to study myelination and demyelination and through the demonstration of changes in relaxation time, metabolic disorders of the brain, muscles, and glands. Because bone does not produce artifact in the images, the posterior fossa and its contents can be studied far better with MRI than with CT scans. This allows blood vessels and the cranial nerves to be imaged. In contrast, the lesser ability of MRI to detect calcification limits its usefulness in the investigation of calcified lesions and acute blood.

Magnetic resonance angiography (MRA) or venography (MRV) is a noninvasive technique used to visualize large extra- and intracranial blood vessels (arterial and venous) without injection of dye. They are not as sensitive as conventional angiography but do not require catheterization. Likewise, an advantage over CTA (see previous section) is the lack of radiation exposure.

Perfusion-weighted imaging is performed using gadolinium-based contrast. The protocol is used in stroke patients to evaluate brain ischemic penumbra. Similarly, diffusion-weighted imaging (DWI) (measuring random motion of water molecules) may show reduced diffusion in areas of cytotoxic edema and is therefore useful in acute stroke and toxic or metabolic brain injuries.

Newer applications for functional assessment of the CNS are being developed. A recently developed MRI technique, MR spectroscopy (MRS) assesses biochemical changes in CNS tissue, measuring signals of increased cellular activity and oxidative metabolism. For example, MRS can be used to identify brain tumors.

Functional MRI (fMRI) is used to localize various brain functions such as language and motor function. Blood oxygenation changes in an area of interest. In evaluation of language, for example, an area of language acquisition during rest and then during a task can identify and lateralize the language cortex. Motor and sensory function can also be identified in this manner. The axonal tracts of neurologic pathways such as the optic radiations, or motor system, can now also be identified which can be helpful for surgical planning. This is called diffusion tensor imaging (DTI). These techniques generally require a team involving a neuropsychologist and radiologist to derive specific paradigms for testing and evaluation of imaging, as well as a cooperative patient.

Table 25–3. Utility of MRI protocols.

Protocol	Useful For
T1	Anatomy, myelination
T2	Pathologic changes; myelination
FLAIR	Pathologic changes
T1 with gadolinium	disruption of blood-brain barrier
Perfusion-weighted imaging	Cerebral blood flow/stroke
DWI	Acute ischemia (stroke)
ADC	Acute cerebral ischemia

ADC, apparent diffusion coefficient; DWI, diffusion-weighted imaging; FLAIR, fluid-attenuated inversion recovery.

Positron Emission Tomography

PET is a nuclear medicine imaging technique that measures the metabolic rate at given sites within the brain, producing three-dimensional reconstructions for localization of CNS function. These scans may be coregistered with a traditional CT scan or MRI allowing more precise localization of functional processes. For measurement of local cerebral metabolism, the radiolabeled substrate most frequently used has been intravenously administered fluorodeoxyglucose.

PET is an additional functional imaging technique used to study cerebral metabolic activity. Pathologic states that have been studied include epilepsy, brain infarction, CNS tumors, and degenerative disorders. It is proving to be very useful in preoperative evaluation for epilepsy surgery. The epileptogenic zone will often be hypermetabolic during seizures and hypometabolic during the time between seizures. PET is most often performed in the interictal state. The information from PET scan complements EEG, SPECT, and MRI findings to aid in the decision about tissue removal. PET scan can occasionally detect focal lesions that are not appreciated on the MRI, thereby leading to successful surgical removal of epileptogenic tissue. PET coregistered with CT scans is used for systemic tumors and is therefore becoming increasingly available for use in evaluation of the CNS.

Single-Photon Emission Computerized Tomography

An application of nuclear medicine imaging, SPECT scans image cerebral blood flow using a radioactive tracer (typically technetium-99m) to produce multiple cuts similar to those obtained in CT scans. This allows virtual three-dimensional visualization of vascular blood flow. It is useful in assessment of patients for epilepsy surgery, aiding in identification of a seizure focus. SPECT scan is most useful in epilepsy patients when the scan is obtained with a seizure and without a seizure. The changes in blood flow between the scans are then compared. In children with brain tumors, SPECT can help in differentiating tumor recurrence from posttreatment changes, in assessing the response to treatment, in directing biopsy, and in planning therapy. Regional cerebral blood flow can be assessed in children with strokes due to vascular stenosis and moyamoya disease.

Ultrasonography

Ultrasonography offers a pictorial display of the varying densities of tissues in a given anatomic region by recording the echoes of ultrasonic waves reflected from it. These waves, modulated by pulsations, are introduced into the tissue by means of a piezoelectric transducer. The many advantages of ultrasonography include the ability to assess a structure and its positioning quickly with easily portable equipment, without ionizing radiation, and at about one-fourth the cost of CT scanning. Sedation is usually not necessary, and the procedure can be repeated as often as needed without risk to the patient. In brain imaging, B-mode and real-time sector scanners are usually used, permitting excellent detail in the coronal and sagittal planes. Contiguous structures can be studied by a continuous sweep and reviewed on videotape. Ultrasonography has been used for in-utero diagnosis of hydrocephalus and other anomalies. In neonates, the thin skull and the open anterior fontanel have facilitated imaging of the brain, and ultrasonography is used to screen and follow infants of less than 32 weeks' gestation or weighing less than 1500 g for intracranial hemorrhage. Other uses in neonates include detection of hydrocephalus, periventricular ischemic lesions, major brain and spine malformations, and calcifications from intrauterine infection with cytomegalovirus (CMV) or *Toxoplasma*. In skilled hands, sonography of the neonatal spine can be used as a screening test for anomalies at the lumbosacral level. Once the fontanels start to close, this modality is no longer useful due to inability to penetrate bone.

Cerebral Angiography

Arteriography remains a useful procedure in the diagnosis of many cerebrovascular disorders, particularly in cerebrovascular accidents or in potentially operable vascular malformations. In some brain tumors, arteriography may be necessary to define the precise location or vascular bed, to differentiate among tumors, or to distinguish tumor from abscess or infarction. Noninvasive CT, CTA, MRI, and MRA scans can diagnose many cases of static or flowing blood disorders (eg, sinus thromboses). If necessary, the more risky invasive arteriography is usually done via femoral artery-aorta catheterization. Since cerebral angiography uses traditional x-ray to produce images, there is significant exposure to ionizing radiation.

Myelography

Radiographic examination of the spine may be indicated in cases of spinal cord tumors, myelitis, or various forms of spinal dysraphism and in the rare instance of herniated disks in children. MRI has largely replaced sonography, CT, and myelography for examination of the spinal cord.

Electromyography & Nerve Conduction Velocity Testing

The term neuromuscular disorder refers to disorders which affect the peripheral nervous system (including nerve roots, nerves, and neuromuscular junction) and/or the muscles.

Electromyography (EMG) and nerve conduction velocity testing (NCV) are used for assessment of neuromuscular disorders such as spinal muscular atrophy, the Guillain-Barre syndrome, defects in neuromuscular transmission such as myasthenia gravis and infantile botulism, myopathies as well as other disorders. NCV can define both acquired and hereditary neuropathies. It can also be used to assess leukodystrophies, disorders associated with central as well as peripheral demyelination.

NCV is performed by introducing a small current into peripheral nerves using small discs overlying the nerves. Recordings are made from the nerves along their course. The conduction velocity of the nerve can then be calculated. EMG records spontaneous and volitional electrical activity of skeletal muscle tissue. It requires placement of tiny needles into selected muscles, detecting activity in resting muscle (which should not show spontaneous activity) and in muscle being voluntarily contracted. While uncomfortable, the tests are not painful and sedation is only rarely necessary.

Bandettini PA: What's new in neuroimaging methods? Annals of New York Academy of Sciences 2009;1156:260–293 [PMID: 19338512].

Beslow et al: Hemorrhagic transformation of childhood arterial ischemic stroke. Stroke 2011;42(4):941–946 [PMID: 21350202].

Bonsu BK, Harper MB: Accuracy and test characteristics of ancillary tests of cerebrospinal fluid for predicting acute bacterial meningitis in children with low white blood cell counts in cerebrospinal fluid. Acad Emerg Med 2005;12:303 [PMID: 15805320].

Cakir B et al: Inborn errors of metabolisms presenting in childhood. J of Neuroimaging 2011;21(2)e117–133 [PMID: 21435076].

Dauud E et al: How MRI can contribute to the diagnosis of acute demyelinating encephalopathies in children. Neurosciences 2011;16(2):137–45 [PMID: 21427663].

Freilich ER, Gaillard WD: Utility of functional MRI in pediatric neurology. Current neurology and neuroscience reports 2010;10 (1):40–46 [PMID: 20425225].

Gaillard WD et al: Guidelines for imaging infants and children with recent onset epilepsy. Epilepsia 2009;50(9):2147–2153 [PMID: 19389145].

Pearl PL: New treatment paradigms in neonatal metabolic epilepsies. J Inherit Metab Dis 2009;32:204–213 [PMID: 19234868].

Rabie M, Jossiphov J, Nevo Y: Electromyography (EMG) accuracy compared to muscle biopsy in childhood. J Child Neurol 2007 Jul;22(7):803–808 [PMID: 17715269].

Spennato P et al: Pseudotumor Cerebri. Childs Nervous System 2011;27(2):215–235 [PMID: 20721668].

Thakur NH, Lowe LH: Borderline low conus of medullaris of infant lumbar sonography: What is the clinical outcome and the role of neuroimaging follow-up? Pediatric Radiology 2011;41(4):483–487 [PMID: 21079942].

Townsend BA et al: Has Pediatric CT at children's hospitals reached its peak? AJ Roentgenology 2010;194(5):1194–1196 [PMID: 20410402].

Towsley K et al: Population based study of neuroimaging findings in children with cerebral palsy. European J of Paediatric Neurology 2011;15(1):29–35 [PMID: 20869285].

Electromyography & Nerve Conduction Velocity Testing

The term neuromuscular disorder refers to disorders which affect the peripheral nervous system (including nerve roots, nerves, and neuromuscular junction) and/or the muscles.

Electromyography (EMG) and nerve conduction study testing (NCS) are used for assessment of neuromuscular disorders such as spinal muscular atrophy, Guillain-Barre syndrome, defects in neuromuscular transmission (such as myasthenia gravis and infantile botulism), and myopathies. It is less informative for primary central nervous system disorders. NCSs can distinguish between primary axonal and demyelinating polyneuropathies, as well as between acquired and inherited processes. In general, in acquired polyneuropathies, nerve involvement tends to be patchy, whereas in inherited disorders, the involvement tends to be uniform. Temporal dispersion and conduction block are hallmarks of an acquired disorder.

The EMG study complements the NCSs, and can distinguish between a primary myopathic or neuropathic disorder. There may be characteristic spontaneous discharges from the muscle membranes, such as myotonia, that can indicate the presence of a small group of disorders. In addition, in the evaluation of a primary neuropathic disorder, the EMG study can characterize the severity, chronicity, and distribution of the neuropathic involvement.

NCSs performed by stimulating the nerves with a low intensity electrical impulse that is conducted along the nerve and recorded by surface electrodes over the distal sensory nerve or muscle. Nerve conduction velocity and amplitude are calculated from this recording. The EMG study is performed by placing a microphone into muscle and recording spontaneous activity in a quiet muscle and motor unit action potentials generated by muscle contraction. EMG records spontaneous and volitional electrical activity of skeletal muscle tissue. Some discomfort is felt as the microphone is placed in the muscle but generally is well-tolerated in the hands of an experienced electromyographer. Sedation is seldom used as the voluntary muscle contraction is difficult to elicit in a sedated patient, and therefore motor unit action potentials difficult to assess. The risks of the study include bleeding and infection, but are rare unless the patient is on anticoagulation or has a primary coagulopathy.

EMG/NCS may be difficult to perform and to interpret in newborns and infants. The motor unit potential is typically very small in an infant, representing the small physical size of the motor unit. It is therefore difficult to differentiate between normal motor unit potentials from myopathic ones in this age group. In addition, because the infant's limbs are much smaller than an adults, small errors in measurement creates a much large error in computed conduction velocities than when larger distances are used. Smaller recording electrodes and stimulators are required for infants due to their small size, as coexcitation of nearby nerves can occur when too high a stimulus intensity is used, resulting in erroneous calculations of amplitude and conduction velocities.

In general, however, this study has been demonstrated to be useful both in the outpatient and inpatient settings, both to confirm a suspected diagnosis, and in the diagnosis of previously unrecognized, significant diagnoses that may alter clinical care. Generally, having a suspected diagnosis in mind before referral of the patient for an EMG/NCS greatly aids the electromyographer in the tailoring the study towards confirmation of that diagnosis.

Change J, Park YG, Choi YC et al: Correlation of electromyogram and muscle biopsy in myopathy of young age. Arch Phys Med Rehabil 2011;92(5):780–784 [PMID: 21530726].

Jones HR Jr: Pediatric electromyography in the acute care setting. Suppl Clin Neurophysiol 2000;53:44–52 [PMID: 12740976].

Perry DL, Tarulli AW, Nardin RA et al: Clinical utility of electrodiagnostic studies in the inpatient setting. Muscle Nerve 2009;40:195–199 [PMID: 19609901].

Pitt M: Paediatric electromyopgrahy in the modern world. Dev Med Child Neurol 2011;53(2):120–124 [PMID: 21087239].

Rabie M, Jossiphov J, Nevo Y: Electromyography (EMG) accuracy compared to muscle biopsy in childhood. J Child Neurol 2007 Jul;22(7):803–808 [PMID: 17715269].

DISORDERS AFFECTING THE NERVOUS SYSTEM IN INFANTS & CHILDREN

ALTERED STATES OF CONSCIOUSNESS

ESSENTIALS OF DIAGNOSIS & TYPICAL FEATURES

- Reduction or alteration in cognitive and affective mental functioning and in arousability or attentiveness.
- Acute onset.

General Considerations

Many terms are used to describe the continuum from full alertness to complete unresponsiveness and deep coma, including clouding, obtundation, somnolence stupor, semicoma light coma, and deep coma. Several scales have been used to grade the depth of unconsciousness (Table 25–4). The commonly used Glasgow Coma Scale is summarized in Table 12–5. Physicians should use one of these tables and provide further descriptions in case narratives (such as, "opens eyes with painful stimulus, but does not respond to voice"). These descriptions help subsequent observers quantify unconsciousness and evaluate changes in the patient's condition.

The neurologic substrate for consciousness is the reticular activating system in the brainstem, up to and including the thalamus and paraventricular hypothalamus. Large lesions of the cortex, especially bilateral lesions, can also cause coma. The term *locked-in syndrome* describes patients who are conscious but have no access to motor or verbal expression because of massive loss of motor function of the pontine portion of the brainstem. *Coma vigil* refers to patients who seem comatose but have some spontaneous motor behavior, such as eye opening or eye tracking, almost always at a reflex level. *Persistent vegetative state* denotes a chronic condition in which there is preservation of the sleep-wake cycle but no awareness and no recovery of mental function.

Treatment

A. Emergency Measures

The clinician's first response is to stabilize the child using the ABCs of resuscitation. The airway must be kept open with positioning; endotracheal intubation is often considered. Breathing and adequate air exchange can be assessed by auscultation. Hand bag respiratory assistance with oxygen may be needed. Circulation must be ensured by assessing pulse and blood pressure. An intravenous line is always necessary. Fluids, plasma, blood, or even a dopamine drip (1–20 mcg/kg/min) may be required in cases of hypotension. Initial intravenous fluids should contain glucose until further assessment disproves hypoglycemia as a cause. An extremely hypothermic or febrile child may require vigorous warming or cooling to save life. The assessment of vital signs may signal the diagnosis. Slow, insufficient respirations suggest poisoning by hypnotic drugs; apnea may indicate diphenoxylate hydrochloride poisoning. Rapid, deep respirations suggest acidosis, possibly metabolic, as with diabetic coma; toxin exposure, such as that due to aspirin; or neurogenic causes, as in Reye syndrome. Hyperthermia may indicate infection or heat stroke; hypothermia may indicate cold exposure, ethanol poisoning, or hypoglycemia (especially in infancy).

Table 25–4. Gradation of coma.

	Deep Coma		Light Coma		
	Grade 4	Grade 3	Grade 2	Grade 1	Stupor
Response to pain	0	+	Avoidance	Avoidance	Arousal unsustained
Tone/posture	Flaccid	Decerebrate	Variable	Variable	Normal
Tendon reflexes	0	+/−	+	+	+
Pupil response	0	+	+	+	+
Response to verbal stimuli	0	0	0	0	+
Other corneal reflex	0	+	+	+	+
Gag reflex	0	+	+	+	+

The signs of impending brain herniation are another priority of the initial assessment. Bradycardia, high blood pressure, and irregular breathing are signs of severely increased intracranial pressure. Third nerve palsy (with the eye deviated down and out, and a "blown" pupil [unilateral pupillary dilation]) is a sign of impending temporal lobe or brainstem herniation. These signs suggest a need for slight hyperventilation reducing cerebral edema, consideration of mannitol, prompt neurosurgical consultation, and head CT. If brainstem herniation or increased pressure is possible, intracranial monitoring may be necessary. Criteria for initiation of intracranial monitoring are still controversial, given the lack of data in this area. This procedure is described in more detail in Chapter 14. Initial treatment of impending herniation includes keeping the patient's head up (15–30 degrees) and providing slight hyperventilation. The use of mannitol, diuretics, corticosteroids, and drainage of cerebrospinal fluid (CSF) are more heroic measures covered in detail in Chapter 14.

A history obtained from parents or witnesses is desirable. Sometimes the only history will be obtained from ambulance attendants. An important point is whether the child is known to have a chronic illness, such as diabetes, hemophilia, epilepsy, or cystic fibrosis. Recent acute illness raises the possibility of coma caused by viral or bacterial meningitis. Trauma is a common cause of coma. Lack of a history of trauma, especially in infants, does not rule it out. Nonaccidental trauma or an unwitnessed fall may have occurred. In coma of unknown cause, poisoning is always a possibility, especially in toddlers. Absence of a history of ingestion of a toxic substance or of medication in the home does not rule out poisoning as a cause.

Often the history is obtained concurrently with a brief pediatric and neurologic screening examination. After the assessment of vital signs, the general examination proceeds with a trauma assessment. Palpation of the head and fontanel, inspection of the ears for infection or hemorrhage, and a careful examination for neck stiffness are indicated. If circumstances suggest head or neck trauma, the head and neck must be immobilized so that any fracture or dislocation will not be aggravated. The skin must be inspected for petechiae or purpura that might suggest bacteremia, infection, bleeding disorder, or traumatic bruising. Examination of the chest, abdomen, and limbs is important to exclude enclosed hemorrhage or traumatic fractures.

Neurologic examination quantifies the stimulus response and depth of coma, such as responsiveness to verbal or painful stimuli. Are the eye movements spontaneous, or is it necessary to do the doll's eye maneuver (rotating the head rapidly to see whether the eyes follow in a patient without neck trauma)? Motor and sensory examinations assess reflex asymmetries, Babinski sign, and evidence of spontaneous posturing or posturing induced by noxious stimuli (eg, decorticate or decerebrate posturing).

If the cause of the coma is not obvious, emergency laboratory tests must be obtained. Table 25–5 lists some of the causes of coma in children. Most comas (90%) in children have a medical (vs structural) cause. Infection is a common cause (30%). An immediate blood glucose (or Dextrostix), complete blood count, urine obtained by catheterization if necessary, pH and electrolytes (including bicarbonate), serum urea nitrogen, and aspartate aminotransferase and ammonia are initial screens. Urine, blood, and even gastric contents must be saved for toxin screen if the underlying cause is not obvious. Blood culture and lumbar puncture often are necessary to rule out CNS infection. However, papilledema is a relative contraindication to lumbar puncture. Often, a blood culture is obtained, antibiotics started, and imaging study of the brain done prior to a diagnostic lumbar puncture. If meningitis is suspected and a lumbar puncture is delayed or believed to be hazardous, antibiotics should be started and the diagnostic lumbar puncture done later. Tests that are helpful in obscure cases of coma include: oxygen and carbon dioxide partial pressures, serum and urine osmolality, porphyrins, lead levels, general toxicology screen, serum amino acids, and urine organic acids. Hashimoto's encephalitis is a controversial, yet potentially treatable consideration. A formal metabolic consultation is also useful in this setting.

If head trauma or increased pressure is suspected, an emergency CT scan or MRI is necessary. CT is usually helpful as an initial screening examination, but MRI is more sensitive in finding anoxic brain injury early in the course. Bone windows on the former study or skull radiographs can be done at the same sitting. The absence of skull fracture does not rule out coma caused by closed head trauma. Injury that results from shaking a child is one example. Treatment of head injury associated with coma is discussed in detail in Chapter 12.

Rarely, an emergency EEG aids in diagnosing the cause of coma. Nonconvulsive status epilepticus or a focal finding as seen with herpes encephalitis (periodic lateralized epileptiform discharges) and focal slowing as seen with stroke or cerebritis are cases in which the EEG might be helpful. The EEG also may correlate with the stage of coma and add prognostic information. An EEG should be ordered if seizures are suspected. If obvious motor seizures have occurred, treatment for status epilepticus is given with intravenous drugs (see later section on Seizure Disorders).

B. General Measures

Vital signs must be monitored and maintained. Most emergency departments and intensive care units have flow sheets that provide space for repeated monitoring of the coma; a coma scale can be a useful tool for this purpose. The patient's response to vocal or painful stimuli and orientation to time, place, and situation are monitored. Posture and movements of the limbs, either spontaneously or in response to pain, are serially noted. Pupillary size, equality, and reaction to light, and movement of the eyes to the doll's eye maneuver or ice water caloric tests should be recorded. Intravenous fluids can be tailored to the situation, as for treatment of acidosis, shock, or hypovolemia. Nasogastric suction is initially important. The bladder should be catheterized for monitoring urine output and for urinalysis.

Table 25–5. Some causes of coma in childhood.

Mechanism of Coma	Likely Cause: Newborn Infant	Likely Cause: Older Child
Anoxia		
Asphyxia	Birth asphyxia, HIE	Carbon monoxide (CO) poisoning
Respiratory obstruction	Meconium aspiration, infection (especially respiratory syncytial virus)	Croup, tracheitis, epiglottitis
Severe anemia	Hydrops fetalis	Hemolysis, blood loss
Ischemia		
Cardiac	Shunting lesions, hypoplastic left heart	Shunting lesions, aortic stenosis, myocarditis
Shock	Asphyxia, sepsis	blood loss, infection
Head trauma (structural cause)	Birth contusion, hemorrhage, nonaccidental trauma (NAT)	Falls, auto accidents, athletic injuries
Infection (most common cause in childhood)	Gram-negative meningitis, enterovirus, herpes encephalitis, sepsis	Bacterial meningitis, viral encephalitis, postinfectious encephalitis, sepsis, typhoid, malaria
Vascular (CVA or stroke, often of unknown cause)	Intraventricular hemorrhage, sinus thrombosis	Arterial or venous occlusion with congenital heart disease, head or neck trauma
Neoplasm (structural cause)	Rare this age. Choroid plexus papilloma with severe hydrocephalus	Brainstem glioma, increased pressure with posterior fossa tumors
Drugs (toxidrome)	Maternal sedatives; injected pudendal and paracervical analgesics	Overdose, salicylates, lithium, sedatives, psychotropic agents
Epilepsy	Constant minor motor seizures; electrical seizure without motor manifestations	Nonconvulsive or, absence status, postictal state; drugs given to stop seizures
Toxins (toxidrome)	Maternal sedatives or injections	Arsenic, alcohol, CO, pesticides, mushroom, lead
Hypoglycemia	Birth injury, diabetic progeny, toxemic progeny	Diabetes, "prediabetes," hypoglycemic agents
Increased intracranial pressure (metabolic or structural cause)	Anoxic brain damage, hydrocephalus, metabolic disorders (urea cycle; amino-, organic acidurias)	Toxic encephalopathy, Reye syndrome, head trauma, tumor of posterior fossa
Hepatic causes	Hepatic failure, inborn metabolic errors in bilirubin conjugation	Hepatic failure
Renal causes, hypertensive encephalopathy	Hypoplastic kidneys	Nephritis, acute (AGN) and chronic, uremia, uremic syndrome
Hypothermia, hyperthermia	Iatrogenic (head cooling)	Cold weather exposure, drowning; heat stroke
Hypercapnia	Congenital lung anomalies, bronchopulmonary dysplasia	Cystic fibrosis (hypercapnia, anoxia)
Electrolyte changes		
Hyper- or hyponatremia	Iatrogenic ($NaHCO_3$ use), salt poisoning (formula errors)	Diarrhea, dehydration
Hyper- or hypocalcemia	SIADH, adrenogenital syndrome, dialysis (iatrogenic)	Lactic acidosis
Severe acidosis, lactic acidosis	epticemia, metabolic errors, adrenogenital syndrome	Infection, diabetic coma, poisoning (eg, aspirin), hyperglycemic nonketotic coma
Purpuric	Disseminated intravascular coagulation (DIC)	DIC, leukemia, thrombotic thrombocytopenic purpura

AGN, acute glomerulonephritis; SIADH, syndrome of inappropriate antidiuretic hormone secretion.
Modified and reproduced, with permission, from Lewis J, Moe PG: The unconscious child. In Conn H, Conn R (editors): Current Diagnosis, 5th ed. WB Saunders, 1977.

Prognosis

About 50% of children with nontraumatic causes of coma have a good outcome. In studies of adults assessed on admission or within the first days after the onset of coma, an analysis of multiple variables was most helpful in assessing prognosis. Abnormal neuro-ophthalmologic signs (eg, the absence of pupillary reaction or of eye movement in response to the doll's eye maneuver or ice water caloric testing and the absence of corneal responses) were unfavorable. Delay in the return of motor responses, tone, or eye opening was also unfavorable. In children, the assessment done on admission is about as predictive as one done in the succeeding days. Approximately two-thirds of outcomes can be successfully predicted at an early stage on the basis of coma severity, extraocular movements, pupillary reactions, motor patterns, blood pressure, temperature, and seizure type. In patients with severe head trauma, a Glasgow Coma Scale ≤ 5, hypothermia, hyperglycemia, and coagulation disorders are factors associated with an increased risk of mortality. Other characteristics, such as the need for assisted respiration, the presence of increased intracranial pressure, and the duration of coma, are not significantly predictive. Published reports suggest that an anoxic (in contrast to traumatic, metabolic, or toxic) coma, such as that caused by near drowning, has a much grimmer outlook.

Ashwal S et al: Use of advanced neuroimaging techniques in the evaluation of pediatric traumatic brain injury. Dev Neurosci 2006;28:309 [PMID: 16943654].

Atabaki SM: Pediatric head injury. Pediatr Rev 2007;28:215 [PMID: 17545333].

Avner JR: Altered states of consciousness. Pediatr Rev 2006;27:331 [PMID: 16950938].

Castro-Gago M, Gómez-Lado C, Maneiro-Freire M, Eirís-Puñal J, Bravo-Mata M: Hashimoto encephalopathy in a preschool girl. Pediatr Neurol 2010 Feb;42(2):143–146 [PMID: 20117754].

Hosain SA et al: Electroencephalographic patterns in unresponsive pediatric patients. Pediatr Neurol 2005;32:162 [PMID: 15730895].

Odetola FO, Clark SJ, Lamarand KE, Davis MM, Garton HJ: Intracranial pressure monitoring in childhood meningitis with coma: A national survey of neurosurgeons in the United States. Pediatr Crit Care Med 2011 Jan 21 [PMID: 21263366].

Posner JB et al: *Diagnosis of Stupor and Coma.* Oxford University Press, 2007.

Shemie SD et al: Diagnosis of brain death in children. Lancet Neurol 2007;6:87 [PMID: 17166805].

Tude Melo JR: Mortality in children with severe head trauma: Predictive factors and proposal for a new predictive scale. Neurosurgery 2010 Dec;67(6):1542–1547 [PMID: 21107185].

Worrall K: Use of the Glasgow Coma Scale in infants. Paediatr Nurs 2004;16:45 [PMID: 15160621].

SEIZURE DISORDERS (EPILEPSIES)

ESSENTIALS OF DIAGNOSIS & TYPICAL FEATURES

- Recurrent unprovoked seizures.
- Often, interictal electroencephalographic changes.

General Considerations

A seizure is a sudden, transient disturbance of brain function, manifested by involuntary motor, sensory, autonomic, or psychic phenomena, alone or in any combination, often accompanied by alteration or loss of consciousness. Seizures can be caused by any factor that disturbs brain function. They may occur after a metabolic, traumatic, anoxic, or infectious insult to the brain (classified as symptomatic seizures), or spontaneously without prior known CNS insult. Genetic mutations are increasingly identified in many patients without prior known cause of seizures.

Repeated seizures without an evident acute symptomatic cause or provocation (eg, fever) are defined as epilepsy. Epilepsy occurs most often in individuals at the extremes of the life span. The incidence is highest in the newborn period and higher in childhood than in later life, with another peak in the elderly. Prevalence flattens out after age 10–15 years. The chance of having a second seizure after an initial unprovoked episode in a child is about 50%. The risk of recurrence after a second unprovoked seizure is 85%. Sixty-five to seventy percent of children with epilepsy will achieve seizure remission with appropriate medication.

Classification

The International League Against Epilepsy (ILAE) has established classifications of seizures and epilepsy syndromes. Seizures are classified as either partial (with localized onset) or generalized (involving the whole brain). Seizures and epilepsy syndromes may be partial at onset and then secondarily generalize (partial seizures with secondary generalization), or generalized from the onset.

Epilepsy syndromes are defined by the nature of the seizures (ie, localized vs generalized), age of onset, EEG findings, and other clinical factors. Epilepsy is classified as symptomatic (the cause is identified or presumed), cryptogenic (undetermined etiology, presumably symptomatic and often due to congenital CNS abnormalities), or idiopathic (often genetic). In general, symptomatic and cryptogenic epilepsy have their onset early in life. Idiopathic (genetic) epilepsy syndromes are usually age specific, occurring at any age from early infancy to adolescence, depending on the specific syndrome. Identification of the specific epilepsy syndrome is helpful in defining prognosis, with idiopathic epilepsy more likely to be controlled and eventually remit than symptomatic epilepsy.

1. Seizures & Epilepsy in Childhood

Classifying the seizure is necessary for accurate diagnosis which will determine the nature of further evaluation and treatment and help in prognostication (Tables 25–6 and 25–7).

Clinical Findings

A. History, Symptoms, and Signs

Seizures are stereotyped paroxysmal clinical events; the key to diagnosis is usually in the history. Not all paroxysmal events

Table 25–6. Seizures by age at onset, pattern, and preferred treatment.

Seizure Type Epilepsy Syndrome	Age at Onset	Clinical Manifestations	Causative Factors	EEG Pattern	Other Diagnostic Studies	Treatment and Comments
Neonatal seizures	Birth–2 wk	Often subtle; sudden limpness or tonic posturing, brief apnea, cyanosis; odd cry; eyes rolling up; blinking or mouthing or chewing movements; nystagmus, twitchiness or clonic movements (focal, multifocal, or generalized). Some seizures are nonepileptic: decerebrate, or other posturings, release from forebrain inhibition. Poor response to drugs.	Neurologic insults (hypoxia/ischemia; intracranial hemorrhage) present more in first 3 d or after 8th day; metabolic disturbances alone between 3rd and 8th days; hypoglycemia, hypocalcemia, hyper- and hyponatremia. Drug withdrawal. Pyridoxine dependency. Other metabolic disorders. CNS infections. Structural abnormalities.	May correlate poorly with clinical seizures. Focal spikes or slow rhythms; multifocal discharges. Electroclinical dissociation may occur: electrical seizure without clinical manifestations.	Lumbar puncture; CSF PCR for herpes, enterovirus; serum Ca^{2+}, PO_4^{3-}, serum and CSF glucose, Mg^{2+}; BUN, amino acid screen, blood ammonia, organic acid screen, TORCHS, other metabolic testing if suspected. Ultrasound or CT/MRI for suspected intracranial hemorrhage and structural abnormalities.	Benzodiazepines, Phenobarbital, IV or IM; if seizures not controlled, add phenytoin IV. Recent experience with levetiracetam and topiramate. Treat underlying disorder. Seizures due to brain damage often resistant to anticonvulsants. When cause in doubt, stop protein feedings until enzyme deficiencies of urea cycle or amino acid metabolism ruled out.
Infantile spasms	3–18 mo, usually about 6 mo	Abrupt, usually but not always symmetrical adduction or flexion of limbs with flexion of head and trunk; or abduction and extensor movements (similar to Moro reflex). Occur in clusters typically upon awakening. Associated irritability and regression in development.	Symptomatic in approximately two-thirds. Acquired CNS injury in approximately one-third; biochemical, infectious, degenerative in approximately one-third; cryptogenic in approximately one-third. With early onset, pyridoxine dependency, inherited metabolic disorders. Tuberous sclerosis in 5–10%. TORCHS, homeobox gene mutations, *ARX*, and other genetic mutations.	Hypsarrhythmia (chaotic high-voltage slow waves or random spikes (90%)); other abnormalities in 10%. Rarely normal at onset. EEG normalization early in course usually correlates with reduction of seizures; not helpful prognostically regarding mental development.	Funduscopic and skin examination, Amino and organic acid screen. Chromosomes TORCHS screen, CT, or MRI scan should be done to (1) establish definite diagnosis, (2) aid in genetic counseling. Trial of pyridoxine. Occasionally, surgical resection of cortical malformation.	ACTH gel (40 IU/d 150 IU/m²/d) IM once daily. Vigabatrin, especially if tuberous sclerosis. B_6 (pyridoxine) trial. In resistant cases, topiramate, zonisamide, valproic acid, lamotrigine, ketogenic diet. Early treatment leads to improved outcome.
Febrile convulsions	3 mo–5 y (maximum 6–18 mo); most common childhood seizure (incidence 2%)	Usually generalized seizures, < 15 min; rarely focal in onset. May lead to status epilepticus. Recurrence risk of second febrile seizure 30% (50% if younger than 1 y of age); recurrence risk is same after status epilepticus.	Nonneurologic febrile illness (temperature rises to 39°C or higher). Risk factors: positive family history, day care, slow development, prolonged neonatal hospitalization.	Normal interictal EEG, especially when obtained 8–10 d after seizure. Therefore, not useful unless complicating features.	Lumbar puncture in infants or whenever suspicion of meningitis exists.	Treat underlying illness, fever. Diazepam orally, 0.3–0.5 mg/kg, divided 3 times daily during illness may be considered. Diastat rectally for prolonged (> 5 min) seizure. Prophylaxis with phenobarbital or valproic acid rarely needed.

Cryptogenic generalized epilepsies of early childhood (Lennox-Gastaut syndrome, Myoclonic-Astatic Epilepsy [Doose Syndrome] and Dravet syndrome)	Any time in childhood (usually 2–7 y)	Mixed seizures dependent on particular syndrome, including tonic, myoclonic (shocklike violent contractions of one or more muscle groups, singly or irregularly repetitive); atonic ("drop attacks") and atypical absence with episodes of absence status epilepticus.	Multiple causes, usually resulting in diffuse neuronal damage. History of infantile spasms; prenatal or perinatal brain damage; viral meningoencephalitis; CNS degenerative disorders; structural cerebral abnormalities (eg, migrational abnormalities). Doose syndrome. Dravet syndrome associated with SCN1A mutation.	Atypical slow (1–2.5 Hz) spike-wave complexes and bursts of high-voltage generalized spikes, often with diffusely slow background frequencies. Electrodecremental and fast spikes during sleep.	As dictated by index of suspicion: genetic testing; inherited metabolic disorders, neuronal ceroid lipofuscinosis, others. MRI scan, WBC lysosomal enzymes. Skin or conjunctival biopsy for electron microscopy, nerve conduction studies if degenerative disease suspected.	Difficult to treat. Topiramate, ethosuximide, felbamate, levetiracetam, zonisamide, valproate, clonazepam, rufinamide, clobazam (approval pending) ketogenic diet, vagus nerve stimulation. Avoid phenytoin, carbamazepine, oxcarbazepine, gabapentin. (Stiripentol used in Europe but not approved in US.)
Childhood absence epilepsy	3–12 y	Lapses of consciousness or vacant stares, lasting about 3–10 s, often in clusters. Automatisms of face and hands; clonic activity in 30–45%. Often confused with complex partial seizures but no aura or postictal confusion. Some risk for developing generalized tonic clonic seizures.	Unknown. Genetic component. Abnormal thalamocortical circuitry.	3/s bilaterally synchronous, symmetrical, high-voltage spikes and waves provoked by hyperventilation. EEG always abnormal. EEG normalization correlates closely with control of seizures.	Hyperventilation often provokes attacks. Imaging studies rarely of value.	Ethosuximide most effective and best tolerated; valproic acid. Lamotrigine, in resistant cases, zonisamide, topiramate, levetiracetam, acetazolamide, ketogenic diet.
Juvenile absence epilepsy	10–15 y	Absence seizures less frequent than in childhood absence epilepsy. May have greater risk of convulsive seizures.	Unknown (idiopathic), possibly genetic.	3-Hz spike wave and atypical generalized discharges.	Not always triggered by hyperventilation.	Same as childhood absence epilepsy but may be more difficult to treat successfully.
Simple partial or focal seizures (motor/sensory/jacksonian)	Any age	Seizure may involve any part of body; may spread in fixed pattern (jacksonian march), becoming generalized. In children, epileptogenic focus often "shifts," and epileptic manifestations may change concomitantly.	Often unknown; birth trauma, inflammatory process, vascular accidents, meningoencephalitis, malformations of cortical development (dysplasia), etc. If seizures are coupled with new or progressive neurologic deficits, a structural lesion (eg, brain tumor) is likely. If epilepsia partialis continua (simple partial status epilepticus), Rasmussen syndrome is likely.	EEG may be normal; focal spikes or slow waves in appropriate cortical region; "rolandic spikes" (centrotemporal spikes) are typical. Possibly genetic.	MRI, repeat if seizures poorly controlled or progressive.	Oxcarbazepine, carbamazepine; lamotrigine, gabapentin, topiramate, levetiracetam, zonisamide, lacosamide, and phenytoin. Valproic acid useful adjunct. If medications fail, surgery may be an option.

(*Continued*)

Table 25–6. Seizures by age at onset, pattern, and preferred treatment. (*Continued*)

Seizure Type Epilepsy Syndrome	Age at Onset	Clinical Manifestations	Causative Factors	EEG Pattern	Other Diagnostic Studies	Treatment and Comments
Complex partial seizures	Any age	Aura progressing to larger event, aura and seizure stereotyped for each patient and related to part of brain seizure originates, eg, temporal lobe seizures may have a sensation of fear, déjà vu; epigastric discomfort, odd smell or taste (usually unpleasant). Seizure may consist of vague stare; facial, tongue, or swallowing movements and throaty sounds; or various complex automatisms. Usually brief, 15–90 s, followed by confusion or sleep.	As above. Temporal lobes especially sensitive to hypoxia; seizure may be a sequela of birth trauma, febrile convulsions, viral encephalitis, especially herpes. Malformations of cortical development (dysplasia) common in medication resistant patients. Remediable causes are small cryptic tumors or vascular malformations. May be genetic.	As above.	MRI; PCR of CSF in acute febrile situation for herpes or enteroviral encephalitis. SPECT, PET scan, video-EEG monitoring when epilepsy surgery considered.	As above.
Benign epilepsy of childhood with centrotemporal spikes (BECTS/rolandic epilepsy)	5–16 y	Simple partial seizures of face, tongue, hand. With or without secondary generalization. Usually nocturnal. Similar seizure patterns may be observed in patients with focal cortical lesions. Almost always remits by puberty.	Seizure history or abnormal EEG findings in relatives of 40% of affected probands and 18%–20% of parents and siblings, suggesting transmission by a single autosomal dominant gene, possibly with age-dependent penetrance.	Centrotemporal spikes or sharp waves ("rolandic discharges") appearing paroxysmally against a normal EEG background.	Seldom need CT or MRI scan.	Often no medication is necessary, especially if seizure is exclusively nocturnal and infrequent. Oxcarbazepine, carbamazepine or others. (See complex partial seizures.)
Juvenile myoclonic epilepsy (of Janz)	Late childhood and adolescence, peaking at 13 y	Mild myoclonic jerks of neck and shoulder flexor muscles after awakening. Usually generalized tonic-clonic seizures as well. Often absence seizures. Intelligence usually normal. Rarely resolves but usually remits on medications.	40% of relatives have myoclonias, especially in females; 15% have the abnormal EEG pattern with clinical attacks.	Interictal EEG shows variety of spike-and-wave sequences or 4-6-Hz multispike-and-wave complexes ("fast spikes").	If course is unfavorable, differentiate from progressive myoclonic syndromes by appropriate studies [eg, biopsies (muscles, liver, etc)]. Imaging may not be necessary.	Lamotrigine, valproic acid, topiramate, levetiracetam, zonisamide.
Generalized tonic-clonic seizures (grand mal) (GTCS)	Any age	Loss of consciousness; tonic-clonic movements, often preceded by vague aura or cry. Incontinence in 15%. Postictal confusion and somnolence. Often mixed with or masking other seizure patterns.	Often unknown. Genetic component. May be seen with metabolic disturbances, trauma, infection, intoxication, degenerative disorders, brain tumors.	Bilaterally synchronous, symmetrical multiple high-voltage spikes, spikes waves (eg, 3/s). EEG often normal in those younger than age 4 y. Focal spikes may become "secondarily generalized."	Imaging; metabolic and infectious evaluation may be appropriate.	Levitiracetam; topiramate, lamotrigine, zonisamide, valproic acid, felbamate. Combinations may be necessary. Carbamazepine, oxcarbazepine or valproic acid; phenytoin may also be effective.

ACTH, adrenocorticotropic hormone; BUN, blood urea nitrogen; CNS, central nervous system; CSF, cerebrospinal fluid; CT, computed tomography; EEG, electroencephalogram; IM, intramuscularly; IV, intravenously; MRI, magnetic resonance imaging; PCR, polymerase chain reaction; PET, positron emission tomography; SPECT, single-photon emission tomography; TORCHS, toxoplasmosis, other infections, rubella, cytomegalovirus, herpes simplex, and syphilis; WBC, white blood cell.

Table 25–7. Benign childhood epileptic syndromes.

Syndrome	Characteristics
Benign idiopathic neonatal convulsions (BINC)	So-called 5th day fits (97% have onset on 3rd–7th d of life); 6% of neonatal convulsions; clonic, multifocal, usually brief; occasional status epilepticus
Benign familial neonatal convulsions (BFNC)	Autosomal dominant; onset in 2–90 d; genes, *KCNQ2* or *KCNQ3*; clonic; 86% recover
Generalized tonic-clonic seizures (GTCS)	Age at onset, 3–11 y; may have family or personal history of febrile convulsions; 50% have 3/s spike-wave EEG; may have concurrent absence seizures
Childhood absence seizures	Incidence higher in girls than in boys; age at onset, 3–12 y (peak 6–7 y); 10–200 seizures per day; 3/s spike-wave EEG; up to 40% may develop GTCS
Juvenile absence seizures	Incidence higher in boys than in girls; age at onset, 10–12 y; uncommon; less frequent seizures; 3–4/s general spike-wave EEG; most have GTCS; some remit
Juvenile myoclonic epilepsy (Janz syndrome)	Age at onset, 12–18 y (average, 15 y); myoclonic jerks upper limbs, seldom fall; 4–6/s general spike-wave EEG; untreated, 90% have GTCS, mostly on waking; 20%–30% have absence seizures; 25%–40% are photosensitive; 10% remission rate (90% do not remit)
Benign epilepsy with centrotemporal spikes (BECTS); "rolandic epilepsy"	Age at onset 3–13 y (most at 4–10 y); 80% have brief, 2–5 min nocturnal (sleep) seizures only; usually simple partial seizures (face, tongue, cheek, hand) sensory or motor; occasionally have GTCS; bilateral independent spikes on EEG; may not need medication if seizures infrequent; remits at puberty
Benign epilepsy of childhood with occipital paroxysms (Panayiotopoulos syndrome)	6% of children with epilepsy; age at onset 3–6 y in 80% of patients (mean age, 5 y; range, 1–12 y); autonomic symptoms and visual aura may suggest migraine

EEG, electroencephalogram.

are epileptic. A detailed description of seizure onset is important in determining if an event is a seizure and if there is localized onset (partial or focal seizure). Events prior to, during, and after the seizure need to be described (although observers often recall little except generalized convulsive activity because of its dramatic appearance). An aura (actually a simple partial seizure) may precede the clinically apparent seizure and indicates focal onset. The patient may describe a feeling of fear, numbness or tingling in the fingers, or bright lights in one visual field. The specific symptoms may help define the location of seizure onset (eg, déjà vu suggests temporal lobe onset).

Often, the child does not recall or cannot define the aura though the family may note alterations in behavior at the onset. Videotapes of events have been extremely useful.

Families may not immediately recall the details of the event but asking specific questions can help provide the details needed to determine the seizure type and, if partial, the site of onset. Did the patient become extremely pale before falling? Was the patient able to respond to queries during the episode? Was the patient unconscious or was there just impaired awareness? Did the patient fall stiffly or gradually slump to the floor? Was there an injury? How long did the tonic stiffening or clonic jerking last? Where in the body did the clonic activity take place? Which direction were head and eyes turned? Postictal states can be helpful in diagnosis. After complex partial and generalized convulsive seizures, postictal sleep typically occurs, but postictal changes are not seen after generalized absence seizures. Was there loss of speech after the seizure (suggesting left temporal lobe seizure) or was the patient able to respond and speak in short order? The parent may report lateralized motor activity (eg, the child's eyes may deviate to one side or the child may experience dystonic posturing of a limb). Motor activity without impaired awareness supports the diagnosis of simple partial seizures. Impaired awareness and automatisms define the event as a complex partial seizure.

In contrast, primary generalized seizures usually manifest with acute loss of consciousness, usually with generalized motor activity. Tonic posturing, tonic-clonic activity, or myoclonus (spasms) may occur. In children with generalized absence seizures, behavioral arrest may be associated with automatisms such as blinking, chewing, or hand movements, making it difficult to differentiate between absence seizures and partial seizures.

Description of the semiology of the event may help determine if the child experienced an epileptic seizure or a nonepileptic event mimicking or misinterpreted as an epileptic seizure. Frequently, the child presenting with a presumed first seizure has experienced unrecognized seizures before the event that brings the child to medical attention. In particular, partial and absence seizures may not be recognized except in retrospect. Thus, careful questioning regarding prior events is important in the child being evaluated for new onset of seizures.

B. Diagnostic Evaluation

The extent and urgency of the diagnostic evaluation is determined, in general, by the child's age, the severity and type of seizure, whether the child is ill or injured, and the clinician's suspicion about the underlying cause. Seizures in early infancy are often symptomatic. Therefore, the younger the child, the more extensive must be the diagnostic assessment (Table 25–8).

It is generally accepted that every child with new onset of unprovoked seizures should be evaluated with an EEG, although this need not be done emergently. An EEG is very unlikely to yield clinically useful information in the child with a febrile seizure. Other diagnostic studies should be used selectively.

Metabolic abnormalities are seldom found in the well child with seizures. Unless there is a high clinical suspicion of serious medical conditions (eg, uremia, hyponatremia, hypocalcemia, etc), "routine" laboratory tests rarely yield clinically significant information. Special studies may be necessary in circumstances that suggest an acute systemic etiology for a seizure, for example, in the presence of apparent renal failure, sepsis, or substance abuse.

Emergent imaging of the brain is usually not necessary in the absence evidence of trauma or of acute abnormalities on examination. Nonurgent MRI should be performed in any child with a significant cognitive or motor impairment, or abnormalities on neurologic examination of unknown etiology, a seizure of partial (focal) onset, or an EEG that does not represent benign partial epilepsy of childhood or primary generalized epilepsy, and should be seriously considered in infants younger than 1 year of age.

The child with a simple febrile seizure or a single unprovoked generalized seizure with normal examination often will not require imaging. Clinically significant abnormalities rarely are found on imaging of children with new onset of idiopathic epilepsy syndromes such as benign focal epilepsy of childhood (BECTS or rolandic epilepsy) and absence epilepsy with a normal neurologic examination and diagnostic EEG. Conversely, in children with symptomatic epileptic syndromes such as infantile spasms and Lennox-Gastaut syndrome, MRI (the preferred study) will be abnormal in as many as 60%–80% of patients. Evidence of localization-related epilepsy is an indication for MRI of the brain. Imaging is not necessary in children with BECTS, but the yield with other focal seizures is 15%–30%, with findings supportive of the diagnosis (eg, focal cortical dysplasia) and useful in defining the prognosis. Other indications for MRI scan include difficulty in controlling seizures, progressive neurologic findings on serial examinations, worsening focal findings on the EEG, or other evidence of progressive neurologic dysfunction, even in the instance where a prior imaging study was normal.

C. Electroencephalography

Appropriate use of EEG requires awareness of its limitations as well as its utility. The limitations of EEG even with epilepsy, for which it is most useful, are considerable. A routine EEG captures electrical activity during a very short period of time, usually 20–30 minutes. Thus, it is useful primarily for defining interictal activity (except for the fortuitous recording of a clinical seizure or in the case seizures that are easily provoked such as childhood absence epilepsy). A seizure is a clinical phenomenon; an EEG showing epileptiform activity may confirm and clarify the clinical diagnosis (for instance, defining an epilepsy syndrome), but it is only occasionally diagnostic.

1. Diagnostic value—The greatest value of the EEG in convulsive disorders is to help classify seizure types and epilepsy syndromes. This can aid in prognostication and in selecting appropriate therapy (see Table 25–6). It is sometimes difficult to distinguish between hypomotor seizures due to generalized absence epilepsy vs localization-related epilepsy. The differing EEG patterns of these seizures will then prove most helpful. The presence of a mixed seizure EEG pattern in a child with clinically generalized convulsive seizures or only focal seizures may lead to identification of specific epilepsy syndromes and help the clinician select anticonvulsants effective for the seizure types identified by the EEG. Similarly, the EEG may help in diagnosing seizures in a young infant with minimal or atypical clinical manifestations; it may show hypsarrhythmia (high-amplitude spikes and slow waves with a chaotic background) in infantile spasms or the 1–4/s slow spike-wave pattern of the Lennox-Gastaut syndrome. The EEG may show focal slowing that, if constant, particularly when corresponding focal seizure manifestations and abnormal neurologic findings, will alert the physician to the presence of a structural lesion. In this case, brain imaging may establish the cause and help determine further investigation and treatment.

The EEG need not be abnormal in a child with epilepsy. Normal EEGs are seen following a first generalized seizure in one-third of children younger than age 4 years. The initial EEG is normal in about 20% of older children with epilepsy and in about 10% of adults with epilepsy. These percentages are reduced when serial tracings are obtained especially if sleep-deprived. Focal spikes and generalized spike-wave discharges are seen in 30% of close nonepileptic relatives of patients with epilepsy.

2. Prognostic value—EEG following febrile seizures is almost always normal and is not clearly predictive of subsequent seizures and therefore is not useful in these situations. Hypsarrhythmia or slow spike and wave patterns support the diagnosis of infantile spasms and Lennox-Gastaut syndrome, respectively. Both are expressions of diffuse brain dysfunction (epileptic encephalopathy) and are generally of grave significance. Central-temporal (rolandic spikes) and occipital spike-wave activity (occipital paroxysms) are the EEG correlates of idiopathic focal epilepsies of childhood.

Following successful treatment, abnormal EEGs may become normal and may aid in the decision to discontinue medications. The normalization of the EEG in childhood absence epilepsy confirms the efficacy of treatment. Normalization can also be seen in infants with infantile spasms who have been successfully treated and, less commonly, in children with epileptic encephalopathies.

EEG should be repeated when the severity and frequency of seizures increase despite adequate anticonvulsant therapy, when the clinical seizure pattern changes significantly, or when progressive neurologic deficits develop. Emergence of new focal or diffuse slowing may indicate a progressive lesion or neurodegenerative disorder.

Table 25–8. Diagnostic evaluation in seizures.

After a first seizure	
Well infant (not neonatal)	Urgent imaging if persistent abnormal neurologic examination (especially Todd paresis), or concern about trauma (rule out nonaccidental trauma). EEG (may be deferred unless concern about nonconvulsive status epilepticus). If clinical suspicion, calcium, BUN, or others.
Well older child	Same as above.
Ill infant	Depending on presentation consider CT, Ca^{2+}, Mg^{2+}, CBC, BUN, glucose, electrolytes, blood culture, lumbar puncture performed acutely. Nonurgent EEG (emergent if concern about nonconvulsive status epilepticus). Possibly MRI.
Ill older child	Depending on presentation consider CT, CBC, BUN, lumbar puncture. Nonurgent EEG. Possibly MRI.
Generalized tonic-clonic seizure	Practice parameter: EEG only. Circumstances may suggest need for toxicology screen, calcium, glucose, CBC, BUN, electrolytes, lumbar puncture, and others if concern about infection (especially HSV).
For new-onset epilepsy (2 or more unprovoked seizures)	
Infant (< 1 y)	Imaging (MRI is preferred study); EEG. Consider evaluation for inherited metabolic disorder: lumbar puncture including CSF (and serum) glucose, lactate, glycine; serum and urine amino and organic acids; high-resolution chromosome analysis; other genetic testing.
Older child	EEG; imaging (MRI). Other evaluation dependant on epilepsy syndrome. Consider CBC and AST before initiation of treatment.
Childhood absence seizure	EEG only.
Symptomatic/cryptogenic generalized epilepsy (Lennox-Gastaut and variants; Dravet syndrome and other myoclonic epilepsies)	EEG. Evaluation for causes of mental retardation: MRI; serum and urine amino and organic acids; chromosomal microarray vs high-resolution chromosome analysis; other genetic testing as indicated per patient, consider biopsy (skin, conjunctiva) for neuronal ceroid lipofuscinosis (NCL). Consider lysosomal enzymes, lumbar puncture including glucose (CSF and serum) lactate, glycine, neurotransmitters, long-chain fatty acids, skin or conjunctival biopsies.
Infantile spasms	Consider tuberous sclerosis complex (including Wood lamp, MRI, renal and cardiac scans). Evaluation as for symptomatic generalized epilepsy.
Cryptogenic focal epilepsy	EEG including video-EEG monitoring if necessary for clarification of diagnosis. MRI with attention to possible focal cortical dysplasia.
Idiopathic focal epilepsy (BECTS)	EEG.

AST, aspartate aminotransferase; BECTS, benign epilepsy with centrotemporal spikes; BUN, blood urea nitrogen; CBC, complete blood count; CSF, cerebrospinal fluid; CT, computed tomography; EEG, electroencephalogram; HSV, herpes simples virus; MRI, magnetic resonance imaging.

The EEG may be helpful in determining when to discontinue anticonvulsant therapy. The presence or absence of epileptiform activity on the EEG prior to withdrawal of anticonvulsants after a seizure-free period of 2 years on medications has been shown to correlate with the degree of risk of seizure recurrence. However, persistent focal epileptiform discharges are common in children with so-called benign epilepsies until they resolve spontaneously in adolescence.

▶ Differential Diagnosis

It is extremely important to be accurate in the diagnosis of epilepsy and not to make the diagnosis without ample proof. To the layperson, epilepsy often has connotations of brain damage and limitation of activity. A person so diagnosed may be excluded from certain occupations in later life. It is often very difficult to change an inaccurate diagnosis of many years' standing.

Misinterpretation of behaviors in children is the most common reason for misdiagnosis. Psychogenic seizures are much less common in children than in adults but must be considered even in the young or cognitively impaired child. The most commonly misinterpreted behaviors are inattention in school-aged children with attention disorders, stereotypies in children with autistic spectrum disorder, sleep-related movements, habit movements such as head-banging and so-called infantile masturbation (sometimes referred to as gratification movements), and gastroesophageal reflux in very young (often impaired) infants.

Some of the common nonepileptic events that mimic seizure disorder are listed in Table 25–9.

Table 25–9. Nonepileptic paroxysmal events.

Breath-holding attacks (cyanotic and pallid) (see below)

Cyanotic: Age 6 mo–3 y. Always precipitated by trauma and fright. Cyanosis; sometimes stiffening, tonic (or jerking-clonic) convulsion (anoxic seizure). Patient may sleep following attack. Family history positive in 30%. Electroencephalogram (EEG) is not useful. No medication treatment is useful but interpretation and reassurance are very important.

Pallid: Usually, there is no apparent precipitant although fright may precipitate. Pallor may be followed by seizure (anoxic-ischemic). Vagally mediated (heart-slowing), like adult syncope. EEG is not useful.

Tics (Tourette syndrome)

Simple or complex stereotyped jerks or movements, coughs, grunts, sniffs. Worse at repose or with stress. May be suppressed during physician visit. Family history often positive for tics or for obsessive compulsive disorder. Diagnosis is clinical. Magnetic resonance imaging (MRI) and EEG are negative. Medications may benefit.

Parasomnias (night terrors, sleep talking, walking, "sit-ups")

Ages 3–10 y. Usually occur in first sleep cycle (30–90 min after going to sleep), with crying, screaming, and autonomic discharge (pupils dilated, perspiring, etc). May last only a few minutes or be more prolonged. Child goes back to sleep and has no recall of event next day. Sleep studies (polysomnogram and EEG) are normal. Sleep talking and walking and short "sit-ups" in bed are fragmentary arousals. If a spell is recorded, EEG shows arousal from deep sleep, but behavior seems wakeful. Child needs to be protected from injury and gradually settled down and taken back to bed. Medications may be considered in rare instances.

Nightmares

Nightmares or vivid dreams occur in subsequent cycles of sleep, often in early morning hours, and generally are partially recalled the next day. The bizarre and frightening behavior may sometimes be confused with complex partial seizures but occurs during REM (rapid eye movement) sleep, whereas epilepsy usually does not. In extreme or difficult cases, an all-night sleep EEG may help differentiate seizures from nightmares. Frontal lobe epilepsy with sleep related "hypermotor" seizures should be considered.

Migraine

On occasion, migraine can be associated with an acute confusional state. Usual migraine prodrome of spots before the eyes, dizziness, visual field defects, followed by headache and then agitated confusion is present. History of other, more typical migraine with severe headache and vomiting but without confusion may aid in diagnosis. Severe headache with vomiting as child comes out of spell may aid in distinguishing the attack from epilepsy. However, partial seizures, while brief, may be associated with more prolonged postictal agitation and confusion. Other seizure manifestations are practically never seen (eg, tonic-clonic movements, falling, complete loss of consciousness). EEG in migraine is usually normal and seldom has epileptiform abnormalities often seen in patients with epilepsy. Migraine and epilepsy are sometimes linked: Benign occipital epilepsy may present with migraine-like visual aura and headache. There may be migraine-caused cortical ischemia which leads to later epilepsy. Postictal headache can be confused with migraine.

Benign nocturnal myoclonus

Common in infants and may last even up to school age. Focal or generalized jerks (the latter also called hypnic or sleep jerks) may persist from onset of sleep on and off all night. A video record for physician review can aid in diagnosis. EEG taken during jerks is normal, proving that these jerks are not epilepsy. Treatment is reassurance.

Shuddering

Shuddering or shivering attacks can occur in infancy and may be a forerunner of essential tremor in later life. Often, family history is positive for tremor. Shivering may be very frequent. EEG is normal. There is no clouding or loss of consciousness.

Gastroesophageal reflux (Sandifer syndrome)

Seen more commonly in children with cerebral palsy or brain damage; reflux of acid gastric contents may cause pain that cannot be described by child. Unusual posturing (dystonic or other) of head and neck or trunk may occur, an apparent attempt to stretch the esophagus or close the opening. There is no loss of consciousness, but eye rolling, apnea, and occasional vomiting may simulate a seizure. An upper gastrointestinal series, cine of swallowing, sometimes even an EEG (normal during episode) may be necessary to distinguish from seizures.

Infantile masturbation/gratification movements

Rarely in infants, repetitive rocking or rubbing motions may simulate seizures. Infant may look out of contact, be poorly responsive to environment, and have autonomic expressions (eg, perspiration, dilated pupils) that may be confused with seizures. Observation by a skilled individual, sometimes even in a hospital setting, may be necessary to distinguish from seizures. EEG is normal between and during attacks. Interpretation and reassurance are the only necessary treatment.

Conversion reaction/psychogenic nonepileptic seizures

Up to 50% of patients with nonepileptic seizures also have epilepsy. Episodes may involve writhing, pelvic thrusting, tonic movements, bizarre jerking and thrashing, or even apparently sudden unresponsiveness. Often, there is ongoing psychological trauma. Children may be developmentally delayed. Spells must often be seen or recorded with a videorecorder to distinguish from epilepsy but are sometimes so bizarre they are easily differentiated. A normal EEG during a spell is a key diagnostic feature. Sometimes, psychogenic seizures can be precipitated by suggestion with injection of normal saline in a controlled situation but this is generally felt to be ethically inappropriate since it involves lying to the patient regarding the reason for the procedure. Combativeness is common; self-injury and incontinence, rare.

Temper tantrums and rage attacks

Child often reports amnesia for events during spell. Attacks are usually precipitated by frustration or anger, often directed either verbally or physically, and subside with behavior modification and isolation. EEGs are generally normal but seldom obtained during an attack. It should be noted that directed violence is very uncommon following partial seizures but severe agitation can occur.

Benign paroxysmal vertigo

Brief attacks of vertigo in which child often appears frightened and pale and clutches parent. Attacks last 5–30 s. Sometimes, nystagmus is identified. There is no loss of consciousness. Usually, child is well and returns to play immediately afterward. Attacks may occur in clusters, and then disappear for months. Attacks are usually seen in infants and preschoolers aged 2–5 y. EEG is normal. If caloric tests can be obtained (often very difficult in this age group), abnormalities with hypofunction of one side are sometimes seen. Medications are usually not desirable or necessary.

Staring spells

Teachers often make referral for absence or "petit mal" seizures in children who stare or seem preoccupied at school. Helpful in the history is the lack of these spells at home (eg, before breakfast, a common time for absence seizures). Lack of other epilepsy in child or family history often is helpful. These children often have difficulties with school and cognitive or learning disabilities. Child can generally be brought out of spell by a firm command or touch. EEG is sometimes necessary to confirm that absence seizures are not occurring. A 24-h ambulatory EEG to record attacks during child's everyday school activities is occasionally necessary.

Complications & Sequelae

A. Psychosocial Impact

Emotional disturbances, especially depression but also including anxiety, anger, and feelings of guilt and inadequacy, often occur in the patient as well as the parents of a child with epilepsy. Actual or perceived stigma as well as issues regarding "disclosure" are common. There is an increased risk of suicide in people with epilepsy. Schools often limit activities of children with epilepsy inappropriately and stigmatize children by these limitations.

Epilepsy with onset in childhood has an impact on adult function. Adults with early onset of epilepsy are less likely to complete high school, have less adequate employment, and are less likely to marry. Persistent epilepsy results in significant dependence; even when epilepsy is successfully treated, patients with long-standing epilepsy often do not become independent due to driving restrictions and safety concerns.

Rarely, psychosis may be seen in patients with epilepsy, usually in older children and adults.

B. Cognitive Delay

Untreated seizures can have an impact on cognition and memory. Clearly, epileptic encephalopathy (ie, regression in cognitive ability and development associated with uncontrolled seizures) does occur, particularly in young children with catastrophic epilepsies such as infantile spasms and Lennox-Gastaut syndrome. Thus, persistent seizures in children under about 3 years of age may be associated with development of cognitive and developmental decline. The impact of persistent partial seizures on development is less clear although persistent temporal lobe seizures in adults is associated with cognitive dysfunction. It is not likely that interictal epileptiform activity contributes to cognitive impairment in most older children, although increased epileptiform burden has been demonstrated to cause mild cognitive problems in some disorders previously thought to be benign such as benign epilepsy with central temporal spikes (BECTS). Continuous epileptiform activity in sleep is associated with Landau-Kleffner syndrome (acquired epileptic aphasia) and the syndrome of Electroencephalographic Status Epilepticus in Slow Wave Sleep (ESES) which are associated with cognitive decline.

Pseudodementia may occur in children with poorly controlled epilepsy because their seizures interfere with their learning. Depression is a common cause of impaired cognitive function in children with epilepsy. Anticonvulsants are less likely to cause such interference at usual therapeutic doses, although phenobarbital topiramate and zonisamide may produce cognitive impairment, reversible on discontinuing the medication.

Cognitive impairment and autistic spectrum disorders may be part of the same pathologic process that causes the seizures and symptoms of these conditions may occasionally be worsened when seizures are frequent or prolonged.

C. Injury and Death

Physical injuries, especially lacerations of the forehead and chin, are frequent in astatic or akinetic seizures (so-called drop attacks), necessitating protective headgear. In all other seizure disorders in childhood, injuries as a direct result of an attack are not as common although drowning, injuries related to working in kitchens, and falls from heights remain a potential risk for all children with active epilepsy. It is therefore extremely important to stress "seizure precautions," in particular, water safety. Bathrooms are a particularly dangerous room for people with uncontrolled epilepsy as the room is usually small and has many hard surfaces. Showers are recommended over bathing as it decreases the likelihood of drowning. Appropriate supervision is recommended.

The greatest fear of a parent of a child with new-onset of epilepsy is the possibility of death or brain injury. There is an increased risk of premature death in patients with symptomatic epilepsy, especially those who have not achieved seizure control Most of the mortality in children with epilepsy is related to the underlying neurologic disorder, not the seizures. Sudden unexpected death with epilepsy (SUDEP) is a very rare event in children. Although children with epilepsy have an increased risk of death, SUDEP is rare (1–2:10,000 patient-years). The greatest risk for SUDEP is in children with medically uncontrolled epilepsy, especially with symptomatic epilepsy (associated with identifiable CNS etiology). There is no current proven strategy to prevent SUDEP other than seizure control. The mechanism for SUDEP is unclear but is probably most commonly related to either cardiac arrhythmia induced by a seizure or sudden respiratory insufficiency. Vigorous attempts to control intractable seizure disorders remain the most important approach. Identifying life-threatening disorders (eg, identifying patients with cardiac arrhythmias, especially prolonged QT syndrome) as the cause of misdiagnosed epilepsy is clearly of utmost importance.

Treatment

The ideal treatment of acute seizures is the correction of specific causes. However, even when a biochemical disorder, a tumor, meningitis, or another specific cause is being treated, anticonvulsant drugs are often still required.

A. First Aid

Caregivers should be instructed to protect the patient against self-injury. Turning the child to the side is useful for preventing aspiration. Thrusting a spoon handle, tongue depressor, or finger into the clenched mouth of a convulsing patient or trying to restrain tonic-clonic movements may cause worse injuries than a bitten tongue or bruised limb and could potentially become a choking hazard. Parents are often concerned that cyanosis will occur during generalized convulsive seizures but it is rare for clinically significant hypoxia to occur. Mouth-to-mouth resuscitation is rarely necessary and is unlikely to be effective.

For prolonged seizures (those lasting over 5 minutes), acute home treatment with benzodiazepines such as rectal diazepam gel (Diastat) or intranasal midazolam may be administered to prevent the development of status epilepticus. Diastat has proven to be safe even when administered by nonmedical professionals, including teachers and day care providers, when appropriately instructed.

B. Antiepileptic Drug (AED) Therapy

1. Drug selection—Treat with the drug appropriate to the clinical situation, as outlined in Table 25–10.

2. Treatment strategy—The child with a single seizure has a 50% chance of recurrence. Thus, it is usually not necessary to initiate AED therapy until the diagnosis of epilepsy is established, that is, there is a second seizure. The seizure type and epilepsy syndrome as well as potential side effects will determine which drug to initiate (see Table 25–10). Start with one drug in moderate dosage and increase the dosage until seizures are controlled. If seizures are not controlled on the maximal tolerated dosage of one major AED, gradually switch to another before using two-drug therapy. Polytherapy (ie, the use of more than two medications concurrently) is rarely sufficiently effective to warrant the considerable risk of adverse side effects from the synergistic impact of multiple medications.

Dosages and usually target serum levels of commonly prescribed AEDs are listed in Table 25–10. Individual variations must be expected, both in tolerance and efficacy. The therapeutic range may also vary somewhat with the method used to determine levels, and published levels are not always reflective of clinical efficacy and tolerability.

For newer drugs, doses, levels, and adverse effects are based on reported clinical experience and not on adequate scientific information from clinical trials in most cases. Some medications do not have FDA approval for children. The package insert for each medication lists indications, potential adverse effects, warnings, and so on. Practitioners should with familiar with current published information as regards specific dosing, as well as potential adverse effects.

3. Counseling—Advise the parents and the patient that the prolonged use of AEDs will not produce significant or permanent mental slowing (although the underlying cause of the seizures might) and that prevention of seizures for 1–2 years substantially reduces the chances of recurrence. Advise them also that AEDs are given to prevent further seizures and that they should be taken as prescribed. Changes in medications or dosages should not be made without the physician's knowledge. Unsupervised sudden withdrawal of AEDs may precipitate severe seizures or even status epilepticus. Medications must be kept where they cannot be ingested by small children or suicidal patients.

Older children should be encouraged to manage their medications on their own, but some degree of supervision by parents is often necessary to guarantee adherence to treatment regimens. Medications are invariably missed on occasions. Making up a single dose is reasonable, but making up multiple doses should be discouraged.

4. Follow-up—Regular follow-up evaluations of the patient are appropriate at intervals that depend on the degree of control, underlying cause of the seizures, and toxic properties of the AEDs used. Blood counts and liver function tests (aspartate aminotransferase; AST) are often obtained periodically in patients taking the older AEDs, such as valproate, phenytoin, and carbamazepine. Routine determination of serum AED levels is not necessary in patients with controlled seizures but levels should be obtained to direct care, for instance, confirming adherence to medication recommendations. Periodic neurologic reevaluation is important. Repeat EEGs are useful for confirming seizure-freedom in children with absence of epilepsy and West syndrome, but otherwise are usually not useful as measures of medication efficacy.

5. Long-term management and discontinuation of treatment—AEDs should be continued until the patient is free of seizures for at least 1–2 years. In about 75% of patients, seizures will not recur following discontinuation of medication after 2 years of remission. Variables such as younger age at onset, normal EEG, idiopathic etiology, and ease of controlling seizures carry a favorable prognosis, whereas symptomatic etiology, later onset, continued epileptiform EEG, difficulty in establishing initial control of the seizures, polytherapy, generalized tonic-clonic or myoclonic seizures, as well as an abnormal neurologic examination are associated with a higher risk of recurrence. Most AEDs (with the exception of barbiturates and clonazepam) can be withdrawn over 6–8 weeks. There does not appear to be an advantage to slower withdrawal.

Recurrent seizures affect up to 25% of children who attempt withdrawal from medications. Recurrence of seizures is most likely within 6–12 months of discontinuing medications. Therefore, seizure safety precautions will need to be reinstituted, including driving restriction. If seizures recur during or after withdrawal, AED therapy should be reinstituted and maintained for at least another 1–2 years. The vast majority of children will again achieve remission of their seizures.

6. Blood levels of AEDs

A. General comments—Most AEDs take two or three times their half-life to reach the target serum levels indicated in Table 25–10. This must be considered when blood levels are assessed after AEDs are started or dosages are changed. Individuals vary in their metabolism and their particular pharmacokinetic characteristics. These and external factors, including, for example, food intake or illness, also affect the blood level. Thus, the level reached on a milligram per kilogram basis varies among patients. Experience and clinical research in the determination of AED blood levels have shown that there is some correlation between (1) drug dose and blood level, (2) blood level and therapeutic effect, and (3) blood level and some toxic effects.

Table 25–10. Guide to AED use (2009).

Medication/Target Dose in Adults [Pediatric Dose mg/kg/d]	Target Serum Levels (mcg/mL)	Idiosyncratic	Dose Related	Age Specific/Other
Carbamazepine 1000–2000 [10–30]	4–12	Dermatologic (rash, including Stevens-Johnson), rare, hematologic, hepatic	Vertigo, visual disturbance (diplopia), leukopenia	Hyponatremia in adults; leukopenia; liver induction; myoclonus in patients with general S/W
Clobazam 5–80 [2 y, 0.5–1; 2–16 y, 5–40]	–		Ataxia, sedation,	Paradoxical reaction with aggressive behavior, withdrawal symptoms with abrupt cessation
Ethosuximide 1000 [15–40]	40–100	Leukopenia, SLE, nephrotic syndrome, rash	Sedation, GI upset	Behavioral
Felbamate 2400–3600 [45–60]	30–100	Aplastic anemia, hepatic failure, rash (rare)	Anorexia, insomnia, headache, irritability	Aplastic anemia; drug interactions
Gabapentin 1800–3600 [30–100]	4–20	Rash (rare)	Somnolence, irritability, weight gain	Renal excretion, no drug interactions
Lacosamide 200–400	–	Prolonged PR interval, hypersensitivity reaction	Dizziness, ataxia, nausea, diplopia	? Interferes with neuronal plasticity
Lamotrigine 300–500 [1–15] (dose depends on concomitant medication)	3–20	Rash, hypersensitivity reaction	Ataxia, diplopia, GI, headache	Rash (1–5% in children), Stevens-Johnson
Levetiracetam 1200–2400 [20–60]	5–50	None reported to date	Somnolence, ataxia	Agitation, aggression, depression
Oxcarbazepine 1200–2400 [15–45]	MHD-10–55	Rash (25% cross-reactivity with CBZ)	CNS, diplopia	Hyponatremia (3% of adults)
Phenytoin 200–600 [4–8]	10–20	Rash (5–10%), hematologic, hepatic, lymphadenopathy others	Cosmetic, CNS, ataxia, nystagmus	Elevated LFTs, induction, reduced vitamin D, cerebellar degeneration?
Phenobarbital 60–120 [2–6]	15–40	Rash, Stevens-Johnson, SLE	Somnolence, irritability	Possible irreversible cognitive effects, liver induction
Primidone 750–2000 [5–20]	4–12	Rash	Sedation, irritability, GI upset	Similar to PB
Rufinamide 400–3200 [10–45]	–	Hypersensitivity reaction	Sedation, headache, behavioral disturbance, shortened QT interval	
Tiagabine 32–56 [0.25–1.25]	5–70	Psychiatric	CNS, tremor, weakness, GE reflux, gait difficulty	
Topiramate 200–400 [5–25]	3–25	Rash (rare), acute glaucoma (rare)	Somnolence, memory disturbance, renal stones anorexia, paresthesia	Language and cognitive disturbance (especially polypharmacy); oligohidrosis
Valproic acid 750–1500 [20–60]	50–150	Hepatic failure; pancreatitis	Tremor, weight gain, alopecia, sedation and cognitive changes, thrombocytopenia, prolonged bleeding time	Hepatic failure (1/500 younger than age 2 on polypharmacy), elevated LFTs; GI upset with syrup; incidence of PCOS unknown, liver enzyme inhibition; teratogenicity
Vigabatrin Max 3000 [40–100]	–	Visual field constriction, sedation, CNS	Psychiatric symptoms (rare), visual field constriction	Especially effective for infantile spasms and tuberous sclerosis
Zonisamide 200–600 [4–10]	10–30	Rash, hematologic, hepatic	Renal stones, anorexia, somnolence	Oligohidrosis in children; cross-sensitivity with sulfa drugs

CBZ, carbamazepine; CNS, central nervous system; GE, gastroesophageal; GI, gastrointestinal; LFT, liver function test; MHD, monohydroxy derivative; PCOS, polycystic ovary syndrome; SLE, systemic lupus erythematosus; S/W, spike and wave discharges.

Note: For newer drugs, doses, levels, and adverse effects are based on reported clinical experience and not on adequate scientific information from clinical trials in most cases. Some medications do not have FDA approval for children. The package insert for each medication lists potential adverse effects, warnings, and other important considerations.

B. Effective levels—The target serum levels listed in Table 25–10 are those within which seizure control without toxicity will be achieved in most patients. The level for any given individual will vary not only with metabolic makeup (including biochemical defects) but also with the nature and severity of the seizures and their underlying cause, and with other medications being taken, among other factors. Seizure control may be achieved at lower levels in some patients, and higher levels may be reached without toxicity in others. When control is achieved at a lower level, the dosage should not be increased merely to move the level into the therapeutic range. Likewise, toxic side effects will be experienced at different levels even within the therapeutic range. Lowering the dosage may relieve the problem, but sometimes the drug must be withdrawn or another added (or both). Some serious toxic effects, including allergic reactions and bone marrow or liver toxicity, are independent of dosage ("idiosyncratic").

C. Interaction of AEDs—Blood levels of older AEDs may be affected by other drugs but this is less often the case with the newer medications. In addition to pharmacokinetic interaction, pharmacodynamic interactions may be observed, with increased side effects despite "therapeutic" levels. Likewise, adverse effects noted with introduction of a second medication may be due to drug interactions and not to toxicity of the newly introduced medication per se.

D. Indications for determination of blood levels—There is rarely an indication for obtaining "routine" blood levels of AEDs. Thus, levels should be determined for specific reasons. After a drug is introduced and seizure control is achieved, it may be useful to determine the effective level for that patient. Blood level monitoring is also useful when expected control on a usual dosage has not been achieved, when seizures recur in a patient with previously well-controlled seizures, or when there is a question of adherence to recommended treatment ("noncompliance"). A low level may indicate inadequate dosage, drug interaction, or nonadherence with the prescribed regimen. A high level may indicate slowed metabolism or excretion or drug interaction.

Blood levels are most commonly obtained when signs and symptoms of toxicity are present, especially when more than one drug is being used or when the dosage of a single drug has been changed. Blood levels may be the only means of detecting intoxication in a comatose patient, very young child, or child with severe cognitive impairment. Toxic levels also occur with drug abuse and in the presence of liver or renal disease. Blood levels are unnecessary when the patient's seizure control is satisfactory and he or she is free of toxic signs or symptoms.

7. Side effects of AEDs—(See also Table 25–10.)

A. Idiosyncratic reactions—Serious **allergic rash** usually necessitates discontinuance of a drug. The risk of significant allergic rash is probably about 5%–10% with carbamazepine, lamotrigine, oxcarbazepine, and phenobarbital, phenytoin. Stevens-Johnson syndrome is a risk in any child with a cutaneous eruption due to AEDs, although the degree of this risk is unclear. Not every rash in a child receiving an AED is drug related. If a useful AED is discontinued and the rash disappears, restarting the drug in a smaller dosage may be warranted to see if the rash recurs.

Hepatic toxicity, pancreatitis, blood dyscrasias, renal stones, and other adverse **systemic effects** have been reported with various medications. It is not clear that routine surveillance is effective in preventing these complications of treatment. Nevertheless, routine laboratory testing is often undertaken by clinicians managing patients with epilepsy.

Many anticonvulsants may have an adverse effect on bone health leading to decreased bone density. Routine surveillance and intervention as well as monitoring vitamin D levels may be indicated. Some authorities are advocating routine supplementation with vitamin D and calcium.

B. Treatment-emergent toxicity—Signs of **dose-related drug toxicity** such as ataxia often disappear with relatively small decreases in medication dose. The exception is phenytoin, where protein binding and so-called zero-order kinetics can make dose adjustments difficult.

Sedation is the most common treatment-emergent side effect of AED treatment. The sedative effect of many of these drugs may be avoided by slowly titrating mediation to a moderate dose over several weeks.

Familiarity with potential side effects can allow **anticipatory counseling.** Gingival hyperplasia secondary to phenytoin is best minimized through good dental hygiene but occasionally requires gingivectomy. The hypertrichosis associated with phenytoin does not regress when the drug is discontinued. The risk of weight gain with valproate and gabapentin and weight loss with topiramate, zonisamide, and felbamate should be discussed on initiation of treatment. Adequate hydration and avoiding overheating on hot days can prevent the hypothermia associated with hypohidrosis in some patients treated with topiramate and zonisamide.

C. Alternative Treatments

1. Adrenocorticotropic hormone (ACTH) and corticosteroids

A. Indications—ACTH is indicated for treatment of infantile spasms. The utility of other immunotherapy is less clear. Duration of ACTH therapy is guided by cessation of clinical seizures and normalization of the EEG. No specific recommendations can be made regarding dosing and duration of therapy, and multiple protocols have been advocated with initial dosing ranging from 20 IU/d to 150 IU/m^2/d. ACTH is often continued in full doses for 2 or more weeks and then, if seizures have ceased, tapered over a variable length of time, usually several weeks. If seizures recur, the dosage is increased to the last effective level. Some neurologists use longer durations of treatment, keeping the patient at the

TABLE 25–11. Children's Hospital Colorado protocols for acth for west syndrome.

1. High dose protocol: based on surface area of child (needs weight and height)
ACTH 80 units/cc: usually 5 cc vial
wk 1: 75 u/m^2 BID
wk 2: 75 u/m^2 QD
day 15–18: 30 u/m^2 in the am
Day 19–21: 15 u/m^2 in the am
Day 22–25: 10 u/m^2 in the am
Day 26–32: 10 u/m^2 every other am for 6 days
For all patients:
1) Teach parents on how to give injections
2) GI prophylaxis with H2 blocker or PPI (Ranitidine, Omperazol, or Prevacid)
3) Urine analysis prior to the start of the ACTH
4) Three times a wk weight check, blood pressure, and dextrosticks; may require daily urine glucose
5) If hypertension, diuretic and low salt diet. Hypertension is usually short-lived and resolves after weaning ACTH.
6) Bactrim prophylaxis BID three times/wk (Monday, Tuesday, and Wednesday)
7) Immunosuppression precautions: Immunizations held; avoid contagion
8) Consider PPD (48 h prior to starting treatment)

effective dosage of ACTH for up to 6 months before attempting withdrawal. There is no strong evidence, however, that longer courses of treatment are more beneficial.

Oral corticosteroids and intravenous immune globulin (IVIG) are occasionally used for pharmacoresistant epilepsy. However, dosing regimens and indications are not well established.

Landau-Kleffner syndrome (acquired epileptic aphasia) is reported to respond to oral steroid treatment. Anecdotal reports of use of immunosuppression in other patients have been published but no controlled clinical trials have been performed.

B. Dosages—For ACTH (Acthar Gel), start with 40–80 IU/d or up to 150 IU/m^2/d intramuscularly in a single morning dose. Parents can be taught to give injections. For prednisone, start with 2–4 mg/kg/d orally in two or three divided doses. (See Table 25–11.)

C. Precautions—Give additional potassium, guard against infections, follow for possible hypertension, and discuss the cushingoid appearance and its disappearance. Do not withdraw oral corticosteroids suddenly. Side effects in some series occur in up to 40% of patients, especially with higher dosages than those listed here (used by some authorities). With long-term use, prophylaxis against *Pneumocystis* infection may be required. Careful and frequent follow-up is necessary. Visiting nurse services can be very helpful in surveillance such as monitoring blood pressure, weight, and potential adverse effects.

2. Ketogenic diet—A diet high in fat and low in protein and carbohydrates will result in ketosis as fatty acids replace glucose as a source of energy for cellular metabolism. Such a diet has been observed to decrease and even control seizures in some children. A ketogenic diet should be considered for children with pharmacoresistant epilepsy, particularly those with symptomatic generalized epilepsies (especially astatic and myoclonic seizures and absence seizures) not responsive to drug therapy. Other seizure types may also respond. This diet should be monitored very carefully to ensure sufficient protein for body maintenance and growth as well as appropriate vitamin and mineral supplementation. The ratio of fat-derived calories to carbohydrate and protein-derived calories is usually 4:1 but can be lowered if needed for tolerance. Adding medium-chain triglycerides to the diet induces ketosis more readily than does a high level of dietary fats and thus requires less carbohydrate restriction. However, medium chain triglycerides are often not well tolerated.

Recent reports suggest efficacy with a modified Atkins diet or a low-glycemic index diet in older and higher functioning children who will not accept the ketogenic diet. A prepared commercial formula is available for children receiving tube feedings.

The mechanism for the anticonvulsant action of the ketogenic diet is not understood. It is the ketosis, not the acidosis, which raises the seizure threshold. There is still some controversy as to whether low glucose, elevated ketones, or some other factors are most important for seizure control.

The ketogenic diet requires close adherence and is often difficult for families as well as the children who cannot participate in family meals or special occasions (eg, birthday parties where cake is served). Full cooperation of all family members is required. However, when seizure control is achieved by this method, acceptance of the diet is usually excellent. Access to other families and patients via Internet has provided support and is particularly useful for providing increased variation of meals for families.

As with all therapies, potential adverse effects can occur with the ketogenic diet. These include acidosis and hypoglycemia, particularly on initiation of the diet. Thus, it is prudent to admit the child for initiation of the diet after screening laboratory studies are performed to rule out underlying metabolic disorders. Renal stones, pancreatitis, and acidosis can occur. In addition, vitamin and minerals need to be followed carefully to avoid deficiencies especially carnitine, iron, and vitamin D.

3. Vagus nerve stimulator (VNS)—The VNS is a pacemaker-like device that is implanted below the clavicle on the left and attached to the left vagus nerve. A cycle of electrical stimulation of the nerve is established (typically 30 seconds of stimulation every 5 minutes), which has an antiepileptic effect, reducing seizures by at least 50% in over half the children so treated. In addition, an emergency mode that is activated by the use of a magnet may interrupt a seizure (ie, an anticonvulsant effect). For patients with sufficient warning of an impending seizure, the device can be activated with abortion of the seizure. Many patients also experience an improvement in learning and behavior with use of this device. With current technology, the battery in the stimulator will last 7 or more years in many patients.

D. Surgery

An evaluation for epilepsy surgery is indicated for all children with medically intractable partial epilepsy. The evaluation and surgery should be performed at a center with expertise in epilepsy surgery and which has a dedicated neurosurgeon as well as a team of physicians and other providers with experience in epilepsy surgery.

The first surgery for treatment of epilepsy took place over 100 years ago, and surgery is now established as an appropriate treatment option for adults and children with epilepsy refractory to medical treatment. Evaluation for possible surgical treatment should begin as soon as it is apparent that a child with focal onset seizures is not responding to standard therapy. Medication resistant ("refractory") epilepsy is usually defined as failure of two or three antiepileptic drugs alone or as combination therapy to control seizures. Advances in technology allow for definition and removal of the epileptogenic focus even in young infants. Many centers now have access to video-EEG monitoring, positron emission tomography (PET), single photon emission computerized tomography (SPECT), and similar noninvasive techniques that can be used to identify lesions such as cortical dysplasias that are amenable to resection. Freedom from seizures is reported in as many as 80% who have been treated surgically. Some patients such as those with Rasmussen encephalitis or extensive perinatal strokes may be candidates for hemispherectomy. Increasingly, surgery is being performed on children with tuberous sclerosis after identification of the epileptogenic tuber.

Corpus callosotomy remains an option for children who are experiencing uncontrolled drop attacks. A marked reduction in injuries due to seizure-related falls is usually seen.

E. General Management of the Child with Epilepsy

1. Education—The initial diagnosis of epilepsy is often devastating for families. The patient and parents must be helped to understand the nature of epilepsy and its management, including etiology, prognosis, safety issues, and treatment options.

Excellent educational materials are available for families of a child with epilepsy, both in print and online. Two excellent web sites are http://www.epilepsyfoundation.org and http://www.epilepsy.com. Materials on epilepsy—including pamphlets, monographs, films, and videotapes suitable for children and teenagers, parents, teachers, and medical professionals—may be purchased through the Epilepsy Foundation: 8301 Professional Place, Landover, MD 20785; (800) 332–1000. The foundation's local chapter and other community organizations are able to provide guidance and other services. Support groups exist in many cities for older children and adolescents and for their parents and others concerned.

2. Privileges and precautions in daily life—"*No seizures and no side effects*" is a motto established by the Epilepsy Foundation. The child should be encouraged to live as normal a life as possible. Children should engage in physical activities appropriate to their age and social group. After seizure control is established, swimming is generally permissible with a buddy system or adequate lifeguard coverage. Scuba diving, gymnastic activities involving heights, and high climbing without safety harness should not be permitted. There are no absolute contraindications to any other sports, although some physicians recommend against contact sports. Physical training and sports are usually to be welcomed rather than restricted. Driving is discussed in the next section.

Emotional disturbances, especially depression, are not uncommon, particularly in adolescents with epilepsy, and need to be treated. Loss of sleep should be avoided as sleep deprivation can be a trigger for seizures. Alcohol intake should be avoided because it may precipitate seizures. Prompt attention should be given to intercurrent illnesses as these can trigger seizures.

Although every effort should be made to control seizures, treatment must not interfere with a child's ability to function normally. A child may do better having an occasional mild seizure than being so heavily sedated that function at home, in school, or at play is impaired. Therapy and medication adjustment often require much art and fortitude on the physician's part. Some patients with infrequent seizures, especially if only nocturnal partial seizures (eg, Rolandic seizures) may not need treatment with AEDs.

3. Driving—Driving becomes important to most young people at age 15 or 16 years. Restrictions for persons with epilepsy and other disturbances of consciousness vary from state to state. In most states, a learner's permit or driver's license will be issued to an individual with epilepsy if he or she has been under a physician's care and free of seizures for at least 1 year provided that the treatment or basic neurologic problems do not interfere with the ability to drive. A guide to this and other legal matters pertaining to persons with epilepsy is published by the Epilepsy Foundation, and its legal department may be able to provide additional information.

4. Pregnancy—Contraception (especially interaction of oral contraceptive with some AEDs), childbearing, potential teratogenicity of AEDs, and the management of pregnancy should be discussed as soon as appropriate with the adolescent young woman with epilepsy. Daily use of vitamin preparations containing folic acid is recommended. For the pregnant teenager with epilepsy, management by an obstetrician conversant with the use of AEDs in pregnancy is appropriate. The patient should be cautioned against discontinuing her medications during pregnancy. The possibility of teratogenic effects of AEDs, such as facial clefts (two to three times increased risk), must be weighed against the risks from seizures. All AEDs appear to have some risk for teratogenicity, although valproate carries a particularly high risk for spinal dysraphism as well as being associated with cognitive issues in children exposed to valproate in utero. Dosing may need to be adjusted frequently during pregnancy as blood volume expands. Frequent AED blood levels may be helpful in making these adjustments.

5. School intervention and seizure response plans— Schools are required by federal law to work with parents to establish a seizure action plan for their child with epilepsy. A template for such a plan is available on the Epilepsy Foundation web site at http://www.epilepsyfoundation.org/programs/upload/snactionplan.pdf. These plans usually require the approval of the child's physician. Schools are sometimes hesitant to administer Diastat or to activate the vagal nerve stimulator. Often, information from the physician especially that obtained from the Epilepsy Foundation web site will relieve anxieties. School authorities should be encouraged to avoid needless restrictions and to address the emotional and educational needs of all children with disabilities, including epilepsy. The local affiliates of the Epilepsy Foundation can often provide support for families in their interactions with the school.

2. Status Epilepticus

Status epilepticus is usually defined as a clinical or electrical seizure lasting at least 15 minutes, or a series of seizures without complete recovery over a 30-minute period. After 30 minutes of seizure activity, hypoxia and acidosis occur, with depletion of energy stores, cerebral edema, and structural damage. Eventually, high fever, hypotension, respiratory depression, and even death may occur. Status epilepticus is a medical emergency. Aggressive treatment of prolonged seizures may prevent development status epilepticus. It is generally recommended that treatment with benzodiazepines at home for prolonged seizures be initiated, 5 minutes after onset of a seizure.

Status epilepticus is classified as (1) convulsive (the common tonic-clonic, or grand mal, status epilepticus) or (2) nonconvulsive (characterized by altered mental status or behavior with subtle or absent motor components). Absence status, or spike-wave stupor, and complex partial status epilepticus are examples of the nonconvulsive type. An EEG may be necessary to aid in diagnosing nonconvulsive status because patients sometimes appear merely stuporous and lack typical convulsive movements.

▶ Clinical Findings

Studies suggest that 25%–75% of children with epilepsy will present with status epilepticus as their initial event. A child with status epilepticus may have a high fever with or without intracranial infection. So-called "benign" febrile seizures may present with recurrent seizures or status epilepticus. The child who presents with status epilepticus as the first febrile seizure is more likely to experience status with subsequent febrile seizures, should they occur. Status epilepticus can be a reflection of an acute or remote insult. Tumor and stroke, which are common causes of status epilepticus in adults, are uncommon causes in childhood. Fifty percent of pediatric status epilepticus is due to acute (25%) or chronic (25%) CNS disorders. Infection and metabolic disorders are common causes of status epilepticus in children. The cause is unknown in 50% of patients. In the child with known epilepsy, medication nonadherence to the prescribed medication regimen should be considered. There is a small number of children with epilepsy who experience frequent episodes of status epilepticus. Status epilepticus occurs most commonly in children aged 5 years and younger (85%). The most common age is 1 year or younger (37%); the distribution is even for each year thereafter (approximately 12% per year).

▶ Treatment

For treatment options, see Table 25–12.

3. Febrile Seizures

Criteria for febrile seizures are (1) age 3 months to 6 years (most occur between ages 6 and 18 months), (2) fever of greater than 38.8°C, and (3) non-CNS infection. More than 90% of febrile seizures are generalized, last less than 5 minutes, and occur early in the illness causing the fever. Febrile seizures occur in 2%–3% of children. Acute respiratory illnesses are most commonly associated with febrile seizures. Gastroenteritis, especially when caused by *Shigella* or *Campylobacter*, and urinary tract infections are less common causes. Roseola infantum is a rare but classic cause. One study implicated viral causes in 86% of cases. Immunizations may be a cause. It is very important, especially in younger children, to exclude CNS infection as a source; these children are not classified as having a febrile seizure.

Rarely febrile seizures may present with status epilepticus. Febrile seizures rarely (1%–3%) lead to recurrent unprovoked seizures (epilepsy) in later childhood and adult life (risk is increased two- to fivefold compared with children who do not have febrile seizures). The chance of later epilepsy is higher if the febrile seizures have complex features, such as duration longer than 15 minutes, more than one seizure in the same day, or focal features. Other adverse factors are an abnormal neurologic status preceding the seizures (eg, cerebral palsy or mental retardation), early onset of febrile seizure (before age 1 year), and a family history of epilepsy. Even with adverse factors, the risk of epilepsy after febrile seizures is still only in the range of 15%–20%, although it is increased if more than one risk factor is present. Recurrent febrile seizures occur in 30%–50% of cases. Therefore, families should be prepared to expect more seizures. In general, recurrence of febrile seizures does not worsen the long-term outlook.

Table 25–12. Status epilepticus treatment.

1. ABCs a. Airway: maintain oral airway; intubation may be necessary. b. Breathing: oxygen. c. Circulation: assess pulse, blood pressure; support with IV fluids, drugs. Monitor vital signs.
2. Start glucose-containing IV (unless patient is on ketogenic diet); evaluate serum glucose; electrolytes, HCO_3^-, CBC, BUN, anticonvulsant levels.
3. Consider arterial blood gases, pH.
4. Give 50% glucose if serum glucose low (1–2 mL/kg).
5. Begin IV drug therapy; goal is to control status epilepticus in 20–60 min. a. Diazepam, 0.3–0.5 mg/kg over 1–5 min (20 mg max); may repeat in 5–20 min; or lorazepam, 0.05–0.2 mg/kg (less effective with repeated doses, longer-acting than diazepam); or midazolam: IV, 0.1–0.2 mg/kg; intranasally, 0.2 mg/kg. b. Phenytoin, 10–20 mg/kg IV (not IM) over 5–20 min; (1000 mg maximum); monitor with blood pressure and ECG. Fosphenytoin may be given more rapidly in the same dosage and can be given IM; order 10–20 mg/kg of "phenytoin equivalent" (PE) c. Phenobarbital, 5–20 mg/kg (sometimes higher in newborns or refractory status in intubated patients).
6. Correct metabolic perturbations (eg, low-sodium, acidosis). Administer fluids judiciously.
7. Other drug approaches in refractory status: a. Repeat phenytoin, phenobarbital (10 mg/kg). Monitor blood levels. Support respiration, blood pressure as necessary. b. Other medications: Valproate sodium, available as 100 mg/mL for IV use; give 15–30 mg/kg over 5–20 min. c. Levetiracetam may be helpful (20–40 mg/kg/dose IV) d. For patients who fail initial intervention consider: midazolam drip: 1–5 mcg/kg/min (even to 20 kg/min); pentobarbital coma; Propofol and general anesthetic.
8. Consider underlying causes: a. Structural disorders or trauma: MRI or CT scan. b. Infection: lumbar puncture, blood culture, antibiotics. c. Metabolic disorders: consider lactic acidosis, toxins, and uremia if child is being treated with chronic AEDs, obtain medication levels. Toxin screen.
9. Initiate maintenance drug treatment with IV medications: phenytoin (10 mg/kg); phenobarbital (5 mg/kg); valproate IV 30 mg/kg; levetiracetam 20–30 mg/kg/. Transition to oral medication when patient can safely take them.

BUN, blood urea nitrogen; CBC, complete blood count; CT, computed tomography; ECG, electrocardiogram; IM, intramuscularly; IV, intravenously; MRI, magnetic resonance imaging.

Generalized epilepsy with febrile seizures plus (GEFS+) is an autosomal dominant form of epilepsy first described in 1997. The most frequently observed GEFS+ phenotype includes childhood onset of multiple febrile seizures persisting beyond the age of 6 years, and unprovoked (afebrile) seizures, including absence, myoclonic, or atonic seizures, and rarely, myoclonic-astatic epilepsy. Originally associated with a point mutation in *SCN1B*, GEFS+ is now known to have other channelopathies.

Clinical Findings

A. Diagnostic Evaluation

The child with a febrile seizure must be evaluated for the source of the fever, in particular to exclude CNS infection. Routine studies such as serum electrolytes, glucose, calcium, skull radiographs, or brain imaging studies are seldom helpful. A white count above 20,000/μL or an extreme left shift may correlate with bacteremia. Complete blood count and blood cultures may be appropriate. Serum sodium is often slightly low but not low enough to require treatment or to cause the seizure. Meningitis and encephalitis must be considered. Signs of meningitis (eg, bulging fontanelle, stiff neck, stupor, and irritability) may all be absent, especially in a child younger than age 18 months.

B. Lumbar Puncture

After controlling the fever and stopping an ongoing seizure, the physician must decide whether to do a lumbar puncture. The fact that the child has had a previous febrile seizure does not rule out meningitis as the cause of the current episode. The younger the child, the more important is the procedure because physical findings are less reliable in diagnosing meningitis. Although the yield is low, a lumbar puncture should probably be done if the child is younger than age 18 months, if recovery is slow, if no other cause for the fever is found, or if close follow-up will not be possible. Occasionally observation in the emergency department for several hours obviates the need for a lumbar puncture. A negative finding does not exclude the possibility of emergence of CNS infection during the same febrile illness. Sometimes a second procedure must be done.

C. EEG

EEG is rarely useful. An EEG may be considered if the febrile seizure is complicated, focal, or otherwise unusual, but has little predictive value. In uncomplicated febrile seizures, the EEG is usually normal. If performed, the EEG should be done at least a week after the illness to avoid transient changes due to fever or the seizure itself. In older children, 3/s spike-wave discharges, suggestive of a genetic propensity to epilepsy, may occur. In the young infant, EEG findings seldom aid in assessing the chance of recurrence of febrile seizures or in long-term prognosis, 2 weeks from the time of the presenting event. Thus, EEG is not recommended for the child with simple febrile seizures.

Treatment & Prognosis

Prophylactic anticonvulsants are not recommended after a febrile seizure.

If febrile seizures are complicated or prolonged, or if medical reassurance fails to relieve family anxiety, anticonvulsant prophylaxis may be indicated and appropriately chosen medication may reduce the incidence of recurrent febrile seizures. Only phenobarbital and valproic acid have demonstrated efficacy in preventing febrile seizures; phenytoin and carbamazepine have been show to be ineffective. Newer antiepileptic drugs have not been studied. Diazepam started at the first onset of fever for the duration of the febrile illness (0.5 mg/kg two or three times per day orally or rectally) may be effective but will sedate a child and possibly complicate the evaluation for a source of the fever. Prophylactic diazepam is also limited by the fact that a seizure is often the first evidence of fever associated with an acute illness. Diastat (rectal diazepam gel) can be used to prevent febrile status epilepticus in the child with a prolonged febrile seizure (one lasting over 5 minutes), often the greatest concern.

Phenobarbital, 3–5 mg/kg/d as a single bedtime dose, is an inexpensive long-term prophylaxis. However, significant behavioral disturbance is seen in about one-third of toddlers treated with phenobarbital. Often, increasing the dosage gradually (eg, starting with 2 mg/kg/d the first week, increasing to 3 mg/kg/d the second week, and so on) decreases side effects and nonadherence. A plasma phenobarbital level in the range of 15–40 mg/mL is desirable. Intermittent use of phenobarbital is not recommended as febrile seizures typically occur at the onset of a febrile illness, and several doses of phenobarbital must be given to obtain adequate blood levels.

Valproate sodium is an alternative with fewer behavioral sequelae but may have greater risks for idiosyncratic side effects in the younger child. In infants, the commonly used liquid suspension has a short half-life and causes more gastrointestinal upset than do the sprinkle capsules. The dosage is 15–60 mg/kg/d in divided doses. Precautionary laboratory studies are necessary. In the infant younger than age 2 years, there is an increased risk of hepatic toxicity. Thrombocytopenia may occur, particularly in the face of an acute illness. The efficacy of newer AEDs in preventing recurrent febrile seizures has not been demonstrated.

Measures to control fever such as sponging or tepid baths, antipyretics, and the administration of antibiotics for proven bacterial illness are reasonable but unproven to prevent recurrent febrile seizures.

Simple febrile seizures do not have any long-term adverse consequences. As noted earlier, there is only a small increase in the risk of developing epilepsy. Cognitive function is not significantly different from that of siblings without febrile seizures.

4. Syncope & Fainting

Fainting is transient loss of consciousness and postural tone due to cerebral ischemia or anoxia. Up to 20%–50% of children (birth–20 years) will faint at some time. There may be a prodrome of dizziness, lightheadedness, nausea, so-called gray-out, sweating, and pallor. One of the most common concerns regarding syncope is the occurrence of convulsive activity. After falling many children stiffen or have jerking motions when unconscious, an anoxic-ischemic seizure mimicking epilepsy, so called "convulsive syncope." Watching or undergoing a venipuncture is a common precipitant of fainting, as are prolonged standing, fatigue, illness, overheating, dehydration, hunger, and athleticism with slow baseline pulse. The family history is positive for similar episodes in 90% of patients.

In infants, cyanotic syncope ("breath-holding" spells) and pallid syncope may occur. In adolescents, there appears to be an association with migraine.

Classification

Ninety-five percent of cases of syncope are of the vasovagal-vasodepressive or neurocardiogenic type (Table 25–13). Vasodilation, cardiac slowing, and hypotension cause transient (1–2 minutes) cerebral ischemia and result in the patient passing out. The patient arouses in 1–2 minutes, but full recovery may take an hour or more. Besides those already listed, rare precipitants include hair grooming, cough, micturition, neck stretching, and emotional stress. More ominous is cardiac syncope, which often occurs during exercise. Angina or palpitations may occur. An obstructive lesion such as aortic stenosis, cardiomyopathy, coronary disease, or arrhythmia may be the cause. Eliciting a typical prodrome of sweating, tunnel vision, and lightheadedness helps to confirm a neurocardiogenic cause, and atypical events should be evaluated for seizure. Other spells that may mimic syncope are listed in Table 25–13.

Clinical Findings

A. Symptoms and Signs

The workup of fainting includes a personal and a detailed family history, and a physical examination with emphasis on blood pressure, cardiac history, and neurologic features. In the adolescent, a blood pressure drop of more than 30 mm Hg after standing for 5–10 minutes or a baseline systolic pressure of less than 80 mm Hg suggests orthostasis.

Table 25–13. Classification of syncope in childhood.

Vasovagal, neurocardiogenic (neurally mediated)
Orthostatic
Athleticism
Pallid and cyanotic breath-holding
Situational (stress, blood drawing)
Cardiac
Obstructive
Arrhythmia
Prolonged QTc
Hypercyanotic (eg, in tetralogy of Fallot)
Nonsyncope mimicker
Migraine with confusion or stupor
Seizure
Hypoglycemia
Hysteria
Hyperventilation
Vertigo

B. Laboratory Findings and Imaging

Hemoglobin should be checked if anemia is suggested by the history. Electrocardiography (ECG) should be done in all patients to assess for a cardiac etiology, especially prolonged QT syndrome. Given the high mortality of purely cardiac causes, primary care physicians should have a low-threshold for cardiology referral, Holter monitoring, and echocardiography. This referral is mandatory if cardiac causes seem likely (ie, fainting during exercise). Tilt testing (though norms are vague) may have a role in frequent recurrent syncope to confirm a vasodepressive cause and avoid more expensive diagnostic investigations. In cases with seizure activity or an atypical history, EEG can be ordered to assess for the possibility of seizures.

Treatment

Treatment consists mostly of giving advice about the benign nature of fainting and about avoiding precipitating situations. The patient should be cautioned to lie down if prodromal symptoms occur. Good hydration and reasonable salt intake are advisable. In some cases, β-blockers or fludrocortisone may have a role. For infantile syncope ("breath-holding"), reassurance as to its benign nature is important. Unfortunately, for the occasional child with frequent spells, no adequate treatment exists.

Abend NS, Gutierrez-Colina AM, Dlugos DJ: Medical treatment of pediatric status epilepticus. Semin Pediatr Neurol 2010;17:169–175 [PMID: 20727486].

Aldenkamp AP et al: Optimizing therapy of seizures in children and adolescents with ADHD. Neurology 2006;67(Suppl 4):S49 [PMID: 17190923].

Arya R, Kabra M, Gulati S: Epilepsy in children with Down syndrome. Epileptic Disord 2011;13(1):1–7 [PMID: 21398208].

Bartha AI et al: Neonatal seizures: Multicenter variability in current treatment practices. Pediatr Neurol 2007;37:85 [PMID: 17675022].

Berg AT, Berkovic SF, Brodie MT: Revised terminology and concepts for organization of seizures and epilepsies: Report of the ILAE Commission on Classification and Terminology, 2005–2009. Epilepsia 2010; 51:676–685 [PMID: 20196795].

Bough KJ, Rho JM: Anticonvulsant mechanisms of the ketogenic diet. Epilepsia 2007;48:43 [PMID: 17241207].

Braakman HM, Vaessen MJ, Hofman PA et al: Cognitive and behavioral complications of frontal lobe epilepsy in children: A review of the literature. Epilepsia 2011;52:849–856 [PMID: 21480882].

Bruhn K et al: Screen sensitivity in photosensitive children and adolescents: Patient-dependant and stimulus-dependant factors. Epileptic Disord 2007;9:57 [PMID: 17307713].

Caraballo RH et al: Ketogenic diet in patients with myoclonic-astatic epilepsy. Epileptic Disord 2006;8:151 [PMID: 16793577].

Ceulemans B: Overall management of patients with Dravet syndrome. Dev Med Child Neurol 2011;53(Suppl 2):19–23 [PMID: 21504428].

Chahine LM, Mikati MA: Benign pediatric localization-related epilepsies. Epileptic Disord 2006;8:243 [PMID: 17150437].

Chin RF et al: Meningitis is a common cause of convulsive status epilepticus with fever. Arch Dis Child 2005;90:66 [PMID: 15613516].

Chu-Shore CJ, Thiele EA: Semin New drugs for pediatric epilepsy. Pediatr Neurol. 2010;17:214–223 [PMID: 21183127].

Deltour L et al: Children with benign epilepsy with centrotemporal spikes (BECTS) show impaired attentional control: Evidence from an attentional capture paradigm. Epileptic Disord 2007;9:32 [PMID: 17307709].

Desai J, Mitchell WG: Does one more medication help? Effect of adding another anticonvulsant in childhood epilepsy. J Child Neurol 2011;26:329–333 [PMID: 21183723].

Hughes JR: Benign epilepsy of childhood with centrotemporal spikes (BECTS): To treat or not to treat, that is the question. Epilepsy Behav 2010;19:197–203 [PMID: 20797913].

Ostrowsky K: Outcome and prognosis of status epilepticus in children. Semin Pediatr Neurol 2010;17:195 [PMID: 20727490].

Dion MH et al: Lamotrigine therapy of epilepsy with Angelman's syndrome. Epilepsia 2007;48:593 [PMID: 17326790].

Evans D et al: Anticonvulsants for preventing mortality and morbidity in full-term newborns with perinatal asphyxia. Cochrane Database Syst Rev 2007:CD001240 [PMID: 17636659].

Ferrie C et al: Panayiotopoulos syndrome: A consensus view. Dev Med Child Neurol 2006;48:236 [PMID: 16483404].

Freeman JM, Kossoff EH: Ketosis and the ketogenic diet, 2010: Advances in treating epilepsy and other disorders. Adv Pediatr 2010;57:315–329 [PMID: 21056745].

Fischer JW, Cho CS: Pediatric syncope: Cases from the emergency department. Emerg Med Clin North Am 2010;28:501–516 [PMID: 20709241].

Gerstner T et al: Valproic acid induced encephalopathy–19 new cases in Germany from 1994 to 2003–a side effect associated to VPA-therapy not only in young children. Seizure 2006;15:443 [PMID: 16787750].

Glauser TA et al: Pharmacokinetics of levetiracetam in infants and young children with epilepsy. Epilepsia 2007;48:1117 [PMID: 17442002].

Glauser TA et al: Topiramate monotherapy in newly diagnosed epilepsy in children and adolescents. J Child Neurol 2007;22:693 [PMID: 17641254].

Grosso S et al: Efficacy and safety of levetiracetam in infants and young children with refractory epilepsy. Seizure 2007;16:345 [PMID: 17368928].

Guillet R, Kwon J: Seizure recurrence and developmental disabilities after neonatal seizures: Outcomes are unrelated to use of phenobarbital prophylaxis. J Child Neurol 2007;22:389 [PMID: 17621516].

Hedera P et al: Identification of a novel locus for febrile seizures and epilepsy on chromosome 21q22. Epilepsia 2006;47:1622 [PMID: 17054683].

Hirtz D et al: Practice parameter: Treatment of the child with a first unprovoked seizure: Report of the Quality Standards Subcommittee of the American Academy of Neurology and the Practice Committee of the Child Neurology Society. Neurology 2003;60:166 [PMID: 12552027].

Holmes GL, Stafstrom CE, Tuberous Sclerosis Study Group: Tuberous sclerosis complex and epilepsy: Recent developments and future challenges. Epilepsia 2007;48:617 [PMID: 17386056].

Jansen FE et al: Epilepsy surgery in tuberous sclerosis: A systematic review. Epilepsia 2007;48:1477 [PMID: 17484753].

Koenig SA et al: Valproic acid-induced hepatopathy: Nine new fatalities in Germany from 1994 to 2003. Epilepsia 2006;47:2027 [PMID: 17201699].

Korinthenberg R, Schreiner A: Topiramate in children with West syndrome: A retrospective multicenter evaluation of 100 patients. J Child Neurol 2007;22:302 [PMID: 17621500].

Kossoff EH et al: A modified Atkins diet is effective for the treatment of intractable pediatric epilepsy. Epilepsia 2006;47:421 [PMID: 16499770].

Kossoff EH et al: Ketogenic diets: An update for child neurologists. J Child Neurol 2009:24:979 [PMID: 19535814].

Loring DW, Meador KJ: No kidding. High risk of cognitive difficulty in new-onset pediatric epilepsy. Neurology 2009 [Epub ahead of print] [PMID: 19675308].

Mancardi MM et al: Familial occurrence of febrile seizures and epilepsy in severe myoclonic epilepsy of infancy (SMEI) patients with SCN1A mutations. Epilepsia 2006;47:1629 [PMID: 17054684].

Obeid M et al: Approach to pediatric epilepsy surgery: State of the art, Part I: General principles and presurgical workup. Eur J Paediatr Neurol 2009:13:102 [PMID: 18692417].

Pellock JM, Hrachovy R, Shinnar S et al: Infantile spasms: A U.S. consensus report. Epilepsia 2010;51:2175–2189 [PMID: 20608959].

Ramos-Lizana J et al: Recurrence risk after withdrawal of antiepileptic drugs in children with epilepsy: A prospective study. Eur J Paediatr Neurol 2009 [Epub ahead of print] [PMID: 19541516].

Rankin PM et al: Pyridoxine-dependent seizures: A family phenotype that leads to severe cognitive deficits, regardless of treatment regime. Dev Med Child Neurol 2007;49:300 [PMID: 17376142].

Rennie J, Boylan G: Treatment of neonatal seizures. Arch Dis Child Fetal Neonatal Ed 2007;92:F148 [PMID: 17337664].

Rho JM, Rogawski MA: The ketogenic diet: Stoking the powerhouse of the cell. Epilepsy Curr 2007;7:58 [PMID: 17505556].

Riviello JJ et al: Practice Parameter: Diagnostic assessment of the child with status epilepticus (an evidence-based review): Report of the Quality Standards Subcommittee of the American Academy of Neurology and the Practice Committee of the Child Neurology Society. Neurology 2006 67:1542 [PMID: 17101884].

Sabaz M et al: The impact of epilepsy surgery on quality of life in children. Neurology 2006;66:557 [PMID: 16505311].

Sadleir LG, Scheffer IE: Febrile seizures. BMJ 2007;334:307 [PMID: 17289734].

Shany E, Berger I: Neonatal Electroencephalography: Review of a Practical Approach. J Child Neurol 2011;26:341–355 [PMID: 21383227].

Shoemaker MT, Rotenberg JS: Levetiracetam for the treatment of neonatal seizures. J Child Neurol 2007;22:95 [PMID: 17608315].

Shostak S, Ottman R: Ethical, legal, and social dimensions of epilepsy genetics. Epilepsia 2006;47:1595 [PMID: 17054679].

Sillanpaa M, Schmidt D: Natural history of treated childhood-onset epilepsy: Prospective, long-term population-based study. Brain 2006;129:617 [PMID: 16401617].

Sillanpää M, Shinnar S: Long-term mortality in childhood-onset epilepsy. N Engl J Med 2010;363:2522–2529 [PMID: 21175314].

Silverstein FS, Jensen FE: Neonatal seizures. Ann Neurol 2007;62:112 [PMID: 17683087].

Singh RK, Gaillard WD: Status epilepticus in children. Curr Neurol Neurosci Rep 2009;9:137 [PMID: 19268037].

Steering Committee on Quality Improvement and Management, Subcommittee on Febrile Seizures: Febriles seizures: Clinical practice guideline for the long-term management of the child with simple febrile seizures. Pediatrics 2008:121:1281 [PMID: 18519501].

Troester M, Rekate HL: Pediatric seizure and epilepsy classification: Why is it important or is it important? Seminars in Pediatric Neurology 2009;16:16 [PMID: 19410152].

Tuchman R: Autism and epilepsy: What has regression got to do with it? Epilepsy Curr 2006;6:107 [PMID: 17260027].

Vining EP: Struggling with Rasmussen's syndrome. Epilepsy Curr 2006;6:20 [PMID: 16477319].

Wheless JW: Managing severe epilepsy syndromes of early childhood. J Child Neurol 2009:24:24S [PMID: 19666880].

Zaccara G et al: Idiosyncratic adverse reactions to antiepileptic drugs. Epilepsia 2007;48:1223 [PMID: 17386054].

Zawadzki L, Stafstrom CE: Status epilepticus treatment and outcome in children: What might the future hold? Semin Pediatr Neurol 2010;17:201–205 [PMID: 20727491].

Zupanc ML: Clinical evaluation and diagnosis of severe epilepsy syndromes of early childhood. J Child Neurol 2009;24:6S [PMID: 19666878].

HEADACHES

ESSENTIALS OF DIAGNOSIS

- The two most common causes of headaches in children are migraine and tension-type headache.
- Diagnosis is based upon a thorough history and physical, excluding secondary causes such as mass or idiopathic intracranial hypertension.
- Warning signs that require further investigation include: headache in a young child, new onset and worsening headache, unexplained fever, awakening with headache or vomiting, headache worse with straining or position change, posterior headaches, neurological deficit, or neurocutaneous stigmata.

Children and adolescents commonly present with headache and it is important to recognize and differentiate the common from the more serious causes. Approximately 11% of children and 28% of adolescents experience recurrent headaches. First, the clinician must determine if the headache is primary or secondary. Symptoms and signs are the center of evaluation; however, red flags (Table 25–14) may prompt further workup and evaluation. Correct diagnosis of headache disorders will guide treatment and management.

Table 25–14. Red flags for children with headaches.

Headache in child less than 5 years
New ("explosive onset") and worsening headache in a previously healthy child
Worst headache of life
Unexplained fever
Night time or early morning awakenings with headache or vomiting
Headache worse with straining
Posterior headaches
Neurological deficit
Postural headache
Worse when lying
Worse when standing
Neurocutaneous stigmata (café au lait spots, hypopigmented macules)

Clinical Findings

Symptoms and Signs

Based on the 2004 International Classification of Headache Disorders-II (IHCD-II), primary headaches are divided into three major categories: migraine, tension-type, and, less commonly in children, trigeminal autonomic cephalgia. Clinical features of migraine without aura and tension-type headache are compared in Table 25–15. Migraine headaches are generally episodic unilateral (commonly bilateral in children), throbbing, severe headaches with a combination of photophobia, phonophobia, nausea, and or vomiting. Tension-type headaches (TTH) are a tight band dull sensation that can occur episodically or daily. TTH are not associated with nausea or vomiting but may have photophobia or phonophobia but not both. Individuals with greater than 15 headaches (migraine or tension-type) per month are considered chronic, and medication overuse must be excluded. Triggers of head pain can include stress, sleep deprivation, dehydration, skipped meals, caffeine, and specific foods (eg, MSG or nitrites). Trigeminal autonomic cephalgia (or cluster headache) is rare in children, but can present as a unilateral severe headache and autonomic dysfunction (watery eye, congestion, facial sweating, miosis, and ptosis).

According to the IHCD-II, migraines include childhood pediatric syndromes such as cyclic vomiting, abdominal migraine, and benign paroxysmal vertigo of childhood. These are precursors to migraines and in an older child with new onset migraines; history of these periodic syndromes/symptoms may be discovered.

Table 25–15. Classification of TTH and migraine.

	Migraine Without Aura	Tension-Type Headache
Duration	1–72 h*	30 min to 7 days
Quality	Throbbing/pounding	Pressure tight band
Severity	Moderate to severe	Mild to moderate
Location	Unilateral/bilateral*	Bilateral
Physical activity	Worsens headache	No effect
Associated factors		
a. Nausea +/− vomiting	a or b	Not present
b. Photo + phonophobia		One feature but not both

*Modified for children based on the IHCD-II classification criteria.

B. Laboratory Findings

Laboratory studies are not routinely needed in children presenting with recurrent headaches. History and examination may prompt basic screening studies for thyroid, anemia, or autoimmune disorders.

C. Imaging

Routine neuroimaging is not indicated for children presenting with recurrent headaches unless there is an abnormal neurological examination, coexistence of seizures, or other red flags notes in Table 25–14. Imaging can also be considered for children with historical features that suggest recent onset of severe headache, change in headache, or features to suggest neurological dysfunction.

Differential Diagnosis

Secondary causes of headache in children include broad categories such as head trauma, infection, vascular, intracranial pressure changes, structural, metabolic, toxic or substance related, and hematologic (Table 25–16). Headaches associated with head trauma are those that start within two weeks of closed head injury. They can have either features of migraines or tension-type headaches. Neck pain and headache after head trauma warrant evaluation for a dissection, especially if examination is for a connective tissue disorder such as Marfans or homocystinemia. Headaches that worsen with lying down or vomiting without nausea are concerns for increased intracranial hypertension from idiopathic intracranial hypertension (IIH), sinus venous clot producing CSF pressure, hydrocephalus, or mass. Headaches that worsen with standing and improve with lying down are suggestive of low pressure headaches caused by a tear in the dura from a preceding LP, penetrating trauma, or surgery.

Medication and substance ingestion and withdrawal are both culprits to secondary headaches. Medications directly related to possible headaches include oral contraceptives, steroids, thyroid replacement, caffeine, cold medicines, ergotamines, vasodilators, overuse of vitamin A or D, sympathomimetics, bronchodilators, atypical antipsychotics, SSRIs, ethanol, antibiotics, and tetracycline. Steroids, vitamin A toxicity, oral contraceptives, and tetracycline are all associated with development of idiopathic intracranial

Table 25–16. Differential diagnosis of headaches.

Primary Causes	Secondary Causes	
• Migraine without aura • Migraine with aura • Childhood pediatric syndromes • Tension-type headache • Trigeminal autonomic cephalgias	• Trauma • Hypertension • Arterial dissection • Medication overuse headache • Idiopathic intracranial hypertension • Intracranial hypotension • Chiari malformation • Seizure • Mass/Neoplasm • Sleep apnea	• Substance withdrawal • Infection • Sinusitis • Hypoxia • Hypercapnia • Mitochondrial disorders • Thyroid dysfunction • Anemia • Asthenopia (eye strain) • Tempomandibular joint dysfunction • Substance use

hypertension. Medications that are commonly associated with medication overuse headache include aspirin, acetaminophen, NSAIDs, Firoinal/fioricet, and triptans. Other toxins such as lead, carbon monoxide, or organic solvent poisoning cannot be overlooked.

Infections both of the CNS or systemically are associated with headaches. Meningitis and encephalitis will present with a combination of fever, seizures, altered mental status, stiff neck, and headache. However, common systemic or other focal infections may cause headaches such as viral upper respiratory infections, strep pharyngitis (especially in younger children), rhinosinusitis (sinus headache), influenza, and Lyme disease. Headaches are frequently misdiagnosed as sinus headaches and physicians should carefully obtain history of pain in the face, ears, or teeth and evaluate for signs of rhinosinusitis on either physical examination or imaging.

Any cause of hypoxia (eg, cardiac, respiratory, altitude, anemia) may cause a bifrontal throbbing headache that may be worsened with exertion, straining, or laying down. Hypercapnea causes a nonspecific headache and may be secondary to sleep apnea or other underlying metabolic or respiratory disorder. Hypothyroidism can cause bilateral nonpulsating continuous mild intensity pain that resolves after thyroid supplementation.

Although eye strain and temporal mandibular joint dysfunction are rare causes of recurrent headaches, they can be simply treated; therefore, when suspected, evaluation by ophthalmology or dentist respectively is indicated. Eye strain or asthenopia causes a mild dull aching soreness of the eyes and usually worsens at school. It can occur with nearsightedness, farsightedness, or an astigmatism. Examination in TMJ dysfunction reveals a click on slow jaw opening and closing in addition to reduced angle of jaw opening.

A thorough history and physical examination helps diagnosing most of these conditions. Several common red flags associated with worrisome secondary causes are listed in Table 25–14. It is not one single symptom or red flag that usually points to a secondary cause; rather, it is a constellation of symptoms.

Complications

Migraines and tension-type headaches are both episodic headache disorders but may transform into more frequent daily headaches. When greater than 15 headaches per month for three or more months, these are considered chronic headaches. Risk factors for chronicity include psychological comorbidity, excessive medication use leading to Medication Overuse Headache, and possibly signs of central sensitization. During migraines, central sensitization is indicated by presence of cutaneous allodynia (eg, pain with combing hair, wearing a pony tail, or touching the skin). These symptoms are currently being investigated and are thought to be associated with worsened prognosis with respect to treatment response and headache chronicity.

Depression and anxiety are both comorbid with headaches and are associated with increased headache burden and disability such as school absenteeism. Equally, children and adolescents with psychiatric disorders also have increased rates of primary headaches.

Treatment

Treatment is divided into two categories: acute and preventative. Management of headaches should emphasize the necessity for early and adequate treatment during a headache, in addition to self-management skills to reduce frequency and disability such as life-style modification and headache diaries. Pharmacologic preventative treatment can be considered if frequency or disability is significant.

Abortive Treatment

Acute treatment for pediatric migraine includes use of simple analgesics and migraine specific medications. Any abortive medication should be given as early as possible after the onset of headache. Of all medications, only almotriptan has been approved by the United States FDA for use in children. Simple analgesics include acetaminophen (15 mg/kg; max dose 1000 mg) and ibuprofen (10 mg/kg; max dose 800 mg).

Studies showing significant benefit for pediatric migraine include rizatriptan, zolmitriptan nasal, sumatriptan nasal, and almotriptan. Occasionally home treatment fails and patients may need IV medications either in an emergency department or infusion center. When a patient fails emergency room treatments, IV dihydroergotamine can be effective with nausea as the most common side effect. All medications used for abortive treatment should be used cautiously to avoid medication overuse headache. Simple analgesics should be limited to 2–3 times per week and migraine-specific medications to approximately six times per month.

During a headache biobehavioral techniques include rest and relaxation. Providing the child with a cool dark room in which to rest may provide added benefit.

Prevention

Any child with headaches should have biobehavioral management as a centerpoint to treatment. These include sleep hygiene; improved fluid intake and elimination of caffeine; nutritional meals; avoidance of skipping meals; regular exercise and stretching, and stress management. Preventative treatment can be considered in individuals with headache frequency of one or more per week. Treatments should be chosen by optimizing wanted side effects and minimizing unwanted side effects (eg, topiramate in an obese child given its side effect of weight loss).

Treatments are categorized into antiepileptic (eg, topiramate, valproic acid, levetiracetam), antihypertensive (eg, β-blockers, calcium channel blockers), antidepressants (eg, amitriptyline), antihistamine/antiseratonergic (eg, cyproheptadine), and neutraceuticals. Only small randomized double blinded or open label studies have tested these agents and there are no FDA-approved preventatives in the United States for the treatment of migraine or tension-type headache in children.

Topiramate is a commonly recommended medication for prevention of headache and if started slowly and at low doses, cognitive side effects can be avoided. Peripheral tingling is uncommon and when present can be usually tolerated by most children. Decreased appetite and weight loss should be monitored at routine appointments. Divalproex sodium has shown efficacy; however, its side effects including weight gain, tremor, hair loss, and teratogenicity warrant caution in adolescent female patients. Amitriptyline is also a commonly used antidepressant for childhood and adolescent migraine. Amitriptyline is usually dosed at nighttime given its side effect of sedation, in addition to other common side effects including constipation, dry mouth, and prolonged QT. Cyproheptadine is a good medication to use in younger children given its small side effect profile of primary increased appetite and sedation. Coenzyme q10, magnesium oxide, and riboflavin have shown efficacy in childhood migraine. They may be a useful option for those children with headaches less than once per week or without significant disability. In addition, these nutraceuticals are helpful for those parents or children who are reluctant to start a once a day medication for their headache and would like "natural' options.

Prognosis

From the few studies regarding long-term prognosis in adolescents presenting with migraines, approximately 25% to 40% of adolescents will have remission of migraine symptoms, 40%–50% have persistence, and 20%–25% convert to tension-type headache. Of those with TTH, 20% convert to migraine. Headache severity at diagnosis is thought to be predictive of headache outcome in the long term.

Abend NS et al: Secondary Headaches in children and adolescents. Seminars in Pediatric Neurology 2010;17:123 [PMID: 20541105].

Anttila P: Tension-type headache in childhood and adolescence. Lancet Neurol 2006;5:268 [PMID: 16488382].

Damen L et al: Prophylactic treatment of migraine in children. Part 1. A systematic review of non-pharmacological trials. Cephalalgia 2006;26:373 [PMID: 16556238].

Eiland LS et al: Pediatric migraine: Pharmacologic agents for prophylaxis. Ann Pharmacother 2007;41:1181 [PMID: 17550953].

Eiland LD et al: The use of triptans for pediatric migraines. Paediatr Drugs 2010;12:379 [PMID: 21028917].

Hershey AD: Current approaches to the diagnosis and management of paediatric migraine. Lancet Neurol 2010;9:190 [PMID: 20129168].

Hershey AD et al: Chronic daily headaches in children. Curr Pain Headache Rep 2006;10:370 [PMID: 16945254].

Lewis DW: Pediatric migraine. Neurol Clin 2009;27:481 [PMID: 19289227].

Lewis DW et al: Efficacy of zolmitriptan nasal spray in adolescent migraine. Pediatrics 2007;120:390 [PMID: 17671066].

Lewis DW et al: Headache evaluation in children and adolescents: When to worry? When to scan? Pediatric Annals 2010;39:399 [PMID: 20666345].

Saadat H, Kain ZN: Hypnosis as a therapeutic tool in pediatrics. Pediatrics 2007;120:179 [PMID: 17606576].

Tepper SJ: Complementary and alternative treatments for childhood headaches. Current pain and headache reports 2008;12:379 [PMID: 18765145].

Wang SJ et al: Chronic daily headache in adolescents: Prevalence, impact and medication overuse. Neurol 2006;66:193 [PMID: 16434652].

PSEUDOTUMOR CEREBRI (IDIOPATHIC INTRACRANIAL HYPERTENSION)

ESSENTIALS OF DIAGNOSIS

- Signs and symptoms of increased intracranial pressure: chronic headache, tinnitus, cranial nerve VI palsy, papilledema, visual loss.

- Normal MRI/MRV of the head.
- Elevated opening pressure on lumbar puncture performed in the lateral decubitus position.

Pathogenesis

The pathogenesis of idiopathic intracranial hypertension is essentially unknown. Multiple risk factors have been identified, but obesity is the most common. Interestingly, multiple medications have been associated with idiopathic intracranial hypertension, including tetracycline, steroids, and retinol.

Clinical Findings

Idiopathic intracranial hypertension is characterized by increased intracranial pressure as documented by a lumbar puncture performed in the lateral decubitus position in the absence of an identifiable intracranial mass, infection, metabolic derangement, or hydrocephalus. Presenting symptoms are headache, tinnitus, and visual loss; signs are those of increased intracranial pressure as outlined in Table 25–17. Visual symptoms are commonly secondary to transient visual obscurations (TVOs), which are transient (less than 1 minute) and reversible alterations of vision in these patients. This must be distinguished from visual field anomalies, which can be permanent. Examination of the patient often reveals papilledema, and occasionally cranial nerve VI palsy; and should include extensive visual field testing.

Differential Diagnosis

The cause of idiopathic intracranial hypertension is usually unknown, but it has been described in association with a variety of inflammatory, metabolic, toxic, and connective tissue disorders (Table 25–18). Assessing for alternative causes of increased intracranial pressure is essential to the diagnosis. MRI (or urgent CT for critically ill patients) may reveal hydrocephalus, tumor, or abscess. MRV may demonstrate a cerebral sinovenous thrombosis (CSVT), requiring hematological evaluation and consideration of anticoagulation. As noted in Table 25–18, medications, endocrinologic disturbances, and rheumatologic anomalies may all predispose patients to idiopathic intracranial hypertension. Lumbar puncture is essential to the diagnosis, as it confirms the presence of increased pressure (above 180–250 mm H_2O), but also assesses for white blood cell count and protein (looking for an infectious mimicker, such as chronic meningitis). In some inflammatory and connective tissue diseases, the CSF protein concentration may be also be increased.

Table 25–17. Signs of increased intracranial pressure.

Acute, subacute
Headache, vomiting
Excessive rate of head growth
Altered behavior
Decreased level of consciousness
Blurred or double vision; loss of vision
Optic disk swelling
Abducens nerve paresis
Chronic
Macrocephaly
Growth impairment
Developmental delay
Optic atrophy
Visual field loss

Table 25–18. Conditions associated with idiopathic intracranial hypertension and idiopathic intracranial hypertension mimickers.

Medications and metabolic-toxic disorders
Hypervitaminosis A, including use of retinoids
Obesity
Steroid therapy
Hormonal therapy
Steroid withdrawal
Tetracycline, minocycline toxicity
Nalidixic acid toxicity
Iron deficiency
Clotting disorders
Hypocalcemia
Hyperparathyroidism or hyperthyroidism
Adrenal insufficiency
Systemic lupus erythematosus
Chronic CO_2 retention
Infectious and parainfectious disorders
Chronic otitis media (lateral sinus thrombosis)
Guillain-Barré syndrome
Lyme disease
Dural sinus thrombosis
Minor head injury

Complications

Vision loss is the main complication of idiopathic intracranial hypertension, as chronic papilledema may lead to permanent optic nerve damage. Vision loss usually occurs in the blind spot and/or nasal aspects of the visual field prior to affecting central vision. Headache, TVOs, cranial nerve VI palsy, and malaise are usually reversible.

Treatment

Treatment of idiopathic intracranial hypertension is aimed at correcting the identifiable predisposing condition and preventing vision loss. The cornerstone of treatment is usually provided by an ophthalmologist: sequential ophthalmologic evaluation to assess optic nerve swelling and visual fields. Some patients may benefit from the use of acetazolamide or topiramate to decrease the volume and pressure of CSF within the CNS. If a program of medical management and ophthalmologic surveillance fail, lumboperitoneal shunt, ventriculoperitoneal shunt, or optic nerve fenestration may be necessary to prevent irreparable visual loss and damage to the optic nerves. Dural venous stenting has limited data in adults with no randomized studies in either adults or children.

Prevention

As idiopathic intracranial hypertension is closely linked to obesity, reducing the prevalence of overweight children is likely the most important factor in preventing this disease.

Prognosis

With appropriate workup and treatment, the majority of patients recover from idiopathic intracranial hypertension without long-term sequela including visual outcome. Reoccurrence risk is greatest within 18 months.

Ball AK, Clarke CE: Idiopathic intracranial hypertension. Lancet Neurol 2006;5:433 [PMID: 16632314].

Bussiere M et al: Unilateral transverse sinus stenting of patients with idiopathic intracranial hypertension. AJNR 2010;31:645 [PMID: 19942702].

De Lucia D et al: Benign intracranial hypertension associated to blood coagulation derangements. Thromb J 2006;4:21 [PMID: 17187688].

Kesler A, Bassan H: Pseudotumor cerebri—idiopathic intracranial hypertension in the pediatric population. Pediatr Endocrinol Rev 2006;3,387 [PMID: 16816807].

Soiberman U et al: Idiopathic intracranial hypertension in children: Visual outcome and risk of recurrence. Childs Nerv Syst 2011 [PMID: 21538129].

Stiebel-Kalish H et al: Puberty as a risk factor for less favorable visual outcome in idiopathic intracranial hypertension. Am J Ophthalmol 2006;142:279 [PMID: 16876509].

Thambisetty M et al: Fulminant idiopathic intracranial hypertension. Neurol 2007;68:229 [PMID: 17224579].

CEREBROVASCULAR DISEASE

Pediatric arterial ischemic stroke is subdivided into two categories: perinatal arterial ischemic stroke (perinatal ischemic stroke) and childhood arterial ischemic stroke (childhood ischemic stroke). Generally, perinatal ischemic stroke is defined as arterial ischemia occurring in a patient younger than age 28 days and older than 28 weeks' gestation. Childhood ischemic stroke is any ischemic stroke occurring in a patient between 28 days and 18 years old.

1. Childhood Arterial Schemic Stroke

Childhood arterial ischemic stroke (AIS) is emerging as a serious and increasingly recognized disorder, affecting 2–8:100,000 children per year. There are numerous adverse outcomes, which include death in 10%, neurologic deficits or seizures in 70%–75%, and recurrent ischemic stroke in up to 20%. It is essential to recognize that childhood AIS represents a neurologic emergency, for which prompt diagnosis can affect treatment considerations and outcome. Unfortunately, most pediatric AIS is not recognized until 24–36 hours after onset; and treatment considerations matter most in the first hours after ischemic stroke onset. When possible, all children who present with ischemic stroke should be transferred to a tertiary care center that specializes in pediatric ischemic stroke management. The evaluation should include a thorough history of prior illnesses, especially those associated with varicella (even in the prior 1–2 years) preceding viral infection, minor head or neck trauma, and familial clotting tendencies. A systematic search for evidence of cardiac, vascular, hematologic, or intracranial disorders should be undertaken (Table 25–19). Although many ischemic strokes are not associated with a single underlying systemic disorder, previously diagnosed congenital heart disease is the most common predisposing illness, followed by hematologic and neoplastic disorders. In many instances the origin is multifactorial, necessitating a thorough investigation even when the cause may seem obvious. Arteriopathy is seen in as many as 80% of "idiopathic" patients, and likely confers an increased recurrence risk.

Clinical Findings

A. Symptoms and Signs

Manifestations of arterial ischemic stroke in childhood vary according to the vascular distribution to the brain structure that is involved. Because many conditions leading to childhood ischemic stroke result in emboli, multifocal neurologic involvement is common. Children may present with acute hemiplegia similarly to ischemic stroke in adults. Symptoms of unilateral weakness, sensory disturbance, dysarthria, and dysphagia may develop over a period of minutes, but at times progressive worsening of symptoms may evolve over several hours. Bilateral hemispheric involvement may lead to a depressed level of consciousness. The patient may also demonstrate disturbances of mood and behavior and experience focal or multifocal seizures. Physical examination of the patient is aimed not only at identifying the specific deficits related to impaired cerebral blood flow, but also at seeking evidence for any predisposing disorder. Retinal hemorrhages, splinter hemorrhages in the nail beds, cardiac murmurs, rash, fever, neurocutaneous stigmata, and signs of trauma are especially important findings.

B. Laboratory Findings and Ancillary Testing

In the acute phase, certain investigations should be carried out emergently with consideration of treatment options. This should include complete blood count, erythrocyte sedimentation rate, C-reactive protein, basic chemistries, blood urea nitrogen, creatinine, prothrombin time/partial

Table 25–19. Etiologic risk factors for ischemic and/or hemorrhagic ischemic stroke.

Cardiac disorders
Cyanotic heart disease
Valvular disease
Rheumatic
Endocarditis
Cardiomyopathy
Cardiac dysrhythmia
Vascular occlusive disorders
Cervical/cerebral arterial dissection
Homocystinuria/homocystinemia
Vasculitis
Meningitis
Polyarteritis nodosa
Systemic lupus erythematosus
Drug abuse (amphetamines)
Varicella
Mycoplasma
Human immunodeficiency virus
Fibromuscular dysplasia
Moyamoya disease
Diabetes
Nephrotic syndrome
Systemic hypertension
Dural sinus and cerebral venous thrombosis
Cortical venous thrombosis
Hematologic disorders
Iron deficiency anemia
Polycythemia
Thrombotic thrombocytopenia
Thrombocytopenic purpura
Hemoglobinopathies
Sickle cell disease
Coagulation defects
Hemophilia
Vitamin K deficiency
Hypercoagulable states
Prothrombin gene mutation
Methylenetetrahydrofolate reductase mutation
Lipoprotein (a)
Factor V Leiden deficiency
Antiphospholipid antibodies
Hypercholesterolemia
Hypertriglyceridemia
Factor VIII elevation
Pregnancy
Systemic lupus erythematosus
Use of oral contraceptives
Antithrombin III deficiency
Protein C and S deficiencies
Leukemia
Intracranial vascular anomalies
Moyamoya
Arteriovenous malformation
Arterial aneurysm
Carotid-cavernous fistula
Focal cerebral arteriopathy

thromboplastin time, chest radiography, ECG, urine toxicology, and imaging (see following section). Subsequent studies can be carried out systemically, with particular attention paid to disorders involving the heart, blood vessels, platelets, red cells, hemoglobin, and coagulation proteins. Twenty percent to fifty percent of all pediatric ischemic stroke patients will have a prothrombotic state. Additional laboratory tests for systemic disorders such as vasculitis, mitochondrial disorders, and metabolic disorders are sometimes indicated.

Examination of CSF is indicated in patients with fever, nuchal rigidity, or obtundation when the diagnosis of intracranial infection requires exclusion. Lumbar puncture may be deferred until a neuroimaging scan (excluding brain abscess or a space-occupying lesion that might contraindicate lumbar puncture) has been obtained. In the absence of infection, rheumatologic disease or intracranial subarachnoid hemorrhage, CSF examination is rarely helpful in defining the cause of the cerebrovascular disorder.

When seizures are prominent, an EEG may be used as an adjunct in the patient's evaluation. An EEG and sequential EEG monitoring may help in patients with severely depressed consciousness.

ECG and echocardiography are useful both in the diagnostic approach to the patient and in ongoing monitoring and management, particularly when hypotension or cardiac arrhythmias complicate the clinical course.

C. Imaging

CT and MRI scans of the brain are helpful in defining the extent of cerebral involvement with ischemia or hemorrhage. CT scans may be normal within the first 12–24 hours of an ischemic stroke and are more useful to assess for hemorrhagic ischemic stroke. A CT scan performed early after the onset of neurologic deficits is valuable in excluding intracranial hemorrhage. This information may be helpful in the early stages of management and in the decision to treat with anticoagulants. Given the high incidence of ischemic stroke mimickers in the pediatric population (complicated migraine, Todd paralysis, encephalitis, etc), urgent MRI with DWI is increasingly used in pediatric stroke centers.

Vascular imaging of the head and neck is an important part of pediatric ischemic stroke management and may include CTA, MRA, or conventional angiography. In studies in which both MRA and cerebral angiography have been used, up to 80% of patients with idiopathic childhood-onset arterial ischemic stroke have demonstrated a vascular abnormality. Vascular imaging is helpful in diagnosing disorders such as transient cerebral arteriopathy, arteriopathy associated with sickle cell disease, moyamoya disease, arterial dissection, aneurysm, fibromuscular dysplasia, and vasculitis. Recent studies have demonstrated that patients with vascular abnormalities on MRA or conventional angiography have a much greater recurrence risk than patients with normal vessels. When vessel imaging is performed, all major vessels should be studied from the aortic arch. If evidence of fibromuscular dysplasia is present in the intracranial or extracranial vessels, renal arteriography is indicated.

Differential Diagnosis

Patients with an acute onset of neurologic deficits must be evaluated for other disorders that can cause focal neurologic deficits. Hypoglycemia, prolonged focal seizures, a prolonged postictal paresis (Todd paralysis), acute disseminated encephalomyelitis, meningitis, hemorrhagic stroke, encephalitis, complicated migraine, ingestion, and brain abscess should all be considered. Migraine with focal neurologic deficits may be difficult to differentiate initially from ischemic stroke. Occasionally the onset of a neurodegenerative disorder (eg, adrenoleukodystrophy or mitochondrial disorder) may begin with the abrupt onset of seizures and focal neurologic deficits. The possibility of drug abuse (particularly cocaine) and other toxic exposures must be investigated diligently in any patient with acute mental status changes.

Treatment

The initial management of ischemic stroke in a child is aimed at providing support for pulmonary, cardiovascular, and renal function. Patients should be administered oxygen and are usually monitored in an intensive care setting. Typically, maintenance fluids without added glucose are indicated to augment vascular volume. Pyrexia should be treated aggressively. Specific treatment of ischemic stroke, including blood pressure management, fluid management, and anticoagulation measures, depends partly on the underlying pathogenesis. Meningitis and other infections should be treated. Sickle cell patients require specialists in hematology to perform urgent exchange transfusion and most patients will require chronic transfusions after hospital discharge. Moyamoya is usually treated with surgical revascularization, while patients with vasculitis are often given anti-inflammatory therapy, such as steroids.

In most idiopathic cases of childhood ischemic stroke, anticoagulation or aspirin therapy is indicated. The Royal College of Physicians Pediatric Ischemic Stroke Working Group recommends aspirin, 5 mg/kg daily, as soon as the diagnosis is made. Aspirin use appears safe but the American Heart Association (AHA) recommends yearly flu-shots and close monitoring for Reye syndrome in pediatric ischemic stroke patients. Other groups, such as the American College of Chest Physicians, recommend initial treatment with anticoagulants, such as low-molecular-weight heparin or unfractionated heparin, for 5–7 days (while excluding cardiac sources and dissection) and then switching to aspirin (3–5 mg/d). Recent AHA guidelines support both of these approaches. In some situations, such as arterial dissection or cardio-embolic events, heparinization is usually considered. In adults with cerebrovascular thrombosis, thrombolytic agents (tissue plasminogen activator) used systemically or delivered directly to a vascular thrombotic lesion using interventional radiologic techniques has been shown to improve outcome in the appropriate patients. Although case reports exist, studies in children have not been completed. AHA guidelines recommend against the thrombolysis, outside of a clinical trial for children, while equivocating in the case of adolescents. Given the time-lag to diagnosis and the lack of evidence in children, tissue plasminogen activator is currently used in less than 2% of U.S. children with ischemic stroke. Cleary, the use of tPA should be limited to practitioner who are familiar with cerebrovascular disease in children.

Long-term management requires intensive rehabilitation efforts and therapy aimed at improving the child's language, educational, and psychological performance. Length of treatment with antithrombotic agents, such as low-molecular-weight heparin and aspirin, is still being studied and depends on the etiology. Constraint therapy may be particularly helpful in cases of hemiparesis.

Prognosis

The outcome of ischemic stroke in infants and children is variable. Roughly one-third may have minimal or no deficits, one-third are moderately affected, and one-third are severely affected. Underlying predisposing conditions and the vascular territory involved all play a role in dictating the outcome for an individual patient. When the ischemic stroke involves extremely large portions of one hemisphere or large portions of both hemispheres and cerebral edema develops, the patient's level of consciousness may deteriorate rapidly, and death may occur within the first few days. In contrast, some patients may achieve almost complete recovery of neurologic function within several days if the cerebral territory is small. Seizures, either focal or generalized, may occur in 30%–50% of patients at some point in the course of their cerebrovascular disorder. Recurrence is up to 20%, and is more prominent in some conditions, such as protein C deficiency, lipoprotein (a) abnormalities, and arteriopathies. Chronic problems with learning, behavior, and activity are common. Long-term follow-up with a multidisciplinary ischemic stroke team and/or pediatric neurologist is indicated.

2. Perinatal Arterial Ischemic Stroke

Perinatal arterial ischemic stroke is more common than childhood ischemic stroke, affecting 1:4000 children. Perinatal ischemic stroke has two distinct presentations: acute and delayed. Most patients with an acute presentation develop neonatal seizures during the first week of life, usually in association with a perinatal event. The seizures in acute perinatal ischemic stroke are often focal motor seizures of the contralateral arm and sometimes leg. The presentation is stereotypical because of the predilection of the ischemic stroke to occur in the middle cerebral artery. The presence of diffusion-weighted abnormalities on an MRI scan confirms an acute perinatal ischemic stroke during the first week of life. Other patients present with delayed symptoms, typically with an evolving hemiparesis at an average of 4–8 months. These patients are termed presumed perinatal arterial ischemic stroke.

Acute treatment of a perinatal ischemic stroke is usually limited to neonates with seizures. Unless an embolic source is identified, aspirin and anticoagulation are almost never prescribed. Management is based on supportive care, identification of comorbid conditions, and treatment of seizures. In acute perinatal ischemic stroke, treatable causes such as infection, cardiac embolus, metabolic derangement, and inherited thrombophilia must be ruled out. In appropriate cases, echocardiography, thrombophilia evaluation, and lumbar puncture are indicated. Supportive management focuses on general measures, such as normalizing glucose levels, monitoring blood pressure, and optimizing oxygenation.

Long-term management of perinatal ischemic stroke usually starts with identifying risk factors, which might include prothrombotic states, cardiac disease, drugs, and dehydration. Although prothrombotic abnormalities with the best evidence of association are factor V Leiden, protein C deficiency, and lipoprotein (a), many practitioners perform an extensive hematologic workup. Maternal risk factors such as infertility, antiphospholipid antibodies, placental infection, premature rupture of membranes, and cocaine exposure are all independently associated with perinatal ischemic stroke.

The prognosis for children who sustain perinatal ischemic strokes has long been considered better than for children or adults with ischemic strokes, presumably because of the plasticity of the neonatal brain. Recent evidence, however, suggests that as patients progress into their school-age years, they may have previously unrecognized cognitive challenges, such as learning deficits or attention-deficit/hyperactivity disorder. Twenty percent to forty percent of patients who experience perinatal ischemic strokes are neurologically normal. Motor impairment affects about 40%–60% of patients and is predominantly hemiplegic cerebral palsy. In acute presentations, MRI can be predictive of motor impairment, as descending corticospinal tract diffusion-weighted MRI signal is associated with a higher incidence of hemiplegia. Language delays, behavioral abnormalities, and cognitive deficits are seen in 20%–40% of infants who experience perinatal ischemic strokes. Patients are also at an increased risk for seizures. Ischemic stroke recurs in 3% of neonates and is usually associated with a prothrombotic abnormality or an underlying illness, such as cardiac malformation or infection. Given the low incidence of recurrence, long-term management is largely rehabilitative, including constraint therapies.

Barnes C et al: Prothrombotic abnormalities in childhood ischaemic ischemic stroke. Thromb Res 2005;1 [PMID: 16039697].

Bernard TJ et al: Treatment of childhood arterial ischemic stroke. Ann Neurol 2008;63:679–696 [PMID: 18496844].

Bernard TJ, Goldenberg NA: Hematol Oncol Clin North Am. 2010 Feb;24(1):167–180 [Review] [PMID: 20113901].

Bernard TJ, Manco-Johnson MJ, Goldenberg NA: The roles of anatomic factors, thrombophilia, and antithrombotic therapies in childhood-onset arterial ischemic stroke. Thromb Res 2011 Jan;127(1):6–12 [PMID: 20947137].

deVeber G: In pursuit of evidence-based treatments for paediatric ischemic stroke: The UK and Chest guidelines. Lancet Neurol 2005;7:432 [PMID: 15963446].

Fullerton H et al: Risk of recurrent childhood arterial ischemic stroke in a population-based cohort: The importance of cerebrovascular imaging. Pediatrics 2007;119:3 [PMID: 17332202].

Goldenberg NA, Bernard TJ, Fullerton HJ, Gordon A, deVeber G: International Pediatric Stroke Study Group. Antithrombotic treatments, outcomes, and prognostic factors in acute childhood-onset arterial ischaemic stroke: A multicentre, observational, cohort study. Lancet Neurol 2009 Dec;8(12):1120–1127 [PMID: 19801204].

Janjua N et al: Thrombolysis for ischemic stroke in children data from the nationwide inpatient sample. Ischemic stroke 2007;38 [PMID: 17431210].

Kirton A et al: Cerebral palsy secondary to perinatal ischemic stroke. Clin Perinatol 2006;367 [PMID: 16765730].

Kirton A et al: Quantified corticospinal tract diffusion restriction predicts ischemic strokeperinatal ischemic stroke outcome. Ischemic stroke 2007;38:3 [PMID: 17272775].

Kurnik K et al: Recurrent thromboembolism in infants and children suffering from symptomatic neonatal arterial ischemic stroke. Ischemic stroke 2003;34:2887 [PMID: 14631084].

Lee J et al: Maternal and infant characteristics associated with perinatal arterial ischemic stroke in the infant. JAMA 2005;293:723 [PMID: 15701914].

Lee J et al: Predictors of outcome in perinatal arterial ischemic stroke: A population-based study. Ann Neurology 2005;58:303 [PMID: 16010659].

Lee M et al: Ischemic stroke prevention trial in sickle cell anemia (STOP): Extended follow-up and final results for the STOP Study Investigators. Blood 2006;108:847 [PMID: 16861341].

Monagle et al: Antithrombotic therapy in children: The seventh ACCP conference on antithrombotic and thrombolytic therapy. Chest 2004;126:645 [PMID: 15383489].

Nelson K et al: Ischemic stroke in newborn infants. Lancet Neurol 2004;3:150 [PMID: 14980530].

Roach ES et al: Management of ischemic stroke in infants and children: A scientific statement from a Special Writing Group of the American Heart Association Ischemic stroke Council and the Council on Cardiovascular Disease in the Young. Ischemic stroke 2008;39:2644–2691 [PMID: 18635845].

Shellhaas R et al: Mimics of childhood ischemic stroke: Characteristics of a prospective cohort. Pediatrics 2006;118:704 [PMID: 16882826].

Srinivasan J et al: Delayed recognition of initial ischemic stroke in children: Need for increased awareness. Pediatrics 2009;124(2):e227–e234 [Epub 2009 Jul 20] [PMID: 19620205].

SLEEP DISORDERS

Sleep disorders can originate from abnormalities within the respiratory system, the neurologic system and as well as the coordination (or lack thereof) between the two systems. In order to understand abnormal sleep, one must understand normal sleep which also changes through development with the child. This is reviewed in Chapter 3 in detail. This discussion focuses on neurologic features of several sleep disorders affecting children. Chapter 3 also discusses behavioral considerations in the treatment of sleep disorders. Respiratory abnormalities that are associated with sleep such as obstructive sleep apnea and sleep-disordered breathing are described in detail in Chapters 18 and 19.

1. Narcolepsy

Narcolepsy, a primary disorder of sleep, affects about 0.05% of the population and is characterized by chronic, inappropriate daytime sleep that occurs regardless of activity or surroundings and is not relieved by increased sleep at night. Onset can occur as early as age 3 years. One half of persons affected by narcolepsy have symptoms in childhood. Of children with narcolepsy, 18% are younger than age 10, and 60% are between puberty and their late teens. Narcolepsy usually interferes severely with normal living.

Associated symptoms are cataplexy, hypnagogic and/or hypnopompic hallucinations (visual or auditory), and sleep paralysis. Cataplexy is a transient partial or total loss of muscle tone, often triggered by laughter, anger, or other emotional upsurge. Consciousness is preserved during these spells and they can last several minutes in duration. Hypnagogic hallucinations are intense dream-like states while falling asleep, whereas hypnopompic hallucinations occur while waking from sleep. Sleep paralysis is a brief loss of voluntary muscle control typically occurring at sleep-wake transitions.

Studies have shown that rapid eye movement (REM) sleep with loss of muscle tone and an EEG low-amplitude mixed frequency pattern occurs soon after sleep onset in patients with narcolepsy, whereas normal subjects experience 80–100 minutes or longer of non-REM (NREM) sleep before the initial REM period. The condition persists throughout life. Nocturnal polysomnography and Multiple Sleep Latency Testing (MSLT) have traditionally been used to diagnose the disorder. HLA subtype DQB1*0602 and DRB1*1501 are associated with narcolepsy (the former is more common than the latter). Recently absence of a hypothalamic neuropeptide, hypocretin was found to be associated with narcolepsy and cataplexy. Spinal fluid (but not plasma) levels of hypocretin-1 are diagnostic (level will be less than one-third of normal controls and can be absent) and have been reported to be absent in up to 95% of patients. It is possible that an autoimmune process may lead to loss of hypocretin containing neurons in the lateral thalamus.

Therapy starts with schedule and behavior modification. CNS stimulants such as amphetamine mixtures (Adderall) or long-acting methylphenidate are typically used to treat excessive daytime somnolence. Modafinil has proven to be effective treatment for narcolepsy or excessive daytime sleepiness associated with narcolepsy in adults and is used at times in children. However, controlled studies in children are lacking. Cataplexy responds to venlafaxine, fluoxetine, or clomipramine. Rarely, acute narcolepsy/cataplexy (autoimmune) responds to IVIG.

2. Benign Neonatal Sleep Myoclonus

Benign neonatal sleep myoclonus (BNSM) is characterized by myoclonic jerks that occur only during sleep and stop abruptly when the child is aroused. It is a benign condition that is frequently confused with epileptic seizures during infancy. Myoclonic jerks usually occur in the first 2 weeks of life, and are usually bilaterally synchronous and symmetrical. Clusters of jerks may last from a few seconds up to 20 minutes. They occur only during sleep and are usually observed at the beginning of the sleep. Waking the child will lead to resolution of the cluster. They resolve spontaneously in the first months of life although may occur as late as 10 months.

3. Nocturnal Frontal Lobe Epilepsy

Nocturnal frontal lobe epilepsy is characterized by paroxysmal arousals from NREM sleep, occasionally with bizarre stereotyped motor movements lasting less than 20 seconds; motor seizures with dystonic or hyperkinetic features lasting 20 seconds to 2 minutes; and episodic nocturnal wanderings which resemble stereotypic agitated somnambulism. NFLE is a heterogeneous disorder which includes both sporadic and familial forms. Autosomal dominant nocturnal frontal lobe epilepsy has been demonstrated to be related to a genetic abnormality affecting nicotinic receptors including two mutant genes coding for the α_4 (*CHRNA4*) and β_2 (*CHRNB2*) subunits of the nicotinic acetyl-choline receptor (nAChR). Lack of definitive epileptiform abnormalities on interictal and at times ictal EEG recordings may lead to misdiagnoses of nocturnal dystonia or a parasomnia, such as night terrors or somnambulism. While antiepileptic drugs may be effective, unresponsiveness to medication is not uncommon.

4. Parasomnias

Parasomnias are abnormal behavioral or physiologic events that occur in association with various sleep stages or the transition between sleeping and waking. The parasomnias of childhood are divided into those occurring in NREM and REM. The NREM parasomnias consist of partial arousals, disorientation, and motor disturbances and include sleepwalking/somnambulism and sleep terrors/pavor nocturnes among others. Several of these types of events are discussed in more detail in Chapter 3.

A. Sleepwalking (Somnambulism)

Somnambulism and somniloquy (sleep talking) are among a group of sleep disturbances known as disorders of arousal which occur in NREM sleep. The onset is abrupt, usually early in the night. It is characterized by coordinated activity (eg, walking and sometimes moving objects seemingly without purpose) in a state of veiled consciousness. The episode is relatively brief and ceases spontaneously. There is poor recall of the event on waking in the morning. Somnambulism may be related to mental activities occurring in stages 3 and 4 of NREM sleep. Incidence has been estimated at only 2%–3%, but up to 15% of cases are reported in children aged 6–16 years. Boys are affected more often than girls and many have recurrent episodes. Psychopathologic features are rarely demonstrated but a strong association (30%) between childhood migraine and somnambulism has been noted. Episodes of somnambulism may be triggered in predisposed children by stresses, including febrile illnesses. No treatment of somnambulism is required, and it is not necessary to seek psychiatric consultation. It is important to educate parents about safety precautions—such as locked doors and safety windows.

B. Night Terrors

Night terrors (pavor nocturnus) are a disorder of arousal from NREM sleep. Most cases occur in children aged 3–8 years, and the disorder rarely occurs after adolescence. It is characterized by sudden (but only partial) waking, with the severely frightened child unable to be fully roused or comforted. Concomitant autonomic symptoms include rapid breathing, tachycardia, and perspiring. The child has no recall of any nightmare. Psychopathologic mechanisms are unclear, but falling asleep after watching scenes of violence on television or hearing frightening stories may play a role. Elimination of such causes and consideration of a sleep study (polysomnogram) to rule out obstructive apnea and complex partial seizures may have a role. Most of the time, watchful waiting and reassurance of the family are sufficient.

5. Restless Legs Syndrome

Restless legs syndrome refers to continuous, bothersome leg movements occurring at rest and producing unpleasant paresthesias (sensory symptoms) that often interfere with restful sleep. Occasionally, anemia (low ferritin) has been noted in adults and children with the disorder; in these cases, improvement has occurred with ferrous sulfate treatment. Avoidance of caffeine, nicotine, alcohol, and some drugs (antidepressants, neuroleptics) has helped in adult series. No pediatric medication studies exist; anecdotally, clonazepam, possibly clonidine, and gabapentin are safe options. DOPA agonists, ropinirole, and pramipexole are used in adults but are unproven in children. This can be familial; therefore, a detailed family history may be helpful.

Ahmed I, Thorpy M: Clinical features, diagnosis, and treatment of Narcolepsy. Clinical chest medicine 2010;31:371–381 [PMID: 20488294].

Cao M, Guilleminault C: Hypocretin and its emerging role as a target for treatment of sleep disorders. Curr Neurol Neurosci Rep 2011;11:227–234 [PMID: 21170610].

Caraballo RH et al: The spectrum of benign myoclonus of early infancy: Clinical and neurophysiologic features in 102 patients. Epilepsia 2009;50:1176–1183 [PMID: 19175386].

Kheirandish-Gozal L: What is "abnormal" in pediatric sleep? Respiratory care 2010;55(10):1366–1374 [PMID: 20875162].

Kotagal S: Parasomnias of childhood. Curr Opin Pediatr 2008; 20:659–665 [PMID: 19005335].

Meltzer LJ et al: Prevalence of diagnosed sleep disorders in pediatric primary care practices. Pediatrics 2010;125(6):e1410–1418 [PMID: 20457689].

Nevsimalova S: Narcolepsy in childhood. Sleep medicine Reviews 2009;13:169–180 [PMID: 19153053].

Picchietti DL et al: Pediatric restless legs syndrome and periodic limb movement disorded: Parent-child pairs. Sleep Medicine 2009;10(9):925–931 [PMID: 19332386].

Sullivan SS: Narcolepsy in adolescents. Adolescent Medicine 2010;21(3):542–555 [PMID: 21302860].

CONGENITAL MALFORMATIONS OF THE NERVOUS SYSTEM

Malformations of the nervous system occur in 1%–3% of living neonates and are present in 40% of infants who die. Developmental anomalies of the CNS may result from a variety of causes, including infectious, toxic, genetic, metabolic, and vascular insults that affect the fetus. The specific type of malformation that results from such insults, however, may depend more on the gestational period during which the insult occurs than on the specific cause. The period of induction, days 0–28 of gestation, is the period during which the neural plate appears and the neural tube forms and closes. Insults during this phase can result in a major absence of neural structures, such as anencephaly, or in a defect of neural tube closure, such as spina bifida, meningomyelocele, or encephalocele. Cellular proliferation and migration characterize neural development that occurs after 28 days' gestation. Lissencephaly, pachygyria, agyria, and agenesis of the corpus callosum may be the result of disruptions (genetic, toxic, infectious, or metabolic) that can occur during the period of cellular proliferation and migration.

1. Abnormalities of Neural Tube Closure

Defects of neural tube closure constitute some of the most common congenital malformations affecting the nervous system, occurring in 1:1000 live births. Spina bifida with associated meningomyelocele or meningocele is commonly found in the lumbar region. Depending on the extent and severity of the involvement of the spinal cord and peripheral nerves, lower extremity weakness, bowel and bladder dysfunction, and hip dislocation may be present. Delivery via cesarean section followed by early surgical closure of meningoceles and meningomyeloceles is usually indicated. Additional treatment is necessary to manage chronic abnormalities of the urinary tract, orthopedic abnormalities such as kyphosis and scoliosis, and paresis of the lower extremities. Hydrocephalus associated with meningomyelocele usually requires ventriculoperitoneal shunting.

A. Arnold-Chiari Malformations

Arnold-Chiari malformation type I consists of elongation and displacement of the caudal end of the brainstem into the spinal canal with protrusion of the cerebellar tonsils through the foramen magnum. In association with this hindbrain malformation, minor to moderate abnormalities of the base of the skull often occur, including basilar impression (platybasia) and small foramen magnum. Arnold-Chiari malformation type I may remain asymptomatic for years, but in older children and young adults it may cause progressive ataxia, paresis of the lower cranial nerves, and progressive vertigo; rarely may it present with apnea or disordered breathing. Posterior cervical laminectomy may be necessary to provide relief from cervical cord compression. Ventriculoperitoneal shunting is required for hydrocephalus.

Arnold-Chiari malformation type II consists of the malformations found in Arnold-Chiari type I plus an associated lumbar meningomyelocele. Hydrocephalus develops in approximately 90% of children with Arnold-Chiari malformation type II. These patients may also have aqueductal stenosis, hydromyelia or syringomyelia, and cortical dysplasias. The clinical manifestations of Arnold-Chiari malformation type II are most commonly caused by the associated hydrocephalus and meningomyelocele. In addition, dysfunction of the lower cranial nerves may be present. Up to 25% of patients may have epilepsy, likely secondary to the cortical dysplasias. Higher lesions of the thoracic or upper lumbar cord are associated with mild mental retardation in about half of patients, while over 85% of patients with lower level lesions have normal intelligence quotients (IQs). Many patients will develop a latex sensitivity or allergy.

Arnold-Chiari malformation type III is characterized by occipital encephalocele, a closure defect of the rostral end of the neural tube. Hydrocephalus is extremely common with this malformation.

B. Diagnosis and Prevention

In general, the diagnosis of neural tube defects is obvious at the time of birth. The diagnosis may be strongly suspected prenatally on the basis of ultrasonographic findings and the presence of elevated α-fetoprotein in the amniotic fluid. All women of childbearing age should take prophylactic folate, which can prevent these defects and decrease the risk of recurrence by 70%.

2. Disorders of Cortical Development

Malformations of cortical development are increasingly recognized with the advent of MRI techniques and the explosion of newly identified genetic syndromes. They are subdivided into disorders based on their etiology: neuronal migration, cortical organization, abnormal proliferation or apoptosis, and unclassified. In this section, we provide some common examples of these subtypes. Lissencephaly is the most common disorder of neuronal migration. Polymicrogyria and schizencephaly are examples of organizational abnormalities. Agenesis of the corpus callosum, described below, is an example of abnormal apoptosis. Finally, some abnormalities such as Dandy-Walker syndrome remained unclassified.

A. Lissencephaly

Lissencephaly is a severe malformation of the brain characterized by an extremely smooth cortical surface with minimal sulcal and gyral development similar to a fetal brain at the end of the first trimester. In addition, lissencephalic brains have a primitive cytoarchitectural construction with a four-layered cerebral mantle instead of the mature six-layered mantle. Pachygyria (thick gyri) and agyria (absence of gyri) may vary in an anterior to posterior gradient, which can be suggestive of the underlying genetic defect. Patients with lissencephaly usually have severe neurodevelopmental delay, microcephaly, and seizures (including infantile spasms); however, there is significant phenotypic heterogeneity, which can depend on the specific mutation. These disorders are auto-somal recessive, except for the X-linked disorders. *LIS1* mutations on chromosome 17 are associated with dysmorphic features (Miller-Dieker syndrome). Another autosomal recessive mutation, involving the *RELN* gene, results in a lissencephaly with severe hippocampal and cerebellar hypoplasia. X-linked syndromes involving mutations in *DCX* (double cortin) and *ARX* (associated with ambiguous genitalia) affect males with lissencephaly and females with band heterotopias or agenesis of the corpus callosum. Lissencephaly in association with hydrocephalus, cerebellar malformations, and muscular dystrophy may occur in Walker-Warburg syndrome (*POMT1* mutation), Fukuyama muscular dystrophy (*fukutin* mutation), and muscle-eye-brain disease (*POMGnT1* mutation). It is particularly important to identify these syndromes not only because clinical tests are available, but also because of their genetic implications. Lissencephaly may also be a component of Zellweger syndrome, a metabolic peroxisomal abnormality associated with the presence of elevated concentrations of very-long-chain fatty acids in plasma. No specific treatment for lissencephaly is available, and seizures are often difficult to control with standard medications.

MRI scans have helped to define several presumed migrational defects that are similar to but anatomically more restricted than lissencephaly. A distinctive example is bilateral perisylvian cortical dysplasia. Patients with this disorder have pseudobulbar palsy, variable cognitive deficits, facial diplegia with dysarthria and drooling, developmental delay, and epilepsy. Seizures are often difficult to control with antiepileptic drugs; some patients have benefited from corpus callosotomy. The cause of this syndrome is as yet unknown, although intrauterine cerebral ischemic injury has been postulated. Therapy is aimed at improving speech and oromotor functions and controlling seizures.

B. Agenesis of the Corpus Callosum

Agenesis of the corpus callosum, once thought to be a rare cerebral malformation, is more frequently diagnosed with modern neuroimaging techniques; occurring in 1:4000 births. The cause of this malformation is unknown. Occasionally it appears to be inherited in either an autosomal dominant or recessive pattern. It has been associated with X-linked patterns (ARX as mentioned earlier). Agenesis of the corpus callosum has been found in some patients with pyruvate dehydrogenase deficiency and in others with nonketotic hyperglycinemia. Most cases are sporadic. Maldevelopment of the corpus callosum may be partial or complete. No specific syndrome is typical of agenesis of the corpus callosum, although many patients have seizures, developmental delay, microcephaly, or mental retardation. Neurologic abnormalities may be related to microscopic cytoarchitectural abnormalities of the brain that occur in association with agenesis of the corpus callosum. The malformation may be found coincidentally by neuroimaging studies in otherwise normal patients and has been described as a coincidental finding at autopsy in neurologically normal individuals. A special form of agenesis of the corpus callosum occurs in Aicardi syndrome. In this X-linked disorder, agenesis of the corpus callosum is associated with other cystic intracerebral abnormalities, early infantile spasms, mental retardation, lacunar chorioretinopathy, and vertebral body abnormalities.

C. Dandy-Walker Syndrome

Despite being described nearly a century ago, the exact definition of the Dandy-Walker syndrome is still debated. Classically, it is characterized by aplasia of the vermis, cystic enlargement of the fourth ventricle, rostral displacement of the tentorium, and absence or atresia of the foramina of Magendie and Luschka. Although hydrocephalus is usually not present congenitally, it develops within the first few months of life. Ninety percent of patients who develop hydrocephalus do so by age 1 year. On physical examination, a rounded protuberance or exaggeration of the cranial occiput often exists. In the absence of hydrocephalus and increased intracranial pressure, few physical findings may be present to suggest neurologic dysfunction. An ataxic syndrome occurs in fewer than 20% of patients and is usually late in appearing. Many long-term neurologic deficits result directly from hydrocephalus. Diagnosis of Dandy-Walker syndrome is confirmed by CT or MRI scanning of the head. Treatment is directed at the management of hydrocephalus.

3. Craniosynostosis

Craniosynostosis, or premature closure of cranial sutures, is usually sporadic and idiopathic. However, some patients have hereditary disorders, such as Apert syndrome and Crouzon disease, that are associated with abnormalities of the digits, extremities, and heart. Occasionally craniosynostosis may be associated with an underlying metabolic disturbance such as hyperthyroidism and hypophosphatasia. The most common form of craniosynostosis involves the sagittal suture and results in scaphocephaly, an elongation of the head in the anterior to posterior direction. Premature closure of the coronal sutures causes brachycephaly, an increase in cranial growth from left to right. Unless many or all cranial sutures close prematurely, intracranial volume will not be compromised, and the brain's growth will not be impaired. Closure of only one or a few sutures will not cause impaired brain growth or neurologic dysfunction. Management of craniosynostosis is directed at preserving normal skull shape and consists of excising the fused suture and applying material to the edge of the craniectomy to prevent reossification of the bone edges. The best cosmetic effect on the skull is achieved when surgery is performed during the first 6 months of life.

4. Hydrocephalus

Hydrocephalus is characterized by an increased volume of CSF in association with progressive ventricular dilation. In communicating hydrocephalus, CSF circulates through the ventricular system and into the subarachnoid space without obstruction. In noncommunicating hydrocephalus, an obstruction blocks the flow of CSF within the ventricular system or blocks the egress of CSF from the ventricular system into the subarachnoid space. A wide variety of disorders, such as hemorrhage, infection, tumors, and congenital malformations, may play a causal role in the development of hydrocephalus. The presence of radialized thumbs and aqueductal stenosis is suggestive of X-linked hydrocephalus due to the clinically testable neural cell adhesion molecule-L1 deficiency.

Clinical features of hydrocephalus include macrocephaly, an excessive rate of head growth, irritability, bulging or full fontanelle, vomiting, loss of appetite, impaired upgaze, impaired extraocular movements, hypertonia of the lower extremities, and generalized hyperreflexia. Without treatment, optic atrophy may occur. In infants, papilledema may not be present, whereas older children with closed cranial sutures can eventually develop swelling of the optic disk. Hydrocephalus can be diagnosed on the basis of the clinical course, findings on physical examination, and CT or MRI scan.

Treatment of hydrocephalus is directed at providing an alternative outlet for CSF from the intracranial compartment. The most common method is ventriculoperitoneal shunting. Other treatment should be directed, if possible, at the underlying cause of the hydrocephalus. For genetic testing, see http://www.genetests.org

Barkovich R et al: A developmental and genetic classification for malformations of cortical development. Neurology 2005;65:1873 [PMID: 16192428].

Doherty D et al: Pediatric perspective on prenatal counseling for myelomeningocele. Birth Defects Res A Clin Mol Teratol 2006;76:645 [PMID: 17001678].

Kotrikova B et al: Diagnostic imaging in the management of craniosynostoses. Eur Radiol 2007;17:1968 [PMID: 17151858].

Liu JS: Molecular genetics of neuronal migration disorders. Curr neurol Neurosci Rep 2011;11:171 [PMID: 21222180].

Paul L et al: Agenesis of the corpus callosum: Genetic, developmental and functional aspects of connectivity. Nat Rev Neurosci 2007;8:287 [PMID: 17375041].

Vertinsky A et al: Macrocephaly, increased intracranial pressure, and hydrocephalus in the infant and young child. Top Magn Reson Imaging 2007;18:31 [PMID: 17607142].

ABNORMAL HEAD SIZE

Bone plates of the skull have almost no intrinsic capacity to enlarge or grow. Unlike long bones, they depend on extrinsic forces to stimulate new bone formation at the suture lines. Although gravity and traction on bone by muscle and scalp probably stimulate some growth, the single most important stimulus for head growth during infancy and childhood is brain growth. Therefore, accurate assessment of head growth is one of the most important aspects of the neurologic examination of young children. A head circumference that is two standard deviations above or below the mean for age requires investigation and explanation.

1. Plagiocephaly

An abnormal skull shape is plagiocephaly ("oblique head"). Flatness of the head (brachycephaly) is a common complaint, and nowadays is usually secondary to supine sleep position ("positional"), not from occipital lambdoid suture craniosynostosis.

Repositioning the head during naps (eg, with a rolled towel under one shoulder), and "tummy time" when awake are remedies. Rarely is a skull film or consultation necessary to rule out craniosynostosis. Most positional nonsynostotic plagiocephaly resolves by age 2 years.

2. Microcephaly

A head circumference more than two standard deviations below the mean for age and sex is by definition microcephaly. More important, however, than a single head circumference measurement is the rate or pattern of head growth over time. Head circumference measurements that progressively drop to lower percentiles with increasing age are indicative of a process or condition that has impaired the brain's capacity to grow. The causes of microcephaly are numerous. Some examples are listed in Table 25–20.

Table 25–20. Causes of microcephaly.

Causes	Examples
Chromosomal	Trisomies 13, 18, 21
Malformation	Lissencephaly, schizencephaly
Syndromes	Rubenstein-Taybi, Cornelia de Lange, Angelman
Toxins	Alcohol, anticonvulsants (?), maternal phenylketonuria (PKU)
Infections (intrauterine)	TORCHS[a]
Radiation	Maternal pelvis, first and second trimester
Placental insufficiency	Toxemia, infection, small for gestational age
Familial	Autosomal dominant, autosomal recessive
Perinatal hypoxia, trauma	Birth asphyxia, injury
Infections (perinatal)	Bacterial meningitis (especially group B streptococci) Viral encephalitis (enterovirus, herpes simplex)
Metabolic	Glut-1 deficiency, PKU, maple syrup urine disease
Degenerative disease	Tay-Sachs, Krabbe

[a]TORCHS is a mnemonic for toxoplasmosis, other infections, rubella, cytomegalovirus, herpes simplex, and syphilis.

Clinical Findings

A. Symptoms and Signs

Microcephaly may be suspected in the full-term newborn and in infants up to age 6 months whose chest circumference exceeds the head circumference (unless the child is very obese). Microcephaly may be discovered when the child is examined because of delayed developmental milestones or neurologic problems, such as seizures or spasticity. There may be a marked backward slope of the forehead (as in familial microcephaly) with narrowing of the bitemporal diameter. The fontanelle may close earlier than expected, and sutures may be prominent.

B. Laboratory Findings

Laboratory findings vary with the cause. Abnormal dermatoglyphics may be present when the injury occurred before 19 weeks' gestation. In the newborn, IgM antibody titers for toxoplasmosis, rubella, CMV, herpes simplex virus, and syphilis may be assessed. Elevated specific IgM titer is indicative of congenital infection. The urine culture for CMV will be positive at birth when this virus is the cause of microcephaly. Eye, cardiac, and bone abnormalities may also be clues to congenital infection. The child's serum and urine amino and organic acid determinations are occasionally diagnostic. The mother may require screening for phenylketonuria. Karyotyping should be considered.

C. Imaging

CT or MRI scans may aid in diagnosis and prognosis. These studies may demonstrate calcifications, malformations, or atrophic patterns that suggest specific congenital infections or genetic syndromes. Plain skull radiographs are of limited value. Genetic counseling should be offered to the family of any infant with significant microcephaly.

Differential Diagnosis

Congenital craniosynostosis involving multiple sutures is easily differentiated by inspection of the head, history, identification of syndromes, hereditary pattern, and sometimes signs and symptoms of increased intracranial pressure. Common forms of craniosynostosis involving sagittal, coronal, and lambdoidal sutures are associated with abnormally shaped heads but do not cause microcephaly. Recognizing treatable causes of undergrowth of the brain such as hypopituitarism or hypothyroidism and severe protein-calorie undernutrition is critical so that therapy can be initiated as early as possible.

Treatment & Prognosis

Except for the treatable disorders already noted, treatment is usually supportive and directed at the multiple neurologic and sensory deficits, endocrine disturbances (eg, diabetes insipidus), and seizures. Many, but not all, children with microcephaly are developmentally delayed. The notable exceptions are found in cases of hypopituitarism (rare) or familial autosomal dominant microcephaly.

3. Macrocephaly

A head circumference more than two standard deviations above the mean for age and sex denotes macrocephaly. Rapid head growth rate suggests increased intracranial pressure, most likely caused by hydrocephalus, extra-axial fluid collections, or neoplasms. Macrocephaly with normal head growth rate suggests familial macrocephaly or true megalencephaly, as might occur in neurofibromatosis. Other causes and examples of macrocephaly are listed in Table 25–21.

Table 25–21. Causes of macrocephaly.

Causes	Examples
Pseudomacrocephaly, pseudohydrocephalus, catch-up growth crossing percentiles	Growing premature infant; recovery from malnutrition, congenital heart disease, postsurgical correction
Increased intracranial pressure	
With dilated ventricles	Progressive hydrocephalus, subdural effusion
With other mass	Arachnoid cyst, porencephalic cyst, brain tumor
Benign familial macrocephaly (idiopathic external hydrocephalus)	External hydrocephalus, benign enlargement of the subarachnoid spaces (synonyms)
Megalencephaly (large brain)	
With neurocutaneous disorder	Neurofibromatosis, tuberous sclerosis, etc
With gigantism	Sotos syndrome
With dwarfism	Achondroplasia
Metabolic	Mucopolysaccharidoses
Lysosomal	Metachromatic leukodystrophy (late)
Other leukodystrophy	Canavan spongy degeneration
Thickened skull	Fibrous dysplasia (bone), hemolytic anemia (marrow), sicklemia, thalassemia

Clinical Findings

Clinical and laboratory findings vary with the underlying process. In infants, transillumination of the skull with an intensely bright light in a completely darkened room may disclose subdural effusions, hydrocephalus, hydranencephaly, and cystic defects. A surgically or medically treatable condition must be ruled out. Thus, the first decision is whether and when to perform an imaging study.

A. Imaging Study Deferred

1. Catch-up growth—Catch-up growth may be evident, as it is in the thriving, neurologically intact premature infant whose rapid head enlargement is most marked in the first weeks of life, or the infant in the early phase of recovery from deprivation dwarfism. As the expected normal size is reached, head growth slows and then resumes a normal growth pattern. If the fontanelle is open, cranial ultrasonography can assess ventricular size and diagnose or exclude hydrocephalus.

2. Familial macrocephaly—This condition may exist when another family member has an unusually large head with no signs or symptoms referable to such disorders as neurocutaneous dysplasias (especially neurofibromatosis) or cerebral gigantism (Sotos syndrome), or when there are no significant mental or neurologic abnormalities in the child.

B. Imaging Study

CT or MRI scans (or ultrasonography, if the anterior fontanelle is open) are used to define any structural cause of macrocephaly and to identify an operable disorder. Even when the condition is untreatable (or does not require treatment), the information gained may permit more accurate diagnosis and prognosis, guide management and genetic counseling, and serve as a basis for comparison should future abnormal cranial growth or neurologic changes necessitate a repeat study. An imaging study is necessary if signs or symptoms of increased intracranial pressure are present (see Table 25–17).

Bishop FS et al: Glutaric aciduria type 1 presenting as bilateral subdural hematomas mimicking nonaccidental trauma. Case report and review of the literature. J Neurosurg 2007;106(Suppl):222 [PMID: 17465389].

Chiu S et al: Early acceleration of head circumference in children with fragile X syndrome and autism. J Dev Behav Pediatr 2007;28:31 [PMID: 17353729].

Fukumoto A et al. Head Circumference and body growth in autism spectrum disorders. Brain Dev 2011;33:569 [PMID: 20934821].

Kaindl A: Many roads lead to primary autosomal recessive microcephaly. Progress in Neurobiology 2010;90:363 [PMID: 19931588].

Losee JE et al: Nonsynostotic occipital plagiocephaly: Factors impacting onset, treatment, and outcomes. Plast Reconstr Surg 2007;119:1866 [PMID: 17440367].

Purugganan OH: Abnormalities in head size. Pediatr Rev 2006;27:473 [PMID: 17142470].

Rogers GF: Deformational plagiocephaly, brachycephaly, and scaphocephaly. Part I: terminology, diagnosis, and etiopathogenesis. J Craniofac Surg 2011;22:9 [PMID: 21187783].

Tarrant A et al: Microcephaly: A radiological review. Pedatr Radiol 2009;39:772 [PMID: 19437006].

NEUROCUTANEOUS DYSPLASIAS

Neurocutaneous dysplasias are diseases of the neuroectoderm and sometimes involve endoderm and mesoderm. Birthmarks—and skin growths appearing later—often suggest a need to look for brain, spinal cord, and eye disease. Hamartomas (histologically normal tissue growing abnormally rapidly or in aberrant sites) are common. The most common dysplasias are dominantly inherited. Benign and even malignant tumors may develop.

Johnson KJ et al: Childhood cancer and birthmarks in the Collaborative Perinatal Project. Pediatrics 2007;119:e1088 [PMID: 17473081].

Kandt RS: Tuberous sclerosis complex and neurofibromatosis type 1: The two most common neurocutaneous diseases. Neurol Clin 2003;21:983 [PMID: 14743661].

Korf BR: The phakomatoses. Clin Dermatol 2005;23:78 [PMID: 15708292].

1. Neurofibromatosis Type 1 (Von Recklinghausen Disease) and Type 2

ESSENTIALS OF DIAGNOSIS & TYPICAL FEATURES

- More than six café au lait spots 5 mm in greatest diameter in prepubertal individuals and over 15 mm in greatest diameter in postpubertal individuals.
- Two or more neurofibromas of any type or one plexiform neurofibroma.
- Freckling in the axillary or inguinal regions.
- Optic glioma.
- Two or more Lisch nodules (iris hamartomas).
- Distinctive bony lesions, such as sphenoid dysplasia or thinning of long bone with or without pseudarthroses.
- First-degree relative (parent, sibling, offspring) with neurofibromatosis type 1 by above criteria.

General Considerations

Neurofibromatosis is a multisystem disorder with a prevalence of 1:3000. Fifty percent of cases are due to new mutations in the *NF1* gene. Forty percent of patients will develop medical complications of the disorder in their lifetime. Two or more positive criteria are diagnostic; others may appear over time. Children with six or more café au lait spots and no other positive criteria should be followed; 95% develop neurofibromatosis type 1.

Clinical Findings

A. Symptoms and Signs

The most common presenting symptoms are cognitive or psychomotor problems; 40% of patients have learning disabilities, and mental retardation occurs in 8%. The family history is important in identifying dominant gene manifestations in parents. Parents should be examined in detail. The history should focus on lumps or masses causing disfigurement, functional problems, or pain. Café au lait spots are seen in most affected children by age 1 year. The typical skin lesion is 10–30 mm, ovoid, and smooth-bordered. Discrete neurofibromas, or lipomas, are more common, are well demarcated, and can occur at any age. Plexiform neurofibromas are more diffuse and can invade normal tissue. They are congenital and are frequently detected during periods of rapid growth. If the face or a limb is involved, there may be associated hypertrophy or overgrowth.

The clinician should ask about visual problems. Strabismus or amblyopia dictates a search for optic glioma, a common tumor in neurofibromatosis. Any progressive neurologic deficit calls for studies to rule out tumor of the spinal cord or CNS. Tumors of cranial nerve VIII (Schwannomas) virtually never occur in neurofibromatosis type 1 but are the rule in neurofibromatosis type 2, a rare autosomal dominant disease. Café au lait spots are less common in neurofibromatosis type 2.

The physician should check blood pressure and examine the spine for scoliosis and the limbs for pseudarthroses. Head measurement often shows macrocephaly. Hearing and vision need to be assessed. The eye examination should include a check for proptosis and iris Lisch nodules. The optic disk should be examined for atrophy or papilledema. Short stature and precocious puberty are occasional findings. An examination for neurologic manifestations of tumors (eg, asymmetrical reflexes or spasticity) is important.

B. Laboratory Findings

Laboratory tests are not likely to be of value in asymptomatic patients. Selected patients require brain MRI with special cuts through the optic nerves to rule out optic glioma. A common finding is hyperintense, nonmass lesions seen on T_2 weighted MRI images. These "unindentified bright objects" ("UBOs") often disappear with time. Hypertension necessitates evaluation of renal arteries for dysplasia and stenosis. Cognitive and school achievement testing may be indicated. Scoliosis or limb abnormalities should be studied by appropriate roentgenograms such as an MRI scan of the spinal cord and roots.

Differential Diagnosis

Patients with McCune-Albright syndrome often have larger café au lait spots with precocious puberty, polyostotic fibrous dysplasia, and hyperfunctioning endocrinopathies. One or two café au lait spots are often seen in normal children. A large solitary café au lait spot is usually innocent, not neurofibromatosis type 1.

Complications

Seizures, deafness, short stature, early puberty, and hypertension occur in less than 25% of patients with neurofibromatosis.

Optic glioma occurs in about 15%. Although the tumor may be apparent at an early age, it rarely causes functional problems and is usually nonprogressive. Patients have a slightly increased risk (5% life risk) for various malignancies. Other tumors may be benign but may cause significant morbidity and mortality because of their size and location in a vital or enclosed space, for example, plexiform neurofibromas.

These "benign" infiltrating tumors can disfigure facially; impair spinal cord, renal, or pelvic-leg function; and are often vexing to treat. PET scans are helpful to detect malignant transformations (to sarcoma). Experimental trials of interferons and mTor inhibitors (rapamycin=sirolimus) are ongoing at many centers.

Strokes from NF-1 cerebral arteropathy are note worthy; arteriopathy of renal arteries can cause reversible hypertension in childhood.

Treatment

Genetic counseling is important. If a parent has neurofibromatosis type 1, the risk to siblings is 50%. The disease may be progressive, with serious complications occasionally seen. Patients sometimes worsen during puberty or pregnancy. Genetic screening of family members is required. Annual or semiannual visits are important in the early detection of school problems or bony or neurologic abnormalities. The following parameters should be recorded at each annual visit:

1. Child's development and progress at school
2. Visual symptoms, visual acuity, and funduscopy until age 7 years (to detect optic pathway glioma, glaucoma)
3. Head circumference (rapid increase might indicate tumor or hydrocephalus)
4. Height (to detect abnormal pubertal development)
5. Weight (to detect abnormal pubertal development)
6. Pubertal development (to detect delayed or precocious puberty due to pituitary or hypothalamic lesion)
7. Blood pressure (to detect renal artery stenosis or pheochromocytoma)
8. Cardiovascular examination (for congenital heart disease, especially pulmonary stenosis)
9. Evaluation of spine (for scoliosis and underlying plexiform neurofibromas)
10. Evaluation of the skin (for cutaneous, subcutaneous, and plexiform neurofibromas)
11. Examination of other systems, depending on specific symptoms

Multidisciplinary clinics at medical centers around the United States are excellent resources. Prenatal diagnosis is probably on the horizon, but the variability of manifestations (trivial to severe) will make therapeutic abortion an unlikely option. Chromosomal linkage studies are under way (chromosome 17q11.2). Information for lay people and physicians is available from the National Neurofibromatosis Foundation (http://www.nf.org).

Al-Otibi M, Rutka JT: Neurosurgical implications of neurofibromatosis type 1 in children. Neurosurg Focus 2006;20:E2 [PMID: 16459992].

Arun D, Gutmann DH: Recent advances in neurofibromatosis type 1. Curr Opin Neurol 2005;17:101 [PMID: 15021234].

Asthagiri AR et al: Neurofibromatosis type 2. Lancet 2009; 373:1974 [Epub May 22].

Ferner RE et al: Guidelines for the diagnosis and management of individuals with neurofibromatosis 1. J Med Genet 2007;44:81 [PMID: 17105749].

Gonzalez G et al: Bilateral segmental neurofibromatosis: A case report and review. Pediatr Neurol 2007;36:51.

Gottfried ON et al: Neurofibromatosis Type 1 and tumorgenesis: Molecular mechanisms and therapeutic implications. Neurosurg Focus 2010;28:E8 [PMID: 20043723].

Jakacki Rl et al: Phase 1 trial of pegylated interferon-alpha-2b in young patients with plexiform neurofibromas. Neurology 2011;76:265 [PMID: 21242495].

Listrnick R et al: Optic pathway gliomas in neruofibromatosis-1: Controversies and recommendations. Ann Neurol 2007;61:189 [PMID: 17387725].

Lorenzo J: Mental, motor, and language development of toddlers with neurofibromatosis type 1. J Pediatr 2011;158:660 [PMID: 21094952].

Rea D et al: Cerebral arteriopathy in children with neurofibromatosis type 1. Pediatrics 2009;124:e476–e483 [PMID: 19706560].

Ruggieri M et al: Earliest clinical manifestations and natural history of neurofibromatosis type 2 (NF2) in childhood: A study of 24 patients. Neuropediatrics 2005;36:21 [PMID: 15776319].

2. Tuberous Sclerosis (Bourneville Disease)

ESSENTIALS OF DIAGNOSIS & TYPICAL FEATURES

- Facial angiofibromas or subungual fibromas.
- Often hypomelanotic macules, gingival fibromas.
- Retinal hamartomas.
- Cortical tubers or subependymal glial nodules, often calcified.
- Renal angiomyolipomas.

General Considerations

Tuberous sclerosis is a dominantly inherited disease. Almost all patients have deletions on chromosome 9 (*TSC1* gene) or 16 (*TSC2* gene). The gene products hamartin and tuberin have tumor-suppressing effects. A triad of seizures, mental retardation, and adenoma sebaceum occurs in only 33% of patients. The disease was earlier thought to have a high rate of mutation. As a result of more sophisticated techniques such as MRI, parents formerly thought not to harbor the gene are now being diagnosed as asymptomatic carriers.

Like neurofibromatosis, tuberous sclerosis is associated with a wide variety of symptoms. The patient may be asymptomatic except for skin findings or may be devastated by severe infantile spasms in early infancy, by continuing epilepsy, and by mental retardation. Seizures in early infancy correlate with later mental retardation.

Clinical Findings

A. Symptoms and Signs

1. Dermatologic features—Skin findings bring most patients to the physician's attention. Ninety-six percent of patients have one or more hypomelanotic macules, facial angiofibromas, ungual fibromas, or shagreen patches. Adenoma sebaceum, the facial skin hamartomas, may first appear in early childhood, often on the cheek, chin, and dry sites of the skin where acne is not usually seen. They often have a reddish hue. The off-white hypomelanotic macules are seen more easily in tanned or dark-skinned individuals than in those with lighter skin. The macules often are oval or "ash leaf" in shape and follow dermatomes. A Wood lamp (ultraviolet light) shows the macules more clearly, a great help in the light-skinned patient. In the scalp, poliosis (whitened hair) is the equivalent. In infancy, the presence of these macules accompanied by seizures is virtually diagnostic of the disease. Subungual or periungual fibromas are more common in the toes. Leathery, orange peel–like shagreen patches support the diagnosis. Café au lait spots are occasionally seen. Fibrous or raised plaques may resemble coalescent angiofibromas.

2. Neurologic features—Seizures are the most common presenting symptom. Up to 20% of patients with infantile spasms (a serious epileptic syndrome) have tuberous sclerosis. Thus, any patient presenting with infantile spasms (and the parents as well) should be evaluated for this disorder. An imaging study of the CNS, such as a CT scan, may show calcified subependymal nodules; MRI may show dysmyelinating white matter lesions or cortical tubers. Virtually any kind of symptomatic seizure (eg, atypical absence, partial complex, and generalized tonic-clonic seizures) may occur.

3. Mental retardation—Mental retardation occurs in up to 50% of patients referred to tertiary care centers; the incidence is probably much lower in randomly selected patients. Patients with seizures are more prone to mental retardation or learning disabilities.

4. Renal lesions—Renal cysts or angiomyolipomas may be asymptomatic. Hematuria or obstruction of urine flow sometimes occurs; the latter requires operation. Ultrasonography of the kidneys should be done in any patient suspected of tuberous sclerosis, both to aid in diagnosis if lesions are found and to rule out renal obstructive disease.

5. Cardiopulmonary involvement—Rarely cystic lung disease may occur. Rhabdomyomas of the heart may be asymptomatic but can lead to outflow obstruction, conduction difficulties, and death. Chest radiographs and echocardiograms can detect these rare manifestations. Cardiac rhabdomyoma may be detected on prenatal ultrasound examination, rhabdomyomas typically regress with age, so symptomatic presentations are typically in the perinatal period or infancy when rhabdomyomas are largest.

6. Eye involvement—Retinal hamartomas are often near the disk.

7. Skeletal involvement—Findings sometimes helpful in diagnosis are cystic rarefactions of the bones of the fingers or toes.

B. Diagnostic Studies

Plain radiographs may detect areas of thickening within the skull, spine, and pelvis, and cystic lesions in the hands and feet. Chest radiographs may show lung honeycombing. More helpful is MRI or CT scanning; the latter can show the virtually pathognomonic subependymal nodular calcifications and sometimes widened gyri or tubers and brain tumors. Contrast material may show the often classically located tumors near the interventricular foramen. Hypomyelinated lesions may be seen with MRI. EEG is helpful in delineating the presence of seizure discharges.

Treatment

Therapy is as indicated by underlying disease (eg, seizures and tumors of the brain, kidney, and heart). Skin lesions on the face may need dermabrasion or laser treatment. Genetic counseling emphasizes identification of the carrier. The risk of appearance in offspring if either parent is a carrier is 50%. The patient should be seen annually for counseling and reexamination in childhood. Identification of the chromosomes (9,16; *TSC1* and *TSC2* genes) may in the future make intrauterine diagnosis possible.

Treatment of refractory epilepsy may lead to surgical extirpation of epileptiform tuber sites.

Recent research (so far, in mice) has suggested the "mammalian target of rapamycin" (mTOR) inhibitors (eg, rapamycin) may inhibit epilepsy in tuberous sclerosis, even shrink dysplasia/tubers, tumors, adenoma sebacea and possibly improve learning.

Davie DM et al: Sirolimus therapy for angiomyolipoma in tuberous sclerosis and sporadic lymphangioleiomyomatosis: A phase 2 trial. Clin Cander Res 2011;17:4071 [PMID: 21525172].

Devlin La et al: Tuberous sclerosis complex: Clinical features, diagnosis, and prevalence within Northern Ireland. Dev Med Child Neurol 2006;48:495 [PMID: 16700943].

Franz DN et al: Tuberous sclerosis complex: Neurological, renal and pulmonary manifestations. Neuropediatrics 2010;41:199 [PMID: 21210335].

Leung AK, Robson WL: Tuberous sclerosis complex: A review. J Pediatr Health Care 2007;21:108 [PMID: 17321910].

Rosser T et al: The diverse clinical manifestations of tuberous sclerosis complex: A review. Semin Pediatr Neurol 2006;13:27 [PMID: 16818173].

Sampason JR: Therapeutic therapy targeting of mTOR in tuberous sclerosis. BiochemSoc Trans 2009;37(Pt 1):259 [PMID: 19143643].

Thiele EA: Managing epilepsy in tuberous sclerosis complex. J Child Neurol 2004;19:680 [PMID: 15563014].

3. Encephalofacial Angiomatosis (Sturge-Weber Disease)

Sturge-Weber disease consists of a facial port wine nevus involving the upper part of the face (in the first division of cranial nerve V), a venous angioma of the meninges in the occipitoparietal regions, and choroidal angioma. The syndrome has been described without the facial nevus (rare, type III, exclusive leptomeningeal angioma).

Clinical Findings

In infancy, the eye may show congenital glaucoma, or buphthalmos, with a cloudy, enlarged cornea. In early stages, the facial nevus may be the only indication, with no findings in the brain even on radiologic studies. The characteristic cortical atrophy, calcifications of the cortex, and meningeal angiomatosis may appear with time, solidifying the diagnosis.

Physical examination may show focal seizures or hemiparesis on the side contralateral the cerebral lesion. The facial nevus may be much more extensive than the first division of cranial nerve V; it can involve the lower face, mouth, lip, neck, and even torso. Hemiatrophy of the contralateral limbs may occur. Mental handicap may result from poorly controlled seizures. Late-appearing glaucoma and rarely CNS hemorrhage occur.

Radiologic studies may show calcification of the cortex; CT scanning may show this much earlier than plain radiographic studies. MRI often shows underlying brain involvement.

The EEG often shows depression of voltage over the involved area in early stages; later, epileptiform abnormalities may be present focally.

The differential diagnosis includes (rare) PHACES syndrome: **P**osterior fossa malformation, segmental (facial) **H**emangioma, **A**rterial abnormalities, **C**ardiac defects, **E**ye abnormalities, and **S**ternal (or ventral) defects; often, only portions of that list are present.

Treatment

Sturge-Weber disease is sporadic. Early control of seizures is important to avoid consequent developmental setback. If seizures do not occur, normal development can be anticipated. Careful examination of the newborn, with ophthalmologic assessment to detect early glaucoma, is indicated. Rarely, surgical removal of the involved meninges and the involved portion of the brain may be indicated, even hemispherectomy.

Adams ME et al: A Spectrum of unusual neuroimaging findings in patients with suspected Sturge-Weber syndrome. AJNR Am J Neuroradiol 2009;30:276 [PMID: 19050205].

Comi AM: Update on Sturge-Weber syndrome: Diagnosis, treatment, quantitative measures, and controversies. Lymphat Res Biol 2007;5:257 [PMID: 18370916].

Heyer GL et al: The neurologic aspect of PHACE: Case report and review of the literature. Pediatr Neurol 2006;35:419 [PMID: 17138012].

Janner D et al: Index of suspicion: Sturge-Weber. Pediatr Rev 2007;28:27 [PMID: 17197457].

Kossoff EH et al: Outcomes of 32 hemispherectomies for Sturge-Weber syndrome worldwide. Neurology 2002;59:1735 [PMID: 12473761].

Kossof EH, Ferenc L, Comi AM: An infantile-onset, severe, yet sporadic seizure pattern in common Sturge-Weber syndrome. Epilepsia 2009 Apr 6 [Epub ahead of print] [PMID: 19389148].

Miyama S, Goto T: Leptomeningeal angiomatosis with infantile spasms. Pediatr Neurol 2004;31:353 [PMID: 15519118].

Oza VS et al: PHACES association: A neurologic review of 17 patients. AJNR Am J Neuroradiol 2008;29:807 [PMID: 18223093].

Park C, Bodensteiner JB: An infant with segmental hemangioma: Sturge-Weber? Semin Pediatr Neurology 2008;15:164 [PMID: 19073319].

Welty LD: Sturge-Weber syndrome: A case study. Neonatal Netw 2006;25:89 [PMID: 16610482].

4. von Hippel-Lindau Disease (Retinocerebellar Angiomatosis)

von Hippel-Lindau disease is a rare, dominantly inherited condition with retinal and cerebellar hemangioblastomas; cysts of the kidneys, pancreas, and epididymis; and sometimes renal cancers. The patient may present with ataxia, slurred speech, and nystagmus due to a hemangioblastoma of the cerebellum or with a medullary spinal cord cystic hemangioblastoma. Retinal detachment may occur from hemorrhage or exudate in the retinal vascular malformation. Rarely a pancreatic cyst or renal tumor may be the presenting symptom.

The diagnostic criteria for the disease are a retinal or cerebellar hemangioblastoma with or without a positive family history, intra-abdominal cyst, or renal cancer.

Fitz EW, Newman SA: Neuro-ophthalmology of von Hippel-Lindau. Curr Neurol Neurosci Rep 2004;4:384 [PMID: 15324605].

Meister et al: Radiological evaluation. Management and surveillance of renal masses in von Hippel-Landau disease. Clin Radiol 2009;64:589 [PMID: 19414081].

Richard S et al: von Hippel-Lindau disease. Lancet 2004;363:1231 [PMID: 15081659].

CENTRAL NERVOUS SYSTEM DEGENERATIVE DISORDERS OF INFANCY & CHILDHOOD

The CNS degenerative disorders of infancy and childhood are characterized by arrest of psychomotor development and loss, usually progressive but at variable rates, of mental and motor functioning and often of vision as well (Tables 25–22 and 25–23). Seizures are common in some disorders, more

Table 25–22. Central nervous system degenerative disorders of infancy.

Disease	Enzyme Defect and Genetics	Onset	Early Manifestations	Vision and Hearing	Somatic Findings
White matter					
Globoid (Krabbe) leukodystrophy	Recessive galactocerebroside β-galactosidase deficiency. Chromosome 14q21–14q31.	Infantile form first 6 mo. Late-onset form 2–6 y. Adolescent and adult forms are rare.	Feeding difficulties. Shrill cry. Irritability. Arching of back.	Optic atrophy, mid to late course. Hyperacusis occasionally.	Head often small. Often underweight.
Metachromatic leukodystrophy	Recessive. Arylsulfatase A deficiency. 22q13. Variant: Saposin B deficiency.	Most common is late-infantile form, presenting at 18–24 mo. Juvenile and adult forms present later.	Incoordination, especially gait disturbance; then general regression. Reverse in juveniles.	Optic atrophy, usually late. Hearing normal.	Macrocephaly. No change in juvenile form.
Pantothenate kinase–associated neurodegeneration (previously Hallervorden-Spatz syndrome)	Autosomal recessive; most common mutation is in PANK2 gene on chromosome 20.	Early onset is by age 10 y.	Rigidity, dystonia, gait disturbance, tremor.	Abnormal ERG. Retinal degeneration.	Dystonia, gait disturbance.
Pelizaeus-Merzbacher disease	X-linked recessive; rare female. Proteolipid protein (myelin) decreased. Xq22.	Birth (perinatal) to 2 y.	Eye rolling often shortly after birth. Head bobbing. Slow loss of intellect.	Slowly developing optic atrophy. Hearing normal. Nystagmus.	Head and body normal.
Diffuse, but primarily gray matter					
Poliodystrophy (Alpers disease or syndrome)	Occasionally familial, recessive. Metabolic forms.	Infancy to adolescence.	Variable: loss of intellect, seizures, incoordination. Vomiting, hepatic failure.	Cortical blindness and deafness.	Head normal initially; may fail to grow.
Tay-Sachs disease and G_{M2} gangliosidosis variants: Sandhoff disease; juvenile; chronic-adult	Recessive. Hexosaminidase deficiencies caused by HEXA gene on chromosome 15q23–24.62,63. Tay-Sachs (93% East European Jewish), hexosaminidase A deficiency. Sandhoff hexosaminidase A and B deficiency. Juvenile partial hexosaminidase A.	Tay-Sachs, and Sandhoff 3–6 mo; others 2–6 y or later.	Variable: shrill cry, loss of vision, infantile spasms, arrest of development. In juvenile and chronic forms: motor difficulties; later, mental difficulties.	Cherry-red macula, early blindness. Hyperacusis early. Strabismus in juvenile form, blindness late.	Head enlarged late. Liver occasionally enlarged. None in juvenile chronic forms.
Niemann-Pick disease and variants	50% Jewish. Recessive. Sphingomyelinase deficiency in types A and C involving the CNS.	First 6 mo. In variants, later onset: often non-Jewish.	Slow development. Protruding belly.	Cherry-red macula in 35%–50%. Blindness late. Deafness occasionally.	Head usually normal. Spleen enlarged more than liver. Occasional xanthomas of skin. Vertical gaze palsy.
Infantile Gaucher disease (glucosylceramide lipidosis)	Recessive. Glucocerebrosidase deficiency.	First 6 mo; rarely, late infancy.	Stridor or hoarse cry; retraction; feeding difficulties.	Occasional cherry-red macula. Convergent squint. Deafness occasionally.	Head usually normal. Liver and spleen equally enlarged.

Motor System	Seizures	Laboratory and Tissue Studies	Course
Early spasticity, occasionally preceded by hypotonia. Prolonged nerve conduction.	Early. Myoclonic and generalized, decerebrate posturing.	CSF protein elevated; usually normal in late onset forms. Sural nerve; nonspecific myelin breakdown. Enzyme deficiency in leukocytes, cultured skin fibroblasts. Demyelination, gliosis with low-signal CT scan, high-signal T_2-weighted MRI.	Rapid. Death usually by 1.5–2 y. Late-onset cases may live 5–10 y. Hematopoietic stem cell transplantation and enzyme replacement therapy is an experimental with variable results.
Combined upper and lower motor neuron signs. Ataxia. Prolonged nerve conduction.	Infrequent, usually late and generalized.	Metachromatic cells in urine: negative sulfatase A test. CSF protein elevated. Urine sulfatide increased. Sural nerve biopsy; metachromasia. Enzyme deficiency in leukocytes, cultured skin fibroblasts. Imaging: Same as globoid leukodystrophy.	Moderately slow. Death in infantile form by 3–8 y, in juvenile form by 10–15 y. Hematopoietic stem cell transplantation is an experimental treatment with variable results.
Extrapyramidal signs, dysarthria, increased deep tendon reflexes.	Variable, EEG may be abnormal.	Axonal degeneration (spheroids). Iron deposits in basal ganglia on MRI: eye-of-the-tiger appearance.	Progressive mental/motor deterioration.
Cerebellar signs early, hyperactive deep reflexes. Spasticity.	Usually only late.	None specific. Brain biopsy: extensive demyelination with small perivascular islands of intact myelin. Point mutations or duplications of PLP gene account for 65%–90% of cases.	Very slow, often seemingly stationary.
Variable: incoordination, spasticity.	Often initial manifestation: myoclonic, akinetic, and generalized.	*POLG1* mutation: multiple deletions, depletions of mitochondrial DNA. Neuronal loss in cortex: may occur very late. Variably increased serum pyruvate, lactate; liver steatosis, cirrhosis late. Muscle and liver biopsy show evidence of mitochondrial dysfunction.	Usually rapid, with death within 1–3 y after onset. Variants in older children, adults.
Initially floppy. Eventual decerebrate rigidity. In juvenile and chronic forms: dysarthria, ataxia, spasticity.	Frequent, in mid and late course. Infantile spasms and generalized.	Blood smears: vacuolated lymphocytes; basophilic hypergranulation. Enzyme deficiencies in serum, leukocytes, culture, skin fibroblasts. High-density thalami on CT scan, low-density white matter.	Moderately rapid. Death usually by 2–5 y. In juvenile form, 5–15 y.
Initially floppy. Eventually spastic. Occasionally extrapyramidal signs. Ataxia, dystonia.	Rare and late.	Blood: vacuolated lymphocytes; increased lipids. X-rays: "mottled" lungs, decalcified bones. "Foam cells" in bone marrow, spleen, lymph nodes. WBC, fibroblast enzyme studies are diagnostic.	Moderately slow. Death usually by 3–5 y.
Opisthotonos early, followed rapidly by decerebrate rigidity.	Rare and late.	Anemia. Increased acid phosphatase. X-rays: thinned cortex, trabeculation of bones. "Gaucher cells" in bone marrow, spleen. Enzyme deficiency in leukocytes or cultured skin fibroblasts.	Very rapid. Experimental enzyme replacement therapy is underway.

(*Continued*)

Table 25–22. Central nervous system degenerative disorders of infancy. (*Continued*)

Disease	Enzyme Defect and Genetics	Onset	Early Manifestations	Vision and Hearing	Somatic Findings
Generalized gangliosidosis and juvenile type (G_{M1} gangliosidoses)	Recessive; β-galactosidase deficiency.	Birth to 6 months in infantile form. 7 mo to 3 y in late infantile or juvenile onset.	Arrest of development. Protruding belly. Coarse facies in infantile (generalized) form. In juvenile form, ataxia and dysarthria.	50% "cherry-red spot." Corneal clouding. Hearing usually normal. In juvenile type. Occasionally retinitis pigmentosa.	Head enlarged early: liver enlarged more than spleen. Gingival hypertrophy. Cardiomyopathy.
Subacute necrotizing encephalomyelopathy (Leigh disease)	Recessive or variable. May have deficiency of pyruvate carboxylase, pyruvate dehydrogenase, cytochrome enzymes.	Infancy to late childhood.	Difficulties in feeding; feeble or absent cry; floppiness; apnea; developmental regression; ataxia. Presentation can be highly variable.	Optic atrophy, often early. Roving eye movements. Ophthalmoplegia.	Head usually normal, occasionally small; cardiac and renal tubular dysfunction occasionally.
Menkes disease (kinky hair disease)	X-linked recessive; defect in copper absorption.	Infancy.	Peculiar facies; secondary hair white, twisted, split; hypothermia.	May show optic disk pallor and micro-cysts of pigment epithelium.	Growth retardation.
Carbohydrate-deficient glycoprotein syndrome	Recessive glycoprotein abnormality; glycosylation faulty.	Infancy.	Failure to thrive, retardation, protein-losing enteropathy.	Strabismus, retinopathy.	Dysmorphic facies. Prominent fat pads. Inverted nipples.
Abetalipoproteinemia (Bassen-Kornzweig disease)	Recessive; primary defect is microsomal triglyceride transfer protein (MTP) on chromosome 4q22–24.	Early childhood.	Diarrhea in infancy.	Retinitis pigmentosa; late ophthalmoplegia.	None.

commonly those with gray matter involvement. Symptoms and signs vary with age at onset and primary sites of involvement of specific types.

These disorders are fortunately rare. An early clinical pattern of decline often follows normal early development. Referral for sophisticated biochemical testing is usually necessary before a definitive diagnosis can be made. Recently, many physicians have been involved in experimental bone marrow transplantation and enzyme-replacement therapy for some of these disorders, with variable results. Patients with metachromatic leukodystrophy, Krabbe disease, and adrenoleukodystrophy are candidates for bone marrow transplantation. Treatment of some lysosomal storage diseases, such as Gaucher disease, with enzyme replacement therapy has shown promising results.

Augestad L et al: Occurrence of and mortality from childhood neuronal ceroid lipofuscinoses in Norway. J Child Neurol 2006;21:917 [PMID: 17092455].

Bindu P et al: Clinical heterogeneity in Hallervorden-Spatz syndrome: A clinicoradiological study in 13 patients from South India. Brain Dev 2006;28:343 [PMID: 16504438].

Brunetti-Pierri N et al: GM1 gangliosidosis: Review of clinical, molecular, and therapeutic aspects. Molecular Genetics and Metabolism 2008;94:391 [PMID: 18524657].

Costello DJ et al: Leukodystrophies: Classification, diagnosis, and treatment. Neurologist 2009;15:319 [PMID: 19901710].

de Bie P et al: Molecular pathogenesis of Wilson and Menkes disease: Correlation of mutations with molecular defects and disease phenotypes. J Med Genet 2007;23 [PMID: 17717039].

Finsterer J: Leigh and Leigh-like syndrome in children and adults. Pediatr Neurol 2008;39:223 [PMID: 1805359].

Fogel B et al: Clinical features and molecular genetics of autosomal recessive cerebellar ataxias. Lancet Neurol 2007;6:245 [PMID: 17303531].

Garbern J: Pelizaeus-Merzbacher disease: Genetic and cellular pathogenesis. Cell Mol Life Sci 2007;64:50 [PMID: 17115121].

Gieselmann V et al: Metachromatic leukodystrophy—An update. Neuropediatrics 2010;41:1 [PMID: 20571983].

Gordon N: Alpers syndrome: Progressive neuronal degeneration of children with liver disease. Dev Med Child Neurol 2006;48:1001 [PMID: 17109792].

Gutierrez J et al: Subacute sclerosing panencephalitis: An update. Dev Med Child neurol 2010;52:901 [PMID: 20561004].

Koehler W: Leukodystrophies with late disease onset: An update. Curr Opin Neurol 2010;23:234 [PMID: 20216214].

Motor System	Seizures	Laboratory and Tissue Studies	Course
Initially floppy, eventually spastic.	Usually late.	Blood: vacuolated lymphocytes. X-rays: dorsolumbar kyphosis, "breaking" of vertebrae. "Foam cells" similar to those in Niemann-Pick disease.	Very rapid. Death within a few years. Slower in juvenile type (to 10 y).
Flaccid and immobile; may become spastic. Spinocerebellar forms; ataxia, myelopathy.	Rare and late tonic seizures.	Increased CSF and blood lactate and pyruvate. High-signal MRI T_2 foci in thalami; globus pallidus, putamen, subthalamic nuclei. May be considered a mitochondrial disorder. DNA, enzyme tests on muscle.	Usually rapid in infants, but may be slow with death after several years. Central hypoventilation a frequent cause of death.
Variable: floppy to spastic.	Myoclonic infantile spasms, status epilepticus.	Defective absorption of copper. Cerebral angiography shows elongated arteries. Hair shows pili torti, split shafts. Copper and ceruloplasmin low.	Moderately rapid. Death usually by 3–4 y.
Variable hypotonia, neuropathy.	Rare.	Normal transferrin decreased. Carbohydrate-deficient transferrin increased. Liver steatosis. Cerebellar hypoplasia.	Cardiomyopathy, thrombosis. Hepatic fibrosis.
Ataxia, late extrapyramidal movement disorder.	None.	Abetalipoproteinemia: acanthocytosis, low serum vitamin E; cerebellar atrophy on imaging.	Progression arrested with vitamin E.

CNS, central nervous system; CSF, cerebrospinal fluid; CT, computed tomography; EEG, electroencephalogram; ERG, electroretinogram; MRI, magnetic resonance imaging; WBC, white blood cell.

Kolter T et al: Sphingolipid metabolism diseases. Biochim Biophys Acta 2006;1758:2057 [PMID: 16854371].

Krupp L et al: Consensus definitions proposed for pediatric multiple sclerosis and related disorders. Neurology 2007;68:S7 [PMID: 17438241].

Rakheja D et al: Juvenile neuronal ceroid-lipofuscinosis (Batten disease): A brief review and update. Current molecular medicine 2007;7:603 [PMID: 17896996].

Roos RA: Huntington's disease: A clinical review. Orphanet J Rare Dis 2010;5:40 [PMID: 21171977].

Sharma et al: Vanishing white matter disease associated with ptosis and myoclonic seizures. J Child Neurol 2011;26:366 [PMID: 21115745].

Sparks S: Inherited disorders of glycosylation. Mol Genet Metab 2006;87:1 [PMID: 16511948].

Van der Knapp MD et al: Megalencephalic leukoencephalopathy with cysts without MLC1 defect. Ann Neurol 2010;67:834 [PMID: 20517947].

Walker F: Huntington's disease. Lancet 2007;369:218 [PMID: 17240289].

Worgall S: Neurological deterioration in late infantile neuronal ceroid lipofuscinosis. Neurology 2007;69:521 [PMID: 17679671].

ATAXIAS OF CHILDHOOD

ESSENTIALS FOR DIAGNOSIS

- Ataxia is most commonly due to cerebellar dysfunction but abnormalities at almost any level of the nervous system can result in motor incoordination.
- It is essential to distinguish between acquired and congenital ataxia as the evaluation, management and outcome is determined by etiology.
- A detailed history and evaluation of truncal vs limb ataxia, mental status, and eye movements can provide the most useful diagnostic points in the formulation of the differential diagnosis.

Pathophysiology

In general, there are two major categories one should consider in the evaluation of ataxia. Acute acquired ataxia is

Table 25–23. Central nervous system degenerative disorders of childhood.[a]

Disease	Enzyme Defect and Genetics	Onset	Early Manifestations	Vision and Hearing	Motor System	Seizures	Laboratory and Tissue Studies	Course
Adrenoleukodystrophy and variants (peroxisomal disease)	X-linked recessive. Neonatal form recessive Xq28. Acyl-CoA synthetase deficiency.	5–10 y. May also present as newborn, adolescent, or adult.	Impaired intellect; behavioral problems.	Cortical blindness and deafness.	Ataxia, spasticity; motor deficits may be asymmetrical or one-sided initially; adrenomyeloneuropathy in adults.	Occasionally.	Hyperpigmentation and adrenocortical insufficiency. ACTH elevated. Accumulation of very-long-chain fatty acids in plasma. Stem cell, marrow transplantation early.	Variable course, many mildly involved. Severe variant with death in 2–5 y.
Neuronal ceroid lipofuscinosis (NCL; cerebromacular degeneration); infantile NCL (INCL); late infantile (LINCL); juvenile NCL (JNCL; Batten disease)	Recessive; multiple gene mutations, polymorphisms.	INCL: 6–24 mo; LINCL: 2–4 y; JNCL: 4–8 y.	Ataxia; visual difficulties; arrested intellectual development. Seizures.	Pigmentary degeneration of macula; optic atrophy; ERG, VER abnormal.	Ataxia; spasticity progressing to decerebrate rigidity.	Often early: myoclonus and later generalized; refractory.	Blood: vacuolated lymphocytes. Biopsy, EM of skin, conjunctiva; WBC: "curvilinear bodies, fingerprint profiles." Molecular testing of *CLN1*, *CLN2*, *CLN3* genes. Protein gene product testing for CLN1 and CLN2.	Moderately slow. Death in 3–8 y.
Subacute sclerosing panencephalitis (Dawson disease)	None. Measles "slow virus" infection. Also reported as result of rubella.	3–22 y; rarely earlier or later.	Impaired intellect; emotional lability; incoordination.	Occasionally chorioretinitis or optic atrophy; hearing normal.	Ataxia; slurred speech; occasionally involuntary movements; spasticity progressing to decerebrate rigidity.	Myoclonic and akinetic seizures relatively early; later, focal and generalized.	CSF protein normal to moderately elevated. High CSF IgG,[b] oligoclonal bands. Elevated CSF (and serum) measles (or rubella) antibody titers. Characteristic EEG. Brain biopsy; inclusion (acidophilic) body encephalitis; culturing of measles virus, perhaps rubella virus.	Variable, death in months to years. Remissions occasional. Treatment: INF-α intrathecal?
Megalencephalic leukodystrophy with subcortical cysts (MLC)	*MLC1* gene defect usually 22q.	Infancy.	Acquired macrocephaly.		Ataxia; spasticity; mild spasticity; dystonia.	Varied; epilepsy.	Characteristic MRI dysmyelination.	Slowly progressive to adulthood; wheelchair bound by teens
Vanishing white matter/ childhood ataxia with CNS hypomyelination (VWM/CACH)	eIF2B 3q27 autosomal recessive.	Fatal infancy variant; other (slower) variants.	Episodic deterioration with fever, head trauma, fear.		Ataxia, spasticity.		MRI: dramatic disappearance of white matter.	Fatal infantile form. Slowly progressive form. Adult variant (autosomal dominant) with ovarian dysgenesis.
Alexander disease	*GFAP* gene mutation autosomal dominant.	Infancy.	Macrocephaly key finding.		As above.		Demyelination; rosenthal fibers characteristic of biopsy.	Fatal infantile. Juvenile: bulbar signs, less retardation.

Multiple sclerosis	None. Diagnosis difficult in childhood.	Adolescent; rare in childhood.	Highly variable: may strike one or more sites of CNS; paresthesias common.	Optic neuritis; diplopia, nystagmus at some time; vestibulocochlear nerves occasionally affected.	Motor weakness; spasticity; ataxia; sphincter disturbances; slurred speech; mental difficulties.	Rare: focal or generalized.	CSF may show slight pleocytosis, elevation of protein and γ-globulin;[b] oligoclonal bands present. CT scan may show areas of demyelination. Auditory, visual, and somatosensory evoked responses often show lesions in respective pathways. Changes in T-cell subsets.	Variable: complete remission possible. Recurrent attacks and involvement of multiple sites are prerequisites for diagnosis.
Cerebrotendinous xanthomatosis	Recessive. Abnormal accumulation of cholesterol.	Late childhood to adolescence.	Xanthomas in tendons; mental deterioration.	Cataracts; xanthelasma.	Cerebellar defects; bulbar paralysis late.	Myoclonus.	Xanthomas may appear in lungs. Xanthomas in tendons (especially Achilles).	Very slowly progressive into middle life. Replace deficient bile acid.
Huntington disease	Dominant. Chromosome 4p CAG repeat.	10% childhood onset.	Hypokinetic; dystonia; rigidity; dementia.	Ophthalmoplegia late.	Rigidity; chorea frequently absent in children.	50% motor seizures "epileptic fits".	CT scan may show "butterfly" atrophy of caudate and putamen.	Moderately rapid with death in 15 y.
Refsum disease (peroxisomal disease)	Recessive. Phytanic acid oxidase deficiency.	5–10 y.	Ataxia; ichthyosis; cardiomyopathy.	Retinitis pigmentosa; nystagmus.	Ataxia; neuropathy; tendon reflexes absent.	None.	Serum phytanic acid elevated. Slow nerve conduction velocity. Elevated CSF protein. Peroxisomal disease.	Treat with low phytanic acid diet.

[a]For late infantile metachromatic leukodystrophy, Pelizaeus-Merzbacher disease, poliodystrophy, Gaucher disease of later onset, and subacute necrotizing encephalomyelopathy, see Table 25–22.

[b]CSF γ-globulin (IgG) is considered elevated in children when IgG is > 9% of total protein (possibly even > 8.3%); definitively elevated when > 14%.

ACTH, adrenocorticotropic hormone; CLN, ceroid lipofuscinosis; CNS, central nervous system; CSF, cerebrospinal fluid; CT, computed tomography; EEG, electroencephalogram; EM, electron microscopy; ERG, electroretinogram; IFN-α, interferon-α; MRI, magnetic resonance imaging; VER, visual evoked response; WBC, white blood cell.

a common reason for emergent neurological consultation. The best approach in the evaluation of these children is obtaining a detailed history of the antecedent events and current symptoms, as well as a detailed examination of associated neurological symptoms. Typically these patients develop symptoms within 72 hours prior to their presentation to medical care, and they have been previously healthy without developmental delay or neurological abnormalities. In contrast, congenital ataxias may be associated with central nervous system abnormalities, genetic abnormalities, or metabolic disorders. In this section, a brief overview of will be provided of the most common causes of acute and congenital ataxia, and the evaluation and the management of each.

ACUTE ATAXIAS OF CHILDHOOD

ESSENTIALS FOR DIAGNOSIS

- Symptoms may include refusal to walk due to ataxia, in addition to sudden development of a wide-based, drunken gait.
- Families may not report unsteadiness of arm movements, ataxia of the trunk, or dysarthria, but these symptoms are essential to localization.
- Serious causes include CNS infections and intracranial mass lesions.

Pathogenesis

Causes of acute ataxia that require emergent evaluation include increased intracranial pressure due to mass lesions. Therefore, any history suggestive of this should be elicited, such as persistent or recurrent headaches, or vision changes such as blurred or double vision. A history of head of neck trauma should prompt evaluation for vertebral artery dissection. Other common causes include accidental or purposeful ingestion. The evaluation of an acutely ataxic patient can be difficult as the patient may refuse to participate in the examination due to the discomfort of being ataxic, causing them to be irritable or hesitant. Therefore, distinguishing between weakness and ataxia can be difficult, but it is essential to making the correct diagnosis.

Clinical Findings

A thorough examination should be performed, with attention to signs suggesting a serious central nervous system disorder, such as mass lesions or central nervous system infections. Changes in mental status are particularly important to observe, as this suggests an ingestion, stroke, acute disseminated encephalomyelitis, or opsoclonus-myoclonus syndrome. The presence of papilledema and cranial nerve palsies suggests an intracranial focal lesion or hydrocephalus. Asymmetry in the examination would be unusual for acute cerebellar ataxia.

Once signs of serious CNS disorders have been sought, localization of the cerebellar lesion should be made. A midline cerebellar lesion may present with dysarthria or truncal titubation. In contrast, a lesion of the cerebellar hemispheres may present with sparse speech, dysmetria, tremor, or hypotonia. A patient with a hemispheric cerebellar lesion will tend to veer to the side of the lesion. A resting tremor, myoclonus, or opsoclonus will suggest a lesion affecting the deep cerebellar nuclei. Patient with cerebellar ataxia will not worsen with closed eyes, as a patient with sensory ataxia would.

Differential Diagnosis

A. Acute cerebellar ataxia

This is the most common cause of acute childhood ataxia, accounting for about 40% of all cases. It occurs most commonly in children aged 2–6 years. The onset is abrupt, and the evolution of symptoms is rapid. In about 70% of patients, a prodromal illness occurs with fever, respiratory or gastrointestinal symptoms, or an exanthem within 3 weeks of onset. Associated viral infections include varicella, rubeola, mumps, echovirus infections, poliomyelitis, infectious mononucleosis, and influenza. Bacterial infections such as scarlet fever and salmonellosis have also been incriminated. Typically, the symptoms evolve rapidly, but the severity can vary between patients. Some patients have such severe ataxia that they cannot walk, and others have only mild unsteadiness. Usually the limbs are not as affected as the trunk. Mental status is normal in these patients, as is sensory and reflex testing.

Laboratory testing—CSF opening pressure, protein, and glucose levels are typically normal, though a mild pleocytosis with lymphocytic predominance can be seen. Any significant elevation in WBC and protein level should prompt an evaluation for meningitis or encephalitis. Autoantibodies against Purkinje cells and other cerebral and cerebellar tissue have been described, but typically are not clinically useful to obtain.

Imaging findings—CT scans are typically normal, as are MR images of the brain. Occasionally focal cerebellar or cerebellopontine demyelinating lesions or enhancement of the meninges can be seen. Decreased regional blood flow in the cerebellum on SPECT without abnormal foci on MRI of the brain has also been reported.

Treatment—Treatment for acute cerebellar ataxia is supportive. IVIg has been used. Steroid use does not result in any improvement. About 80%–90% of patients recover without sequelae within 6–8 weeks, though some may demonstrate residual behavioral changes, learning problems, eye movement abnormalities, and speech problems.

B. Toxic cerebellar syndrome

Ataxia due to toxins or medications accounts for as many as 32.5% of acute cases. Substances such as anticonvulsants, benzodiazepines, alcohol, and antihistamines, and less commonly organic chemicals and heavy metals, can cause ataxia. In these cases, ataxia is usually accompanied by mental status changes, including lethargy, confusion, inappropriate speech and behavior, and in some cases, nystagmus or pupillary changes.

Laboratory testing—Urine toxicology screen may not detect specific medications, and therefore a detailed history is always helpful is guiding testing for specific medications. For phenytoin, the toxic level in serum is usually above 25 mcg/mL; for phenobarbital, above 50 mcg/mL; and for primidone, above 14 mcg/mL.

Imaging findings—Imaging is usually normal for patients with toxic cerebellar syndrome.

Treatment—Treatment is guided by the ingested agent, and requires toxicological consolation.

C. Acute demyelinating encephalomyelitis

Ataxia is a common feature of acute demyelinating encephalomyelitis (ADEM), and like acute cerebellar ataxia, can occur after a viral infection or vaccination. However, this entity may be distinguished from acute cerebellar ataxia by the accompanying change in mental status or other associated difficulties such as seizures, cranial nerve palsies, or hemiparesis. These clinical events arise from presumed immune-mediated demyelination of the central nervous system.

Laboratory findings—Lumbar puncture findings may be normal or mildly abnormal, with mild pleocytosis and elevation of the CSF protein in 25%–50% of cases. Typically oligoclonal bands are not seen in clinically isolated syndromes, but elevated IgG indices and presence of oligoclonal bands are more often observed in children who subsequently develop multiple sclerosis.

Imaging findings—MRI of the brain can show multiple; large asymmetrically located areas of demyelination in the cerebral white matter and deep gray matter such as the basal ganglia or thalamus. Acute lesions may enhance after administration of contrast, suggesting breakdown of the blood-brain barrier in those regions.

Treatment—There is no standard treatment for ADEM, as, to date, there have been no randomized controlled trials for the treatment of ADEM in children. Steroid treatment has been the most widely reported therapy for ADEM, typically at high doses. However, the specific schedules and formulations have been variable between centers and providers. Most pediatric groups have used IV methylprednisoline 10–30 mg/kg/day to a maximum dose of 1 g/day, followed by an oral steroid taper for 4–6 weeks with full recovery reported in 50%–80% of patients.

D. Posterior circulation stroke

Though rare, this should be considered as an etiology for ataxia if a history of neck trauma or family history of vascular abnormalities is present. Workup and management are discussed in the stroke section of this chapter.

E. Paraneoplastic syndromes

Acute ataxia can occasionally be seen in the entity known as opsoclonus-myoclonus syndrome (OMS). In its classic form, patients will present with ataxia; rapid chaotic conjugate, multidirectional eye movements (opsoclonus); and nonepileptic jerking of the head, extremities, and face (myoclonus). Some patients may additionally have sleep disturbance, cognitive dysfunction, and behavioral disruption. It is a rare disorder, with an incidence estimated to be 0.18 cases per million children per year in a prospective survey of United Kingdom pediatric neurology centers. Atypical presentations can result in initial erroneous diagnoses, such of as acute cerebellar ataxia, Guillain-Barre syndrome, and epileptic seizures. However, making the diagnosis has significant implications for treatment and prognosis. Forty-eight percent of patients with OMS have a neuroblastoma detected. Traditional methods to detect neuroblastoma with urine catecholamines or metaiodobenzylguanidine scans may be insensitive in patients with opsoclonus-myoclonus syndrome. Therefore, CT or MRI of the entire torso should be obtained in all patients with (OMS). Sometimes repeat testing is necessary to attain the diagnosis. In patients without a neuroblastoma, few will have an identifiable cause, though parainfectious or postinfectious processes have been implicated in some cases.

Laboratory testing—Readily available biomarkers would greatly facilitate the diagnosis of OMS. However, only in rare patients have autoantibodies against intracellular antigens been found, such as with anti-Hu or anti-*N*-methyl-D-aspartate receptor antibodies. None of these antibodies appear to be sensitive for the majority of patients. Relative CSF B-cell expansion has been proposed as a candidate biomarker for OMS, but more data need to be gathered regarding the sensitivity of this biomarker and its relationship to clinical severity. Laboratory evaluation for neuroblastoma or other malignancies should be pursued, with urine catecholamines.

Imaging—All patients with OMS should undergo CT or MRI of the entire torso to evaluate for occult malignancies.

Treatment—Gold standard treatment for OMS includes corticosteroids and adrenocorticotropic hormone, but no standard formulation or dosing is available, and the short-term benefits do not appear to predict a favorable long-term outcome. Additionally, relapses with dose tapering are common. Therefore, with the poor long-term outcome and the side effects of steroid use, new approaches have been used for treatment, including use of cyclophosphamide, chemotherapy to treat an identified neuroblastoma-associated OMS, and IVIG with ACTH and rituximab.

The long-term outcome for these patients is generally poor for patients both with and without neuroblastoma. From pooled data, 75%–80.6% of patients with OMS had abnormal neurological findings at follow-up, including eye movement abnormalities, dysarthria, ataxia, and myoclonus. In addition, all patients had cognitive impairment, including language, attention, memory, and intellectual disability.

F. Sensory ataxia

Ataxia can result from loss of sensory input to the cerebellum due to posterior column of the spinal cord, nerve root, or peripheral nerve lesions. Etiologies may include Guillain-Barre syndrome (acute inflammatory demyelinating polyneuropathy) or its variant, Miller-Fisher syndrome; or toxins. These patients, in addition to ataxia, will demonstrate decreased reflexes, a Romberg sign, loss of proprioception and vibratory sensation, and a high steppage gait.

Laboratory testing—Testing for suspected Guillain-Barre syndrome should include a lumbar puncture. The CSF findings may show elevated protein with normal cells, known as albuminocytologic dissociation, but very early in the course can be normal in as many as 20% of children. Antibodies against GQ1b should be obtained if Miller-Fisher syndrome is suspected. Electrophysiologic testing with nerve conduction studies may also be helpful, though acutely there may be little in the way of abnormalities.

Imaging—MR imaging of the spine may show enhancement of the nerve roots in Guillain-Barre syndrome.

Special testing—Electromyography/nerve conduction study may be useful to identify a demyelinating polyneuropathy. Nerve conduction velocities will be slowed into the demyelinating range (motor conduction velocities in the upper extremities ≤ 38 m/s) in a patchy, nonuniform fashion. The sural sensory response is typically spared early in the disease. Conduction block and temporal dispersion are hallmarks of this acquired polyneuropathy.

Treatment—Both IVIg and plasmapheresis have been used in treatment of GBS. IVIg is typically used in a regimen of 0.4 g/kg daily for 5 days. The typical regimen for PE is a total exchange of about 5 plasma volumes over a 2 week time period. A Cochrane review of the use of IVIg and PE showed no significant difference between the two treatments with respect to diability after 4 weeks, duration of mechanical ventilation, mortality, or residual disability. Steroid treatment has not been showed to be beneficial in GBS.

G. Basilar migraine

A basilar migraine may present with ataxia. Typically, other accompanying neurological signs are present, such as vertigo, nausea, vomiting, cranial nerve dysfunction, and headache. The patient's first episode may be concerning for a focal lesion and may prompt workup for a stroke. However, the description of positive visual phenomenon, such as flashing lights, suggests the migrainous nature of the episodes. Subsequent episodes, in the context of the history, are much easier to identify as basilar migraines.

H. Mass lesions

Posterior fossa tumors arise from the cerebellum or the brainstem and typically present with slowly progressive ataxia and symptoms of increased intracranial pressure. About 45%–60% of all childhood brain tumors are posterior fossa tumors. Therefore, in any patient in which there is a history of nocturnal headaches, chronic headaches, nocturnal emesis, focal neurological deficits, visual changes, or other signs concerning for mass lesion should have neuroimaging performed immediately.

I. Functional ataxia

In functional ataxia, the patient appears to lurch and stagger when walking, the gait is not wide-based, and falls are rare. The findings on the neurological examination do not indicate neuroanatomic localization, and therefore suggest a functional ataxia.

Blaes F, Pike MG, Lang B: Autoantibodies in childhood opsoclonus-myoclonus syndrome. J Neuroimmunol 2008;201–202:221–226 [PMID: 18687475].

Burke MJ, Cohn SL: Rituximab for treatment of opsoclonus-myoclonus syndrome in neuroblastoma. Pediatr Blood Cancer 2008;50(3):679–680 [PMID: 16900484].

Chemli J, Ketata S, Dalhoumi A et al: Opsoclonus-myoclonus syndrome associated with Mycoplasma pneumoniae infection. Arch Pediatr 2007;14(8):1003–1006 [PMID: 17543509].

Dalmau J, Rosenfeld MR: Paraneoplastic syndromes of the CNS. Lancet Neurol 2008;7(4):327–340 [PMID: 18339348].

De Bruecker Y, Claus F, Demaerel P et al: MRI findings in acute cerebellitis. Eur Radiol 2004;14(8):1478–1483 [PMID: 14968261].

Glatz K, Meinck HM, Wildemann B: Parainfectious opsoclonus-myoclonus syndrome: High dose intravenous immunoglobulins are effective. J Neurol Neurosurg Psychiatry 2003;74(2): 279–280 [PMID: 12531974].

Go T: Intravenous immunoglobulin therapy for acute cerebellar ataxia. Acta Paediatr 2003;92(4):504–506 [PMID: 12801122].

Gorman MP: Update on diagnosis, treatment, and prognosis in opsoclonus-myoclonus-ataxia syndrome. Curr Opin Pediatr 2010;22(6):745–750 [PMID: 20871403].

Hughes RA, Raphael JC, Swan AV, van Doorn PA. Intravenous immunoglobulin for Guillain-Barre syndrome. Cochrane Database Syst Rev 2006(1):CD002063 [PMID: 16437439].

Kalra V, Sankhyan N, Sharma S, Gulati S, Choudhry R, Dhawan B: Outcome in childhood Guillain-Barre syndrome. Indian J Pediatr 2009;76(8):795–799 [PMID: 19381495].

Ketelslegers IA, Neuteboom RF, Boon M, Catsman-Berrevoets CE, Hintzen RQ: A comparison of MRI criteria for diagnosing pediatric ADEM and MS. Neurology 2010 4;74(18):1412–1415 [PMID: 20335562].

Ketelslegers IA, Visser IE, Neuteboom RF, Boon M, Catsman-Berrevoets CE, Hintzen RQ: Disease course and outcome of acute disseminated encephalomyelitis is more severe in adults than in children. Mult Scler 2011;17(4):441–448 [PMID: 21148017].

Krug P, Schleiermacher G, Michon J et al: Opsoclonus-myoclonus in children associated or not with neuroblastoma. Eur J Paediatr Neurol 2010;14(5):400–409 [PMID: 20110181].

Kubota M, Takahashi Y: Steroid-responsive chronic cerebellitis with positive glutamate receptor delta 2 antibody. J Child Neurol 2008;23(2):228–230 [PMID: 18263760].

Leen WG, Weemaes CM, Verbeek MM, Willemsen MA, Rotteveel JJ: Rituximab and intravenous immunoglobulins for relapsing postinfectious opsoclonus-myoclonus syndrome. Pediatr Neurol 2008;39(3):213–217 [PMID: 18725071].

Markakis I, Alexiou E, Xifaras M, Gekas G, Rombos A: Opsoclonus-myoclonus-ataxia syndrome with autoantibodies to glutamic acid decarboxylase. Clin Neurol Neurosurg 2008;110(6):619–621 [PMID: 18433986].

Neuteboom RF, Boon M, Catsman Berrevoets CE et al: Prognostic factors after a first attack of inflammatory CNS demyelination in children. Neurology 2008;71(13):967–973 [PMID: 18672475].

Pang KK, de Sousa C, Lang B, Pike MG: A prospective study of the presentation and management of dancing eye syndrome/opsoclonus-myoclonus syndrome in the United Kingdom. Eur J Paediatr Neurol 2010;14(2):156–161 [PMID: 19423368].

Pavone P, Pettoello-Mantovano M, Le Pira A et al: Acute disseminated encephalomyelitis: A long-term prospective study and meta-analysis. Neuropediatrics 2010;41(6):246–255 [PMID: 21445814].

Pohl KR, Pritchard J, Wilson J: Neurological sequelae of the dancing eye syndrome. Eur J Pediatr 1996;155(3):237–244 [PMID: 8929735].

Pranzatelli MR, Tate ED, Crowley JM, Toennies B, Creer M: Neurometabolic effects of ACTH on free amino compounds in opsoclonus-myoclonus syndrome. Neuropediatrics 2008;39(3):164–171 [PMID: 18991196].

Pranzatelli MR, Tate ED, Travelstead AL et al: Rituximab (anti-CD20) adjunctive therapy for opsoclonus-myoclonus syndrome. J Pediatr Hematol Oncol 2006;28(9):585–593 [PMID: 17006265].

Pranzatelli MR, Tate ED, Verhulst SJ et al: Pediatric dosing of rituximab revisited: Serum concentrations in opsoclonus-myoclonus syndrome. J Pediatr Hematol Oncol 2010;32(5):e167–e172 [PMID: 20606544].

Rostasy K: Promising steps towards a better understanding of OMS. Neuropediatrics 2007;38(3):111 [PMID: 17985256].

Ryan MM, Engle EC: Acute ataxia in childhood. J Child Neurol 2003;18(5):309–316 [PMID: 12822814].

Tate ED, Allison TJ, Pranzatelli MR, Verhulst SJ: Neuroepidemiologic trends in 105 U.S. cases of pediatric opsoclonus-myoclonus syndrome. J Pediatr Oncol Nurs 2005;22(1):8–19 [PMID: 15574722].

Tenembaum S, Chitnis T, Ness J, Hahn JS: Acute disseminated encephalomyelitis. Neurology 2007;68(16 Suppl 2):S23–S36 [PMID: 17438235].

Uchibori A, Sakuta M, Kusunoki S, Chiba A: Autoantibodies in postinfectious acute cerebellar ataxia. Neurology 11 2005;65(7):1114–1116 [PMID: 16217070].

Van der Stappen A, De Cauwer H, van den Hauwe L: MR findings in acute cerebellitis. Eur Radiol 2005;15(5):1071–1072 [PMID: 15378339].

Wilken B, Baumann M, Bien CG, Hero B, Rostasy K, Hanefeld F: Chronic relapsing opsoclonus-myoclonus syndrome: Combination of cyclophosphamide and dexamethasone pulses. Eur J Paediatr Neurol 2008;12(1):51–55 [PMID: 17625938].

Wilson J: Neuroimmunology of dancing eye syndrome in children. Dev Med Child Neurol 2006;48(8):693–696 [PMID: 16836785].

Wong A: An update on opsoclonus. Curr Opin Neurol 2007;20(1):25–31 [PMID: 17215685].

CONGENITAL CAUSES OF CHRONIC AND EPISODIC ATAXIAS

ESSENTIALS OF DIAGNOSIS

- Establishing an inheritance pattern and temporal course is useful in determining the diagnosis.
- The findings of spasticity, ophthalmologic abnormalities, eye movement abnormalities, peripheral nervous system involvement, and seizures can be helpful in the evaluation of these patients.

Pathogenesis

In considering congenital causes of ataxia, it is probably easiest for the general pediatrician to classify them by the disease progression, either progressive or intermittent/episodic. For instance, Friedreich's ataxia and ataxia-telangeictasia are both progressive ataxias, with worsening of the ataxia over years. In contrast, in metabolic disorders such as maple syrup urine disease and channelopathies such as episodic ataxia type 1, ataxia occurs episodically and occasionally in response to a trigger. Further defining the ataxias by inheritance pattern is also useful in determining an etiology (see Table 25–24).

Clinical findings

Similar to the evaluation of a patient with acute onset of ataxia, the examination of a patient with congenital causes of ataxia should include localization of signs to the cerebellum,

Table 25–24. Miscellaneous causes of subacute/chronic ataxias.

Title	Causes	Lab Aids
Developmental coordination disorder (DCD) (*DSM-IV*)	Unknown (prematurity, LBW) 2%–5% incidence	Motor achievement, ADHD scales; 50% +
Cerebral palsy, ataxia variant	Prenatal, HIE	MRI scan
Celiac disease	AB binding to neurons	Anti-gliadin AB, etc
Vitamin E deficiency (AVED)	Malabsorption vitamin E	Vitamin E level
Ataxia telangiectasia	Genetic, "ataxin" lack	A-Fetoprotein, etc
Wilson disease	Maldistribution of Cu	Ceruloplasmin
Bassen-Kornzweig disease	Abetalipoproteinemia	Beta lipoprotein
NH_3 cycle disorder	Hyperammonemia	NH_3, AA, UA
Leigh syndrome	Mitochondrial disorder, PDH, complex II, IV, etc	POLG genetic studies, lactate
Other mitochondrial	Mitochondrial, nuclear DNA aberrations	CoQ10 assay, mitochondrial genome
Refsum syndrome	Phytanic acid excess	Phytanic acid
Biotinidase deficiency	Biotin lack, genetic	Serum biotinidase

AA, serum amino acids; AVED, ataxia with vitamin E deficiency; DSM-IV, Diagnostic and Statistical Manual of Mental Disorders, Fourth Edition; HIE, hypoxic ischemic encephalopathy; LBW, low birth weight; MRI, magnetic resonance imaging; PDH, pyruvate dehydrogenase; UA, urine organic acids.

either the hemispheres or the vermis. Therefore, the presence of ataxia in the trunk and limbs should be noted, of nystagmus, of the quality of eye movements, and of reflexes. Many of the patients may have multisystemic involvement, which may provide diagnostic clues to the etiology.

Differential diagnosis

Intermittent/episodic ataxias

A. Inborn errors of metabolism

Inborn errors of metabolism should be considered when ataxia is either intermittent or progressive. Acute exacerbation or worsening after high protein ingestion, a long period of fasting, febrile illness, or other physical stress is suggestive of a metabolic disorder. Disorders in this category are broad and beyond the scope of this text, but may include aminoacidopathies such as maple syrup urine disease, urea cycle defects such as ornithine transcarbamylase deficiency, lactic acidosis such as in Leigh disease, leukodystrophies, lysosomal disorders such as metchromatic leukodystrophy, peroxisomal disorders, and disorders of glycosylation. Because some of these etiologies, such as maple syrup urine disease, can be treatable, diagnostic studies to consider include MRI of the brain, thyroid studies, vitamins E and B12, serum ammonia, ceruloplasmin, serum amino acids, urine organic acids, serum lactate and pyruvate, serum biotinidase, EMG/NCS, serum cholesterol, very long chain fatty acids, phytanic acid, transferring isoelectric focusing, and lysosomal enzyme profile on leukocytes.

B. Channelopathies

Channelopathies are a broad category of neurological disorders, and result from altered function of a voltage-gated ion channel which subsequently alters membrane excitability in neurons. This group includes the episodic ataxias and familial hemiplegic migraines. There are 6 recognized genetic forms of episodic ataxia (EA) at this time. They are generally inherited in an autosomal dominant fashion, with episodes of ataxia lasting from seconds to minutes. In some patients, the episodes of ataxia are precipitated by stress, exercise, startle, or fatigue. EA2 is the most common episodic ataxia. It is allelic with familial hemiplegic migraine and spinocerebellar ataxia 6, both of which can also result in ataxia. Typically the attacks in EA2 are more prolonged, lasting from hours to days.

Progressive ataxias

A. Autosomal dominant hereditary ataxias

At this time, there are 29 described dominantly inherited spinocerebellar ataxias. The initial manifestation in infants can by hypotonia and delayed motor development, while in children the symptoms may include nystagmus, truncal and gait ataxia, spasticity, extensor plantar responses, and cognitive delay. Neurological symptoms are progressive, with wheelchair-dependence later the in disorder. In addition, in contrast to the autosomal recessive hereditary ataxias, they may exhibit diverse neurological symptoms, such as retinopathy, optic atrophy, extrapyramidal or pyramidal signs, peripheral neuropathy, cognitive impairment, or epilepsy. The neuroimaging findings can be relatively nonspecific for the various subtypes. However, three general patterns of atrophy on imaging have been described on brain MRI: pure cerebellar atrophy, olivopontocerebellar atrophy, and global brain atrophy. Because many of the spinocerebellar ataxias have overlapping clinical and radiographic phenotypes and there is significant intrafamilial and interfamilial variability in the clinical presentation, confirmation by genetic testing of the subtype of spinocerebellar ataxia needs to be performed. Treatment in these patients is typically symptomatic, with use of acetazolamine for ataxia, and the use of baclofen for spasticity.

B. Autosomal recessive hereditary ataxias

Most autosomal recessive ataxias are early onset, before 20 years of age. These patients, like those with autosomal dominant forms, also develop spinocerebellar ataxia, with poor balance with falls, difficulty with hand coordination, dysarthria, vertigo, and diplopia. In addition, they are generally associated with peripheral neuropathy, with loss of proprioception and vibratory sense. Areflexia is more commonly seen in autosomal recessive ataxias. Unlike the autosomal dominant inherited disorders, they typically do not exhibit other neurological symptoms, such as seizures, but they do tend to involve systems outside of the nervous system. The two most commonly encountered autosomal recessive hereditary ataxias that may be seen by the general pediatrician are Friedreich ataxia and ataxia-telangiectasia and will be discussed below.

Friedreich ataxia—Friedreich ataxia is the most common of the autosomal recessive ataxias, with a prevalence of about 1 in 30,000–50,000, and a carrier rate of 1 in 85. Typically, patients present at the ages of 5 to 25 years, with progressive gait and limb ataxia, dysarthria, loss of proprioception and vibration, areflexia, abnormal eye movements, and pyramidal weakness of the feet with upgoing toes. In addition, patients develop systemic symptoms, and may have associated pes cavus, cardiomyopathy, diabetes, and scoliosis.

LABORATORY TESTING—The diagnosis is made by performing genetic testing. Ninety eight percent of patients have a triplet GAA expansion in the frataxin gene on chromosome 9q13. In general, a greater number of repeats predicts an earlier onset of disease, more severe systemic manifestations, and more severe ataxia.

IMAGING—Neuroimaging does not show progressive cerebellar degeneration, unlike the other inherited ataxias. Mild atrophy of the cervical spinal cord may be seen.

TREATMENT—Because of the multisystem involvement in Friedreich ataxia, yearly screening needs to be performed with an x-ray to track the scoliosis; serum glucose and hemoglobin A1C to monitor for the onset of diabetes, and echocardiogram to monitor for hypertrophic cardiomyopathy. Current evidence suggests that frataxin has a role in mitochondrial iron handling and respiratory chain function. Therefore, treatment trials have targeted antioxidant protection. Trials have demonstrated that coenzyme Q10 and vitamin E can result in improvement in cardiac symptoms, and low dose idebenone can reduce cardiac hypertrophy. However, none of these have resulted in improvement in neurological symptoms, and therefore treatment of the progressive neurological symptoms remains symptomatic.

Ataxia-telangiectasia—Ataxia-telangiectasia is a multisystem disorder arising from a defect in DNA repair. Patients with classic ataxia-telangiectasia present with slurred speech, truncal ataxia, and oculomotor apraxia between the ages of 1 and 4 years. Choreoathetosis is found in nearly all patients with ataxia-telangiectasia. Deep tendon reflexes are decreased or absent in older patients. Plantar reflexes are upgoing or absent. Nonneurologic manifestations include oculocutaneous telangiectasias, recurrent sinopulmonary infections, and hypersensitivity to inonizing radiation with increased susceptibility to cancers, usually leukemia or lymphoma. Premature aging with strands of gray hair and insulin-resistant diabetes mellitus may also be features. After Friedreich ataxia, this is the most common autosomal recessive ataxia, with an estimated prevalence of 1:40,000 to 1:100,000 live births. Greater than 99% of individuals with classic ataxia-telangiectasias have mutations in the ATM gene.

LABORATORY TESTING—The serum alpha-fetoprotein level which is typically elevated in these patients to 10 ng/mL or higher, and can remain normal in unaffected children until age 24 months. Immunodeficiencies of IgA and IgE are common. To establish a diagnosis, an immunoblotting assay of the ATM protein level should be performed. Patients with absent or trace amounts of the ATM protein have a definitive diagnosis of ataxia-telangiectasia. Molecular genetic testing of the ATM gene can identify the disease-causing mutations.

IMAGING—Though a small cerebellum can be seen in older patients on neuroimaging, it is typically not seen in children.

TREATMENT—To establish the extent of systemic involvement in ataxia-telangectasia, screening should be performed at diagnosis. This should include screening for infectious and oncologic involvement with chest x-ray, pulmonary function testing, CBC with differential, immunoglobulin levels, B/T levels, and T cell function. In addition, screening for diabetes should be performed with a urinalysis, fasting blood glucose, and hemoglobin A1C. Neurological evaluation should be performed regularly to monitor for disease progression, including ocular coordination, and MRI of the cerebellum. Patients should report any easy bruising, weight loss, or localized swelling to their physician as this may be an early manifestation of malignancy.

Treatment is symptomatic in these patients, though several compounds are under investigation in clinical trials. IVIg replacement should be considered in patients with frequent and severe infections and very low IgG levels, as well as aggressive pulmonary toilet. The neurological manifestations are treated symptomatically, to minimize drooling and ataxia. Most patients will require a wheelchair by 10 years of age. Contractures and scoliosis can limit function, and physical therapy instituted early and continuously can minimize the development of both. Though steroids may decrease the neurological symptoms, discontinuation of steroids results in return of the neurological symptoms. Mutation-targeted therapy such as with antisense oligonucleotides appears promising.

C. X-linked cerebellar ataxias

Fragile X tremor ataxia syndrome has not been documented to occur before 50 years of age, but will be included here as a rare cause of an X-linked inherited ataxia. Patients typically exhibit tremor or ataxia, in inverse relationship to the number of CGG triplet repeat expansions they harbor. In addition, they may also present with varying combinations of parkinsonism, autonomic dysfunction, polyneuropathy, and cognitive deficits.

Babady NE, Carelle N, Wells RD et al: Advancements in the pathophysiology of Friedreich's Ataxia and new prospects for treatments. Mol Genet Metab Sep–Oct 2007;92(1–2):23–35 [PMID: 17596984].

Bencze KZ, Kondapalli KC, Cook JD et al: The structure and function of frataxin. Crit Rev Biochem Mol Biol 2006;41(5):269–291 [PMID: 16911956].

Du L, Damoiseaux R, Nahas S et al: Nonaminoglycoside compounds induce readthrough of nonsense mutations. J Exp Med 2009;206(10):2285–2297 [PMID: 19770270].

Du L, Pollard JM, Gatti RA: Correction of prototypic ATM splicing mutations and aberrant ATM function with antisense morpholino oligonucleotides. Proc Natl Acad Sci U S A 2007;104(14):6007–6012 [PMID: 17389389].

Fogel BL, Perlman S: Clinical features and molecular genetics of autosomal recessive cerebellar ataxias. Lancet Neurol 2007;6:245–257 [PMID: 17303531].

Jen JC, Wan J, Palos TP, Howard BD, Baloh RW: Mutation in the glutamate transporter AAT1 causes episodic ataxia, hemiplegia, and seizures. Neurology 2005;65(4):529–534] [PMID: 16116111].

Lynch DR, Farmer JM, Wilson RB: Mortality in Friedreich Ataxia. Tex Heart Inst J 2007;34(4):502–503; author reply 503–504 [PMID: 18172544].

Kullman DM: Neurological channelopathies. Annu Rev Neurosci 2010;33:151–172.

Koeppen AH: Friedreich ataxia: Pathology, pathogenesis, and molecular genetics. J Neurol Sci 2011;15:303(1–2):1–12 [PMID: 20331364].

Mateo I, Llorca J, Volpini V, Corral J, Berciano J, Combarros O: Expanded GAA repeats and clinical variation in Friedreich ataxia. Acta Neurol Scand 2004;109(1):75–78 [PMID: 14653855].

Matsuoka S, Ballif BA, Smogorzewska A et al: ATM and ATR substrate analysis reveals extensive protein networks responsive to DNA damage. Science 2007;316(5828):1160–1166 [PMID: 17525332].

Manto M, Marmolino D: Cerebellar ataxias. Curr Opin Neurol 2009;22:419–429.

Parker CC, Evans OB: Metabolic disorders causing childhood ataxia. Semin Pediatr Neurol 2003;10(3):193–199 [PMID: 14653407].

Payne RM, Pride PM, Babbey CM: Cardiomyopathy of Friedreich ataxia: Use of mouse models to understand human disease and guide therapeutic development. Pediatr Cardiol 2011;32(3):366–378 [PMID: 21360265].

Poretti A, Wolf NI, Bolthauser E: Differential diagnosis of cerebellar atrophy in childhood. Eur J Paediatr Neurol 2008;12(3):155–167 [PMID: 17869142].

Ryan DP, Ptacek LJ: Episodic neurological channelopathies. Neuron 2010;68:282–292 [PMID: 20955935].

Wan J, Khanna R, Sandusky M, Papazian DM, Jen JC, Baloh RW: CACNA1A mutations causing episodic and progressive ataxia alter channel trafficking and kinetics. Neurology 2005;64(12):2090–2097 [PMID: 15985579].

Watase K, Barrett CF, Miyazaki T et al: Spinocerebellar ataxia type 6 knockin mice develop a progressive neuronal dysfunction with age-dependent accumulation of mutant CaV2.1 channels. Proc Natl Acad Sci U S A 2008;105(33):11987–11992 [PMID: 18687887].

EXTRAPYRAMIDAL DISORDERS

Extrapyramidal disorders are characterized by the presence in the waking state of one or more of the following features: dyskinesias, athetosis, ballismus, tremors, rigidity, and dystonias.

For the most part, the precise pathologic and anatomic localization of these disorders is not understood. Motor pathways synapsing in the striatum (putamen and caudate nucleus), globus pallidus, red nucleus, substantia nigra, and the body of Luys are involved; this system is modulated by pathways originating in the thalamus, cerebellum, and reticular formation.

1. Sydenham Post-Rheumatic Chorea

Sydenham chorea is characterized by an acute onset of choreiform movements and variable degrees of psychological disturbance. It is frequently associated with rheumatic endocarditis and arthritis. Although the disorder follows infections with group A β-hemolytic streptococci, the interval between infection and chorea may be greatly prolonged; throat cultures and antistreptolysin O titers may therefore (rarely!) be negative. Chorea has also been associated with hypocalcemia; with vascular lupus erythematosus; and with toxic, viral, infectious, parainfectious, and degenerative encephalopathies. Paraneoplastic chorea is not seen in children.

Clinical Findings

A. Symptoms and Signs

Chorea, or rapid involuntary movements of the limbs and face, is the hallmark physical finding. In addition to the jerky incoordinate movements, the following are noted: emotional lability, waxing and waning ("milkmaid's") grip, darting tongue, "spooning" of the extended hands and their tendency to pronate, and knee jerks slow to return from the extended to their prestimulus position ("hung up"). Hemichorea occurs in 20% of patients with Sydenham chorea.

B. Laboratory Findings

Anemia, leukocytosis, and an increased erythrocyte sedimentation rate and C-reactive protein may be present. The antistreptolysin O or anti-DNase titer (or both) are usually elevated, and C-reactive protein is present. Throat culture is sometimes positive for group A β-hemolytic streptococci.

ECG and echocardiography are often essential to detect cardiac involvement. Antineuronal antibodies are present in most patients but are not specific for this disease. Antiphospholipid antibody (APA) may be elevated (more so with lupus, causative of the chorea?). Specialized radiologic procedures (MRI and SPECT) may show basal ganglia abnormalities.

Differential Diagnosis

The diagnosis of Sydenham chorea is usually not difficult. Tics, drug-induced extrapyramidal syndromes, Huntington chorea, and hepatolenticular degeneration (Wilson disease), as well as other rare movement disorders, can usually be ruled out on historical and clinical grounds. Immunologic linkages among chorea, tics, and obsessive-compulsive disorder are being studied in pediatric patients. Thus, other causes of chorea in childhood include dyskinetic, "extrapyramidal" cerebral palsy, benign hereditary chorea, kernicterus, Lupus, postpump cardiac surgery, and, for unilateral chorea, stroke, and tumor. These other causes of chorea can often be ruled out by laboratory tests, such as antinuclear antibody for lupus, thyroid screening tests, serum calcium for hypocalcemia, and immunologic and virologic tests for (rare) HIV, parvovirus B19, and Epstein-Barr virus infection. Relapse of herpes encephalitis rarely manifests as choreoathetosis. Anti-N-methyl-D-aspartate receptor (anti-NMDAR) encephalitis may cause chorea or other dyskinesias; detection of NMDAR antibodies is diagnostic.

Treatment

There is no specific treatment. Dopaminergic blockers such as haloperidol (0.5 mg/d to 3–6 mg/d) and pimozide (2–10 mg/d) have been used. Parkinsonian side effects such as rigidity and masked facies, and with high doses tardive dyskinesia, rarely occur in childhood. Other drugs have been used with success in individual cases; these include the anticonvulsant sodium valproate (50–60 mg/kg/d in divided doses) and prednisone (high-dose IV, or orally 0.5–2 mg/kg/d in divided doses). IVIG has been successful in severe cases. Emotional lability and depression sometimes warrant administration of antidepressants. All patients should be given antistreptococcal rheumatic fever prophylaxis, possibly through child-bearing age.

Prognosis

Sydenham chorea is a self-limited disease that may last from a few weeks to months. Relapse of chorea may occur with nonspecific stress or illness—or with breakthrough streptococcal infections (if penicillin prophylaxis is not done). One-third of patients relapse one or more times, but the ultimate outcome does not appear to be worse in those with recurrences. In older studies, eventual valvular heart disease occurs in about one-third of patients, particularly if other rheumatic manifestations appear. Psychoneurotic disturbances occur in a significant percentage of patients.

Barash J et al: Corticosteroid treatment in patients with Sydenham's chorea. Pediatr Neurol 2005;32:205 [PMID: 15730904].

Cardoso F: Sydenham's chorea. Curr Treat Options Neurol 2008;230 [PMID: 18579027].

Citak EC et al: Functional brain imaging in Sydenham's chorea and streptococcal tic disorders. J Child Neurol 2004;19:387 [PMID: 15224712].

Demiroren K et al: Sydenham's chorea: A clinical follow-up on 65 patients. Child Neurol 2007;22:550 [PMID: 17690060].

Fong CY, de Sousa C: Childhood chorea-encephalopathy associated with human parvovirus B19 infection. Dev Med Child Neurol 2006;48:526 [PMID: 16700948].

Garvey MA et al: Treatment of Sydenham's chorea with intravenous immunoglobulin, plasma exchange, or prednisone. J Child Neurol 2005;20:424 [PMID: 15968928].

Kullnat MW, Morse RP: Choreoathetosis after herpes simplex encephalitis with basal ganglia involvement in MRI. Pediatrics 2008;121:e1003–e1007 [PMID: 18378549].

Panzar J, Dalmau J: Movement disorders in paraneoplastic and autoimmune disease. Curr Opin Neurol 2011;24:346 [PMID: 21577108].

Pavone P et al: Autoimmune neuropsychiatric disorders associated with streptococcal infection: Sydenham chorea, PANDAS, and PANDAS variants. J Child Neurol 2006;21:727 [PMID: 16970875].

Singer HS et al: Serial immune markers do not correlate with clinical exacerbations in pediatric autoimmune neuropsychiatric disorders associated with streptococcal infections. Pediatrics 2008;121:1198 [PMID: 18519490].

Van Immerzeel TD et al: Beneficial use of immunoglobulins in the treatment of Sydenham chorea. Eur J Pediatr 2010:169:1151 [PMID: 20349351].

Walker AR et al: Rheumatic chorea: Relationship to systemic manifestations and response to corticosteroids. J Pediatr 2008; 151:679 [PMID: 18035153].

Zomorrodi A, Wald ER: Sydenham's chorea in western Pennsylvania. Pediatrics 2006;117:e675 [PMID: 16533893].

2. Tics (Habit Spasms)

Clinical Findings

Tics, or habit spasms, are quick repetitive but irregular movements, often stereotyped, and briefly suppressible. Coordination and muscle tone are not affected. A premonitory urge ("I had to do it") is unique to tics. Transient tics of childhood (12%–24% incidence in school-aged children) last from 1 month to 1 year and seldom need treatment. Many children with tics have a history of encephalopathic past events, neurologic soft signs, and school problems. Facial tics such as grimaces, twitches, and blinking predominate, but the trunk and extremities are often involved and twisting or flinging movements may be present. Vocal tics are less common; 90% of tics are "above the neck."

Tourette syndrome is characterized by multiple fluctuating motor and vocal tics with no obvious cause lasting more than 1 year. Tics evolve slowly, new ones being added to or replacing old ones. Coprolalia and echolalia are relatively infrequent. Complex motor Tics are coordinated sequenced movements mimicking normal motor acts or gestures; ear scratching, head shaking, twisting, and "giving the finger" are examples. Self-injurious behavior is common in Tourette syndrome.

The usual age for all tic disorders at onset is 2–11 years (median age 6), and the familial incidence is 35%–50%. The disorder occurs in all ethnic groups. Tics may be triggered by stimulants such as methylphenidate and dextroamphetamine. An imbalance of or hypersensitivity to neurotransmitters, especially dopaminergic and adrenergic, has been hypothesized. No single chromosome/gene defect is causative; many "hot spots" have been identified. Either parent can transmit the disease.

In mild cases, tics are self-limited and wane with time. Most pediatric tic patients have transient tics of childhood (tics last less than one year), or chronic motor tics (> 1 year). When attention is paid to one tic, it may disappear only to be replaced by another that is often worse. If the tic and its underlying anxiety or compulsive neuroses are severe, psychiatric evaluation and treatment are needed.

Important comorbidities are attention-deficit/hyperactivity disorder and obsessive-compulsive disorder. Learning disabilities, migraine (25%), sleep difficulties, anxiety states, and mood swings are also common. REM sleep is decreased, arousals common. Tics may persist into sleep. Medications such as methylphenidate, amphetamines, and atomoxetine should be carefully titrated to treat attention-deficit/hyperactivity disorder and avoid worsening tics. Fluoxetine, clomipramine, or other selective serotonin reuptake inhibitors (SSRIs) may be useful for obsessive-compulsive disorder and rage episodes in patients with tics.

Table 25–25. Medications for Tourette syndrome and tics.

Dopamine blockers (many are antipsychotics)[a]
Pimozide (Orap)
Aripiprazole (Abilify)[a]
Olanzapine (Zyprexa)[a]
Risperidone (Risperdal)
Serotonergic drugs[b]
Fluoxetine (Prozac)
Anafranil (Clomipramine) (a trycyclic) for > 10 y old
Noradrenergic drugs[c]
Clonidine (Catapres)
Guanfacine (Tenex)
Other
Selegiline (Eldepryl)[d]
Baclofen (Lioresal)
Pergolide (Permax)[d]
Clonazepam (Klonopin)
Levetiracetam (Keppra)
Topiramate (Topamax)

[a]Some off-label use.
[b]Useful for obsessive-compulsive disorder.
[c]Useful for attention-deficit/hyperactivity disorder.
[d]Dopamine-modulating.

Treatment

The most effective medications for treating Tourette syndrome are dopamine blockers; these drugs, however, have a small risk of tardive dyskinesia, and are thus reserved for use in difficult to control tic patients. And many pediatric patients can manage without drug treatment or with less hazardous medications. Medications are generally reserved for patients with disabling symptoms; treatment may be relaxed or discontinued when the symptoms abate (Table 25–25). Nonpharmacologic treatment of Tourette syndrome includes education of patients, family members, and school personnel. In some cases, restructuring the school environment to prevent tension and teasing may be necessary. Supportive counseling, either at or outside school, should be provided. Medications usually do not eradicate the tics. The goal of treatment should be to reduce the tics to tolerable levels without inducing undesirable side effects. Medication dosage should be increased at weekly intervals until a satisfactory response is obtained. Often a single dose at bedtime is sufficient. The two neuroleptic agents used most often are pimozide and risperidone. Sleepiness and weight gain are the most common side effects; rare are prolonged QT interval (ECG), akathisia, and tardive dyskinesia. Clonidine, guanfacine (probably the two most safe drugs), and dopamine modulators have been used in individual patients with some success. Sometimes these agents are used in combination (eg, clonidine with pimozide). Clonazepam has the virtue of safety, but sleepiness and slowing of thinking are drawbacks. Topiramate has shown benefit in one controlled animal trial; human experience is limited. Levetiracetam failed in a controlled trial, but showed benefit in open trials. Tetrabenazine is being utilized for Tourette's syndrome in some university centers. IVIG has been unsuccessful. Habit reversal therapy ("HRT") is controversial, very labor intensive, variably successful.

Sydenham chorea is a well-documented pediatric autoimmune disorder associated with streptococcal infections (pediatric autoimmune neuropsychiatric disorder associated with streptococcal infection; PANDAS). Patients with tic disorders occasionally have obsessive-compulsive disorder precipitated or exacerbated by streptococcal infections. Less definite (much less frequent) are tic flare-ups with streptococcal infection.

Active prospective antibody (antineuronal and antistreptococcal) and clinical studies are in progress. Research centers have used experimental treatments (IVIG, plasmapheresis, and corticosteroids) in severe cases. At present, most patients with a tic do not worsen with group A streptococcal infections; with rare exceptions, penicillin prophylaxis is not necessary.

Awaad Y, Michon AM, Minarik S: Use of levetiracetam to treat tics in children and adolescents with Tourette syndrome. Mov Disord 2005;20:714 [PMID: 15704204].

Bate KS et al: The efficacy of habit reversal therapy for tics, habit disorders, and stuttering: A meta-analytic review. Clin Psychol Rev 2001;31:865 [PMID: 21549664].

Bubl E et al: Aripiprazole in patients with Tourette syndrome. World J Biol Psychiatry 2006;7:123 [PMID: 16684686].

Goodman WK et al: Obsessive-compulsive disorder in Tourette syndrome. J Child Neurol 2006;21:704 [PMID: 16970872].

Guo H, Ou-Yang Y: Curative effect and possible mechanisms of topiramate in treatment of Tourette syndrome in rats. Zhongguo Dang Dai Er Ke Za Zhi 2008;10:509 [PMID: 18706175].

Himle MB et al: Brief review of habit reversal training for Tourette syndrome. J Child Neurol 2006;21:719 [PMID: 16970874].

Hoekstra J et al: Lack of effect of intravenous immunoglobulins on tics: A double-blind placebo-controlled study. J Clin Psychiatry 2004;65:537 [PMID: 14119917].

Jankovic J, Kurlan R: Tourette syndrome: Evolving concepts. Mov Disord 2011;26:1149 [PMID: 21484868].

Kurlan R: Clinical practice: Tourette syndrome. N Engl J Med 2010;363:2332 [PMID: 21142535].

Mell LK et al: Association between streptococcal infection and obsessive-compulsive disorder, Tourette syndrome and tic disorder. Pediatrics 2005;116:56 [PMID: 15995031].

Piacentini J et al: Behavior therapy for children with Tourette disorder: A randomized controlled trial. JAMA 2010;303:1929 [PMID: 20483969].

Pringsheim T, Steeves T: Pharmacological treatment for Attention Deficit Hyperactivity Disorder (ADHD) in children with comorbid tic disorders. Cochrane Database Syst Rev 2011;Apr 13;(4):CD007990 [PMID: 21491404].

Singer HS: Tourette syndrome and other tic disorders. Handb Clin Neurol 2011;100:641 [PMID: 21496613].

Qasaymeh MM, Mink JW: New treatments for tic disorders. Curr Treat Options Neurol 2006;8:465 [PMID: 17032567].

Smith-Hicks CL et al: A double blind randomized placebo control trial of levetiracetam in Tourette Syndrome. Mov Disord 2007;22:1764 [PMID: 17566124].

3. Paroxysmal Dyskinesias/Chronic Dystonia

Paroxysmal dyskinesias are sudden-onset, short-duration choreoathetosis or dystonia episodes (a sustained muscle contraction, of limb or torso, frequently twisting or with abnormal posture). Most often these episodes are of familial or genetic origin. Episodes may occur spontaneously or be set off by actions ("kinesigenic," or movement-induced) such as rising from a chair, reaching for a glass, or walking. Sometimes only hard sustained exercise will induce the dyskinesia. (Nocturnal dyskinesia/dystonic episodes are currently thought to be frontal lobe seizures.)

Table 25–26. Paroxysmal movement disorders (genetics).

Name	PKD[a]	PNKD[b]	PED[c]
Duration	Few minutes	2–10 min	5–40 min
Occurrence	Frequent	Occasional	Hyperventilation, exercise
Precipitants	Stress	Alcohol, caffeine, stress	Stress
Treatment	Anticonvulsants	Meds problematic, clonazepam?	Acetazolamide

[a]Paroxysmal kinesigenic dyskinesia.
[b]Paroxysmal non-kinesigenic dyskinesia.
[c]Paroxysmal exercise-induced dyskinesia.

The diagnosis is clinical. Onset is usually in childhood; average age, 12 years. The patient is alert and often disconcerted during an episode.

Episodes may last seconds to 5–20 minutes and occur several times daily or monthly. Laboratory work is normal. EEG is normal between or during an attack; brain imaging is normal. Inheritance is usually autosomal dominant. Anticonvulsants (eg, carbamazepine) usually prevent further attacks. Patients often grow out of this disease in one or two decades (Table 25–26).

Nonkinesigenic dyskinesia is often secondary to an identifiable brain lesion, less or not responsive to medications, and nongenetic.

Disorders of ion channels underlie many of the genetic cases; some cases are linked to epilepsy and hemiplegic migraine. Chromosome loci are known for the latter. Chronic dystonia in childhood is often "cerebral palsy" a "secondarily caused" movement disorder often from perinatal vicissitudes.

Other chronic dystonias may have unidentifiable genetic cause: autosomal dominant. DYT-1 is the most common.

The diagnosis of chronic persistent dystonia may be aided by spinal fluid neurotransmitter (DYT5) and readily available genetic chromosome studies. Any child with dystonia of unknown cause should have a trial of lowish-dose L-dopa; a prompt improvement suggests DYT5—a genetic cause with favorable outcome! Long-term oral L-dope is curative. Rarely, transient dyskinesia (eg, dystonia) may be precipitated by fever. While the cause of persistent dystonia is often genetic, underlying biochemical and structural causes (eg, Wilson disease, basal ganglia tumor or other pathology, hypoxic ischemic encephalopathy (HIE), glutaric aciduria, etc) must be ruled out. Treatment for chronic dystonia may be specific if a syndrome cause is identified (eg, 1-DODA for DYT5). Nonspecific treatment may be physical therapy (eg, for cerebral palsy) or medication trials with anticholinergics trihexyphenidyl (Artane), tetrabenozine, bocoten or botulism injections (eg, for a focal foot, or neck dystonia), or even chronic deep brain stimulation.

Persistent chorea (rarely) may be a benign lifelong genetic disease. Treatment is complex: L-dopa, anticholinergics (trihexyphenidyl, large doses), tetrabenazine ($$), and baclofen are primary medications.

A common cause (reversible) of transient dystonia in childhood (adolescent) is a drug reaction to antipsychotic (eg, chlorpromazine) or antiemetics (phenothiazines, metaclopromide).

Bruno MK et al: Genotype-phenotype correlations of paroxysmal nonkinesigenic dyskinesia. Neurology 2007;68:1782 [PMID: 17515540].

Chaila EC et al: Broadening the phenotype of childhood-onset dopa-responsive dystonia. Arch Neurol 2006;63:1185 [PMID: 16908750].

Fernandez-Alvarez E: Dystonia. The pediatric perspective. Eur J Neurol 2010;17:1:46 [PMID: 20590808].

Haridas A et al: Pallidal deep brain stimulation for primary dystonia in children. Neurosurgery 2011;68:738 discussion 743 [PMID: 21164379].

Jankovic J: Treatment of dystonia. Lancet Neurol 2006;5:864 [PMID: 16987733].

Kleiner-Fisman G et al: Benign hereditary chorea: Clinical, genetic and pathological findings. Ann Neurol 2003;54:244 [PMID: 12891678].

Sanger TD et al: Definition and classification of hyperkinetic movements in childhood. Mov Disord 2010;25:1538 [PMID: 20589866].

Li Z et al: Childhood paroxysmal kinesigenic dyskinesia: Report of seven cases with onset at an early age. Epilepsy Behav 2005;6:435 [PMID: 15820356].

Tarsy D, Simon DK: Dystonia. N Engl J Med 2006;355:818 [PMID: 16928997].

4. Tremor

The most common cause of persisting tremors in childhood is essential tremor; average age of onset is 12 years. Tremor is the third most common movement disorder, after restless legs and tics. Of those with this lifelong malady, 4.6% have onset in childhood (2–16 years). A genetic dominant inheritance is probable; 20%–80% afflicted report a relative with tremors. Tremor, a mild fine motor and cosmetic handicap, is worsened by anxiety, fatigue, stress, physical activity, and caffeine, and transiently improved by alcohol. Comorbidities include attention-deficit/hyperactivity disorder, dystonia, and possibly Tourette syndrome. Hand/arm tremor is the major manifestation; voice and head tremors are rare. Sometimes, "shuddering attacks" in infancy are a forerunner.

Laboratory studies are normal. No single chromosome/gene defect is known. Subtle abnormalities (eg, increased cerebellar blood flow) can be found in 25% in research studies. Progression is usually minimal. Some patients develop other movement disorders over a lifetime. Helpful medications (rarely needed long term) include propranolol or primidone.

Differential diagnosis includes birth asphyxia, Wilson disease, hyperthyroidism, and hypocalcemia; history and laboratory tests rule out these rare possibilities.

Recent research studies in adults utilizing proton MRS (magnetic resonance spectroscopy) suggest decreased nerve cells in the cerebellar cortex and increased harmane, a neurotoxin, at the same site. The latter suggests a possible environmental contribution to essential tremor.

Ferrara J, Jankovic J: Epidemiology and management of essential tremor in children. Paediatr Drugs 2009;11:293 [PMID: 19725596].

Jankovic J et al: Essential tremor among children. Pediatrics 2004;114:1203 [PMID: 15520096].

Keller S, Dure LS: Tremor in childhood. Semin Pediatr Neurol 2009;16:60 [PMID: 19501333].

Louis ED, Zheng W: Blood harmane is correlated with cerebellar metabolism in essential tremor. Neurology 2007;69:515 [PMID: 17679670].

Schlaggar BL, Mink JW: Movement disorders in children. Pediatr Rev 2003;24:39 [PMID: 15972843].

5. Wilson Disease

(See also Chapter 22.) Wilson disease, a treatable, reversible genetic disease (AR), must be ruled out with any significant neurologic or psychiatric disease in school-age children (adolescents, especially). Any juvenile movement disorder or psychosis demands serum ceruloplasm, liver function panel, and possibly 24-hour urine copper laboratory assessment. Half of patients with Wilson disease present with or have neuropsychiatric diseases; early symptoms may be as nonspecific as school work deterioration or mild tremor. MRI may show hyperintense basal ganglia. Kayser-Fleischer rings (slit-lamp eye examination) are usually present (and virtually diagnostic) in neurologically involved patients.

Harris MK et al: Movement disorders. Med Clin N Am 2009;93:371 [PMID: 19272514].

MaK CM, Lam CW: Diagnosis of Wilson's disease: A comprehensive review. Crit Rev Clin Lab Sc 2008;45:263 [PMID: 18568852].

CEREBRAL PALSY

The term *cerebral palsy* is a nonspecific term used to describe a chronic, static impairment of muscle tone, strength, coordination, or movements. The term implies that the condition is nonprogressive and originated from some type of cerebral insult or injury before birth, during delivery, or in the perinatal period. Other neurologic deficits or disorders (eg, blindness, deafness, or epilepsy) often coexist. Some form of cerebral palsy occurs in about 0.2% of neonatal survivors. The fundamental course, severity, precise manifestations, and prognosis vary widely.

The most common forms of cerebral palsy (75% of cases) involve spasticity of the limbs. A variety of terms denote the specific limb or combination of limbs affected: monoplegia (one limb); hemiplegia (arm and leg on same side of body, but arm more affected than leg); paraplegia (both legs affected with arms unaffected); quadriplegia (all four limbs affected equally).

Ataxia is the second most common form of cerebral palsy, accounting for about 15% of cases. The ataxia frequently affects fine coordinated movements of the upper extremities, but may also involve lower extremities and trunk. A dyskinetic movement disorder usually in the form of choreoathetosis or dystonia accounts for 5% of cases and persistent hypotonia without spasticity for 1%.

Depending on the type and severity of the motor deficits, associated neurologic deficits or disorders may occur: seizures in up to 50%, mild mental retardation in 26%, and severe retardation in up to 27%. Disorders of language, speech, vision, hearing, and sensory perception are found in varying degrees and combinations.

The findings on physical examination are variable and are predominantly those of spasticity, hyperreflexia, and, less often ataxia, and/or involuntary movements. Microcephaly is frequently present. In patients with hemiplegia, the affected arm and leg may be smaller and shorter than the unaffected limbs. Cataracts, retinopathy, and congenital heart defects may be indicative of congenital infections such as CMV and rubella.

Appropriate laboratory studies depend on the history and physical findings. MRI scans may be helpful in understanding the full extent of cerebral injury, and occasionally neuroimaging results suggest specific etiologies (eg, periventricular calcifications in congenital CMV infections or brain malformations such as pachygyri or lissencephaly). Other diagnostic tests that may be considered include genetic studies based on history or MRI findings and to diagnose or "rule out" rare metabolic causes; urine amino acids and organic acids; and blood amino acids, lactate, pyruvate, and ammonia concentrations.

The determination that a child has cerebral palsy is based in part on excluding other neurologic disorders and following the child for a sufficient amount of time to ascertain the usually static, nonprogressive nature of the disorder.

Treatment and management are directed at assisting the child to attain maximal physical functioning and potential physical, occupational, and speech therapy; orthopedic monitoring and intervention and special educational assistance may all contribute to an improved outcome. Medications and injections (eg, botulinum toxin) for spasticity and seizures are needed in many children. A new treatment, constraint-induced movement therapy is being studied in controlled trials. Also important is the general support of the parents and family with counseling, educational programs, and support groups.

The prognosis for patients with cerebral palsy depends greatly on the child's IQ, severity of the motor deficits, and degree of incapacity. Aspiration, pneumonia, or other intercurrent infections are the most common causes of death.

In contrast, patients with mild cerebral palsy may improve with age. Some patients experience resolution of their motor deficits by age 7 years. Many children with normal intellect have normal life spans and are able to lead productive, satisfying lives.

The cause is often obscure or multifactorial. No definite etiologic diagnosis is possible in 25% of cases. The incidence is high among infants small for gestational age or with extreme prematurity. Intrauterine hypoxia is a frequent cause. Other known causes are intrauterine bleeding, infections, toxins, congenital malformations, obstetric complications (including birth hypoxia), neonatal infections, kernicterus, neonatal hypoglycemia, metabolic disorders, and a small number of genetic syndromes.

Blair E: Epidemiology of the cerebral palsies. Orthop Clin North Am 2010;41:441 [PMID: 20868877].

Carroll Je, Mays RW: Update on stem cell therapy for cerebral palsy. Expert Opin Biol Ther 2011;11:463 [PMID: 21299445].

Delgado MR et al: Practice Parameter: Pharmacologic treatment of spasticity in children and adolescents with cerebral palsy (an evidence-based review). Neurology 2010;74:336 [PMID: 20101040].

Deon LL, Gaebler-Spira D: Assessment and treatment of movement disorders in children with cerebral palsy. Orthop Clin North Am 2010;41:507 [PMID: 20868881].

Garvey MA et al: Cerebral palsy: New approaches to therapy. Curr Neurol Neurosci Rep 2007;7:147 [PMID: 17324366].

Hoare BJ et al: Constraint-induced movement therapy in the treatment of the upper limb in children with hemiplegic cerebral palsy. Cochrane Database Syst Rev 2007;2:CD004149 [PMID: 17443542].

Novacheck TF et al: Examination of the child with cerebral palsy. Orthop Clin North Am 2010;41:469 [PMID: 20868879].

Pidcock FS: The emerging role of therapeutic botulinum toxin in the treatment of cerebral palsy. J Pediatr 2004;145(Suppl):S33 [PMID: 15292885].

Rethlefsen SA: Classification systems in cerebral palsy. Orthop Clin North Am 2010;41:457 [PMID: 20868878].

Russman BS, Ashwal S: Evaluation of the child with cerebral palsy. Semin Pediatr Neurol 2004;11:47 [PMID: 15132253].

Wood E: The child with cerebral palsy: Diagnosis and beyond. Semin Pediatr Neurol 2006;13:286 [PMID: 17178359].

INFECTIONS & INFLAMMATORY DISORDERS OF THE CENTRAL NERVOUS SYSTEM

Infections of the CNS are among the most common neurologic disorders encountered by pediatricians. Although infections are among the CNS disorders most amenable to treatment, they also have a very high potential for causing catastrophic destruction of the nervous system. It is imperative for the clinician to recognize infections early in order to treat and prevent massive tissue destruction.

Clinical Findings

A. Symptoms and Signs

Patients with CNS infections, whether caused by bacteria, viruses, or other microorganisms, present with similar manifestations. Systemic signs of infection include fever, malaise, and impaired heart, lung, liver, or kidney function. General features suggesting CNS infection include headache, stiff neck, fever or hypothermia, changes in mental status (including hyperirritability evolving into lethargy and coma), seizures, and focal sensory and motor deficits. Meningeal irritation is manifested by the presence of Kernig and Brudzinski signs. In very young infants, signs of meningeal irritation may be absent, and temperature instability and hypothermia are often more prominent than fever. In young infants, a bulging fontanelle and an increased head circumference are common. Papilledema may eventually develop, particularly in older children and adolescents. Cranial nerve palsies may develop acutely or gradually during the course of neurologic infections. No specific clinical sign or symptom is reliable in distinguishing bacterial infections from infections caused by other microbes.

During the initial clinical assessment, conditions that predispose the patient to infection of the CNS should be sought. Infections involving the sinuses or other structures in the head and neck region can result in direct extension of infection into the intracranial compartment. Open head injuries, recent neurosurgical procedures, immunodeficiency, and the presence of a mechanical shunt may predispose to intracranial infection.

B. Laboratory Findings

When CNS infections are suspected, blood should be obtained for a complete blood count, general chemistry panel, and culture. Most important, however, is obtaining CSF. In the absence of focal neurologic deficits or signs of brainstem herniation, CSF should be obtained immediately from any patient in whom serious CNS infection is suspected. When papilledema or focal motor signs are present, a lumbar puncture may be delayed until a neuroimaging procedure has been done to exclude space-occupying lesions. Treatment must be started even if lumbar puncture is delayed. It is generally safe to obtain spinal fluid from infants with nonfocal neurologic examination even if the fontanelle is bulging. Spinal fluid should be examined for the presence of red and white blood cells, protein concentration, glucose concentration, bacteria, and other microorganisms; a sample should be cultured. In addition, serologic, immunologic, and nucleic acid detection (PCR) tests may be performed on the spinal fluid in an attempt to identify the specific organism. Spinal fluid that contains a high proportion of polymorphonuclear leukocytes, a high protein concentration, and a low glucose concentration strongly suggests bacterial infection (see Chapter 42). CSF containing predominantly lymphocytes, a high protein concentration, and a low glucose concentration suggests infection with mycobacteria, fungi, uncommon bacteria, and some viruses such as lymphocytic choriomeningitis virus, herpes simplex virus, mumps virus, and arboviruses (see Chapters 40 and 43). CSF that contains a high proportion of lymphocytes, normal or only slightly elevated protein concentration, and a normal glucose concentration is most suggestive of viral infections, although partially treated bacterial meningitis and parameningeal infections may also result in this type of CSF formula. Typical CSF findings in a variety of infectious and inflammatory disorders are shown in Table 25–2.

In some cases, brain biopsy may be needed to identify the presence of specific organisms and clarify the diagnosis. Herpes simplex virus infections can be confirmed using the PCR test to assay for herpes DNA in spinal fluid. This test has 95% sensitivity and 99% specificity. Brain biopsy may be needed to detect the rare PCR-negative case of herpes simplex and various parasitic infections, or in a suspected parainfectious or postinfectious cause with ambiguous spinal fluid findings (eg, vasculitis).

C. Imaging

Neuroimaging with CT and MRI scans may be helpful in demonstrating the presence of brain abscess, meningeal inflammation, or secondary problems such as venous and arterial infarctions, hemorrhages, and subdural effusions when these are suspected. In addition, these procedures may identify sinus or other focal infections in the head or neck region that are related to the CNS infection. CT bone windows may demonstrate bony abnormalities such as basilar fractures.

EEGs may be helpful in the assessment of patients who have had seizures at the time of presentation. The changes are often nonspecific and characterized by generalized slowing. In some instances, such as herpes simplex virus or focal enterovirus infection, periodic lateralized epileptiform discharges (PLEDs) may be seen early in the course and may be one of the earliest study abnormalities to suggest the diagnosis. EEGs may also show focal slowing over regions of infarcts or (rare) abscesses.

BACTERIAL MENINGITIS

Bacterial infections of the CNS may present acutely (symptoms evolving rapidly over 1–24 hours), subacutely (symptoms evolving over 1–7 days), or chronically (symptoms evolving over more than 1 week). Diffuse bacterial infections involve the leptomeninges, superficial cortical structures, and blood vessels. Although the term *meningitis* is used to describe these infections, it should not be forgotten that the brain parenchyma is also inflamed and that blood vessel walls may be infiltrated by inflammatory cells that result in endothelial cell injury, vessel stenosis, and secondary ischemia and infarction. Overall clinical characteristics of bacterial meningitis (and viral meningoencephalitis) are outlined in Table 25–27.

Pathologically, the inflammatory process involves all intracranial structures to some degree. Acutely, this inflammatory

Table 25–27. Encephalitis.

Definition: brain inflammation (usually acute)
Clinical: (fever, headache) seizures, motor paralysis, impaired consciousness
Laboratory: CSF cells, protein increased; culture/PCR; serology CSF/blood
Radiographic: swelling (focal), dysmyelination, infarcts
Pathologic: perivascular cells, gray matter, even neuronophagia; edema, dysmyelination, gliosis
Infectious: (95%) enteroviruses, *Mycoplasma*, herpes, EBV, other viral
Unusual: bacteria, fungi, protozoa
Some causes are mosquito- or tick-borne; seasonal.
Para-/Postinfectious (ADEM): (25%) during or after respiratory infection or exanthem; most often no etiologic agent is identified
Treatment: supportive
Herpes: acyclovir
ADEM: steroids, IVIG, plasma exchange
Broad Spectrum Antibiotics until cultures are negative

ADEM, acute disseminated encephalomyelitis; CSF, cerebrospinal fluid; EBV, Epstein-Barr virus; IVIG, intravenous immune globulin; PCR, polymerase chain reaction.
Data from Lewis P, Glaser CA: Encephalitis. Pediatr Rev 2005;26:347.

process may result in cerebral edema or impaired CSF flow through and out of the ventricular system, resulting in hydrocephalus.

Treatment

A. Specific Measures

(See also Chapters 39, 40, and the section on bacterial infections in Chapter 42.)

While awaiting the results of diagnostic tests, the physician should start broad-spectrum antibiotic coverage as noted in the following discussion. After specific organisms are identified, antibiotic therapy can be tailored based on antibiotic sensitivity patterns. Bacterial meningitis in children younger than age 3 months is treated initially with cefotaxime (or ceftriaxone if the child is older than age 1 month) and ampicillin; the latter agent is used to treat *Listeria* and enterococci infections, which rarely affect older children. Children older than 3 months are given ceftriaxone or cefotaxime *plus* vancomycin. Due to the prevalence of penicillin-resistant pneumococci in the US, individuals greater than 1 month of age should be treated with vancomycin. Rifampin and dexamethasome use should be considered on a case by case basis. Therapy may be narrowed when organism sensitivity allows. Duration of therapy is 7 days for meningococcal infections, 10 days for *Haemophilus influenzae* or pneumococcal infection, and 14–21 days for other organisms. Slow clinical response or the occurrence of complications may prolong the need for therapy.

B. General and Supportive Measures

Children with bacterial meningitis are often systemically ill. The following complications should be looked for and treated aggressively: hypovolemia, hypoglycemia, hyponatremia, acidosis, septic shock, increased intracranial pressure, seizures, disseminated intravascular coagulation, and metastatic infection (eg, pericarditis, arthritis, or pneumonia). Children should initially be monitored closely (cardiorespiratory monitor, strict fluid balance and frequent urine specific gravity assessment, daily weights, and neurologic assessment every few hours), not fed until neurologically very stable, isolated until the organism is known, rehydrated with isotonic solutions until euvolemic, and then given intravenous fluids containing dextrose and sodium at no more than maintenance rate (assuming no unusual losses occur).

Complications

Abnormalities of water and electrolyte balance result from either excessive or insufficient production of antidiuretic hormone and require careful monitoring and appropriate adjustments in fluid administration. Monitoring serum sodium every 8–12 hours during the first 1–2 days, and urine sodium if the inappropriate secretion of antidiuretic hormone is suspected, usually uncovers significant problems.

Seizures occur in up to 30% of children with bacterial meningitis. Seizures tend to be most common in neonates and less common in older children. Persistent focal seizures or focal seizures associated with focal neurologic deficits strongly suggest subdural effusion, abscess, or vascular lesions such as arterial infarct, cortical venous infarcts, or dural sinus thrombosis. Because generalized seizures in a metabolically compromised child may have severe sequelae, early recognition and therapy are critical; some practitioners prefer phenytoin for acute management because it is less sedating than phenobarbital.

Subdural effusions occur in as many as 50% of young children with *S pneumoniae* meningitis. Subdural effusions are often seen on CT scans of the head during the course of meningitis. They do not require treatment unless they are producing increased intracranial pressure or progressive mass effect. Although subdural effusions may be detected in children who have persistent fever, such effusions do not usually have to be sampled or drained if the infecting organism is *H influenzae*, meningococcus, or pneumococcus. These are usually sterilized with the standard treatment duration, and slowly waning fever during an otherwise uncomplicated recovery may be followed clinically. Under any other circumstance, however, aspiration of the fluid for documentation of sterilization or for relief of pressure should be considered. Interestingly, prognosis is not worsened by subdural effusions.

Cerebral edema can participate in the production of increased intracranial pressure, requiring treatment with dexamethasone, osmotic agents, diuretics, or hyperventilation; continuous pressure monitoring may be needed.

Long-term sequelae of meningitis result from direct inflammatory destruction of brain cells, vascular injuries, or secondary gliosis. Focal motor and sensory deficits, visual impairment, hearing loss, seizures, hydrocephalus, and a variety of cranial nerve deficits can result from meningitis. Sensorineural hearing loss in *H influenzae* meningitis occurs in approximately 5%–10% of patients during long-term follow-up. Recent studies have suggested that early addition of dexamethasone to the antibiotic regimen may modestly decrease the risk of hearing loss in some children with *bacterial* meningitis (see Chapter 42).

In addition to the variety of disorders mentioned earlier in this section, some patients with meningitis develop mental retardation and severe behavioral disorders that limit their function at school and later performance in life.

BRAIN ABSCESS

Clinical Findings

Patients with brain abscess often appear to have systemic illness similar to patients with bacterial meningitis, but in addition they show signs of focal neurologic deficits, papilledema, and other evidence of increased intracranial pressure or a mass lesion. Symptoms may be present for a week or more; children with bacterial meningitis usually present within a few days. Conditions predisposing to development of brain abscess include penetrating head trauma; chronic infection of the middle ear, mastoid, or sinuses (especially the frontal sinus); chronic dental or pulmonary infection; cardiovascular lesions allowing right-to-left shunting of blood (including arteriovenous malformations); and endocarditis. Sinus infections more characteristically cause subdural-epidural, orbital and forehead abscesses or empyemas, or cellulitis rather than intrabrain abscesses. Recent reports have identified a predisposition to brain abscess in patients with congenital heart disease and acute immunosuppression, with a fungal cause in the latter, and *Citrobacter* infection in infants.

When brain abscess is strongly suspected, a neuroimaging procedure such as CT or MRI scans with contrast enhancement should be done prior to lumbar puncture. (CT scan can miss an epidural collection.) If a brain abscess is identified, lumbar puncture may be dangerous and rarely alters the choice of antibiotic or clinical management since the CSF abnormalities usually reflect only parameningeal inflammation or are often normal. With spread from contiguous septic foci, streptococci and anaerobic bacteria are most common. Staphylococci most often enter from trauma or spread from distant or occult infections. Enteric organisms may form an abscess from chronic otitis. Unfortunately, cultures from a large number of brain abscesses remain negative.

The diagnosis of brain abscess is based primarily on a strong clinical suspicion and confirmed by a neuroimaging procedure. Strongly positive inflammatory markers (erythrocyte sedimentation rate, C-reactive protein) are useful in screening. Normal results would be unlikely in patients with brain abscess. EEG changes are nonspecific but frequently demonstrate focal slowing in the region of brain abscess.

Differential Diagnosis

Differential diagnosis of brain abscess includes any condition that produces focal neurologic deficits and increased intracranial pressure, such as neoplasms, subdural effusions, cerebral infarctions, and certain infections (herpes simplex, cysticercosis, and toxocariasis).

Treatment

When a primary source or contiguous foci is suspected use 3rd generation cephalosporin (Cefotaxime or Ceftriaxone) plus metronidazole. Penicillin G is an alternative to a cephalosporin. In posttraumatic and postsurgical cases, Naficillin or oxacillin plus 3rd generation cephalosporin (cefotaxime or ceftriaxone). Vancomycin should be considered as a substitute for naficillin or oxacillin when methicillin-resistant *Staphlococcus aureus* is suspected. Cefotaxime is a good alternative to penicillin. Treatment may include neurologic consultation and anticonvulsant and edema therapy if necessary. In their early stages, brain abscesses are areas of focal cerebritis and can be treated with antibiotic therapies alone. Encapsulated abscesses require surgical drainage.

Prognosis

The surgical mortality rate in the treatment of brain abscess is lower than 5%. Untreated cerebral abscesses lead to irreversible tissue destruction and may rupture into the ventricle, producing catastrophic deterioration in neurologic function and death. Because brain abscesses are often associated with systemic illness and systemic infections, the death rate is frequently high in these patients.

VIRAL INFECTIONS

Viral infections of the CNS can involve primarily meninges (meningitis) (see Chapter 40) or cerebral parenchyma (encephalitis) (see Table 25–27). All patients, however, have some degree of involvement of both the meninges and cerebral parenchyma (meningoencephalitis). Many viral infections are generalized and diffuse, but some viruses, notably herpes simplex and some enteroviruses, characteristically cause prominent focal disease. Focal cerebral involvement is clearly evident on neuroimaging procedures. Some viruses have an affinity for specific CNS cell populations. Poliovirus and other enteroviruses can selectively infect anterior horn cells (poliomyelitis) and some intracranial motor neurons.

Although most viral infections of the nervous system have an acute or subacute course in childhood, chronic infections can occur. Subacute sclerosing panencephalitis, for example, represents a chronic indolent infection caused by altered measles virus and is characterized clinically by progressive neurodegeneration and seizures.

Inflammatory reactions within the nervous system may occur during the convalescent stage of systemic viral infections. Parainfectious or postinfectious inflammation of the CNS results in several well-recognized disorders: acute disseminated encephalomyelitis (ADEM; 25% of encephalitis), transverse myelitis, optic neuritis, polyneuritis, and Guillain-Barré syndrome. MRI findings in ADEM are distinctive:

demyelinating lesions, seen on T_2 and FLAIR images, are key to the diagnosis. Small and large white matter lesions can mimic findings in multiple sclerosis (MS) but, unusually for MS, may involve gray matter such as cortex, basal ganglia, especially thalamus. Radiologic changes are usually florid when the patient is first seen but occasionally emerge only days to weeks later. Thus, serial or repeat scans may be necessary.

In cases of ADEM, corticosteroids are beneficial. Current practice is to administer high dose therapy, followed by oral prednisone taper over 4–6 weeks. Most pediatric groups initially utilize intravenous methylprednisolone (10–30 mg/kg/d up to a maximum dose of 1 g/d) or Dexamethasone (1 mg/kg/d) for 3–5 days (no comparative dose studies are available). In refractory patients, IVIG or plasmapheresis (or both) may be effective. Rarely, ADEM relapses (biphasic acute disseminated encephalomyelitis; biDEM or BDEM). Recurrence more than 3 months after treatment should raise strong suspicion of MS. Congenital viral infections can also affect the CNS. CMV, herpes simplex virus, varicella, and (rare now, because of immunization) rubella virus are the most notable causes of viral brain injury in utero.

Treatment of CNS viral infections is usually limited to symptomatic and supportive measures, except for herpes simplex virus, and some cases of varicella zoster virus infections where acyclovir is used. West Nile virus, new in the United States, is an arthropod-borne flavivirus. It is found in mosquitoes, birds, and horses, and in 1991 accounted for 27% of hospitalized patients with encephalitis and muscle weakness in New York. Fourteen percent had encephalitis alone, and 6% had aseptic meningitis. CSF antibody studies and PCR (57% positive for viral RNA) were diagnostic aids. The infection is now endemic as far as the western United States, particularly in California.

This disease is often asymptomatic or mild in pediatric patients; paralysis and death occur mostly in the elderly.

ENCEPHALOPATHY OF HUMAN IMMUNODEFICIENCY VIRUS INFECTION

Neurologic syndromes associated directly with HIV infection include subacute encephalitis, meningitis, myelopathy, polyneuropathy, and myositis. In addition, secondary opportunistic infections of the CNS occur in patients with HIV-induced immunosuppression. *Pneumocystis, Toxoplasma,* and CMV infections are particularly common. Progressive multifocal leukoencephalopathy, a secondary papillomavirus infection, and herpes simplex and varicella-zoster infections also occur frequently in patients with HIV infection. Various fungal (especially cryptococcal), mycobacterial, and bacterial infections have been described.

Neurologic abnormalities in these patients can also be the result of noninfectious neoplastic disorders. Primary CNS lymphoma and metastatic lymphoma to the nervous system are the most frequent neoplasms of the nervous system in these patients. See Chapters 33, 39, and 41 for diagnosis and management of HIV infection.

OTHER INFECTIONS

A wide variety of other microorganisms, including *Toxoplasma,* mycobacteria, spirochetes, rickettsiae, amoebae, and mycoplasmas, can cause CNS infections. CNS involvement in these infections is usually secondary to systemic infection or other predisposing factors. Appropriate cultures and serologic testing are required to confirm infections by these organisms. Parenteral antimicrobial treatment for these infections is discussed in Chapter 39.

NONINFECTIOUS INFLAMMATORY DISORDERS OF THE CENTRAL NERVOUS SYSTEM

The differential diagnosis of bacterial, viral, and other microbial infections of the CNS includes disorders that cause inflammation but for which no specific causal organism has been identified. Sarcoidosis, Behçet disease, systemic lupus erythematosus, other collagen-vascular disorders, and Kawasaki disease are examples. In these disorders, CNS inflammation usually occurs in association with characteristic systemic manifestations that allow proper diagnosis. Management of CNS involvement in these disorders is the same as the treatment of the systemic illness.

OTHER PARAINFECTIOUS ENCEPHALOPATHIES

In association with systemic infections or other illnesses, CNS dysfunction may occur in the absence of direct CNS inflammation or infection. Reye syndrome is a prominent example of this type of encephalopathy that often occurs in association with varicella virus or other respiratory or systemic viral infections. In Reye syndrome, cerebral edema and cerebral dysfunction occur, but there is no evidence of any direct involvement of the nervous system by the associated microorganism or inflammation. Cerebral edema in Reye syndrome is accompanied by liver dysfunction and fatty infiltration of the liver. As a result of efforts to discourage use of aspirin in childhood febrile illnesses, the number of patients with Reye syndrome has markedly decreased. The precise relationship, however, between aspirin and Reye syndrome is unclear.

Anti-NMDA receptor encephalitis occurs in children with or without a tumor—thus sometimes paraneopicotic, sometimes not. Behavioral changes, aphasia, seizures, and movement disorders are prominent. Detection of antibody is diagnostic, immunotherapy therapy sometimes successful.

MULTIPLE SCLEROSIS

Multiple sclerosis (MS) can begin in childhood; 3%–10% of individuals with MS have symptom onset before age 18 years. Formation of a Pediatric MS Study Group led to a supplementary issue of *Neurology,* summarizing pediatric MS and related disorders. (See Krupp and Hertz citation, included in the references below.) Essential points follow:

- Multiple sclerosis may start with Clinically Isolated Symptoms (CIS) of CNS demyelination. Examples include optic neuritis; transverse myelitis; or brainstem, cerebellar, or hemispheric dysfunction; without fever or encephalopathy (whereas ADEM usually has both).

- Atypical clinical features (think of *other* diagnoses) include fever and involvement of the peripheral nervous system or other organ systems. Aberrant (for MS) laboratory results might include elevated erythrocyte sedimentation rate or marked CSF pleocytosis.
- A diagnosis of MS demands multiple episodes of CNS demyelination, separated in time and space. MRI (many fine-tuned criteria) and spinal fluid changes (oligoclonal bands, IgG index) are key laboratory tests. At present, there are several sophisticated MRI criteria to separate pediatric MS diagnosis from alternatives (eg, ADEM).
- Differential diagnosis includes especially ADEM. Excellent tables, examples, and criteria abound in the supplementary issue of *Neurology*. Many other infections, metabolic disorders, and degenerative diseases can mimic MS.
- Acute treatment (mainly corticosteroids; sometimes IVIg or plasmapheresis) and prevention or modulation of relapses is extrapolated from adult studies; pediatric trials are in their infancy. Immunomodulatory treatment to prevent relapses in children includes interferon-B or glatimer acetate (injections); or an oral agent that is in trials (fingolimod). Natalizumab is utilized in refractory patients.

CNS inflammatory demyelination syndromes

Monophasic Illness (Knupp, Dale ref)	
ADEM	Encephalopathy (behavior, consciousness change) fever
CIS	No encephalopathy (mono or multifocal lesions)
NMO	Long segment myelitis, optic neuritis, NMO-IgG +
Relapsing ADEM	Rare > 3 mo interval (again, multi-location demyelinating lesions)
Relapsing NMO	As above (NMO- IgG + optic neuritis. (NMO Antibody may be absent at initial illness)
Pediatric MS	Two or more multi-demyelinating events with lesions separated in time and space

ADEM, acute disseminated encephalomyelitis; CIS, clinically isolated syndrome; MS, multiple sclerosis; NMO, neuromyelitis optica.

Adame N et al: Sinogenic intracranial empyema in children. Pediatrics 2005;116:e461 [PMID: 16190693].

Avery RA et al: Prediction of Lyme meningitis in children from a Lyme disease-endemic region. Pediatrics 2006;117:e1 [PMID: 16396843].

Chang LY et al: Neurodevelopment and cognition in children after enterovirus 71 infection. N Engl J Med 2007;356:1226 [PMID: 17377160].

Chavez-Bueno S, McCracken GH Jr: Bacterial meningitis in children. Pediatr Clin North Am 2005;52:795 [PMID: 15925663].

Chitnis T et al: Pediatric multiple sclerosis. Neurol Clin 2011;29:481 [PMID: 21439455].

Christie LJ et al: Pediatric encephalitis: What is the role of Mycoplasma pneumoniae? Pediatrics 2007;120:305 [PMID: 17671056].

Collongues N et al: Long-term follow-up of neuromyelitis optica with a pediatric onset. Neurology 2010;75:1084 [PMID: 20855851].

Cortese I et al: Evidence-based guideline update: Plasmapheresis in neurologic disorders: report of the Therapeutics and Technology Assessment Subcommittee of the American Adademy of Neurology. Neurology 2011;18:76:294 [PMID: 21242498].

Dale RC et al: Pediatric central nervous system inflammatory demyelination: acute disseminated encephalomyelitis, clinically isolated syndromes, neuromyelitis optica, and multiple sclerosis. Curr Opin Neurol 2009;22:233 [PMID: 19434783].

Dale RC et al: Cerebrospinal fluid B-cell expansion in longitudinally extensive transverse myelitis associated with neuromyelitis optica immunoglobulin G. Dev Med Child Neurol 2011;June 17:d0i:10.1111 [PMID: 21679355].

Davis LE et al: West Nile virus neuroinvasive disease. Ann Neurol 2006;60:286 [PMID: 16983682].

De Cauwer HG et al: Differential diagnosis between viral and bacterial meningitis in children. Eur J Emerg Med 2007;14:343 [PMID: 17968200].

Feigin RD: Use of corticosteroids in bacterial meningitis. Pediatr Infect Dis J 2004;23:355 [PMID: 15071293].

Florance NR et al: Anti-N-methyl-D-aspartate receptor (NMDAR) encephalitis in children and adolescents. Ann Neurol 2009;66:11 [PMID: 19670433].

Frohman EM, Wingerchuk DM: Clinical practice. Transverse myelitis. N Engl J Med 2010;363:564–572 [PMID: 20818891].

Goodkin HP et al: Intracerebral abscess in children: Historical tends at Children's Hospital Boston. Pediatrics 2004;113:1765 [PMID: 15173504].

Grose C: The puzzling picture of acute necrotizing encephalopathy after influenza A and B virus infection in young children. Pediatr Infect Dis J 2004;23:253 [PMID: 15014302].

Hayes EB: West Nile virus disease in children. Pediatr Infect Dis J 2006;25:1065 [PMID: 17072131].

Helperin JJ et al: Practice parameter: Treatment of nervous system Lyme disease (and evidence-based review). Neurology 2007;69:91 [PMID: 17522387].

Huang MC et al: Long-term cognitive and motor deficits after enterovirus 71 brainstem encephalitis in children. Pediatrics 2006;118:e1785 [PMID: 17116698].

Huppke P et al: Neuromyelitis optica and NMO-IgG in European pediatric patients. Neurology 2010;75:1740 [PMID: 21060098].

Kennedy PG: Neurological infection. Lancet Neurol 2004;3:13 [PMID: 14693102].

Khurana DS et al: Acute disseminated encephalomyelitis in children: Discordant neurologic and neuroimaging abnormalities and response to plasmapheresis. Pediatrics 2004;116:431 [PMID: 16061599].

Krupp LB, Hertz DP (editors): Pediatric multiple sclerosis and related disorders. Neurology 2007;68(Suppl 2) [PMID: 17438241].

Kuntz Nl et al: Treatment of multiple sclerosis in children and adolescents. Expert Opin Pharmacother 2010;11:505 [PMID: 20163265].

Lebas A et al: Expanding spectrum of encephalitis with NMDA receptor antibodies in young children. J Child Neurol 2010;25:742 [PMID: 19833974].

Lewis P, Glaser CA: Encephalitis. Pediatr Rev 2005;26:353 [PMID: 16199589].

Lim BC et al: Relapsing demyelination CNS disease in a Korean pediatric population: Multiple sclerosis versus neuromyelitis optica. Mult Scler 2011;17:67 [PMID: 20858690].

Lindsey NP et al: West Nile virus disease in children, United States, 1999–2007. Pediatrics 2009;123(6):e1084.

Mata S, Lolli F: Neuromyelitis optica: An update. J Neurol Sci 2011;303(1–2):13 [PMID: 21300379].

Pasquinelli L: Enterovirus infections. Pediatr Rev 2006;27:e14 [PMID: 16473836].

Silvia MT, Licht DJ: Pediatric central nervous system infections and inflammatory white matter disease. Pediatr Clin North Am 2005;52:1107 [PMID: 16009259].

Sonneville R, Klein IF, Wolff M: Update on investigation and management of postinfectious encephalitis. Curr Opin Neurol 2010;23:300 [PMID: 20442573].

Tenembaum SN: Disseminated encephalomyelitis in children. Clin Neurol Neurosurg 2008;110(9):928 [PMID: 18272282].

Torok M: Neurological infections: Clinical advances and emerging threats. Lancet Neurol 2007;6:16 [PMID: 17166795].

Van de Beek D et al: Corticosteroids for acute bacterial meningitis. Cochrane Database Syst Rev 2007;1:CD004405 [PMID: 17253505].

Whitley RJ, Kimberlin DW: Herpes simplex encephalitis: Children and adolescents. Semin Pediatr Infect Dis 2005;16:17 [PMID: 15685145].

Yeh EA et al: Multiple sclerosis therapies in pediatric patients with refractory multiple sclerosis. Arch Neurol 2011;68:437 [PMID: 21149803].

Yeh EA, Waubant E et al: Multiple sclerosis therapies in pediatric patients with refractory multiple sclerosis. Arch Neurol 2011;68:437.

Yeh EA, Weinstock-Guttman B: Fingolimod: An oral disease-modifying therapy for relapsing multiple sclerosis. Adv Ther 2011;28:270 [PMID: 21394595].

Yeh Ea, Weinstock-Guttman B: Natalizumab in pediatric multiple sclerosis patients. Ther Adv Neurol Disord 2010;3:293 [PMID: 21179619].

SYNDROMES PRESENTING AS ACUTE FLACCID PARALYSIS

Flaccid paralysis evolving over hours or a few days suggests involvement of the lower motor neuron complex (see section on Floppy Infant Syndrome, later). Anterior horn cells (spinal cord) may be involved by viral infection (paralytic poliomyelitis) or by paraviral or postviral immunologically mediated disease (acute transverse myelitis). The nerve trunks (polyneuritis) may be diseased as in Guillain-Barré syndrome or affected by toxins (diphtheria or porphyria). The neuromuscular junction may be blocked by tick toxin or botulinum toxin. The paralysis rarely will be due to metabolic (periodic paralysis) or inflammatory muscle disease (myositis). A lesion compressing the spinal cord must be ruled out. The back often is tender to percussion at that site. Plain films may show disk or bone erosion; MRI, a displaced or compressed spinal cord. Several examples with pertinent discussions are included in a recent issue of *Pediatrics in Review* (2007, volume 28; see references at the end of this section).

▶ Clinical Findings

A. Symptoms and Signs

Features assisting diagnosis are age, a history of preceding or waning illness, the presence (at time of paralysis) of fever, rapidity of progression, cranial nerve findings, and sensory findings (Table 25–28). The examination may show long tract findings (pyramidal tract), causing increased reflexes and a positive Babinski sign. The spinothalamic tract may be interrupted, causing loss of pain and temperature. Back pain, even tenderness to percussion, may occur, as well as bowel and bladder incontinence. Often the paralysis is ascending, symmetrical, and painful (muscle tenderness or myalgia). Laboratory findings occasionally are diagnostic.

B. Laboratory Findings (See Table 25–28)

Examination of CSF is helpful. Imaging studies of the spinal column (plain radiographs) and spinal cord (MRI) are occasionally essential. Viral cultures (CSF, throat, and stool) and titers aid in diagnosing poliomyelitis. A high sedimentation rate may suggest tumor or abscess; the presence of antinuclear antibody may suggest lupus arteritis.

EMG and nerve conduction studies (NCSs) can be helpful in diagnosing polyneuropathy. NCSs in Guillain-Barre syndrome are helpful: the first changes are delayed or absent H or F reflexes. Later, motor NCS show prolonged distal latency, conduction block or temporal dispersion, with these changes in 50% of patients by 2 weeks and 85% by 3 weeks. EMG findings of fibrillation potentials and increased compound muscle action potential with high-frequency stimulation are suggestive of botulism. Rarely, elevation of muscle enzymes or even myoglobinuria may aid in diagnosis of myopathic paralysis. Porphyrin urine studies and heavy-metal assays (arsenic, thallium, and lead) can reveal those rare toxic causes of polyneuropathic paralysis.

▶ Differential Diagnosis

The child who has been well and becomes paralyzed often has polyneuritis. Acute transverse myelitis sometimes occurs in an afebrile child. The child who is ill and febrile at the time of paralysis often has acute transverse myelitis or poliomyelitis. Acute epidural spinal cord abscess (or other compressive lesion) must be ruled out. Poliomyelitis is very rare among the immunized population in the United States. Enterovirus 71 and West Nile disease are two new causes. Paralysis due to tick bites occurs seasonally (spring and summer). The tick is usually found in the occipital hair. Removal is curative.

Paralysis due to botulinum toxin occurs most commonly in those younger than age 6 months (see Chapter 42). Intravenous drug abuse can lead to myelitis and paralysis. Furthermore, chronic myelopathy occurs with two human immunodeficiency virus infections: HTLV-I and HTLV-III (now called HIV-1).

Table 25–28. Acute flaccid paralysis in children.

	Poliomyelitis (Paralytic, Spinal, and Bulbar), with or without Encephalitis	Guillain-Barré Syndrome (AIDP)	Botulism	Tick-Bite Paralysis	Transverse Myelitis and Neuromyelitis Optica (NMO)
Etiology	Poliovirus types I, II, and III; other enteroviruses, eg, EV-71; vaccine strain poliovirus (rare); West Nile virus: epidemic in birds; mosquitoes infect horses, humans. EV-71 is hand-foot-mouth disease, rarely paralytic.	Likely delayed hypersensitivity—with T-cell-mediated antiganglioside antibodies. Mycoplasmal and viral infections (EBV, CMV), *Campylobacter jejuni*, hepatitis B.	*Clostridium botulinum* toxin. Block at neuromuscular junction. Under age 1, toxin synthesized in bowel by organisms in ingested spores or honey. At older ages toxin ingested in food. Rarely from wound infection.	Probable interference with transmission of nerve impulse caused by toxin in tick saliva.	Usually unknown; multiple viruses (herpes, EBV, varicella, hepatitis A) often postviral (see Guillain-Barré syndrome). Antibodies to Aquaporin in NMO.
History	None, or inadequate polio immunization. Upper respiratory or GI symptoms followed by brief respite. Bulbar paralysis more frequent after tonsillectomy. Often in epidemics, in summer and early fall.	Nonspecific respiratory or GI symptoms in preceding 5–14 d common. Any season, though slightly lower incidence in summer.	Infancy: dusty environment (eg, construction area), honey. Older: food poisoning. Multiple cases hours to days after ingesting contaminated food.	Exposure to ticks (dog tick in eastern United States; wood ticks). Irritability 12–24 h before onset of a rapidly progressive ascending paralysis.	Rarely symptoms compatible with multiple sclerosis or optic neuritis. Progression from onset to paraplegia often rapid, usually without a history of bacterial infection.
Presenting complaints	Febrile at time of paralysis. Meningeal signs, muscle tenderness, and spasm. Asymmetrical weakness widespread or segmental (cervical, thoracic, lumbar). Bulbar symptoms early or before extremity weakness; anxiety; delirium.	Symmetrical weakness of lower extremities, which may ascend rapidly to arms, trunk, and face. Verbal child may complain of paresthesias. Fever uncommon. Facial weakness early. Miller-Fisher variant presents as areflexia, ataxia, and ophthalmoplegia (rare).	Infancy: constipation, poor suck and cry. "Floppy." Apnea. Lethargy. Choking (cause of SIDS). Bulbar palsy. Older: blurred vision, diplopia, ptosis, choking, and weakness.	Rapid onset and progression of ascending flaccid paralysis; often accompanied by pain and paresthesias. Paralysis of upper extremities 2nd day after onset. Sometimes acute ataxia presentation.	Root and back pain in about 30%–50% of cases. Sensory loss below level of lesion accompanying rapidly developing paralysis. Sphincter difficulties common. Fever (58%).
Findings	Flaccid weakness, usually asymmetrical. Cord level: Lumbar: legs, lower abdomen. Cervical: shoulder, arm, neck, diaphragm. Bulbar: respiratory, lower cranial nerves. Encephalopathy accompanies paralysis in West Nile.	Flaccid weakness, symmetrical, usually greater proximally, but may be more distal or equal in distribution. Rarely cranial nerves IX–XI, III–VI. Miller-Fisher variant: ophthalmoplegia, ataxia. Bulbar involvement may occur. Slight distal impairment of position, vibration, touch; difficult to assess in young children.	Infants: Flaccid weakness. Alert. Eye, pupil, facial weakness. Deep tendon reflexes decreased. Absent suck, gag. Constipation. Older: paralysis accommodation, eye movements. Weak swallow. Respiratory paralysis.	Flaccid, symmetrical paralysis. Cranial nerve and bulbar (respiratory) paralysis, ataxia, sphincter disturbances, and sensory deficits may occur. Some fever. Diagnosis rests on finding tick, which is especially likely to be on occipital scalp.	Paraplegia with areflexia below level of lesion early; later, may have hyperreflexia. Sensory loss below and hyperesthesia or normal sensation above level of lesion. Paralysis of bladder and rectum. Optic neuritis rarely may be present. Test for NMO antibody justified; in "usual" TM will be negative.
CSF	Pleocytosis (20–500 + cells) with PMN predominance in 1st few days, later monocytic preponderance. Protein frequently elevated (50–150 mg/dL). CSF IgM-positive in West Nile.	Cytoalbuminologic dissociation; 10 or fewer mononuclear cells with high protein after 1st week. Normal glucose. IgG may be elevated. West Nile will have cells; nerves can be involved in a myeloradiculitis.	Normal.	Normal.	Usually no manometric block; CSF may show increased protein, pleocytosis with predominantly mononuclear cells, increased IgG.

EMG/NCS	EMG shows denervation after 10–21 d. Nerve conduction normal. Amplitude reduced in West Nile.	NCSs may be normal early (within 1st week). Earliest changes slowed to absent F or H reflexes. Demyelinating changes are typically seen 7–10 d after onset of symptoms.	EMG distinctive: BSAP (brief small abundant potentials). High-frequency stimulation shows increase in CMAP. Helpful but not diagnostic.	Nerve conduction slowed; returns rapidly to normal after removal of tick.	Normal early. Denervation at level of lesion after 10–21 d.
Other studies	Virus in stool and throat. Serial serologic titers IgG, IgM in West Nile. Hyponatremia 30% in West Nile.	Search for specific cause such as infection, intoxication, autoimmune disease. Antiganglioside antibodies to GM_1 (GQ1b in Miller-Fisher).	Infancy: stool culture, toxin. Rare serum toxin positive. Older: serum (or wound) toxin.	Leukocytosis, often with moderate eosinophilia.	Normal spine x-rays do not exclude spinal epidural abscess. MRI to rule out cord-compressive lesions. Cord usually swollen and distorted in myelitis.
Course and prognosis	Paralysis usually maximal 3–5 d after onset. Transient bladder paralysis may occur. Outlook varies with extent and severity of involvement. ***Note:*** Mortality greatest from respiratory failure and superinfection. West Nile paralysis may be permanent.	Course progressive over a few days to about 2 wk. ***Note:*** Threat greatest from respiratory failure (10%), autonomic crises (eg, widely variable blood pressure, arrhythmia), and superinfection. Majority recover completely. Plasmapheresis may have a role. IVIG. Relapses occasionally occur.	Infancy: supportive. Penicillin. Botulism immune globulin intravenous (BIGIV). Respiratory support, gavage feeding. Avoid aminoglycosides. Older: penicillin, antitoxin, prolonged respiratory support. Prognosis: excellent. Fatality 3%.	Total removal of tick is followed by rapid improvement and recovery. Otherwise, mortality rate due to respiratory paralysis is very high.	Large degree of functional recovery possible. Corticosteroids are of controversial benefit in shortening duration of acute attack or altering the overall course. Plasmapheresis, IVIG: anecdotal benefit.

[a]AMAN is acute motor axonal neuropathy (uncommon variant in the United States).

AIDP, acute inflammatory demyelinating neuropathy; CMAP, compound muscle action potentials; CMV, cytomegalovirus; CSF, cerebrospinal fluid; EBV, Ebstein–Barr virus; EMG, electromyogram; EV-71, enterovirus 71; GI, gastrointestinal; IVIG, intravenous immune globulin; MRI, magnetic resonance imaging; NCS, nerve conduction studies; PMN, polymorphonuclear neutrophil; SIDS, sudden infant death syndrome.

Complications

A. Respiratory Weakness and Failure

Early and careful attention to oxygenation is essential. Administration of oxygen, intubation, mechanical respiratory assistance, and careful suctioning of secretions may be required. Increasing anxiety and a rise in diastolic and systolic blood pressures are early signs of hypoxia. Cyanosis is a late sign. Deteriorating spirometric findings (forced expiratory volume in 1 second and total vital capacity) may indicate the need for controlled intubation and respiratory support and is an important mode of monitoring as blood gases may be normal even in late stages of respiratory failure.

B. Infections

Pneumonia is common, especially in patients with respiratory paralysis. Antibiotic therapy is best guided by results of cultures. Bladder infections occur when an indwelling catheter is required because of bladder paralysis. Recovery from myelitis may be delayed by urinary tract infection.

C. Autonomic Crisis

This may be a cause of death in Guillain-Barré syndrome. Strict attention to vital signs to detect and treat hypotension or hypertension and cardiac arrhythmias in an intensive care setting is advisable, at least early in the course and in severely ill patients.

Treatment

Most of these syndromes have no specific treatment, and therefore, supportive treatment is of the essence. Ticks causing paralysis must be removed. Other therapies include the use of erythromycin in *Mycoplasma* infections and botulism immune globulin in infant botulism. Recognized associated disorders (eg, endocrine, neoplastic, or toxic) should be treated by appropriate means. Supportive care also involves pulmonary toilet, adequate fluids and nutrition, bladder and bowel care, prevention of decubitus ulcers, and in many cases, psychiatric support.

A. Corticosteroids

Corticosteroids have no role in treatment of Guillain-Barré syndrome. Autonomic symptoms (eg, hypertension) in polyneuritis may require treatment.

B. Plasmapheresis, Intravenous Immunoglobulin

Plasma exchange or IVIG has been beneficial in moderate or severe cases of Guillain-Barré syndrome.

C. Physical Therapy

Rehabilitative measures are best instituted when acute symptoms have subsided and the patient is stable.

D. Antibiotics

Appropriate antibiotics and drainage are required for epidural abscess.

Alper G et al: Idiopathic acute transverse myelitis in children: An analysis and discussion of MRI findings. Mult Scler 2011;17:74 [PMID: 20858691].

Banwell BL: The long (-itudinally extensive) and the short of it: Transverse myelitis in children. Neurology 2007;68:1447 [PMID: 17470744].

Borchers At, Gershwin ME. Transverse myelitis. Autoimmun Rev 2011;May 18 [PMID: 21621005].

Combiath DR et al: Treatment for guillain-barre syndrome. Ann Neurol 2009;66:569 (letter).

Cortese I et al: Evidence-based guideline update: Plasmapheresis in neurologic disorders: Report of the Therapeutics and Technology Assessment Subcommittee of the American Academy of Neurology. Neurology 2011;76:294 [PMID: 21242498].

Dalakas MC: Intravenous immunoglobulin in autoimmune neuromuscular diseases. JAMA 2004;291:2367 [PMID: 15150209].

Defresne P et al: Acute transverse myelitis in children: Clinical course and prognostic factors. J Child Neurol 2003;18:401 [PMID: 12886975].

De Goede CG et al: Acquired transverse myelopathy in children in the United Kingdom—a 2 year prospective study. Eur J Paediatr Neurol 2010;14:479 [PMID: 20089428].

Dimario FJ Jr: Intravenous immunoglobulin in the treatment of childhood Guillain-Barré syndrome: A randomized trial. Pediatrics 2005;116:226 [PMID: 15995056].

Francisco AM, Arnon SS: Clinical mimics of infant botulism. Pediatrics 2007;119:826 [PMID: 17403857].

Frohman EM, Wingerchuk DM: Transverse myelitis. N Engl J Med 2010;363:564 [PMID: 23818891].

Greenberg BM et al: Idiopathic transverse myelitis. Neurology 2007;68:1614 [PMID: 17485649].

Hughes RA, Cornblath DR: Guillain-Barré syndrome. Lancet 2005;366:1653 [PMID: 16271648].

Hughes RA, Swan AV, Van Doom PA: Intravenous immunoglobulin for Guillain-Barre syndrome. Cochrane Database Syst Rev 2010;Jun 16:CD002063 [PMID: 20556755].

Kincaid O, Lipton HL: Viral myelitis: An update. Curr Neurol Neurosci Rep 2006;6:469 [PMID: 17074281].

Korinthenberg R et al: Clinical presentation and course of childhood Guillain-Barre syndrome: A prospective multicentre study. Neuropediatrics 2007;38(1):10–17.

Linn JJ et al: Risk factors and outcomes of Guillain-Barre syndrome with acute myelitis. Pediatr Neurol 2011;44:110 [PMID: 21215910].

Li Z, Turner RP: Pediatric tick paralysis: Discussion of two cases and literature review. Pediatr Neurol 2004;31:304 [PMID: 15464647].

Mori M, Kuwabara S: Fisher syndrome. Curr Treat Options Neurol 2011;13:71 [PMID: 21104459].

Risko W: Infant botulism. Pediatr Rev 2006;27:36 [PMID: 16473839].

Roodbol J et al: Recognizing Guillain-Barre syndrome in preschool children. Neurology 2011;76:807 [PMID: 21357832].

Sejvar JJ et al: West Nile virus-associated flaccid paralysis. Emerg Infect Dis 2005;11:1021 [PMID: 16022775].

Shahar E: Current therapeutic options in severe Guillain-Barré syndrome. Clin Neuropharmacol 2006;29:45 [PMID: 16518134].

Thompson JA et al: Infant botulism in the age of botulism immune globulin. Neurology 2005;64:2029 [PMID: 15917401].

Tsiodras S et al: *Mycoplasma pneumoniae*-associated myelitis: A comprehensive review. Eur J Neurol 2006;13:112 [PMID: 16490040].

Walgaard C et al: Early recognition of poor prognosis in Guillain-Barre syndrome. Neurology 2011;968–975 [PMID: 21403108].

Wang KC et al: The rescue effect of plasma exchange for neuromyelitis optica. J clin Neuroscl 2011;18(1):43 [PMID: 20888238].

Wingerchuk DM: Diagnosis and treatment of neuromyelitis optica. Neurologist 2007;13:2 [PMID: 17215722].

DISORDERS OF CHILDHOOD AFFECTING MUSCLES

ESSENTIALS OF DIAGNOSIS & TYPICAL FEATURES

- Usually painless, symmetric proximal more than distal muscle weakness (positive Gowers sign, excessive lordosis with walking, waddling gait).
- Preserved deep tendon reflexes compared with muscle weakness.
- Normal to elevated serum creatine kinase (CK) levels.
- Generally normal NCSs; myopathic findings on EMG.

DIAGNOSTIC STUDIES

Serum Enzymes

Serum creatine kinase (CK) levels reflect muscle damage or "leaks" from muscle into plasma. Generally, CK levels are normal to mildly elevated in myopathies, and markedly elevated in muscular dystrophies, up to 50–100 times, as in Duchenne muscular dystrophy. Medications and activity level may affect CK levels, for instance after an EMG or muscle biopsy procedure. Corticosteroids may suppress levels despite very active muscle disease, for example, as in polymyositis.

Electrophysiologic Studies

Nerve conduction study (NCS) and needle electromyography (EMG) are often helpful in grossly differentiating myopathic from neurogenic processes. Generally, NCSs are normal in muscle disorders. In demyelinating polyneuropathies, NCSs may show slowing of conduction velocities or conduction block. EMG involves inserting a needle electrode into muscle to record muscle electrical potentials. The examination includes assessment of abnormal spontaneous activity (eg, fibrillation and fasciculation potentials, myotonic discharges, myokymic discharges, and complex repetitive discharges) and motor unit action potentials (MUAPs). In the myopathies, MUAPs during contraction characteristically are of short duration, polyphasic, and increased in number for the strength of the contraction (increased interference pattern). In neuropathic processes, MUAPs are polyphasic, are of large amplitude, and show decreased recruitment.

Muscle Biopsy

A muscle biopsy can be helpful in the diagnosis of a muscle disorder, if properly executed. It is important to biopsy an affected muscle and consider the timing of the biopsy. The biopsied muscle should be chosen based upon the degree of weakness (ie, weaker muscles will show more pathology than strong muscles). Imaging with MRI or ultrasound may guide the choice of an appropriate site. Biopsies performed in the newborn period may be of limited utility as pathologic changes may not be evident in immature muscle. Care should be taken to avoid sites of prior needle EMG examinations or injections as this may cause spurious areas of focal inflammation pathologically. Findings common to the muscular dystrophies include variation in the size and shape of muscle fibers, increase in connective tissue, interstitial infiltration of fatty tissue, areas of degeneration and regeneration, focal areas of inflammatory changes, and centralized nuclei. Myopathies typically do not have the vigorous cycles of degeneration/regeneration and inflammation is seen in dystrophies.

Immunostaining for proteins of the sarcolemmal membrane, surrounding collagen matrix, and intracellular components of the myofiber is a valuable tool. For instance, demonstration of absent collagen VI is virtually diagnostic of Ullrich congenital muscular dystrophy. In the past, absent dystrophin staining at the sarcolemmal membrane on muscle biopsy was diagnostic of Duchenne muscular dystrophy, but mutation analysis of the dystrophin gene is the preferred initial step given the ready availability of commercial testing.

Genetic Testing & Carrier Detection

Mutation analysis for Duchenne and Becker muscular dystrophy is considered the initial step in diagnosis, though it should be noted that readily available commercial testing is not exhaustive, and an initial negative result does not exclude the diagnosis. Full characterization of the mutation is critical, as newer treatments targeting specific mutations are emerging. Carrier testing should be offered to all mothers, not only for genetic counseling purposes but also because carriers are at increased risk for developing cardiomyopathy.

Genetic testing for other myopathies and muscular dystrophies should be guided by the clinical findings, serum CK levels, and muscle biopsy results. Commercially available tests are available for many of these disorders (see Table 25–29).

Genetic counseling is particularly important for families of patients with spinal muscular atrophy. Testing for the survival motor neuron (SMN)1 gene deletion has a sensitivity

Table 25–29. Muscular dystrophies, myopathies, myotonias, and anterior horn diseases of childhood.

Disease	Genetic Pattern	Age at Onset	Early Manifestation	Involved Muscles	Reflexes
Muscular dystrophies					
Duchenne muscular dystrophy (pseudohypertrophic infantile)	X-linked recessive; Xp21; 30%–50% have no family history and are spontaneous mutations.	2–6 y; rarely in infancy.	Clumsiness, easy fatigability on walking, running, and climbing stairs. Walking on toes; waddling gait with excessive lumbar lordosis. Motor delays. Positive Gowers maneuver.	Proximal (pelvic and shoulder girdle) muscles; pseudohypertrophy of gastrocnemius, triceps brachii, and vastus lateralis. Second decade, progressive scoliosis, cardiomyopathy and respiratory weakness develop.	Knee jerks +/– or 0; ankle jerks + to ++
Becker muscular dystrophy (late onset)	X-linked recessive; Xp21.	Variable: childhood to adulthood.	Similar to Duchenne.	Similar to Duchenne.	Similar to Duchenne
Limb-girdle muscular dystrophy	Autosomal dominant, autosomal recessive, and X-linked forms.	Variable; early childhood to adulthood.	Weakness, with distribution according to type. Waddling gait, difficulty climbing stairs. Excessive lumbar lordosis.	Slowly progressive, symmetric proximal muscle involvement; characteristically involves shoulder and pelvic muscles.	Usually present
Facioscapulohumeral muscular dystrophy (Landouzy-Déjérine)	Most are autosomal dominant inherited deletions of D4Z4 on 4q35; sporadic cases in 10%–30% cases.	Usually late in 1st–5th decade depending on size of deletion.	Diminished facial movements with inability to close eyes, smile, or whistle. Difficulty in raising arms over heard.	Face, shoulder girdle muscles (biceps, triceps), often asymmetric. Deltoid and forearm spared. 75% have sensorineural hearing loss; 60% Coats disease; 89% mental retardation.	Present
Congenital myopathies					
Myotubular myopathy	X-linked recessive; Xq27.	Neonatal period.	Floppy infant; severe hypotonia and respiratory insufficiency.	Ptosis, ophthalmoplegia; severe symmetric distal and proximal weakness.	+ to -
Central core myopathy	Most autosomal dominant, some autosomal recessive, 19q13, RYR1.	Infancy to adulthood.	Reduced fetal movements; hypotonia; ankle contractures.	Nonprogressive proximal weakness of legs more than arms, mild facial weakness, normal eye movements.	+ to -
Metabolic myopathies					
Pompe disease	Autosomal recessive; 17q23.	Classic infantile presentation: present by 6 mo of age.	Severe hypotonia, hepatomegaly, cardiomyopathy, hypoventilation.	Proximal more than distal muscles, bulbar and respiratory muscles.	0
		Juvenile: 2–18 y.	Proximal muscle weakness.	Recurrent respiratory infections; nocturnal hypoventilation.	
Ion channel disorders					
Hyperkalemic periodic paralysis	Autosomal dominant 17q35.	Childhood, usually by 1st decade.	Episodic flaccid weakness, precipitated by rest after exercise, stress, fasting or cold.	Proximal and symmetric muscles, distal muscles may be involved if exercised.	Normal, may be 0 with episode

Muscle Biopsy Findings	Other Diagnostic Tests	Treatment	Prognosis
Areas of degeneration and regeneration, variation in fiber size, inflammatory changes, proliferation of connective tissue. Immunostaining for dystrophin absent.	Myopathic EMG. CK levels can be up to 50–100× normal, but decrease with increasing disease severity, reflecting replacement of muscle with fat/connective tissue. Genetic testing will show deletion 60% of time, while 5%–15% are duplications, and 20%–30% are point mutations, intronic deletions, or repeats.	Corticosteroids may prolong extend independent ambulation by 2.5 y if started between age 4 and 8 y; management is largely supportive. Close pulmonary and cardiac follow-up should be maintained due to risk of cardiorespiratory failure in 2nd–3rd decade of life. Osteoporosis should be treated with calcium and vitamin D.	Patients are wheelchair-bound by ~12 y old. Death from cardiorespiratory causes usually occurs by the early 20s.
Same as above except dystrophin immunostaining is reduced, not absent.	As above.	As above.	Variable. Patients may remain ambulant 15–20 y after 1st symptoms. Near-normal life expectancies.
Necrosis and fiber splitting, increased endomysial connective tissue and inflammation, absent immunostaining for various DGC proteins by subtype.	Myopathic EMG. CK often > 5000 IU/L. MRI of the legs may show selective involvement (eg, peroneal muscles in Miyoshi myopathy).	Physical therapy. Echocardiogram to screen for cardiomyopathy. PFTs to screen to respiratory weakness. No curative treatment available.	Variable by subtype.
Nonspecific myopathic changes: variation in fiber size, moderate increased endomysial connective tissue, mild inflammatory changes.	Nonspecific chronic myopathic changes. CK mild to moderately elevated (< 1500 IU/L).	No curative treatments available. Management of pain important. Identify and treat hearing loss, retinal telangiectasias, respiratory insufficiency (1% cases). Ongoing clinical trials with β2-agonists. Studies show possible benefit with creatine monohydrate and exercise.	Variable and inversely related to age at symptom onset. Life-threatening bulbar, respiratory and cardiac problems rare, so life expectancy normal.
Small rounded myotube-like myofibers. Patchy central clearing with radial spokes.	Normal to mildly elevated CK. Myopathic EMG with fibrillations and complex repetitive discharges.	No curative treatment. Respiratory, nutritional support. Liver and peritoneal hemorrhage reported in cases.	Generally death before 5 mo of age.
Variable myofiber size; oxidative staining shows central cores absent of mitochondrial activity.	High CK, mild myopathic changes on EMG, muscle MRI shows increased T1 signal.	Physical therapy. Respiratory follow-up required. Avoid inhalational anesthetics and succinylcholine due to risk of malignancy hyperthermia.	Weakness is nonprogressive. Life expectancy normal.
Cytoplasmic lysosomal vacuoles stain positive with acid phosphatase.	High CK in infants (< 10 × normal). Mildly high CK in teens.	Enzyme replacement therapy with alglucosidase alfa (Myozyme). Respiratory and nutritional support. Monitor cardiomyopathy. As above.	Significant but variable with treatment, with improved survival, cardiorespiratory status and motor skills. Variable, some become nonambulatory and most require ventilatory support.
Hyperkalemic periodic paralysis.	CK normal to 300 IU/L; attacks associated with high serum K^+; NCS show increased CMAP amplitude after 5 min exercise.	Many attacks are brief and do not need treatment; treat acute attack with carbohydrates; if needed, chronic treatment with acetazolamide.	Attacks may be more frequent with increasing age.

(Continued)

Table 25–29. Muscular dystrophies, myopathies, myotonias, and anterior horn diseases of childhood. (*Continnued*)

Disease	Genetic Pattern	Age at Onset	Early Manifestation	Involved Muscles	Reflexes
Congenital muscular dystrophies (CMD)					
CMD with CNS involvement: includes laminin α_2 (merosin) deficiency, Ullrich CMD	Autosomal recessive, autosomal dominant.	Birth to 1st mo.	Hypotonia, generalized weakness. Contractures proximally and lax hypermobility distally.	Generalized and respiratory muscle weakness.	0 to +
CMD with CNS involvement: Fukayama (FCMD), Walker-Warburg (WW), Muscle-eye-brain (MEB)	Recessive; 6 genes identified (including *POMT*). Associated with abnormalities of glycosylation of α-dystroglycan.	Birth to 9 mo.	Severe weakness; profound motor delay; severe mental. retardation. MEB with severe congenital myopia, retinal hypoplasia.	Severe generalized weakness.	Variable
Benign congenital hypotonia (Oppenheim)	Variable.	Variable.	Hypotonia only. Deep tendon reflexes positive. Laboratory tests, biopsy normal.	Somatic muscles (respiratory muscles spared).	Normal to decreased
Myotonic disorders					
Myotonic dystrophy type 1 (DM1)	Autosomal dominant, expanded CTG triple repeat on chromosome 19q13.	Congenital presentation.	Decreased fetal movement, respiratory insufficiency, difficulties in feeding, sucking, and swallowing.	Generalized weakness; Facial and pharyngeal involvement prominent; mental retardation.	Decreased to 0
		Typical teen to adult onset (2nd–4th decade).	Complaints of difficulty opening jars, releasing objects, manipulating small objects.	Distal more than proximal weakness; involved hands and feet. Slow release of hand grip or eyelid closure (myotonia); cataracts; insulin resistance, cardiac conduction defects.	+ to ++
Myotonic dystrophy type 2 (DM2)	Autosomal dominant expanded CCTG repeat on chromosome 3q21.	~8–60 y old.	Complaints of difficult climbing stairs, arising from stairs.	Mild facial weakness, with proximal > distal and legs > arms (usually hip flexors and leg extensors); grip myotonia.	+ to ++
Myotonia congenita (Thomsen)	Autosomal dominant on chromosome 7q35 on CLCN1 gene.	Early infancy to adulthood.	Muscle hypertrophy. Difficulty in relaxing muscles after contracting them, especially with cold or stress.	Mild fixed proximal muscle weakness or mild functional difficulties (like climbing stairs).	Normal
Myotonia congenital (Becker)	Autosomal recessive on chromosome 7q35 on CLCN1 gene.	4–12 y	Myotonia, relaxes with exercise. Muscle hypertrophy of legs and gluteals.	Mild distal muscle weakness; limitations from myotonia (inability to voluntarily relax muscle.	Normal
Spinal muscular atrophy					
SMA type 1 (Werdnig-Hoffman)	Autosomal recessive, rare cohorts with autosomal dominant or X-linked inheritance, 5q.	1st 6 mo of life.	Hypotonia, "floppy" infant, with alert look, fasciculations may be noted of tongue.	Severe progressive, symmetric proximal and respiratory muscle weakness; face spared.	0

Muscle Biopsy Findings	Other Diagnostic Tests	Treatment	Prognosis
Laminin α_2 deficiency: absent/reduced laminin α_2 staining. Ullrich CMD: reduced/absent COLVI.	CK normal to 10 × normal. Laminin α_2 deficiency: mild neuropathy. Skin changes in Ullrich CMD: follicular hyperkeratosis.	Most never walk or lose ability to walk early. Respiratory support required early.	Variable: death by 1st–2nd decade secondary to respiratory failure.
Variability in fiber size, internalized nuclei, decreased immunostaining of α-dystroglycan.	CK 400–4000 IU/L, myopathic EMG, small evoked response on electroretinogram, MRI shows white matter changes, migrational abnormalities, lissencephaly, cerebellar hypoplasia.	No curative treatment. Respiratory and nutritional support. Treatment of seizures.	Variable, but generally poor with death by 2nd decade secondary to respiratory failure.
Normal histochemical and immunohistochemical studies.	Use of this diagnosis is shrinking with increasingly sophisticated biochemical and genetic studies.	Supportive. Physical therapy.	Good (by definition). Few documented long-term studies.
Mild myopathic changes, centralized nuclei, variation in fiber size, ring fibers.	Usually normal CK. Electrical myotonia on EMG. Cataracts on slit lamp exam. Reduced testosterone levels. ECG shows conduction defects, like ventricular arrhythmias. Insulin resistance. Sleep study shows hypercapnia and hypoventilation.	No curative treatment. Patients should avoid medications that predispose to arrhythmia such as quinine, amitriptyline, and digoxin. Should be closely followed by pulmonologist with sleep studies, by cardiologist for risk of arrhythmia, by endocrinologist for insulin resistance, and by ophthalmologist for cataracts. May have GI hypomotility with constipation and pseudoobstruction.	Reduced survival to age 65; mean survival to 60 y. 50% patients are wheelchair bound before death.
Mild myopathic changes: variability in fiber size, centralized nuclei.	Mildly elevated CK. Electrical myotonia on EMG. Cataracts seen in 100%, cardiac arrhythmias in 20% (less than DM1), insulin resistance in 20%, hearing loss 20%.	No curative treatment. Supportive are same as DM1.	More benign prognosis than DM1.
Usually normal, though there may be absence of 2B fibers.	Myotonia and mild myopathic changes on EMG; CK may be slightly elevated 3–4× normal.	Symptomatic treatment with quinine, mexiletine, dilantin, carbamazepine. May improve with exercise. Worsened with β_2-agonists, monocarboxylic amino acids, depolarizing muscle relaxants.	Normal life expectancy; muscle stiffness may interfere with activity but improves with exercise.
Same as above.	Same as above.	Same as above.	Same as above.
Large areas of grouped muscle fiber atrophy, most larger fibers are type I.	EMG shows fibrillation and fasciculation potentials, large amplitude motor unit potentials. Normal to mildly elevated CK.	No curative treatments. Respiratory and nutritional support. Clinical trials underway with sodium phenylbutyrate, valproic acid, and riluzole.	No independent sitting or standing. Life expectancy < 2 y without respiratory or nutritional support

(*Continued*)

Table 25–29. Muscular dystrophies, myopathies, myotonias, and anterior horn diseases of childhood. (*Continued*)

Disease	Genetic Pattern	Age at Onset	Early Manifestation	Involved Muscles	Reflexes
SMA type 2		1st 18 mo.	Motor delays.	Progressive symmetric proximal muscles, mild to moderate respiratory weakness, limited cough and secretion control.	0 to +
SMA type 3 (Kugelberg-Welander)		Recognized after 18 mo of age.	Motor delays, difficulty with climbing stairs, may achieve independent walking but may lose this.	Progressive symmetric proximal muscle weakness, +/– tremor of hands.	0 to +
SMA type 4		Adulthood.	Clumsy gait.	Mild progressive proximal muscle weakness.	0 to ++

of 95% and a specificity of 100%. Carrier testing, along with genetic counseling, should also be offered, as the carrier rate is 1 in 25 to 1 in 50, depending upon ethnicity.

Complications

Though skeletal muscle weakness may be profound in muscle disorders, the greatest morbidity and mortality arises from cardiorespiratory complications. Advances in supportive care, especially in critical care management of these patients, have had a tremendous impact in the care of these patients. Noninvasive ventilation, better management of secretions, and generation of effective cough are a few examples. Other complications include delayed gastrointestinal motility which can lead to debilitating constipation or pseudoobstruction. Contractures are a particularly frustrating complication which can limit mobility of these patients, cause pain, and affect quality of life. Some DMD patients may have a nonprogressive mental retardation with IQ scores one standard deviation below normal means.

Treatment

Treatment for patients with muscle disorders is predominantly supportive, and medications altering disease progression is, at this time, limited. Patients with Duchenne muscular dystrophy (DMD)/Becker muscular dystrophy (BMD) should be offered treatment with corticosteroids (prednisone/prednisolone and deflazacort) which have been shown to extend the period of independent ambulation by approximately 2.5 years, and to preserve respiratory strength and cardiac function into the second decade. Instituting steroid treatment between 4 and 8 years, when motor function plateaus or is in decline, appears to have the greatest impact on muscle strength and cardiorespiratory function, according to recent practice parameter guidelines. Additional promising treatments targeting the mutation more specifically have been developed over the last decade and are currently in clinical trials, including exon-skipping and read-through strategies that target specific mutations.

In the past, the prognosis for infantile Pompe disease was uniformly grim, with death by age 1 year, but enzyme replacement therapy with recombinant alglucosidase alpha has changed the outlook for many of these patients. Published short-term studies of infants with Pompe disease show significant improvement after treatment with alglucosidase alpha; with improved survival, respiratory performance, cardiomyopathy, and attainment of motor skills.

Until curative treatments for muscle diseases are available, the emphasis on management ought to be on slowing the progressive deterioration in muscle strength and cardiorespiratory function, and to improve quality of life.

Aartsma-Rus A et al: Entries in the Leiden Duchenne muscular dystrophy mutation database: An overview of mutation types and paradoxical cases that confirm the reading-frame rule. Muscle Nerve 2006;34:135–144 [PMID: 16770791].

American Association of Neuromuscular & Electrodiagnostic Medicine: Diagnostic criteria for late-onset (childhood and adult) Pompe disease. Muscle Nerve 2009;40:140–160 [PMID: 19533647].

Angelini C: The role of corticosteroids in muscular dystrophy: A critical appraisal. Muscle Nerve 2007;36:424–435 [PMID: 17541998].

Bushby K, Finkel R, Birnkrant Dj et al: Diagnosis and management of Duchenne muscular dystrophy part 1. Lancet Neurol 2010;9(2):77–93 [PMID: 19945913].

Bushby K, Finkel R, Birnkrant Dj et al: Diagnosis and management of Duchenne muscular dystrophy part 2. Lancet Neurol 2010;9(2):177–189 [PMID: 19945914].

Cossu G, Sampaolesi M: New therapies for Duchenne muscular dystrophy: Challenges, prospects and clinical trials. Trends Mol Med 2007;13:520–526 [PMID: 17983835].

Finder JD: A 2009 perspective on the 2004 American Thoracic Society statement, "respiratory care of the patient with Duchenne muscular dystrophy." Pediatrics 2009;123(Suppl 4):S239–S241 [PMID: 19420152].

Muscle Biopsy Findings	Other Diagnostic Tests	Treatment	Prognosis
As above.	EMG also shows fibrillation potentials and large amplitude motor unit potentials, but fasciculations not as common as in SMA type 1; tremor of fingers.	No curative treatments. Mild to moderate respiratory weakness, sleep-disordered breathing, and limited cough and secretion control require close follow-up with pulmonologist.	Will achieve independent sitting but not standing. 75% alive at 25 y old.
As above.	EMG similar to SMA type 2.	No curative treatments.	Independent ambulation may be achieved, but this skill may be lost. Normal life expectancy.
As above.	EMG similar to SMA type 2; tremor of hands often noted.	No curative treatment. Physical therapy and assistive devices. No pulmonary issues.	Slow progression of muscle weakness. Normal life expectancy.

ASA, acetylsalicylic acid; CK, creatine kinase; CPT, carnitine palmityl transferase; CSF, cerebrospinal fluid; CT, computed tomography; ECG, electrocardiogram; EMG, electromyogram; MRI, magnetic resonance imaging; PCR, polymerase chain reaction; SIDS, sudden infant death syndrome.

Gauld LM: Airway clearance in neuromuscular weakness. Dev Med Child Neurol 2009;51:350–355 [PMID: 19379290].

Kinali M et al: Congenital myasthenic syndromes in childhood: Diagnostic and management challenges. J Neuroimmunol 2008;201–202:6–12 [PMID: 18707767].

Kirschner J, Bonnemann CG: The congenital and limb-girdle muscular dystrophies. Arch Neurol 2004;61:189–199 [PMID: 14967765].

Kishnani PS et al: A retrospective, multinational, multicenter study on the natural history of infantile-onset Pompe disease. J Pediatr 2006;148:671–676 [PMID: 16737883].

Kishnani PS et al: Pompe disease diagnosis and management guideline. Genet Med 2006;8:267–288 [PMID: 16702877].

Kishnani PS et al: Recombinant human acid [alpha]-glucosidase: Major clinical benefits in infantile-onset Pompe disease. Neurology 2007;68:99–109 [PMID: 17151339].

Kolb SJ, Kissel JT: Spinal muscular atrophy. Arch Neurol 2011 [Epub ahead of print] [PMID: 21482919].

Moxley RT 3rd et al: Practice parameter: Corticosteroid treatment of Duchenne dystrophy: Report of the Quality Standards Subcommittee of the American Academy of Neurology and the Practice Committee of the Child Neurology Society. Neurology 2005;64:13–20 [PMID: 15642897].

Muntoni F et al: Dystrophin and mutations: One gene, several proteins, multiple phenotypes. Lancet Neurol 2003;2:731–740 [PMID: 14636778].

Schara U et al: Myotonic dystrophies type 1 and 2: A summary on current aspects. Semin Pediatr Neurol 2006;13:71 [PMID: 17027856].

Swoboda KJ et al: Perspectives on clinical trials in spinal muscular atrophy. J Child Neurol 2007;22:957–966 [PMID: 17761650].

Tawil R et al: Facioscapulohumeral muscular dystrophy. Muscle Nerve 2006;34:1 [PMID: 16508966].

Wang CH et al: Consensus statement for standard of care in spinal muscular atrophy. J Child Neurol 2007;22:1027–1049 [PMID: 17761659].

Wang CH et al: Consensus statement on standard of care for congenital muscular dystrophies. J Child Neurol 2010;25(12):1559–1581 [PMID: 21078917].

Yang ML, Finkel RS: Overview of paediatric neuromuscular disorders and related pulmonary issues. Paediatr Resp Rev 2010;11(1):9–17 [PMID: 20113986].

BENIGN ACUTE CHILDHOOD MYOSITIS

Benign acute childhood myositis (myalgia cruris epidemica) is characterized by transient severe muscle pain and weakness affecting mainly the calves and occurring 1–2 days following an upper respiratory tract infection. Although symptoms involve mainly the gastrocnemius muscles, all skeletal muscles appear to be invaded directly by virus; recurrent episodes are due to different viral types. By seroconversion or isolation of the virus, acute myositis has been shown to be largely due to influenza types B and A and occasionally due to parainfluenza and adenovirus.

Agyeman P et al: Influenza-associated myositis in children. Infection 2004;32:199 [PMID: 15293074].

MYASTHENIC SYNDROMES

ESSENTIALS OF DIAGNOSIS & TYPICAL FEATURES

- Asymmetric, variable weakness, usually coming on or increasing with use (fatigue).
- Involves extraocular, bulbar, and respiratory muscles.
- Positive response to neostigmine and edrophonium.

General Considerations

Myasthenic syndromes are characterized by easy fatigability of muscles, particularly the extraocular, bulbar, and respiratory muscles. In the neonatal period, however, or in early infancy, the weakness may be so constant and general that an affected infant may present nonspecifically as a "floppy infant." Three general categories of myasthenic syndromes are recognized: transient neonatal myasthenia, autoimmune myasthenia gravis, and congenital myasthenia.

Clinical Findings

A. Symptoms and Signs

1. Neonatal (transient) myasthenia—This disorder occurs in 12%–19% of infants born to myasthenic mothers as a result of passive transfer of maternal acetylcholine receptor antibody across the placenta. Neonates present before the third day of life with bulbar weakness, difficulty feeding, weak cry, and hypotonia.

2. Juvenile myasthenia gravis—Like the adult form of myasthenia gravis, juvenile myasthenia gravis is characterized by fatiguable and asymmetric weakness. However, more than half of patients present with ocular symptoms (ptosis or ophthalmoplegia), unlike adult patients who typically present with limb weakness. Weakness may remain limited to the extraocular muscles in 10%–15% of patients, but approximately half of children develop systemic or bulbar symptoms within 2 years and 75% within 4 years. Symptoms of weakness tend to recur and remit, and can be precipitate by illness or medications such as aminoglycoside antibiotics. Typical signs include difficulty chewing foods like meat, dysphagia, nasal voice, ptosis, ophthalmoplegia, and proximal limb weakness. Other autoimmune disorders such as rheumatoid arthritis and thyroid disease may be associated findings.

3. Congenital myasthenic syndromes—These syndromes are a heterogenous group of hereditary, nonimmune disorders of presynaptic, synaptic, or postsynaptic neuromuscular transmission. Patients present with symptoms similar to that of myasthenia gravis, but onset is earlier, before the age of 2 years, and can vary from mild motor delay to dramatic episodic apnea. Serum acetylcholine receptor antibody testing is negative. Response to anticholinesterases is variable, depending on the type of congenital myasthenic syndrome, and some forms may paradoxically worsen. The distinction between this group of disorders and myasthenia gravis is important, as these patients will not benefit from a thymectomy, steroids, or immunosuppressants, but it may be clinically difficult to distinguish between the two.

B. Laboratory Findings

1. Anticholinesterase inhibitor testing

A. NEOSTIGMINE TEST—In newborns and very young infants, the neostigmine test may be preferable to the edrophonium (Tensilon) test because the longer duration of its response permits better observation, especially of sucking and swallowing movements. There is a delay of about 10 minutes before the effect may be manifest. The physician should be prepared to suction secretions, and administer atropine if necessary.

B. EDROPHONIUM TEST—Testing with edrophonium is used in older children who are capable of cooperating in certain tasks and who exhibit easily observable clinical signs, such as ptosis, ophthalmoplegia, or dysarthria. Maximum improvement occurs within 2 minutes. Both cholinesterase inhibitor tests can be limited by patient cooperation and lack of an easily observable clinical sign.

2. Antibody testing—Serum acetylcholine receptor binding, blocking, and modulating antibodies typically, though not always, are found in autoimmune juvenile myasthenia gravis. Though not specifically studied in the pediatric population, in the general myasthenia gravis population at large, about 40% of the seronegative patients have muscle-specific receptor tyrosine kinase (MuSK) antibodies. Serum acetylcholine receptor antibodies or MuSK antibodies are often found in the neonatal and juvenile forms. In juveniles, thyroid studies are appropriate.

3. Genetic testing—Commercially available genetic testing is limited for patients with congenital myasthenic syndromes.

C. Electrophysiologic Studies

Electrophysiologic studies may be helpful when myasthenic syndromes are considered. Repetitive stimulation of a motor nerve at slow rates of 2–3 Hz with recording over an appropriately chosen muscle reveals a progressive fall in compound muscle action potentials by the fourth to fifth repetition in myasthenic patients. At higher rates of stimulation of 50 Hz, there may be a transient repair of this defect before the progressive decline is seen. Both studies may be technically difficult to perform in infants and younger children as repetitive stimulation can be painful and requires cooperation. If this study is negative, single-fiber EMG in older cooperative children may be helpful diagnostically, but it is technically challenging and time intensive, and requires concentration on the part of the child. Stimulated single-fiber EMG may be performed by trained electromyographers.

D. Imaging

Chest radiograph and CT scanning in older children may show thymic hyperplasia. Thymomas are rare in children.

Treatment

A. General and Supportive Measures

In the newborn or in a child in myasthenic or cholinergic crisis (see the following section Complications), supportive care is essential and the child should be monitored in a critical care setting. A careful search for signs of respiratory failure is crucial: simple bedside tests include evaluation of cough and counting to 20 in a single breath. An inability to do either signals respiratory failure. Neck flexion weakness, nasal speech, and drooling are other important signs to observe. Management of secretions and respiratory assistance should be monitored by trained critical care staff.

B. Treatment

1. Anticholinesterase inhibitors

A. Pyridostigmine bromide—Pyridostigmine is the first-line treatment in patients with juvenile myasthenia gravis and mild weakness. Anticholinesterase inhibitors do not modify disease progression but transiently improve muscle strength. For younger children, the starting dose is 0.5–1 mg/kg every 4–6 hours. In older children, the initial dose is 30–60 mg every 4–6 hours. The maximal daily dose is 7 mg/kg/d with an absolute maximum dose of 300 mg/d. The dosage must be adjusted for each patient based on clinical symptoms and side effects.

B. Neostigmine—Fifteen milligrams of neostigmine are roughly equivalent to 60 mg of pyridostigmine bromide. Neostigmine often causes gastric hypermotility with diarrhea, but it is the drug of choice in newborns, in whom prompt treatment may be lifesaving. It may be given parenterally.

2. Immunomodulatory treatment—Patients with more severe weakness not responding to cholinesterase inhibitors alone require long-term treatment with immunomodulation. There are four therapeutic options in this category: (1) plasmapheresis, (2) intravenous immunoglobulins (IVIg), (3) steroids, and (4) immunosuppressants. The mainstay of treatment is steroids, but some patients who either cannot tolerate or do not respond to steroids require treatment with other immunosuppressants such as azathioprine, cyclosporine, or mycophenolate mofetil. Both plasmapheresis and IVIg may be given on a long-term basis, depending on the severity of symptoms, as well as in the acute setting, with myasthenic crises. Special note must be made to the use of steroids, which can transiently worsen symptoms before any benefit is noted, particularly with large starting doses.

Complications

1. Myasthenic crisis—Respiratory failure can develop swiftly due to critical weakness of respiratory muscle, bulbar muscles or both, resulting in a myasthenic crisis. Crises are generally not fatal as long as patients receive timely respiratory support and appropriate immunotherapy. Particular vigilance, however, needs to be maintained as crises can occur in the setting of medical illnesses or surgical procedures. Patients and their caregivers should also be alerted that certain medications can exacerbate myasthenia gravis, including aminoglycoside antibiotics, muscle relaxants, and anesthetics.

2. Cholinergic crisis—Cholinergic crisis may result from overmedication with anticholinesterase drugs. The resulting weakness may be similar to that of myasthenic crises, and the muscarinic side effects (diarrhea, sweating, lacrimation, miosis, bradycardia, and hypotension) are often absent or difficult to evaluate. If suspected, cholinesterase inhibitors should be discontinued immediately, and improvement afterwards suggests cholinergic crisis. As in myasthenic crisis, supportive respiratory care and appropriate immunotherapy should be given.

C. Surgical Measures

Data for efficacy of thymectomy in the pediatric population are few. Some studies suggest that thymectomy within 2 years of diagnosis results in a higher rate of remission in Caucasian children. Experienced surgical and postsurgical care are prerequisites.

Prognosis

Prognosis for neonatal (transient) myasthenia is generally good, with complete resolution of symptoms in 2–3 weeks. However, immediate treatment with appropriate respiratory support in the acute presentation period is crucial, primarily because of the risk of secretion aspiration. No further treatment is required thereafter. The prognosis for congenital myasthenic syndromes is variable by subtype. Some subtypes show improvement in weakness with age. Others demonstrate life-threatening episodic apnea, including those with rapsyn mutations, fast-channel mutations, and choline acetyltransferase mutations. Patients with juvenile myasthenia gravis generally do well, with greater spontaneous remission rates than adult patients. Improvements in respiratory and critical care support has improved prognosis for these patients.

Chiang L et al: Juvenile myasthenia gravis. Muscle & Nerve 2009; 39(4):423–431 [PMID: 19229875].

Cortese I, Chaudhry V, So YT et al: Evidence-based guideline update: Plasmapheresis in neurologic disorders: Report of the Therapeutics and Technology Assessment Subcommittee of the American Academy of Neurology. Neurology 2011;76(3): 294–300.

Hennessey IA, Long AM, Hughes I et al: Thymectomy for inducing remission in juvenile myasthenia gravis. Pediatr Surg Int 2011;27(6):591–594 [PMID: 21243366].

Juel VC, Massey JM: Autoimmune myasthenia gravis: Recommendations for treatment and immunologic modulation. Curr Treat Opt Neurol 2005;7:3 [PMID: 15610702].

Keesey JC: Clinical evaluation and management of myasthenia gravis. Muscle Nerve 2004;29(4):484–505 [PMID: 15052614].

Kinali M et al: Congenital myasthenic syndromes in childhood: Diagnostic and management challenges. J Neuroimmunol 2008; 201–202:6–12 [PMID: 180707767].

Mehndiratta MM, Pandey S, Kuntzer T: Acetylcholinesterase inhibitor treatment for myasthenia gravis. Cochrane Database Syst Rev 2011;16(2):CD006986 [PMID: 21328290].

PERIPHERAL NERVE PALSIES

Facial Weakness

Facial asymmetry may be present at birth or may develop later, either suddenly or gradually, unilaterally or bilaterally. Nuclear or peripheral involvement of the facial nerves results in sagging or drooping of the mouth and inability to close one or both eyes, particularly when newborns and infants cry. Inability to wrinkle the forehead may be demonstrated in infants and young children by getting them to follow a light moved vertically above the forehead. Loss of taste of the anterior two-thirds of the tongue on the involved side may be demonstrated in cooperative children by age 4 or 5 years. Playing with a younger child and the judicious use of a tongue blade may enable the physician to note whether the child's face puckers up when something sour (eg, lemon juice) is applied with a swab to the anterior tongue. Ability to wrinkle the forehead is preserved, owing to bilateral innervation, in supranuclear facial paralysis.

Injuries to the facial nerve at birth occur in 0.25%–6.5% of consecutive live births. Forceps delivery is the cause in some cases; in others, the side of the face affected may have abutted in utero against the sacral prominence. Often, no cause can be established.

Acquired peripheral facial weakness (Bell palsy) of sudden onset and unknown cause is common in children. It often follows a viral illness (postinfectious) or physical trauma (eg, cold). It may be a presenting sign of Lyme disease, infectious mononucleosis, herpes simplex, or Guillain-Barré syndrome and is usually diagnosable by the history, physical examination, and appropriate laboratory tests. Chronic cranial nerve VII palsy may be a sign of brainstem tumor.

Bilateral facial weakness in early life may be due to agenesis of the facial nerve nuclei or muscles (part of Möbius syndrome) or may even be familial. Myasthenia gravis, polyneuritis (Miller-Fisher syndrome), and myotonic dystrophy or other congenital myopathies must be considered.

Asymmetrical crying facies, in which one side of the lower lip depresses with crying (ie, the normal side) and the other does not, is usually an innocent form of autosomal dominant inherited congenital malformation. The defect in the parent (the asymmetry often improves with age) may be almost inapparent. EMG suggests congenital absence of the depressor angularis muscle of the lower lip. Forceps pressure is often erroneously incriminated as a cause of this innocent congenital anomaly. Occasionally other major (eg, cardiac septal defects) congenital defects accompany the palsy. Congenital unilateral lower lip paralysis with asymmetric crying facies, most often attributed to congenital absence of the depressor anguli oris, is associated with major malformations, most commonly heart defects, in 10% of cases.

In the vast majority of cases of isolated peripheral facial palsy—both those due to birth trauma and those acquired later—improvement begins within 1–2 weeks, and near or total recovery of function is observed within 2 months. In severe palsy with inefficient blinking, methylcellulose drops, 1%, should be instilled into the eyes to protect the cornea during the day; at night the lid should be taped down with cellophane tape. Upward massage of the face for 5–10 minutes three or four times a day may help maintain muscle tone. Prednisone therapy (2–4 mg/kg orally for 5–7 days) likely does not aid recovery. In the older child, acyclovir or valacyclovir (herpes antiviral agent) therapy or antibiotics (Lyme disease) may have a role in Bell palsy.

In the few children with permanent and cosmetically disfiguring facial weakness, plastic surgical intervention at age 6 years or older may be of benefit. New procedures, such as attachment of facial muscles to the temporal muscle and transplantation of cranial nerve XI, are being developed.

Akcakus M et al: Asymmetric crying facies associated with congenital hypoparathyroidism and 22q11 deletion. Turk J Pediatr 2004;46:191 [PMID: 15214756].

Ashtekar CS et al: Best evidence topic report. Do we need to give steroids in children with Bell's palsy? Emerg Med J 2005;22:505 [PMID: 15983089].

Gilden DH: Clinical practice. Bell's palsy. N Engl J Med 2004;351:1323 [PMID: 15385659].

Hato N et al: Valcyclovir and prednisolone treatment for Bell's palsy: A multicenter, randomized, placebo-controlled study. Otol Neurotology 2007;28:408 [PMID: 17414047].

Kawaguchi K et al: Reactivation of herpes simplex virus type 1 and varicella-zoster virus and therapeutic effects of combination therapy with prednisolone and valacyclovir in patients with Bell's palsy. Laryngoscope 2007;117:147 [PMID: 17202945].

Salinas RA et al: Corticosteroids for Bell's palsy (idiopathic facial paralysis). Cochrane Database Syst Rev 2004;(4):CD001942 [PMID: 15495021].

Sapin SO et al: Neonatal asymmetric crying facies: A new look at an old problem. Clin Pediatr (Phila) 2005;44:109 [PMID: 15735828].

Terada K et al: Bilateral facial nerve palsy associated with Epstein-Barr virus infection with a review of the literature. Scand J Infect Dis 2004;36:75 [PMID: 15000569].

Vorstman JA, Kuiper H: Peripheral facial palsy in children: Test for Lyme borreliosis only in the presence of other clinical signs. Ned Tijdschr Geneeskd 2004;148:655 [PMID: 15106315].

CHRONIC POLYNEUROPATHY

ESSENTIALS OF DIAGNOSIS & TYPICAL FEATURES

- Insidious onset of weakness and fatigability of the limbs, sometimes with pain or numbness; decreased strength and reflexes.

General Considerations

Polyneuropathy is usually insidious in onset and slowly progressive. Children present with disturbances of gait and easy fatigability in walking or running, and slightly less often, weakness or clumsiness of the hands. Pain, tenderness, or paresthesias are mentioned less frequently. Neurologic examination discloses muscular weakness, greatest in the distal portions of the extremities, with steppage gait and depressed or absent deep tendon reflexes. Cranial nerves are sometimes affected. Sensory deficits occur in a stocking-and-glove distribution. The muscles may be tender, and trophic changes such as glassy or parchment skin and absent sweating may occur. Rarely, thickening of the ulnar and peroneal nerves may be felt. In sensory neuropathy, the patient may not feel minor trauma or burns, and thus allows trauma to occur.

Known causes include (1) toxins (lead, arsenic, mercurials, vincristine, and benzene); (2) systemic disorders (diabetes mellitus, chronic uremia, recurrent hypoglycemia, porphyria, polyarteritis nodosa, and lupus erythematosus); (3) inflammatory states (chronic inflammatory demyelinating polyneuropathy and neuritis associated with mumps or diphtheria); (4) hereditary, often degenerative conditions, which in some classifications include certain storage diseases, leukodystrophies, spinocerebellar degenerations with neurogenic components, and Bassen-Kornzweig syndrome; and (5) hereditary sensory or combined motor and sensory neuropathies. Polyneuropathies associated with malignancies, vitamin deficiencies, or excessive vitamin B_6 intake are not reported or are exceedingly rare in children.

The most common chronic motor neuropathy of insidious onset often has no identifiable cause. This chronic inflammatory demyelinating neuropathy (CIDP) is assumed to be immunologically mediated and may have a relapsing course. Sometimes facial weakness occurs. CSF protein levels are elevated. Nerve conduction velocity is slowed, and findings on nerve biopsy are abnormal. Immunologic abnormalities are seldom demonstrated, although nerve biopsy findings may show round cell infiltration. Corticosteroids, repeated IVIG, and, occasionally, immunosuppressants may give long-term benefit.

Clinical Findings

Hereditary neuropathy is the most common documented cause of chronic neuropathy in childhood. A careful genetic history (pedigree) and examination and electrical testing (motor and sensory nerve conduction and EMG) of patient and relatives are keys to diagnosis. Genetic tests are available for many of the variants. Nerve biopsy is rarely necessary.

Other hereditary neuropathies may have ataxia as a prominent finding, often overshadowing the neuropathy. Examples are Friedreich ataxia, dominant cerebellar ataxia, and Marinesco-Sjögren syndrome. Finally, some hereditary neuropathies are associated with identifiable and occasionally treatable metabolic errors (see Tables 25–22 and 25–23). These disorders are described in more detail in Chapter 36.

Laboratory diagnosis of chronic polyneuropathy is made by measurement of motor and sensory nerve conduction velocities. EMG may show a neurogenic pattern. CSF protein levels are often elevated, sometimes with an increased IgG index. Nerve biopsy, with teasing of the fibers and staining for metachromasia, may demonstrate loss of myelin, and to a lesser degree, loss of axons and increased connective tissue or concentric lamellas (so-called onion-skin appearance) around the nerve fiber. Muscle biopsy may show the pattern associated with denervation. Other laboratory studies directed toward specific causes mentioned above include screening for heavy metals and for metabolic, renal, or vascular disorders.

Treatment & Prognosis

Therapy is directed at specific disorders whenever possible. Corticosteroid therapy is used first when the cause is unknown or neuropathy is considered to be due to chronic inflammation (this is not the case in acute Guillain-Barré syndrome [AIDP; acute inflammatory demyelinating neuropathy]). Prednisone is initiated at 2–4 mg/kg/d orally, with tapering to the lowest effective dose; it may need to be reinstituted when symptoms recur. (Prednisone should probably not be used for treatment of hereditary neuropathy.) Immunomodulating therapy may be safer or "steroid-sparing"; IVIG, plasmapheresis, mycophenolate mofetil, and rituximab are choices.

The long-term prognosis varies with the cause and the ability to offer specific therapy. In the corticosteroid-dependent group, residual deficits are more frequent.

Finsterer J: Treatment of immune-mediated, dysimmune neuropathies. Acta Neurol Scand 2005;112:115 [PMID: 16008538].

Fudge E et al: Chronic inflammatory demyelinating polyradiculoneuropathy in two children with type 1 diabetes mellitus. Pediatr Diabetes 2005;6:244 [PMID: 16390395].

Gorson KC et al: Efficacy of mycophenolate mofetil in patients with chronic immune demyelinating polyneuropathy. Neurology 2004;63:715 [PMID: 15326250].

Kararizou E et al: Polyneuropathies in teenagers: A clinicopathological study of 45 cases. Neuromuscul Disord 2006;16:304 [PMID: 16616844].

Pareyson D: Differential diagnosis of Charcot-Marie-Tooth disease and related neuropathies. Neurol Sci 2004;25:72 [PMID: 15221625].

Ropper AH: Current treatments for CIDP. Neurology 2003; 60(Suppl 3):S16 [PMID: 12707418].

Rossignol E et al: Evolution and treatment of childhood chronic inflammatory polyneuropathy. Pediatr Neurol 2007;36:88 [PMID: 17275659].

Ruts L et al: Distinguishing acute-onset CIDP from Guillain-Barré syndrome with treatment related fluctuations. Neurology 2005;65:138 [PMID: 16009902].

van Doorn PA: Treatment of Guillain-Barré syndrome and CIDP. J Peripher Nerv Syst 2005;10:113 [PMID: 15958124].

Visudtibhan A: Cyclosporine in chronic inflammatory demyelinating polyradiculoneuropathy. Pediatr Neurol 2005;33:368 [PMID: 16243226].

MISCELLANEOUS NEUROMUSCULAR DISORDERS

FLOPPY INFANT SYNDROME

ESSENTIALS OF DIAGNOSIS & TYPICAL FEATURES

- In early infancy, decreased muscular activity, both spontaneous and in response to postural reflex testing and to passive motion.
- In young infants, "frog posture" or other unusual positions at rest.
- In older infants, delay in motor milestones.

General Considerations

In the young infant, ventral suspension (ie, supporting the infant with a hand under the chest) normally results in the infant's holding its head slightly up (45 degrees or less), the back straight or nearly so, the arms flexed at the elbows and slightly abducted, and the knees partly flexed. The "floppy" infant droops over the hand like an inverted U. The normal newborn attempts to keep the head in the same plane as the body when pulled up from supine to sitting by the hands (traction response). Marked head lag is characteristic of the floppy infant. Hyperextensibility of the joints is not a dependable criterion.

The usual reasons for seeking medical evaluation in older infants are delays in walking, running, or climbing stairs or motor difficulties and lack of endurance. Hypotonia or decreased motor activity is a frequent presenting complaint in neuromuscular disorders but may also accompany a variety of systemic (nonneuromuscular) conditions or, rarely, may be due to certain disorders of connective tissue.

1. Paralytic Group

The hypotonic infant who is weak (appearing paralyzed) usually has a lesion of the lower motor neuron complex (Table 25–30). The child has significant lack of movement against gravity (eg, fails to kick the legs, hold up the arms, or attempt to stand when held) or in response to stimuli such as tickling or slight pain. Spinal muscular atrophy type 1 (Werdnig-Hoffman disease) is the most common cause. Neuropathy is rare. Botulism and myasthenia gravis (rare) are neuromuscular junction causes. Myotonic dystrophy and rare myopathies (eg, central core myopathy) are muscle disease entities.

In anterior horn cell or muscle disease, weakness is proximal (ie, in shoulders and hips); finger movement is preserved. Tendon reflexes are absent or depressed; strength (to noxious stimuli) is decreased (paralytic). Intelligence is preserved. Fine motor, language, and personal and social milestones are normal, as measured, for example, on a Denver Developmental Screening Test (DDST, or Denver II) (see Chapter 3).

A. Myopathies

The congenital myopathies, muscular dystrophies, myotonic syndromes, and periodic paralysis were discussed earlier in this chapter (see Table 25–30).

B. Glycogenoses with Muscle Involvement

Glycogen storage diseases are described in Chapter 36. Patients with type II disease (Pompe disease, due to a deficiency of acid maltase) are most likely to present as floppy infants. Muscle cramps on exertion or easy fatigability, rather than floppiness in infancy, is the presenting complaint in type V disease (McArdle phosphorylase deficiency) or in the glycogenosis due to phosphofructokinase deficiency or phosphohexose isomerase inhibition.

C. Myasthenia Gravis

Neonatal transient and congenital persistent myasthenia gravis, with patients presenting as paralytic floppy infants, is described earlier in this chapter.

D. Arthrogryposis Multiplex (Congenital Deformities about Multiple Joints)

This symptom complex, sometimes associated with hypotonia, may be of neurogenic or myopathic origin (or both) and may be associated with a variety of other anomalies. Orthopedic aspects are discussed in Chapter 26.

E. Spinal Cord Lesions

Severe hypotonia in newborns following breech extraction with stretching or actual tearing of the lower cervical to upper thoracic spinal cord is rarely seen today, owing to improved obstetric delivery. Klumpke lower brachial plexus paralysis may be present; the abdomen is usually exceedingly soft, and the lower extremities are flaccid. Urinary retention is present initially; later, the bladder may function autonomously. MRI of the cervical cord should define the lesion. After a few weeks, spasticity of the lower limbs becomes obvious. Treatment is symptomatic and consists of bladder and skin care and eventual mobilization on crutches or in a wheelchair.

2. Nonparalytic Group

The nonparalytic hypotonic infant often has a damaged brain (Table 25–31). Rarely, tendon reflexes may be depressed or absent; usually, brisk reflexes (with hypotonia) point to "suprasegmental" or cerebral dysfunction. Intrauterine or perinatal insults to brain or upper cord, while sometimes difficult to document, are major causes. (Occasionally, severe congenital myopathies presenting in the newborn period simulate nonparalytic hypotonia.) Persisting severe hypotonia is ominous.

Table 25–30. Floppy infant: paralytic causes.

Disease	Genetic	Early Manifestations
Spinal muscular atrophy (SMA) SMA type 1	Autosomal recessive; diagnose by SMN deletion exon 7, 8 (98% of cases). Rarely, X-linked SMA, a new (also fatal) variant with diaphragmatic paralysis.	In-utero movements decreased in one-third. Gradual weakness, delay in gross motor milestones. Weak cry. Abdominal breathing. Poor limb motion ("no kicking"). No deep tendon reflexes. Fasciculations of tongue. Normal personal-social behavior.
SMA type 2	Autosomal recessive; same as above. EMG helpful.	Onset before age 1 y usual. Progression slower than SMA type 1. Hand tremors common.
Infantile botulism	Acquired, younger than age 1 y (mostly before age 6 mo); botulism spore in stool makes toxin.	Poor feeding. Constipation. Weak cry. Failure to thrive. Lethargy. Facial weakness, ptosis, ocular muscle palsy. Inability to suck, swallow. Apnea. Source: soil dust (outdoor construction workers or family gardeners may bring it home on clothes), honey. EMG helpful, RMNS.
Myasthenia gravis Neonatal transient	12% of infants born from a myasthenic mother.	Floppiness. Poor sucking and feeding; choking. Respiratory distress. Weak cry. Autoimmune antibodies from mother.
Congenital	Mother normal. Rare autosomal recessive (autosomal dominant).	As above; may improve and later exacerbate. Multiple syndromes (rare).
Myotonic dystrophy type 1	Autosomal dominant: in 99% mother transmits gene. DNA testing 98% accurate.	Polyhydramnios; failure of suck, respirations. Facial diplegia. Ptosis. Arthrogryposis. Thin ribs. Later, developmental delay. Examine mother for myotonia, physiognomy. EMG variable in infant.
Neonatal congenital myopathy Nemaline, central core, "minimal change," etc	Autosomal recessive or dominant.	Virtually all of the rare myopathies may have a severe (even fatal) neonatal or early infant form. Clinical features often include respiratory failure. Muscle biopsy for definitive diagnosis.
Congenital muscular dystrophy Fukayama (FCMD)	Autosomal recessive.	Early onset. Facial weakness. Joint contractures. Severe mental retardation. Seizures. Brain structural abnormalities; MRI helpful.
Ullrich CMD	Generally autosomal dominant.	Severe weakness. No mental retardation. Proximal joint contractures with distal joint laxity.
Infantile neuropathy Hypomyelinating (rare)	HSMN most common cause.	Demyelinating or axonal; a rare cause. Rule out mimicking SMA (deletion study). EMG, NCV are key studies. Nerve biopsy.
Benign congenital hypotonia	Unknown cause.	Diagnosis of exclusion. Family history variable. Mild to moderate hypotonia with weakness. (This term being used less with increasing genetic, microscopy advances.) Improves with time.

AD, autosomal dominant; AR, autosomal recessive; EMG, electromyogram; HSMN, hereditary sensory motor neuropathy; MRI, magnetic resonance imaging; NCV, nerve conduction velocity; RMNS, repetitive motor nerve stimulation; SMN, survival motor neuron.

Table 25–31. Floppy infant: nonparalytic causes.

	Causes	Manifestations
Central nervous system disorders		
Atonic diplegia (prespastic diplegia)	Intrauterine, perinatal asphyxia, cord injury.	Limpness, stupor; poor suck, cry, Moro reflex, and grasp; later, irritability, increased tone and reflexes.
Choreoathetosis	As above; kernicterus.	Hypotonic early; movement disorder emerges later (6–18 mo).
Ataxic cerebral palsy	Same as choreoathetosis.	Same as choreoathetosis.
Syndromes with hypotonia (CNS origin)		
Trisomy 21	Genetic.	All have hypotonia early.
Prader-Willi syndrome	Genetic deletion 15q11.	Hypotonia, hypomentia, hypogonadism, obesity ("H_3O").
Marfan syndrome	Autosomal dominant.	Arachnodactyly.
Dysautonomia	Autosomal recessive.	Respiratory infections, corneal anesthesia.
Turner syndrome	45X, or mosaic.	Somatic stigmata (see Chapter 36).
Degenerative disorders		
Tay-Sachs disease	Autosomal recessive.	Cherry-red spot on macula.
Metachromatic leukodystrophy	Autosomal recessive.	Deep tendon reflexes increased early, polyneuropathy late; mental retardation.
Systemic diseases[a]		
Malnutrition	Deprivation, cystic fibrosis, celiac disease.	
Chronic illness	Congenital heart disease; chronic pulmonary disease (eg, bronchopulmonary dysplasia); uremia, renal acidosis.	
Metabolic disease	Mitochondrial; Lowe, Pompe, Leigh disease; hypercalcemia.	
Endocrinopathy	Hypothyroid.	

[a]See elsewhere in text for manifestations.
CNS, central nervous system.

Tone will often vary. Spasticity and other forms of cerebral palsy may emerge; hypertonia and hypotonia may occur at varying times or sites in the same infant. Associated choreoathetoid or ataxic movements and developmental delay can clarify the diagnosis. Tendon reflexes are usually increased; pathologic infant reflexes (Babinski and tonic neck) may persist or worsen.

The creatine kinase level and the EMG are usually normal. Prolonged nerve conduction velocities (rare in this situation) point to polyneuritis or leukodystrophy. Muscle biopsy evaluation, using special stains and histographic analysis, often shows a reduction in size of type II fibers associated with decreased voluntary motor activity.

Limpness in the neonatal period and early infancy and subsequent delay in achieving motor milestones are the presenting features in a large number of children with a variety of CNS disorders, including mental retardation, as in trisomy 21. In many such cases, no specific diagnosis can be made. Close observation and scoring of motor patterns and adaptive behavior, as by the DDST, are helpful.

Anagnostou E et al: Type I spinal muscular atrophy can mimic sensory-motor axonal neuropathy. J Child Neurol 2005;20:147 [PMID: 15794183].

Birdi K et al: The floppy infant: Retrospective analysis of clinical experience (1990–2000) in a tertiary care facility. J Child Neurol 2005;20:803 [PMID: 16417874].

Clemmens MR, Bell L: Infant botulism presenting with poor feeding and lethargy: A review of 4 cases. Pediatr Emerg Care 2007;23:492 [PMID: 17666936].

Darras BT, Jones HR Jr: Neuromuscular problems of the critically ill neonate and child. Semin Pediatr Neurol 2004;11:147 [PMID: 15259868].

Howell RR et al: Diagnostic challenges for Pompe disease: An underrecognized cause of floppy baby syndrome. Genet Med 2006;8:289 [PMID: 16702878].

Kim CT et al: Neuromuscular rehabilitation and electrodiagnosis. 4. Pediatric issues. Arch Phys Med Rehabil 2005:86(3 Suppl 1): S28 [PMID: 15761797].

Kroksmark AK et al: Myotonic dystrophy: Muscle involvement in relation to disease type and size of expanded CTG-repeat sequence. Dev Med Child Neurol 2005;47:478 [PMID: 15991869].

Lee JS et al: Mitochondrial respiratory complex 1 deficiency simulating spinal muscular atrophy. Pediatr Neurol 2007;36:45 [PMID: 17162196].

Paro-Panjan D, Neubauer D: Congenital hypotonia: Is there an algorithm? J Child Neurol 2005;19:439 [PMID: 15446393].

Premasiri MK, Lee YS: The myopathology of floppy and hypotonic infants in Singapore. Pathology 2003;35:409 [PMID: 14555385].

Richer LP et al: Diagnostic profile of neonatal hypotonia: An 11-year study. Pediatr Neurol 2001;25:32 [PMID: 11483393].

Thompson JA et al: Infant botulism in the age of botulism immune globulin. Neurology 2005;64:2029 [PMID: 15917401].

Vasta I et al: Can clinical signs identify newborns with neuromuscular disorders? J Pediatr 2005;146:73 [PMID: 1564482].

Web Resources

American Association of Child and Adolescent Psychiatry: http://www.aacap.org

Contains practice parameters and relevant information about childhood psychiatric conditions.

American Academy of Neurology: http://www.aan.com

Provides both adult and child neurology practice parameters.

American Epilepsy Society: http://www.aesnet.org

Includes general information about epilepsy, and a comprehensive section about antiepileptic drugs.

Child Neurology Foundation: http://www.childneurologyfoundation.org/index.html

Describes resources and tests related to child neurology, and provides a comprehensive list of child neurology–related website links.

Child Neurology Society: http://www.childneurologysociety.org

Provides research updates, organizational information, and has child neurology–specific practice parameters.

Cure CMD: http://curecmd.org/

Epilepsy Foundation of America: http://www.epilepsyfoundation.org

Includes tutorials about epilepsy and living with epilepsy.

Families of SMA: http://www.fsma.org/

Gene tests: http://www.genetests.org

Provides detailed information about available genetic testing, research, literature/disorder reviews, and resources for most genetically determined neurologic disorders.

Muscular Dystrophy Association: http://www.mda.org

Contains research updates, organizational information, and detailed information regarding neuromuscular disorders.

National Institute of Neurological Disorders and Stroke: http://www.ninds.nih.gov

Provides brief descriptions of neurologic disorders, related research, research opportunities, and relevant organizations.

National Ataxia Foundation http://www.ataxia.org/

Resource for providers and patients with ataxia including research and support groups.

Neurofibromatosis Foundation: http://www.nf.org

Provides detailed information for parents and providers about neurofibromatosis.

Provides information about spinal muscular atrophy for families and providers, including ongoing research, conferences, and literature.

Provides resources about congenital muscular dystrophy for families and providers, including registry data, recent literature, and current clinical trials.

Washington University, St. Louis, Neuromuscular Disease Center: http://neuromuscular.wustl.edu

Includes detailed descriptions of neuromuscular disorders and differential diagnoses.

Tuberous Sclerosis Association: http://www.tsalliance.org

Contains detailed information for parents and providers about Tuberous Sclerosis.

We Move: worldwide education and awareness for movement disorders: http://wemove.org

Descriptions of movement disorders, related research and research opportunities.

26 Orthopedics

Mark A. Erickson, MD
Conor Merritt, BS
John D. Polousky, MD

Orthopedics is the medical discipline that deals with disorders of the musculoskeletal system. Patients with orthopedic problems generally present with one or more of the following complaints: pain, swelling, loss of function, or deformity. While the history reveals the patient's expectation, physical examination and radiographic imaging are vitally important features of orthopedic diagnosis.

DISTURBANCES OF PRENATAL ORIGIN

ESSENTIALS OF DIAGNOSIS & TREATMENT

- Conditions are present at birth.
- Multiple organ systems may be involved.
- Treatment is aimed at maximizing function.

CONGENITAL AMPUTATIONS & LIMB DEFICIENCIES

Congenital amputations may be due to teratogens (eg, drugs or viruses), amniotic bands, or metabolic diseases (eg, maternal diabetes). Limb deficiencies are generally caused by vascular disruption defects. The most common form of limb deficiency is congenital longitudinal deficiency of the fibula. Children with congenital limb deficiencies, such as absence of the femur, tibia, or fibula, have a high incidence of other congenital anomalies, including genitourinary, cardiac, and palatal defects. Deficiencies usually consist of a partial absence of structures in the extremity along one side. For example, in radial club hand, the entire radius is absent, but the thumb may be either hypoplastic or completely absent. The effect on structures distal to the deficiency varies. Complex tissue defects are virtually always associated with longitudinal bone deficiency since associated nerves and muscles are not completely represented when a bone is absent.

Treatment

Limb lengthening and/or contralateral limb shortening can be used to treat less severe deficiencies. More severe deficiencies are treated with a prosthesis to compensate for the length discrepancy. For certain severe anomalies, operative treatment to remove a portion of the malformed extremity (eg, foot) is indicated to allow for early prosthetic fitting. In these instances, early prosthetic fitting allows for maximization of function.

Typically, a lower extremity prosthesis would be fit at about one year of age allowing the child to begin ambulation at an appropriate developmental age. The prosthesis is well accepted since it becomes necessary for balancing and walking. In unilateral upper extremity amputation, the child benefits from the use of a passive mitten type prosthesis starting as early as 6 months of age. Early fitting has the advantage of instilling an accustomed pattern of proper length and bimanual manipulation. Although myoelectric prostheses have a technologic appeal, the majority of patients find the simplest construct to be the most functional. Children quickly learn how to function with their prostheses and can lead active lives.

Gold NB, Westgate MN, Holmes LB: Anatomic and etiological classification of congenital limb deficiencies. Am J Med Genet Part A 2011;155:1225–1235.

Klaassen Z et al: Supernumerary and absent limbs and digits of the lower limb: A review of literature. Clinical Anatomy 2011;24:570–575.

Walker JL et al: Adult outcomes following amputation or lengthening for fibular deficiency. J Bone Joint Surg Am 2009;91(4): 797–804 [PMID: 19339563].

DEFORMITIES OF THE EXTREMITIES

1. Metatarsus Varus

Metatarsus varus, a common congenital foot deformity, is characterized by inward deviation of the forefoot. When the deformity is more rigid, it is characterized by a vertical crease in the medial aspect of the arch. Angulation occurs at the base of the fifth metatarsal causing prominence of this bone. Most flexible deformities are secondary to intrauterine positioning and usually resolve spontaneously. Several investigators have noticed that 10%–15% of children with metatarsus varus have hip dysplasia; therefore, a careful hip examination is necessary. The etiology determining the rigidity of the deformity is unknown. However, if the deformity is rigid and cannot be manipulated past the midline, it is worthwhile to perform serial casting, with cast changes in 1–2 week intervals, to correct the deformity. Corrective shoes do not live up to their name; however, they can be used to maintain the correction obtained by casting.

Sankar WN, Weiss J, Skaggs DL: Orthopaedic conditions in the newborn. J Am Acad Orthop Surg 2009;17(2):112–122 [PMID: 19202124].

2. Clubfoot (Talipes Equinovarus)

Classic talipes equinovarus, or clubfoot, requires three features for diagnosis: (1) plantar flexion of the foot at the ankle joint (equinus), (2) inversion deformity of the heel (varus), and (3) medial deviation of the forefoot (varus). Clubfoot occurs in approximately 1:1000 live births. The three major categories of clubfoot are idiopathic, neurogenic, and those associated with syndromes such as arthrogryposis and Larsen syndrome. Infants with a clubfoot should be examined carefully for associated anomalies, especially of the spine. Idiopathic club feet may be hereditary.

Treatment

Manipulation of the foot to stretch the contracted tissues on the medial and posterior aspects, followed by casting to hold the correction is the preferred treatment. When instituted shortly after birth, correction is rapid. If treatment is delayed, the foot tends to become more rigid within a matter of days. After full correction is obtained, a night brace is necessary for long-term maintenance of correction. Casting treatment requires patience and experience, but fewer patients require surgery when attention is paid to details of the Ponseti technique. If the foot is rigid and resistant to cast treatment, surgical release and correction are appropriate. Fifteen percent to fifty percent of patients require a surgical release.

Dobbs MB, Gurnett CA: Update on clubfoot: Etiology and treatment. Clin Orthop Relat Res 2009;467(5):1146–1153 [PMID: 19224303].

3. Developmental Dysplasia of the Hip Joint

Dysplasia is the term used to describe abnormal growth or development. Dysplasia of the hip encompasses a spectrum of conditions where an abnormal relationship exists between the proximal femur and the acetabulum. In the most severe condition, the femoral head is not in contact with the acetabulum and is classified as a *dislocated hip*. In a *dislocatable hip,* the femoral head is within the acetabulum but can be dislocated with a provocative maneuver. A *subluxatable hip* is one in which the femoral head comes partially out of the joint with a provocative maneuver. *Acetabular dysplasia* is used to denote insufficient acetabular development and is a radiographic diagnosis.

Congenital dislocation of the hip more commonly affects the left hip, occurring in approximately 1%–3% of newborns. At birth, both the acetabulum and femur are underdeveloped. Dysplasia is progressive with growth unless the instability is corrected. If the dislocation is corrected in the first few weeks of life, the dysplasia can be completely reversible and a normal hip will more likely develop. If the dislocation or subluxation persists with age, the deformity will worsen until it is not completely reversible, especially after the walking age. For this reason, it is important to diagnose the deformity and institute treatment early.

Clinical Findings

Clinical diagnosis of dislocations in newborns is dependent on demonstrating the instability of the joint by placing the infant on his or her back and obtaining complete relaxation. The examiner's long finger is then placed over the greater trochanter and the thumb over the inner side of the thigh. Both hips are flexed 90 degrees and then slowly abducted from the midline, one hip at a time. With gentle pressure, an attempt is made to lift the greater trochanter forward. A feeling of slipping as the head relocates is a sign of instability (Ortolani sign). When the joint is more stable, the deformity must be provoked by applying slight pressure with the thumb on the medial side of the thigh as the thigh is adducted, thus slipping the hip posteriorly and eliciting a palpable clunk as the hip dislocates (Barlow sign). Limited hip abduction of less than 60 degrees while the knee is in 90 degrees of flexion is believed to be the most sensitive sign for detecting a dysplastic hip. Clinical signs of instability are more reliable than radiographs for diagnosing developmental dislocation of the hip in the newborn. Ultrasonography is most useful in newborns, and can be helpful for screening high-risk infants, such as those with breech presentation or positive family history. Asymmetrical skinfolds are present in about 25% of normal newborns and therefore are not particularly helpful to diagnosing hip dislocation.

The signs of instability become less evident after the first month of life. Contractures begin to develop about the hip joint, limiting abduction to less than 90 degrees. It is important to hold the pelvis level to detect asymmetry of abduction. If the knees are at unequal heights when the hips and knees are flexed, the dislocated hip will be on the side with the lower knee. Radiological examination becomes more valuable after the first 6 weeks of life, with lateral displacement of the femoral head being the most reliable sign. An acetabular index or angle can be measured on pelvis radiographs by drawing one line horizontally through the tri-radiate cartilage, and another line starting at the tri-radiate cartilage and extending to the outer edge of the acetabulum. A normal angle would be less than 30 degrees. In mild cases, increased steepness of acetabular alignment (acetabular angle > 35 degrees) may be the only abnormality.

If dysplasia of the hip has not been diagnosed before the child begins to walk, there will be a painless limp and a lurch to the affected side. When the child stands on the affected leg, a dip of the pelvis will be evident on the opposite side, due to weakness of the gluteus medius muscle. This is called the Trendelenburg sign and accounts for the unusual swaying gait. In children with bilateral dislocations, the loss of abduction is almost symmetrical and may be deceiving. In children with incomplete abduction during the first few months of life, a radiograph of the pelvis is indicated. As a child with bilateral dislocation of the hips begins to walk, the gait is waddling. The perineum is widened as a result of lateral displacement of the hips, and there is flexion contracture as a result of posterior displacement of the hips. This flexion contracture contributes to marked lumbar lordosis, causing the greater trochanters to be easily palpable in their elevated position. Treatment is still possible in the first 2 years of life, but the results are not as good as with early treatment. In patients older than 2 years, osteotomies are often necessary to create a more normal orientation and shape of the hip joint.

Treatment

Most unstable hips undergo spontaneous correction by 2–6 weeks of age. A Pavlik harness, which maintains reduction by placing the hip in a flexed and abducted position, can be easily used to treat dislocation or dysplasia diagnosed in the first few weeks or months of life. In order to be safely treated in a Pavlik harness, hips must be manually reducible with only gentle manipulation. Forced abduction, or reduction requiring extremes of motion for stability, can lead to avascular necrosis of the femoral head and is contraindicated. The use of double or triple diapers is ineffective. An orthopedic surgeon with experience managing the problem is best to supervise treatment.

In the first 4 months of life, reduction can be obtained by simply flexing and abducting the hip with a Pavlik harness; no other manipulation is usually necessary. In late cases, preoperative traction for 2–3 weeks relaxes soft tissues about the hip. Following traction, in which the femur is brought down opposite the acetabulum, reduction can typically be achieved, without force, under general anesthesia. A hip spica cast is used for 3 months after reduction. If the hip is not stable within a reasonable range of motion after closed reduction, open reduction is indicated. If reduction is done at an older age, operations to correct the deformities of the acetabulum and femur, as well as open reduction, may be necessary. Older children are more likely to experience complications from more extensive procedures.

4. Torticollis

Injury to the sternocleidomastoid muscle during delivery or disease affecting the cervical spine in infancy, such as congenital vertebral anomalies, may cause torticollis. When contracture of the sternocleidomastoid muscle causes torticollis, the chin is rotated to the side opposite of the affected muscle, causing the head to tilt toward the side of the contracture. A mass felt in the midportion of the sternocleidomastoid muscle is not a true tumor but a fibrous transformation within the muscle.

If the deformity is left untreated, a striking facial asymmetry can persist. Passive stretching is effective treatment in most cases. If the deformity does not correct with passive stretching during the first year of life, surgical release of the muscle origin and insertion can be an effective treatment option. Excising the "tumor" of the sternocleidomastoid muscle is unnecessary and creates an unsightly scar.

Torticollis is occasionally associated with congenital deformities of the cervical spine. Radiographs of the spine are indicated in most cases where such anomalies are suspected. In addition, there is a 15%–20% incidence of associated hip dysplasia.

Acute torticollis may follow upper respiratory infection or mild trauma in children. Upper respiratory infections may lead to swelling in the upper cervical spine, particularly at the C1-C2 region. This swelling renders the C1-C2 articulation susceptible to rotatory subluxation, which commonly presents as a clinical picture of torticollis. Rotatory subluxation of the upper cervical spine requires computed tomography for accurate imaging. Traction or a cervical collar usually results in resolution of the symptoms within 1 or 2 days. Other causes of torticollis include spinal cord or cerebellar tumors, syringomyelia, and rheumatoid arthritis.

Sankar WN, Weiss J, Skaggs DL: Orthopaedic conditions in the newborn. J Am Acad Orthop Surg 2009;17(2):112–122 [PMID: 19202124].

GENERALIZED DISORDERS OF SKELETAL OR MESODERMAL TISSUES

1. Arthrogryposis Multiplex Congenita (Amyoplasia Congenita)

Clinical Findings & Diagnosis

Arthrogryposis multiplex congenita consists of incomplete fibrous ankylosis (usually bilateral) of many or all joints of the body. Upper extremity contractures usually consist of adduction of the shoulders; extension of the elbows; flexion of the wrists; and stiff, straight fingers with poor muscle control of the thumbs. Common deformities of the lower extremities include dislocation of the hips, extension contractures of the knees, and severe club feet. The joints are fusiform and the joint capsules decreased in volume due to lack of movement during fetal development. Muscle development is poor, and may be represented only by fibrous bands. Various investigations have attributed the basic defect to an abnormality of muscle or lower motor neurons.

Treatment

Passive mobilization of joints is the early treatment. Prolonged casting results in further stiffness and is not indicated. Removable splints combined with vigorous therapy is the most effective conservative treatment; however, surgical release of the affected joints is often necessary. Clubfoot associated with arthrogryposis is very stiff and nearly always requires surgical correction. Knee surgery, including capsulotomy, osteotomy, and tendon lengthening, is used to correct deformities. In young children, a dislocated hip may be reduced operatively by a medial approach. Multiple operative hip procedures are contraindicated, as they may further stiffness with consequent impairment of motion. Affected children are often able to walk if the dislocations and contractures are reduced surgically. The long-term prognosis for physical and vocational independence is guarded. These patients have normal intelligence, but they have such severe physical restrictions that gainful employment is hard to find.

Bamshad M, Van Heest AE, Pleasure D: Arthrogryposis: A review and update. J Bone Joint Surg Am 2009(Suppl 4):40–46 [PMID: 19571066].

2. Marfan Syndrome

Marfan syndrome is a connective tissue disorder characterized by unusually long fingers and toes (arachnodactyly); hypermobility of the joints; subluxation of the ocular lenses; other eye abnormalities, including cataract, coloboma, megalocornea, strabismus, and nystagmus; a high-arched palate; a strong tendency to scoliosis (60% of all those diagnosed); pectus carinatum (an outward protrusion of the sternum); and thoracic aortic aneurysms due to weakness of the media of the vessels (see Chapter 37). Fibrillin-1 gene mutations are commonly associated with Marfan syndrome. Serum mucoproteins may be decreased, and urinary excretion of hydroxyproline increased. The condition is easily confused with homocystinuria, because the phenotypic presentation is nearly identical. The two diseases are differentiated by detecting homocystine in the urine of patients with homocystinuria.

Treatment is usually supportive and includes management of blood pressure and restriction of physical activity. Scoliosis may involve more vigorous treatment by bracing or spine fusion. The long-term prognosis has improved for patients since the development of better treatment of their aortic aneurysms.

Lebreiro A et al: Marfan syndrome clinical manifestations, pathophysiology, and new outlook on drug therapy. Rev Port Cardiol 2010;(29):1021–1036.

Yuan SM, Jing H: Marfan syndrome: An overview. San Paulo Med J 2010;128(6):360–366.

3. Klippel-Feil Syndrome

Klippel-Feil syndrome is characterized by failure of segmentation of some or all of the cervical vertebrae. Multiple congenital spinal anomalies may be present, with hemivertebrae and scoliosis. The neck is short and stiff, the hairline is low, and the ears are low-set. Congenital scoliosis, cervical rib, spina bifida, torticollis, web neck, high scapula, renal anomalies, and deafness are commonly associated defects. Renal ultrasound as well as a hearing test are indicated if there is evidence of abnormal renal function. Spinal arthrodesis is indicated if progressive scoliotic deformities develop.

4. Sprengel Deformity

Sprengel deformity is a congenital condition where one or both scapulas are elevated and hypoplastic. The deformity prevents the arm from raising completely on the affected side, and torticollis may be an associated finding. The deformity occurs alone or in association with Klippel-Feil syndrome. If the deformity is functionally limiting, the scapula may be surgically relocated lower in the thorax. Excision of the upper portion of the scapula improves cosmetic appearance but has little effect on function.

Mooney JF 3rd, White DR, Glazier S: Previously unreported structure in Sprengel deformity. J Pediatr Orthop 2009;29(1):26–28 [PMID: 19098640].

5. Osteogenesis Imperfecta

Osteogenesis imperfecta is a rare genetic connective tissue disease characterized by multiple and recurrent fractures. The severe fetal type (osteogenesis imperfecta congenita) is distinguished by multiple intrauterine or perinatal fractures. Moderately affected children have numerous fractures and are dwarfed as a result of bony deformities and growth retardation. Cortical thickness is reduced in the shafts of the long bones, and accessory skull bones that are completely surrounded by cranial sutures (wormian bones) are present in the skull. Blue sclerae, thin skin, hyperextensibility of ligaments, otosclerosis with significant hearing loss, and hypoplastic and deformed teeth are characteristic of osteogenesis imperfecta. Intelligence is not affected. In the moderately affected children, fractures begin to occur at variable times after the perinatal period, resulting in fewer fractures and deformities relative to severe cases. Affected patients are sometimes suspected of having suffered abuse. Osteogenesis imperfecta should be ruled out in any case of nonaccidental trauma.

Molecular genetic studies have identified more than 150 mutations of the *COL1A1* and *COL1A2* genes, which encode for type I procollagen. The likelihood of a second affected child to be born to parents without this mutation is negligible as spontaneous mutations are felt to be responsible.

Bisphosphonates have been shown to decrease the incidence of fractures. Surgical treatment involves correction of deformity of the long bones. Multiple intramedullary rods have been used to prevent deformity from fracture malunion. Patients are often confined to wheelchairs during adulthood.

Basel D, Steiner RD: Osteogenesis imperfecta: Recent findings shed new light on this once well-understood condition. Gene Med 2009;11(6):375–385 [PMID: 195334842].

6. Osteopetrosis (Osteitis Condensans Generalisata, Marble Bone Disease, Albers-Schönberg Disease)

Osteopetrosis is a rare disorder of osteoclastic resorption of bone, resulting in abnormally dense bones. The reduced marrow spaces result in anemia. There are two types: a milder autosomal dominant type and a more malignant autosomal recessive type. The findings may appear at any age. Radiologic examination shows increased bone density and transverse bands in the shafts, clubbing of ends, and vertical striations of long bones. Thickening about the cranial foramina is present, and heterotopic calcification of soft tissues is possible. Diminished life expectancy is seen in severe infantile forms.

Treatment is largely symptomatic. The most severe autosomal recessive forms of osteopetrosis can be treated successfully by hematopoietic stem cell transplantation.

Michou L, Brown JP: Genetics of bone diseases Paget's disease, fibrous dysplasia, OSTEOPETROSIS, and osteogenesis imperfecta. Joint Bone Spine 2011;(78):252–258.

7. Achondroplasia (Classic Chondrodystrophy)

Achondroplasia is the most common form of short-limbed dwarfism. The upper arms and thighs are proportionately shorter than the forearms and legs. Skeletal dysplasia is suspected based on abnormal stature, disproportion, dysmorphism, or deformity. Measurement of height is an excellent clinical screening tool. Findings frequently include bowing of the extremities, a waddling gait, limitation of motion of major joints, relaxation of the ligaments, short stubby fingers of almost equal length, frontal bossing, midface hypoplasia, otolaryngeal system dysfunction, moderate hydrocephalus, depressed nasal bridge, and lumbar lordosis. Intelligence and sexual function are normal. While this disorder has an autosomal dominant transmission pattern, 80% of cases result from a random mutation in the fibroblast growth factor receptor-3 (*FGFR3*) gene. Radiographs demonstrate short, thick tubular bones and irregular epiphysial plates. The ends of the bones are thick, with broadening and cupping. Epiphysial ossification may be delayed. Due to diminished growth in the spinal pedicles, the spinal canal is narrowed (congenital stenosis), and a herniated disk in adulthood may lead to acute paraplegia. Growth hormone is given to some children with bone dysplasia. Limb lengthening is possible, but controversial.

Shirley ED, Ain MC. Achondroplasia: Manifestations and Treatment. J Am Acad Orthop Surg 2009;(17):231–241.

8. Osteochondrodystrophy (Morquio Disease)

Morquio disease is an autosomal recessive disorder affecting mucopolysaccharide storage. Skeletal abnormalities include shortening of the spine, kyphosis, scoliosis, shortened extremities, pectus carinatum, genu valgum or "knock knees", and a hypoplastic odontoid with atlantoaxial instability. Appearance is generally normal at birth, with deformities developing between ages 1 and 4 years as a result of abnormal deposition of mucopolysaccharides. Increased urinary glycoseaminoglycan levels are associated with increased severity.

Radiographs demonstrate wedge-shaped flattened vertebrae and irregular, malformed epiphyses. The ribs are broad and have been likened to canoe paddles. The lower extremities are more severely involved than the upper extremities.

The major treatment issue revolves around prevention of cervical myelopathy. Bone marrow transplantation has been successful in alleviating some symptoms. Prognosis depends on age of onset.

Valayannopoulos V et al: Mucopolysaccharidosis VI. Orphanet Journal of Rare Diseases 2010. http://www.ojrd.com/content/5/1/5.

GROWTH DISTURBANCES OF THE MUSCULOSKELETAL SYSTEM

SCOLIOSIS

Scoliosis is characterized by lateral curvature of the spine associated with rotation of the involved vertebrae and classified by its anatomic location, in either the thoracic or lumbar spine, with rare involvement of the cervical spine. The convexity of the curve is designated right or left. A right thoracic scoliosis would denote a thoracic curve with convexity to the right. This is the most common type of idiopathic curve. Kyphosis or posterior curvature of the spine is normal in the thoracic area, although excessive curvature is pathologic. Anterior curvature of the spine, or lordosis, is normal in the lumbar and cervical spine regions.

Eighty percent of cases of scoliosis are idiopathic. Idiopathic scoliosis typically develops around age 8 to 10, with progression occurring during periods of rapid skeletal growth. In rare instances, infantile scoliosis may be seen in children age 3 years or younger. Idiopathic infantile scoliosis, occurring in children age 0–3 years, is much more common in Great Britain than in the United States. In infantile scoliosis, if the rib-vertebral angle of Mehta is less than

20 degrees, the curve will likely resolve spontaneously. If the angle is greater, the curve will likely progress.

Idiopathic scoliosis is about four or five times more common in girls. The disorder is usually asymptomatic in the adolescent years, but severe curvature can progress during adulthood causing pain or, in extreme cases, diminished pulmonary function as a result of reduced lung volumes due to deformity of the rib cage. The screening examination for scoliosis is performed by having the patient bend forward 90 degrees with the hands joined in the midline. Asymmetry of the height of the ribs or paravertebral muscles on one side indicates rotation of the trunk associated with lateral curvature. Because 30% of family members are also affected, siblings of an affected child should be examined.

Neurofibromatosis, Marfan syndrome, cerebral palsy, muscular dystrophy, poliomyelitis, and myelodysplasia are among several diseases that may be present with an associated scoliosis.

Congenital vertebral anomalies such as hemiverebra or unilateral vertebral bar account for 5% to 7% of all scoliosis. These curves are more rigid than the more common idiopathic curve and will often increase with skeletal growth, especially during adolescence.

Olisthetic scoliosis may result from pressure on the spinal cord or roots by infectious processes or herniation of the nucleus pulposus; the underlying cause must be sought. Secondary curvature will resolve as the primary problem is treated.

Clinical Findings

A. Symptoms and Signs

Scoliosis in adolescents does not typically cause significant pain. If a patient has significant pain, then the source of the pain should be sought in order to rule out the possibility of some other disorder such as infection or tumor. Deformity of the rib cage and asymmetry of the waistline are clinically evident for curvatures of 30 degrees or more. Lesser curves may be detected through the forward bending test, which is designed to detect early abnormalities of rotation that may not be apparent when the patient is standing erect.

B. Imaging

Radiographs taken of the entire spine in the standing position in both the anteroposterior and lateral planes are the most valuable for diagnosis. Usually a primary curve is evident with compensatory curvature to balance the body. At times two primary curvatures may be seen (usually in the right thoracic and left lumbar regions). A left thoracic curvature should be suspected of being secondary to neurologic disease and prompt a more meticulous neurologic examination. If the curvatures of the spine are balanced (compensated), the head is centered over the center of the pelvis. If the spinal alignment is uncompensated, the head will be displaced to one side, which produces an unsightly deformity. Rotation of the spine may be measured with a scoliometer. Rotation is associated with a marked rib hump as the lateral curvature increases in severity.

Treatment

Treatment of scoliosis depends on the curve magnitude, skeletal maturity, and risk of progression. Treatment is indicated for any curvature that demonstrates progression on serial radiologic examination. Definitive spinal fusions should be delayed as long as possible in young children through the use of casting, bracing, and growth modulating surgeries such as growing rods or vertical expandable prosthetic titanium ribs (VEPTR).

Scoliosis is measured on standing anteroposterior x-rays of the spine and the measurement standard is the Cobb angle. Curvatures of less than 20 degrees typically do not require treatment unless they show progression. Bracing is controversial, but often used for curvatures of 20–40 degrees in a skeletally immature child. Recent studies have shown bracing to be effective for female patients with a Cobb angle of 25–35 degrees. Bracing and casting may be a beneficial way to prevent the progression of scoliosis without the negative quality of life effects associated with other treatments. Curvatures greater than 40 degrees are resistant to treatment by bracing. Thoracic curvatures greater than 70 degrees have been correlated with poor pulmonary function in adult life leading our treatment algorithms toward preventing the progression to this extreme. Surgical intervention should be geared to maximize pulmonary function, while improving spinal alignment. Curvatures reaching the magnitude of 40–60 degrees are indicated for surgical correction as they are highly likely to continue to progress, ultimately reaching the 70 degree threshold in adulthood.

The surgical procedure for scoliosis has two fundamental components, the deformity correction and the spinal fusion. Spinal instrumentation (rods, screws, hooks, etc) are applied to the region of the spine to be corrected. The instrumentation is then used to manually reposition the spine intraoperatively. Surgical fusion involves decortication of the bone over the laminas and spinous processes, with the addition of bone graft. The instrumentation is then secured/tightened in order to maintain postoperative correction, with activity restriction for several months until the bone fusion is solid. Treatment requires a team approach and is best done in centers with full support facilities.

Prognosis

Compensated small curves that do not progress may cause minor deformities but are well tolerated throughout life. Patients should be counseled about the genetic transmission of scoliosis and cautioned that their children's backs should be examined as part of routine physicals. Early detection allows for simple brace treatment. Severe scoliosis may require correction by spinal fusion, although fusionless techniques are being developed.

SLIPPED CAPITAL FEMORAL EPIPHYSIS

Slipped capital femoral epiphysis (SCFE) is caused by displacement of the proximal femoral epiphysis due to disruption of the growth plate. The head of the femur is usually displaced medially and posteriorly relative to the femoral neck. This condition is most commonly seen in adolescent, obese males. While the cause is unclear, some authorities have experimentally shown that the strength of the perichondrial ring stabilizing the epiphyseal area is sufficiently weakened by hormonal changes during adolescence such that the overload of excessive body weight can produce a pathologic fracture through the growth plate. Hormonal studies in these children are usually normal, although SCFE is associated with hypothyroidism.

Clinically, SCFE is classified as stable or unstable. SCFE is considered stable if the child is able to bear weight on the affected extremity. In unstable SCFE, the child is unable to bear weight. An increased rate of avascular necrosis is correlated with the inability to bear weight.

Acute SCFE occasionally occurs following a fall or direct trauma to the hip. More commonly, vague symptoms occur over a protracted period in an otherwise healthy child who presents with pain and limp. The pain can be referred into the thigh or the medial side of the knee, making examination of the hip joint important in any obese child complaining of knee pain. Physical examination consistently reveals a limitation of internal rotation of the hip. The diagnosis may be clearly apparent only in the lateral radiographic view.

Initial management consists of making the patient non–weight-bearing on crutches and immediate referral to an orthopedic surgeon. Treatment is based on the same principles that govern treatment of any fracture of the femoral neck: the head of the femur is internally fixed to the neck of the femur and the fracture line allowed to heal.

The long-term prognosis is guarded because most of these patients continue to be overweight and overstress their hip joints. Follow-up studies have shown a high incidence of premature degenerative arthritis, even in those who do not develop avascular necrosis. The development of avascular necrosis almost guarantees a poor prognosis, because new bone does not readily replace the dead bone at this late stage of skeletal development. About 30% of patients have bilateral involvement, which may occur as late as 1 or 2 years after the primary episode.

Gholve PA, Cameron DB, Millis MB: Slipped capital femoral epiphysis update. Curr Opin Pediatr 2009;21(1):39–45 [PMID: 19242240].

GENU VARUM & GENU VALGUM

Genu varum (bowleg) is normal from infancy through 3 years of age. The alignment then changes to genu valgum (knock-knee) until about age 8 years, at which time adult alignment is attained. If bowing persists beyond age 2, increases rather than decreases, occurs in only one leg, or if a patient is knock-kneed in association with short stature, the patient should be referred to an orthopedist. Genu varum is usually secondary to tibial rotation, while genu valgum may be caused by skeletal dysplasia or rickets.

Bracing may be appropriate. An osteotomy may be necessary for severe problems such as occurs in Blount disease (proximal tibial epiphysial dysplasia).

Fabry G: Clinical practice: Static, axial, and rotational deformities of the lower extremities in children. Eur J Pediatr 2010;529–534.

TIBIAL TORSION

"Toeing in" in small children is a common parental concern. Tibial torsion refers to rotation of the leg between the knee and the ankle. Internal rotation amounts to about 20 degrees at birth but decreases to neutral rotation by age 16 months. The deformity may be accentuated by laxity of the knee ligaments, which allows excessive internal rotation of the leg in small children. This condition is largely self-limiting and usually resolves spontaneously with further growth and development. Treatment is focused on educating the families to the benign nature and expected resolution with observation.

FEMORAL ANTEVERSION

Toeing in beyond age 2 or 3 years is usually secondary to femoral anteversion, characterized by more internal rotation of the hip than external rotation. This femoral alignment decreases toward neutral during growth. Little is gained by active treatment with shoes or braces. Active external rotation exercises, such as skating or bicycle riding, are encouraged. Osteotomy for rotational correction is rarely required. Children who have no external rotation of hip in extension are candidates for orthopedic consultation. However, the vast majority go on to resolve spontaneously.

Lincoln TL, Suen PW: Common rotational variations in children. J Am Acad Orthop Surg 2003;11:312 [PMID: 14565753].

COMMON FOOT PROBLEMS

When a child begins to stand and walk, the longitudinal arch of the foot is flat with a medial bulge over the inner border of the foot. The forefeet are mildly pronated or rotated inward, with a slight valgus alignment of the knees. As the child grows and joint laxity decreases, the long arch is better supported and more normal relationships occur in the lower extremities. (See also sections on Metatarsus Varus and Clubfoot [Talipes Equinovarus] earlier.)

1. Flatfoot

Flatfoot is normal in infants. If the heel cord is of normal length, full dorsiflexion is possible when the heel is in the neutral position. As long as the heel cord is of normal length and a longitudinal arch is noted when the child is sitting in a non–weight-bearing position, a normal arch will generally develop. Around 15% of flatfeet do not resolve spontaneously. There is usually a familial incidence of relaxed flatfeet in children who have no apparent arch. In any child with a shortened heel cord or stiffness of the foot, other causes of flatfoot such as tarsal coalition (congenital fusion of the tarsal bones) should be ruled out by a complete orthopedic examination and radiographs.

For an ordinary relaxed flatfoot, no active treatment is indicated unless calf or leg pain is present. In children who have leg pains attributable to flatfoot, a supportive shoe, such as a good-quality sports shoe, is useful. An orthotic that holds the heel in neutral position and supports the arch may relieve discomfort if more support is needed. An arch insert should not be prescribed unless passive correction of the arch is easily accomplished; otherwise, the skin over the medial side of the foot will be irritated.

Fabry G: Clinical practice: Static, axial, and rotational deformities of the lower extremities in children. Eur J Pediatr 2010;529–534.

2. Talipes Calcaneovalgus

Talipes calcaneovalgus is characterized by excessive dorsiflexion at the ankle and eversion of the foot. This condition is due to intrauterine position and is often present at birth. Treatment consists of passive exercises, stretching the foot into plantar flexion. In rare instances, it may be necessary to use plaster casts to help with manipulation and positioning. Complete correction is the rule.

This disorder can be associated with posteromedial bowing of the tibia.

3. Cavus Foot

Cavus foot consists of an unusually high longitudinal arch of the foot. It may be hereditary or associated with neurologic conditions such as poliomyelitis, hereditary sensory motor neuropathies, and diastematomyelia (congenital splitting of the spinal cord). Typically there is an associated contracture of the toe extensors, producing a claw toe deformity in which the metatarsal phalangeal joints are hyperextended and the interphalangeal joints acutely flexed. Cavus foot presents with diffuse and localized pain in the lower legs commonly caused by an inflexible foot deformity. Any child presenting with cavus feet should receive a careful neurologic examination as well as radiographs and magnetic resonance imaging (MRI) of the spine.

Conservative therapy is ineffective. In symptomatic cases, surgery may be necessary to lengthen the contracted extensor and flexor tendons and to release the plantar fascia and other tight plantar structures. Associated varus heel deformities cause more problems than the high arch.

Fabry G: Clinical practice: Static, axial, and rotational deformities of the lower extremities in children. Eur J Pediatr 2010;529–534.

4. Bunions (Hallux Valgus)

Adolescents may present with lateral deviation of the great toe associated with a prominence over the head of the first metatarsal, with an unknown etiology. Around 60% of patients have a family history of this condition. The deformity is painful with shoe wear and almost always relieved by fitting shoes that are wide enough in the toe area. Since further growth tends to cause recurrence of the deformity, surgery should be avoided in the adolescent.

Therapeutic treatments are aimed at correcting the muscular and weight bearing forces that act on the joint. While conservative treatment provides symptomatic relief, it does not reverse the natural history, as these deformities will typically continue to progress until corrected surgically. A high percentage of these patients ultimately have surgery in adulthood due to a continued progression of the deformity.

Glasoe WM, Nuckley DJ, Ludewig PM: Hallux valgus and the first metatarsal arch segment: A theoretical biomechanical perspective. Physical Therapy 2010;(90):110–120.

DEGENERATIVE PROBLEMS (ARTHRITIS, BURSITIS, & TENOSYNOVITIS)

ESSENTIALS OF DIAGNOSIS & TREATMENT

- Chronic conditions.
- Overuse syndromes.
- Rule out more serious conditions first.
- Activity restriction is the treatment.

Degenerative arthritis may follow childhood skeletal problems, such as infection, SCFE, avascular necrosis, trauma, or hemarthroses in patients with hemophilia. Early, effective treatment of these disorders can prevent arthritis. Overuse in young athletes can also cause degenerative changes to the soft tissues around the joints. Young boys throwing excessive numbers of pitches, especially curve balls, may develop "Little League" elbow, consisting of degenerative changes around the humeral condyles associated with pain, swelling, and limitation of motion (see Chapter 27). Limitation of the number of pitches thrown by little league pitchers is the key to prevention.

Acute bursitis is uncommon in childhood, and other causes should be ruled out before this diagnosis is accepted.

Tenosynovitis is most common in the knees and feet. Children taking dancing lessons, particularly toe dancing, may have pain around the flexor tendon sheaths in the toes or ankles. Rest is effective treatment. Around the knee, the patellar ligament may be irritated, with associated swelling in the infrapatellar fat pad. Synovitis in this area is usually due to overuse and is treated by rest and nonsteroidal anti-inflammatory drugs. Corticosteroid injections are contraindicated.

TRAUMA

ESSENTIALS OF DIAGNOSIS & TREATMENT

- Directed physical examination (eg, swelling, tenderness, deformity, instability).
- Radiographic examination.
- Rule out physeal fracture.
- Early motion for sprains and strains.
- Reduction and immobilization for fractures.

SOFT TISSUE TRAUMA (SPRAINS, STRAINS, & CONTUSIONS)

A sprain is the stretching of a ligament and a strain is a stretch of a muscle or tendon. Contusions are generally due to tissue compression, with damage to blood vessels within the tissue and the formation of hematoma.

In a severe sprain, the ligament is completely disrupted resulting in instability of the joint. Incomplete tearing of the ligament, with local pain and swelling but no joint instability, is considered a mild or moderate sprain.

The initial treatment of any sprain consists of ice, compression, and elevation. Brief splinting followed by early range of motion exercises of the affected joint protect against further injury and relieves swelling and pain. Ibuprofen and other nonsteroidal anti-inflammatory drugs are useful for pain. Rest, ice, and elevation are usually sufficient for mild or moderate sprains. If more severe trauma occurs, resulting in complete tearing of a ligament, instability of the joint may be demonstrated by gross examination or by stress testing with radiographic documentation. Such deformity of the joint may cause persistent instability resulting from inaccurate apposition of the ligament ends during healing. If instability is evident, surgical repair of the torn ligament may be indicated. If a muscle is torn at its tendinous insertion, it also should be repaired surgically.

1. Ankle Sprains

The history will indicate that the injury was by either forceful inversion or eversion. The more common inversion injury results in tearing or injury to the lateral ligaments, whereas an eversion injury will injure the medial ligaments of the ankle. The injured ligaments can be identified by careful palpation for point tenderness around the ankle. The joint should be supported or immobilized in the functional position (right angle). Use of an air splint produces joint rest, and the extremity can be protected by using crutches. Functional rehabilitation to include edema control, range of motion, strengthening, and restoration of proprioceptive sensation can prevent long-term disability. Re-injury is common. Continued injury can lead to chronic ankle instability.

Kemler E, Port I, Backx F, Dijk CN: A systematic review on the treatment of acute ankle sprain brace versus other functional treatment types. Sports Medicine 2011;41:185–197.

2. Knee Sprains

Sprains of the collateral and cruciate ligaments are uncommon in children. These ligaments are so strong that it is more common to injure the growth plates, which are the weakest structures in the region of the knees of children. In adolescence, as the physes start to close, rupture of the anterior cruciate ligament can result from a rotational injury. If the injury produces avulsion of the tibial spine, anatomic reduction and fixation are often required.

Effusion of the knee after trauma deserves referral to an orthopedic specialist. The differential diagnosis includes torn ligament, torn meniscus, and osteochondral fracture. Nontraumatic effusion should be evaluated for inflammatory conditions (eg, juvenile rheumatoid arthritis) or patellar malalignment.

Vaquero J, Vidal C, Cubillo A: Intra-articular traumatic disorders of the knee in children and adolescents. Clin Orthop Relat Res 2005;432:97 [Review] [PMID: 15738809].

3. Internal Derangements of the Knee

Meniscal injuries are uncommon in children younger than 12 years of age. Clicking or locking of the knee may occur in young children as a result of a discoid lateral meniscus, which is a rare congenital anomaly. As the child approaches adolescence, internal damage to the knee from a torsion weight-bearing injury may result in locking of the knee if tearing and displacement of a meniscus occurs. Osteochondritis dissecans also presents as swelling and mechanical symptoms of the knee in adolescence. Posttraumatic synovitis may mimic a meniscal lesion. Epiphysial injury should be suspected in any severe injury to the knee or when there is tenderness on both sides of the femoral metaphysis after injury. Stress films will sometimes demonstrate separation of the distal femoral epiphysis.

Kapur S et al: Acute knee dislocation review of an elusive entity. Curr Probl Diagn Radiol 2009;237–250.

4. Back Sprains

Sprains of the ligaments and muscles of the back are unusual in children but may occur as a result of violent trauma from automobile accidents or athletic injuries. Sprains usually cause lateral and midline pain over musculature. Back pain in a child may be the only symptom of significant disease and warrants clinical investigation. Inflammation, infection, renal disease, or tumors can cause back pain in children, and sprain should not be accepted as a routine diagnosis.

Gurd DP: Back pain in the young athlete. Sports Med Arthrosc Rev 2011;19:7–16.

5. Contusions

Muscle contusions with hematoma formation produce the familiar "charley horse" injury. Treatment includes application of ice, compression, and rest. Exercise should be avoided for 5–7 days. Local heat may hasten healing once the acute phase of tenderness and swelling has passed.

6. Myositis Ossificans

Ossification within muscle occurs when sufficient trauma causes a hematoma that later heals in the manner of a fracture. Contusions of the quadriceps of the thigh or the triceps of the arm are the most common injuries.

Disability is great, with local swelling, heat and extreme pain with the slightest provocation of the adjacent joint. The limb should be rested until the local reaction has subsided (5–7 days). When local heat and tenderness have decreased, gentle active exercises may be initiated. Passive stretching exercises are not indicated as they may stimulate the ossification reaction. If an extremity experiences a severe injury with a hematoma, it should be splinted and further activity should be avoided until the acute reaction has subsided. If additional trauma causes recurrent injury, ossification may reach spectacular proportions and resemble an osteosarcoma. Surgery to excise the ossification may restart the process and lead to an even more severe reaction and should not be attempted before 9 months to 1 year after injury.

TRAUMATIC SUBLUXATIONS & DISLOCATIONS

Joint dislocation is always associated with severe damage to the joint capsule and associated ligaments. In contrast to fracture reduction, which may be safely postponed, dislocations must be reduced immediately in order to minimize further joint damage. Dislocations can usually be reduced by gentle sustained traction. Often, no anesthetic is needed for several hours after the injury due to the protective anesthesia produced by the injury. A thorough neurovascular examination should be performed and documented pre- and postreduction. Radiographs should be obtained postreduction to document congruency and assess for the presence of associated fractures. Following reduction, the joint should be splinted for transportation of the patient.

The dislocated joint should be treated by immobilization, followed by graduated active exercises through a full range of motion. Vigorous passive manipulation of the joint by a therapist may be harmful.

1. Subluxation of the Radial Head (Nursemaid's Elbow)

Infants may sustain subluxation of the radial head as a result of being lifted or pulled by the hand. The child appears with the elbow fully pronated and painful. The usual complaint is that the child's elbow will not bend. Radiographic findings are normal, but there is point tenderness over the radial head. When the elbow is placed in full supination and slowly moved from full extension to full flexion, a click may be palpated at the level of the radial head. The relief of pain is remarkable, as the child usually stops crying immediately. The elbow may be immobilized in a sling for comfort for a day. Occasionally, symptoms last for several days, requiring more prolonged immobilization.

A pulled elbow may be a clue to battering. This should be considered during examination, especially if the problem is recurrent.

2. Recurrent Dislocation of the Patella

Complete patellar dislocations nearly always dislocate laterally. Pain is severe, and the patient will present with the knee slightly flexed and an obvious bony mass lateral to the knee joint associated with a flat area over the anterior knee. Radiologic examination confirms the diagnosis. The patella may be reduced by extending the knee and placing slight pressure on the patella while gentle traction is exerted on the leg. When subluxation of the patella occurs symptoms may be more subtle, and the patient will complain that the knee "gives out" or "jumps out of place."

Recurrent dislocations more commonly occur in loose-jointed individuals, especially adolescent girls. Factors that affect risk for recurrence include length of patellar tendon, the depth of trochlear groove, and position of the patella in relation to the trochlear groove.

For first-time dislocation, initial treatment after reduction should be nonoperative, consisting of physical therapy to strengthen the quadriceps, hips, and core stabilizers. Surgery is reserved for individuals with reparable osteochondral injuries, loose bodies, and recurrent dislocation following appropriate nonoperative therapy. Around one-third of patients report a repeated dislocation after rehabilitation.

Kapur S et al: Acute knee dislocation review of an elusive entity. Curr Probl Diagn Radiol 2009;237–250.

Smith TO et al: Clinical outcomes of rehabilitation for patients following lateral patellar dislocation. Physiotherapy 2010;(96):269–281.

FRACTURES

1. Epiphysial Separations

Epiphysial separations or fractures are more common than ligamentous injuries in children since the ligaments of the joints are generally stronger than their associated growth plates. Radiographs should be taken whenever a dislocation is suspected in order to rule out epiphysial fracture. Radiographs of the opposite extremity, especially for injuries around the elbow, are valuable for comparison. Fractures across the growth plate may produce bony bridges that will cause premature cessation of growth or angular deformities of the extremity. These bridges are due to the trauma to the growth plate and can occur even with adequate reductions.

Reduction of a fractured epiphysis should be done under anesthesia to align the growth plate with the least amount of force. Epiphysial fractures around the shoulder, wrist, and fingers can usually be treated by closed reduction, but fractures of the epiphyses around the elbow often require open reduction. In the lower extremity, accurate reduction of the epiphysial plate is necessary to prevent joint deformity when a joint surface is involved. If angular deformities result, corrective osteotomy may be necessary.

Dwek JR: The radiographic approach to child abuse. Clin Orthop Relat Res 2011;469:776–789.

2. Torus Fractures

Torus fractures consist of "buckling" of the cortex due to compression of the bone. They are most common in the distal radius or ulna. Alignment is usually satisfactory, and simple immobilization for 3 weeks is sufficient.

3. Greenstick Fractures

Greenstick fractures involve frank disruption of the cortex on one side of the bone but no discernible cleavage plane on the opposite side. Bone ends are not separated making these fractures angulated but not displaced. Reduction is achieved by straightening the arm into normal alignment, and maintained by a snugly fitting cast. It is necessary to obtain radiographs of greenstick fractures again in 7–10 days to make certain that the reduction has been maintained in the cast. A slight angular deformity can be corrected by remodeling of the bone. The farther the fracture is from the growing end of the bone, the longer the time required for remodeling. The fracture can be considered healed when no tenderness is present and a bony callus is seen on a radiograph.

4. Fracture of the Clavicle

Clavicular fractures are very common injuries in infants and children. The patient can be immobilized in a sling for comfort. The healing callus will be apparent when the fracture has consolidated, but this unsightly lump will generally resolve over a period of months to a year via bone remodeling.

5. Supracondylar Fractures of the Humerus

Supracondylar fractures tend to occur in children age 3–6 years and are the most common elbow fracture in children. The proximity to the brachial artery in the distal arm creates a potential danger when dealing with these types of fractures. Absence of a distal pulse is a strong indicator of a secondary arterial injury. Swelling may be severe as these injuries are usually associated with a significant amount of trauma. Most often, these fractures are treated by closed reduction and percutaneous pinning performed under general anesthesia. Complications associated with supracondylar fractures include Volkmann ischemic contracture of the forearm due to vascular compromise and cubitus varus (decreased carrying angle, "gunstock deformity") secondary to poor reduction. The "gunstock deformity" of the elbow may be somewhat unsightly but does not usually interfere with joint function.

White L: A systematic review of vascular injuries in pediatric supracondylar humerus fractures and results of a POSNA questionnaire. J Pediatr Orthop 2010;30:328–335.

6. General Comments on Other Fractures in Children

Reduction of fractures in children can usually be accomplished by simple traction and manipulation; open reduction is indicated if a satisfactory alignment is not obtained. Remodeling of the fracture callus generally produces an almost normal appearance of the bone over a matter of months. The younger the child, the more remodeling is possible. Angular deformities remodel reliably while rotational malalignment does not remodel well.

There should be suspicion of child abuse whenever the age of a fracture does not match the history given or when the severity of the injury is more than the alleged accident would have produced. In suspected cases of battering in which no fracture is present on the initial radiograph, a repeat radiograph 10 days later is in order. Bleeding beneath the periosteum will be calcified by 7–10 days, and the radiographic appearance is diagnostic of severe closed trauma characteristic of a battered child.

INFECTIONS OF THE BONES & JOINTS

ESSENTIALS OF DIAGNOSIS & TREATMENT

- Movement of the extremity causes pain.
- Soft tissue swelling.

- Elevated erythrocyte sedimentation rate (ESR) and C-reactive protein (CRP).
- Surgical drainage of abscess, plus antibiotics.
- Antibiotic therapy for early osteomyelitis without abscess.

OSTEOMYELITIS

Osteomyelitis is an infectious process that usually starts in the spongy or medullary bone and extends into compact or cortical bone. Commonly preceded by trauma, the lower extremities are more likely to be affected. Osteomyelitis is most commonly caused by hematogenous spread of bacteria from other infected or colonized areas (eg, pyoderma or upper respiratory tract) but it may occur as a result of direct invasion from the outside (exogenous), through a penetrating wound (nail), or open fracture. *Staphylococcus aureus* is the most common infecting organism and has a tendency to infect the metaphyses of growing bones. Anatomically, the arterial supply to the metaphysis in the long bones includes end arteries just below the growth plate which turn sharply end in venous sinusoids, causing relative stasis that predisposes to bacterial localization. In the infant (younger than age 1 year), there is direct vascular communication with the epiphysis across the growth plate. Bacterial spread occurs from the metaphysis to the epiphysis and into the joint. In the older child, the growth plate provides an effective barrier and the epiphysis is usually not infected. Infection spreads retrograde from the metaphysis into the diaphysis, and by rupture through the cortical bone, down along the diaphysis beneath the periosteum.

1. Exogenous Osteomyelitis

All wounds must be carefully examined and cleansed to avoid osteomyelitis by direct extension. Osteomyelitis is a common occurrence from pressure sores in insensate areas, such as in patients with spina bifida. Copious irrigation is necessary, and all nonviable skin, subcutaneous tissue, fascia, and muscle must be excised. In extensive or contaminated wounds, antibiotic coverage is indicated. Contaminated lacerations should be left open and secondary closure performed 3–5 days later. Leaving the wound open allows infection to stay at the surface rather than extend inward to the bone. Further necrotic tissue should be excised if present at the time of delayed closure. Puncture wounds are especially prone to causing osteomyelitis and should be carefully debrided.

Initially, broad-spectrum antibiotics should be administered for contaminated wounds, but the final choice of antibiotics is directed by culture results. A tetanus toxoid booster may be indicated. Gas gangrene is best prevented by adequate debridement.

After exogenous osteomyelitis has become established, treatment becomes more complicated, requiring extensive surgical debridement and antibiotics, initially by the intravenous route.

2. Hematogenous Osteomyelitis

Hematogenous osteomyelitis is the most common infection of the bone in children. It most often occurs in the metaphyseal region of tubular bones and is usually caused by pyogenic bacteria; 85% of cases are due to staphylococci. Streptococci (group B streptococcus in young infants, *Streptococcus pyogenes* in older children) are a less common cause of osteomyelitis. *Pseudomonas aeruginosa* is common in cases of nail puncture wounds. Children with sickle cell anemia are especially prone to osteomyelitis caused by *Salmonella* spp.

Clinical Findings

A. Symptoms and Signs

Osteomyelitis may be subtle in infants, presenting as irritability, diarrhea, or failure to feed properly; temperature may be normal or slightly low; and white blood cell count may be normal or only slightly elevated. There may be pseudoparalysis of the involved limb. The manifestations are more striking in older children, with severe local tenderness and pain, often, but not invariably, high fever, rapid pulse, and elevated white blood cell count, ESR, and CRP. Osteomyelitis of a lower extremity often occurs around the knee joint in children age 7–10 years. Tenderness is most marked over the metaphysis of the bone where the process has its origin. For a child who refuses to bear weight, osteomyelitis is high in the differential diagnosis.

B. Laboratory Findings

Blood cultures are often positive early. The most significant test is the aspiration of pus. It is useful to insert a needle into the bone in the area of suspected infection and aspirate any fluid present. Fluid should be stained for organisms and cultured. Even edema fluid can be useful for determining the causative organism. Elevation of the ESR above 50 mm/h is typical for osteomyelitis. CRP is elevated earlier than the ESR.

C. Imaging

Osteomyelitis should be diagnosed clinically before significant plain radiographic findings are present. Plain film findings progress from nonspecific local swelling, to elevation of the periosteum, with formation of new bone from the cambium layer of the periosteum occurring after 3–6 days. As infection becomes chronic, areas of cortical bone are isolated by pus spreading down the medullary canal, causing rarefaction and demineralization of the bone. Isolated pieces of cortex become ischemic and form sequestra (dead bone fragments). These radiographic findings are specific, but late. Bone scan is sensitive (before plain radiographic findings are apparent) but nonspecific and should be interpreted in the clinical context. MRI can demonstrate early edema and subperiosteal abscess and is helpful to confirm and localize disease prior to plain film changes.

Treatment

A. Specific Measures

Intravenous antibiotics should be started as soon as the diagnosis of osteomyelitis is made and diagnostic specimens have been obtained. Transition to oral antibiotics occurs when tenderness, fever, the white cell count, and the CRP are all decreasing and is facilitated by a positive culture. Agents that cover *S aureus* and *Streptococcus pyogenes* (eg, oxacillin, nafcillin, cefazolin, and clindamycin) are appropriate for most cases. Alternative antistaphylococcal therapy (eg, vancomycin) may be needed if methicillin-resistant and clindamycin-resistant *Staphylococcus aureus* is suspected or isolated. Consultation with an infectious disease specialist can be helpful. For specific recommendations and for possible *Pseudomonas* infection, see Chapter 42.

Acute osteomyelitis is usually treated for a minimum of 4–6 weeks and until normalization of the physical exam and inflammatory markers. Chronic infections are treated for months. Following surgical debridement, *Pseudomonas* foot infections usually respond to 1–2 weeks of antibiotic treatment.

B. General Measures

Splinting minimizes pain and decreases spread of the infection through lymphatic channels in the soft tissue. The splint should be removed periodically to allow active use of adjacent joints and prevent stiffening and muscle atrophy. In chronic osteomyelitis, splinting may be necessary to guard against fracture of the weakened bone.

C. Surgical Measures

Aspiration of the metaphysis for culture and Gram stain is the most useful diagnostic measure in any case of suspected osteomyelitis. If frank pus is aspirated from the bone, surgical drainage is indicated. If the infection has not shown a significant response within 24 hours, surgical drainage is also indicated. It is important that all devitalized soft tissue be removed and adequate exposure of the bone obtained to permit free drainage. Excessive amounts of bone should not be removed when draining acute osteomyelitis as it will not be completely replaced by the normal healing process. Bone damage is limited by surgical drainage, whereas failure to evacuate pus in acute cases may lead to widespread damage.

Prognosis

When osteomyelitis is diagnosed in the early clinical stages and prompt antibiotic therapy is begun, the prognosis is excellent. If the process has been unattended for a week to 10 days, there is almost always some permanent loss of bone structure, as well as the possibility of future growth abnormality due to physeal injury.

Conrad DA: Acute hematogenous osteomyelitis. American Academy of Pediatrics 2011;31:464–471.

Harik NS, Smeltzer MS: Management of acute hematogenous osteomyelitis in children. Expert Rev Anti Infect Ther 2010;8(2):175–181.

PYOGENIC ARTHRITIS

The source of pyogenic arthritis varies according to the child's age. Infantile pyogenic arthritis often develops from adjacent osteomyelitis. In older children, it presents as an isolated infection, usually without bony involvement. In teenagers with pyogenic arthritis, an underlying systemic disease or an organism (eg, gonococcus) that has an affinity for joints is often the cause.

The infecting organism similarly varies with age: group B *Streptococcus* and *S aureus* in those younger than age 4 months; *Haemophilus influenza* B and *S aureus* in those aged 4 months to 4 years; and *S aureus* and *S pyogenes* in older children and adolescents. *Streptococcus pneumoniae* and *Neisseria meningitis* are occasionally implicated, and *Neisseria gonorrhoeae* is a cause in adolescents. *H influenza* B is now uncommon because of effective immunization. *Kingella kingae* is a gram-negative bacterium that occasionally causes pyarthrosis in children under 5 years of age.

The initial effusion of the joint rapidly becomes purulent. An effusion of the joint may accompany osteomyelitis in the adjacent bone, but a white cell count exceeding 50,000/μL in the joint fluid indicates a purulent infection involving the joint. Generally, spread of infection is from the bone into the joint, but unattended pyogenic arthritis may also affect adjacent bone. The ESR is often above 50 mm/h.

Clinical Findings

A. Symptoms and Signs

In older children, signs may be striking, with fever, malaise, vomiting, and restriction of motion. In infants, paralysis of the limb due to inflammatory pseudoparalysis may be evident. Infection of the hip joint in infants should be suspected if decreased abduction of the hip is present in an infant who is irritable or feeding poorly. A history of umbilical catheter treatment in the newborn nursery should alert the physician to the possibility of pyogenic arthritis of the hip.

B. Imaging

Early distention of the joint capsule is nonspecific and difficult to measure by plain radiograph. In infants with unrecognized pyogenic arthritis, dislocation of the joint may follow within a few days as a result of distention of the capsule by pus. Destruction of the joint space, resorption of epiphysial cartilage, and erosion of the adjacent bone of the metaphysis occur later. The bone scan shows increased flow and increased uptake about the joint. MRI and ultrasound imaging are useful adjuncts for detecting joint effusions, which can be helpful in assessing potential joint sepsis.

Treatment

Aspiration of the joint is the key to diagnosis. Surgical drainage followed by the appropriate antibiotic therapy provides the best treatment for pyogenic arthritis. Antibiotics can be selected based on the child's age and results of the Gram stain and culture of aspirated pus. Reasonable empiric therapy in infants and young children is nafcillin or oxacillin plus a third-generation cephalosporin. An antistaphylococcal agent alone is usually adequate for children older than age 5 years, unless gonococcal or meningococcal infection is suspected. Alternative antistaphylococcal therapy (eg, clindamycin or vancomycin) may be needed if methicillin-resistant *Staphylococcus aureus* is suspected or isolated. Consultation with an infectious disease specialist can be helpful.

For staphylococcal infections, a minimum of 3 weeks of therapy and until examination and inflammatory markers are normal is recommended; for other organisms, a minimum of 2 weeks and until examination and inflammatory markers are normal is usually sufficient. Oral therapy may be begun when clinical signs and inflammatory markers have improved markedly. It is not necessary to give intra-articular antibiotics since good levels are achieved in the synovial fluid with parenteral administration.

Prognosis

The prognosis for the patient with pyogenic arthritis is excellent if the joint is drained before damage to the articular cartilage has occurred. If infection is present for more than 24 hours, dissolution of the proteoglycans in the articular cartilage takes place, with subsequent arthrosis and fibrosis of the joint. Damage to the growth plate may occur, especially within the hip joint, where the epiphyseal plate is intracapsular.

Jesus AA et al: Pediatric hereditary autoinflammatory syndromes. Jornal de Pediatria 2010;86(5):353–366.

TUBERCULOUS ARTHRITIS

Tuberculous arthritis is now a rare disease in the United States, afflicting children in poor social circumstances such as homeless families, or children who have immigrated from tuberculosis-endemic regions or who are in contact with adults with tuberculosis risk factors. Generally, the infection may be ruled out by negative skin testing. The intervertebral discs are the most commonly affected sites of involvement in children, resulting in gibbus or dorsal angular deformity at the affected site. MRI is effective in showing the number of lesions, their location and size and whether or not necrosis has occurred.

Treatment is by local drainage of the abscess, followed by antituberculous therapy. Prolonged immobilization in a plaster cast or prolonged bed rest is necessary to promote healing. Spinal fusion may be required to preserve stability of the vertebral column.

Lu M: Imaging diagnosis of spinal intramedullary tuberculoma: Case reports and literature review. American Paraplegia Society 2009;159–162.

DISKITIS

Diskitis is pyogenic infectious spondylitis in children. Although many infections are culture-negative, *Staphylococcus aureus* is considered to be the most frequent etiologic pathogen. The typical clinical presentation includes back pain and malaise over a several weeks to months duration. Younger children, less than 5 years, may not be able to focalize their complaints and commonly present with "abdominal" pain. Supportive treatment and appropriate antibiotics are likely to lead to rapid relief of symptoms and signs without recurrence.

Gouliouris T, Aliyu SH, Brown NM: Spondylodiscitis update on diagnosis and management. Journal of Antimicrobial Chemotherapy 2010;65:11–24.

TRANSIENT (TOXIC) SYNOVITIS OF THE HIP

The most common cause of limping and hip pain in children in the United States is transient synovitis. This acute inflammatory reaction often follows an upper respiratory or gastrointestinal infection and is generally self-limited. In questionable cases, aspiration of the hip yields only yellowish fluid, rather than pyogenic arthritis. Generally, toxic synovitis of the hip is not associated with elevation of the ESR, white blood cell count, or temperature above 38.3°C. Classically affecting children aged 3–10 years, it is more common in boys than girls. The hip joint experiences limitation of motion, particularly internal rotation, and radiographic changes are nonspecific, with some swelling apparent in the soft tissues around the joint.

Rest and nonsteroidal anti-inflammatory medications are the preferred treatments. Nonsteroidal anti-inflammatory drugs shorten the course of the disease, although even with no treatment, the disease usually runs its course in days. Radiographic follow-up is essential as toxic synovitis may be the precursor of avascular necrosis of the femoral head (described in the next section) in a small percentage of patients. Radiographs can be obtained at 6 weeks, or earlier if either a persistent limp or pain is present.

Fabry G: The hip from birth to adolescence. Eur J Pediatr 2010;169:143–148.

VASCULAR LESIONS & AVASCULAR NECROSIS (OSTEOCHONDROSES)

ESSENTIALS OF DIAGNOSIS & TREATMENT

- Diagnosis made by characteristic radiographic findings.
- Radiographic resolution lags behind symptomatic resolution.
- Treatment for most cases is supportive.

Osteochondrosis due to vascular lesions may affect various growth centers. Table 26–1 indicates the common sites and the typical ages at presentation.

In contrast to other body tissues that undergo infarction, bone removes necrotic tissue and replaces it with living bone through creeping substitution (a process where necrotic bone is replaced by viable bone). This replacement of necrotic bone may be so complete that a normal bone results. Adequacy of replacement depends on the patient's age, the presence or absence of associated infection, the congruity of the involved joint, and other physiologic and mechanical factors.

Rapid growth of the secondary ossification centers in the epiphyses in relation to their blood supply subject them to avascular necrosis. Despite the number of different names referring to avascular necrosis of the epiphyses, the process is identical: necrosis of bone followed by replacement (see Table 26–1).

Even though the pathologic and radiographic features of avascular necrosis of the epiphyses are well known, the cause is not generally agreed upon. Necrosis may follow known causes such as trauma or infection, but idiopathic lesions usually develop during periods of rapid growth of the epiphyses.

Table 26–1. The osteochondroses.

Ossification Center	Eponym	Typical Age (y)
Capital femoral	Legg-Calvé-Perthes disease	4–8
Tarsal navicular	Köhler bone disease	6
Second metatarsal head	Freiberg disease	12–14
Vertebral ring	Scheuermann disease	13–16
Capitellum	Panner disease	9–11
Tibial tubercle	Osgood-Schlatter disease	11–13
Calcaneus	Sever disease	8–9

AVASCULAR NECROSIS OF THE PROXIMAL FEMUR (LEGG-CALVÉ-PERTHES DISEASE)

Necrosis results if the vascular supply to the proximal femur is interrupted.

Clinical Findings

A. Symptoms and Signs

The highest incidence of Legg-Calvé-Perthes disease occurs between 4 and 8 years of age. Persistent pain is the most common symptom, and the patient may present with limp or limitation of motion.

B. Laboratory Findings

Laboratory findings, including studies of joint aspirates, are normal.

C. Imaging

Radiographic findings correlate with progression of the disease and the extent of necrosis. Effusion of the joint associated with slight widening of the joint space and periarticular swelling are the early findings. Decreased bone density in and around the joint is apparent after a few weeks. The necrotic ossification center appears denser than the surrounding viable structures, and the femoral head is collapsed or narrowed.

As replacement of the necrotic ossification center occurs, rarefaction of the bone begins in a patchwork fashion, producing alternating areas of rarefaction and relative density, referred to as "fragmentation" of the epiphysis.

Widening of the femoral head may be associated with flattening, or coxa plana. If infarction has extended across the growth plate, a radiolucent lesion will be evident within the metaphysis. If the growth center of the femoral head has been damaged and normal growth arrested, shortening of the femoral neck results.

Eventually, complete replacement of the epiphysis develops as living bone replaces necrotic bone by creeping substitution. The final shape of the head depends on the extent of the necrosis and collapse of weakened bone.

Differential Diagnosis

Differential diagnosis must include inflammation and infection and dysplasia. Transient synovitis of the hip may be distinguished from Legg-Calvé-Perthes disease by serial radiographs.

Treatment

Protection of the joint by minimizing impact is the principal treatment. If the joint is deeply seated within the acetabulum and normal joint motion is maintained, a reasonably good hip can result. Little benefit has been shown from bracing. Surgical treatment is controversial.

Prognosis

The prognosis for complete replacement of the necrotic femoral head in a child is excellent, but the functional result depends on the amount of deformity that has developed. Better outcomes are observed for patients with an onset of symptoms before the age of 6. Generally a poorer prognosis is expected for patients who develop the disease late in childhood, those with more completed involvement of the epiphysial center, those with metaphysial defects and those who have more complete involvement of the femoral head.

OSTEOCHONDRITIS DISSECANS

In osteochondritis dissecans, a wedge-shaped necrotic area of bone and cartilage develops adjacent to the articular surface. The fragment of bone may break off from the host bone and displace into the joint as a loose body. If it remains attached, the necrotic fragment may be completely replaced through creeping substitution.

The pathologic process is the same as that for avascular necrosing lesions of ossification centers. Joint damage may occur because of the proximity of these lesions to adjacent articular cartilage.

The knee (medial femoral condyle), the elbow joint (capitellum), and the talus (superior lateral dome) are the most common sites for these lesions. Joint pain is the usual presenting complaint; however, local swelling or locking may be present, particularly if a fragment is free in the joint. Laboratory studies are normal.

Treatment consists of protection of the involved area from mechanical damage. Stable/attached lesions are generally treated with activity modification and immobilization for 3–6 months. Unstable/dislodged lesions are treated surgically with arthroscopic drilling, in order to bring new blood flow to the area, and fixation to stabilize the lesion. For some marginal lesions, it may be worthwhile to drill the necrotic fragment to encourage more rapid vascular in growth and replacement. If a fragment is free within the joint as a loose body, it must be removed. If large areas of a weight-bearing joint are involved, secondary degenerative arthritis may result. Adolescents have less favorable outcomes with nonoperative therapy.

Polousky JD: Juvenile osteochondritis dissecans. Sports Med Arthrosc Rev 2011;19:56–63.

NEUROLOGIC DISORDERS INVOLVING THE MUSCULOSKELETAL SYSTEM

ORTHOPEDIC ASPECTS OF CEREBRAL PALSY

Early physical therapy encouraging completion of normal developmental patterns may benefit patients with cerebral palsy. This therapy is most effective during the first few years of life, and should be discontinued when no improvement is apparent.

Bracing and splinting are of questionable benefit, although night splints may be useful in preventing equinus deformity of the ankle, the most common deformity found in this population, or adduction contractures of the hips. Orthopedic surgery is useful for treating joint contractures that interfere with function. Muscle transfers are effective in carefully selected patients with cerebral palsy, and most orthopedic procedures are directed at tendon lengthening or bony stabilization by osteotomy or arthrodesis.

Flexion and adduction of the hip due to hyperactivity of the adductors and flexors may produce a progressive paralytic dislocation of the hip. This can lead to pain and dysfunction, with treatment being difficult and unsatisfactory. The principal preventive measure is abduction bracing, supplemented by release of the adductors and hip flexors in order to prevent dislocation. In severe cases, osteotomy of the femur may be necessary to correct bony deformities of femoral anteversion and coxa valga that are invariably present. Patients with a predominantly athetotic pattern are poor candidates for any surgical procedure or bracing due to largely unpredictable results.

Surgeons must examine patients on several occasions before any operative procedure as it is difficult to predict the surgical outcome in individuals diagnosed with cerebral palsy. Follow-up care with a physical therapist can maximize the anticipated long-term gains and should be arranged before surgery.

ORTHOPEDIC ASPECTS OF MYELODYSPLASIA

Early closure of the sac in patients born with spina bifida is the rule, although there has been some hesitancy to provide treatment to all of these patients due to the extremely poor prognosis associated with congenital hydrocephalus, high levels of paralysis, and associated congenital anomalies in some cases. A high percentage of these children have hydrocephalus, which may be evident at birth or shortly thereafter, requiring shunting. Careful urologic evaluation and follow-up must be obtained to prevent complications from bladder dysfunction.

Patients should be examined early by an orthopedic surgeon. The level of neurologic involvement determines the muscle imbalance that will be present to produce deformity with growth. The involvement is often asymmetrical and tends to change during the first 12–18 months of life. Associated musculoskeletal problems may include clubfoot, congenital dislocation of the hip, arthrogryposis-type changes of the lower extremities, and congenital scoliosis and kyphosis. Spina bifida lesions are most common at the L3–L4 level and tend to affect the hip joint, with progressive dislocation occurring during growth due to unopposed hip flexion and adduction forces. Foot deformities are complicated by the fact that sensation is generally absent; these deformities may be in any direction depending on the muscle imbalance present. Spinal deformities develop in a high percentage of these children, with scoliosis present in approximately 40%.

Ambulation may require long leg braces. In children who have a reasonable likelihood of walking, operative treatment consists of reduction of the hip, alignment of the feet in the weight-bearing position as well as stabilization of the scoliosis. In children who lack active quadriceps function and extensor power of the knee, the likelihood of ambulation is greatly decreased. In such patients, aggressive surgery to the foot and hip region is usually not indicated as it may result in stiffening of the joints and prevent sitting.

The overall treatment of the child with spina bifida should be coordinated in a multidisciplinary clinic where various medical specialists work with therapists, social workers, and teachers to provide the best possible care.

NEOPLASIA OF THE MUSCULOSKELETAL SYSTEM

The poor prognosis of malignant tumors arising in the bone or other tissues derived from the mesoderm makes neoplastic diseases of the musculoskeletal system a serious problem. Fortunately, few benign lesions undergo malignant transformation. Accurate diagnosis depends on correlation of the clinical, radiographic, and microscopic findings. Complaints about the knee should be investigated for tumor, although the usual causes of knee pain are traumatic, infectious, or developmental in origin.

Hashefi M: Ultrasound in the diagnosis of noninflammatory musculoskeletal conditions. Seminars in Ultrasound CT and MRI 2011;74–90.

Osteochondroma

Osteochondroma is the most common benign bone tumor in children. It usually presents as a pain-free mass. When present, pain is caused by bursitis or tendinitis due to irritation by the tumor. Lesions may be single or multiple. Pathologically, the lesion is a bone mass capped with cartilage. These masses result from a developmental defect of the growth plate and tend to grow during childhood and adolescence in proportion to the child's growth. Males are more affected than females.

Generally, the tumors are present on radiographs in the metaphyseal region of long bones and may be pedunculated or sessile. The cortex of the underlying bone "flows" into the base of the tumor.

An osteochondroma should be excised if it interferes with function, is frequently traumatized, or is large enough to be deforming. The prognosis is excellent. Malignant transformation is very rare.

Gunay C et al: Spinal osteochondroma a report on six patients and a review of the literature. Orthopeadic Surgery 2010;130:1459–1465.

Osteoid Osteoma

Osteoid osteoma classically produces night pain that can be relieved by nonsteroidal anti-inflammatory drugs. On physical examination, there usually is tenderness over the lesion. An osteoid osteoma in the upper femur may cause referred pain to the knee.

The radiographic lesion consists of a radiolucent nidus surrounded by dense osteosclerosis that may obscure the nidus. Bone scan shows intense uptake in the lesion. CT scans are confirmatory and delineate the nidus well.

Surgical excision or radiofrequency ablation of the nidus is curative and may be done using computed tomography imaging and minimally invasive technique. The prognosis is excellent, with no known cases of malignant transformation, although the lesion has a tendency to recur if incompletely excised. The etiology remains unclear.

Enchondroma

Enchondroma (nest of benign cartilage within long bones) is usually a silent lesion unless it produces a pathologic fracture. On radiograph it is radiolucent, usually in a long bone. Speckled calcification may be present. The classic lesion looks as though someone dragged his or her fingernails through clay, making streaks in the bones. Enchondroma is treated by surgical curettage and bone grafting. The prognosis is excellent. Malignant transformation may occur but is very rare in childhood.

Chondroblastoma

The presenting complaint in chondroblastoma (benign chondral origin lesions typically in the epiphyses [joint ends] of long bones) is pain around a joint. This neoplasm may produce a pathologic fracture. On radiograph, the lesion is radiolucent and usually located in the epiphysis. With little to no reactive bone, calcification is unusual. The lesion is treated by surgical curettage and bone grafting. The prognosis is excellent if complete curettage is performed. There is no known malignant transformation.

Kim J, Kumar R, Raymond AK: Non-epiphyseal chondroblastoma arising in the iliac bone, and complicated by an aneurysmal bone cyst. Skeletal Radiol 2010;39:583–587.

Nonossifying Fibroma

Nonossifying fibroma, or benign cortical defect, is nearly always an incidental finding on radiograph. Nonossifying fibroma is a radiolucent lesion eccentrically located in the metaphyseal region of the bone. Usually a thin sclerotic border is evident. Multiple lesions may be present. The most frequent sites are the distal femur and proximal tibia. In general, no treatment is needed because these lesions heal as they ossify with maturation and growth. Rarely, pathologic fractures result from large lesions.

Osteosarcoma

In osteosarcoma, the presenting complaint is usually pain in a long bone; however, the patient may present with, loss of function, mass, or limp. Pathologic fracture is common. The malignant osseous tumor produces a destructive, expanding, and invasive lesion. A triangle may be adjacent to the tumor produced by elevated periosteum and subsequent tumor ossification. The lesion may contain calcification and violates the cortex of the bone. Femur, tibia, humerus, and other long bones are the sites usually affected.

Surgical excision (limb salvage) or amputation is indicated based on the extent of the tumor. Adjuvant chemotherapy is routinely used prior to surgical excision. The prognosis is improving, with 60%–70% long-term survival rates being reported in modern series. Death usually occurs as a result of lung metastasis.

Heare T, Hensley MA, Dell'Orfano S: Bone tumors: Osteosarcoma and Ewing's sarcoma. Curr Opin Pediatr 2009;21(3):365–672 [PMID: 19421061].

Ewing Sarcoma

In Ewing sarcoma, the presenting complaint is usually pain and tenderness, but fever and leukocytosis may be present. Osteomyelitis is the main differential diagnosis. The lesion may be multicentric. Ewing sarcoma is radiolucent and destroys the cortex, frequently in the diaphysial region. Reactive bone formation may occur about the lesion, seen as successive layers of so-called onion skin layering.

Treatment is with multiagent chemotherapy, radiation, and surgical resection. Large tumor size, pelvic lesions, and inadequate response to chemotherapy portend a poor prognosis.

MISCELLANEOUS DISEASES OF BONE AND JOINT

ESSENTIALS OF DIAGNOSIS & TREATMENT

- Rule out malignant process.
- Rule out pathologic fracture.
- Beware of associated endocrine abnormalities.
- Treatment based on symptoms and location.

FIBROUS DYSPLASIA

Dysplastic fibrous tissue replacement of the medullary canal is accompanied by the formation of metaplastic bone in areas with fibrous dysplasia. Three forms of the disease are recognized: monostotic, polyostotic, and polyostotic with endocrine disturbances (precocious puberty in females, hyperthyroidism, and hyperadrenalism [Albright syndrome]).

Clinical Findings

A. Symptoms and Signs

The lesion or lesions may be asymptomatic. If present, pain is probably due to pathologic fractures. In females, endocrine disturbances may be present in the polyostotic variety and associated with café au lait spots.

B. Laboratory Findings

Laboratory findings are normal unless endocrine disturbances are present, in which case secretion of gonadotropic, thyroid, or adrenal hormones may be increased.

C. Imaging

The lesion begins centrally within the medullary canal, usually of a long bone, and expands slowly. Pathologic fracture may occur. If metaplastic bone predominates, the contents of the lesion have the density of bone. The disease is often asymmetrical, and limb length disturbances may occur as a result of stimulation of epiphysial cartilage growth. Marked deformity of the bone may result, and a shepherd's crook deformity of the upper femur is a classic feature of the disease.

Differential Diagnosis

The differential diagnosis includes other fibrous lesions of bone as well as destructive lesions such as unicameral bone cyst, eosinophilic granuloma, aneurysmal bone cyst, nonossifying fibroma, enchondroma, and chondromyxoid fibroma.

Treatment

If the lesion is small and asymptomatic, no treatment is needed. If the lesion is large and produces or threatens pathologic fracture, curettage and bone grafting are indicated.

Prognosis

Unless the lesions affect epiphysial growth, the prognosis for patients with fibrous dysplasia is good. Lesions tend to enlarge during the growth period but are stable during adult life. Malignant transformation is rare.

UNICAMERAL BONE CYST

Unicameral bone cysts occur in the metaphysis of a long bone, usually in the femur or humerus. A cyst begins in the medullary canal adjacent to the epiphysial cartilage. It probably results from some fault in enchondral ossification (the process where bone is formed from cartilaginous precursors).

The cyst is considered active as long as it abuts onto the metaphysial side of the epiphysial cartilage, and there is a risk of growth arrest with or without treatment. When a border of normal bone exists between the cyst and the epiphysial cartilage, the cyst is inactive. The lesion is usually identified when a pathologic fracture occurs, producing pain. Laboratory findings are normal. On radiograph, the cyst is identified centrally within the medullary canal, producing expansion of the cortex and thinning over the widest portion of the cyst. Treatment consists of curettage and bone grafting. The cyst may heal after a fracture.

Mik G et al: Results of a minimally invasive technique for treatment of unicameral bone cysts. Clin Orthop Relat Res 2009 Aug 4 [Epub ahead of print] [PMID: 19653053].

ANEURYSMAL BONE CYST

Aneurysmal bone cyst is similar to unicameral bone cyst, except it contains blood rather than clear fluid. It usually occurs in a slightly eccentric position in a long bone, expanding the cortex of the bone but not breaking the cortex. Involvement of the flat bones of the pelvis is less common. On radiographs, the lesion appears somewhat larger than the width of the epiphysial cartilage, distinguishing it from a unicameral bone cyst.

Chromosomal abnormalities have been associated with aneurysmal bone cysts. The lesion may appear aggressive histologically, and it is important to differentiate it from osteosarcoma or hemangioma. Treatment is by curettage and bone grafting. The prognosis is good.

INFANTILE CORTICAL HYPEROSTOSIS (CAFFEY SYNDROME)

Infantile cortical hyperostosis is a benign disease of unknown cause that has its onset before age 6 months and is characterized by irritability; fever; and nonsuppurating, tender, painful swellings. Swellings may involve almost any bone of the body and are frequently widespread. Classically, swellings of the mandible and clavicle occur in 50% of patients; swellings of the ulna, humerus, and ribs also occur. The disease is limited to the shafts of bones and does not involve subcutaneous tissues or joints. It is self-limited but may persist for weeks or months. Anemia, leukocytosis, an increased ESR, and elevation of the serum alkaline phosphatase concentration are usually present. Cortical hyperostosis is demonstrable by a typical radiographic appearance and may be diagnosed on physical examination by an experienced pediatrician. In rare instances, a biopsy may be needed to confirm the diagnosis.

Fortunately, the disease appears to be decreasing in frequency. Indomethacin may be useful for treatment. The prognosis is good, and the disease usually terminates without deformity.

GANGLION

A ganglion is a smooth, small cystic mass connected by a pedicle to the joint capsule, usually on the dorsum of the wrist. It may also occur in the tendon sheath over the flexor or extensor surfaces of the fingers. These ganglia can be excised if they interfere with function or cause persistent pain.

BAKER CYST

A Baker cyst is a herniation of the synovium in the knee joint into the popliteal region. In children, the diagnosis may be made by aspiration of mucinous fluid, but the cyst nearly always disappears with time. Whereas Baker cysts may be indicative of intra-articular disease in the adult, they occur without internal derangement in children and rarely require excision.

Sit M, Higgs JB: Non-popliteal synovial rupture. Journal of Clinical Radiology 2009;15:185–189.

Sports Medicine

27

Quynh B. Hoang, MD, FAAP, CAQSM
Rachel A. Coel, MD, PhD, FAAP, CAQSM
Armando Vidal, MD
Pamela E. Wilson, MD
K. Brooke Pengel, MD, FAAP, CAQSM

Sports medicine as a separate discipline has grown since the 1980s in response to an expanding body of knowledge in the areas of exercise physiology, biomechanics, and musculoskeletal medicine. As more children participate in recreational and competitive activities, pediatric health care providers are encountering more young athletes in their practice. Familiarity with the common medical and orthopaedic issues faced by athletically active children and knowledge of which injuries necessitate referral to a sports medicine specialist are essential.

BASIC PRINCIPLES

Pediatric Injury Patterns

Although young athletes have injuries and issues similar to those of adults, there are many injuries that are unique to the pediatric and adolescent athlete. An understanding of the differences between adult and pediatric injury patterns is important to foster an appropriate index of suspicion for situations unique to pediatrics.

Components of a long bone include the diaphysis, metaphysis, and epiphysis. In the pediatric bone architecture, the presence of cartilaginous growth plates and apophyses predispose children to unique injury patterns that are different from their adult counterparts. Open growth plates or physes and their various stages of development are important factors to consider when treating young athletes. The physes are located at the ends of the long bones and are the primary ossification centers where length is added to the immature skeleton. The physis is a weak link in the musculoskeletal complex and has a high risk of fracture during periods of rapid growth. The surrounding soft tissues, including ligaments and tendons, are relatively stronger than the physis. The epiphyses are secondary centers of ossification that also contribute to long bone formation and, like the adjacent articular cartilages, are vulnerable to trauma. Injuries that involve the epiphysis can lead to joint deformity. The apophyses are secondary centers of ossification that add contour but not length to the bone. The apophysis is the attachment site of the muscle-tendon unit and is vulnerable to both acute and chronic overuse traction injury during times of rapid growth. Unlike injuries to the physis and epiphysis, however, apophyseal injuries do not result in long-term growth disturbance. Recognizing injuries to growth centers is important because of the risk for partial or complete physeal arrest. Complications of growth plate injury can lead to limb length discrepancy or angular deformity.

Strength Training

Strength is defined as the peak force that can be generated during a single maximal contraction. Strength training uses progressive resistance to improve an athlete's ability to resist or exert force. This can be achieved by a variety of techniques, including body weight, free weight, or machine resistance. The benefits of strength training include improved performance, endurance, and muscular strength. Strength training can be safely started in prepubescent athletes as early as 7 and 8 years old if designed appropriately with a focus on lighter resistance, increased repetitions, proper technique and mechanics, coordination, and building self-confidence. Children mature at varying paces and strength training programs should be individualized to accommodate for these unique differences. All strength training regimens should be modified as needed to remain age-appropriate and pain-free. Tanner staging (see Chapter 34) helps to define readiness for progression to more strenuous programs. Power lifting and maximal weight lifting should be restricted to athletes who have reached or passed Tanner stage V. To prevent injuries, care should be taken to instruct children on the proper use of weight-training equipment at home. Children and adults with disabilities can benefit from weight-training programs modified to meet their specific needs.

Faigenbaum AD et al: Youth resistance training: Updated position statement paper from the national strength and conditioning association. J Strength Cond Res 2009;23(Suppl):S60–S79 [PMID: 19620931].

Myer GD et al: When to initiate integrative neuromuscular training to reduce sports-related injuries and enhance health in youth? Current Sports Medicine Reports 2011;10(3):155–166.

FITNESS AND CONDITIONING

Compared to children who are sedentary, physically active youth tend to develop greater agility and skills and maintain better fitness throughout their lifetime. Young children and adolescents should participate in 60 minutes or more of physical activity each day. To improve overall fitness and reduce the risk of injury, children and adolescents should focus on 3 different components of exercise:

1. Resistance (strength) training (progressive resistive loads in a variety of modalities)
2. Neuromuscular conditioning (mixture of basic fundamental and specialized motor control exercises aimed at improving general health and sports performance)

   Examples: core strength exercises, agility, plyometrics
3. Integrative training (curriculum of diverse skills, increasing fitness, and appropriate rest periods)

   Examples: developing fundamental skills and technique, learning proper movement mechanics, aerobic and anaerobic conditioning

Periodization is a training concept that emphasizes variations in the volume and intensity of training throughout the year in a conditioning program. Continuously varying the specific type and goals of training provides adequate recovery from each strenuous exercise session and avoids overtraining, burnout, and overuse injuries.

Myer GD et al: When to initiate integrative neuromuscular training to reduce sports-related injuries and enhance health in youth? Current Sports Medicine Reports 2011;10(3):155–166.

SPORTS NUTRITION

Proper nutrition in young athletes focuses on maintaining an appropriate energy balance, creating healthy eating and hydration habits, and avoiding harmful food, drink, and supplement choices. Keeping an adequate nutritional intake will increase lean muscle mass, maximizing strength, endurance, immunity, and training benefit. Athletes should be encouraged to balance caloric intake with energy expenditure, eat whole grains, avoid processed foods, focus on healthy fats and proteins, and maintain proper hydration. Carbohydrates should compose 55%–60% of a young athlete's diet, with fat and protein making up 25%–30% and 12%–15% respectively. Hydration can come mainly from water if the exercise lasts less than 1 hour, after which time a carbohydrate-containing sports drink is appropriate. Water or sports drinks should be consumed every 15–20 minutes during prolonged exercise greater than 1 hour or in hot playing conditions. A light snack and hydration are recommended prior to and immediately after an extended workout. To avoid excessive caloric and sugar intake, sports drinks are not recommended at meals or times other than prolonged exercise. The average athlete eats a well-balanced diet not necessitating nutritional supplementation. However, if food allergies or improper dietary intake is confirmed, an athlete may benefit from a daily multivitamin. In general, nutritional sports supplements are not recommended and extreme caution is suggested when considering their use. The supplement industry is not well-regulated and contamination with toxic and banned substances has been noted in the past. Similarly, energy drinks are not recommended for use in any youth under the age of 18 years due to high levels of caffeine and other stimulants contained in such beverages.

ACSM, ADA, DOC: Nutrition and athletic performance. Medicine and Science in Sports and Exercise 2009;709–731.

Kleinman R (editor): *Pediatric Nutrition Handbook*, 6th edition. 2009:AAP.

Montain S: Hydration recommendations for sport 2008. Current Sports Medicine Reports 2008;187–192.

PREPARTICIPATION PHYSICAL EVALUATION

The ultimate goal of the preparticipation physical evaluation (PPE) is to promote the health and safety of athletes. Its primary objectives are to screen for conditions that may be life threatening or disabling and for conditions that may predispose to injury or illness. Secondary objectives of the PPE include: establishing a medical home, determining the general health of the individual, assessing fitness for specific sports, and counseling on injury prevention and health related issues. The ideal timing of the examination is at least 6–8 weeks before training starts. This allows time to further evaluate, treat, or rehabilitate any identified problems.

Preparticipation History

The medical history is the most important part of the encounter, identifying 65%–77% of medical and musculoskeletal conditions. Therefore, obtaining a thorough and accurate history is essential in identifying conditions that may affect a child's ability to safely participate in sports. Many key elements should be explored with the athlete. An updated standardized PPE form, endorsed by six medical societies including the American Academy of Pediatrics, is available in the fourth edition of the PPE monograph (Bernhardt DT, 2010) or on the internet. Figure 27–1A contains examples of the essential questions contained in a preparticipation history. The history includes the following areas:

PREPARTICIPATION HISTORY

Name ______________________________ DOB __________ Age ______ Sex (M or F)

Primary Physician ____________________ Sports ______________________________

Allergies (medications, latex, foods, bees, etc) ______________________________

Medications (Include prescription, nonprescription, supplements and vitamins) ______________________________

____

Answer questions by checking yes (Y)/no (N)/don't know (?)

	Y	N	?
General Health			
1. Have you had any injuries or illnesses?			
2. Have you ever been hospitalized?			
3. Do you think you are too thin or overweight?			
4. Have you ever used anything to gain or lose weight?			
5. Any problems exercising in the heat: heat cramps, heat exhaustion, or heat stroke?			
6. Ever had frostbite?			
7. Any vision problems?			
8. Do you wear glasses, contact lens, or eye protection?			
9. Any dental appliances?			
10. Have you had any surgeries?			
11. Any organs missing?			
12. Immunizations (tetanus/hepatitis B) are they current?			
13. Any concerns about participating in sports?			
Cardiac/Respiratory History			
1. Has any family member died suddenly, had heart disease before age 50 or other heart problems?			
2. Do you have any dizziness, chest pain, a racing heart, or shortness of breath with exercise?			
3. Have you ever passed out?			
4. Do you have a heart murmur, high blood pressure, or any heart condition?			
5. Can you exercise as much as your friends?			
6. Any history of asthma, problems breathing, coughing with exercise?			
Neurologic History			
1. Any history of a head injury/concussion: being knocked out, dazed, or having memory loss?			
2. Have you ever had a seizure or convulsion?			
3. Any never problems: stingers, burners, pinched serves numbness?			
4. Any problems with headaches?			
Musculoskeletal History			
1. Do you have a history of sprains, strains or fractures?			
2. Any hip, knee or ankle injuries?			
3. Any shoulder, elbow, wrist hand or finger injuries?			
4. Any back or neck problems?			
5. Ever have to be in a splint, east or use crutches?			
6. Do you use any special equipment when competing (braces, orthotics, pads, etc)			
Females Only			
1. Any problems with menstruation: cramps, irregularity, etc?			
2. When was your last period? ______________________________			

COMMENT ON YES ANSWERS

____

____

____

____

____

____

▲ **Figure 27–1.** A: Preparticipation Physical Evaluation form.

PREPARTICIPATION PHYSICAL EVALUATION
HISTORY FORM

(Note: This form is to be filled out by the patient and parent prior to seeing the physician. The physician should keep this form in the chart.)

Date of Exam ______________________________

Name ______________________________ Date of birth ______________

Sex ______ Age ______ Grade ______ School ______________ Sport(s) ______________

Medicines and Allergies: Please list all of the prescription and over-the-counter medicines and supplements (herbal and nutritional) that you are currently taking

____

____

____

Do you have any allergies? ☐ Yes ☐ No If yes, please identify specific allergy below.
☐ Medicines ☐ Pollens ☐ Food ☐ Stinging Insects

Explain "Yes" answers below. Circle questions you don't know the answers to.

GENERAL QUESTIONS	Yes	No
1. Has a doctor ever denied or restricted your participation in sports for any reason?		
2. Do you have any ongoing medical conditions? If so, please identify below: ☐ Asthma ☐ Anemia ☐ Diabetes ☐ Infections Other: ______		
3. Have you ever spent the night in the hospital?		
4. Have you ever had surgery?		
HEART HEALTH QUESTIONS ABOUT YOU	**Yes**	**No**
5. Have you ever passed out or nearly passed out DURING or AFTER exercise?		
6. Have you ever had discomfort, pain, tightness, or pressure in your chest during exercise?		
7. Does your heart ever race or skip beats (irregular beats) during exercise?		
8. Has a doctor ever told you that you have any heart problems? If so, check all that apply: ☐ High blood pressure ☐ A heart murmur ☐ High cholesterol ☐ A heart infection ☐ Kawasaki disease Other: ______		
9. Has a doctor ever ordered a test for your heart? (For example, ECG/EKG, echocardiogram)		
10. Do you get lightheaded or feel more short of breath than expected during exercise?		
11. Have you ever had an unexplained seizure?		
12. Do you get more tired or short of breath more quickly than your friends during exercise?		
HEART HEALTH QUESTIONS ABOUT YOUR FAMILY	**Yes**	**No**
13. Has any family member or relative died of heart problems or had an unexpected or unexplained sudden death before age 50 (including drowning, unexplained car accident, or sudden infant death syndrome)?		
14. Does anyone in your family have hypertrophic cardiomyopathy, Marfan syndrome, arrhythmogenic right ventricular cardiomyopathy, long QT syndrome, short QT syndrome, Brugada syndrome, or catecholaminergic polymorphic ventricular tachycardia?		
15. Does anyone in your family have a heart problem, pacemaker, or implanted defibrillator?		
16. Has anyone in your family had unexplained fainting, unexplained seizures, or near drowning?		
BONE AND JOINT QUESTIONS	**Yes**	**No**
17. Have you ever had an injury to a bone, muscle, ligament, or tendon that caused you to miss a practice or a game?		
18. Have you ever had any broken or fractured bones or dislocated joints?		
19. Have you ever had an injury that required x-rays, MRI, CT scan, injections, therapy, a brace, a cast, or crutches?		
20. Have you ever had a stress fracture?		
21. Have you ever been told that you have or have you had an x-ray for neck instability or atlantoaxial instability? (Down syndrome or dwarfism)		
22. Do you regularly use a brace, orthotics, or other assistive device?		
23. Do you have a bone, muscle, or joint injury that bothers you?		
24. Do any of your joints become painful, swollen, feel warm, or look red?		
25. Do you have any history of juvenile arthritis or connective tissue disease?		

MEDICAL QUESTIONS	Yes	No
26. Do you cough, wheeze, or have difficulty breathing during or after exercise?		
27. Have you ever used an inhaler or taken asthma medicine?		
28. Is there anyone in your family who has asthma?		
29. Were you born without or are you missing a kidney, an eye, a testicle (males), your spleen, or any other organ?		
30. Do you have groin pain or a painful bulge or hernia in the groin area?		
31. Have you had infectious mononucleosis (mono) within the last month?		
32. Do you have any rashes, pressure sores, or other skin problems?		
33. Have you had a herpes or MRSA skin infection?		
34. Have you ever had a head injury or concussion?		
35. Have you ever had a hit or blow to the head that caused confusion, prolonged headache, or memory problems?		
36. Do you have a history of seizure disorder?		
37. Do you have headaches with exercise?		
38. Have you ever had numbness, tingling, or weakness in your arms or legs after being hit or falling?		
39. Have you ever been unable to move your arms or legs after being hit or falling?		
40. Have you ever become ill while exercising in the heat?		
41. Do you get frequent muscle cramps when exercising?		
42. Do you or someone in your family have sickle cell trait or disease?		
43. Have you had any problems with your eyes or vision?		
44. Have you had any eye injuries?		
45. Do you wear glasses or contact lenses?		
46. Do you wear protective eyewear, such as goggles or a face shield?		
47. Do you worry about your weight?		
48. Are you trying to or has anyone recommended that you gain or lose weight?		
49. Are you on a special diet or do you avoid certain types of foods?		
50. Have you ever had an eating disorder?		
51. Do you have any concerns that you would like to discuss with a doctor?		
FEMALES ONLY		
52. Have you ever had a menstrual period?		
53. How old were you when you had your first menstrual period?		
54. How many periods have you had in the last 12 months?		

Explain "yes" answers here

____

____

____

____

____

____

____

____

I hereby state that, to the best of my knowledge, my answers to the above questions are complete and correct.

Signature of athlete ______________ Signature of parent/guardian ______________ Date ______

▲ **Figure 27–1.** B: Preparticipation examination.

PREPARTICIPATION PHYSICAL EVALUATION

THE ATHLETE WITH SPECIAL NEEDS: SUPPLEMENTAL HISTORY FORM

Date of Exam ______________________

Name ______________________ Date of birth ______________________

Sex ______ Age ______ Grade ______ School ______________________ Sport(s) ______________________

1. Type of disability		
2. Date of disability		
3. Classification (if available)		
4. Cause of disability (birth, disease, accident/trauma, other)		
5. List the sports you are interested in playing		
	Yes	**No**
6. Do you regularly use a brace, assistive device, or prosthetic?		
7. Do you use any special brace or assistive device for sports?		
8. Do you have any rashes, pressure sores, or any other skin problems?		
9. Do you have a hearing loss? Do you use a hearing aid?		
10. Do you have a visual impairment?		
11. Do you use any special devices for bowel or bladder function?		
12. Do you have burning or discomfort when urinating?		
13. Have you had autonomic dysreflexia?		
14. Have you ever been diagnosed with a heat-related (hyperthermia) or cold-related (hypothermia) illness?		
15. Do you have muscle spasticity?		
16. Do you have frequent seizures that cannot be controlled by medication?		

Explain "yes" answers here

____

____

____

____

____

Please indicate if you have ever had any of the following.

	Yes	No
Atlantoaxial instability		
X-ray evaluation for atlantoaxial instability		
Dislocated joints (more than one)		
Easy bleeding		
Enlarged spleen		
Hepatitis		
Osteopenia or osteoporosis		
Difficulty controlling bowel		
Difficulty controlling bladder		
Numbness or tingling in arms or hands		
Numbness or tingling in legs or feet		
Weakness in arms or hands		
Weakness in legs or feet		
Recent change in coordination		
Recent change in ability to walk		
Spina bifida		
Latex allergy		

Explain "yes" answers here

____

____

____

____

____

I hereby state that, to the best of my knowledge, my answers to the above questions are complete and correct.

Signature of athlete ______________________ Signature of parent/guardian ______________________ Date ______________

▲ **Figure 27–1.** B: Preparticipation examination. (*Continued*)

PREPARTICIPATION PHYSICAL EVALUATION
PHYSICAL EXAMINATION FORM

Name ______________________________ Date of birth ______________

PHYSICIAN REMINDERS

1. Consider additional questions on more sensitive issues
   - Do you feel stressed out or under a lot of pressure?
   - Do you ever feel sad, hopeless, depressed, or anxious?
   - Do you feel safe at your home or residence?
   - Have you ever tried cigarettes, chewing tobacco, snuff, or dip?
   - During the past 30 days, did you use chewing tobacco, snuff, or dip?
   - Do you drink alcohol or use any other drugs?
   - Have you ever taken anabolic steroids or used any other performance supplement?
   - Have you ever taken any supplements to help you gain or lose weight or improve your performance?
   - Do you wear a seat belt, use a helmet, and use condoms?
2. Consider reviewing questions on cardiovascular symptoms (questions 5–14).

EXAMINATION				
Height	Weight	☐ Male ☐ Female		
BP / (/)	Pulse	Vision R 20/	L 20/	Corrected ☐ Y ☐ N

MEDICAL	NORMAL	ABNORMAL FINDINGS
Appearance • Marfan stigmata (kyphoscoliosis, high-arched palate, pectus excavatum, arachnodactyly, arm span > height, hyperlaxity, myopia, MVP, aortic insufficiency)		
Eyes/ears/nose/throat • Pupils equal • Hearing		
Lymph nodes		
Heart[a] • Murmurs (auscultation standing, supine, +/- Valsalva) • Location of point of maximal impulse (PMI)		
Pulses • Simultaneous femoral and radial pulses		
Lungs		
Abdomen		
Genitourinary (males only)[b]		
Skin • HSV, lesions suggestive of MRSA, tinea corporis		
Neurologic[c]		
MUSCULOSKELETAL		
Neck		
Back		
Shoulder/arm		
Elbow/forearm		
Wrist/hand/fingers		
Hip/thigh		
Knee		
Leg/ankle		
Foot/toes		
Functional • Duck-walk, single leg hop		

[a]Consider ECG, echocardiogram, and referral to cardiology for abnormal cardiac history or exam.
[b]Consider GU exam if in private setting. Having third party present is recommended.
[c]Consider cognitive evaluation or baseline neuropsychiatric testing if a history of significant concussion.

☐ Cleared for all sports without restriction

☐ Cleared for all sports without restriction with recommendations for further evaluation or treatment for ______________________________

☐ Not cleared

- ☐ Pending further evaluation
- ☐ For any sports
- ☐ For certain sports ______________________________

Reason ______________________________

Recommendations ______________________________

I have examined the above-named student and completed the preparticipation physical evaluation. The athlete does not present apparent clinical contraindications to practice and participate in the sport(s) as outlined above. A copy of the physical exam is on record in my office and can be made available to the school at the request of the parents. If conditions arise after the athlete has been cleared for participation, the physician may rescind the clearance until the problem is resolved and the potential consequences are completely explained to the athlete (and parents/guardians).

Name of physician (print/type) ______________________________ Date ______________

Address ______________________________ Phone ______________

Signature of physician ______________________________, MD or DO

HE0503 9-2681/0410

▲ **Figure 27–1.** B: Preparticipation examination. (*Continued*)

PREPARTICIPATION PHYSICAL EVALUATION
CLEARANCE FORM

Name ______________________ Sex ☐ M ☐ F Age __________ Date of birth __________

☐ Cleared for all sports without restriction

☐ Cleared for all sports without restriction with recommendations for further evaluation or treatment for ______________________

____

☐ Not cleared

☐ Pending further evaluation

☐ For any sports

☐ For certain sports ______________________

Reason ______________________

Recommendations ______________________

____

____

____

____

____

I have examined the above-named student and completed the preparticipation physical evaluation. The athlete does not present apparent clinical contraindications to practice and participate in the sport(s) as outlined above. A copy of the physical exam is on record in my office and can be made available to the school at the request of the parents. If conditions arise after the athlete has been cleared for participation, the physician may rescind the clearance until the problem is resolved and the potential consequences are completely explained to the athlete (and parents/guardians).

Name of physician (print/type) ______________________ Date __________

Address ______________________ Phone __________

Signature of physician ______________________, MD or DO

EMERGENCY INFORMATION

Allergies ______________________

____

____

____

____

____

Other information ______________________

____

____

____

____

____

____

____

____

____

▲ **Figure 27–1.** B: Preparticipation examination. (*Continued*)

A. Cardiovascular History

The routine use of ECG and echocardiography in the preparticipation cardiovascular screening in athletes remains a highly debated topic in sports medicine and sports cardiology. Currently, the American Heart Association recommends against its usage in asymptomatic athletes due to its low sensitivity, high false-positive rate, limited resources, lack of trained physicians to interpret the ECG, and poor cost effectiveness because of the low prevalence of disease. In 2007, the American Heart Association (AHA) updated its consensus statement on cardiovascular screening stating its position to this effect. According to the AHA, the goal of the preparticipation physical evaluation is to reduce cardiovascular risk associated with physical activity. It recommends cardiovascular screening be incorporated into the PPE and that the evaluation be standardized to include a twelve point screen:

Personal Medical History:

1. Chest pain or discomfort with exercise
2. Syncope or near syncope associated with exercise
3. Excessive shortness or breath or fatigue associated with exertion
4. History of heart murmur
5. History of elevated blood pressure

Family Medical History:

6. Premature death before age 50 year due to heart disease
7. Disability from heart disease in a close relative less than 50 year of age
8. Knowledge of specific cardiac conditions: hypertrophic or dilated cardiomyopathy, long QT syndrome, other ion channelopathies, Marfan syndrome, or arrhythmias

Physical Exam:

9. Auscultation of heart murmur in supine and standing position
10. Palpation of radial and femoral pulses
11. Physical stigmata of Marfan syndrome
12. Brachial blood pressure taken in seated position

Sudden cardiac arrest is the leading cause of death in young athletes, accounting for 75% of all sudden deaths. Addressing these areas may help identify potentially life-threatening cardiac lesions. In the United States, the most common causes of sudden cardiac death on the playing field are hypertrophic cardiomyopathy (HCM) and congenital coronary artery anomalies, with HCM accounting for one-third of sudden cardiac death in young athletes. Any athletes with cardiovascular symptoms require further evaluation before allowing them to participate in sports. Any activity restrictions or sports disqualification for an athlete should be made in consultation with a cardiologist.

B. History of Hypertension

Any history of hypertension requires investigation for secondary causes of hypertension and target organ disease. Athletes should also be asked about the use of stimulants (ie, caffeine, nicotine) and a family history of hypertension. The diagnosis of hypertension in children less than 18 years of age is based on gender, age, height, and the blood pressure must be measured on three separate occasions. Blood pressure measurements with values from 90% to 95% of gender, age, and height-based norms are considered prehypertension; values from 95% to 5 mm Hg above the 99% of norms are defined as stage I hypertension; and values > 5 mm Hg above the 99% of norms are defined as stage 2 hypertension. Athletes who have stage 2 hypertension or end-organ damage should not be cleared to participate in competitive sports until their blood pressure is evaluated, treated, and under control.

C. Central Nervous System

A history of frequent or exertional headaches, seizure disorders, concussion or head injuries, recurrent stingers or burners, or cervical cord neuropraxia may affect an athlete's ability to participate in sports. These conditions require further evaluation, rehabilitation, or informed decision-making prior to clearance for sports participation.

D. History of Chronic Diseases

Diseases such as reactive airway disease, exercise-induced asthma, diabetes, renal disease, liver disease, chronic infections, or hematologic diseases should be noted.

E. Surgical History

Surgical history may influence participation in certain sports. Full recovery with no long-term impact on athletic performance is required prior to clearance.

F. Infectious Mononucleosis

Ask about infectious mononucleosis in the last four weeks. The risk for splenic rupture is highest within the first three weeks of illness and can occur in the absence of trauma. Therefore, physical activity should be avoided during the first three to four weeks after the infection starts. The athlete may return to play once clinical symptoms are resolved and risk for splenic rupture is assessed as minimal. The use of serial abdominal ultrasound to assess spleen size to aid in return to play decisions is debatable. Parameters for spleen size based on ethnicity, sex, height, and weight have not yet been established so determining when spleen size has normalized based on imaging becomes difficult.

G. Musculoskeletal Limitations and Prior Injuries

The physician should inquire about joints with limited range of motion, muscle weakness, and prior injuries that may affect future performance. Chronic pain or soreness long after activity may reflect overuse syndromes that should be evaluated.

H. Menstrual History in Females

The physician should pay particular attention to the so-called female athletic triad: amenorrhea, eating disorders, and osteoporosis.

I. Nutritional Issues

The physician should record methods the athlete uses to maintain, gain, or lose weight.

J. Medication History

Inquire about the use of prescription, over-the-counter medications, and supplements. Not only will medications reveal problems omitted in the medical history but the information will also provide data on current medications whose side effects may suggest activity modifications. Documenting drug use may provide the opportunity to explore with the patient the drawbacks of performance-enhancing compounds such as anabolic steroids, creatine, stimulants, and narcotics.

Armsey TD, Hosey RG: Medical aspects of sports: Epidemiology of injuries, preparticipation examination and drugs in sports. Clin Sports Med 2004;23:255 [PMID: 15183571].

Bernhardt DT, Roberts WO: *Preparticipation Physical Evaluation.* 4th Ed. American Academy of Pediatrics 2010.

Burrows M et al: The components of the female athlete triad do not identify all physically active females at risk. J Sports Sci 2007;25:12 [PMID: 17786682].

Gregory AJ, Fitch RW: Sports medicine: Performance-enhancing drugs. Pediatr Clin North Am 2007;54:797–806 [PMID: 17723878].

Maron BJ: Sudden death in young athletes. N Engl J Med 2003; 349(11):1064–1075.

Maron BJ et al: Profile and frequency of sudden death in 1463 young competitive athletes: From a 25 year U.S. national registry: 1980–2005. Circulation 2006;114:II(18):830.

Maron BJ et al: Recommendations and considerations related to preparticipation screening for cardiovascular abnormalities in competitive athletes: 2007 update: A scientific statement from the American Heart Association Council on Nutrition, Physical Activity and Metabolism: endorsed by the American College of Cardiology Foundation. Circulation 2007;115(12).

Maron BJ et al: Cardiovascular preparticipation screening of competitive athletes. A statement for health professionals from the Sudden Death Committee and Congenital Cardiac Defects Committee, American Heart Association. Circulation 1996;94(4):850–856.

National Blood Pressure Education Program Working Group on High Blood Pressure in Children and Adolescents: The fourth report on the diagnosis, evaluation and treatment of high blood pressure in children and adults. Pediatrics 2004;114:555–576.

Putukian M, O'Connor FG, Stricker P: Mononucleosis and athletic participation: An evidence-based subject review. Clin J Sport Med 2008;18(4):309–315.

Physical Examination

The physical examination should be focused on the needs of the athlete. It may be the only time an athlete has contact with medical personnel and can be used to promote wellness along with screening for physical activity. Figure 27–1B is an example of a preparticipation physical examination form endorsed in the fourth edition of the Preparticipation Physical Evaluation monograph (Bernhardt DT: 2010). The examination should include routine vital signs, including blood pressure measurements obtained in the upper extremity. The cardiovascular examination should include palpation of pulses, auscultation for murmurs while sitting and standing, evaluation for physical stigmata of Marfan syndrome, and assessment of any cardiovascular symptoms as previously described. The musculoskeletal examination is used to determine strength, range of motion, flexibility, and previous injuries. Included is a quick guide that can be used to screen for musculoskeletal abnormalities (Table 27–1). The remainder of the examination should emphasize the following areas:

A. Skin

Are there any contagious lesions such as herpes or impetigo?

B. Vision

Are there any visual problems? Is there any evidence of retinal problems? Are both eyes intact?

C. Abdomen

Is there any evidence of hepatosplenomegaly?

D. Genitourinary System

Are any testicular abnormalities or hernias present?

E. Neurologic System

Are there any problems with coordination, gait, or mental processing?

F. Sexual Maturity

What is the individual's Tanner stage?

Recommendations for Participation

After completing the medical evaluation, the physician can make recommendations about sports clearance. The options are:

- Cleared for all sports without restrictions
- Cleared for all sports without restrictions with recommendations for further evaluation or treatment
- Not cleared: pending further evaluation, for any sports, or for certain sports

Table 27–1. The screening sports examination.[a]

General evaluation	Have patient stand in front of examiner; evaluate both front and back along with posture. Look at general body habitus. Look for asymmetry in muscle bulk, scars, or unusual postures. Watch how patient moves when instructed.
Neck evaluation	Evaluate range of motion (ROM) by having patient bend head forward (chin to chest), rotate from side to side and laterally bend (ear to shoulder). Observe for asymmetry, lack of motion, or pain with movement.
Shoulder and upper extremity evaluation	Observe clavicles, shoulder position, scapular position, elbow position, and fingers. ROM screening: Fully abduct arms with palms in jumping jack position. Internally and externally rotate shoulder. Flex and extend wrist, pronate and supinate wrist, flex and extend fingers. Do the following manual muscle testing: Have patient shrug shoulders (testing trapezius). Abduct to 90 degrees (testing deltoid). Flex elbow (testing biceps). Extend elbow over head (testing triceps). Test wrist flexion and extension. Have patient grasp fingers.
Back evaluation	General inspection to look for scoliosis or kyphosis. ROM screening: Bend forward touching toes with knees straight (spine flexion and hamstring range). Rotation, side bending, and spine extension.
Gait and lower extremity evaluation	General observation while walking. Have patient walk short distance normally (look at symmetry, heel-toe gait pattern, look at all joints involved in gait and leg lengths, any evidence of joint effusions or pain). Have patient toe-walk and heel-walk for short distance and check tandem walking (balance beam walking).

[a]If any abnormalities are found, a more focused evaluation is required.

Table 27–2 is a composite of recommendations for sports participation organized by body system. Recommendations for sports participation in specific medical conditions can be found on the American Academy of Pediatrics (AAP) website.

Anderson BR, Vetter VL: Return to play? Practical considerations for young athletes with cardiovascular disease. Br J Sports Med 2009;43:690 [PMID: 19734504].

Ansved T: Muscular dystrophies: Influence of physical conditioning on the disease evolution. Curr Opin Clin Nutr Metab Care 2003;6:435 [PMID: 12806128].

Bernhardt DT, Roberts WO: *Preparticipation Physical Evaluation*. 4th Ed. American Academy of Pediatrics 2010.

Firoozi S et al: Risk of competitive sport in young athletes with heart disease. Heart 2003;89:710 [PMID: 12807837].

Glover DW, Glover DW, Maron BJ: Evolution in the process of screening United States high school student-athletes for cardiovascular disease. Am J Cardiol 2007;100:1709–1712 [PMID: 18036373].

Howard GM et al: Epilepsy and sports participation. Curr Sports Med Rep 2004;3:15 [PMID: 14728909].

Maron BJ et al: Recommendations and considerations related to preparticipation screening for cardiovascular abnormalities in competitive athletes: 2007 update: A scientific statement from the American Heart Association Council on Nutrition, Physical Activity, and Metabolism. Circulation 2007;115:1643–1655 [PMID: 17353433].

Murphy NA, Carbone PS: Council on Children with Disabilities: Clinical report: Promoting the participation of children with disabilities in sports, recreation and physical activity. Pediatr 2008;121:1057–1061 [PMID: 18450913].

Platt LS: Medical and orthopaedic conditions in Special Olympics athletes. J Athl Train 2001;36:74 [PMID: 16404438].

Rice SG and the Council on Sports Medicine and Fitness, American Academy of Pediatrics: Medical conditions affecting sports participation. Pediatrics 2008;121(4):841–848.

Tucker A, Grady M: Role of the adolescent preparticipation physical examination. Phys Med Rehabil Clin N Am 2008;19:217–234 [PMID: 18395645].

Winell J, Burke SW: Sports participation of children with Down syndrome. Orthop Clin North Am 2003;34:439 [PMID: 12975593].

Ansved T: Muscular dystrophies: Influence of physical conditioning on the disease evolution. Curr Opin Clin Nutr Metab Care 2003;6:435 [PMID: 12806128].

Braith RW: Exercise for those with chronic heart failure. Phys Sportsmed 2002;31:29.

Birrer RB, Sedaghat V: Exercise and diabetes mellitus: Optimizing performance in patients who have type 1 diabetes. Phys Sportsmed 2003;30:29.

Disabella V, Sherman C: Your guide to exercising with asthma. Phys Sportsmed 1998;26:85.

Draznin MB: Type 1 diabetes and sports participation: Strategies for training and competing safely. Phys Sportsmed 2000;28:49.

Firoozi S et al: Risk of competitive sport in young athletes with heart disease. Heart 2003;89:710 [PMID: 12807837].

Howard GM et al: Epilepsy and sports participation. Curr Sports Med Rep 2004;3:15.

Howe WB: Preventing infectious disease in sports. Phys Sportsmed 2003;31:23.

MacKnight JM: Infectious mononucleosis: Ensuring safe return to sport. Phys Sportsmed 2002;31:27.

Table 27–2. Recommendations and considerations for participation in sports.

Disorders	Considerations and Recommendations	References
Cardiac		
Anticoagulation treatment	Need to avoid all contact sports.	
Aortic stenosis	Individualize treatment based on extent of disease and systolic gradient: Mild: < 20 mm Hg, all sports if asymptomatic. Moderate: limited sports. Severe: no competitive sports.	
Arrhythmias	Long-QT syndrome, malignant ventricular arrhythmias, symptomatic Wolff-Parkinson-White syndrome, advanced heart block, family history of sudden death or previous sudden cardiac event, and implantation of a cardioverter-defibrillator. May participate: qualified yes. Consult with cardiologist.	Rice 2008
Arrhythmogenic right ventricular cardiomyopathy	May participate: qualified no. Consult with cardiologist.	Rice 2008
Carditis	May participate: qualified no. May result in sudden death with exertion.	Rice 2008
Congenital heart disease	May participate: qualified yes. Consult with cardiologist. Mild, moderate and severe disease for cardiac lesions are defined by the 36th Bethesda Conference. Those with mild lesions may fully participate in most cases. Those with moderate or severe lesions or who have undergone surgery need further evaluation.	Maron 2005
Coronary artery anomalies	May participate: qualified no. Consult with cardiologist.	Rice 2008
Ehlers-Danlos syndrome, vascular form	May participate: qualified no. Consult with cardiologist.	Rice 2008
Heart failure	Screen patient with LVEF < 30% for ischemia. Use AHA risk stratification criteria to define exercise capacity.	Braith 2002
Heart implants	No jumping, swimming, or contact sports.	
Hypertrophic cardiomyopathy	May participate: qualified no. Athletes should not participate in sports except possibly low-intensity forms (eg, golf, bowling). Consult with cardiologist.	Maron 2002a, b
Hypertension	May participate: qualified yes. Those with hypertension > 5 mm Hg above 99th percentile for age, gender, and height should avoid heavy weightlifting and power lifting, bodybuilding, and high-static component sports.	Rice 2008
Marfan syndrome	Aortic root dilation is associated with mitral valve prolapse and regurgitation. May participate: qualified yes. Participate in sports with minimal physical demands.	Salim et al 2001
Mitral valve prolapse	May participate: qualified yes. No restrictions unless there is a history of syncope, positive family history of sudden death, arrhythmias with exercise, or moderate regurgitation.	
Syncope	Unexplained syncopal episodes during exercise must be evaluated by ECG, echocardiograph, Holter and tilt test prior to resumption of any activities.	Firoozi 2002
Vasculitis/vascular disease	Kawasaki disease, pulmonary hypertension. May participate: qualified yes. Consult with cardiologist.	Rice 2008

(Continued)

Table 27–2. Recommendations and considerations for participation in sports. (*Continued*)

Disorders	Considerations and Recommendations	References
Endocrine		
Diabetes mellitus type 1	No restrictions to activity, however: Short-term exercise = no insulin changes. Vigorous exercise may require 25% reduction in insulin with 15–30 g of carbohydrates before and every 30 min during exercise. Strenuous exercise = may require up to an 80% reduction in insulin with extra carbohydrates. Generally monitor blood glucose closely.	Birrer et al 2003, Draznin 2000
Eye		
Detached retina	Do not participate in strenuous sports regardless of contact risk.	Moeller 1996
Functionally one eyed	Defined as having best corrected visual acuity worse than 20/40 in the poorest seeing eye. Consider avoiding contact sports, although if patient does participate use of eye protection is mandatory.	Vinger 2000
Genitourinary		
One testicle	Need to wear protective cups in collision and contact sports.	
Solitary kidney	May participate: qualified yes. Protective equipment may reduce risk of injury to remaining kidney sufficiently to allow participation in most sports.	Rice 2008
Hematologic		
Hemophilia	Avoid contact and collision sports.	
Sickle cell disease	May participate: qualified yes. If illness status permits, all sports may be played. However, any sport or activity that entails over-exertion, overheating, dehydration, or chilling should be avoided. Participation at high altitude poses risk for sickle cell crisis.	Rice 2008
Sickle cell trait	May participate: yes. Under normal environmental conditions, no increased risk of sudden death or other medical problems. Ensure acclimatization to extreme environment conditions (eg, altitude, heat, humidity) and adequate hydration during participation to reduce risk of heat illness and/or rhabdomyolysis.	Rice 2008
Infectious disease		
Fever	May participate: no. Cardiopulmonary effort is increased while maximum exercise capacity is decreased during febrile illnesses. Risk of heat illness is also increased.	Rice 2008
Enterovirus	Coxsackievirus causes respiratory and GI symptoms but more importantly can cause myocarditis. Anyone with systemic symptoms such as fever or myalgias should avoid strenuous exercise.	Primos 1996
Infectious mononucleosis	Splenic rupture is most important consideration. Risk of spleen rupture highest during first three weeks of illness. No athletic participation during the first three to four weeks after the infection starts. Too early a return to sports increases risk of splenic rupture or could cause EBV reactivation and relapse. If symptoms resolve by third week, light activities can be started during the fourth week with graded increases in intensity. Full contact activity participation may resume at week five.	Putukian 2008

(*Continued*)

Table 27–2. Recommendations and considerations for participation in sports. (*Continued*)

Disorders	Considerations and Recommendations	References
Skin infections	Herpes simplex, molluscum contagiosum, warts, staphylococcal and streptococcal infections, impetigo, scabies and tinea. May participate: qualified yes. During contagious periods, participation in gymnastics or cheerleading with mats, martial arts, wrestling, or other collision, contact or limited contact sports is not allowed.	Rice 2008
Sinusitis	Similar considerations as cold (see below) except diving should be restricted until symptoms resolve.	
Streptococcus group A	Restrict from activity until afebrile and on antibiotics for > 24 h.	O'Kane 2002
Upper respiratory infections (including common cold)	"Neck check," with symptoms (fevers, myalgias, arthralgias, etc) above the neck participation can be allowed; however, if they migrate below that level activity should be limited.	Primos 1996
Neurologic		
Epilepsy	Majority of sports are safe for those with good seizure control; contact sports are allowed with proper protection. Definitely wear a helmet. Fitness may reduce number of seizures. Swimming and water sports should be supervised. Sports such as free climbing, hang gliding, and scuba are not recommended.	Howard 2004
Herniated disk (with cord compression)	Avoid contact and collision sports.	
Muscle disease or myopathy	Exercise within physical limits. Low- to moderate-intensity activity is appropriate for patients with slow progressive disorders. Patients with disorders that are rapidly progressing should avoid high-resistance and eccentric muscle activity. With eccentric exercise, muscles elongate during contraction and oppose the force of gravity (eg, lowering of weights), resulting in high levels of tension in the muscle. Modification of exercise with intercurrent illness is also necessary.	Tarnopolsky 2002, Ansved 2003
Spinal stenosis	Avoid contact and collision sports.	
Orthopedic		
Scoliosis	No restrictions unless severe.	
Spondylolisthesis	Grade 2 and above should avoid contact sports or sports with lumbar hyperextension.	
Spondylolysis	No restrictions if pain-free.	
Respiratory		
Asthma	No activity restrictions. Use common sense about when to use medications.	Disabella et al 1998
Pneumothorax	Can occur in sports, especially in males. Increased risk for recurrence; should consider not participating in strenuous and contact sports.	
Tuberculosis	Active infection: not allowed to participate because of exposure to other athletes.	

(*Continued*)

Table 27–2. Recommendations and considerations for participation in sports. (*Continued*)

Disorders	Considerations and Recommendations	References
Other		
Cerebral palsy	Full participation with modifications.	
Developmental disabilities	Athletes with developmental disabilities often have associated medical problems including diabetes, obesity, and hypokinesia.	Platt 2001
Down syndrome	10%–20% have atlantoaxial instability. All athletes need to be cleared with a lateral view radiograph including flexion and extension. If abnormal no contact sports should be allowed. Evaluation of underlying congenital heart disorders should be considered in this population.	Platt 2001, Winell 2003
Remote spinal cord injury or spina bifida	Full participation. Consider modification of equipment to accommodate activity or modification of activity to accommodate disability. Consider how modification affects performance. Be aware of thermoregulatory dysfunction, medications, and pressure areas.	

AHA, American Heart Association; EBV, Epstein-Barr virus; ECG, electrocardiogram; GI, gastrointestinal; LVEF, left ventricular ejection fraction; WPW, Wolff-Parkinson-White syndrome.

Maron BJ: Hypertrophic cardiomyopathy: Practical steps for preventing sudden death. Phys Sportsmed 2002a;30:19 [PMID: 11984027].

Maron BJ: The young competitive athlete with cardiovascular abnormalities: Causes of sudden death, detection by preparticipation screening, and standards for disqualification. Card Electrophysiol Rev 2002b;6:100.

Maron BJ, Zipes DP et al: 36th Bethesda Conference. Eligibility recommendations for competitive athletes with cardiovascular abnormalities. J Am Coll Cardiol 2005;45(8):1318–1321.

Moeller JL: Contraindications to athletic participation: Spinal, systemic, dermatologic, paired-organ, and other issues. Phys Sportsmed 1996;24:56.

O'Kane JW: Upper respiratory infection. Phys Sportsmed 2002;30:39.

Platt LS: Medical and orthopaedic conditions in Special Olympics athletes. J Athl Train 2001;36:74 [PMID: 16404438].

Primos WA: Sports and exercise during acute illness: Recommending the right course for patients. Phys Sportsmed 199624:44.

Putukian M, O'Connor FG, Stricker P: Mononucleosis and athletic participation: An evidence-based subject review. Clin J Sport Med 2008;18(4):309–315.

Rice SG and the Council on Sports Medicine and Fitness, American Academy of Pediatrics: Medical conditions affecting sports participation. Pediatrics 2008;121(4):841–848.

Salim MA, Alpert BS: Sports and Marfan syndrome. Phys Sportsmed 2001;29:80.

Tarnopolsky MS: Metabolic myopathies and physical activity: When fatigue is more than simple exertion. Phys Sportsmed 2002;30:37.

Terrell T et al: Blunt trauma reveals a single kidney: A disqualification dilemma. Phys Sportsmed 1997;25:75.

Vinger PF: A practical guide for sports eye protection. Phys Sportsmed 2000;28:49.

Winell J, Burke SW: Sports participation of children with Down syndrome. Orthop Clin North Am 2003;34:439 [PMID: 12975593].

REHABILITATION OF SPORTS INJURIES

Participation in sports benefits children not only by promoting physical activity but also by the acquisition of motor and social skills. All sports participation, however, carries an inherent risk of injury. Injuries are classified as either acute or chronic. Chronic injuries occur over time as a result of overuse, repetitive microtrauma, and inadequate repair of injured tissue. When the demands of exercise exceed the body's ability to recover, overuse injury may occur. Overuse injury accounts for up to 50% of all injuries in pediatric sports medicine. Risk factors for overuse include year round participation, participation in more than one sport at time, poor mechanics, and training errors such as increasing exercise volume, load, frequency, or intensity too quickly. To avoid overuse injury, athletes should train with a regular variety of resistances, power, speed, agility, skills, and distance. Adequate periods of rest and recovery should be incorporated into every training regimen in order to ensure proper healing of stressed tissues.

Acute injuries or macrotrauma are one-time events that can cause alterations in biomechanics and physiology. Response to an acute injury occurs in predictable phases.

The first week is characterized by an acute inflammatory response. During this time, initial vasoconstriction is followed by vasodilation. Chemical mediators of inflammation are released, resulting in the classical physical findings of local swelling, warmth, pain, and loss of function. This phase is essential in healing of the injury. The proliferative phase occurs over the next 2–4 weeks and involves repair and clean-up. Fibroblasts infiltrate and lay down new collagen. Lastly, the maturation phase allows for repair and regeneration of the damaged tissues.

The management of acute sports injuries focuses on optimizing healing and restoring function. The goals of immediate care are to minimize the effects of the injury by reducing pain and swelling, to educate the athlete about the nature of the injury and how to treat it, and to maintain the health and fitness of the rest of the body. The treatment for an acute injury is captured in the acronym PRICE:

- **P**rotect the injury from further damage (taping, splints, braces)
- **R**est the area
- **I**ce
- **C**ompression of the injury
- **E**levation immediately

Nonsteroidal anti-inflammatory drugs (NSAIDs) may reduce the inflammatory response and reduce discomfort. These medications may be used immediately after the injury. When safely and appropriately managed, therapeutic use of physical modalities, including early cold and later heat, hydrotherapy, massage, electrical stimulation, iontophoresis, and ultrasound, can enhance recovery in the acute phase.

The recovery phase can be lengthy and requires athlete participation. Physical therapy prescription is a common treatment modality. Initial treatment is focused on joint range of motion and flexibility. Range-of-motion exercises should follow a logical progression of starting with passive motion, then active assistive and finally active movement. Active range of motion is initiated once normal joint range has been reestablished. Flexibility exercises are sport-specific and aimed at reducing tightness of musculature. Strength training can begin early in this phase of rehabilitation. Initially only isometric exercises (static muscle contraction against stable resistance without movement of a joint or change in length of a muscle) are encouraged. As recovery progresses and flexibility increases, isotonic (change in length of a muscle without varying resistance) and isokinetic (change in length of a muscle against variable resistance without varying speed) exercises can be added to the program. These should be done at least three times per week.

As the athlete approaches near-normal strength and is pain-free, the final maintenance phase can be introduced. During this phase the athlete continues to build strength and work on endurance. The biomechanics of sport-specific activity need to be analyzed and retraining incorporated into the exercise program. Generalized cardiovascular conditioning should continue during the entire rehabilitation treatment. Typically, return-to-play guidelines after an injury include the attainment of full joint range of motion, nearly full and symmetric strength, full speed, and nearly full sport-specific agility and skill.

Present trends in injury rehabilitation and prevention focus on core stability training and dynamic warm-up and stretching. Core exercises emphasize isometric holds that activate the core and pelvis and utilize light single limb movements to challenge endurance over protracted time periods. Programs should be age-appropriate and modified as needed to exercise in a pain-free range. The development of back pain during a core program signifies poor technique, overly complicated curriculum, or a prior back injury. Exercise programs can be obtained from the website resource: http://www.webexercises.com

Dynamic warm-up and stretching programs concentrate on controlled, full active range of motion of each joint for an overall excitatory effect prior to exercise. In contrast to traditional static stretching regimens, an appropriate dynamic curriculum will incorporate aerobic activity with dynamic flexibility and sport-specific movement preparation. The aim is to initiate light perspiration and increase heart rate, peripheral circulation, and connective tissue suppleness through simple excitatory activity. Areas of focus include joint range of motion, proprioception, coordination, balance, flexibility, muscular contraction, and stimulation of the central nervous system and energy resources. Static stretching is appropriate after exercise is complete.

http://www.webexercises.com

Brooks GP et al: Musculoskeletal injury in the young athlete: Overview of rehabilitation for nonoperative injuries. UpToDate May 2011.

Faccioni A: Dynamic warm-up routines for sports. Faccioni Speed and Conditioning Consultancy 2004 [web PDF].

COMMON SPORTS MEDICINE ISSUES & INJURIES

INFECTIOUS DISEASES

Infectious diseases are common in both recreational and competitive athletes. These illnesses have an effect on basic physiologic function and athletic performance. Physicians, parents, and coaches can adopt the guidelines listed in Table 27–3.

Active skin infections are common reasons to exclude athletes from sports participation. Herpes simplex, staphylococcal, molluscum, and tinea skin infections are commonly seen and most easily transmitted in sports with skin-to-skin contact and shared equipment usage. In particular, athletes are at high risk for infection with community-associated methicillin-resistant *Staphylococcus aureus* (CA-MRSA). Recent reports of outbreaks in sports teams have prompted

Table 27–3. Sports participation guidelines: infectious diseases.

Bacterial dermatoses (including impetigo, furuncles, cellulitis, folliculitis, and abscesses)
Athlete may participate when: no new lesions for 48 h, no moist or draining lesions, and has completed oral antibiotics for at least 72 h.
Diarrhea, infectious
May participate: No
May increase risk of dehydration and heat illness. No participation is permitted unless symptoms are mild and athlete is fully hydrated.
Fever
May participate: No
Cardiopulmonary effort increases with fever and maximum exercise capacity is reduced. Heat illness also more likely to occur.
Hepatitis, infectious
May participate: Qualified yes
Minimal risk to others. May participate in all sports if health allows. Use universal precautions when handling blood or bodily fluids. Athlete should have skin lesions covered properly.
Herpes gladiatorum
Transmission occurs by skin-to-skin contact. Athlete may participate when: free of systemic symptoms, have no new lesions for 72 h, and have been on oral antiviral treatment for 120 h. Any open wounds must be properly covered.
Human immunodeficiency virus infection
May participate: Yes
Minimal risk to others. May participate in all sports if health allows. Use universal precautions when handling blood or bodily fluids. Athletes should have skin lesions covered properly with an occlusive dressing. They should also be instructed to report bleeding wounds.
Infectious mononucleosis
Splenomegaly is present in almost all cases and risk of splenic rupture is highest in the first 3 weeks of illness. Once clinical symptoms resolve, gradual return to activity 3 weeks after symptom onset is reasonable. Contact sports should be avoided until 4 weeks post-illness onset.
Methicillin-resistant *Staphylococcus aureus* (MRSA) skin infections
Athletes with suspected MRSA should be cultured and treated accordingly with antibiotics. Abscesses should be treated with incision and drainage. Athlete may return to sport when: no new lesions for 48 h, no moist or draining lesions, and have been on oral antibiotics for at least 72 h.
Molloscum contagiosum
Require appropriate covering for participation.
Streptococcal pharyngitis
Athletes can resume activity once treatment has been provided for 24 h and they are afebrile.
Warts
Require appropriate covering for participation.

many sports organizations to adopt specific protocols to deal with the problem. Transmission is primarily by skin-to-skin contact and clinical manifestations are most commonly skin infections and soft tissue abscesses. Early treatment of CA-MRSA soft tissue infections by incision and drainage followed by appropriate antibiotic treatment is important to prevent significant morbidity and possible mortality.

Benjamin HJ, Nikore V, Takagishi J: Practical management: Community-associated methicillin-resistant *Staphylococcus aureus* (CA-MRSA): The latest sports epidemic. Clin J Sport Med 2007;17:393–397 [PMID: 17873553].

Selected Issues for the Adolescent Athlete and the Team Physician: A Consensus Statement. Med Sci Sports Exerc Nov 2008;40(11):1997–2012.

Rice SG and the Council on Sports Medicine and Fitness, American Academy of Pediatrics: Medical conditions affecting sports participation. Pediatrics 2008;121(4):841–848.

HEAD & NECK INJURIES

Head and neck injuries occur most commonly in contact and individual sports. The sports with the highest incidence of brain injury are football, bicycling, baseball, and horseback riding. Concussions most commonly occur in football, ice hockey, rugby, boxing, basketball, lacrosse, soccer, and baseball/softball. The optimal treatment of these injuries has not been established and multiple guidelines have been developed. As a general rule, treatment of injuries in young children should be as conservative as possible because of their developing central nervous systems.

1. Concussion

Concussion is a complex process that occurs when a direct blow to the body or head translates forces into the brain. Even in the presence of neurologic symptoms, concussions are usually not associated with structural changes in brain tissue detectable by standard imaging studies. Instead, they may cause metabolic and vascular changes in cerebral tissues. Consequently, there are complex alterations in physiologic function, such as catecholamine surges and failure of cerebral blood flow autoregulation leading to the common symptoms we ascribe to this type of injury. Confusion, headache, visual disturbance, posttraumatic amnesia, and balance problems are common symptoms. It is important to note that concussion does not have to involve loss of consciousness. Concussion should be suspected in any athlete with somatic, cognitive, or behavioral complaints as listed in Table 27–4. In the acute setting, computed tomography (CT) is rarely indicated beyond the first 24 hours after injury. CT should be considered during initial evaluation if the patient displays altered mental status, prolonged loss of consciousness, repeated vomiting, severe headache, signs of basilar skull fracture, or has a reported history of severe mechanism of injury. Symptoms associated with concussions usually follow a predictable pattern and most resolve in 7–10 days. Younger athletes and females tend to have a longer recovery interval. Acute management of concussion includes physical and cognitive rest. In young athletes, interventions may

Table 27–4. Concussion: symptom checklist.

Headache
Confusion
Amnesia
posttraumatic
retrograde
Dizziness
Balance problems
Nausea
Vomiting
Visual disturbances
Light sensitivity
Noise sensitivity
Ringing in the ears
Fatigue or excessive sleepiness
Sleep abnormalities
Memory problems
Concentration difficulties
Irritability
Behavioral changes

include modified school attendance, decreased school work, reduction in technological stimulation (television, internet, computer games, cellular phone use), proper nutrition and hydration, and adequate rest and sleep. Before athletes are allowed to return to sports participation, symptoms should be resolved both at rest and during exercise, and a graded return-to-play protocol should be completed.

Return to play is a six-step progression with each step lasting 24 hours: (1) when asymptomatic at rest for 24 hours, then progress to (2) light aerobic exercise, followed by (3) sport-specific exercise, then begin (4) noncontact drills, followed by (5) contact practice drills, and finally (6) release to game play. If any symptoms recur during any of the steps, the athlete should not move to the next stage and should rest until symptom-free. Once symptom-free for at least 24 hours, the step-wise return to play protocol may resume, starting at the previous step where the athlete was asymptomatic. Commonly, it is recommended that an athlete follow-up with a medical provider for clearance for return to contact or collision sports. Many states have passed legislation requiring medical assessment of concussed youth and medical clearance for safe return-to-play. Notably, an athlete should not be cleared for return to physical activity on the same day of their suspected concussion injury. Likewise, athletes should not be cleared for play while still suffering from the residual symptoms of their concussion.

Preseason testing may provide a baseline to help practitioners assess acute concussive status. Among commonly used assessment tools are the Standardized Assessment of Concussion (SAC), Balance Error Scoring System (BESS), computerized testing, and symptoms checklist (Table 27–4). Neuropsychology testing is advocated for athletes with severe or prolonged symptoms. Recent findings related to multiple concussions in athletes indicate that one concussion episode places an athlete at a higher risk for a repeat concussion and that children with repeat concussions may have more severe injuries with protracted recovery times. In general, conservative return to play guidelines should be used in children.

Kuppermann N et al: Identification of children at very low risk of clinically-important brain injuries after head trauma: A prospective cohort study. The Lancet 2009;374:1160–1170.

McCrory P et al: Consensus statement on concussion in sports—The 3rd international conference on concussion in sports held in Zurich, November 2008. PM R 2009;1:406–420 [PMID: 19627927].

Randolph C: Baseline neuropsychological testing in managing sport-related concussion: Does it modify risk? Current Sports Medicine Reports 2011;10(1):21–26.

Schatz P, Moser RS: Current issues in pediatric sports concussion. Clin Neuropsychologist 2011:1–16.

2. Second Impact Syndrome

Second impact syndrome is a rare but potentially deadly complication of head injuries. There is not universal agreement on the existence of this reported phenomenon. Athletes who sustain a second head injury while still healing from a prior brain injury are at risk for a loss of vascular autoregulation, catecholamine surge, increased cerebral blood pressure, and subsequent malignant cerebral edema without intracranial hematoma. Consequences include massive brain swelling and herniation leading to seizure, coma, and possibly death. There appears to be an age-related susceptibility to second impact syndrome, with younger athletes and particularly high school athletes most vulnerable. The highest incidence has been seen in football.

Byard RW, Vink R: The second impact syndrome. Forensic Sci Med Pathol 2009;5:36–38.

Thomas M et al: Epidemiology of sudden death in young, competitive athletes due to blunt trauma. Pediatrics 2011;128:e1–e8.

Wetjen NM, Pichelmann MA, Atkinson JLD: Second impact syndrome: Concussion and second injury brain complications. J Am Coll Surg 2010;211(4):553–557.

3. Atlantoaxial Instability

Atlantoaxial instability is common in children with Down syndrome because of hypotonia and ligamentous laxity, especially including the annular ligament of C1. Consequently, this condition causes increased mobility at C1 and C2. Most cases are asymptomatic. Lateral cervical neck films in flexion, extension, and neutral position evaluate the atlanto-dens interval (ADI). ADI is normally less than 2.5 mm, but up to 4.5 mm is acceptable in this population. Children with an ADI greater than 4.5 mm should be restricted from contact and collision activities, as well as any sport requiring excessive neck flexion or extension.

Dimberg EL: Management of common neurologic conditions in sports. Clin Sports Med 2005;24:637 [PMID: 16004923].

Klenck C, Gebke K: Practical management: Common medical problems in disabled athletes. Clin J Sport Med 2007;17(1):55–60.

Winell J: Sports participation of children with Down syndrome. Orthop Clin North Am 2003;34:439 [PMID: 12974493].

4. Burners or Stingers

ESSENTIALS OF DIAGNOSIS & TYPICAL FEATURES

- Symptoms appear on the same side as an injury to the neck and shoulder.
- Burning pain or numbness in the shoulder and arm.
- Weakness may be present.

Burners or stingers are common injuries in contact sports, especially football. The two terms are used interchangeably to describe transient unilateral pain and paresthesias in the upper extremity. These cervical radiculopathies or brachial plexopathies typically occur when the head is laterally bent and the shoulder depressed, causing a compressive injury to a cervical nerve root on the symptomatic upper extremity, or a traction injury to the brachial plexus of the ipsilateral shoulder. Symptoms include immediate burning pain and paresthesias down one arm generally lasting only minutes. Unilateral weakness in the muscles of the upper trunk—supraspinatus, deltoid, and biceps—also tends to resolve quickly, but can persist for weeks. The most important part of the workup is a thorough neurologic assessment to differentiate this injury from a more serious brain or cervical spine injury. The key distinguishing feature of the stinger is its unilateral nature. If symptoms persist or include headache, change in mental status, or severe neck pain, then a diagnostic evaluation should include a careful neurological examination and possibly cervical spine radiographs including flexion/extension views, magnetic resonance imaging (MRI) scans, and electromyography (EMG).

Treatment consists of removal from play and observation. The athlete can return to play once symptoms have resolved, neck and shoulder range of motion is pain-free, reflexes and strength are normal, and the Spurling test is negative. The Spurling test is performed by having the head extended, rotated, and flexed to the ipsilateral shoulder while applying an axial load. Restriction of same day return to play should be considered in athletes with a history of multiple stingers, particularly if sustained in the same season. Preventative strategies include always wearing well-fitting protective gear, proper blocking and tackling techniques, and maintaining neck and shoulder strength. Long-term complications are possible, including permanent neurologic injury or repeated occurrence of stingers, which would necessitate further workup and possible lifetime exclusion from contact or collision sports.

Rihn JA et al: Cervical spine injuries in American football. Sports Medicine 2009;39(9):697–708.

Standaert CJ, Herring SA: Expert opinion and controversies in musculoskeletal and sports medicine: Stingers. Arch Phys Med Rehabil 2009; 90:402–406 [PMID: 19254603].

SPINE INJURIES

As children have become more competitive in sports, spine injuries have become more common. Sports with a fairly high incidence of back injuries include golf, gymnastics, football, dance, wrestling, and weightlifting. Back pain lasting more than 2 weeks indicates a possible structural problem that should be investigated.

Acute injury to the spine often results from an axial load injury. Patients present with focal tenderness of the thoracic or thoracolumbar spine. Evaluation includes plain radiography that may demonstrate anterior wedging of the thoracic vertebra, representing a compression fracture. When significant spinal tenderness or any neurological abnormalities are present, radiographs are often followed by computed tomography (CT) or MRI. Treatment of minor compression fractures includes pain control, bracing, rest from high-risk sports, and physical therapy. With appropriate rehabilitation, athletes can usually return to contact activity within 8 weeks.

1. Spondylolysis

ESSENTIALS OF DIAGNOSIS & TYPICAL FEATURES

- Injury to the pars interarticularis.
- Usually presents as back pain with extension.

Spondylolysis is an injury to the pars interarticularis of the vertebral complex, resulting in a stress reaction or an acquired stress fracture. The pars interarticularis is the bony connection between the inferior and superior articulating facets. Injuries to the pars interarticularis, or pars defects for short, are present in 4%–6% of the population. The incidence of pars defects in athletes such as gymnasts, dancers, divers, and wrestlers is significantly increased because of the repetitive flexion/extension motions combined with rotation. Repetitive overload results in stress fractures. Spondylolysis occurs at L5 in 85% of cases. The athlete presents with midline low back pain that is aggravated by extension, such as arching the back in gymnastics. There may be palpable tenderness over the lower lumbar vertebrae, with pain on the single leg hyperextension test (Stork test). Tight hamstrings are another common physical finding. Evaluation includes anteroposterior (AP) and lateral radiographs of the lumbar spine. Although oblique radiographic views of the lumbar spine are helpful to look for the so-called Scottie dog sign, they are falling out of favor because they do not improve diagnostic accuracy and increases radiation exposure. Single photon emission computed tomography scan, CT scan, and MRI can be useful to determine the presence of an active spondylolytic lesion. Bone/SPECT scan show stress reaction or pars injury before other radiographic changes. CT provides excellent definition of bony anatomy and can document healing. MRI is an alternative to detect pars interarticularis problems. With the use of high magnetic field strength and fat saturation techniques, high resolution MRI images can now show subtle bone marrow edema of early stress injuries and are being used more in some centers.

There is currently no gold standard for the treatment of spondylolysis. Management includes refraining from hyperextension and high-impact sporting activities; stretching of the hamstrings; and core and back stabilization exercises. Athletes can cross-train with low-impact activity and neutral or flexion-based physical therapy. Bracing is controversial. Outcome studies show similar results regarding return to sports and bony healing whether or not braces are worn. Return to play is often delayed 8–12 weeks or longer based on clinical signs of healing. Most symptomatic spondylolysis improves with nonoperative treatment, with our without radiologic evidence of healing. Surgery is reserved for refractory cases.

2. Spondylolisthesis

ESSENTIALS OF DIAGNOSIS & TYPICAL FEATURES

- Bilateral pars interarticularis injury resulting in forward slippage of one vertebra over the one below it.
- Usually presents as back pain with extension.
- Hyperlordosis, possible step-off.

When a bilateral pars stress fracture (spondylolysis) occurs, slippage of one vertebra over another causes a spondylolisthesis. Patients present with hyperlordosis, kyphosis, pain with hyperextension and in severe cases, a palpable step-off. A standing lateral radiograph is used to make the diagnosis and to monitor for any progression of slippage. These injuries are graded from 1 to 4 based on the percentage of slippage: grade 1 (0%–24%), grade 2 (25%–49%), grade 3 (50%–74%), and grade 4 (75%–100%).

Treatment is often symptom-based. Asymptomatic athletes with less than 25% slippage often have no restrictions and are followed on a routine basis for radiograph assessment. Management of symptomatic spondylolisthesis requires a period of activity modifications, particularly protection from spine extension and impact activities, coupled with a regimen of stretching of the hamstrings and core and back stabilization exercises. Bracing may also be considered. Surgical intervention is considered for slippage > 50%, progressive spondylolisthesis, or intractable pain despite nonoperative treatment. If surgery is required, the athlete must understand that he or she cannot return to activities for at least a year and may not be able return to previous sporting activities.

3. Disk Herniation

ESSENTIALS OF DIAGNOSIS & TYPICAL FEATURES

- Back pain worse with flexion and sitting.
- Radiculopathy can be present.
- Positive straight leg raise.

Discogenic back pain accounts for a small percentage of back injuries in children. These injuries are almost unheard of in preadolescence. Back pain can originate from disk bulging, disk herniation, or disk degeneration. Most injuries occur at L4–L5 and L5–S1 vertebrae. In adolescents most disk herniations are central rather than posterolateral. Symptoms include back pain, which may be increased with activities such as bending, sitting, and coughing. Although not as common as in adults, radicular symptoms of pain down the leg can also occur and are often associated with large disk herniations. Evaluation includes physical and neurologic examinations, including straight leg testing, sensory testing, and checking reflexes. If symptoms persist, evaluation usually begins with radiographs and an MRI, which is the imaging test of choice for diagnosing disc herniation. Electromyography may also be considered in the presence of radiculopathy.

Treatment usually is conservative as most disk herniations, even if large, improve spontaneously. The athlete can rest the back for a short period and then begin a structured exercise program of extension and isometrics followed by flexion exercises. If symptoms persist, a short course of steroids may be indicated. Surgery is recommended for significant or progressive radiculopathy, or if neurologic compromise persists.

Curtis C, d'Hemecourt P: Diagnosis and management of back pain in adolescents. Adolesc Med State Art Rev 2007;18:140–164 [PMID: 18605395].

Eddy D et al: A review of spine injuries and return to play. Clin J Sport Med 2005;15:453 [PMID: 16278551].

Selected Issues for the Adolescent Athlete and the Team Physician: A Consensus Statement. Med Sci Sports Exerc Nov 2008;40(11):1997–2012.

SHOULDER INJURIES

Shoulder injury is usually a result of acute trauma or chronic overuse. Acute injuries around the shoulder include contusions, fractures, sprains (or separations), and dislocations. The age of the patient affects the injury pattern, as younger patients are more likely to sustain fractures instead of sprains. Sprains (ligaments) and strains (muscle and tendon) are generally defined as low grade soft tissue injuries that do not result in functional compromise of a structure.

1. Fracture of the Clavicle

ESSENTIALS OF DIAGNOSIS & TYPICAL FEATURES

- Injury by fall on shoulder or outstretched hand.
- Severe pain in the shoulder.
- Deformity over clavicle.

Clavicular fractures occur from a fall or direct trauma to the shoulder. Focal swelling, deformity, and tenderness are present over the clavicle. The diagnosis is made by radiographs of the clavicle; the fractures are most common in the middle third of the bone.

Initial treatment is focused on pain control and protection with a sling and swathe. Early range of motion is permitted, based on pain level. Progressive rehabilitation is important. Athletes cannot return to contact sports for 8–10 weeks. Absolute surgical indications for acute clavicular fractures include open fractures or neurovascular compromise. Fracture nonunion is unusual in young patients. However, there is recent evidence in the adult population recommending surgical stabilization for fractures that are very displaced or shortened. The role of acute surgical stabilization in the pediatric and adolescent population in regards to shortening is still being defined. Patients with recurrent fractures or nonunion typically will also require surgical fixation.

2. Acromioclavicular Separation

ESSENTIALS OF DIAGNOSIS & TYPICAL FEATURES

- Injury with fall on shoulder.
- Severe pain in the shoulder.
- Deformity over acromioclavicular joint.

A fall on the point of the shoulder is the most common cause of acromioclavicular separation. Tearing of the acromioclavicular joint capsule and possibly the coracoclavicular ligaments occurs. The injury is classified by the extent of the injuries to these ligaments. Athletes present with focal soft tissue swelling and tenderness over the acromioclavicular joint. More severe injuries are associated with deformity. Patients have a positive cross-arm test, in which pain is localized to the acromioclavicular joint. Radiographs are necessary in this setting to assess the degree of injury and to evaluate for a coexisting fracture or growth plate injury.

Treatment is supportive, with rest and immobilization in a sling followed by progressive rehabilitation. Return to activity can be accomplished in 1–6 weeks depending on the severity of the injury and the persistence of symptoms. Full range of motion and full strength must be achieved prior to being cleared to return to sports.

3. Fracture of the Humerus

ESSENTIALS OF DIAGNOSIS & TYPICAL FEATURES

- Injury with significant fall on outstretched arm.
- Severe pain in proximal humerus.
- Swelling and/or deformity over proximal humerus.

Fractures of the humerus occur from a severe blow or fall on the shoulder. Pain and swelling are localized to the proximal humeral region. The fractures can include the physes or may be extraphyseal. A significant amount of displacement and angulation can be tolerated in this location because of the young athlete's potential for remodeling and because of the intrinsic range of motion of the shoulder. Careful assessment of the brachial plexus and radial nerves are needed to rule out associated nerve damage.

Treatment consists of a sling for 4–6 weeks followed by progressive rehabilitation.

4. Acute Traumatic Anterior Shoulder Instability (Anterior Shoulder Dislocation/Subluxation)

ESSENTIALS OF DIAGNOSIS & TYPICAL FEATURES

- Injury with an abducted and externally rotated arm.
- Severe pain in the shoulder.
- Squared-off shoulder on examination.
- Reduced range of motion of the shoulder.

Acute traumatic anterior shoulder instability occurs when significant force is applied to the abducted and externally rotated shoulder. Most often, the humeral head is dislocated in an anterior and inferior direction. The patient has severe pain and a mechanical block to motion. Some patients will spontaneously reduce within seconds or minutes of their injury. Most patients, however, require immediate closed reduction on the field or in the emergency room. Radiographs are helpful to confirm the position of the humeral head as well as to evaluate for coexisting fracture. MRI may be required for accurate visualization of fractures and cartilaginous injury.

Optimal follow-up treatment for glenohumeral dislocation in young athletes has not been established. Initially, the shoulder is immobilized for comfort. Range-of-motion exercises and progressive rehabilitation are initiated. Prolonged immobilization does not decrease the risk of recurrence, and is discouraged. Because of the high risk of recurrence, options for treatment should be individualized, with consideration given to both nonoperative and surgical management.

5. Rotator Cuff Injury

ESSENTIALS OF DIAGNOSIS & TYPICAL FEATURES

- Injury can be acute or chronic.
- Pain is described as diffuse or anterior and lateral.
- Overhead activities exacerbate the pain.

Shoulder injuries are often a consequence of repetitive overuse and tissue failure. Rotator cuff tendonitis and bursitis are the most commonly observed rotator cuff injuries in youth sports. Rotator cuff tears in children and adolescents are exceedingly rare. These overuse injuries typically occur in sports requiring repetitive overhead motions. Muscle imbalances and injury can cause the position of the humeral head to be abnormal, which may cause entrapment of the supraspinatus tendon under the acromial arch. Patients with nontraumatic shoulder instability due to ligamentous and capsular laxity (also known as multidirectional instability) are prone to overuse rotator cuff injury. These athletes present with chronic pain in the anterior and lateral shoulder, which is increased with overhead activities. Diagnostic workup includes plain radiographs and an outlet view to look for anatomic variability. The rehabilitation of this injury is geared toward reduction of inflammation, improved flexibility, and core stabilization and strengthening of the scapular stabilizers and rotator cuff muscles. A biomechanics evaluation can assist athletes in the recovery process by building sport-specific skills and eliminating substitution patterns. Surgery is rarely indicated.

6. Little League Shoulder

ESSENTIALS OF DIAGNOSIS & TYPICAL FEATURES

- Participation in a throwing sport.
- Pain with throwing.
- Pain in the lateral aspect of the humerus.
- Swelling around the shoulder.
- Widening of the proximal humeral physis on radiographs.

Proximal humeral epiphysitis, or "Little League shoulder," is an overuse injury that occurs in children aged 11–14 years who play overhead sports such as baseball. The patient presents with activity-related pain in the lateral aspect of the proximal humerus. Examination often shows tenderness over the proximal humerus. Absence of findings on office examination does not preclude this diagnosis. The hallmark feature is pain with throwing. Radiographs show widening, sclerosis, and irregularity of the proximal humeral physis. Comparison views are often helpful when considering this diagnosis.

Treatment consists of rest from throwing or other aggravating activity. Physical therapy is initiated during the rest period. Return to play can only be considered after a period of rest has significantly decreased the pain and the athlete has proceeded through a progressive throwing program. Healing can take several months. Signs of radiographic healing may lag behind the athlete's clinical progress and normal radiographs are not necessarily required to return an athlete to play. Permanent sequelae such as fracture, growth arrest, or deformity is extremely rare but can occur in chronic cases that are not treated appropriately.

Mariscalco MW, Saluan P: Upper extremity injuries in the adolescent athlete. Sports Med Arthroscopy Review 2011;19:17–26 [PMID: 21293234].

Brophy RH, Marx RG: The treatment of traumatic anterior instability of the shoulder: Nonoperative and surgical treatment. Arthroscopy 2009;25:298–304 [PMID: 19245994].

Sciascia A et al: The pediatric overhead athlete: What is the problem? Clin J Sports Med 2006;16:6 [PMID: 17119360].

ELBOW INJURIES

Injuries in the elbow are quite common with both chronic and acute etiologies (eg, the chronic overuse "Little League elbow"). The term *Little League elbow* is used loosely to encompass a variety of causes of elbow pain in young throwing athletes. These injuries include medial epicondylitis, apophysitis, medial epicondyle avulsion fracture, and osteochondritis dessicans of the capitellum. It is intended, however, to refer to medial epicondyle apophysitis, an overuse elbow injury resulting from repetitive valgus stress from overhead throwing.

When evaluating the elbow, consider dividing the examination into specific anatomic areas as discussed below.

1. Medial Epicondyle Apophysitis (Little League Elbow)

ESSENTIALS OF DIAGNOSIS & TYPICAL FEATURES

- Participation in a throwing sport.
- Pain over the medial epicondyle, especially with pitching.
- Swelling of medial elbow.

Little League elbow is a traction injury to the medial epicondylar physis that develop in young overhead throwing athletes, particularly baseball pitchers. The biomechanical forces generated around the elbow during throwing, namely repetitive valgus stress, can result in shearing, inflammation, traction, and abnormal bone development. The symptoms are primarily swelling, pain, performance difficulties, and weakness. The pain localizes to the medial epicondyle, which may be tender to palpation, and worsened with valgus stress. Wrist flexion and forearm pronation may increase symptoms. The physician should inquire about the exposure to throwing, including pitch counts, the number of practices and games, and the duration of the season. Workup includes elbow radiographs, with comparison films of the unaffected side, to look for widening of the apophysis. Rarely, MRI is used to confirm the diagnosis.

Treatment of the injury includes complete rest from throwing activities. It is not uncommon for a player to be restricted from throwing for up to 6 weeks. Competition can be resumed once the player is asymptomatic and has progressed through a graduated, age-appropriate throwing program. The key approach for this injury is prevention. Children should be properly conditioned and coached in correct throwing biomechanics. Guidelines for Little League pitching limits in youth baseball have been developed and are outlined in Table 27–5.

Table 27–5. Guidelines for pitching limits in youth baseball.

Age (y)	Pitches per Day
7-8	50
9-10	75
11-12	85
13-16	95
17-18	105

2. Panner Disease

ESSENTIALS OF DIAGNOSIS & TYPICAL FEATURES

- Participation in a throwing sport.
- Pain over the lateral elbow.
- Swelling and flexion contracture.

Panner disease refers to osteochondrosis of the capitellum that results from overuse injury. The lesion involves disordered ossification of the capitellum, which is the lower end of the humerus that articulates with the radius. This condition occurs in children aged 5–12 years who play sports that involve overhead throwing and in gymnasts. The repetitive lateral compressive forces from loading the elbow in these sports compromises the blood supply to the growing epiphysis, leading to degeneration of the ossification center, or osteochondrosis. The child may have dull aching in the lateral elbow that worsens with throwing. Swelling and reduced elbow extension usually are present. Radiocapitellar compression test will also elicit pain—with elbow fully extended, arm is actively pronated and supinated. Radiographs show an abnormal, flattened capitellum, with fragmentation and areas of sclerosis. Treatment is conservative, using rest, ice, and splinting. Avoid activities that load the elbow for three to six months. The child can return to play once symptoms resolve and there is evidence of healing on follow-up radiographs. The natural history of this condition is one of complete resolution of symptoms and, ultimately, normal ossification of the capitellum.

3. Ulnar Collateral Ligament Tear

ESSENTIALS OF DIAGNOSIS & TYPICAL FEATURES

- Sudden forceful tensile stress on ligament from a fall or from valgus stress to elbow during overhead throw.
- Feeling a pop or sensation of elbow giving out.
- Medial elbow pain.
- Tenderness distal to medial epicondyle.

Once the medial epicondylar physis closes in a skeletally mature athlete, valgus forces are then transmitted to the ulnar collateral ligament, resulting in a sprain or tear. Patients present with medial elbow pain and are often unable to fully extend the elbow. Examination reveals tenderness just distal to the medial epicondyle and there may be instability with valgus stressing. Treatment is conservative, including rest, ice, and physical therapy directed at range of motion and strengthening. Surgery may be suggested for those with persistent pain or instability and who desire to continue participating in overhead sports.

4. Osteochondritis Dissecans

ESSENTIALS OF DIAGNOSIS & TYPICAL FEATURES

- Participation in a throwing sport.
- Pain over the lateral elbow, especially with pitching.
- Tenderness over radiocapitellar joint.
- Elbow flexion contracture.

Lateral elbow pain in a slightly older throwing athlete, usually aged 13–15 years, can be secondary to osteochondritis dissecans (OCD), which is a more worrisome diagnosis than Panner disease. It is an injury to the subchondral bone and its overlying articular cartilage. Valgus compressive forces can lead to avascular necrosis of the capitellum, which can ultimately result in the formation of loose bodies in the joint. The athlete presents with lateral pain, swelling, lack of full extension, and occasionally locking. Radiographs show lucency of the capitellum with surrounding sclerotic bone. MRI can more fully delineate the lesion. The prognosis for high-grade lesions is guarded.

The child should be seen by an orthopedic specialist with expertise in upper extremity injuries. Treatment is based on classification and can be either conservative or surgical. For early or stable OCD lesions, particularly in skeletally immature individuals, management includes throwing activity restrictions and range of motion exercises. More advanced lesions or those with persistent symptoms despite conservative treatment may require surgical intervention.

5. Lateral Epicondylitis

Lateral epicondylitis (also known as tennis elbow) is common in skeletally mature athletes participating in racquet sports. It is a tendinopathy of the extensor muscles in the forearm, which inserts onto the lateral epicondyle causing lateral elbow pain. The pain is increased by wrist extension. Initial treatment is aimed at inflammation control. Stretching and strengthening of forearm muscles are the primary interventions during the subsequent phases. Stroke mechanics may need to be altered and a forearm brace used to decrease the forces in the extensor muscles.

6. Posterior Elbow Pain

Posterior elbow pain is uncommon. Etiologies include dislocations, fractures, triceps avulsions, olecranon apophysitis, and olecranon bursitis.

Benjamin HJ et al: Little League elbow. Clin Sports Med 2005;15:1 [PMID: 15654190].

Gerbino PG: Elbow disorders in throwing athletes. Orthop Clin North Am 2003;34:417 [PMID: 12974491].

Hang DW et al: A clinical and roentgenographic study of Little League elbow. Am J Sports Med 2004;32:79 [PMID: 14754727].

Harris SS, Anderson SJ: *Care of the Young Athlete.* 2nd Ed. American Academy of Pediatrics 2010.

http://www.littleleague.org

Kobayashi K, Burton KJ et al: Lateral compression injuries in the pediatric elbow: Panner's disease and osteochondritis dissecans of the capitellum. J Am Acad Orthop Surg 2004;12:246–254.

HAND & WRIST INJURIES

The hand is the most common area of injury in children and accounts for a large proportion of emergency room visits. All hand and wrist injuries have the potential for serious long-term disability and deserve thorough evaluation. A thorough neurovascular examination as well as evaluation of rotational or angular deformity or malalignment is critical. Examples of complications include loss of range of motion, dysfunction, deformity, limb length discrepancy, and arthritis.

1. Distal Phalanx Injury

Tuft injury requires splinting for 3–6 weeks or until the patient is pain-free. If there is significant displacement, then a surgical K-wire can be used for reduction. **Nail bed injury** often requires nail bed suturing, splinting, and drainage of subungual hematomas. Nail avulsions should be replaced into the nail fold, and if not possible, a substitute material should be interposed into the nail bed as a stent. Patients with nail bed injuries should be advised that nail regrowth may appear irregular or may not occur at all.

2. Distal Interphalangeal Injury

Mallet finger or extensor tendon avulsion occurs more commonly in ball-handling sports. The mechanism of injury is an axial load or forced flexion against an actively extending finger, causing avulsion fracture or rupture of the extensor digitorum tendon. Athletes present with a flexion contracture at the distal interphalangeal (DIP) joint and inability to actively extend the distal phalanx. Conservative treatment is splinting in extension for 4 weeks for fractures and 6–8 weeks for tendon rupture. Surgery may be required if the initial fracture involves greater than 30% of the joint space or poor healing with loss of function occurs.

Jersey finger, or flexor tendon avulsion, occurs in contact sports, particularly American football. The mechanism of injury is forced extension against an actively flexed finger. The fourth ("ring") finger is the most commonly injured digit. Athletes present with tenderness, swelling, and inability to flex at the DIP. The examiner can test the function of the flexor tendon by holding the proximal interphalangeal joint in extension while having the injured athlete attempt flexion at the DIP joint. The injured finger should be splinted in a comfortable position and immediately referred to an orthopedic surgeon, as definitive treatment is often surgical.

3. Thumb Injury

Gamekeeper's thumb is an injury to the ulnar collateral ligament from forced abduction of the thumb metacarpophalangeal (MCP) joint. It is a common skiing injury to those who fall while holding on to their ski poles. Patients will complain of pain over the medial aspect of the MCP joint and pain with apposition or pinching. If a radiograph shows an avulsed fragment that is displaced less than 2 mm, a thumb spica cast can be used. If there is no fragment, less than 35 degrees of lateral joint space opening, or less than 15 degrees difference in joint space opening compared to the uninjured thumb, a spica cast for 4–6 weeks is indicated. Surgery is required for more serious injuries.

4. Hand Fractures

All finger fractures should be assessed for growth plate involvement, rotation, angulation, and displacement. If stable and not displaced, these fractures can be splinted for 3–4 weeks and buddy-taped for immediate return to sports. However, spiral or oblique fractures of the middle phalanx, intra-articular fractures, and severely angulated physeal fractures are considered unstable and should be referred to an orthopedic surgeon.

Boxer's fracture is a neck fracture of the fourth or fifth metacarpal, typically caused by poor punching technique or punching into a hard surface. Less than 40 degrees of angulation in the fourth or fifth metacarpals is acceptable. Assessment of displacement and rotational deformity is critical, as displaced or rotated fractures require reduction and fixation. Prior to definitive treatment with hand-based casting for 4 weeks, boxer's fractures may be temporarily immobilized with an ulnar gutter splint with the MCP joints flexed to 70 degrees.

5. Wrist Injury

Most swollen wrists without evidence of gross deformity or instability can be splinted temporarily for several days. Radial and ulnar fractures, which are fairly common in children, must be ruled out. Particular attention should be paid to the growth plates and the scaphoid bone. Typically, distal radius and ulna fractures require casting for 3–6 weeks in either a short or long arm cast, depending on the involvement of one or both bones and the severity of displacement or angulation. Torus, or buckle, fractures may be placed in a rigid wrist brace or short arm cast for 3–4 weeks. Scaphoid fractures are caused by a force applied to a hyperextended wrist, most commonly a fall onto an outstretched hand. Despite normal radiographs, if evidence of snuffbox tenderness and swelling is present, there is tenderness along the volar aspect of the scaphoid, or there is pain with radial wrist deviation or active wrist range of motion, the wrist must be further evaluated, either by magnetic resonance imaging acutely or immobilized for 10 days and then reassessed both clinically and with follow-up radiographs. A nondisplaced scaphoid fracture requires at least 6 weeks of immobilization in a thumb spica cast. Nonunion can occur, particularly in fractures of the proximal pole of the scaphoid, related to the poor blood supply of this carpal bone. Displacement requires operative management. Gymnast's wrist is chronic wrist pain due to repetitive overloading of the distal radial physis. Athletes complain of dorsal wrist pain, worsened with weightbearing on the affected upper extremity or active extension of the wrist. This overuse stress injury may cause long-term growth abnormalities or degenerative wrist joint changes, which may ultimately require surgical intervention. Athletes should be placed in a rigid wrist brace or short arm cast for 4 weeks and undergo a period of relative rest and activity modification.

http://emedicine.medscape.com/article/827104-overview#a0199

Anz AW et al: Pediatric scaphoid fractures. J Am Acad Orthop Surg 2009;17:77–87 [PMID: 19202121].

Carson S et al: Pediatric upper extremity injuries. Pediatr Clin North Am 2006; 53:41–67 [PMID: 16487784].

Cornwall R, Ricchetti ET: Pediatric phalanx fractures: Unique challenges and pitfalls. Clin Orthop Relat Res 2006 Apr;445:146–156 [PMID: 16505727].

Fetter-Zarzeka A, Joseph MM: Hand and fingertip injuries in children. Ped Emer Care 2002;18:341–345.

Mariscalco MW, Saluan P: Upper extremity injuries in the adolescent athlete. Sports Med Arthrosc Rev 2011;19(1):17–26.

HIP INJURIES

Because the pelvis and hip articulate with both the lower extremities and the spine, this area is rich in ligaments, muscle attachments, and nerves. Injuries in young children are rare, but sprains, strains, and avulsion fractures can occur. Additionally, athletes can be susceptible to overuse injury involving the hip.

1. Hip Avulsion Fractures

ESSENTIALS OF DIAGNOSIS & TYPICAL FEATURES

- Fractures at apophyseal areas.
- Pain with weight bearing.
- Focal pain over the site of injury.

Avulsion fractures around the hip in adolescents occur at apophyseal regions such as the ischial tuberosity, anterior superior iliac spine, anterior inferior iliac spine, and iliac crest. The mechanism of injury is a forceful, unbalanced muscle contraction that causes avulsion of the muscle tendon insertion. The athlete presents with a history of an acute traumatic incident; often a "pop" is felt and the athlete is immediately unable to bear weight. Range of motion of the hip is limited secondary to pain and focal tenderness is present over the apophysis.

Treatment is conservative. Surgical management is rarely required even in displaced fractures. The athlete is typically placed on crutches for the first couple of weeks for pain control and to normalize gait. After the acute phase, an athlete can progress to weight bearing as tolerated. The rehabilitation phase focuses on regaining motion, flexibility training and pelvic, and core strengthening. Progressive return to activity can often be accomplished in 4–6 weeks, if full range of motion, full strength, and sport-specific skills have been achieved.

2. Slipped Capital Femoral Epiphysis

ESSENTIALS OF DIAGNOSIS & TYPICAL FEATURES

- Pain in the hip or knee, or both.
- Loss of internal rotation of the hip.
- Radiographs in the frog-leg position show widening of the physis and epiphyseal slippage.

Slipped capital femoral epiphysis occurs in children aged 11–16 years. The physis is weakened during times of rapid growing and is susceptible to shearing failure either acutely secondary to a traumatic injury or insidiously from chronic overload. Patients complain of groin, thigh, or knee pain and often have a limp. Examination shows painful range of motion of the hip, limited internal rotation, and obligatory external rotation when the hip is flexed. Radiographs include AP and frog-leg lateral films, which demonstrate widening of the physis and epiphyseal slippage or displacement of the femoral head relative to the femoral neck.

Treatment consists of immediate non–weight-bearing and urgent referral to an orthopedic specialist for open reduction and internal fixation. Failure to identify this injury can result in permanent hip deformity and damage resulting in early arthritis. Rehabilitation is a component of the postsurgical treatment. Return to activity is progressive over months. (See also Chapter 26.)

3. Acetabular Labral Tears

Acetabular labral tears are an increasingly recognized cause of anterior hip and groin pain in athletes. The majority of hip labral tears occur as a result of some underlying hip disorder such as femoroacetabular impingement (FAI) or hip dysplasia. Because of the stress and range of motion requirements for most athletics, these injuries tend to present and be more symptomatic in the athletic population. Athletes with this injury typically do not report an acute traumatic event that precipitated their symptoms. Symptoms often develop insidiously rather than acutely. Athletes present with deep anterior hip or groin pain that worsens with activity and is resistant to treatment. Radiographic findings can be normal. An MRI arthrogram is used to demonstrate the tear. Treatment typically starts conservatively and requires rest. Ultimately, treatment is tailored to the athlete's particular needs and symptoms. Arthroscopy to repair the tear and address any underlying structural issue that caused the tear is often required.

4. Adductor Strain

An adductor strain or a groin pull is generally caused by forced abduction during running, falling, twisting, or tackling. Sports that require quick directional changes place athletes at risk for these types of injuries. The associated pain is in the adductor muscle. There is often pain with hip adduction or flexion and tenderness over the adductor tubercle. Treatment includes rest, ice, and protection—often with crutches, and strengthening of the muscle when it heals.

5. Hamstring Strain

ESSENTIALS OF DIAGNOSIS & TYPICAL FEATURES

- Mechanism is forced knee extension.
- Pain with tearing or popping sensation in the posterior leg.
- Pain with resisted knee extension.

Hamstring strain is a common injury in athletes. The majority of these injuries occur in the muscle belly and can be treated successfully with nonoperative management. The mechanism of injury is forced extension of the knee or directional changes. Typically, the athlete with a hamstring strain suddenly stops playing and grabs the back of the knee. There are three grades of injury. Examination reveals pain on palpation of the muscle and occasionally a defect. Pain also occurs with knee flexion against resistance.

Initial treatment is focused on minimizing swelling, bruising, and pain. The thigh should be iced and compression applied. In moderate and severe injuries, crutches may be needed for a short duration. The athlete can walk as soon as he or she can tolerate the activity. It is particularly important to stretch the hamstring because, as a two-joint muscle, it is more susceptible to injury than other types of muscle. Eccentric strengthening is an important component of rehabilitation.

6. Quadriceps Contusion

Quadriceps contusion is caused by a direct injury to the muscle that causes bruising, swelling, and pain. The amount of damage is directly related to the amount of force. The anterior and lateral thigh regions are most commonly injured, often in contact sports such as football and lacrosse.

Treatment is rest, ice, and protection for the first 24 hours. The knee should be kept in a fully flexed position. Two to 3 days after the injury, range-of-motion exercises may begin in both flexion and extension. Once 120 degrees of motion has been established and movement does not cause pain, the athlete may return to competitive activity. If the muscle remains firm on examination after 2 weeks, then radiographs of the thigh should be obtained to rule out **myositis ossificans**, an abnormal deposition of calcium in the muscle that may be induced by aggressive stretching of the muscle too early in the clinical course.

7. Hip Dislocation

ESSENTIALS OF DIAGNOSIS & TYPICAL FEATURES

- Usually produces posterior dislocation.
- Leg is flexed, adducted, and internally rotated.
- Hip pain is severe.
- This is an on-site emergency and must be treated quickly.

The hip is a very constrained joint and is inherently very stable. Therefore, hip dislocations are very rare and typically occur only in high energy or forceful injuries. Most hip dislocations occur in the posterior direction. Athletes with this injury typically have severe pain and any motion of the hip or leg is poorly tolerated. Classically, these athletes present with an acutely painful hip following a major impact and the hip is locked in flexion, adduction, and internal rotation. Hip dislocations in skeletally mature athletes are often associated with acetabular and femoral neck fractures. The preadolescent, skeletally immature competitor may have an isolated dislocation without fracture. Hip radiographs and advanced imaging such as a CT or MRI scan are needed to completely evaluate the injury.

This injury is an emergency. The athlete should be transported immediately to the nearest facility that has an orthopedic surgeon available. Severe bleeding, avascular necrosis, and nerve damage can result with delay in relocation. Most athletes can be relocated in a closed fashion. Once reduction has been established in an uncomplicated case, protected weight bearing on crutches for 6 weeks is recommended followed by another 6 weeks of range-of-motion and strengthening exercises. An athlete may return gradually to competition after 3 months, when strength and motion are normal.

Surgery can be necessary if there is an associated fracture, labral tear, loose body, or if a concentric reduction cannot be achieved in a closed fashion.

8. Pelvic Apophysitis

Pelvic apophysitis occurs in competitive adolescent athletes who typically are participating consistently, often year round, in their sport. Common locations are the ischial tuberosity and iliac crest. The athlete presents with pain over the apophysis and pain with resisted hip motion specific to the muscle insertion. Radiographs can show irregularity over the apophysis, or be normal. Treatment consists of relative rest, progressive rehabilitation focusing on flexibility, and pelvis and core stabilization.

9. Iliotibial Band Syndrome

ESSENTIALS OF DIAGNOSIS & TYPICAL FEATURES

- Overuse running injury.
- Pain over lateral knee or hip.
- Positive Ober test.

Iliotibial band syndrome and associated trochanteric bursitis result when the bursa and IT band become inflamed because of repetitive friction from the underlying greater trochanter. This condition can cause pain when the hip is flexed as a result of reduced flexibility of the iliotibial band and gluteus medius tendons. The bursa is a structure that normally allows for improved motion by reducing friction but becomes pathologic in this condition. Movement is painful and may be limited. Iliotibial band syndrome is best evaluated in a side-lying position and pain is reproduced when the hip is actively flexed from a fully extended hip (Ober test).

Initial treatment is to alter the offending activity and then start a stretching program geared at the iliotibial band and hip abductors. Core and pelvic stabilization are also important. Ultrasound can be beneficial and corticosteroid injections may be used after conservative treatment has failed.

10. Femoral Neck Fractures

Femoral neck fractures (stress fractures) are generally the result of repetitive microtrauma. They commonly occur in running athletes who have increased their mileage. Athletes with this type of injury present with persistent pain in the groin and pain with internal and external rotation. Symptoms often are present with sports, but as the fracture progresses, symptoms often develop during activities of daily living. Athletes with a history of previous stress fracture, disordered eating, or any disorder of calcium metabolism and groin pain should alert the provider to the possibility of this diagnosis. Special attention should be given to the female athlete triad of eating disorders, amenorrhoea, or oligomenorrhoea, and low bone density and the risk of stress fracture in this population.

On physical examination, range of motion may be limited in hip flexion and internal rotation. A limp may be present. Pain with hopping on the affected leg is universally present. If plain radiographs are negative, an MRI or a bone scan is indicated.

Treatment is based on the type of fracture. A tension-sided fracture (on the superior aspect of the femoral neck) generally requires internal fixation to prevent femoral displacement and reduce the risk of avascular necrosis. A compression fracture (on the inferior aspect of the femoral neck) is less likely to be displaced; treatment is conservative and involves resting the hip until it heals. Cardiovascular conditioning can be maintained easily through nonimpact exercises and activity.

Cooper DE: Severe quadriceps muscle contusions in athletes. Am J Sports Med 2004;32:820 [PMID: 15090402].

Jacoby L, Yi-Meng Y, Kocher MS: Hip problems and arthroscopy: Adolescent hip as it relates to sports. Clinics in Sports Medicine 2011;30;435–451 [PMID: 21419965].

Kovacevic D, Mariscalco M, Goodwin RC: Injuries about the hip in the adolescent athlete. Sports Med Arthroscopy Review 2011;19:64–74 [PMID: 21293240].

KNEE INJURIES

Knee injuries are one of the most common sports-related problems. The knee is stabilized through a variety of ligaments, tendons, and the menisci. Knee injuries can be divided into two groups: those resulting from acute or chronic causes. Acute injuries occur during a well-defined traumatic incident. The mechanism of injury is an important historical feature, although many young patients have difficulty describing the details of the inciting event. The onset of rapid swelling after a traumatic event indicates the presence of a hemarthrosis and likely internal derangements such as fracture, rupture of the anterior cruciate ligament (ACL), meniscal tear, or patellar dislocation.

1. Anterior Knee Pain

The most common knee complaint is anterior knee pain. This complaint can have multiple etiologies but should always include hip pathology as a possible source. Patellofemoral dysfunction (defined below) is a common cause of anterior knee pain. The differential diagnosis of anterior knee pain is extensive and requires a thorough examination. The following are the most common knee diagnoses responsible for anterior knee pain.

A. Patellofemoral Overuse Syndrome

Patellofemoral overuse syndrome occurs during running and sports that involve repetitive stress in the lower extremity. The athlete presents with activity-related pain in the anterior knee. In young athletes, it is occasionally associated with swelling and crepitus of the knee joint.

Evaluation of these injuries is comprehensive and requires a "top-down" evaluation of the athlete's leg from the hip to the foot. Most athletes with this condition, regardless of level or physical condition, typically have hip/core weakness that results in altered knee biomechanics. A comprehensive evaluation of hip alignment and rotation, muscle development, tightness in the hamstrings and iliotibial band, and foot mechanics is necessary to fully understand and treat the cause of this disorder. Most athletes with this complaint often have a multifactorial cause for their symptoms.

Treatment should be geared toward identifying the cause. Often athletes are overtraining and need to modify current activities. Cross-training may help. Addressing hip and pelvic stability is now a mainstay of treatment for this disorder. Stretching and strengthening of the hamstrings and quadriceps are recommended. Use of braces providing proprioceptive feedback during competition is controversial.

B. Patellar Tendonitis ("Jumper's Knee")

This overuse injury is caused by repetitive loading of the quadriceps during running or jumping. This diagnosis is common in jumping sports such as basketball and volleyball. Tenderness is located directly over the patellar tendon at its insertion site at the inferior pole of the patella.

C. Osgood-Schlatter Disease (Tibial Tubercle Apophysitis)

ESSENTIALS OF DIAGNOSIS & TYPICAL FEATURES

- Activity-related anterior knee pain in adolescents.
- Swelling and pain over tibial tubercle.
- Progressive fragmentation of tibial tubercle apophysis.

This condition is caused by the recurrent traction on the tibial tubercle apophysis (growth plate) that occurs in jumping and running sports. Fragmentation and microfractures of the tibial tubercle occur during its time of rapid growth. The condition occurs in the preteen and adolescent years and is most common in boys aged 12–15 years and girls aged 11–13 years. Pain is localized to the tibial tubercle and is aggravated by activities using eccentric quadriceps muscle movement. The pain can become so severe that routine activity must be curtailed. Radiographs typically demonstrate fragmentation or irregular ossification of the tibial tubercle.

Typically the condition resolves spontaneously as the athlete reaches skeletal maturity. In the interim, pain control using NSAIDs is indicated. Physical therapy and stretching the hamstrings and application of ice after workouts is helpful.

D. Sinding-Larsen-Johansson Disease (Apophysitis of the Inferior Pole of the Patella)

This condition involves a process similar to that in Osgood-Schlatter disease, but occurs in younger athletes between ages 9 and 12 years. Traction from the patellar tendon on the inferior pole of the patella results in fragmentation of the inferior patella that is often obvious on a lateral knee radiograph. Treatment and prognosis is similar to Osgood-Schlatter disease.

Treatment

The treatment of the above knee disorders is similar. As with many injuries, control of pain and inflammation is essential. This begins with relative rest from offending activity and application of ice. Alignment problems and mechanics across the anterior knee can be improved with an effective rehabilitation program that includes flexibility and strengthening. Quadriceps, pelvic, and core strengthening are all important components of this program. Orthotics, in theory, can have an impact on mechanics across the knee joint if they correct excessive pronation or supination.

Knee bracing is controversial and the major benefits are proprioceptive feedback and patellar tracking. Return to activity is often based on symptoms.

2. Posterior Knee Pain

Posterior knee pain often results from an injury to the gastrocnemius-soleus complex caused by overuse. Other causes include a Baker cyst (benign synovial fluid filled cyst in the posterior aspect of the knee), tibial stress fracture, or tendonitis of the hamstring. Treatment is rest, ice, and strengthening exercises after symptoms have improved. Intra-articular injuries such as meniscal tears and cartilage injuries can also cause posterior knee pain and should be considered if symptoms do not improve.

3. Meniscal Injuries

ESSENTIALS OF DIAGNOSIS & TYPICAL FEATURES

- Medial or lateral knee pain.
- Effusion and joint line tenderness.
- Feeling of locking or of the knee giving way.
- Positive McMurray test.

The meniscus of the knee cushions forces in the knee joint, increases nutrient supply to the cartilage, and stabilizes the knee. Most injuries are related to directional changes on a weight-bearing extremity. **Medial meniscus injuries** have a history of tibial rotation in a weight-bearing position. This injury happens frequently in ball-handling sports. **Lateral meniscus injuries** occur with tibial rotation with a flexed knee, as in exercises such as squatting or certain wrestling maneuvers. These injuries are uncommon in children younger than age 10 years.

Clinical Findings

The athlete with such an injury has a history of knee pain, swelling, snapping, or locking and may report a feeling of the knee giving way. Physical examination often reveals effusion, joint line tenderness, and a positive McMurray hyperflexion-rotation test. The McMurray test is performed by having the examiner place his/her fingers across the joint lines while flexing the knee maximally. The knee is then rotated while it is brought out into extension. A positive test is evoked when the patient reports pain and the examiner feels an associated click or catch along the joint line. The diagnostic test of choice is MRI of the knee, although standard knee radiographs should be included. It is important to note that the increased vascularity of the meniscus in the pediatric population often causes increased signal changes on MRI that can be confused with a tear. Therefore, an MRI diagnosis of a meniscal tear in a young athlete needs to be correlated with the patient's clinical symptoms and exam.

Treatment

Treatment of these injuries is typically surgical because of the limited ability of the meniscus to heal without surgical intervention. Nonoperative management can be considered if the tear is minor and symptoms are minimal. Surgery can entail repairing the tear or removing the torn portion of the meniscus. Typically, every attempt is made to preserve the meniscal tissue in young athletes because of their favorable healing rates and the long-term concern over the development of arthritis in meniscal deficient patients. Menisectomy (removal of torn tissue) patients can often return to sports 3–6 weeks after surgery. Meniscal repair patients require a period of 6 weeks of crutch protection followed by physical therapy. Return to sport after a repair is typically 3–4 months.

4. Medial & Lateral Collateral Ligament Injuries

ESSENTIALS OF DIAGNOSIS & TYPICAL FEATURES

- Pain on the medial or lateral portion of the knee.
- Tenderness along the ligament.
- Positive valgus stress test at 0 and 30 degrees.

The medial and lateral collateral ligaments are positioned along either side of the knee and act to stabilize the knee during varus and valgus stress. Medial injuries occur either with a blow to the lateral aspect of the knee, as seen in a football tackle, or with a noncontact rotational stress.

Clinical Findings

The athlete may feel a pop or lose sensation along the medial aspect of the knee. The examination reveals a mild effusion and tenderness medially along the course of the ligament. A valgus stress test performed in 20–30 degrees of flexion reproduces pain and possibly instability.

Medial collateral ligament (MCL) injuries are graded on a scale of 1–3. Grade 1 injury represents a stretching injury. Grade 2 injury involves partial disruption of the ligament. Grade 3 injury is a complete disruption of the ligament. Radiographs are useful, especially in the skeletally immature athlete, to look for distal femoral or proximal tibial bone injury. MRI scans are used if grade 3 injury or concomitant intra-articular derangement is suspected.

Treatment

Treatment is almost always conservative. Initial injuries should be iced and elevated. A protective brace is worn and full knee motion in the brace can be permitted within a few days. Weight bearing is allowed and a strengthening program can be started. The athlete should use the brace until pain and range of motion have improved. The use of a functional brace is often required when a player returns to competition. Bracing is temporary until the ligament heals completely and the athlete has no subjective feelings of instability. Return to sports is variable and is dependent on the severity of the tear and other associated injuries. Most isolated, low-grade MCL injuries can return to play in 3–5 weeks.

5. Anterior Cruciate Ligament Injuries

ESSENTIALS OF DIAGNOSIS & TYPICAL FEATURES

- Pain and effusion of the knee.
- Pain along the lateral joint line.
- Positive Lachman test.

The anterior cruciate ligament (ACL) consists of two bundles that prevent anterior subluxation and rotation of the tibia. Most ACL injuries are noncontact and occur with deceleration, twisting, and cutting motions. ACL injuries can also occur with knee hyperextension or from a direct blow to the knee—typically on the lateral side—which causes an extreme valgus stress with both ACL and MCL disruption.

Clinical Findings

The athlete often reports hearing or feeling a "pop" followed by swelling that occurs within hours of the injury. Evaluation of the knee begins with examination of the uninjured knee. The Lachman test provides the most accurate information about knee stability in relation to the ACL. The Lachman test is performed by holding the knee in 30 degrees of flexion while supporting the tibia and femur. The tibia is pulled anteriorly and the degree of excursion and the firmness of the endpoint are assessed and compared to the contralateral side. All other structures of the knee should be examined to rule out concomitant injuries. Imaging of the knee includes plain radiographs and an MRI scan. In skeletally immature athletes, a tibial spine avulsion is frequently seen on radiographs rather than a midsubstance ACL tear.

Treatment

Initial treatment focuses on controlling swelling and pain. Structured physical therapy can be instituted early to assist in regaining range of motion and strength. Conservative treatment includes bracing, strengthening, and restricting physical activity. Knee braces enhance proprioception and control terminal extension. Conservative management can be complicated by continued instability and damage to meniscal cartilage.

Surgical reconstruction is typically indicated for young athletes in cutting sports and is also required for persistent instability. Surgery can be performed 2–6 weeks following the injury if the swelling and motion of the knee have improved. Recent advances in surgical treatment of the skeletally immature athlete have been helpful in dealing with the complicated management of young athletes with ACL tears. Rehabilitation of the knee starts immediately after surgery. A structured ACL physical therapy protocol is initiated with the goals of building strength, muscle reeducation, endurance, agility, and coordination. Return to cutting and pivoting sports can be achieved by 6 months after surgery if certain criteria are met.

6. Posterior Cruciate Ligament Injuries

ESSENTIALS OF DIAGNOSIS & TYPICAL FEATURES

- Pain and swelling of the knee.
- Increased pain with knee flexion.
- Positive posterior Drawer test.

The posterior cruciate ligament (PCL) runs from the medial femoral condyle to the posterior tibial plateau and has two bundles. Its main function is to prevent posterior tibial subluxation. Injury to the PCL is uncommon; it occurs when the individual falls on a flexed knee with the ankle in plantarflexion or with forced hyperflexion of the knee. The most common sports in which PCL injuries are sustained are football and hockey.

Clinical Findings

The athlete presents with swelling and pain in the posterior and lateral knee. The examination begins with the uninjured knee and proceeds to the injured side. Confirmatory testing includes the posterior drawer test, performed with the patient supine, the knee flexed to 90 degrees, and the foot stabilized. Grading is based on the amount of translation. Grade 1 (mild) is up to 5 mm, grade 2 (moderate) is 5–10 mm, and grade 3 (severe) is more than 10 mm. Grade 3 injuries are typically indicative that another ligament is injured in addition to the PCL and should alert the provider to an associated injury. Diagnostic imaging includes plain radiographs and MRI scan.

Treatment

Isolated PCL injuries are almost universally treated nonoperatively. The exception is bony avulsions of the PCL off the femur or tibia. Generally surgical fixation is recommended for these injuries. Ligamentous PCL injuries in isolation are remarkably well tolerated in athletes and can be treated with bracing and a progressive rehabilitation program. PCL injuries with injury to other structures are complex and often require surgical stabilization. Surgical stabilization of these injuries is complicated and return to sports at the previous level is uncertain after combined injuries that involve the PCL.

Kyist J: Rehabilitation following anterior cruciate ligament injury: Current recommendations for sports participation. Sports Med 2004;34:269 [PMID: 15049718].

Lord J, Winell JJ: Overuse injuries in pediatric athletes. Curr Opin Pediatr 2004;16:47–50 [PMID: 14758113].

Schub D, Saluan P: Anterior cruciate ligament injuries in the young athlete: evaluation and treatment. Sports Med Arthroscopy Review 2011;19:34–43 [PMID: 21293236].

FOOT & ANKLE INJURIES

Injuries in the lower leg, ankle, and foot are quite common in pediatric athletes. The types of injuries sustained depend on the age group. Young children tend to have diaphyseal injuries, in contrast to older children in rapid growth, who tend to have epiphyseal and apophyseal injuries. Skeletally mature adolescents are prone to adult-pattern ligamentous injury. Although fractures of the ankle are possible with inversion and eversion mechanisms, the most common acute injury involving the ankle is the lateral ankle sprain.

1. Ankle Sprain

ESSENTIALS OF DIAGNOSIS & TYPICAL FEATURES

- Mechanism is usually inversion and plantarflexion.
- Swelling and pain in the ankle over the ligament.
- Bruising over the ankle.

When a ligament is overloaded, tearing occurs. These injuries are graded on a scale of 1–3. Grade 1 injury is a stretch without instability; grade 2 is a partial tear with some instability; and grade 3 is a total disruption of the ligament with instability of the joint. The ankle has three lateral ligaments (anterior talofibular, calcaneofibular, and posterior talofibular) and a medial deltoid ligament. Inversion of the foot generally damages the anterior talofibular ligament, whereas eversion injures the deltoid ligament. Lateral ankle sprains are far more common than medial ankle sprains because the deltoid ligament is stronger mechanically than the lateral ligaments. However, medial ankle sprains may have more severe complications, including syndesmotic tearing and instability of the ankle joint requiring surgical stabilization. High ankle sprains involve injury to the tibiofibular syndesmosis, ligamentous structures supporting the integrity of the ankle mortise joint. These typically require longer healing times than low-grade ankle sprains.

Clinical Findings

Physical examination often reveals swelling, bruising, and pain. Diagnostic testing should be done when a bony injury is suspected. Obtaining radiographs is especially important when evaluating skeletally immature athletes who are more prone to growth plate injury.

The adult Ottawa Ankle Rules are used to determine whether obtaining x-rays are necessary, and do not pertain to patients younger than age 18 years. Tenderness over the malleoli, tenderness beyond ligament attachments, and excessive swelling are reasons to obtain radiographs.

Differential Diagnosis

Other injuries to consider include injuries to the fifth metatarsal, which can occur with an inversion mechanism. In this injury, the athlete presents with localized swelling and tenderness over the base of the fifth metatarsal. Fractures at the base of the fifth metatarsal can be divided into avulsion, Jones, and diaphyseal fractures. Tibiofibular syndesmosis tears occur most commonly with dorsiflexion and external rotation. Radiographs are required and the squeeze test is positive. Fractures of the malleoli, fibula, talar dome, or calcaneus may also mimic ankle sprain.

Treatment

Appropriate treatment of ligamentous ankle injuries is imperative to ensure full recovery and should begin immediately after the injury. Phase 1 care involves immediate compressive wrapping and icing to control swelling and inflammation. Protected weight bearing is encouraged as tolerated in the early phase of rehabilitation. Severe ankle sprains may benefit from a short period of treatment in a lower leg walking boot or cast. Phase 2 begins when the athlete can ambulate without pain. Supervised physical therapy prescription may be beneficial. During this time, ankle range of motion is emphasized, along with isometric contractions of the ankle dorsiflexors. Once 90% of strength has returned, active isotonic (eccentric and concentric exercises) and isokinetic exercises can be added. Phase 3 is designed to increase strength, improve proprioception, and add ballistic activity (more complex movement patterns) as well as sport-specific agility and function. The "foot alphabet" and "balance board" are excellent methods to improve ankle range of motion and proprioception. To restore range of motion, the patient is asked to actively move the ankle by drawing letters of the alphabet with the toes. To restore proprioception, the ability to maintain proper balance and control, balance exercises are performed on a balance board (or wobble board). This could also be done by having the patient stand on one leg while playing catch with a ball. This program can be effective in returning athletes to activity within a few weeks, although up to 6 weeks may be required for return to full activity. The athlete should wear a protective brace for 3–4 months, continue phase 3 home exercises, and ice after exercising.

2. Sever Disease

ESSENTIALS OF DIAGNOSIS & TYPICAL FEATURES

- Activity-related heel pain in preadolescents.
- Pain localized to the calcaneal apophysis and Achilles insertion.
- Positive calcaneal squeeze test.

Sever disease, or calcaneal apophysitis, occurs in athletes aged 8–12 years who are typically involved in high-impact activities, such as gymnastics and soccer. Causes include overuse, improper footwear, and tightness in the calf musculature and Achilles tendon. Pain occurs about the heel and at the point of muscle tendon insertion onto the growth center of the calcaneus. The athlete presents with activity-related heel pain and examination reveals focal tenderness over the apophysis. Tenderness created by pressing forcefully on the lateral and medial heel constitutes a positive "calcaneal squeeze test." Treatment is symptomatic and consists of relative rest, heel cord stretching, eccentric calf strengthening, ice massage, heel cups, NSAIDs for pain control, and progression to activity as tolerated based on pain level. Heel cups are rubber or gel infused shoe inserts that provide heel lift and cushion to decrease both tension and impact on the calcaneal apophysis. Refractory cases may benefit from brief immobilization and partial or nonweightbearing in a walking boot or cast followed by supervised physical therapy.

3. Plantar Fasciitis

Plantar fasciitis is a common problem that manifests as heel pain in the adolescent or older athlete. It typically occurs in runners who log more than 30 miles per week and in athletes who have tight Achilles tendons or wear poorly fitting shoes. It is also common in people with cavus feet and in those who are overweight. The pain is worse upon first standing up in the morning and taking a few steps. A bone spur is often found on examination. Treatment involves local massage, stretching of the gastrocnemius-soleus-Achilles complex, NSAIDs, arch supports, and local steroid injections. Runners may need to cut back on their weekly mileage until these measures eliminate pain.

Bahr R: Prevention of ankle sprains in adolescent athletes. Clin J Sports Med 2007;17:4 [PMID: 17620800].

Gillespie H: Osteochondroses and apophyseal injuries of the foot in the young athlete. Current Sports Medicine Reports 2010;9(5):266–268.

Pontell D, Hallivis R, Dollard MD: Sports injuries in the pediatric and adolescent foot and ankle: Common overuse and acute presentations. Clin Podiatr Med Surg 2006;23:209–231 [PMID: 16598916].

Seah R, Mani-Babu S: Managing ankle sprains in primary care: What is best practice? A systematic review of the last 10 years of evidence. Br Med Bull online August 14, 2010.

PREVENTION

As in all activities, most sports-related injuries can be prevented by education, reducing dangerous behaviors, use of protective equipment, and proper training. Early recognition of injuries, treatment, and appropriate rehabilitation are also crucial to ensure safe sports participation. Protective equipment should be properly fitted and maintained by an individual with training and instruction. Helmets should be used in football, baseball, hockey, bicycling, skiing, in-line skating, skateboarding, or any sport with risk of head injury. Eye protection should be used in sports that have a high incidence of eye injuries. Proper protective padding should be identified and used, including chest pads for catchers; shin guards in soccer; shoulder, arm, chest, and leg padding in hockey; and wrist and elbow protectors in skating. Other primary prevention strategies should also be addressed by coaches, parents, and physicians in order to ensure the safety of children participating in sports. These include inspecting playing fields for potential hazards, adapting rules to the developmental level of the participants, and matching opponents equally in skill level and size.

The use of the preparticipation history and physical examination can identify potential problems and allow for prevention and early intervention. Proper training techniques reduce injuries by encouraging flexibility, promoting endurance, and teaching correct biomechanics. Sports education reinforces the concepts of fitness and a healthy lifestyle along with sport-specific training. Early identification of an injury allows the athlete to modify techniques and avoid micro- and macrotrauma. Once an injury has occurred, it needs to be identified properly and appropriate measures used to minimize morbidity. Rehabilitation of the injury starts as soon as it has been identified. Early and appropriate care offers the athlete an optimal chance for full recovery and return to full participation.

Emery CA: Injury prevention and future research. Med Sport Sci 2005;49:170–191 [PMID: 16247266].

Rehabilitation Medicine

28

Pamela E. Wilson, MD
Gerald H. Clayton, PhD

Rehabilitation medicine is the multispecialty discipline involved in diagnosis and therapy of individuals with congenital and acquired disabilities. The goals of rehabilitation medicine are to maximize functional capabilities and improve quality of life. Disabilities are described using the World Health Organization's International Classification of Function, Health, and Disability. Three aspects are evaluated in every patient: (1) the impact of the disability on body structure and function, (2) the impact of the disability on activity and participation in society, and (3) the environmental factors with an impact on the individual's function. These three areas are the common framework for discussion of a disabling condition and its therapy.

PEDIATRIC BRAIN INJURY

General Considerations

There are an estimated 475,000 emergency department visits for brain injuries per year among children from birth through 14 years of age, with 3000 deaths and 37,000 hospitalizations. Children with brain injuries may have long-term deficits and disabilities that must be identified and treated. There are two ways to classify the injury to the brain and classically these are grouped into primary and secondary injury.

Primary injury occurs at the time of trauma causing focal and diffuse damage. *Focal damage* includes skull fracture, parenchymal bruising or contusion, extraparenchymal or intraparenchymal hemorrhage, blood clots, tearing of blood vessels, or penetrating injury. *Diffuse damage* includes diffuse axonal injury and edema. Consequences of primary injury, either focal or diffuse, include cellular disruption with release of excitatory amino acids, opiate peptides, and inflammatory cytokines.

Secondary injury is the loss of cellular function accompanying primary injury that results in loss of cerebrovascular regulation, altered cellular homeostasis, or cell death and functional dysregulation. A primary injury can initiate the processes of secondary programmed cell death (apoptosis), which further exacerbates the primary injury. Secondary injury may develop hours or days after the initial insult. It appears to be precipitated by elevated intracranial pressure, cerebral edema, and release of neurochemical mediators. Current treatment paradigms are focused on treating and preventing secondary injury.

Clinical Classification & Severity Scores for Head Injury

Traumatic brain injury is usually categorized as open or closed. *Open* injuries are the result of penetration of the skull by missile or sharp object, or deformation of the skull with exposure of the underlying intracranial tissues. *Closed* injuries are the result of blunt trauma to the head, which causes movement (intracranial acceleration or deceleration and rotational forces) and compression of brain tissue. Brain contusions are referred to as *coup* (occurring at the site of injury) or *contra-coup* (occurring on the side of the brain opposite the injury). Rating the severity of injury and eventual outcomes is important in medical management. Included below are several common scales.

A. Glasgow Coma Scale

The Glasgow Coma Scale (GCS) is the most commonly used system to assess the depth and duration of impaired consciousness in the acute setting. The score is derived from three areas of evaluation: motor responsiveness (maximum score 6), verbal performance (maximum score 5), and eye opening to stimuli (maximum score 6). The scale has been modified for use in infants and children younger than 5 years of age, allowing for their lack of verbal responsiveness and understanding (see Table 12–5). Cumulative scores on the GCS define injury as mild (13–15), moderate (9–12), and severe (≤ 8). The concept of posttraumatic amnesia is used to gauge severity of injury and is an adjunct to the GCS, termed the GCS-E (extended). Posttraumatic amnesia is defined as the period of time after an injury during which new memory cannot be incorporated and the person appears confused or disoriented. Amnesia can be retrograde, anterograde, or both. A complicating factor in the use of either of these tools is the utilization of anesthesia, paralytics, and intubation in the acute care setting.

B. Rancho Los Amigos Levels of Cognitive Function

The Rancho Los Amigos Levels of Cognitive Function (LCFS or "Rancho") is used to gauge the overall severity of cognitive deficit and can be used serially during recovery as a rough gauge of improvement. The scale has 10 levels of functioning ranging from "no response" to "purposeful, appropriate."

Common Sequelae of Brain Injury

Depending on the severity of brain injury, there may be deficits in cognition and behavior, as well as physical impairments. Injuries can also produce changes in sensory and motor function, emotional stability, social behavior, speed of mental processing, memory, speech, and language. The consequences of mild brain injuries may be difficult to discern. Small intraparenchymal injuries, easily identified by computed tomographic (CT) or magnetic resonance imaging (MRI) scans, may not cause obvious signs or symptoms. The following are common problems associated with brain injury.

A. Seizures

Seizures occurring in the first 24 hours after injury are referred to as *immediate seizures*. Those occurring during the first week are *early seizures*, and those starting more than 1 week after injury are referred to as *late seizures*. Seizure prophylaxis with medications is recommended in the first week after brain injury in children at high risk for seizures and in very young children. Younger children are at a higher risk for early seizures than are older children and adults. Seizure prophylaxis is also recommended for 1 week after any penetrating brain trauma. Seizure prophylaxis is probably not effective for prevention of late-onset seizures. Late-developing seizures may require long-term treatment.

B. Neuromotor Deficits/Movement Disorders

Neuromotor deficits after brain injury include movement disorders, spasticity, paralysis, and weakness. The type of disorder will be influenced by the areas damaged from the trauma. The most common movement disorders are tremors and dystonias. These deficits can result in impaired ambulation, coordination, impaired ability to use upper extremities, and speech problems. Physical therapy is the primary means of treating these problems.

C. Communication Disorders

Language and communication disorders are fairly common. Aphasia which is difficulty in understanding and producing written and spoken language, is categorized as either fluent, nonfluent, or global. Individuals with fluent aphasia or Wernick type disorder can produce speech, but have little content associated. The nonfluent aphasias or Brocas type have a paucity of speech and may have word finding difficulties. Global aphasias have extensive injuries and the most severe language disorders.

D. Paroxysmal Autonomic Instability Associated with Dystonia

Severe brain injuries may be associated with autonomic dysfunction of the thalamus and hypothalamus, which causes a constellation of symptoms known as paroxysmal autonomic instability associated with dystonia (PAID). Symptoms of PAID are tachycardia, tachypnea, sweating, hyperthermia, agitation, and posturing. Common medications used to treat PAID include dopamine agonists (eg, bromocriptine), β-blockers (eg, propranolol), and α-agonists (eg, clonidine).

E. Cognitive and Behavioral Deficits

After brain injury, cognitive and behavioral deficits are a frequent occurrence. Cognitive disorders depend on the location and severity of the injury. Damage to the frontal lobes can cause executive function problems along with initiation delays. Neuropsychiatric sequelae are common and depression, anxiety disorders, and posttraumatic stress disorders (PTSD) are present in one-third of those injured. Testing from a neuropsychologist may help to identify the problem areas and develop interventional programs including school modifications and behavioral strategies.

F. Hypothalamic-Pituitary-Adrenal Axis Dysfunction

Dysfunction of the hypothalamic-pituitary-adrenal axis is common after head injury. The syndrome of inappropriate secretion of antidiuretic hormone (SIADH) and diabetes insipidus (DI) from a posterior pituitary injury can result in significant electrolyte and osmolality imbalance. Amenorrhea that typically resolves spontaneously is common in females. Injury near the onset of puberty can complicate normal development, and endocrine status should be monitored closely.

G. Cranial Nerve Injuries

The sensory and motor components of the cranial nerves are often damaged, resulting in a wide variety of deficits not centrally mediated. The most common injured nerves are I, IV, VII, and VIII. Hyposmia or anosmia (cranial nerve I) can occur if the shearing forces at the cribriform plate disrupt the afferent olfactory nerves. Injury to cranial nerves IV (trochlear) is common as it has the longest intracranial length. Superior oblique injuries typically cause a head tilt and vertical diplopia. Facial nerve injuries (cranial nerve VII) are common especially with temporal bone fractures. This impacts the ability to use the facial muscles, causes dryness in the eye and salivary glands along with decreasing taste in the anterior part of the tongue. The cochlear nerve (VIII) is also frequently damaged in temporal bone fractures and can result in vertigo and dizziness.

Developmental Considerations

Much of what we know of traumatic brain injury is based on adult experience. The confounding effects of age and the etiologies unique to the pediatric population (eg, child abuse) make care of the pediatric head-injured patient very complex.

The assumption that younger children will fare better than older children or adults after a brain injury is a myth. The fact that, in a child, a significant amount of development and synaptic reorganization has yet to occur does not guarantee an improved chance for functional recovery. Indeed, disruption of developmental processes, especially in very young infants or neonates, may be catastrophic as these processes often cannot be resumed once disrupted.

The mechanism of injury plays an important role in determining the severity of brain injury in very young children. Mechanisms associated with nonaccidental injury such as shaking often result in global diffuse injury. The weak neck musculature, large head–body mass ratio, immature blood-brain barrier, and high intracranial fluid–brain mass ratio all contribute to widespread damage.

During puberty, major hormonal changes have an impact on the outcome of brain injury. Behavioral problems may be pronounced in brain-injured adolescents. Precocious puberty and precocious development of sexual activity may occur in preadolescents and should be carefully monitored.

Careful consideration should be given to the developmental progress of the brain-injured child and adolescent. Delays can be anticipated after moderate and severe brain injuries related to abnormalities of cognition and behavior. It is critical to identify developmental disabilities as early as possible so that appropriate therapy can be started in order to maximize the child's residual capabilities. Educational programs should include an individualized educational program (IEP) to support the child with significant remediation and assistance needs during their school years. Programs should also include a 504 plan (named for Section 504 of the Rehabilitation Act and the Americans with Disabilities Act). The 504 plan identifies the accommodations necessary in regular school settings for students with lesser disabilities so that they may be educated in a setting with their peers.

Treatment

The primary goal of rehabilitation after childhood brain injury is to maximize functional independence. Rehabilitative care can be divided into three phases: acute, subacute, and long term. The acute and subacute phases typically occur in the inpatient setting while the long-term phase is an outpatient endeavor.

A. Acute Care

Therapy in the acute phase consists mainly of medical, surgical, and pharmacological measures to decrease brain edema, treat increased intracranial pressure, and normalize serum laboratory values. Nutrition is essential in the healing process and either parenteral nutrition or supplemental enteral feedings are employed. Current research suggests that transitioning to enteral nutrition (eg, nasogastric tube feeding) as soon as possible after brain injury is associated with improved outcomes. Placement of a gastrostomy tube for supplemental enteral feeding is often performed in patients with severe brain injuries when recovery will be protracted and swallowing function is inadequate for safe oral feeding.

B. Subacute Care

Therapy in the subacute phase is characterized by early, intensive participation in rehabilitative therapies promoting functional recovery. Treatment should be planned after consultation with physical therapy, occupational therapy, speech-language specialists, and neuropsychologists. Nursing staff members are a primary interface with the patient and often serve as educators for family-directed care. Most children and adolescents with brain injuries can be discharged home to continue with treatment on an outpatient basis.

C. Long-Term Care

Long-term follow-up starts immediately after discharge. Medical issues must be thoroughly and regularly reviewed to ensure that changing needs are met. Annual multidisciplinary evaluation is important, especially as the child approaches school age. Neuropsychological testing may be required to define cognitive and behavioral deficits and plan strategies to deal with them in the educational environment. Therapies should be flexible, providing strategies to maximize independence and facilitate the child's involvement in changing environments.

Medication is often required for cognitive and behavioral issues. Attention deficit and fatigue associated with brain injury may be amenable to treatment with stimulants such as methylphenidate and modafinil. Dopaminergic agents such as amantadine, levodopa, and bromocriptine can be useful in improving cognition, processing speed, and agitation. Antidepressants such as selective serotonin reuptake inhibitors can be helpful in treating depression and mood lability. Anticonvulsants can be useful as mood stabilizers and in treating agitation and aggression. Tegretol and valproic acid are typical agents for this purpose.

Attention and arousal can also be successfully addressed by utilizing behavioral techniques to reinforce desired behaviors as well as identifying environmental situations that optimize those behaviors. Gains made in the behavioral realm often have a positive impact on therapies designed to address physical issues.

Prognosis & Outcomes

Directly after brain injury, poor pupillary reactivity, low blood pH, absence of deep tendon reflexes, and low GCS all correlate with poor outcome. An increased number of intracranial lesions and increased depth and duration of coma are also associated with poor functional recovery. Children younger than 1 year of age tend to have worse outcomes.

Functional outcome assessment is important for judging the efficacy of rehabilitation therapy. Global multidomain measures (eg, FIM/WeeFIM, FRESNO) are used to provide a functional "snapshot in time" of select functions—motor function and mobility, self-care, cognition, socialization, and communication. Sensitive and specific domain-specific outcome tools are important to follow for functional recovery that may occur in small increments.

Outcome associated with mild brain injury is often quite favorable. Most patients recover normal function within a short time. A small percentage develop persistent problems such as chronic headache, poor focusing ability, altered memory, and vestibular abnormalities. Differentiating between musculoskeletal and central nervous system (CNS) etiologies is important.

In children, recovery may not be fully achieved for many months or years after the initial injury. The impact of the injury on developmental processes and its future consequences are difficult to predict. Long-term follow-up is required, particularly as the child approaches school age.

Atabaki SM: Pediatric head injury. Pediatr Rev 2007;28:215 [PMID: 17545333].

Blackman JA et al: Paroxysmal autonomic instability with dystonia after brain injury. Arch Neurol 2004;61:321 [PMID: 15023807].

Pangilinan PH et al: Neuropharmacology in pediatric brain injury: A review. PMR 2010 Dec;2(12) [PMID: 21145525].

Walker PA et al: Modern approaches to pediatric brain injury therapy. J Trauma 2009 Aug;67(Suppl 2) [PMID: 19667844].

SPINAL CORD INJURY

General Considerations

Epidemiologic studies of spinal cord injuries (SCI) suggest that there will be about 10,000 new injuries per year and that 20% will be in children younger than age 20 years. Motor vehicle accidents are the leading cause of SCI in all ages. Falls are common causes in young children. The phenomenon of SCI without obvious radiologic abnormality (SCIWORA) can be present in 20%–40% of young children. Children from birth to 2 years tend to have high-level injuries to the cervical spine because of the anatomical features of the spine in this age group. The facets tend to be shallower and oriented horizontally, and the boney spine is more flexible than the spinal cord. In addition, the head is disproportionately large and the neck muscles are weak.

SCI is classified using the American Spinal Injury Association classification (ASIA class). This classification evaluates motor and sensory function, defines the neurologic level of the injury, and assesses the completeness of the deficit. The 72-hour ASIA examination is used in predicting recovery. A complete lesion identified on ASIA examination at 72 hours predicts a very poor recovery potential. The ASIA classification is as follows:

1. ASIA class A is a complete SCI, with no motor or sensory function in the lowest sacral segments.
2. ASIA class B is an incomplete injury, with preserved sensory function but no motor function in the sacral segments.
3. ASIA class C is an incomplete lesion in which the strength of more than 50% of key muscles below the injury level is graded less than 3/5 on manual muscle testing.
4. ASIA class D is an incomplete lesion in which the strength of more than 50% of key muscles below the injury level is graded greater than 3/5 on manual muscle testing.
5. ASIA class E is an injury in which full motor and sensory function is preserved.

Clinical Findings

A. Clinical Patterns of Spinal Cord Injury

1. Brown-Séquard injury—The cord is hemisected causing motor paralysis, loss of proprioception and vibration on the ipsilateral side, and loss of pain and temperature on the contralateral side.

2. Central cord syndrome—Injury is to the central part of the cord and results in greater weakness in the arms than the legs.

3. Anterior cord syndrome—Disruption of the anterior spinal artery causes motor deficits and loss of pain and temperature sensation. Proprioception and fine touch is spared.

4. Conus medullaris syndrome—Injury or tumor of the conus can cause minimal motor impairment but significant sensory, bowel, and bladder abnormalities.

5. Cauda equina syndrome—Injury to the nerve roots produces flaccid bilateral weakness in the legs, sensory abnormalities in the perineum, and lower motor neuron bowel and bladder dysfunction.

B. Imaging

The diagnosis and anatomic description of SCI is made mainly through imaging techniques. Initial studies should include radiographs of the entire spine (including cervical spine) and special studies for boney structures. MRI imaging is required to evaluate soft tissues. CT scans, including three-dimensional reconstructions, may be used to further define the injured elements.

Treatment

A. Initial Management

The two primary precepts of SCI treatment are early identification and immediate stabilization of the spine. The approach used to stabilize the spine is determined by the type of injury, location of injury, and underlying condition of the spinal cord. Stabilizing the spine may prevent further damage to the spinal cord. External traction devices such as halo traction and orthotics are often used. Some injuries require internal stabilization. The benefit of corticosteroid administration in pediatric SCI has not been established but treatment is usually initiated based on adult data from the National Acute Spinal Cord Injury Study. The initial loading dose is 30 mg/kg over 15 minutes, followed by 5.4 mg/kg for the next 23 hours if started within 3 hours of injury. If started within 3–8 hours of injury, corticosteroids should be continued for 48 hours.

B. Functional Expectations after Spinal Cord Injury

The lesions associated with SCI have a predictable impact on motor and sensory function. It is helpful to understand these concepts when discussing functional expectations with patients and parents (Table 28–1).

C. Special Clinical Problems Associated with Spinal Cord Injury

1. Autonomic hyperreflexia or dysreflexia—This condition occurs in spinal injuries above the T6 level. Noxious stimuli in the injured patient cause sympathetic vasoconstriction below the level of injury. Vasoconstriction produces hypertension and then a compensatory, vagally mediated bradycardia. Symptoms include hypertension, bradycardia, headaches, and diaphoresis. This response may be severe enough to be life threatening. Treatment requires identification and relief of the underlying noxious stimulus. Bowel, bladder, and skin problems are the most common noxious stimuli causing this syndrome. The patient should be placed in an upright position and antihypertensive medication used if conservative measures fail. Nifedipine (oral or sublingual) and nitrates have been used in treatment of this condition.

2. Hypercalcemia—Hypercalcemia often occurs in male adolescents within the first 2 months of becoming paraplegic or tetraplegic. The serum calcium level rises significantly in response to immobilization. Patients complain of abdominal pain and malaise. Behavioral problems may occur. Initial treatment is focused on hydration and forced diuresis using fluids and furosemide to increase urinary excretion of calcium. In severe cases, especially in older children, calcitonin and etidronate may be required.

Table 28–1. Functional expectations related to spinal cord injury.

Level of Injury and Key Muscle Function	Functional Skills
C1–C4 (no upper extremity function)	Dependent for all skills, can use voice-activated computer, mouth stick; can drive power wheelchair with technology devices such as sip and puff, chin drive, or head array
C5 (biceps function)	Can assist with ADLs, power wheelchair with joy stick, push manual wheelchair short distances, use modified push rims
C6 (wrist extension)	More ADL skills; can push manual wheelchair indoors, perform level transfers; hand function augmented with adapted equipment
C7 (elbow extension)	ADLs independent; hand function augmented with adapted equipment; can push manual wheelchair indoor and outdoor
C8 (finger flexors) T1 (little finger abduction)	ADLs independent; independent manual wheelchair skills; increased transfer skills
T2–T12 (chest, abdominal, and spinal extensors)[a]	ADLs independent; independent manual wheelchair skills; improved transfer; standing with braces
L1 and L2 (hip flexors)	Standing and walking with long leg braces, KAFO, and RGO; swing-through gait; manual wheelchair main form of mobility
L3 (knee extension)	Home and limited community ambulation; long or short leg braces
L4 (ankle dorsiflexion)	Community ambulation with short leg braces, AFO
L5 (long toe extensors) S1 (ankle plantar flexors)	Community ambulation; may be slower than peers and have some endurance issues

[a]Level defined by sensory dermatome.
ADLs, activities of daily living; AFO, ankle-foot orthosis; KAFO, braces named for the joints being supported (ie, knee-ankle-foot orthosis); RGO, reciprocal gait orthosis.

3. Thermoregulation problems—These problems are most common and most severe in higher level injuries and usually result in a poikilothermic state. The ability to vasoconstrict and vasodilate below the injury level is impaired. The person with an SCI above T6 is particularly susceptible to environmental temperature and is at risk for hypothermia and hyperthermia.

4. Deep vein thrombosis—Thrombosis is a common complication of SCI, especially in postpubescent children. Deep vein thrombosis should be suspected in children with any unilateral extremity swelling, palpable cords in the calf muscles, fevers, erythema, or leg pain. Diagnosis is confirmed by Doppler ultrasound, and full evaluation may require spiral CT scan or ventilation-perfusion scan if pulmonary embolus is suspected. Preventative measures include elastic stockings and compression devices. Anticoagulation prophylaxis may be required using medications such as heparin (100–150 U/kg intravenous) and low-molecular-weight heparins (0.5 mg/kg subcutaneously, every 12 hours).

5. Heterotopic ossification—This complication occurs in both spinal cord and traumatic brain injuries. Ectopic calcium deposits usually appear around joints in the first 6 months after injury. They may cause swelling, decreased range of motion, pain with motion, palpable firm masses, fever, elevated sedimentation rate, and abnormal triple phase bone scan. Nonsteroidal anti-inflammatory drugs or bisphosphonates such as Etidronate therapy should be started at the time of diagnosis. Surgical removal of ectopic deposits is controversial and usually performed only in cases of extreme loss of motion, pressure sores, or severe pain.

Bilston LE, Brown J: Pediatric spinal injury type and severity are age and mechanism dependent. Spine 2007;32:2339 [PMID: 17906576].

Bracken MB: Steroids for acute spinal cord injury. Cochrane Database Sys Rev 2002;(3):CD001046 [PMID: 12137616].

Krassioukov A et al: A systematic review of the management of autonomic dysreflexia after spinal cord injury. Arch Phys Med and Rehabil 2009 April;90(4):682 [PMID: 19345787].

Yucosoy L et al: SCIWORA in MRI era. Clin Neurol Neurosurg 2008 May;110(5) [PMID: 18353536].

BRACHIAL PLEXUS LESIONS

General Considerations

The brachial plexus is the complex nervous connection between the spinal cord and the muscles of the upper extremity and scapular area. The nerve roots forming the plexus derive from the fifth cervical through the first thoracic nerves. These nerve roots form trunks that further divide into divisions and then into cords. The upper trunk (C5 and C6) is the most common area injured and results in the classic **Erb palsy.** Injury to the lower trunk (C7–T1) produces a **Klumpke palsy.** Most brachial plexus lesions will spontaneously resolve within a few months. Those with persistent deficits may require interventions.

Clinical Findings

Erb palsy has been described as the "waiter's tip posture" and is characterized by shoulder weakness with internal rotation and adduction of the upper arm. The elbow is extended and the wrist flexed. There is good preservation of hand function. Klumpke palsy is characterized by good shoulder function but decreased or absent hand function. Brachial plexus injuries may also cause a Horner syndrome (unilateral miosis, ptosis, and facial anhidrosis) due to disruption of cervical sympathetic nerves. Associated bone and nerve injuries are common in brachial plexus injury. The physical examination should include inspection of the humerus and clavicle for fractures. There may be injuries of the phrenic and facial nerves.

The diagnosis of a brachial plexus lesion should be based on the history and clinical examination. Diagnostic testing helps confirm, localize, and classify the lesion. Electromyography is helpful 3–4 weeks after the injury. This test not only is used diagnostically but can track recovery. MRI, myelography, and CT scan can help to locate the lesion and determine its extent.

Treatment & Prognosis

Primary surgery to the nerves of the plexus is indicated for children who have no spontaneous recovery of biceps function by 6–9 months. Secondary procedures to maximize function include muscle transfers and orthopedic interventions. Physical therapy is the major treatment for brachial plexus injury and includes stretching, bracing, and functional training.

The currently accepted method of predicting recovery is based on the spontaneous recovery of the biceps. Children in whom antigravity function returns within 2 months of injury will probably have nearly full recovery of function. If antigravity function is delayed until 6 months of age, recovery will probably be limited. If antigravity function is absent at 6–9 months of age, there will be no recovery of function and surgery should be considered. The presence of a Horner syndrome suggests a poor outcome.

Hale HB et al: Current concepts in the management of brachial plexus birth palsy. J Hand Surg Am 2010 Feb;35(2):322 [PMID: 20141905].

Malessy MJ et al: Obstetrical brachial plexus injuries. Nuerosurg Clin N Am 2009 Jan;20(1):1 [PMID: 19064174].

COMMON REHABILITATION PROBLEMS

1. Neurogenic Bladder

The function of the bladder is to hold and expel urine. The muscles of the bladder include the detrusor and urethral sphincters. During the first year of life the bladder is a reflex-driven system that empties spontaneously. After the first year control begins to develop, and most children achieve continence by age 5 years. Children with damage to the central or peripheral nervous system may develop neurogenic bladder. Neurogenic bladder is usually classified as noted below:

1. *Uninhibited* neurogenic bladder occurs after upper motor neuron injuries at the level of the brain or spinal cord that result in failure to inhibit detrusor contractions. This results in a hyperreflexive voiding pattern.
2. *Reflex* neurogenic bladder results from damage to the sensory and motor nerves above the S3 and S4 level. The bladder empties reflexively but coordination may not be present and dyssynergia (contraction of the bladder musculature against a closed sphincter) can occur. Increased intravesicular pressure and vesicourethral reflux may be consequences of dyssynergia.
3. *Autonomous* neurogenic bladder is a flaccid bladder and is associated with lower motor neuron damage. Bladder volumes are usually increased and overflow incontinence can occur.
4. *Motor paralytic* neurogenic bladder results from injury to the motor nerves of the S2–S4 roots. Sensation is intact but there is motor dysfunction. The child has the sensation to void but has difficulty with the voluntary contractions.
5. *Sensory paralytic* neurogenic bladder results when sensory roots are disrupted. Affected patients do not have sensation of the full bladder but are able to initiate voiding.

The diagnosis of neurogenic bladder requires a complete history and physical examination. The type of neurologic damage should be identified as this will help to predict anticipated voiding issues. The upper tracts should be assessed by several techniques, including ultrasound, intravenous pyelogram, and renogram (isotope) studies. Lower tract testing includes urinalysis, postvoid residuals, urodynamics, cystography, and cystoscopy.

Treatment

Treatment is geared to the type of bladder dysfunction. The simplest methods are those employing behavioral strategies. Timed voiding can be effective for children with uninhibited bladders. In this technique, children are reminded verbally or use a cueing device (watch with a timer) to void every 2–3 hours before bladder capacity is reached. The Credé and Valsalva maneuvers are used in patients with an autonomous bladder to assist in draining a flaccid bladder. There is a risk of increasing intravesicular pressure during these maneuvers, which can provoke vesicoureteral reflux. These maneuvers should never be used in a patient with a reflex neurogenic bladder.

Medications are often employed to treat neurogenic bladder. Anticholinergics are commonly used to reduce detrusor contractions, decrease the sense of urgency, and increase bladder capacity. Medications include oxybutynin, tolterodine, and hyoscyamine. The side effects of these medications include sleepiness, nausea, and constipation. Families often find these effects unacceptable and frequently abandon treatment.

External methods are also used to improve continence and function. Absorbent pads and diapers, external catheters, internal catheters, and intermittent catheterization are some typical methods. Surgical procedures to protect the upper tracts from urinary reflux are often used. A young child with a high-pressure bladder is at particular risk for reflux and may need medication, intermittent catheterization, or vesicostomy to prevent hydrostatic renal damage and infection. An older child may require bladder augmentation or an intestinal conduit from bladder to skin surface to relieve bladder distention (Mitrofanoff procedure). If an incompetent urethral sphincter causes urinary leakage, injections, slings, or implants may be used to increase the urethral barrier. Recently, electrical stimulation of sacral roots has been used to initiate voiding. Biofeedback training is also used to improve voiding.

2. Neurogenic Bowel

Control of bowel function depends on an intact autonomic (sympathetic and parasympathetic) and somatic nervous system. Interruption of any of these pathways can result in retention and/or incontinence. Goals of treatment for patients with neurogenic bowel are to establish a predictable and reliable bowel habit, and prevent incontinence and complications. There are two types of neurogenic bowel dysfunction: upper motor and lower motor dysfunction. The upper neuron bowel results from damage above the conus. Affected patients usually have reflex bowel contractions of high amplitude, absence of sensation, and no voluntary sphincter control. Patients with the lower motor neuron bowel have no sphincter control and no anocutaneous reflex. It has been described as a flaccid bowel. In general, establishing a bowel program is easier in patients with upper motor neuron lesions.

Treatment

Diet is important in either type of neurogenic bowel. Fiber and fluids are critical elements. Stool consistency should be on the soft side, although some patients try to keep themselves constipated to prevent accidents. A predictable and scheduled bowel program is essential. Bowel movements should be scheduled to occur with meals, as the gastrocolic reflex can trigger defecation.

Laxative and stool softening medications are usually included in a comprehensive bowel program. Stool softeners such as docusate retain stool water. Mineral oil is an acceptable stool softener in patients not at risk for pulmonary aspiration. Bulking agents such as Metamucil increase fiber and water content of stool and reduce transit time. Stimulants such as senna fruit extract or bisacodyl increase peristalsis. Osmotic agents such as polyethylene glycol keep stools soft by retaining stool water. Suppositories and enemas are often used when other methods have not been successful. Upper motor neuron bowel management programs may include digital rectal stimulation. Newer surgical options include sacral nerve stimulators and techniques to provide flushing of the colon. Cecostomy button or antegrade continence enema is employed when other conservative methods have not been able to achieve desired goals.

3. Spasticity

Spasticity is a velocity-dependent increase in muscle tone and a loss of isolated muscle function. Whereas tone is the resistance felt in a muscle as it is moved in space, spasticity occurs when there is damage to the CNS from trauma or injury. It is included in the upper motor neuron syndrome (hyperactive and exaggerated reflexes, increased tone, clonus, positive Babinski sign). Spasticity is evaluated using the Ashworth Scale, with 0 indicating no increase in muscle tone and 4 indicating complete rigidity of the extremity.

Treatment

Treatment is goal directed and influenced by the functional status of the client. Spasticity has both positive and negative effects on quality of life. The positive aspects include the ability to use spasticity for functional tasks along with maintaining muscle strength. Negatively spasticity can interfere with positioning and hygiene, can affect function, and can cause pain.

Options for therapy range from conservative to aggressive. A pyramidal approach starts from a base of prevention of nociceptive input and aggressive physical therapy. Children should be positioned properly and have appropriate equipment to support this strategy. Physical therapy is designed to reduce the long-term effects of spasticity by stretching and range-of-motion exercises. Heat and cold are useful in improving tone, but their effects are not long lived. Casting of both upper and lower extremities can decrease tone and increase range of motion. Constraint therapy can be used to try to improve upper extremity function.

The next step on the pyramid is the use of medications, mainly baclofen, diazepam, dantrolene, and tizanidine. Baclofen (a direct $GABA_B$ agonist) is a first-line medication, which produces effects at the spinal cord level. Side effects are mainly sleepiness and weakness. Seizure threshold may be reduced by baclofen. Baclofen can be delivered directly to the CNS through an intrathecal pump. It has been used successfully in children with brain injury, cerebral palsy, and SCI. Diazepam is an allosteric modulator of postsynaptic $GABA_A$ receptors in both the brain and the spinal cord. It can cause drowsiness and dependence. Dantrolene decreases the release of calcium in muscle. Side effects include weakness and, rarely, hepatotoxicity. Tizanidine is a newer agent and works at the α_2-adrenergic receptors presynaptically. It can cause dry mouth and sedation, and liver function tests can be elevated.

Relief of focal spasticity can be achieved by using chemodenervation techniques. Botulinum toxin A and B can be injected in selected muscles to improve range of motion, thus improving function and hygiene as well as reducing pain and deformity. More recently, botulinum toxins have been used to treat drooling, hyperhydrosis, and chronic pain. These toxins block the release of acetylcholine at the neuro-muscular junction. The effects are temporary, lasting only 3–6 months, and repeat injections are often needed. Phenol injections are another option for treatment of local spasticity and are technically more challenging. Phenol denatures proteins in both myelinated and unmyelinated fibers and produces neurolysis or myolysis, depending on the site of injection. The effects may last longer than botulinum toxins. Injections carry a risk of sensory dysesthesia if mixed nerves are injected.

Surgical options include orthopedic procedures geared toward improving function and ambulation and alleviating deformities produced over time by spasticity. Contractures are common in the Achilles tendon, hamstrings, and adductors. Upper extremity contractures occur in the elbow, wrist, and finger flexors. Scoliosis is fairly common and bracing or surgery may be needed. Gait analysis may be helpful in evaluating the child with functional spasticity as a guide for the use of orthotics, therapy, and surgery. Neurosurgical techniques such as selective dorsal rhizotomy are used in a very select group of children to permanently alter spasticity patterns and improve ambulation.

Nijman RJ: Diagnosis and management or urinary incontinence and functional fecal (encoporesis) in children. Gastroenterol Clin N Amer 2008 Sept;37(3):731 [PMID: 18794006].

Tilton A et al: Pharmacologic treatment of spasticity in children. Semin Pediatr Neurol 2010 Dec;17(4):261 [PMID: 21183133].

Rheumatic Diseases

29

Jennifer B. Soep, MD

JUVENILE IDIOPATHIC ARTHRITIS

ESSENTIALS OF DIAGNOSIS & TYPICAL FEATURES

- Arthritis, involving pain, swelling, warmth, tenderness, morning stiffness, and/or decreased range of motion of one or more joints, lasting at least 6 weeks.
- May have associated systemic manifestations, including fever, rash, uveitis, serositis, anemia, and fatigue.

Juvenile idiopathic arthritis (JIA) is characterized by chronic arthritis in one or more joints for at least 6 weeks. There are four main subtypes of JIA: oligoarticular, polyarticular, systemic, and enthesitis-associated. The exact cause of JIA is not known, but there is substantial evidence that it is an autoimmune process with genetic susceptibility factors.

Clinical Findings

A. Symptoms and Signs

The most common type of JIA is the oligoarticular form, which constitutes 30% of patients and is characterized by arthritis of four or fewer joints. This type of JIA often affects medium to large joints. Because the arthritis is often asymmetrical, children may develop a leg-length discrepancy in which the involved leg grows longer due to increased blood flow and growth factors. The synovitis is usually mild and may be painless. Systemic features are uncommon except for inflammation in the eye. Up to 20% of children with this type of JIA develop insidious, asymptomatic uveitis, which may cause blindness if untreated. The activity of the eye disease does not correlate with that of the arthritis. Therefore, routine ophthalmologic screening with slit-lamp examination must be performed at 3-month intervals if the antinuclear antibody (ANA) test is positive, and at 6-month intervals if the ANA test is negative, for at least 4 years after the onset of arthritis, as this is the period of highest risk.

Polyarticular disease is defined as arthritis involving five or more joints. This type of JIA affects 25% of patients. Both large and small joints are involved, typically in a symmetrical pattern. Systemic features are not prominent, although low-grade fever, fatigue, rheumatoid nodules, and anemia may be present. This group is further divided into rheumatoid factor (RF)–positive and RF–negative disease. The former resembles adult rheumatoid arthritis with more chronic, destructive arthritis.

The systemic form, previously known as Still disease, comprises 5% of patients with JIA. The arthritis can involve any number of joints and affects both large and small joints, but may be absent at disease onset. One of the classic features is a high fever, often as high as 39–40°C, typically occurring one to two times per day. In between fever spikes, the temperature usually returns to normal or subnormal. Ninety percent of patients have a characteristic evanescent, salmon-pink macular rash that is most prominent on pressure areas and when fever is present. Other systemic features that may be present, but are not specific for JIA, include hepatosplenomegaly, lymphadenopathy, leukocytosis, and serositis.

Enthesitis-associated arthritis is most common in males, older than 10 years of age, and is typically associated with lower extremity, large joint arthritis. The hallmark of this form is inflammation of tendinous insertions (enthesopathy), such as the tibial tubercle or the heel. Low back pain and sacroiliitis are also commonly seen in this form of arthritis which comprises approximately 25% of patients with JIA.

There are two additional subtypes of JIA. Children with psoriatic arthritis (5%) may have typical psoriasis, but may also present prior to the onset of the classic thick scaly plaques and have more subtle changes such as nail pitting (see Chapter 15). Patients with psoriatic arthritis may also present with dactylitis or "sausage digit" which is painful swelling of an entire finger or toe. Undifferentiated JIA, comprising 10% of patients, includes children with chronic arthritis that do not meet criteria for any of the other subgroups or meet more than 1 criterion and therefore could be classified into multiple subgroups.

B. Laboratory Findings

There is no diagnostic test for JIA. A normal erythrocyte sedimentation rate (ESR) does not exclude the diagnosis of JIA. However, patients with systemic JIA typically have significantly elevated markers of inflammation, including ESR, C-reactive protein (CRP), white blood cell count, and platelets. RF is positive in about 5% of patients, usually when the onset of polyarticular disease occurs after age 8 years. A newer test, anti–cyclic citrullinated peptide (CCP) antibody, has a very high specificity for rheumatoid arthritis and may be detectable prior to the RF. ANAs are associated with an increased risk of iridocyclitis in patients with oligoarticular disease. A positive ANA test is also fairly common in patients with the late-onset RF–positive form of the disease. Carriage of HLAB27 antigen is associated with an increased risk of developing enthesitis-associated arthritis.

Table 29–1 lists the general characteristics of joint fluid in various conditions. The main indication for joint aspiration and synovial fluid analysis is to rule out infection. A positive Gram stain or culture is the only definitive test for infection. A leukocyte count over 2000/μL suggests inflammation; this may be due to infection, rheumatologic diseases, leukemia, or reactive arthritis. A very low glucose concentration (< 40 mg/dL) or very high polymorphonuclear leukocyte count (> 60,000/μL) is highly suggestive of bacterial arthritis.

C. Imaging Studies

In the early stages of the disease, only soft tissue swelling and possibly periarticular osteoporosis may be seen. Magnetic resonance imaging (MRI) of involved joints may show early joint damage and, if obtained with gadolinium, can confirm the presence of synovitis. Later in the course of the disease, particularly in patients with RF–positive disease, plain films may demonstrate joint space narrowing due to cartilage thinning and erosive changes of the bone related to chronic inflammation.

Table 29–1. Joint fluid analysis.

Disorder	Cells/μL	Glucose[a]
Trauma	More red cells than white cells; usually < 2000 white cells	Normal
Reactive arthritis	3000–10,000 white cells, mostly mononuclear cells	Normal
Juvenile idiopathic arthritis and other inflammatory arthritides	5000–60,000 white cells, mostly neutrophils	Usually normal or slightly low
Septic arthritis	> 60,000 white cells, > 90% neutrophils	Low to normal

[a]Normal value is ≥ 75% of the serum glucose value.

Differential Diagnosis

Table 29–2 lists the most common causes of limb pain in childhood. JIA is a diagnosis of exclusion; therefore, it is important to rule out other causes of the clinical signs and symptoms prior to settling on this diagnosis. The differential diagnosis is often quite broad, including orthopedic conditions, infectious diseases, and malignancies. A few key features can help distinguish these different entities, including the timing of the pain and associated signs and symptoms. In inflammatory conditions, patients frequently have increased

Table 29–2. Differential diagnosis of limb pain in children.

Orthopedic
- Stress fracture
- Chondromalacia patellae
- Osgood-Schlatter disease
- Slipped capital femoral epiphysis
- Legg-Calvé-Perthes disease
- Hypermobility syndrome

Reactive arthritis
- Henoch-Schönlein purpura
- Transient synovitis
- Rheumatic fever
- Poststreptococcal arthritis

Infections
- Bacterial
  - Lyme arthritis
  - Osteomyelitis
  - Septic arthritis
  - Discitis
- Viral
  - Parvovirus
  - Epstein-Barr virus
  - Hepatitis B arthritis

Rheumatologic
- Juvenile idiopathic arthritis
- Systemic lupus erythematosus
- Dermatomyositis

Neoplastic
- Leukemia
- Lymphoma
- Neuroblastoma
- Osteoid osteoma
- Bone tumors (benign or malignant)

Pain syndromes
- Growing pains
- Fibromyalgia
- Complex regional pain syndrome

symptoms in the morning with associated stiffness. In contrast, patients with an orthopedic abnormality typically have increased symptoms later in the day and with activity. Growing pains, a common cause of leg pain in childhood, are characterized by poorly localized pain at night, which frequently wakes the child from sleep; no objective signs of inflammation; and no daytime symptoms. Patients with growing pains often ask to be massaged, which is not typical of those with arthritis.

It is particularly important to establish the diagnosis in the case of monoarticular arthritis. Bacterial arthritis is usually acute and monoarticular except for arthritis associated with gonorrhea, which may be associated with a migratory pattern and hemorrhagic pustules, usually on the distal extremities. Fever, leukocytosis, and increased ESR with an acute process in a single joint demand synovial fluid examination and culture to identify the pathogen. Pain in the hip or lower extremity is a frequent symptom of childhood cancer, especially leukemia, neuroblastoma, and rhabdomyosarcoma. Infiltration of bone by tumor and a joint effusion may be seen. Radiographs of the affected site and examination of the blood smear for unusual cells and thrombocytopenia are necessary. An elevated lactate dehydrogenase value should also raise concern about an underlying neoplastic process. In doubtful cases, bone marrow examination is indicated.

In cases of reactive arthritis, a preceding illness is identified in approximately half of cases. Patients often have acute onset of arthritis, and there may be a migratory pattern. The duration of symptoms is a very important distinction between reactive arthritides and JIA. Symptoms associated with reactive arthritis typically resolve within 4–6 weeks. In contrast, to meet criteria for chronic arthritis, symptoms must be present for at least 6 weeks.

The arthritis of rheumatic fever is migratory, transient, and often more painful than that of JIA. Rheumatic fever is very rare in children younger than 5 years of age (see Chapter 21). In suspected cases, evidence of rheumatic carditis should be sought based on examination and electrocardiographic findings. Evidence of recent streptococcal infection is essential to the diagnosis. The fever pattern in rheumatic fever is low grade and persistent compared with the spiking fever that characterizes the systemic form of JIA. Lyme arthritis resembles oligoarticular JIA, but the former usually occurs as discrete, recurrent episodes of arthritis lasting 2–6 weeks and children should have a history of being in an endemic area. The typical bull's-eye rash, erythema chronicum migrans, occurs in 70%–80% of patients. For children suspected of having Lyme disease, testing for antibodies against *Borrelia burgdorferi* should be performed, with confirmatory testing by Western blot (see Chapter 42).

▶ Treatment

The objectives of therapy are to restore function, relieve pain, maintain joint motion, and prevent damage to cartilage and bone.

A. Nonsteroidal Anti-Inflammatory Medications

First-line therapy is nonsteroidal anti-inflammatory drugs (NSAIDs). A wide range of agents is available but only a few are approved for use in children, including naproxen (10 mg/kg per dose twice daily), ibuprofen (10 mg/kg per dose three to four times daily), and meloxicam (0.125 mg/kg once daily). NSAIDs are generally well tolerated in children, as long as they are taken with food. The average time to symptomatic improvement is 1 month, but in some patients a response is not seen for 8–12 weeks.

B. Disease-Modifying and Biologic Agents

For patients with JIA who fail to respond to NSAIDs, weekly methotrexate is the second-line medication of choice. Symptomatic response usually begins within 3–4 weeks. The low dosages used (5–10 mg/m^2/wk or 1 mg/kg/wk as a single dose) are generally well tolerated. Potential side effects include nausea, vomiting, hair thinning, stomatitis, bone marrow suppression, and hepatotoxicity. A complete blood count and liver function tests should be obtained every 2–3 months. Several additional disease-modifying agents are available for use in patients with persistently active disease or those intolerant to methotrexate. Leflunomide is an antipyrimidine medication that has been shown to be as effective as methotrexate. Side effects may include diarrhea and alopecia. Biological modifying medications that inhibit tumor necrosis factor, a cytokine known to play an important role in the pathogenesis of JIA, include etanercept, infliximab, and adalimumab. These drugs are generally quite effective in controlling disease and preventing cartilage and bone damage, and have been associated with healing based on radiologic changes. However, their potential long-term effects are unknown, they are very expensive, and require parenteral administration. Newer biologic agents, including anakinra, rituximab, abatacept, and tocilizumab, have demonstrated some efficacy in patients who have not responded to other treatments.

C. Corticosteroids

Steroids are reserved for children with severe involvement, primarily patients with systemic disease. Local steroid joint injections may be helpful in patients who have arthritis in one or a few joints. Triamcinolone hexacetonide is a long-acting steroid that can be used for injections and is often associated with at least several months of disease control.

D. Uveitis

Iridocyclitis should be closely monitored by an ophthalmologist (see Chapter 16). Typically treatment is initiated with corticosteroid eye drops and dilating agents to prevent scarring between the iris and the lens. In patients who fail topical treatments, methotrexate, cyclosporine, and/or a tumor-necrosis factor inhibitor such as infliximab or adalimumab may be used.

E. Rehabilitation

Physical and occupational therapies are important to focus on range of motion, stretching, and strengthening. These exercises, as well as other modalities such as heat, water therapy, and ultrasound, can help control pain, maintain and restore function, and prevent deformity and disability. Young children with oligoarticular disease affecting asymmetrical lower extremity joints can develop a leg-length discrepancy, which may require treatment with a shoe lift on the unaffected side.

Prognosis

The course and prognosis for JIA is variable, depending on the subtype of disease. Children with persistent oligoarticular JIA have the highest rate of clinical remission, while patients with RF-positive disease are the least likely to achieve this status and are at highest risk for chronic, erosive arthritis that may continue into adulthood. The systemic features associated with systemic arthritis tend to remit within months to years. The prognosis in systemic disease is worse in patients with persistent systemic disease after 6 months, thrombocytosis, and more extensive arthritis.

Beukelman T et al: 2011 American College of Rheumatology recommendations for the treatment of juvenile idiopathic arthritis: initiation and safety monitoring of therapeutic agents for the treatment of arthritis and systemic features. Arthritis Care Res 2011;63:465–482 [PMID: 21452260]. Available at: http://emedicine.medscape.com/article/1007276-overview.

Hayward K, Wallace CA: Recent developments in anti-rheumatic drugs in pediatrics: Treatment of juvenile idiopathic arthritis. Arthritis Res Ther 2009;11:216 [PMID: 19291269].

Perry DC, Bruce C: Evaluating the child who presents with an acute limp. BMJ 2010;341:c4250 [PMID: 20729271].

Prakken B, Albani S, Martini A: Juvenile idiopathic arthritis. Lancet 2011;377:2138–2149 [PMID: 21684384]. Available at: www.arthritis.org.

SYSTEMIC LUPUS ERYTHEMATOSUS

ESSENTIALS OF DIAGNOSIS & TYPICAL FEATURES

- Multisystem inflammatory disease of the joints, serosal linings, skin, kidneys, blood, and central nervous system.
- Autoantibodies such as ANA, double-stranded DNA, and anti-Smith antibodies are present and related to the pathogenesis of disease.

Pathogenesis

Systemic lupus erythematosus (SLE) is the prototype of immune complex diseases; its pathogenesis is related to the formation of antibody-antigen complexes that exist in the circulation and deposit in the involved tissues. The spectrum of symptoms is due to tissue-specific autoantibodies, as well as damage to the tissue by lymphocytes, neutrophils, and complement evoked by the deposition of immune complexes. Autoreactive T lymphocytes that have escaped clonal deletion and unregulated B-lymphocyte production of autoantibodies may initiate the disease.

Clinical Findings

A. Symptoms and Signs

The onset of pediatric SLE is most common in girls between the ages of 9 and 15 years. Signs and symptoms depend on the organs affected by immune complex deposition. The American College of Rheumatology has established criteria to aid in the diagnosis of SLE; four of the following 11 criteria are necessary to establish the diagnosis:

1. Malar rash—photosensitive, so-called butterfly rash on the cheeks and nasal bridge
2. Discoid rash—annular, scaly rash on the scalp, face, and extremities that can lead to scarring
3. Photosensitivity—increased rash or other disease symptoms in response to sunlight exposure
4. Mucous membrane ulcers—painless ulcers on the hard palate and/or nasal septum
5. Arthritis—nonerosive arthritis of large and small joints, typically in a symmetrical distribution
6. Serositis—pericarditis and/or pleuritis, often associated with chest pain and difficulty breathing
7. Renal abnormalities—proteinuria (> 0.5 g/d) and/or cellular casts
8. Neurologic abnormalities—seizures and/or psychosis
9. Blood count abnormalities—low white blood cell count (< 4000/mm^3), Coombs test–positive anemia, and/or thrombocytopenia (< 100,000/mm^3)
10. Positive ANA—seen in almost 100% of patients with SLE
11. Autoantibodies—positive double-stranded DNA antibody, anti-Smith antibody, anticardiolipin antibodies, lupus anticoagulant, and/or false-positive blood test for syphilis

Other common signs and symptoms include fever, fatigue, weight loss, anorexia, Raynaud phenomenon, myositis, vasculitis, chorea, neuropathies, depression, and cognitive changes.

B. Laboratory Findings

Complete blood count abnormalities are common, including leukopenia, anemia, and thrombocytopenia. Approximately 15% of patients are Coombs test–positive, but many patients develop anemia due to other causes, including chronic disease and blood loss. Patients with significant renal involvement may have electrolyte disturbances, elevated kidney function tests, and hypoalbuminemia. The ESR is frequently elevated during active disease. In contrast, many patients with active SLE have a normal CRP. When the CRP is elevated, it is important to investigate possible infectious causes, particularly bacterial infections. It is critical to monitor the urinalysis in patients with SLE for proteinuria and hematuria, as the renal disease may be otherwise clinically silent. In immune complex diseases, complement is consumed; therefore, levels of C3 and C4 are depressed with active disease.

The ANA test is positive in almost 100% of patients, usually at titers of 1:320 or above. In patients with suspected SLE, it is important to obtain a full ANA profile—including antibodies directed against double-stranded DNA, Smith, ribonucleic protein, and Sjogren's specific antibody A and B antibodies—to better characterize their serologic markers of disease. Because approximately 50%–60% of pediatric SLE patients have antiphospholipid antibodies and are therefore at increased risk of thrombosis, it is important to screen all patients with SLE for anticardiolipin antibodies and lupus anticoagulant.

Differential Diagnosis

Because there is such a wide spectrum of disease with SLE, the differential diagnosis is quite broad, including systemic JIA, mixed connective tissue disease (MCTD), rheumatic fever, vasculitis, malignancies, and bacterial and viral infections. A negative ANA test essentially excludes the diagnosis of SLE. Anti–double-stranded DNA and Smith antibodies are very specific for SLE. The preceding diagnostic criteria, which are very helpful in establishing the diagnosis of SLE, have a specificity and sensitivity of 96%.

MCTD, an overlap syndrome with features of several collagen-vascular diseases, shares many features with SLE. The symptom complex is diverse and often includes arthritis, fever, skin tightening, Raynaud phenomenon, muscle weakness, and rash. The ANA test is typically positive in very high titers. The ANA profile is negative except for antibodies directed against ribonucleic protein.

Treatment

The treatment of SLE should be tailored to the organ system involved so that toxicities may be minimized. Prednisone is the mainstay of treatment and has significantly lowered the mortality rate in SLE. Patients with severe, life-threatening, or organ-threatening disease are typically treated with intravenous pulse methylprednisolone, 30 mg/kg per dose (maximum of 1000 mg) daily for 3 days, and then switched to 2 mg/kg/d of prednisone. The dosage should be adjusted using clinical and laboratory parameters of disease activity, and the minimum amount of corticosteroid to control the disease should be used. Skin manifestations, arthritis, and fatigue may be treated with antimalarials such as hydroxychloroquine, 5–7 mg/kg/d orally. Pleuritic pain or arthritis can often be managed with NSAIDs.

If disease control is inadequate with prednisone or if the dose required produces intolerable side effects, a steroid-sparing agent, such as mycophenolate mofetil, azathioprine, or cyclophosphamide, should be added. More recently, rituximab, a monoclonal antibody directed against the B-cell surface marker CD20, has been used for persistent active disease, particularly in patients with hematologic manifestations. Patients who have evidence of antiphospholipid antibodies should be treated with a baby aspirin every day to help prevent thrombosis. Thrombotic events due to these antibodies require long-term anticoagulation.

The toxicities of the regimens must be carefully considered. Growth failure, osteoporosis, Cushing syndrome, adrenal suppression, and aseptic necrosis are serious side effects of chronic use of prednisone. When high doses of corticosteroids are used (> 2 mg/kg/d), there is a high risk of infection. Cyclophosphamide can cause bladder epithelial dysplasia, hemorrhagic cystitis, and sterility. Azathioprine has been associated with liver damage and bone marrow suppression. Immunosuppressant treatment should be withheld if the total white blood cell count falls below 3000/μL or the neutrophil count falls below 1000/μL. Retinal damage from hydroxychloroquine has not been observed with recommended dosages.

Prognosis

The prognosis in SLE relates to the presence of renal involvement or infectious complications of treatment. Nonetheless, the survival rate has improved from 51% at 5 years in 1954 to 90% today. The disease has a natural waxing and waning cycle; the disease may flare at any time and spontaneous remission may rarely occur.

Brunner HI, Huggins J, Klein-Gitelman MS: Pediatric SLE—towards a comprehensive management plan. Nature Reviews Rheumatology 2011;7:225–233 [PMID: 21386795].

Marks SD, Tullus K: Modern therapeutic strategies for paediatric systemic lupus erythematosus and lupus nephritis. Acta Paediatr 2010;99:967–974 [PMID: 20222881].

Tucker LB: Making the diagnosis of systemic lupus erythematosus in children and adolescents. Lupus 2007;16:546 [PMID: 17711886].

DERMATOMYOSITIS

ESSENTIALS OF DIAGNOSIS & TYPICAL FEATURES

- Pathognomonic skin rashes.
- Weakness of proximal muscles and occasionally of pharyngeal and laryngeal groups.
- Pathogenesis related to vasculitis.

Clinical Findings

A. Symptoms and Signs

The predominant symptom is proximal muscle weakness, particularly affecting pelvic and shoulder girdle muscles. Tenderness, stiffness, and swelling may be found. Pharyngeal involvement, manifested as voice changes and difficulty swallowing, is associated with an increased risk of aspiration. Intestinal vasculitis can be associated with ulceration and perforation of involved areas. Flexion contractures and muscle atrophy may produce significant residual deformities. Calcinosis may follow the inflammation in muscle and skin.

Several characteristic rashes are seen in dermatomyositis. Patients often have a heliotrope rash with a reddish-purple hue on the upper eyelids, along with a malar rash that may be accompanied by edema of the eyelids and face. Gottron papules are shiny, erythematous, scaly plaques on the extensor surfaces of the knuckles, elbows, and knees. Nail-fold abnormalities, including dilation, thrombosis, and dropout of periungual capillaries, may identify patients with a worse prognosis.

B. Laboratory Findings/Imaging Studies/Special Tests

Determination of muscle enzyme levels, including aspartate aminotransferase, alanine aminotransferase, lactate dehydrogenase, creatine phosphokinase, and aldolase, is helpful in confirming the diagnosis, assessing disease activity, and monitoring the response to treatment. Even in the face of extensive muscle inflammation, the ESR and CRP are frequently normal. An MRI scan of the quadriceps muscle can be used in equivocal cases to confirm the presence of inflammatory myositis. Electromyography is useful to distinguish myopathic from neuropathic causes of muscle weakness. Muscle biopsy is indicated in cases of myositis without the pathognomonic rash.

Treatment

Treatment is aimed at suppression of the inflammatory response and prevention of the loss of muscle function and joint range of motion. Acutely, it is very important to assess the adequacy of the ventilatory effort and swallowing and to rule out intestinal vasculitis. Corticosteroids are the initial therapy of choice. Treatment is usually initiated with prednisone, 2 mg/kg/d, and continued until signs and symptoms of active disease are controlled; the dosage is then gradually tapered. In severe cases, intravenous pulse methylprednisolone for 3 days is indicated. Therapy is guided by the physical examination findings and muscle enzyme values. Methotrexate is often used concomitantly to achieve better control of the disease and minimize the steroid side effects. If patients continue to have active disease, additional steroid-sparing agents, such as cyclosporine, and, in severe cases, cyclophosphamide, should be started.

Hydroxychloroquine and intravenous immunoglobulin may be helpful in managing the skin manifestations. As the rashes are photosensitive, sun protection is very important. Physical and occupational therapy should be initiated early in the course of disease. Initially, passive range-of-motion exercises are performed to prevent loss of motion. Later, once the muscle enzymes have normalized, a graduated program of stretching and strengthening exercises is introduced to restore normal strength and function.

Prognosis

Most patients have a monocyclic course; 10%–20% of patients have more chronic or recurrent symptoms. Factors that influence the outcome include the rapidity of symptom onset, extent of weakness, presence of cutaneous or gastrointestinal vasculitis, timeliness of diagnosis, initiation of therapy, and response to treatment. Dermatomyositis in children is not associated with an increased risk of cancer as it is in adults.

Feldman BM et al: Juvenile dermatomyositis and other idiopathic inflammatory myopathies of childhood. Lancet 2008;371:2201 [PMID: 18586175].

Stringer E, Bohnsack J, Bowyer SL et al: Treatment approaches to juvenile dermatomyositis (JDM) across North America: The Childhood Arthritis and Rheumatology Research Alliance (CARRA) JDM Treatment Survey. J Rheumatol 2010;37:1953–1961 [PMID: 20595275].

VASCULITIS

ESSENTIALS OF DIAGNOSIS & TYPICAL FEATURES

- Cutaneous involvement with nonblanching, tender skin lesions.
- Frequently with systemic inflammation, particularly in the lungs and kidneys.
- Gold-standard for diagnosis is demonstration of vasculitis on biopsy.

The vasculitides are a group of conditions that involve inflammation of blood vessels. They are classified by the size of the blood vessels affected (Table 29–3). The two most common forms of vasculitis in childhood, Henoch-Schonlein Purpura (HSP) (see Chapter 30) and Kawasaki Disease (see Chapter 20), are acute, self-limited forms of vasculitis. In contrast, there are idiopathic, chronic forms of vasculitis, such as granulomatosis with polyangiitis (GPA) and microscopic polyangiitis (MPA), that are rare in childhood.

Table 29–3. Classification of vasculitides by vessel size involved.

Large vessel
Takayasu arteritis
Giant cell arteritis
Medium vessel
Kawasaki disease
Granulomatosis with polyangiitis (previously called Wegener granulomatosis)
Polyarteritis nodosa
Churg-Strauss syndrome
Small vessel
Henoch-Schonlein purpura
Microscopic polyarteritis

Clinical Findings

Symptoms and Signs

Signs and symptoms vary by disease, but most children with chronic forms of vasculitis have persistent fever, fatigue, weight loss, and signs of pulmonary, renal, musculoskeletal, gastrointestinal, and/or skin inflammation.

Granulomatosis with polyangiitis (previously called Wegener granulomatosis) often causes nephritis and involves the lungs, manifesting as chronic cough, hemorrhage, and/or cavitating lesions. This form of vasculitis also frequently affects the upper respiratory tract, causing chronic otitis media, sinusitis, and/or inflammation of the trachea; saddle nose deformity may occur.

Children with polyarteritis nodosa (PAN) often present with skin lesions such as purpura, nodules or ulcers, and evidence of organ involvement with abdominal pain, testicular pain, hypertension, hematuria and/or neurologic symptoms. Microscopic polyangiitis (MPA) typically presents with pulmonary-renal syndrome with features of pulmonary hemorrhage and rapidly progressive kidney inflammation.

B. Laboratory Findings/Imaging Studies/Special Tests

Patients with vasculitis often have elevated inflammatory markers. If they have significant renal involvement, they may have elevated renal function tests and abnormal urinary sediment. Anemia is common, due to chronic disease and/or renal insufficiency. A low hemoglobin may also be an indicator of pulmonary hemorrhage in a patient with cough, hemoptysis, respiratory distress, and/or infiltrates on chest x-ray.

Antineutrophil cytoplasmic antibodies (ANCA) may be present in patients with small vessel vasculitis. Cytoplasmic ANCA (c-ANCA) is usually directed against proteinase 3 and is quite sensitive and specific for GPA and is positive in 80%–95% of patients with active disease. Perinuclear ANCA (p-ANCA) is typically directed against myeloperoxidase and is associated with MPA and can also be seen in HSP, Churg-Strauss, and inflammatory bowel disease.

The diagnosis is made based on a typical clinical presentation and laboratory findings. If the diagnosis remains uncertain, then attempting to definitively establish the diagnosis with a biopsy of involved tissue is warranted. A biopsy in patients with GPA typically demonstrates necrotizing granulomatous vasculitis. Biopsies of involved areas will confirm the presence of vasculitis in small vessels in patients with MPA and small and medium arteries in PAN. If a biopsy is not feasible, additional imaging studies such as an angiogram, which can demonstrate characteristic patterns of inflammation in affected blood vessels, should be considered.

Treatment

The treatment of the various forms of chronic vasculitis is based on the severity of illness and the organs involved. Typically, corticosteroids are the initial therapy. Patients with severe disease are usually treated with intravenous pulse methylprednisolone, 30 mg/kg per dose (maximum of 1000 mg) daily for 3 days, and then switched to 2 mg/kg/d of prednisone. The dosage is then gradually tapered as tolerated based on clinical and laboratory markers of disease activity. Patients are usually treated with other immunosuppressant medications to gain and maintain control of the disease and minimize the steroid side effects. Standard treatment has included cyclophosphamide for induction, followed by maintenance with methotrexate, azathioprine, or mycophenolate. More recent studies in patients with GPA suggest that rituximab can be used for induction therapy with potentially fewer side effects and risks than cyclophosphamide.

Prognosis

Immunosuppressive medications have improved survival and remission rates for patients with chronic vasculitis. Conditions such as GPA had been almost always fatal; since introducing the regimen of high dose steroids and cyclophosphamide (or other cytotoxic agents), patients with vasculitides have greatly improved outcomes, with five year survival ranging from 50% to 100%. Because relapses are common when therapy is weaned or stopped, maintenance immunosuppression is commonly used in these disorders.

Gedalia A, Cuchacovich R: Systemic vasculitis in childhood. Curr Rheumatol Rep 2009;11:402–409 [PMID: 19922729].

O'Neil K: Progress in pediatric vasculitis. Curr Opin Rheumatol 2009;21:538–546 [PMID: 19568171].

RAYNAUD PHENOMENON

Raynaud phenomenon is an intermittent vasospastic disorder of the extremities. As much as 10% of the adult population has this disorder, and onset in childhood is not uncommon. The classic triphasic presentation is cold-induced pallor, then cyanosis, followed by hyperemia, but incomplete forms are frequent. In adults older than 35 years who are ANA-positive, Raynaud phenomenon may be a harbinger of rheumatic disease. This progression is rarely seen in childhood. Evaluation should include a detailed history with review of systems relevant to rheumatic disease and examination for nail-fold capillary abnormalities. In the absence of positive findings, Raynaud phenomenon is likely to be idiopathic.

Treatment involves education about keeping the extremities and core body warm and the role of stress, which may be a precipitant. In very symptomatic patients, treatment with calcium channel blockers such as nifedipine can be effective.

Pope JE: The diagnosis and treatment of Raynaud phenomenon: A practical approach. Drugs 2007;67:57 [PMID: 17352512].

NONINFLAMMATORY PAIN SYNDROMES

1. Complex Regional Pain Syndrome

Complex regional pain syndrome, previously known as reflex sympathetic dystrophy, is a painful condition that is frequently confused with arthritis. Prevalence and recognition of the condition appear to be increasing. Severe extremity pain leading to nearly complete loss of function is the hallmark of the condition. Evidence of autonomic dysfunction is demonstrated by pallor or cyanosis, temperature differences (with the affected extremity cooler than surrounding areas), and generalized swelling. On examination, marked cutaneous hyperesthesia to even the slightest touch is often evident. Results of laboratory tests are normal, without evidence of systemic inflammation. Radiographic findings are normal except for late development of osteoporosis. Bone scans may be helpful and may demonstrate either increased or decreased blood flow to the painful extremity.

The cause of this condition remains elusive. Treatment includes physical therapy to focus on restoration of function, maintenance of range of motion, and pain relief. NSAIDs can be helpful for pain control, and in patients with more chronic disease, gabapentin is frequently effective. Persistent disease may respond to local nerve blocks. Counseling is helpful to identify potential psychosocial stressors and to assist with pain management. Long-term prognosis is good if recovery is rapid; recurrent episodes imply a less favorable prognosis.

Tan EC et al: Complex regional pain syndrome type I in children. Acta Paediatr 2008;97:848 [PMID: 18410465]. Available at: http://childhoodrnd.org/index.php.

2. Fibromyalgia

Fibromyalgia is a chronic pain syndrome characterized by diffuse musculoskeletal pain, fatigue, sleep disturbance, and chronic headaches. Weather changes, fatigue, and stress exacerbate symptoms. Patients have a normal examination except for characteristic trigger points at the insertion of muscles, especially along the neck, spine, and pelvis.

Treatment centers on physical therapy, nonnarcotic pain medications, improving sleep, and counseling. Low-dose amitriptyline or trazodone can help with sleep and may produce remarkable reduction in pain. Physical therapy should emphasize a graded rehabilitative approach to stretching and exercise and promote regular aerobic exercise. Pregabalin recently became the first medication to be approved by the Food and Drug Administration for the treatment of fibromyalgia. Use of the drug is associated with decreased pain in adults with fibromyalgia, and studies are planned to test the safety and efficacy of its use in children with the condition. The prognosis for children with fibromyalgia is not clear, and long-term strategies may be necessary to enable them to cope with the condition.

Buskila D: Pediatric fibromyalgia. Rheum Dis Clin North Am 2009;35:253 [PMID: 19647140]. Available at: www.myalgia.com.

3. Hypermobility Syndrome

Ligamentous laxity, which previously was thought to occur only in Ehlers-Danlos syndrome or Down syndrome, is now recognized as a common cause of joint pain. Patients with hypermobility present with episodic joint pain and occasionally with swelling that lasts a few days after increased physical activity. Depending on the activity, almost any joint may be affected. Five criteria have been established: (1) passive opposition of the thumb to the flexor surface of the forearm, (2) passive hyperextension of the fingers so that they are parallel to the extensor surface of the forearm, (3) hyperextension of the elbow, (4) hyperextension of the knee, and (5) palms on floor with knees extended. Results of laboratory tests are normal. The pain associated with the syndrome is produced by improper joint alignment caused by the laxity during exercise. Treatment consists of a graded conditioning program designed to provide muscular support of the joints to compensate for the loose ligaments and to train patients to protect their joints from hyperextension.

Tofts LJ et al: The differential diagnosis of children with joint hypermobility: A review of the literature. Pediatr Rheumatol Online J 2009;7:1 [PMID: 19123951].

Hematologic Disorders

30

Daniel R. Ambruso, MD
Taru Hays, MD
Neil A. Goldenberg, MD, PhD
Rachelle Nuss, MD

NORMAL HEMATOLOGIC VALUES

The normal ranges for peripheral blood counts vary significantly with age. Normal neonates show a relative polycythemia with a hematocrit concentration of 45%–65%. The reticulocyte count at birth is relatively high at 2%–8%. Within the first few days of life, erythrocyte production decreases, and the values for hemoglobin and hematocrit fall to a nadir at about 6–8 weeks. During this period, known as physiologic anemia of infancy, normal infants have hemoglobin values as low as 10 g/dL and hematocrits as low as 30%. Thereafter, the normal values for hemoglobin and hematocrit gradually increase until adult values are reached after puberty. Premature infants can reach a nadir hemoglobin level of 7–8 g/dL at 8–10 weeks.

Newborns have larger red cells than children and adults, with a mean corpuscular volume (MCV) at birth of more than 94 fL. The MCV subsequently falls to a nadir of 70–84 fL at about age 6 months. Thereafter, the normal MCV increases gradually until it reaches adult values after puberty.

The normal number of white blood cells is higher in infancy and early childhood than later in life. Neutrophils predominate in the differential white count at birth and in the older child. Lymphocytes predominate (up to 80%) between about ages 1 month and 6 years.

Normal values for the platelet count are 150,000–400,000/μL and vary little with age.

BONE MARROW FAILURE

Failure of the marrow to produce adequate numbers of circulating blood cells may be congenital or acquired and may cause pancytopenia (aplastic anemia) or involve only one cell line (single cytopenia). Constitutional and acquired aplastic anemias are discussed in this section and the more common single cytopenias in later sections. Bone marrow failure caused by malignancy or other infiltrative disease is discussed in Chapter 31. It is important to remember that many drugs and toxins may affect the marrow and cause single or multiple cytopenias.

Suspicion of bone marrow failure is warranted in children with pancytopenia and in children with single cytopenias who lack evidence of peripheral red cell, white cell, or platelet destruction. Macrocytosis often accompanies bone marrow failure. Many of the constitutional bone marrow disorders are associated with a variety of congenital anomalies.

CONSTITUTIONAL APLASTIC ANEMIA (FANCONI ANEMIA)

ESSENTIALS OF DIAGNOSIS & TYPICAL FEATURES

- Progressive pancytopenia.
- Macrocytosis.
- Multiple congenital anomalies.
- Increased chromosome breakage in peripheral blood lymphocytes.

General Considerations

Fanconi anemia is a syndrome characterized by defective DNA repair that is caused by a variety of genetic mutations. Inheritance is autosomal recessive, and the disease occurs in all ethnic groups. Hematologic manifestations usually begin with thrombocytopenia or neutropenia and subsequently progress over the course of months or years to pancytopenia. Typically the diagnosis is made between ages 2 and 10 years.

Clinical Findings

A. Symptoms and Signs

Symptoms are determined principally by the degree of hematologic abnormality. Thrombocytopenia may cause purpura, petechiae, and bleeding; neutropenia may cause severe or recurrent infections; and anemia may cause weakness, fatigue, and pallor. Congenital anomalies are present in at least 50% of patients. The most common include abnormal pigmentation of the skin (generalized hyperpigmentation, café au lait or hypopigmented spots), short stature with delicate features, and skeletal malformations (hypoplasia, anomalies, or absence of the thumb and radius). More subtle anomalies are hypoplasia of the thenar eminence or a weak or absent radial pulse. Associated renal anomalies include aplasia, horseshoe kidney, and duplication of the collecting system. Other anomalies are microcephaly, microphthalmia, strabismus, ear anomalies, and hypogenitalism.

B. Laboratory Findings

Thrombocytopenia or leukopenia typically occurs first, followed over the course of months to years by anemia and progression to severe aplastic anemia. Macrocytosis is virtually always present, is usually associated with anisocytosis and an elevation in fetal hemoglobin levels, and is an important diagnostic clue. The bone marrow reveals hypoplasia or aplasia. The diagnosis is confirmed by the demonstration of an increased number of chromosome breaks and rearrangements in peripheral blood lymphocytes. The use of diepoxybutane to stimulate these breaks and rearrangements provides a sensitive assay that is virtually always positive in children with Fanconi anemia, even before the onset of hematologic abnormalities.

Specific molecular markers or genes (Fanc-A, B, C, and others) found in different ethnic populations are identified in research laboratories and are not available as routine clinical tests.

Differential Diagnosis

Because patients with Fanconi anemia frequently present with thrombocytopenia, the disorder must be differentiated from idiopathic thrombocytopenic purpura (ITP) and other more common causes of thrombocytopenia. In contrast to patients with ITP, those with Fanconi anemia usually exhibit a gradual fall in the platelet count. Counts less than 20,000/μL are often accompanied by neutropenia or anemia, along with phenotypical features. Fanconi anemia may also be manifested initially by pancytopenia, and must be differentiated from acquired aplastic anemia and other disorders, such as acute leukemia. Examination of the bone marrow and chromosome studies of peripheral blood lymphocytes (chromosomal breakage) will usually distinguish between these disorders.

Complications

The most important complications of Fanconi anemia are those related to thrombocytopenia and neutropenia. Endocrine dysfunction may include growth hormone deficiency, hypothyroidism, or impaired glucose metabolism. In addition, persons with Fanconi anemia have a significantly increased risk of developing malignancies, especially acute nonlymphocytic leukemia, head and neck cancers, genital cancers, and myelodysplastic syndromes. Death is usually the result of thrombocytopenic hemorrhage, overwhelming infection, or malignancy.

Treatment

Attentive supportive care is critical. Patients with neutropenia who develop fever require prompt evaluation and parenteral broad-spectrum antibiotics. Transfusions are important, but should be used judiciously, especially in the management of thrombocytopenia, which frequently becomes refractory to platelet transfusions as a consequence of alloimmunization. Transfusions from family members should be discouraged because of the negative effect on the outcome of bone marrow transplantation. At least 50% of patients with Fanconi anemia respond, albeit incompletely, to oxymetholone, and many recommend institution of androgen therapy before transfusions are needed. However, oxymetholone is associated with hepatotoxicity, hepatic adenomas, and masculinization, and is particularly troublesome for female patients.

Successful bone marrow transplantation cures the aplastic anemia and is an important treatment option for children with Fanconi anemia who have a human leukocyte antigen (HLA)–identical sibling donor. Before transplantation, the prospective donor must be screened for Fanconi anemia by chromosome-breakage testing.

Prognosis

Many patients succumb to bleeding, infection, or malignancy in adolescence or early adulthood. The long-term outlook after successful bone marrow transplantation is uncertain, particularly with regard to the risk of subsequently developing malignancies.

Alter BP: Cancer in Fanconi anemia, 1927–2001. Cancer 2003;97:425 [PMID: 12518367].

Dokal I: Inherited aplastic anemias/bone marrow failure syndromes. Blood Rev 2008;22:141 [PMID: 18164793].

Green A: Fanconi anemia. Hematol Oncol Clin North Am 2009;23(2):193 [PMID: 19327579].

ACQUIRED APLASTIC ANEMIA

ESSENTIALS OF DIAGNOSIS & TYPICAL FEATURES

- Weakness and pallor.
- Petechiae, purpura, and bleeding.

- Frequent or severe infections.
- Pancytopenia with hypocellular bone marrow.

General Considerations

Acquired aplastic anemia is characterized by peripheral pancytopenia with a hypocellular bone marrow. Approximately 50% of cases in childhood are idiopathic. Other cases are secondary to idiosyncratic reactions to drugs such as phenylbutazone, sulfonamides, nonsteroidal anti-inflammatory drugs (NSAIDs), and anticonvulsants. Toxic causes include exposure to benzene, insecticides, and heavy metals. Infectious causes include viral hepatitis (usually non-A, non-B, non-C), infectious mononucleosis, and human immunodeficiency virus (HIV). In immunocompromised children, aplastic anemia has been associated with human parvovirus B19. Immune mechanisms of marrow suppression are suspected in most cases.

Clinical Findings

A. Symptoms and Signs

Weakness, fatigue, and pallor result from anemia; petechiae, purpura, and bleeding occur because of thrombocytopenia; and fevers due to generalized or localized infections are associated with neutropenia. Hepatosplenomegaly and significant lymphadenopathy are unusual.

B. Laboratory Findings

Anemia is usually normocytic, with a low reticulocyte count. The white blood cell count is low, with a marked neutropenia. The platelet count is typically below 50,000/μL, and is frequently below 20,000/μL. Bone marrow biopsy shows a marked decrease in cellularity typically less than 20% of normal in severe aplastic anemia.

Differential Diagnosis

Examination of the bone marrow usually excludes pancytopenia caused by peripheral destruction of blood cells or by infiltrative processes such as acute leukemia, storage diseases, and myelofibrosis. Many of these other conditions are associated with hepatosplenomegaly. Preleukemic conditions also may present with pancytopenia and hypocellular bone marrows. Cytogenetic analysis of the marrow is helpful, because a clonal abnormality may predict the subsequent development of leukemia. Since congenital anomalies may not be apparent in some children with Fanconi anemia, patients with newly diagnosed aplastic anemia should be studied for chromosome breaks and rearrangements in peripheral blood lymphocytes.

Complications

Acquired aplastic anemia is characteristically complicated by infection and hemorrhage, which are the leading causes of death. Other complications are those associated with therapy.

Treatment

Comprehensive supportive care is most important in the management of acute acquired aplastic anemia. Febrile illnesses require prompt evaluation and usually parenteral antibiotics. Red blood cell transfusions alleviate symptoms of anemia. Platelet transfusions may be lifesaving, but they should be used sparingly because many patients eventually develop platelet alloantibodies and become refractory to platelet transfusions.

Bone marrow transplantation is generally considered the treatment of choice for severe aplastic anemia when an HLA-identical sibling donor is available. Because the likelihood of success with transplantation is influenced adversely by multiple transfusions, HLA typing of family members should be undertaken as soon as the diagnosis of aplastic anemia is made. Increasingly patients who lack HLA-identical siblings are able to find matched donors through cord blood banks or the National Marrow Donor Program.

An alternative to bone marrow transplantation from an HLA-identical sibling donor is immunomodulation, usually with antithymocyte globulin and cyclosporine or tacrolimus. Responses are very good. Most patients show hematologic improvement and become transfusion-independent.

Prognosis

Children receiving early bone marrow transplantation from an HLA-identical sibling have a long-term survival rate of greater than 80%. Sustained, complete remissions may be seen in 65%–80% of patients receiving immunosuppressive therapy. However, both therapies are associated with an increased risk of myelodysplastic syndromes, acute leukemia, and other malignancies in long-term survivors.

Guinan EC: Acquired aplastic anemia in childhood. Hematol Oncol Clin N Am 2009;23:171 [PMID: 19327578].

Leguit RJ: The pathology of bone marrow failure. Histopathology 2010;57:655 [PMID: 20727024].

ANEMIAS

APPROACH TO THE CHILD WITH ANEMIA

Anemia is a relatively common finding, and identifying the cause is important. Even though anemia in childhood has many causes, the correct diagnosis can usually be established with relatively little laboratory cost. Frequently the cause is identified with a careful history. Nutritional causes should be sought by inquiry about dietary intake; growth and development; and symptoms of chronic disease, malabsorption, or blood loss. Hemolytic disease may be associated with a history of jaundice (including neonatal jaundice) or by a family history of anemia, jaundice, gallbladder disease, splenomegaly, or splenectomy. The child's ethnic background may suggest the possibility of certain hemoglobinopathies or of deficiencies of red cell enzymes, such as glucose-6-phosphate dehydrogenase (G6PD). The review of systems may reveal clues to a previously unsuspected systemic disease associated with anemia. The patient's age is important because some causes of anemia are age-related. For example, patients with iron-deficiency anemia and β-globin disorders present more commonly at ages 6–36 months than at other times in life.

The physical examination may also reveal clues to the cause of anemia. Poor growth may suggest chronic disease or hypothyroidism. Congenital anomalies may be associated with constitutional aplastic anemia (Fanconi anemia) or with congenital hypoplastic anemia (Diamond-Blackfan anemia). Other disorders may be suggested by the findings of petechiae or purpura (leukemia, aplastic anemia, hemolytic-uremic syndrome), jaundice (hemolysis or liver disease), generalized lymphadenopathy (leukemia, juvenile rheumatoid arthritis, HIV infection), splenomegaly (leukemia, sickle hemoglobinopathy syndromes, hereditary spherocytosis, liver disease, hypersplenism), or evidence of chronic or recurrent infections.

The initial laboratory evaluation of the anemic child consists of a complete blood count (CBC) with differential and platelet count, review of the peripheral blood smear, and a reticulocyte count. The algorithm in Figure 30–1 uses limited laboratory information, together with the history and physical examination, to reach a specific diagnosis or to focus additional laboratory investigations on a limited diagnostic category (eg, microcytic anemia, bone marrow failure, pure red cell aplasia, or hemolytic disease). This diagnostic scheme depends principally on the MCV to determine whether the anemia is microcytic, normocytic, or macrocytic, according to the percentile curves of Dallman and Siimes (Figure 30–2).

Although the incidence of iron deficiency in the United States has decreased significantly with improvements in infant nutrition, it remains an important cause of microcytic anemia, especially at ages 6–24 months. A trial of therapeutic iron is appropriate in such children, provided the dietary history is compatible with iron deficiency and the physical examination or CBC does not suggest an alternative cause for the anemia. If a trial of therapeutic iron fails to correct the anemia and microcytosis, further laboratory evaluation is warranted.

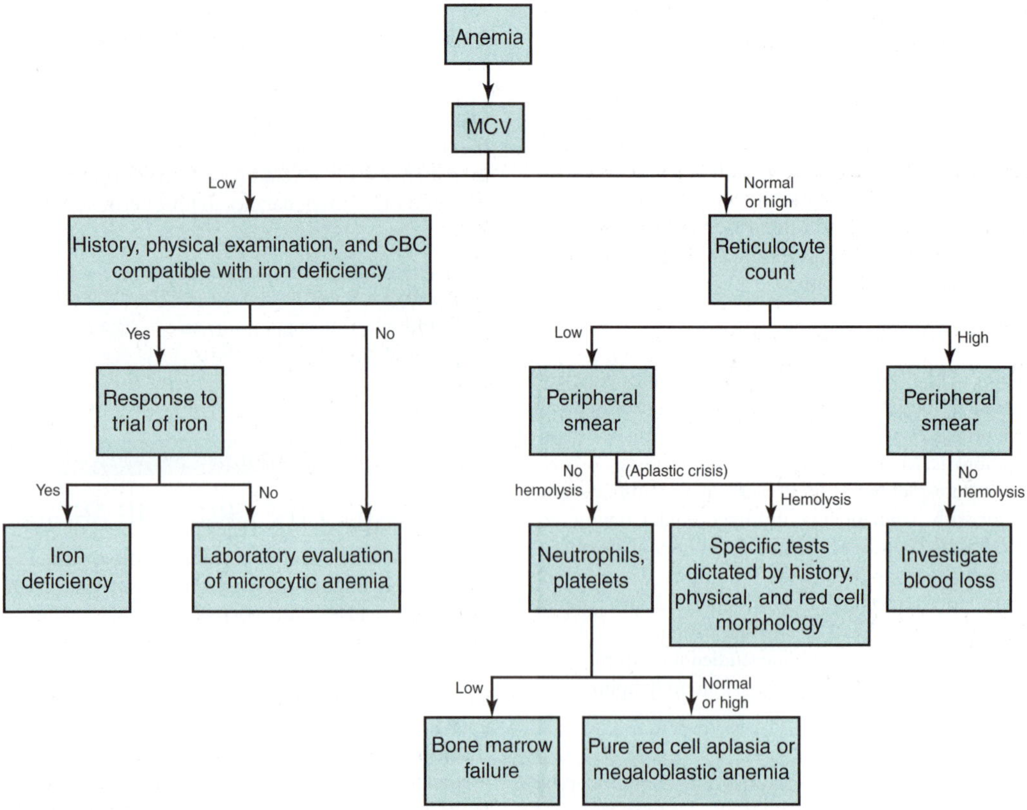

▲ **Figure 30–1.** Investigation of anemia.

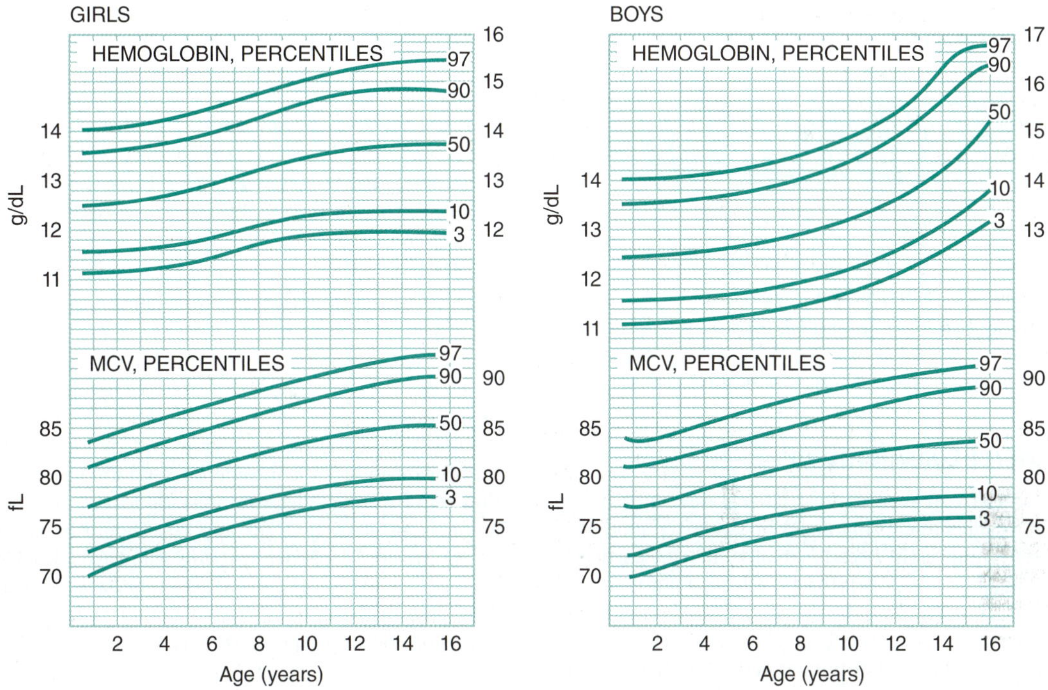

▲ **Figure 30–2.** Hemoglobin and red cell volume in infancy and childhood. (Reproduced, with permission, from Dallman PR, Siimes MA: Percentile curves for hemoglobin and red cell volume in infancy and childhood. J Pediatr 1979;94:26.)

Another key element of Figure 30–1 is the use of both the reticulocyte count and the peripheral blood smear to determine whether a normocytic or macrocytic anemia is due to hemolysis. Typically hemolytic disease is associated with an elevated reticulocyte count, but some children with chronic hemolysis initially present during a period of a virus-induced aplasia when the reticulocyte count is not elevated. Thus, review of the peripheral blood smear for evidence of hemolysis (eg, spherocytes, red cell fragmentation, sickle forms) is important in the evaluation of children with normocytic anemias and low reticulocyte counts. When hemolysis is suggested, the correct diagnosis may be suspected by specific abnormalities of red cell morphology or by clues from the history or physical examination. Autoimmune hemolysis is usually excluded by direct antiglobulin testing. Review of blood counts and the peripheral blood smears of the mother and father may suggest genetic disorders such as hereditary spherocytosis. Children with normocytic or macrocytic anemias, with relatively low reticulocyte counts and no evidence of hemolysis on the blood smear, usually have anemias caused by inadequate erythropoiesis in the bone marrow. The presence of neutropenia or thrombocytopenia in such children suggests the possibility of aplastic anemia, malignancy, or severe folate or vitamin B_{12} deficiency, and usually dictates examination of the bone marrow.

Pure red cell aplasia may be congenital (Diamond-Blackfan anemia), acquired, and transient (transient erythroblastopenia of childhood); a manifestation of a systemic disease such as renal disease or hypothyroidism; or associated with malnutrition or mild deficiencies of folate or vitamin B_{12}.

Perkins SL: Pediatric red cell disorders and pure red cell aplasia. Am J Clin Pathol 2004;122 (Suppl S70) [PMID: 15690644].

PURE RED CELL APLASIA

Infants and children with normocytic or macrocytic anemia, a low reticulocyte count, and normal or elevated numbers of neutrophils and platelets should be suspected of having pure red cell aplasia. Examination of the peripheral blood smear in such cases is important because signs of hemolytic disease suggest chronic hemolysis complicated by an aplastic crisis due to parvovirus infection. Appreciation of this phenomenon is important because chronic hemolytic disease may not be diagnosed until the anemia is exacerbated by an episode of red cell aplasia and subsequent rapidly falling hemoglobin level. In such cases, cardiovascular compromise and congestive heart failure may develop quickly.

1. Congenital Hypoplastic Anemia (Diamond-Blackfan Anemia)

ESSENTIALS OF DIAGNOSIS & TYPICAL FEATURES

- Age: birth to 1 year.
- Macrocytic anemia with reticulocytopenia.
- Bone marrow with erythroid hypoplasia.
- Short stature or congenital anomalies in one-third of patients.

General Considerations

Diamond-Blackfan anemia is a relatively rare cause of anemia that usually presents in infancy or early childhood. Early diagnosis is important because treatment with corticosteroids results in increased erythropoiesis in about two-thirds of patients, thus avoiding the difficulties and complications of long-term chronic transfusion therapy. The cause is unclear; both autosomal dominant and autosomal recessive modes of inheritance occur.

Clinical Findings

A. Symptoms and Signs

Signs and symptoms are generally those of chronic anemia, such as pallor; congestive heart failure sometimes follows. Jaundice, splenomegaly, or other evidence of hemolysis are usually absent. Short stature or other congenital anomalies are present in one-third of patients. A wide variety of anomalies have been described; those affecting the head, face, and thumbs are the most common.

B. Laboratory Findings

Diamond-Blackfan anemia is characterized by severe macrocytic anemia and marked reticulocytopenia. The neutrophil count is usually normal or slightly decreased, and the platelet count is normal, elevated, or decreased. The bone marrow usually shows a marked decrease in erythroid precursors but is otherwise normal. In older children, fetal hemoglobin levels are usually increased and there is evidence of persistent fetal erythropoiesis, such as the presence of the i antigen on erythrocytes. In addition, the level of adenosine deaminase in erythrocytes is elevated.

Differential Diagnosis

The principal differential diagnosis is transient erythroblastopenia of childhood. Children with Diamond-Blackfan anemia generally present at an earlier age, often have macrocytosis, and have evidence of fetal erythropoiesis and an elevated level of red cell adenosine deaminase. In addition, short stature and congenital anomalies are not associated with transient erythroblastopenia. Lastly, transient erythroblastopenia of childhood usually resolves within 6–8 weeks of diagnosis, whereas Diamond-Blackfan anemia is a lifelong affliction. Other disorders associated with decreased red cell production such as renal failure, hypothyroidism, and the anemia of chronic disease need to be considered.

Treatment

Oral corticosteroids should be initiated as soon as the diagnosis of Diamond-Blackfan anemia is made. Two-thirds of patients will respond to prednisone, 2 mg/kg/d, and many of those who respond subsequently tolerate significant tapering of the dose. Patients who are unresponsive to prednisone require chronic transfusion therapy, which inevitably causes transfusion-induced hemosiderosis and the need for chelation with parenteral deferoxamine. Bone marrow transplantation is an alternative therapy that should be considered for transfusion-dependent patients who have HLA-identical siblings. Hematopoietic growth factors have been used in some cases with limited success. Unpredictable spontaneous remissions occur in up to 20% of patients.

Prognosis

The prognosis for patients responsive to corticosteroids is generally good, particularly if remission is maintained with low doses of alternate-day prednisone. Patients dependent on transfusion are at risk for the complications of hemosiderosis, including death from congestive heart failure, cardiac arrhythmias, or hepatic failure. This remains a significant threat, particularly during adolescence, when compliance with nightly subcutaneous infusions of deferoxamine is often difficult to ensure.

Berndt A: Successful transplantation of CD34+ selected peripheral blood stem cells from an unrelated donor in an adult patient with Diamond-Blackfan anemia and secondary hemochromatosis. Bone Marrow Transplant 2005;35:99 [PMID: 15516941].

Lipton J: Diamond-Blackfan anemia: Diagnosis, treatment and molecular pathogenesis. Hematol Oncol Clin North Am 2009;23(2):261 [PMID: 19327583].

Vlachos A: Diagnosing and treating Diamond-Blackfan anemia: Results of international clinical concensus conference. Br J Haematol 2009;145(3):428 [PMID: 18671700].

2. Transient Erythroblastopenia of Childhood

ESSENTIALS OF DIAGNOSIS & TYPICAL FEATURES

- Age: 6 months to 4 years.
- Normocytic anemia with reticulocytopenia.

- Absence of hepatosplenomegaly or lymphadenopathy.
- Erythroid precursors initially absent from bone marrow.

General Considerations

Transient erythroblastopenia of childhood is a relatively common cause of acquired anemia in early childhood. The disorder is suspected when a normocytic anemia is discovered during evaluation of pallor or when a CBC is obtained for another reason. Because the anemia is due to decreased red cell production, and thus develops slowly, the cardiovascular system has time to compensate. Therefore, children with hemoglobin levels as low as 4–5 g/dL may look remarkably well. The disorder is thought to be autoimmune in most cases, because IgG from some patients has been shown to suppress erythropoiesis in vitro.

Clinical Findings

Pallor is the most common sign, and hepatosplenomegaly and lymphadenopathy are absent. The anemia is normocytic, and the peripheral blood smear shows no evidence of hemolysis. The platelet count is normal or elevated, and the neutrophil count is normal or, in some cases, decreased. Early in the course, no reticulocytes are identified. The Coombs test is negative, and there is no evidence of chronic renal disease, hypothyroidism, or other systemic disorder. Bone marrow examination shows severe erythroid hypoplasia initially; subsequently, erythroid hyperplasia develops along with reticulocytosis, and the anemia resolves.

Differential Diagnosis

Transient erythroblastopenia of childhood must be differentiated from Diamond-Blackfan anemia, particularly in infants younger than age 1 year. In contrast to Diamond-Blackfan anemia, transient erythroblastopenia is not associated with macrocytosis, short stature, or congenital anomalies, or with evidence of fetal erythropoiesis prior to the phase of recovery. Also in contrast to Diamond-Blackfan anemia, transient erythroblastopenia is associated with normal levels of red cell adenosine deaminase. Transient erythroblastopenia of childhood must also be differentiated from chronic disorders associated with decreased red cell production, such as renal failure, hypothyroidism, and other chronic states of infection or inflammation. As with other single cytopenias, the possibility of malignancy (ie, leukemia) should always be considered, particularly if fever, bone pain, hepatosplenomegaly, or lymphadenopathy is present. In such cases, examination of the bone marrow is generally diagnostic. Confusion may sometimes arise when the anemia of transient erythroblastopenia is first identified during the early phase of recovery when the reticulocyte count is high. In such cases, the disorder may be confused with the anemia of acute blood loss or with hemolytic disease. In contrast to hemolytic disorders, transient erythroblastopenia of childhood is not associated with jaundice or peripheral destruction of red cells.

Treatment & Prognosis

By definition, this is a transient disorder. Some children require red cell transfusions if cardiovascular compromise is present. Resolution of the anemia is heralded by an increase in the reticulocyte count, which generally occurs within 4–8 weeks of diagnosis. Transient erythroblastopenia of childhood is not treated with corticosteroids because of its short course.

NUTRITIONAL ANEMIAS

1. Iron-Deficiency Anemia

ESSENTIALS OF DIAGNOSIS & TYPICAL FEATURES

- Pallor and fatigue.
- Poor dietary intake of iron (ages 6–24 months).
- Chronic blood loss (age > 2 years).
- Microcytic hypochromic anemia.

General Considerations

Long considered the most common cause of anemia in pediatrics, iron deficiency has decreased substantially in incidence due to improved nutrition and the increased availability of iron-fortified infant formulas and cereals. Thus, the current approach to anemia in childhood must take into consideration a relatively greater likelihood of other causes.

Normal-term infants are born with sufficient iron stores to prevent iron deficiency for the first 4–5 months of life. Thereafter, enough iron needs to be absorbed to support the needs of rapid growth. For this reason, nutritional iron deficiency is most common between 6 and 24 months of life. A deficiency earlier than age 6 months may occur if iron stores at birth are reduced by prematurity, small birth weight, neonatal anemia, or perinatal blood loss or if there is subsequent iron loss due to hemorrhage. Iron-deficient children older than age 24 months should be evaluated for blood loss. Iron deficiency, in addition to causing anemia, has adverse effects on multiple organ systems. Thus, the importance of identifying and treating iron deficiency extends past the resolution of any symptoms directly attributable to a decreased hemoglobin concentration.

Clinical Findings

A. Symptoms and Signs

Symptoms and signs vary with the severity of the deficiency. Mild iron deficiency is usually asymptomatic. In infants with more severe iron deficiency, pallor, fatigue, irritability, and delayed motor development are common. Children whose iron deficiency is due in part to ingestion of unfortified cow's milk may be fat and have poor muscle tone. A history of pica is common.

B. Laboratory Findings

The severity of anemia depends on the degree of iron deficiency, and the hemoglobin level may be as low as 3–4 g/dL in severe cases. Red cells are microcytic and hypochromic, with a low MCV and low mean corpuscular hemoglobin. The red blood cell distribution width is typically elevated, even with mild iron deficiency. The reticulocyte count is usually normal or slightly elevated, but the reticulocyte index or absolute reticulocyte count is decreased. Iron studies show a decreased serum ferritin and a low serum iron, elevated total iron-binding capacity, and decreased transferrin saturation. These laboratory abnormalities are usually present with moderate to severe iron deficiency, but mild cases may be associated with variable laboratory results. The peripheral blood smear shows microcytic, hypochromic red blood cells with anisocytosis, and occasional target, teardrop, elliptical, spherocytic and fragmented red cells. Leukocytes are normal, and very often the platelet count is increased with normal morphology.

The bone marrow examination is not helpful in the diagnosis of iron deficiency in infants and small children because little or no iron is stored as marrow hemosiderin at these ages.

Differential Diagnosis

The differential diagnosis is that of microcytic, hypochromic anemia. The possibility of thalassemia (α-thalassemia, β-thalassemia, and hemoglobin E disorders) should be considered, especially in infants of African, Mediterranean, or Asian ethnic background. In contrast to infants with iron deficiency, those with thalassemia generally have an elevated number of erythrocytes (the index of the MCV divided by the red cell number is usually less than 13) and are less likely, in mild cases, to have an elevated red blood cell distribution width. Thalassemias are associated with normal or increased levels of serum iron and ferritin and with normal iron-binding capacity. The hemoglobin electrophoresis in β-thalassemia minor typically shows an elevation of hemoglobin A_2 levels, but coexistent iron deficiency may lower the percentage of hemoglobin A_2 into the normal range. Hemoglobin electrophoresis will also identify children with hemoglobin E, a cause of microcytosis common in Southeast Asians. In contrast, the hemoglobin electrophoresis in α-thalassemia trait is normal. Lead poisoning has also been associated with microcytic anemia, but anemia with lead levels less than 40 mg/dL is often due to coexistent iron deficiency.

The anemia of chronic inflammation or infection is normocytic but in late stages may be microcytic. This anemia is usually suspected because of the presence of a chronic systemic disorder. The level of serum iron is low, but the iron-binding capacity is normal or decreased, and the serum ferritin level is normal or elevated. Relatively mild infections, particularly during infancy, may cause transient anemia. As a result, caution should be exercised when the diagnosis of mild iron deficiency is entertained in infants and young children who have had recent viral or bacterial infections. Ideally, screening tests for anemia should not be obtained within 3–4 weeks of such infections.

Treatment

The recommended oral dose of elemental iron is 6 mg/kg/d in three divided daily doses. Mild cases may be treated with 2 mg/kg/d given once daily before breakfast. Parenteral administration of iron is rarely necessary. Iron therapy results in an increased reticulocyte count within 3–5 days, which is maximal between 5 and 7 days. The hemoglobin level begins to increase thereafter. The rate of hemoglobin rise is inversely related to the hemoglobin level at diagnosis. In moderate to severe cases, an elevated reticulocyte count 1 week after initiation of therapy confirms the diagnosis and documents compliance and response to therapy. When iron deficiency is the only cause of anemia, adequate treatment usually results in a resolution of the anemia within 4–6 weeks. Treatment is generally continued for a few additional months to replenish iron stores.

Collard KJ: Iron homeostasis in the neonate. Pediatrics 2009;123(4):1208 [PMID: 19336381].

Jain S: Evaluation of microcytic anemia. Clin Pediatr 2009;48(1):7 [PMID: 18832550].

2. Megaloblastic Anemias

ESSENTIALS OF DIAGNOSIS & TYPICAL FEATURES

- Pallor and fatigue.
- Nutritional deficiency or intestinal malabsorption.
- Macrocytic anemia.
- Megaloblastic bone marrow changes.

General Considerations

Megaloblastic anemia is a macrocytic anemia caused by deficiency of cobalamin (vitamin B_{12}), folic acid, or both. Cobalamin deficiency due to dietary insufficiency may occur in infants who are breast fed by mothers who are strict vegetarians or who have pernicious anemia. Intestinal malabsorption is the usual cause of cobalamin deficiency in children and occurs with Crohn disease, chronic pancreatitis, bacterial overgrowth of the small bowel, infection with the fish tapeworm (*Diphyllobothrium latum*), or after surgical resection of the terminal ileum. Deficiencies due to inborn errors of metabolism (transcobalamin II deficiency and methylmalonic aciduria) also have been described. Malabsorption of cobalamin due to deficiency of intrinsic factor (pernicious anemia) is rare in childhood.

Folic acid deficiency may be caused by inadequate dietary intake, malabsorption, increased folate requirements, or some combination of the three. Folate deficiency due to dietary deficiency alone is rare but occurs in severely malnourished infants and has been reported in infants fed with goat's milk not fortified with folic acid. Folic acid is absorbed in the jejunum, and deficiencies are encountered in malabsorptive syndromes such as celiac disease. Anticonvulsion medications (eg, phenytoin and phenobarbital) and cytotoxic drugs (eg, methotrexate) also have been associated with folate deficiency, caused by interference with folate absorption or metabolism. Finally, folic acid deficiency is more likely to develop in infants and children with increased requirements. This occurs during infancy because of rapid growth and also in children with chronic hemolytic anemia. Premature infants are particularly susceptible to the development of the deficiency because of low body stores of folate.

Clinical Findings

A. Symptoms and Signs

Infants with megaloblastic anemia may show pallor and mild jaundice as a result of ineffective erythropoiesis. Classically, the tongue is smooth and beefy red. Infants with cobalamin deficiency may be irritable and may be poor feeders. Older children with cobalamin deficiency may complain of paresthesias, weakness, or an unsteady gait and may show decreased vibratory sensation and proprioception on neurologic examination.

B. Laboratory Findings

The laboratory findings of megaloblastic anemia include an elevated mean corpuscular volume (MCV) and mean corpuscular hemoglobin (MCH). The peripheral blood smear shows numerous macro-ovalocytes with anisocytosis and poikilocytosis. Neutrophils are large and have hypersegmented nuclei. The white cell and platelet counts are normal with mild deficiencies, but may be decreased in more severe cases. Examination of the bone marrow typically shows erythroid hyperplasia with large erythroid and myeloid precursors. Nuclear maturation is delayed compared with cytoplasmic maturation, and erythropoiesis is ineffective. The serum indirect bilirubin concentration may be slightly elevated.

Children with cobalamin deficiency have a low serum vitamin B_{12} level, but decreased levels of serum vitamin B_{12} may also be found in about 30% of patients with folic acid deficiency. The level of red cell folate is a better reflection of folate stores than is the serum folic acid level. Serum levels of metabolic intermediates (methylmalonic acid and homocysteine) may help establish the correct diagnosis. Elevated methylmalonic acid levels are consistent with cobalamin deficiency, whereas elevated levels of homocysteine occur with both cobalamin and folate deficiency.

Differential Diagnosis

Most macrocytic anemias in pediatrics are not megaloblastic. Other causes of an increased MCV include drug therapy (eg, anticonvulsants, anti-HIV nucleoside analogues), Down syndrome, an elevated reticulocyte count (hemolytic anemias), bone marrow failure syndromes (Fanconi anemia, Diamond-Blackfan anemia), liver disease, and hypothyroidism.

Treatment

Treatment of cobalamin deficiency due to inadequate dietary intake is readily accomplished with oral supplementation. Most cases, however, are due to intestinal malabsorption and require parenteral treatment. In severe cases, parenteral therapy may induce life-threatening hypokalemia and require supplemental potassium. Folic acid deficiency is treated effectively with oral folic acid in most cases. Children at risk for the development of folic acid deficiencies, such as premature infants and those with chronic hemolysis, are often given folic acid prophylactically.

ANEMIA OF CHRONIC DISORDERS

Anemia is a common manifestation of many chronic illnesses in children. In some instances, causes may be mixed. For example, children with chronic disorders involving intestinal malabsorption or blood loss may have anemia of chronic inflammation in combination with nutritional deficiencies of iron, folate, or cobalamin. In other settings, the anemia is due to dysfunction of a single organ (eg, renal failure, hypothyroidism), and correction of the underlying abnormality resolves the anemia.

1. Anemia of Chronic Inflammation

Anemia is frequently associated with chronic infections or inflammatory diseases. The anemia is usually mild to moderate in severity, with a hemoglobin level of 8–12 g/dL. In general, the severity of the anemia corresponds to the severity of the underlying disorder, and there may be microcytosis, but not hypochromia. The reticulocyte count is low. The anemia is thought to be due to inflammatory cytokines that inhibit erythropoiesis, and shunting of iron into, and impaired iron release from, reticuloendothelial cells. High levels of hepcidin, a peptide produced in the liver during infection or inflammation, reduce iron absorption by the gut and release from macrophages. Levels of erythropoietin are relatively low for the severity of the anemia. The serum iron concentration is low, but in contrast to iron deficiency, anemia of chronic inflammation is not associated with elevated iron-binding capacity and is associated with an elevated serum ferritin level. Treatment consists of correction of the underlying disorder, which, if controlled, generally results in improvement in hemoglobin level.

Ganz T: Hepcidin and iron regulation, 10 years later. Blood 2011;117:4425 [PMID: 21346250].

2. Anemia of Chronic Renal Failure

Severe normocytic anemia occurs in most forms of renal disease that have progressed to renal insufficiency. Although white cell and platelet production remain normal, the bone marrow shows significant hypoplasia of the erythroid series and the reticulocyte count is low. The principal mechanism is deficiency of erythropoietin, a hormone produced in the kidney, but other factors may contribute to the anemia. In the presence of significant uremia, a component of hemolysis may also be present. Recombinant human erythropoietin (epoetin alfa) and iron correct the anemia, largely eliminating the need for transfusions.

3. Anemia of Hypothyroidism

Some patients with hypothyroidism develop significant anemia. Occasionally, anemia is detected before the diagnosis of the underlying disorder. A decreased growth velocity in an anemic child suggests hypothyroidism. The anemia is usually normocytic or macrocytic, but it is not megaloblastic and, hence not due to deficiencies of cobalamin or folate. Replacement therapy with thyroid hormone is usually effective in correcting the anemia.

CONGENITAL HEMOLYTIC ANEMIAS: RED CELL MEMBRANE DEFECTS

The congenital hemolytic anemias are divided into three categories: defects of the red cell membrane; hemoglobinopathies; and disorders of red cell metabolism. Hereditary spherocytosis and elliptocytosis are the most common red cell membrane disorders. The diagnosis is suggested by the peripheral blood smear, which shows characteristic red cell morphology (eg, spherocytes, elliptocytes). These disorders usually have an autosomal dominant inheritance, and the diagnosis may be suggested by a family history. The hemolysis is due to the deleterious effect of the membrane abnormality on red cell deformability. Decreased cell deformability leads to entrapment of the abnormally shaped red cells in the spleen. Many patients have splenomegaly, and splenectomy usually alleviates the hemolysis.

1. Hereditary Spherocytosis

ESSENTIALS OF DIAGNOSIS & TYPICAL FEATURES

- Anemia and jaundice.
- Splenomegaly.
- Positive family history of anemia, jaundice, or galltones.
- Spherocytosis with increased reticulocytes.
- Increased osmotic fragility.
- Negative direct antiglobulin test (DAT).

General Considerations

Hereditary spherocytosis is a relatively common inherited hemolytic anemia that occurs in all ethnic groups but is most common in persons of northern European ancestry, in whom the incidence is about 1:5000. The disorder is a heterogeneous one, marked by variable degrees of anemia, jaundice, and splenomegaly. In some persons, the disorder is mild and there is no anemia because erythroid hyperplasia fully compensates for hemolysis. Severe cases are transfusion-dependent prior to splenectomy. The hallmark of hereditary spherocytosis is the presence of microspherocytes in the peripheral blood. The disease is inherited in an autosomal dominant fashion in about 75%–80% of cases; the remaining cases are thought to be autosomal recessive or to be caused by new mutations.

Hereditary spherocytosis is usually the result of a partial deficiency of spectrin, an important structural protein of the red cell membrane skeleton. Spectrin deficiency weakens the attachment of the cell membrane to the underlying membrane skeleton and causes the red cell to lose membrane surface area. This process creates spherocytes that are poorly deformable and have a shortened life span because they are trapped in the microcirculation of the spleen and engulfed by splenic macrophages. The extreme heterogeneity of hereditary spherocytosis is related directly to variable degrees of spectrin deficiency. In general, children who inherit spherocytosis in an autosomal dominant fashion have less spectrin deficiency and mild or moderate hemolysis. In contrast, those with nondominant forms of spherocytosis tend to have greater deficiency of spectrin and more severe anemia.

Clinical Findings

A. Symptoms and Signs

Hemolysis causes significant neonatal hyperbilirubinemia in 50% of affected children. Splenomegaly subsequently develops in the majority and is often present by age 5 years. Jaundice is variably present and in many patients may be noted only during infection. Patients with significant chronic anemia may complain of pallor, fatigue, or malaise. Intermittent exacerbations of the anemia are caused by increased hemolysis, splenic sequestration or by aplastic crises, and may be associated with severe weakness, fatigue, fever, abdominal pain, or even heart failure.

B. Laboratory Findings

Most patients have mild chronic hemolysis with hemoglobin levels of 9–12 g/dL. In some cases, the hemolysis is fully compensated and the hemoglobin level is in the normal range. Rare cases of severe disease require frequent transfusions. The anemia is usually normocytic and hyperchromic, and many patients have an elevated mean corpuscular hemoglobin concentration. The peripheral blood smear shows numerous microspherocytes and polychromasia. The reticulocyte count is elevated, often higher than might be expected for the degree of anemia. White blood cell and platelet counts are usually normal. The osmotic fragility is increased, particularly after incubation at 37°C for 24 hours. Serum bilirubin usually shows an elevation in the unconjugated fraction. The DAT is negative.

▶ Differential Diagnosis

Spherocytes are frequently present in persons with immune hemolysis. Thus, in the newborn, hereditary spherocytosis must be distinguished from hemolytic disease caused by ABO or other blood type incompatibilities. Older patients with autoimmune hemolytic anemia frequently present with jaundice and splenomegaly and with spherocytes on the peripheral blood smear. The DAT is positive in most cases of immune hemolysis and negative in hereditary spherocytosis. Occasionally, the diagnosis is confused in patients with splenomegaly from other causes, especially when hypersplenism increases red cell destruction and when some spherocytes are noted on the blood smear. In such cases, the true cause of the splenomegaly may be suggested by signs or symptoms of portal hypertension or by laboratory evidence of chronic liver disease. In contrast to children with hereditary spherocytosis, those with hypersplenism typically have some degree of thrombocytopenia or neutropenia.

▶ Complications

Severe jaundice may occur in the neonatal period and, if not controlled by phototherapy, may occasionally require exchange transfusion. Intermittent or persistent splenomegaly occurs in 10%–25% of patients and may require removal. Splenectomy is associated with an increased risk of overwhelming bacterial infections, particularly with pneumococci. Gallstones occur in 60%–70% of adults who have not undergone splenectomy and may form as early as age 5–10 years.

▶ Treatment

Supportive measures include the administration of folic acid to prevent the development of red cell hypoplasia due to folate deficiency. Acute exacerbations of anemia, due to increased rates of hemolysis or to aplastic crises caused by infection with human parvovirus, may be severe enough to require red cell transfusions. Splenectomy is performed in many cases and always results in significant improvement. The procedure increases the survival of the spherocytic red cells and leads to complete correction of the anemia in most cases. Patients with more severe disease may show some degree of hemolysis after splenectomy. Except in unusually severe cases, the procedure should be postponed until the child is at least age 5 years because of the greater risk of postsplenectomy sepsis prior to this age. All patients scheduled for splenectomy should be immunized with pneumococcal, *Haemophilus influenzae* type b, and meningococcal vaccines prior to the procedure, and some clinicians recommend daily penicillin prophylaxis afterward. Asplenic patients with fever should be promptly evaluated for severe infection. The need for splenectomy in mild cases is controversial. Splenectomy in the middle childhood years prevents the subsequent development of cholelithiasis and eliminates the need for the activity restrictions recommended for children with splenomegaly. However, these benefits must be weighed against the risks of the surgical procedure and the subsequent lifelong risk of postsplenectomy sepsis.

▶ Prognosis

Splenectomy eliminates signs and symptoms in all but the most severe cases and reduces the risk of cholelithiasis. The abnormal red cell morphology and increased osmotic fragility persist without clinical consequence.

An X: Disorders of red cell membrane. Br J Haematol 2008;141:367 [PMID: 18341630].

2. Hereditary Elliptocytosis

Hereditary elliptocytosis is a heterogeneous disorder that ranges in severity from an asymptomatic state with almost normal red cell morphology to severe hemolytic anemia. Most affected persons have numerous elliptocytes on the peripheral blood smear, but mild or no hemolysis. Those with hemolysis have an elevated reticulocyte count and may have jaundice and splenomegaly. These disorders are caused by mutations of red cell cytoskeletal proteins (spectrin and ankyrin), and most have an autosomal dominant inheritance. Because most patients are asymptomatic, no treatment is indicated. Patients with significant degrees of hemolytic anemia may benefit from folate supplementation or splenectomy.

Some infants with hereditary elliptocytosis present in the neonatal period with moderate to marked hemolysis and significant hyperbilirubinemia. This disorder has been termed transient infantile pyknocytosis because such infants exhibit bizarre erythrocyte morphology with elliptocytes, budding red cells, and small misshapen cells that defy description.

The MCV is low, and the anemia may be severe enough to require red cell transfusions. Typically, one parent has hereditary elliptocytosis, usually mild or asymptomatic. The infant's hemolysis gradually abates during the first year of life, and the erythrocyte morphology subsequently becomes more typical of hereditary elliptocytosis.

CONGENITAL HEMOLYTIC ANEMIAS: HEMOGLOBINOPATHIES

The hemoglobinopathies are an extremely heterogeneous group of congenital disorders that may occur in all ethnic groups. The relatively high frequency of these genetic variants is related to the malaria protection afforded to heterozygous individuals. The hemoglobinopathies are generally classified into two major groups. The first, the thalassemias, are caused by quantitative deficiencies in the production of globin chains. These quantitative defects in globin synthesis cause microcytic and hypochromic anemias. The second group of hemoglobinopathies consists of those caused by structural abnormalities of globin chains. The most important of these, hemoglobins S, C, and E, are all the result of point mutations and single amino acid substitutions in β-globin. Many, but not all, infants with hemoglobinopathies are identified by routine neonatal screening.

Figure 30–3 shows the normal developmental changes that occur in globin-chain production during gestation and the first year of life. At birth, the predominant hemoglobin is fetal hemoglobin (hemoglobin F), which is composed of two α-globin chains and two γ-globin chains. Subsequently, the production of γ-globin decreases and the production of β-globin increases so that adult hemoglobin (two α chains and two β chains) predominates after 2–4 months. Because α-globin chains are present in both fetal and adult hemoglobin, disorders of α-globin synthesis (α-thalassemia) are clinically manifest in the newborn as well as later in life. In contrast, patients with β-globin disorders such as β-thalassemia and sickle cell disease are generally asymptomatic during the first 3–4 months of age and present clinically after γ-chain production—and therefore fetal hemoglobin levels—have decreased substantially.

1. α-Thalassemia

ESSENTIALS OF DIAGNOSIS & TYPICAL FEATURES

- Predominately African, Mediterranean, Middle Eastern, Chinese, or Southeast Asian ancestry.
- Microcytic, hypochromic anemia of variable severity.
- Generally Bart's hemoglobin detected by neonatal screening.

General Considerations

Most of the α-thalassemia syndromes are the result of deletions of one or more of the α-globin genes on chromosome 16 although nondeletional α+ mutations also occur. Excess non-α globin chains damage the red cell causing extravascular hemolysis. Normal diploid cells have four α-globin genes; thus, the variable severity of the α-thalassemia syndromes is related to the number of gene deletions (Table 30–1). The severity of the α-thalassemia syndromes varies among affected ethnic groups, depending on the genetic abnormalities prevalent in the population. In persons of African ancestry, α-thalassemia is usually caused by the deletion of only one of the two α-globin genes on each chromosome. Thus, in the African population, heterozygous individuals are silent

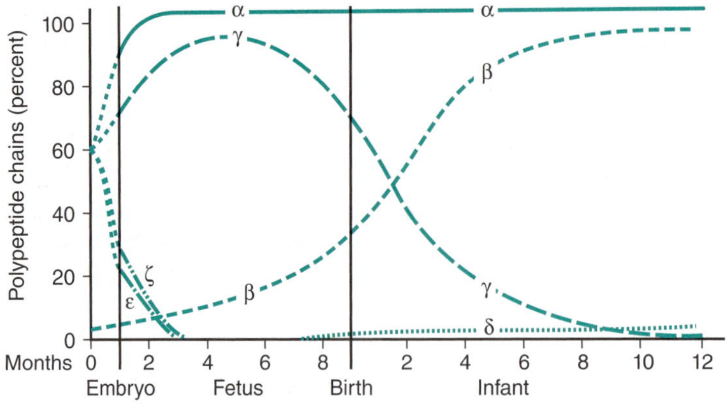

▲ **Figure 30–3.** Changes in hemoglobin polypeptide chains during human development. (Reproduced, with permission, from Miller DR, Baehner RL: *Blood Diseases of Infancy and Childhood*, 6th ed. Mosby, 1989.)

Table 30–1. The α-thalassemias.

Usual Genotypes[a]	α-Gene Number	Clinical Features	Hemoglobin Electrophoresis[b]	
			Birth	> 6 mo
αα/αα	4	Normal	N	N
–α/αα	3	Silent carrier	0%–3% Hb Bart's	N
–/αα or -α/-α	2	α-Thal trait	2%–10% Hb Bart's[c]	N
–/–α	1	Hb H disease	15%–30% Hb Bart's	Hb; H present
–/–	0	Fetalhydrops	> 75% Hb Bart's	—

[a]α indicates presence of α-globin gene, – indicates deletion of α-globin gene.
[b]N = normal results, Hb = hemoglobin, Hb Bart's = γ_4, Hb H = β_4.
[c]The level of Hb Bart's does not directly correlate with the number of deleted α genes.

carriers and homozygous individuals have α-thalassemia trait. In Asians, deletions of one or of both α-globin genes on the same chromosome are common; heterozygous individuals are either silent carriers or have α-thalassemia trait, and homozygous individuals or compound heterozygous individuals have α-thalassemia trait, hemoglobin H disease, or hydrops fetalis. Thus, the presence of α-thalassemia in a child of Asian ancestry may have important implications for genetic counseling, whereas this is not usually the case in families of African ancestry.

Clinical Findings

The clinical findings depend on the number of α-globin genes deleted. Table 30–1 summarizes the α-thalassemia syndromes.

Persons with three α-globin genes (one-gene deletion) are asymptomatic and have no hematologic abnormalities. Hemoglobin electrophoresis in the neonatal period shows 0%–3% Bart's hemoglobin, which is a variant hemoglobin composed of four γ-globin chains. Hemoglobin electrophoresis after the first few months of life is normal. Thus, this condition is usually suspected only in the context of family studies or when a small amount of Bart's hemoglobin is detected by neonatal screening for hemoglobinopathies.

Persons with two α-globin genes (two-gene deletion) are typically asymptomatic. The MCV is usually less than 100 fL at birth. Hematologic studies in older infants and children show a normal or slightly decreased hemoglobin level with a low MCV and a slightly hypochromic blood smear with some target cells.

Persons with one α-globin gene (three-gene deletion) have a mild to moderately severe microcytic hemolytic anemia (hemoglobin level of 7–10 g/dL), which may be accompanied by hepatosplenomegaly and some bony abnormalities caused by the expanded medullary space. The reticulocyte count is elevated, and the red cells show marked hypochromia and microcytosis with significant poikilocytosis and some basophilic stippling. Incubation of red cells with brilliant cresyl blue (hemoglobin H preparation) shows inclusion bodies formed by denatured hemoglobin H.

The deletion of all four α-globin genes causes severe intrauterine anemia and asphyxia and results in hydrops fetalis and fetal demise or neonatal death shortly after delivery. Extreme pallor and massive hepatosplenomegaly are present. Hemoglobin electrophoresis reveals a predominance of Bart's hemoglobin with a complete absence of normal fetal or adult hemoglobin.

Differential Diagnosis

α-Thalassemia trait (two-gene deletion) must be differentiated from other mild microcytic anemias, including iron deficiency and β-thalassemia minor (see next section). In contrast to children with iron deficiency, children with α-thalassemia trait show normal or increased levels of ferritin and serum iron. In contrast to children with β-thalassemia minor, children with α-thalassemia trait have a normal hemoglobin electrophoresis after age 4–6 months. Finally, the history of a low MCV (96 fL) at birth or the presence of Bart's hemoglobin on the neonatal hemoglobinopathy screening test suggests α-thalassemia.

Children with hemoglobin H disease may have jaundice and splenomegaly, and the disorder must be differentiated from other hemolytic anemias. The key to the diagnosis is the decreased MCV and the marked hypochromia on the blood smear. With the exception of β-thalassemia, most other significant hemolytic disorders have a normal or elevated MCV and the red blood cells are not hypochromic. Infants with hydrops fetalis due to severe α-thalassemia must be distinguished from those with hydrops due to other causes of anemia, such as alloimmunization.

Complications

The principal complication of α-thalassemia trait is the needless administration of iron, given in the belief that a mild microcytic anemia is due to iron deficiency. Persons with hemoglobin H disease may have intermittent exacerbations of their anemia in response to oxidant stress or infection, which occasionally require blood transfusions. Splenomegaly may exacerbate the anemia and may require splenectomy. Women pregnant with hydropic α-thalassemia fetuses are subject to increased complications of pregnancy, particularly toxemia and postpartum hemorrhage.

Treatment

Persons with α-thalassemia trait require no treatment. Those with hemoglobin H disease should receive supplemental folic acid and avoid the same oxidant drugs that cause hemolysis in persons with G6PD deficiency, because exposure to these drugs may exacerbate their anemia. The anemia may also be exacerbated during periods of infection, and transfusions may be required. Hypersplenism may develop later in childhood and require surgical splenectomy. Genetic counseling and prenatal diagnosis should be offered to families at risk for hydropic fetuses.

Cunningham MJ: Update on thalassemia: Clinical care and complications. Hematol Oncol Clin North Am 2010;24:215 [PMID: 20113904].

Harteveld CL: α-thalassemia. Orphanet J Rare Dis 2010;5:13 [PMID: 20507641].

Lal A: Heterogeneity of hemoglobin H disease in childhood. N Engl J Med 2011;364:710 [PMID: 21345100].

2. β-Thalassemia

ESSENTIALS OF DIAGNOSIS & TYPICAL FEATURES

β-Thalassemia minor:

- Normal neonatal screening test.
- Predominantly African, Mediterranean, Middle Eastern, or Asian ancestry.
- Mild microcytic, hypochromic anemia.
- No response to iron therapy.
- Elevated level of hemoglobin A_2.

β-Thalassemia intermedia:

- Ancestry as above.
- Microcytic, hypochromic anemia that usually becomes symptomatic after the first few years of life with hepatosplenomegaly.

β-Thalassemia major:

- Neonatal screening shows hemoglobin F only.
- Mediterranean, Middle Eastern, or Asian ancestry.
- Severe microcytic, hypochromic anemia with marked hepatosplenomegaly.

General Considerations

In contrast to the four α-globin genes, only two β-globin genes are present in diploid cells, one on each chromosome 11. Excess non-β globin chains damage the red cells causing extravascular hemolysis. Some β-thalassemia genes produce no β-globin chains and are termed β^0-thalassemia. Other β-globin genes produce some β-globin, but in diminished quantities, and are termed β^{++}-thalassemia. Individuals heterozygous for one β-thalassemia gene have β-thalassemia minor. Homozygous individuals generally have β-thalassemia major (Cooley anemia), a severe transfusion-dependent anemia. Individuals with β-thalassemia intermedia, which is more severe than thalassemia minor but is not generally transfusion-dependent, are usually heterozygous for two β^+ mutations, have both β^0 and + mutations, or have an alternative mutation such as E in conjunction with a severe β^+ or β^0 mutation. Thalassemia major is the most common worldwide cause of transfusion-dependent anemia in childhood. In addition, β-thalassemia genes interact with genes for structural β-globin variants such as hemoglobin S and hemoglobin E to cause serious disease in compound heterozygous individuals. These disorders are discussed further in the sections dealing with sickle cell disease and with hemoglobin E disorders.

Clinical Findings

A. Symptoms and Signs

Persons with β-thalassemia minor are usually asymptomatic with a normal physical examination. The time to presentation for those with β-thalassemia intermedia is variable. Those with β-thalassemia major are normal at birth but develop significant anemia during the first year of life. If the disorder is not identified and treated with blood transfusions, such children grow poorly and develop massive hepatosplenomegaly and enlargement of the medullary space with thinning of the bony cortex. The skeletal changes (due to ineffective erythropoiesis) cause characteristic facial deformities (prominent forehead and maxilla) and predispose the child to pathologic fractures.

B. Laboratory Findings

Children with β-thalassemia minor have normal neonatal screening results but subsequently develop a decreased MCV with or without mild anemia. The peripheral blood smear typically shows hypochromia, target cells, and sometimes basophilic stippling. Hemoglobin electrophoresis performed after 6–12 months of age is usually diagnostic when levels of hemoglobin A_2, hemoglobin F, or both are elevated. β-Thalassemia major is often initially suspected when hemoglobin A is absent on neonatal screening. Such infants are hematologically normal at birth, but develop severe anemia after the first few months of life. The peripheral blood smear typically shows a severe hypochromic, microcytic anemia with marked anisocytosis and poikilocytosis. Target cells are prominent, and nucleated red blood cells often exceed the number of circulating white blood cells. The hemoglobin level usually falls to 5–6 g/dL or less, and the reticulocyte count is elevated, but the reticulocyte index is normal to decreased. Platelet and white blood cell counts may be increased, and the serum bilirubin level is elevated. The bone marrow shows marked erythroid hyperplasia, but this finding is rarely needed for diagnosis. Hemoglobin electrophoresis shows only fetal hemoglobin and hemoglobin A_2 in children with homozygous β^0-thalassemia.

Those with β^+-thalassemia genes make a variable amount of hemoglobin A, depending on the mutation, but have a marked increase in fetal hemoglobin and hemoglobin A_2 levels. The diagnosis of homozygous β-thalassemia, intermedia or minor, may also be supported by testing both parents.

Differential Diagnosis

β-Thalassemia minor must be differentiated from other causes of mild microcytic, hypochromic anemias, principally iron deficiency and α-thalassemia. In contrast to patients with iron-deficiency anemia, those with β-thalassemia minor typically have an elevated number of red blood cells, and the index of the MCV divided by the red cell count is under 13. Generally, the finding of an elevated hemoglobin A_2 level is diagnostic; however, the A_2 level is lowered by coexistent iron deficiency. Thus, in children thought to be iron-deficient, hemoglobin electrophoresis with quantitation of hemoglobin A_2 is sometimes deferred until after a course of iron therapy.

β-Thalassemia major is rarely confused with other disorders. Hemoglobin electrophoresis and family studies readily distinguish it from hemoglobin E/β-thalassemia, which is the other increasingly important cause of transfusion-dependent thalassemia.

Complications

The principal complication of β-thalassemia minor is the unnecessary use of iron therapy in a futile attempt to correct the microcytic anemia. Children with β-thalassemia major who are inadequately transfused experience poor growth and recurrent infections and may have hepatosplenomegaly, thinning of the cortical bone, and pathologic fractures. Without treatment, most children die within the first decade of life. The principal complications of β-thalassemia major in transfused children are hemosiderosis, splenomegaly, and hypersplenism. Transfusion-related hemosiderosis requires chelation therapy with deferoxamine, given parentally, or deferasirox (Exjade), given orally, to prevent cardiac, hepatic, and endocrine dysfunction. Noncompliance with chelation in adolescents and young adults may lead to death from congestive heart failure, cardiac arrhythmias, or hepatic failure. Even with adequate transfusions, many patients develop splenomegaly and some degree of hypersplenism. This may require surgical splenectomy because of the increasing transfusion requirements, but the procedure increases the risk of thrombosis, pulmonary hypertension, and overwhelming septicemia.

Treatment

β-Thalassemia minor requires no specific therapy, but the diagnosis may have important genetic implications for the family. The time to presentation for those with β-thalassemia intermedia is variable. For β-thalassemia major, two treatments are available: chronic transfusion with iron chelation and stem cell transplantation. Programs of blood transfusion are generally targeted to maintain a nadir hemoglobin level of 9–10 g/dL. This approach gives increased vigor and well-being, improved growth, and fewer overall complications. However, maintenance of good health currently requires iron chelation. Small doses of supplemental ascorbic acid may enhance the efficacy of iron chelation. Patients who undergo splenectomy to reduce transfusion requirements, and hence iron loading, should receive pneumococcal vaccine prior to the procedure and prophylactic penicillin and urgent treatment of all febrile illness after splenectomy. Chronic transfusion is infrequently indicated for individuals with β-thalassemia intermedia.

Bone marrow or umbilical cord blood transplantation is an important therapeutic option for children with β-thalassemia major who have an HLA-identical sibling donor. The probability of hematologic cure is greater than 90% when transplantation is performed prior to the development of hepatomegaly or portal fibrosis.

Angelucci E: Hematopoietic stem cell transplantation in thalassemia. Hematology Am Soc Hematol Educ Program 2010;2010:456 [PMID: 21239835].

Taher AT: Optimal management of β thalassemia intermedia. Br J Haematology 2011;152:512 [PMID: 21250971].

3. Sickle Cell Disease

ESSENTIALS OF DIAGNOSIS & TYPICAL FEATURES

- Neonatal screening test usually with hemoglobins FS, FSC, or FSA (S > A).
- Predominantly African, Mediterranean, Middle Eastern, Indian, or Caribbean ancestry.
- Anemia, elevated reticulocyte count, usually jaundice.
- Recurrent episodes of musculoskeletal or abdominal pain.
- Often hepatomegaly and splenomegaly that resolves.
- Increased risk of bacterial sepsis.

General Considerations

Sickle cell disease encompasses a family of disorders with manifestations secondary to sickling, a change in red cell morphology. Sickle cell anemia, the most severe sickling disorder, is caused by homozygosity for the sickle gene and is the most common form of sickle cell disease. Other clinically important sickling disorders are compound heterozygous conditions in which the sickle gene interacts with genes for hemoglobins C, D_{Punjab}, O_{Arab}, C_{Harlem}, or β-thalassemia.

Overall, sickle cell disease occurs in about 1 of every 400 African-American infants. Eight percent of African Americans are heterozygous carriers of the sickle gene and are said to have sickle cell trait.

The protean clinical manifestations of sickle hemoglobinopathies can be linked directly or indirectly to the propensity of deoxygenated hemoglobin S to polymerize. Polymerization of sickle hemoglobin distorts erythrocyte morphology, decreases red cell deformability, causes a marked reduction in red cell life span, increases blood viscosity, and predisposes to episodes of vaso-occlusion.

Clinical Findings

A. Symptoms and Signs

These are related to the hemolytic anemia and to tissue ischemia and organ dysfunction caused by vaso-occlusion and are most severe in children with sickle cell anemia or sickle β^0-thalassemia. Physical findings are normal at birth, and symptoms are unusual before age 3–4 months because high levels of fetal hemoglobin inhibit sickling. A moderately severe hemolytic anemia may be present by age 1 year. This causes pallor, fatigue, and jaundice, and predisposes to the development of gallstones during childhood and adolescence. Intense congestion of the spleen with sickled cells may cause splenomegaly in early childhood and results in functional asplenia as early as age 3 months in sickle cell anemia. This places children at great risk for overwhelming infection with encapsulated bacteria, particularly pneumococci. Up to 30% of patients experience one or more episodes of acute splenic sequestration, characterized by sudden enlargement of the spleen with pooling of red cells, acute exacerbation of anemia, and, in severe cases, shock and death. Acute exacerbation of anemia also occurs with aplastic crises, usually caused by infection with human parvovirus and other viruses.

Recurrent episodes of vaso-occlusion and tissue ischemia cause acute and chronic problems. Dactylitis, or hand-and-foot syndrome, is the most common initial symptom of the disease and occurs in up to 50% of children with sickle cell anemia before age 3 years. Recurrent episodes of abdominal and musculoskeletal pain may occur throughout life. Overt strokes occur in about 11% of children with sickle cell anemia and tend to be recurrent. Recurrence is significantly reduced with chronic red cell transfusions. The so-called acute chest syndrome, characterized by fever, pleuritic chest pain, and acute pulmonary infiltrates with hypoxemia, is caused by pulmonary infection, infarction, or fat embolism from ischemic bone marrow. All tissues are susceptible to damage from vaso-occlusion, and multiple organ dysfunction is common by adulthood in those with sickle cell anemia or sickle β^0-thalassemia. The common manifestations of sickle cell disease are listed in Table 30–2. Manifestations generally develop less frequently in those with SC and S β^+-thalassemia.

Table 30–2. Common clinical manifestations of sickle cell disease.

	Acute	Chronic
Children	Bacterial sepsis or meningitis[a] Splenic sequestration[a] Aplastic crisis Vaso-occlusive events Dactylitis Bone infarction Acute chest syndrome[a] Stroke[a] Priapism	Functional asplenia Delayed growth and development Avascular necrosis of the hip Hyposthenuria Cholelithiasis
Adults	Bacterial sepsis[a] Aplastic crisis Vaso-occlusive events Bone infarction Acute chest syndrome[a] Stroke[a] Priapism Acute multiorgan failure syndrome[a]	Leg ulcers Proliferative retinopathy Avascular necrosis of the hip Cholecystitis Chronic organ failure[a] Liver Lung Kidney Decreased fertility

[a]Associated with significant mortality rate.

B. Laboratory Findings

Children with sickle cell anemia generally show a baseline hemoglobin level of 7–10 g/dL. This value may fall to life-threatening levels at the time of a splenic sequestration or aplastic crisis; often this occurs in association with parvovirus B19 infection. The baseline reticulocyte count is elevated markedly. The anemia is usually normocytic or macrocytic, and the peripheral blood smear typically shows the characteristic sickle cells as well as numerous target cells. Patients with sickle β-thalassemia also generally have a low MCV and hypochromia. Those with sickle β^+-thalassemia tend to have less hemolysis and anemia. Persons with sickle hemoglobin C disease have fewer sickle forms and more target cells, and the hemoglobin level may be normal or only slightly decreased because the rate of hemolysis is much less than in sickle cell anemia.

Most infants with sickle hemoglobinopathies born in the United States are identified by neonatal screening. Results indicative of possible sickle cell disease require prompt confirmation with hemoglobin electrophoresis. Children with sickle cell anemia and with sickle β^0-thalassemia have only hemoglobins S and F. Persons with sickle β^+-thalassemia have a preponderance of hemoglobin S with a lesser amount of hemoglobin A. Persons with sickle hemoglobin C disease have equal amounts of hemoglobins S and C. The use of solubility tests to screen for the presence of sickle hemoglobin should be avoided because a negative result is frequently encountered in infants with sickle cell disease, and because a positive result in an older child does not differentiate sickle cell trait from sickle cell disease. Thus, hemoglobin electrophoresis is always necessary to accurately identify a sickle disorder.

Differential Diagnosis

Hemoglobin electrophoresis and sometimes hematologic studies of the parents are usually sufficient to confirm sickle cell disease, although DNA testing is available. It is critical to determine whether the child with only F and S hemoglobins on newborn screening has sickle cell anemia, sickle β^0 thalassemia or is a compound heterozygote for sickle hemoglobin and pancellular hereditary persistence of fetal hemoglobin. Such children, when older, typically have 30% fetal hemoglobin and 70% hemoglobin S, but they do not have significant anemia or develop vaso-occlusive episodes.

Complications

Repeated tissue ischemia and infarction causes damage to virtually every organ system. Table 30–2 lists the most important complications. Patients who require multiple transfusions are at risk of developing transfusion-related hemosiderosis and infections as well as red cell alloantibodies.

Treatment

The cornerstone of treatment is enrollment in a program involving patient and family education, comprehensive outpatient care, and appropriate treatment of acute complications. Important to the success of such a program are psychosocial services, blood bank services, and the ready availability of baseline patient information in the setting in which acute illnesses are evaluated and treated.

Management of sickle cell anemia and sickle β^0-thalassemia includes daily prophylactic penicillin, which should be initiated by age 2 months and continued at least until age 5 years. The routine use of penicillin prophylaxis in sickle hemoglobin C disease and sickle β^+-thalassemia is controversial. Pneumococcal conjugate and polysaccharide vaccines should be administered to all children who have sickle cell disease. Other routine immunizations, including yearly vaccination against influenza, should be provided. All illnesses associated with fever greater than 38.5°C should be evaluated promptly, bacterial cultures performed, parenteral broad-spectrum antibiotics (eg, ceftriaxone) administered, and careful inpatient or outpatient observation conducted.

Treatment of painful vaso-occlusive episodes includes the maintenance of adequate hydration (with avoidance of overhydration), correction of acidosis if present, administration of adequate analgesia, maintenance of normal oxygen saturation, and the treatment of any associated infections.

Red cell transfusions play an important role in management. Transfusions are indicated to improve oxygen-carrying capacity during acute severe exacerbations of anemia, as occurs during episodes of splenic sequestration or aplastic crisis. Red cell transfusions are not indicated for the treatment of chronic steady-state anemia, which is usually well tolerated, or for uncomplicated episodes of vaso-occlusive pain. Simple or partial exchange transfusion to reduce the percentage of circulating sickle cells is indicated for some severe acute vaso-occlusive events and may be lifesaving. These events include stroke, moderate to severe acute chest syndrome, and acute life-threatening failure of other organs. Transfusions may also be used prior to high-risk procedures such as surgery with general anesthesia and arteriograms with ionic contrast materials. Some patients who develop severe vaso-occlusive complications may benefit from chronic transfusion therapy. The most common indications for transfusions are stroke and an abnormal transcranial Doppler assessment indicating an increased risk for stroke. Extended matching for red cell antigens is controversial but reduces incidence of alloimmunization.

Successful stem cell transplantation cures sickle cell disease, but to date its use has been limited because of the risks associated with the procedure, the inability to predict in young children the severity of future complications, and the paucity of HLA-identical sibling donors. Daily administration of oral hydroxyurea increases levels of fetal hemoglobin, decreases hemolysis, and significantly reduces episodes of pain in children with sickle cell anemia, including some evidence for a reduction in acute chest syndrome, hospitalization rates, and transfusions. The hematologic effects and short-term toxicity of hydroxyurea in children are similar to those in adults. Thus, hydroxyurea is being increasingly prescribed for children and adolescents with sickle cell anemia and sickle β^0-thalassemia; efficacy in SC and β^+-thalassemia has not been formally studied.

Prognosis

Early identification by neonatal screening of infants with sickle cell disease, combined with comprehensive care that includes prescription of prophylactic penicillin, instruction on splenic palpation, and education on the need to urgently seek care when fever occurs, has markedly reduced mortality in childhood. Most patients now live well into adulthood, but eventually succumb to complications.

Lasalle-Williams M: Extended red blood cell antigen matching for transfusions in sickle cell disease: A review of a 14-year experience from a single center. Transfusion 2011 Feb 18 [Epub ahead of print] [PMID: 21332724].

Prabhakar H: Sickle cell disease in the United States: Looking back and forward at 100 years of progress in management and survival. Am J Hematol 2010;85:346 [PMID: 20425797].

Wang WC: Hydroxycarbamide in very young children with sickle-cell anaemia: A multicentre, randomized, controlled trial (BABY HUG). Lancet 2011;377:1663 [PMID: 21571150].

Ware RE: How do I use hydroxyurea to treat young patients with sickle anemia. Blood 2010;115:5300 [PMID: 20223921].

4. Sickle Cell Trait

Individuals who are heterozygous for the sickle gene have sickle cell trait. Infants with sickle cell trait are identified by neonatal screening that shows hemoglobin FAS (A > S). Accurate identification of older persons with sickle cell trait depends on hemoglobin electrophoresis, which typically shows about 60% hemoglobin A and about 40% hemoglobin S. No anemia or hemolysis is present, and the physical examination is normal. Persons with sickle cell trait are generally healthy with normal life expectancy.

However, sickle trait erythrocytes are capable of sickling, with acidemia and hypoxemia. Thus, the kidney may be affected with the most common manifestation of sickle trait being hyposthenuria. Painless hematuria, usually microscopic, affects about 4% of those with sickle trait and does not progress to significant renal dysfunction. Less than 40 individuals have been reported with an exceedingly rare malignancy, renal medullary carcinoma, and all but one have had sickle trait. The incidence of bacteriuria and pyelonephritis may be increased during pregnancy, but overall rates of maternal and infant morbidity and mortality are not affected by sickle cell trait.

Exertion at moderate altitudes rarely precipitates splenic infarction. Whether or not the risk of sudden unexplained death during strenuous exercise, as occurs during military basic training, is increased in men with sickle cell trait is controversial. In general, exercise tolerance seems to be normal; the incidence of sickle cell trait in black professional football players is similar to that of the general African-American population.

There is no reason to restrict strenuous activity for individuals with sickle cell trait. As is true for all individuals performing strenuous activity, it is important to be conditioned, dress appropriately, have access to fluids, rest reasonably, and moderate activity in extreme heat and humidity. Sickle cell trait is most significant for its genetic implications.

5. Hemoglobin C Disorders

Hemoglobin C is detected by neonatal screening. Two percent of African Americans are heterozygous for hemoglobin C and are said to have hemoglobin C trait. Such individuals have no symptoms, anemia, or hemolysis, but the peripheral blood smear may show some target cells. Identification of persons with hemoglobin C trait is important for genetic counseling, particularly with regard to the possibility of sickle hemoglobin C disease in offspring.

Persons with homozygous hemoglobin C have a mild microcytic hemolytic anemia and may develop splenomegaly. The peripheral blood smear shows prominent target cells. As with other hemolytic anemias, complications of homozygous hemoglobin C include gallstones and aplastic crises.

Steinberg MH, Nagel RH: Hemoglobin SC and hemoglobin C disorders. In Steinberg MH, Forget BG, Higgs DR, Weatherall DJ (editors): *Disorders of Hemoglobin, 2nd edition.* Lippincott-Raven 2009:539–531.

6. Hemoglobin E Disorders

Hemoglobin E is the second most common hemoglobin variant worldwide, with a gene frequency up to 60% in northeast Thailand and Cambodia. Persons heterozygous for hemoglobin E show hemoglobin FAE by neonatal screening and are asymptomatic and usually not anemic, but they may develop mild microcytosis. Persons homozygous for hemoglobin E are also asymptomatic but may have mild anemia; the peripheral blood smear shows microcytosis and some target cells.

Compound heterozygotes for hemoglobin E and β^0-thalassemia are normal at birth and, like infants with homozygous E, show hemoglobin FE on neonatal screening. Unlike homozygotes, they subsequently develop mild to severe microcytic hypochromic anemia. Such children may exhibit jaundice, hepatosplenomegaly, and poor growth if the disorder is not recognized and treated appropriately. In some cases, the anemia becomes severe enough to require lifelong transfusion therapy. Even without regular transfusions, hemosiderosis may occur. In certain areas of the United States, hemoglobin E/β^0-thalassemia has become a more common cause of transfusion-dependent anemia than homozygous β-thalassemia.

Olivieri NF: HbE/β-thalassemia: Basis of marked clinical diversity. Hematol Oncol Clin North Am 2010;24:1055 [PMID: 21075280].

7. Other Hemoglobinopathies

Hundreds of other human globin-chain variants have been described. Some, such as hemoglobins D and G, are relatively common. Heterozygous individuals, who are frequently identified during the course of neonatal screening programs for hemoglobinopathies, are generally asymptomatic and usually have no anemia or hemolysis. The principal significance of most hemoglobin variants is the potential for disease in compound heterozygous individuals who also inherit a gene for β-thalassemia or sickle hemoglobin. For example, children who are compound heterozygous for hemoglobins S and D_{Punjab} ($D_{Los\ Angeles}$) have sickle cell disease.

CONGENITAL HEMOLYTIC ANEMIAS: DISORDERS OF RED CELL METABOLISM

Erythrocytes depend on the anaerobic metabolism of glucose for the maintenance of adenosine triphosphate levels sufficient for homeostasis. Glycolysis also produces the 2,3-diphosphoglycerate levels needed to modulate the oxygen affinity of hemoglobin. Glucose metabolism via the hexose monophosphate shunt is necessary to generate sufficient reduced nicotinamide adenine dinucleotide phosphate (NADPH) and reduced glutathione to protect red cells against oxidant damage. Congenital deficiencies of many glycolytic pathway enzymes have been associated with hemolytic anemias. In general, the morphologic abnormalities present on the peripheral blood smear are nonspecific, and the inheritance of these disorders is autosomal recessive or X-linked. Thus, the possibility of a red cell enzyme defect should be considered during the evaluation of a patient with a congenital hemolytic anemia in the following instances: when the peripheral blood smear does not show red cell morphology typical of membrane or hemoglobin defects (eg, spherocytes, sickle forms, target cells); when hemoglobin disorders are excluded by hemoglobin electrophoresis and by isopropanol precipitation tests; and when family studies do not suggest an autosomal dominant disorder. The diagnosis is confirmed by finding a low level of the deficient enzyme.

The two most common disorders of erythrocyte metabolism are G6PD deficiency and pyruvate kinase deficiency.

1. Glucose-6-Phosphate Dehydrogenase (G6PD) Deficiency

ESSENTIALS OF DIAGNOSIS & TYPICAL FEATURES

- African, Mediterranean, or Asian ancestry.
- Neonatal hyperbilirubinemia.
- Sporadic hemolysis associated with infection or with ingestion of oxidant drugs or fava beans.
- X-linked inheritance.

General Considerations

Deficiency of G6PD is the most common red cell enzyme defect that causes hemolytic anemia. The disorder has X-linked recessive inheritance and occurs with high frequency among persons of African, Mediterranean, and Asian ancestry. Hundreds of different G6PD variants have been characterized. In most instances, the deficiency is due to enzyme instability; thus, older red cells are more deficient than younger ones, and are unable to generate sufficient NADH to maintain the levels of reduced glutathione necessary to protect the red cells against oxidant stress. Thus, most persons with G6PD deficiency do not have a chronic hemolytic anemia; instead, they have episodic hemolysis at times of exposure to the oxidant stress of infection or of certain drugs or food substances. The severity of the disorder varies among ethnic groups; G6PD deficiency in persons of African ancestry usually is less severe than in other ethnic groups.

Clinical Findings

A. Symptoms and Signs

Infants with G6PD deficiency may have significant hyperbilirubinemia and require phototherapy or exchange transfusion to prevent kernicterus. The deficiency is an important cause of neonatal hyperbilirubinemia in infants of Mediterranean or Asian ancestry, but less so in infants of African ancestry. Older children with G6PD deficiency are asymptomatic and appear normal between episodes of hemolysis. Hemolytic episodes are often triggered by infection or by the ingestion of oxidant drugs such as antimalarial compounds and sulfonamide antibiotics (Table 30–3). Ingestion of fava beans may trigger hemolysis in children of Mediterranean or Asian ancestry but usually not in children of African ancestry. Episodes of hemolysis are associated with pallor, jaundice, hemoglobinuria, and sometimes cardiovascular compromise.

Table 30–3. Some common drugs and chemicals that can induce hemolytic anemia in persons with G6PD deficiency.

Acetanilide	Niridazole
Doxorubicin	Nitrofurantoin
Furazolidone	Phenazopyridine
Methylene blue	Primaquine
Nalidixic acid	Sulfamethoxazole

Reproduced, with permission, from Beutler E: Glucose-6-phosphate dehydrogenase deficiency. N Engl J Med 1991;324:171.

B. Laboratory Findings

The hemoglobin concentration, reticulocyte count, and peripheral blood smear are usually normal in the absence of oxidant stress. Episodes of hemolysis are associated with a variable fall in hemoglobin. "Bite" cells or blister cells may be seen, along with a few spherocytes. Hemoglobinuria is common, and the reticulocyte count increases within a few days. Heinz bodies may be demonstrated with appropriate stains. The diagnosis is confirmed by the finding of reduced levels of G6PD in erythrocytes. Because this enzyme is present in increased quantities in reticulocytes, the test is best performed at a time when the reticulocyte count is normal or near normal.

Complications

Kernicterus is a risk for infants with significant neonatal hyperbilirubinemia. Episodes of acute hemolysis in older children may be life-threatening. Rare G6PD variants are associated with chronic hemolytic anemia; the clinical course of patients with such variants may be complicated by splenomegaly and by the formation of gallstones.

Treatment

The most important treatment issue is avoidance of drugs known to be associated with hemolysis (see Table 30–3). For some patients of Mediterranean, Middle Eastern, or Asian ancestry, the consumption of fava beans must also be avoided. Infections should be treated promptly and antibiotics given when appropriate. Most episodes of hemolysis are self-limiting, but red cell transfusions may be lifesaving when signs and symptoms indicate cardiovascular compromise.

2. Pyruvate Kinase Deficiency

Pyruvate kinase deficiency is an autosomal recessive disorder observed in all ethnic groups but is most common in northern Europeans. The deficiency is associated with a chronic hemolytic anemia of varying severity. Approximately one-third of those affected present in the neonatal period with jaundice and hemolysis that require phototherapy or exchange transfusion. Occasionally, the disorder causes hydrops fetalis and neonatal death. In older children, the hemolysis may require red cell transfusions or be mild enough to go unnoticed for many years. Jaundice and splenomegaly frequently occur in the more severe cases. The diagnosis of pyruvate kinase deficiency is occasionally suggested by the presence of echinocytes on the peripheral blood smear, but these findings may be absent prior to splenectomy. The diagnosis depends on the demonstration of low levels of pyruvate kinase activity in red cells.

Treatment of pyruvate kinase depends on the severity of the hemolysis. Blood transfusions may be required for significant anemia, and splenectomy may be beneficial. Although the procedure does not cure the disorder, it ameliorates the anemia and its symptoms. Characteristically, the reticulocyte count increases and echinocytes become more prevalent after splenectomy, despite the decreased hemolysis and increased hemoglobin level.

Tavazzi D: Red blood cell enzyme disorders: An overview. Pediatr Ann 2008;37:303 [PMID: 18543541].

ACQUIRED HEMOLYTIC ANEMIA

1. Autoimmune Hemolytic Anemia

ESSENTIALS OF DIAGNOSIS & TYPICAL FEATURES

- Pallor, fatigue, jaundice, and dark urine.
- Splenomegaly.
- Positive DAT.
- Reticulocytosis and spherocytosis.

General Considerations

Acquired autoimmune hemolytic anemia (AIHA) is rare during the first 4 months of life but is one of the more common causes of acute anemia after the first year. It may arise as an isolated problem or may complicate an infection (hepatitis, upper respiratory tract infections, mononucleosis, or cytomegalovirus infection); systemic lupus erythematosus and other autoimmune syndromes; immunodeficiency states, including autoimmune lymphoproliferative syndrome (ALPS); or, very rarely, malignancies.

Clinical Findings

A. Symptoms and Signs

The disease usually has an acute onset manifested by weakness, pallor, dark urine, and fatigue. Jaundice is a prominent finding, and splenomegaly is often present. Some cases have a more chronic, insidious onset. Clinical evidence of an underlying disease may be present.

B. Laboratory Findings

The anemia is normochromic and normocytic and may vary from mild to severe (hemoglobin concentration < 5 g/dL). The reticulocyte count and index are usually increased but occasionally are normal or low. Spherocytes and nucleated red cells may be seen on the peripheral blood smear. Although leukocytosis and elevated platelet counts are a common finding, thrombocytopenia occasionally occurs. Other laboratory data consistent with hemolysis are present, such as increased indirect and total bilirubin, lactic dehydrogenase, aspartate aminotransferase, and urinary urobilinogen. Intravascular hemolysis is indicated by hemoglobinemia or hemoglobinuria. Examination of bone marrow shows marked erythroid hyperplasia and hemophagocytosis, but is seldom required for the diagnosis.

Serologic studies are helpful in defining pathophysiology, planning therapeutic strategies, and assessing prognosis (Table 30–4). In almost all cases, the direct and indirect antiglobulin (DAT and IAT) tests are positive. Further evaluation allows distinction into one of three syndromes. The presence of IgG and no or low level of complement activation on the patient's red blood cells, maximal in vitro antibody activity at 37°C, and either no antigen specificity or an Rh-like specificity constitute warm autoimmune hemolytic anemia with extravascular destruction by the reticuloendothelial system. In contrast, the detection of complement alone on red blood cells, optimal reactivity in vitro at 4°C, and I or i antigen specificity are diagnostic of cold autoimmune hemolytic anemia with intravascular hemolysis. Although cold agglutinins are relatively common (~10%) in normal individuals, clinically significant cold antibodies exhibit in vitro reactivity at 30°C or above. Warm reactive IgM antibodies are rare.

Paroxysmal cold hemoglobinuria presents a different category of disease. The laboratory evaluation is identical to cold autoimmune hemolytic anemia except for antigen specificity (P) and the exhibition of an in vitro hemolysin. Paroxysmal cold hemoglobinuria is almost always associated with significant infections, such as *Mycoplasma*, Epstein-Barr virus, and cytomegalovirus.

Differential Diagnosis

Autoimmune hemolytic anemia must be differentiated from other forms of congenital or acquired hemolytic anemias.

Table 30–4. Classification of autoimmune hemolytic anemia (AIHA) in children.

Syndrome	Warm AIHA	Cold AIHA	Paroxysmal Cold Hemoglobinuria
Specific antiglobulin test IgG Complement	 Strongly positive. Negative or mildly positive.	 Negative. Strongly positive.	 Negative. Strongly positive.
Temperature at maximal reactivity (in vitro)	37°C.	4°C.	4°C.
Antigen specificity	May be panagglutinin or may have an Rh-like specificity.	I or i.	P.
Other	. . .	. . .	Positive biphasic hemolysin test.
Pathophysiology	Extravascular hemolysis, destruction by the RES (eg, spleen). Rarely an intravascular component early in the course.	Intravascular hemolysis (may have extravascular component).	Intravascular hemolysis (may have extravascular component).
Prognosis	May be more chronic (> 3 mo) with significant morbidity and mortality. May be associated with a primary disorder (lupus, immunodeficiency, etc).	Generally acute (< 3 mo). Good prognosis: often associated with infection.	Acute, self-limited. Associated with infection.
Therapy	Responds to RES blockade, including steroids (prednisone, 2 mg/kg/d), IVIG (1 g/kg/d for 2 d), or splenectomy.	May not respond to RES blockade. Severe cases may benefit from plasmapheresis.	Usually self-limited. Symptomatic management.

IVIG, intravenous immune globulin; RES, reticuloendothelial system.

The DAT discriminates antibody-mediated hemolysis from other causes, such as hereditary spherocytosis. The presence of other cytopenias and antibodies to platelets or neutrophils suggests an autoimmune (eg, lupus) syndrome, immunodeficiency (eg, ALPS, congenital immunodeficiency), or Evans syndrome. Up to one-third of patients diagnosed as Evans syndrome may have ALPS.

Complications

The anemia may be very severe and result in cardiovascular collapse, requiring emergency management. The complications of an underlying disease, such as disseminated lupus erythematosus or an immunodeficiency state, may be present.

Treatment

Medical management of the underlying disease is important in symptomatic cases. Defining the clinical syndrome provides a useful guide to treatment. Most patients with warm autoimmune hemolytic anemia (in which hemolysis is mostly extravascular) respond to prednisone (2 mg/kg/d). After the initial treatment, the dose of corticosteroids may be decreased slowly. Patients may respond to 1 g of intravenous immune globulin (IVIG) per kilogram per day for 2 days, but fewer patients respond to IVIG than to prednisone. Although the rate of remission with splenectomy may be as high as 50%, particularly in warm autoimmune hemolytic anemia, this should be carefully considered in younger patients and withheld until other treatments have failed. In severe cases, unresponsive to more conventional therapy, immunosuppressive agents such as mycophenolate, sirolimus, cyclosporine, cyclophosphamide, azathioprine, or busulfan may be tried alone or in combination with corticosteroids. The initial three may induce less myelosuppression and be helpful when hemolysis is associated with Evans syndrome or ALPS. In severe cases, rituximab may be a successful alternative; however, this drug should be avoided in AIHA associated with ALPS. Transplantation has been used in a small number of cases.

Patients with cold autoimmune hemolytic anemia and paroxysmal cold hemoglobinuria are less likely to respond to corticosteroids or IVIG. Because these syndromes are most apt to be associated with infections and have an acute, self-limited course, supportive care alone may be sufficient. Plasma exchange may be effective in severe cold autoimmune (IgM) hemolytic anemia because the offending antibody has an intravascular distribution.

Supportive therapy is crucial. Patients with cold-reacting antibodies, particularly paroxysmal cold hemoglobinuria, should be kept in a warm environment. Transfusion may be necessary because of the complications of severe anemia but should be used only when there is no alternative. In most patients, cross-match compatible blood will not be found, and the least incompatible unit may be identified. Transfusion must be conducted carefully, beginning with a test dose (see Transfusion Medicine section, later in this chapter). Identification of the patient's phenotype for minor red cell alloantigens may be helpful in avoiding alloimmunization or in providing appropriate transfusions if alloantibodies arise after initial transfusions. Patients with severe intravascular hemolysis may have associated disseminated intravascular coagulation (DIC), and heparin therapy should be considered in such cases.

Prognosis

The outlook for autoimmune hemolytic anemia in childhood usually is good unless associated diseases are present (eg, congenital immunodeficiency, ALPS, AIDS, lupus erythematosus), in which case hemolysis is likely to have a chronic course. In general, children with warm (IgG) autoimmune hemolytic anemia are at greater risk for more severe and chronic disease with higher morbidity and mortality rates. Hemolysis and positive antiglobulin tests may continue for months or years. Patients with cold autoimmune hemolytic anemia or paroxysmal cold hemoglobinuria are more likely to have acute, self-limited disease (< 3 months). Paroxysmal cold hemoglobinuria is almost always associated with infection (eg, *Mycoplasma* infection, CMV, and EBV).

Aladjidi N: New insights into childhood autoimmune hemolytic anemia: A French national observational study of 265 children. Haematologica 2011;96:655 [PMID: 21228033].

Notarangelo LD: Primary immunodeficiencies (PIDs) presenting with cytopenias. Hematology Am Soc Hematol Educ Program 2009;139 [PMID: 20008192].

Petz LD: Unusual problems regarding autoimmune hemolytic anemias. In Petz LD, Garratty G (editors): *Acquired Immune Hemolytic Anemias,* 2nd ed. Churchill Livingstone, 2004:341–344.

Rao VK: Use of rituximab for refractory cytopenias associated with autoimmune lymphoproliferative syndrome (ALPS). Pediatr Blood Cancer 2009;52:847 [PMID: 19214977].

2. Nonimmune Acquired Hemolytic Anemia

Hepatic disease may alter the lipid composition of the red cell membrane. This usually results in the formation of target cells and is not associated with significant hemolysis.

Occasionally, hepatocellular damage is associated with the formation of spur cells and brisk hemolytic anemia. Renal disease may also be associated with significant hemolysis; hemolytic-uremic syndrome is one example. In this disorder, hemolysis is associated with the presence, on the peripheral blood smear, of echinocytes, helmet cells, fragmented red cells, and spherocytes.

A microangiopathic hemolytic anemia with fragmented red cells and some spherocytes may be observed in several conditions associated with intravascular coagulation and fibrin deposition within vessels. This occurs with DIC complicating severe infection, but may also occur when the intravascular coagulation is localized, as with giant cavernous hemangiomas (Kasabach-Merritt syndrome). Fragmented red cells may also be seen with mechanical damage (eg, associated with artificial heart valves).

POLYCYTHEMIA & METHEMOGLOBINEMIA

CONGENITAL ERYTHROCYTOSIS (FAMILIAL POLYCYTHEMIA)

In pediatrics, polycythemia is usually secondary to chronic hypoxemia. However, several families with congenital erythrocytosis have been described. The disorder differs from polycythemia vera in that only red blood cells are affected; the white blood cell and platelet counts are normal. It occurs as an autosomal dominant or recessive disorder. There are usually no physical findings except for plethora and splenomegaly. The hemoglobin level may be as high as 27 g/dL. Patients usually have no symptoms other than headache and lethargy. Studies in a number of families have revealed (1) abnormal hemoglobin with altered oxygen affinity, (2) reduced red cell diphosphoglycerate, (3) autonomous increase in erythropoietin production, or (4) hypersensitivity of erythroid precursors to erythropoietin.

Treatment is not indicated unless symptoms are marked. Phlebotomy is the treatment of choice.

SECONDARY POLYCYTHEMIA

Secondary polycythemia occurs in response to hypoxemia. The most common cause of secondary polycythemia in children is cyanotic congenital heart disease. It also occurs in chronic pulmonary disease such as cystic fibrosis. Persons living at extremely high altitudes, as well as some with methemoglobinemia, develop polycythemia. It has on rare occasions been described without hypoxemia in association with renal tumors, brain tumors, Cushing disease, or hydronephrosis.

Polycythemia may occur in the neonatal period; it is particularly exaggerated in infants who are preterm or small for gestational age. In these infants, polycythemia is sometimes associated with other symptoms. It may occur in infants of diabetic mothers, in Down syndrome, and as a complication of congenital adrenal hyperplasia.

Iron deficiency may complicate polycythemia and aggravate the associated hyperviscosity. This complication should always be suspected when the MCV falls below the normal range. Coagulation and bleeding abnormalities, including thrombocytopenia, mild consumption coagulopathy, and elevated fibrinolytic activity, have been described in severely polycythemic cardiac patients. Bleeding at surgery may be severe.

The ideal treatment of secondary polycythemia is correction of the underlying disorder. When this cannot be done, phlebotomy may be necessary to control symptoms. Iron sufficiency should be maintained. Adequate hydration of the patient and phlebotomy with plasma replacement may be indicated prior to major surgical procedures. These measures prevent the complications of thrombosis and hemorrhage. Isovolumetric exchange transfusion is the treatment of choice in severe cases.

METHEMOGLOBINEMIA

Methemoglobin is continuously formed at a slow rate by the oxidation of heme iron to the ferric state. Normally, it is enzymatically reduced back to hemoglobin. Methemoglobin is unable to transport oxygen and causes a shift in the dissociation curve of the residual oxyhemoglobin. Cyanosis is produced with methemoglobin levels of approximately 15% or greater. Levels of methemoglobin increase by several mechanisms.

1. Hemoglobin M

The designation M is given to several abnormal hemoglobins associated with methemoglobinemia. Affected individuals are heterozygous for the gene, which is transmitted as an autosomal dominant disorder. The different types of hemoglobin M result from different amino acid substitutions in α-globin or β-globin. Hemoglobin electrophoresis at the usual pH will not always demonstrate the abnormal hemoglobin, and isoelectric focusing may be needed. The patient has cyanosis but is otherwise usually asymptomatic. Exercise tolerance may be normal, and life expectancy is not affected. This type of methemoglobinemia does not respond to any form of therapy.

2. Congenital Methemoglobinemia Due to Enzyme Deficiencies

Congenital methemoglobinemia is caused most frequently by congenital deficiency of the reducing enzyme diaphorase I (coenzyme factor I). It is transmitted as an autosomal recessive trait. Affected patients may have as much as 40% methemoglobin but usually have no symptoms, although a mild compensatory polycythemia may be present. Patients with methemoglobinemia associated with a deficiency of diaphorase I respond readily to treatment with ascorbic acid and methylene blue (see next section), but treatment is not usually indicated.

3. Acquired Methemoglobinemia

Several compounds activate the oxidation of hemoglobin from the ferrous to the ferric state, forming methemoglobin. These include the nitrites and nitrates (contaminated water), chlorates, and quinones. Drugs in this group are the aniline dyes, sulfonamides, acetanilid, phenacetin, bismuth subnitrate, and potassium chlorate. Poisoning with a drug or chemical containing one of these substances should be suspected in any infant or child who presents with sudden cyanosis. Methemoglobin levels in such cases may be extremely high and can produce anoxia, dyspnea, unconsciousness, circulatory failure, and death. Young infants and newborns are more susceptible to acquired methemoglobinemia because their red cells have difficulty reducing hemoglobin, probably because their NADH methemoglobin reductase is transiently deficient. Infants with metabolic acidosis from diarrhea and dehydration or other causes also may develop methemoglobinemia.

Patients with the acquired form of methemoglobinemia respond dramatically to methylene blue in a dose of 1–2 mg/kg intravenously. For infants and young children, a smaller dose (1–1.5 mg/kg) is recommended. Ascorbic acid administered orally or intravenously also reduces methemoglobin, but the response is slower.

DISORDERS OF LEUKOCYTES

NEUTROPENIA

ESSENTIALS OF DIAGNOSIS & TYPICAL FEATURES

- Increased frequency of infections.
- Ulceration of oral mucosa and gingivitis.
- Decreased absolute neutrophil count; normal numbers of red cells and platelets.

General Considerations

Neutropenia is an absolute neutrophil (granulocyte) count of less than 1500/μL in childhood, or less than 1100/μL between ages 1 month and 2 years. During the first few days of life, an absolute neutrophil count of less than 3500/μL may be considered neutropenia in term infants. Neutropenia results from absent or defective myeloid stem cells; ineffective or suppressed myeloid maturation; decreased production of hematopoietic cytokines (eg, granulocyte colony-stimulating factor [G-CSF] or granulocyte-macrophage colony-stimulating factor [GM-CSF]); decreased marrow release; increased neutrophil apoptosis; destruction or consumption; or, in pseudoneutropenia, from an increased neutrophil marginating pool (Table 30–5). A decrease in neutrophil mass diminishes delivery of these cells to areas where the balance favors bacterial proliferation and invasion.

The most severe types of congenital neutropenia include reticular dysgenesis (congenital aleukocytosis), Kostmann syndrome (severe neutropenia with maturation defect in the marrow progenitor cells), Shwachman syndrome (neutropenia with pancreatic insufficiency), neutropenia with immune deficiency states, cyclic neutropenia, and myelokathexis or dysgranulopoiesis. Genetic mutations for Chédiak-Higashi syndrome, Kostmann syndrome, Shwachman syndrome, and cyclic neutropenia have been identified. Neutropenia may also be associated with storage and metabolic diseases and immunodeficiency states. The most common causes of acute neutropenia are viral infection or drugs resulting in decreased neutrophil production in the marrow, increased peripheral

Table 30–5. Classification of neutropenia of childhood.

Congenital neutropenia with stem cell abnormalities
Reticular dysgenesis
Cyclic neutropenia
Congenital neutropenia with abnormalities of committed myeloid progenitor cells
Neutropenia with immunodeficiency disorders (T cells and B cells)
Severe congenital neutropenia (Kostmann syndrome)
Chronic idiopathic neutropenia of childhood
Myelokathexis with dysmyelopoiesis
Chédiak-Higashi syndrome
Shwachman-Diamond syndrome
Cartilage-hair hypoplasia
Dyskeratosis congenital
Fanconi anemia
Organic acidemias (eg, propionic, methylmalonic)
Glycogenosis Ib
Osteopetrosis
Acquired neutropenias affecting stem cells
Malignancies (leukemia, lymphoma) and preleukemic disorders
Drugs or toxic substances
Ionizing radiation
Aplastic anemia
Acquired neutropenias affecting committed myeloid progenitors or survival of mature neutrophils
Ineffective granulopoiesis (vitamin B_{12}, folate, and copper deficiency)
Infection
Immune (neonatal alloimmune or autoimmune; autoimmune or chronic benign neutropenia of childhood)
Hypersplenism

turnover, or both. Severe bacterial infections may be associated with neutropenia. Although rare, neonatal alloimmune neutropenia can be severe and associated with risk for infection. Autoimmune neutropenia occurs with autoimmune disorders or, in the newborn, as a result of passive transfer of antibody from the mother to the fetus. Malignancies, osteopetrosis, marrow failure syndromes, and hypersplenism usually are not associated with isolated neutropenia.

Clinical Findings

A. Symptoms and Signs

Acute severe bacterial or fungal infection is the most significant complication of neutropenia. Although the risk is increased when the absolute neutrophil count is less than 500/µL, the actual susceptibility is variable and depends on the cause of neutropenia, marrow reserves, and other factors. The most common types of infection include septicemia, cellulitis, skin abscesses, pneumonia, and perirectal abscesses. Sinusitis, aphthous ulcers, gingivitis, and periodontal disease also cause significant problems. In addition to local signs and symptoms, patients may have chills, fever, and malaise. In most cases, the spleen and liver are not enlarged. *Staphylococcus aureus* and gram-negative bacteria are the most common pathogens.

B. Laboratory Findings

Neutrophils are absent or markedly reduced in the peripheral blood smear. In most forms of neutropenia or agranulocytosis, the monocytes and lymphocytes are normal and the red cells and platelets are not affected. The bone marrow usually shows a normal erythroid series, with adequate megakaryocytes, but a marked reduction in the myeloid cells or a significant delay in maturation of this series may be noted. Total cellularity may be decreased.

In the evaluation of neutropenia (eg, persistent, intermittent, cyclic), attention should be paid to the duration and pattern of neutropenia, the types of infections and their frequency, and phenotypic abnormalities on physical examination. A careful family history and blood counts from the parents are useful. If an acquired cause, such as viral infection or drug, is not obvious as an acute cause and no other primary disease is present, white blood cell counts, white cell differential, and platelet and reticulocyte counts should be completed twice weekly for 6 weeks to determine the possibility of cyclic neutropenia. Bone marrow aspiration and biopsy are most important to characterize the morphologic features of myelopoiesis. Measuring the neutrophil counts in response to corticosteroid infusion may document the marrow reserves. Other tests that aid in the diagnosis include measurement of neutrophil antibodies, immunoglobulin levels, antinuclear antibodies, and lymphocyte phenotyping to detect immunodeficiency states. Cultures of bone marrow are important for defining the numbers of stem cells and progenitors committed to the myeloid series or the presence of inhibitory factors. Cytokine levels in plasma or mononuclear cells can be measured directly. Some neutropenia disorders have abnormal neutrophil function, but severe neutropenia may preclude collection of sufficient cells to complete assays. Recent studies have documented abnormalities in an antiapoptotic gene, *HAX1,* and the elastase gene, *ELA2,* in Kostmann syndrome and *ELA2* mutations in cyclic neutropenia. A mutation for Shwachman syndrome has been described. Increased apoptosis in marrow precursors or circulating neutrophils has been described in several congenital or genetic disorders.

Treatment

Underlying disorders should be identified and treated or associated agents should be eliminated. Infections should be aggressively assessed and treated. Prophylactic antimicrobial therapy is not indicated for afebrile, asymptomatic patients, but may be considered in rare cases with recurrent infections. Recombinant G-CSF will increase neutrophil counts in most patients; GM-CSF may be considered, but is less extensively used. Patients may be started on 3–5 mcg/kg/d of G-CSF (filgrastim) given subcutaneously or intravenously once a day. Depending on the counts, the dose may be adjusted. The dose should be regulated to keep the absolute neutrophil count below 10,000/μL. Some patients maintain adequate counts with G-CSF given every other day or three times a week. Treatment will decrease infectious complications, but may have little effect on periodontal disease. However, not all patients with neutropenia syndromes require G-CSF (eg, chronic benign neutropenia of childhood). Patients with cyclic neutropenia may have a milder clinical course as they grow older. Immunizations should be given if the immune system is normal. Hematopoietic stem cell transplantation may be considered for patients with severe complications, especially those with severe congenital neutropenia.

Prognosis

The prognosis varies greatly with the cause and severity of the neutropenia. In severe cases with persistent agranulocytosis, the prognosis is poor in spite of antibiotic therapy; in mild or cyclic forms of neutropenia, symptoms may be minimal and the prognosis for normal life expectancy excellent. G-CSF has the potential to prolong life expectancy. Up to 50% of patients with Shwachman syndrome may develop aplastic anemia, myelodysplasia, or leukemia during their lifetime. Patients with Kostmann syndrome also have a potential for leukemia, as do patients with neutropenia associated with some immune disorders. Hematopoietic stem cell transplantation may be the only curative therapy for some disorders.

Boztug K: Genetic etiologies of severe congenital neutropenia. Curr Opin Pediatr 2011;23:21 [PMID: 21206270].

Carlsson G: Hematopoietic stem cell transplantation in severe congenital neutropenia. Pediatr Blood Cancer 2011;56:444 [PMID: 21072829].

Chou JY: Neutropenia in type Ib glycogen storage disease. Curr Opin Hematol 2010;17:36 [PMID: 19741523].

Newburger PE: Cyclic neutropenia and severe congenital neutropenia in patients with a shared ELANE mutation and paternal haplotype: Evidence for phenotype determination by modifying genes. Pediatr Blood Cancer 2010;55:314 [PMID: 20582973].

Zeidler C: Clinical implications of ELA2-, HAX1-, and G-CSF-receptor (CSF3R) mutations in severe congenital neutropenia. Br J Haematol 2009;144:459 [PMID: 19120359].

NEUTROPHILIA

Neutrophilia is an increase in the absolute neutrophil count in the peripheral blood to greater than 7500–8500/μL for infants, children, and adults. To support the increased peripheral count, neutrophils may be mobilized from bone marrow storage or peripheral marginating pools. Neutrophilia occurs acutely in association with bacterial or viral infections, inflammatory diseases (eg, juvenile rheumatoid arthritis, inflammatory bowel disease, Kawasaki disease), surgical or functional asplenia, liver failure, diabetic ketoacidosis, azotemia, congenital disorders of neutrophil function (eg, chronic granulomatous disease, leukocyte adherence deficiency), and hemolysis. Drugs such as corticosteroids, lithium, and epinephrine increase the blood neutrophil count. Corticosteroids cause release of neutrophils from the marrow pool, inhibit egress from capillary beds, and postpone apoptotic cell death. Epinephrine causes release of the marginating pool. Acute neutrophilia has been reported after stress, such as from electric shock, trauma, burns, surgery, and emotional upset. Tumors involving the bone marrow, such as lymphomas, neuroblastomas, and rhabdomyosarcoma, may be associated with leukocytosis and the presence of immature myeloid cells in the peripheral blood. Infants with Down syndrome have defective regulation of proliferation and maturation of the myeloid series and may develop neutrophilia. At times this process may affect other cell lines and mimic myeloproliferative disorders or acute leukemia.

The neutrophilias must be distinguished from myeloproliferative disorders such as chronic myelogenous leukemia and juvenile chronic myelogenous leukemia. In general, abnormalities involving other cell lines, the appearance of immature cells on the blood smear, and the presence of hepatosplenomegaly are important differentiating characteristics.

DISORDERS OF NEUTROPHIL FUNCTION

Neutrophils play a key role in host defenses. Circulating in capillary beds, they adhere to the vascular endothelium adjacent to sites of infection and inflammation. Moving between endothelial cells, the neutrophil migrates toward the offending agent. Contact with a microbe that is properly opsonized with complement or antibodies triggers ingestion, a process in which cytoplasmic streaming results in the formation of pseudopods that fuse around the invader, encasing it in a phagosome. During the ingestion phase, the oxidase enzyme system assembles and is activated, taking oxygen from the surrounding medium and reducing it to form toxic oxygen metabolites critical to microbicidal activity. Concurrently, granules from the two main classes (azurophil and specific) fuse and release their contents into the phagolysosome. The concentration of toxic oxygen metabolites (eg, hydrogen peroxide, hypochlorous acid, hydroxyl radical) and other compounds (eg, proteases, cationic proteins, cathepsins, defensins) increases dramatically, resulting in the death and dissolution of the microbe. Complex physiologic and biochemical processes support and control these functions. Defects in any of these processes may lead to inadequate cell function and an increased risk of infection.

Classification

Table 30–6 summarizes congenital neutrophil function defects. Recently reported is variant CGD with p40phox deficiency manifested by inflammatory bowel disease. Also described is a syndrome of severe neutrophil dysfunction

Table 30–6. Classification of congenital neutrophil function deficits.

Disorder	Clinical Manifestations	Functional Defect	Biochemical Defect	Inheritance (Chromosome; Gene)
Chédiak-Higashi syndrome	Oculocutaneous albinism, photophobia, nystagmus, ataxia. Recurrent infections of skin, respiratory tract, and mucous membranes with gram-positive and gram-negative organisms. Many patients die during lymphoproliferative phase with hepatomegaly, fever, which may be a viral-associated hemophagocytic syndrome secondary to Epstein-Barr virus infection. Older patients may develop degenerative CNS disease.	Neutropenia. Neutrophils, monocytes, lymphocytes, platelets, and all granule-containing cells have giant granules. Most significant defect is in chemotaxis. Also milder defects in microbicidal activity and degranulation.	Gene deficit identified. Alterations in membrane fusion with formation of giant granules. Other biochemical abnormalities in cAMP and cGMP, microtubule assembly.	Autosomal recessive (1q42.1-.2; *CHS1*)
Leukocyte adherence deficiency I	Recurrent soft-tissue infections, including gingivitis, otitis, mucositis, periodontitis, skin infections. Delayed separation of the cord in newborn and problems with wound healing.	Neutrophilia. Diminished adherence to surfaces, leading to decreased chemotaxis.	Absence or partial deficiency of CD11/CD18 cell surface adhesive glycoproteins.	Autosomal recessive (12q22.3; *ITGB2*)
Leukocyte adherence deficiency II	Recurrent infections, mental retardation, craniofacial abnormalities, short stature.	Neutrophilia. Deficient "rolling" interactions with endothelial cells. Red cells have Bombay phenotype.	Deficient fucosyl transferase results in deficient sialyl Lewis X antigen, which interacts with P selectin. P selectin on endothelial cells is required for neutrophil rolling, a prerequisite for adherence and diapedesis.	Autosomal recessive (11p11.2; *SLC35C1*)
Chronic granulomatous disease	Recurrent purulent infections with catalase-positive bacteria and fungi. May involve skin, mucous membranes. Patients also develop deep infections (lymph nodes, lung, liver, bones) and sepsis.	Neutrophilia. Neutrophils demonstrate deficient bactericidal activity but normal chemotaxis and ingestion. Defect in the oxidase enzyme system, resulting in absence or diminished production of oxygen metabolites toxic to microbes.	Several molecular defects in oxidase components. Absent cytochrome b558 with decreased expression of either (1) or (2):	
			(1) gp91-phox	X-linked in 60%–65% of cases (Xp21.1; *CYBB*)
			(2) p22-phox	Autosomal recessive in < 5% of cases (16q24; *CYBA*)
			Absent p47-phox or p67-phox (cytosolic components).	Autosomal recessive in 30% of cases (7q11.23; *NCF1* and 1q25; *NCF2*, respectively)
Myeloperoxidase deficiency	Generally healthy. Fungal infections when deficiency associated with systemic diseases (eg, diabetes).	Diminished capacity to enhance hydrogen peroxide-mediated microbicidal activity. Decreased killing of *Candida*.	Diminished or absent myeloperoxidase; post-translational defect in processing protein.	Autosomal recessive (17q22-23)
Specific granule deficiency	Recurrent skin and deep tissue infections.	Neutropenia. Neutrophils have band-shaped or bilobed nuclei. Decreased chemotaxis and bactericidal activity.	Failure to produce specific granules or their contents during myelopoiesis. Defect in transcription factor.	Autosomal recessive (14q11.2; *CEBPε*)

cAMP, cyclic adenosine monophosphate; cGMP, cyclic guanosine monophosphate; CNS, central nervous system.

and severe infections associated with a mutation in a GTPase signaling molecule, Rac2. New syndromes of innate immune dysfunction include defects in interferon and interleukin-12 receptor and signaling pathways, leading to monocyte and macrophage dysfunction and toll-like receptor signaling pathways (interleukin-1 receptor-associated [IRAK] deficiency) associated with recurrent bacterial infections. Leukocyte adhesion deficiency (LAD) III is a disorder characterized by severe bleeding, impaired leukocyte adhesion, and endothelial inflammation and is associated with mutations of *FERMT3* gene, which encodes for a protein, Kindlin-3, critical for intracellular function of β integrins. Other congenital or acquired causes of mild to moderate neutrophil dysfunction include metabolic defects (eg, glycogen storage disease, diabetes mellitus, renal disease, and hypophosphatemia), viral infections, and certain drugs. Neutrophils from newborn infants have abnormal adherence, chemotaxis, and bactericidal activity. Cells from patients with thermal injury, trauma, and overwhelming infection have defects in cell motility and bactericidal activity similar to those seen in neonates.

Clinical Findings

Recurrent bacterial or fungal infections are the hallmark of neutrophil dysfunction. Although patients will have infection-free periods, episodes of pneumonia, sinusitis, cellulitis, cutaneous and mucosal infections (including perianal or peritonsillar abscesses), and lymphadenitis are frequent. As with neutropenia, aphthous ulcers of mucous membranes, severe gingivitis, and periodontal disease are also major complications. In general, *S aureus* or gram-negative organisms are commonly isolated from infected sites; other organisms may be specifically associated with a defined neutrophil function defect. In some disorders, fungi account for an increasing number of infections. Deep or generalized infections, such as osteomyelitis, liver abscesses, sepsis, meningitis, and necrotic or gangrenous soft-tissue lesions, occur in specific syndromes (eg, leukocyte adherence deficiency or chronic granulomatous disease). Patients with severe neutrophil dysfunction may die in childhood from severe infections or associated complications. Table 30–6 summarizes pertinent laboratory findings.

Treatment

The mainstays of management of these disorders are anticipation of infections and aggressive attempts to identify the foci and the causative agents. Surgical procedures to achieve these goals may be both diagnostic and therapeutic. Broad-spectrum antibiotics covering the range of possible organisms should be initiated without delay, switching to specific antimicrobial agents when the microbiologic diagnosis is made. When infections are unresponsive or they recur, granulocyte transfusions may be helpful.

Chronic management includes prophylactic antibiotics. Trimethoprim–sulfamethoxazole and some other antibiotics (eg, rifampin) enhance the bactericidal activity of neutrophils from patients with chronic granulomatous disease. Some patients with Chédiak-Higashi syndrome improve clinically when given ascorbic acid. Recombinant γ-interferon decreases the number and severity of infections in patients with chronic granulomatous disease. Demonstration of this activity with one patient group raises the possibility that cytokines, growth factors, and other biologic response modifiers may be helpful in other conditions in preventing recurrent infections. Bone marrow transplantation has been attempted in most major congenital neutrophil dysfunction syndromes, and reconstitution with normal cells and cell function has been documented. Combining genetic engineering with autologous bone marrow transplantation may provide a future strategy for curing these disorders.

Prognosis

For mild to moderate defects, anticipation and conservative medical management ensure a reasonable outlook. For severe defects, excessive morbidity and significant mortality still exist. In some diseases, the development of noninfectious complications, such as the lymphoproliferative phase of Chédiak-Higashi syndrome or inflammatory syndromes in chronic granulomatous disease, may influence prognosis.

Ambruso DR: Human neutrophil immunodeficiency syndrome is associated with an inhibitory Rac2 mutation. Proc Natl Acad Sci USA 2000;97:4654 [PMID: 10758162].

Ambruso DR, Johnston RB Jr: Chronic granulomatous disease of childhood and common variable immunodeficiency. In Chernick V, Boat TF (editors): *Kendig's Disorders of the Respiratory Tract in Children.* WB Saunders, 2012.

Dinauer MC: Disorders of neutrophil function: An overview. Methods Mol Biol 2007;412:489 [PMID: 18453130].

Froissart R: Glucose-6-phophatase deficiency. Orphanet J Rare Dis 2011;6:27 [PMID: 21599942].

Kuhns DB: Residual NADPH oxidase and survival in chronic granulomatous disease. N Engl J Med 2010;363:2600 [PMID: 21190454].

LYMPHOCYTOSIS

From the first week up to the fifth year of life, lymphocytes are the most numerous leukocytes in human blood. The ratio then reverses gradually to reach the adult pattern of neutrophil predominance. An absolute lymphocytosis in childhood is associated with acute or chronic viral infections, pertussis, syphilis, tuberculosis, and hyperthyroidism. Other noninfectious conditions, drugs, and hypersensitivity and serum sickness–like reactions cause lymphocytosis.

Fever, upper respiratory symptoms, gastrointestinal complaints, and rashes are clues in distinguishing infectious from noninfectious causes. The presence of enlarged liver, spleen, or lymph nodes is crucial to the differential diagnosis, which includes acute leukemia and lymphoma. Most cases of infectious mononucleosis are associated with hepatosplenomegaly or adenopathy. The absence of anemia and thrombocytopenia helps to differentiate these disorders. Evaluation of the morphology of lymphocytes on peripheral blood smear is crucial. Infectious causes, particularly infectious mononucleosis, are associated with atypical features in the lymphocytes, such as basophilic cytoplasm, vacuoles, finer and less-dense chromatin, and an indented nucleus. These features are distinct from the characteristic morphology associated with lymphoblastic leukemia. Lymphocytosis in childhood is most commonly associated with infections and resolves with recovery from the primary disease.

EOSINOPHILIA

Eosinophilia in infants and children is an absolute eosinophil count greater than 300/μL. Marrow eosinophil production is stimulated by the cytokine interleukin-5. Allergies, particularly eczema, are the most common primary causes of eosinophilia in children. Eosinophilia also occurs in drug reactions, with tumors (Hodgkin and non-Hodgkin lymphomas and brain tumors), and with immunodeficiency and histiocytosis syndromes. Increased eosinophil counts are a prominent feature of many invasive parasitic infections. Gastrointestinal disorders such as chronic hepatitis, ulcerative colitis, Crohn disease, and milk precipitin disease may be associated with eosinophilia. Increased blood eosinophil counts have been identified in several families without association with any specific illness. Rare causes of eosinophilia include the hypereosinophilic syndrome, characterized by counts greater than 1500/μL and organ involvement and damage (hepatosplenomegaly, cardiomyopathy, pulmonary fibrosis, and central nervous system injury). This is a disorder of middle-aged adults and is rare in children. Eosinophilic leukemia has been described, but its existence as a distinct entity is very rare.

Eosinophils are sometimes the last type of mature myeloid cell to disappear after marrow ablative chemotherapy. Increased eosinophil counts are associated with graft-versus-host disease after bone marrow transplantation, and elevations are sometimes documented during rejection episodes in patients who have solid organ grafts.

BLEEDING DISORDERS

Bleeding disorders may occur as a result of (1) quantitative or qualitative abnormalities of platelets, (2) quantitative or qualitative abnormalities in plasma procoagulant factors, (3) vascular abnormalities, or (4) accelerated fibrinolysis. The coagulation cascade and fibrinolytic system are shown in Figures 30–4 and 30–5.

The most critical aspect in evaluating the bleeding patient is obtaining detailed personal and family bleeding histories, including bleeding complications associated with dental interventions, surgeries, suture placement and removal, and trauma. Excessive mucosal bleeding is suggestive of a platelet disorder, von Willebrand disease (vWD),

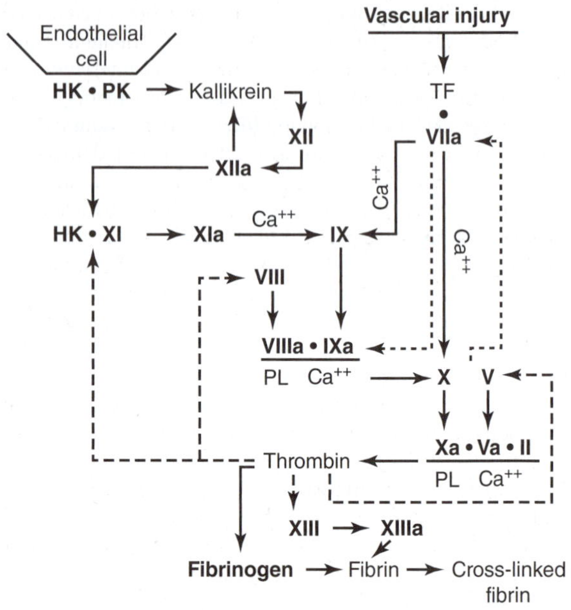

▲ **Figure 30–4.** The procoagulant system and formation of a fibrin clot. Vascular injury initiates the coagulation process by exposure of tissue factor (TF); the dashed lines indicate thrombin actions in addition to clotting of fibrinogen. The dotted lines associated with VIIa indicate the feedback activation of the VII-TF complex by Xa and IXa. Ca++, calcium; HK, high-molecular-weight kininogen; PK, prekallikrein; PL, phospholipid. (Reproduced, with permission, from Goodnight SH, Hathaway WE [editors]: *Disorders of Hemostasis & Thrombosis: A Clinical Guide*, 2nd ed. McGraw-Hill, 2001.)

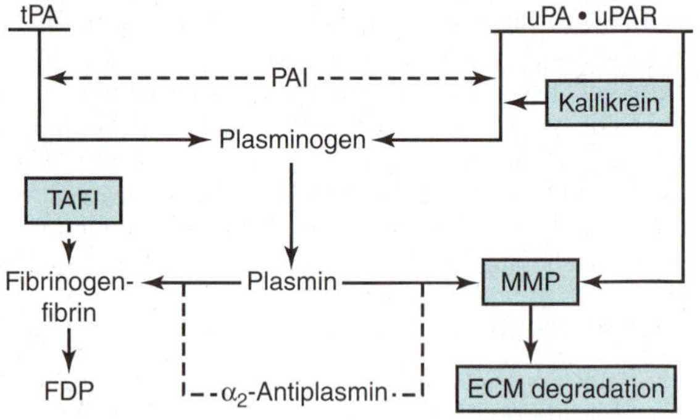

▲ **Figure 30–5.** The fibrinolytic system. Solid arrows indicate activation; dashed line arrows indicate inhibition. ECM, extracellular matrix; FDP, fibrinogen-fibrin degradation products; MMP, matrix metalloproteinases; PAI, plasminogen activator inhibitor; TAFI, thrombin activatable fibrinolysis inhibitor; tPA, tissue plasminogen activator; uPA, urokinase; uPAR, cellular urokinase receptor. (Reproduced, with permission, from Goodnight SH, Hathaway WE [editors]: *Disorders of Hemostasis & Thrombosis: A Clinical Guide*, 2nd ed. McGraw-Hill, 2001.)

dysfibrinogenemia, or vasculitis. Bleeding into muscles and joints may be associated with a plasma procoagulant factor abnormality. In either scenario, the abnormality may be congenital or acquired. A thorough physical examination should be performed with special attention to the skin, oro- and nasopharynx, liver, spleen, and joints. Screening and diagnostic evaluation in patients with suspected bleeding disorders should initially include the following laboratory testing:

1. Prothrombin time (PT) to assess clotting function of factors VII, X, V, II, and fibrinogen.
2. Activated partial thromboplastin time (aPTT) to assess clotting function of high molecular weight kininogen, prekallikrein, XII, XI, IX, VIII, X, V, II, and fibrinogen.
3. Platelet count and size determined as part of a CBC.
4. Platelet functional assessment by platelet function analyzer-100 (PFA-100), or template bleeding time.
5. Fibrinogen functional level by clotting assay.

The following laboratory tests may also be useful:

1. Thrombin time to measure the generation of fibrin from fibrinogen following conversion of prothrombin to thrombin, as well as the antithrombin effects of fibrin-split products and heparin. The thrombin time may be prolonged in the setting of a normal fibrinogen concentration if the fibrinogen is dysfunctional (ie, dysfibrinogenemia).
2. Euglobulin lysis time (ELT), if available, to evaluate for accelerated fibrinolysis if the preceding workup is nonrevealing despite documented history of pathologic bleeding. If the ELT is shortened, assessment of plasminogen activator inhibitor-1 and α_2-antiplasmin is warranted, as congenital deficiency in these fibrinolytic inhibitors may cause hyperfibrinolysis. In ill patients, measurement of fibrin degradation products may assist in the diagnosis of DIC.

Goodnight SH, Hathaway WE (editors): *Disorders of Hemostasis & Thrombosis: A Clinical Guide*, 2nd ed. McGraw-Hill, 2001:41–51.

ABNORMALITIES OF PLATELET NUMBER OR FUNCTION

Thrombocytopenia in the pediatric age range is often immune-mediated (eg, ITP, neonatal auto- or alloimmune thrombocytopenia, heparin-induced thrombocytopenia), but is also caused by consumptive coagulopathy (eg, DIC, Kasabach-Merritt syndrome), acute leukemias, rare disorders such as Wiskott-Aldrich syndrome and type 2b vWD, and artifactually in automated cytometers (eg, Bernard-Soulier syndrome), where giant forms may not be enumerated as platelets by automated cell counters.

1. Idiopathic Thrombocytopenic Purpura

ESSENTIALS OF DIAGNOSIS & TYPICAL FEATURES

- Otherwise healthy child.
- Decreased platelet count.
- Petechiae, ecchymoses.

General Considerations

Acute ITP is the most common bleeding disorder of childhood. It occurs most frequently in children aged 2–5 years and often follows infection with viruses, such as rubella, varicella, measles, parvovirus, influenza, EBV, or acute and chronic HIV. Most patients recover spontaneously within a few months. Chronic ITP (> 6 months' duration) occurs in 10%–20% of affected patients. The thrombocytopenia results from clearance of circulating IgM- or IgG-coated platelets by the reticuloendothelial system. The spleen plays a predominant role in the disease by forming the platelet cross-reactive antibodies and sequestering the antibody-bound platelets.

Clinical Findings

A. Symptoms and Signs

Onset of ITP is usually acute, with the appearance of multiple petechiae and ecchymoses. Epistaxis is also common at presentation. No other physical findings are usually present. Rarely, concurrent infection with EBV or CMV may cause hepatosplenomegaly or lymphadenopathy, simulating acute leukemia.

B. Laboratory Findings

1. Blood—The platelet count is markedly reduced (usually < 50,000/μL and often < 10,000/μL), and platelets frequently are of larger size on peripheral blood smear, suggesting accelerated production of new platelets. The white blood count and differential are normal, and the hemoglobin concentration is preserved unless hemorrhage has been significant.

2. Bone marrow—The number of megakaryocytes is increased. Erythroid and myeloid cellularity is normal.

3. Other laboratory tests—Platelet-associated IgG or IgM, or both, may be demonstrated on the patient's platelets or in the serum. PT and aPTT are normal.

Differential Diagnosis

Table 30–7 lists common causes of thrombocytopenia. ITP is a diagnosis of exclusion. Family history or the finding of predominantly giant platelets on the peripheral blood

Table 30–7. Common causes of thrombocytopenia.

Increased Turnover			Decreased Production	
Antibody-Mediated	**Coagulopathy**	**Other**	**Congenital**	**Acquired**
Idiopathic thrombocytopenic purpura	Disseminated intravascular coagulopathy	Hemolytic-uremic syndrome	Fanconi anemia	Aplastic anemia
Infection	Sepsis	Thrombotic thrombocytopenic purpura	Wiskott-Aldrich syndrome	Leukemia and other malignancies
Immunologic diseases	Necrotizing enterocolitis Thrombosis Cavernous hemangioma	Hypersplenism Respiratory distress syndrome Wiskott-Aldrich syndrome	Thrombocytopenia with absent radii Metabolic disorders Osteopetrosis	Vitamin B_{12} and folate deficiencies

smear is helpful in separating from thrombocytopenia that is hereditary. Bone marrow examination should be performed if the history is atypical (ie, the child is not otherwise healthy, or if there is a family history of bleeding), if abnormalities other than purpura and petechiae are present on physical examination, or if other cell lines are affected on the CBC. The importance of performing a bone marrow examination prior to using corticosteroids in the treatment for ITP is controversial.

Complications

Severe hemorrhage and bleeding into vital organs are the feared complications of ITP. Intracranial hemorrhage is the most serious (but rarely seen) complication, occurring in less than 1% of affected children. The most important risk factors for hemorrhage are a platelet count less than 10,000/μL and mean platelet volume less than 8 fL.

Treatment

A. General Measures

Treatment is optional in most children in the absence of bleeding. Aspirin and other medications (eg, NSAIDs such as Advil, Naproxin, etc) that compromise platelet function should be avoided. Bleeding precautions (eg, restriction from physical contact activities and use of helmets) should be observed. Platelet transfusion should be avoided except in circumstances of life-threatening bleeding, in which case emergent splenectomy is to be pursued. In this setting, administration of corticosteroids and IVIG is also advisable.

B. Corticosteroids

Patients with clinically significant but non–life-threatening bleeding (ie, epistaxis, hematuria, and hematochezia) and those with a platelet count of less than 10,000/μL may benefit from prednisone at 1–2 mg/kg/day for 2–3 weeks with a maximum dose of 60–80 mg/day. A higher dose initially (3–5 mg/kg/day) for 3–7 days may lead to faster count recovery. The dosage is then tapered and stopped. No further prednisone is given regardless of the platelet count unless significant bleeding recurs, at which time prednisone is administered in the smallest dose that achieves resolution of bleeding episodes (usually 2.5–5 mg twice daily). Follow-up continues until the steroid can again be discontinued, spontaneous remission occurs, or other therapeutic measures are instituted. Toxicity (Cushingoid facies, weight gain, change in behavior, hyperglycemia, and hypertension) is usually mild for short treatment courses.

C. Intravenous Immunoglobulin (IVIG)

IVIG is the treatment of choice for severe, acute bleeding, and may also be used as an alternative or adjunct to corticosteroid treatment in both acute and chronic ITP of childhood. IVIG may be effective even when the patient is resistant to corticosteroids; responses are prompt and may last for several weeks. Most patients receive 1 g/kg/d for 1–2 days. Infusion time is typically 4–6 hours. Platelets may be given simultaneously during life-threatening hemorrhage but are rapidly destroyed. Adverse effects of IVIG are common, including transient neurologic complications (eg, headache, nausea, and aseptic meningitis) in one-third of patients. These symptoms may mimic those of intracranial hemorrhage and necessitate radiologic evaluation of the brain. A transient decrease in neutrophil number may also be seen.

D. Anti-Rh(D) Immunoglobulin

This polyclonal immunoglobulin binds to the D antigen on red blood cells. The splenic clearance of anti-D–coated red cells interferes with removal of antibody-coated platelets, resulting in improvement in thrombocytopenia. This approach is effective only in Rh(+) patients with a functional spleen. The time required for platelet increase is slightly longer than with IVIG. However, approximately 80% of Rh(+) children with acute or chronic ITP respond well. Significant hemolysis may occur transiently with an average hemoglobin concentration decrease of 0.8 g/dL. However, severe hemolysis occurs in 5% of treated children, and clinical and laboratory evaluation following administration is warranted in all patients. Rh(D) immunoglobulin is less expensive and infused more rapidly than IVIG, but is more expensive than corticosteroids.

E. Splenectomy

Many children with chronic ITP have platelet counts greater than 30,000/μL. Up to 70% of such children spontaneously recover with a platelet count greater than 100,000/μL within 1 year. For the remainder, corticosteroids, IVIG, and anti-D immunoglobulin are typically effective treatment for acute bleeding. Splenectomy produces a response in 70%–90%, but it should be considered only after persistence of significant thrombocytopenia for at least 1 year. Preoperative treatment with corticosteroids, IVIG, or anti-D immunoglobulin is usually indicated. Postoperatively, the platelet count may rise to 1 million/μL, but is not often associated with thrombotic complications in the pediatric age group. The risk of overwhelming infection (predominantly with encapsulated organisms) is increased after splenectomy, particularly in the young child. Therefore, the procedure should be postponed, if possible, until age 5 years. Administration of pneumococcal, *H influenzae* type b and meningococcal vaccines at least 2 weeks prior to splenectomy is recommended. Daily penicillin prophylaxis should be started postoperatively and continued for 1–3 years.

F. Rituximab (Anti-CD20 Monoclonal Antibody)

The efficacy of treating childhood chronic ITP in several series and a phase I/II trial has been demonstrated; remission was observed in 40%. Because of significant adverse events, this therapy may be reserved for refractory cases with significant bleeding.

G. New Agents

Thrombopoietin receptor agonists are undergoing clinical trials in pediatric patients with ITP with promising results.

Prognosis

Ninety percent of children with ITP will have a spontaneous remission. Features associated with the development of chronic ITP include female gender, age greater than 10 years at presentation, insidious onset of bruising, and the presence of other autoantibodies. Older child- and adolescent-onset ITP is associated with an increased risk of chronic autoimmune diseases or immunodeficiency states. Appropriate screening by history and laboratory studies (eg, antinuclear antibody) is warranted.

Blanchette V: Childhood immune thrombocytopenic purpura: Diagnosis and management. Pediatr Clin North Am 2008;55:393 [PMID: 18381093].

Imbach P: Childhood ITP: 12 months follow-up data from the prospective registry I of the Intercontinental Childhood ITP Study Group (ICIS). Pediatr Blood Cancer 2006;46:351 [PMID: 16086422].

Rodeghiero F: First-line therapies for immune thrombocytopenic purpura: Re-evaluating the need to treat. Eur J Haematol Suppl 2008;69:19–26 [PMID: 18211569].

2. Thrombocytopenia in the Newborn

Thrombocytopenia is one of the most common causes of neonatal hemorrhage and should be considered in any newborn with petechiae, purpura, or other significant bleeding. Defined as a platelet count less than 150,000/μL, thrombocytopenia occurs in approximately 0.9% of unselected neonates. Several specific entities may be responsible (see Table 30–7); however, half of such neonates have alloimmune thrombocytopenia. Infection and DIC are the most common causes of thrombocytopenia in ill full-term newborns and in preterm newborns. In the healthy neonate, antibody-mediated thrombocytopenia (alloimmune or maternal autoimmune), viral syndromes, hyperviscosity, and major-vessel thrombosis are frequent causes of thrombocytopenia. Management is directed toward the underlying etiology.

A. Thrombocytopenia Associated with Platelet Alloantibodies (Neonatal Alloimmune Thrombocytopenia)

Platelet alloimmunization occurs in 1 out of approximately 350 pregnancies. Unlike in Rh incompatibility, 30%–40% of affected neonates are first-born. Thrombocytopenia is progressive over the course of gestation and worse with each subsequent pregnancy. Alloimmunization occurs when a platelet antigen of the infant differs from that of the mother and the mother is sensitized by fetal platelets that cross the placenta into the maternal circulation. In Caucasians, alloimmune thrombocytopenia is most often due to human platelet antigen (HPA)-1a incompatibility. Sensitization of a mother homozygous for HPA-1b to paternally acquired fetal HPA-1a antigen results in severe fetal thrombocytopenia in 1 in 1200 fetuses. Only 1 in 20 HPA-1a–positive fetuses of HPA-1a–negative mothers develop alloimmunization. Other platelet-specific alloantigens may be etiologic. The presence of antenatal maternal platelet antibodies on more than one occasion and their persistence into the third trimester is predictive of severe neonatal thrombocytopenia; a weak or undetectable antibody does not exclude thrombocytopenia. Severe intracranial hemorrhage occurs in 10%–30% of affected neonates as early as 20 weeks' gestation. Petechiae or other bleeding manifestations are usually present shortly after birth. The disease is self-limited, and the platelet count normalizes within 4 weeks.

If alloimmunization is associated with clinically significant bleeding, transfusion of platelet concentrates harvested from the mother is more effective than random donor platelets in increasing the platelet count. Transfusion with HPA-matched platelets from unrelated donors or treatment with IVIG or methylprednisolone to acutely block macrophage uptake of sensitized cells has also been successful in raising the platelet count and achieving hemostasis. If thrombocytopenia is not severe and bleeding is absent, observation alone is often appropriate.

Intracranial hemorrhage in a previous child secondary to alloimmune thrombocytopenia is the strongest risk factor for severe fetal thrombocytopenia and hemorrhage in a subsequent pregnancy. Amniocentesis or chorionic villus sampling to obtain fetal DNA for platelet antigen typing is sometimes performed if the father is heterozygous for HPA-1a. If alloimmunization has occurred with a previous pregnancy, irrespective of history of intracranial hemorrhage, screening cranial ultrasound for hemorrhage should begin at 20 weeks' gestation and be repeated regularly. In addition, cordocentesis should be performed at approximately 20 weeks' gestation, with prophylactic transfusion of irradiated, leukoreduced, maternal platelet concentrates. If the fetal platelet count is less than 100,000/μL, the mother should be treated with weekly IVIG. Delivery by elective cesarean section is recommended if the fetal platelet count is less than 50,000/μL, to minimize the risk of intracranial hemorrhage associated with birth trauma.

B. Thrombocytopenia Associated with Idiopathic Thrombocytopenic Purpura in the Mother (Neonatal Autoimmune Thrombocytopenia)

Infants born to mothers with ITP or other autoimmune diseases (eg, antiphospholipid antibody syndrome or systemic lupus erythematosus) may develop thrombocytopenia as a result of transfer of antiplatelet IgG from the mother to the infant. Unfortunately, maternal and fetal platelet counts and maternal antiplatelet antibody levels are unreliable predictors of bleeding risk. Antenatal corticosteroid administration to the mother is generally instituted once maternal platelet count falls below 50,000/μL, with or without a concomitant course of IVIG.

Most neonates with neonatal autoimmune thrombocytopenia do not develop clinically significant bleeding, and thus treatment for thrombocytopenia is not often required. The risk of intracranial hemorrhage is 0.2%–2%. If diffuse petechiae or minor bleeding are evident, a 1- to 2-week course of oral prednisone, 2 mg/kg/d, may be helpful. If the platelet count remains consistently less than 20,000/μL or if severe hemorrhage develops, IVIG should be given (1 g/kg daily for 1–2 days). Platelet transfusions are only indicated for life-threatening bleeding, and may only be effective after removal of antibody by exchange transfusion. The platelet nadir is typically between the fourth and sixth day of life and improves significantly by 1 month; full recovery may take 2–4 months. Platelet recovery may be delayed in breast-fed infants because of transfer of IgG to the milk.

C. Neonatal Thrombocytopenia Associated with Infections

Thrombocytopenia is commonly associated with severe generalized infections during the newborn period. Between 50% and 75% of neonates with bacterial sepsis are thrombocytopenic. Intrauterine infections such as rubella, syphilis, toxoplasmosis, CMV, herpes simplex (acquired intra- or post-partem), enteroviruses, and parvovirus are often associated with thrombocytopenia. In addition to specific treatment for the underlying disease, platelet transfusions may be indicated in severe cases.

D. Thrombocytopenia Associated with Kaposiform Hemangioendotheliomas (Kasabach-Merritt Syndrome)

A rare but important cause of thrombocytopenia in the newborn is kaposiform hemangioendotheliomas, a benign neoplasm with histopathology distinct from that of classic infantile hemangiomas. Intense platelet sequestration in the lesion results in peripheral thrombocytopenia and may rarely be associated with a DIC-like picture and hemolytic anemia. The bone marrow typically shows megakaryocytic hyperplasia in response to the thrombocytopenia. Corticosteroids, α-interferon, and vincristine are all useful for reducing the size of the lesion and are indicated if significant coagulopathy is present, the lesion compresses a vital structure, or the lesion is cosmetically unacceptable. If consumptive coagulopathy is present, heparin or aminocaproic acid may be useful. Depending on the site, embolization may be an option. Surgery is often avoided because of the high risk of hemorrhage.

Hall GW: Kasabach-Merritt syndrome: Pathogenesis and management. Br J Haematol 2001;112:851 [PMID: 11298580].

Kaplan RN: Differential diagnosis and management of thrombocytopenia in childhood. Pediatr Clin North Am 2004;51:1109 [PMID: 15275991].

3. Disorders of Platelet Function

Individuals with platelet function defects typically develop abnormal bruising and mucosal bleeding similar to that occurring in persons with thrombocytopenia. Historically, platelet function has been screened by measuring the bleeding time. If this is prolonged, in vitro platelet aggregation is studied using agonists, such as adenosine diphosphate, collagen, arachidonic acid, and ristocetin, and simultaneous comparison with a normal control subject. While labor-intensive, platelet aggregometry remains important in selected clinical situations. The PFA-100 has become available to evaluate platelet dysfunction and vWD, and has replaced the template bleeding time in many clinical laboratories. Unfortunately, none of these screening tests of platelet function is uniformly predictive of clinical bleeding severity.

Platelet dysfunction may be inherited or acquired, with the latter being more common. Acquired disorders of platelet function may occur secondary to uremia, cirrhosis, sepsis, myeloproliferative disorders, congenital heart disease, and viral infections. Many pharmacologic agents decrease platelet function. The most common offending agents in the pediatric population are aspirin and other NSAIDs, synthetic penicillins, and valproic acid. In acquired platelet dysfunction, the PFA-100 closure time is typically prolonged with collagen-epinephrine, while normal with collagen-ADP.

The inherited disorders are due to defects in platelet-vessel interaction, platelet-platelet interaction, platelet granule content or release (including defects of signal transduction), thromboxane and arachidonic acid pathway, and platelet-procoagulant protein interaction. Individuals with hereditary platelet dysfunction generally have a prolonged bleeding time with normal platelet number and morphology by light microscopy. PFA-100 closure time, in contrast to that in acquired dysfunction, is typically prolonged with both collagen-ADP and collagen-epinephrine.

Congenital causes of defective platelet–vessel wall interaction include Bernard-Soulier syndrome. This condition is characterized by increased platelet size and decreased platelet number. The molecular defect in this autosomal recessive disorder is a deficiency or dysfunction of glycoprotein Ib-V-IX complex on the platelet surface resulting in impaired von Willebrand factor (vWF) binding, and hence, impaired platelet adhesion to the vascular endothelium.

Glanzmann thrombasthenia is an example of platelet-platelet dysfunction. In this autosomal recessive disorder, glycoprotein IIb-IIIa is deficient or dysfunctional. Platelets do not bind fibrinogen effectively and exhibit impaired aggregation. As in Bernard-Soulier syndrome, acute bleeding is treated by platelet transfusion.

Disorders involving platelet granule content include storage pool disease and Quebec platelet disorder. In individuals with storage pool disease, platelet-dense granules lack adenosine dinucleotide phosphate and adenosine trinucleotide phosphate and are often found to be low in number by electron microscopy. These granules are also deficient in Hermansky-Pudlak, Chédiak-Higashi, and Wiskott-Aldrich syndromes. Whereas deficiency of α-granules results in the gray platelet syndrome, Quebec platelet disorder is characterized by a normal platelet α-granule number, but with abnormal proteolysis of α-granule proteins and deficiency of platelet α-granule multimerin. α-Granule abnormality in this disorder also results in increased serum levels of urokinase-type plasminogen activator. Epinephrine-induced platelet aggregation is markedly impaired.

Platelet dysfunction has also been observed in other congenital syndromes, such as Down and Noonan syndromes, without a clear understanding of the molecular defect.

Treatment

Acute bleeding in many individuals with acquired or selected congenital platelet function defects responds to therapy with desmopressin acetate, likely due to an induced release of vWF from endothelial stores and/or upregulated expression of glycoprotein Ib-V-IX on the platelet surface. If this therapy is ineffective, or if the patient has Bernard-Soulier syndrome or Glanzmann syndrome, the mainstay of treatment for bleeding episodes is platelet transfusion, possibly with HLA type-specific platelets. Recombinant VIIa has variable efficacy and may be helpful in platelet transfusion-refractory patients.

Israels SJ: Inherited disorders of platelet function and challenges to diagnosis of mucocutaneous bleeding. Haemophilia 2010;16 (Suppl 5):152 [PMID: 20590875].

INHERITED BLEEDING DISORDERS

Table 30–8 lists normal values for coagulation factors. The more common factor deficiencies are discussed in this section. Individuals with bleeding disorders should avoid exposure to medications that inhibit platelet function. Participation in contact sports should be considered in the context of the severity of the bleeding disorder.

1. Factor VIII Deficiency (Hemophilia A, Classic Hemophilia)

ESSENTIALS OF DIAGNOSIS & TYPICAL FEATURES

- Bruising, soft-tissue bleeding, hemarthrosis.
- Prolonged activated partial thromboplastin time (aPTT).
- Reduced factor VIII activity.

General Considerations

Factor VIII activity is reported in units per milliliter, with 1 U/mL equal to 100% of the factor activity found in 1 mL of normal plasma. The normal range for factor VIII activity is 0.50–1.50 U/mL (50%–150%). Hemophilia A occurs predominantly in males as an X-linked disorder. One-third of cases are due to a new mutation. The incidence of factor VIII deficiency is 1:5000 male births.

Clinical Findings

A. Symptoms and Signs

Patients with severe hemophilia A (< 1% plasma factor VIII activity) have frequent spontaneous bleeding episodes involving skin, mucous membranes, joints, muscles, and viscera. In contrast, patients with mild hemophilia A (5%–40% factor VIII activity) bleed only at times of trauma or surgery. Those with moderate hemophilia A (1% to < 5% factor VIII activity) typically have intermediate bleeding manifestations.

Table 30–8. Physiologic alterations in measurements of the hemostatic system.

Measurement	Normal Adults	Fetus (20 wk)	Preterm (25–32 wk)	Term Infant	Infant (6 mo)	Pregnancy (term)	Exercise (acute)	Aging (70–80 y)
Platelets								
Count μL/10^3	250	107–297	293	332	—	260	↑ 18%–40%	225
Size (fL)	9.0	8.9	8.5	9.1	—	9.6	↑	—
Aggregation ADP	N	+	↓	↓	—	↑	↓ 15%	—
Collagen	N	↓	↓	↓	—	N	↓ 60%	N
Ristocetin	N	—	↑	↑	—	—	↓ 10%	—
BT (min)	2–9	—	3.6 ± 2	3.4 ± 1.8	—	9.0 ± 1.4	—	5.6
Procoagulant system								
PTT*	1	4.0	3	1.3	1.1	1.1	↓ 15%	↓
PT*	1.00	2.3	1.3	1.1	1	0.95	N	—
TCT*	1	2.4	1.3	1.1	1	0.92	N	—
Fibrinogen mg/dL	278 (0.61)	96 (50)	250 (100)	240 (150)	251 (160)	450 (100)	↓ 25%	↑ 15%
II, U/mL	1 (0.7)	0.16 (0.10)	0.32 (0.18)	0.52 (0.25)	0.88 (0.6)	1.15 (0.68–1.9)	—	N
V, U/mL	1.0 (0.6)	0.32 (0.21)	0.80 (0.43)	1.00 (0.54)	0.91 (0.55)	0.85 (0.40–1.9)	—	N
VII, U/mL	1.0 (0.6)	0.27 (0.17)	0.37 (0.24)	0.57 (0.35)	0.87 (0.50)	1.17 (0.87–3.3)	↑ 200%	↑ 25%
VIIIc, U/mL	1.0 (0.6)	0.50 (0.23)	0.75 (0.40)	1.50 (0.55)	0.90 (0.50)	2.12 (0.8–6.0)	↑ 250%	1.50
vWF, U/mL	1.0 (0.6)	0.65 (0.40)	1.50 (0.90)	1.60 (0.84)	1.07 (0.60)	1.7	↑ 75–200%	↑
IX, U/mL	1.0 (0.5)	0.10 (0.05)	0.22 (0.17)	0.35 (0.15)	0.86 (0.36)	0.81–2.15	↑ 25%	1.0–1.40
X, U/mL	1.0 (0.6)	0.19 (0.15)	0.38 (0.20)	0.45 (0.3)	0.78 (0.38)	1.30	—	N
XI, U/mL	1.0 (0.6)	0.13 (0.08)	0.2 (0.12)	0.42 (0.20)	0.86 (0.38)	0.7	—	N
XII, U/mL	1.0 (0.6)	0.15 (0.08)	0.22 (0.09)	0.44 (0.16)	0.77 (0.39)	1.3 (0.82)	—	↑ 16%
XIII, U/mL	1.04 (0.55)	0.30	0.4	0.61 (0.36)	1.04 (0.50)	0.96	—	—
PreK, U/mL	1.12 (0.06)	0.13 (0.08)	0.26 (0.14)	0.35 (0.16)	0.86 (0.56)	1.18	—	↑ 27%
HK, U/mL	0.92 (0.48)	0.15 (0.10)	0.28 (0.20)	0.64 (0.50)	0.82 (0.36)	1.6	—	↑ 32%

Anticoagulant system								
AT-U/mL	1.0	0.23	0.35	0.56	1.04	1.02	↑ 14%	N
α_2-MG, U/mL	1.05 (0.79)	0.18 (0.10)	—	1.39 (0.95)	1.91 (1.49)	1.53 (0.85)	—	—
C1IN, U/mL	1.01	—	—	0.72	1.41	—	—	—
PC, U/mL	1.0	0.10	0.29	0.50	0.59	0.99	N	N
Total PS, U/mL	1.0 (0.6)	0.15 (0.11)	0.17 (0.14)	0.24 (0.1)	0.87 (0.55)	0.89	—	N
Free, PS, U/mL	1.0 (0.5)	0.22 (0.13)	0.28 (0.19)	0.49 (0.33)	—	0.25	—	—
Heparin	1.01	0.10 (0.06)	0.25 (0.10)	0.49 (0.33)	0.97 (0.59)	—	—	↓ 15%
Cofactor II, U/mL	(0.73)							
TFPI, ng/mL	73	21	20.6	38	—	—	—	—
Fibrinolytic system								
Plasminogen U/mL	1.0	0.20	0.35 (0.20)	0.37 (0.18)	0.90	1.39	↓ 10%	N
tPA, ng/mL	4.9	—	8.48	9.6	2.8	4.9	↑ 300%	N
α_2-AP, U/mL	1.0	1.0	0.74 (0.5)	0.83 (0.65)	1.11 (0.83)	0.95	N	N
PAI-1, U/mL	1.0	—	1.5	1.0	1.07	4.0	↓ 5%	N
Overall fibrinolysis	N	↑	↑	↓	—	↓	↑	↓

Except as otherwise indicated values are mean ±2 standard deviation (SD) or values in parentheses are lower limits (−2 SD or lower range); +, positive or present; ↓, decreased; ↑, increased; N, normal or no change; *, values as ratio or subject/mean of reference range; α_2-MG, α_2-macroglobulin; α_2-AP, α_2-antiplasmin; ADP, adenosine diphosphate; AT, antithrombin; BT, bleeding time; C1IN, C1 esterase inhibitor; HK, high molecular weight kininogen; PAI, plasminogen activator inhibitor; PC, protein C; PreK, prekallikrein; PS, protein S; PT, prothrombin time; PTT, partial thromboplastin time; TCT, thrombin clotting time; TFPI, tissue factor pathway inhibitor; tPA, tissue plasminogen activator; vWF, von Willebrand factor. Overall fibrinolysis is measured by euglobulin lysis time.

Adapted, with permission, from Goodnight SH, Hathaway WE (editors): *Disorders of Hemostasis & Thrombosis: A Clinical Guide,* 2nd ed. McGraw-Hill, 2001.

The most crippling aspect of factor VIII deficiency is the tendency to develop recurrent hemarthroses that incite joint destruction.

B. Laboratory Findings

Individuals with hemophilia A have a prolonged aPTT, except in some cases of mild deficiency. The PT is normal. The diagnosis is confirmed by finding decreased factor VIII activity with normal vWF activity. In two-thirds of families of hemophilic patients, the females are carriers and some are mildly symptomatic. Carriers of hemophilia can be suspected by determination of the ratio of factor VIII activity to vWF antigen and definitely diagnosed by molecular genetic techniques. In a male fetus or newborn with a family history of hemophilia A, cord blood sampling for factor VIII activity is accurate and important in subsequent care.

Complications

Intracranial hemorrhage is the leading disease-related cause of death among patients with hemophilia. Most intracranial hemorrhages in moderate to severe deficiency are spontaneous (ie, not associated with trauma). Hemarthroses begin early in childhood and, particularly when recurrent, can result in joint destruction (ie, hemophilic arthropathy). Large intramuscular hematomas can lead to a compartment syndrome with resultant neurologic compromise. Although these complications are most common in severe hemophilia A, they may be experienced by individuals with moderate or mild disease. A serious complication of hemophilia is the development of an acquired circulating antibody to factor VIII after treatment with factor VIII concentrate. Such factor VIII inhibitors develop in 15%–25% of patients with severe hemophilia A, and most commonly among patients with large deletions in the factor VIII gene. The type of treatment product as a risk factor for inhibitor development is under study. Inhibitors may be amenable to desensitization with regular factor VIII infusion (immune tolerance therapy) with or without immunosuppressive therapy. In recent years, the "bypassing agent" recombinant factor VIIa has become a therapy of choice for treatment of acute hemorrhage in patients with hemophilia A and a high-titer inhibitor.

In prior decades, therapy-related complications in hemophilia A have included infection with the human immunodeficiency virus, hepatitis B virus, and hepatitis C virus. Through more stringent donor selection, the implementation of sensitive screening assays, the use of heat or chemical methods for viral inactivation, and the development of recombinant products, the risk of these infections is minimal. Inactivation methods do not eradicate viruses lacking a lipid envelope, however, so that transmission of parvovirus and hepatitis A remains a concern with the use of plasma-derived products. Immunization with hepatitis A and hepatitis B vaccines is recommended for all hemophilia patients.

Treatment

The general aim of management is to raise the factor VIII activity to prevent or stop bleeding. Some patients with mild factor VIII deficiency may respond to desmopressin via release of endothelial stores of factor VIII and vWF into plasma; however, most patients require administration of exogenous factor VIII to achieve hemostasis. The in vivo half-life of factor VIII is generally 8–12 hours but may exhibit considerable variation among individuals depending on comorbid conditions. Non–life-threatening, non–limb-threatening hemorrhage is treated initially with 20–30 U/kg of factor VIII, to achieve a rise in plasma factor VIII activity to 40%–60%. Large joint hemarthrosis and life- or limb-threatening hemorrhage is treated initially with approximately 50 U/kg of factor VIII, targeting a rise to 100% factor VIII activity. Subsequent doses are determined according to the site and extent of bleeding and the clinical response. Doses are rounded to the nearest whole vial size. In circumstances of suboptimal clinical response, recent change in bleeding frequency, or comorbid illness, monitoring the plasma factor VIII activity response may be warranted. For most instances of non–life-threatening hemorrhage in experienced patients with moderate or severe hemophilia A, treatment can be administered at home, provided adequate intravenous access exists and close contact is maintained with the hemophilia clinician team.

Prophylactic factor VIII infusions (eg, two or three times weekly) may prevent the development of arthropathy in severe hemophiliacs, and this approach is becoming more common in pediatric hemophilia care.

Prognosis

The development of safe and effective therapies for hemophilia A has resulted in improved long-term survival in recent decades. In addition, more aggressive management and the coordination of comprehensive care through hemophilia centers have greatly improved quality of life and level of function.

Blanchette VS: Meeting unmet needs in inhibitor patients. Haemophilia 2010;16(Suppl 3):46–51 [PMID: 20586802].

Gringeri A; ESPRIT Study Group: A randomized clinical trial of prophylaxis in children with hemophilia A (the ESPRIT Study). J Thromb Haemost 2011;9:700–710 [PMID: 21255253].

2. Factor IX Deficiency (Hemophilia B, Christmas Disease)

The mode of inheritance and clinical manifestations of factor IX deficiency are the same as those of factor VIII deficiency. Hemophilia B is 15%–20% as prevalent as hemophilia A. As in factor VIII deficiency, factor IX deficiency is associated with a prolonged aPTT, but the PT and thrombin time are normal. However, the aPTT is slightly less sensitive to factor IX deficiency than factor VIII deficiency. Diagnosis of hemophilia B is made by assaying factor IX activity, and severity is determined similarly to factor VIII deficiency. In general, clinical bleeding severity correlates less well with factor activity in hemophilia B than in hemophilia A.

The mainstay of treatment in hemophilia B is exogenous factor IX. Unlike factor VIII, about 50% of the administered dose of factor IX diffuses into the extravascular space. Therefore, 1 U/kg of plasma-derived factor IX concentrate or recombinant factor IX is expected to increase plasma factor IX activity by approximately 1%. Factor IX typically has a half-life of 20–22 hours in vivo, but due to variability, therapeutic monitoring may be warranted. As for factor VIII products, viral-inactivation techniques for plasma-derived factor IX concentrates appear effective in eradicating enveloped viruses. Only 1%–3% of persons with factor IX deficiency develop an inhibitor to factor IX, but patients may be at risk for anaphylaxis when receiving exogenous factor IX. The prognosis for persons with factor IX deficiency is comparable to that of patients with factor VIII deficiency. Gene therapy research efforts are ongoing for both hemophilias.

Aledort LM: Optimizing the treatment of haemophilia B: Laboratory and clinical perspectives. Haemophilia 2010;16 (Suppl 6):1–2 [PMID: 20561350].

Santagostino E: Prophylaxis in haemophilia B patients: Unresolved issues and pharmacoeconomic implications. Haemophilia 2010;16(Suppl 60):13–17 [PMID: 20561353].

3. Factor XI Deficiency (Hemophilia C)

Factor XI deficiency is a genetic, autosomally transmitted coagulopathy, typically of mild to moderate clinical severity. Cases of factor XI deficiency account for less than 5% of all hemophilia patients. Homozygotes generally bleed at surgery or following severe trauma, but do not commonly have spontaneous hemarthroses. In contrast to factor VIII and IX deficiencies, factor XI activity is least predictive of bleeding risk. Although typically mild, pathologic bleeding may be seen in heterozygous individuals with factor XI activity as high as 60%. The aPTT is often considerably prolonged. In individuals with deficiency of both plasma and platelet-associated factor XI, the PFA-100 may also be prolonged. Management typically consists of perioperative prophylaxis and episodic therapy for acute hemorrhage. Treatment includes infusion of fresh frozen plasma (FFP); platelet transfusion may also be useful for acute hemorrhage in patients with deficiency of platelet-associated factor XI. Desmopressin has been used in some cases. The prognosis for an average life span in patients with factor XI deficiency is excellent.

Gomez K: Factor XI deficiency. Haemophilia 2008;14(6):1183–1189 [PMID: 18312365].

4. Other Inherited Bleeding Disorders

Other hereditary single clotting factor deficiencies are rare. Transmission is generally autosomal. Homozygous individuals with a deficiency or structural abnormality of prothrombin, factor V, factor VII, or factor X may have excessive bleeding.

Persons with dysfibrinogenemia (ie, structurally or functionally abnormal fibrinogen) may develop recurrent venous thromboembolic episodes or bleeding. Immunologic assay of fibrinogen is normal, but clotting assay may be low and the thrombin time prolonged. The PT and aPTT may be prolonged. Cryoprecipitate, which is rich in fibrinogen, is the treatment of choice, given the present lack of availability of a plasma-derived or recombinant fibrinogen product in the United States.

Afibrinogenemia resembles hemophilia clinically but has an autosomal recessive inheritance. Affected patients can experience a variety of bleeding manifestations, including mucosal bleeding, ecchymoses, hematomas, hemarthroses, and intracranial hemorrhage, especially following trauma. Fatal umbilical cord hemorrhage has been reported in neonates. The PT, aPTT, and thrombin time are all prolonged. A severely reduced fibrinogen concentration in an otherwise well child is confirmatory of the diagnosis. As in dysfibrinogenemia, cryoprecipitate infusion is used for surgical prophylaxis and for acute hemorrhage.

Todd T: A review of long-term prophylaxis in the rare inherited coagulation factor deficiencies. Haemophilia 2010;16(4):569–583 [PMID: 19906159].

VON WILLEBRAND DISEASE

ESSENTIALS OF DIAGNOSIS & TYPICAL FEATURES

- Easy bruising and epistaxis from early childhood.
- Menorrhagia.
- Prolonged PFA-100 (or bleeding time); normal platelet count; absence of acquired platelet dysfunction.
- Reduced activity or abnormal structure of vWF.

General Considerations

vWD is the most common inherited bleeding disorder among Caucasians, with a prevalence of 1%. vWF is a protein present as a multimeric complex in plasma, which binds factor VIII and is a cofactor for platelet adhesion to the endothelium. An estimated 70%–80% of all patients with vWD have classic vWD (type 1), which is caused by a partial quantitative deficiency of vWF. vWD type 2 involves a qualitative deficiency of (ie, dysfunctional) vWF, and vWD type 3 is characterized by a nearly complete deficiency of vWF. The majority (> 80%) of individuals with type 1 disease are asymptomatic. vWD is most often transmitted as an autosomal dominant trait, but can be autosomal recessive. The disease can also be acquired, developing in association with hypothyroidism, Wilms tumor, cardiac disease, renal disease, or systemic lupus erythematosus, and in individuals receiving valproic acid. Acquired vWD is most often caused by the development of an antibody to vWF or increased turnover of vWF.

Clinical Findings

A. Symptoms and Signs

A history of increased bruising and excessive epistaxis is often present. Prolonged bleeding also occurs with trauma or at surgery. Menorrhagia is often a presenting finding in females.

B. Laboratory Findings

PT is normal, and aPTT is sometimes prolonged. Prolongation of the PFA-100 or bleeding time is usually present since vWF plays a role in platelet adherence to endothelium. Platelet number may be decreased in type 2b vWD. Factor VIII and vWF antigen are decreased in types 1 and 3, but may be normal in type 2 vWD. vWF activity (eg, ristocetin cofactor or collagen binding) is decreased in all types. Since normal vWF antigen levels vary by blood type (type O normally has lower levels), blood type must be determined. Complete laboratory classification requires vWF multimer assay. The diagnosis requires confirmation of laboratory testing and bleeding history is often helpful when present.

Treatment

The treatment to prevent or halt bleeding for most patients with vWD types 1 and 2 is desmopressin acetate, which causes release of vWF from endothelial stores. Desmopressin may be administered intravenously at a dose of 0.3 mcg/kg diluted in at least 20–30 mL of normal saline and given over 20–30 minutes. This dose typically elicits a three- to fivefold rise in plasma vWF. A high-concentration desmopressin nasal spray (150 mcg/spray), different than the preparation used for enuresis, may alternatively be used. Because response to vWF is variable among patients, factor VIII and vWF activities are typically measured before and 60 minutes after infusion, if no recent response has been measured. Desmopressin may cause fluid shifts, hyponatremia, and seizures in children younger than 2 years of age. Because release of stored vWF is limited, tachyphylaxis often occurs with desmopressin.

If further therapy is indicated, vWF-replacement therapy (eg, plasma-derived concentrate) is recommended; such therapy is also used in patients with type 1 or 2a vWD who exhibit suboptimal laboratory response to desmopressin, and for all individuals with type 2b or 3 vWD. Antifibrinolytic agents (eg, ε-aminocaproic acid) may be useful for control of mucosal bleeding. Topical thrombin and fibrin glue may also be of benefit, although antibodies that inhibit clotting proteins have been described. Estrogen-containing contraceptive therapy may be helpful for menorrhagia.

Prognosis

With the availability of effective treatment and prophylaxis for bleeding, life expectancy in vWD is normal.

Halimeh S: Long-term secondary prophylaxis in children, adolescents and young adults with von Willebrand disease. Results of a cohort study. Thromb Haemost 2011 Apr;105(4):597–604 [PMID: 21301780].

Mikhail S: von Willebrand disease in the pediatric and adolescent population. J Pediatr Adolesc Gynecol 2010;23(6 Suppl):S3–S10 [PMID: 20934894].

ACQUIRED BLEEDING DISORDERS

1. Disseminated Intravascular Coagulation

ESSENTIALS OF DIAGNOSIS & TYPICAL FEATURES

- Presence of disorder known to trigger DIC.
- Evidence for consumptive coagulopathy (prolonged aPTT, PT, or thrombin time; increase in FSP [fibrin-fibrinogen split products]; decreased fibrinogen or platelets).

General Considerations

DIC is an acquired pathologic process characterized by tissue factor–mediated diffuse coagulation activation in the host. DIC involves dysregulated, excessive thrombin generation, with consequent intravascular fibrin deposition and consumption of platelets and procoagulant factors. Microthrombi, composed of fibrin and platelets, may produce tissue ischemia and end-organ damage. The fibrinolytic system is frequently activated in DIC, leading to plasmin-mediated destruction of fibrin and fibrinogen; this results in fibrin-fibrinogen degradation products (FDPs) which exhibit anticoagulant and platelet-inhibitory functions. DIC commonly accompanies severe infection and other critical illnesses in infants and children. Conditions known to trigger DIC include endothelial damage (eg, endotoxin, virus), tissue necrosis (eg, burns), diffuse ischemic injury (eg, shock, hypoxia acidosis), and systemic release of tissue procoagulants (eg, certain cancers, placental disorders).

Clinical Findings

A. Symptoms and Signs

Signs of DIC may include (1) signs of shock, often including end-organ dysfunction, (2) diffuse bleeding tendency (eg, hematuria, melena, purpura, petechiae, persistent oozing from needle punctures or other invasive procedures), and (3) evidence of thrombotic lesions (eg, major vessel thrombosis, purpura fulminans).

B. Laboratory Findings

Tests that are most sensitive, easiest to perform, most useful for monitoring, and best reflect the hemostatic capacity of the patient are the PT, aPTT, platelet count, fibrinogen, and fibrin-fibrinogen split products. The PT and aPTT are typically prolonged and the platelet count and fibrinogen concentration may be decreased. However, in children, the fibrinogen level may be normal until late in the course. Levels of fibrin-fibrinogen split products are increased, and elevated levels of D-dimer, a cross-linked fibrin degradation byproduct, may be helpful in monitoring the degree of activation of both coagulation and fibrinolysis. However, D-dimer is nonspecific and may be elevated in the context of a triggering event (eg, severe infection) without concomitant DIC. Often, physiologic inhibitors of coagulation, especially antithrombin III and protein C, are consumed, predisposing to thrombosis. The specific laboratory abnormalities in DIC may vary with the triggering event and the course of illness.

Differential Diagnosis

DIC can be difficult to distinguish from coagulopathy of liver disease (ie, hepatic synthetic dysfunction), especially when the latter is associated with thrombocytopenia secondary to portal hypertension and hypersplenism. Generally, factor VII activity is decreased markedly in liver disease (due to deficient synthesis of this protein, which has the shortest half-life among the procoagulant factors), but only mildly to moderately decreased in DIC (due to consumption). Factor VIII activity is often normal or even increased in liver disease, but decreased in DIC.

Treatment

A. Therapy for Underlying Disorder

The most important aspect of therapy in DIC is the identification and treatment of the triggering event. If the pathogenic process underlying DIC is reversed, often no other therapy is needed for the coagulopathy.

B. Replacement Therapy for Consumptive Coagulopathy

Replacement of consumed procoagulant factors with FFP and of platelets via platelet transfusion is warranted in the setting of DIC with hemorrhagic complications, or as periprocedural bleeding prophylaxis. Infusion of 10–15 mL/kg FFP typically raises procoagulant factor activities by approximately 10%–15%. Cryoprecipitate can also be given as a rich source of fibrinogen; one bag of cryoprecipitate per 3 kg in infants or one bag of cryoprecipitate per 6 kg in older children typically raises plasma fibrinogen concentration by 75–100 mg/dL.

C. Anticoagulant Therapy for Coagulation Activation

Continuous intravenous infusion of unfractionated heparin is sometimes given in order to attenuate coagulation activation and consequent consumptive coagulopathy. The rationale for heparin therapy is to maximize the efficacy of, and minimize the need for, replacement of procoagulants and platelets; however, clinical evidence demonstrating benefit of heparin in DIC is lacking. Unfractionated heparin dosing and monitoring is listed on page 939.

D. Specific Factor Concentrates

A nonrandomized pilot study of antithrombin concentrate in children with DIC and associated acquired antithrombin deficiency demonstrated favorable outcomes, suggesting that replacement of this consumed procoagulant may be of benefit. Protein C concentrate has also shown promise in two small pilot studies of meningococci-associated DIC with purpura fulminans. Activated protein C has reduced mortality in septic adults in a large randomized multicenter trial; efficacy in pediatrics is controversial.

2. Liver Disease

The liver is the major synthetic site of prothrombin, fibrinogen, high-molecular-weight kininogen, and factors V, VII, IX, X, XI, XII, and XIII. In addition, plasminogen and the physiologic anticoagulants (antithrombin III, protein C, and protein S) are hepatically synthesized. α_2-Antiplasmin, a regulator of fibrinolysis, is also produced in the liver. Deficiency of factor V and the vitamin K–dependent factors (II, VII, IX, and X) is most often a result of decreased hepatic synthesis and is manifested by a prolonged PT and often a prolonged aPTT. Extravascular loss and increased consumption of clotting factors may contribute to PT and aPTT prolongation. Fibrinogen production is often decreased, or an abnormal fibrinogen (dysfibrinogen) containing excess sialic acid residues may be synthesized, or both. Hypofibrinogenemia or dysfibrinogenemia is associated with prolongation of thrombin time and reptilase time. FDPs and D-dimers may be present because of increased fibrinolysis, particularly in the setting of chronic hepatitis or cirrhosis. Thrombocytopenia secondary to hypersplenism may occur. DIC and coagulopathy of liver disease also mimic vitamin K deficiency; however, vitamin K deficiency has normal factor V activity. Treatment of acute bleeding in the setting of coagulopathy of liver disease consists of replacement with FFP and platelets.

Desmopressin may shorten the bleeding time and aPTT in patients with chronic liver disease, but its safety has not been well established. Recombinant VIIa also is efficacious for life-threatening hemorrhage.

3. Vitamin K Deficiency

The newborn period is characterized by physiologically depressed activity of the vitamin K–dependent factors (II, VII, IX, and X). If vitamin K is not administered at birth, a bleeding diathesis previously called hemorrhagic disease of the newborn, now termed vitamin K deficiency bleeding (VKDB), may develop. Outside of the newborn period, vitamin K deficiency may occur as a consequence of inadequate intake, excess loss, inadequate formation of active metabolites, or competitive antagonism.

One of three patterns is seen in the neonatal period:

1. Early VKDB of the newborn occurs within 24 hours of birth and is most often manifested by cephalohematoma, intracranial hemorrhage, or intra-abdominal bleeding. Although occasionally idiopathic, it is most often associated with maternal ingestion of drugs that interfere with vitamin K metabolism (eg, warfarin, phenytoin, isoniazid, and rifampin). Early VKDB occurs in 6%–12% of neonates born to mothers who take these medications without receiving vitamin K supplementation. The disorder is often life-threatening.
2. Classic VKDB occurs at 24 hours to 7 days of age and usually is manifested as gastrointestinal, skin, or mucosal bleeding. Bleeding after circumcision may occur. Although occasionally associated with maternal drug usage, it most often occurs in well infants who do not receive vitamin K at birth and are solely breast fed.
3. Late neonatal VKDB occurs on or after day 8. Manifestations include intracranial, gastrointestinal, or skin bleeding. This disorder is often associated with fat malabsorption (eg, in chronic diarrhea) or alterations in intestinal flora (eg, with prolonged antibiotic therapy). Like classic VKDB, late VKDB occurs almost exclusively in breast-fed infants.

The diagnosis of vitamin K deficiency is suspected based on the history, physical examination, and laboratory results. The PT is prolonged out of proportion to the aPTT (also prolonged). The thrombin time becomes prolonged late in the course. The platelet count is normal. This laboratory profile is similar to the coagulopathy of acute liver disease, but with normal fibrinogen level and absence of hepatic transaminase elevation. The diagnosis of vitamin K deficiency is confirmed by a demonstration of noncarboxylated proteins in the absence of vitamin K in the plasma and by clinical and laboratory responses to vitamin K. Intravenous or subcutaneous treatment with vitamin K should be given immediately and not withheld while awaiting test results. In the setting of severe bleeding, additional acute treatment with FFP or recombinant factor VIIa may be indicated.

4. Uremia

Uremia is frequently associated with acquired platelet dysfunction. Bleeding occurs in approximately 50% of patients with chronic renal failure. The bleeding risk conferred by platelet dysfunction associated with metabolic imbalance may be compounded by decreased vWF activity and procoagulant deficiencies (eg, factor II, XII, XI, IX) due to increased urinary losses of these proteins in some settings of renal insufficiency. In accordance with platelet dysfunction, uremic bleeding is typically characterized by purpura, epistaxis, menorrhagia, or gastrointestinal hemorrhage. Acute bleeding may be managed with infusion of desmopressin acetate, factor VIII concentrates containing vWF, or cryoprecipitate with or without coadministration of FFP. Red cell transfusion may be required. Prophylactic administration of erythropoietin before the development of severe anemia appears to decrease the bleeding risk. Recombinant VIIa may be useful in refractory bleeding.

Levi M: Guidelines for the diagnosis and management of disseminated intravascular coagulation. British Committee for Standards in Haematology. Br J Haematol 2009;145:24–33 [PMID: 19222477].

Shearer MJ: Vitamin K deficiency bleeding (VKDB) in early infancy. Blood Rev 2009;23:49–59 [PMID: 18804903].

Witmer CM: Off-label recombinant factor VIIa use and thrombosis in children: A multi-center cohort study. J Pediatr 2011;158:820–825 [PMID: 21146180].

VASCULAR ABNORMALITIES ASSOCIATED WITH BLEEDING

1. Henoch-Schönlein Purpura (Anaphylactoid Purpura)

ESSENTIALS OF DIAGNOSIS & TYPICAL FEATURES

- Purpuric cutaneous rash.
- Migratory polyarthritis or polyarthralgias.
- Intermittent abdominal pain.
- Nephritis.

General Considerations

Henoch-Schönlein purpura (HSP), the most common type of small vessel vasculitis in children, primarily affects boys 2–7 years of age. Occurrence is highest in the spring and fall, and upper respiratory infection precedes the diagnosis in two-thirds of children.

Leukocytoclastic vasculitis in HSP principally involves the small vessels of the skin, gastrointestinal tract, and kidneys, with deposition of IgA immune complexes. The most common and earliest symptom is palpable purpura, which results from extravasation of erythrocytes into the tissue surrounding the involved venules. Antigens from group A β-hemolytic streptococci and other bacteria, viruses, drugs, foods, and insect bites have been proposed as inciting agents.

Clinical Findings

A. Symptoms and Signs

Skin involvement may be urticarial initially, progresses to a maculopapules, and coalesces to a symmetrical, palpable purpuric rash distributed on the legs, buttocks, and elbows. New lesions may continue to appear for 2–4 weeks, and may extend to involve the entire body. Two-thirds of patients develop migratory polyarthralgias or polyarthritis, primarily of the ankles and knees. Intermittent, sharp abdominal pain occurs in approximately 50% of patients, and hemorrhage and edema of the small intestine can often be demonstrated. Intussusception may develop. From 25% to 50% of those affected develop renal involvement in the second or third week of illness with either a nephritic or, less commonly, nephrotic picture. Hypertension may accompany the renal involvement. In males, testicular torsion may also occur, and neurologic symptoms are possible due to small vessel vasculitis.

B. Laboratory Findings

The platelet count is normal or elevated, and other screening tests of hemostasis and platelet function are typically normal. Urinalysis frequently reveals hematuria, and sometimes proteinuria. Stool may be positive for occult blood. The antistreptolysin O (ASO) titer is often elevated and the throat culture positive for group A β-hemolytic streptococci. Serum IgA may be elevated.

Differential Diagnosis

The rash of septicemia (especially meningococcemia) may be similar to skin involvement in HSP, although the distribution tends to be more generalized. The possibility of trauma should be considered in any child presenting with purpura. Other vasculitides should also be considered. The lesions of thrombotic thrombocytopenic purpura are not palpable.

Treatment

Generally, treatment is supportive. NSAIDs may be useful for the arthritis. Corticosteroid therapy may provide symptomatic relief for severe gastrointestinal or joint manifestations but does not alter skin or renal manifestations. If culture for group A β-hemolytic streptococci is positive or if the ASO titer is elevated, a therapeutic course of penicillin is warranted.

Prognosis

The prognosis for recovery is generally good, although symptoms frequently (25%–50%) recur over a period of several months. In patients who develop renal manifestations, microscopic hematuria may persist for years. Progressive renal failure occurs in less than 5% of patients with HSP, with an overall fatality rate of 3%.

McCarthy HJ: Clinical practice: Diagnosis and management of Henoch-Schönlein purpura. Eur J Pediatr 2010;169:643–650 [PMID: 20012647].

2. Collagen Disorders

Mild to life-threatening bleeding occurs with some types of Ehlers-Danlos syndrome, the most common inherited collagen disorder. Ehlers-Danlos syndrome is characterized by joint hypermobility, skin extensibility, and easy bruising. Coagulation abnormalities may sometimes be present, including platelet dysfunction and deficiencies of coagulation factors VIII, IX, XI, and XIII. However, bleeding and easy bruising, in most instances, relates to fragility of capillaries and compromised vascular integrity. Individuals with Ehlers-Danlos syndrome types 4 and 6 are at risk for aortic dissection and spontaneous rupture of aortic aneurysms. Surgery should be avoided for patients with Ehlers-Danlos syndrome, as should medications that induce platelet dysfunction.

De Paepe A: Bleeding and bruising in patients with Ehlers-Danlos syndrome and other collagen vascular disorders. Br J Haematol 2004;127:491 [PMID: 15566352].

THROMBOTIC DISORDERS

General Considerations

Although uncommon in children, thrombotic disorders are being recognized with increasing frequency, particularly with heightened physician awareness and improved survival in pediatric intensive care settings. Several clinical conditions have a potential association with thrombotic events in childhood (see Clinical Risk Factors, below).

Clinical Findings

Initial evaluation of the child who has thrombosis includes an assessment for potential triggering factors, as well as a family history of thrombosis and early cardiovascular or cerebrovascular disease.

A. Clinical Risk Factors

Clinical risk factors are present in more than 90% of children with acute venous thromboembolism (VTE). These conditions include the presence of an indwelling vascular catheter, cardiac disease, infection, trauma, surgery, immobilization, collagen-vascular or chronic inflammatory disease, renal disease, sickle cell anemia, and malignancy. Prospective findings employing serial radiologic evaluation as screening indicate that the risk of VTE is nearly 30% for short-term central venous catheters placed in the internal jugular veins.

Retrospective data suggest that approximately 8% of children with cancer develop symptomatic VTE.

1. Inherited thrombophilia (hypercoagulability) states

A. Protein C deficiency—Protein C is a vitamin K–dependent protein that is normally activated by thrombin bound to thrombomodulin and inactivates activated factors V and VIII. In addition, activated protein C promotes fibrinolysis. Two phenotypes of hereditary protein C deficiency exist. Heterozygous individuals with autosomal dominant protein C deficiency often present with VTE as young adults, but the disorder may manifest during childhood or in later adulthood. In mild protein C deficiency, anticoagulant prophylaxis is typically limited to periods of increased prothrombotic risk. Homozygous or compound heterozygous protein C deficiency is rare but phenotypically severe. Affected children generally present within the first 12 hours of life with purpura fulminans (Figure 30–6) and/or VTE. Prompt protein C replacement by infusion of protein C concentrate or (if unavailable) FFP every 6–12 hours, along with therapeutic heparin administration, is recommended. Subsequent management requires chronic anticoagulation with warfarin, sometimes along with routine protein C concentrate infusion in order to permit lower warfarin dosing. Recurrent VTE is common, especially during periods of subtherapeutic anticoagulation or in the presence of conditions associated with increased prothrombotic risk.

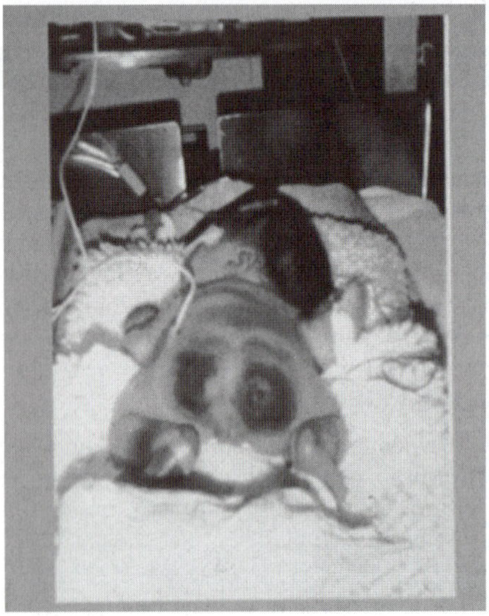

▲ **Figure 30–6.** Purpura fulminans in an infant with severe protein C deficiency.

B. Protein S deficiency—Protein S is a cofactor for protein C. Neonates with homozygous protein S deficiency have a course similar to those with homozygous or compound heterozygous protein C deficiency. Lifelong warfarin therapy is indicated in homozygous/severe deficiency, or in heterozygous individuals who have experienced recurrent VTE. Efforts must be made to distinguish from these conditions from acquired deficiency, which can be antibody-mediated or secondary to an increase in C4b-binding protein induced by inflammation.

C. Antithrombin deficiency—Antithrombin is the most important physiologic inhibitor of thrombin and inhibits activated factors IX, X, XI, and XII. Antithrombin deficiency is transmitted in an autosomal dominant pattern and is associated with VTE, typically with onset in adolescence or young adulthood. Therapy for acute VTE involves replacement with antithrombin concentrate and therapeutic anticoagulation. The efficiency of heparin may be significantly diminished in the setting of severe antithrombin deficiency often requires supplementation of antithrombin via concentrate. Patients with homozygous/severe deficiency or recurrent VTE are maintained on lifelong warfarin.

D. Factor V Leiden mutation—An amino acid substitution in the gene coding for factor V results in factor V Leiden, a factor V polymorphism that is resistant to inactivation by activated protein C. The most common cause of activated protein C resistance in Caucasians, factor V Leiden is present in approximately 5% of the Caucasian population, 20% of Caucasian adults with deep vein thrombosis, and 40%–60% of those with a family history of VTE. VTE occurs in both heterozygous and homozygous individuals. In the former case, thrombosis is typically triggered by a clinical risk factor (or else develops in association with additional thrombophilia traits), whereas in the latter case, it is often spontaneous. Population studies suggest that the risk of incident VTE is increased two- to sevenfold in the setting of heterozygous factor V Leiden, 35-fold among heterozygous individuals taking the oral contraceptives, and 80-fold in those homozygous for factor V Leiden.

E. Prothrombin mutation—The 20210 glutamine to alanine mutation in the prothrombin gene is a relatively common polymorphism in Caucasians that enhances its activation to thrombin. In heterozygous form, this mutation is associated with a two- to threefold increased risk for incident VTE. This mutation also appears to modestly increase the risk for recurrent VTE.

F. Other inherited disorders—Qualitative abnormalities of fibrinogen (dysfibrinogenemias) are usually inherited in an autosomal dominant manner. Most individuals with dysfibrinogenemia are asymptomatic. Some patients experience bleeding, while others develop venous or arterial thrombosis. The diagnosis is suggested by a prolonged thrombin time with a normal fibrinogen concentration. Hyperhomocysteinemia can be an inherited or an acquired condition and is associated with an increased risk for both arterial and venous thromboses. In children, it may also serve as a risk factor for ischemic arterial stroke. However, hyperhomocysteinemia is quite uncommon in the setting of dietary folate supplementation (as in the United States), and is observed almost uniquely in cases of renal insufficiency or metabolic disease (eg, homocystinuria). Furthermore, methylene tetrahydrofolate reductase receptor mutations do not appear to constitute a risk factor for thrombosis in U.S. children if homocysteine is not elevated.

Lipoprotein(a) is a lipoprotein with homology to plasminogen. In vitro studies suggest that lipoprotein(a) may both promote atherothrombosis and inhibit fibrinolysis. Some evidence to date suggests that elevated plasma concentrations of lipoprotein(a) are associated with an increased risk of VTEs and ischemic arterial stroke in children.

Increased factor VIII activity is a risk factor for incident VTE and is common among children with acute VTE. Elevation in factor VIII may persist in the long-term follow-up of these patients, and can be inherited.

2. Acquired disorders

A. Antiphospholipid antibodies—The development of antiphospholipid antibodies is the most common form of acquired thrombophilia in children. Antiphospholipid antibodies, which include the lupus anticoagulant, anticardiolipin antibodies, and β_2-glycoprotein-1 antibodies (among others) are common in acute childhood VTE. The lupus anticoagulant is demonstrated in vitro by its inhibition of phospholipid-dependent coagulation assays (eg, aPTT and dilute Russell viper venom time), whereas immunologic techniques (eg, enzyme-linked immunosorbent assays) are often used to detect anticardiolipin and β_2-glycoprotein-1 antibodies. Although common in persons with autoimmune diseases such as systemic lupus erythematosus, antiphospholipid antibodies may also develop following certain drug exposures, infection, acute inflammation, and lymphoproliferative diseases. Sometimes VTE and antiphospholipid antibodies may predate other signs of lupus for long periods of time. Viral illness is a common precipitant in children, and in many cases, the inciting infection may be asymptomatic.

If an antiphospholipid antibody persists for 12 weeks following the acute thrombotic event, the diagnosis of this syndrome is confirmed. Optimal duration of anticoagulation in this setting is unclear, such that current pediatric treatment guidelines recommend a 3-month to lifelong course.

B. Deficiencies of intrinsic anticoagulants—Acquired deficiencies of proteins C and S and antithrombin may occur in the clinical context of antibodies (eg, protein S antibodies in acute varicella) or in excessive consumption, including sepsis, DIC, major-vessel or extensive VTE, and post–bone marrow transplant sinusoidal obstruction syndrome (formerly termed hepatic veno-occlusive disease). Pilot studies in children have suggested a possible therapeutic role for antithrombin or protein C concentrates in sepsis-associated DIC (eg, meningococcemia) and severe posttransplant sinusoidal obstruction syndrome.

C. Acute phase reactants—As part of the acute phase response, elevations in plasma fibrinogen concentration, plasma factor VIII, and platelet count may occur, all of which may contribute to an acquired prothrombotic state.

Reactive thrombocytosis is rarely associated with VTEs in children when the platelet count is less than 1 million/μL.

B. Symptoms and Signs

Presenting features of thrombosis vary with the anatomic site, extent of vascular involvement, degree of vaso-occlusion, and presence of end-organ dysfunction. The classic presentation of deep venous thrombosis of an upper or lower extremity is painful acute or subacute extremity swelling, while that for pulmonary embolism commonly involves dyspnea and pleuritic chest pain, and in cerebral sinovenous thrombosis (CSVT) often includes severe or persistent headache, with or without neurologic deficit in otherwise well children. It is not infrequently preceded by sign/symptoms of otitis media progressing to mastoiditis. Arterial thrombosis of the lower extremity (eg, neonatal umbilical artery catheter–associated) as well as vasospasm without identified thrombosis, often manifests with diminished distal pulses and dusky discoloration of the limb.

C. Laboratory Findings

A comprehensive laboratory investigation for thrombophilia (ie, hypercoagulability) is recommended by the International Society on Thrombosis and Haemostasis in order to disclose possible underlying congenital or acquired abnormalities that may affect acute or long-term management. Testing evaluates for intrinsic anticoagulant deficiency (proteins C and S and antithrombin), procoagulant factor excess (eg, factor VIII), proteins and genetic mutations mediating enhanced procoagulant activity or reduced sensitivity to inactivation (antiphospholipid antibodies; factor V Leiden and prothrombin 20210 polymorphisms), biochemical mediators of endothelial damage (homocysteine), and markers or regulators of fibrinolysis (eg, D-dimer, plasminogen activator inhibitor-1, and lipoprotein[a]). Interpretation of procoagulant factor and intrinsic anticoagulant levels should take into account the age dependence of normal values for these proteins. Among these VTE risk factors, antiphospholipid antibodies and elevated levels of homocysteine and lipoprotein(a) have also been demonstrated as risk factors for arterial thrombotic and ischemic events.

D. Imaging

Appropriate radiologic imaging is essential to objectively document the thrombus and to delineate the type (venous vs arterial), occlusiveness, and extent (proximal and distal termini) of thrombosis. Depending on site, typical imaging modalities include compression ultrasound with Doppler, computed tomographic (CT) venography, magnetic resonance venography, and conventional angiography.

Treatment

Current guidelines for the treatment of first-episode VTE in children have been largely based on adult experience and include therapeutic anticoagulation for at least 3 months. During the period of anticoagulation, bleeding precautions should be followed, as previously described (see Treatment under Idiopathic Thrombocytopenic Purpura, earlier); in CVST, presentation with postthrombotic hemorrhage often does not preclude anticoagulant therapy. Initial therapy for acute VTE employs continuous intravenous unfractionated heparin or subcutaneous injections of low-molecular-weight heparin (LMWH) for at least 7 days, monitored by anti-Xa activity level to maintain anticoagulant levels of 0.3–0.7 or 0.5–1.0 IU/mL, respectively. Subsequent extended anticoagulant therapy is given with LMWH or daily oral warfarin, the latter agent monitored by the PT to maintain an international normalized ratio (INR) of 2.0–3.0 (2.5–3.5 in the presence of an antiphospholipid antibody). During warfarin treatment, the INR optimally should be within the therapeutic range for two consecutive days before discontinuation of heparin. Warfarin pharmacokinetics are affected by acute illness, numerous medications, and changes in diet, and can necessitate frequent monitoring. In children, warfarin dose is determined by age. LMWH offers the advantage of infrequent need for monitoring but is far more expensive than warfarin. Anatomic contributions to venous stasis (eg, mastoiditis or depressed skull fracture as risk factors for CVST; congenital left iliac vein stenosis in DVT of proximal left lower extremity with May-Thurner anomaly) should be addressed to optimize response to anticoagulation. In cases of limb- or life-threatening VTEs, including major proximal pulmonary embolus, and in cases of progressive VTE despite therapeutic anticoagulation, thrombolytic therapy (eg, tissue-type plasminogen activator) may be considered. A recent cohort study has indicated that initial thrombolytic therapy may also reduce the risk of the postthrombotic syndrome (PTS) in children with veno-occlusive deep venous thrombosis of the proximal limbs in whom adverse prognostic biomarkers (ie, elevated factor VIII and D-dimer levels) are present at diagnosis; however, the safety and efficacy of this approach must be further evaluated in larger studies. In adolescent females, estrogen-containing contraceptives are relatively contraindicated in those with prior VTE, particularly if an additional genetic cause for impairment of protein C pathway is disclosed.

Prognosis

Registries and cohort studies have suggested that recurrent VTE occurs in approximately 10% of children within 2 years. Persistent thrombosis is evident following completion of a standard therapeutic course of anticoagulation in up to 30% of children, with unclear clinical importance. Approximately one in four children with deep venous thrombosis involving the extremities develop post thrombotic syndrome, a condition of venous insufficiency of varying severity characterized by chronic skin changes, edema, and dilated collateral superficial venous formation, and often accompanied by functional limitation (pain with activities or at rest). The presence of homozygous anticoagulant deficiencies, multiple thrombophilia traits, or persistent antiphospholipid antibodies following VTE diagnosis has been associated with increased risk of recurrent VTE, leading to consideration of extended anticoagulation in these instances. Complete veno-occlusion and elevated levels of factor VIII and D-dimer at VTE diagnosis have been identified as prognostic factors for PTS among children with deep venous thrombosis affecting the limbs. In CSVT failure to provide antithrombotic therapy has been associated with adverse neurologic outcome.

Goldenberg NA: The "age" of understanding VKA dose. Blood 2010;116:5789–5790 [PMID: 21183695].

Goldenberg NA: Post-thrombotic syndrome in children: A systematic review of frequency of occurrence, validity of outcome measures, and prognostic factors. Haematologica 2010;95:1952–1959 [PMID: 20595095].

Monagle P: Antithrombotic therapy in neonates and children: American College of Chest Physicians Evidence-Based Clinical Practice Guidelines (8th Edition). Chest 2008;133(Suppl 6):887S–968S [PMID: 18574281].

Raffini L: Dramatic increase in venous thromboembolism in children's hospitals in the United States from 2001 to 2007. Pediatrics 2009;124:1001–1008 [PMID: 19736261].

SPLENIC ABNORMALITIES

SPLENOMEGALY & HYPERSPLENISM

The differential diagnosis of splenomegaly includes the general categories of congestive splenomegaly, chronic infections, leukemia and lymphomas, hemolytic anemias, reticuloendothelioses, and storage diseases (Table 30–9).

Splenomegaly due to any cause may be associated with hypersplenism and the excessive destruction of circulating red cells, white cells, and platelets. The degree of cytopenia is variable and, when mild, requires no specific therapy. In other cases, the thrombocytopenia may cause life-threatening bleeding, particularly when the splenomegaly is secondary to portal hypertension and associated with esophageal varices or the consequence of a storage disease. In such

Table 30–9. Causes of chronic splenomegaly in children.

Cause	Associated Clinical Findings	Diagnostic Investigation
Congestive splenomegaly	History of umbilical vein catheter or neonatal omphalitis; signs of portal hypertension (varices, hemorrhoids, dilated abdominal wall veins); pancytopenia; history of hepatitis or jaundice	Complete blood count, platelet count, liver function tests, ultrasonography
Chronic infections	History of exposure to tuberculosis, histoplasmosis, coccidiomycosis, other fungal disease; chronic sepsis (foreign body in bloodstream; subacute infective endocarditis)	Appropriate cultures and skin tests, ie, blood cultures; PPD, fungal serology and antigen tests, chest film; HIV serology
Infectious mononucleosis	Fever, fatigue, pharyngitis, rash, adenopathy, hepatomegaly	Atypical lymphocytes on blood smear, monospot, EBV antibody titers
Leukemia, lymphoma, Hodgkin disease	Evidence of systemic involvement with fever, bleeding tendencies, hepatomegaly, and lymphadenopathy; pancytopenia	Blood smear, bone marrow examination, chest film, gallium scan, LDH, uric acid
Hemolytic anemia	Anemia, jaundice; family history of anemia, jaundice, and gallbladder disease in young adults	Reticulocyte count, Coombs test, blood smear, osmotic fragility test, hemoglobin electrophoresis
Reticuloendothelioses (histiocytosis X)	Chronic otitis media, seborrheic or petechial skin rashes, anemia, infections, lymphadenopathy, hepatomegaly, bone lesions	Skeletal radiographs for bone lesions; biopsy of bone, liver, bone marrow, or lymph node
Storages diseases	Family history of similar disorders, neurologic involvement, evidence of macular degeneration, hepatomegaly	Biopsy of liver or bone marrow in search for storage cells
Splenic cyst	Evidence of other infections (postinfectious cyst) or congenital anomalies; peculiar shape of spleen	Radionuclide scan, ultrasonography
Splenic hemangioma	Other hemangiomas, consumptive coagulopathy	Radionuclide scan, arteriography, platelet count, coagulation screen

EBV, Epstein-Barr virus; HIV, human immunodeficiency virus; LDH, lactic dehydrogenase; PPD, purified protein derivative.

cases, treatment with surgical splenectomy or with splenic embolization may be warranted. Although more commonly associated with acute enlargement, rupture of an enlarged spleen can be seen in more chronic conditions such as Gaucher disease.

Stone DL: Life threatening splenic hemorrhage in two patients with Gaucher's disease. Am J Hematol 2000;64:140 [PMID: 10814997].

ASPLENIA & SPLENECTOMY

Children who lack normal splenic function are at risk for sepsis, meningitis, and pneumonia due to encapsulated bacteria such as pneumococci and *H influenzae*. Such infections are often fulminant and fatal because of inadequate antibody production and impaired phagocytosis of circulating bacteria.

Congenital asplenia is usually suspected when an infant is born with abnormalities of abdominal viscera and complex cyanotic congenital heart disease. Howell-Jolly bodies are usually present on the peripheral blood smear, and the absence of splenic tissue is confirmed by technetium radionuclide scanning. The prognosis depends on the underlying cardiac lesions, and many children die during the first few months. Prophylactic antibiotics, usually penicillin, and pneumococcal conjugate, HiB and meningococcal vaccines are recommended.

The risk of overwhelming sepsis following surgical splenectomy is related to the child's age and to the underlying disorder. Because the risk is highest when the procedure is performed earlier in life, splenectomy is usually postponed until after age 5 years. The risk of postsplenectomy sepsis is also greater in children with malignancies, thalassemias, and reticuloendothelioses than in children whose splenectomy is performed for ITP, hereditary spherocytosis, or trauma. Prior to splenectomy, children should be immunized against *Streptococcus pneumoniae, H influenzae*, and *Neisseria meningitidis*. Additional management should include penicillin prophylaxis and prompt evaluation for fever 38.8°C or above or signs of severe infection.

Children with sickle cell anemia develop functional asplenia during the first year of life, and overwhelming sepsis is the leading cause of early deaths in this disease. Prophylactic penicillin reduces the incidence of sepsis by 84%.

Pickering L: American Academy of Pediatrics: Immunization in special circumstances. Red Book 2000;25:66.

TRANSFUSION MEDICINE

DONOR SCREENING & BLOOD PROCESSING: RISK MANAGEMENT

Minimizing the risks of transfusion begins by screening volunteer donors with a questionnaire that will protect the recipient from transmission of infectious agents as well as other risks of transfusions. In addition, information defining high-risk groups whose behavior increases the possible transmission of HIV, hepatitis, and other diseases is provided, with the request that persons in these groups not donate blood. Positive responses may result in temporary or permanent deferral from donation.

Before blood components can be released for transfusion, donor blood is screened for hepatitis B surface antigen; antibodies to hepatitis B core antigen, hepatitis C, HIV-1 and 2, and human T-cell lymphotropic virus (HTLV) I and II; and a serologic test for syphilis (Table 30–10). Screening donor blood for viral genome (nucleic acid amplification [NAT]

Table 30–10. Transmission risks of infectious agents for which screening of blood products is routinely performed.

Disease Entity	Transmission	Screening and Processing Procedures	Approximate Risk of Transmission
Syphilis	Low risk: fresh blood drawn during spirochetemia can transmit infection. Organism not able to survive beyond 72 h during storage at 4°C.	Donor history. RPR or VDRL.	< 1:100,000
Hepatitis A	Units drawn during prodrome could transmit virus. Because of brief viremia during acute phase, absence of asymptomatic carrier phase, and failure to detect transmission in multiple transfused individuals, infection by this agent is unlikely.	Donor history.	1:1,000,000
Hepatitis B	Prolonged viremia during various phases of the disease and asymptomatic carrier state make HBV infection a significant risk of transfusion. Incidence has markedly decreased with screening strategies.	Donor history, education, and self-exclusion. Hepatitis B surface antigen (HBsAg). Surrogate test for non-A, non-B hepatitis (hepatitis-B core antibody) has helped screen out population at risk for transmitting HBV.	1:500,000–1:200,000
Hepatitis C	Over two-thirds of cases of non-A, non-B post-transfusion hepatitis may be due to this agent. Virus has characteristics similar to those of HBV which are responsible for risk from transfusion.	Donor history. Surrogate tests: hepatitis B core antibody (anti-HBc), anti-HCV. Nucleic acid testing for viral genome required.	1:2,000,000
Non-A, non-B, non-C hepatitis	Agents other than HAV, HBV, HCV, Epstein-Barr virus, and cytomegalovirus, which can cause post-transfusion hepatitis.	Donor history. Surrogate tests: anti-HBc.	Undefined
Human immunodeficiency virus (HIV-1, HIV-2) infection	Retroviruses spread by sexual contact, parenteral (including transfusion) and vertical routes.	Donor history, education, and self-exclusion. Anti-HIV by EIA screening test. Western blot confirmatory. Nucleic acid testing for viral genome required.	1:2,000,000
Human T-cell lymphotropic virus I and II (HTLVI and II) infection	Retroviruses spread by sexual contact, parenteral (including transfusion) and vertical modes.	Donor history. Anti-HTLV-I and II by enzyme immunoassay screening test. Western blot confirmatory.	1:3,000,000
Chagas disease	Transmitted by insect vector, blood transfusion (all components), organ transplantation, food contaminated with parasites, and mother to fetus.	History, detection of antibody in donor serum or plasma.	< 1:25,000
West Nile Virus	Seasonal transmission through mosquito vector. Transmitted by blood transfusion and organ transplantation.	History, nucleic acid testing for viral genome.	< 1:10,000 (undefined for nucleic acid testing)

HIV, human immunodeficiency virus; EIA, enzyme-linked immunosorbent assay; HAV, HBV, HCV, hepatitis A virus, hepatitis B virus, hepatitis C virus, respectively; HTLV, human T-cell lymphotropic virus; RPR, rapid plasma reagin; VDRL, syphilis test.

testing) was mandated for HIV, HCV, and West Nile virus. NAT testing for other viruses may be added in the future, and screening for Chagas disease was accepted in 2007. Positive tests are repeated.

Upon confirmation of a screening test, the unit in question is destroyed and the donor is notified and deferred from future donations. Many of the screening tests used are very sensitive and have a high rate of false-positive results. As a result, confirmatory tests have been developed to check the initial screening results and separate the false-positives from the true-positives. Recently, bacterial culture of platelet concentrates was added to the testing paradigm.

With these approaches, the risk of an infectious complication from blood components has been minimized (see Table 30–10), with the greatest risk being posttransfusion hepatitis (see sections on hepatitis C virus and non-A, non-B, non-C hepatitis in Chapter 22). Autologous donation is recognized by some centers as a safe alternative to homologous blood. Issues of donor size make the techniques of autologous donation difficult to apply to the pediatric population.

Primary CMV infections are significant complications of blood transfusion in transplant recipients, neonates, and immunodeficient individuals. Transmission of CMV can be avoided by using seronegative donors, apheresis platelet concentrates collected by techniques ensuring low numbers of residual white cells, or red cell or platelet products leukocyte-depleted by filtering (< 5 million white blood cells per packed red cell unit or apheresis platelet concentrate equivalent).

STORAGE & PRESERVATION OF BLOOD & BLOOD COMPONENTS

Whole blood is routinely fractionated into packed red cells, platelets, and FFP or cryoprecipitate for most efficient use of all blood components. The storage conditions and biologic characteristics of the fractions are summarized in Table 30–11. The conditions provide the optimal environment to maintain appropriate recovery, survival, and function and are different for each blood component. For example, red cells undergo dramatic metabolic changes during their 35- to 42-day storage, with a decrease in 2,3-diphosphoglycerate (DPG) by day 14 of storage, a decrease in adenosine triphosphate, a gradual loss of intracellular potassium, an in vivo recovery of ≥ 80% transfused cells in red cells by day of storage outdate. Fortunately, these changes are reversed readily in vivo within hours to days after the red cells are transfused. However, in certain clinical conditions, these effects may define the type of components used. For example, blood less than 7–10 days old would be preferred for exchange transfusion in neonates or replacement of red cells in persons with severe cardiopulmonary disease to ensure adequate oxygen-carrying capacity. Storage time is not an issue when administering transfusions to those with chronic anemia.

If extracellular potassium in older packed red cells may present a problem, one may use blood less than 10 days old, making packed cells out of an older unit of whole blood, or washing blood stored as packed cells. Regardless of the blood's age, over 70%–80% of the red cells will circulate after transfusion and approximate normal survival in the circulation.

Platelets are stored at 22°C for a maximum of 5 days; criteria for 7-day storage are being developed. At the extremes of storage, there should be at least a 60% recovery, a survival time that approximates turnover of fresh autologous platelets, and normalization of the bleeding time or PFA-100 in proportion to the peak platelet count. Frozen components, red cells, FFP, and cryoprecipitate are outdated at 10 years, 1 year, and 1 year, respectively. Frozen red cells retain the same biochemical and functional characteristics as the day they were frozen. FFP contains 80% or more of all of the clotting factors of fresh plasma. Factors VIII and XIII and fibrinogen are concentrated in cryoprecipitate.

PRETRANSFUSION TESTING

Both the donated blood and the recipient are tested for ABO and Rh(D) antigens and screened for auto- or alloantibodies in the plasma. The cross-match is required on any component that contains red cells. In the major cross-match, washed donor red cells are incubated with the serum from the patient, and agglutination is detected and graded. The antiglobulin phase of the test is then performed; Coombs reagent, which will detect the presence of IgG or complement on the surface of the red cells, is added to the mixture, and agglutination is evaluated. In the presence of a negative antibody screen in the recipient, a negative immediate spin cross-match test confirms the compatibility of the blood and antiglobulin phase is not required. Further testing is required if the antibody screen or the cross-match is positive, and blood should not be given until the nature of the reactivity is delineated. An incompatible cross-match is evaluated first with a DAT or Coombs test to detect IgG or complement on the surfaces of the recipient's red cells. The indirect antiglobulin test is also used to determine the presence of antibodies that will coat red cells or activate complement, and additional studies are completed to define the antibody.

TRANSFUSION PRACTICE

General Rules

Several rules should be observed in administering any blood component:

1. In final preparation of the component, no solutions should be added to the bag or tubing set except for normal saline (0.9% sodium chloride for injection, USP), ABO-compatible plasma, or other specifically approved

Table 30–11. Characteristics of blood and blood components.

Component	Storage Conditions	Composition and Transfusion Characteristics	Indications	Risks and Precautions	Administration
Whole blood	4°C for 35 days. RBC characteristics: • *Survival*: recovery decreases during storage, but is always > 70%–80%. Cells that circulate approximate normal survival. • *Function*: 2,3-DPG levels fall to undetectable after second week of storage. This defect is repaired within 12 h of transfusion. • *Electrolytes*: with storage, potassium increases in plasma. This rises to high levels after 2 wk of storage.	Contains RBCs and many plasma compounds of whole blood. Leukocytes and platelets lose activity or viability after 1–3 days under these conditions. Procoagulant clotting factors (particularly VIII and V) deteriorate rapidly during storage. Each unit has about 500 mL volume and Hct 36%–40%.	Oxygen-carrying capacity (anemia). Volume replacement for massive blood loss or severe shock.	Must be ABO-identical and cross-match-compatible. Infections. Febrile or hemolytic transfusion reactions. Alloimmunization to red cell, white cell, or platelet antigens.	During acute blood loss, as rapidly as tolerated. In other settings, 2–4 h. 10 mL/kg will raise Hct by 5% and support volume.
Packed red cells	Same as for whole blood. Special preservative solutions allow storage for 42 d.	Contains RBCs; most plasma removed in preparation. Status of leukocytes, clotting factors, and platelets same as for whole blood. Hct about 70%, volume 200–250 mL. May request tighter pack to give Hct 80%–90%.	Oxygen carrying capacity. Acute trauma or bleeding or situations requiring intensive cardiopulmonary support (Hct < 25%–30%). Chronic anemia (Hct < 21%).	Same as for whole blood.	May be given as patient will tolerate, based on cardiovascular status over 2–4 h. Dose of 3 mL packed RBC/kg will raise Hct by 3%. If cardiovascular status is stable, give 10 mL/kg over 2–4 h. If unstable, use smaller volume or do packed RBC exchange.
Washed or filtered red cells	When cells are washed, there is a 24-h outdate. Up to that time, they have the same characteristics as for packed red cells.	Same as for packed red cells.	Same as packed red cells. Depending on technique used and extent of reduction of white blood cells, leukoreduced red cells may achieve the following: • Decrease in febrile reactions. • Decrease transmission of CMV. • Decrease incidence of alloimmunization to white cell antigens.	Same as whole blood. Removal of white cells diminishes the risk of febrile reactions. Filtration with high-efficiency white cell filters may decrease rate of alloimmunization to white cell antigens and transmission of CMV.	Same as for packed red cells.
Frozen red cells	Packed red cells frozen in 40% glycerol solution at less than −65°C. After storage for 10 y, cells retain the same biochemical characteristics, function, and capacity for survival as on the day they were frozen; when thawed, 24-h outdate.	Same as for packed red cells.	Same as packed red cells. Useful for avoiding febrile reactions, decreasing transmission of CMV, autologous blood donation, and developing an inventory of rare red cell blood groups.	Same as for whole blood. Risk of CMV transmission is at same level as using seronegative components.	Same as for packed red cells.

Fresh frozen plasma	Plasma from whole blood stored at less than −18°C for up to 1 y.	Contains > 80% of all procoagulant and anticoagulant plasma proteins.	Replacement of plasma procoagulant and anticoagulant plasma proteins. May provide "other" factors, eg, treatment of TTP.	Need not be cross-matched; should be type compatible. Volume overload, infectious diseases, allergic reactions. Solvent detergent-treated plasma or donor-retested plasma units have decreased risk for viral transmission.	As rapidly as tolerated by patient, but not > 4 h. Dose: 10–15 mL/kg will increase level of all clotting factors by 10%–20%.
Cryoprecipitate	Produced by freezing fresh plasma to less than −65°C, then allowed to thaw 18 h at 4°C. After centrifugation, cryoprecipitable proteins are separated. May be stored at less than −18°C for up to 1 y.	Contains factor VIII, fibrinogen, and fibronectin at concentrations greater than those of plasma. Also contains factor XIII, VIII > 80 IU/pack, fibrinogen 100–350 mg/pack.	Treatment of acquired or congenital deficiencies of fibrinogen. Useful in making biologic glues that contain fibrinogen. Commercial clotting factor concentrates are the treatment of choice for factor VIII deficiency and von Willebrand disease because sterilization procedures further reduce the risk of viral transmission.	Same as for fresh frozen plasma. ABO agglutinogens may also be concentrated and can give positive direct agglutination test if not type-specific.	Cryoprecipitate can be given as a rapid infusion. Dose: ½ pack/kg body weight will increase factor VIII level by 80%–100% and fibrinogen by 200–250 mg/dL.
Platelet concentrates from whole blood donation	Separated from platelet-rich plasma and stored with gentle agitation at 22–24°C for 5 d. Containers currently in use are plastic and allow for gas exchange, diffusion of CO_2 helps keep pH > 6, a major factor in keeping platelets viable and functional.	Each unit contains about 5×10^{10} platelets. *Survival*: Although there may be some loss with storage, 60%–70% recovery should be achieved, with stored platelets able to correct platelet function test in proportion to the peak counts reached.	Treatment of thrombocytopenia or platelet function defects.	No cross-match necessary. Should be ABO type-specific. Other risks as for whole blood.	Can be taken during rapid transfusion or as defined by cardiovascular status, not more than 4 h. Dose: 10 mL/kg should increase platelet count by at least 50,000/µL.
Platelet concentrates by apheresis techniques	Same as random donor units.	Platelet content is equivalent to 6–10 units of concentrates from whole blood (3×10^{11} platelets), can be made relatively free of leukocytes, which is important for avoiding alloimmunization.	As above, particularly useful in treating patients who have insufficient production and also may have a problem with alloisoimmunization.	Same as above.	As above.
Granulocytes	Although they may be stored stationary at 22–24°C, transfuse as soon as possible after collection.	Contains at least 1×10^{10} granulocytes, but also platelets and red cells. When donors given 10 mcg/kg G-CSF subcutaneously and 8 mg Decadron orally 12–15 h before collection, yield increases to $> 5 \times 10^{10}$ granulocytes.	Severely neutropenic individuals (< 500/µL) with poor marrow reserves and suspected bacterial or fungal infections not responding to 48–72 h of parenteral antibiotics. Also in patients with neutrophil dysfunction.	Same as for platelets. Pulmonary leukostasis reactions. Severe febrile reactions.	Given in an infusion over 2–4 h. Dose: 1 unit daily for newborns and infants, 1×10^9 granulocytes/kg.

CMV, cytomegalovirus; DPG, diphosphoglycerate; G-CSF, granulocyte colony-stimulating factor; Hct, hematocrit; RBC, red blood cell.

expanders. Hypotonic solutions cause hemolysis of red cells, and, if these are transfused, a severe reaction will occur. Any reconstitution should be completed by the blood bank.

2. Transfusion products should be protected from contact with any calcium-containing solution (eg, lactated Ringer); recalcification and reversal of the citrate effect will cause clotting of the blood component.
3. Blood components should not be warmed to a temperature greater than 37°C. If a component is incubated in a water bath, it should be enclosed in a watertight bag to prevent bacterial contamination of entry ports.
4. Whenever a blood bag is entered, the sterile integrity of the system is violated, and that unit should be discarded within 4 hours if left at room temperature or within 24 hours if the temperature is 4–6°C.
5. Transfusions of products containing red cells should not exceed 4 hours. Blood components in excess of what can be infused during this time period should be stored in the blood bank until needed.
6. Before transfusion, the blood component should be inspected visually for any unusual characteristics, such as the presence of flocculent material, hemolysis, or clumping of cells, and mixed thoroughly.
7. The unit and the recipient should be identified properly.
8. The administration set includes a standard 170- to 260-micron filter. Under certain clinical circumstances, an additional microaggregate filter may be used to eliminate small aggregates of fibrin, white cells, and platelets that will not be removed by the standard filter.
9. The patient should be observed during the entire transfusion and especially during the first 15 minutes. With the onset of any adverse symptoms or signs the transfusion should be stopped, an evaluation initiated immediately and the reaction reported promptly to the transfusion service.
10. When cross-match–incompatible red cells or whole blood unit(s) must be given to the patient (as with autoimmune hemolytic anemia), a test dose of 10% of the total volume (not to exceed 50 mL) should be administered over 15–20 minutes; the transfusion is then stopped and the patient observed. If no adverse effects are noted, the remainder of the volume can be infused carefully.
11. Blood for exchange transfusion in the newborn period may be cross-matched with either the infant's or the mother's serum. If the exchange is for hemolysis, 500 mL of whole blood stored for less than 7 days will be adequate. If replacement of clotting factors is a key issue, packed red cells (7 days old) reconstituted with ABO type-specific FFP may be considered. Based on posttransfusion platelet counts, platelet transfusion may be considered. Other problems to be anticipated are acid-base derangements, hyponatremia, hyperkalemia, hypocalcemia, hypoglycemia, hypothermia, and hypervolemia or hypovolemia.

Choice of Blood Component

Several principles should be considered when deciding on the need for blood transfusion. Indications for blood or blood components must be well defined, and the patient's medical condition, not just the laboratory results, should be the basis for the decision. Specific deficiencies exhibited by the patient (eg, oxygen-carrying capacity, thrombocytopenia) should be treated with appropriate blood components and the use of whole blood minimized. Information about specific blood components is summarized in Table 30–11.

A. Whole Blood

Whole blood may be used in patients who require replacement of oxygen-carrying capacity and volume. More specifically, it may be considered during massive blood loss, after initial response to replace volume with crystalloid and oxygen carrying capacity. Doses vary depending on volume considerations (see Table 30–11). In acute situations, the transfusion may be completed rapidly to support blood volume.

B. Packed Red Cells

Packed red cells (which include leukocyte-poor, filtered, or frozen deglycerolized products) prepared from whole blood by centrifugal techniques are the appropriate choice for almost all patients with deficient oxygen-carrying capacity. Exact indications will be defined by the clinical setting, the severity of the anemia, the acuity of the condition, and any other factors affecting oxygen transport.

C. Platelets

The decision to transfuse platelets depends on the patient's clinical condition, the status of plasma phase coagulation, the platelet count, the cause of the thrombocytopenia, and the functional capacity of the patient's own platelets. In the face of decreased production, clinical bleeding, and platelet counts less than 10,000/μL, the risk of severe, spontaneous bleeding is increased markedly; and in the absence heparin-induced thrombocytopenia, thrombotic thrombocytopenic purpura, or antibody-mediated thrombocytopenia transfusion may be considered. Under certain circumstances, especially with platelet dysfunction or treatment that inhibits the procoagulant system, transfusions at higher platelet counts may be necessary.

Transfused platelets are sequestered temporarily in the lungs and spleen before reaching their peak concentrations, 45–60 minutes after transfusion. A significant proportion of the transfused platelets never circulate but remain sequestered in the spleen. This phenomenon results in reduced recovery; under best conditions, only 60%–70% of the transfused platelets are accounted for when peripheral platelet count increments are used as a measure of response.

In addition to cessation of bleeding, two variables indicate the effectiveness of platelet transfusions. The first is platelet recovery, as measured by the maximum number of platelets circulating in response to transfusion. The practical measure is the platelet count at 1 hour after transfusion. In the absence of immune or drastic nonimmune factors that markedly decrease platelet recovery, one would expect a 7000/μL increment for each random donor unit and a 40,000–70,000/μL increment for each single-donor apheresis unit in a large child or adolescent. For infants and small children, 10 mL/kg of platelets will increase the platelet count by at least 50,000/μL. The second variable is the survival of transfused platelets. Normally, if the recovery is great enough, transfused platelets will approach a normal half-life in the circulation. In the presence of increased platelet destruction, the life span may be shortened to a few days or a few hours. Frequent platelet transfusions may be required to maintain adequate hemostasis.

A particularly troublesome outcome in patients receiving long-term platelet transfusions is the development of a refractory state characterized by poor (≤ 20%) recovery or no response to platelet transfusion (as measured at 1 hour). Most (70%–90%) of these refractory states result from the development of alloantibodies directed against HLA antigens on the platelet. Platelets have class I HLA antigens, and the antibodies are primarily against HLA A or B determinants. A smaller proportion of these alloantibodies (< 10%) may be directed against platelet-specific alloantigens. The most effective approach to prevent HLA sensitization is to use leukocyte-depleted components (< 5 million leukocytes per unit of packed red cells or per apheresis or 6–10 random donor unit concentrates). For the alloimmunized, refractory patient, the best approach is to provide HLA-matched platelets for transfusion. Reports have suggested that platelet cross-matching procedures using HLA-matched or unmatched donors may be helpful in identifying platelet concentrates most likely to provide an adequate response.

D. Fresh Frozen Plasma

The indication for FFP is replacement of plasma coagulation factors in clinical situations in which a deficiency of one or more clotting factors exists and associated bleeding manifestations are present. In some hereditary factor deficiencies, such as factor VIII deficiency or vWD, commercially prepared concentrates contain these factors in higher concentrations and, because of viral inactivation, impose less infectious risk and are more appropriate than plasma. Treatment with FFP is indicated for decreased liver production of clotting factors or generalized consumption (DIC) when INR > 1.5.

E. Cryoprecipitate

This component may be used for acquired or congenital disorders of hypofibrinogenemia or afibrinogenemia. Although cryoprecipitate is a rich source for factor VIII or vWF, commercial concentrates that contain these factors are more appropriate (see preceding section). The dose given depends on the protein to be replaced. Cryoprecipitate can be given in a rapid transfusion over 30–60 minutes and is currently under investigation.

F. Granulocytes

With better supportive care over the past 20 years, the need for granulocytes in neutropenic patients with severe bacterial infections has decreased. Indications still remain for severe bacterial or fungal infections unresponsive to vigorous medical therapy in either newborns or older children with bone marrow failure, or patients with neutrophil dysfunction. Newer mobilization schemes using G-CSF and steroids in donors result in granulocyte collections with at least 50 billion neutrophils. This may provide a better product for patients requiring granulocyte support.

G. Apheresis Products and Procedures

Apheresis equipment allows one or more blood components to be collected while the rest are returned to the donor. Apheresis platelet concentrates, which have as many platelets as 6–10 units of platelet concentrates from whole blood donations, are one example; granulocytes are another. Apheresis techniques can also be used to collect hematopoietic stem cells that have been mobilized into the blood by cytokines (G-CSF or GM-CSF) given alone or after chemotherapy or mononuclear cells for immunotherapy. These stem cells are used for allogeneic or autologous bone marrow transplantation. Blood cell separators can be used for the collection of single-source plasma or removal of a blood component that is causing disease. Examples include red cell exchange in sickle cell disease and plasmapheresis in Goodpasture syndrome or in Guillain-Barré syndrome.

Adverse Effects

The noninfectious complications of blood transfusions are outlined in Table 30–12. Most complications present a significant risk to the recipient.

Allain JP: Transfusion-transmitted infectious diseases. Biologicals 2009;37:71 [PMID: 19231236].

Dodd R: Transfusion medicine and safety. Biologicals 2009;37:62 [PMID: 19230706].

Fasano R: Blood component therapy. Pediatr Clin North Am 2008;55:421 [PMID: 18381094].

Slichter SJ: Platelet transfusion therapy. Hematol Oncol Clin North Am 2007;21:697 [PMID: 17666286].

Table 30–12. Adverse events following transfusions.

Event	Pathophysiology	Signs and Symptoms	Management
Acute hemolytic transfusion reaction	Preformed alloantibodies (most commonly to ABO) and infrequently autoantibodies cause rapid intravascular hemolysis of transfused cells with activation of clotting (DIC), activation of inflammatory mediators, and acute renal failure.	Fever, chills, nausea, chest pain, back pain, pain at transfusion site, hypotension, dyspnea, oliguria, hemoglobinuria.	The risk of this type of reaction overall is low (1:30,000–1:70,000), but the mortality rate is high (up to 40%). Stop the transfusion; maintain renal output with intravenous fluids and diuretics (furosemide or mannitol); treat DIC with heparin; and institute other appropriate supportive measures.
Delayed hemolytic transfusion reaction	Formation of alloantibodies after transfusion and resultant destruction of transfused red cells, usually by extravascular hemolysis.	Jaundice, anemia. A small percentage may develop chronic hemolysis.	Detection, definition, and documentation (for future transfusions). Supportive care. Risk, < 5% of transfused patients may develop alloantibody; hemolysis, 1:2500.
Febrile reactions	Usually caused by leukoagglutinins in recipient, cytokines, or other biologically active compounds.	Fever. May also involve chills.	Supportive. Consider leukocyte-poor products for future. Risk per transfusion, 1:200–1:17 per transfusion.
Allergic reactions	Most causes not identified. In IgA-deficient individuals, reaction occurs as a result of antibodies to IgA.	Itching, hives, occasionally chills and fever. In severe reactions, may see signs of anaphylaxis: dyspnea, pulmonary edema.	Mild to moderate reactions: diphenhydramine. More severe reactions: epinephrine subcutaneously and steroids intravenously. Risk for mild to moderate allergic reactions,1:100. Severe anaphylactic reactions, 1:50,000.
Transfusion-related acute lung injury	Acute lung injury occurring within 6 h after transfusion. Two sets of factors interact to produce the syndrome. Patient factors: infection, surgery, cytokine therapy. Blood component factors: lipids, antibodies, cytokines. Two groups of factors interact during transfusion to result in lung injury indistinguishable from ARDS.	Tachypnea, dyspnea, hypoxia. Diffuse interstitial markings. Cardiac evaluation normal.	May consider younger products: packed red blood cells ≤ 2 wk, platelets ≤ 3 d, washing components to prevent syndrome. Management: supportive care. Risk, 1:2000–1:3000 per transfusion. Current preventative procedures include avoiding donors at risk for alloimmunization: use of male-only FFP or white blood cell antibody-negative apheresis FFP or platelet products.
Dilutional coagulopathy	Massive blood loss and transfusion with replacement with fluids or blood components and deficient clotting factors.	Bleeding.	Replacement of clotting factors or platelets with appropriate blood components.
Bacterial contamination	Contamination of units results in growth of bacteria or production of clinically significant levels of endotoxin.	Chills, high fever, hypotension, other symptoms of sepsis or endotoxemia.	Stop transfusion; make aggressive attempts to identify organism; provide vigorous support.1:10:000–1:000,000
Graft-versus-host disease	Lymphocytes from donor transfused in an immunoincompetent host.	Syndrome can involve a variety of organs, usually skin, liver, gastrointestinal tract, and bone marrow.	Preventive management: irradiation (> 1500 cGy) of cellular blood components transfused to individuals with congenital or acquired immunodeficiency syndromes, intrauterine transfusion, very premature infants, and when donors are relatives of the recipient.
Iron overload	There is no physiologic mechanism to excrete excess iron. Target organs include liver, heart, and endocrine organs. In patients receiving red cell transfusions over long periods of time, there is an increase in iron burden.	Signs and symptoms of dysfunctional organs affected by the iron.	Chronic administration of iron chelator such as deferoxamine given intravenously or Exjade given orally.

ARDS, adult respiratory distress syndrome; DIC, disseminated intravascular coagulation.

REFERENCES

Goodnight SH, Hathaway WE (editors): *Disorders of Hemostasis and Thrombosis: A Clinical Guide,* 2nd ed. McGraw-Hill, 2001.

Hillyer CD et al (editors): *Blood Banking and Transfusion Medicine, Basic Principles and Practice.* Churchill Livingstone, 2006.

Petz LD, Garratty G (editors): *Acquired Immune Hemolytic Anemias,* 2nd ed. Churchill Livingstone, 2004.

Roback JD et al: *Technical Manual,* 16th ed. AABB, 2008.

Neoplastic Disease

31

Doug K. Graham, MD, PhD
Ralph R. Quinones, MD
Amy K. Keating, MD
Kelly Maloney, MD
Nicholas K. Foreman, MD, MRCP
Roger H. Giller, MD
Brian S. Greffe, MD

Each year approximately 150 out of every 1 million children younger than age 20 years are diagnosed with cancer. For children between the ages of 1 and 20 years, cancer is the fourth leading cause of death, behind unintentional injuries, homicides, and suicides. However, combined-modality therapy, including surgery, chemotherapy, and radiation therapy, has improved survival dramatically, such that the overall 5-year survival rate of pediatric malignancies is now greater than 75%. It is estimated that by the year 2020, 1 in 600 adults will be a survivor of childhood cancer.

Because pediatric malignancies are rare, cooperative clinical trials have become the mainstay of treatment planning and therapeutic advances. The Children's Oncology Group (COG), representing the amalgamation of four prior pediatric cooperative groups (Children's Cancer Group, Pediatric Oncology Group, Intergroup Rhabdomyosarcoma Study Group, and the National Wilms Tumor Study Group), offers current therapeutic protocols and strives to answer important treatment questions. A child or adolescent newly diagnosed with cancer should be enrolled in a cooperative clinical trial whenever possible. Because many protocols are associated with significant toxicities, morbidity, and potential mortality, treatment of children with cancer should be supervised by a pediatric oncologist familiar with the hazards of treatment, preferably at a multidisciplinary pediatric cancer center.

Advances in molecular genetics, cell biology, and tumor immunology have contributed and are crucial to the continued understanding of pediatric malignancies and their treatment. Continued research into the biology of tumors will lead to the identification of targeted therapy for specific tumor types with, it is hoped, fewer systemic effects.

Research in supportive care areas, such as prevention and management of infection, pain, and emesis, has improved the survival and quality of life for children undergoing cancer treatment. Long-term studies of childhood cancer survivors are yielding information that provides a rationale for modifying future treatment regimens to decrease morbidity. A guide for caring for childhood cancer survivors is now available to medical providers as well as families and details suggested examinations and late effects by type of chemotherapy received.

Cure Search. Children's Oncology Group. Available at: http://www.survivorshipguidelines.org

Ries LAG et al: SEER Cancer Statistics Review, 1975–2000. Available at: http://seer.cancer.gov/csr/1975_2000

MAJOR PEDIATRIC NEOPLASTIC DISEASES

ACUTE LYMPHOBLASTIC LEUKEMIA

ESSENTIALS OF DIAGNOSIS & TYPICAL FEATURES

- Bone marrow aspirate or biopsy specimen contains more than 25% lymphoblasts.
- Pallor, petechiae, purpura (50%), bone pain (25%).
- Hepatosplenomegaly (60%), lymphadenopathy (50%).
- Single or multiple cytopenias: neutropenia, thrombocytopenia, anemia (99%).
- Leukopenia (15%) or leukocytosis (50%), often with lymphoblasts identifiable on blood smear.
- Diagnosis confirmed by bone marrow examination.

General Considerations

Acute lymphoblastic leukemia (ALL) is the most common malignancy of childhood, accounting for about 25% of all cancer diagnoses in patients younger than age 15 years. The worldwide incidence of ALL is about 1:25,000 children per year, including 3000 children per year in the United States. The peak age at onset is 4 years; 85% of patients are diagnosed between ages 2 and 10 years. Children with Down syndrome have a 14-fold increase in the overall rate of leukemia.

ALL results from uncontrolled proliferation of immature lymphocytes. Its cause is unknown, and genetic factors may play a role. Leukemia is defined by the presence of more than 25% malignant hematopoietic cells (blasts) in the bone marrow aspirate. Leukemic blasts from the majority of cases of childhood ALL have an antigen on the cell surface called the common ALL antigen (CALLA). These blasts derive from B-cell precursors early in their development, called B-precursor ALL. Less commonly, lymphoblasts are of T-cell origin or of mature B-cell origin. Over 70% of children receiving aggressive combination chemotherapy and early presymptomatic treatment to the central nervous system (CNS) are now cured of ALL.

Clinical Findings

A. Symptoms and Signs

Presenting complaints of patients with ALL include those related to decreased bone marrow production of red blood cells (RBCs), white blood cells (WBCs), or platelets and to leukemic infiltration of extramedullary (outside bone marrow) sites. Intermittent fevers are common, as a result of either cytokines induced by the leukemia itself or infections secondary to leukopenia. Many patients present due to bruising or pallor. About 25% of patients experience bone pain, especially in the pelvis, vertebral bodies, and legs.

Physical examination at diagnosis ranges from virtually normal to highly abnormal. Signs related to bone marrow infiltration by leukemia include pallor, petechiae, and purpura. Hepatomegaly or splenomegaly occurs in over 60% of patients. Lymphadenopathy is common, either localized or generalized to cervical, axillary, and inguinal regions. The testes may occasionally be unilaterally or bilaterally enlarged secondary to leukemic infiltration. Superior vena cava syndrome is caused by mediastinal adenopathy compressing the superior vena cava. A prominent venous pattern develops over the upper chest from collateral vein enlargement. The neck may feel full from venous engorgement. The face may appear plethoric, and the periorbital area may be edematous. A mediastinal mass can cause tachypnea, orthopnea, and respiratory distress. Leukemic infiltration of cranial nerves may cause cranial nerve palsies with mild nuchal rigidity. The optic fundi may show exudates of leukemic infiltration and hemorrhage from thrombocytopenia. Anemia can cause a flow murmur, tachycardia, and, rarely, congestive heart failure.

B. Laboratory Findings

A complete blood count (CBC) with differential is the most useful initial test because 95% of patients with ALL have a decrease in at least one cell type (single cytopenia): neutropenia, thrombocytopenia, or anemia with most patients having a decrease in at least two blood cell lines. The WBC count is low or normal (= 10,000/μL) in 50% of patients, but the differential shows neutropenia (absolute neutrophil count < 1000/μL) along with a small percentage of blasts amid normal lymphocytes. In 30% of patients the WBC count is between 10,000/μL and 50,000/μL; in 20% of patients it is over 50,000/μL, occasionally higher than 300,000/μL. Blasts are usually readily identifiable on peripheral blood smears from patients with elevated WBC counts. Peripheral blood smears also show abnormalities in RBCs, such as teardrops. Most patients with ALL have decreased platelet counts (< 150,000/μL) and decreased hemoglobin (< 11 g/dL) at diagnosis. In approximately 1% of patients diagnosed with ALL, CBCs and peripheral blood smears are entirely normal but patients have bone pain that leads to bone marrow examination. Serum chemistries, particularly uric acid and lactate dehydrogenase (LDH), are often elevated at diagnosis as a result of cell breakdown.

The diagnosis of ALL is made by bone marrow examination, which shows a homogeneous infiltration of leukemic blasts replacing normal marrow elements. The morphology of blasts on bone marrow aspirate can usually distinguish ALL from acute myeloid leukemia (AML). Lymphoblasts are typically small, with cell diameters of approximately two erythrocytes. Lymphoblasts have scant cytoplasm, usually without granules. The nucleus typically contains no nucleoli or one small, indistinct nucleolus. Immunophenotyping of ALL blasts by flow cytometry helps distinguish precursor B-cell ALL from T-cell ALL or AML. Histochemical stains specific for myeloblastic and monoblastic leukemias (myeloperoxidase and nonspecific esterase) distinguish ALL from AML. About 5% of patients present with CNS leukemia, which is defined as a cerebrospinal fluid (CSF) WBC count greater than 5/μL with blasts present on cytocentrifuged specimen.

C. Imaging

Chest radiograph may show mediastinal widening or an anterior mediastinal mass and tracheal compression secondary to lymphadenopathy or thymic infiltration, especially in T-cell ALL. Abdominal ultrasound may show kidney enlargement from leukemic infiltration or uric acid nephropathy as well as intra-abdominal adenopathy. Plain radiographs of the long bones and spine may show demineralization, periosteal elevation, growth arrest lines, or compression of vertebral bodies.

Differential Diagnosis

The differential diagnosis, based on the history and physical examination, includes chronic infections by Epstein-Barr virus (EBV) and cytomegalovirus (CMV), causing lymphadenopathy, hepatosplenomegaly, fevers, and anemia. Prominent petechiae and purpura suggest a diagnosis of immune thrombocytopenic purpura. Significant pallor could be caused by transient erythroblastopenia of childhood, autoimmune hemolytic anemias, or aplastic anemia. Fevers and joint pains, with or without hepatosplenomegaly and lymphadenopathy, suggest juvenile rheumatoid arthritis (JRA). The diagnosis of leukemia usually becomes straightforward once the CBC reveals multiple cytopenias and leukemic blasts. Serum LDH levels may help distinguish JRA from leukemia, as the LDH is usually normal in JRA. An elevated WBC count with lymphocytosis is typical of pertussis; however, in pertussis the lymphocytes are mature, and neutropenia is rarely associated.

Treatment

A. Specific Therapy

Intensity of treatment is determined by specific prognostic features present at diagnosis, the patient's response to therapy, and specific biologic features of the leukemia cells. The majority of patients with ALL are enrolled in clinical trials designed by clinical groups and approved by the National Cancer Institute; the largest group is COG (Children's Oncology Group). The first month of therapy consists of induction, at the end of which over 95% of patients exhibit remission on bone marrow aspirates by morphology. The drugs most commonly used in induction include oral prednisone or dexamethasone, intravenous vincristine, daunorubicin, intramuscular or intravenous asparaginase, and intrathecal methotrexate. For T-cell ALL, intravenous cyclophosphamide may be added during induction.

Consolidation is the second phase of treatment, during which intrathecal chemotherapy along with continued systemic therapy and sometimes cranial radiation therapy are given to kill lymphoblasts "hiding" in the meninges. Several months of intensive chemotherapy follows consolidation, often referred to as intensification. This intensification has led to improved survival in pediatric ALL.

Maintenance therapy can include daily oral mercaptopurine, weekly oral methotrexate, and, often, monthly pulses of intravenous vincristine and oral prednisone or dexamethasone. Intrathecal chemotherapy, either with methotrexate alone or combined with cytarabine and hydrocortisone, is usually given every 2–3 months.

Chemotherapy has significant potential side effects. Patients need to be monitored closely to prevent drug toxicities and to ensure early treatment of complications. The duration of treatment ranges between 2.2 years for girls and 3.2 years for boys in COG trials. Treatment for ALL is tailored to prognostic, or risk, groups. A child aged 1–9 years with a WBC count below 50,000/μL at diagnosis and without poor biologic features [t(9;22) or t(4;11)] is considered to be at "standard risk" and receives less intensive therapy than a "high-risk" patient who has a WBC count at diagnosis over 50,000/μL or is 10 years of age or greater. Also important is the patient's response to treatment determined by minimal residual disease (MRD) monitoring. This risk-adapted treatment approach has significantly increased the cure rate among patients with less favorable prognostic features by allowing for early intensification while minimizing treatment-related toxicities in those with favorable features. Bone marrow relapse is usually heralded by an abnormal CBC, either during treatment or following completion of therapy.

The CNS and testes are sanctuary sites of extramedullary leukemia. Currently, about one-third of all ALL relapses are isolated to these sanctuary sites. Systemic chemotherapy does not penetrate these tissues as well as it penetrates other organs. Thus, presymptomatic intrathecal chemotherapy is a critical part of ALL treatment, without which many more relapses would occur in the CNS, with or without bone marrow relapse. The majority of isolated CNS relapses are diagnosed in an asymptomatic child at the time of routine intrathecal injection, when CSF cell count and differential shows an elevated WBC with leukemic blasts. Occasionally, symptoms of CNS relapse develop: headache, nausea and vomiting, irritability, nuchal rigidity, photophobia, changes in vision, and cranial nerve palsies. Currently, testicular relapse occurs in less than 5% of boys. The presentation of testicular relapse is usually unilateral painless testicular enlargement, without a distinct mass. Routine follow-up of boys both on and off treatment includes physical examination of the testes.

Bone marrow transplantation, now called hematopoietic stem cell transplantation (HSCT), is rarely used as initial treatment for ALL, because most patients are cured with chemotherapy alone. Patients whose blasts contain certain chromosomal abnormalities, such as t(9;22) or hypodiploidy (< 44 chromosomes), and patients with a very slow response to therapy may have a better cure rate with early HSCT from a human leukocyte antigen (HLA)-DR–matched sibling donor, or perhaps a matched unrelated donor, than with intensive chemotherapy alone. HSCT cures about 50% of patients who relapse, provided that a second remission is achieved with chemotherapy before transplant. Children who relapse more than 1 year after completion of chemotherapy (late relapse) may be cured with intensive chemotherapy without HSCT.

Several new biologic agents, including tyrosine kinase inhibitors and immunotoxins, are currently in various stages of research, development and in chemotherapeutic trials. Some of these therapies may prove relevant for future treatment of poor risk or relapsed ALL.

Several years ago, Imatinib, a tyrosine kinase inhibitor (TKI), directed against the Philadelphia chromosome (Ph+) protein product, was combined in a backbone of intensive ALL therapy for Ph+ ALL in pediatric patients. The preliminary results of this trial showed a 3 year event-free survival (EFS) of 78% compared to about 50% in historical controls. An ongoing trial for COG in Ph+ ALL is incorporating a newer, more targeted TKI, Dasatinib, into a very similar intensive chemotherapy background with the goal of improving EFS further for this select group of patients. As more is understood about the biology of ALL, further therapy will likely include more of these targeted agents.

B. Supportive Care

Tumor lysis syndrome, which consists of hyperkalemia, hyperuricemia, hyperphosphatemia, should be anticipated when treatment is started. Maintaining brisk urine output with intravenous fluids plus/minus alkalinization of urine with intravenous sodium bicarbonate, and treating with oral allopurinol are appropriate steps in managing tumor lysis syndrome. Rasburicase is indicated for severe tumor lysis syndrome with initial high uric acid values or high WBC at presentation. Serum levels of potassium, phosphorus, and uric acid should be monitored. If superior vena caval or superior mediastinal syndrome is present, general anesthesia is contraindicated temporarily and until there has been some decrease in the mass. If hyperleukocytosis (WBC count > 100,000/μL) is accompanied by hyperviscosity with symptoms of respiratory distress and/or mental status changes, leukophoresis may be indicated to rapidly reduce the number of circulating blasts and minimize the potential thrombotic or hemorrhagic CNS complications. Throughout the course of treatment, all transfused blood and platelet products should be irradiated to prevent graft-versus-host disease from the transfused lymphocytes. Whenever possible, blood products should be leukodepleted to minimize CMV transmission, transfusion reactions, and sensitization to platelets.

Due to the immunocompromised state of the patient with ALL, bacterial, fungal, and viral infections are serious and can be life-threatening or fatal. During the course of treatment, fever (temperature = 38.3°C) and neutropenia (absolute neutrophil count < 500/μL) require prompt assessment, blood cultures from each lumen of a central line, and prompt treatment with empiric broad-spectrum antibiotics. Patients receiving ALL treatment must receive prophylaxis against *Pneumocystis jiroveci* (formerly *Pneumocystis carinii*). Trimethoprim–sulfamethoxazole given twice each day on 2 or 3 consecutive days per week is the drug of choice. Patients who are nonimmune to varicella are at risk for very serious—even fatal—infection. Such patients should receive varicella-zoster immune globulin (VZIG) within 72 hours after exposure and treatment with intravenous acyclovir for active infection.

Prognosis

Cure rates depend on specific prognostic features present at diagnosis, biologic features of the leukemic blast, and the response to therapy. Two of the most important features are WBC count and age. Children aged 1–9 years whose diagnostic WBC count is less than 50,000/μL, standard risk ALL, have an EFS in the 90% range, while children 10 years of age or older have an EFS of approximately 88%. Minimal residual disease (MRD) measurements are now frequently used to determine both the rapidity of response as well as the depth of remission attained at the end of inductin (first 4–6 weeks of therapy). Patients with very low levels of MRD at the end of induction will likely have a superior EFS as compared to other patients with similar initial risk factors but a higher MRD level. On the flip side, by identifying patients with higher MRD at end induction, more intensified therapy can be delivered in order to reduce the MRD and thus, improve the EFS.

Certain chromosomal abnormalities present in the leukemic blasts at diagnosis influence prognosis. Patients with t(9;22), the Philadelphia chromosome, had a poor chance of cure in the past but as discussed earlier in this chapter, now have improved outcome with the incorporation of a directed TKI. Likewise, infants younger than age 6 months with t(4;11) have a poor chance of cure with conventional chemotherapy. In contrast, patients whose blasts are hyperdiploid (containing > 50 chromosomes instead of the normal 46) with trisomies of chromosomes 4, and 10, and patients whose blasts have a t(12;21) and *ETV6-AML1* rearrangement have a greater chance of cure, approaching 95%–97% EFS, than do children without these characteristics.

Advani AS, Hunger SP, Burnett AK: Acute leukemia in adolescents and young adults. Semin Oncol 2009;36(3):213 [PMID: 19460579].

Gaynon PS et al: Long term results of the children's cancer group studies for childhood acute lymphoblastic leukemia 1983–2002: A Children's Oncology Group report. Leukemia 2010:24(2):285 [PMID: 20016531].

Nguyen K et al: Factors influencing survival after relapse from acute lymphoblastic leukemia: A children's oncology group study. Leukemia 2008;22(12):2142 [PMID: 18818707].

Pui CH, Robison LL, Look AT: Acute lymphoblastic leukemia. Lancet 2008;371(9617):1030 [PMID: 18358930].

Schultz KR et al: Improved early event-free survival with imatinib in Philadelphia chromosome-positive Acute Lymphoblastic Leukemia: A children's oncology group study. JCO 2009:27(31): 5175 [PMID: 19805687].

Vrooman LM, Silverman LB: Childhood acute lymphoblastic leukemia: Update on prognostic factors. Curr Opin Pediatr 2009;21(1): 1 [PMID: 19242236].

ACUTE MYELOID LEUKEMIA

ESSENTIALS OF DIAGNOSIS & TYPICAL FEATURES

- Bone marrow aspirate or biopsy shows 20% or more leukemic blasts.
- Fatigue, bleeding, or infection.
- Adenopathy, hepatosplenomegaly, skin nodules (M4 and M5 subtypes).
- Cytopenias: neutropenia (69%), anemia (44%), thrombocytopenia (33%).

General Considerations

Approximately 500 new cases of AML occur per year in children and adolescents in the United States. Although AML accounts for only 25% of all leukemias in this age group, it is responsible for at least one-third of deaths from leukemia in children and teenagers. Congenital conditions associated with an increased risk of AML include Diamond-Blackfan anemia; neurofibromatosis; Down syndrome; Wiskott-Aldrich, Kostmann, and Li-Fraumeni syndromes; as well as chromosomal instability syndromes such as Fanconi anemia. Acquired risk factors include exposure to ionizing radiation, cytotoxic chemotherapeutic agents, and benzenes. However, the vast majority of patients have no identifiable risk factors. Historically, the diagnosis of AML was based almost exclusively on morphology and immunohistochemical staining of the leukemic cells. AML has eight subtypes (M0–M7) according to the French-American-British (FAB) classification (Table 31–1). Immunophenotypic, cytogenetic, and molecular analyses are increasingly important in confirming the diagnosis of AML and subclassifying it into biologically distinct subtypes that have therapeutic and prognostic implications. Recently the World Health Organization (WHO) classification was published to describe AML as AML with recurrent genetic abnormalities with a list of genetic abnormalities sufficient to diagnose AML and then AML not otherwise specified with morphologic descriptions of AML including similar to the FAB classification. Cytogenetic clonal abnormalities occur in 80% of patients with AML and are often predictive of outcome.

Aggressive induction therapy currently results in a 75%–85% complete remission rate. However, long-term survival has improved only modestly to approximately 50%, despite the availability of several effective agents, improvements in supportive care, and increasingly intensive therapies.

Clinical Findings

The clinical manifestations of AML commonly include anemia (44%), thrombocytopenia (33%), and neutropenia (69%). Symptoms may be few and innocuous or may be life-threatening. The median hemoglobin value at diagnosis is 7 g/dL, and platelets usually number fewer than 50,000/μL. Frequently the absolute neutrophil count is under 1000/μL, although the total WBC count is over 100,000/μL in 25% of patients at diagnosis.

Hyperleukocytosis may be associated with life-threatening complications. Venous stasis and sludging of blasts in small vessels cause hypoxia, hemorrhage, and infarction, most notably in the lung and CNS. This clinical picture is a medical emergency requiring rapid intervention, such as leukophoresis, to decrease the leukocyte count. CNS leukemia is present in 5%–15% of patients at diagnosis, a higher rate of initial involvement than in ALL. Certain subtypes,

Table 31–1. FAB subtypes of acute myeloid leukemia.

FAB Classification	Common Name	Distribution in Childhood (Age)		Cytogenetic Associations	Clinical Features
		< 2 y	> 2 y		
M0	Acute myeloid leukemia, minimally differentiated	1%		inv (3q26), t(3;3)	
M1	Acute myeloblastic leukemia without maturation	17%	23%		
M2	Acute myeloblastic leukemia with maturation	26%		t(8;21), t(6;9); rare	Myeloblastomas or chloromas
M3	Acute promyelocytic leukemia	4%		t(15;17); rarely, t(11;17) or (5;17)	Disseminated intravascular coagulation
M4	Acute myelomonoblastic leukemia	30%	24%	11q23, inv 3, t(3;3), t(6;9)	Hyperleukocytosis, CNS involvement, skin and gum infiltration
M4Eo	Acute myelomonoblastic leukemia with abnormal eosinophils			inv16, t(16;16)	
M5	Acute monoblastic leukemia	46%	15%	11q23, t(9;11), t(8;16)	Hyperleukocytosis, CNS involvement, skin and gum infiltration
M6	Erythroleukemia	2%			
M7	Acute megakaryoblastic leukemia	7%	5%	t(1;22)	Down syndrome frequent (< age 2 y)

CNS, central nervous system; FAB, French-American-British classification.

such as M4 and M5, have a higher likelihood of meningeal infiltration than do other subtypes. Additionally, clinically significant coagulopathy may be present at diagnosis in patients with M3, M4, or M5 subtypes. This problem manifests as bleeding or an abnormal disseminated intravascular coagulation screen and should be at least partially corrected prior to initiation of treatment, which may transiently exacerbate the coagulopathy.

Treatment

A. Specific Therapy

AML is less responsive to treatment than ALL and requires more intensive chemotherapy. Toxicities from therapy are common and likely to be life-threatening; therefore, treatment should be undertaken only at a tertiary pediatric oncology center.

Current AML protocols rely on intensive administration of anthracyclines, cytarabine, and etoposide for induction of remission. After remission is obtained patients who have a matched sibling donor undergo allogeneic HSCT, while those without an appropriate related donor are treated with additional cycles of aggressive chemotherapy for a total of 6–9 months. Inv16 and t(8;21) herald a more responsive subtype of AML. In patients with a rapid response to induction chemotherapy, intensive chemotherapy alone may be curative in patient's whose blasts harbor theses cytogenetic abnormalities. Additional recognized genetic risk factors that carry a poor outcome for children with AML include monosomy 7 and Flt3 internal tandem duplications (ITD). HSCT is recommended for all these patients, using either a related or unrelated donor. Trials with risk grouping are ongoing as more is understood about the varying biologic factors.

The biologic heterogeneity of AML is becoming increasingly important therapeutically. The M3 subtype, associated with t(15;17) demonstrated either cytogenetically or molecularly, is currently treated with all *trans*-retinoic acid in addition to chemotherapy with high-dose cytarabine and daunorubicin. All *trans*-retinoic acid leads to differentiation of promyelocytic leukemia cells and can induce remission, but cure requires conventional chemotherapy as well. The use of arsenic trioxide has also been investigated in the treatment of this subtype of AML with favorable results. This subtype has an increased event-free survival over other AML subtypes.

Another biologically distinct subtype of AML occurs in children with Down syndrome, M7, or megakaryocytic AML. Using less intensive treatment, remission induction rate and overall survival of these children are dramatically superior to non–Down syndrome children with AML. It is important that children with Down syndrome receive appropriate treatment specifically designed to be less intensive.

As with ALL, newer biologic agents with more specific targeting are available and undergoing clinical trails. One such agent, sorafenib, appears to be active against AML with Flt3 ITDs. Combining sorafenib with AML therapy has been useful in relapsed disease and is now moving in to upfront trials.

Clofarabine, a newer nucleoside analogue, also has activity in AML and is currently undergoing trials in relapsed and refractory patients with promising results.

B. Supportive Care

Tumor lysis syndrome rarely occurs during induction treatment of AML. Nevertheless, when the diagnostic WBC cell count is greater than 100,000/μL or significant adenopathy or organomegaly is present, one should maintain brisk urine output, and follow potassium, uric acid, and phosphorous laboratory values closely. Hyperleukocytosis (WBC > 100,000/μL) is a medical emergency and, in a symptomatic patient, requires rapid intervention such as leukophoresis to rapidly decrease the number of circulating blasts and thereby decrease hyperviscosity. Delaying transfusion of packed RBCs until the WBC can be decreased to below 100,000/μL avoids exacerbating hyperviscosity. It is also important to correct the coagulopathy commonly associated with M3, M4, or M5 subtypes prior to beginning induction chemotherapy. As with the treatment of ALL, all blood products should be irradiated and leukodepleted; *Pneumocystis* prophylaxis must be administered during treatment and for several weeks afterward; and patients not immune to varicella must receive VZIG within 72 hours of exposure and prompt treatment with intravenous acyclovir for active infection.

Onset of fever (temperature ≥ 38.3°C) or chills associated with neutropenia requires prompt assessment, blood cultures from each lumen of a central venous line, other cultures such as throat or urine as appropriate and prompt initiation of broad-spectrum intravenous antibiotics. Infections in this population of patients can rapidly become life-threatening. Because of the high incidence of invasive fungal infections, there should be a low threshold for initiating antifungal therapy. Filgrastim (granulocyte colony-stimulating factor) may be used to stimulate granulocyte recovery during the treatment of AML and results in shorter periods of neutropenia and hospitalization. It must be stressed that the supportive care for this group of patients is as important as the leukemia-directed therapy and that this treatment should be carried out only at a tertiary pediatric cancer center.

Prognosis

Published results from various centers show a 50%–60% survival rate at 5 years following first remission for patients who do not have matched sibling hematopoietic stem cell donors. Patients with matched sibling donors fare slightly better, with 5-year survival rates of 60%–70% after allogeneic HSCT.

As treatment becomes more sophisticated, outcome is increasingly related to the subtype of AML. Currently, AML in patients with t(8;21), t(15;17), inv 16, or Down syndrome has the most favorable prognosis, with 65%–75% long-term survival using modern treatments, including chemotherapy alone. The least favorable outcome occurs in AML patients with monosomy 7 or 5, 7q, 5q–, 11q23 cytogenetic abnormalities, or Flt 3 mutations.

Gibson BE, Webb DK, Howman AJ, De Graaf SS, Harrison CJ, Wheatley K: Results of a randomized trial in children with Acute Myeloid Leukaemia: Medical Research Council AML12 trial. Br J Haematol 2011 Nov;155(3):366–376 [PMID: 21902686].

Meshinchi S, Arceci RJ: Prognostic factors and risk-based therapy in pediatric acute myeloid leukemia. Oncologist 2007;12:341 [PMID: 17405900].

Neudorf S et al: Allogeneic bone marrow transplantation for children with acute myelocytic leukemia in first remission demonstrates a role for graft versus leukemia in the maintenance of disease-free survival. Blood 2004;103:3655 [PMID: 14751924].

Sternherz PG et al: Clofarabine induced durable complete remission in heavily pretreated adolescents with relapsed and refractory leukemia. J Pediatr Hematol Oncol 2007;29:656 [PMID: 17805046].

Vardiman J et al: The 2008 revision of the World Health Organization (WHO) classification of myeloid neoplasms and acute leukemia: Rationale and important changes. Blood 2009;114:937.

MYELOPROLIFERATIVE DISEASES

ESSENTIALS OF DIAGNOSIS & TYPICAL FEATURES

- Leukocytosis with predominance of immature cells.
- Often indolent course.
- Fever, bone pain, respiratory symptoms.
- Hepatosplenomegaly.

Myeloproliferative diseases in children are relatively rare. They are characterized by ineffective hematopoiesis that results in excessive peripheral blood counts. The three most important types are chronic myelogenous leukemia (CML), which accounts for less than 5% of the childhood leukemias, transient myeloproliferative disorder in children with Down syndrome, and juvenile myelomonocytic leukemia (Table 31–2).

1. Chronic Myelogenous Leukemia

General Considerations

CML with translocation of chromosomes 9 and 22 (the Philadelphia chromosome, Ph+) is identical to adult Ph+CML. Translocation 9;22 results in the fusion of the *BCR* gene on chromosome 22 and the *ABL* gene on chromosome 9. The resulting fusion protein is a constitutively active tyrosine kinase that interacts with a variety of effector proteins and allows for deregulated cellular proliferation, decreased adherence of cells to the bone marrow extracellular matrix, and resistance to apoptosis. The disease usually progresses within 3 years to an accelerated phase and then to a blast crisis. It is generally accepted that Ph+ cells have an increased susceptibility to the acquisition of additional molecular changes that lead to the accelerated and blast phases of disease.

Clinical Findings

Patients with CML may present with nonspecific complaints similar to those of acute leukemia, including bone pain, fever, night sweats, and fatigue. However, patients can also be asymptomatic. Patients with a total WBC count of more than 100,000/μL may have symptoms of leukostasis, such as dyspnea, priapism, or neurologic abnormalities. Physical findings may include fever, pallor, ecchymoses, and hepatosplenomegaly. Anemia, thrombocytosis, and leukocytosis are frequent laboratory findings. The peripheral smear is usually diagnostic, with a characteristic predominance of myeloid cells in all stages of maturation, increased basophils and relatively few blasts.

Table 31–2. Comparison of JMML, CML, and TMD.

	CML	TMD	JMML
Age at onset	> 3 y	< 3 mo	< 2 y
Clinical presentation	Nonspecific constitutional complaints, massive splenomegaly, variable hepatomegaly	DS features, often no or few symptoms; or hepatosplenomegaly, respiratory symptoms	Abrupt onset; eczematoid skin rash, marked lymphadenopathy, bleeding tendency, moderate hepatosplenomegaly, fever
Chromosomal alterations	t(9;22)	Constitutional trisomy 21, but usually no other abnormality	Monosomy or del (7q) in 20% of patients
Laboratory features	Marked leukocytosis (> 100,000/μL), normal to elevated platelet count, decreased to absent leukocyte alkaline phosphatase, usually normal muramidase	Variable leukocytosis, normal to high platelet count, large platelets, myeloblasts	Moderate leukocytosis (> 10,000/μL), thrombocytopenia, monocytosis (> 1000/μL), elevated fetal hemoglobin, normal to diminished leukocyte alkaline phosphatase, elevated muramidase

CML, chronic myelogenous leukemia; DS, Down syndrome; JMML, juvenile myelomonocytic leukemia; TMD, transient myeloproliferative disorder.

Treatment & Prognosis

Historically, hydroxyurea or busulfan has been used to reduce or eliminate Ph+ cells. However, HSCT is the only consistently curative intervention. Reported survival rates for patients younger than age 20 years transplanted in the chronic phase from matched-related donors are 70%–80%. Unrelated stem cell transplants result in survival rates of 50%–65%.

The understanding of the molecular mechanisms involved in the pathogenesis of CML has led to the rational design of molecularly targeted therapy. Imatinib mesylate (Gleevec) is a tyrosine kinase inhibitor that has had dramatic success in the treatment of CML, with most adults and children achieving cytogenetic remission. There are now newer, more targeted TKIs including dasatinib, irlotinib. These medications in adults have an increased incidence of molecular remissions and may be all that is required for long-term survival in adults. The durability of the remission for children with TKIS therapy alone is unclear but is now the accepted upfront therapy.

2. Transient Myeloproliferative Disorder

Transient myeloproliferative disorder is unique to patients with trisomy 21 or mosaicism for trisomy 21. It is characterized by uncontrolled proliferation of blasts, usually of megakaryocytic origin, during early infancy and spontaneous resolution. The pathogenesis of this process is not well understood, although mutations in the *GATA1* gene have recently been implicated as initial events.

Although the true incidence is unknown, it is estimated to occur in up to 10% of patients with Down syndrome. Despite the fact that the process usually resolves by 3 months of age, organ infiltration may cause significant morbidity and mortality.

Patients can present with hydrops fetalis, pericardial or pleural effusions, or hepatic fibrosis. More frequently, they are asymptomatic or only minimally ill. Therefore, treatment is primarily supportive. Patients without symptoms are not treated, and those with organ dysfunction receive low doses of chemotherapy or leukophoresis (or both) to reduce peripheral blood blast counts. Although patients with transient myeloproliferative disorder have apparent resolution of the process, approximately 30% go on to develop acute megakaryoblastic leukemia (AML M7) within 3 years.

3. Juvenile Myelomonocytic Leukemia

Juvenile myelomonocytic leukemia (JMML) accounts for approximately one-third of the myelodysplastic and myeloproliferative disorders in childhood. Patients with neurofibromatosis type 1 (NF-1) are at higher risk of JMML than the general population. It typically occurs in infants and very young children and is occasionally associated with monosomy 7 or a deletion of the long arm of chromosome 7.

Patients with JMML present similarly to those with other hematopoietic malignancies, with lymphadenopathy, hepatosplenomegaly, skin rash, or respiratory symptoms. Patients may have stigmata of NF-1 with neurofibromas or café au lait spots. Laboratory findings include anemia, thrombocytopenia, leukocytosis with monocytosis, and elevated fetal hemoglobin.

The results of chemotherapy for children with JMML have been disappointing, with estimated survival rates of less than 30%. Approximately 40%–45% of patients are projected to survive long term using HSCT, although optimizing conditioning regimens and donor selection may improve these results.

Crispino JD: GATA1 mutations in Down syndrome: Implications for biology and diagnosis of children with transient myeloproliferative disorder and acute megakaryoblastic leukemia. Pediatr Blood Cancer 2005;44:40 [PMID: 15390312].

Gassas A et al: A basic classification and a comprehensive examination of pediatric myeloproliferative syndromes. J Pediatr Hematol Oncol 2005;27:192 [PMID: 15838389].

Lee SJ et al: Impact of prior imatinib mesylate on the outcome of hematopoietic cell transplantation for chronic myeloid leukemia. Blood 2008;112(8):3500 [PMID: 18664621].

Mundschau G et al: Mutagenesis of GATA1 is an initiating event in Down syndrome leukemogenesis. Blood 2003;101:4298 [PMID: 12560215].

Passmore SJ et al: Paediatric myelodysplastic syndromes and juvenile myelomonocytic leukaemia in the UK: A population-based study of incidence and survival. Br J Haematol 2003;121:758 [PMID: 12780790].

Pulsipher MA: Treatment of CML in pediatric patients: Should imatinib mesylate (STI-571, Gleevec) or allogeneic hematopoietic cell transplant be front-line therapy? Pediatr Blood Cancer 2004;43:523 [PMID: 15382266].

Snyder DS: New approved dasatinib regimen available for clinical use. Expert Rev Anticancer Ther 2009;9(3):285 [PMID: 19275507].

Suttorp M: Innovative approaches of targeted therapy for CML of childhood in combination with paediatric haematopoietic SCT. Bone Marrow Transplant 2008;42(Suppl 2):S40 [PMID: 18978743].

Vardiman JW: Chronic myelogenous leukemia, *BCR-ABL1+*. Am J Clin Pathol 2009;132(2):250 [PMID: 19605820].

BRAIN TUMORS

ESSENTIALS OF DIAGNOSIS & TYPICAL FEATURES

- Classic triad: morning headache, vomiting, and papilledema.
- Increasing head circumference, cranial nerve palsies, dysarthria, ataxia, hemiplegia, papilledema, hyperreflexia, macrocephaly, cracked pot sign.
- Seizures, personality change, blurred vision, diplopia, weakness, decreased coordination, precocious puberty.

General Considerations

The classic triad of morning headache, vomiting, and papilledema is present in fewer than 30% of children at presentation. School failure and personality changes are common in older children. Irritability, failure to thrive, and delayed development are common in very young children with brain tumors. Recent-onset head tilt can result from a posterior fossa tumor.

Brain tumors are the most common solid tumors of childhood, accounting for 1500–2000 new malignancies in children each year in the United States and for 25%–30% of all childhood cancers. In general, children with brain tumors have a better prognosis than do adults. Favorable outcome occurs most commonly with low-grade and fully resectable tumors. Unfortunately, cranial irradiation in young children can have significant neuropsychological, intellectual, and endocrinologic sequelae.

Brain tumors in childhood are biologically and histologically heterogeneous, ranging from low-grade localized lesions to high-grade tumors with neuraxis dissemination. High-dose systemic chemotherapy is used frequently, especially in young children with high-grade tumors, in an effort to delay, decrease, or completely avoid cranial irradiation. Such intensive treatment may be accompanied by autologous HSCT or peripheral stem cell reconstitution.

The causes of most pediatric brain tumors are unknown. The risk of developing astrocytomas is increased in children with neurofibromatosis or tuberous sclerosis. Several studies show that some childhood brain tumors occur in families with increased genetic susceptibility to childhood cancers in general, brain tumors, or leukemia and lymphoma. A higher incidence of seizures has been observed in relatives of children with astrocytoma. The risk of developing a brain tumor is increased in children who received cranial irradiation for treatment of meningeal leukemia. All children with gliomas and meningiomas should be screened for NF-1. In children with meningiomas, without the skin findings of NF-1, neurofibromatosis type 2 and Von Hippel-Lindau syndrome should be considered. Inherited germline mutations are possible in atypical teratoid/rhabdoid tumors (AT/RTs) and in choroid plexus carcinomas. Careful family histories should be taken in these tumors and genetic counseling considered.

Because pediatric brain tumors are rare, they are often misdiagnosed or diagnosed late; most pediatricians see no more than two children with brain tumors during their careers.

Clinical Findings

A. Symptoms and Signs

Clinical findings at presentation vary depending on the child's age and the tumor's location. Children younger than age 2 years more commonly have infratentorial tumors. Children with such tumors usually present with nonspecific symptoms such as vomiting, unsteadiness, lethargy, and irritability. Signs may be surprisingly few or may include macrocephaly, ataxia, hyperreflexia, and cranial nerve palsies. Because the head can expand in young children, papilledema is often absent. Measuring head circumference and observing gait are essential in evaluating a child for possible brain tumor. Eye findings and apparent visual disturbances such as difficulty tracking can occur in association with optic pathway tumors such as optic glioma. Optic glioma occurring in a young child is often associated with neurofibromatosis.

Older children more commonly have supratentorial tumors, which are associated with headache, visual symptoms, seizures, and focal neurologic deficits. Initial presenting features are often nonspecific. School failure and personality changes are common. Vaguely described visual disturbance is often present, but the child must be directly asked. Headaches are common, but they often will not be predominantly in the morning. The headaches may be confused with migraine.

Older children with infratentorial tumors characteristically present with symptoms and signs of hydrocephalus, which include progressively worsening morning headache and vomiting, gait unsteadiness, double vision, and papilledema. Cerebellar astrocytomas enlarge slowly, and symptoms may worsen over several months. Morning vomiting may be the only symptom of posterior fossa ependymomas, which originate in the floor of the fourth ventricle near the vomiting center. Children with brainstem tumors may present with facial and extraocular muscle palsies, ataxia, and hemiparesis; hydrocephalus occurs in approximately 25% of these patients at diagnosis.

B. Imaging and Staging

In addition to the tumor biopsy, neuraxis imaging studies are obtained to determine whether dissemination has occurred. It is unusual for brain tumors in children and adolescents to disseminate outside the CNS.

Magnetic resonance imaging (MRI) has become the preferred diagnostic study for pediatric brain tumors. MRI provides better definition of the tumor and delineates indolent gliomas that may not be seen on computed tomography (CT) scan. In contrast, a CT scan can be done in less than 10 minutes—as opposed to the 30 minutes required for an MRI scan—and is still useful if an urgent diagnostic study is necessary or to detect calcification of a tumor. Both scans are generally done with and without contrast enhancement. Contrast enhances regions where the blood-brain barrier is disrupted. Postoperative scans to document the extent of tumor resection should be obtained within 48 hours after surgery to avoid postsurgical enhancement.

Imaging of the entire neuraxis and CSF cytologic examination should be part of the diagnostic evaluation for patients with tumors such as medulloblastoma, ependymoma, and pineal region tumors. Diagnosis of neuraxis drop metastases (tumor spread along the neuraxis) can be accomplished by gadolinium-enhanced MRI incorporating sagittal and axial views. MRI of the spine should be obtained preoperatively in all children with midline tumors of the fourth ventricle or cerebellum. A CSF sample should be obtained during the diagnostic surgery. Lumbar CSF is preferred over ventricular CSF for cytologic examination. Levels of biomarkers in the blood and CSF, such as human chorionic gonadotropin and α-fetoprotein, may be helpful at diagnosis and in follow-up. Both human chorionic gonadotropin and α-fetoprotein should be obtained from the blood preoperatively for all pineal and suprasellar tumors.

The neurosurgeon should discuss staging and sample collection with an oncologist before surgery in a child newly presenting with a scan suggestive of brain tumor.

C. Classification

About 50% of the common pediatric brain tumors occur above the tentorium and 50% in the posterior fossa. In the very young child, posterior fossa tumors are more common. Most childhood brain tumors can be divided into two categories according to the cell of origin: (1) glial tumors, such as astrocytomas and ependymomas, or (2) nonglial tumors, such as medulloblastoma and other primitive neuroectodermal tumors. Some tumors contain both glial and neural elements (eg, ganglioglioma). A group of less common CNS tumors does not fit into either category (ie, craniopharyngiomas, AT/RTs, germ cell tumors, choroid plexus tumors, and meningiomas). Low- and high-grade tumors are found in most categories. Table 31–3 lists the locations and frequencies of the common pediatric brain tumors.

Table 31–3. Location and frequency of common pediatric brain tumors.

Location	Frequency of Occurrence (%)
Hemispheric	**37**
Low-grade astrocytoma	23
High-grade astrocytoma	11
Other	3
Posterior fossa	**49**
Medulloblastoma	15
Cerebellar astrocytoma	15
Brainstem glioma	15
Ependymoma	4
Midline	**14**
Craniopharyngioma	8
Chiasmal glioma	4
Pineal region tumor	2

Table 31–4. Prognostic factors in children with medulloblastoma.

Factor	Favorable	Unfavorable
Extent of disease	Nondisseminated	Disseminated
Histologic features	Undifferentiated, desmoplastic	Large cell, anaplastic
Age	≥ 4 y	< 4 y

Astrocytoma is the most common brain tumor of childhood. Most are juvenile pilocytic astrocytoma (WHO grade I) found in the posterior fossa with a bland cellular morphology and few or no mitotic figures. Low-grade astrocytomas are in many cases curable by complete surgical excision alone. Chemotherapy is effective in low-grade astrocytomas.

Medulloblastoma and related primitive neuroectodermal tumors are the most common high-grade brain tumors in children. These tumors usually occur in the first decade of life, with a peak incidence between ages 5 and 10 years and a female-male ratio of 2.1:1.3. The tumors typically arise in the midline cerebellar vermis, with variable extension into the fourth ventricle. Neuraxis dissemination at diagnosis affects from 10% to 46% of patients. Prognostic factors are outlined in Table 31–4. Determination of risk using histology may soon be replaced by molecular classifications.

Brainstem tumors are third in frequency of occurrence in children. They are frequently of astrocytic origin and often are high grade. Children with tumors that diffusely infiltrate the brainstem and involve primarily the pons have a long-term survival rate of less than 15%. Brainstem tumors that occur above or below the pons and grow in an eccentric or cystic manner have a somewhat better outcome. Exophytic tumors in this location may be amenable to surgery. Generally, brainstem tumors are treated without a tissue diagnosis.

Other brain tumors such as ependymomas, germ cell tumors, choroid plexus tumors, and craniopharyngiomas are less common, and each is associated with unique diagnostic and therapeutic challenges.

Treatment

A. Supportive Care

Dexamethasone should be started prior to initial surgery (0.5–1.0 mg/kg initially, then 0.25–0.5 mg/kg/d in four divided doses). Anticonvulsants (usually phenytoin, 4–8 mg/kg/d) should be started if the child has had a seizure or if the surgical approach is likely to induce seizures. Because postoperative treatment of young children with high-grade brain tumors incorporates increasingly more intensive systemic chemotherapy, consideration should also be given to the use of prophylaxis for prevention of oral candidiasis and

Pneumocystis infection. Dexamethasone and phenytoin potentially reduce the effectiveness of chemotherapy and should be discontinued as soon after surgery as possible.

Optimum care for the pediatric patient with a brain tumor requires a multidisciplinary team including subspecialists in pediatric neurosurgery, neuro-oncology, neurology, endocrinology, neuropsychology, radiation therapy, and rehabilitation medicine, as well as highly specialized nurses, social workers, and staff in physical therapy, occupational therapy, and speech and language science.

B. Specific Therapy

The goal of treatment is to eradicate the tumor with the least short- and long-term morbidity. Long-term neuropsychological morbidity becomes an especially important issue related to deficits caused by the tumor itself and the sequelae of treatment. Meticulous surgical removal of as much tumor as possible is generally the preferred initial approach. Technologic advances in the operating microscope, the ultrasonic tissue aspirator, and the CO_2 laser (which is less commonly used in pediatric brain tumor surgery); the accuracy of computerized stereotactic resection; and the availability of intraoperative monitoring techniques such as evoked potentials and electrocorticography have increased the feasibility and safety of surgical resection of many pediatric brain tumors. Second-look surgery after chemotherapy is increasingly being used when tumors are incompletely resected at initial surgery.

Radiation therapy for pediatric brain tumors is in a state of evolution. For tumors with a high probability of neuraxis dissemination (eg, medulloblastoma), craniospinal irradiation is still standard therapy in children older than age 3 years. In others (eg, ependymoma), craniospinal irradiation has been abandoned because neuraxis dissemination at first relapse is rare. Conformal radiation and the use of three-dimensional treatment planning is now routine.

Chemotherapy is effective in treating low-grade and malignant astrocytomas and medulloblastomas. There is an initial report supporting the effectiveness of chemotherapy in AT/RTs. The therapy used in this study was prolonged and intensive. The utility of chemotherapy in ependymoma is being re-explored in national trials. A series of brain tumor protocols for children younger than age 3 years involved administering intensive chemotherapy after tumor resection and delaying or omitting radiation therapy. The results of these trials have generally been disappointing but have taught valuable lessons regarding the varying responses to chemotherapy of different tumor types. Current trials give shorter courses of more intense chemotherapy with stem cell rescue often followed by conformal radiotherapy. Conformal techniques allow the delivery of radiation to strictly defined fields and may limit side effects.

Perhaps the most exciting development in pediatric neuro-oncology is the development of biologically and clinically relevant subclassifications in both medulloblastoma and ependymoma. This development will drive a new generation of targeted therapy aimed at these biologically defined groups. The definition of four defined biologically defined entities in medulloblastoma, including the Wnt and SHH groups, is the best example of this.

In older children with malignant glioma, the current approach is surgical resection of the tumor and combined-modality treatment with irradiation and intensive chemotherapy. In patients with glioblastoma, the use of high-dose chemotherapy and autologous bone marrow or peripheral stem cell reconstitution is being studied. Initial results have been mixed, but the toxicity of such therapy remains a concern. Surgery is not indicated for diffuse brainstem gliomas. Traditional treatment of these tumors has been local irradiation. Hyperfractionation to increase the dose from the conventional 54 Gy to 72–78 Gy showed no apparent benefit in a recent Children's Cancer Group (CCG) study. New approaches are needed for this prognostically poor tumor.

The treatment of low-grade astrocytomas is evolving. Increasing numbers of young children are receiving antitumor chemotherapeutic agents such as carboplatin and vincristine after incomplete resection of these tumors. The role of irradiation after subtotal resection even in older children is being questioned.

Prognosis

Despite improvements in surgery and radiation therapy, the outlook for cure remains poor for children with high-grade glial tumors. For children with high-grade gliomas, an early CCG study showed a 45% progression-free survival rate for children who received radiation therapy and chemotherapy. A follow-up CCG study in which all patients had chemotherapy and radiation therapy showed a 5-year progression-free survival rate of 36%. There is a possibility of effective salvage therapy with high-dose chemotherapy for children who relapse. In addition, the extent of resection appeared to correlate positively with prognosis, with a 3-year progression-free survival rate of 17% for patients receiving biopsy only, 29%–32% for patients receiving partial or subtotal resections, and 54% for those receiving 90% resections. Biologic factors that may affect survival are being increasingly recognized. The prognosis for diffuse pontine gliomas remains very poor, with no benefit from high-dose chemotherapy plus radiation therapy versus radiation alone.

The 5- and even 10-year survival rate for low-grade astrocytomas of childhood is 60%–90%. However, prognosis depends on both site and grade. A child with a pilocytic astrocytoma of the cerebellum has a considerably better prognosis than a child with a fibrillary astrocytoma of the cerebral cortex. Recently, a new entity of low-grade tumor of childhood, the pilomyxoid astrocytoma has been recognized. Pilomyxoid astrocytomas seem to have a worse prognosis than juvenile pilocytic astrocytomas. For recurrent or progressive low-grade astrocytoma of childhood, relatively moderate chemotherapy may improve the likelihood of survival.

Conventional craniospinal irradiation for children with low-stage medulloblastoma results in survival rates of 60%–90%. Ten-year survival rates are lower (40%–60%). Chemotherapy allows a reduction in the craniospinal radiation dose while preserving survival rates for average-risk patients (86% survival at 5 years on the most recent COG average-risk protocol). However, even reduced-dose craniospinal irradiation has an adverse effect on intellect, especially in children younger than age 7 years. Five-year survival rates for high-risk medulloblastoma have been 25%–40%, but a recent trial reported at the American Society of Clinical Oncology (ASCO) conference in 2007 suggests a dramatically improved prognosis for patients receiving intensive chemotherapy and irradiation. Children with supratentorial primitive neuroectodermal tumors also benefit from the addition of chemotherapy to craniospinal irradiation.

The previously poor prognosis for children with AT/RTs seems improved by intensive multimodality therapy. A single center study suggests an improved outcome for ependymoma using conformational radiation techniques. This awaits confirmation by a national study.

Major challenges remain in treating brain tumors in children younger than age 3 years and in treating brainstem gliomas and malignant gliomas. The increasing emphasis is on the quality of life of survivors, not just the survival rate.

Armstrong GT et al: Long-term outcomes among adult survivors of childhood central nervous system malignancies in the Childhood Cancer Survivor Study. J Natl Cancer Inst 2009;101:946 [PMID: 19535780].

Chi SN et al: Intensive multimodality treatment for children with newly diagnosed CNS atypical teratoid rhabdoid tumor. J Clin Oncol 2009;20:385 [PMID: 19064966].

Jakacki R et al: Outcome for metastatic (M+) medulloblastoma (MB) treated with carboplatin during craniospinal radiotherapy (CSRT) followed by cyclophosphamide (CPM) and vincristine: Preliminary results of COG 99701. J Clin Oncol 2007;25:A2017.

Korshunov A et al: Molecular staging of intracranial ependymoma in children and adults. J Clin Oncol 2010;28:3182 [PMID: 20516456].

Merchant TE et al: Conformal radiotherapy after surgery for paediatric ependymoma: A prospective study. Lancet Oncol 2009;10:258 [PMID: 19274783].

Packer RJ et al: Phase III study of craniospinal radiation therapy followed by adjuvant chemotherapy for newly diagnosed average-risk medulloblastoma. J Clin Oncol 2006;24:4202 [PMID: 16943538].

Northcott PA et al: Medulloblastoma comprises four distinct molecular variants. J Clin Oncol 2011;29:1408 [PMID: 20823417].

LYMPHOMAS & LYMPHOPROLIFERATIVE DISORDERS

The term *lymphoma* refers to a malignant proliferation of lymphoid cells, usually in association with and arising from lymphoid tissues (ie, lymph nodes, thymus, spleen). In contrast, the term *leukemia* refers to a malignancy arising from the bone marrow, which may include lymphoid cells. Because lymphomas can involve the bone marrow, the distinction between the two can be confusing. The diagnosis of lymphoma is a common one among childhood cancers, accounting for 10%–15% of all malignancies. The most common form is Hodgkin disease, which represents nearly half of all cases. The remaining subtypes, referred to collectively as non-Hodgkin lymphoma, are divided into four main groups: lymphoblastic, small noncleaved cell, large B-cell, and anaplastic large cell lymphomas.

In contrast to lymphomas, lymphoproliferative disorders (LPDs) are quite rare in the general population. Most are polyclonal, nonmalignant (though often life-threatening) accumulations of lymphocytes that occur when the immune system fails to control virally transformed lymphocytes. However, a malignant monoclonal proliferation can also arise. The posttransplant LPDs arise in patients who are immunosuppressed to prevent solid organ or bone marrow transplant rejection, particularly liver and heart transplant patients. Spontaneous LPDs occur in immunodeficient individuals and, less commonly, in immunocompetent persons.

1. Hodgkin Disease

ESSENTIALS OF DIAGNOSIS & TYPICAL FEATURES

- Painless cervical (70%–80%) or supraclavicular (25%) adenopathy; mediastinal mass (50%).
- Fatigue, anorexia, weight loss, fever, night sweats, pruritus, cough.

General Considerations

Children with Hodgkin disease have a better response to treatment than do adults, with a 75% overall survival rate at more than 20 years following diagnosis. Although adult therapies are applicable, the management of Hodgkin disease in children younger than age 18 years frequently differs. Because excellent disease control can result from several different therapeutic approaches, selection of staging procedures (radiographic, surgical, or other procedures to determine additional locations of disease) and treatment are often based on the potential long-term toxicity associated with the intervention.

Although Hodgkin disease represents 50% of the lymphomas of childhood, only 15% of all cases occur in children aged 16 years or younger. Children younger than age 5 years account for 3% of childhood cases. There is a 4:1 male predominance in the first decade. Notably, in underdeveloped countries the age distribution is quite different, with a peak incidence in younger children.

Hodgkin disease is subdivided into four histologic groups, and the distribution in children parallels that of adults: lymphocyte-predominant (10%–20%); nodular sclerosing (40%–60%) (increases with age); mixed cellularity (20%–40%); and lymphocyte-depleted (5%–10%). Prognosis is independent of sub classification, with appropriate therapy based on stage (see later discussion of staging).

Clinical Findings

A. Symptoms and Signs

Children with Hodgkin disease usually present with painless cervical adenopathy. The lymph nodes often feel firmer than inflammatory nodes and have a rubbery texture. They may be discrete or matted together and are not fixed to surrounding tissue. The growth rate is variable, and involved nodes may wax and wane in size over weeks to months.

As Hodgkin disease nearly always arises in lymph nodes and spreads to contiguous nodal groups, a detailed examination of all nodal sites is mandatory. Lymphadenopathy is common in children, so the decision to perform biopsy is often difficult or delayed for a prolonged period. Indications for consideration of early lymph node biopsy include lack of identifiable infection in the region drained by the enlarged node, a node greater than 2 cm in size, supraclavicular adenopathy or abnormal chest radiograph, and lymphadenopathy increasing in size after 2 weeks or failing to resolve within 4–8 weeks.

Constitutional symptoms occur in about one-third of children at presentation. Symptoms of fever greater than 38.0°C, weight loss of 10% in the previous 6 months, and drenching night sweats are defined by the Ann Arbor staging criteria as B symptoms. The A designation refers to the absence of these symptoms. B symptoms are of prognostic value, and more aggressive therapy is usually required for cure. Generalized pruritus and pain with alcohol ingestion may also occur.

Half of patients have asymptomatic mediastinal disease (adenopathy or anterior mediastinal mass), although symptoms due to compression of vital structures in the thorax may occur. A chest radiograph should be obtained when lymphoma is being considered. The mediastinum must be evaluated thoroughly before any surgical procedure is undertaken to avoid airway obstruction or cardiovascular collapse during anesthesia and possible death. Splenomegaly or hepatomegaly is generally associated with advanced disease.

B. Laboratory Findings

The CBC is usually normal, although anemia, neutrophilia, eosinophilia, and thrombocytosis may be present. The erythrocyte sedimentation rate and other acute-phase reactants are often elevated and can serve as markers of disease activity. Immunologic abnormalities occur, particularly in cell-mediated immunity, and anergy is common in patients with advanced-stage disease at diagnosis. Autoantibody phenomena such as hemolytic anemia and an idiopathic thrombocytopenic purpura–like picture have been reported.

C. Staging

Staging of Hodgkin disease determines treatment and prognosis. The most common staging system is the Ann Arbor classification that describes extent of disease by I–IV and symptoms by an A or a B suffix (eg, stage IIIB). A systematic search for disease includes chest radiography; CT scan of the chest, abdomen, and pelvis; and bilateral bone marrow aspirates and biopsies. Technetium bone scanning may show bony involvement and is usually reserved for patients with bone pain, as bone involvement is rare. Gallium scanning defines gallium-avid tumors and is most useful in evaluating residual mediastinal disease at the completion of treatment. Positron emission tomography is increasingly used in the staging and follow-up of patients with Hodgkin disease, often replacing gallium scanning.

The staging laparotomy in pediatrics is rarely performed because almost all patients are given systemic chemotherapy rather than radiation therapy. This shift in favored therapy is due to the toxicities of high-dose, extended-field radiation in children and the complications of laparotomy, including postsplenectomy sepsis.

D. Pathologic Findings

The diagnosis of Hodgkin disease requires the histologic presence of the Reed-Sternberg cell or its variants in tissue. Reed-Sternberg cells are germinal-center B cells that have undergone malignant transformation. Nearly 20% of these tumors in developed countries are positive for EBV, and there is building evidence to implicate EBV in the development of Hodgkin disease.

Treatment & Prognosis

To achieve long-term disease-free survival while minimizing treatment toxicity, Hodgkin disease is increasingly treated by chemotherapy alone—and less often by radiation therapy.

Several combinations of chemotherapeutic agents are effective, and treatment times are relatively short compared with pediatric oncology protocols for leukemia. A current COG study is addressing whether only 9 weeks of therapy with AV-PC (Adriamycin [doxorubicin], vincristine, prednisone, and cyclophosphamide) is sufficient to induce a complete response in patients with low-risk Hodgkin disease. Two additional drugs, bleomycin and etoposide, are currently added in the treatment of intermediate-risk patients for a total of 4–6 months of therapy for patients with intermediate-risk disease. The removal of involved field irradiation in patients with intermediate-risk Hodgkin disease who respond early to chemotherapy is being investigated. Combined-modality therapy with chemotherapy and irradiation is used in advanced disease.

Current treatment gives children with stage I and stage II Hodgkin disease at least a 90% disease-free likelihood of survival 5 years after diagnosis, which generally equates with cure. Two-thirds of all relapses occur within 2 years after diagnosis, and relapse rarely occurs beyond 4 years. In more advanced disease (stages III and IV), 5-year event-free survival rates range from over 60% to 90%. With more patients being long-term survivors of Hodgkin disease, the risk of secondary malignancies, both leukemias and solid tumors, is becoming more apparent and is higher in patients receiving radiation therapy. Therefore, elucidating the optimal treatment strategy that minimizes such risk should be the goal of future studies.

Patients with relapsed Hodgkin disease are often salvageable using chemotherapy and radiation therapy. An increasingly popular alternative is autologous HSCT, which may improve survival rates. Allogeneic HSCT is also used, but carries increased risks of complications and may not offer added survival benefit.

Buglio D et al: Novel small-molecule therapy of Hodgkin lymphoma. Expert Rev Anticancer Ther 2007;7:735 [PMID: 17492936].

Freed J et al: Current approaches to the management of pediatric Hodgkin lymphoma. Paediatr Drugs 2010;85 [PMID: 20218745].

Jaglowski SM et al: Lymphomas in adolescents and young adults. Semin Oncol 2009;36:381 [PMID: 19835736].

Keller FG et al: What is the best treatment for children with limited-stage Hodgkin lymphoma? Curr Hematol Malig Rep 2009;4:129 [PMID: 20425426].

2. Non-Hodgkin Lymphoma

ESSENTIALS OF DIAGNOSIS & TYPICAL FEATURES

- Cough, dyspnea, orthopnea, swelling of the face, lymphadenopathy, mediastinal mass, pleural effusion.
- Abdominal pain, abdominal distention, vomiting, constipation, abdominal mass, ascites, hepatosplenomegaly.
- Adenopathy, fevers, neurologic deficit, skin lesions.

General Considerations

Non-Hodgkin lymphomas (NHLs) are a diverse group of cancers accounting for 5%–10% of malignancies in children younger than age 15 years. About 500 new cases arise per year in the United States. The incidence of NHLs increases with age. Children aged 15 years or younger account for only 3% of all cases of NHLs, and the disease is uncommon before age 5 years. There is a male predominance of approximately 3:1. In equatorial Africa, NHLs cause almost 50% of pediatric malignancies.

Most children who develop NHL are immunologically normal. However, children with congenital or acquired immune deficiencies (eg, Wiskott-Aldrich syndrome, severe combined immunodeficiency syndrome, X-linked lymphoproliferative syndrome, HIV infection, immunosuppressive therapy following solid organ or marrow transplantation) have an increased risk of developing NHLs. It has been estimated that their risk is 100–10,000 times that of age-matched control subjects.

Animal models suggest a viral contribution to the pathogenesis of NHL, and there is evidence of viral involvement in human NHL as well. In equatorial Africa, 95% of Burkitt lymphomas contain DNA from the EBV. But in North America, less than 20% of Burkitt tumors contain the EBV genome. The role of other viruses (eg, human herpesviruses 6 and 8), disturbances in host immunologic defenses, chronic immunostimulation, and specific chromosomal rearrangements as potential triggers in the development of NHL is under investigation.

Unlike adult NHL, virtually all childhood NHLs are rapidly proliferating, high-grade, diffuse malignancies. These tumors exhibit aggressive behavior but are usually very responsive to treatment. Nearly all pediatric NHLs are histologically classified into four main groups: lymphoblastic lymphoma (LL), small noncleaved cell lymphoma (Burkitt lymphoma [BL] and Burkitt-like lymphoma [BLL]), large B-cell lymphoma (LBCL), and anaplastic large cell lymphoma (ALCL). Immunophenotyping and cytogenetic features, in addition to clinical presentation, are increasingly important in the classification, pathogenesis, and treatment of NHLs. Comparisons of pediatric NHLs are summarized in Table 31–5.

Clinical Findings

A. Symptoms and Signs

Childhood NHLs can arise in any site of lymphoid tissue, including lymph nodes, thymus, liver, and spleen. Common extralymphatic sites include bone, bone marrow, CNS, skin, and testes. Signs and symptoms at presentation are determined by the location of lesions and the degree of dissemination. Because NHL usually progresses very rapidly, the duration of symptoms is quite brief, from days to a few weeks. Nevertheless, children present with a limited number of syndromes, most of which correlate with cell type.

Children with LL often present with symptoms of airway compression (cough, dyspnea, orthopnea) or superior vena cava obstruction (facial edema, chemosis, plethora, venous engorgement), which are a result of mediastinal disease. *These symptoms are a true emergency necessitating rapid diagnosis and treatment.* Pleural or pericardial effusions may further compromise the patient's respiratory and cardiovascular status. CNS and bone marrow involvement are not common at diagnosis. When bone marrow contains more than 25% lymphoblasts, patients are diagnosed with ALL.

Table 31–5. Comparison of pediatric non-Hodgkin lymphomas.

	Lymphoblastic Lymphoma	Small Noncleaved Cell Lymphoma (BL and BLL)	Large B-Cell Lymphoma	Anaplastic Large Cell Lymphoma
Incidence (%)	30–40	35–50	10–15	10–15
Histopathologic features	Indistinguishable from ALL lymphoblasts	Large nucleus with prominent nucleoli surrounded by very basophilic cytoplasm that contains lipid vacuoles	Large cells with cleaved or noncleaved nuclei	Large pleomorphic cells
Immunopheno-type	Immature T cell	B cell	B cell	T cell or null cell
Cytogenetic markers	Translocations involving chromosome 14q11 and chromosome 7; interstitial deletions of chromosome 1	t(8;14), t(8;22), t(2;8)	Many	t(2;5)
Clinical presentation	Intrathoracic tumor, mediastinal mass (50%–70%), lymphadenopathy above diaphragm (50%–80%)	Intra-abdominal tumor (90%), jaw involvement (10–20% sporadic BL, 70% endemic BL), bone marrow involvement	Abdominal tumor most common; unusual sites: lung, face, brain, bone, testes, muscle	Lymphadenopathy, fever, weight loss, night sweats, extranodal sites including viscera and skin
Treatment	Similar to ALL therapy; 24 mo duration	Intensive administration of alkylating agents and methotrexate; CNS prophylaxis; 3–9 mo duration	Similar to therapy for BL/BLL	Similar to therapy for lymphoblastic lymphoma or BL/BLL

ALL, acute lymphoblastic leukemia; BL, Burkitt lymphoma; BLL, Burkitt-like lymphoma; CNS, central nervous system.

Most patients with BL and BLL present with abdominal disease. Abdominal pain, distention, a right lower quadrant mass, or intussusception in a child older than age 5 years suggests the diagnosis of BL. Bone marrow involvement is common (~65% of patients). BL is the most rapidly proliferating tumor known and has a high rate of spontaneous cell death as it outgrows its blood supply. Consequently, children presenting with massive abdominal disease frequently have tumor lysis syndrome (hyperuricemia, hyperphosphatemia, and hyperkalemia). These abnormalities can be aggravated by tumor infiltration of the kidney or urinary obstruction by tumor. Although similar histologically, numerous differences exist between cases of BL occurring in endemic areas of equatorial Africa and the sporadic cases of North America (Table 31–6).

Table 31–6. Comparison of endemic and sporadic Burkitt lymphoma.

	Endemic	Sporadic
Incidence	10 per 100,000	0.9 per 100,000
Cytogenetics	Chromosome 8 breakpoint upstream of c-*myc* locus	Chromosome 8 breakpoint within c-*myc* locus
EBV association	≥ 95%	≤ 20%
Disease sites at presentation	Jaw (58%), abdomen (58%), CNS (19%), orbit (11%), marrow (7%)	Jaw (7%), abdomen (91%), CNS (14%), orbit (1%), marrow (20%)

CNS, central nervous system; EBV, Epstein-Barr virus.

Large cell lymphomas are similar clinically to the small noncleaved cell lymphomas, although unusual sites of involvement are quite common, particularly with ALCL. Skin lesions, focal neurologic deficits, and pleural or peritoneal effusions without an obvious associated mass are frequently seen.

B. Diagnostic Evaluation

Diagnosis is made by biopsy of involved tissue with histology, immunophenotyping, and cytogenetic studies. If mediastinal disease is present, general anesthesia must be avoided if the airway or vena cava is compromised by tumor. In these cases samples of pleural or ascitic fluid, bone marrow, or peripheral nodes obtained under local anesthesia may confirm the diagnosis. Major abdominal surgery and intestinal resection should be avoided in patients with an abdominal mass that is likely to be BL, as the tumor will regress rapidly with the initiation of chemotherapy. The rapid growth of these tumors and the associated life-threatening complications demand that further studies be done expeditiously so that specific therapy is not delayed.

After a thorough physical examination, a CBC, liver function tests, and a biochemical profile (electrolytes, calcium, phosphorus, uric acid, renal function) should be obtained. An elevated LDH reflects tumor burden and can serve as a marker of disease activity. Imaging studies should include a chest radiograph and chest CT scan, an abdominal ultrasound or CT scan, and possibly a gallium or positron emission tomography scan. Bone marrow and CSF examinations are also essential.

Treatment

A. Supportive Care

The management of life-threatening problems at presentation is critical. The most common complications are superior mediastinal syndrome and acute tumor lysis syndrome. Patients with airway compromise require prompt initiation of specific therapy. Because of the risk of general anesthesia in these patients, it is occasionally necessary to initiate corticosteroids or low-dose emergency radiation therapy until the mass is small enough for a biopsy to be undertaken safely. Response to steroids and radiation therapy is usually prompt (12–24 hours).

Tumor lysis syndrome should be anticipated in all patients who have NHL with a large tumor burden. Maintaining a brisk urine output (> 5 mL/kg/h) with intravenous fluids and diuretics is the key to management. Allopurinol will reduce serum uric acid, and alkalinization of urine will increase its solubility. Rasburicase is an effective intravenous alternative to allopurinol and is increasingly used for patients with high risk of tumor lysis based on tumor burden or in patients who do not have an optimal response to allopurinol. Because phosphate precipitates in alkaline urine, alkali administration should be discontinued if hyperphosphatemia occurs. Renal dialysis is occasionally necessary to control metabolic abnormalities. Every attempt should be made to correct or minimize metabolic abnormalities before initiating chemotherapy; however, this period of stabilization should not exceed 24–48 hours.

B. Specific Therapy

Systemic chemotherapy is the mainstay of therapy for NHLs. Nearly all patients with NHL require intensive intrathecal chemotherapy for CNS prophylaxis. Surgical resection is not indicated unless the entire tumor can be resected safely, which is rare. Partial resection or debulking surgery has no role. Radiation therapy does not improve outcome, so its use is confined to exceptional circumstances.

Therapy for LL is generally based on treatment protocols designed for ALL and involves dose-intensive, multiagent chemotherapy. The duration of therapy is 2 years. Treatment of BL and BLL using alkylating agents and intermediate- to high-dose methotrexate administered intensively but for a relatively short time produce the highest cure rates. LBCL is treated similarly, whereas ALCL has been treated with both BL and LL protocols.

Monoclonal antibodies such as rituximab (anti-CD20) allow for more targeted therapy of lymphomas and have been successful in improving outcomes in adults. Studies employing this type of therapy in children are underway in those with newly diagnosed as well as relapsed or refractory B-cell NHL. Molecular profiling of pediatric lymphomas has identified other potential biologic targets. Developing therapeutics against biologic targets may improve outcomes for patients, particularly those patients with advanced stage disease, while reducing the potential for late effects.

Prognosis

A major predictor of outcome in NHL is the extent of disease at diagnosis. Ninety percent of patients with localized disease can expect long-term, disease-free survival. Patients with extensive disease on both sides of the diaphragm, CNS involvement, or bone marrow involvement in addition to a primary site have a 70%–80% failure-free survival rate. Relapses occur early in NHL; patients with LL rarely have recurrences after 30 months from diagnosis, whereas patients with BL and BLL very rarely have recurrences beyond 1 year. Patients who experience relapse may have a chance for cure by autologous or allogeneic HSCT.

Gore L et al: Emerging non-transplant-based strategies in treating pediatric non-Hodgkin's lymphoma. Curr Hematol Malig Rep 2010;5:177 [PMID: 20640605].

Klapper W et al: Molecular profiling of pediatric mature B-cell lymphoma treated in population-based prospective clinical trials. Blood 2008;112:1374 [PMID: 1850988].

Okur FV et al: Stem cell transplantation in childhood non-Hodgkin's lymphoma. Curr Hematol Malig Rep 2010;2:192 [PMID: 20661786].

Yuston JT et al: Biology and treatment of Burkitt's lymphoma. Curr Opin Hematol 2007;14:375 [PMID: 17534164].

3. Lymphoproliferative Disorders

LPDs can be thought of as a part of a continuum with lymphomas. Whereas LPDs represent inappropriate, often polyclonal proliferations of nonmalignant lymphocytes, lymphomas represent the development of malignant clones, sometimes arising from recognized LPDs.

A. Posttransplantation Lymphoproliferative Disorders

Posttransplantation lymphoproliferative disorders (PTLDs) arise in patients who have received substantial immunosuppressive medications for solid organ or bone marrow transplantation. In these patients, reactivation of latent EBV infection in B cells drives a polyclonal proliferation of these cells that is fatal if not halted. Occasionally a true lymphoma develops, often bearing a chromosomal translocation.

LPDs are an increasingly common and significant complication of transplantation. The incidence of PTLD ranges from approximately 2% to 15% of transplant recipients, depending on the organ transplanted and the immunosuppressive regimen.

Treatment of these disorders is a challenge for transplant physicians and oncologists. The initial treatment is reduction in immunosuppression, which allows the patient's own immune cells to destroy the virally transformed lymphocytes. However, this is only effective in approximately half of the patients. For those patients who do not respond to reduced immune suppression, chemotherapy of various regimens may succeed. The use of anti-B-cell antibodies, such as rituximab (anti-CD20), for the treatment of PTLDs has been promising in clinical trials.

B. Spontaneous Lymphoproliferative Disease

Immunodeficiencies in which LPDs occur include Bloom syndrome, Chédiak-Higashi syndrome, ataxia-telangiectasia, Wiskott-Aldrich syndrome, X-linked lymphoproliferative syndrome, congenital T-cell immunodeficiencies, and HIV infection. Treatment depends on the circumstances, but unlike PTLD, few therapeutic options are often available. Castleman disease is an LPD occurring in pediatric patients without any apparent immunodeficiency. The autoimmune lymphoproliferative syndrome (ALPS) is characterized by widespread lymphadenopathy with hepatosplenomegaly, and autoimmune phenomena. ALPS results from mutations in the Fas ligand pathway that is critical in regulation of apoptosis.

Everly MJ et al: Posttransplant lymphoproliferative disorder. Ann Pharmacother 2007;41:1850 [PMID: 17940127].

Gheorghe G et al: Posttransplant Hodgkin lymphoma preceded by polymorphic posttransplant lymphoproliferative disorder: Report of a pediatric case and review of the literature. J Pediatr Hematol Oncol 2007;29:112 [PMID: 17279008].

Giulina LB et al: Treatment with rituximab in benign and malignant hematologic disorders in children. J Pediatr 2007;150:338 [PMID: 17382107].

Gross TG: Post-transplant lymphoproliferative disease in children following solid organ transplant and rituximab—the final answer? Pediatr Transplant 2007;11:575 [PMID: 17663676].

Kerkar N et al: The changing face of post-transplant lymphoproliferative disease in the era of molecular EBV monitoring. Pediatr Transplant 2010;14:504 [PMID: 20070559].

NEUROBLASTOMA

ESSENTIALS OF DIAGNOSIS & TYPICAL FEATURES

- Bone pain, abdominal pain, anorexia, weight loss, fatigue, fever, irritability.
- Abdominal mass (65%), adenopathy, proptosis, periorbital ecchymosis, skull masses, subcutaneous nodules, hepatomegaly, spinal cord compression.

General Considerations

Neuroblastoma arises from neural crest tissue of the sympathetic ganglia or adrenal medulla. It is composed of small, fairly uniform cells with little cytoplasm and hyperchromatic nuclei that may form rosette patterns. Pathologic diagnosis is not always easy, and neuroblastoma must be differentiated from the other "small, round, blue cell" malignancies of childhood (Ewing sarcoma, rhabdomyosarcoma, peripheral neuroectodermal tumor, and lymphoma).

Neuroblastoma accounts for 7%–10% of pediatric malignancies and is the most common solid neoplasm outside the CNS. Fifty percent of neuroblastomas are diagnosed before age 2 years and 90% before age 5 years.

Neuroblastoma is a biologically diverse disease with varied clinical behavior ranging from spontaneous regression to progression through very aggressive therapy. Unfortunately, despite significant advances in our understanding of this tumor at the cellular and molecular level, the overall survival rate in advanced disease has changed little in 20 years, with 3-year event-free survival being less than 15%.

Clinical Findings

A. Symptoms and Signs

Clinical manifestations vary with the primary site of malignant disease and the neuroendocrine function of the tumor. Many children present with constitutional symptoms such as fever, weight loss, and irritability. Bone pain suggests metastatic disease, which is present in 60% of children older than 1 year of age at diagnosis. Physical examination may reveal a firm, fixed, irregularly shaped mass that extends beyond the midline. The margins are often poorly defined. Although most children have an abdominal primary tumor (40% adrenal gland, 25% paraspinal ganglion), neuroblastoma can arise wherever there is sympathetic tissue. In the posterior mediastinum, the tumor is usually asymptomatic and discovered on a chest radiograph obtained for other reasons. Patients with cervical neuroblastoma present with a neck mass, which is often misdiagnosed as infection. Horner syndrome (unilateral ptosis, myosis, and anhydrosis) or heterochromia iridis (differently colored irises) may accompany cervical neuroblastoma. Paraspinous tumors can extend through the spinal foramina, causing cord compression. Patients may present with paresis, paralysis, and bowel or bladder dysfunction.

The most common sites of metastases are bone, bone marrow, lymph nodes (regional as well as disseminated), liver, and subcutaneous tissue. Neuroblastoma has a predilection for metastasis to the skull, in particular the sphenoid bone and retrobulbar tissue. This causes periorbital ecchymosis and proptosis. Liver metastasis, particularly in the newborn, can be massive. Subcutaneous nodules are bluish in color and associated with an erythematous flush followed by blanching when compressed, probably secondary to catecholamine release.

Neuroblastoma may also be associated with unusual paraneoplastic manifestations. Perhaps the most striking example is opsoclonus-myoclonus, also called dancing eyes/dancing feet syndrome. This phenomenon is characterized by the acute onset of rapid and chaotic eye movements, myoclonic jerking of the limbs and trunk, ataxia, and behavioral disturbances. This process, which often persists after therapy is complete, is thought to be secondary to cross-reacting antineural antibodies. Intractable, chronic watery diarrhea is associated with tumor secretion of vasoactive intestinal peptides. Both of these paraneoplastic syndromes are associated with favorable outcomes.

B. Laboratory Findings

Anemia is present in 60% of children with neuroblastoma and can be due to chronic disease or marrow infiltration. Occasionally, thrombocytopenia is present, but thrombocytosis is a more common finding, even with metastatic disease in the marrow. Urinary catecholamines (vanillylmandelic acid and homovanillic acid) are elevated in at least 90% of patients at diagnosis and should be measured prior to surgery.

C. Imaging

Plain radiographs of the primary tumor may show stippled calcifications. Metastases to bone appear irregular and lytic. Periosteal reaction and pathologic fractures may also be seen. CT scanning provides more information, including the extent of the primary tumor, its effects on surrounding structures, and the presence of liver and lymph node metastases. Classically, in tumors originating from the adrenal gland, the kidney is displaced inferolaterally, which helps to differentiate neuroblastoma from Wilms tumor. MRI is useful in determining the presence of spinal cord involvement in tumors that appear to invade neural foramina.

Technetium bone scanning is obtained for the evaluation of bone metastases, because the tumor usually takes up technetium. Metaiodobenzyl-guanidine (MIBG) scanning is also performed to detect metastatic disease.

D. Staging

Staging of neuroblastoma is performed according to the International Neuroblastoma Staging System (INSS) (Table 31–7). A biopsy of the tumor is performed to determine the biologic characteristics of the tumor. In addition, bilateral bone marrow aspirates and biopsies must be performed to evaluate marrow involvement.

Tumors are classified as favorable or unfavorable based on histologic characteristics. Amplification of the *MYCN* protooncogene is a reliable marker of aggressive clinical behavior with rapid disease progression. Tumor cell DNA content is also predictive of outcome. Hyperdiploidy is a favorable finding, whereas diploid DNA content is associated with a worse outcome.

Table 31–7. International Neuroblastoma Staging System.

Stage	Description
1	Localized tumor with complete gross excision, with or without microscopic residual disease; representative ipsilateral lymph nodes negative for tumor microscopically.
2A	Localized tumor with incomplete gross excision; representative ipsilateral nonadherent lymph nodes negative for tumor microscopically.
2B	Localized tumor with or without complete gross excision, with ipsilateral nonadherent lymph nodes positive for tumor. Enlarged lymph nodes must be negative microscopically.
3	Unresectable unilateral tumor infiltrating across the midline, with or without regional lymph node involvement; or localized unilateral tumor with contralateral regional lymph node involvement; or midline tumor with bilateral extension by infiltration (unresectable) or by lymph node involvement. The midline is defined as the vertebral column. Tumors originating on one side and crossing the midline must infiltrate to or beyond the opposite side of the vertebral column.
4	Any primary tumor with dissemination to distant lymph nodes, bone, bone marrow, liver, skin, or other organs, except as defined for stage 4S.
4S	Localized primary tumor, as defined for stage 1, 2A, or 2B, with dissemination limited to skin, liver, or bone marrow, and limited to infants younger than age 1 y. Marrow involvement should be $< 10\%$ of nucleated cells.

Treatment & Prognosis

Patients are treated based on a risk stratification system adopted by the COG based on INSS stage, age, *MYCN* status, histology, cytogenetic findings, and DNA index. The mainstay of therapy is surgical resection coupled with chemotherapy. The usually massive size of the tumor often makes primary resection impossible. Under these circumstances, only a biopsy is performed. Following chemotherapy, a second surgical procedure may allow for resection of the primary tumor. Radiation therapy is sometimes also necessary. Effective chemotherapeutic agents in the treatment of neuroblastoma include cyclophosphamide, doxorubicin, etoposide, cisplatin, vincristine, and topotecan. About 80% of patients achieve complete or partial remission, although in advanced disease, remission is seldom durable.

For low-risk disease (stage 1 and 2, with good biologic features), surgical resection alone may be sufficient to affect a cure. Infants younger than 1 year with stage 4S disease may need little if any therapy, although chemotherapy may be initiated because of bulky disease causing mechanical complications. In intermediate-risk neuroblastoma (subsets of patients with stage 3 and 4 disease) the primary treatment approach is surgical combined with chemotherapy. High-risk patients (the majority with stage 3 and 4 disease) require multimodal therapy, including surgery, irradiation, chemotherapy, and autologous HSCT. The administration of *cis*-retinoic acid, a differentiating agent, can prolong disease-free survival in advanced-stage neuroblastoma when administered in the setting of minimal residual disease (MRD) after HSCT.

A recent cooperative clinical trial concluded that administration of ch14.18 (a monoclonal antibody specific for the predominant antigen on neuroblastoma cells) and cytokines improves outcome in the high-risk population following HSCT. All patients with high-risk disease are offered this therapy. The current COG trial for high-risk patients is comparing single versus tandem HSCT in this population. Fenretinide, a synthetic retinoid, and radiolabeled MIBG are also under investigation.

For children with stage 1, 2, or 4S disease, the 5-year survival rate is 70%–90%. Infants younger than 460 days old have a greater than 80% likelihood of long-term survival. Children older than age 1 year with stage 3 disease have an intermediate prognosis (approximately 40%–70%). Older patients with stage 4 disease have a poor prognosis (5%–50% survival 5 years from diagnosis), although patients 12–18 months old with hyperdiploidy and nonamplified *MYCN* have an excellent prognosis.

George RE et al: Hyperdiploidy plus nonamplified *MYCN* confers a favorable prognosis in children 12–18 months old with disseminated neuroblastoma: A Pediatric Oncology Group Study. J Clin Oncol 2005;23:6466 [PMID: 16116152].

London WB et al: Evidence for an age cutoff greater than 365 days for neuroblastoma risk group stratification in the Children's Oncology Group. J Clin Oncol 2005;23:6459 [PMID: 16116153].

Matthay KK et al: Opsoclonus myoclonus syndrome in neuroblastoma: A report from a workshop on the dancing eyes syndrome at the advances in neuroblastoma meeting in Genoa, Italy, 2004. Cancer Lett 2005;228:275 [PMID: 15922508].

Mattay KK et al: Long-term results for children with high-risk neuroblastoma treated on a randomized trial of myeloablative therapy followed by 13-cis-retinoic acid: A Children's Oncology Group Study. J Clin Oncol 2009;27:1007 [PMID: 19171716].

Schmidt ML et al: Favorable prognosis for patients 12–18 months of age with stage 4 nonamplified *MYCN* neuroblastoma: A Children's Cancer Group Study. J Clin Oncol 2005;23:6474 [PMID: 16116154].

National Cancer Institute: http://www.cancer.gov/cancertopics/types/neuroblastoma

WILMS TUMOR (NEPHROBLASTOMA)

ESSENTIALS OF DIAGNOSIS & TYPICAL FEATURES

- Asymptomatic abdominal mass or swelling (83%).
- Fever (23%), hematuria (21%).
- Hypertension (25%), genitourinary malformations (6%), aniridia, hemihypertrophy.

General Considerations

Approximately 460 new cases of Wilms tumor occur annually in the United States, representing 5%–6% of cancers in children younger than age 15 years. After neuroblastoma, this is the second most common abdominal tumor in children. The majority of Wilms tumors are of sporadic occurrence. However, in a few children, Wilms tumor occurs in the setting of associated malformations or syndromes, including aniridia, hemihypertrophy, genitourinary malformations (eg, cryptorchidism, hypospadias, gonadal dysgenesis, pseudohermaphroditism, and horseshoe kidney), Beck-with-Wiedemann syndrome, Denys-Drash syndrome, and WAGR syndrome (Wilms tumor, aniridia, ambiguous genitalia, mental retardation).

The median age at diagnosis is related both to gender and laterality, with bilateral tumors presenting at a younger age than unilateral tumors, and males being diagnosed earlier than females. Wilms tumor occurs most commonly between ages 2 and 5 years; it is unusual after age 6 years. The mean age at diagnosis is 4 years.

Clinical Findings

A. Symptoms and Signs

Most children with Wilms tumor present with increasing size of the abdomen or an asymptomatic abdominal mass incidentally discovered by a parent and/or health care provider. The mass is usually smooth and firm, well demarcated, and rarely crosses the midline, though it can extend inferiorly into the pelvis. About 25% of patients are hypertensive at presentation. Gross hematuria is an uncommon presentation, although microscopic hematuria occurs in approximately 25% of patients.

B. Laboratory Findings

The CBC is usually normal, but some patients have anemia secondary to hemorrhage into the tumor. Blood urea nitrogen and serum creatinine are usually normal. Urinalysis may show some blood or leukocytes.

C. Imaging and Staging

Ultrasonography or CT of the abdomen should establish the presence of an intrarenal mass. It is also essential to evaluate the contralateral kidney for presence and function as well as synchronous Wilms tumor. The inferior vena cava needs to be evaluated by ultrasonography with Doppler flow for the presence and extent of tumor propagation. The liver should be imaged for the presence of metastatic disease. Chest CT scan should be obtained to determine whether pulmonary metastases are present. Approximately 10% of patients will have metastatic disease at diagnosis. Of these, 80% will have pulmonary disease and 15% liver metastases. Bone and brain metastases are extremely uncommon and usually associated with the rarer, more aggressive renal tumor types, such as clear cell sarcoma or rhabdoid tumor; hence, bone scans and brain imaging are not routinely performed. The clinical stage is ultimately decided at surgery and confirmed by the pathologist.

Treatment & Prognosis

In the United States, treatment of Wilms tumor begins with surgical exploration of the abdomen via an anterior surgical approach to allow for inspection and palpation of the contralateral kidney. The liver and lymph nodes are inspected and suspicious areas biopsied or excised. En bloc resection of the tumor is performed. Every attempt is made to avoid tumor spillage at surgery as this may increase the staging and treatment. Because therapy is tailored to tumor stage, it is imperative that a surgeon familiar with the staging requirements perform the operation.

In addition to the staging, the histologic type has implications for therapy and prognosis. Favorable histology (FH; see later discussion) refers to the classic triphasic Wilms tumor and its variants. Unfavorable histology (UH) refers to the presence of diffuse anaplasia (extreme nuclear atypia) and is present in 5% of Wilms tumors. Only a few small foci of anaplasia in a Wilms tumor give a worse prognosis to patients with stage II, III, or IV tumors. Loss of heterozygosity of chromosomes 1p and 16q are adverse prognostic factors in those with favorable histology. Following excision and pathologic examination, the patient is assigned a stage that defines further therapy.

Improvement in the treatment of Wilms tumor has resulted in an overall cure rate of approximately 90%. The National Wilms Tumor Study Group's fourth study (NWTS-4) demonstrated that survival rates were improved by intensifying therapy during the initial treatment phase while shortening overall treatment duration (24 weeks vs 60 weeks of treatment).

Table 31–8 provides an overview of the current treatment recommendations in NWTS-5. Patients with stage III or IV Wilms tumor require radiation therapy to the tumor bed and to sites of metastatic disease. Chemotherapy is optimally begun within 5 days after surgery, whereas radiation therapy should be started within 10 days. Stage V (bilateral Wilms tumor) disease dictates a different approach, consisting of possible bilateral renal biopsies followed by chemotherapy and second-look renal-sparing surgery. Radiation therapy may also be necessary.

Using these approaches, 4-year overall survival rates through NWTS-4 are as follows: stage I FH, 96%; stage II–IV FH, 82%–92%; stage I–III UH (diffuse anaplasia), 56%–70%; stage IV UH, 17%. Patients with recurrent Wilms tumor have a salvage rate of approximately 50% with surgery, radiation therapy, and chemotherapy (singly or in combination). HSCT is also being explored as a way to improve the chances of survival after relapse.

Table 31–8. Treatment of Wilms tumor.

Stage/Histologic Subtype	Treatment
I–II FH and I UH	18 wk (dactinomycin and vincristine)
III–IV FH and II–IV focal anaplasia	24 wk (dactinomycin, vincristine, and doxorubicin) with radiation
II–IV UH (diffuse anaplasia)	24 wk (vincristine, doxorubicin, etoposide, and cyclophosphamide) with radiation

FH, favorable histology; UH, unfavorable histology.

Future Considerations

Although progress in the treatment of Wilms tumor has been extraordinary, important questions remain to be answered. Questions have been raised regarding the role of prenephrectomy chemotherapy in the treatment of Wilms tumor. Presurgical chemotherapy seems to decrease tumor rupture at resection but may unfavorably affect outcome by changing staging. Future studies will be directed at minimizing acute and long-term toxicities for those with low-risk disease and improving outcomes for those with high-risk and recurrent disease.

Buckley KS: Pediatric genitourinary tumors. Curr Opin Oncol 2010:23(3):297 [PMID: 21460723].

Davidoff AM: Wilm's tumor. Curr Opin Pediatr 2009;21(3):357 [PMID: 19417665].

Davidoff AM et al: The feasibility and outcome of nephron-sparing surgery for children with bilateral Wilms tumor. The St Jude Children's Research Hospital experience: 1999–2006. Cancer 2008;112(9):2060 [PMID: 18361398].

Gratias EJ, Dome JS: Current and emerging chemotherapy treatment strategies for Wilms tumor in North America. Paediatr Drugs 2008;10(2):115 [PMID: 18345721].

Grundy PE et al: Loss of heterozygosity for chromosomes 1p and 16q is an adverse prognostic factor in favorable-histology Wilms tumor: A report from the National Wilms Tumor Study Group. J Clin Oncol 2005;23:7312 [PMID: 16129848].

Wright KD, Green DM, Daw NC: Late effects of treatment of Wilms tumor. Pediatr Hematol Oncol 2009;26(6):407 [PMID: 19657990].

National Cancer Institute: http://www.cancer.gov/cancertopics/types/wilms

BONE TUMORS

ESSENTIALS OF DIAGNOSIS & TYPICAL FEATURES

- Bone pain.
- Mass lesion noted on examination.

Primary malignant bone tumors are uncommon in childhood with only 650–700 new cases per year. Osteosarcoma accounts for 60% of cases and occurs mostly in adolescents and young adults. Ewing sarcoma is the second most common malignant tumor of bony origin and occurs in toddlers to young adults. Both tumors have a male predominance.

The cardinal signs of bone tumor are pain at the site of involvement, often following slight trauma, mass formation, and fracture through an area of cortical bone destruction.

1. Osteosarcoma

General Considerations

Although osteosarcoma is the sixth most common malignancy in childhood, it ranks third among adolescents and young adults. This peak occurrence during the adolescent growth spurt suggests a causal relationship between rapid bone growth and malignant transformation. Further evidence for this relationship is found in epidemiologic data showing patients with osteosarcoma to be taller than their peers, osteosarcoma occurring most frequently at sites where the greatest increase in length and size of bone occurs, and osteosarcoma occurring at an earlier age in girls than boys, corresponding to their earlier growth spurt. The metaphyses of long tubular bones are primarily affected. The distal femur accounts for more than 40% of cases, with the proximal tibia, proximal humerus, and mid and proximal femur following in frequency.

Clinical Findings

A. Symptoms and Signs

Pain over the involved area is the usual presenting symptom with or without an associated soft tissue mass. Patients generally have symptoms for several months prior to diagnosis. Systemic symptoms (fever, weight loss) are rare. Laboratory evaluation may reveal elevated serum alkaline phosphatase or LDH levels.

B. Imaging and Staging

Radiographic findings show permeative destruction of the normal bony trabecular pattern with indistinct margins. In addition, periosteal new bone formation and lifting of the bony cortex may create a Codman triangle. A soft tissue mass plus calcifications in a radial or sunburst pattern are frequently noted. MRI is more sensitive in defining the extent of the primary tumor and has mostly replaced CT scanning. The most common sites of metastases are the lung (≤ 20% of newly diagnosed cases) and the additional boney sites (10%). CT scan of the chest and bone scan are essential for detecting metastatic disease. Bone marrow aspirates and biopsies are not indicated.

Despite the rather characteristic radiographic appearance, a tissue sample is needed to confirm the diagnosis. Placement of the incision for biopsy is of critical importance. A misplaced incision could preclude a limb salvage procedure and necessitate amputation. The surgeon who will carry out the definitive surgical procedure should perform the biopsy. A staging system for osteosarcoma based on local tumor extent and presence or absence of distant metastasis has been proposed, but it has not been validated.

Treatment & Prognosis

Historical studies showed that over 50% of patients receiving surgery alone developed pulmonary metastases within 6 months after surgery. This suggests the presence of micrometastatic disease at diagnosis. Adjuvant chemotherapy trials showed improved disease-free survival rates of 55%–85% in patients followed for 3–10 years.

Osteosarcomas are highly radioresistant lesions; for this reason, radiation therapy has no role in its primary management. Chemotherapy is often administered prior to definitive surgery (neoadjuvant chemotherapy). This permits an early attack on micrometastatic disease and may also shrink the tumor, facilitating a limb salvage procedure. Preoperative chemotherapy also makes detailed histologic evaluation of tumor response to the chemotherapy agents possible. If the histologic response is poor (> 10% viable tumor tissue), postoperative chemotherapy can be changed accordingly. Chemotherapy may be administered intra-arterially or intravenously, although the benefits of intra-arterial chemotherapy are disputed. Agents having efficacy in the treatment of osteosarcoma include doxorubicin, cisplatin, high-dose methotrexate, and ifosfamide.

Definitive cure requires en bloc surgical resection of the tumor with a margin of uninvolved tissue. Amputation, limb salvage, and rotationplasty (Van Ness rotation) are equally effective in achieving local control of osteosarcoma. Contraindications to limb-sparing surgery include major involvement of the neurovascular bundle by tumor; immature skeletal age, particularly for lower extremity tumors; infection in the region of the tumor; inappropriate biopsy site; and extensive muscle involvement that would result in a poor functional outcome.

Postsurgical chemotherapy is generally continued until the patient has received 1 year of treatment. Relapses are unusual beyond 3 years, but late relapses do occur. Histologic response to neoadjuvant chemotherapy is an excellent predictor of outcome. Patients with localized disease having 90% tumor necrosis have a 70%–85% long-term, disease-free survival rate. Other favorable prognostic factors include distal skeletal lesions, longer duration of symptoms, age older than 20 years, female gender, and near-diploid tumor DNA index. Patients with metastatic disease at diagnosis or multifocal bone lesions do not fair well, despite advances in chemotherapy and surgical techniques.

2. Ewing Sarcoma

General Considerations

Ewing sarcoma accounts for only 10% of primary malignant bone tumors; fewer than 200 new cases occur each year in the United States. It is a disease primarily of white males, almost never affects blacks, and occurs mostly in the second decade of life. Ewing sarcoma is considered a "small, round, blue cell" malignancy. The differential diagnosis includes rhabdomyosarcoma, lymphoma, and neuroblastoma. Although most commonly a tumor of bone, it may also occur in soft tissue (extraosseous Ewing sarcoma or peripheral neuroectodermal tumor [PNET]).

Clinical Findings

A. Symptoms and Signs

Pain at the site of the primary tumor is the most common presenting sign, with or without swelling and erythema. No specific laboratory findings are characteristic of Ewing sarcoma, but an elevated LDH may be present and is of prognostic significance. Associated symptoms include fevers and weight loss.

B. Imaging and Staging

The radiographic appearance of Ewing sarcoma overlaps with osteosarcoma, although Ewing sarcoma usually involves the diaphyses of long bones. The central axial skeleton gives rise to 40% of Ewing tumors. Evaluation of a patient diagnosed as having Ewing sarcoma should include an MRI of the primary lesion to define the extent of local disease as precisely as possible. This is imperative for planning future surgical procedures or radiation therapy. Metastatic disease is present in 25% of patients at diagnosis. The lung (38%), bone (particularly the spine) (31%), and the bone marrow (11%) are the most common sites for metastasis. CT scan of the chest, bone scan, and bilateral bone marrow aspirates and biopsies are all essential to the staging workup.

A biopsy is essential in establishing the diagnosis. Histologically, Ewing sarcoma consists of sheets of undifferentiated cells with hyperchromatic nuclei, well-defined cell borders, and scanty cytoplasm. Necrosis is common. Electron microscopy, immunocytochemistry, and cytogenetics may be necessary to confirm the diagnosis. A generous tissue biopsy specimen is often necessary for diagnosis but should not delay starting chemotherapy.

A consistent cytogenetic abnormality, t(11;22), has been identified in Ewing sarcoma and PNET and is present in 85%–90% of tumors. These tumors also express the protooncogene c-*myc*, which may be helpful in differentiating Ewing sarcoma from neuroblastoma, in which c-*myc* is not expressed.

Treatment & Prognosis

Therapy usually commences with the administration of chemotherapy after biopsy and is followed by local control measures. Depending on many factors, including the primary site of the tumor and the response to chemotherapy, local control can be achieved by surgery, radiation therapy, or a combination of these methods. Following local control, chemotherapy continues for approximately 1 year. Effective treatment for Ewing sarcoma uses combinations of dactinomycin, vincristine, doxorubicin, cyclophosphamide, etoposide, and ifosfamide. Recent data showed that giving chemotherapy every 2 weeks, rather than every 3 weeks, improved the event-free survival for localized Ewing sarcoma.

Patients with small localized primary tumors have a 50%–70% long-term, disease-free survival rate. For patients with metastatic disease and large pelvic primary tumors, survival is poor. Autologous HSCT is being investigated for the treatment of these high-risk patients.

Bernstein M et al: Ewing's sarcoma family of tumors: Current management. Oncologist 2006;11:503 [PMID: 16720851].

Geller DS, Gorlick R: Osteosarcoma: A review of diagnosis, management and treatement strategies. Clin Adv Hematol Oncol 2010;8(10):705 [PMID: 2137869].

Grimer RJ et al: Surgical options for children with osteosarcoma. Lancet Oncol 2005;6:85 [PMID: 15683817].

Heare T et al: Bone tumors. Curr Opin Pediatr 2009;21(3):365 [PMID: 19421061].

Meyer JS et al: Imaging guidelines for children with Ewing sarcoma and osteosarcoma: A report from the Children's Oncology Group Bone Tumor Committee. Pediatr Blood Cancer 2008;51(2):163 [PMID: 18454470].

Subbiah V et al: Ewing's sarcoma: Standard and experimental treatment options. Curr Treat Options Oncol 2009;10(1–2):126 [PMID: 19533369].

RHABDOMYOSARCOMA

ESSENTIALS OF DIAGNOSIS & TYPICAL FEATURES

- Painless, progressively enlarging mass; proptosis; chronic drainage (nasal, aural, sinus, vaginal); cranial nerve palsies.
- Urinary obstruction, constipation, hematuria.

General Considerations

Rhabdomyosarcoma is the most common soft tissue sarcoma occurring in childhood and accounts for 10% of solid tumors in childhood. The peak incidence occurs at ages 2–5 years; 70% of children are diagnosed before age 10 years. A second smaller peak is seen in adolescents with extremity tumors. Males are affected more commonly than females.

Rhabdomyosarcoma can occur anywhere in the body. When rhabdomyosarcoma imitates striated muscle and cross-striations are seen by light microscopy, the diagnosis is straightforward. Immunohistochemistry, electron microscopy, or chromosomal analysis is sometimes necessary to make the diagnosis. Rhabdomyosarcoma is further classified into subtypes based on pathologic features: embryonal

(60%–80%), of which botryoid is a variant; alveolar (about 15%–20%); undifferentiated sarcoma (8%); pleomorphic, which is seen in adults (1%); and other (11%). These subtypes occur in characteristic locations and have different metastatic potentials and outcomes.

Although the pathogenesis of rhabdomyosarcoma is unknown, in rare cases a genetic predisposition has been determined. Li-Fraumeni syndrome is an inherited mutation of the *p53* tumor suppressor gene that results in a high risk of bone and soft tissue sarcomas in childhood plus breast cancer and other malignant neoplasms before age 45 years. Two characteristic chromosomal translocations [t(2;13) and t(1;13)] have been described in alveolar rhabdomyosarcoma. The t(1;13) translocation appears to be a favorable prognostic feature in patients with metastatic alveolar rhabdomyosarcoma, whereas t(2;13) is associated with poor outcomes.

Clinical Findings

A. Symptoms and Signs

The presenting symptoms and signs of rhabdomyosarcoma result from disturbances of normal body function due to tumor growth (Table 31–9). For example, patients with orbital rhabdomyosarcoma present with proptosis, whereas patients with rhabdomyosarcoma of the bladder can present with hematuria, urinary obstruction, or a pelvic mass.

B. Imaging

A plain radiograph and a CT and/or MRI scan should be obtained to determine the extent of the primary tumor and to assess regional lymph nodes. A chest CT scan is obtained to rule out pulmonary metastasis, the most common site of metastatic disease at diagnosis. A skeletal survey and a bone scan are obtained to determine whether bony metastases are present. Bilateral bone marrow biopsies and aspirates are obtained to rule out bone marrow infiltration. Additional studies may be warranted in certain sites. For example, in parameningeal primary tumors, a lumbar puncture is performed to evaluate CSF for tumor cells.

Treatment

Optimal management and treatment of rhabdomyosarcoma is complex and requires combined modality therapy. When feasible, the tumor should be excised, but this is not always possible because of the site of origin and size of tumor. When only partial tumor resection is feasible, the operative procedure is usually limited to biopsy and sampling of lymph nodes. Debulking of unresectable tumor may improve outcomes. Chemotherapy can often convert an inoperable tumor to a resectable one. A second-look procedure to remove residual disease and confirm the clinical response to chemotherapy and radiation therapy is generally performed at about week 20 of therapy.

Radiation therapy is an effective method of local tumor control for both microscopic and gross residual disease. It is generally administered to all patients, the only exception being those with a localized tumor that has been completely resected. All patients with rhabdomyosarcoma receive chemotherapy, even when the tumor is fully resected at diagnosis. The exact regimen and duration of chemotherapy are determined by primary site, group, and tumor node metastasis classification. Vincristine, dactinomycin, and cyclophosphamide have shown the greatest efficacy in the treatment of rhabdomyosarcoma. Newer agents such as irinotecan are also being used in the upfront treatment of metastatic rhabomyosarcoma based on good responses in relapsed disease. Newer treatment strategies for high-risk patients include different drug combinations and dosing schedules

Table 31–9. Characteristics of rhabdomyosarcoma.

Primary Site	Frequency (%)	Symptoms and Signs	Predominant Pathologic Subtype
Head and neck	**35**		Embryonal
Orbit	9	Proptosis	
Parameningeal	16	Cranial nerve palsies; aural or sinus obstruction with or without drainage	
Other	10	Painless, progressively enlarging mass	
Genitourinary	**22**		Embryonal (botryoid variant in bladder and vagina)
Bladder and prostate	13	Hematuria, urinary obstruction	
Vagina and uterus	2	Pelvic mass, vaginal discharge	
Paratesticular	7	Painless mass	
Extremities	**18**	Adolescents, swelling of affected body part	Alveolar (50%), undifferentiated
Other	25	Mass	Alveolar, undifferentiated

with hematopoietic growth factor support, hyperfractionated radiation therapy, and autologous HSCT.

Prognosis

The age of the patient, the extent of tumor at diagnosis, the primary site, the pathologic subtype, and the response to treatment all influence the long-term, disease-free survival rate from the time of diagnosis. Children with localized disease at diagnosis have a 70%–75% 3-year disease-free survival rate, whereas children with metastatic disease at presentation have a worse outcome (39% 3-year disease-free survival).

Hayes-Jordan A, Andrassy R: Rhabdomyosarcoma in children. Curr Opin Pediatr 2009;21(3):373 [PMID: 19448544].

Joshi D et al: Age is an independent prognostic factor in rhabdomyosarcoma: A report from the Soft Tissue Sarcoma Committee of the Children's Oncology Group. Pediatr Blood Cancer 2004;42:64 [PMID: 14752797].

Raney RB et al: Results of treatment of fifty-six patients with localized retroperitoneal and pelvic rhabdomyosarcoma: A report from the Intergroup Rhabdomyosarcoma Study-IV, 1991–1997. Pediatr Blood Cancer 2004;42:618 [PMID: 15127417].

Raney RB et al: Rhabdomyosarcoma and undifferentiated sarcoma in the first two decades of life: A selective review of Intergroup Rhabdomyosarcoma Study Group experience and rational for Intergroup Rhabdomyosarcoma Study V. J Pediatr Hematol Oncol 2001;23(4):215 [PMID: 11846299].

Rodeberg D, Paidas C: Childhood rhabdomyosarcoma. Semin Pediatr Surg 2006;15(1):57 [PMID: 16458847].

National Cancer Institute: http://www.cancer.gov/cancertopics/types/childrhabdomyosarcoma

RETINOBLASTOMA

General Considerations

Retinoblastoma is a neuroectodermal malignancy arising from embryonic retinal cells that accounts for 3% of malignant disease in children younger than age 15 years. It is the most common intraocular tumor in pediatric patients and causes 5% of cases of childhood blindness. In the United States, 200–300 new cases occur per year. This is a malignancy of early childhood, with 90% of the tumors diagnosed before age 5 years. Bilateral involvement occurs in 20%–30% of children and typically is diagnosed at a younger age (median age 14 months) than unilateral disease (median age 23 months).

Retinoblastoma is the prototype of hereditary cancers due to a mutation in the retinoblastoma gene (*RB1*), which is located on the long arm of chromosome 13 (13q14). This gene is a tumor-suppressor gene that normally controls cellular growth. When the gene is inactivated, as in retinoblastoma, cellular growth is uncontrolled. Uncontrolled cell growth leads to tumor formation. Inactivation of both *RB1* alleles within the same cell is required for tumor formation.

Retinoblastoma is known to arise in heritable and nonheritable forms. Based on the different clinical characteristics of the two forms, Knudson proposed a "two-hit" hypothesis for retinoblastoma tumor development. He postulated that two independent events were necessary for a cell to acquire tumor potential. Mutations at the *RB1* locus can be inherited or arise spontaneously. In heritable cases, the first mutation arises during gametogenesis, either spontaneously (90%) or through transmission from a parent (10%). This mutation is present in every retinal cell and in all other somatic and germ cells. Ninety percent of persons who carry this germline mutation will develop retinoblastoma. For tumor formation, the loss of the second *RB1* allele within a cell must occur; loss of only one allele is insufficient for tumor formation. The second mutation occurs in a somatic (retinal) cell. In nonheritable cases (60%), both mutations arise in a somatic cell after gametogenesis has taken place.

Clinical Findings

A. Symptoms and Signs

Children with retinoblastoma generally come to medical attention while the tumor is still confined to the globe. Although present at birth, retinoblastoma is not usually detected until it has grown to a considerable size. Leukocoria (white pupillary reflex) is the most common sign (found in 60% of patients). Parents may note an unusual appearance of the eye or asymmetry of the eyes in a photograph. The differential diagnosis of leukocoria includes *Toxocara canis* granuloma, astrocytic hamartoma, retinopathy of prematurity, Coats disease, and persistent hyperplastic primary vitreous. Strabismus (in 20% of patients) is seen when the tumor involves the macula and central vision is lost. Rarely (in 7% of patients), a painful red eye with glaucoma, a hyphema, or proptosis is the initial manifestation. A single focus or multiple foci of tumor may be seen in one or both eyes at diagnosis. Bilateral involvement occurs in 20%–30% of children.

B. Diagnostic Evaluation

Suspected retinoblastoma requires a detailed ophthalmologic examination under general anesthesia. An ophthalmologist makes the diagnosis of retinoblastoma by the appearance of the tumor within the eye without pathologic confirmation. A white to creamy pink mass protruding into the vitreous matter suggests the diagnosis; intraocular calcifications and vitreous seeding are virtually pathognomonic of retinoblastoma. A CT scan of the orbits and MRI of the orbits/brain detects intraocular calcification, evaluates the optic nerve for tumor infiltration, and detects extraocular extension of tumor. A single focus or multiple foci of tumor may be seen in one or both eyes at diagnosis. Metastatic disease of the marrow and meninges can be ruled out with bilateral bone marrow aspirates and biopsies plus CSF cytology.

Treatment

Each eye is treated according to the potential for useful vision, and every attempt is made to preserve vision. The choice of therapy depends on the size, location, and number of intraocular lesions. Absolute indications for enucleation include no vision, neovascular glaucoma, inability to examine the treated eye, and inability to control tumor growth with conservative treatment. External beam irradiation has been the mainstay of therapy. A total dose of 35–45 Gy is administered. However, many centers are investigating the role of systemic chemotherapy for the treatment of retinoblastoma confined to the globe and the elimination of external beam radiotherapy is now accepted. Cryotherapy, photocoagulation, and radioactive plaques can be used for local tumor control. Patients with metastatic disease receive chemotherapy.

Children with retinoblastoma confined to the retina (whether unilateral or bilateral) have an excellent prognosis, with 5-year survival rates greater than 90%. Mortality is correlated directly with extent of optic nerve involvement, orbital extension of tumor, and massive choroid invasion. Patients who have disease in the optic nerve beyond the lamina cribrosa have a 5-year survival rate of only 40%. Patients with meningeal or metastatic spread rarely survive, although intensive chemotherapy and autologous HSCT have produced long-term survivors.

Patients with the germline mutation (heritable form) have a significant risk of developing second primary tumors. Osteosarcomas account for 40% of such tumors. Second malignant neoplasms occur in both patients who have and those who have not received radiation therapy. The 30-year cumulative incidence for a second neoplasm is 35% in patients who received radiation therapy and 6% in those who did not receive radiation therapy. The risk continues to increase over time. Although radiation contributes to the risk, it is the presence of the retinoblastoma gene itself that is responsible for the development of nonocular tumors in these patients.

Abramson DH, Sxhefler AC: Update on retinoblastoma. Retina 2004;24:828 [PMID: 15579980].

Canty CA: Retinoblastoma: An overview for advanced practice nurses. J Am Acad nurse Pract 2009;21(3):149 [PMID: 19302690].

Kiss S, Leiderman YI, Mukai S: Diagnosis, classification and treatment of retinoblastoma. Int Ophthalmol Clin 2008;48(2):135 [PMID: 18427266].

Lin P, O'Brien JM: Frontiers in the management of retinoblastoma. Am J Ophthalmol 2009;148(2):192 [PMID: 19477707].

Rodriguez-Galindo C et al: Treatment of intraocular retinoblastoma with vincristine and carboplatin. J Clin Oncol 2003;15:2019 [PMID: 12743157].

Sastre X et al: Proceedings of the consensus meetings from the International Retinoblastoma Staging Working Group on the pathology guidelines for the examination of enucleated eyes and evaluation of prognostic risk factors in retinoblastoma. Arch Pathol Lab Med 2009;133(8):1199 [PMID: 19653709].

Shields C et al: Continuing challenges in the management of retinoblastoma with chemotherapy. Retina 2004;24:849 [PMID: 15579981].

HEPATIC TUMORS (SEE ALSO CHAPTER 22)

Two-thirds of liver masses found in childhood are malignant. Ninety percent of hepatic malignancies are either hepatoblastoma or hepatocellular carcinoma. Hepatoblastoma accounts for the vast majority of liver tumors in children younger than age 5 years, hepatocellular carcinoma for the majority in children aged 15–19 years. The features of these hepatic malignancies are compared in Table 31–10. Of the benign tumors, 60% are hamartomas or vascular tumors such as hemangiomas. There is mounting evidence for a strong association between prematurity and the risk of hepatoblastoma.

Table 31–10. Comparison of hepatoblastoma and hepatocellular carcinoma in childhood.

	Hepatoblastoma	Hepatocellular Carcinoma
Median age at presentation	1 y (0–3 y)	12 y (5–18 y)
Male-female ratio	1.7:1	1.4:1
Associated conditions	Hemihypertrophy, Beckwith-Wiedemann syndrome, prematurity, Gardner syndrome	Hepatitis B virus infection, hereditary tyrosinemia, biliary cirrhosis, α_1-antitrypsin deficiency
Pathologic features	Fetal or embryonal cells; mesenchymal component (30%)	Large pleomorphic tumor cells and tumor giant cells
Solitary hepatic lesion	80%	20%–50%
Unique features at diagnosis	Osteopenia (20%–30%), isosexual precocity (3%)	Hemoperitoneum, polycythemia
Laboratory features		
Hyperbilirubinemia	5%	25%
Elevated AFP	> 90%	50%
Abnormal liver function tests	15%–30%	> 30%–50%

AFP, α-fetoprotein.

Children with hepatic tumors usually come to medical attention because of an enlarging abdomen. Approximately 10% of hepatoblastomas are first discovered on routine examination. Anorexia, weight loss, vomiting, and abdominal pain are associated more commonly with hepatocellular carcinoma. Serum α-fetoprotein is often elevated and is an excellent marker for response to treatment.

Imaging studies should include abdominal ultrasound, CT scan, or MRI. Malignant tumors have a diffuse hyperechoic pattern on ultrasonography, whereas benign tumors are usually poorly echoic. Vascular lesions contain areas with varying degrees of echogenicity. Ultrasound is also useful for imaging the hepatic veins, portal veins, and inferior vena cava. CT scanning and, in particular, MRI are important for defining the extent of tumor within the liver. CT scanning of the chest should be obtained to evaluate for metastatic spread. Because bone marrow involvement is extremely rare, bone marrow aspirates and biopsies are not indicated.

The prognosis for children with hepatic malignancies depends on the tumor type and the resectability of the tumor. Complete resectability is essential for survival. Chemotherapy can decrease the size of most hepatoblastomas. Following biopsy of the lesion, neoadjuvant chemotherapy is administered prior to attempting complete surgical resection. Monitoring the rate of decline of the alpha fetoprotein levels can help indicate favorable versus poor responders to chemotherapy. Chemotherapy can often convert an inoperable tumor to a completely resectable one and can also eradicate metastatic disease. Approximately 50%–60% of hepatoblastomas are fully resectable, whereas only one-third of hepatocellular carcinomas can be completely removed. Even with complete resection, only one-third of patients with hepatocellular carcinoma are long-term survivors. A recent CCG/Pediatric Oncology Group trial has shown cisplatin, fluorouracil, and vincristine to be as effective as but less toxic than cisplatin and doxorubicin in treating hepatoblastoma. The current open Children's Oncology Group trial is using cisplatin, fluorouracil, vincristine, and doxorubicin along with the cardioprotectant dexrazoxane in intermediate and high risk patients. Other drug combinations that have demonstrated benefit include carboplatin plus etoposide and doxorubicin plus ifosfamide. Liver transplantation has been shown to be a successful surgical option in patients whose tumors are considered to be unresectable.

Faraj W et al: Liver transplantation for hepatoblastoma. Liver Transpl 2008;14:1614 [PMID: 18975296].

Feusner J, Plaschkes J: Hepatoblastoma and low birth weight: A trend or chance observation? Med Pediatr Oncol 2002;39:508 [PMID: 12228908].

Katzenstein HM et al: Hepatocellular carcinoma in children and adolescents: Results from the Pediatric Oncology Group and the Children's Cancer Group intergroup study. J Clin Oncol 2002;12:2789 [PMID: 12065555].

Katzenstein HM et al: Treatment of unresectable and metastatic hepatoblastoma: A Pediatric Oncology Group Phase II study. J Clin Oncol 2002;20:3438 [PMID: 12177104].

Malogolowkin MH et al: Intensified platinum therapy is an ineffective strategy for improving outcome in pediatric patients with advanced hepatoblastoma. J Clin Oncol 2006;24:2879 [PMID: 16782927].

LANGERHANS CELL HISTIOCYTOSIS

ESSENTIALS OF DIAGNOSIS & TYPICAL FEATURES

- Seborrheic skin rashes.
- Diaper rash.
- Draining ears.
- Bone pain.

General Considerations

Langerhans cell histiocytosis (LCH; formerly called histiocytosis X) is a rare and poorly understood spectrum of disorders. It can occur as an isolated lesion or as widespread systemic disease involving virtually any body site. Eosinophilic granuloma, Hand-Schüller-Christian disease, and Letterer-Siwe disease are all syndromes encompassed by this disorder. LCH is not a true malignancy, but instead is a clonal, reactive proliferation of normal histiocytic cells, perhaps resulting from an immunoregulatory defect.

The distinctive pathologic feature is proliferation of histiocytic cells beyond what would be seen in a normal inflammatory process. Langerhans histiocytes have typical features: on light microscopy, the nuclei are deeply indented (coffee bean–shaped) and elongated, and the cytoplasm is pale, distinct, and abundant. Additional diagnostic characteristics include Birbeck granules on electron microscopy, expression of CD1 on the cell surface, and positive immunostaining for S-100 protein.

Clinical Findings

Because LCH encompasses a broad spectrum of diseases; its presentation can be variable, from a single asymptomatic lesion to widely disseminated disease.

Patients with localized disease present primarily with lesions limited to bone. Occasionally found incidentally on radiographs obtained for other reasons, these lesions are well-demarcated and frequently found in the skull, clavicles, ribs, and vertebrae. These lesions can be painful. Patients can also present with localized disease of the skin, often as a diaper rash that does not resolve.

Bony lesions, fever, weight loss, otitis media, exophthalmos, and diabetes insipidus occur in a small number of children with the disease. Children with this multifocal disease, formerly called Hand-Schüller-Christian disease, commonly present with generalized symptoms and organ dysfunction.

Children with disseminated LCH (formerly called Letterer-Siwe disease) typically present before age 2 years with a seborrheic skin rash, fever, weight loss, lymphadenopathy, hepatosplenomegaly, and hematologic abnormalities.

Diagnosis is made with biopsy of the involved organ. The workup should include a CBC, liver and kidney function tests, a skeletal survey or technetium bone scan, and a urinalysis with specific gravity to rule out diabetes insipidus.

Treatment & Prognosis

The outcome in LCH is extremely variable, but the process usually resolves spontaneously. Isolated lesions may need no therapy at all. Intralesional corticosteroids, curettage, and low-dose radiation therapy are useful local treatment measures for symptomatic focal lesions. Patients with localized disease have an excellent prognosis.

Multifocal disease is often treated with systemic chemotherapy. Prednisone and vinblastine are used for mutlifocal disease or disease involving other organs such as liver, spleen, hematopoietic system. The agents are given repeatedly or continuously until lesions heal; the drugs can then be reduced and finally stopped. A common therapeutic protocol for LCH is LCH III. Other active chemotherapeutic agents include 6-mercaptopurine, methotrexate, and etoposide. HSCT can also be used with success in refractory cases.

Multifocal disease is less predictable, but most cases resolve without sequelae. Age, degree of organ involvement, and response to therapy are the most important prognostic factors. Infants with disseminated disease tend to do poorly, with mortality rates approaching 50%. New treatment approaches for patients who do not respond to conventional chemotherapy have been evaluated in small studies. 2-Chlorodeoxyadenosine (2-CDA) has been used with some success. Therapeutic strategies targeting the dysregulated immune response using interferon-α or etanercept (anti–tumor necrosis factor-α) have also been reported.

Cooper N et al: The use of reduced-intensity stem cell transplantation in haemophagoacytic lymphohistiocytosis and Langerhans cell histiocytosis. Bone Marrow transplant 2008;42(Suppl 2):S47 [PMID: 18978744].

Gasent Blesa JM et al: Langerhans cell histiocytosis. Clin Transl Oncol 2008;10(11):688 [PMID: 19015065].

Henter JI et al: Successful treatment of Langerhan's cell histiocytosis with etanercept. N Engl J Med 2001;345:1577 [PMID: 11794238].

Jubran RF et al: Predictors of outcome in children with Langerhans cell histiocytosis. Pediatr Blood Cancer 2005;45:37 [PMID: 15768381].

Rodriquez-Galindo C et al: Treatment of children with Langerhans cell histiocytosis with 2-chlorodeoxyadenosine. Am J Hematol 2002;69:179 [PMID: 11891804].

Satter EK, High WA: Langerhans cell histiocytosis: A review of the current recommendations of the Histiocyte Society. Pediatr Dermatol 2008;25(3):291 [PMID: 18577030].

Weitzman S, Egeler RM: Langerhans cell histiocytosis: Update for the pediatrician. Curr Opin Pediatr 2008;20(1):23 [PMID: 18197035]. www.histiocytesociety.org

HEMATOPOIETIC STEM CELL TRANSPLANT

Amy K. Keating, MD, Roger H. Giller, MD, & Ralph R. Quinones, MD

GENERAL CONSIDERATIONS

Hematopoietic stem cell transplant (HSCT) is considered standard therapy for a variety of malignancies, hematopoietic disorders (aplastic anemia, hemoglobinopathies), storage diseases, and severe immunodeficiencies. In most instances, high doses of chemotherapy and/or radiation are given to the HSCT patient for myeloablation prior to infusion of stem cells which rescue marrow function. HSCT can be divided into two main categories: autologous, infusion of the patient's own hematopoietic stem cells, or allogeneic, infusion of another individual's (donor) hematopoietic stem cells. Stem cells can be obtained from bone marrow, peripheral blood, or umbilical cord blood.

The rationale for HSCT in patients with nonmalignant disorders is to use the transplanted donor stem cells to replace the defective hematopoietic or lymphoid elements of the recipient. For children with oncologic disorders, the rationale for HSCT is multifaceted. The extremely high doses of chemotherapy and/or radiation optimize tumor kill by overcoming potential cancer cell chemoresistance. Additionally, in patients who receive an allogeneic HSCT, the donor lymphoid cells may recognize the cancer as foreign and provide an immunologic attack on the malignancy, a concept known as the graft-versus-tumor (GVT) effect.

Autologous transplantation, often referred to as "stem cell rescue," is restricted to the treatment of certain pediatric malignancies: neuroblastoma, lymphoma, selected brain tumors, germ cell tumors, and Ewing sarcoma. Relapse of the malignancy continues to be the greatest obstacle in autologous transplantation, likely due to limitations in achieving systemic cancer control prior to transplant and lack of GVT effect.

Allogeneic transplantation rescues hematopoiesis with stem cells from another person, either within the immediate family or an unrelated individual from a volunteer bank. Allogeneic HSCT patients require additional therapy to provide immunosuppression both to prevent rejection of donor cells and to reduce risk of graft versus host disease (GVHD).

The selection of a suitable donor, who matches the recipient most closely at the HLA antigens, HLA-A, B, C, DR, and potentially DQ, is critical, as these mediate graft rejection and GVHD. Each child expresses one set of paternal and one set of maternal HLA antigens. Thus, the probability of one child inheriting any specific combination and matching another sibling for an allogeneic transplant is one in four. Large worldwide registries for bone marrow and umbilical cord blood donors have been developed; however, finding a closely matched unrelated donor can be challenging, especially for underrepresented minorities.

Supportive care in the initial weeks after transplant includes management of chemotherapy side effects, prevention and treatment of infection, nutritional support, and immunosuppression to lessen the potential development of GVHD in allogeneic HSCT recipients. Additionally, because a post-HSCT patient will not have a functioning marrow for several weeks following preparative therapy, they will need blood product support. These blood products should be leukocyte-depleted to reduce the risk of CMV transmission and irradiated to prevent GVHD from contaminating lymphocytes that remain even in leukocyte-reduced blood products.

HSCT COMPLICATIONS

HSCT patients are profoundly immunocompromised for many months following transplantation and infections from bacteria, viruses, fungi, and protozoa account for significant morbidity and mortality. During the early phase (0–1 month after transplant), when there is profound neutropenia and mucosal disruption, bacteria from the patient's aerodigestive tract are common culprits in bacteremia. Additionally, the presence of a central venous catheter makes gram-positive bacteremia an important consideration. Therefore, empiric antibiotic coverage and intravenous immune globulin supplementation are used to decrease the risk of bacterial sepsis. Acyclovir prophylaxis is used to prevent the reactivation of herpes simplex virus that may occur early in up to 70% of seropositive patients, while antifungal therapies are routinely used to prevent infections from fungi, particularly Candida and Aspergillus.

In the intermediate phase (1–6 months after transplant), the HSCT patient usually has adequate neutrophil counts and yet remains significantly compromised due to reduced T-lymphocyte cell quantity and function. Because of this relative T-cell defect a child after transplant is susceptible to sudden, overwhelming illness from viral pathogens. CMV reactivation or new infection is relatively common and can result in retinitis, enteritis, and pneumonia. Treatment with foscarnet and ganciclovir is usually successful if CMV infection is recognized early. Common community acquired viruses, such as respiratory syncytial virus, adenovirus, influenza, parainfluenza, and human metapneumovirus, can also be life-threatening; therefore, prevention is critical through frequent hand washing and contact restriction, and treatment with available antiviral therapies, such as inhaled ribavirin, can be lifesaving in this population. Prophylactic administration of acyclovir helps limit reactivation of herpes simplex virus and varicella-zoster virus (shingles) while trimethoprim–sulfamethoxazole, dapsone, or pentamidine prophylaxis reduces, but does not eliminate, *P jiroveci* pneumonia. The late phase (6–12 months after transplant) is characterized by dysfunction of the reticuloendothelial system, leading to infections from encapsulated bacteria such as *Pneumococcus,* and ongoing inadequate lymphocyte function, resulting in poor control of viral infection and reactivation. Patients on immunosuppressive treatment for GVHD have increased and protracted risk of all types of infections.

Graft versus host disease results when donor lymphocytes recognize the HSCT patient tissues as foreign and mount an immunologic attack. Despite the use of immunosuppressive agents, anti–T-cell antibodies, and T-cell depletion of the donor graft, 20%–70% of allogeneic HSCT patients experience some degree of acute GVHD. Factors influencing GVHD risk include the degree of HLA match, stem cell source, patient age, and donor sex. Acute GVHD generally occurs within the first 100 days after transplant and presents with a maculopapular skin rash, secretory diarrhea, and cholestatic jaundice. Chronic GVHD occurs after day 100 and may involve multiple organ systems. Sclerotic skin, malabsorption, weight loss, keratoconjunctivitis sicca, oral mucositis, chronic lung disease, and cholestatic jaundice are common manifestations. Treatment for GVHD consists of further use of immunosuppressive agents.

Long-term follow-up of HSCT patients is essential. Patients are at risk for numerous complications, including pulmonary disease, cataracts, endocrine dysfunction affecting growth and fertility, cardiac dysfunction, avascular necrosis of bone, developmental delay, and secondary malignancies. Although HSCT has many challenges, it represents an important advance in curative treatment for a variety of serious pediatric illnesses.

MacMillan ML et al: Transplant outcomes in bone marrow failure syndromes and hemoglobinopathies. Semin Hematol 2010 Jan;47(1):37–45 [Review] [PMID: 20109610].

Peters C et al: Stem cell source and outcome after hematopoietic stem cell transplantation (HSCT) in children and adolescents with acute leukemia. Pediatr Clin North Am 2010 Feb;57(1):27–46 [Review] [PMID: 20307710].

Rocha V et al: Pediatric related and unrelated cord blood transplantation for malignant diseases. Bone Marrow Transplant 2009 Nov;44(10):653–659 [Epub 2009 Oct 5] [Review] [PMID: 19802021].

LATE EFFECTS OF PEDIATRIC CANCER THERAPY

Late effects of treatment by surgery, radiation, and chemotherapy have been identified in survivors of pediatric cancer. Current estimates are that 1 in every 640 adults between the ages of 20 and 39 years is a pediatric cancer survivor. One recent study found that 60% of survivors of pediatric cancer diagnosed between 1970 and 1986 have at least one chronic condition. Virtually any organ system can demonstrate sequelae related to previous cancer therapy. This has necessitated the creation of specialized oncology clinics whose function is to identify and provide treatment to these patients.

The Childhood Cancer Survivor Study, a pediatric multi-institutional collaborative project, was designed to investigate the various aspects of late effects of pediatric cancer therapy in a cohort of over 13,000 survivors of childhood cancer.

GROWTH COMPLICATIONS

Children who have received cranial irradiation are at highest risk of developing growth complications. Growth complications of cancer therapy in the pediatric survivor are generally secondary to direct damage to the pituitary gland, resulting in growth hormone deficiency. However, new evidence in children treated for ALL suggests that chemotherapy alone may result in an attenuation of linear growth without evidence of catch-up growth once therapy is discontinued. Up to 90% of patients who receive more than 30 Gy of radiation to the CNS will show evidence of growth hormone deficiency within 2 years. Approximately 50% of children receiving 24 Gy will have growth hormone problems. The effects of cranial irradiation appear to be age-related, with children younger than age 5 years at the time of therapy being particularly vulnerable. These patients usually benefit from growth hormone therapy. Currently, there is no evidence that such therapy causes a recurrence of cancer.

Spinal irradiation inhibits vertebral body growth. In 30% of treated children, standing heights may be less than the fifth percentile. Asymmetrical exposure of the spine to radiation may result in scoliosis.

Growth should be monitored closely, particularly in young survivors of childhood cancer. Follow-up studies should include height, weight, growth velocity, scoliosis examination, and, when indicated, growth hormone testing.

ENDOCRINE COMPLICATIONS

Thyroid dysfunction, manifesting as hypothyroidism, is common in children who received total body irradiation, cranial irradiation, or local radiation therapy to the neck and/or mediastinum. Particularly at risk are children with brain tumors who received more than 3000 cGy and those who received more than 4000 cGy to the neck region. The average time to develop thyroid dysfunction is 12 months after exposure, but the range is wide. Therefore, individuals at risk should be monitored yearly for at least 7 years from the completion of therapy. Although signs and symptoms of hypothyroidism may be present, most patients will have a normal thyroxine level with an elevated thyroid-stimulating hormone level. These individuals should be given thyroid hormone replacement because persistent stimulation of the thyroid from an elevated thyroid-stimulating hormone level may predispose to thyroid nodules and carcinomas. In a recent report from the Childhood Cancer Survivor Study, thyroid cancer occurred at 18 times the expected rate for the general population in pediatric cancer survivors who received radiation to the neck region. Hyperthyroidism, although rare, also occurs in patients who have received neck irradiation.

Precocious puberty, delayed puberty, and infertility are all potential consequences of cancer therapy. Precocious puberty, more common in girls, is usually a result of cranial irradiation causing premature activation of the hypothalamic-pituitary axis. This results in premature closure of the epiphysis and decreased adult height. Luteinizing hormone analogue and growth hormone are used to halt early puberty and facilitate continued growth.

Gonadal dysfunction in males is usually the result of radiation to the testes. Patients who receive testicular irradiation as part of their therapy for ALL, abdominal irradiation for Hodgkin disease, or total body irradiation for HSCT are at highest risk. Radiation damages both the germinal epithelium (producing azoospermia) and Leydig cells (causing low testosterone levels and delayed puberty). Alkylating agents such as ifosfamide and cyclophosphamide can also interfere with male gonadal function, resulting in oligospermia or azoospermia, low testosterone levels, and abnormal follicle-stimulating hormone (FSH) and luteinizing hormone (LH) levels. Determination of testicular size, semen analysis, and measurement of testosterone, FSH, and LH levels will help identify abnormalities in patients at risk. When therapy is expected to result in gonadal dysfunction, pretherapy sperm banking should be offered to adolescent males.

Exposure of the ovaries to abdominal radiation may result in delayed puberty with a resultant increase in FSH and LH and a decrease in estrogen. Girls receiving total body irradiation as preparation for HSCT and those receiving craniospinal irradiation are at particularly high risk for delayed puberty as well as premature menopause. In patients at high risk for development of gonadal complications, a detailed menstrual history should be obtained, and LH, FSH, and estrogen levels should be monitored if indicated.

No studies to date have confirmed an increased risk of spontaneous abortions, stillbirths, premature births, congenital malformations, or genetic diseases in the offspring of childhood cancer survivors. Women who have received abdominal irradiation may develop uterine vascular insufficiency or fibrosis of the abdominal and pelvic musculature or uterus, and their pregnancies should be considered high risk.

CARDIOPULMONARY COMPLICATIONS

Pulmonary dysfunction generally manifests as pulmonary fibrosis. Therapy-related factors known to cause pulmonary toxicities include certain chemotherapeutic agents, such as bleomycin, the nitrosoureas, and busulfan, as well as lung or total body irradiation. Pulmonary toxicity due to chemotherapy is related to the total cumulative dose received. Pulmonary function tests in patients with therapy-induced toxicity show restrictive lung disease, with decreased carbon monoxide diffusion and small lung volumes. Individuals exposed to these risk factors should be counseled to refrain from smoking and to give proper notification of the treatment history if they should require general anesthesia.

Cardiac complications usually result from exposure to anthracyclines (daunorubicin, doxorubicin, and mitoxantrone), which destroy myocytes and lead to inadequate myocardial growth as the child ages, and eventually result in congestive heart failure. The incidence of anthracycline cardiomyopathy increases in a dose-dependent fashion. A recent report indicates that survivors receiving cumulative doses larger than 360 mg/m^2 were more than 40 times more likely to die of cardiac disease. In a recent study, complications from these agents appeared 6–19 years following administration of the drugs. Pregnant women who have received anthracyclines should be followed closely for signs and symptoms of congestive heart failure, as peripartum cardiomyopathy has been reported.

Radiation therapy to the mediastinal region, which is a common component of therapy for Hodgkin disease, has been linked to an increased risk of coronary artery disease; chronic restrictive pericarditis may also occur in these patients.

Current recommendations include an echocardiogram and electrocardiogram every 1–5 years, depending on the age at therapy, total cumulative dose received, and presence or absence of mediastinal irradiation. Selective monitoring with various modalities is indicated for those who were treated with anthracyclines when they were younger than age 4 years or received more than 500 mg/m^2 of these drugs. Biomarkers such as cardiac troponins and brain naturetic peptides may be useful in assessing cardiotoxicity of anthracyclines.

RENAL COMPLICATIONS

Long-term renal side effects stem from therapy with cisplatin, alkylating agents (ifosfamide and cyclophosphamide), or pelvic irradiation. Patients who have received cisplatin may develop abnormal creatinine clearance, which may or may not be accompanied by abnormal serum creatinine levels, as well as persistent tubular dysfunction with hypomagnesemia. Alkylating agents can cause hemorrhagic cystitis, which may continue after chemotherapy has been terminated and has been associated with the development of bladder carcinoma. Ifosfamide can also cause Fanconi syndrome, which may result in clinical rickets if adequate phosphate replacement is not provided. Pelvic irradiation may result in abnormal bladder function with dribbling, frequency, and enuresis.

Patients seen in long-term follow-up who have received nephrotoxic agents should be monitored with urinalysis, appropriate electrolyte profiles, and blood pressure. Urine collection for creatinine clearance or renal ultrasound may be indicated in individuals with suspected renal toxicity.

NEUROPSYCHOLOGICAL COMPLICATIONS

Pediatric cancer survivors who have received cranial irradiation for ALL or brain tumors appear to be at greatest risk for neuropsychological sequelae. The severity of cranial irradiation effects varies among individual patients and depends on the dose and dose schedule, the size and location of the radiation field, the amount of time elapsed after treatment, the child's age at therapy, and the child's gender. Girls may be more susceptible than boys to CNS toxicity because of more rapid brain growth and development during childhood.

Auditory complications can be seen in childhood cancer survivors exposed to platinum-based chemotherapy and/or temporal or posterior fossa radiation. Difficulty hearing sounds, tinnitus, or hearing loss requiring an aid have been reported.

The main effects of CNS irradiation appear to be related to attention capacities, ability with nonverbal tasks and mathematics, and short-term memory. Recent studies support the association between treatment with high-dose systemic methotrexate, triple intrathecal chemotherapy, and, more recently, dexamethasone and more significant cognitive impairment.

Additionally, pediatric cancer patients have been reported as having more behavior problems and as being less socially competent than a sibling control group. Adolescent survivors of cancer demonstrate an increased sense of physical fragility and vulnerability manifested as hypochondriasis or phobic behaviors.

A recent report from Childhood Cancer Survivor Study noted that when compared to population norms, childhood cancer survivors and siblings report positive psychological health, good health-related quality of life, and life satisfaction. There are, however, subgroups that could be targeted for intervention.

SECOND MALIGNANCIES

Approximately 3%–12% of children receiving cancer treatment will develop a new cancer within 20 years of their first diagnosis. This is a 10-fold increased incidence when compared with age-matched control subjects. Particular risk factors include exposure to alkylating agents, epipodophyllotoxins (etoposide), and radiation therapy, primary diagnosis of retinoblastoma or Hodgkin disease, or the presence of an inherited genetic susceptibility syndrome (Li-Fraumeni syndrome or NF). In a recent report, the cumulative estimated incidence of second malignant neoplasms for the cohort of the Childhood Cancer Survivor Study was 3.2% at 20 years from diagnosis.

Second hematopoietic malignancies (acute myelogenous leukemia) occur as a result of therapy with epipodophyllotoxins or alkylating agents. The schedule of drug administration (etoposide) and the total dose may be related to the development of this secondary leukemia.

Children receiving radiation therapy are at risk for developing second malignancies, such as sarcomas, carcinomas, or brain tumors, in the field of radiation. A recent report examining the incidence of second neoplasms in a cohort of pediatric Hodgkin disease patients showed the cumulative risk of a second neoplasm to be as high as 8% at 15 years from diagnosis. The most common solid tumor was breast cancer (the majority located within the radiation field) followed by thyroid cancer. Girls aged 10–16 years when they received radiation therapy were at highest risk and had an actuarial incidence that approached 35% by age 40 years.

Chow EJ et al: Decreased adult height in survivors of childhood acute lymphoblastic leukemia: A report from the Childhood Cancer Survivor Study. J Pediatr 2007;150:370 [PMID: 17382112].

Green DM et al: Fertility of female survivors of childhood cancer: A report from the childhood cancer survivor study. J Clin Oncol 2009;27:2677 [PMID: 19364965].

Henderson TO et al: Secondary sarcomas in childhood cancer survivors: A report from the Childhood Cancer Survivor Study. J Natl Cancer Inst 2007;99:300 [PMID: 17312307].

Oeffinger KC et al: Chronic health conditions in adult survivors of childhood cancer. N Engl J Med 2006;355:1572 [PMID: 17035650].

Schultz KA et al: Behavioral and social outcomes in adolescent survivors of childhood cancer: A report from the Childhood Cancer Survivor Study. J Clin Oncol 2007;25:3649 [PMID: 17704415].

Trachtenberg BH et al: Anthracycline-associated cardiotoxicity in survivors of childhood cancer. Pediatr Cardiol 2011;32:342.

Whelan K et al: Auditory complications in childhood cancer survivors: A report from the Childhood Cancer Survivor Study. Pediatr Blood Cancer 2011;57:126.

Zeltzer LK et al: Psychological outcomes and health-related quality of life in adult childhood cancer survivors: A report from the childhood cancer survivor study. Cancer Epidemiol Biomarkers Prev 2008;17:435 [PMID: 18268128].

32 Pain Management & Pediatric Palliative & End-of-Life Care

Brian S. Greffe, MD
Jeffrey L. Galinkin, MD
Nancy A. King, MSN, RN, CPNP

Children experience pain to at least the same level as adults. Multiple studies have shown that neonates and infants perceive pain and have memory of these painful experiences. Frequently, children are underprescribed and underdosed for opioid and nonopioid analgesics due to excessive concerns of respiratory depression and/or poor understanding of the need for pain medications in children. Few data are available to guide the dosing of many pain medications and the majority of pain medications available on the market today are unlabeled for use in pediatric patients.

PAIN ASSESSMENT

Standardizing pain measurements require the use of appropriate pain scales. At most institutions, pain scales are stratified by age (Table 32–1) and are used throughout the institution from operating room to medical floor to clinic, creating a common language around a patient's pain. Pain assessment by scales has become the "5th vital sign" in hospital settings and is documented at least as frequently as heart rate and blood pressure at many pediatric centers around the world. There are many pain scales available, all of which have advantages and disadvantages (Figures 32–1 and 32–2, and Table 32–2, for example). It is less important what type of scale is used, but that they are used on a consistent basis.

Special Populations

Noncommunicative patients such as neonates and the cognitively impaired are often difficult to assess for pain. For these patients, using an appropriate assessment tool (see Table 32–1) on a frequent basis (every 1–2 hours) is essential in ensuring adequate pain control. For these populations, increasing pain score trends are often a sign of discomfort.

ACUTE PAIN

Definition Etiology

Acute pain is caused by an identifiable source. In most cases, it is self-limiting and treatment is a reflection of severity and type of injury. In children, the majority of acute pain is caused by trauma or, if in a hospital setting, an iatrogenic source such as surgery.

Treatment

Treatment of acute pain is dependent on the disposition of the individual patient. For outpatient care, the mainstay of treatment is nonsteroidal anti-inflammatory drugs (NSAIDs) (Table 32–3). Acetaminophen is the most commonly used NSAID. Acetaminophen is administered via the oral or rectal routes. Acetaminophen is more predictable in its effects as an oral dose. It has also been found that round-the-clock administration (oral 10–15 mg/kg, rectal 20 mg/kg) is better than PRN dosing for both minor pain or as an adjunct for major pain. The toxicity of acetaminophen is low in clinically used doses. However, the use of acetaminophen combined with many over-the-counter and prescription-combination products has been a frequent cause of toxicity. Liver damage or failure can occur with doses exceeding 200 mg/kg/d. Other oral analgesics available in suspension are ibuprofen (10–15 mg/kg) and naproxen (10–20 mg/kg).

When pain is more severe, oral opioids can be added for short-term use (Table 32–4). Many of these opioids come formulated with an NSAID, that is, oxycodone/acetaminophen (Percocet) and hydrocodone/acetaminophen (Lortab). When using these combination drugs, the dose of drug is based on the opioid component. Other concomitantly administered similar NSAIDs should be discontinued. The most commonly used oral opioids are oxycodone, hydrocodone, and codeine. The use of codeine is least recommended due to its metabolism. Codeine is metabolized to morphine via the cytochrome P-450 2D4 isoenzyme. From 1% to 10% people (Asians 1%–2%, African Americans 1%–3%, Caucasians 5%–10%) are poor metabolizers as a result of a genetic polymorphism. Thus, patients with this defect get no effect from this drug. A very small percentage of patients (primarily from East Africa) are ultrarapid metabolizers. These patients convert 10–15 times the amount of parent

Table 32–1. Pain scales—description and age-appropriate use.

Name of Scale	Type	Description	Age Group
Numeric	Self-report	Verbal 0–10 scale; 0 = no pain, 10 = worst pain you could ever imagine	Children who understand the concept of numbers, rank, and order; approximately > 8 y
Bieri and Wong-Baker scales	Self-report	6 faces that range from no pain to the worst pain you can imagine	Younger children who have difficulty with numeric scale; cognitive age 3–7 y
FLACC	Behavioral observer	5 categories: face, legs, activity, cry, and consolability; range of total score is 0–10; score ≥ 7 is severe pain. Figures 32-1 and 32-2 and Table 32-2	Nonverbal children > 1 y
CRIES, NIPS, PIPP	Behavioral observer	Rates a set of standard criteria and gives a score	Nonverbal infant < 1 y

CRIES, ***C****rying* ***r****equires* O_2 saturation, ***i****ncreased vital signs*, ***e****xpression*, and ***s****leeplessness*; FLACC, ***F****ace*, ***L****egs*, ***A****ctivity*, ***C****rying*, ***C****onsolability*; NIPS, Neonatal Infant Pain Scale; PIPP, Premature Infant Pain Profile.

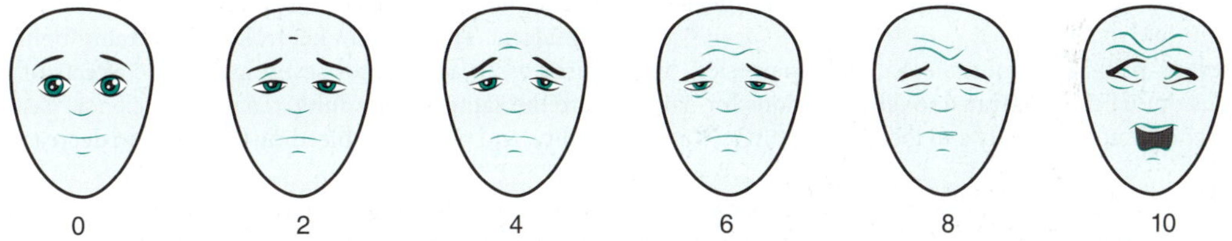

▲ **Figure 32–1.** Bieri Faces Pain Scale, revised. (Bieri D et al: The Faces Pain Scale for the self-assessment of the severity of pain experienced by children: Development, initial validation, and preliminary investigations for ratio scale properties. Pain 1990;41:139.)

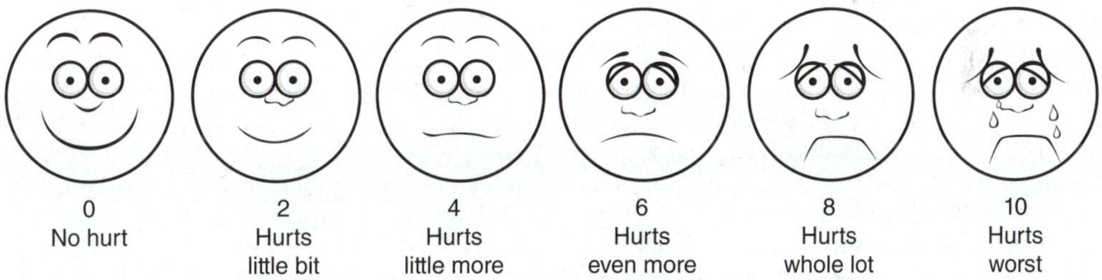

▲ **Figure 32–2.** Wong-Baker Pain Scale. (From Hockenberry MJ, WilsonD: Wong's essentials of pediatric nursing, ed 8, St. Louis, 2009, Mosby. Used with permission. Copyright Mosby)

Table 32–2. FLACC pain assessment tool.

Categories	Score 0	Score 1	Score 2
Face	No particular expression or smile	Occasional grimace or frown, withdrawn, disinterested	Frequent to constant frown, clenched jaw, quivering chin
Legs	Normal position or relaxed	Uneasy, restless, tense	Kicking, or legs drawn up
Activity	Lying quietly, normal position, moves easily	Squirming, shifting back and forth, tense	Arched, rigid, or jerking
Cry	No cry (awake or asleep)	Moans or whimpers, occasional complaint	Crying steadily, screams or sobs, frequent complaints
Consolability	Content, relaxed	Reassured by occasional touching, hugging, or being talked to, distractible	Difficult to console or comfort

Table 32–3. Suggested doses for nonopioid analgesics.

	Route	Dosage Guidelines	Half-life	Duration
Acetaminophen	PO	10–15 mg/kg/dose every 4–6 h, maximum dose 4000 mg/d	Neonates: 2–5 h Adults: 2–3 h	4 h
	PR	40 mg/kg loading dose, followed by 10–20 mg/kg/dose every 6 h		
	IV	12.5 mg/kg every 4 h or 15 mg/kg every 6 h	5–10 min	4–6 h
Ibuprofen	PO	4–10 mg/kg/dose every 6–8 h, maximum dose 40 mg/kg/d, no greater than 2400 mg/d	Children 1–7 y: 1–2 h Adults: 2–4 h	6–8 h
Ketorolac	IV	0.5 mg/kg/dose every 6 h, maximum of 30 mg/dose, maximum course of 8 doses	Children: ~ 6 h Adults: ~ 5 h	4–6 h

drug to active compound which can result in clinical toxicity. Morphine, oxycodone, and hydrocodone are all available as suspensions, are active as administered, and are metabolized by multiple routes.

For severe pain not amenable to oral analgesics, an intravenous opioid can be titrated to effect; options for pain relief are dependent on severity and location of pain and age. Intravenous opioids used as bolus dose, continuous infusion, and as part of a patient-controlled analgesia (PCA) infusion have a long track record of both safe and efficacious use in children. The NSAID ketorolac or acetaminophen can be used as an adjunct for severe pain. Side effects of ketorolac are the same as for adults: renal insufficiency, gastric irritability, and prolonged bleeding times due to decreased platelet

Table 32–4. Suggested doses of oral and intravenous opioids in infants and children.

Opioid Drug	Route	Dosage Guidelines	Onset	Duration
Fentanyl	IV intermittent	0.5–1 mcg/kg/dose (best for intermittent short duration analgesia; titrate to effect)	1–3 min	30–60 min
Hydromorphone	IV	Children: 0.015 mg/kg/dose every 3–6 h Adolescents: 1–4 mg every 3–6 h	15 min	4–5 h
Methadone	IV	0.1 mg/kg/dose every 4 h for 2–3 doses, then every 6–12 h	10–20 min	6–8 h (22–48 h after repeated doses)
Morphine	IV intermittent	0.05–0.1 mg/kg/dose every 2–4 h	Neonates: 7–8 h 1–3 mo: 6 h 6 mo–2.5 y: 3 h 3–19 y: 1–2 h Adults: 2–4 h	2–4 h
Codeine	PO	0.5–1 mg/kg/dose every 4–6 h, maximum of 60 mg/dose	30–60 min	4–6 h
Hydromorphone	PO	Children: 0.03–0.1 mg/kg/dose every 4–6 h Adolescents: 1–4 mg every 3–4 h	15–30 min	4–5 h
Hydrocodone (in Vicodin, Lortab elixir)	PO	Children: 0.15–0.2 mg/kg/dose every 4–6 h Adolescents: 1–2 tabs every 4–6 h (limited due to acetaminophen content; see acetaminophen recommendations in text)	10–20 min	3–6 h
Methadone	PO	0.1 mg/kg/dose every 4–6 h for 2–3 doses, then every 6–12 h	30–60 min	6–8 h (22–48 h after repeated doses)
Morphine	PO-IR	0.2–0.5 mg/kg/dose every 4–6 h	15–60 min	3–5 h
	PO-ER	0.3–0.6 mg/kg/dose every 12 h	1–2 h	8–12 h
Oxycodone	PO	0.1–0.2 mg/kg/dose every 4–6 h	15–30 min	4–5 h

Data from Polaner DM: Acute pain management in infants and children. In Perkins RM et al (editors): *Pediatric Hospital Medicine*, 2nd ed. Lippincott Williams and Wilkins, 2008:743–754.

adhesiveness. Patients with bleeding concerns should not receive ketorolac.

PCA pumps can be used in children as young as 6 years with proper instruction and coaching (Table 32–5). Morphine and hydromorphone are the most commonly used drugs for PCA management in the United States. Whenever PCA is used, it is imperative to assess patients frequently (at least hourly) to ensure adequate pain relief.

CHRONIC PAIN MANAGEMENT

Assessment

Chronic pain is a pain that persists past the usual course of an acute illness or beyond the time that is expected for an acute injury. In children, this is an increasingly recognized problem. It is estimated that chronic pain may affect as much as 10%–15% of the population. The most common problems include headache, chronic abdominal pain, myofascial pain, fibromyalgia, juvenile rheumatoid arthritis, complex regional pain syndrome, phantom limb pain, and pain associated with cancer. Chronic pain in children often has multiple other contributing factors, including psychological issues, psychosocial factors, sociologic factors, and family dynamics. Associating pain with a single physical cause can lead the physician to investigate the patient with repeated invasive testing, laboratory tests, and procedures and to overprescribe medications. A multidimensional assessment to chronic pain is optimal and often required.

Treatment

When possible, a multidisciplinary team approach is standard of care for treating chronic pain in children. All children evaluated for chronic pain should be seen on their initial visit by all primary members of the team to establish a management strategy. Team members should include a pain physician, a pediatric psychologist and/or a psychiatrist, occupational and physical therapists (OT/PT), advanced pain nurses (APNs), and a social worker. The majority of pediatric chronic pain management programs in the United States base their approach on combined intensive rehabilitation and intensive psychotherapy relying minimally on invasive procedures and pharmacotherapy.

A. Tolerance, Dependence, and Addiction

Physiologic and psychological responses to opioids are similar between adults and children. A consensus paper by the American Academy of Pain Medicine, American Pain Society, and American Society of Addiction Medicine defined important differences between normal and pathologic responses to opioids. The definitions of tolerance dependence and addiction are listed below.

1. Tolerance—A state of adaptation in which exposure to a drug induces changes that result in a diminution of one or more of the drug's effects over time. Tolerance develops at different rates for different opioid effects, that is, tolerance to sleepiness and respiratory depression occurs earlier than that to constipation and analgesia.

2. Dependence—A state of adaptation that is manifested by a drug class–specific withdrawal syndrome that can be produced by abrupt cessation, rapid dose reduction, decreasing blood level of the drug, and/or administration of an antagonist.

3. Addiction—A primary, chronic, neurobiologic disease, with genetic, psychosocial, and environmental factors influencing its development and manifestations. It is characterized by behaviors that include one or more of the following:

- Loss of **C**ontrol over use of drug
- **C**raving and **C**ompulsive use of drug
- Use despite adverse **C**onsequences

Addiction is rare when opioids are used appropriately for acute pain on both inpatient and outpatient settings. It should be emphasized that tolerance and dependence do not equal addiction.

B. Withdrawal

1. Recognition—Withdrawal symptoms can be expected to occur for all patients after 1 week of opioid treatment. Signs

Table 32–5. PCA dosing recommendations.

	Morphine	Fentanyl	Hydromorphone
Solution	1 mg/mL	Solution 10 mcg/mL	0.1 mg/mL or 1 mg/mL
Initial dose	15-20 mcg/kg (max 1.5 mg)	0.25 mcg/kg	3-4 mcg/kg (max 0.3 mg)
Lockout time	8-10 min	8-10 min	8-10 min
Basal infusion	0-20 mcg/kg/h	0-1 mcg/kg/h	0-4 mcg/kg/h
Maximum starting dose (for nonopioid tolerant patients)	100 mcg/kg/h	1-2 mcg/kg/h	20 mcg/kg/h

of withdrawal in older children include agitation, irritability, dysphoria, tachycardia, tachypnea, nasal congestion, temperature instability, and feeding intolerance. In neonates with withdrawal (neonatal abstinence syndrome), common symptoms include neurologic excitability, gastrointestinal dysfunction, autonomic signs (increased sweating, nasal stuffiness, fever, mottling, poor weight gain), and skin excoriation secondary to excessive rubbing.

2. Treatment

- Make a schedule/plan in conjunction with patient and family.
- Factor in duration of time on opioid.
- Consider switching to once-a-day opioid (see methadone dosing in Table 32–4).
- Decrease the dose by 10%–25% every 1–2 days.
- Look for signs of withdrawal.
- Consider adding lorazepam 0.05–0.1 mg/kg every 6–8 hours.
- Consider adding clonidine patch 0.1 mg/d (changed every fifth day).

Richard J et al: A prospective evaluation of opioid weaning in opioid-dependent pediatric critical care patients. Anesthesia and Analgesia 2006;102:1045–1050.

PEDIATRIC PALLIATIVE & END-OF-LIFE CARE

INTRODUCTION

It has been estimated that almost 55,000 children die each year in the United States. At least 50% of these children die during the newborn period or within the first year of life. Many of these children, particularly those older than 1 year of age, suffer from illnesses that are clearly life-limiting. Thousands more children are diagnosed with life-limiting illnesses, resulting in a chronic condition that may last for many years, even decades. Furthermore, children who are diagnosed with life-threatening illnesses that may be curable, such as cancer, continue to live with the potential of a recurrence of their malignancy for many years. The above populations are those where palliative and end-of-life care could play an important role during the illness of these patients.

Although commonly used interchangeably, *palliative care* and *end-of-life care* are not synonymous terms. Palliative care aims to prevent, relieve, reduce, or soothe the symptoms produced by potential life-limiting illnesses or their treatments and to maintain the patient's quality of life along the entire continuum of treatment. Provision of palliative care does not imply imminent death nor does it prohibit aggressive curative treatment modalities. Rather, it acknowledges the uncertainty and potential for suffering inherent in a potentially life-limiting condition such as cancer. Understanding how a family defines quality of life and suffering for their child is imperative and provides a framework for decision making between care provider and the family throughout treatment.

While a child is doing well with treatment, the primary focus will be on achieving cure or stabilization of the disease. Palliative care goals at this time focus on promoting quality of life in preparation for survivorship in the face of a potentially life-limiting illness. Some of these goals include helping a family come to terms with the diagnosis, addressing issues of treatment-related pain and distress, facilitating reintegration into the social realms of school and community, and promoting as much normalcy in the child's life as possible. When it becomes clear that the chances for cure are poor or present an unreasonable cost to the child's quality of life, the goals of palliative care will shift toward end-of-life care. The focus will still be on promoting quality of life but now in preparation for a comfortable and dignified end of life with increasingly less attention given to the treatment or cure of the disease itself.

Palliative care not only comprises support in the pain and symptom management of the disease but also addresses equally the psychosocial, emotional, and spiritual needs of the patient with a potential life-limiting illness and their family.

CHILDREN WHO MAY BENEFIT FROM PALLIATIVE CARE INTERVENTIONS

In a recent review by Himelstein et al, conditions that are appropriate for palliative care were divided into four groups as follows:

- Conditions for which curative treatment is possible but may fail such as advanced or progressive cancer and complex and severe congenital or acquired heart disease
- Conditions requiring intensive long-term treatment aimed at maintaining the quality of life such as HIV/AIDS, cystic fibrosis, and muscular dystrophy
- Progressive conditions in which treatment is exclusively palliative after diagnosis such as progressive metabolic disorders and certain chromosomal abnormalities
- Conditions involving severe, nonprogressive disability, causing extreme vulnerability to health complications such as severe cerebral palsy and anoxic brain injury

The United States Congress mandated in 2010 that palliative care will be covered concurrently with curative therapies for children with terminal conditions who are receiving Medicaid. Based on the *Patient Protection and Affordable Care Act*, a voluntary election to receive hospice care for a child does not constitute a waiver of any rights of the child to be provided with, or to have payments made for services that are related to the treatment of the child's condition. This significant milestone in pediatric palliative care should open the door to concurrent care being covered by private insurance companies in the future.

PAIN MANAGEMENT IN PEDIATRIC PALLIATIVE CARE

Optimal pain management is critical when providing pediatric palliative care. (See the section on Pain Management earlier, for definitions and guidelines for treatment.) As end of life approaches, dosing of comfort medications may eventually exceed normally prescribed doses. The goal at all times must be to achieve and maintain comfort. When pain management at the end of life is provided with this goal at the forefront and in concert with careful ongoing assessment and documentation of the child's symptoms, there should be no reason to fear that this action is tantamount to euthanasia which is a conscious action intended to hasten death.

QUALITY-OF-LIFE ADJUNCTS & SYMPTOM MANAGEMENT IN PEDIATRIC PALLIATIVE CARE

When offering treatment to children with a life-limiting illness particularly at the end of life, certain nonpain symptoms and signs may develop more quickly in children when compared to the adult population. A thorough and complete history and physical examination should be obtained. It is critical to determine how much distress the symptom causes the child and how much it interferes with child and family's routine when deciding upon treatment. Areas of management should include drug treatment, nursing care, and psychosocial support. Symptoms that commonly occur during disease progression and at the end of life in children with a life-limiting condition are listed in Table 32–6, with suggestions for management.

Table 32–6. Symptom management in pediatric palliative care.

Symptom	Etiology	Management
Nausea and vomiting	Chemotherapy, narcotics, metabolic	Diphenhydramine, hydroxyzine, 5-HT_3 inhibitors, prokinetic agents for GI motility
Anorexia	Cancer, pain, abnormal taste, GI alterations, metabolic changes, drugs, psychological factors	Treat underlying condition, exercise, dietary consultation, appetite stimulants (dronabinol, megestrol, steroid, medical marijuana if age appropriate)
Constipation/diarrhea	Narcotics, chemotherapy, malabsorption, drug related	Laxatives (must be initiated whenever starting narcotics), loperamide for diarrhea, peripheral opioid antagonists (methylnaltrexone, alvimopan)
Dyspnea	Airway obstruction; decrease in functional lung tissue due to effusion, infection, metastases; impaired chest wall movement; anemia	Treatment of specific cause (surgery to alleviate obstruction, red blood cell transfusion, chemotherapy/radiation therapy for metastatic disease), nonpharmacologic management (reassurance, position of comfort, improvement of air circulation using electric fan, oxygen, and relaxation therapy), pharmacologic management with opioids given IV/SQ as continuous infusion, nebulized morphine in older patients, concomitant use of anxiolytics (lorazepam, midazolam) if agitation
Terminal respiratory congestion	Airway/oral secretions at the end of life, resulting in rattling, noisy, gurgling breath sounds	Repositioning, anticholinergics such as hyoscine IV/SQ/PO or transdermal scopolamine
Pressure sores	Direct tissue damage, tissue fragility, immobility, diminished response to pain or irritation	Prevention (avoidance of trauma, relieve pressure, good hygiene), treatment with local hygiene, debridement, use of appropriate wound dressings, antibiotics, analgesics
Bone pain	Bony metastases, leukemic infiltration of bone marrow	Palliative radiation, bone-seeking isotopes, bisphosphonates, chemotherapy, analgesics
Agitation	Present in conjunction with pain, dyspnea, terminal phase of illness	Benzodiazepines (midazolam), barbiturates to achieve complete sedation in terminal restlessness
Pruritus	Urticaria, postherpetic neuralgia, cholestasis, uremia, opioids	Antihistamines (cholestasis, uremia, opioids), 5-HT_3 receptor antagonists (cholestasis, opioids)
Hematologic	Marrow infiltration by malignant cells (leukemia)	Transfusions (red blood cells, platelets) to relieve symptoms, hemostatics (Amicar)

Complementary and Alternative Modalities

It is not unusual for families seek complementary or alternative modalities (CAM) for their child when mainstream treatment has failed or is unavailable. Children with chronic conditions such as cancer, asthma, sickle cell disease, and epilepsy have a higher incidence of CAM usage compared to the general pediatric population (Post-White, 2009). As children approach end of life, many families opt to try some form of CAM. Most often, these treatments are aimed at improving physical or spiritual quality of life. Sometimes the goal is a desperate hope to find a treatment when other options have failed or an attempt to find something perceived as less toxic than mainstream treatments to induce remission, support the child's ability to fight the disease, or prolong life. Parents report using CAM gives them a sense of control and hope. The most common modalities reported in pediatrics are prayer/meditation, relaxation techniques, massage, chiropractic care including acupuncture, and nutritional supplements (Post-White et al, 2009). The use of CAM in children is influenced primarily by parental use and acceptance of CAM. Culturally accepted beliefs and practices also play an important role. In Asia, the use of meditation and prayer as a method to control pain is well supported by the medical community. In Europe, the use of homeopathic remedies is commonplace.

Studies of the effectiveness of CAM use in children have been small and the data is often conflicting. There is generally an acceptance for the lack of harm associated with mind-body techniques such as prayer, meditation, touch and sensory modalities, and relaxation. Acupuncture and acupressure are gaining more acceptance in the Western medical community and may be beneficial in some children for relief of pain, nausea, and other symptoms. Touch and sensory modalities such as massage, Healing Touch, and aromatherapy can induce a relaxation response in some children which can be very helpful. The use of supplements including botanicals and vitamins has been of more concern due to the lack of dosing information for pediatrics and the potential for serious drug interactions and toxicities. Treatments touted as alternative "cures" are likely not beneficial and can have very dangerous consequences. The cost of CAM, particularly botanicals and alternative medicine treatments, can be prohibitive and the cost is rarely covered by insurance. Hospice providers frequently incorporate relaxation and mind/body/spirit modalities into their programs.

It is important for the health care provider to ask parents and adolescents about CAM usage and to be open to discussion with the family about modalities they are using or may wish to consider. Parents consistently have reported in studies their desire to inform and discuss CAM with their health care provider, but may be reluctant to do so if they are unsure what response they will get from the provider. Providing families with clear information about the treatment they are considering or using and any contraindications is key. In some cases, recommendation of complementary techniques such as massage, mind/body modalities, and acupuncture/acupressure may be appropriate.

PSYCHOSOCIAL ASPECTS OF PEDIATRIC PALLIATIVE CARE

Pediatric palliative care is unique in that caregivers must be familiar with children's normal emotional and spiritual development. Working with a child at his or her level of development through the use of both oral and expressive communication will allow the child to be more open with respect to hopes, dreams, and fears. A child's understanding of death will depend also on his or her stage of development. Children understand death as a changed state by 3 years of age, universality by 5–6 years of age, and personal mortality by 8–9 years of age. Table 32–7 gives a broad overview of children's concepts of death and offers some helpful interventions.

CHILDREN'S CONCEPT OF DEATH

As end of life approaches, psychosocial support is invaluable to the child and family. Children may need someone to talk to outside of the family unit who can respond to their questions and concerns openly and honestly. Parents may need guidance and support in initiating discussions with or responding to questions from their child about death and dying. Children and adolescents may have specific tasks they wish to complete before they die. Some want to have input into funeral and memorial service plans and disposition of their body. Parents often need support in making funeral arrangements, handling financial concerns, talking with siblings and other family members, and coping with their own grief.

It is important to recognize that grief is not an illness but a normal, multidimensional, unique, dynamic process presenting as pervasive distress due to a perceived loss. Once parents have accepted the reality of the loss of the child, they must then complete the other tasks of grief such as experiencing the pain of their loss and adjusting to an environment without their child in order to move on with their lives. Parents who lose a child are at high risk for complicated grief reactions such as absent grief, delayed grief, and prolonged or unresolved grief. Siblings are also at risk for complicated grief and require special attention.

SPIRITUAL & CULTURAL SUPPORT

Health care decisions are often intertwined with a family's culture and belief system. Understanding the influences of a family's beliefs and culture allows the practitioner to provide sensitive, appropriate care, particularly at the end of life. Interaction with members of the family's faith and cultural communities can often be instrumental in helping both the care team and the community support of the family. Allowance for specific prayers, rituals, or other activities may help facilitate procedures and discussions.

Table 32–7. Children's concepts of death.

Age Group and Cognitive Development	Cognitive Understanding of Death	Response to Stress	Helpful Interventions
Infancy: Sense of self is directly related to having needs met	None	Lethargy, irritability, failure to thrive	Maintain routines Prompt response to physical and emotional caretaking needs Cuddling, holding, rocking
Toddler: Egocentric, concrete thinking; see objects and events in relationship to their usefulness to self	None but beginning to perceive implications of separation	Irritability, change in sleep-wake patterns, clinginess, regression, tantrums	Maintain routines Keep familiar people and objects at hand Prompt response to physical and emotional caretaking needs Accept need for increased physical and emotional comfort but continue to encourage acquisition of developmental skills
Preschool: Beginning to understand concept of time but limited sense of time permanence, curious, still quite concrete in thinking	View death as deliberately caused Magical thinking about causes of illness and death Death is not a permanent state	Oppositional behaviors, regression, sleep-wake changes, nightmares, somatic complaints Beginning to identify meaning and context of emotions	Simple, concrete explanations to questions—find out what it is they want to know Reassurance that death and illness are not the result of their thoughts or wishes Keep familiar people and objects at hand Play is a powerful tool to help children process events and emotions and as distraction from stressful situations
School age: Beginning of ability to apply logic; accept points of view other than their own	Death is seen in context of experience (pets, grandparents, what is seen on TV or in movies) Can understand that death is permanent	Oppositional behaviors, nightmares, sleep disruption, withdrawal, sadness Can verbally identify own feelings of fear, sadness, happiness	Ascertain how they perceive and understand what is happening and respond accordingly to their questions Acknowledge that feelings of sadness, fear, and anger are normal Allow age-appropriate control whenever possible Maintain as much normalcy in routine as possible Play is very important for expression of emotions and release of stress, amenable to directed play
Preadolescence and adolescence: Gaining mastery over themselves as individuals by exploring their own moral, ethical, and spiritual beliefs; increased reliance on peers for emotional support and information	Adult awareness of death but still may be highly experiential in understanding	Anger, withdrawal, sadness, depression, somatic complaints May have difficulty asking for emotional help	Set the tone for open, honest communication Allow the young person as much control as possible in decisions about his or her own health care Be willing to discuss and respect wishes and desires for disposition of belongings, funeral planning, what happens to his or her body Assist the young person in accomplishing important life tasks and activities that give meaning to his or her existence or leave behind a legacy

Families who speak a foreign language probably suffer from inadequate support the most. Every effort should be made to find and utilize a qualified interpreter, particularly for any discussion that involves delivering difficult news or making critical decisions. Many times, the role of interpreter is imposed upon a bilingual family member or friend who may not understand medical terminology well enough to translate clearly or who may deliberately translate the information inaccurately in an attempt to protect the family.

WITHDRAWAL OF MEDICAL LIFE SUPPORT

Medical technology has enabled many children with serious health conditions to enjoy a good quality of life. When technological support no longer enables a child's quality and enjoyment of life or there are no viable options to restore quality of life to the child, it may be appropriate to discontinue it. Feeding tubes, ventilators, dialysis, parenteral nutrition, and implanted cardiac pacemakers are examples of medical modalities that may need to be re-evaluated when a child's condition deteriorates or in the case of a catastrophic injury.

There are 5 circumstances in which withdrawal of medical support and technology can be considered in children (Tournay, 2000) (see table).

Brain death	All reversible causes excluded, meets established criteria for determination of brain death
Persistent vegetative state (PVS)	Child totally dependent for all cares, has no ability to interact meaningfully with his environment. Lack of cortical peaks in the somatosensory evoked potential may be helpful in making prognosis of PVS (Tournay, 2000)
Treatment will delay death without significantly relieving the suffering caused by the condition	No chance for cure, invasiveness of the treatment may prolong life but does not diminish or increases suffering
Child's life may be saved, but at the cost of physical and mental impairment that makes life intolerable for the child	Important to understand how child and family defines "intolerable life"
Additional treatment with potential benefit will cause further suffering	Burden of suffering outweighs the potential for benefit

At these times, it will be necessary to have a gentle but frank and honest discussion with the family that includes listening to their understanding of the child's situation and prognosis. Helping them identify and define what quality of life means to their child and to the family and what would be an intolerable life for the child is important. It is critical to present in a clear and understandable format the child's medical condition, test results, and the treatments that have been tried, what the expectations are for the child's ability to survive or function and interact with his environment, and why it is believed that current or additional interventions will be futile or induce further suffering. These discussions should be conducted with sensitivity and without need for an immediate answer from the parents. It often takes several such discussions for families to come to a decision that they themselves will be able to live with and families should not be rushed into decision making. The family may request additional testing or retesting to assure themselves they are making the right decision for their child. When feasible, these requests should be honored. Spiritual support may be very helpful to families during this process and should be offered.

Once the family has made the decision to withdraw support, it is helpful to explain what the anticipated course will be following withdrawal, what the child will look like during that time and what the plan of care will be to ensure there is no suffering. Create a plan with the family for time and place of withdrawal, who they would like to be there with them, any specific requests for environment such as music, a favorite movie playing, or a book being read, and who they would like to perform the withdrawal. Offering the opportunity for rituals, prayer, or private time prior to or during the withdrawal is appropriate. If death is anticipated to happen quickly after withdrawal, any specific religious requirements for the body after death should be arranged in advance. In all cases of withdrawal, the family should be offered support during the process and after the death occurs.

ADVANCE CARE PLANNING

Advance care planning allows patients and families to make known their wishes about what to do in case of serious or life-threatening problems. Himelstein et al describe advance care planning as a four-step process. First, those individuals considered decision makers are identified and included in the process. Second, an assessment of the patient and family understanding of the illness and prognosis is made and the impending death is described in terms that the child and family can understand. Third, on the basis of their understanding of the illness and prognosis, the goals of care are determined regarding current and future intervention—curative, uncertain, or primarily focused on providing comfort. Finally, shared decisions about the current and future use or abandonment of life-sustaining techniques and aggressive medical interventions are made. In the event of a disagreement between parents or parents and patient regarding these techniques or interventions, it may be prudent to involve the hospital's ethics committee in order to resolve these issues.

Some states permit parents to sign an advanced directive that asserts their decision not to have resuscitative attempts made in the event of a cardiac or respiratory arrest outside of the hospital. When an advanced directive is in place, emergency responders are not required to provide cardiopulmonary resuscitation (CPR) if called to the scene. Some school districts will respect an advanced directive on school property, many will not. If a child with an advanced directive in place wishes to go to school, a discussion between the medical team and school officials should be arranged to determine the best plan should the child have a cardiac or respiratory arrest at school.

Parents, and occasionally the child, may bring up the possibility of donating organs or body tissues after death. Although the tissues that may be donated by a child may be limited in some instances by the type of disease (eg, cancer), some parents find immense comfort in knowing their child was able to benefit another. If the parents have not discussed donation with the physician by the time of death and donation is possible, the physician should offer the opportunity to the family.

Autopsy is another subject many physicians find difficult to approach with a family, but it is an important option to discuss. In cases of anticipated death from natural causes, autopsies are generally not mandatory; however, information obtained from an autopsy may be useful for parental peace of mind or medical research. If death at home is to be followed by an autopsy, special arrangements for transporting and receiving the body will need to be made with the mortuary or the coroner.

REFERENCES

Andersson T et al: Drug-metabolizing enzymes: Evidence for clinical utility of pharmacogenomic tests. Clin Pharmacol Ther 78:559–581 [PMID: 16338273].

Becker G, Blum HE: Novel opioid antagonists for opioid-induced bowel dysfunction and postoperative ileus. Lancet 2009;373: 1198.

Berde CB, Sethna N: Analgesics for the treatment of pain in children. N Engl J Med 2002 Oct 3;347(14):1094–1103.

Goldman A et al (editors): *Oxford Textbook of Palliative Care for Children*. Oxford University Press, 2006.

Heit HA: Addiction, physical dependence, and tolerance: Precise definitions to help clinicians evaluate and treat chronic pain patients. J Pain Palliat Care Pharmacother 2003;17:15–29 [PMID: 14640337].

Hendrickson K, McCorkle R: A dimensional analysis of the concept: Good death of a child with cancer. J Pediatr Oncol Nurs 2008 May–Jun;25(3):127–138 [PMID: 18413698].

Himelstein B et al: Pediatric palliative care. N Engl J Med 2004; 350:1752 [PMID: 15103002].

Knapp C et al: Innovative pediatric palliative care programs in four countries. J Palliat Care 2009;25:132.

McGrath PA, Ruskin DA: Caring for children with chronic pain: Ethical considerations. Paediatr Anaesth 2007 Jun;17(6):505–508 [PMID: 17498011].

Moody K et al: Pediatric palliative care. Prim Care Clin Office Pract 2011;38:327–361.

Ott M: Mind-body therapies for the pediatric oncology patient: Matching the right therapy with the right patient. Journal of Pediatric Oncology Nursing 2006;223(5):254–257.

Post-White J, Fitzgerald M, Hageness S, Sencer S: Complementary and alternative medicine use in children with cancer and general and specialty pediatrics. Journal of Pediatric Oncology Nursing 2009;26(1):7–15.

Storey P, Knight C: Alleviating psychological and spiritual pain in the terminally ill. In American Academy of Hospice and Palliative Care Medicine (editor): *Hospice/Palliative Care Training for Physicians: A Self-Study Program*. Mary Ann Liebert, Inc., 2003.

Thompson LA et al: Pediatricians' perceptions of and preferred timing for pediatric palliative care. Pediatrics 2009;123:e777.

Tournay AE: Withdrawal of medical treatment in children. Western Journal of Medicine 2000;173,407–411.

Widger K, Picot C: Parents' perceptions of the quality of pediatric and perinatal end-of-life care. Pediatr Nurs 2008;34(1): 53–58.

Wong DL, Baker CM: Smiling faces as anchor for pain intensity scales. Pain 2001;89:295–300.

Woodruff R (editor): *Palliative Medicine*. Oxford University Press, 2005.

Web Resources

www.ampainsoc.org/advocacy/pediatric.htm

Education on Palliative and End of Life Care (EPEC; adult focused): www.epec.net

Initiative for Pediatric Palliative Care (IPPC): www.ippcweb.org

National Hospice and Palliative Care Organization (NHPCO)—Children's Project on Palliative/Hospice Services (ChiPPs): www.nhpco.org

End of Life Nursing Education Consortium Pediatric Palliative Care Course: module seminars available for viewing online at www.Cure4Kids.org . Upcoming Pediatric ELNEC courses may be found at www.aacn.nchc.edu

33

Immunodeficiency

Pia J. Hauk, MD
Richard B. Johnston, Jr., MD
Andrew H. Liu, MD

Immunodeficiencies that present in childhood comprise rare disorders that have been characterized by a combination of clinical patterns, immunologic laboratory tests, and often molecular identification of the mutant gene. Children with primary immunodeficiency (PID) commonly present with recurrent and/or severe bacterial infections, failure to thrive, and/or developmental delay as a result of infection. Immunodeficiency should be considered when infections are recurrent, severe, persistent, resistant to standard treatment, or caused by opportunistic organisms. Because delayed diagnosis of PIDs is common, heightened diagnostic suspicion is warranted.

The human immune system consists of the phylogenetically more primitive innate immune system and the adaptive immune system, both of which contain humoral and cellular components. For the purpose of clinical categorization, PIDs are commonly divided into four main groups: antibody deficiencies, combined T- and B-cell immunodeficiencies, phagocyte disorders, and complement deficiencies. Understanding the role each part of the immune system plays in host defense allows critical evaluation for possible immunodeficiency as the cause of recurrent infections.

IMMUNODEFICIENCY EVALUATION: PRIMARY CONSIDERATIONS

When evaluating for a possible PID, other conditions that increase susceptibility to infections have to be considered, such as allergic rhinitis, asthma, cystic fibrosis, foreign body aspiration, and conditions that interfere with skin barrier function. Common causes of secondary or acquired immunodeficiency need to be excluded. These include malnutrition, aging, certain drugs (chemotherapy, immunosuppressive medications, glucocorticoids, disease-modifying antirheumatic drugs, rituximab), protein loss via gastroenteropathy or kidney disease, and other diseases associated with impaired immunity (bone marrow and blood cell malignancies, and certain chronic infections, including AIDS). If a single site is involved, anatomic defects and foreign bodies may be present. Figure 33–1 outlines when PIDs should be considered.

Key clinical patterns can indicate the presence of a PID and the category of immune impairment. Frequency, severity, and age of onset of infections are important clues. The Modell Foundation warning signs for PID are shown in Figure 33–2. Children who meet two or more of these signs should be screened for PID. The type of infections should guide initial investigation, as antibody, complement, and phagocyte defects predispose mainly to bacterial infections, but diarrhea, superficial candidiasis, opportunistic infections, and severe herpesvirus infections are more characteristic of T-lymphocyte immunodeficiency. Combined immunodeficiency syndromes will present with a combination of infections typical for B- and T-lymphocyte deficiencies. Table 33–1 classifies PID into four main host immunity categories based on age of onset, infections with specific pathogens, affected organs, and other special features. Finally, male gender increases the likelihood of an X-linked (XL) PID, while consanguinity increases the likelihood of an autosomal recessive (AR) form of PID.

Research on deficiencies of the innate immune response is an evolving field. Pattern-recognition receptors (PRRs) are important for the recognition of pathogen-associated molecular patterns specific for different microbes, initiation of the innate immune response, and cross talk with adaptive immunity. They are expressed on the surface or in the cytoplasm of cells of the innate immune system, dependent on where specific microbes are encountered. Four classes of PRRs have been identified. Toll-like receptors (TLRs) recognize a spectrum of bacteria, viruses, selected fungi, and protozoa. C-type lectin receptors (CLRs) that include dectin-1 and mannose-binding lectin are involved in recognition of bacteria and fungi. Cytoplasmic PRRs include nucleotide-binding oligomerization domain (NOD) leucine-rich-repeat containing receptors (NLRs) that recognize peptidoglycan structures on bacteria, and retinoic acid-inducible gene I protein (RIG-1) helicase receptors that recognize viral

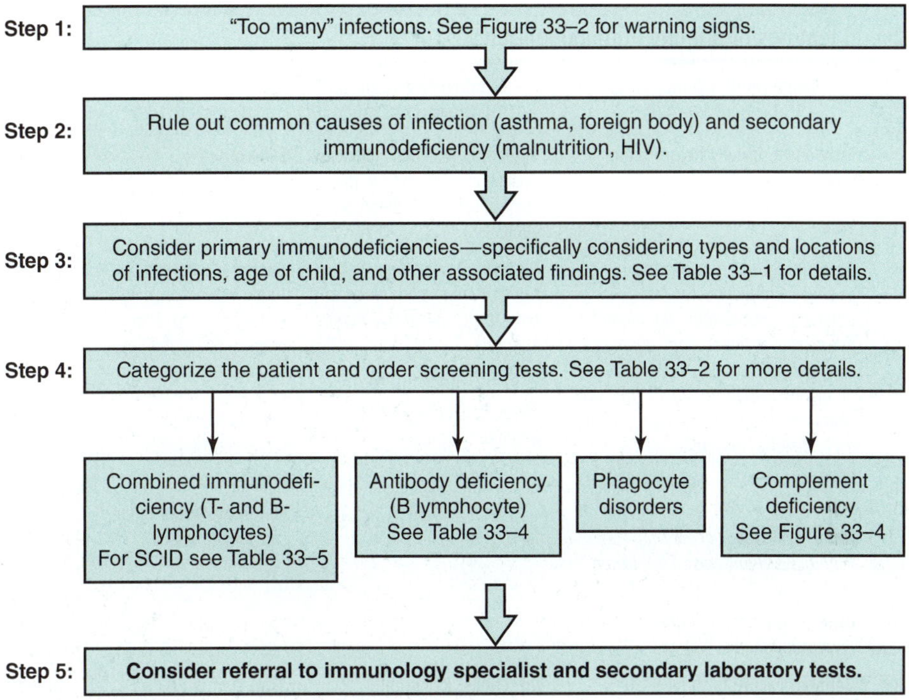

▲ **Figure 33–1.** General approach to primary immunodeficiencies.

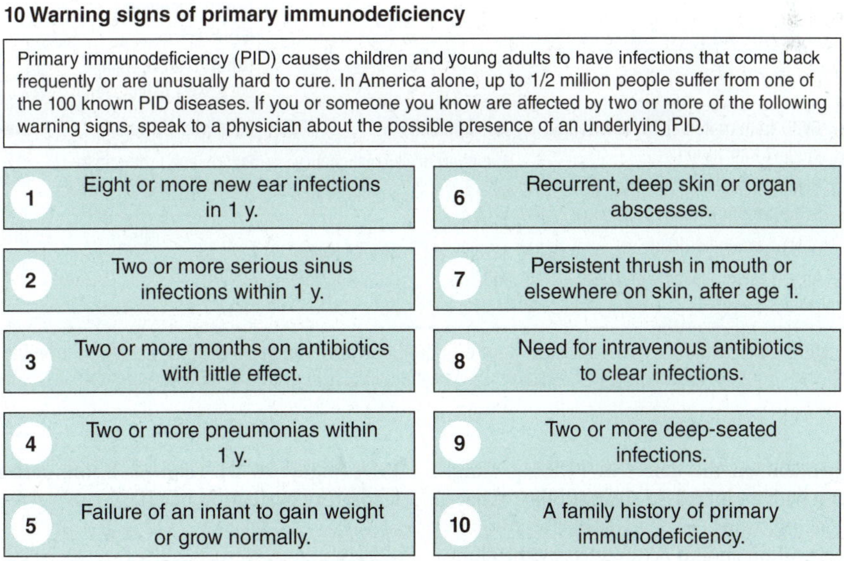

▲ **Figure 33–2.** Warning signs of primary immunodeficiency. (Data from the Jeffrey Modell Foundation.)

Table 33–1. Clinical features of primary immunodeficiencies.

Characteristic	Combined Deficiency (T- and B-Lymphocyte Defect)	Antibody Deficiency (B-Lymphocyte Defect)	Phagocyte Defect	Complement Defect
Age at onset of infections	Early onset, usually before 6 mo	Onset after maternal antibodies decline, usually after 3-6 mo; some later in childhood or adults	Early onset	Any age
Specific pathogens	**Bacteria:** *Streptococcus pneumoniae, Campylobacter fetus, Staphylococcus aureus, Haemophilus influenzae, Pseudomonas aeruginosa, Mycoplasma hominis, Ureaplasma urealyticum, Listeria monocytogenes, Salmonella* spp, enteric flora, atypical mycobacteria, and BCG **Viruses:** CMV, EBV, varicella, RSV, enterovirus, rotavirus **Fungi/protozoa:** *Candida albicans, Aspergillus fumigatus, Toxoplasma gondii* **Other:** *Pneumocystis carinii, Cryptosporidium*	**Bacteria:** *S pneumoniae, C fetus, H influenzae, P aeruginosa, U urealyticum, S aureus, M hominis* **Viruses:** Enteroviruses **Fungi/protozoa:** *Giardia lamblia*	**Bacteria:** *S aureus, enteric flora, Burkholderia* spp, *Aspergillus* spp, *P aeruginosa, Salmonella* spp, *Serratia* spp, *Nocardia asteroides, Klebsiella* spp, nontuberculous mycobacteria, and BCG **Viruses:** None **Fungi/protozoa:** C albicans, A fumigatus	**Bacteria:** *Neisseria meningitidis and gonorrhoeae, S pneumoniae, S aureus, P aeruginosa, H influenzae* **Viruses:** None **Fungi/protozoa:** None common
Affected organs and infections	**General:** Failure to thrive **Infections:** Severe infections (meningitis, septicemia, sinopulmonary), recurrent candidiasis, protracted diarrhea	**Infections:** Recurrent sinopulmonary, pneumonia, meningitis **GI:** Chronic malabsorption, IBD-like symptoms **Other**: Arthritis	**Skin:** Dermatitis, abscesses, cellulitis **Lymph nodes:** Suppurative adenitis **Oral cavity:** Periodontitis, ulcers **Lungs:** Pneumonia, abscesses **Other:** Liver & brain abscesses, osteomyelitis	**Infections:** Meningitis, disseminated gonococcal infection, septicemia, pneumonia
Special features	GVHD from maternal T cells or blood product transfusion Disseminated infection after BCG or live polio immunization Absent lymphoid tissue Absent thymic shadow on chest radiograph	Autoimmunity Lymphoreticular malignancy Postvaccination polio or BCG infection Chronic enteroviral encephalitis	Poor wound healing Pyloric and urethral stenosis, IBD	**Autoimmune disorders:** SLE, vasculitis, dermatomyositis, scleroderma, glomerulonephritis **Other**: Hereditary angioedema, aHUS

aHUS, atypical hemolytic uremic syndrome; BCG, bacille Calmette-Guérin; CMV, cytomegalovirus; EBV, Epstein-Barr virus; GVHD, graft-versus-host disease; IBD, inflammatory bowel disease; RSV, respiratory syncytial virus; SLE, systemic lupus erythematosus.

nucleic acids. Dependent on the defect in PRR signaling, patients may present with an increased susceptibility of bacterial, viral, or fungal infections.

Laboratory investigation should be directed by the clinical presentation and the suspected category of host immunity impairment. A complete blood cell count (CBC) with cell differential and measurement of quantitative immunoglobulins (Igs) will identify the majority of patients with PID, as antibody deficiencies account for at least 50% of PIDs (Figure 33–3). Table 33–2 summarizes the approach to laboratory evaluation of PID.

Antibodies & Immunoglobulins

The initial laboratory screening for antibody deficiency includes the measurement of serum Igs: IgG, IgM, IgA, and IgE, which have age-dependent normal ranges (Table 33–3). Normal IgG, IgM, and IgA and increased IgE levels are

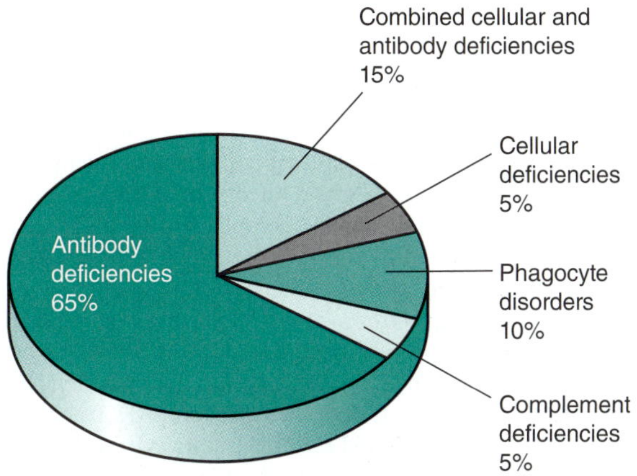

▲ Figure 33–3. Relative frequencies of primary immunodeficiencies. (Adapted, with permission, from Stiehm ER et al [editors]: *Immunologic Disorders in Infants and Children*, 5th ed. Elsevier, 2004.)

indicative of atopy. Some patients may have normal Ig levels but fail to make protective antibodies to certain microbes; other patients have subnormal Ig levels, but make protective antibodies. Specific antibodies include isohemagglutinins, naturally occurring IgM antibodies that are detectable by age 6 months except in children with blood group AB. Specific IgG antibodies to protein antigens (tetanus, diphtheria, rubella, mumps) and polysaccharide antigens (*Haemophilus influenzae, Streptococcus pneumoniae*) can be measured after immunization. The response to polysaccharide antigens develops during the second year of life, but protein-conjugated vaccines elicit an earlier response in immunocompetent children. Assessing the antibody response to pneumococcal polysaccharide antigens can be helpful in the face of repeated pneumococcal infections. The gold standard is comparison of pre- and postimmunization titers.

Obtaining a CBC with differential and T- and B-lymphocyte counts are recommended if an initial screen reveals very low concentrations of all Ig classes. Certain types of hypogammaglobulinemia are characterized by low levels of or absent B-lymphocytes, such as X-linked (XL) Bruton agammaglobulinemia. Protein electrophoresis can help identify monoclonal gammopathy as seen in XL lymphoproliferative syndrome, which can be complicated by fatal Epstein-Barr virus (EBV) infection, and in heavy-chain diseases. Serum albumin should be measured in patients with hypogammaglobulinemia to exclude secondary deficiencies due to protein loss through bowel or kidneys. IgG or IgA subclass measurements may be abnormal in patients with varied immunodeficiency syndromes, but they are rarely helpful in an initial evaluation.

T Lymphocytes

The initial laboratory screening for a T-lymphocyte deficiency includes a CBC with cell differential to evaluate for a decreased absolute lymphocyte count (< 1000/μL) and enumeration of absolute numbers of T cells and their subsets, B cells, and natural killer (NK) cells (Table 33–2). T-cell function can be analyzed by in-vitro lymphocyte

Table 33–2. Laboratory evaluation for primary immunodeficiency.

Suspected Defect	Screening Evaluation	Secondary Evaluation	Advanced Evaluation
B-lymphocyte defect	Quantitative immunoglobulins (IgG, IgM, IgA, IgE)	B-lymphocyte enumeration panel ($CD19^+/20^+$ B cells) Antibody response to prior or repeat immunizations (tetanus, diphtheria, *H influenzae*) Isohemagglutinins	DNA analysis for specific genetic mutations Screen for memory B cells (IgM^- IgD^- $CD27^+/CD20^+$ B cells)
Combined T- and B-lymphocyte defect	CBC, absolute lymphocyte count, HIV testing	T- and B-lymphocyte, NK-cell enumeration (T = $CD3^+$, $CD4^+$, or $CD8^+$; B = $CD19^+/D20^+$; NK = $CD56^+/CD16^+$) Lymphocyte proliferation assay to mitogens and antigens Delayed-type hypersensitivity skin test	DNA analysis for specific genetic mutations ADA or PNP levels of RBC Cytotoxicity studies
Phagocyte disorder	WBC count with differential	DHR flow cytometry assay Nitroblue tetrazolium reduction assay	Bactericidal assays, CD11/18 analysis Chemotaxis assay
Complement deficiency	CH50	AH50	Individual complement levels and function

CD, cluster of differentiation; ADA, adenosine deaminase; DHR, dihydrorhodamine; HIV, human immunodeficiency virus; PNP, purine nucleoside phosphorylase; RBC, red blood cell; WBC, white blood cell.

Adapted, with permission, from Cunningham-Rundles C: Immune deficiency: office evaluation and treatment. Allergy Asthma Proc 2003;24:409–15 [PMID: 14763242].

Table 33–3. Normal values for immunoglobulins by age.

Age	IgG (mg/dL)	IgM (mg/dL)	IgA (mg/dL)
Newborn	1031 ± 200	11 ± 7	2 ± 3
1-3 mo	430 ± 119	30 ± 11	21 ± 13
4-6 mo	427 ± 186	43 ± 17	28 ± 18
7-12 mo	661 ± 219	55 ± 23	37 ± 18
13-24 mo	762 ± 209	58 ± 23	50 ± 24
25-36 mo	892 ± 183	61 ± 19	71 ± 34
3-5 y	929 ± 228	56 ± 18	93 ± 27
6-8 y	923 ± 256	65 ± 25	124 ± 45
9-11 y	1124 ± 235	79 ± 33	131 ± 60
12-16 y	946 ± 124	59 ± 20	148 ± 63
Adults	1158 ± 305	99 ± 27	200 ± 61

Adapted, with permission, from Stiehm ER et al: *Immunologic Disorders of Infants and Children*, 5th ed. Elsevier, 2004.

proliferation assays to mitogens that stimulate all T cells and by specific antigens that stimulate only antigen-specific T cells. Borderline function must be interpreted based on clinical correlation. T-lymphocyte function is often also studied in vivo by delayed hypersensitivity skin tests to specific antigens, including *Candida albicans*, tetanus, or mumps, but a negative result is not helpful, as it may be due to young age, chronic illness, vitamin D deficiency, or poor test technique. T-lymphocyte deficiencies will often not manifest as skin-test anergy until the impairment is severe, for example, as in AIDS. It is important to evaluate a patient's specific antibody production because proper B-lymphocyte function and antibody production are dependent on adequate T-lymphocyte function. Therefore, most T-lymphocyte deficiencies manifest as combined T- and B-lymphocyte deficiencies.

Phagocyte Immunity

The initial laboratory screening for phagocyte disorders, mainly impaired neutrophil function, should include a CBC and cell differential to look for neutropenia. A blood smear can detect Howell-Jolly bodies in erythrocytes, indicative of asplenia, and abnormalities in lysosomal granules in neutrophils. An abnormality of the neutrophil respiratory burst, which would lead to impaired neutrophil bactericidal activity, can be tested by nitroblue tetrazolium (NBT) reduction. The dihydrorhodamine (DHR) flow cytometry assay assesses the same function more quantitatively. Leukocyte adhesion molecules can be studied by flow cytometry. Assays to study neutrophil phagocytosis of bacteria and phagocytic microbicidal activity are available in specialized laboratories. The clinical symptom pattern that suggests a possible defect of phagocytic cell function should dictate which tests are used.

Complement Pathways (Figure 33–4)

Testing for total hemolytic complement activity with the CH50 assay screens for most of the diseases of the complement system. A normal CH50 titer depends on the ability of all 11 components of the classical pathway and membrane attack complex to interact and then lyse antibody-coated sheep erythrocytes. Alternative complement pathway deficiencies are identified by subnormal lysis of rabbit erythrocytes in the AH50 assay. For both assays, the patient's serum must be separated and frozen at –70°C within 30–60 minutes after collection to prevent loss of activity. Measuring levels of individual components is not necessary when both CH50 and AH50 are normal. If both the CH50 and AH50 are low, a deficiency in their shared terminal pathway (C3, C5, C6, C7, C8, or C9) would be the most common explanation. If the CH50 is low but the AH50 is normal, the deficiency must affect C1, C4, C2, or components of the lectin pathway. If the AH50 is low but the CH50 is normal, a deficiency in factors D or B or properdin should be suspected.

Pattern Recognition Receptors

Selected laboratories offer tests to assess TLR function upon stimulation with ligands for different TLRs that have been identified. Mannose binding lectin levels can be measured in clinical laboratories. However, expression or function of PRRs and associated gene mutations are studied mostly in a research setting at the current time.

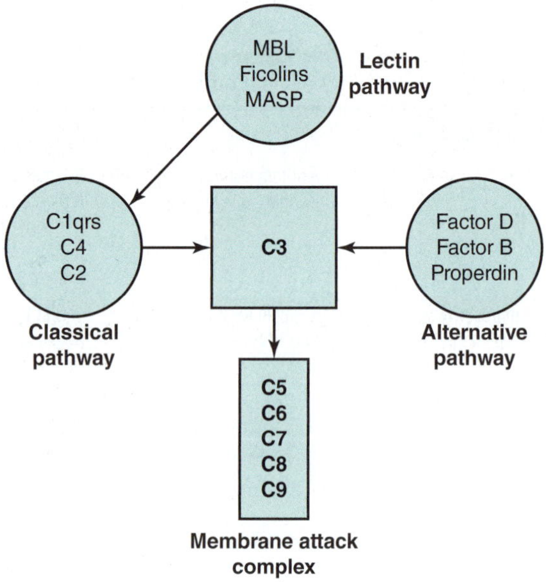

▲ **Figure 33–4.** Pathways of complement activation and the central functional role of C3. MASP, MBL-associated serine protease; MBL, mannose-binding lectin.

Netea MG, van der Meer JWM: Immunodeficiency and genetic defects of pattern-recognition receptors. N Engl J Med 2011;364:1–69 [PMID: 21208109].

ANTIBODY DEFICIENCY SYNDROMES

ESSENTIALS OF DIAGNOSIS & TYPICAL FEATURES

- Recurrent bacterial infections, typically due to encapsulated pyogenic bacteria.
- Low immunoglobulin levels.
- Inability to make specific antibodies to vaccine antigens or infections.

General Considerations

Antibody deficiency syndromes include both congenital and acquired forms of hypogammaglobulinemia with low levels of one or more of the immunoglobulins IgM, IgG, and IgA. Deficiencies result in recurrent bacterial infections, typically with encapsulated bacteria, including pneumonia, otitis, sinusitis, meningitis, cellulitis, and sepsis. As a group, antibody deficiencies represent nearly half of all PIDs. They can be divided into: (1) early defects of B cell development, with absent B cells and severe hypogammaglobulinemia; (2) hyper-IgM syndromes with defects in Ig class switching; (3) common variable immunodeficiency (CVID), with insufficient antibody production; and (4) specific antibody deficiencies. Table 33–4 outlines primary antibody deficiency syndromes, laboratory findings, and genetic inheritance in these disorders.

1. X-Linked Agammaglobulinemia

ESSENTIALS OF DIAGNOSIS & TYPICAL FEATURES

- Infections early in life, usually after age 4 months.
- Typical bacterial infections include infections with encapsulated bacteria, for example, *H influenzae, S pneumoniae, Staphylococcus aureus*, and *Pseudomonas aeruginosa,* but also *Mycoplasma* species.
- Risk for severe enteroviral infections and, rarely, polio due to live polio vaccine.
- Failure to thrive and absent lymphoid tissue on examination.
- Very low levels of Igs and B lymphocytes.

General Considerations

X-linked agammaglobulinemia (XLA) accounts for 85% of congenital hypogammaglobulinemia and occurs in about 1:200,000 male births. Children with XLA typically present with infections after 4 months of age, when maternally derived IgG levels have declined. XLA is caused by a gene mutation on the X chromosome (Xq21.33–q22) that affects the expression of a B-cell–specific tyrosine kinase (*BTK*), halting the maturation of B cells and resulting in low or absent B-cell numbers and serum Igs. Early detection and diagnosis of XLA allow Ig replacement therapy to start before a potentially life-threatening infection can occur.

Clinical Findings

A. Symptoms and Signs

Sinopulmonary infections due to *H influenzae* and *S pneumoniae* are common, but deep tissue infections and arthritis due to *Mycoplasma* or *Ureaplasma* species can occur. Recurrent pulmonary infections may lead to bronchiectasis. Antibody-deficient patients are also at risk for polio due to oral polio vaccine strains, resulting in paralysis, and echoviruses causing chronic encephalitis. At presentation, male infants have scant or absent lymphoid tissue, including tonsils, adenoids, and lymph nodes. A small proportion also has a history of poor growth.

B. Laboratory Findings

Most patients have low levels of or absent Igs M, G, A, and E, and, despite a normal leukocyte count, few or no B lymphocytes. T lymphocyte numbers and function are normal. Genetic testing for a *BTK* gene mutation confirms the diagnosis in affected males. Female carriers can be detected by genetic testing or screening for *BTK* protein expression in platelets followed by mutation analysis if needed.

Differential Diagnosis

The differential diagnosis includes other causes of antibody deficiency and combined immunodeficiencies (Tables 33–4 and 33–5). Additional causes of recurrent infections and low Ig levels include protein loss through renal or gastrointestinal disease, but patients with these disorders present with normal numbers of B lymphocytes and, typically, an isolated IgG deficiency.

Conley ME et al: Primary B cell immunodeficiencies: Comparisons and contrasts. Annu Rev Immunol 2009;27:199–227 [PMID: 19302039].

Davies EG, Thrasher AJ: Update on the hyper immunoglobulin M syndromes. Br J Haematol 2010;149:167–180 [PMID: 20180797].

Driessen G, van der Burg M: Educational paper: Primary antibody deficiencies. Eur J Pediatr 2011;170:693–702 [PMID: 21544519].

Table 33–4. Antibody deficiency disorders.

Disease	Serum Ig	Circulating B Cells	Genetic Mutation	Mode of Inheritance	Clinical features
Defects in early B cell development					
X-linked agammaglobulinemia	All isotypes low or absent	Profoundly decreased	*BTK* gene	XL	Severe bacterial infections
Autosomal recessive agammaglobulinemia	All isotypes low or absent	Profoundly decreased	μ (IGHM), *Igα* (CD79A), *Igβ*(CD79B), *λ5* (IGLL1, CD179B), *BLNK* or *LRRC8A* genes	AR	Severe bacterial infections
Ig heavy-chain gene deletions	IgG_1 or IgG_2, IgG_4 absent, in some cases IgE and IgA_1 or IgA_2 absent	Normal or decreased	Chromosomal deletion at 14q32	AR	Not always symptomatic
Κ chain deficiency	Ig(κ) decreased: Antibody response normal or decreased	Normal or decreased k-bearing cells	Point mutations at chromosome 2p11 in some patients	AR	None
Hyper-IgM syndromes with defects in Ig class switch recombination					
CD40 ligand (CD154) deficiency	Low IgG, IgA; normal or elevated IgM	Normal	*CD40L* gene	XL	Bacterial and opportunistic infections, neutropenia; T cell defect
CD40 deficiency	Low IgG, IgA; normal or elevated IgM	Normal	*CD40* gene	AR	Bacterial and opportunistic infections
NFκB-signaling defects	Low IgG and/or IgA and/or specific antipolysaccharide antibodies	Normal	*IKBKG (NEMO)* gene *NFKBIA* gene	XL AR	Bacterial and opportunistic infections
AID deficiency	Low IgG, IgA; normal or elevated IgM	Normal	*AICDA* gene	AR, AD (AID C terminal defect)	Bacterial infections, enlarged lymph nodes
UNG deficiency	Low IgG, IgA; normal or elevated IgM	Normal	*UNG* gene	AR	Bacterial infections, enlarged lymph nodes
Common variable immunodeficiency					
Heterogeneous group of disorders	Normal or low IgM, low IgG, low IgA, poor specific antibody production	Normal or decreased	Variable; *TACI (AD), ICOS (AR), CD19 (AR)* genes	AD and AR	Recurrent infections, autoimmune disorders (TACI)
Selective immunoglobulin deficiencies					
IgG subclass deficiency	Decrease in one or more IgG isotypes	Normal	Defects of isotype differentiation	Unknown	Not always symptomatic
IgA deficiency	Decrease in IgA_1 and IgA_2	Normal	Failure of terminal differentiation in IgA-positive B cells	Variable	Autoimmune or allergic disorders, some have infections
Specific antibody deficiency	Normal	Normal	Unknown	Unknown	Inability to make antibody to specific antigens
Transient hypogammaglobulinemia of infancy	IgG and IgA decreased, but IgM usually normal	Normal	Differentiation defect: Delayed maturation of helper function	Unknown	Not always symptomatic, may have respiratory infections, otitis media

AD, autosomal dominant; AID/*AICDA*, activation-induced cytidine deaminase; AR, autosomal recessive; BTK, Bruton tyrosine kinase; ICOS, inducible costimulator; Ig (κ), immunoglobulin of κ light-chain type; *IKBKG*, I kappa B kinase gene; NFκB, nuclear factor kappa-light-chain-enhancer of activated B cells; *NFKBIA gene*, NFκB inhibitor alpha gene; TACI, transmembrane activator and calcium-modulator and cyclophilin ligand inter-actor; UNG, uracil-DNA glycosylase; XL, X-linked.

Table 33–5. Severe combined immunodeficiency variants.

Gene	Locus	Gene Product and Function	Presence of			Inheritance
			T Cell	B Cell	NK Cell	
IL2RG	xq13.1	Common γ chain of IL-2, 4, 7, 9, 15, 21 cytokine receptors; necessary to activate *JAK3* for intracellular signaling	–	+	–	XL
ADA	20q13.11	Part of the purine salvage pathway; necessary for removal of toxic metabolites that inhibit all lymphoid cells	–	–	–	AR
JAK3	19p13.1	A tyrosine kinase important for differentiation of lymphoid cells	–	+	–	AR
IL7R	5p13	IL-7 receptor is necessary for T-cell development and activates *JAK3*	–	+	+	AR
RAG1/RAG2	11p13	DNA recombinases, which mediate DNA recombination during B- and T-cell development	–	–	+	AR
CD3δ	11q23	Essential for T-cell development	–	+	+	AR
CD45	1q31–32	Tyrosine kinase, important for regulation of other kinases in T- and B-cell antigen receptor development	–	+	+	AR
Artemis	20q13.11	Involved in repairing DNA double-strand breaks that occur during recombination	–	–	+	AR

–, absent; +, present; AR, autosomal recessive; IL, interleukin; NK, natural killer; XL, X-linked.
Adapted, with permission, from Kalman L et al: Mutations in genes for T-cell development: IL7R, CD45, IL2RG, JAK3, RAG1, RAG2, ARTEMIS, and ADA and severe combined immunodeficiency: HuGE review. Genet Med 2004;6:16 [PMID: 15461463].

Treatment

Current therapy consists of lifelong Ig replacement therapy. In addition to preventing infections, Ig replacement usually results in resolution of inflammatory arthritis and improves growth. Because the severity of infections varies and antibiotics are widely used, the diagnosis is often delayed for years, but XLA should be considered in males with recurrent infections regardless of severity. Early diagnosis can prevent permanent disability and premature death.

2. Autosomal Recessive Congenital Agammaglobulinemia

General Considerations

Autosomal recessive congenital agammaglobulinemia is rare, accounting for less than 15% of all congenital hypogammaglobulinemia, and occurs in both male and female children. In the most common form, it is caused by mutations of the IgM heavy-chain gene on chromosome 14q32. These mutations result in abnormal or absent IgM expression and abnormal development of B cells with decreased or absent antibody production.

Clinical Findings

A. Symptoms and Signs

Similarly to patients with XLA, children present with recurrent and severe bacterial infections, typically before age 6 months. Infections include pneumonia, otitis, sinusitis, meningitis, cellulitis, and sepsis. Chronic central nervous system (CNS) infections by enteroviruses have been observed.

B. Laboratory Findings

Patients usually have low numbers of circulating B lymphocytes and low levels of or absent immunoglobulins. Specific antibody function is poor. When the diagnosis is suspected, the detection of a mutation in the μ heavy chain can confirm the most common type. Additional mutations include mutations of the genes encoding the Igα and Igβ molecules, the λ5 surrogate light chain, and *BLNK* or *LRRC8* genes.

Differential Diagnosis

The differential diagnosis is similar to that of XLA and includes XLA for male patients.

Treatment

Treatment and prognosis are similar to those outlined for XLA.

3. Hyper-IgM Syndromes

Hyper-IgM (HIGM) syndromes are a heterogeneous group of genetic disorders (Table 33–4) with impaired Ig class switching from IgM to production of IgG, IgA, or IgE associated with normal or elevated serum IgM. If signaling through CD40 is affected, patients present also with opportunistic bacterial infections. Deficiencies of AID or UNG differ from CD40L and CD40 deficiencies in that the patients have large lymph nodes with germinal centers and are not susceptible to opportunistic infections. Patients with HIGM syndrome are at increased risk of autoimmune diseases. Treatment with Ig replacement decreases infections and often normalizes IgM levels. XL CD40L deficiency and NFκB signaling defects will be addressed further in section "Other combined immunodeficiency disorders."

4. Common Variable Immunodeficiency

ESSENTIALS OF DIAGNOSIS & TYPICAL FEATURES

- Recurrent sinopulmonary infections, also infections with *Giardia lamblia* and *Campylobacter jejuni*.
- Decreased levels of IgG and IgA; poor specific antibody responses.
- Often associated with autoimmune diseases.

General Considerations

Common variable immunodeficiency (CVID) is a diagnosis of exclusion after other causes of hypogammaglobulinemia have been eliminated. The onset may be at any age, and the incidence approaches 1:30,000. Many cases are sporadic, but a small percentage of patients have autosomal dominant or recessive inheritance, and some cases are associated with specific HLA-DR/DQ alleles (Table 33–4).

Clinical Findings

A. Symptoms and Signs

Patients have recurrent infections, most often of the sinopulmonary tract, but chronic gastrointestinal infections may manifest with recurrent diarrhea. Patients with CVID are at risk for developing bronchiectasis, autoimmune diseases (idiopathic thrombocytopenic purpura, autoimmune hemolytic anemia, rheumatoid arthritis, and inflammatory bowel disease), and malignancies (especially gastric carcinoma and lymphoma).

B. Laboratory Findings

Laboratory findings are variable, but typically reveal low levels of IgG and IgA, normal numbers of B lymphocytes, low numbers of memory B lymphocytes (evaluated by flow cytometry), and abnormal specific antibody levels and responses. Some patients have evidence of T-lymphocyte abnormalities as well. Chronic gastrointestinal tract infections are often due to *G lamblia* or *C jejuni*.

Although CVID is typically a diagnosis of exclusion, recent research has revealed multiple specific genetic mutations in patients with CVID. One example is a mutation in a member of the tumor necrosis factor receptor family, identified as transmembrane activator and calcium-modulator and cyclophilin ligand interactor (TACI), which mediates isotype switching in B lymphocytes. TACI mutations were recently found in 10%–15% of patients with CVID, as well as in some relatives of CVID patients with IgA deficiency. The mutations appear to be autosomal dominant, with variable penetrance of clinical immunodeficiency and autoimmune disease, and impairment of T-regulatory cell function.

Differential Diagnosis

When a patient presents with recurrent infections, low immunoglobulin levels, and potentially autoimmune symptoms, many different diagnoses must be considered, including other causes of low immunoglobulin levels (loss and abnormal production) and autoimmune diseases. CVID patients have normal numbers of B lymphocytes despite their poor specific antibody responses, which differentiates them from patients with XLA and autosomal recessive agammaglobulinemia. Patients with CVID also lack the specific mutations responsible for those other disorders. However, CVID patients often have decreased numbers of memory B cells ($IgM^-/IgD^-/CD27^+/CD20^+$ B cells).

Treatment

Treatment includes lifelong Ig replacement therapy and routine assessment for bronchiectasis, autoimmune disorders, and malignancies. The prognosis can be good and depends on the time to diagnosis and implementation of Ig replacement therapy. Other complications include B-cell hyperplasia in the gut that may be severe enough to resemble Crohn disease, and gastric atrophy with achlorhydria, sometimes followed by pernicious anemia. Lymphoreticular proliferation can occur after EBV infection and is not always malignant.

5. Acquired Hypogammaglobulinemia

Acquired forms of hypogammaglobulinemia are common and may develop at any age. Causes of secondary hypogammaglobulinemia (nephrotic syndrome and protein-losing enteropathy) should be excluded by measuring serum albumin. The loss of albumin (MW 69323 Da) is usually paralleled by a loss of IgG (MW 150,000 Da). Generally, acquired forms are not treated with Ig replacement therapy because, although immunoglobulin levels are low, antibody function is adequately protective. Morphologic disorders or associated syndromes may point to a specific diagnosis.

6. Transient Hypogammaglobulinemia

Serum IgG levels normally decrease during an infant's first 4–6 months of life as maternal IgG transmitted in utero is metabolized. Transient hypogammaglobulinemia represents a delay in the onset of immunoglobulin synthesis that results in a prolonged nadir. Symptomatic patients present with recurrent infections, including upper respiratory tract infections, otitis, and sinusitis. The diagnosis is suspected in infants and young children with low levels of IgG and IgA (usually two standard deviations below normal for age), but normal levels of IgM and normal numbers of circulating B lymphocytes. Importantly, affected children have normal specific antibody responses and T-lymphocyte function. Apart from appropriate antibiotics, no treatment is required. Infants with severe infections and hypogammaglobulinemia could be given Ig replacement, but benefits and risk must be considered and this is rarely necessary. Recovery occurs between 18 and 30 months of age, and the prognosis for affected children is excellent provided infections are treated promptly and appropriately.

7. Selective Immunoglobulin Deficiencies

Selective IgA deficiency is the most common immune abnormality, found in approximately 1:700 persons. It is defined by a serum IgA level less than 7 mg/dL. Serum IgM, IgG, specific antibodies, and B- and T-lymphocyte numbers and function are normal. IgA is primarily effective in its secreted form on mucosal surfaces. Therefore, symptomatic patients with low serum IgA develop upper respiratory tract infections, diarrhea, or both, but most people are asymptomatic.

Associations also exist with inflammatory bowel disease, allergic disease, asthma, and autoimmune disorders (thyroiditis, arthritis, vitiligo, thrombocytopenia, and diabetes). IgA replacement is currently not feasible. For the majority of symptomatic IgA-deficient patients, antibiotics and appropriate autoimmune therapies are sufficient. Caution must be exercised, as IgA-deficient patients are at risk for developing anti-IgA antibodies with blood product exposure, and the administration of blood products can result in anaphylaxis. Therefore, when blood products are needed, washed packed red blood cells and volume expanders without blood products are recommended.

The possibility that deficiency of an IgG subclass (eg, abnormally low serum IgG2, IgG3, or IgG4) might predispose to recurrent upper respiratory tract infections in patients with normal total serum immunoglobulin levels is not well established. Normally, IgG1 comprises over 60% of total IgG, IgG2 over 10%, IgG3 about 5%, and IgG4 may be undetectable in up to 20% of healthy persons. Additionally, serum levels are age-related. It has been difficult to establish a link between IgG subclass deficiencies and any consistent pattern of infections. IgG replacement should be reserved for patients with defects in specific antibody production and recurrent infections, which is rarely seen in patients with selective IgA or IgG subclass deficiencies.

Treatment of Hypogammaglobulinemia

The mainstay of therapy for hypogammaglobulinemia is replacement with IgG, but appropriate management of infections is also important. Curative therapy with bone marrow transplantation (BMT) has been successful in patients with XL HIGM syndrome. Replacement IgG is usually given by intravenous infusions at a dose of 400–600 mg/kg every 3–4 weeks to maintain trough serum IgG levels above 500–800 mg/dL (a higher trough level is targeted for patients with established pulmonary disease). Subcutaneous replacement is available, but requires more frequent injections and may limit maximum dosing. The aim of treatment is to *prevent* future infections and minimize any progression of chronic lung disease (bronchitis or bronchiectasis). Despite the passive immunity provided by replacement IgG, infections remain a persistent risk for affected patients. The prognosis also depends on timely and appropriate antibiotic therapy. Typical infecting organisms include encapsulated bacteria, but *Ureaplasma* and *Mycoplasma* species must also be considered. Infusions are generally well tolerated, with most reactions being mild, including headache, back and limb pain, anxiety, and chest tightness. Rare systemic reactions can occur, including tachycardia, shivering, fever, and, in severe cases, anaphylactoid shock. These adverse symptoms can be prevented by pretreatment with corticosteroids, antihistamines, and nonsteroidal anti-inflammatory drugs. For patients with congenital hypogammaglobulinemia, replacement therapy is currently lifelong. As a precautionary measure, patients with agammaglobulinemia or hypogammaglobulinemia should not receive live vaccines, but nonlive vaccines may be beneficial, particularly in patients with CVID.

Berger M: Principles of and advances of immunoglobulin replacement therapy for primary immunodeficiency. Immunol Allergy Clin N Am 2008;28:413–437 [PMID: 18424340].

SEVERE COMBINED IMMUNODEFICIENCY DISEASES

ESSENTIALS OF DIAGNOSIS & TYPICAL FEATURES

- Onset in first year of life.
- Recurrent infections caused by bacteria, viruses, fungi, and opportunistic pathogens.
- Chronic diarrhea and failure to thrive.
- Absent lymphoid tissue.

General Considerations

Severe combined immunodeficiency diseases (SCID) encompass congenital diseases caused by different genetic mutations that result in severe deficiency of T- and B-lymphocytes. Despite differences in underlying mutations, affected patients present similarly, with recurrent infections caused by bacteria, viruses, fungi, and opportunistic pathogens. Patients often suffer from chronic diarrhea and failure to thrive and typically die within the first year of life without treatment. Children with atypical SCID usually survive longer due to mutations in SCID-associated genes with residual protein function. SCID must be considered in the differential diagnosis in any infant with diarrhea and hypogammaglobulinemia.

Clinical Findings

A. Symptoms and Signs

Common presentations include persistent cough, tachypnea, or hypoxia secondary to underlying *Pneumocystis carinii* infection, or persistent oral or diaper candidiasis. Physical examination is notable for a lack of lymphoid tissue including tonsils and lymph nodes. A chest radiograph usually demonstrates an absent thymic shadow.

B. Laboratory Findings

Laboratory evaluation often reveals lymphopenia and some degree of hypogammaglobulinemia. Occasionally, an infant with SCID will present with normal numbers of lymphocytes resulting from transfusion-related engraftment or maternal T-lymphocyte engraftment via peripartum transfusion. NK cells and B-lymphocyte numbers may be decreased, normal, or elevated. Numbers of $CD31^+/CD45RA^+/CD4^+$ recent thymic emigrant T cells reflect thymic T cell output and are usually decreased in SCID patients. Additionally, in-vitro lymphocyte assays show poor response to mitogens, and specific antibodies are absent. Antenatal diagnosis is possible. Once the diagnosis of SCID is suspected, genetic testing should be pursued to confirm the diagnosis and the mutation present for both prognostic and genetic counseling purposes. Clinical presentation and treatment are generally similar. The variants of SCID can be organized by the presence or absence of specific lymphocytes, including T, B, and NK cells (Table 33–5).

Differential Diagnosis

The differential diagnosis of SCID includes other causes of recurrent and severe infections and abnormal immune responses, most notably HIV disease. Other causes of hypogammaglobulinemia or agammaglobulinemia may be considered but can usually be ruled out in the presence of abnormal T-lymphocyte numbers and function. The infection spectrum and severity of presentation in children with SCID is more severe and of earlier onset than that seen with agammaglobulinemia. Symptoms of congenital abnormalities with combined immunodeficiency features are discussed later in this chapter (see section on Genetic Syndromes Associated with Immunodeficiency).

Treatment

When SCID is suspected, *Pneumocystis* prophylaxis with trimethoprim–sulfamethoxazole and replacement Ig therapy should be initiated. *Patients with suspected SCID should only be transfused with irradiated blood products and should not receive any live vaccines.* Confirmation of the diagnosis should include screening for SCID subtypes listed in Table 33–5. BMT offers the best possibility of cure, with use of a human leukocyte antigen (HLA)-matched sibling offering the highest chance of success. In affected patients without HLA-identical donors, HLA haploidentical bone marrow cells from family members or HLA-matched unrelated donors are used. For most patients, myeloablation is not necessary as the patient is without T lymphocytes. Additionally, most patients do not require prophylaxis for graft-versus-host disease (GVHD) unless the donor is unrelated. T-lymphocyte reconstitution takes approximately 4 months, but only about 50% of patients regain full B-lymphocyte function, with the majority requiring long-term Ig replacement. For months posttransplantation, patients are susceptible to many serious infections, and prophylaxis is usually continued. Additionally, any signs or symptoms of infection must be promptly investigated and aggressively treated. The highest rate of success is in the youngest patients prior to developing infections (> 95% survival), but overall rates of survival range from 50% to 100% depending on the underlying mutation. XL SCID and ADA deficiency have been treated with gene therapy. Normal gene function was transduced in XL SCID patients, but due to insertion of the retroviral vector near an oncogene, some patients developed lymphoproliferative disorders. At this time, safer vectors are being sought.

Van der Burg M, Gennery AR: Educational paper: The expanding clinical and immunologic spectrum of severe combined immunodeficiency. Eur J Pediatr 2011;170:561–572 [PMID: 21479529].

1. X-Linked Severe Combined Immunodeficiency

XL SCID, the most common form (40%) of SCID, results from mutations in *IL2RG* (IL-2 receptor gene) that encodes the common γ chain. The γ-chain protein is shared by multiple cell surface receptors for cytokines that are essential for T-lymphocyte maturation, including IL-2, IL-4, IL-7, IL-9, IL-15, and IL-21. Within the first 3 months of life, male infants present with diarrhea, cough, and rash. Laboratory evaluation reveals low T-lymphocyte numbers, normal numbers of B lymphocytes (which do not produce functional antibody), and absent NK cells.

2. Adenosine Deaminase Deficiency

Adenosine deaminase deficiency (ADA) is an AR form of SCID caused by absence of adenosine deaminase, which is important for removal of toxic metabolites formed in lymphocytes, including adenosine, 2′-deoxyadenosine, and 2′*O*-methyladenosine. Increased levels of these metabolites result in lymphocyte death. Subsequently, affected patients develop complete absence of T-lymphocyte function and progressive decrease in immunoglobulin production. ADA SCID is distinguished from other variants of SCID by the following findings: the most profound lymphopenia (< 500/mm^3); skeletal abnormalities, including chondro-osseous dysplasia (flared costochondral junctions and bone-in-bone anomalies in vertebrae); and deficiency of all types of lymphocytes. Diagnosis is suspected in patients with profound lymphopenia and recurrent infections. The diagnosis is confirmed with a red blood cell assay for ADA activity. The genetic mutation is on chromosome 20q13.2–13.11. In addition to BMT, restoration of immune competence can occur in some patients with weekly infusions of polyethylene glycol–stabilized ADA enzyme conjugate. Gene therapy of stem cells with an ADA-incorporating retroviral vector has been successful, but the vector caused oncogenic adverse effects.

3. Janus Kinase 3 Deficiency

Another form of AR SCID is due to mutations in the gene encoding janus kinase 3, which is important for intracellular signaling through the common γ chain. The clinical presentation and lymphocyte phenotype most closely resembles X-linked SCID, with low T and NK lymphocytes, and normal or elevated, nonfunctional B lymphocytes.

4. Interleukin-7-Receptor-α-Chain Deficiency

IL-7-receptor-α-chain (IL-7R α) deficiency SCID is transmitted by AR inheritance. The IL-7 receptor is important for T-lymphocyte maturation and mutations result in low T-lymphocyte numbers, but normal numbers of dysfunctional B lymphocytes and NK cells.

5. Recombinase-Activating Gene Deficiencies

Another form of autosomal recessive SCID is due to mutations in recombinase-activating genes (*RAG1* and *RAG2*), which encode proteins critical for assembling antigen receptor genes for both T- and B-lymphocytes. Several mutations in these genes have been described. The clinical presentation is similar to that of other forms of SCID, but the lymphocyte phenotype differs, as patients with SCID due to *RAG1* or *RAG2* mutations lack both T- and B-lymphocytes, but maintain normal or elevated numbers of NK cells.

Omenn syndrome is an autosomal AR syndrome characterized by SCID, eczematoid rash, hepatosplenomegaly, lymphadenopathy, and alopecia. The disease is caused by mutations in *RAG1, RAG2,* or Artemis mutations (see below). Laboratory evaluation reveals absent B lymphocytes, normal to elevated T-lymphocyte numbers with restricted function, and normal functional NK cells. Additionally, affected patients often have eosinophilia and elevated levels of IgE. The syndrome is typically fatal, although BMT has been used successfully.

6. CD3-δ-Chain Deficiency

CD3-δ-chain (CD3δ) deficiency is a rare form of AR SCID. Homozygous defects in the CD3δ chain halt T-lymphocyte maturation. Clinical presentation and lymphocyte phenotype are similar to IL-7Rα deficiency, but CD3δ-chain deficiency differs from other forms of SCID in that these patients have a normal-appearing thymic silhouette on chest radiograph.

7. CD45 Deficiency

Another rare form of AR SCID is due to mutations in the gene for CD45. CD45 is a tyrosine phosphatase important for regulating signal transduction. Affected patients have a similar presentation to other forms of SCID and a lymphocyte phenotype with low to absent T and NK cells, but normal B lymphocytes.

8. Artemis Deficiency

Artemis is a DNA repair factor important for repairing cuts in the double-stranded DNA essential for the assembly of antigen receptors for T- and B-lymphocytes. Inheritance is AR, and clinical presentation and lymphocyte phenotype are similar to those seen in *RAG1* and *RAG2* deficiencies.

9. ZAP-70 Deficiency

Deficiency of zeta-chain–associated protein (ZAP)-70 results in a rare form of AR SCID. ZAP-70 is a tyrosine kinase critical for T-lymphocyte signaling and activation. Clinical presentation is similar to that of other forms of SCID, but most affected patients have palpable lymph nodes and visible thymic silhouette. Lymphocyte evaluation reveals absence of CD8$^+$ T lymphocytes, normal but nonfunctional CD4$^+$ T lymphocytes, normal numbers of poorly functioning B lymphocytes, and normal numbers and function of NK cells.

OTHER COMBINED IMMUNODEFICIENCY DISORDERS

Combined immunodeficiencies include defects that directly impair both T- and B-lymphocytes, as well as T-lymphocyte–specific defects, because proper B-lymphocyte function and antibody production are dependent on T-lymphocyte help. Therefore, most T-lymphocyte deficiencies manifest as combined impairments.

Kersseboom R et al: Educational paper: Syndromic forms of primary immunodeficiency. Eur J Pediatr 2011;170:295–308 [PMID: 21337117].

1. Wiskott-Aldrich Syndrome

ESSENTIALS OF DIAGNOSIS & TYPICAL FEATURES

- Immunodeficiency with recurrent infections.
- Microplatelet thrombocytopenia.
- Eczema.
- Occurs only in males.

General Considerations

Wiskott-Aldrich syndrome (WAS) is an XL recessive disease characterized by immunodeficiency, microplatelet thrombocytopenia, and eczema. The syndrome results from mutations of the gene encoding WASP at X11p. WASP is a protein involved in the rearrangement of actin and is important in interactions between T lymphocytes and antigen-presenting cells.

Clinical Findings

A. Symptoms and Signs

Common presenting symptoms include mucosal bleeding, bloody diarrhea, cerebral hemorrhage, and severe infections with polysaccharide-encapsulated bacteria, but the clinical presentation can vary from classic severe WAS to mild thrombocytopenia without immunodeficiency, or X-linked thrombocytopenia (XLT), depending on the mutation. Early deaths are due to bleeding and infections, but malignancies and autoimmune syndromes can develop over time. Survival beyond adolescence is rare in patients not receiving treatment, although XLT is sometimes diagnosed in adults.

B. Laboratory Findings

Laboratory findings that suggest the diagnosis are a low platelet count, small platelets, low or absent isohemagglutinins, and reduced antibody responses to polysaccharide antigens (*S pneumoniae* and *H influenzae*). IgM may be low; IgG is usually normal; IgA and IgE are often high. The diagnosis can be confirmed by genetic testing for a mutation of the *WASP* gene or by assessing WASP expression. Genetic testing can also be used for carrier screening.

Differential Diagnosis

In addition to WAS and XLT, the differential diagnosis in a patient with a low platelet count must include other causes of platelet consumption, destruction, and abnormal production, such as idiopathic thrombocytopenic purpura, leukemia or myelodysplasia, drug adverse effect, and infection. WAS can be differentiated from these other conditions by small-sized platelets on smear evaluation, the presence of eczema and other atopic features, and documented immune dysfunction. Additionally, there is a continuous spectrum between WAS and XLT that lacks immunodeficiency. Subsequently, a scoring system has been developed to help clinicians distinguish WAS from XLT.

Treatment

Treatment includes infection prophylaxis with antibiotics (including trimethoprim–sulfamethoxazole for *P carinii* pneumonia) and IVIG replacement therapy for patients with deficient antibody responses. Splenectomy to reduce thrombocytopenia has been helpful in some patients with XLT, but must be followed by antibiotic prophylaxis because of the increased risk of septicemia and sudden death. Platelet transfusions should be avoided unless severe bleeding has occurred. Finally, BMT using the best-matched donor offers the possibility of a definitive cure, but is associated with morbidity and mortality.

2. 22q11.2 Deletion Syndrome (DiGeorge Syndrome)

ESSENTIALS OF DIAGNOSIS & TYPICAL FEATURES

- Congenital heart defects.
- Hypocalcemia and seizures.
- Distinctive craniofacial features.
- Thymic hypoplasia.

General Considerations

DiGeorge syndrome or 22q11.2 deletion syndrome is an AD syndrome, resulting in defective development of the third and fourth pharyngeal pouches. There is considerable variability in phenotype based on the location and extent of the deletion, but deletions that include the *TBX1* gene appear relevant. Overlapping syndromes include velocardiofacial syndrome and Shprintzen syndrome. The incidence is about 1:4000 births, and the abnormal chromosome is usually inherited from the mother. The associated immunodeficiency is secondary to the aplastic or hypoplastic thymus, where T-lymphocyte maturation occurs. Surprisingly, most patients have no or only mild immune defects. The term *partial DiGeorge syndrome* is commonly applied to these patients with impaired rather than absent thymic function.

Clinical Findings

A. Symptoms and Signs

Clinical characteristics include congenital heart defects, hypocalcemia due to hypoparathyroidism, distinctive craniofacial features, renal anomalies, and thymic hypoplasia. Presentation usually results from cardiac failure or from hypocalcemia 24–48 hours postpartum. The diagnosis is sometimes made during the course of cardiac surgery when no thymus is found in the mediastinum. Infections commonly present as recurrent ENT infections. Additional important clinical issues include delayed speech, cognitive impairment, and behavioral problems. Patients have an increased risk to develop schizophrenia and autoimmune disorders.

B. Laboratory Findings

Laboratory evaluation typically reveals normal to decreased numbers of T lymphocytes with preserved T-lymphocyte function and normal B-lymphocyte function. In the rare patient with absent or dysfunctional T lymphocytes, B-lymphocyte function and antibody production may be abnormal. Over time, T-lymphocyte numbers normalize in the majority of patients who have low numbers of T lymphocytes at initial presentation. The diagnosis is confirmed via fluorescence in situ hybridization (FISH) chromosomal analysis for the microdeletion on chromosome 22, or microarray based comparative genomic hybridization.

Treatment

Treatment of the 22q11.2 deletion syndrome may require surgery for cardiac defects, and vitamin D, calcium, or parathyroid hormone replacement to correct hypocalcemia and treat seizures. Transfusion products should be irradiated. Both thymic grafts and BMT have been used successfully in patients with absent T-lymphocyte immunity. Prior to giving live vaccines, T-cell numbers and function should be assessed if not done earlier, to prevent vaccine-related side effects.

3. Ataxia-Telangiectasia

Ataxia-telangiectasia (A-T) is a rare, neurodegenerative, AR-inherited disorder caused by mutations in the ataxia telangiectasia mutated (*ATM*) gene located on chromosome 11q22–23 that encodes the ATM protein, a protein kinase involved in repair of double-stranded DNA and cell cycle regulation. A-T is characterized by progressive cerebellar ataxia, telangiectasia, and variable immunodeficiency. Children usually present as toddlers with slurred speech and balance problems, and also with sinopulmonary infections. Telangiectasias of the conjunctivae and exposed areas (eg, nose, ears, and shoulders) follow later during childhood. Respiratory tract infections promoted by respiratory muscle weakness, swallowing dysfunction and recurrent aspirations, and malignancies, including carcinomas and lymphomas, are the major causes of death between the second and fourth decade of life. Abnormal findings in A-T include elevated serum α-fetoprotein levels that increase over time and are used diagnostically; immunoglobulin deficiencies, including low levels of IgA, IgE, or IgG; and defective ability to repair radiation-induced DNA fragmentation. There is no definitive treatment, although Ig replacement and aggressive antibiotics have been used with limited success. Heterozygotes have an increased risk for breast cancer.

Similarly to A-T, the **Nijmegen breakage** syndrome is a disorder associated with impaired DNA repair and mutations in the *NBS1* gene that shows more severe clinical features, including microcephaly and facial dysmorphisms, small stature, immunodeficiency, and increased risk for lymphoid malignancies.

4. X-Linked Hyper-IgM Syndrome

X-linked HIGM syndrome or CD40L deficiency is the most common and most severe form of hyper-IgM syndrome and involves a mutation in the gene encoding for CD40L (CD154). CD40L is expressed on activated T lymphocytes and necessary for T cells to induce immunoglobulin isotype switching in B cells. Unlike the AR forms of hyper-IgM syndrome, the mutation results in both antibody and cell-mediated deficiencies, as the interaction between CD40L on T cells and CD40 on B cells and antigen-presenting cells is important for both antibody production and T-cell activation. Affected males have normal numbers of B lymphocytes, low levels of IgG and IgA, but normal or elevated levels of IgM. Typically, male infants present with recurrent bacterial and opportunistic infections such as *P carinii* pneumonia or *Cryptosporidium* diarrhea. Additionally, affected males have a high frequency of sclerosing cholangitis, increased liver and biliary tract carcinomas, neutropenia, and autoimmune syndromes, including thrombocytopenia, arthritis, and inflammatory bowel disease. Conservative treatment includes Ig replacement and antibiotic prophylaxis. Because the prognosis is still quite poor, BMT has been used with initial success.

5. NFκB Signaling Defects

Immunodeficiency due to mutations in the gene for nuclear factor-κB–essential modulator (NEMO; *IKBKG* gene) is an XL syndrome in which male patients manifest ectodermal dysplasia (abnormal, conical teeth, fine sparse hair, and abnormal or absent sweat glands) and defects of T- and B-lymphocytes. Nuclear factor-κB (NFκB) is involved in signaling through CD40 on B cells, and NEMO mutations result in abnormal immunoreceptor signaling. Many mutations are fatal in utero for male infants. Female carriers may have incontinentia pigmenti. Surviving males present with early serious infections, including opportunistic infections with *P carinii* and atypical mycobacteria. Laboratory evaluation reveals hypogammaglobulinemia that may present as HIGM syndrome and poor specific antibody production, but normal numbers of T- and B-lymphocytes. Functional evaluation of lymphocytes demonstrates variable response. Because patients with confirmed NEMO mutations are quite rare, the best treatment course is unknown, but aggressive antibiotic therapy in combination with Ig replacement as well as BMT has been used. The prognosis is dependent on the severity of immunodeficiency, with most deaths due to infection. Mutations in the *NFKBIA* gene that encodes IκBα (nuclear factor of kappa light polypeptide gene enhancer in B-cells inhibitor alpha) result in an AD inherited defect with similar clinical presentation.

6. Combined Immunodeficiency with Defective Expression of Major Histocompatibility Complex Types I & II

Major histocompatibility complex class I (MHC I) deficiency or bare lymphocyte syndrome type I is an AR combined immunodeficiency. Affected patients have abnormal expression of the transporter associated with antigen processing (TAP). TAP proteins are important for intracellular transport and expression of MHC I on cell surfaces. Patients with bare lymphocyte syndrome type I present with recurrent sinopulmonary and skin infections. The diagnosis is confirmed by demonstrating an absence of MHC I expression.

Major histocompatibility complex class II (MHC II) deficiency or bare lymphocyte syndrome type II is a rare AR combined immunodeficiency in which cells lack MHC II expression due to mutations in *CIITA*, *RFX-5*, *RXAP*, or *RFZANK* genes. Clinical presentation includes recurrent viral, bacterial, and fungal infections. Patients with bare lymphocyte syndrome type II have normal numbers of T- and B-lymphocytes, but low $CD4^+$ lymphocyte numbers, abnormal lymphocyte function, and hypogammaglobulinemia. They also have a high incidence of sclerosing cholangitis. When this diagnosis is suspected, demonstration of absent MHC II molecules confirms the disorder. Severe cases are fatal without BMT, but milder phenotypes may be managed with Ig replacement and aggressive use of antibiotics.

Reith W, Mach B: The bare lymphocyte syndrome and the regulation of MHC expression. Annu Rev Immunol 2001;19:331–373 [PMID: 11244040].

7. Purine Nucleoside Phosphorylase Deficiency

Purine nucleoside phosphorylase (PNP) deficiency is an immunodeficiency due to defects in the gene encoding PNP, which is important in the purine salvage pathway. Deficiency of PNP causes toxic metabolites that result in T-lymphocyte death, but in many patients B lymphocytes are spared. This AR disease not only results in recurrent and serious infections, but affected patients also have concomitant neurologic (developmental delay, ataxia, and spasticity) and autoimmune disorders. Infections present at variable ages. Laboratory evaluation reveals low numbers of or absent T lymphocytes and a variable B-lymphocyte deficiency. Without BMT, this disease is fatal due to infection or malignancy.

PHAGOCYTE DISORDERS

Phagocyte defects include abnormalities of both numbers (neutropenia) and function of polymorphonuclear neutrophils. Functional defects consist of impairments in adhesion, chemotaxis, bacterial killing, or, less often, of combinations of these.

1. Neutropenia

The presence of neutropenia should be considered when evaluating recurrent infections. The diagnosis and treatment of neutropenia is discussed in Chapter 30. Additionally, some PID syndromes are associated with neutropenia (eg, XLA).

Bouma G et al: Recent advances in the understanding of genetic defects of neutrophil number and function. Br J Haematol 2010;151:312–326 [PMID: 20813010].

Boxer LA, Newburger PE: Disorders of phagocyte function and leukopenia. In Kleigman RM et al (editors): *Nelson Textbook of Pediatrics*, 19th ed. 2011, 741–752.

2. Chronic Granulomatous Disease

ESSENTIALS OF DIAGNOSIS & TYPICAL FEATURES

- Recurrent infections with catalase-positive bacteria and fungi.
- X-linked and autosomal recessive forms.
- Caused by abnormal phagocytosis-associated generation of microbicidal oxygen metabolites (respiratory burst) by neutrophils, monocytes, and macrophages.

General Considerations

Chronic granulomatous disease (CGD) is caused by a defect in any of several genes encoding proteins in the enzyme complex nicotinamide adenine dinucleotide phosphate (NADPH) oxidase, which results in defective superoxide and hydrogen peroxide generation during ingestion of microbes. Most cases (probably 75%) are inherited as an X-linked recessive trait; the rest are AR in inheritance.

Clinical Findings

A. Symptoms and Signs

The typical clinical presentation is characterized by recurrent abscess formation in subcutaneous tissue, lymph nodes, lungs, and liver, and by pneumonia and eczematous and purulent skin rashes. Infecting organisms are typically catalase-positive bacteria, which can break down their own hydrogen peroxide and thus avoid death when captured in a CGD phagocytic vacuole. (Streptococci, pneumococci, and

H influenzae lack catalase and are not unusually pathogenic in CGD.) Aspergillosis is also common and a frequent cause of death. Lymphadenopathy and hepatosplenomegaly are found on physical examination, and granulomas are seen in histopathologic sections. Granulomatous inflammation can narrow the outlet of the stomach or bladder in these patients, leading to vomiting or urinary obstruction.

B. Laboratory Findings

Patients typically present with serious infection, positive microbial cultures, and neutrophilia. The most common infecting organisms are *S aureus, Aspergillus* species, *Burkholderia cepacia*, and *Serratia marcescens*. (Culture of either of the last two should suggest this diagnosis.) Patients also present with granulomas of lymph nodes, skin, liver, and genitourinary tract. The erythrocyte sedimentation rate may be elevated without obvious infection. The diagnosis is confirmed by demonstrating lack of hydrogen peroxide production using the DHR flow cytometry assay or lack of superoxide production using the NBT test. Both tests can demonstrate carrier status of X-linked disease.

Differential Diagnosis

The differential diagnosis includes other phagocyte abnormalities or deficiencies described in this section, as well as the rare neutrophil granule deficiency. Other immunodeficient states leading to severe bacterial or fungal infections should be considered, but none have the striking abscess formation and deficient phagocytosis-associated respiratory burst that characterize CGD.

Treatment

Daily intake of an antimicrobial agent such as trimethoprim–sulfamethoxazole is indicated in all patients; and an oral antifungal agent like itraconazole and regular subcutaneous injections of INF-γ can greatly reduce the risk of severe infections. BMT has been successful in some cases, but the risk of death is high unless the patient's condition is stable. Gastric or GU obstruction can be relieved by short-term steroid therapy.

Johnston RB Jr: Clinical aspects of chronic granulomatous disease. Curr Opin Hematol 2001;8:17–22 [PMID: 11138621].

3. Leukocyte Adhesion Defects Types I & II

ESSENTIALS OF DIAGNOSIS & TYPICAL FEATURES

- Recurrent serious infections.
- "Cold" abscesses without pus formation.
- Poor wound healing.
- Gingival or periodontal disease (or both).

General Considerations

The ability of phagocytic cells to enter peripheral sites of infection is critical for effective host defense. In leukocyte adhesion defect (LAD), defects in proteins required for leukocyte adherence to and migration through blood vessel walls prevent these cells from arriving at the sites of infection. LAD I is an AR disease caused by mutations in the common chain of the β_2 integrin family (CD18) located on chromosome 21q22.3. These mutations result in impaired neutrophil migration, adherence, and antibody-dependent phagocytosis. LAD II is a rare AR disease caused by an inborn error in fucose metabolism that results in abnormal expression of leukocyte sialyl-Lewis X (CD15s), which binds to selectins on the vessel endothelium. The resulting phenotype is similar to LAD I, with recurrent infections, lack of pus formation, poor wound healing, and periodontal disease. LAD II patients also have developmental delays, short stature, dysmorphic facies, and the Bombay (hh) blood group.

Clinical Findings

A. Symptoms and Signs

Patients present with variably severe phenotypes, including recurrent serious infections, lack of pus formation, poor wound healing, and gingival and periodontal disease. The hallmark is little inflammation and absent neutrophils on histopathologic evaluation of infected sites (ie, "cold" abscesses), especially when concurrent with neutrophilia, an expression of poor adherence to vessel walls. The most severe phenotype manifests with infections in the neonatal period, including delayed separation of the umbilical cord with associated omphalitis.

B. Laboratory Findings

Laboratory evaluation often demonstrates a striking neutrophilia. Diagnosis of suspected cases is confirmed by flow cytometry analysis for CD18 (LAD I) or CD15s (LAD II).

Treatment

Treatment includes aggressive antibiotic therapy. Fucose supplementation in LAD II has been reported with some success.

4. Glucose-6-Phosphate Dehydrogenase Deficiency

Rare forms of X-linked glucose-6-phosphate dehydrogenase deficiency with associated hemolytic anemia affect leukocytes as well as erythrocytes and result in recurrent infections due to an abnormal neutrophil respiratory burst, probably due to NAD/NADPH deficiency.

5. Myeloperoxidase Deficiency

Leukocyte myeloperoxidase (MPO) is important for intracellular destruction of *C albicans*. Although deficiency is quite common, only a very few patients with concurrent diabetes have had severe candidal infections. Diagnosis can be confirmed with assays measuring MPO levels in leukocytes.

COMPLEMENT DEFICIENCIES

Complement contributes to innate immunity and facilitates antibody-mediated immunity through opsonization, lysis of target cells, and recruitment of phagocytic cells. The complement system includes three interactive pathways of enzymatic reactions: classical, alternative, and lectin (see Figure 33–4). All three pathways generate cleavage of C3 and result in promotion of inflammation, elimination of pathogens, and enhancement of the immune response. Activation of the complement system occurs through microbial products, tissue enzymes, and surface-bound IgG and IgM antibodies or pentraxins, for example, C-reactive protein.

1. Complement Component Deficiencies

Deficiencies of individual complement components (C1–C9) are inherited as autosomal co-dominant traits, each parent contributing one null gene. Serum levels of the deficient component are about half normal in the parents and zero or almost zero in the patients. Deficiencies of C1, C2, or C4 predispose to increased infections but are particularly associated with autoimmune disorders such as systemic lupus erythematosus. Patients with homozygous C2 deficiency can present at any age in childhood with bacteremia or meningitis due to *S pneumoniae* or *H influenzae*. Primary C3 deficiency presents with severe pyogenic infections since C3 is critical for opsonization in both the classical and alternative pathways. Deficiency of the control protein factor I, which acts to break up the C3-cleaving complex formed in the classical or alternative pathway, leads to unbridled consumption of C3 and, thereby, severe bacterial infections. Deficiency of a terminal complement component in the membrane attack complex (C5, C6, C7, C8, and C9) or of properdin (an X-linked alternative pathway control protein) results in recurrent neisserial meningitis or disseminated gonococcal infection. Survivors of either of these serious neisserial infections should be screened for complement deficiency, first with a CH50 assay and later with an AH50 assay if the CH50 is normal.

Mannose-binding lectin (MBL) and ficolins-1, 2, and 3 serve as the recognition components of the lectin pathway, which recognizes microbial surface carbohydrates. Deficiency of MBL has been linked to increased risk of infections in infancy and in patients who have another defect of host defense. Ficolin-3 deficiency has been associated with severe infections.

Johnston RB Jr: The complement system and disorders of the complement system. In Kliegman RM et al (editors): *Nelson Textbook of Pediatrics*, 19th ed. 2011, 753–756.

Tebruegge M, Curtis N: Epidemiology, etiology, pathogenesis, and diagnosis of recurrent bacterial meningitis. Clin Microbiol Rev 2008;21:519 [PMID: 18625686].

Ram S et al: Infections of people with complement deficiencies and patients who have undergone splenectomy. Clin Microbiol Rev 2010;23:740–780 [PMID: 20930072].

2. Hereditary Angioedema Due to C1 Inhibitor Deficiency

ESSENTIALS OF DIAGNOSIS & TYPICAL FEATURES

- Recurrent episodes of angioedema often triggered by trauma.
- No associated urticaria or pruritus.
- Onset at any age but more common after puberty.

General Considerations

Hereditary angioedema is an autosomal dominant disorder caused by deficiency of C1 inhibitor (C1-INH), which controls activation of the classical complement pathway, coagulation factors XIa and XIIa, and kallikrein. There is no increased susceptibility to infection. Acquired forms can occur with B-lymphocyte malignancies, factor XII mutations, or use of an angiotensin-converting enzyme inhibitor as medication.

Clinical Findings

A. Symptoms and Signs

Affected patients can experience edema of skin and bowel and potentially life-threatening edema of the airway. Typical sites of swelling include the face, extremities, and genitals. Trauma, accidental or due to surgery, childbirth, or dental work, may induce edema. Typical problems include episodic intestinal obstruction and dental procedure–induced upper airway obstruction. The edema is usually nonpainful (unless it involves the bowel) and lasts 48–72 hours. There is no associated urticaria, redness, or pruritus. Age of onset is variable, and there is often a positive family history.

B. Laboratory Findings

Initial screening tests for C1-INH deficiency show a decreased CH50 or low levels of C4 and C2. C1q is usually normal. The diagnosis is confirmed by low or absent levels of C1-INH (type I, 85% of cases) or poor or absent C1-INH function (type II).

Differential Diagnosis

Other causes of acquired angioedema, including that associated with certain medications (most notably angiotensin-converting enzyme modifying drugs), autoimmune diseases, and lymphoproliferative diseases, should be considered. A normal level of C1q in hereditary angioedema usually distinguishes this form from the acquired forms.

Treatment

Intravenous C1-INH concentrate is the treatment of choice for the emergency management of acute edema (eg, laryngeal or diffuse facial edema, severe abdominal attacks). Treatment with this concentrate can also be used for long-term prophylaxis when attacks occur monthly or have been life-threatening, or for preparation for surgery or dental work. Fresh frozen plasma may be used as a substitute in the acute situation. The synthetic androgen oxandrolone prevents attacks by increasing C1-INH levels, and this is approved for cautious use in children. Antihistamines, adrenalin, and steroids have no therapeutic value.

Morgan PB: Hereditary angioedema—therapies old and new. N Engl J Med 2010;363:581–583 [PMID: 20818894].

Zuraw BL: Hereditary angioedema. N Engl J Med 2008;359:1027–1036 [PMID: 18768946].

3. Factor H Deficiency & Atypical Hemolytic Uremic Syndrome (aHUS)

The effects of factor H deficiency are like those of factor I deficiency because factor H helps dismantle the alternative pathway C3-cleaving enzyme. Levels of C3, factor B, CH50, and AP50 are all decreased. Some patients have sustained serious infections, and many have had glomerulonephritis or atypical hemolytic uremic syndrome (aHUS). Mutations in genes encoding membrane control protein, factor I, factor B, C3, or the endothelial anti-inflammatory protein thrombomodulin, or autoantibodies to factor H, have also been associated with HUS. In a child with HUS, it seems advisable to screen for a complement deficiency, first with the CH50 assay. With an associated complement disorder the prognosis is less favorable, and recognizing the presence of a complement deficiency should alert the physician to the associated increased risk of infection or autoimmune disease, or both.

Noris M, Remuzzi G: Atypical hemolytic-uremic syndrome. N Engl J Med 2009;361:1676–1687 [PMID: 19846853].

OTHER WELL-DEFINED IMMUNODEFICIENCY SYNDROMES

1. Hyper-IgE Syndrome

Hyper-IgE syndrome (HIES), also known as Job syndrome, is a rare PID characterized by elevated levels of IgE (> 2000 IU/mL), neonatal eczematoid rash, recurrent infections with *S aureus*, recurrent pneumonia with pneumatocele formation, and typical facies. Mutations in a specific transcription factor, signal transducer and activator of transcription 3 (*STAT3*), underlie sporadic and AD forms of HIES. Additional clinical findings of HIES include retained primary teeth, scoliosis, hyperextensibility, high palate, and osteoporosis. In addition to staphylococcal infections, affected patients also have increased incidence of infections due to *Streptococcus* spp, *Pseudomonas* spp, *C albicans*, and even opportunistic infections with *P carinii*. Autosomal recessive HIES is associated with mutations in dedicator of cytokinesis 8 (*DOCK8*) and tyrosine kinase 2 (*TYK2*) genes. Patients with AR HIES have an increased susceptibility to viral infections including recurrent molluscum contagiosum, warts, and herpes simplex infections. Increased susceptibility to mycobacterial infections is found in patients with *TYK2* mutations. Laboratory evaluation reveals normal to profoundly elevated levels of IgE and occasionally eosinophilia. However, atopic dermatitis and parasite infection are much more common causes of elevated IgE. Diagnosis is often difficult due to variable presentation, which may become progressively severe with increasing age, but genetic testing for *STAT3, DOCK8,* and *TYK2* mutations will help to confirm the diagnosis of HIES particularly at a young age. All patients with HIES have impaired T_H17 cell function, and measurement of T_H17+ cells in the peripheral blood can be used as screening test if HIES is suspected. The mainstay of treatment is prophylactic and symptomatic antibiotic use in combination with good skin care. Ig replacement has been used with some success to decrease infections and possibly modify IgE levels.

Woellner C et al: Mutations in STAT3 and diagnostic guidelines for hyper-IgE syndrome. J Allergy Clin Immunol 2010;125:424–432 [PMID: 20159255].

Rezaei N et al: Primary immunodeficiency diseases associated with increased susceptibility to viral infections and malignancies. J Allergy Clin Immunol 2011;127:1329–1341 [PMID: 21514636].

2. Immune Dysregulation, Polyendocrinopathy, Enteropathy, X-Linked Syndrome

Immune dysregulation, polyendocrinopathy, enteropathy, X-linked (IPEX) syndrome is a rare disease that usually manifests with severe diarrhea and insulin-dependent diabetes mellitus within the first months of life. Affected males also have severe eczema, food allergy, autoimmune cytopenias, lymphadenopathy, splenomegaly, and recurrent infections. Most die before 2 years of age due to malnutrition or sepsis. IPEX syndrome results from mutations in the *FOXP3* gene that encodes a protein essential for developing regulatory T lymphocytes. Leukocyte counts and immunoglobulin levels are generally normal. Immunosuppression and nutritional supplementation produce temporary improvements, but the prognosis is poor and most cases result in early death. BMT has been attempted with variable success. More recently, IPEX-like syndromes have been described as associated with mutations of the gene encoding CD25, the high affinity IL-2 receptor (IL2R) which is constitutively expressed on regulatory T cells. If IPEX or IPEX-like syndromes are suspected, the presence of $FOXP3^+/CD25^+$ regulatory T cells should be assessed not only in affected boys, but also in girls. Genetic testing for FOXP3 mutations will be helpful to identify affected patients and carriers of the gene mutation.

Torgerson T, Ochs HD: Immune dysregulation, polyendocrinopathy, enteropathy, X-linked: Forkhead box protein 3 mutations and lack of regulatory T cells. J Allergy Clin Immunol 2007;120:744 [PMID: 17942886].

3. X-Linked Lymphoproliferative Syndrome

X-linked lymphoproliferative syndrome is an immunodeficiency that usually develops following EBV infection. Affected males develop fulminant infectious mononucleosis with hemophagocytic syndrome, multiple organ system failure, and bone marrow aplasia. The mutated gene (*SH2D1A/SAP/DSHP*) encodes a signaling protein used by T lymphocytes and NK cells called SLAM-adapter protein (SAP). Affected boys are immunologically normal prior to EBV infection and during acute infection they produce antibody to EBV. In most instances, infection with EBV is fatal. Patients who survive the initial episode or who are never infected with EBV in childhood develop lymphomas, vasculitis, hypogammaglobulinemias (with elevated IgM), or CVID in later life. Genetic analysis for a mutation of the SAP (*SH2D1A*) gene, and testing for SAP protein expression are available. Mutations in the genes encoding for the X-linked inhibitor of apoptosis (XIAP), a potent regulator of lymphocyte homeostasis, and for IL-2-inducible T-cell kinase (ITK) have been described to present as an XLP-like syndrome. Testing for mutations of the gene encoding for XIAP (*BIRC4*) and XIAP protein expression will help to establish the diagnosis. A decreased number of naïve, $CD45RA^+$ T cells is indicative of ITK deficiency, and further genetic analysis can establish the diagnosis.

Rezaei N et al: Primary immunodeficiency diseases associated with increased susceptibility to viral infections and malignancies. J Allergy Clin Immunol 2011;127:1329–1341 [PMID: 21514636].

4. Chronic Mucocutaneous Candidiasis

There are two forms of chronic mucocutaneous candidiasis (CMC). The first type is an AD disorder that is characterized by isolated candidal infections of the skin, nails, and mucous membranes. Systemic disease is not characteristic, but case reports of intracranial mycotic aneurysms exist. Primary CMC most commonly occurs as an isolated syndrome, but can be associated with endocrine or autoimmune disorders. CMC has been associated with a defect in T_H17 cells and mutations in *CARD9* and *Dectin-1* genes.

An AR form of CMC with associated autoimmunity, also known as autoimmune polyendocrinopathy, candidiasis, ectodermal dysplasia (APECED) syndrome, is characterized by recurrent candidal infections, abnormal T-lymphocyte response to *Candida*, autoimmune endocrinopathies, and ectodermal dystrophies. APECED is caused by mutations in the gene for an important transcription regulator protein called autoimmune regulator (AIRE) that is critical for normal thymocyte development. Treatment includes antifungal therapy in combination with therapy for associated endocrinopathies.

Morzes-Vasconcelos D et al: Primary immune deficiency disorders presenting as autoimmune diseases: IPEX and APECED. J Clin Imm 2008;28:S11–S19 [PMID: 18264745].

5. Autoimmune Lymphoproliferative Syndrome

Autoimmune lymphoproliferative syndrome (ALPS) results from mutations of genes important for regulating programmed lymphocyte death (apoptosis). Most commonly, the defect is in Fas (CD95) or Fas ligand, but other defects in the Fas pathway have also been described (eg, caspase 10). Clinical presentation includes lymphadenopathy, splenomegaly, and autoimmune disorders (autoimmune hemolytic anemia, neutropenia, thrombocytopenia, and sometimes arthritis). Occasionally, patients have frequent infections. The diagnosis is suspected when T-lymphocyte subsets by flow cytometry demonstrate elevated numbers of $CD3^+CD4^-CD8^-$ (double negative) T lymphocytes. Several different types of ALPS are distinguished by the response of lymphocytes to Fas-induced apoptosis. Patients are often heterozygous, and inheritance is mostly autosomal dominant. Treatment with prednisone often controls the lymphadenopathy. Infections should be treated appropriately. In some cases, BMT has been curative. Affected patients are also at risk for lymphoma. Mutations affecting another apoptosis-related protein, caspase 8, cause an ALPS variant syndrome in which the susceptibility to infection by herpes simplex virus also increases.

Magerus-Chatinet et al: FAS-L, IL-10, and double-negative CD4-CD8- TCR alpha/beta+ T cells are reliable markers of autoimmune lymphoproliferative syndrome (ALPS) associated with FAS loss of function. Blood 2009;113:3027 [PMID: 19176318].

6. WHIM Syndrome

WHIM (warts, hypogammaglobulinemia, infection, myelokathexis) syndrome is a rare AD immunodeficiency caused by gain-of-function mutations in the gene encoding the chemokine receptor CXCR4. Patients have an increased susceptibility to viral infections including HPV-, EBV-, and HSV-infections, also recurrent bacterial infections. Laboratory evaluation reveals peripheral blood neutropenia in context of bone marrow hypercellularity, decreased B cell numbers and hypogammaglobulinemia, and T cell lymphopenia with normal CD4+/CD8+ ratio.

Kawai T, Malech HL: WHIM syndrome: Congenital immune deficiency disease. Curr Opin Hematol 2009;16:20–26 [PMID: 19057201].

7. Diseases Due to Defective Interferon-γ & Interleukin-12 Pathways

IL-12 is a powerful inducer of interferon-γ (IFN-γ) production by T cells and NK cells. IFN-γ, and therefore the IFN-γ –IL-12 axis, is critical for macrophage activation and resistance to mycobacterial infections. Individuals with inherited deficiency in macrophage receptors for IFN-γ or lymphocyte receptors for IL-12, or in IL-12 itself, suffer a profound and selective susceptibility to infection by nontuberculous mycobacteria such as *Mycobacterium avium* complex or bacille Calmette-Guérin (BCG). About half of these patients have had disseminated salmonellosis. Treatment with supplemental IFN-γ is effective unless the IFN-γ receptor is not functional. Long-term mycobacterial prophylaxis should be considered in these individuals.

Rosenzweig SD, Holland SM: Congenital defects in the interferon-gamma/interleukin-12 pathway. Curr Opin Pediatr 2004;16:3.

8. Defects in Pattern-Recognition Receptors

Defects of PRRs are associated with altered cytokine production and increased susceptibility to specific microbes. The clinical presentation of affected patients is most severe during infancy and early childhood with improvement of infections while patients get older, suggesting that adaptive immune responses compensate for defects in innate immunity. Toll-like receptors and members of the interleukin-1 receptor (IL-1R) family signal through IL-1R associated kinases (IRAK) 1 and 4 while using the adaptor molecule MyD88, leading to activation of NF-κB and inflammatory cytokine production. Patients with AR deficiencies in MyD88 and IRAK-4 are predisposed to severe bacterial infections that are not associated with a high fever or significant increase in C-reactive protein at the beginning of the infection. Laboratory results may reveal a decreased antibody response to polysaccharide antigens, increased IgG and IgG4 concentrations, and decreased IL-6 production upon whole blood stimulation through most TLR- and IL-1R agonists. TLR3 deficiency increases susceptibility to infections with herpes simplex infections, while polymorphisms of TLR5 predispose to Legionella pneumonia infections. Chronic mucocutaneous fungal infections have been linked to defects in the dectin-1/CARD9 pathway. Bacterial infections, specifically with Neisseria meningitis, but also viral and fungal infections can occur in context of mannose-binding lectin deficiency

GENETIC SYNDROMES ASSOCIATED WITH IMMUNODEFICIENCY

Several described genetic syndromes have associated immunodeficiency that is often identified after the syndrome has been diagnosed. Usually, the immune defect is not the major presenting clinical problem.

Ming JE, Stiehm ER: Genetic syndromic immunodeficiencies with antibody defects. Immunol Allergy Clin N Am 2008:715–736 [PMID: 18940571].

1. Bloom Syndrome

Characteristics of Bloom syndrome include growth retardation, sunlight sensitivity, and telangiectasias of the face. The syndrome results from mutations in the *Blm*-gene that encodes a RecQ-helicase involved in DNA repair. Affected patients present with growth retardation, microcephaly, and sun-sensitive rashes. They have an increased risk of malignancy and life-threatening infections. B- and T-cell numbers are low. Serum Igs are decreased, and T-lymphocyte function is abnormal.

2. Transcobalamin Deficiency

Transcobalamin deficiency is a rare AR disease due to defective cellular transport of cobalamin associated with mutations in the *TCN2* gene. Patients present with megaloblastic anemia, diarrhea, poor growth, neurologic abnormalities, hypogammaglobulinemia and poor specific antibody production.

Nissen PH et al: Transcobalamin deficiency caused by compound heterozygosity for two novel mutations in the TCN2 gene: A study of two affected siblings, their brother, and their parents. J Inherit Metab Dis 2010 [PMID: 20607612].

3. Immunodeficiency, Centromeric Instability, Facial Anomalies Syndrome

Immunodeficiency, centromeric instability, facial anomalies (ICF) syndrome is a rare AR condition caused by abnormal DNA methyltransferase. In half of the patients, a mutation can be detected in the *DNMT3B* gene. Unlike other chromosome instability syndromes, ICF syndrome does not have an associated hypersensitivity to sunlight. Affected patients have severe respiratory, gastrointestinal, and skin infections due to low or absent immunoglobulins and abnormal T-lymphocyte numbers and function.

4. Trisomy 21

Patients with trisomy 21 or Down syndrome have increased susceptibility to respiratory infection. Immunodeficiency is variable, and abnormal numbers and function of T- and B-lymphocytes have been reported. Additionally, patients have an increased incidence of autoimmune diseases.

5. Turner Syndrome

Turner syndrome (partial or complete absence of one X chromosome) is associated with increased risk of otitis media, respiratory infections, and malignancies. Immune defects are variable but may include abnormal T-lymphocyte numbers and function and hypogammaglobulinemia.

6. Chédiak-Higashi Syndrome

Chédiak-Higashi syndrome is a rare autosomal recessive disease caused by mutations in a lysosomal trafficking regulator (*LYST*) gene. The neutrophils of affected individuals have giant lysosomes, impaired chemotaxis, neutropenia, and abnormal NK-cell cytotoxicity. Patients present with recurrent infections (particularly periodontitis), partial oculocutaneous albinism, and neuropathy. Most patients progress to generalized lymphohistiocytic infiltration syndrome, which is a common cause of death. Treatment strategies address infections and neuropathy and the use of immunosuppression attempts to slow lymphoproliferative progression.

7. Griscelli Syndrome

Characterized by partial albinism, neutropenia, thrombocytopenia, and lymphohistiocytosis, Griscelli syndrome is a rare AR syndrome resulting from mutations in the myosin *VA* gene. Affected patients have recurrent and serious infections caused by fungi, viruses, and bacteria. Immunologic evaluation demonstrates variable immunoglobulin levels and antibody function with impaired T-lymphocyte function. BMT can correct the immunodeficiency. Griscelli syndrome is distinguished from Chédiak-Higashi syndrome by the lack of granules in white blood cells.

8. Netherton Syndrome

Patients with the AR Netherton syndrome present with trichorrhexis (brittle hair), ichthyosiform rash, and allergic diseases. A subset of patients develops recurrent infections. Immune function is variable but may include hypo- or hypergammaglobulinemia, abnormal T-lymphocyte function, or abnormal phagocyte function. The disease results from mutations in a serine protease inhibitor encoded on the *SPINK5* gene.

9. Cartilage-Hair Hypoplasia

Cartilage-hair hypoplasia is an AR form of chondrodysplasia manifesting with short-limbed short stature, hypoplastic hair, defective immunity, and poor erythrogenesis. The immune defect is characterized by mild to moderate lymphopenia and abnormal lymphocyte function, but normal antibody function. Affected patients have increased susceptibility to infections and increased risk of lymphoma. The disorder results from mutation in the *RMRP* gene that encodes the RNA component of an RNase MRP complex. BMT can restore cell-mediated immunity but does not correct the cartilage or hair abnormalities.

Endocrine Disorders

34

Philip S. Zeitler, MD, PhD
Sharon H. Travers, MD
Kristen Nadeau, MD
Jennifer M. Barker, MD
Megan Moriarty Kelsey, MD
Michael S. Kappy, MD, PhD

GENERAL CONCEPTS

The classic concept that *endocrine* effects are the result of substances secreted into the blood with effects on a distant target cell has been updated to account for other ways in which hormonal effects occur. Specifically, some hormone systems involve the stimulation or inhibition of metabolic processes in neighboring cells (eg, within the pancreatic islets or cartilage). This phenomenon is termed *paracrine*. Other hormone effects reflect the action of hormones on the same cells that produced them. This action is termed *autocrine*. The discoveries of local production of insulin, glucagon, ghrelin, somatostatin, cholecystokinin, and many other hormones in the brain and gut support the concept of paracrine and autocrine processes in these tissues.

Another significant discovery in endocrine physiology was an appreciation of the role of specific hormone receptors in target tissues, without which the hormonal effects cannot occur. For example, in the complete androgen insensitivity syndrome (AIS), androgen receptors are defective, and the 46,XY individual develops varying degrees of undervirilization of the external genitalia and internal (wolffian) duct system despite the presence of testes and adequate testosterone production. Similarly, in nephrogenic diabetes insipidus or Albright hereditary osteodystrophy (AHO) (pseudohypoparathyroidism [PHP]), affected children have defective antidiuretic hormone or parathyroid hormone (PTH) receptor function, respectively, and show the metabolic effects of diabetes insipidus or hypoparathyroidism despite more-than-adequate hormone secretion. Alternatively, abnormal activation of a hormone receptor leads to the effects of the hormone without its abnormal secretion. Examples of this phenomenon include McCune-Albright syndrome (precocious puberty and hyperthyroidism), testotoxicosis (familial male precocious puberty), and hypercalciuric hypocalcemia (see relevant sections later).

HORMONE TYPES

Hormones are of three main chemical types: peptides and proteins, steroids, and amines. The peptide hormones include the releasing factors secreted by the hypothalamus, the hormones of the anterior and posterior pituitary gland, pancreatic islet cells, parathyroid glands, lung (angiotensin II), heart, and brain (atrial and brain natriuretic hormones) and local growth factors such as insulin-like growth factor 1 (IGF-1). Steroid hormones are secreted primarily by the adrenal cortex, gonads, and kidney (active vitamin D [1,25$(OH)_2$ D3]). The amine hormones are secreted by the adrenal medulla (epinephrine) and the thyroid gland (triiodothyronine [T_3] and thyroxine [T_4]).

As a rule, peptide hormones and epinephrine act after binding to specific receptors on the surface of their target cell. The metabolic effects of these hormones are usually stimulation or inhibition of the activity of preexisting enzymes or transport proteins (posttranslational effects). The steroid hormones, thyroid hormone, and active vitamin D, in contrast, act more slowly and bind to cytoplasmic receptors inside the target cell and subsequently to specific regions on nuclear DNA, where they direct a read-out of specific protein(s). Their metabolic effects are generally caused by stimulating or inhibiting the synthesis of new enzymes or transport proteins (transcriptional effects), thereby increasing or decreasing the amount rather than the activity of these proteins in the target cell.

Metabolic processes that require rapid response, such as blood glucose or calcium homeostasis, are usually controlled by peptide hormones and epinephrine, while processes that respond more slowly, such as pubertal development and metabolic rate, are controlled by steroid hormones and thyroid hormone. The control of electrolyte homeostasis is intermediate and is regulated by a combination of peptide and steroid hormones (Table 34–1).

Table 34–1. Hormonal regulation of metabolic processes.

First Level (Most Direct)			
Metabolite or Other Parameter	**Stimulus**	**Endocrine Gland**	**Hormone**
Glucose	Hyperglycemia	Pancreatic beta cell	Insulin
Glucose	Hypoglycemia	Pancreatic alpha cell	Glucagon
Glucose	Hypoglycemia	Adrenal medulla	Epinephrine
Calcium	Hypercalcemia	Thyroid C cell	Calcitonin (?)
Calcium	Hypocalcemia	Parathyroid	PTH
Sodium/plasma osmolality	Hypernatremia/hyperosmolality	Hypothalamus with posterior pituitary gland as reservoir	ADH
Plasma volume	Hypervolemia	Heart	ANH
Second Level: Sodium and Potassium Balance			
Metabolite or Other Parameter	**Abnormality**	**Endocrine Gland**	**Hormone**
Sodium/potassium	Hyponatremia }	Kidney	Renin (an enzyme)
	Hyperkalemia }	Liver and others	Angiotensin I
	Hypovolemia }	Lung	Angiotensin II
		Adrenal cortex	Aldosterone
Third Level (Most Complex)			
Hypothalamic-Releasing Hormone	**Tropic Hormone (Pituitary Gland)**	**Endocrine Target Tissue**	**Endocrine Gland Hormone**
CRH	ACTH	Adrenal cortex	Cortisol
GHRH	GH	Liver et al tissues	IGF-1
GnRH	LH	Testis	Testosterone
GnRH	FSH/LH	Ovary	Estradiol/progesterone
TRH	TSH	Thyroid gland	T_4 and T_3

ACTH, adrenocorticotropic hormone; ADH, antidiuretic hormone; ANH, atrial natriuretic hormone; CRH, corticotropin-releasing hormone; FSH, follicle-stimulating hormone; GH, growth hormone; GHRH, growth hormone–releasing hormone; GnRH, gonadotropin-releasing hormone; IGF-1, insulin-like growth factor 1; LH, luteinizing hormone; PTH, parathyroid hormone; T_3, triiodothyronine; T_4, thyroxine; TRH, thyrotropin-releasing hormone; TSH, thyroid-stimulating hormone.

FEEDBACK CONTROL OF HORMONE SECRETION

Hormone secretion is regulated, for the most part, by feedback in response to changes in the internal environment. When the metabolic imbalance is corrected, stimulation of the hormone secretion ceases and may even be inhibited. Overcorrection of the imbalance stimulates secretion of a counter-balancing hormone or hormones, so that homeostasis is maintained within relatively narrow limits.

Hypothalamic-pituitary control of hormonal secretion is also regulated by feedback. End-organ failure (endocrine gland insufficiency) leads to decreased circulating concentrations of endocrine gland hormones and thence to increased secretion of the respective hypothalamic releasing and pituitary hormones (see Table 34–1; Figure 34–1). If restoration of normal circulating concentration of hormones occurs, feedback inhibition at the pituitary and hypothalamus results in cessation of the previously stimulated secretion of releasing and pituitary hormones and restoration of their circulating concentrations to normal.

Similarly, if there is autonomous endocrine gland hyperfunction (eg, McCune-Albright syndrome, Graves disease, or adrenal tumor), the specific hypothalamic releasing and pituitary hormones are suppressed (see Figure 34–1).

Bethin K, Fuqua JS: General concepts and physiology. In: Kappy MS, Allen DB, Geffner ME (editors): *Pediatric Practice-Endocrinology*. McGraw-Hill, 2010: 1–22.

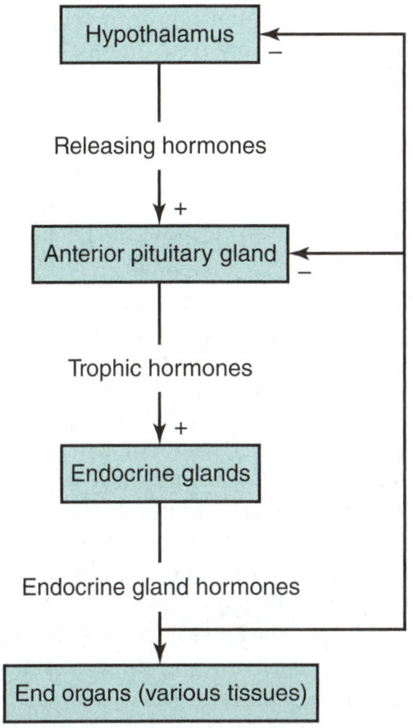

▲ **Figure 34–1.** General scheme of the hypothalamus-pituitary-endocrine gland axis. Releasing hormones synthesized in the hypothalamus are secreted into the hypophyseal portal circulation. Trophic hormones are secreted by the pituitary gland in response, and they in turn act on specific endocrine glands to stimulate the secretion of their respective hormones. The endocrine gland hormones exert their respective effects on various target tissues (end organs) and exert a negative feedback (feedback inhibition) on their own secretion by acting at the level of the pituitary and hypothalamus. This system is characteristic of those hormones listed in Table 34–1 (third level).

DISTURBANCES OF GROWTH

Disturbances of growth and development are the most common problems evaluated by a pediatric endocrinologist. While most cases represent normal developmental variants, it is critical to identify abnormal growth patterns, as deviations from the norm can be the first or only manifestation of an endocrine disorder. Height velocity is the most critical parameter in evaluating a child's growth. A persistent increase or decrease in height percentiles between age 2 years and the onset of puberty always warrants evaluation. Similarly, substantial deviations from target height may be indications of underlying endocrine or skeletal disorders. It is more difficult to distinguish normal from abnormal growth in the first 2 years of life, as infants may have catch-up or catch-down growth during this period. Similarly, the variable timing of the onset of puberty makes early adolescence another period during which evaluation of growth abnormalities may require careful consideration.

Appropriate standards must be used to evaluate growth. The National Center for Health Statistics provides standard cross-sectional growth charts for North American children (see Chapter 2). Normal growth standards may vary with country of origin. Growth charts are available for some ethnic groups in North America and for some syndromes with specific growth disturbance such as Turner or Down syndromes.

TARGET HEIGHT & SKELETAL MATURATION

A child's growth and height potential is determined largely by genetic factors. The target (midparental) height of a child is calculated from the mean parental height plus 6.5 cm for boys or minus 6.5 cm for girls. This calculation helps identify a child's genetic growth potential. Most children achieve an adult height within 8 cm of the midparental height. Another parameter that determines growth potential is skeletal maturation or bone age. Beyond the neonatal period, bone age is evaluated by comparing a radiograph of the child's left hand and wrist with the standards of Greulich and Pyle. Delayed or advanced bone age is not diagnostic of any specific disease, but the extent of skeletal maturation allows determination of remaining growth potential as a percentage of total height and allows prediction of ultimate height.

SHORT STATURE

It is important to distinguish normal variants of growth (familial short stature and constitutional growth delay) from pathologic conditions (Table 34–2). Pathologic short stature is more likely in children whose growth velocity is abnormal (crossing major height percentiles on the growth curve) or who are significantly short for their family. Children with chronic illness or nutritional deficiencies may have poor linear growth, but this is typically associated with inadequate weight gain. In contrast, endocrine causes of short stature are usually associated with normal or excessive weight gain.

1. Familial Short Stature & Constitutional Growth Delay

Children with familial short stature typically have normal birth weight and length. In the first 2 years of life, their linear growth velocity decelerates as they near their genetically determined percentile. Once the target percentile is reached, the child resumes normal linear growth parallel to the growth curve, usually between 2 and 3 years of age. Skeletal maturation and timing of puberty are consistent with chronologic age. The child grows along his/her own growth percentile and the final height is short but appropriate for the family (Figure 34–2). For example, an infant boy of a

Table 34–2. Causes of short stature.

A. Genetic-familial short stature
B. Constitutional growth delay
C. Endocrine disturbances
1. Growth hormone (GH) deficiency
   a. Hereditary
      (1) Growth hormone–releasing hormone (GHRH) receptor mutation
      (2) GH gene deletion
      (3) Congenital hypopituitarism—GH deficiency in combination with deficiency of other anterior pituitary hormones
   b. Idiopathic—with and without associated abnormalities of midline structures of the central nervous system
      (1) Isolated GH deficiency
      (2) Combined pituitary hormone deficiency
   c. Acquired
      (1) Transient—eg, psychosocial short stature
      (2) Organic—tumor, irradiation of the central nervous system, infection, or trauma
2. GH resistance/Insulin-like growth factor 1 (IGF-1) deficiency
3. Hypothyroidism
4. Excess cortisol—Cushing disease and Cushing syndrome (including iatrogenic causes)
5. Diabetes mellitus (poorly controlled)
6. Pseudohypoparathyroidism
7. Rickets

D. Intrauterine growth restriction
1. Intrinsic fetal abnormalities—chromosomal disorders
2. Syndromes (eg, Russell-Silver, Noonan, Bloom, de Lange, Cockayne)
3. Congenital infections
4. Placental abnormalities
5. Maternal abnormalities
   a. Hypertension/toxemia
   b. Drug use
   c. Malnutrition

E. Inborn errors of metabolism
1. Mucopolysaccharidosis
2. Other storage diseases

F. Intrinsic diseases of bone
1. Defects of growth of tubular bones or spine (eg, achondroplasia, metatropic dwarfism, diastrophic dwarfism, metaphyseal chondrodysplasia)
2. Disorganized development of cartilage and fibrous components of the skeleton (eg, multiple cartilaginous exostoses, fibrous dysplasia with skin pigmentation)

G. Short stature associated with chromosomal defects
1. Autosomal (eg, Down syndrome, Prader-Willi syndrome)
2. Sex chromosomal (eg, Turner syndrome-XO)

H. Chronic systemic diseases, congenital defects, and cancers
(eg, chronic infection and infestation, inflammatory bowel disease, hepatic disease, cardiovascular disease, hematologic disease, central nervous system disease, pulmonary disease, renal disease, malnutrition, cancers, collagen-vascular disease)

I. Psychosocial short stature (deprivation dwarfism)

mother who is 5 ft 0 in and father who is 5 ft 5 in (calculated midparental height 5 ft 5 in) may have a birth length at the 50th percentile. However, this child's length percentile will drift downward during the first 2 years of life and will settle in at the fifth percentile where it will stay.

Children with constitutional growth delay do not necessarily have short parents but have a growth pattern similar to those with familial short stature. The difference is that children with constitutional growth delay have a delay in skeletal maturation and a delay in the onset of puberty. In these children, growth continues beyond the time the average child stops growing, and final height is appropriate for target height (Figure 34–3). There is often a history of other family members being "late bloomers."

2. Growth Hormone Deficiency

Human growth hormone (GH) is produced by the anterior pituitary gland. Secretion is stimulated by growth hormone–releasing hormone (GHRH) and inhibited by somatostatin. GH is secreted in a pulsatile pattern in response to sleep, exercise, and hypoglycemia and has direct growth-promoting and metabolic effects (Figure 34–4). GH also promotes growth indirectly by stimulating production of insulin-like growth factors, primarily IGF-1.

Growth hormone deficiency (GHD) is characterized by decreased growth velocity and delayed skeletal maturation in the absence of other explanations. Laboratory tests indicate subnormal GH secretion or action. GHD may be isolated or coexist with other pituitary hormone deficiencies and may be congenital (septo-optic dysplasia or ectopic posterior pituitary), genetic (GH or GHRH gene mutation), or acquired (craniopharyngioma, germinoma, histiocytosis, or cranial irradiation). Idiopathic GHD is the most common deficiency state with an incidence of about 1:4000 children. Patients have been described with a GH resistance syndrome caused by mutations in the GH receptor or other components of the GH signaling pathway. The presentation of GH resistance is similar to that of GHD, but short stature is often severe, with little or no response to GH therapy. Some mutations, such as Laron dwarfism, are accompanied by facial and skeletal dysmorphology.

Infants with GHD have normal birth weight with only slightly reduced length, suggesting that GH is a minor contributor to intrauterine growth. GH deficient infants may present with hypoglycemia, particularly when associated with other pituitary deficiencies such as central adrenal insufficiency. Micropenis may be a feature of newborn males with gonadotropin and GH deficiency. Isolated GHD and hypopituitarism may be unrecognized until late in infancy or childhood as growth retardation may be delayed until later childhood. Regardless of onset, the primary manifestation of idiopathic or acquired GHD is subnormal growth velocity (Figure 34–5). Because GH promotes lipolysis, many GH deficient children have truncal adiposity.

Laboratory tests to assess GH status may be difficult to interpret. Children with normal short stature have a broad range of GH secretion patterns and there is significant overlap between normal and GH deficient children. Random samples for measurement of serum GH are of no value in the diagnosis of GHD, as GH secretion is pulsatile. Serum

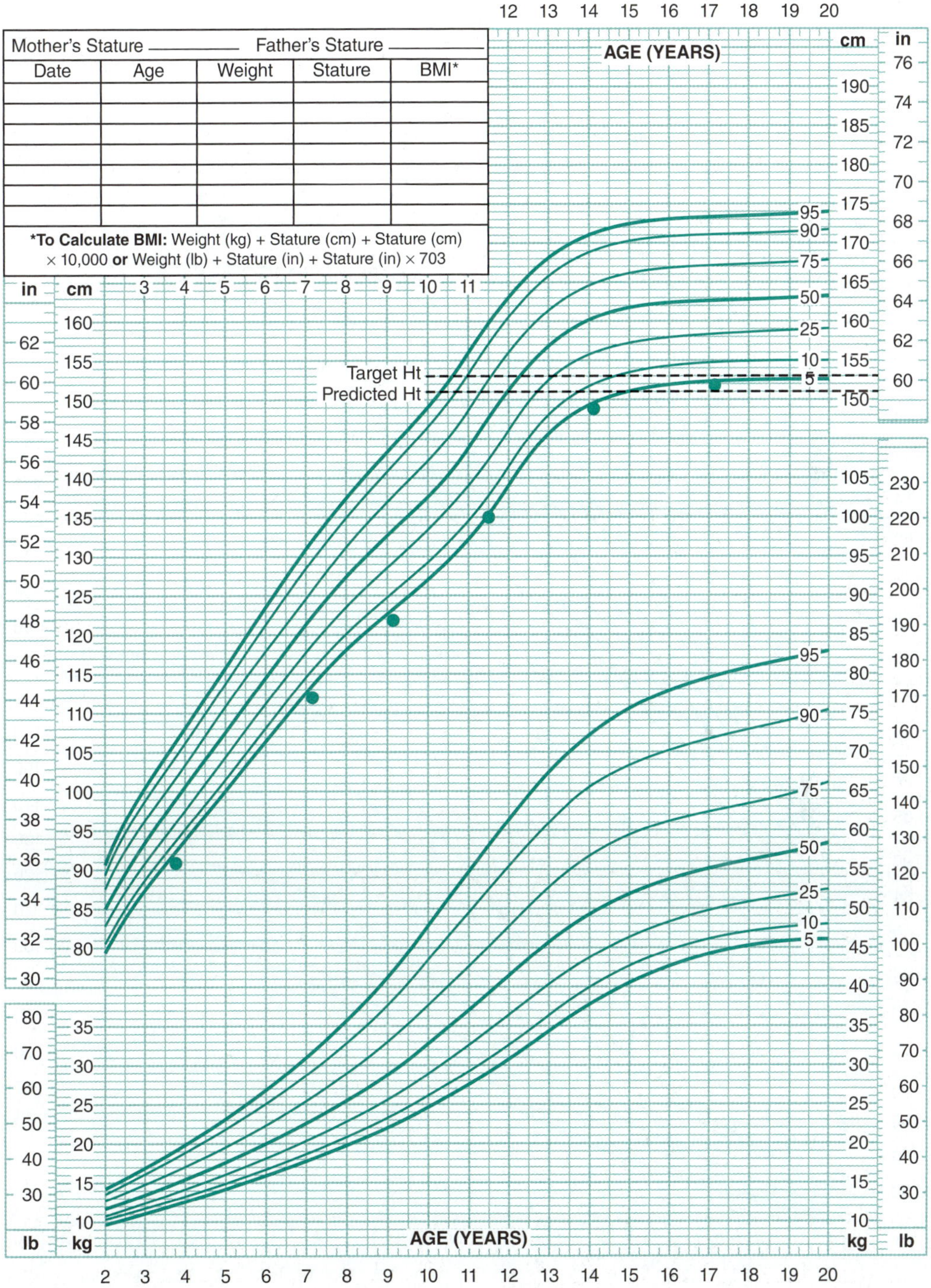

▲ **Figure 34–2.** Typical pattern of growth in a child with familial short stature. After attaining an appropriate percentile during the first 2 years of life, the child will have normal linear growth parallel to the growth curve. Skeletal maturation and the timing of puberty are consistent with chronologic age. The height percentile the child has been following is maintained, and final height is short but appropriate for the family.

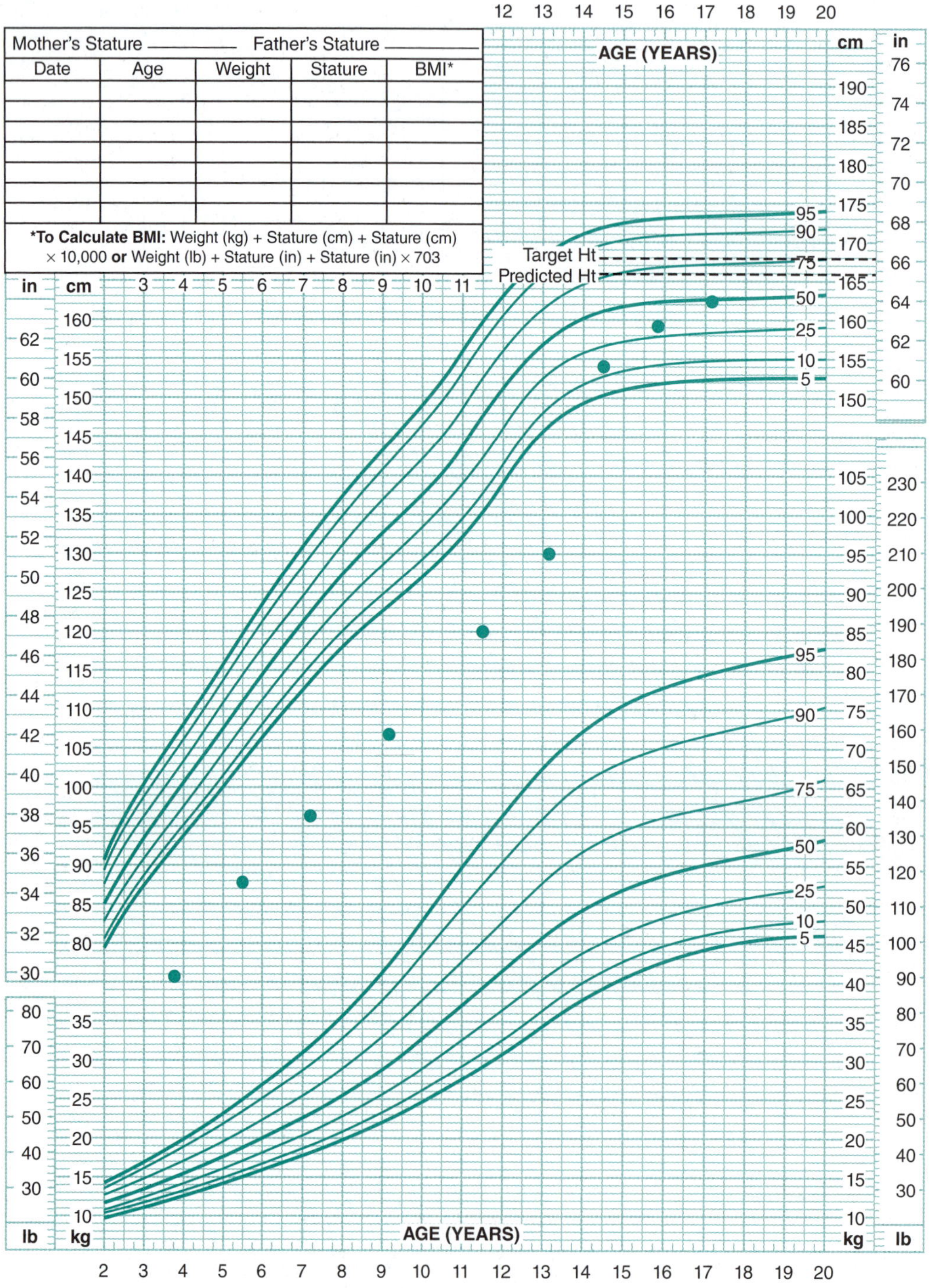

▲ **Figure 34–3.** Typical pattern of growth in a child with constitutional growth delay. Growth slows during the first 2 years of life, similarly to children with familial short stature. Subsequently the child will have normal linear growth parallel to the growth curve. However, skeletal maturation and the onset of puberty are delayed. Growth continues beyond the time the average child has stopped growing, and final height is appropriate for target height.

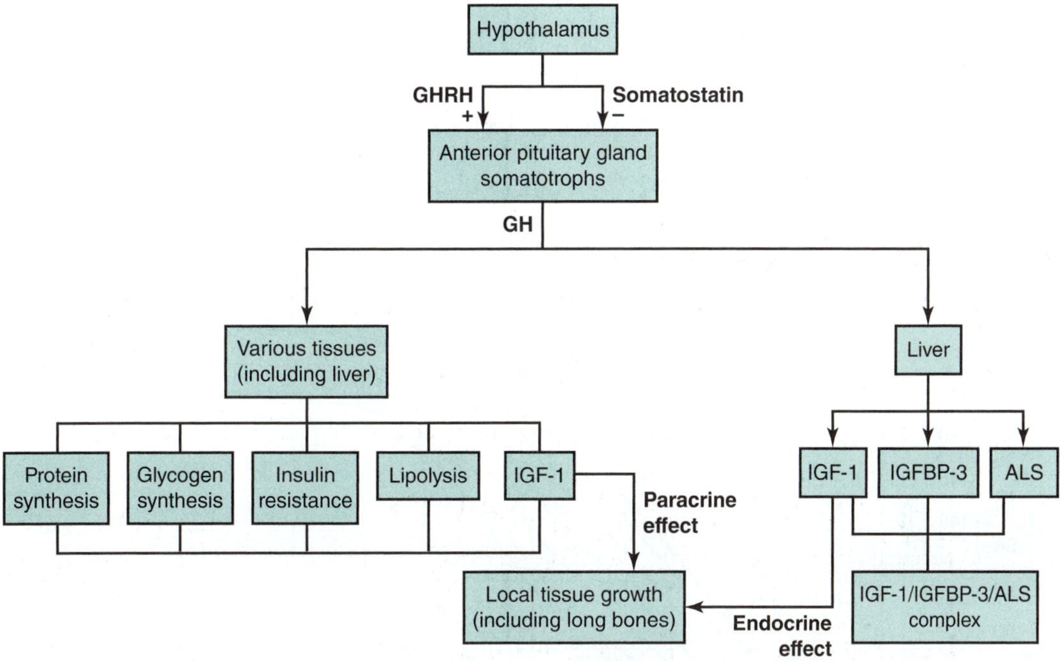

▲ **Figure 34–4.** The GHRH/GH/IGF-1 system. The effects of GH on growth are partly due to its direct anabolic effects in muscle, liver, and bone. In addition, GH stimulates many tissues to produce IGF-1 locally, which stimulates the growth of the tissue itself (paracrine effect of IGF-1). The action of GH on the liver results in the secretion of IGF-1 (circulating IGF-1), which stimulates growth in other tissues (endocrine effect of IGF-1). The action of growth hormone on the liver also enhances the secretion of IGF-binding protein 3 (IGFBP-3) and acid-labile subunit (ALS), which form a high-molecular-weight complex with IGF-1. The function of this complex is to transport IGF-1 to its target tissues, but the complex also serves as a reservoir and possible inhibitor of IGF-1 action. In various chronic illnesses, the direct metabolic effects of GH are inhibited; the secretion of IGF-1 in response to GH is blunted, and in some cases IGFBP-3 synthesis is enhanced, resulting in marked inhibition in the growth of the child. IGF-1, insulin-like growth factor 1; GH, growth hormone; GHRH, growth hormone–releasing hormone.

concentrations of IGF-1 give reasonable estimations of GH secretion and action in the adequately nourished child (see Figure 34–4), and is often used as a first step in the evaluation for GHD. IGF-binding protein 3 (IGFBP-3) is less sensitive marker of GH deficiency, but may be useful in the underweight child or in children under 4 years of age, since it is less affected by age or nutritional status. Provocative studies using such agents as insulin, arginine, levodopa, clonidine, or glucagon are traditionally done to clarify GH secretion, but are not physiologic and are often poorly reproducible, ultimately limiting their value in the clarification of GH secretion. When results of GH tests are equivocal, a trial of GH treatment may help determine whether an abnormally short child will benefit from GH. Currently, the recommended treatment schedule for GHD is subcutaneous recombinant GH given 7 days per week with total weekly dose of 0.15–0.3 mg/kg.

GH therapy is approved by the U.S. Food and Drug Administration (FDA) for children with GHD and growth restriction associated with chronic renal failure, for girls with Turner syndrome, children with Prader-Willi and Noonan's syndromes, and children born small for gestational age (SGA) who fail to demonstrate catch-up growth by age 4. GH therapy has also been approved for children with idiopathic short stature whose current height is more than 2.25 standard deviations below the norm for age. Final height improvement may be 5–7 cm in this population. This last indication is controversial and the role of GH for idiopathic short stature is still unclear. Side effects of recombinant GH are uncommon but include benign intracranial hypertension and slipped capital femoral epiphysis. With early diagnosis and treatment, children with GHD reach normal or near-normal adult height. Recombinant IGF-1 is used to treat children with GH resistance or IGF-1 deficiency.

3. Small for Gestational Age/Intrauterine Growth Restriction

SGA infants have birth weights below the 10th percentile for the population's birth weight–gestational age relationship.

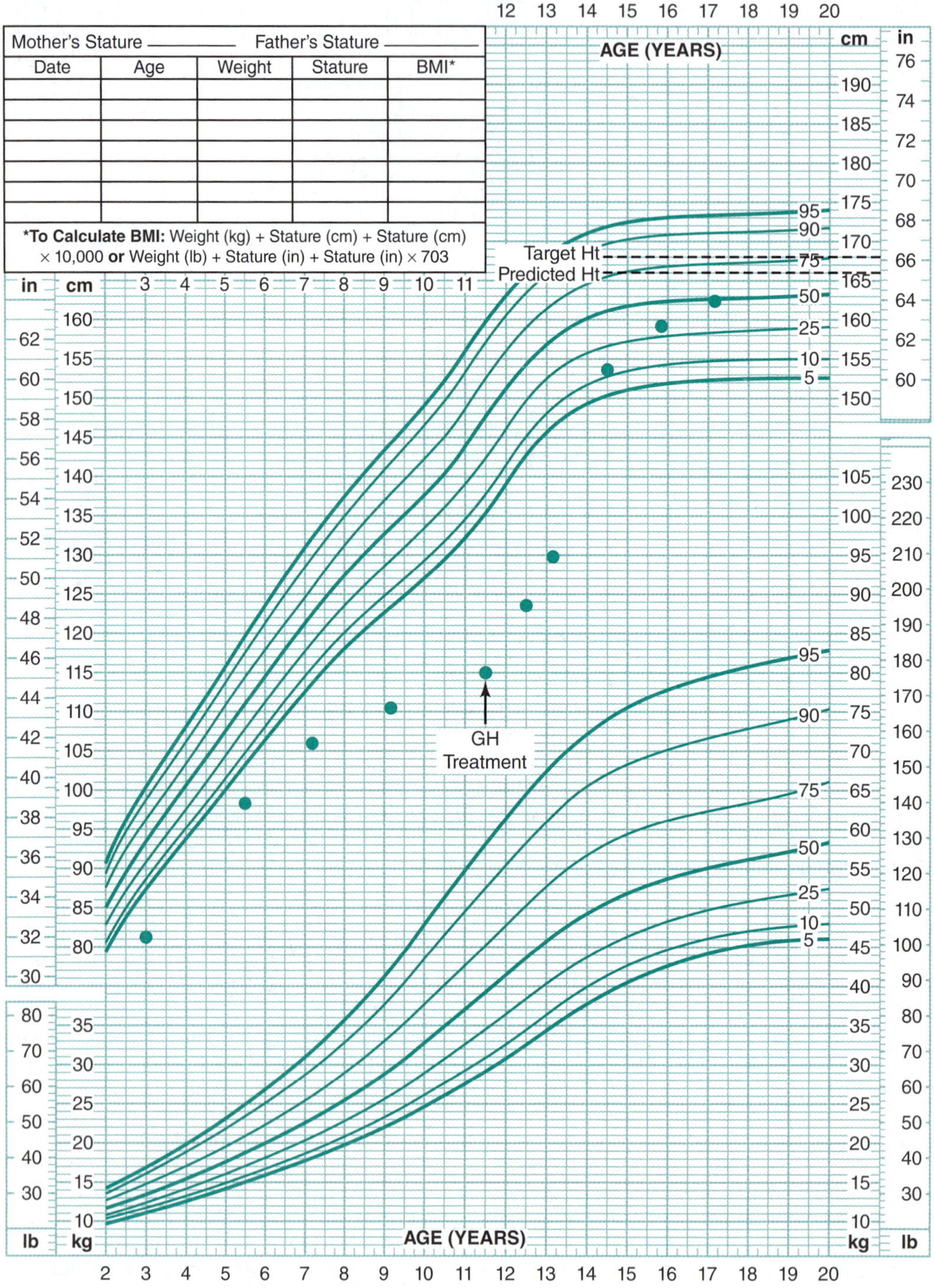

▲ **Figure 34–5.** Typical pattern of growth in a child with acquired growth hormone deficiency (GHD). Children with acquired GHD have an abnormal growth velocity and fail to maintain height percentile during childhood. Other phenotypic features (central adiposity and immaturity of facies) may be present. Children with congenital GHD will cross percentiles during the first 2 years of life, similarly to the pattern seen in familial short stature and constitutional delay, but will fail to attain a steady height percentile subsequently.

SGA infants include constitutionally small infants growing at their potential and infants with intrauterine growth restriction (IUGR).

SGA/IUGR may be a result of poor maternal environment, intrinsic fetal abnormalities, congenital infections, or fetal malnutrition. Intrinsic fetal abnormalities causing SGA/IUGR (often termed primordial short stature) include Russell-Silver, Seckel, Noonan, Bloom, and Cockayne syndromes, and progeria. Many children with mild SGA/IUGR and no intrinsic fetal abnormalities exhibit catch-up growth during the first 3 years. However, 15%–20% remains short throughout life, particularly those whose growth restriction in utero occurred over several months rather than just the last 2–3 months of gestation. Catch-up growth may also be inadequate in preterm SGA/IUGR infants with poor postnatal nutrition. Children who do not show catch-up growth may have normal growth velocity, but they will follow a lower height percentile than expected for the family. In contrast to children with constitutional growth delay, those with SGA/IUGR have skeletal maturation that corresponds to chronologic age or is only mildly delayed.

GH therapy for SGA/IUGR children with growth delay is FDA approved and appears to be effective in increasing growth velocity and final adult height.

4. Disproportionate Short Stature

There are more than 200 sporadic and genetic skeletal dysplasias that may cause disproportionate short stature. Measurements of arm span and upper-to-lower body segment ratio are helpful in determining whether a child has normal body proportions. If disproportionate short stature is found, a skeletal survey may be useful to detect specific radiographic features characteristic of some disorders. The effect of GH on most of these rare disorders is unknown.

5. Short Stature Associated with Syndromes

Short stature is associated with many syndromes, including Turner, Down, Noonan, and Prader-Willi. Girls with Turner syndrome often have recognizable features such as micrognathia, webbed neck, low posterior hairline, edema of hands and feet, multiple pigmented nevi, and an increased carrying angle. However, in some girls short stature is the only obvious manifestation. Consequently, any girl with unexplained short stature should have a chromosomal evaluation. Although girls with Turner syndrome are not usually GH deficient, GH therapy can improve final height by an average of 6.0 cm. Duration of GH therapy is a significant predictor of long-term height gain; consequently, it is important that Turner syndrome be diagnosed early and GH started as soon as possible.

GH is approved for treatment of growth failure in Prader-Willi syndrome. Many affected individuals are GH deficient and GH improves growth, body composition, and physical activity. A few deaths have been reported in Prader-Willi children receiving GH, all of which occurred in very obese children, children with respiratory impairments, sleep apnea, or unidentified respiratory infections. The role of GH, if any, in these deaths is unknown. However, as a precaution, it is recommended that all Prader-Willi patients be evaluated for upper airway obstruction and sleep apnea prior to starting GH therapy.

Children with Down syndrome should be evaluated for GHD only if their linear growth is abnormal compared with the Down syndrome growth chart.

6. Psychosocial Short Stature (Psychosocial Dwarfism)

Psychosocial short stature refers to growth retardation associated with emotional deprivation. Undernutrition probably contributes to growth retardation in some of these children. Other symptoms include bizarre eating and drinking habits, bowel and bladder incontinence, social withdrawal, and delayed speech. GH secretion in children with psychosocial short stature is diminished, but GH therapy is usually not beneficial. Foster home placement or a change in the psychological environment at home usually results in improved growth and normalization of GH secretion, personality, and eating behaviors.

Clinical Evaluation

Laboratory investigation should be guided by the history and physical examination. Data included in history and physical include size at birth, pattern of growth since birth, familial growth patterns, pubertal stage, dysmorphic features, body segment proportion, and psychological health. In a child with poor weight gain as the primary disturbance, history of chronic illness and nutritional assessment are indicated. The following laboratory tests may be useful as guided by history and clinical judgment:

1. Radiograph of left hand and wrist for bone age
2. Complete blood count (to detect chronic anemia or infection)
3. Erythrocyte sedimentation rate (often elevated in collagen-vascular disease, cancer, chronic infection, and inflammatory bowel disease)
4. Urinalysis, blood urea nitrogen, and serum creatinine (occult renal disease)
5. Serum electrolytes, calcium, and phosphorus (renal tubular disease and metabolic bone disease)
6. Stool examination for fat, or measurement of serum tissue transglutaminase (malabsorption or celiac disease)
7. Karyotype (girls) and/or Noonan's testing
8. Thyroid function tests: thyroxine (T4) and thyroid-stimulating hormone (TSH)
9. IGF-1 (IGFBP-3 is an alternative for children < 4 or in malnourished individuals)

Clayton PE et al: Management of the child born small for gestational age through to adulthood: A consensus statement of the International Societies of Pediatric Endocrinology and the Growth Hormone Research Society. J Clin Endocrinol Metab 2007;92:804 [PMID: 17200164].

Collett-Solberg PF: Update in growth hormone therapy in children. J Clin Endocrinol Metab 2011;96:573 [PMID: 21378219].

Rosenbloom AL: Mecasermin (recombinant human insulin-like growth factor 1). Adv Ther 2009;26:40 [PMID: 19198769].

TALL STATURE

Although growth disturbances are usually associated with short stature, potentially serious pathologic conditions may be associated with tall stature and excessive growth (Table 34–3). Excessive GH secretion is rare, generally associated with a functioning pituitary adenoma. GH excess leads to gigantism if the epiphyses are open and to acromegaly if the epiphyses are closed. The diagnosis is confirmed by finding elevated random GH and IGF-1 levels and failure of GH suppression during oral glucose tolerance test.

Because the upper limit of acceptable height in both sexes is increasing, concerns about excessive growth in girls are less frequent currently than in the past. When such concerns arise, the family history, growth curve, pubertal stage, and assessment of skeletal maturation allow prediction of final adult height. Reassurance, counseling, and education may alleviate family and personal concerns. Rarely, when the predicted height is excessive and unacceptable, estrogen therapy may be used to accelerate bone maturation and shorten the growth period.

Sotos JF, Argente J: Overgrowth disorders associated with tall stature. Adv Pediatr 2008;55:213 [PMID: 19048732].

DISORDERS OF THE POSTERIOR PITUITARY GLAND

The posterior pituitary (neurohypophysis) is an extension of the ventral hypothalamus. Its two principal hormones—oxytocin and arginine vasopressin—are synthesized in the supraoptic and paraventricular nuclei of the ventral hypothalamus. After synthesis, these peptide hormones are packaged in granules with specific neurophysins and transported via the axons to their storage site in the posterior pituitary. Vasopressin is essential for water balance; it acts primarily on the kidney to promote reabsorption of water from urine. Oxytocin is most active during parturition and breast feeding and is not discussed further here.

Table 34–3. Causes of tall stature.

A. Constitutional (familial)

B. Endocrine causes

1. Growth hormone excess (pituitary gigantism)
2. Precocious puberty
3. Hypogonadism

C. Nonendocrine causes

1. Klinefelter syndrome
2. XYY males
3. Marfan syndrome
4. Cerebral gigantism (Sotos syndrome)
5. Homocystinuria

ARGININE VASOPRESSIN (ANTIDIURETIC HORMONE) PHYSIOLOGY

Vasopressin release is controlled primarily by serum osmolality and intravascular volume. Release is stimulated by minor increases in plasma osmolality (detected by osmoreceptors in the anterolateral hypothalamus) and large decreases in intravascular volume (detected by baroreceptors in the cardiac atria). Disorders of vasopressin release and action include (1) central (neurogenic) diabetes insipidus, (2) nephrogenic diabetes insipidus (see Chapter 24), and (3) the syndrome of inappropriate secretion of antidiuretic hormone (see Chapter 45).

CENTRAL DIABETES INSIPIDUS

ESSENTIALS OF DIAGNOSIS & TYPICAL FEATURES

- Polydipsia, polyuria (> 2 L/m^2/d), nocturia, dehydration, and hypernatremia.
- Inability to concentrate urine after fluid restriction (urine specific gravity < 1.010; urine osmolality < 300 mOsm/kg).
- Plasma osmolality > 300 mOsm/kg with urine osmolality < 600 mOsm/kg.
- Low plasma vasopressin with antidiuretic response to exogenous vasopressin.

General Considerations

Central diabetes insipidus (DI) is an inability to synthesize and release vasopressin. Without vasopressin the kidneys cannot concentrate urine, causing excessive urinary water loss. Genetic causes of central DI are rare and include mutations in the vasopressin gene (mostly in the neurophysin portion of the vasopressin precursor) and the *WFS1* gene that causes DI, diabetes mellitus, optic atrophy, and deafness (Wolfram or DIDMOAD syndrome). Transcription factor mutations, such as PROP1 and PIT1, that are known to be associated with other anterior pituitary hormone deficiencies are not typically associated with DI. Midline brain abnormalities, such as septo-optic dysplasia and holoprosencephaly, are also associated with central DI. Traumatic brain injury or neurosurgery in or near the hypothalamus or pituitary can cause transient or permanent DI. Traumatic DI often has three phases. Initially, transient DI is caused by edema in the hypothalamus or pituitary area. In 2–5 days, unregulated release of vasopressin from dying neurons causes the syndrome of inappropriate secretion of antidiuretic hormone (SIADH). Finally, permanent DI occurs if a sufficient number of vasopressin neurons are destroyed.

Tumors and infiltrative diseases of the hypothalamus and pituitary may cause DI. In children with craniopharyngioma, DI usually develops after neurosurgical intervention. In contrast, germinomas often present with DI. Germinomas may be undetectable for several years; consequently, children with unexplained DI should have regularly repeated magnetic resonance imaging (MRI). Infiltrative diseases such as histiocytosis and lymphocytic hypophysitis can cause DI. In these conditions, as in germinomas, MRI scans characteristically show thickening of the pituitary stalk. Infections involving the base of the brain also cause transient DI.

Clinical Findings

Onset of DI is often abrupt, characterized by polyuria, nocturia, enuresis, and intense thirst. Children with DI typically crave cold water. Hypernatremia, hyperosmolality, and dehydration occur if insufficient fluid intake due to lack of access or impaired thirst mechanism does not keep up with urinary losses. In infants, symptoms may also include failure to thrive, vomiting, constipation, and unexplained fevers. Some infants may present with severe dehydration, circulatory collapse, and seizures. Vasopressin deficiency may be masked in patients with panhypopituitarism due to the impaired excretion of free water associated with adrenal insufficiency. Treating these patients with glucocorticoids may unmask their DI.

DI is confirmed when serum hyperosmolality is associated with urine hypoosmolarity. If the history indicates that the child can go through the night comfortably without drinking, outpatient testing is appropriate. Oral fluid intake is prohibited after midnight. Osmolality, sodium, and specific gravity of the first morning void are obtained. If urine specific gravity is greater than 1.015, DI is excluded. If urine is not concentrated, a blood sample is obtained within a few minutes of the urine collection for osmolality, sodium, creatinine, and calcium concentration.

If screening results are unclear or if symptoms preclude safely withholding fluids at home, a water deprivation test performed in the hospital is indicated. In this test, fluid is withheld and the child is monitored. Serum osmolality greater than 290 mOsm/kg associated with inappropriately dilute urine; osmolality less than 600 mOsm/kg is diagnostic for DI. Low serum vasopressin concentration and an antidiuretic response to vasopressin administration at the end of the test distinguishes central from nephrogenic DI. Children with central DI should have a head MRI scan with contrast to look for tumors or infiltrative processes. The posterior pituitary "bright spot" on MRI is often absent in DI.

Decreased ability to concentrate urine also occurs in hypercalcemic disorders and renal tubular abnormalities (eg, Fanconi syndrome). Primary polydipsia must be distinguished from DI. Children with primary polydipsia tend to have lower serum sodium levels and usually can concentrate their urine with overnight fluid deprivation. Some may have secondary nephrogenic DI due to dilution of the renal medullary interstitium and decreased renal concentrating ability, but this resolves with restriction of fluid intake.

Treatment

Central DI is treated with oral or intranasal desmopressin acetate (DDAVP). The aim of therapy is to provide antidiuresis that allows uninterrupted sleep and approximately 1 hour of diuresis before the next dose. Children hospitalized with acute-onset DI can be managed with intravenous vasopressin. Due to the amount of antidiuresis, intravenous fluids will need to be restricted to two-thirds the maintenance rate and electrolytes closely monitored to avoid water intoxication. Infants with DI should not be treated with DDAVP. Treatment with DDAVP in association with the volume of formula or breast milk needed to ensure adequate caloric intake could cause water intoxication. For this reason, infants are treated with extra free water, rather than DDAVP, to maintain normal hydration. A formula with a low renal solute load and chlorothiazides may be helpful in infants with central DI.

Cheetham T, Baylis PH: Diabetes insipidus in children: Pathophysiology, diagnosis and management. Paediatr Drugs 2002;4:785 [PMID: 12431131].

Ghirardello S et al: The diagnosis of children with central diabetes insipidus. J Pediatr Endocrinol Metab 2007;20:359 [PMID: 17451074].

Kelberman D et al: Genetic regulation of pituitary gland development in human and mouse. Endo Rev 2009;30:790 [PMID: 19837867].

Rivkees SA et al: The management of central diabetes insipidus in infancy: Desmopressin, low renal solute load formula, thiazide diuretics. J Pediatr Endocrinol Metab 2007;20:459 [PMID: 17550208].

Wise-Faberowski L et al: Perioperative management of diabetes insipidus in children. J Neurosurg Anesthesiol 2004;16:14 [PMID: 14676564].

THYROID GLAND

FETAL DEVELOPMENT OF THE THYROID

The fetal thyroid synthesizes thyroid hormone as early as the 10th week of gestation. Thyroid hormone appears in the fetal serum by the 11th week of gestation and progressively increases throughout gestation. The fetal pituitary-thyroid axis functions largely independently of the maternal pituitary-thyroid axis because maternal TSH cannot cross the placenta. However, maternal thyroid hormone can cross the placenta in limited amounts.

At birth, there is a TSH surge peaking at about 70 mU/L within 30–60 minutes. Thyroid hormone serum level increases rapidly during the first days of life in response to this TSH surge. The TSH level decreases to childhood levels within a few weeks. The physiologic neonatal TSH surge can produce a false-positive newborn screen for hypothyroidism (ie, high TSH) if the blood sample for the screen is collected on the first day of life.

PHYSIOLOGY

Hypothalamic thyrotropin-releasing hormone (TRH) stimulates the anterior pituitary gland to release TSH. In turn, TSH stimulates the thyroid gland to take up iodine, and to synthesize and release the active hormones, thyroxine (T_4) and triiodothyronine (T_3). This process is regulated by negative feedback involving the hypothalamus, pituitary, and thyroid (see Figure 34–1).

T_4 is the predominant thyroid hormone secreted by the thyroid gland. Most circulating T_3 and T_4 are bound to thyroxine-binding globulin (TBG), albumin, and prealbumin. Less than 1% of T_3 and T_4 exist as free T_3 (FT_3) and free T_4 (FT_4). T_4 is deiodinated in the tissues to either T_3 (active) or reverse T_3 (inactive). In peripheral tissues, T_3 binds to high-affinity nuclear thyroid hormone receptors in the cytoplasm and translocates to the nucleus, exerting its biologic effects by modifying gene expression.

The T_4 level is low in hypothyroidism. It may also be low in premature infants, malnutrition, severe illness, and following therapy with T_3. It is not clear whether premature infants with low T_4 benefit from treatment. T_4 is also low in situations that affect TBG. TBG levels are decreased in familial TBG deficiency, nephrosis, and in patients receiving androgens. In sepsis, TBG cleavage is increased. Treatment with certain medications (heparin, furosemide, salicylates, and phenytoin) results in abnormal binding to TBG. However, since these effects involve primarily TBG levels, and not thyroid function per se, TSH and FT_4 levels remain in the normal range.

T_3 and T_4 levels are high in hyperthyroidism and may be elevated in conditions associated with increased TBG levels (congenital TBG excess, pregnancy, estrogen therapy) and increased thyroid hormone binding to transport proteins.

HYPOTHYROIDISM (CONGENITAL & ACQUIRED)

ESSENTIALS OF DIAGNOSIS & TYPICAL FEATURES

- Growth retardation, decreased physical activity, weight gain, constipation, dry skin, cold intolerance, and delayed puberty.
- Neonates with congenital hypothyroidism often look normal but may have thick tongue, large fontanels, poor muscle tone, hoarseness, umbilical hernia, jaundice, and intellectual retardation.
- T4, FT4, and T3 resin uptake are low; TSH levels are elevated in primary hypothyroidism.

General Considerations

Thyroid hormone deficiency may be congenital or acquired (Table 34–4). It can be due to defects in the thyroid gland (primary hypothyroidism) or in the hypothalamus or pituitary (central hypothyroidism).

Congenital hypothyroidism occurs in about 1:3000–1:4000 infants. Untreated, it causes severe neurocognitive

Table 34–4. Causes of hypothyroidism.

A. Congenital
1. Aplasia, hypoplasia, or maldescent of thyroid
a. Embryonic defect of thyroid development
2. Inborn errors of thyroid hormone synthesis, secretion, or recycling (due to autosomal recessive mutations)
a. Iodide transport defect
b. Organification defect
(1) Mutation in iodine peroxidase
(2) Mutation in pendrin: Pendred syndrome, associated with congenital sensorineural deafness
c. Coupling defect
d. Iodotyrosine deiodinase defect
e. Abnormal iodinated polypeptide (thyroglobulin)
f. Inability to convert T_4 to T_3
3. Maternal antibody-mediated (inhibit TSH binding to receptor)
4. TSH receptor defect
5. Thyroid hormone receptor defect
6. In-utero exposures
a. Radioiodine
b. Goitrogens (propylthiouracil, methimazole)
c. Iodine excess
7. Iodide deficiency (endemic cretinism)
B. Acquired (juvenile hypothyroidism)
1. Autoimmune (lymphocytic) thyroiditis
2. Thyroidectomy or radioiodine therapy for
a. Thyrotoxicosis
b. Thyroid cancer
3. Irradiation to the thyroid
4. Thyrotropin deficiency
a. Isolated
b. Associated with other anterior pituitary hormone deficiencies
5. TRH deficiency due to hypothalamic injury or disease
6. Medications
a. Iodides
(1) Excess (eg, amiodarone)
(2) Deficiency
b. Lithium
c. Cobalt
7. Large hemangiomas
8. Idiopathic

T_3, triiodothyronine; T_4, thyroxine; TRH, thyrotropin-releasing hormone; TSH, thyroid-stimulating hormone.

impairment. Most cases are sporadic resulting from hypoplasia or aplasia of the thyroid gland or failure of the gland to migrate to its normal anatomic location (ie, lingual or sublingual thyroid gland). Another cause of congenital hypothyroidism is dyshormonogenesis due to enzymatic defects in thyroid hormone synthesis. Since antithyroid drugs, including propylthiouracil (PTU) and methimazole, freely cross the placenta, goitrous hypothyroid newborns may be born to hyperthyroid mothers treated with these drugs during pregnancy.

Low T_4 levels may also be caused by decreased TSH secretion associated with prolonged glucocorticoid use, dopamine, or somatostatin. Cabbage, soybeans, aminosalicylic acid, thiourea derivatives, resorcinol, phenylbutazone, cobalt, and excessive iodine intake can cause goiter and hypothyroidism during pregnancy. Many of these agents cross the placenta and should be used with caution during pregnancy. Iodine deficiency also causes hypothyroidism. In severe maternal iodine deficiency, both the fetus and the mother are T_4-deficient, with irreversible brain damage in the fetus.

Juvenile hypothyroidism, particularly if goiter is present, is usually a result of chronic lymphocytic (Hashimoto) thyroiditis.

Several hundred patients with resistance to thyroid hormone have been described and present with elevations in T_4 and/or FT_4, with normal TSH. There is often a family history of the disorder. Clinical manifestations are highly variable due to differential expression of thyroid hormone receptor isoforms in different tissues

Clinical Findings

A. Symptoms and Signs

Even when the thyroid gland is completely absent, most newborns with congenital hypothyroidism appear normal at birth and gain weight normally for the first few months of life without treatment. Since congenital hypothyroidism must be treated as early as possible to prevent intellectual impairment, the diagnosis should be based on the newborn screening test and not on signs or symptoms. Jaundice associated with an unconjugated hyperbilirubinemia may be present in newborns with congenital hypothyroidism. Some infants may have obvious findings of thick tongue, hypotonia, large fontanelles, constipation, umbilical hernia, hoarse cry, and dry skin.

Juvenile hypothyroidism often presents with short stature and abnormal weight gain. Other findings include delayed epiphyseal development, delayed closure of fontanels, and retarded dental eruption. The skin may be dry, thick, scaly, coarse, pale, cool, or mottled, or have a yellowish tinge. The hair may be dry, coarse, or brittle. Lateral thinning of the eyebrows may occur. Musculoskeletal findings include hypotonia and a slow relaxation component of deep tendon reflexes (best appreciated in the ankles). Muscular hypertrophy (Kocher-Debré-Semélaigne syndrome) is not commonly seen in congenital hypothyroidism. Other findings include physical and mental sluggishness, nonpitting myxedema, constipation, large tongue, hypothermia, bradycardia, hoarse voice or cry, umbilical hernia, and transient deafness. Puberty may be delayed. Metromenorrhagia may occur in older girls. Sometimes, hypothyroidism induces pseudopuberty. Galactorrhea can also occur, due to stimulation of prolactin secretion.

In hypothyroidism resulting from enzymatic defects, ingestion of goitrogens, or chronic lymphocytic thyroiditis, the thyroid gland may be enlarged. Thyroid enlargement in children is usually symmetrical, and the gland is moderately firm and not nodular. In chronic lymphocytic thyroiditis, however, the thyroid frequently has a cobblestone surface.

B. Laboratory Findings

Total T_4 and FT_4 levels are decreased. T_3 resin uptake (T_3RU) is low. In primary hypothyroidism, the serum TSH level is elevated. In central hypothyroidism, the TSH level may be low or inappropriately normal. Circulating autoantibodies to thyroid peroxidase and thyroglobulin may be present. Serum prolactin may be elevated, resulting in galactorrhea. Serum GH may be decreased, with subnormal GH response to stimulation in children with severe primary hypothyroidism, as well as low IGF-1 or IGFBP-3 levels, or both.

C. Imaging

Thyroid imaging, while helpful in establishing the cause of congenital hypothyroidism, does not affect the treatment plan and is not necessary. Bone age is delayed. Centers of ossification, especially of the hip, may show multiple small centers or a single stippled, porous, or fragmented center (epiphyseal dysgenesis). Cardiomegaly is common. Longstanding primary hypothyroidism may be associated with thyrotrophic hyperplasia characterized by an enlarged sella or pituitary gland.

D. Screening Programs for Neonatal Hypothyroidism

All newborns should be screened for congenital hypothyroidism shortly after birth as most do not have suggestive physical findings. Depending on the state, the newborn screen measures either the total T_4 or TSH level. Abnormal newborn screening results should be confirmed immediately with a T_4 and TSH level. Treatment should be started as soon as possible. Initiation of treatment in the first month of life and good compliance during infancy usually results in a normal neurocognitive outcome.

E. Conditions Associated with Hypothyroidism

Children with Down syndrome, Turner syndrome, and autoimmune diseases such as celiac disease, vitiligo, alopecia, and type 1 diabetes are at an increased risk for the development of acquired autoimmune hypothyroidism.

A detailed family history may reveal the presence of multiple autoimmune diseases in the family members of the affected individual. Individuals at a high risk based on a chromosomal disorder or other autoimmune disease benefit from careful monitoring of growth and development, routine screening (in the case of Down syndrome, Turner syndrome, and type 1 diabetes), and a low threshold for measurement of thyroid function.

Central hypothyroidism is associated with other disorders of the hypothalamus and pituitary including congenital defects such as septo-optic dysplasia and acquired defects such as tumors in the hypothalamic/pituitary region.

Treatment

Levothyroxine (75–100 mcg/m^2/d) is the drug of choice for acquired hypothyroidism. In neonates with congenital hypothyroidism, the initial dose is 10–15 mcg/kg/d. Serum total T_4 or FT_4 concentrations are used to monitor the adequacy of initial therapy because the normally high neonatal TSH may not normalize for several days to weeks. Subsequently, T_4 and TSH are used in combination, as elevations of serum TSH are sensitive early indicators of the need for increased medication or better compliance.

American Academy of Pediatrics et al: Update of newborn screening and therapy for congenital hypothyroidism. Pediatrics 2006;117:2290 [PMID: 16740880].

Delahunty C et al: Levels of neonatal thyroid hormone in preterm infants and neurodevelopmental outcomes at 5 ½ years: Millennium cohort study. J Clin Endocrinol Metabl 2010;95:4898–4908 [PMID: 20719832].

LaFranchi SH, Austin J: How should we be treating children with congenital hypothyroidism. J Pediatr Endocrinol Metab 2007;20:559 [PMID: 17642417].

Kempers MJ et al: Intellectual and motor development of young adults with congenital hypothyroidism diagnosed by neonatal screening. J Clin Endocrinol Metab 2006;91:418 [PMID: 16303842].

Kratzsch J, Pulzer F: Thyroid gland development and defects. Best Prac Res Clin Endocrinol Metab 2008;22:57–75 [PMID: 18279780].

Ng SM, Anand D, Weindling AM: High versus low dose of initial thyroid hormone replacement for congenital hypothyroidism. Cochrane Database Syst Rev 2009;21:CD006972 [PMID: 19160309].

Obregon MJ et al: The effects of iodine deficiency on thyroid hormone deiodination. Thyroid 2005;15:917 [PMID: 16131334].

Selva KA et al: Neurodevelopmental outcomes in congenital hypothyroidism: Comparison of initial T_4 dose and time to reach target T_4 and TSH. J Pediatr 2005;147:775 [PMID: 16356430].

Simpser T, Rapaport R: Update on some aspects of neonatal thyroid disease. J Clin Res Pediatr Endocrinol 2010;2:95–99 [PMID: 21274321].

Woo HC et al: Congenital hypothyroidism with a delayed thyroid-stimulating hormone elevation in very premature infants: Incidence and growth and developmental outcomes. J Pediatr 2011;158:538–542.

THYROIDITIS

1. Chronic Lymphocytic Thyroiditis (Chronic Autoimmune Thyroiditis, Hashimoto Thyroiditis)

ESSENTIALS OF DIAGNOSIS & TYPICAL FEATURES

- Firm, freely movable, nontender, diffusely enlarged thyroid gland.
- Thyroid function is usually normal but may be elevated or decreased depending on the stage of the disease.

General Considerations

Chronic lymphocytic thyroiditis is the most common cause of goiter and acquired hypothyroidism in childhood. It is more common in girls, and the incidence peaks during puberty. The disease is caused by an autoimmune attack on the thyroid. Increased risk of thyroid autoimmunity (and other endocrine autoimmune disorders) is associated with certain histocompatibility alleles.

Clinical Findings

A. Symptoms and Signs

The thyroid is characteristically enlarged, firm, freely movable, nontender, and symmetrical. It may be nodular. Onset is usually insidious. Occasionally patients note a sensation of tracheal compression or fullness, hoarseness, and dysphagia. No local signs of inflammation or systemic infection are present. Most patients are euthyroid. Some patients are symptomatically hypothyroid, and few patients are symptomatically hyperthyroid.

B. Laboratory Findings

Laboratory findings vary. Serum concentrations of TSH, T_4, FT_4, and T_3RU are usually normal. Some patients are hypothyroid with an elevated TSH and low thyroid hormone levels. A few patients are hyperthyroid with a suppressed TSH and elevated thyroid hormone levels. Thyroid antibodies (antithyroglobulin, antithyroid peroxidase) are frequently elevated. Thyroid uptake scan adds little to the diagnosis. Surgical or needle biopsy is diagnostic but seldom necessary.

Treatment

There is controversy about the need to treat chronic lymphocytic thyroiditis with normal thyroid function. Full replacement doses of thyroid hormone may decrease the size of the thyroid, but may also result in hyperthyroidism. Hypothyroidism commonly develops over time. Consequently, patients require lifelong surveillance. Children with documented hypothyroidism should receive thyroid hormone replacement.

2. Acute (Suppurative) Thyroiditis

Acute thyroiditis is rare. The most common causes are group A streptococci, pneumococci, *Staphylococcus aureus*, and anaerobes. Oropharyngeal organisms are thought to reach the thyroid via a patent foramen cecum and thyroglossal duct remnant. Thyroid abscesses may form. The patient is toxic with fever and chills. The thyroid gland is enlarged and exquisitely tender with associated erythema, hoarseness, and dysphagia. Thyroid function tests are typically normal. Patients have a leukocytosis, "left shift," and elevated erythrocyte sedimentation rate. Specific antibiotic therapy should be administered.

3. Subacute (Nonsuppurative) Thyroiditis

Subacute thyroiditis (de Quervain thyroiditis) is rare. It is thought to be caused by viral infection with mumps, influenza, echovirus, coxsackievirus, Epstein-Barr virus, or adenovirus. Presenting features are similar to acute thyroiditis—ever, malaise, sore throat, dysphagia, and thyroid pain that may radiate to the ear. The thyroid is firm and enlarged. Sedimentation rate is elevated. In contrast to acute thyroiditis, the onset is generally insidious and serum thyroid hormone concentrations may be elevated.

HYPERTHYROIDISM

ESSENTIALS OF DIAGNOSIS & TYPICAL FEATURES

- Nervousness, emotional lability, hyperactivity, fatigue, tremor, palpitations, excessive appetite, weight loss, increased perspiration, and heat intolerance.
- Goiter, exophthalmos, tachycardia, widened pulse pressure, systolic hypertension, weakness, and smooth, moist, warm skin.
- TSH is suppressed. Thyroid hormone levels (T_4, FT_4, T_3, T_3RU) are elevated.

General Considerations

In children, most cases of hyperthyroidism are due to Graves disease, caused by antibodies directed at the TSH receptor that stimulate thyroid hormone production. Hyperthyroidism may also be due to acute, subacute, or chronic thyroiditis; autonomous functioning thyroid nodules; tumors producing TSH; McCune-Albright syndrome; exogenous thyroid hormone excess; and acute iodine exposure.

Clinical Findings

A. Symptoms and Signs

Hyperthyroidism is more common in females than males. In children, it most frequently occurs during adolescence. The course of hyperthyroidism tends to be cyclic, with spontaneous remissions and exacerbations. Symptoms include worsening school performance, poor concentration, fatigue, hyperactivity, emotional lability, nervousness, personality disturbance, insomnia, weight loss (despite increased appetite), palpitations, heat intolerance, increased perspiration, diarrhea, polyuria, and irregular menses. Signs include tachycardia, systolic hypertension, increased pulse pressure, tremor, proximal muscle weakness, and moist, warm, skin. Accelerated growth and development may occur. Thyroid storm is a rare condition characterized by fever, cardiac failure, emesis, delirium, coma, and death. Most cases of Graves disease are associated with a diffuse firm goiter. A thyroid bruit and thrill may be present. Many cases are associated with exophthalmos, but severe ophthalmopathy is rare.

B. Laboratory Findings

TSH is suppressed. T_4, FT_4, T_3, FT_3, and T_3RU are elevated except in rare cases in which only the serum T_3 is elevated (T3 thyrotoxicosis). The presence of thyroid-stimulating immunoglobulin (TSI) confirms the diagnosis of Graves disease. TSH receptor–binding antibodies (TRaB) are usually elevated.

C. Imaging

In Graves disease, radioactive iodine uptake by the thyroid is increased, whereas in subacute and chronic thyroiditis it is decreased. An autonomous hyperfunctioning nodule takes up iodine and appears as a "hot nodule" while the surrounding tissue has decreased iodine uptake. In children with hyperthyroidism, bone age may be advanced. In infants, accelerated skeletal maturation may be associated with premature fusion of the cranial sutures. Long-standing hyperthyroidism causes osteoporosis.

Differential Diagnosis

Hypermetabolic states (severe anemia, chronic infections, pheochromocytoma, and muscle-wasting disease) may resemble hyperthyroidism clinically but differ in thyroid function tests.

Treatment

A. General Measures

In untreated hyperthyroidism, strenuous physical activity should be avoided. Bed rest may be required in severe cases.

B. Medical Treatment

1. β-Adrenergic blocking agents—These agents are adjuncts to therapy. They can rapidly ameliorate symptoms such as nervousness, tremor, and palpitations, and are indicated in severe disease with tachycardia and hypertension. β_1-Specific agents such as atenolol are preferred because they are more cardioselective.

2. Antithyroid agents (PTU and methimazole)—Antithyroid agents are frequently used in the initial treatment of childhood hyperthyroidism. These drugs interfere with thyroid hormone synthesis, and usually take a few weeks to produce a clinical response. Adequate control is usually achieved within a few months. If medical therapy is unsuccessful, more definitive therapy, such as radioablation of the thyroid or thyroidectomy, should be considered.

In response to reports of severe hepatoxicity related to PTU, recent recommendations state that PTU should not be used in infants, children, or adolescents, except when methimazole is contraindicated due to hypersensitivity or pregnancy.

A. INITIAL DOSAGE—Methimazole is initiated at a dose of 10–60 mg/d (0.5–1 mg/kg/d) given once a day. Initial dosing is continued until FT_4 or T_4 have normalized and signs and symptoms have subsided.

B. MAINTENANCE—The optimal dose of antithyroid agent for maintenance treatment remains unclear. Recent studies suggest that 10–15 mg/d of methimazole provides adequate long-term control in most patients with a minimum of side effects. If the TSH becomes elevated, many providers decrease the dose of the antithyroid agent. Some providers continue the same dose of antithyroid agent and add exogenous thyroid hormone replacement. Treatment usually continues for 2 years with the goal of inducing remission. If thyroid hormone levels are stable, a trial off medication could be considered at that point.

C. TOXICITY—If rash, vasculitis, arthralgia, arthritis, granulocytopenia, or hepatitis occur, the drug must be discontinued.

3. Iodide—Large doses of iodide usually produce a rapid but short-lived blockade of thyroid hormone synthesis and release. This approach is recommended only for acute management of severely thyrotoxic patients.

C. Radiation Therapy

Radioactive iodine ablation of the thyroid is usually reserved for children with Graves disease who do not respond to antithyroid agents, develop adverse effects from the antithyroid agents, fail to achieve remission after several years of medical therapy, or have poor medication adherence. With recent concerns regarding potential hepatotoxicity of antithyroid medications, some pediatric endocrinologists advocate radioablation as first-line therapy for children with Graves disease. Antithyroid agents should be discontinued 4–7 days prior to radioablation to allow radioiodine uptake by the thyroid. ^{131}I is administered orally which concentrates in the thyroid and results in gradual ablation of the gland. In the first 2 weeks following radioablation, hyperthyroidism may worsen as thyroid tissue is destroyed and thyroid hormone is released. Therapy with a β-adrenergic antagonist may be necessary for a few months until FT_4 and T_4 fall into the normal range. In most cases, hypothyroidism develops and thyroid hormone replacement is needed. Long-term follow-up studies have not shown any increased incidence of thyroid cancer, leukemia, infertility, or birth defects when ablative doses of ^{131}I were used.

D. Surgical Treatment

Subtotal and total thyroidectomy are infrequently used in children with Graves disease. Surgery is indicated for extremely large goiters, goiters with a suspicious nodule, very young or pregnant patients, or patients refusing radioiodine ablation. Before surgery, a β-adrenergic blocking agent is given to treat symptoms, and antithyroid agents are given for several weeks to minimize the surgical risks associated with hyperthyroidism. Iodide (eg, Lugol solution, 1 drop every 8 hours, or saturated solution of potassium iodide, 1–2 drops daily) is given for 1–2 weeks prior to surgery to reduce thyroid vascularity and inhibit release of thyroid hormone. Surgical complications include hypoparathyroidism, recurrent laryngeal nerve damage, and rarely, death. An experienced thyroid surgeon is crucial to good surgical outcome. After thyroidectomy, patients become hypothyroid and need thyroid hormone replacement.

Course & Prognosis

Partial remissions and exacerbations may continue for several years. Treatment with an antithyroid agent results in prolonged remissions in one-third to two-thirds of children.

Bauer AJ: Approach to the pediatric patient with Graves' disease: When is definitive therapy warranted? J Clin Endocrinol Metab 2011;96:580–588 [PMID: 21378220].

Lee JA et al: The optimal treatment for pediatric Graves' disease is surgery. J Clin Endocrinol Metab 2007;92:80 [PMID: 17341575].

Rivkees SA, Dinauer C: An optimal treatment for pediatric Graves' disease is radioiodine. J Clin Endocrinol Metab 2007;92:797 [PMID: 17341574].

Rivkees SA, Mattison DR: Ending propylthiouracil-induced liver failure in children. N Engl J Med 2009;360:1574 [PMID: 19357418].

Neonatal Graves Disease

Transient congenital hyperthyroidism (neonatal Graves disease) occurs in about 1% of infants born to mothers with Graves disease. It occurs when maternal TSH receptor antibodies cross the placenta and stimulate excess thyroid hormone production in the fetus and newborn. Neonatal Graves disease can be associated with irritability, IUGR, poor weight gain, flushing, jaundice, hepatosplenomegaly, and thrombocytopenia. Severe cases may result in cardiac failure and death. Hyperthyroidism may develop several days after birth, especially if the mother was treated with PTU (which crosses the placenta). Symptoms develop as PTU levels decline in the newborn. Thyroid studies should be obtained at birth and repeated within the first week. Immediate management should focus on the cardiac manifestations. Temporary treatment may be necessary with iodide, antithyroid agents, β-adrenergic antagonists, or corticosteroids. Hyperthyroidism gradually resolves over 1–3 months as maternal antibodies decline. As TSH receptor antibodies may still be present in the serum of previously hyperthyroid mothers after thyroidectomy or radioablation, neonatal Graves disease should be considered in all infants of mothers with a history of hyperthyroidism.

Lewis KA et al: Neonatal Graves disease associated with severe metabolic abnormalities. Pediatrics 2011;128(1):e232–e236 [PMID: 21646263].

Papendieck P et al: Thyroid disorders of neonates born to mothers with Graves' disease. J Pediatr Endocrinol Metab 2009;22:547 [PMID: 19694202].

Polak M et al: Fetal and neonatal thyroid function in relation to maternal Graves' disease. Best Pract Res Clin Endocrinol Metab 2004;18:289 [PMID: 15157841].

THYROID CANCER

Thyroid cancer is rare in childhood. Children usually present with a thyroid nodule or an asymptomatic asymmetrical neck mass. Dysphagia and hoarseness are unusual symptoms. Thyroid function tests are usually normal. A "cold" nodule is often seen on a technetium or radioiodine uptake scan of the thyroid. Fine-needle aspiration biopsy of the nodule assists in the diagnosis.

The most common thyroid cancer is papillary thyroid carcinoma, a well-differentiated carcinoma arising from the thyroid follicular cell. Children frequently present with local metastases to the cervical lymph nodes and occasionally with pulmonary metastasis. Despite its aggressive presentation, children with papillary thyroid carcinoma have a relatively good prognosis, with a 20-year survival rate greater than 90%. Treatment consists of total thyroidectomy and removal of all involved lymph nodes, usually followed by radioiodine ablation to destroy residual thyroid remnant and metastatic tissue left behind after surgery. Thyroid hormone replacement is started to suppress TSH secretion and stimulation of residual thyroid tissue. Since papillary thyroid carcinoma in children is associated with a high recurrence rate, regular follow-up with serum thyroglobulin levels (a tumor marker), neck ultrasound, and radioiodine whole body scan are required.

Follicular thyroid carcinoma, medullary thyroid carcinoma, anaplastic carcinoma, and lymphoma are less common thyroid malignancies. Medullary thyroid carcinoma, due to autosomal dominant mutations in the RET protooncogene, arises from the thyroid C cells, which secrete calcitonin. It can occur sporadically or can be inherited in multiple endocrine neoplasia (MEN) type 2 and familial medullary thyroid carcinoma. It is associated with elevated serum calcitonin levels. In affected families, all members should be screened for the mutation, and those identified with the mutation should be treated with prophylactic thyroidectomy in early childhood.

Corrias A et al: Diagnostic features of thyroid nodules in Pediatrics. Arch Pediatr Adolesc Med 2010:164:714–719 [PMID: 20679162].

Dinauer CA, Breuer C, Rivkees SA: Differentiated thyroid cancer in children: Diagnosis and management. Curr Opin Oncol 2008;20:59 [PMID: 18043257].

Dotto J, Nose V: Familia thyroid carcinoma: A diagnostic algorithm. Adv Anat Pathol 2008;15:332 [PMID: 18948764].

Kloos RT et al: Medullary thyroid cancer: Management guidelines of the American Thyroid Association. Thyroid 2009;19:565 [PMID: 19469690].

Leboulleux S et al: Follicular cell-derived thyroid cancer in children. Horm Res 2005;63:145 [PMID: 15802922].

Rachmiel M et al: Evidence-based review of treatment and follow up of pediatric patients with differentiated thyroid carcinoma. J Pediatr Endocrinol Metab 2006;19:1377 [PMID: 17252690].

DISORDERS OF CALCIUM & PHOSPHORUS METABOLISM

Serum calcium concentration is tightly regulated by the coordinated actions of the parathyroid glands, kidney, liver, and small intestine. Low serum calcium concentrations, detected by calcium-sensing receptors on the surface of parathyroid cells, stimulate parathyroid hormone (PTH) release. PTH in turn promotes release of calcium and phosphorus from bone, reabsorption of calcium from urinary filtrate, and excretion of phosphorus in the urine. Another essential cofactor in calcium homeostasis is 1,25-dihydroxy vitamin D (calcitriol). The first step in production of this active form of vitamin D occurs in the liver where dietary vitamin D is hydroxylated to 25-hydroxy vitamin D. The final step in formation of calcitriol is 1-hydroxylation, which takes place in the kidney under control of PTH. The primary effect of calcitriol is to promote the absorption of calcium from the intestines. In concert with PTH, however, it also facilitates calcium and phosphorus mobilization from bones. Deficiencies or excesses of PTH or calcitriol, abnormalities in their receptors, or abnormalities of vitamin D metabolism lead to clinically significant aberrations in calcium homeostasis. Although calcitonin, released from the thyroid gland C cells, also reduces serum calcium concentration, changes in its serum concentration rarely cause clinically relevant disease.

HYPOCALCEMIC DISORDERS

A normal serum calcium concentration is approximately 8.9–10.2 mg/dL. The normal concentration of ionized calcium is approximately 1.1–1.3 mmol/L. Serum calcium levels in newborns are slightly lower than normal and may be as low as 7 mg/dL in premature infants. Fifty to sixty percent of calcium in the serum is protein-bound and metabolically fairly inactive. Thus, measurement of ionized serum calcium, the metabolically active form, is helpful if serum proteins are low or in conditions such as acidosis that cause abnormal calcium binding to protein.

ESSENTIALS OF DIAGNOSIS & TYPICAL FEATURES

- Tetany with facial and extremity numbness, tingling, cramps, spontaneous muscle contractures, carpopedal spasm, positive Trousseau and Chvostek signs, loss of consciousness, and convulsions.
- Diarrhea, prolongation of electrical systole (QT interval), and laryngospasm.
- In hypoparathyroidism or PHP: defective nails and teeth, cataracts, and ectopic calcification in the subcutaneous tissues and basal ganglia.

General Considerations

Hypocalcemia is a consistent feature of conditions such as hypoparathyroidism, pseudohypoparathyroidism (PHP), transient tetany of the newborn, and severe vitamin D deficiency rickets and may be present in rare disorders of vitamin D action (receptor defects). Hypocalcemia may also occur as a result of intestinal malabsorption of calcium, chronic renal disease, tumor lysis syndrome, rhabdomyolysis, or as the result of an activating mutation in the calcium-sensing receptor of the parathyroid glands and kidneys (hypercalciuric hypocalcemia). (See Table 34–5.)

Deficient PTH *secretion* may be due to deficient parathyroid tissue (DiGeorge syndrome), autoimmunity, or sometimes, magnesium deficiency. Decreased PTH *action* may be due to magnesium deficiency, vitamin D deficiency, or defects in the PTH receptor (PHP). Occasionally, PTH deficiency is idiopathic. Table 34–6 summarizes the characteristics of disorders of PTH secretion and action.

Autoimmune parathyroid destruction with subsequent hypoparathyroidism may be isolated, or associated with other autoimmune disorders in the APECED syndrome (autoimmune polyendocrinopathy-candidiasis-ectodermal dystrophy, or APS-1). Hypoparathyroidism may also result from unavoidable surgical removal in patients with thyroid cancer. Other features of the DiGeorge syndrome (a deletion of 22.q11) include congenital absence of the thymus (with thymus-dependent immunologic deficiency) and cardiovascular anomalies, especially coarctation of the aorta.

Autosomal dominant hypocalcemia, also called familial hypercalciuric hypocalcemia, is associated with a gain-of-function mutation in the calcium receptor, which causes a low serum PTH despite hypocalcemia, and excessive urinary loss of calcium. A family history of hypocalcemia may be the clue that differentiates this condition from other causes of hypocalcemia.

Transient neonatal hypoparathyroidism (transient tetany of the newborn) is caused both by a relative deficiency of PTH secretion and PTH action (see Table 34–6). The early form of this condition (first 2 weeks of life) occurs in newborns with birth asphyxia. In mothers with hyperparathyroidism, maternal hypercalcemia may suppress fetal PTH secretion and cause early transient neonatal hypoparathyroidism. Likewise, women with gestational diabetes may have relative hyperparathyroidism in the third trimester and their infants may experience transient hypoparathyroidism. Associated hypomagnesemia often aggravates the symptoms associated with hypocalcemia. The late form of neonatal hypoparathyroidism (after 2 weeks of age) occurs in infants receiving high-phosphate formulas (whole cow's milk is a well-known example). Phosphate binds calcium and produces functional hypocalcemia.

Tumor lysis syndrome and rhabdomyolysis cause cellular destruction that liberates large amounts of intracellular phosphate that complex with serum calcium, producing functional hypocalcemia. Malabsorption states such as celiac disease impair the absorption of calcium, vitamin D, and magnesium, all of which cause hypocalcemia (see Table 34–6). Hypomagnesemia, due to losses from the gastrointestinal tract or kidney, may cause or augment the severity of hypocalcemia by impairing the release of PTH.

Rickets is a term describing the characteristic clinical and bony radiologic features associated with vitamin D deficiency (see Chapter 11). Vitamin D deficiency, caused by lack of sunlight exposure or dietary deficiency, is the most common cause of rickets. Occult vitamin D deficiency is probably more common than is currently recognized. This concern forms the basis for the 2008 recommendation by the American Association of Pediatrics that breast-fed infants receive vitamin D supplementation of at least 400 IU/d, or supplementation of breast feeding women with 3–4000 IU/d. Rickets can also be caused by defects in the metabolism of vitamin D (see Table 34–5), including liver disease (impaired 25-hydroxylation), kidney disease [impaired 1-hydroxylation of 25-(OH) vitamin D], genetic deficiency of 1α-hydroxylase (vitamin D–dependent rickets), or end-organ resistance to vitamin D (vitamin D–resistant rickets).

Familial hypophosphatemic rickets has skeletal findings similar to those of vitamin D–related rickets. The defect in this condition is abnormal renal phosphate loss related to abnormal fibroblast growth factor 23 (FGF23) regulation.

Table 34–5. Hypocalcemia associated with rickets and other disorders.

Condition	Pathogenesis	Disease States/Inheritance	Clinical Features	Initial Biochemical Findings			
				Serum Calcium	Serum Phosphorus	Serum Alkaline Phosphatase	Other
Malabsorption	Impairment in intestinal absorption in any or all of the following: calcium, vitamin D, and magnesium	Cystic fibrosis, celiac or other intestinal disease, liver disease, Shwachman syndrome	Failure to thrive, poor weight gain, steatorrhea, superimposed vitamin D deficiency rickets	Low or normal	Low or normal	Variable: usually high in vitamin D deficiency, but may be low with concomitant zinc deficiency	Potentially low magnesium levels, potentially low 25-OH vitamin D
Chronic renal insufficiency	Decreased renal phosphate excretion, decreased 1-hydroxylase activity	Obstruction, glomerulonephritis, dysplastic kidneys	Uremia, growth failure, acidosis	Low or normal	Elevated	Elevated or normal	Elevated PTH levels in long-standing cases, low 1,25-OH vitamin D
Rhabdomyolysis	Muscle damage with liberation of large amounts of intracellular phosphate	Crush injuries of muscles, Pompe disease, carnitine deficiency	Hypocalcemic tetany, cardiac arrhythmia, risk of renal failure	Low	Elevated	Normal	Myoglobinuria
Tumor lysis syndrome	Release of intracellular phosphate and potassium	Initiation of chemotherapy for ALL, Burkitt lymphoma, or other malignancies	Hypocalcemic tetany, cardiac arrhythmia, risk of renal failure	Low	Elevated	Normal	Hyperkalemia, elevated uric acid
Vitamin D–deficiency rickets	Deficient dietary vitamin D intake, vitamin D malabsorption; other risk factors include dark skin and lack of sunlight exposure	May cluster in families due to shared risk factors	Characteristic skeletal changes appear early, poor growth, symptomatic hypocalcemia is a late Finding	Normal until late in course	Low or normal	Elevated	Elevated PTH levels, low 25-OH vitamin D
Vitamin D–dependent rickets	Mutation in 1-hydroxylase enzyme required for synthesis of fully active 1,25-OH vitamin D	Autosomal recessive inheritance	Skeletal changes of rickets, symptomatic hypocalcemia	Low	Low or normal	Elevated	Elevated PTH, low 1,25-OH vitamin D
Vitamin D–resistant rickets	Mutation in 1,25 OH vitamin D receptor	Autosomal recessive inheritance	Severe skeletal changes of rickets, total alopecia, symptomatic hypocalcemia	Low	Low or normal	Elevated	Elevated PTH, elevated 1,25-OH vitamin D
Hypophosphatemic rickets	Excessive loss of phosphate in the urine Abnormal fibroblast growth factor 23 (FGF23) regulation	X-linked dominant	Skeletal changes primarily in the lower extremities—genu varum or valgus, short stature	Normal or low	Very low	Usually high	Normal PTH levels initially, abnormally high urinary phosphate excretion

ALL, acute lymphoblastic leukemia; PTH, parathyroid hormone.

Table 34–6. Hypocalcemia associated with disorders of parathyroid hormone secretion or action.

				Initial Biochemical Findings[a]			
Condition	Pathogenesis	Inheritance Pattern	Clinical Features	Serum Calcium	Serum Phosphorus	Serum Alkaline Phosphatase	Serum PTH
Isolated hypoparathyroidism	Trauma, surgical destruction, isolated autoimmune destruction, rare familial forms	None; reports in familial forms of inheritance as X-linked recessive, autosomal recessive, or autosomal dominant	Symptoms of hypocalcemia	Low	High	Normal or low	Low, low 1,25-OH vitamin D
DiGeorge syndrome	Deletion in chromosome 22	Majority represent new mutations	Symptoms of hypocalcemia, cardiac anomalies, immune disorder	Low	High	Normal or low	Low, low 1,25-OH vitamin D
APS type 1	Autoimmune destruction	Autosomal recessive	Mucocutaneous candidiasis, Addison disease; potential for autoimmune destruction in other endocrine glands	Low	High	Normal or low	Low, low 1,25-OH vitamin D
PHP type IA	Mutation in stimulatory G protein; resistance to PTH action	Autosomal dominant	AHO phenotype, short stature, variable hypocalcemia, may have resistance to other hormones using G protein signaling	Low or normal	Elevated or normal	Variable	Very Elevated, low 1,25-OH vitamin D
PPHP	Mutation in stimulatory G protein	Autosomal dominant—frequently found within same families with PHP type IA	AHO phenotype, biochemical parameters are normal	Normal	Normal	Normal	Normal
Transient tetany of the newborn–early	Deficiency in PTH secretion or action	Sporadic—associated with difficult deliveries, infants of diabetic mothers, or maternal hyperparathyroidism	Onset of symptoms of hypocalcemia within 2 wk of birth	Low	Normal or low	Normal or low	Normal or low, low 1,25-OH vitamin D
Transient tetany of the newborn–late onset	Deficiency in PTH secretion or action	Sporadic—associated with infant formulas that have a high phosphate content	Onset of symptoms of hypocalcemia after 2 wk of age	Low	Normal or low	Normal or low	Normal or low, low 1,25-OH vitamin D
Familial hypercalciuric hypocalcemia	Gain of functional mutation of calcium-sensing receptor	Autosomal dominant	Symptoms of hypocalcemia, family history	Low	High	Normal or low	Low, low 1,25-OH vitamin D

[a]Urinary calcium excretion (calcium-creatinine ratio) is low in all but familial hypercalciuric hypocalcemia.
AHO, Albright hereditary osteodystrophy; APS, autoimmune polyglandular syndrome; PHP, pseudohypoparathyroidism; PPHP, pseudopseudohypoparathyroidism; PTH, parathyroid hormone.

Dietary deficiency of calcium may also cause rickets but more often causes osteopenia.

Clinical Findings

A. Symptoms and Signs

Prolonged hypocalcemia from any cause is associated with tetany, photophobia, blepharospasm, and diarrhea. The symptoms of tetany are numbness, muscle cramps, twitching of the extremities, carpopedal spasm, and laryngospasm. Tapping the face in front of the ear causes facial spasms (Chvostek sign). Some patients with hypocalcemia exhibit bizarre behavior, irritability, loss of consciousness, and convulsions. Retarded physical and mental development may be present. Headache, vomiting, increased intracranial pressure, and papilledema may occur. In early infancy, respiratory distress may be a presenting finding.

B. Laboratory Findings

In rickets, calcium levels may be low or normal (see Tables 34–5 and 34–6). Phosphate levels in hypocalcemia disorders may be low, normal, or high depending on the cause of the hypocalcemia. Magnesium levels may also be low. PTH levels are reduced in many hypocalcemic conditions, but may be elevated in PHP or severe vitamin D deficiency. Measurement of urinary excretion of calcium as the calcium-creatinine ratio can assist in diagnosis and monitoring of therapy in children on calcitriol therapy.

C. Imaging

Soft tissue and basal ganglia calcification may occur in idiopathic hypoparathyroidism and PHP. Various skeletal changes are associated with rickets, including cupped and irregular long bone metaphyses. Torsional deformities can result in genu varum (bowleg). Accentuation of the costochondral junction gives the rachitic rosary appearance seen on the chest wall.

Differential Diagnosis

Tables 34–5 and 34–6 outline the features of disorders associated with hypocalcemia. In individuals with hypoalbuminemia, the total serum calcium may be low and yet the functional serum ionized calcium is normal. Ionized calcium is the test of choice for hypocalcemia in patients with low serum albumin.

Treatment

A. Acute or Severe Tetany

Hypocalcemia is corrected acutely by administration of intravenous calcium gluconate or calcium chloride; 10 mg/kg is the usual dose in acute treatment. Intravenous calcium infusions should not exceed 50 mg/min because of possible cardiac arrhythmia. Cardiac monitoring should be performed during calcium infusion.

B. Maintenance Management of Hypoparathyroidism or Chronic Hypocalcemia

The objective of treatment is to maintain the serum calcium and phosphate at near-normal levels without excess urinary calcium excretion.

1. Diet—Diet should be high in calcium with added calcium supplements starting at a dose of 50–75 mg of elemental calcium per kilogram of body weight per day divided in three to four doses. The dose may be changed based on response of serum level and urinary calcium excretion. Therapy should be monitored to prevent hypercalcemia. Supplemental calcium can often be discontinued in patients with rickets after vitamin D therapy has stabilized.

2. Vitamin D supplementation—A variety of vitamin D preparations are available. Ergocalciferol (vitamin D_2) and cholecalciferol (vitamin D_3) are the most commonly used oral preparations. Calcitriol (1,25-dihydroxy vitamin D_3) is also available. Cholecalciferol is slightly more active than ergocalciferol in therapy of most vitamin D deficiency states. If there is impaired metabolism of dietary vitamin D to 25-OH Vitamin D as seen in hepatic dysfunction, or to its active end product, 1,25-dihydroxy vitamin D, or impaired PTH function, supplementation with calcitriol is recommended. Selection and dosage of vitamin D supplements varies with the underlying condition and the response to therapy. Monitoring of therapy is essential to avoid toxicity.

3. Monitoring—Dosage of calcium and vitamin D must be tailored for each patient. Monitoring serum calcium, urine calcium, and serum alkaline phosphatase levels at 1- to 3-month intervals is necessary to ensure adequate therapy and to prevent hypercalcemia and nephrocalcinosis.

The major goals of monitoring in vitamin D deficiency are to ensure (1) maintenance of serum calcium and phosphorus concentrations within normal ranges, (2) normalization of alkaline phosphatase activity for age, (3) regression of skeletal changes, and (4) maintenance of an age-appropriate urine calcium-creatinine ratio. The ratio should be less than 0.8 in newborns, 0.3–0.6 in children, and less than 0.25 in adolescents (when using creatinine and calcium measured in milligrams per deciliter).

Monitoring goals are somewhat different in hypophosphatemic rickets. Serum calcium and alkaline phosphatase, and urinary calcium to creatinine ratio should be maintained within normal limits. Monitoring of serum PTH is necessary to ensure that secondary hyperparathyroidism does not develop from excessive phosphate treatment or inadequate calcitriol replacement.

PSEUDOHYPOPARATHYROIDISM (RESISTANCE TO PARATHYROID HORMONE ACTION)

In PHP, PTH production is adequate, but target organs (renal tubule, bone, or both) fail to respond because of receptor resistance. Resistance to PTH action is due to a heterozygous inactivating mutation in the stimulatory G protein subunit associated with the PTH receptor, which leads to impaired signaling. Resistance to other G protein–dependent hormones such as TSH, GHRH, and follicle-stimulating hormone (FSH)/luteinizing hormone (LH), may also be present.

There are several types of PHP with variable biochemical and phenotypic features (see Table 34–6). Biochemical abnormalities in PHP (hypocalcemia and hyperphosphatemia) are similar to those seen in hypoparathyroidism, but the PTH levels are elevated. PHP may be accompanied by a characteristic phenotype known as Albright hereditary osteodystrophy (AHO), which includes short stature; round, full facies; irregularly shortened fourth metacarpal; a short, thick-set body; delayed and defective dentition; and mild mental retardation. Corneal and lenticular opacities and ectopic calcification of the basal ganglia and subcutaneous tissues (osteoma cutis) may occur with or without abnormal serum calcium levels. Treatment is the same as for hypoparathyroidism.

Pseudopseudohypoparathyroidism (PPHP) describes individuals with the AHO phenotype, but normal calcium homeostasis. PHP and PPHP can occur in the same cohort. Genomic imprinting is probably responsible for the different phenotypic expression of disease. Heterozygous loss of the maternal allele causes PHP and heterozygous loss of the paternal allele causes PPHP.

Allgrove J: A practical approach to rickets. Endocr Dev 2009;16:115–132 [Epub 2009 Jun 3] [Review] [PMID: 19494664].

Gattineni J, Baum M: Regulation of phosphate transport by fibroblast growth factor 23 (FGF23): Implications for disorders of phosphate metabolism. Pediatr Nephrol 2010 Apr;25(4):591–601 [Review] [PMID: 19669798].

Hendy GN, Guarnieri V, Canaff L: Calcium-sensing receptor and associated diseases. Prog Mol Biol Transl Sci 2009;89:31–95 [Epub 2009 Oct 7] [Review] [PMID: 20374733].

Kelley A, Levine M: Disorders of bone and mineral metabolism. In Kappy MS, Allen DB, Geffner ME (editors): *Pediatric Practice Endocrinology* 2009:191–256.

Koo WWK: Neonatal calcium, magnesium and phosphorus disorders. In Lifshitz F (editor): *Pediatric Endocrinology,* 5th ed. Informa Healthcare 2007:497.

Malloy PJ, Feldman D: Genetic disorders and defects in vitamin D action. Endocrinol Metab Clin North Am 2010 Jun;39(2):333–346 [PMID: 20511055].

Shaw N: A practical approach to hypocalcaemia in children. Endocr Dev 2009;16:73–92 [Review] [PMID: 19494662].

HYPERCALCEMIC STATES

Hypercalcemia is defined as a serum calcium level > 11 mg/dL. Severe hypercalcemia is a level > 13.5 mg/dL.

ESSENTIALS OF DIAGNOSIS & TYPICAL FEATURES

- Abdominal pain, polyuria, polydipsia, hypertension, nephrocalcinosis, failure to thrive, renal stones, intractable peptic ulcer, constipation, uremia, and pancreatitis.
- Bone pain or pathologic fractures, subperiosteal bone resorption, renal parenchymal calcification or stones, and osteitis fibrosa cystica.
- Impaired concentration, altered mental status, mood swings, and coma.

General Considerations

More than 80% of hypercalcemic children or adolescents have either hyperparathyroidism or a malignant tumor. Table 34–7 summarizes the differential diagnosis of childhood hypercalcemia.

Hyperparathyroidism is rare in childhood and may be primary or secondary. The most common cause of primary hyperparathyroidism is parathyroid adenoma. Diffuse parathyroid hyperplasia or multiple adenomas may occur in families. Familial hyperparathyroidism may be an isolated disease, or it may be associated with MEN type 1, or rarely type 2A. Hypercalcemia of malignancy is associated with

Table 34–7. Hypercalcemic states.

A. Primary hyperparathyroidism
1. Parathyroid hyperplasia
2. Parathyroid adenoma
3. Familial, including MEN types 1 and 2
4. Ectopic PTH secretion

B. Hypercalcemic states other than primary hyperparathyroidism associated with increased intestinal or renal absorption of calcium
1. Hypervitaminosis D (including idiopathic hypercalcemia of infancy)
2. Familial hypocalciuric hypercalcemia
3. Lithium therapy
4. Sarcoidosis
5. Phosphate depletion
6. Aluminum intoxication

C. Hypercalcemic states other than hyperparathyroidism associated with increased mobilization of bone minerals
1. Hyperthyroidism
2. Immobilization
3. Thiazides
4. Vitamin A intoxication
5. Malignant neoplasms
   a. Ectopic PTH secretion or PTH-related protein (PTHRP)
   b. Prostaglandin-secreting tumor and perhaps prostaglandin release from subcutaneous fat necrosis
   c. Tumors metastatic to bone
   d. Myeloma

MEN, multiple endocrine neoplasia; PTH, parathyroid hormone.

solid and hematologic malignancies and is due either to local destruction of bone by tumor or to ectopic secretion of PTH-related protein. When ectopic PTH-related protein is present, calcium is elevated, serum PTH is suppressed, and serum PTH–related protein is elevated. Chronic renal disease with impaired phosphate excretion is the most common secondary cause of hyperparathyroidism.

Iqbal CW, Wahoff DC: Diagnosis and management of pediatric endocrine neoplasms. Curr Opin Pediatr 2009 Jun;21(3):379–385 [Review] [PMID: 19421059].

Waller S: Parathyroid hormone and growth in chronic kidney disease. Pediatr Nephrol 2011 Feb;26(2):195–204 [Epub 2010 Aug 9] [Review] [PMID: 20694820].

Toke J, Patócs A, Balogh K, Gergics P, Stenczer B, Rácz K, Tóth M: Parathyroid hormone-dependent hypercalcemia. Wien Klin Wochenschr 2009;121(7–8):236–245 [Review] [PMID: 19562279].

Clinical Findings

A. Symptoms and Signs

1. Due to hypercalcemia—Manifestations include hypotonicity and muscle weakness; apathy, mood swings, and bizarre behavior; nausea, vomiting, abdominal pain, constipation, and weight loss; hyperextensibility of joints; and hypertension, cardiac irregularities, bradycardia, and shortening of the QT interval. Coma occurs rarely. Calcium deposits occur in the cornea or conjunctiva (band keratopathy) and are detected by slitlamp examination. Intractable peptic ulcer and pancreatitis occur in adults but rarely in children.

2. Due to increased calcium and phosphate excretion—Loss of renal concentrating ability causes polyuria, polydipsia, and calcium phosphate deposition in renal parenchyma or as urinary calculi with progressive renal damage.

3. Due to changes in the skeleton—Initial findings include bone pain, osteitis fibrosa cystica, subperiosteal bone absorption in the distal clavicles and phalanges, absence of lamina dura around the teeth, spontaneous fractures, and moth-eaten appearance of the skull on radiographs. Later, there is generalized demineralization with high risk of subperiosteal cortical bone.

B. Imaging

Bone changes may be subtle in children. Technetium sestamibi scintigraphy is preferred over conventional procedures (ultrasound, computed tomography [CT], and MRI) for localizing parathyroid tumors.

Treatment

A. Symptomatic

Initial management is vigorous hydration with normal saline and forced calcium diuresis with a loop diuretic such as furosemide (1 mg/kg given every 6 hours). If response is inadequate, glucocorticoids or calcitonin may be used. Bisphosphonates, standard agents for the management of acute hypercalcemia in adults, are being used more often in refractory pediatric hypercalcemia.

B. Chronic

Treatment options vary with the underlying cause. Resection of parathyroid adenoma or subtotal removal of hyperplastic parathyroid glands is the preferred treatment. Postoperatively, hypocalcemia due to the rapid remineralization of chronically calcium-deprived bones may occur. A diet high in calcium and vitamin D is recommended immediately postoperatively and is continued until serum calcium concentrations are normal and stable. Treatment of secondary hyperparathyroidism from chronic renal disease is primarily directed at controlling serum phosphorus levels with phosphate binders. Pharmacologic doses of calcitriol are used to suppress PTH secretion. Long-term therapy for hypercalcemia of malignancy is the treatment of the underlying disorder.

Course & Prognosis

The prognosis after resection of a single adenoma is excellent. The prognosis following subtotal parathyroidectomy for diffuse hyperplasia or removal of multiple adenomas is usually good and depends on correction of the underlying defect. In patients with multiple sites of parathyroid adenoma or hyperplasia, MEN is likely, and other family members may be at risk. Genetic counseling and DNA analysis to determine the specific gene defect are indicated.

FAMILIAL HYPOCALCIURIC HYPERCALCEMIA (FAMILIAL BENIGN HYPERCALCEMIA)

Familial hypocalciuric hypercalcemia is distinguished by low to normal urinary calcium excretion as a result of high renal reabsorption of calcium. PTH is normal or slightly elevated. In most cases, the genetic defect is a mutation in the membrane-bound calcium-sensing receptor expressed on parathyroid and renal tubule cells. It is inherited as an autosomal dominant trait with high penetrance. There is a low rate of new mutations. Most patients are asymptomatic, and treatment is unnecessary. A severe form of symptomatic neonatal hyperparathyroidism may occur in infants homozygous for the receptor mutation.

HYPERVITAMINOSIS D

Vitamin D intoxication is almost always the result of ingestion of excessive amounts of vitamin D. Signs, symptoms, and treatment of vitamin D–induced hypercalcemia are the same as those in other hypercalcemic conditions. Treatment depends on the stage of hypercalcemia. Severe hypercalcemia requires hospitalization and aggressive intervention. Due to the storage of vitamin D in the adipose tissue, several months of a low-calcium, low–vitamin D diet may be required.

IDIOPATHIC HYPERCALCEMIA OF INFANCY (WILLIAMS SYNDROME)

Williams syndrome is an uncommon disorder of infancy characterized by elfin-appearing facies and hypercalcemia in infancy. Other features include failure to thrive, mental and motor retardation, cardiovascular abnormalities (primarily supravalvular aortic stenosis), irritability, purposeless movements, constipation, hypotonia, polyuria, polydipsia, and hypertension. A gregarious and affectionate personality is the rule in children with the syndrome. Hypercalcemia may not appear until several months after birth. Treatment consists of restriction of dietary calcium and vitamin D (Calcilo formula) and, in severe cases, moderate doses of glucocorticoids or even bisphosphonates.

A defect in the metabolism of, or responsiveness to, vitamin D is postulated as the cause of Williams syndrome. Elastin deletions localized to chromosome 7 have been identified in more than 90% of patients. Fluorescent in situ hybridization analysis (FISH) may be the best initial diagnostic tool. The risk of hypercalcemia generally resolves by age 4 and dietary restrictions can be relaxed.

Cagle AP, Waguespack SG, Buckingham BA, Shankar RR, Dimeglio LA: Severe infantile hypercalcemia associated with Williams syndrome successfully treated with intravenously administered pamidronate. Pediatrics 2004 Oct;114(4):1091–1095 [PMID: 15466114].

IMMOBILIZATION HYPERCALCEMIA

Abrupt immobilization, particularly in a rapidly growing adolescent, may cause hypercalcemia and hypercalciuria. Abnormalities often appear 1–3 weeks after immobilization. Medical or dietary intervention may be required in severe cases.

HYPOPHOSPHATASIA

Hypophosphatasia is a rare autosomal recessive condition characterized by deficiency of alkaline phosphatase activity in serum, bone, and tissues. Enzyme deficiency leads to poor skeletal mineralization with clinical and radiographic features similar to rickets. Six different clinical forms are identified. The perinatal form is characterized by severe skeletal deformity and death within a few days of birth. The infantile form includes failure to thrive, hypotonia, and craniosynostosis. The childhood form manifests with variable skeletal findings, reduced bone mineral density, and premature loss of deciduous teeth. Serum calcium levels may be elevated. The diagnosis of hypophosphatasia is made by demonstrating elevated urinary phosphoethanolamine associated with low serum alkaline phosphatase. Therapy is generally supportive. Children who survive the neonatal period may experience gradual improvement. Calcitonin may be of value for the acute treatment of hypercalcemia.

Bringhurst RF, Demay MB, Krane SM, Kronenberg HM: Bone and Mineral Metabolism in Health and Disease. Khosla Sandeep: Approach to Hypercalcemia and Hypocalcemia. Potts JT Jr: Diseases of the Parathyroid Gland: In Lameson JL (editor): *Harrison's Endocrinology*. 2nd ed. McGraw-Hill, 2010.

Diaz R: Calcium disorders in children and adolescents. In Lifshitz F (editor): *Pediatric Endocrinology*, 5th ed. Informa Healthcare 2007:475.

Lietman SA, Germain-Lee EL, Levine MA: Hypercalcemia in children and adolescents. Curr Opin Pediatr 2010 Aug;22(4):508–515 [Review] [PMID: 20601885].

Varghese J, Rich T, Jimenez C: Benign familial hypocalciuric hypercalcemia. Endocr Pract 2011 Mar–Apr;17(Suppl 1):13–17 [Review] [PMID: 21478088].

GONADS (OVARIES & TESTES)

DEVELOPMENT & PHYSIOLOGY

The fetal gonads develop from bipotential anlagen in the genital ridge. In infants with a Y chromosome, the transcription factor SRY located on the short arm of the Y at location YP11.3 directs the formation of testes from the bipotential gonads. Without expression of SRY, ovaries develop; however, a 46,XX complement of chromosomes is necessary for the development of normal ovaries. WT1 and many other transcription factors, including but not limited to SF1, DAX1, WNT4, and SOX9, are also important in gonadal differentiation. Two pairs of internal reproductive structures, the müllerian and wolffian ducts, develop in both sexes (Figure 34–6). Once testicular differentiation has

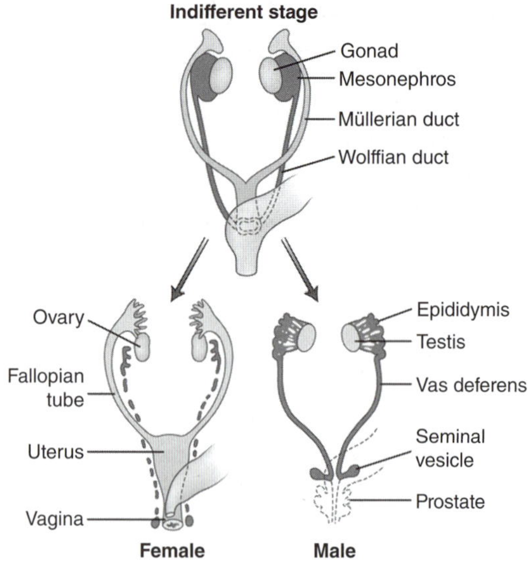

▲ **Figure 34–6.** Differentiation of internal reproductive ducts. (Reprinted, with permission from Kronenberg H [editor]: *Williams Textbook of Endocrinology*, 11th ed. Saunders Elsevier, 2008.)

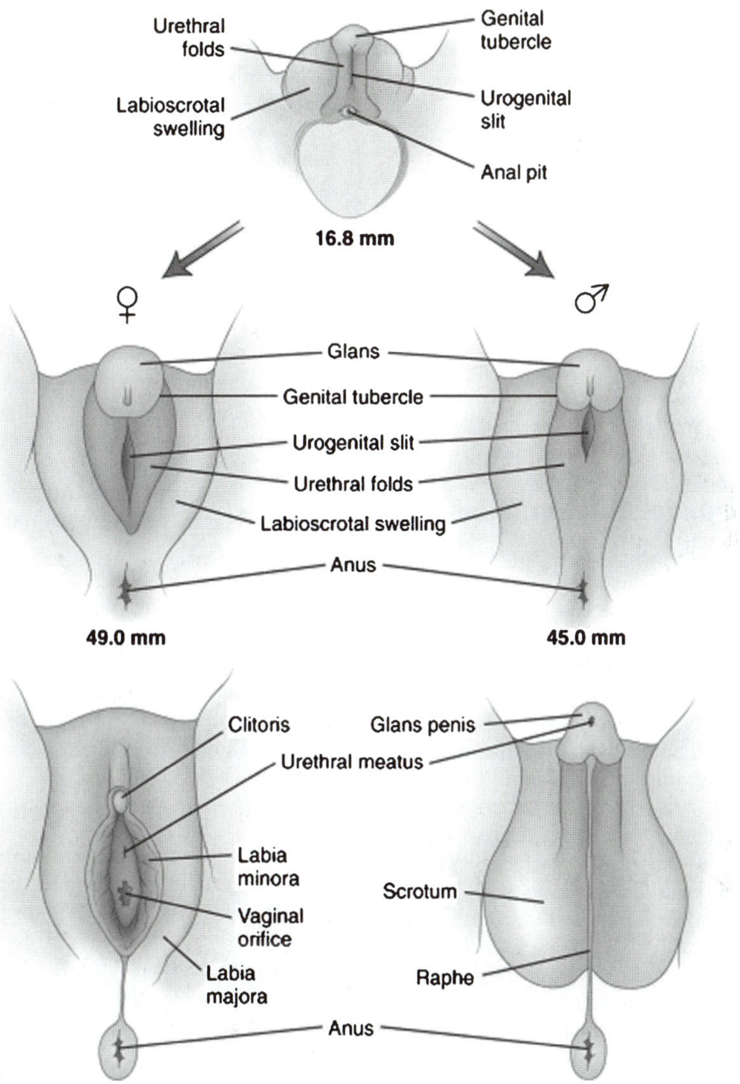

▲ **Figure 34–7.** Differentiation of external genitalia ducts. (Adapted from Spaulding MH: The development of the external genitalia in the human embryo. Contrib Embryol 1921;13:69–88)

been determined, the fetal testes produce two substances critical for male differentiation of these ducts. Antimüllerian hormone (AMH) promotes the regression of müllerian structures, and high local concentrations of testosterone from the Leydig cells of the testes stimulate growth of the wolffian structures. These structures become the epididymis, vas deferens, and seminal vesicle. In the absence of testes, as in a XX fetus, the lack of AMH production permits the müllerian structures to develop into the paired fallopian tubes, the midline uterus, and the upper portion of the vagina. The wolffian structures, without exposure to high local concentrations of testosterone, regress.

The external genitalia (Figure 34–7) develop from sexually indifferent structures called the genital tubercle (precursor of the penis or clitoris), the labioscrotal swellings (precursors of the scrotum or labia majora), and the urethral folds (precursors of the penile urethra or labia minora). Normal development of male external genitalia depends on an adequate circulating concentration of testosterone, which is converted to dihydrotestosterone (DHT) in the target tissues by the enzyme 5α-reductase. Sexual differentiation of the external genitalia is completed at about 12 weeks' gestation. Excessive androgen exposure of a female infant prior to 12 weeks' gestation will lead to variable degrees of masculinization of the external genitalia including posterior labial fusion and formation of penile urethra. Exposure after 12 weeks will only result in clitoromegaly.

DISORDERS OF SEXUAL DEVELOPMENT

Disorders of Sexual Development (DSD) is now the preferred terminology replacing terms such as "intersex" and "pseudohermaphrodite," as these contain pejorative elements. DSD result from incomplete or disordered genital or gonadal development that cause a discordance between genetic sex, gonadal sex, and phenotypic sex. When an infant is born with genital ambiguity, immediate consultation with pediatric endocrinology, urology, and, if possible, psychiatry/psychology and genetics is required. Disorders of sexual development stem from alterations in three main processes: gonadal differentiation, steroidogenesis, or androgen action.

1. Disorders of Gonadal Differentiation

These abnormalities include XY gonadal dysgenesis, mosaicism involving the Y chromosome, XX sex reversal, and true hermaphroditism. Gonadal dysgenesis occurs as a result of abnormal gonadal development. Individuals with complete 46,XY gonadal dysgenesis have streak gonads and normal female external genitalia. As streak gonads do not produce AMH or testosterone, internal reproductive structures are also female. Affected individuals typically present as girls with delayed puberty and amenorrhea. Partial XY gonadal dysgenesis is associated with incomplete testis determination resulting in a phenotype of varying degrees of virilization. Mutations in the transcription factors SRY, WT1, SF1, and SOX9 have all been implicated in 46,XY gonadal dysgenesis. It is important to recognize that some of these mutations are associated with abnormalities separate from sexual development. For example, WT1 mutations are associated with increased risk of Wilms tumor and nephropathy.

Mosaicism occurs when cells with two or more karyotypes are found in the same individual. The most common form of mosaicism is 45,X/46,XY. The majority of these individuals have normal male external genitalia but some may have ambiguity due to abnormal testicular formation. These individuals may also share some features of Turner syndrome such as short stature. XX sex reversal, characterized by masculine or ambiguous genital development in an XX individual, can be caused by translocation of the *SRY* gene to the X chromosome. A true hermaphrodite is defined as having both ovarian and testicular tissue and most often has a karyotype of 46,XX. Dysgenetic gonads have an increased risk for neoplastic transformation; therefore, if gonads are intra-abdominally located, gonadectomy is recommended.

2. Disorders of Steroidogenesis (Figure 34–8)

Testosterone biosynthesis in the testicular leydig cells depends on the function of multiple enzymes which are responsible for conversion of intermediary metabolites. Enzymatic defects in this pathway result in decreased or absent testosterone synthesis and in affected XY individuals, there will be reduced or lack of virilization of the external genitalia. Wolffian duct derivatives can be absent, hypoplastic, or normal depending on the degree of the enzyme inactivity. Sertoli cell production of AMH is preserved so müllerian development is also inhibited. Disorders in this category include StAR deficiency, 3β-hydroxysteroid dehydrogenase deficiency, P-450 C_{17} hydroxylase deficiency, and 17β-hydroxysteroid dehydrogenase deficiency. Additionally, defects in conversion of testosterone to dihydrotestosterone (DHT) from 5α-reductase deficiency also results in undervirilization. In this disorder, if the enzyme defect is incomplete, the external genitalia may masculinize at puberty when testosterone production increases. Since the gonads and adrenal gland share common enzymes of steroid hormone production, some of the enzymatic defects associated with male undervirilization may also affect production of cortisol and aldosterone, leading to cortisol deficiency and salt wasting (see later section on the Adrenal Cortex).

In an XX individual, the most common disorder in this category is congenital adrenal hyperplasia (CAH) secondary to 21-hydroxylase deficiency. In the classic salt-losing form of this disorder, infant girls present with genital ambiguity but have normal uterus and ovaries. A less common form of CAH is 3β-hydroxysteroid dehydrogenase deficiency and presents similarly.

3. Disorders of Androgen Action

Androgen Insensitivity Syndrome (AIS) is caused by a mutation in the androgen receptor gene located on the proximal, long arm of the X chromosome at Xq11–12. In complete androgen insensitivity syndrome (CAIS), there is no androgen action; thus, 46,XY affected individuals have female external genitalia with a short, blind-ending vagina. The production of AMH in these individuals leads to müllerian regression and the absence of testosterone action leads to absent or rudimentary wolffian structures. Gonads are located either intra-abdominally or in the inguinal canal. Some of these individuals present when surgery for an inguinal hernia reveals testis in the hernia sack. With partial androgen insensitivity syndrome (PAIS), the degree of virilization and ambiguity depends on the degree of abnormality in androgen binding.

4. Miscellaneous Syndromes

Syndromes such as VATER (vertebral defects, anal atresia, tracheoesophageal fistula with esophageal atresia, and radial and renal anomalies), WAGR (Wilms tumor, aniridia, genitourinary malformations, and mental retardation), and Smith-Lemli-Opitz produce a wide variety of congenital anomalies, including disordered sexual development. Maternal exposure to androgens or androgen antagonists is a rare cause of DSD in newborns.

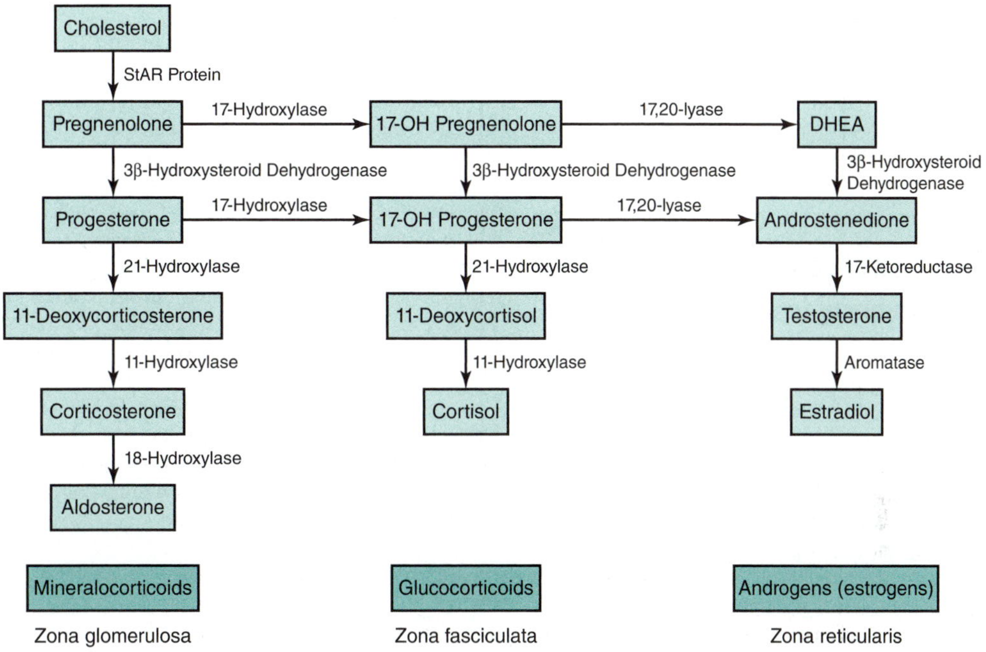

▲ **Figure 34–8.** The corticosteroid hormone synthetic pathway. The pathways illustrated are present in differing amounts in the steroid-producing tissues: adrenal glands, ovaries, and testes. In the adrenal glands, mineralocorticoids from the zona glomerulosa, glucocorticoids from the zona fasciculata, and androgens (and estrogens) from the zona reticularis are produced. The major adrenal androgen is androstenedione, because the activity of 17-ketoreductase is relatively low. The adrenal gland does secrete some testosterone and estrogen, however. The pathways leading to the synthesis of mineralocorticoids and glucocorticoids are not present to any significant degree in the gonads; however, the testes and ovaries each produce both androgens and estrogens. Further metabolism of testosterone to dihydrotestosterone occurs in target tissues of the action of the enzyme 5α-reductase. DHEA, dehydroepiandrosterone.

5. Evaluation

A complete family and maternal history should be completed focusing on previous affected offspring, neonatal deaths, history of consanguinity, and maternal exposure to any drugs or hormones. On physical examination, dysmorphic features, other congenital anomalies, and hyperpigmentation of nipples and labia/scrotum should be noted. The genital examination should include measuring the width and length of the stretched phallus and noting the position of the urethral meatus. The normal stretched penile length (SPL) is greater than 2.5 cm (and diameter greater than 0.9 cm) in term infants, greater that 2 cm in 34-week infants, greater than 1.5 cm in 30-week infants, and greater than 0.8 cm in 25-week infants. The labioscrotal and inguinal regions should be palpated for presence of gonads. The labioscrotal area should also be evaluated for the degree of fusion and rugation.

In all infants, karyotype and FISH studies for SRY should be done initially. Additional laboratory evaluation is usually based on these results. A pelvic ultrasound can be helpful to evaluate for the presence of a uterus and gonads; however, ultrasound findings can be unreliable so should be done in an institution which has expertise in pediatric imaging. Sometimes, laparoscopic examination is necessary to delineate internal structures. If a virilized female is suspected, studies to evaluate for 21-hydroxylase deficiency, the most common form of congenital adrenal hyperplasia, should be sent.

It is important that gender assignment be avoided until expert evaluation by a multidisciplinary team is performed. The team should develop a plan for diagnosis, gender assignment, and treatment options before making any recommendations. Open communications with the parents is essential and their participation in decision making encouraged.

Houk CP, Lee PA: Intersexed states: Diagnosis and management. Endocrinol Metab Clin North Am 2005;34:791 [PMID: 16085171].

Houk CP, Hughes IA, Ahmed SF, Lee PA: Writing Committee for the International Intersex Consensus Conference Participants. Summary of consensus statement on intersex disorders and their management. Pediatrics 2006;118(2):753–757 [PMID: 16882833].

Lambert SM, Vilain EJ, Kolon TF: A practical approach to ambiguous genitalia in the newborn period. Urol Clin N Am 2010;37(2):195–205 [PMID: 20569798].

Oakes MB, Eyvazzadeh AD, Quint E, Smith YR: Complete androgen insensitivity syndrome—A review. J Pediatr Adolesc Gynecol 2008;21(6):305–310 [PMID: 19064222].

ABNORMALITIES IN FEMALE PUBERTAL DEVELOPMENT & OVARIAN FUNCTION

1. Precocious Puberty in Girls

Precocious puberty is defined as pubertal development occurring below the age limit set for normal onset of puberty. Puberty is considered precocious in girls if the onset of secondary sexual characteristics occurs before age 8 years in Caucasian girls and 7 years for African-American and Hispanic girls. Precocious puberty is more common in girls than in boys. This disparity is explained by the large number of girls with central idiopathic precocity, a rare condition in boys. Girls showing signs of puberty between 6 and 8 years of age often have a benign, slowly progressing form that requires no intervention. The age of pubertal onset may be advanced by obesity.

Central (gonadotropin-releasing hormone [GnRH]–dependent) precocious puberty involves activation of the hypothalamic GnRH pulse generator, an increase in gonadotropin secretion, and a resultant increase in production of sex steroids (Table 34–8). The sequence of hormonal and physical events in central precocious puberty is identical to that of normal puberty. Central precocious puberty in girls is generally idiopathic but may be secondary to a central nervous system (CNS) abnormality that disrupts the prepubertal restraint on the GnRH pulse generator. Such CNS abnormalities include, but are not limited to, hypothalamic hamartomas, CNS tumors, cranial irradiation, hydrocephalus, and trauma. Peripheral precocious puberty (GnRH-independent) occurs independent of gonadotropin secretion. In girls, peripheral precocious puberty can be caused by ovarian or adrenal tumors, ovarian cysts, congenital adrenal hyperplasia, McCune-Albright syndrome, or exposure to exogenous estrogen. Estrogen-secreting ovarian or adrenal tumors are rare. Girls with these tumors typically present with markedly elevated estrogen levels and rapidly progressive pubertal changes. McCune-Albright syndrome is a triad of irregular café au lait lesions, polyostotic fibrous dysplasia, and GnRH-independent precocious puberty. It is caused by an activating mutation in the gene encoding the α-subunit of Gs, the G protein that stimulates adenyl cyclase. Endocrine cells with this mutation have autonomous hyperfunction and secrete excess amounts of their respective hormones.

Table 34–8. Causes of precocious pubertal development.

A. Central (GnRH-dependent) precocious puberty
1. Idiopathic
2. Central nervous system abnormalities
a. Acquired—abscess, chemotherapy, radiation, surgical trauma
b. Congenital—arachnoid cyst, hydrocephalus, hypothalamic hamartoma, septo-optic dysplasia, suprasellar cyst
c. Tumors—astrocytoma, craniopharyngioma, glioma
B. Peripheral (GnRH-independent) precocious puberty
1. Congenital adrenal hyperplasia
2. Adrenal tumors
3. McCune-Albright syndrome
4. Familial male-limited gonadotropin independent precocious puberty
5. Gonadal tumors
6. Exogenous estrogen—oral (contraceptive pills) or topical
7. Ovarian cysts (females)
8. HCG-secreting tumors (eg, hepatoblastomas, choriocarcinomas) (males)

GnRH, gonadotropin-releasing hormone; HCG, human chorionic gonadotropin.

Clinical Findings

A. Symptoms and Signs

Female central precocious puberty usually starts with breast development, followed by pubic hair growth and menarche. However, the order may vary. Girls with ovarian cysts or tumors generally have signs of estrogen excess such as breast development and possibly vaginal bleeding. Adrenal tumors or CAH produce signs of adrenarche (ie, pubic hair, axillary hair, acne, and sometimes, increased body odor). Children with precocious puberty usually have accelerated growth and skeletal maturation, and may temporarily be tall for age. However, because skeletal maturation advances at a more rapid rate than linear growth, final adult stature may be compromised.

B. Laboratory Findings

One of the first steps in evaluating a child with early pubertal development is obtaining a radiograph of the left hand and wrist to determine skeletal maturity (bone age). An estradiol level can also be drawn to rule out an ovarian tumor or cyst. If the bone age is advanced, further evaluation is warranted. In central precocious puberty, the basal serum concentrations of FSH and LH may still be in the prepubertal range. Thus, documentation of the maturity of the hypothalamic-pituitary axis depends on demonstrating a pubertal LH response after stimulation with a GnRH agonist. In peripheral precocious puberty, basal serum FSH and LH are low, and the LH response to GnRH stimulation is suppressed by feedback inhibition of the hypothalamic-pituitary axis by the autonomously secreted gonadal steroids (see Figure 34–1). In girls with an ovarian cyst or tumor, estradiol levels will be markedly elevated. In girls with signs of adrenarche and an advanced bone age, androgen levels (testosterone, androstenedione, dehydroepiandrosterone-sulfate) and possibly adrenal intermediate metabolites (such as 17-hydroxyprogesterone) should be measured.

C. Imaging

When a diagnosis of central precocious puberty is made, a MRI of the brain should be done to evaluate for CNS lesions. It is unlikely that an abnormality will be found in girls 6–8 years of age, so the need for an MRI in this age group should be individually assessed. In girls whose laboratory tests suggest peripheral precocious puberty, an ultrasound of the ovaries and adrenal gland is indicated.

Treatment

Girls with central precocious puberty can be treated with GnRH analogues that downregulate pituitary GnRH receptors and thus decrease gonadotropin secretion. Currently, the two most common GnRH analogues used are (1) leuprolide, which is given as a monthly intramuscular injection or (2) histrelin subdermal implant, which is replaced annually. With treatment, physical changes of puberty regress or cease to progress and linear growth slows to a prepubertal rate. Projected final heights often increase as a result of slowing of skeletal maturation. After stopping therapy, pubertal progression resumes, and ovulation and pregnancy have been documented. Therapy is instituted for both psychosocial and final height considerations.

Treatment of peripheral precocious puberty is dependent on the underlying cause. In a girl with an ovarian cyst, intervention is generally not necessary, as the cyst usually regresses spontaneously. Serial ultrasounds are recommended to document this regression. Treatment with glucocorticoids is indicated for congenital adrenal hyperplasia. Surgical resection is indicated for the rare adrenal or ovarian tumor.

In McCune-Albright syndrome, therapy with antiestrogens (eg, tamoxifen), agents that block estrogen synthesis (ketoconazole), or aromatase inhibitors (eg, letrozole) may be effective. Regardless of the cause of precocious puberty or the medical therapy selected, attention to the psychological needs of the patient and family is essential.

2. Benign Variants of Precocious Puberty

Benign premature thelarche (benign early breast development) occurs most commonly in girls younger than 2 years of age. Girls present with isolated breast development without other signs of puberty such as linear growth acceleration and pubic hair development. The breast development is typically present since birth and often waxes and wanes in size. It may be unilateral or bilateral. Benign thelarche is thought to be caused by greater ovarian hormone production during infancy. Treatment is parental reassurance regarding the self-limited nature of the condition. Observation of the child every few months is also indicated. Onset of thelarche after age 36 months or in association with other signs of puberty requires evaluation.

Benign premature adrenarche (benign early adrenal maturation) is manifested by early development of pubic hair, axillary hair, acne, and/or body odor. Benign premature adrenarche is characterized by normal linear growth and no or minimal bone age advancement. The timing of true puberty is not affected, and no treatment is required. Approximately 15% of girls with premature adrenarche are at risk for developing polycystic ovarian syndrome during puberty.

Carel JC et al: Consensus statement on the use of gonadotropin-releasing hormone analogs in children. Pediatrics 2009;123(4):e752–762 [PMID: 19332438].

Nathan BM, Palmert MR: Regulation and disorders of pubertal timing. Endocrinol Metab Clin North Am 2005;34:617 [PMID: 16085163].

Pasquino AM et al: Long-term observation of 87 girls with idiopathic central precocious puberty treated with gonadotropin-releasing hormone analogs: Impact on adult height, body mass index, bone mineral content, and reproductive function. J Clin Endocrinol Metab 2008;93:190 [PMID: 7940112].

3. Delayed Puberty

Delayed puberty in girls should be evaluated if there are no pubertal signs by age 13 years or menarche by 16 years. Failure to complete pubertal development to Tanner stage V within 4 years of onset is also considered delay. Primary amenorrhea refers to the absence of menarche, and secondary amenorrhea refers to the absence of menses for at least 6 months after regular menses have been established. The most common cause of delayed puberty is constitutional growth delay (Table 34–9). This growth pattern, characterized by short stature, normal growth velocity, and a delay in skeletal maturation, is described in detail earlier in this chapter. The timing of puberty is commensurate to the bone

Table 34–9. Cause of delayed puberty or amenorrhea.

A. Constitutional growth delay
B. Hypogonadism
1. Primary ovarian insufficiency
    a. Gonadal dysgenesis (Turner syndrome, true gonadal dysgenesis)
    b. Premature ovarian failure
        (1) Autoimmune disease
        (2) Surgery, radiation, chemotherapy
    c. Galactosemia
2. Central hypogonadism
    a. Hypothalamic or pituitary tumor, infection, irradiation
    b. Congenital hypopituitarism
    c. Kallmann syndrome
    d. Functional (chronic illness, undernutrition, exercise, hyperprolactinemia
C. Anatomic
1. Müllerian agenesis (Mayer-Rokitansky-Küster-Hauser syndrome)
2. Complete androgen resistance

age, not the chronologic age. Girls may also have delayed puberty from any condition that delays growth and skeletal maturation, such as hypothyroidism and GHD.

Primary hypogonadism in girls refers to a primary abnormality of the ovaries. The most common diagnosis in this category is Turner syndrome, in which the lack of or an abnormal second X chromosome leads to early loss of oocytes and accelerated stromal fibrosis. Other types of primary ovarian insufficiency are less common, including 46,XY gonadal dysgenesis, 46,XX gonadal dysgenesis, galactosemia, and autoimmune ovarian failure. Radiation and chemotherapy can also cause primary ovarian insufficiency. Girls who are premutation carriers for fragile X syndrome are also at increased risk of premature ovarian failure.

Central hypogonadism refers to a hypothalamic or pituitary deficiency of GnRH or FSH/LH, respectively. Central hypogonadism can be functional (reversible), caused by stress, undernutrition, prolactinemia, excessive exercise, or chronic illness. Permanent central hypogonadism is typically associated with conditions that cause multiple pituitary hormone deficiencies, such as congenital hypopituitarism, CNS tumors, or cranial irradiation. Isolated gonadotropin deficiency is rare but may occur in Kallmann syndrome, which is also characterized by hyposmia or anosmia. In either primary or central hypogonadism, signs of adrenarche are generally present.

Delayed menarche or secondary amenorrhea may result from primary ovarian failure or central hypogonadism, or may be the consequence of hyperandrogenism, anatomic obstruction precluding menstrual outflow, or müllerian agenesis. This latter disorder is called Mayer-Rokitansky-Küster-Hauser syndrome and is characterized by an absent vagina and various uterine abnormalities, with or without renal and skeletal anomalies.

Girls with complete AIS (androgen receptor defect) typically present with primary amenorrhea, breast development, and absence of sexual hair. The affected individual (46,XY) has functioning testes that produce antimüllerian hormone during fetal life. Thus, no müllerian duct (oviduct or uterus) development occurs. External genitalia are female because of the lack of androgen action. At puberty, if the gonads have not been removed, testosterone produced in the testes is aromatized to estrogen resulting in breast development.

Clinical Evaluation

The history should ascertain whether and when puberty commenced, level of exercise, nutritional intake, stressors, sense of smell, symptoms of chronic illness, and family history of delayed puberty. Past growth records should be assessed to determine if height and weight velocity have been appropriate. Physical examination includes body proportions, breast and genital development, and stigmata of Turner syndrome. Pelvic examination or pelvic ultrasonography should be considered, especially in girls with primary amenorrhea.

A bone age radiograph should be obtained first. If the bone age is lower than that consistent with pubertal onset (< 12 years in girls), evaluations should focus on finding the cause of the bone age delay. If short stature and normal growth velocity are present, constitutional growth delay is likely. If growth rate is abnormal, laboratory studies may include a complete blood count, erythrocyte sedimentation rate, chemistry panel, and renal and liver function tests to look for unsuspected chronic medical illness. Evaluation for hypothyroidism and GHD may also be indicated. Measurement of FSH and LH may not be helpful in the setting of delayed bone age since prepubertal levels are normally low. Determination of a karyotype should be considered if there is short stature, or any stigmata of Turner syndrome.

If the patient has attained a bone age of more than 12 years and there are minimal or no signs of puberty on physical examination, FSH and LH levels will distinguish between primary ovarian failure and central hypogonadism. Primary ovarian failure is also called hypergonadotropic hypogonadism, as there is lack of estrogen feedback to the brain with elevated FSH and LH. If gonadotropins are elevated, a karyotype is the next step, as Turner syndrome is the most common cause of female hypergonadotropic hypogonadism. Central hypogonadism is characterized by low gonadotropin levels, and evaluation is geared toward determining if the hypogonadism is functional or permanent. Laboratory tests should be directed toward identifying chronic disease and hyperprolactinemia. Cranial MRI may be helpful.

In girls with adequate breast development and amenorrhea, a progesterone challenge may be helpful to determine if sufficient estrogen is being produced. Girls who are producing estrogen have a withdrawal bleed after 5–10 days of oral progesterone, whereas those who are estrogen-deficient have little or no bleeding. The exception is girls with an absent uterus (androgen insensitivity or Mayer-Rokitansky-Küster-Hauser syndrome). They have sufficient estrogen but cannot have withdrawal bleeding. The most common cause of amenorrhea in girls with sufficient estrogen is polycystic ovarian syndrome. Girls who are estrogen-deficient should be evaluated similarly to those who have delayed puberty.

Treatment

Replacement therapy in hypogonadal girls begins with estrogen alone at the lowest available dosage. Oral preparations such as estradiol or topical patches are used. Cyclic estrogen–progesterone therapy is started 12–18 months later, and eventually the patient may be switched over to a birth control pill for convenience. Progesterone therapy is needed to counteract the effects of estrogen on the uterus, as unopposed estrogen promotes endometrial hyperplasia. Estrogen is also necessary to promote bone mineralization and prevent osteoporosis.

Bondy CA: Care of girls and women with Turner syndrome: A guideline of the Turner Syndrome Study Group. J Clin Endocrinol Metab 2007;92:10 [PMID: 17047017].

Nelson LM: Clinical practice: Primary ovarian insufficiency. N Engl J Med 2009;360:606 [PMID: 19196677].

4. Secondary Amenorrhea

See discussion of amenorrhea in Chapter 4.

ABNORMALITIES IN MALE PUBERTAL DEVELOPMENT & TESTICULAR FUNCTION

1. Precocious Puberty in Boys

Puberty is considered precocious in boys if secondary sexual characteristics appear before age 9 years. While the frequency of central precocious puberty is much lower in boys than girls, boys are more likely to have an associated CNS abnormality (see Table 34–8).

Several types of gonadotropin-independent (peripheral) precocious puberty occur in boys (see Table 34–8). Increased adrenal androgen production from an adrenal tumor or from a virilizing form of CAH will cause pubertal changes in boys. Familial male-limited gonadotropin-independent puberty (familial testotoxicosis) is a condition in which a mutated LH receptor on the Leydig cell is autonomously activated, resulting in testicular production of testosterone despite prepubertal LH levels. McCune-Albright syndrome can also occur in boys. Leydig cell tumors of the testis cause rapid onset of unilateral testicular enlargement and physical signs of testosterone excess. Human chorionic gonadotropin (HCG)–secreting tumors such as teratomas, CNS germinomas, and hepatoblastomas also cause early puberty in boys, as HCG stimulates testosterone production from Leydig cells.

Clinical Findings

A. Symptoms and Signs

In precocious development, increased linear growth rate and growth of pubic hair are the most common presenting signs. Testicular size may differentiate central precocity, in which the testes enlarge, from gonadotropin-independent causes such as CAH, in which the testes usually remain small (< 2 cm in the longitudinal axis). However, in familial testotoxicosis and HCG mediated precocious puberty, there is some testicular enlargement but not to the degree as seen in central precocity. Tumors of the testis are associated with either asymmetrical or unilateral testicular enlargement.

B. Laboratory Findings

Elevated testosterone levels verify early pubertal status but do not differentiate the source. As in girls, basal serum LH and FSH concentrations may not be in the pubertal range in boys with central precocious puberty, but the LH response to GnRH stimulation testing is pubertal. Sexual precocity caused by CAH is usually associated with abnormal plasma dehydroepiandrosterone, androstenedione, 17-hydroxyprogesterone (in CAH due to 21-hydroxylase deficiency), 11-deoxycortisol (in CAH due to 11-hydroxylase deficiency), or a combination of these steroids (see later section on the Adrenal Cortex). Serum β-HCG concentrations can signify the presence of an HCG-producing tumor (eg, CNS dysgerminoma or hepatoma) in boys who present with precocious puberty and testicular enlargement but suppressed gonadotropins following GnRH testing.

C. Imaging

In all boys with central precocious puberty, cranial MRI should be obtained to evaluate for a CNS abnormality. If testing suggests peripheral precocious puberty, and laboratory studies are not consistent with CAH, ultrasonography may be useful in detecting hepatic, adrenal, and testicular tumors.

Treatment

Treatment of central precocious puberty in boys is with GnRH analogues, similar to treatment in girls. Boys with McCune-Albright syndrome or familial testotoxicosis can be treated with agents that block steroid synthesis (ketoconazole), or with a combination of antiandrogens (spironolactone) and aromatase inhibitors (anastrazole or letrozole) which block the conversion of testosterone to estrogen.

2. Delayed Puberty

Boys should be evaluated for delayed puberty if they have no secondary sexual characteristics by 14 years of age or if more than 5 years have elapsed since the first signs of puberty without completion of genital growth.

The most common cause of delayed puberty in boys, as in girls, is constitutional growth delay, a normal variant of growth that is described in detail earlier in this chapter. Hypogonadism in boys may be primary, due to absence, malfunction, or destruction of testicular tissue, or central, due to pituitary or hypothalamic insufficiency. Primary testicular insufficiency may be due to anorchia, Klinefelter syndrome (47,XXY), or other sex chromosome abnormalities, enzymatic defects in testosterone synthesis, or inflammation or destruction of the testes following infection (mumps), autoimmune disorders, radiation, trauma, or tumor.

Central hypogonadism may accompany panhypopituitarism, Kallmann syndrome (GnRH deficiency with anosmia), or isolated LH or FSH deficiencies. Destructive lesions in or near the anterior pituitary (especially craniopharyngioma and glioma) or infection may also result in hypothalamic or pituitary dysfunction. Prader-Willi syndrome and Laurence-Moon syndrome (Bardet-Biedl syndrome) are frequently associated with LH and FSH deficiency in boys and girls secondary to GnRH deficiency. Deficiencies in gonadotropins may be partial or complete. Functional or reversible gonadotropin may occur with chronic illness, malnutrition, hyperprolactinemia, hypothyroidism, or excessive exercise.

Clinical Evaluation

The history should focus on whether and when puberty has started, testicular descent, symptoms of chronic illness, nutritional intake, sense of smell, and family history of delayed puberty. Physical examination should include body proportions, height and weight, pubertal stage, and testicular location, size, and consistency. Testes less than 2 cm in length are prepubertal; testes more than 2.5 cm in length suggest early pubertal growth.

A radiograph of the left hand and wrist to assess bone age should be the first step in evaluating a boy with delayed puberty. If bone age is delayed (< 12 years) and growth velocity is normal, constitutional growth delay is the most likely diagnosis.

Laboratory evaluation includes LH and FSH levels (especially if bone age is > 12 years). Elevated gonadotropin levels indicate primary hypogonadism or testicular failure. The most common cause of primary hypogonadism in boys is Klinefelter syndrome; however, the usual presentation of this disorder is not delayed puberty but failure to complete puberty with a discrepancy noted between testicular size (small) and degree of virilization. If gonadotropin values are low, the working diagnosis is central hypogonadism and further evaluation should focus on looking for pituitary hormone deficiencies, chronic disease or undernutrition (or both), hyperprolactinemia, and CNS abnormalities.

Treatment

Boys with simple constitutional delay may be offered a short (4–6 months) course of low-dose depot testosterone (50–75 mg/mo) to stimulate their pubertal appearance and "jump-start" their endogenous development. In adolescents with permanent hypogonadism, treatment with depot testosterone, beginning with 50–75 mg intramuscularly each month, may be used until growth is complete. Thereafter, adult dosing (150–200 mg every 2–3 weeks) may be used. An alternative to intramuscular injections is testosterone gel, either in single-dose packets or in a pump set to dispense a preset dose. Gel is applied daily after showering. Specific therapy for GnRH deficiency with pulsatile subcutaneous GnRH may promote fertility in patients with hypothalamic-pituitary insufficiency. However, the inconvenience of treatment and the need for repeated doses for long periods of time have limited its application in pediatrics.

3. Cryptorchidism

Cryptorchidism (undescended testis) is very common, affecting 2%–4% of full-term male newborns and up to 30% of premature infants. Short-term postnatal endogenous testosterone secretion decreases the incidence of cryptorchidism to 1% by 3 months of age. After six months of age, spontaneous descent occurs only very rarely. Consequently, intervention is typically considered beginning at this time.

Infertility and testicular malignancy are major risks of cryptorchidism. Fertility is impaired by approximately 33% after unilateral cryptorchidism and by 66% after bilateral disease. The cancer risk for adults after cryptorchidism in childhood is reported to be 5–10 times greater than normal. However, histologic changes clearly occur as early as age 6 months in children with undescended testes.

The cause of most cases of cryptorchidism is not completely understood. Cryptorchidism can occur in an isolated fashion or associated with other findings. Abnormalities in the hypothalamic-pituitary-gonadal axis predispose to cryptorchidism. Androgen biosynthesis or receptor defects also predispose to cryptorchidism and undervirilization.

The diagnosis of bilateral cryptorchidism in an apparently normal male newborn should never be made until the possibility that the child is actually a fully virilized female with potentially fatal salt-losing CAH has been considered.

Clinical Findings

In infants between 2 and 6 months of age, LH, FSH, and testosterone levels help determine whether testes are present. After this time, an HCG stimulation test can be done to confirm the presence or absence of functional abdominal testes. Ultrasonography, CT scanning, and MRI may detect testes in the inguinal region, but these studies are not completely reliable in finding abdominal testes.

Differential Diagnosis

In palpating the testis, the cremasteric reflex that causes the testis to retract into the inguinal canal or abdomen (pseudocryptorchidism) may be elicited. To prevent retraction during examination, the fingers first should be placed across the abdominal ring and the upper portion of the inguinal canal to obstruct testicular ascent. Examination while the child is in the squatting position or in a warm bath is helpful. No treatment for retractile testes is necessary, and the prognosis for testicular descent and function is excellent.

Treatment

The current recommendation for treatment of cryptorchidism is that surgical orchidopexy be performed by an experienced surgeon if descent has not occurred by 6–12 months of age. The recommended timing of surgical intervention is based on the assumption that early surgery to relocate the testis into the low-temperature environment of the scrotum will allow normal germ cell development and decrease the risk for future infertility and cancer. However, in a certain number of cases, there is a primary abnormality of the testis which is thought to be responsible for the undescent and future risks. Hormonal therapy with HCG to induce descent of the testis only has a success rate of about 20%, and even less when retractile testes are excluded. HCG doses range from 250 to 1000 international units and are given twice weekly for 5 weeks. In the future, there may be a role for therapy with a GnRH analogue in addition to surgery as preliminary studies suggest that this treatment stimulates germ cell development and thus may improve future fertility.

4. Gynecomastia

Gynecomastia is a common, self-limited condition that may occur in up to 75% of normal pubertal boys. Adolescent gynecomastia typically resolves within 2 years but may not totally resolve if the degree of gynecomastia is extreme (> 2 cm of tissue). Gynecomastia may sometimes occur as part of Klinefelter syndrome, or it may occur in boys who are taking drugs such as antidepressants or marijuana. Medical therapy using antiestrogens and aromatase inhibitors have been used but generally the results are not deemed satisfactory. Surgical intervention is a reasonable option for prolonged and/or severe cases (see Chapter 4).

Hutson JM, Balic A, Nation T, Southwell B: Cryptorchidism. Semin Pediatr Surg 2010;19(3):215–224 [PMID: 20610195].

Husmann DA: Testicular descent: A hypothesis and review of current controversies. Pediatr Endocrinol Rev 2009;6:491 [PMID: 19550384].

Layman LC: Hypogonadotropic hypogonadism. Endocrinol Metab Clin North Am 2007;36:283 [PMID: 17543719].

ADRENAL CORTEX

The adult adrenal cortex has a regional distribution of terminal steroid production. The outermost zona glomerulosa is the predominant source of aldosterone. The middle zona fasciculata makes cortisol and small amounts of mineralocorticoids. The innermost zona reticularis produces mainly androgens and estrogens. A fetal zone, or provisional cortex, that predominates during fetal development produces glucocorticoids, mineralocorticoids, androgens, and estrogens. The fetal zone is relatively deficient in 3β-hydroxysteroid dehydrogenase (see Figure 34–8); hence placentally produced progesterone is the major precursor used in fetal adrenal production of cortisol and aldosterone.

The adrenal cortical production of cortisol is under the control of pituitary adrenocorticotropic hormone (ACTH; see Figure 34–1 and Table 34–1), which is in turn regulated by the hypothalamic peptide, corticotropin-releasing hormone (CRH). The complex interaction of CNS influences on CRH secretion, coupled with negative feedback of serum cortisol, leads to a diurnal pattern of ACTH and cortisol release. ACTH concentration is greatest during the early morning hours with a smaller peak in the late afternoon and a nadir at night. The pattern of serum cortisol concentration follows this pattern with a lag of a few hours. In the absence of cortisol feedback, there is dramatic CRH and ACTH hypersecretion.

Glucocorticoids are critical for gene expression in a many cell types. In excess, glucocorticoids are both catabolic and antianabolic; that is, they promote the release of amino acids from muscle and increase gluconeogenesis while decreasing incorporation of amino acids into muscle protein. They also antagonize insulin activity and facilitate lipolysis. Glucocorticoids help maintain blood pressure by promoting peripheral vascular tone and sodium and water retention.

Mineralocorticoids (primarily aldosterone in humans) promote sodium retention and stimulate potassium excretion in the distal renal tubule. Although ACTH can stimulate aldosterone production, the predominant regulator of aldosterone secretion is the volume- and sodium-sensitive renin-angiotensin-aldosterone system. Elevations of serum potassium also directly influence aldosterone release from the cortex.

Androgen (dehydroepiandrosterone and androstenedione) production by the zona reticularis is insignificant before puberty. At the onset of puberty, androgen production increases and may be an important factor in the dynamics of puberty in both sexes. The adrenal gland is a major source of androgen in the pubertal and adult female.

ADRENOCORTICAL INSUFFICIENCY (ADRENAL CRISIS, ADDISON DISEASE)

The leading causes of adrenal insufficiency are hereditary enzyme defects (congenital adrenal hyperplasia), autoimmune destruction of the glands (Addison disease), central adrenal insufficiency caused by intracranial neoplasm or its treatment, or congenital midline defects associated with optic nerve hypoplasia (septo-optic dysplasia). Rare forms of familial adrenal insufficiency occur in association with cerebral sclerosis and spastic paraplegia (adrenoleukodystrophy) or in association with achalasia and alacrimia in the triple A syndrome or Allgrove syndrome. Addison disease may be familial and has been described in association with hypoparathyroidism, mucocutaneous candidiasis, hypothyroidism, pernicious anemia, hypogonadism, and diabetes mellitus as one of the polyglandular autoimmune syndromes. Less commonly, the gland is destroyed by tumor, calcification, or hemorrhage (Waterhouse-Friderichsen syndrome). Adrenal disease secondary to opportunistic infections (fungal or tuberculous) is reported in AIDS. In children, central adrenal insufficiency due to anterior pituitary tumor is rare. Salt-losing disorders can occur from homozygous mutations affecting the aldosterone synthase enzyme (CYP11B2) or from partial or complete unresponsiveness of the mineralocorticoid receptor to aldosterone action (pseudohypoaldosteronism). A transient autosomal dominant form of pseudohypoaldosteronism has been reported in infancy. It is speculated to be secondary to a maturation disorder of function or number of aldosterone receptors and usually resolves by the first year of life.

Acute illness, surgery, trauma, or hyperthermia may precipitate an adrenal crisis in patients with adrenal insufficiency. Patients with primary adrenal insufficiency are at greater risk for life-threatening crisis than patients with central ACTH deficiency because mineralocorticoid secretion and low-level autonomous cortisol secretion remain intact in central ACTH deficiency.

Clinical Findings

A. Symptoms and Signs

1. Acute form (adrenal crisis)—Manifestations include nausea, vomiting, diarrhea, abdominal pain, dehydration, fever (sometimes followed by hypothermia), weakness, hypotension, circulatory collapse, confusion, and coma. Increased pigmentation may be associated with primary adrenal insufficiency caused by melanocyte-stimulating activity of the hypersecreted parent molecule, ACTH.

2. Chronic form—Manifestations include fatigue, hypotension, weakness, failure to gain weight, weight loss, salt craving (primary insufficiency), vomiting, and dehydration. Diffuse tanning with increased pigmentation over pressure points, scars, and mucous membranes may be present in primary adrenal insufficiency. A small heart may be seen on chest radiograph.

B. Laboratory Findings

1. Suggestive of adrenocortical insufficiency—In primary adrenal insufficiency, serum sodium and bicarbonate levels, arterial partial pressure of carbon dioxide, blood pH, and blood volume are decreased. Serum potassium and urea nitrogen levels are increased. Urinary sodium level and the ratio of urinary sodium to potassium are inappropriate for the degree of hyponatremia. In central adrenal insufficiency, serum sodium levels may be mildly decreased as a result of impaired water excretion. Eosinophilia and moderate lymphopenia occur in both forms of insufficiency.

2. Confirmatory tests

A. ACTH (COSYNTROPIN) STIMULATION TEST—In primary adrenal insufficiency (originating in the gland itself), plasma cortisol and aldosterone concentrations do not increase significantly over baseline 60 minutes after an intravenous dose of ACTH (250 mcg). To diagnose central adrenal insufficiency, a low dose of ACTH is given (1 mcg).

B. BASELINE SERUM ACTH CONCENTRATION—Values are elevated in primary adrenal failure and low in central adrenal insufficiency.

C. URINARY FREE CORTISOL AND 17-HYDROXYCORTICOSTEROID EXCRETION—Values are decreased.

D. CRH TEST—This test assesses responsiveness of the entire hypothalamic-pituitary-adrenal axis. After administration of ovine CRH, serum concentrations of ACTH and cortisol are measured over 2 hours. Verification of an intact axis or localization of the site of impairment is possible with careful interpretation of results.

Differential Diagnosis

Acute adrenal insufficiency must be differentiated from severe acute infections, diabetic coma, various disturbances of the CNS, and acute poisoning. In the neonatal period, adrenal insufficiency may be clinically indistinguishable from respiratory distress, intracranial hemorrhage, or sepsis. Chronic adrenocortical insufficiency must be differentiated from anorexia nervosa, certain muscular disorders (myasthenia gravis), salt-losing nephritis, and chronic debilitating infections, and must be considered in cases of recurrent spontaneous hypoglycemia.

Treatment

A. Acute Insufficiency (Adrenal Crisis)

1. Hydrocortisone sodium succinate—Hydrocortisone sodium succinate is given initially at a dose of 50 mg/m^2 intravenously over 2–5 minutes or intramuscularly; thereafter, it is given intravenously, 12.5 mg/m^2, every 4–6 hours until stabilization is achieved and oral therapy can be tolerated.

2. Fluids and electrolytes—In primary adrenal insufficiency, 5%–10% glucose in normal saline, 10–20 mL/kg intravenously, is given over the first hour and repeated if necessary to reestablish vascular volume. Normal saline is continued thereafter at 1.5–2 times the maintenance fluid requirements. Intravenous boluses of glucose (10% glucose, 2 mL/kg) may be needed every 4–6 hours to treat hypoglycemia. In central adrenal insufficiency, routine fluid management is generally adequate after restoration of vascular volume and institution of cortisol replacement.

3. Fludrocortisone—When oral intake is tolerated, fludrocortisone, 0.05–0.15 mg daily, is started and continued as necessary every 12–24 hours for primary adrenal insufficiency.

4. Inotropic agents—Rarely, inotropic agents such as dopamine and dobutamine are needed. However, adequate cortisol replacement is critical because pressor agents may be ineffective in adrenal insufficiency.

5. Waterhouse-Friderichsen syndrome with fulminant infections—The use of adrenocorticosteroids and norepinephrine in the treatment or prophylaxis of fulminant infections remains controversial. Corticosteroids may augment the generalized Shwartzman reaction in fatal cases of meningococcemia. However, corticosteroids should be considered if there is possible adrenal insufficiency, particularly if there is hypotension and circulatory collapse.

B. Maintenance Therapy

Following initial stabilization, the most effective substitution therapy is hydrocortisone, combined with fludrocortisone in primary adrenal insufficiency. Overtreatment should be avoided as it causes obesity, growth retardation, and other cushingoid features. Additional hydrocortisone, fludrocortisone, or sodium chloride, singly or in combination, may be necessary with acute illness, surgery, trauma, or other stress reactions. Supportive adrenocortical therapy should be given whenever surgical operations are performed in patients who have at some time received prolonged therapy with adrenocorticosteroids.

1. Glucocorticoids—A maintenance dosage of 6–10 mg/m^2/day of hydrocortisone (or equivalent) is given orally in two or three divided doses. The dosage of all glucocorticoids is increased to 30–50 mg/m^2/day during intercurrent illnesses or other times of stress.

2. Mineralocorticoids—In primary adrenal insufficiency, fludrocortisone is given, 0.05–0.15 mg orally daily as a single dose or in two divided doses. Periodic monitoring of blood pressure is recommended to avoid overdosing.

3. Salt—The child should be given ready access to table salt. Frequent blood pressure determinations in the recumbent position should be made to check for hypertension. In the infant, supplementation of 3–5 mEq Na^+/kg/day by adding the injectable solution (4 mg/mL) to formula or breast milk is generally required until table foods are introduced.

C. Corticosteroids in Patients with Adrenocortical Insufficiency Who Undergo Surgery

1. Before operation—Hydrocortisone sodium succinate, 30–50 mg/m^2 IM or intravenously 1 hour before surgery.

2. During operation—Hydrocortisone sodium succinate, 25–100 mg intravenously with 5%–10% glucose in saline as a continuous drip throughout surgery.

3. During recovery—Hydrocortisone sodium succinate, 12.5 mg/m^2 intravenously every 4–6 hours until oral doses are tolerated. The oral dose of three to five times the maintenance dose is continued until the acute stress is over, at which time the patient can be returned to the maintenance dose.

Course & Prognosis

The course of acute adrenal insufficiency is rapid, and death may occur within a few hours, particularly in infants, unless adequate treatment is given. Spontaneous recovery is unlikely. Patients who have received long-term treatment with adrenocorticosteroids may exhibit adrenal collapse if they undergo surgery or other acute stress. Pharmacologic doses of glucocorticoids during these episodes may be needed throughout life. In all forms of acute adrenal insufficiency, the patient should be observed carefully once the crisis has passed and evaluated with laboratory tests to assess the degree of permanent adrenal insufficiency.

Patients with chronic adrenocortical insufficiency who receive adequate therapy can lead normal lives.

Akirav EM, Ruddle NH, Herold KC: The role of AIRE in human autoimmune disease. Nat Rev Endocrinol 2011 Jan;7(1):25–33 [Epub 2010 Nov 23] [PMID: 21102544].

Ferraz-de-Souza B, Achermann JC: Disorders of adrenal development. Endocr Dev 2008;13:19–32 [PMID: 18493131].

Michels AW, Eisenbarth GS: Immunologic endocrine disorders. J Allergy Clin Immunol 2010 Feb;125(Suppl 2):S226–S237 [PMID: 20176260].

Michels AW, Gottlieb PA: Autoimmune polyglandular syndromes. Nat Rev Endocrinol 2010 May;6(5):270–277 [Epub 2010 Mar 23] [PMID: 20309000].

Reisch N, Arlt W: Fine tuning for quality of life: 21st century approach to treatment of Addison's disease. Endocrinol Metab Clin North Am 2009;38(2):407–418, ix–x [PMID: 19328419].

CONGENITAL ADRENAL HYPERPLASIAS

ESSENTIALS OF DIAGNOSIS & TYPICAL FEATURES

- Genital virilization in females, with labial fusion, urogenital sinus, enlargement of the clitoris, or other evidence of androgen action.
- Salt-losing crises in infant males or isosexual precocity in older males with infantile testes.
- Increased linear growth and advanced skeletal maturation.
- Elevation of plasma 17-hydroxyprogesterone concentrations in the most common form; may be associated with hyponatremia, hyperkalemia, and metabolic acidosis, particularly in newborns.

General Considerations

Autosomal recessive mutations in the enzymes of adrenal steroidogenesis in the fetus cause abnormal cortisol biosynthesis with increased ACTH secretion. ACTH excess subsequently results in adrenal hyperplasia with increased production of adrenal hormone precursors which are conveyed through the unblocked androgen pathway with resulting increase in androgen production. Increased pigmentation, especially of the scrotum, labia majora, and nipples, is common with excessive ACTH secretion. CAH is most commonly (> 90% of patients) the result of homozygous or compound heterozygous mutations in the cytochrome P-450 C21 (CYP21A2) gene causing 21-hydroxylase deficiency (see Figure 34–8). In its severe form, excess adrenal androgen production starting in the first trimester of fetal development causes virilization of the female fetus and life-threatening hypovolemic, hyponatremic shock (adrenal crisis) in the newborn. Other enzyme defects that less commonly result in CAH include 11-hydroxylase, 3 beta hydroxysteroid dehydrogenase, 20,22-desmolase, 17 α hydroxylase, and P450 oxidoreductase (POR) deficiencies. The clinical syndromes associated with these defects are shown in Figure 34–8 and Table 34–10.

Studies of patients with 21-hydroxylase deficiency indicate that the clinical type (salt-wasting or non–salt-wasting) is usually consistent within a kindred and that a close genetic linkage exists between the 21-hydroxylase gene and the human leukocyte antigen complex on chromosome 6. Prenatal diagnosis is now possible by allele-specific PCR or direct sequencing of the fetal CYP21A2 gene. This can be done when there is a known index case in the family. Population studies indicate that the defective gene is present in 1:250–1:100 people and that the worldwide incidence of the disorder is 1:15,000 with increased incidence is certain ethnic groups. Mass screening for this enzyme defect, using a microfilter paper technique to measure serum 17-hydroxyprogesterone, has been established in all 50 U.S. states and many other countries worldwide.

Nonclassic presentations of 21-hydroxylase deficiency have been reported with increasing frequency. Affected persons have a normal phenotype at birth but may develop evidence of virilization during later childhood, adolescence, or early adulthood. In these cases, results of hormonal studies are characteristic of 21-hydroxylase deficiency with cosyntropin stimulated 17-OHP levels being intermediate between those of nonaffected individuals and those with the classic form of the disease. Many individuals with the nonclassic form of the disease can be asymptomatic or only mildly symptomatic and do not need treatment. However, they can carry a severe CYP21A2 mutation and produce offspring with the classic form. Thus, it is recommended that these individuals should receive genetic counseling.

Clinical Findings

A. Symptoms and Signs

1. In females—Abnormality of the external genitalia varies from mild enlargement of the clitoris to complete fusion of the labioscrotal folds, forming an empty malrotated scrotum, a penile urethra, a penile shaft, and with clitoral enlargement sufficient to form a normal-sized glans (see Figure 34–7). Signs of adrenal insufficiency (salt loss) may occur in the first days of life but more typically appear in the second or third week. Rarely, signs of adrenal insufficiency do not occur for months or years. With milder enzyme defects, salt loss may not occur, and virilization predominates (simple virilizing form). In untreated non–salt-losing 21-hydroxylase or 11-hydroxylase deficiency, growth rate and skeletal maturation are accelerated and patients appear muscular. Pubic hair appears early (often before the second birthday),

Table 34–10. Clinical and laboratory findings in adrenal enzyme defects resulting in congenital adrenal hyperplasia.

Enzyme Deficiency[a]	Urinary 17-Ketosteroids	Elevated Plasma Metabolite	Plasma Androgens	Aldosterone	Hypertension/ Salt Loss	External Genitalia
StAR Protein	↓↓↓	–	↓↓↓	↓↓↓	–/+	Males: ambiguous Females: normal
3β-Hydroxysteroid dehydrogenase	↑↑ (DHEA)	17-OH pregnenolone (DHEA)	↑ (DHEA)	↓↓↓	–/+	Males: ambiguous Females: possibly virilized
17α-Hydroxylase/17-20 lyase	↓↓↓	Progesterone	↓↓	Normal to	±/	Males: ambiguous Females: normal
21-Hydroxylase[a]	↑↑↑	17-OHP	↑↑	↓↓	–/+	Males: normal Females: virilized
11-Hydroxylase	↑↑	11-Deoxycortisol	↑↑ ↓↓	(↑ Deoxycorticosterone)	+/–	Males: normal Females: virilized
P450 oxidoreductase	↓↓	17-OHP (mild elevation)	↓↓	Normal or mildly elevated	+/–	Males: ambiguous Females: ambiguous

[a]Children with "simple virilizing (non–salt-wasting)" forms of 21-hydroxylase deficiency congenital adrenal hyperplasia (CAH) may have normal aldosterone production and serum electrolytes, but some children have normal aldosterone production and serum electrolytes at the expense of elevated plasma renin activity and are, by definition, compensated salt-wasters. These children usually receive mineralocorticoid as well as glucocorticoid treatment. Children with 21-hydroxylase deficiency CAH should therefore have documented normal plasma renin activity in addition to normal serum electrolytes before they are considered non–salt-wasters.

DHEA, dehydroepiandrosterone; 17-OHP, 17-hydroxyprogestrone.

acne may be excessive, and the voice may deepen. Excessive pigmentation may develop. Isosexual central precocious puberty may occur if treatment is not initiated before the bone age is significantly advanced. Final adult height is often compromised.

2. In males—The male infant usually appears normal at birth but may present with salt-losing crisis in the first 2–4 weeks of life. In milder forms, salt-losing crises may not occur. In this circumstance, enlargement of the penis and increased pigmentation may be noted during the first few months. Other symptoms and signs are similar to those of affected females. The testes are not enlarged except in the rare male in whom aberrant adrenal cells (adrenal rests) are present in the testes, producing unilateral or asymmetrical bilateral enlargement. In the rare isolated defect of StAR protein, 17α hydroxylase, or 3β-hydroxysteroid dehydrogenase activity, ambiguous genitalia may be present because of impaired androgen production (see Figure 34–8). Individuals with PORD present with skeletal malformations similar to the Antler Bixley syndrome in addition to genital ambiguity. Rare cases of 17α hydroxylase mutations affecting only the 17–20 lyase functions of the enzyme have been reported. In those cases, patients present with isolated androgen deficiency and normal cortisol and aldosterone levels.

B. Laboratory Findings

1. Blood—Hormonal studies are essential for accurate diagnosis. Findings characteristic of the enzyme deficiencies are shown in Table 34–10.

2. Genetic studies—Rapid chromosomal diagnosis should be obtained in any newborn with ambiguous genitalia.

3. Urine—The diagnosis of PORD is best done by CG/MS analysis of urinary steroid metabolytes, as serum steroids can be misleading. Pathonogmonic findings include: Increased pregnenolone and progesterone metabolites, increased 17-OHP metabolites, and decreased androgen metabolites

C. Imaging

Ultrasonography, CT scanning, and MRI may be useful in defining pelvic anatomy or enlarged adrenals or in localizing an adrenal tumor. Contrast-enhanced radiographs of the vagina and pelvic ultrasonography may be helpful in delineating the internal anatomy in a newborn with ambiguous genitalia.

Treatment

A. Medical Treatment

Treatment goals in CAH are to replace deficient steroids with the smallest dose of glucocorticoid that will produce normalization of growth velocity and skeletal maturation by adequately suppressing excess build-up of androgen precursors. Excessive glucocorticoids cause the undesirable side effects of Cushing syndrome. Mineralocorticoid replacement sustains normal electrolyte homeostasis, but excessive mineralocorticoids cause hypertension and hypokalemia. Undervirilized males with the less frequent forms of CAH may require adult androgen replacement therapy in addition to glucocorticoid and mineralocorticoid replacement.

1. Glucocorticoids—Supraphysiologic doses of hydrocortisone are often needed to suppress androgen excess in CAH. Initially, parenteral or oral hydrocortisone (30–50 mg/m^2/day) suppresses abnormal adrenal steroidogenesis within 2 weeks. When adrenal suppression has been accomplished, as evidenced by normalization of serum 17-hydroxyprogesterone, patients are placed on maintenance doses of 10–15 mg/m^2/day in three divided doses. Dosage is adjusted to maintain normal growth rate and skeletal maturation. Various serum and urine androgens have been used to monitor therapy, including 17-hydroxyprogesterone, androstenedione, and urinary pregnanetriol. No one test is universally accepted. In adolescent girls, normal menses are a sensitive index of the adequacy of therapy. Therapy should be continued throughout life in both males and females because of the possibility of malignant degeneration of the hyperplastic adrenal gland. In pregnant females with CAH, suppression of adrenal androgen secretion is critical to avoid virilization of the fetus, particularly a female fetus. Hydrocortisone is the preferred choice for glucocorticoid replacement therapy in pregnant women with CAH because it does not cross the placenta.

2. Mineralocorticoids—Fludrocortisone, 0.05–0.15 mg, is given orally once a day or in two divided doses. Periodic monitoring of blood pressure and plasma renin is recommended to adjust dosing.

B. Surgical Treatment

For affected females, consultation with a urologist or gynecologist experienced in female genital reconstruction should be arranged as soon as possible during infancy.

Course & Prognosis

When therapy is initiated in early infancy, abnormal metabolic effects and progression of masculinization can be avoided. Treatment with glucocorticoids permits normal growth, development, and sexual maturation. If not adequately controlled, CAH results in sexual precocity and masculinization throughout childhood. Affected individuals will be tall as children but short as adults because of a rapid rate of skeletal maturation and premature closure of the epiphyses. If treatment is delayed or inadequate until somatic development is completed (12–14 years as determined by bone age), true central sexual precocity may occur in males and females.

Patient education stressing lifelong therapy is important to ensure compliance in adolescence and later life.

Virilization and multiple surgical genital reconstructions are associated with a high risk of psychosexual disturbances in female patients. Ongoing psychological evaluation and support is a critical component of care.

Nicole Reisch, Wiebke Arlt, Nils Krone: Health problems in congenital adrenal hyperplasia due to 21-hydoxylase deficiency. Horm Res Paediatr 2011 May 15 [Epub ahead of print] [PMID: 21597280].

Nimkarn S, New MI: Prenatal diagnosis and treatment of congenital adrenal hyperplasia due to 21-hydroxylase deficiency. Mol Cell Endocrinol 2009;300(1–2):192–196 [PMID: 19101608].

Speiser PW, Azziz R, Baskin LS et al: Congenital adrenal hyperplasia due to steroid 21-hydroxylase deficiency: An Endocrine Society clinical practice guideline. J Clin Endocrinol Metab 2010;95:4133–4160 [PMID: 20823466].

ADRENOCORTICAL HYPERFUNCTION (CUSHING DISEASE, CUSHING SYNDROME)

ESSENTIALS OF DIAGNOSIS & TYPICAL FEATURES

- Truncal adiposity, thin extremities, moon facies, muscle wasting, weakness, plethora, easy bruising, purple striae, decreased growth rate, and delayed skeletal maturation.
- Hypertension, osteoporosis, and glycosuria.
- Elevated serum corticosteroids, low serum potassium, eosinopenia, and lymphopenia.

General Considerations

Cushing syndrome may result from excessive secretion of adrenal steroids autonomously (adenoma or carcinoma), excess pituitary ACTH secretion (Cushing disease), ectopic ACTH secretion, or chronic exposure to exogenous glucocorticoid medications. In children younger than 12 years, Cushing syndrome is usually iatrogenic (secondary to exogenous ACTH or glucocorticoids). It may rarely be due to adrenal tumor, adrenal hyperplasia, pituitary adenoma, or extrapituitary ACTH-producing tumor.

Clinical Findings

A. Symptoms and Signs

1. Excess glucocorticoid—Manifestations include adiposity, most marked on the face, neck, and trunk (a fat pad in the interscapular area is characteristic); fatigue; plethoric facies; purplish striae; easy bruising; osteoporosis; hypertension; glucose intolerance; back pain; muscle wasting and weakness; and marked retardation of growth and skeletal maturation.

2. Excess mineralocorticoid—Patients have hypokalemia, mild hypernatremia with water retention, increased blood volume, edema, and hypertension.

3. Excess androgen—Hirsutism, acne, and varying degrees of virilization are present. Menstrual irregularities occur in older girls.

B. Laboratory Findings

1. Blood

a. Plasma cortisol—Values are elevated, with loss of normal diurnal variation. Determination of cortisol level between midnight and 2 AM may be a sensitive indicator of the loss of diurnal variation.

b. Serum chloride and potassium—Both values are usually low, but serum sodium and bicarbonate concentrations may be elevated with metabolic alkalosis.

c. Serum ACTH—ACTH concentration is decreased in adrenal tumor and increased with ACTH-producing pituitary or extrapituitary tumors.

d. CBC—Polymorphonuclear leukocytosis with lymphopenia and eosinopenia are common. Polycythemia occurs.

2. Salivary cortisol—This is a less invasive means by which to measure serial cortisol values, and the tests may be performed at home. Salivary cortisol obtained at midnight is a highly specific and sensitive test for hypercortisolism.

3. 24-Hour urinary free cortisol excretion—This value is elevated. It is considered the most useful initial test to document hypercortisolism, although midnight salivary cortisol is considered a reasonable and more practical alternative.

4. Response to dexamethasone suppression testing—The suppression of adrenal function by a small dose (0.5 mg) of dexamethasone is reduced in adrenal hyperfunction; larger doses (4–16 mg/d in four divided doses) of dexamethasone cause suppression of adrenal activity when the disease is due to ACTH hypersecretion, whereas hypercortisolism due to adenomas and adrenal carcinomas is rarely suppressed.

5. CRH test—The CRH stimulation test, in conjunction with petrosal sinus sampling, is effective in distinguishing pituitary and ectopic sources of ACTH excess and for lateralization of pituitary sources prior to surgery.

C. Imaging

Pituitary imaging may demonstrate a pituitary adenoma. Adrenal imaging by CT scan may demonstrate adenoma or bilateral hyperplasia. Radionuclide studies of the adrenals may be useful in complex cases. Osteoporosis, evident first in the spine and pelvis, with compression fractures may occur in advanced cases. Skeletal maturation is usually delayed.

Differential Diagnosis

Children with exogenous obesity accompanied by striae and hypertension are often suspected of having Cushing syndrome. The child's height, growth rate, and skeletal maturation are helpful in differentiating the two. Children with Cushing syndrome have a poor growth rate, relatively short stature, and delayed skeletal maturation, while those with exogenous obesity usually have a normal or slightly increased growth rate, normal to tall stature, and advanced skeletal maturation. The color of the striae (purplish in Cushing syndrome, pink in obesity) and the distribution of the obesity assist in differentiation. The urinary-free cortisol excretion (in milligrams per gram of creatinine) may be mildly elevated in obesity, but midnight salivary cortisol is normal.

Treatment

In all cases of primary adrenal hyperfunction due to tumor, surgical removal is indicated if possible. Glucocorticoids should be administered parenterally in pharmacologic doses during and after surgery until the patient is stable. Supplemental oral glucocorticoids, potassium, salt, and mineralocorticoids may be necessary until the suppressed contralateral adrenal gland recovers, sometimes over a period of several months. The use of mitotane, a DDT derivative that is toxic to the adrenal cortex, and aminoglutethimide, an inhibitor of steroid synthesis, have been suggested, but their efficacy in children with adrenal tumors has not been determined. Pituitary microadenomas may respond to pituitary surgery or irradiation.

Prognosis

If the tumor is malignant, the prognosis is poor if it cannot be completely removed. If it is benign, cure is to be expected following proper preparation and surgery.

Biller BM et al: Treatment of adrenocorticotropin-dependent Cushing's syndrome: A consensus statement. J Clin Endocrinol Metab 2008;93(7):2454–2462 [PMID: 18413427].

Clutter WE: Screening for Cushing's syndrome in an era of epidemic obesity. Mo Med 2011 Mar–Apr;108(2):104–106 [PMID: 21568231].

Mancini T, Porcelli T, Giustina A: Treatment of Cushing disease: Overview and recent findings. Ther Clin Risk Manag 2010 Oct 21;6:505–516 [PMID: 21063461].

Nieman LK et al: The diagnosis of Cushing's syndrome: An Endocrine Society Clinical Practice Guideline. J Clin Endocrinol Metab 2008;93(5):1526–1540 [PMID: 18334580].

Savage MO et al: Work-up and management of paediatric Cushing's syndrome. Curr Opin Endocrinol Diabetes Obes 2008;15(4):346–351 [PMID: 18594275].

PRIMARY HYPERALDOSTERONISM

Primary hyperaldosteronism may be caused by an adrenal adenoma or adrenal hyperplasia. It is characterized by paresthesias, tetany, weakness, nocturnal enuresis, periodic paralysis, low serum potassium and elevated serum sodium levels, hypertension, metabolic alkalosis, and production of large volume, alkaline urine with low specific gravity. The specific gravity does not respond to vasopressin. Glucose tolerance test is frequently abnormal. Plasma and urinary aldosterone are elevated. In contrast to renal disease or Bartter syndrome, plasma renin activity is suppressed, creating a high aldosterone-renin ratio. In patients with adrenal tumor, ACTH may further increase the excretion of aldosterone. Marked improvement after the administration of an aldosterone antagonist such as spironolactone may be of diagnostic value.

Treatment is with glucocorticoids (glucocorticoid remediable hyperaldosteronism or familial hyperaldosteronism type 1), spironolactone (familial hyperaldosteronism type 2), or subtotal or total adrenalectomy for hyperplasia, and surgical removal if a tumor is present.

Rossi GP, Seccia TM, Pessina AC: Primary aldosteronism—part I: Prevalence, screening, and selection of cases for adrenal vein sampling. J Nephrol 2008;21(4):447–454 [PMID: 18651532].

Rossi GP, Seccia TM, Pessina AC: Primary aldosteronism—part II: Subtype differentiation and treatment. J Nephrol 2008;21(4):455–462 [PMID: 18651533].

USES OF GLUCOCORTICOIDS & ADRENOCORTICOTROPIC HORMONE IN TREATMENT OF NONENDOCRINE DISEASES

Glucocorticoids are used for their anti-inflammatory and immunosuppressive properties in a variety of conditions in childhood. Pharmacologic doses are necessary to achieve these effects, and side effects are common. Numerous synthetic preparations possessing variable ratios of glucocorticoid to mineralocorticoid activity are available (Table 34–11).

Actions

Glucocorticoids exert a direct or permissive effect on virtually every tissue of the body; major known effects include the following:

1. Gluconeogenesis in the liver
2. Stimulation of fat breakdown (lipolysis) and redistribution of body fat
3. Catabolism of protein with an increase in nitrogen and phosphorus excretion
4. Decrease in lymphoid and thymic tissue and a decreased cellular response to inflammation and hypersensitivity
5. Alteration of CNS excitation
6. Retardation of connective tissue mitosis and migration; decreased wound healing
7. Improved capillary tone and increased vascular compartment volume and pressure

Table 34–11. Potency equivalents for adrenocorticosteroids.

Adrenocorticosteroid	Trade Names	Potency/mg Compared with Cortisol (Glucocorticoid Effect)	Potency/mg Compared with Cortisol (Sodium-Retaining Effect)
Glucocorticoids			
Hydrocortisone (cortisol)	Cortef	1	1
Cortisone	Cortone Acetate	0.8	1
Prednisone	Meticorten, others	4-5	04
Methylprednisolone	Medrol, Meprolone	5-6	Minimal
Triamcinolone	Aristocort, Kenalog Kenacort, Atolone	5-6	Minimal
Dexamethasone	Decadron, others	25-40	Minimal
Betamethasone	Celestone	25	Minimal
Mineralocorticoid			
Fludrocortisone	Florinef	15-20	300-400

Side Effects of Therapy

When prolonged use of pharmacologic doses of glucocorticoids is necessary, clinical manifestations of Cushing syndrome are common. Side effects may occur with the use of synthetic exogenous agents by any route, including inhalation and topical administration, or with the use of ACTH. Use of a larger dose of glucocorticoids given once every 48 hours (alternate-day therapy) lessens the incidence and severity of some of the side effects (Table 34–12).

Tapering of Pharmacologic Doses of Steroids

Prolonged use of pharmacologic doses of glucocorticoids causes suppression of ACTH secretion and consequent adrenal atrophy. The abrupt discontinuation of glucocorticoids

Table 34–12. Side effects of glucocorticoid use.

A. **Endocrine and metabolic effects**
1. Hyperglycemia and glycosuria (chemical diabetes)
2. Cushing syndrome
3. Persistent suppression of pituitary-adrenal responsiveness to stress with resultant hypoadrenocorticism

B. **Effects on electrolytes and minerals**
1. Marked retention of sodium and water, producing edema, increased blood volume, and hypertension (more common in endogenous hyperadrenal states)
2. Potassium loss with symptoms of hypokalemia
3. Hypocalcemia, tetany

C. **Effects on protein metabolism and skeletal maturation**
1. Negative nitrogen balance, with loss of body protein and bone protein, resulting in osteoporosis, pathologic fractures, and aseptic bone necrosis
2. Suppression of growth, retarded skeletal maturation
3. Muscular weakness and wasting
4. Osteoporosis

D. **Effects on the gastrointestinal tract**
1. Excessive appetite and intake of food
2. Activation or production of peptic ulcer
3. Gastrointestinal bleeding from ulceration or from unknown cause (particularly in children with hepatic disease)
4. Fatty liver with embolism, pancreatitis, nodular panniculitis

E. **Lowering of resistance to infectious agents; silent infection; decreased inflammatory reaction**
1. Susceptibility to fungal infections; intestinal parasitic infections
2. Activation of tuberculosis; false-negative tuberculin reaction
3. Stimulation of activity of herpes simplex virus

F. **Neuropsychiatric effects**
1. Euphoria, excitability, psychotic behavior, and status epilepticus with electroencephalographic changes
2. Increased intracranial pressure with pseudotumor cerebri syndrome

G. **Hematologic and vascular effects**
1. Bleeding into the skin as a result of increased capillary fragility
2. Thrombosis, thrombophlebitis, cerebral hemorrhage

H. **Miscellaneous effects**
1. Myocarditis, pleuritis, and arteritis following abrupt cessation of therapy
2. Cardiomegaly
3. Nephrosclerosis, proteinuria
4. Acne (in older children), hirsutism, amenorrhea, irregular menses
5. Posterior subcapsular cataracts; glaucoma

may result in adrenal insufficiency. ACTH secretion generally does not restart until the administered steroid has been given in subphysiologic doses (< 6 mg/m^2/d orally) for several weeks.

If pharmacologic glucocorticoid therapy has been given for less than 10–14 days, the drug can be discontinued abruptly (if the condition for which it was prescribed allows) because adrenal suppression will be short-lived. However, it is advisable to educate the patient and family about the signs and symptoms of adrenal insufficiency in case problems arise.

If tapering is necessary in treating the condition for which the glucocorticoid is prescribed, a reduction of 25%–50% every 2–7 days is sufficiently rapid to permit observation of clinical symptomatology. An alternate-day schedule (single dose given every 48 hours) will allow for a 50% decrease in the total 2-day dosage while providing the desired pharmacologic effect. If tapering is not required for the underlying disease, the dosage can be rapidly decreased safely to the physiologic range. Although a rapid decrease in dose to the physiologic range will not lead to frank adrenal insufficiency (because adequate exogenous cortisol is being provided), some patients may experience a steroid withdrawal syndrome, characterized by malaise, insomnia, fatigue, and loss of appetite. These symptoms may necessitate a two- or three-step decrease in dose to the physiologic range.

Once a physiologic equivalent dose (8–10 mg/m^2/day hydrocortisone or equivalent) is achieved and the patient's underlying disease is stable, the dose can be decreased to 4–5 mg/m^2/day given only in the morning. This will allow the adrenal axis to recover. After this dose has been given for 4–6 weeks, assessment of endogenous adrenal activity is estimated by obtaining fasting plasma cortisol concentrations between 7 and 8 AM prior to the morning steroid dose. When an alternate-day schedule is followed, plasma cortisol is measured the morning before treatment. Plasma cortisol concentration in the physiologic range (> 10 mg/dL) indicates return of basal physiologic adrenal rhythm. Exogenous steroids may then be discontinued safely, although it is advisable to continue giving stress doses of glucocorticoids when appropriate until recovery of the response to stress has been documented.

After basal physiologic adrenal function returns, the adrenal reserve or capacity to respond to stress and infection can be estimated by the low-dose ACTH stimulation test, in which 1 mcg of synthetic ACTH (cosyntropin) is administered intravenously. Plasma cortisol is measured prior to (zero time) and at 45–60 minutes after the infusion. A plasma cortisol concentration greater than 18 mg/dL at 60 minutes indicates a satisfactory adrenal reserve.

Even if the results of testing are normal, patients who have received prolonged treatment with glucocorticoids may develop signs and symptoms of adrenal insufficiency during acute stress, infection, or surgery for months to years after treatment has been stopped. Careful monitoring, and the use of stress doses of glucocorticoids, should be considered during severe illnesses and surgery.

Allen DB: Effects of inhaled steroids on growth, bone metabolism, and adrenal function. Adv Pediatr 2006;53:101–110 [PMID: 17089864].

Gulliver T, Eid N: Effects of glucocorticoids on the hypothalamic-pituitary-adrenal axis in children and adults. Immunol Allergy Clin North Am 2005;25:541 [PMID: 16054542].

Zöllner EW: Hypothalamic-pituitary-adrenal axis suppression in asthmatic children on inhaled corticosteroids (part 2)—the risk as determined by gold standard adrenal function tests: A systematic review. Pediatr Allergy Immunol 2007;18(6):469–474 [PMID: 17680905].

Zöllner EW: Hypothalamic-pituitary-adrenal axis suppression in asthmatic children on inhaled corticosteroids: Part 1. Which test should be used? Pediatr Allergy Immunol 2007;18(5):401–409 [PMID: 17561933].

ADRENAL MEDULLA PHEOCHROMOCYTOMA

Pheochromocytoma is an uncommon tumor, and only 10% of reported cases occur in pediatric patients. The tumor can be located wherever chromaffin tissue (adrenal medulla, sympathetic ganglia, or carotid body) is present, possibly from decreased apoptosis of neural crest cells during development. It may be multiple, recurrent, and sometimes malignant. Familial forms include pheochromocytomas associated with the dominantly inherited neurofibromatosis type 1, MEN type 2, and von Hippel-Lindau syndromes, as well as mutations of the succinate dehydrogenase genes. Neuroblastomas, ganglioneuromas, and other neural tumors, as well as carcinoid tumors, may secrete pressor amines and mimic pheochromocytoma.

The symptoms of pheochromocytoma are generally caused by excessive secretion of epinephrine or norepinephrine and most commonly include headache, sweating, tachycardia, and hypertension. Other symptoms are anxiety, hypertension, dizziness, weakness, nausea and vomiting, diarrhea, dilated pupils, blurred vision, abdominal and precordial pain, and vasomotor instability (flushing and postural hypotension). Sustained symptoms may lead to cardiac, renal, optic, or cerebral damage.

Laboratory diagnosis is possible in more than 90% of cases. Serum and urine catecholamines are elevated, but abnormalities may be limited periods of symptomatology or paroxysm. Plasma-free metanephrine level (phenoxybenzamine, tricyclic antidepressants, and β-adrenoreceptor blockers can create false-positive results) is the most sensitive test and the gold standard for diagnosis. Levels three times the normal range are diagnostic. Intermediate values may require additional testing, with urinary vanillylmandelic acid and urinary total metanephrines providing the highest specificity. Provocative tests using histamine, tyramine, or glucagon and the phentolamine tests may be abnormal but are dangerous and are rarely necessary. After demonstrating a tumor biochemically, imaging methods including CT or MRI are used to localize the tumor. When available, functional ligands such as (123)I-MIBG, [^{18}F]DA positron emission tomography scanning, and somatostatin receptor scintigraphy (with either [^{123}I]Tyr3-octreotide or [^{111}In] DTPA-octreotide) are useful in further diagnostic evaluation.

Laparoscopic tumor removal is the treatment of choice; however, the procedure must be undertaken with great caution and with the patient properly stabilized. Oral phenoxybenzamine or intravenous phentolamine is used preoperatively. Profound hypotension may occur as the tumor is removed but may be controlled with an infusion of norepinephrine, which may have to be continued for 1–2 days.

Unless irreversible secondary vascular changes have occurred, complete relief of symptoms is to be expected after recovery from removal of a benign tumor. However, prognosis is poor in patients with metastases, which occur more commonly with large, extra-adrenal pheochromocytomas.

Armstrong R et al: Phaeochromocytoma in children. Arch Dis Child 2008;93(10):899–904 [PMID: 18499773].

Havekes B et al: Update on pediatric pheochromocytoma. Pediatr Nephrol 2009;24(5):943–950 [PMID: 18566838].

Karagiannis A et al: Pheochromocytoma: An update on genetics and management. Endocr Relat Cancer 2007;14(4):935–956 [PMID: 18045948].

Kinney MA et al: Perioperative management of pheochromocytoma. J Cardiothorac Vasc Anesth 2002;16:359 [PMID: 12073213].

Pozo J et al: Sporadic pheochromocytoma in childhood: Clinical and molecular variability. J Pediatr Endocrinol Metab 2005;18:527 [PMID: 16042317].

Diabetes Mellitus

35

Marian Rewers, MD, PhD
H. Peter Chase, MD
George S. Eisenbarth, MD, PhD

ESSENTIALS OF DIAGNOSIS & TYPICAL FEATURES

- Polyuria, polydipsia, and weight loss.
- Hyperglycemia and glucosuria often with ketonemia/ketonuria.

GENERAL CONSIDERATIONS

Type 1 diabetes (T1D) is the most common type of diabetes mellitus in people younger than 20 years; however, it can develop at any age and most of the cases are diagnosed after age 20. While the classical presentation included significant weight loss and ketoacidosis, most patients diagnosed today present with milder symptoms and obesity is not uncommon at presentation. T1D is further divided into T1a (autoimmune) (~95% of the cases) and T1b (idiopathic) diabetes. T1a diabetes is marked by presence of autoantibodies to islet cell autoantigens (insulin, GAD65, IA-2, and ZnT8) and/or high risk HLA haplotypes (DR4,DQ8 and DR3/DQ2). Insulin production, measured by fasting or stimulated C-peptide levels, is usually low. In the United States, T1D affects an estimated 1.5 million people including 160,000–200,000 patients younger than 20 (~20,000 diagnosed annually).

Type 2 diabetes (T2D) is a heterogeneous phenotype diagnosed most often in persons older than 40 who are usually obese and initially not insulin-dependent. T2D is rare before age 10, but has increased in frequency in older children, following the epidemic of obesity. T2D is responsible for vast majority of the 26 million cases of diabetes in the United States, but only an estimated 16,000 patients younger than 20 (~5000 diagnosed annually).

Monogenic forms of diabetes can by diagnosed at any age, account for < 1% of childhood cases, but for the majority of those diagnosed before the 9th month of life. Maturity-onset diabetes of the young (MODY) presents as a nonketotic and usually non-insulin-dependent diabetes in absence of obesity or islet autoantibodies. Strong family history of early-onset diabetes is common. The most frequent forms are due to mutations in glucokinase or hepatic nuclear factor 1 or 2 genes. Glucokinase mutations rarely require therapy; other forms respond to oral hypoglycemic agents or insulin. Neonatal diabetes is transient in about half of the cases. If persistent, it presents significant clinical challenge. Some infants respond better to sulfonylurea than insulin.

Pathogenesis

A. Type 1 Diabetes

Type 1 diabetes results from autoimmune damage to the insulin-producing β cells of the pancreatic islets. This damage occurs gradually—over months or years—and symptoms do not appear until about 80% of the pancreatic islets have been destroyed. The genetic predisposition is primarily defined by the HLA region; more than 30 additional loci have been implicated.

All ethnic groups are affected; the rates are the highest in children of European ancestry, followed by African Americans and Hispanics, and the lower rates in Asians and Native Americans.

About 6% of siblings or offspring of persons with type 1 diabetes also develop diabetes (compared with prevalence in the general population of 0.2–0.3%). However, fewer than 10% of children newly diagnosed with T1D have a parent or sibling with the disease. More than 90% of children with T1D carry at least one of the high-risk HLA haplotypes: DR4,DQ8 or DR3/DQ2 and 40% of the U.S. children diagnosed below the age of 10 have both (one from each parent), compared with only 2.5% of the general population.

The incidence of T1D has increased dramatically worldwide, doubling every ~20 years in all ethnic groups, pointing to powerful environmental determinants. Despite much research focusing on early childhood infections and diet, the environmental factor(s) initiating or sustaining the insult are poorly defined. There is no effective prevention, as of late 2011.

Autoantibodies to insulin, GAD, IA-2, ZnT8, and other antigens are present for months to years prior to diagnosis in the serum of patients who develop T1a diabetes. These antibodies are not mediating β-cell destruction, but offer a useful screening tool. The β-cell damage is mediated by T lymphocytes. Immunosuppression at different checkpoints of the autoimmune process can slow down the damage but has no durable effect when stopped. Immunomodulation, including induction of tolerance to islet autoantigens, with or without immunosuppression is an area of intensive research.

B. Type 2 Diabetes

Type 2 diabetes has a strong genetic component, although the inherited defects vary in different families. Obesity, particularly central, and lack of exercise are major causes, but rarely sufficient alone to cause diabetes in the youth. Most of the pediatric patients come from low socioeconomical strata of the society and dysfunctional families; some present with psychiatric disorders. Obesity, T2D, and associated insulin resistance adversely affect cardiovascular health. Acanthosis nigricans, a thickening and darkening of the skin over the posterior neck, armpits, or elbows, is present in many obese children and rarely helps in the diagnosis of type 2 diabetes.

Prevention

A. Type 1 Diabetes

Free antibody screening is now available for families having a relative with type 1 diabetes as well as new-onset patients (1-800-425-8361). Intervention trials on antibody-positive first-degree relatives have begun in an effort to try to prevent type 1 diabetes.

B. Type 2 Diabetes

The prevention of type 2 diabetes was evaluated in a large study of adults with impaired glucose tolerance: normal fasting blood glucose < 126 mg/dL and elevated (140–199 mg/dL) blood glucose 2 hours after 75 g load of oral glucose—the Diabetes Prevention Program. The study found that 30 minutes of exercise per day (5 d/wk) and a low-fat diet reduced the risk of diabetes by 58%. Taking metformin also reduced the risk of type 2 diabetes by 31%.

Clinical Findings

The classic symptoms of polyuria, polydipsia, and weight loss in a child are unique to diabetes. Unfortunately, these symptoms are often missed by primary care providers or even emergency department staff. The frequency of diabetic ketoacidosis in the U.S. children has not improved in the past 20 years and approaches 40%—a sign of poor provider and community awareness. More than half of DKA patients have been seen by a provider in days preceding diagnosis and obvious symptoms and signs were missed. In contrast, less than 20% of newly diagnosed children in Scandinavia or Canada present in DKA. This embarrassing statistic could be greatly improved with better history taking and point of care urine analysis. Initial diagnosis can be easily confirmed by blood glucose and ketones measurement using widely available and inexpensive meters.

The clinical presentation of DKA includes abdominal pain, nausea, and vomiting that can mimic an acute abdomen. The patients are mildly to moderately dehydrated (5%–10%), may have Kussmaul respiration, and become progressively somnolent and obtunded. As the distribution of diagnosis has shifted to younger age, infants, toddlers, and preschool age children are at particular risk. They often have symptoms of minor infection or gastrointestinal upset. Heavy diaper in a dehydrated child without diarrhea should always flash alarm. Blood or urine glucose levels can be checked in a few seconds, which could be lifesaving. Blood glucose higher than 200 mg/dL in a child is always abnormal and must be promptly and meticulously followed in consultation with a pediatric endocrinology service. If the presentation is mild and an outpatient diabetes education service is available, hospitalization is usually not necessary.

Transient, "stress" or steroid-induced hyperglycemia can occur with illness. In a well child, the diagnosis must not be based on a single plasma glucose test or borderline results obtained using a glucose meter. Our center routinely tests such children for islet autoantibodies to rule out ongoing islet autoimmunity; the quality of commercial assays for the autoantibodies varies widely and absence of at least three autoantibodies (to insulin, GAD, and IA-2) provides 80% negative predictive value. If HbA_{1c} is normal, we recommend home monitoring of blood glucose for several days. In children progressing to overt diabetes, hyperglycemia after dinner is usually the initial abnormality detectable by self-blood glucose monitoring at home.

In presence of typical symptoms, a random blood glucose level above 200 mg/dL (11 mmol/L) confirmed on a CLIA-certified instrument is sufficient to make the diagnosis of diabetes. An oral glucose tolerance test is rarely necessary in children. In borderline or asymptomatic cases, a fasting plasma glucose level over 126 mg/dL (7 mmol/L) or a plasma glucose level above 200 mg/dL (11.1 mmol/L) two hours after an oral glucose load (1.75 g glucose/kg up to a maximum of 75 g) on two separate days confirms the diagnosis. Impaired (not yet diabetic) fasting glucose values are 100–125 mg/dL (5.5–6.9 mmol/L) and impaired 2-hour values are 140–200 mg/dL (7.8–11.1 mmol/L). Children with impaired fasting glucose or impaired glucose tolerance are at high risk of T2D and require careful follow-up and lifestyle modification with weight loss, if obese.

Treatment

Major variables in T1D treatment are (1) insulin therapy, (2) diet, (3) exercise, (4) psychosocial support, and (5) blood glucose and ketone monitoring. All must be considered to obtain safe and effective metabolic control.

At present, the safest recommendation for glycemic control in children is to achieve the lowest HbA_{1c}, if possible < 7.5%, that can be sustained without severe hypoglycemia or frequent moderate hypoglycemia. Each child should have targets individually determined.

Intensive diabetes management includes: (1) three or more insulin injections per day, or insulin pump therapy; (2) four or more blood glucose determinations per day; (3) carbohydrate counting; and (4) frequent contact with diabetes health care provider. This approach was shown in the Diabetes Control and Complications Trial to improve HbA_{1c} to ~7% and to reduce the risk for retinal, renal, cardiovascular, and neurologic complications of diabetes.

A. Patient and Family Education

Education about diabetes for all family members is essential for the home management of diabetes. The use of an educational book (see *Understanding Diabetes* in References) can be very helpful to the family. All caregivers need to learn about diabetes, how to give insulin injections, perform home blood glucose monitoring, and handle acute complications. Although teenagers can be taught to perform many of the tasks of diabetes management, they do better when supportive, not overbearing, parents continue to be involved in management of their disease. Children younger than age 12 years cannot reliably administer insulin without adult supervision because they lack fine motor control and may not understand the importance of accurate dosage.

B. Insulin

Insulin has three key functions: (1) it allows glucose to pass into the cell for oxidative utilization; (2) it decreases the physiologic production of glucose, particularly in the liver; and (3) it turns off lipolysis and ketone production.

1. Treatment of new-onset diabetes—Children presenting in DKA (pH < 7.30 or bicarbonate < 15 in presence of hyperglycemia and ketosis/ketonemia) require intravenous insulin in addition to replacement of fluids and electrolytes (see section Ketonuria, Ketonemia, and Ketoacidosis). Regular insulin is given as a continuous drip at a rate 0.05–0.1 U/kg/h to achieve drop in blood glucose of ~100 mg/dL per hour. Giving an IV insulin bolus of starting insulin drip before completion of the initial fluid bolus has been associated with brain edema. Fast-acting insulin analogs have no advantage over regular insulin when given IV.

In children who present without DKA and have adequate oral intake, the initial insulin dose can be administered subcutaneously as 0.2 U/kg of short-acting insulin (Regular) or, preferentially, rapid-acting analog: lispro (Humalog), aspart (NovoLog), or glulisine (Apidra). At the same time, 0.2–0.3 U/kg of intermediate-(NPH) or long-acting insulin analog: glargine (Lantus) of detemir (Levemir) can be administered subcutaneously to limit the need for multiple insulin injections. This usually suffices for the initial 12–24 hours preceding systematic diabetes education.

The dose is adjusted with each injection during the first week. The rule of thumb is to start insulin at the low end of estimated daily requirements and titrate it up based on frequent (q 2–4 h) blood glucose monitoring. The initial daily dose of insulin is higher in presence of ketosis, infection, obesity, or steroid treatment. It also varies with age and severity of onset. A total subcutaneous daily dose of 0.3–0.7 U/kg/day may suffice in prepubertal children, while pubertal or overweight children and those with initial HbA_{1c} > 12% commonly require 1.0–1.5 U/kg/day of insulin during the initial week of treatment.

The insulin dose peaks about one week after diagnosis and decreases slightly with waning glucotoxicity and voracious appetite. Approximately 3–6 weeks after diagnosis, most school-children and adolescents experience a partial remission or "honeymoon period." Temporary decrease in the insulin dose during this period is necessary to avoid severe hypoglycemia. The remission is rarely complete and tends to last longer in older children.

2. Long-term insulin dosage—Children usually receive a rapid-acting insulin to cover food intake or high blood glucose and a longer-acting insulin to suppress endogenous hepatic glucose production. This is achieved by combining insulins with the desired properties. Understanding the onset, peak, and duration of insulin activity is essential (Table 35–1).

Nearly all children diagnosed with T1D at our center receive a basal-bolus multiple daily injection (MDI) treatment. It usually consists of 3–4 injections (boluses) of rapid-acting

Table 35–1. Kinetics of insulin action.

Type of Insulin	Begins Working	Main Effect	All Gone
Rapid-acting			
Regular	30 min	95 min	6–9 h
Humalog, NovoLog, Apidra	10–15 min	55 min	4 h
Intermediate-acting			
NPH (neutral protamine Hagedorn)	2–4 h	6–8 h	12–15 h
Long-acting			
Lantus or Levemir	3–4 h	6–18 h	18–26 h
Premixed (available in various combinations)			
75/25 (75% NPH + 25% Humalog)	15 min	1–8 h	12–15 h
NPH/Regular	30 min	Variable	12–18 h

analog before meals and 1–2 injections of long-acting analog insulin. The dose of premeal rapid-acting insulin is calculated based on anticipated carbohydrate content of the meal and additional insulin to correct for high blood glucose, if needed. Sliding scales for dosing of rapid-acting insulin are helpful initially, while families learn carbohydrate counting. This shortcut assumes that the content of carbohydrates does not vary in a meal, for example, dinner, from day to day and may lead to significant under- and overdosing.

Children younger than age 4 years usually need 1 or 2 units of rapid-acting insulin to cover meals. Children aged 4–10 years may require up to 4 units of rapid-acting insulin to cover breakfast and dinner, whereas 4–10 units of rapid-acting insulin are used in older children. Families gradually learn to make small weekly adjustments in insulin dosage based on home blood glucose testing. Rapid-acting analogs (lispro, aspart, or glulisin) are given 10–20 minutes before eating to account for delay in insulin action. If slower human regular insulin is used, the injections should be given 30–60 minutes before meals—rarely a practical option. In young children who eat unpredictably, it is often necessary to wait until after the meal to decide on the appropriate dose of rapid-acting insulin. It is a compromise between safety from hypoglycemia and tolerating hyperglycemia after most of the meals.

A long-acting analog insulin glargine (Lantus) or detemir (Levemir) is given once or twice a day to maintain basal insulin levels between meals. Daily adjustments in long-acting insulin dose usually are not needed. However, decreases should be made for heavy activity (eg, sports, hikes, or overnight events).

In the past, most children would receive two injections per day of a rapid-acting insulin and an intermediate-acting insulin (NPH), often mixed just before injection. About two-thirds of the total dosage would be given before breakfast and the remainder before dinner. This regiment has been shown to be inferior in achieving recommended HbA_{1c} levels and avoiding hypoglycemia, compared with the basal-bolus regiment described above. Analog insulin (glargine, detemir) works more efficiently than NPH. When changing a patient from NPH insulin to an analog, initially only 50% of the daily units of long-acting insulin is recommended.

3. Insulin pump treatment—Continuous subcutaneous insulin (insulin pump) therapy is the best way to restore the body's physiologic insulin profile. The pump delivers a variable programmed basal rate that corresponds to the diurnal variation in insulin needs. Prepubertal children require higher basal rate in the early part of night, while postpubertal patients who experience the 'dawn phenomenon' require higher rates in the morning. The user initiates bolus doses before meals and to correct hyperglycemia. Most pumps can receive wireless transmission of test results from glucose meters, but the patient or caregiver must still manually enter the amount of carbohydrate being consumed. The pump calculates the amount of insulin needed for a meal or correction based on previously entered parameters which include: insulin-to-carbohydrate ratios, insulin sensitivity factor, glycemic target, and duration of insulin action (set at 3–4 hours to protect from accumulating too much insulin). The user may override the suggestion or press a button to initiate the bolus.

Most clinical trials have demonstrated better HbA_{1c} and less severe hypoglycemia with pump therapy, compared to MDI. Pump therapy can improve the quality of life in children who have trouble with or fear of injections or who desire greater flexibility in their lifestyle, for example, with sleeping in, sports, or irregular eating. Insulin pumps can be particularly helpful in young children or infants who have multiple meals and snacks and require multiple small doses of rapid-acting insulin. The newer generation of insulin pumps can deliver as little as 0.025 U/h, but higher rates using diluted insulin may be needed for uninterrupted flow.

Compliance problems include infrequent blood glucose testing, not reacting to elevated blood glucose, incorrect carbohydrate counting or missing the boluses altogether. Side effects of insulin pump treatment include failures of insulin delivery because of a displaced or obstructed infusion set. Insulin pump treatment is significantly more expensive than regimens based on injections. For some patients, pumps may be too difficult to operate or comply with the multiple testing and carbohydrate counting requirements, or be unacceptable because of body image issues or extreme physical activity (swimming, contact sports).

Disposable pumps are already available and much smaller "patch" pumps are in development. In the near future, one may expect a "closed-loop" system allowing the insulin pump to be directed automatically by a continuous glucose sensor with minimal human input. A number of issues, however, remain to be solved, including the biocompatibility of the sensors and infusion sets, limitations of the systemic versus intraportal administration of insulin, lack of counterbalancing delivery of glucagon, and optimal delivery algorithms for various meals and activities.

4. Treatment of type 2 diabetes—Treatment of type 2 diabetes in children varies with the severity of the disease. If the HbA_{1c} is still near normal, modification of lifestyle (preferably for the entire family) is the first line of therapy. This must include reducing caloric intake (portion size and of high fat, fast food meals) and increasing exercise. If the HbA_{1c} is mildly elevated (6.2–8.0%), but ketone levels are not increased, an oral hypoglycemia agent can be tried. Metformin is usually tried along with modification of lifestyle, starting with a dose of 250–500 mg once daily. If needed, and if gastrointestinal adaptation has occurred, the dose can be gradually increased to 1 g twice daily. If the presentation is more severe, with ketosis, the initial treatment is similar to that of type 1 diabetes (including intravenous or subcutaneous insulin). Of note, 10% of children with T2D present in DKA. Oral hypoglycemic agents may be tried at a later date, particularly if weight loss has been successful.

C. Diet

A thorough dietary history should be obtained including the family's dietary habits and traditions, the child's typical meal times, and patterns of food intake. Nutritional management in children with diabetes does not require a restrictive diet, just a healthy dietary regimen that the children and their families can benefit from. Insulin pump and MDI therapy utilize carbohydrate counting in which the grams of carbohydrate to be eaten are counted and a matching dose of insulin is administered. This plan allows for the most freedom and flexibility in food choices, but it requires expert education and commitment and may not be suitable for many families or situations, for example, school lunches and teenagers.

Exchange planning teaches that it is not necessary to count precise grams. Exchanges are taught as either 10- or 15-g servings of carbohydrate. The exchange plan can enable a more consistent daily intake of carbohydrate. The constant carbohydrate meal plan was used often in the past with insulin regimens based on NPH and regular insulin, where carbohydrate intake and the amount of insulin were kept relatively constant from day to day. It has been perceived as too restrictive and a potential source of conflict.

D. Exercise

Regular aerobic exercise is important for children with diabetes. Exercise fosters a sense of well-being; helps increase insulin sensitivity; and helps maintain proper weight, blood pressure, and HDL-cholesterol levels.

Hypoglycemia during exercise or in the 2–12 hours after exercise can be prevented by careful monitoring of blood glucose before, during, and after exercise; reducing the dosage of the insulin active at the time of (or after) the exercise; and by providing extra snacks. Fifteen grams of glucose usually covers about 30 minutes of exercise. The use of drinks containing 5%–10% dextrose, such as Gatorade, during the period of exercise is often beneficial. Preexercise bolus insulin dosages as well as the basal dosages during (and sometimes after) the exercise should be reduced; the longer and more vigorous the activity, the greater the reduction in insulin dose.

E. Psychological Care

The diagnosis of T1D changes lives of the affected families and brings on relentless challenges. It is impossible to take "vacation" from diabetes without some unpleasant consequences. The stress imposed on the family around the time of initial diagnosis may lead to feelings of shock, denial, sadness, anger, fear, and guilt. Meeting with a counselor to express these feelings at the time of diagnosis helps with long-term adaptation. Children with T1D and their parents often experience difficult adjustment. Persisting adjustment problems may mark underlying dysfunction of the family or psychopathology of the child or caregiver. Young people with T1D are more frequently diagnosed with and treated for psychiatric disorders, disordered eating, neurocognitive, learning problems, and poor coping skills, than the general population.

Routine assessment should be made of developmental adjustment to and understanding of diabetes management, including diabetes-related knowledge, insulin adjustment skills, goal setting, problem-solving abilities, regimen adherence, and self-care autonomy and competence. This is especially important during late childhood and prior to adolescence. General family functioning also needs to be assessed and diabetes-related functioning: communication, parental involvement and support, and roles and responsibilities for self-care behaviors, especially when there is evidence of cultural, language, or family problems. Training parents in effective behavior management skills, especially at diagnosis and prior to adolescence, should emphasize appropriate family involvement and support, effective problem-solving and self-management skills, and realistic expectations. Adolescents should be encouraged to assume increasing responsibility for diabetes management but with continuing, mutually agreed parental involvement and support. The transition to adult diabetes care should be negotiated and planned between adolescents, their parents, and the diabetes team well in advance of the actual transfer.

F. Home Blood Glucose Measurements

All families must be able to monitor blood glucose levels at least four times daily—and more frequently in patients who have glucose-control problems or intercurrent illnesses. Blood glucose levels can be monitored using any of the available meters, which generally have an accuracy of 90% or better. Target levels when no food has been eaten for 2 or more hours vary according to age (Table 35–2). At least half of the values must be below the upper limit to have a good HbA_{1c}.

The frequency of SMBG is associated with improved HbA_{1c} in patients with T1D. Patient acceptance of SMBG may be enhanced by including the opportunity for testing alternative sites in addition to the fingertips, for example, the forearm; alternative sites, however, may be slower to reflect falling blood glucose.

Table 35–2. Ideal glucose levels after 2 or more hours of fasting.

Age (y)	Glucose Level
4 or younger	80–200 mg/dL (4.6–11 mmol/L)
5–11	70–180 mg/dL (3.9–10 mmol/L)
12 or older	70–150 mg/dL (3.9–8.3 mmol/L)

Blood glucose results, insulin dosage, and events, for example, illness, parties, exercise, menses, and episodes of hypoglycemia or ketonuria/ketosis should be recorded in a logbook or downloaded and evaluated at regular intervals by the family to look for patterns and make changes in insulin dosage. If more than 50% of the values are above the desired range for age or more than 14% below the desired range, the insulin dosage usually needs to be adjusted. This is particularly useful at the time of consultation or troubleshooting.

Some families are able to make these changes independently, whereas others need help from the health care provider by fax or email to keep insulin dose up to date between visits. Children with diabetes should be evaluated by a diabetes provider every 3 months. This provides an opportunity to check compliance, adjust insulin dose according to growth, HbA_{1c}, and blood glucose patterns as well as to carry out routine review of systems, physical examination, and tests (see Table 35–3).

Home continuous glucose monitoring (CGM) is now routinely available and can tremendously improve diabetes management, if used most of the time. Subcutaneous glucose levels are obtained every 1–5 minutes from a sensor placed under the skin. As with insulin pump therapy, intensive education and follow-up, usually at a specialty diabetes center, is required.

Table 35–3. Checklist of good diabetes management in children and adolescents.

Variable	Frequency of Measurement	Tests and Values
Blood glucose	At least 4 times daily	See Table 35-2
Hemoglobin A_{1c}	Every 3 mo	< 7.5%
Blood pressure	Every 3 mo	Less than 95th percentile for age
Blood lipid panel	Within 1 year after diagnosis (age 2 y and older); if normal, repeat q 5 y	LDL < 100 mg/dL (2.6 mmol/L), HDL > 35 mg/dL (0.9 mmol/L), Triglycerides < 150 mg/dL (1.7 mmol/L).
Urine microalbumin	Annually after 3-5 y of diabetes (age 10 y and older)	AER < 20 mcg/min A/C ratio < 30 mg/g
Ophthalmology referral	Annually after 3-5 y of diabetes (age 10 y and older)	Retinal photographs
Signs of other endocrinopathy	Evaluate thyroid at least annually; Autoantibody screening every 1-2 years	TSH: 0.5-5.0 IU/mL T4: 4.5-10 mcg/dL TPO Ab Transglutaminase IgA Ab 21-hydroxylase Ab

A/C, albumin/creatinine; TSH, thyroid-stimulating hormone; T4, thyroxine; TPO, thyroid peroxidase autoantibodies; LDL, low-density lipoprotein; HDL, high-density lipoprotein; AER, albumin excretion rate.

G. Prevention of Chronic Complications

Elevated HbA_{1c} predicts long-term microvascular and macrovascular complications. HbA_{1c} values ~7%, compared to values ~9%, result in greater than 50% reductions in the eye, kidney, cardiovascular, and neurologic complications of diabetes. Normal values vary among laboratories but are usually below 6.2%. In diabetes, the desired ranges are less than 7.5% in children and less than 7% in adults. Higher levels may be acceptable in younger children at risk of severe hypoglycemia. Low HbA_{1c} values are generally associated with a greater risk for hypoglycemia.

The HbA_{1c} level reflects the average blood glucose levels over the previous 3 months and should be measured every 3 months. However, in the DCCT, HbA_{1c} 7% (53 mmol/mol) corresponded to a higher average blood glucose concentration (measured seven times a day) of 192 mg/dL in the conventionally treated patients compared with 163 mg/dL in the intensively treated patients. HbA_{1c} can only be one of the measures of optimal glycemic control, along with hypoglycemia and quality of life.

The long-term prognosis of children diagnosed with T1D has improved tremendously over the past 20 years, primarily due to better control of blood glucose and blood pressure. While life expectancy is now only 3 years shorter in these patients, compared to the general population, the risk of cardiovascular disease is still 4–10 times higher, especially in diabetic women. A checklist of routine tests is presented in Table 35–3.

Elevated blood pressure is one of the strongest predictors of both micro- and macrovascular diseases and treatment of blood pressure is critical in reducing these complications in adults and presumably in children and adolescents as well. Blood pressure should be checked and reviewed at each clinic visit. Hypertension is defined as systolic or diastolic blood pressure (measured on at least 3 separate days) above the 95th percentile for the child's age, sex, and height. Care should be taken to ensure use of the appropriate size cuff in children to avoid inaccurate readings. If elevated blood pressure is confirmed, nondiabetic causes of hypertension should first be excluded. Angiotensin-converting enzyme inhibitors are the first-line agents; if not tolerated well, angiotensin II receptor blockers can be used.

Lipid profiles are generally favorable in children with T1D. The screening for dyslipidemia should commence after the age of 2 years and should be repeated every 5 years thereafter if normal. Good glycemic control should be established in newly diagnosed patients prior to screening, but it should not be delayed more than 1 year after diagnosis. Children with LDL levels 130–159 mg/dL (3.4–4.1 mmol/L) should obtain glucose control, dietary, and exercise counseling for 6 months with consideration of pharmacologic therapy if this fails; statin therapy in addition to diet and lifestyle changes are recommended if LDL is > 160 mg/dL (4.1 mmol/L). The treatment goals are LDL < 100 mg/dL (2.6 mmol/L), HDL > 35 mg/dL (0.9 mmol/L), and triglycerides < 150 mg/dL

(1.7 mmol/L). The use of lipid-lowering drugs in children has been the subject of much discussion. The American Heart Association recommends initiating therapy with statins at the lowest dose at age > 10 years in boys, Tanner stage II or higher, and preferably after menarche in girls.

Microalbuminuria is the first clinical manifestation of diabetic nephropathy and may be reversible with diligent glycemic and blood pressure control. Microalbuminuria is defined as: urinary albumin excretion rate between 20 and 200 mg/min or urinary albumin/creatinine ratio 2.5–25 mg/mmol or 30–300 mg/g (spot urine) in males and 3.5–25 mg/mmol in females. Screening for microalbuminuria with a random spot urine sample should occur annually in children once they are 10 years of age and have had diabetes for more than 3–5 years. If values are abnormal, borderline, or increasing, two timed overnight collections should occur and abnormal results should be repeated. The diagnosis of microalbuminuria requires documentation of 2 out of 3 abnormal samples over a period of 3–6 months. Once persistent microalbuminuria is confirmed, non-diabetic-related causes of renal disease should be excluded. Following this evaluation, treatment with an ACE inhibitor should be started, even if the blood pressure is normal. Patients should be counseled about the importance of glycemic control and smoking cessation, if applicable. Patients with type 2 diabetes should have microalbuminuria assessed soon after diagnosis and then annually.

The first dilated ophthalmologic examination should be obtained by an ophthalmologist or optometrist trained in diabetes-specific retinal examination once the child is ≥ 10 year old and has had diabetes for 3–5 years. The frequency of subsequent examination is generally every 1–2 years, depending on the patient risk profile and advice of the eye care provider. While rare in children, proliferative retinopathy does occur in adolescents with long duration and poor control of diabetes. Laser treatment to coagulate proliferating capillaries prevents bleeding and leakage of blood into the vitreous fluid or behind the retina. This treatment preserves useful vision.

Thyroid-stimulating hormone (TSH) level should be measured yearly in all patients. Thyroid peroxidase autoantibody (TPO) is usually the first test to become abnormal in the autoimmune thyroiditis present in up to 20% of children with type 1 diabetes. If TPO is positive, we recommend screening with TSH and free T4 every 6–12 months.

Transglutaminase autoantibodies offer a sensitive and specific screening test for celiac disease, present in up to 10% of children with T1D as well as in 3% of their siblings. Risk of celiac disease is most strongly associated with the HLA-DR3,DQ2 haplotype. We recommend routine screening for transglutaminase autoantibodies at diagnosis of diabetes and, if negative, re-testing every 1–2 year. About half of celiac disease cases develop several years after diagnosis of T1D. Most of the biopsy-confirmed cases are "asymptomatic" at the time of screening, but report improved health status upon initiation of gluten-free diet. Untreated celiac disease may lead to severe hypoglycemia, increased bone turnover, and decreased bone mineralization, among many other long-term complications.

The 21-hydroxylase autoantibody, a marker of increased risk of Addison disease, is present in approximately 1.3% of patients with type 1 diabetes, although Addison disease develops (usually slowly) in only about one-third of these antibody-positive individuals.

Acute Complications

A. Hypoglycemia

Hypoglycemia (or insulin reaction) is defined as a blood glucose level below 60 mg/dL (3.3 mmol/L). For preschool children, values below 70 mg/dL (3.9 mmol/L) should be cause for concern. The common symptoms of hypoglycemia are hunger, weakness, shakiness, sweating, drowsiness (at an unusual time), headache, and behavioral changes. In the DCCT study, 10% of patients with standard management and 25% of those with intensive insulin management had one or more severe hypoglycemic reactions each year. Children learn to recognize hypoglycemia at different ages but can often report "feeling funny" as young as age 4–5 years. School personnel, sports coaches, and baby-sitters must be trained to recognize and treat hypoglycemia. If low blood glucose is not treated immediately with simple sugar, the hypoglycemia may result in loss of consciousness and seizures; brain damage or death can occur with prolonged hypoglycemia.

Consistency in daily routine, correct insulin dosage, regular blood glucose monitoring, controlled snacking, compliance of patients and parents, and good education are all important in preventing severe hypoglycemia. In addition, insulin should not be injected prior to getting into a hot tub, bath, or shower. The heat will increase circulation to the skin and cause more rapid insulin uptake. The use of insulin analogs has helped to reduce the occurrence of hypoglycemia.

The treatment of mild hypoglycemia involves giving 4 oz of juice, a sugar-containing soda drink, or milk, and waiting 10 minutes. If the blood glucose level is still below 60 mg/dL (3.3 mmol/L), the liquids are repeated. If the glucose level is above 60 mg/dL, solid foods are given. Moderate hypoglycemia, in which the person is conscious but incoherent, can be treated by squeezing one-half tube of concentrated glucose (eg, Insta-Glucose or cake frosting) between the gums and lips and stroking the throat to encourage swallowing.

Families are advised to have glucagon in the home and in their travel pack to treat severe hypoglycemia by giving subcutaneous or intramuscular injections of 0.3 mL (30 units in an insulin syringe) for children younger than age 5 years, 0.5 mL (50 units) to those older than age 5 years, and 1 mL (100 units) to those heavier than 100 lb. Smaller doses of glucagon (2 units + number of units equal to the age of the child, eg, 2 + 10 = 12 units in a 10 year-old) can be used to prevent severe hypoglycemia during nondiabetic illness (gastroenteritis, respiratory infections).

Some patients, usually those who have had diabetes for more than 10 years or those tolerating routinely blood glucose 50–80 mg/dL, fail to recognize the symptoms of low blood glucose (hypoglycemic unawareness). For these individuals, glucose control must be liberalized to prevent severe hypoglycemia. The use of continuous glucose monitoring should be considered.

B. Sick Day and Diabetic Ketoacidosis (DKA)

Families must be educated to check blood or urine ketone levels during any illness (including vomiting even once) or any time a fasting blood glucose level is above 240 mg/dL (13.3 mmol/L), or a randomly measured glucose level is above 300 mg/dL (16.6 mmol/L). If moderate or significant ketonuria is detected, or the blood ketone (β-hydroxybutyrate—using the Precision Xtra meter) is above 1.0 mmol/L, the health care provider should be called. Usually 10%–20% of the total daily insulin dosage is given subcutaneously as rapid-acting analog or regular insulin every 3–4 hours until blood glucose normalizes. This prevents ketonuria and ketonemia from progressing to ketoacidosis and allows most patients to receive treatment at home by telephone management. Water is the oral fluid of choice if blood glucose is > 250 mg/dL; at lower levels of glycemia, one should switch to Gatorade/Poweraid.

Ketonuria/ketonemia secondary to fasting or acute gastrointestinal upset and associated with normal or low blood glucose does not require supplemental insulin treatment. Of note, the brain uses β-hydroxybutyrate as the alternate fuel to glucose in the setting of hypoglycemia. Overtreatment with insulin during a sick day that begins with hyperglycemia and ketosis may lead to loss of consciousness and/or seizures due to severe hypoglycemia.

Diabetic ketoacidosis

Acidosis (venous blood pH < 7.30 or bicarbonate < 15 mEq/L) is now present in up to 40% of newly diagnosed children in the United States. The clinical presentation of DKA includes abdominal pain, nausea, and vomiting that can mimic an acute abdomen. The patients are mildly to moderately dehydrated (5–10%), may have Kussmaul respiration, and become progressively somnolent and obtunded.

Acidosis may also occur in those with known diabetes who miss insulin injections, do not check blood or urine ketone levels, or fail to seek help when ketones are elevated. Repeated episodes of ketoacidosis signify that counseling may be indicated, and that a responsible adult must take over the diabetes management. If for any reason this is not possible, a change in the child's living situation may be necessary.

Treatment of diabetic ketoacidosis (DKA) is based on four physiologic principles: (1) restoration of fluid volume, (2) intravenous insulin to inhibit lipolysis and return to glucose utilization, (3) replacement of electrolytes, and (4) correction of acidosis. Mild DKA is defined as a venous blood pH of 7.2–7.3; moderate DKA, a pH of 7.10–7.19; and severe DKA, a pH below 7.10. Patients with severe DKA should be hospitalized in a pediatric intensive care unit, if available in the area. Laboratory tests at the start of treatment should include venous blood pH, glucose, and an electrolyte panel. More severe cases may benefit from determination of blood osmolality, calcium and phosphorus, and urea nitrogen levels. Severe and moderate episodes of DKA generally require hourly determinations of serum glucose, electrolytes, and venous pH levels, whereas these parameters can be measured every 2 hours if the pH level is 7.20–7.30.

1. Restoration of fluid volume—Dehydration is judged by estimated loss of body weight, dryness of oral mucous membranes, low blood pressure, and tachycardia. Initial treatment is with normal saline (0.9%), 10–20 mL/kg during the first hour (can be repeated in severely dehydrated patients during the second hour). The total volume of fluid in the first 4 hours of treatment should not exceed 20–40 mL/kg because of the danger of cerebral edema. After initial reexpansion, 0.45%–0.9% saline is given at 1.5 times maintenance to replace losses over 24–36 hours. When blood glucose level falls below 250 mg/dL (13.9 mmol/L), 5% dextrose is added to the intravenous fluids. If blood glucose level decreases below 120 mg/dL (6.6 mmol/L), 10% dextrose can be added.

2. Inhibition of lipolysis and return to glucose utilization—Insulin turns off fat breakdown and ketone formation. Regular insulin is given intravenously at a rate of 0.05–0.1 U/kg/h. The insulin solution should be administered by pump and can be made by diluting 30 units of regular insulin in 150 mL of 0.9% saline (1 U/5 mL). If necessary, the insulin dosage can be reduced, but it should not be discontinued before the venous blood pH reaches 7.30 and there is sufficient level of insulin from subcutaneous injections. The half-life of intravenous insulin is 6 minutes, whereas subcutaneous rapid-acting analog insulins take 10–15 minutes, and regular insulin takes 30–60 minutes, to begin activity. We recommend to continue intravenous insulin for at least 30 minutes after the initial subcutaneous insulin injection.

3. Replacement of electrolytes—In patients with DKA, both sodium and potassium pass into the urine and are depleted. In addition, serum sodium concentrations may be falsely lowered by hyperglycemia, causing water to be drawn into the intravenous space, and by hyperlipidemia if fat replaces some of the water in the serum used for electrolyte analysis. Sodium is usually replaced adequately by the use of 0.45%–0.9% saline in the rehydration fluids.

Serum potassium levels may be elevated initially because of inability of potassium to stay in the cell in the presence of acidosis (even though total body potassium is low). Potassium should not be given until the serum potassium level is known to be < 5.0 mEq/L and urine output is confirmed. It is then usually given at a concentration of 40 mEq/L, with half of the potassium (20 mEq/L) either as potassium acetate or potassium chloride and the other half as potassium phosphate (20 mEq/L). Hypocalcemia can occur if all of the potassium is given as the phosphate salt; hypophosphatemia occurs if none of the potassium is of the phosphate salt.

4. Correction of acidosis—Acidosis corrects spontaneously as the fluid volume is restored and insulin facilitates aerobic glycolysis are inhibits ketogenesis. Bicarbonate is not given, except for truly extreme situations.

5. Management of cerebral edema—Some degree of cerebral edema has been shown by computed tomography scan to be common in DKA. Associated clinical symptoms are rare, unpredictable, and may be associated with demise. Cerebral edema may be related to the degree of dehydration, cerebral hypoperfusion, acidosis, and hyperventilation at the time of presentation. In general, it is recommended that no more than 40 mL/kg of fluids be given in the first 4 hours of treatment and the following fluid replacement does not exceed 1.5 times maintenance. Cerebral edema is more common when the serum sodium is noted to be falling rather than rising. Early neurologic signs may include headache, excessive drowsiness, and dilated pupils. Prompt initiation of therapy should include elevation of the head of the bed, mannitol (1 g/kg over 30 minutes), and fluid restriction. If the cerebral edema is not recognized and treated early, over 50% of patients will die or have permanent brain damage.

In summary, modern diabetes care can lead to excellent health outcomes. Tremendous progress in biotechnology (insulin analogs), insulin pumps, and continuous glucose sensing has made the prevention of acute and long-term complications achievable. However, comprehensive and continuing education of patients and their families remains the foundation of healthy and quality life with diabetes.

REFERENCES

American Diabetes Association: Clinical practice recommendations. Diabetes Care 2009;32(Suppl 1):S13.

Chan C, Rewers M: Diabetes in Childhood. In Holt RIG, Cockram C, Flyvbjerg A, Goldstein BJ (editors): *Textbook of Diabetes*, 4th ed. Wiley-Blackwell 2010;859–874.

Dabelea D, Mayer-Davis EG: SEARCH for diabetes in youth study: The value of national diabetes registries. Imperatore Curr Diab Rep 2010;10:362–369.

Diabetes Control and Complications Trial/Epidemiology of Diabetes Interventions and Complications (DCCT/EDIC) Research Group: Modern-day clinical course of type 1 diabetes mellitus after 30 years' duration. Arch Intern Med 2009;169:1307.

Eisenbarth GS (editor): Type 1 Diabetes: Cellular, Molecular, & Clinical Immunology. http://www.barbaradaviscenter.org

ISPAD: Clinical Practice Consensus Guidelines 2009 Compendium. Pediatric Diabetes 2009;10(Suppl 12):1–210.

Monogenic Forms of Diabetes: Neonatal Diabetes Mellitus and Maturity-onset Diabetes of the Young. Available at: http://diabetes.niddk.nih.gov/pubs/mody

Rewers M, Gottlieb P: Immunotherapy for the prevention and treatment of type 1 diabetes: Human trials and a look into the future. Diabetes Care 2009;32:1769–1782.

Understanding Diabetes and Understanding Insulin Pumps and Continuous Glucose Monitors by H. Peter Chase. Available at: http://www.barbaradaviscenter.org

36 Inborn Errors of Metabolism

Janet A. Thomas, MD
Johan L.K. Van Hove, MD, PhD, MBA

Disorders in which single gene defects cause clinically significant blocks in metabolic pathways are called inborn errors of metabolism. Once considered rare, the number of recognized inborn errors has increased dramatically and they are now recognized to affect 1:1500 children. Many of these disorders can be treated effectively. Even when treatment is not available, correct diagnosis permits parents to make informed decisions about future offspring.

The pathology in metabolic disorders usually results from accumulation of enzyme substrate behind a metabolic block or deficiency of a reaction product. In some cases, the accumulated enzyme substrate is diffusible and has adverse effects on distant organs; in other cases, as in lysosomal storage diseases, the substrate primarily accumulates locally. The clinical manifestations of inborn errors vary widely with both mild and severe forms of virtually every disorder. Many patients do not match the classic phenotype because mutations are not identical in different patients, even though they occur in the same gene.

A first treatment strategy is to enhance the reduced enzyme activity. Gene replacement is a long-term goal, but problems of gene delivery to target organs and control of gene action make this an unrealistic option at present. Enzyme replacement therapy using intravenously administered recombinant enzyme has been developed as an effective strategy in lysosomal storage disorders. Organ transplantation (liver or bone marrow) can provide a source of enzyme for some conditions. Pharmacologic doses of a cofactor such as a vitamin can sometimes be effective in restoring enzyme activity. Residual activity can be increased by pharmacologically promoting transcription (transcriptional upregulation) or by stabilizing the protein product through therapy with chaperones. Alternatively, some strategies are designed to cope with the consequences of enzyme deficiency. Strategies used to avoid substrate accumulation include restriction of precursor in the diet (eg, low-phenylalanine diet for phenylketonuria), avoidance of catabolism, inhibition of an enzyme in the synthesis of the precursor (eg, NTBC in tyrosinemia type I (see Hereditary tyrosinemia), or removal of accumulated substrate pharmacologically (eg, glycine therapy for isovaleric acidemia) or by dialysis. An inadequately produced metabolite can also be supplemented (eg, glucose administration for glycogen storage disease type I).

Inborn errors can manifest at any time, can affect any organ system, and can mimic many common pediatric problems. This chapter focuses on when to consider metabolic disorder in the differential diagnosis of common pediatric problems. A few of the more important disorders are then discussed in detail.

DIAGNOSIS

SUSPECTING INBORN ERRORS

Inborn errors must be considered in the differential diagnosis of critically ill newborns, children with seizures, neurodegeneration, recurrent vomiting, Reye-like syndrome, parenchymal liver disease, cardiomyopathy, unexplained metabolic acidosis, hyperammonemia, and hypoglycemia. Mental retardation, developmental delay, and failure to thrive are often present, but have little specificity. Inborn errors should be suspected when (1) symptoms accompany changes in diet, (2) the child's development regresses, (3) the child shows specific food preferences or aversions, or (4) the family has a history of parental consanguinity or problems suggestive of inborn error such as retardation or unexplained deaths in first- and second-degree relatives.

Physical findings associated with inborn errors include alopecia or abnormal hair, retinal cherry-red spot or retinitis pigmentosa, cataracts or corneal opacity, hepatomegaly or splenomegaly, coarse features, skeletal changes (including gibbus), neurologic regression, and intermittent or progressive ataxia or dystonia. Other features that may be important in the context of a suspicious history include failure to thrive, microcephaly, rash, jaundice, hypotonia, and hypertonia.

Finding an immediate cause of symptoms does not rule out an underlying inborn error. For example, renal tubular acidosis and cirrhosis may be due to an underlying inborn error. Acute crises may be brought on by intercurrent infections in some inborn errors. Some inborn errors suggest a diagnosis of nonaccidental trauma (eg, glutaric acidemia type I) or poisoning (eg, methylmalonic acidemia). In addition, children with inborn errors may be at higher risk for child abuse or neglect because of their frustrating irritability.

LABORATORY STUDIES

Table 36–1 lists common clinical and laboratory features of different groups of inborn errors. Table 36–2 lists the most common laboratory tests used to diagnose these diseases and offers suggestions about their use.

Laboratory studies are almost always needed for the diagnosis of inborn errors. Serum electrolytes and pH should be used to estimate anion gap and acid-base status. Serum lactate, pyruvate, and ammonia levels are available in most hospitals, but care is needed in obtaining samples appropriately. Amino acid, acylcarnitine, and organic acid studies must be performed at specialized facilities to ensure accurate analysis and interpretation. An increasing number of inborn errors are diagnosed with DNA sequencing, but interpretation of private mutations, that is, mutations only seen in this particular family, can be problematic. Knowing the causative mutation in the family allows prenatal diagnosis to be done by molecular analysis. This can be done on any material that contains fetal DNA such as chorionic villi, amniotic cells, or fetal blood obtained through umibilical cord blood sampling.

The physician should know what conditions a test can detect and when it can detect them. For example, urine organic acids may be normal in patients with medium-chain acyl-CoA dehydrogenase deficiency or biotinidase deficiency; glycine may be elevated only in cerebrospinal fluid (CSF) in patients with glycine encephalopathy. A result that is normal in one physiologic state may be abnormal in another. For instance, the urine of a child who becomes hypoglycemic upon prolonged fasting should be positive for ketones. In such a child, the absence of ketones in the urine suggests a defect in fatty acid oxidation.

Samples used to diagnose metabolic disease may be obtained at autopsy. Samples must be obtained in a timely fashion and may be analyzed directly or stored frozen until a particular analysis is justified by the results of postmortem examination, new clinical information, or developments in the field. Studies of other family members may help establish the diagnosis of a deceased patient. It may be possible to demonstrate that parents are heterozygous carriers of a particular disorder or that a sibling has the condition.

COMMON CLINICAL SITUATIONS

1. Mental Retardation

Some inborn errors can cause mental retardation without other distinguishing characteristics. Measurements of serum amino acids, urine organic acids, and serum uric acid should be obtained in every patient with nonspecific mental retardation. Urine screens for mucopolysaccharides and succinylpurines, and serum testing for carbohydrate-deficient glycoproteins are useful because these disorders do not always have specific physical findings. Absent speech can point to disorders of creatine. Abnormalities of the brain detected by magnetic resonance imaging can suggest specific groups of disorders (eg, cortical migrational abnormalities in peroxisomal biogenesis disorders).

2. Acute Presentation in the Neonate

Acute metabolic disease in the neonate is most often a result of disorders of protein or carbohydrate metabolism and may be clinically indistinguishable from sepsis. Prominent symptoms include poor feeding, vomiting, altered mental status or muscle tone, jitteriness, seizures, and jaundice. Acidosis, alkalosis, or altered mental status out of proportion to systemic symptoms should increase suspicion of a metabolic disorder. Laboratory measurements should include electrolytes, ammonia, lactate, glucose, blood pH, and urine ketones and reducing substances. Amino acids in CSF should be measured if glycine encephalopathy is suspected. Serum and urine amino acid, urine organic acid, and serum acylcarnitine analysis should be performed urgently. Neonatal cardiomyopathy or ventricular arrhythmias should be investigated with serum acylcarnitine analysis.

3. Vomiting & Encephalopathy in the Infant or Older Child

Electrolytes, ammonia, glucose, urine pH, urine reducing substances, and urine ketones should be measured in all patients with vomiting and encephalopathy before any treatment affects the results. Samples for serum amino acids, serum acylcarnitine profile, and urine organic acid analysis should be obtained early. In the presentation of a Reye-like syndrome (ie, vomiting, encephalopathy, and hepatomegaly), amino acids, acylcarnitines, carnitine levels, and organic acids should be assessed immediately. Hypoglycemia with inappropriately low urine or serum ketones suggests the diagnosis of fatty acid oxidation defects.

4. Hypoglycemia

Duration of fasting, presence or absence of hepatomegaly, and Kussmaul breathing provide clues to the differential diagnosis of hypoglycemia. Serum insulin, cortisol, and growth

Table 36–1. Presenting clinical and laboratory features of inborn errors.

	Defects of Carbohydrate Metabolism	Defects of Amino Acid Metabolism†	Organic Acid Disorders¶	Defects of Fatty Acid Oxidation	Defects of Purine Metabolism	Lysosomal Storage Diseases	Disorders of Peroxisomes	Disorders of Energy Metabolism
Neurodevelopmental								
Mental/developmental retardation	+	+++	+++	–	++	+++	+++	+++
Developmental regression	–	–	+	–	+	+++	+++	+++
Acute encephalopathy	+++	+++	+++	+++	–	–	–	+
Seizures	+	+++	+++	+	–	+++	++	+++
Ataxia/movement disorder	–	+	++	–	+++	–	–	+++
Hypotonia	+	++	++	+++	–	+	+++	+++
Hypertonia	–	++	+++	–	++	+	–	++
Abnormal behavior	–	++	++	–	++	++	–	+
Growth								
Failure to thrive	+++	+++	+++	+	–	+	–	++
Short stature	++	–	+	–	–	++	–	++
Macrocephaly	–	–	+	–	–	++	++	–
Microcephaly	+	++	+++	–	–	+	–	++
General								
Vomiting/anorexia	++	+++	+++	+	–	–	++	+
Food aversion or craving	++	+++	+++	–	–	–	–	–
Odor	–	++	++	–	–	–	–	–
Dysmorphic features	–	+	+	–	–	++	++	–
Congenital malformations	–	++	++	–	–	–	++	+
Organ-specific								
Hepatomegaly	+++	–	++	+++	–	+++	+++	+
Liver disease/cirrhosis	++	+	–	+	–	–	+	++
Splenomegaly	–	–	–	–	–	++	+	–
Skeletal dysplasia	–	–	–	–	–	++	++	–
Cardiomyopathy	+	–	+	+++	–	++	–	+++
Tachypnea/hyperpnea	++	++	++	++	–	–	–	+
Rash	–	++	++	–	–	–	–	–
Alopecia or abnormal hair	–	+	++	–	–	–	+	–
Cataracts or corneal opacity	++	–	–	–	–	++	–	+
Retinal abnormality	–	+	+	+	–	++	++	++
Frequent infections	++	–	++	–	++	–	–	–
Deafness	–	–	+	–	–	++	–	+++

(*Continued*)

Table 36–1. Presenting clinical and laboratory features of inborn errors. (*Continued*)

	Defects of Carbohydrate Metabolism	Defects of Amino Acid Metabolism†	Organic Acid Disorders¶	Defects of Fatty Acid Oxidation	Defects of Purine Metabolism	Lysosomal Storage Diseases	Disorders of Peroxisomes	Disorders of Energy Metabolism
Laboratory								
Hypoglycemia	+++	+	++	+++	–	–	–	+
Hyperammonemia	–	++	++	++	–	–	–	–
Metabolic acidosis	++	++	+++	++	–	–	–	+++
Respiratory alkalosis	–	++	–	–	–	–	–	–
Elevated lactate/pyruvate	++	–	+++	++	–	–	–	+++
Elevated liver enzymes	++	++	++	+++	–	+	+	+
Neutropenia or thrombocytopenia	+	–	+	–	+	+	–	+
Hyperketosis	+++	++	+++	–	–	–	–	+
Hypoketosis	–	–	+	+++	–	–	–	–

†Includes disorders of the urea cycle but not maple syrup urine disease.
¶Includes maple syrup urine disease and disorders of pyruvate oxidation.
+++, most conditions in group; ++, some; +, one or few; –, not found.

Table 36–2. Obtaining and handling samples to diagnose inborn errors.

Test	Comments
Acid-base status	Accurate estimation of anion gap must be possible. Samples for blood gases should be kept on ice and analyzed immediately.
Blood ammonia	Sample should be kept on ice, and analyzed immediately, artefactual elevation common.
Blood lactic acid and pyruvic acid	Sample should be collected without a tourniquet, kept on ice, and analyzed immediately. Conversion of lactic to pyruvic acid must be prevented. Normal values are for the fasting, rested state, with postprandial values 50% higher.
Amino acids	Blood and urine should be examined. CSF amino acids should be measured for encephalopathies such as non-ketotic hyperglycinemia. Normal values are for the fasting state. Growth of bacteria in urine should be prevented.
Organic acids	Urine preferred for analysis. Serum or CSF organic acids are rarely indicated and often miss diagnoses.
Carnitine and acylcarnitine profile	Blood or plasma may be analyzed for total, free, and esterified carnitine; normal values are for the healthy, nonfasted state. Acylcarnitine profile in blood identifies compounds esterified to carnitine. Rarely urine and bile studies may be needed. Profiling in cultured fibroblasts after fat loading can be helpful in diagnosis of certain conditions.
Urine mucopolysaccharides	Variations in urine protein concentration may cause errors in screening tests. Diagnosis requires knowing which mucopolysaccharides are increased. Some patients with Morquio disease and many with Sanfilippo disease do not have abnormal mucopolysacchariduria.
Enzyme assays	Specific assays must be requested. Exposure to heat may cause loss of enzyme activity. Enzyme activity in whole blood may become normal after transfusion or vitamin therapy. Leukocyte or fibroblast pellets should be kept frozen prior to assays. Fibroblasts may be grown from skin biopsies taken up to 72 h after death. Tissues such as muscle, liver, and kidney should be taken as soon as possible after death (< 2 h), frozen immediately, and kept at −70°C until assayed.

CSF, cerebrospinal fluid.

hormone should be obtained on presentation. Urine ketones, urine organic acids, plasma lactate, serum acylcarnitine profile, carnitine levels, ammonia, and uric acid should be measured. Ketone body production is usually not efficient in the neonate, and ketonuria in a hypoglycemic or acidotic neonate suggests an inborn error. In the older child, inappropriately low urine ketone levels suggest an inborn error of fatty acid oxidation. Assessment of ketone generation requires simultaneous measurements of quantitative serum 3-hydroxybutyrate, acetoacetate, and free fatty acids in relation to a sufficient duration of fasting and age. Metabolites obtained during the acute episode can be very helpful and avoid the need for a formal fasting test.

5. Hyperammonemia

Symptoms of hyperammonemia may appear and progress rapidly or insidiously. Decreased appetite, irritability, and behavioral changes appear first with vomiting, ataxia, lethargy, seizures, and coma appearing as ammonia levels increase. Tachypnea inducing respiratory alkalosis due to a direct effect on respiratory drive is characteristic. Physical examination cannot exclude the presence of hyperammonemia, and serum ammonia should be measured whenever hyperammonemia is possible. Severe hyperammonemia may be due to urea cycle disorders, organic acidemias, or fatty acid oxidation disorders (such as carnitine-acylcarnitine translocase deficiency) or, in the premature infant, transient hyperammonemia of the newborn. The cause can usually be ascertained by measuring quantitative serum amino acids (eg, citrulline), plasma carnitine and acylcarnitine esters, and urine organic acids and orotic acid. Respiratory alkalosis is usually present in urea cycle defects and transient hyperammonemia of the newborn, while acidosis is characteristic of hyperammonemia due to organic acidemias.

6. Acidosis

Inborn errors may cause chronic or acute acidosis at any age, with or without an increased anion gap. Inborn errors should be considered when acidosis occurs with recurrent vomiting or hyperammonemia and when acidosis is out of proportion to the clinical status. Acidosis due to an inborn error can be difficult to correct. The main causes of anion gap metabolic acidosis are lactic acidosis, ketoacidosis (including abnormal ketone body production such as in β-ketothiolase deficiency), methylmalonic aciduria or other organic acidurias, intoxication (ethanol, methanol, ethylene glycol, and salicylate), and uremia. Causes of non–anion gap metabolic acidosis include loss of base in diarrhea or renal tubular acidosis (isolated renal tubular acidosis or renal Fanconi syndrome). If renal bicarbonate loss is found, then a distinction must be made between isolated renal tubular acidosis and a more generalized renal tubular disorder or renal Fanconi syndrome by testing for renal losses of phosphorus and amino acids. Inborn errors associated with renal tubular acidosis or renal Fanconi syndrome include cystinosis, tyrosinemia type I, carnitine palmitoyltransferase I, galactosemia, hereditary fructose intolerance, Lowe syndrome, and mitochondrial diseases. Serum glucose and ammonia levels and urinary pH and ketones should be examined. Samples for amino acids and organic acids should be obtained at once and may be evaluated immediately or frozen for later analysis, depending on how strongly an inborn error is suspected. It is useful to test blood lactate and pyruvate levels in the chronically acidotic patient even if urine organic acid levels are normal. Lactate and pyruvate levels are difficult to interpret in the acutely ill patient, but in the absence of shock, high levels of lactic acid suggest primary lactic acidosis.

MANAGEMENT OF METABOLIC EMERGENCIES

Patients with severe acidosis, hypoglycemia, and hyperammonemia may be very ill; initially mild symptoms may worsen quickly, and coma and death may ensue within hours. With prompt and vigorous treatment, however, patients can recover completely, even from deep coma. All oral intake should be stopped. Sufficient glucose should be given intravenously to avoid or minimize catabolism in a patient with a known inborn error who is at risk for crisis. Most conditions respond favorably to glucose administration, although a few (eg, primary lactic acidosis due to pyruvate dehydrogenase deficiency) do not. After exclusion of fatty acid oxidation disorders, immediate institution of intravenous fat emulsions (eg, intralipid) can provide crucial caloric input. Severe or increasing hyperammonemia should be treated pharmacologically or with dialysis (see Disorders of the Urea Cycle), and severe acidosis should be treated with bicarbonate. More specific measures can be instituted when a diagnosis is established.

NEWBORN SCREENING

Criteria for screening newborns for a disorder include its frequency, its consequences if untreated, the ability of therapy to mitigate consequences, the cost of testing, and the cost of treatment. With the availability of tandem mass spectrometry, newborn screening has expanded greatly to now include 20 core conditions and multiple secondary conditions screened by most states. In general, amino acidopathies, organic acidurias, and disorders of fatty acid oxidation are the disorders for which screening now occurs. Most states also screen for hypothyroidism, congenital adrenal hyperplasia, hemoglobinopathies, biotinidase deficiency, galactosemia, and cystic fibrosis. Screening for severe combined immune deficiency has been recently added. Screening should occur for all infants between 24 and 72 hours of life or before hospital discharge.

Some screening tests measure a metabolite (eg, phenylalanine) that becomes abnormal with time and exposure to diet. In such instances, the disease cannot be detected reliably until intake of the substrate is established. Other tests measure enzyme activity and can be performed at any time (eg, for biotinidase deficiency). Transfusions may cause false-negative results in this instance, and exposure of the sample to heat may cause false-positive results. Technologic advances have extended the power of newborn screening but have brought additional challenges. For example, although tandem mass spectrometry can detect many more disorders in the newborn period, consensus on diagnosis and treatment for some conditions is still under development.

Screening tests are not diagnostic, and diagnostic tests must be undertaken when an abnormal screening result is obtained. Further, because false-negative results occur, a normal newborn screening test does not rule out a condition.

The appropriate response to an abnormal screening test depends on the condition in question and the predictive value of the test. For example, when screening for galactosemia by enzyme assay, complete absence of enzyme activity is highly predictive of classic galactosemia. Failure to treat may rapidly lead to death. In this case, treatment must be initiated immediately while diagnostic studies are pending. In phenylketonuria, however, a diet restricted in phenylalanine is harmful to the infant whose screening test is a false-positive, while diet therapy produces an excellent outcome in the truly affected infant if treatment is established within the first weeks of life. Therefore, treatment for phenylketonuria should only be instituted when the diagnosis is confirmed. Physicians should review American College of Medical Genetics recommendations, state laws and regulations, and consult with their local metabolic center to arrive at appropriate strategies for each hospital and practice.

Dietzen DJ et al: National academy of clinical biochemistry laboratory medicine practice guidelines: Follow-up testing for metabolic disease identified by expanded newborn screening using tandem mass spectrometry; executive summary. ClinChem 2009;55:1615 [PMID: 19574465].

Garcia-Cazorla A et al: Mental retardation and inborn errors of metabolism. J Inherit Metab Dis 2009;32:597 [PMID: 19685154].

Garcia-Cazorla A et al: Inborn errors of metabolism and motor disturbances in children. J Inherit Metab Dis 2009;32:618 [PMID: 19731074].

Levy PA: An overview of newborn screening. J Dev Behav Pediatr 2010;31:622 [PMID: 20814260].

Lindner M et al: Efficacy and outcome of expanded newborn screening for metabolic diseases: Report of 10 years from South-West Germany. Orphanet J Rare Dis 2011;6:44 [PMID: 21689452].

Van Hove JL et al: Acute nutrition management in the prevention of metabolic illness: A practical approach with glucose polymers. Mol Genet Metab 2009;97:1 [PMID: 19367873].

Wolf et al: Epilepsy and inborn errors of metabolism in children. J Inherit Metab Dis 2009;32:609 [PMID: 19642011].

DISORDERS OF CARBOHYDRATE METABOLISM

GLYCOGEN STORAGE DISEASES

ESSENTIALS OF DIAGNOSIS & TYPICAL FEATURES

- Types 0, I, III, VI, and IX manifest with hypoglycemia in infants.
- Types II, V, and VII manifest with rhabdomyolysis or muscle weakness.
- Types IV and IX manifest with hepatic cirrhosis.

Glycogen is a highly branched polymer of glucose that is stored in liver and muscle. Different enzyme defects affect its biosynthesis and degradation. The hepatic forms of the glycogenoses cause growth failure, hepatomegaly, and severe fasting hypoglycemia. They include glucose-6-phosphatase deficiency (type I; von Gierke disease), debrancher enzyme deficiency (type III), hepatic phosphorylase deficiency (type VI), and phosphorylase kinase deficiency (type IX), which normally regulates hepatic phosphorylase activity. Glycogen synthase deficiency (GSD0) causes hypoglycemia usually after about 12 hours fasting, and can cause mild postprandial hyperglycemia and hyperlactatemia. There are two forms of glucose-6-phosphatase deficiency: in type Ia, the catalytic glucose-6-phosphatase is deficient, and in type Ib, the glucose-6-phosphate transporter is deficient. The latter form also has neutropenia. Glycogenosis type IV, brancher enzyme deficiency, usually presents with progressive liver cirrhosis, as well as some rare forms of phosphorylase kinase deficiency.

The myopathic forms of glycogenosis affect skeletal muscle. Skeletal myopathy with weakness or rhabdomyolysis may be seen in muscle phosphorylase deficiency (type V), phosphofructokinase deficiency (type VII), and acid maltase deficiency (type II; Pompe disease). The infantile form of Pompe disease also has hypertrophic cardiomyopathy and macroglossia. The gluconeogenetic disorder fructose-1,6-bisphosphatase deficiency presents with major lactic acidosis and delayed hypoglycemia on fasting.

Diagnosis

Initial tests include glucose, lactate, triglycerides, cholesterol, uric acid, transaminases, and creatine kinase. Functional testing includes responsiveness of blood glucose and lactate to fasting; for myopathic forms, an ischemic exercise test is helpful. Most glycogenoses can now be diagnosed by molecular analysis. Other diagnostic studies include enzyme assays of leukocytes, fibroblasts, liver, or muscle. Disorders diagnosable from analysis of red or white blood cells include deficiency of debrancher enzyme (type III) and phosphorylase kinase (type IX). Pompe disease can usually be diagnosed by assaying acid maltase in a blood spot with confirmation in fibroblasts.

Treatment

Treatment is designed to prevent hypoglycemia and avoid secondary metabolite accumulations such as elevated lactate in glycogenosis type I. In the most severe hepatic forms, the special diet must be strictly monitored with restriction of free sugars and measured amounts of uncooked cornstarch, which slowly releases glucose in the intestinal lumen. Good results have been reported following continuous nighttime carbohydrate feeding or uncooked cornstarch therapy. Late complications even after years of treatment include focal segmental glomerulosclerosis, hepatic adenoma or carcinoma, and gout. Enzyme replacement therapy in Pompe disease corrects the cardiomyopathy, but the response in skeletal myopathy is variable with optimal results seen in patients treated early and who have mutations that allow formation of some residual protein which is detected as cross-reacting material on Western blotting. Immunomodulation is used for patients whose treatment response declines due to antibodies to the recombinant enzyme.

Bhattacharya K: Dietary dilemmas in the management of glycogen storage disease type 1. J Inherit Metab Dis 2011;34:621 [PMID: 21491105].

Chou JY et al: Glycogen storage disease type I and G6Pase-β deficiency: Etiology and therapy. Nat Rev Endocrinol 2010;6:676 [PMID: 20975743].

Kishnani PS et al: Glycogen storage disease type III diagnosis and management guidelines. Genet Med 2010;12:446 [PMID: 20631546].

Quinlivan R et al: Pharmacological and nutritional treatment for McArdle disease (glycogen storage disease type V). Cochrane Database Syst Rev 2010;12:CD003458 [PMID: 21154353].

Rake JP et al: Guidelines for management of glycogen storage disease type I—European Study on Glycogen Storage Disease Type I (ESGSD I). Eur J Pediatr 2002;161(Suppl 1):S112 [PMID: 12373584].

Visser G et al: Consensus guidelines for management of glycogen storage disease type 1b—European Study on Glycogen Storage Disease Type 1. Eur J Pediatr 2002;161(Suppl 1):S120 [PMID: 12373585].

Patient and parent support group web site with useful information for families: Available at: http://www.agsdus.org

GALACTOSEMIA

ESSENTIALS OF DIAGNOSIS & TYPICAL FEATURES

- Severely deficient neonates present with vomiting, jaundice, and hepatomegaly on initiation of lactose-containing feedings.
- Renal Fanconi syndrome, cataracts of the ocular lens, hepatic cirrhosis, and sepsis occur in untreated children.
- Delayed, apraxic speech and ovarian failure occur frequently even with treatment. Developmental delay, tremor, and ataxia occur less frequently.

Classic galactosemia is caused by almost total deficiency of galactose-1-phosphate uridyltransferase. Accumulation of galactose-1-phosphate causes hepatic parenchymal disease and renal Fanconi syndrome. Onset of the severe disease is marked in the neonate by vomiting, jaundice (both direct and indirect), hepatomegaly, and rapid onset of liver insufficiency after initiation of milk feeding. Hepatic cirrhosis is progressive. Without treatment, death frequently occurs within a month, often from *Escherichia coli* sepsis. Cataracts usually develop within 2 months in untreated cases, but usually reverse with treatment. With prompt institution of a galactose-free diet, the prognosis for survival without liver disease is excellent. Even when dietary restriction is instituted early, patients with galactosemia are at increased risk for speech and language deficits and ovarian failure. Some patients develop progressive mental retardation, tremor, and ataxia. Milder variants of galactosemia with better prognosis exist.

The disorder is autosomal recessive with an incidence of approximately 1:40,000 live births.

Diagnosis

In infants receiving foods containing galactose, laboratory findings include liver dysfunction particularly PT prolongation, together with proteinuria and aminoaciduria. Absence of reducing substances in urine does not exclude the diagnosis. Galactose-1-phosphate is elevated in red blood cells. When the diagnosis is suspected, galactose-1-phosphate uridyltransferase should be assayed in erythrocytes. Blood transfusions give false-negative results and sample deterioration false-positive results.

Newborn screening by demonstrating enzyme deficiency in red cells with the Beutler test or by demonstrating increased serum galactose allows timely institution of treatment.

Treatment

A galactose-free diet should be instituted as soon as the diagnosis is made. Compliance with the diet must be monitored by following galactose-1-phosphate levels in red blood cells. Appropriate diet management requires not only the exclusion of milk but an understanding of the galactose content of foods. Avoidance of galactose should be life-long with appropriate calcium replacement, intake of which tends to be low due to the restriction of dairy products.

Fridovich-Keil, JL et al: Ovarian function in girls and women with GALT-deficiency galactosemia. J Inherit Metab Dis 2011;34:357 [PMID: 20978943].

Hoffmann B et al: Cross-sectional analysis of speech and cognitive performance in 32 patients with classic galactosemia. J Inherit Metab Dis 2011;34:421 [PMID: 21347587].

Ridel KR et al: An updated review of the long-term neurological effects of galactosemia. Pediatr Neurol 2005;33:153 [PMID: 16087312].

Patient and parent support group web site with useful information for families: Available at: http://www.galactosemia.org

HEREDITARY FRUCTOSE INTOLERANCE

Hereditary fructose intolerance is an autosomal recessive disorder in which deficient activity of fructose-1-phosphate aldolase causes hypoglycemia and tissue accumulation of fructose-1-phosphate on fructose ingestion. Other abnormalities include failure to thrive, vomiting, jaundice, hepatomegaly, proteinuria, and renal Fanconi syndrome. The untreated condition can progress to death from liver failure.

Diagnosis

The diagnosis is suggested by finding fructosuria or an abnormal transferrin glycoform in the untreated patient. Diagnosis is made by sequencing the HFI gene. An alternative method for diagnosis is enzyme assay of fructose-1-phosphate aldolase in liver biopsy.

Treatment

Treatment consists of strict dietary avoidance of fructose. Vitamin supplementation is usually needed. Drugs and vitamins dispensed in a sucrose base should be avoided. Treatment monitoring can be done with transferrin glycoform analysis. If diet compliance is poor, physical growth retardation may occur. Growth will resume when more stringent dietary restrictions are reinstituted. If the disorder is recognized early, the prospects for normal development are good. As affected individuals grow up, they may recognize the association of nausea and vomiting with ingestion of fructose-containing foods and selectively avoid them.

Wong D: Hereditary fructose intolerance. Mol Genet Metab 2005;85:165 [PMID: 16086449].

Web site with useful information for families: http://www.bu.edu/aldolase

DISORDERS OF ENERGY METABOLISM

The most common disorders of central mitochondrial energy metabolism are pyruvate dehydrogenase deficiency and deficiencies of respiratory chain components. Disorders of the Krebs cycle include deficiencies in fumarase, 2-ketoglutarate dehydrogenase, and succinyl-CoA ligase. In many, but not all patients, lactate is elevated in either blood or CSF. In pyruvate dehydrogenase deficiency, the lactate-pyruvate ratio is normal, whereas in respiratory chain disorders, the ratio is often increased. Care must be taken to distinguish an elevated lactate level that is due to these conditions (called primary lactic acidoses) from elevated lactate that is a consequence of hypoxia, ischemia, or sampling problems. Table 36–3 lists some causes of primary lactic acidosis.

Patients with a defect in the pyruvate dehydrogenase complex often have agenesis of the corpus callosum or Leigh syndrome (lesions in the globus pallidus, dentate nucleus, and periaqueductal gray matter). They can have mild facial dysmorphism. Recurrent altered mental status, recurrent ataxia, and recurrent acidosis are typical of many disturbances of pyruvate metabolism. The most common genetic defect is in the X-linked E_1-α component, with males carrying milder mutations and females carrying severe mutations leading to periventricular cystic brain lesions.

The respiratory chain disorders are frequent (1:5000), and involve a heterogenous group of genetic defects that produce a variety of clinical syndromes (now > 50) of varying severity and presentation. The disorders can affect multiple organs. The following set of symptoms (not intended as a comprehensive listing) can indicate a respiratory chain disorder:

1. General: Failure to thrive
2. Brain: Progressive neurodegeneration, Leigh syndrome, myoclonic seizures, brain atrophy, and subcortical leukodystrophy
3. Eye: Optic neuropathy, retinitis pigmentosa, and progressive external ophthalmoplegia

Table 36–3. Causes of primary lactic acidosis in childhood.

Defects of the pyruvate dehydrogenase complex
E_1 (pyruvate decarboxylase) deficiency
E_2 (dihydrolipoyl transacetylase) deficiency
E_3 (lipoamide dehydrogenase) deficiency
E3-binding protein X deficiency
Pyruvate decarboxylase phosphate phosphatase deficiency
Abnormalities of gluconeogenesis
Pyruvate carboxylase deficiency
Isolated
Biotinidase deficiency
Holocarboxylase synthetase deficiency
Fructose-1,6-diphosphatase deficiency
Glucose-6-phosphatase deficiency (von Gierke disease)
Defects in the mitochondrial respiratory chain
Complex I deficiency
Complex IV deficiency (cytochrome C oxidase deficiency; frequent cause of Leigh disease)
Complex V (ATPase) deficiency (frequent cause of Leigh disease)
Complex II deficiency
Complex III deficiency
Combined deficiencies: due to defects in mitochondrial DNA maintenance (deletions or depletion) or in mitochondrial translation (eg, mitochondrial tRNA defects)
Coenzyme Q10 deficiency
Other respiratory chain disorders
Defects in the Krebs cycle
Succinyl-CoA ligase deficiency

4. Ears: Nerve deafness
5. Muscle: Myopathy with decreased endurance or rhabdomyolysis
6. Kidney: Renal Fanconi syndrome, proteinuria (in CoQ deficiency)
7. Endocrine: Diabetes mellitus and hypoparathyroidism
8. Intestinal: Pancreatic or liver insufficiency or pseudoobstruction
9. Skin: Areas of hypopigmentation
10. Heart: Cardiomyopathy, conduction defects, and arrhythmias

Respiratory chain disorders are among the more common causes of static, progressive, or self-limited neurodevelopmental problems in children. Patients may present with nonspecific findings such as hypotonia, failure to thrive, or renal tubular acidosis, or with more specific features such as ophthalmoplegia or cardiomyopathy. Symptoms are often combined in recognizable clinical syndromes with ties to specific genetic causes. Ragged red fibers and mitochondrial abnormalities may be noted on histologic examination of muscle. Thirteen of the more than 100 genes that control activity of the respiratory chain are part of the mitochondrial genome. Therefore, inheritance of defects in the respiratory chain may be mendelian or maternal.

Diagnosis

Pyruvate dehydrogenase deficiency is diagnosed by enzyme assay in leukocytes or fibroblasts. Confirmation can be obtained by molecular analysis. Diagnosis of respiratory chain disorders is based on a convergence of clinical, biochemical, morphologic, enzymatic, and molecular data. Classic pathologic features of mitochondrial disorders are the accumulation of mitochondria, which produces ragged red fibers in skeletal muscle biopsy, and abnormal mitochondrial shapes and inclusions inside mitochondria on electron microscopy. However, these findings are only present in 5% of children. Enzyme analysis on skeletal muscle or liver tissue is complicated by an overlap between normal and affected range. Blue native PAGE analyzes the assembly of the respiratory chain enzyme complexes. Mitochondrial DNA analysis in blood or tissue may identify a diagnostic mutation. A rapidly increasing number of nuclear genes (now > 100) causing respiratory chain defects are recognized. Children with defects in mtDNA maintenance (such as mitochondrial DNA polymerase γ, *POLG1* gene) often present with liver disease and neurodegeneration and are diagnosed by sequencing the causative nuclear genes. Although diagnostic criteria have been published, the cause of respiratory chain defects still cannot be defined in many patients. In some instances, the genetics and prognosis may be clear, but in many cases neither prognosis nor genetic risk can be predicted. Due to the high complexity of this group of disorders, many patients require a high degree of expertise and multiple studies to arrive at a final diagnosis.

Treatment

A ketogenic diet is useful in pyruvate dehydrogenase deficiency. In rare patients with primary coenzyme Q deficiency, coenzyme Q treatment is very effective. Other treatments are of theoretical value, with little data on efficacy. Thiamine and lipoic acid have been tried in patients with pyruvate dehydrogenase complex deficiencies, and coenzyme Q and riboflavin have been helpful in some patients with respiratory chain defects. Dichloroacetic acid has limited clinical response in pyruvate dehydrogenase deficiency and has adverse effects. Transcriptional upregulation in partial deficiencies of nuclear origin offers new hope for the treatment of respiratory chain defects.

Blok MJ et al: The unfolding clinical spectrum of POLG mutations. J Med Genet 2009;46:776 [PMID: 19578034].

Kisler JE et al: Mitochondrial disease in childhood: A clinical approach to investigation and management. Dev Med Child Neurol 2010;52:422 [PMID: 20163433].

Marin-Valencia I et al: Pyruvate carboxylase deficiency: Mechanisms, mimics and anaplerosis. Mol Genet Metab 2010;101:9 [PMID: 20598931].

Schon EA et al: Therapeutic prospects for mitochondrial disease. Trends Mol Med 2010;16:268 [PMID: 20556877].

Tucker EJ et al: Recent advances in the genetics of mitochondrial encephalopathies. Curr Neurol Neurosci Rep 2010;10:277 [PMID: 20446063].

Wong LJ et al: Current molecular diagnostic algorithm for mitochondrial disorders. Mol Genet Metab 2010;100:111 [PMID: 20359921].

Patient and parent support group web site with useful information for families: http://www.umdf.org

DISORDERS OF AMINO ACID METABOLISM

DISORDERS OF THE UREA CYCLE

Ammonia is derived from the catabolism of amino acids and is converted to an amino group in urea by enzymes of the urea cycle. Patients with severe defects (often those enzymes early in the urea cycle) usually present in infancy with severe hyperammonemia, vomiting, and encephalopathy, which is rapidly fatal. Patients with milder genetic defects may present with vomiting and encephalopathy after increased protein ingestion or infection. Although defects in argininosuccinic acid synthetase (citrullinemia) and argininosuccinic acid lyase (argininosuccinic acidemia) may cause severe hyperammonemia in infancy, the usual clinical course is chronic with mental retardation. Ornithine transcarbamylase deficiency is X-linked; the others are autosomal recessive. Age at onset of symptoms varies with residual enzyme activity, protein intake, growth, and stresses such as infection.

Even within a family, males with ornithine transcarbamylase deficiency may differ by decades in the age of symptom onset. Many female carriers of ornithine transcarbamylase deficiency have protein intolerance. Some develop migraine-like symptoms after protein loads, and others develop potentially fatal episodes of vomiting and encephalopathy after protein ingestion, infections, or during labor and delivery. Trichorrhexis nodosa is common in patients with argininosuccinic aciduria.

Diagnosis

Blood ammonia should be measured in any acutely ill newborn in whom a cause is not obvious. In urea cycle defects, early hyperammonemia is associated with hyperventilation and respiratory alkalosis. Serum citrulline is low or undetectable in carbamoyl phosphate synthetase and ornithine transcarbamylase deficiency, high in argininosuccinic acidemia, and very high in citrullinemia. Large amounts of argininosuccinic acid are found in the urine of patients with argininosuccinic acidemia. Urine orotic acid is increased in infants with ornithine transcarbamylase deficiency. Citrullinemia and argininosuccinic acidemia can be diagnosed in utero by appropriate enzyme assays in uncultured CVS material or in amniocytes, but carbamoyl phosphate synthetase and ornithine transcarbamylase deficiency can be diagnosed in utero only by molecular methods.

Treatment

During treatment of acute hyperammonemic crisis, protein intake should be stopped, and glucose and lipids should be given to reduce endogenous protein breakdown from catabolism. Arginine is given intravenously. It is an essential amino acid for patients with urea cycle defects and increases the excretion of waste nitrogen in citrullinemia and argininosuccinic acidemia. Sodium benzoate and sodium phenylacetate are given intravenously to increase excretion of nitrogen as hippuric acid and phenylacetylglutamine. Additionally, hemodialysis or hemofiltration is indicated for severe or persistent hyperammonemia, as is usually the case in the newborn. Peritoneal dialysis and exchange transfusion are ineffective. Long-term treatment includes low-protein diet, oral administration of arginine or citrulline, and sodium benzoate or sodium phenylbutyrate (a prodrug of sodium phenylacetate). Symptomatic heterozygous female carriers of ornithine transcarbamylase deficiency should also receive such treatment. Liver transplantation may be curative and is indicated for patients with severe disorders.

The outcome of urea cycle disorders depends on the genetic severity of the condition (residual activity) and the severity and prompt treatment of hyperammonemic episodes. Many patients with urea cycle defects, no matter what the enzyme defect, develop permanent neurologic and intellectual impairments, with cortical atrophy and ventricular dilation seen on computed tomographic scan. Rapid identification and treatment of the initial hyperammonemic episode improves outcome.

Braissant O: Current concepts in the pathogenesis of urea cycle disorders. Mol Genet Metab 2010;100(Suppl 1):S3 [PMID: 20227314].

Enns G: Nitrogen sparing therapy revisited 2009. Mol Genet Metab 2010;100(Suppl 1):S65 [PMID: 20202877].

Meyburg J, Hoffmann GF: Liver, liver cell and stem cell transplantation for the treatment of urea cycle defects. Mol Genet Metab 2010;100(Suppl 1):S77 [PMID: 20156696].

Scaglia F: New insights in nutritional management and amino acid supplementation in urea cycle disorders. Mol Genet Metab 2010;100(Suppl 1):S72 [PMID: 20299258].

Summar ML et al: Diagnosis, symptoms, frequency and mortality of 260 patients with urea cycle disorders from a 21-year, multicentre study of acute hyperammonaemic episodes. Acta Paediatr 2008;97:1420 [PMID: 18647279].

Patient and parent support group web site with useful information for families: http://www.nucdf.org

Urea Cycle Disorders Consortium: http://rarediseasesnetwork.epi.usf.edu/ucdc/about/index.htm

PHENYLKETONURIA & THE HYPERPHENYLALANINEMIAS

ESSENTIALS OF DIAGNOSIS & TYPICAL FEATURES

- Mental retardation, hyperactivity, seizures, light complexion, and eczema characterize untreated patients.
- Newborn screening for elevated serum phenylalanine identifies most infants.
- Disorders of cofactor metabolism also produce elevated serum phenylalanine level.
- Early diagnosis and treatment with phenylalanine-restricted diet prevents mental retardation.

Probably the best-known disorder of amino acid metabolism is the classic form of phenylketonuria caused by decreased activity of phenylalanine hydroxylase, the enzyme that converts phenylalanine to tyrosine. In classic phenylketonuria, there is little or no phenylalanine hydroxylase activity. In the less severe hyperphenylalaninemia there may be significant residual activity. Rare variants can be due to deficiency of dihydropteridine reductase or defects in biopterin synthesis.

Phenylketonuria is an autosomal recessive trait, with an incidence in Caucasians of approximately 1:10,000 live births. On a normal neonatal diet, affected patients develop hyperphenylalaninemia. Patients with untreated phenylketonuria exhibit severe mental retardation, hyperactivity, seizures, a light complexion, and eczema.

Success in preventing severe mental retardation in phenylketonuric children by restricting phenylalanine starting in early infancy led to screening programs to detect the disease early. Because the outcome is best when treatment is begun in the first month of life, infants should be screened during the first few days. A second test is necessary when newborn screening is done before 24 hours of age, and should be completed by the third week of life.

Diagnosis & Treatment

The diagnosis of phenylketonuria is based on finding elevated serum phenylalanine and an elevated phenylalanine/tyrosine ratio in a child on a normal diet. The condition must be differentiated from other causes of hyperphenylalaninemia by examining pterins in urine and dihydropteridine reductase activity in blood.

Determination of carrier status and prenatal diagnosis of phenylketonuria or pterin defects is possible using molecular methods.

A. Phenylalanine Hydroxylase Deficiency: Classic Phenylketonuria and Hyperphenylalaninemia

In phenylketonuria, serum phenylalanine levels are persistently elevated above 1200 μM (20 mg/dL) on a regular diet, with normal or low serum levels of tyrosine, and normal pterins. Poor phenylalanine tolerance persists throughout life. Treatment to decrease phenylalanine levels is always indicated. Hyperphenylalaninemia is diagnosed in infants whose serum phenylalanine levels are usually 240–1200 μM (4–20 mg/dL), and pterins are normal while receiving a normal protein intake. Treatment to reduce phenylalanine levels is indicated if phenylalanine levels consistently exceed 600 μM (10 mg/dL). In contrast, in the rare case of transient hyperphenylalaninemia, serum phenylalanine levels are elevated early, but progressively decline toward normal. Dietary restriction is only temporary, if required at all.

Treatment of all forms of phenylketonuria is aimed at maintaining phenylalanine levels less than 360 μM (6 mg/dL). Treatment can consist of dietary restriction of phenylalanine, increasing enzyme activity with pharmacologic doses of R-tetrahydrobiopterin, or new methods to interfere with phenylalaine absorption or to breakdown phenylalanine.

Dietary restriction of phenylalanine intake to amounts that permit normal growth and development is the most common therapy and results in good outcome if instituted in the first month of life and carefully maintained. Metabolic formulas deficient in phenylalanine are available but must be supplemented with normal milk and other foods to supply enough phenylalanine to permit normal growth and development. Serum phenylalanine concentrations must be monitored frequently while ensuring that growth, development, and nutrition are adequate. This monitoring is best done in experienced clinics. Children with classic phenylketonuria who receive treatment promptly after birth and achieve phenylalanine and tyrosine homeostasis will develop well physically and can be expected to have normal or near-normal intellectual development.

Phenylalanine restriction should continue throughout life. Patients who discontinued diet after treatment for several years have developed subtle changes in intellect and behavior, and risk neurologic damage. Counseling should be given during adolescence particularly to girls about the risk of maternal phenylketonuria (see below), and women's diets should be monitored closely prior to conception and throughout pregnancy. Late treatment may still be of benefit in reversing behaviors such as hyperactivity, irritability, and distractibility, but does not reverse the mental retardation.

Treatment with R-tetrahydrobiopterin results in improved phenylalanine tolerance in up to 60% of patients with a deficiency in phenylalanine hydroxylase. The best results and the most frequent responsiveness are seen in patients with hyperphenylalaninemia. Provision of high doses of large neutral amino acids results in a moderate reduction in phenylalanine and is used as an adjunctive treatment in some adults with phenylketonuria. Treatment trials with pegylated phenylalanine ammonia lyase administration to decrease phenylalanine levels show promise.

B. Biopterin Defects: Dihydropteridine Reductase Deficiency and Defects in Biopterin Biosynthesis

In these patients, serum phenylalanine levels vary. The pattern of pterin metabolites is abnormal. Clinical findings include myoclonus, tetraplegia, dystonia, oculogyric crises, and other movement disorders. Seizures and psychomotor regression occur even with diet therapy, probably because the enzyme defect also causes neuronal deficiency of serotonin and dopamine. These deficiencies require treatment with levodopa, carbidopa, 5-hydroxytryptophan, and folinic acid. Tetrahydrobiopterin may be added for some biopterin synthesis defects.

C. Tyrosinemia of the Newborn

Serum phenylalanine levels are lower than those associated with phenylketonuria and are accompanied by marked hypertyrosinemia. Tyrosinemia of the newborn usually occurs in premature infants and is due to immaturity of 4-hydroxyphenylpyruvic acid oxidase, resulting in increase in tyrosine and its precursor phenylalanine. The condition resolves spontaneously within 3 months, almost always without sequelae.

D. Maternal Phenylketonuria

Offspring of phenylketonuric mothers may have transient hyperphenylalaninemia at birth. Elevated maternal phenylalanine causes mental retardation, microcephaly, growth retardation, and often congenital heart disease or other malformations in the offspring. The risk to the fetus is lessened considerably by maternal phenylalanine restriction with maintenance of phenylalanine levels below 360 μM (6 mg/dL) throughout pregnancy and optimally started before conception.

American College of Obstetricians and Gynecologists Committee on Genetics: ACOG Committee Opinion No. 449: Maternal phenylketonuria. Obstet Gynecol 2009;114:1432 [PMID: 20134300].

Blau N et al: Optimizing the use of sapropterin (BH(4)) in the management of phenylketonuria. Mol Genet Metab 2009;96:158 [PMID: 19208488].

Blau N et al: Phenylketonuria. Lancet 2010;376:1417 [PMID: 20971365].

de Groot MJ et al: Pathogenesis of cognitive dysfunction in phenylketonuria: Review of hypotheses. Mol Genet Metab 2010;99 (Suppl 1):S86 [PMID: 20123477].

Feillet F, Agostoni C: Nutritional issues in treating phenylketonuria. J Inherit Metab Dis 2010;33:659 [PMID: 20151202].

Feillet F et al: Outcomes beyond phenylalanine: An international perspective. Mol Genet Metab 2010;99(Suppl 1):S79 [PMID: 20123476].

Longo N. Disorders of biopterin metabolism. J Inherit Metab Dis 2009;32:333 [PMID: 19234759].

Patient and parent support group web site with useful information for families: http://www.pkunews.org and www.pkunetwork.org

HEREDITARY TYROSINEMIA

Type I hereditary tyrosinemia is an autosomal recessive condition caused by deficiency of fumarylacetoacetase. It presents with acute or progressive hepatic parenchymal damage, renal tubular dysfunction with generalized aminoaciduria, hypophosphatemic rickets, or neuronopathic crises. Tyrosine and methionine are increased in blood and tyrosine metabolites and δ-aminolevulinic acid in urine. The key diagnostic metabolite is elevated succinylacetone in urine. Liver failure may be rapidly fatal in infancy or somewhat more chronic, with a high incidence of liver cell carcinoma in long-term survivors. Tyrosinemia type II presents with corneal ulcers and keratotic lesions on palms and soles and very high serum tyrosine levels (> 600 μM).

Diagnosis

Similar clinical and biochemical findings may occur in other liver diseases such as galactosemia and hereditary fructose intolerance. Increased succinylacetone occurs only in fumarylacetoacetase deficiency, and is diagnostic. Diagnosis is confirmed by mutation analysis or by enzyme assay in liver tissue. Prenatal diagnosis is possible. Tyrosinemia type II is diagnosed by molecular methods.

Treatment

A diet low in phenylalanine and tyrosine ameliorates liver disease, but does not prevent carcinoma development. Pharmacologic therapy to inhibit the upstream enzyme 4-hydroxyphenylpyruvate dehydrogenase using 2-(2-nitro-4-trifluoromethylbenzoyl)-1,3-cyclohexanedione (NTBC) decreases the production of toxic metabolites, maleylacetoacetate and fumarylacetoacetate. It improves the liver disease and renal disease, prevents acute neuronopathic attacks, and greatly reduces the risk of hepatocellular carcinoma. Liver transplantation is effective therapy. Tyrosinemia type II symptoms respond well to treatment with dietary tyrosine restriction.

Held PK: Disorders of tyrosine catabolism. Mol Genet Metab 2006;88:103 [PMID: 16773741].

Masurel-Paulet A et al: NTBC treatment in tyrosinaemia type I: Long-term outcome in French patients. J Inherit Metab Dis 2008;31:81 [PMID: 18214711].

Meissner T et al: Richner-Hanhart syndrome detected by expanded newborn screening. Pediatr Dermatol 2008;25:378 [PMID: 18577048].

MAPLE SYRUP URINE DISEASE (BRANCHED-CHAIN KETOACIDURIA)

ESSENTIALS OF DIAGNOSIS & TYPICAL FEATURES

- Typical presentation is infantile encephalopathy.

Maple syrup urine disease is due to deficiency of the enzyme catalyzing oxidative decarboxylation of the branched-chain keto acid derivatives of leucine, isoleucine, and valine. Accumulated keto acids of leucine and isoleucine cause the characteristic odor. Only leucine and its corresponding keto acid have been implicated in causing central nervous system dysfunction. Many variants of this disorder have been described, including mild, intermittent, and thiamine-dependent forms. All are autosomal recessive traits.

Patients with classic maple syrup urine disease are normal at birth but after about 1 week develop feeding difficulties, coma, and seizures. Unless diagnosis is made and dietary restriction of branched-chain amino acids is begun, most will die in the first month of life. Nearly normal growth and development may be achieved if treatment is begun before about age 10 days, which is facilitated by newborn screening.

Diagnosis

Amino acid analysis shows marked elevation of branched-chain amino acids including alloisoleucine, a diagnostic transamination product of the keto acid of isoleucine. Urine organic acids demonstrate the characteristic keto acids. The magnitude and consistency of metabolite changes are altered in mild and intermittent forms. Prenatal diagnosis is possible by enzyme assay in cultured amniocytes or chorionic villi, and by molecular analysis of the mutation is known.

Treatment

Dietary leucine restriction and avoidance of catabolism are the cornerstones of treatment. Infant formulas deficient in branched-chain amino acids must be supplemented with normal foods to supply enough branched-chain amino acids to permit normal growth. Serum levels of branched-chain amino acids must be monitored frequently to deal with changing protein requirements. Acute episodes must be aggressively treated to prevent catabolism and negative nitrogen balance. Very high leucine levels may require hemodialysis.

Simon E et al: Maple syrup urine disease: Favorable effect of early diagnosis by newborn screening on the neonatal course of the disease. J Inherit Metab Dis 2006;29:532 [PMID: 16817013].

Knerr I et al: Advances and challenges in the treatment of branched-chain amino/keto acid metabolic defects. J Inherit Metab Dis 2011;Feb 3 [Epub ahead of print] [PMID: 21290185].

Strauss KA et al: Classical maple syrup urine disease and brain development: Principles of management and formula design. Mol Genet Metab 2010;99:333 [PMID: 20061171].

Patient and parent support group web site with useful information for families: http://www.msud-support.org

HOMOCYSTINURIA

ESSENTIALS OF DIAGNOSIS & TYPICAL FEATURES

- Consider in a child of any age with a marfanoid habitus, dislocated lenses, or thrombosis.
- Newborn screening allows early diagnosis and treatment resulting in a normal outcome.

Homocystinuria is most often due to deficiency of cystathionine β-synthase (CBS), but may also be due to deficiency of methylenetetrahydrofolate reductase (MTHR) or to defects in the biosynthesis of methyl-B_{12}, the coenzyme for methionine synthase. All inherited forms of homocystinuria are autosomal recessive traits.

About 50% of patients with untreated CBS deficiency are mentally retarded, and most have arachnodactyly, osteoporosis, and a tendency to develop dislocated lenses and thromboembolic phenomena. Mild variants of CBS deficiency present with thromboembolic events. Patients with severe remethylation defects usually exhibit failure to thrive and a variety of neurologic symptoms, including brain atrophy, microcephaly, and seizures in infancy and early childhood. Very mild elevations of homocysteine, such as caused by a polymorphism of MTHFR resulting in a heat sensitive protein, are increasingly recognized as a factor in the etiology of vascular disease leading to myocardial infarction and stroke.

Diagnosis

Diagnosis is made by demonstrating elevated total serum homocysteine or by identifying homocystinuria in a patient who is not severely deficient in vitamin B_{12}. Serum methionine levels are usually high in patients with CBS deficiency and often low in patients with remethylation defects. Cystathionine levels are low in CBS deficiency. When the remethylation defect is due to deficiency of methyl-B_{12}, megaloblastic anemia or hemolytic uremic syndrome may be present, and an associated deficiency of adenosyl-B_{12} may cause methylmalonic aciduria. Mutation analysis or studies of cultured fibroblasts can make a specific diagnosis.

Treatment

About 50% of patients with CBS deficiency respond to large oral doses of pyridoxine. Pyridoxine nonresponders are treated with dietary methionine restriction and oral administration of betaine, which increases methylation of homocysteine to methionine and improves neurologic function. Early treatment prevents mental retardation, lens dislocation, and thromboembolic manifestations, which justifies the screening of newborn infants. Large doses of vitamin B_{12} (eg, 1–5 mg hydroxycobalamin administered daily intramuscularly or subcutaneously) are indicated in some patients with defects in cobalamin metabolism.

Baric I: Inherited disorders in the conversion of methionine to homocysteine. J Inherit Metab Dis 2009;32:459 [PMID: 19585268].

Mudd SH: Hypermethioninemias of genetic and non-genetic origin: A review. Am J Med Genet C Semin Med Genet 2011;157:3 [PMID: 21308989].

NONKETOTIC HYPERGLYCINEMIA

ESSENTIALS OF DIAGNOSIS & TYPICAL FEATURES

- Severely affected newborns have apnea, hypotonia, lethargy, myoclonic seizures, and hiccups.
- Mental and motor retardation in most patients.
- Mildly affected children have developmental delay, hyperactivity, mild chorea, and seizures.
- Electroencephalography (EEG) shows burst suppression.
- CSF glycine is elevated.

Inherited deficiency of various subunits of the glycine cleavage enzyme causes nonketotic hyperglycinemia. Glycine accumulation in the brain disturbs neurotransmission of the glycinergic receptors and the *N*-methyl-d-aspartate type of glutamate receptor. In its most severe form, also termed glycine encephalopathy, the condition presents in the newborn as hypotonia, lethargy proceeding to coma, myoclonic seizures, and hiccups, with a burst suppression pattern on EEG. Respiratory depression may require ventilator assistance in the first 2 weeks, followed by spontaneous recovery. The majority of patients develop severe mental retardation and seizures. Some patients have agenesis of the corpus callosum or posterior fossa malformations. Most patients have restricted diffusion on MRI in the already myelinated long tracts at birth. Some patients present with seizures, developmental delay, and mild chorea later in infancy or in childhood. All forms of the condition are autosomal recessive.

Diagnosis

Nonketotic hyperglycinemia should be suspected in any neonate or infant with seizures, particularly those with burst suppression pattern on EEG. Diagnosis is confirmed by demonstrating a large increase in glycine in nonbloody CSF, with an abnormally high ratio of CSF glycine to serum glycine. Molecular analysis is diagnostic in more than 90% of cases. Enzyme analysis on liver tissue can confirm the diagnosis. Prenatal diagnosis is possible by molecular analysis if both mutations are known or by enzyme assay on uncultured chorionic villus samples.

Treatment

In patients with mild disease, treatment with sodium benzoate (to normalize serum glycine levels) and dextromethorphan or ketamine (to block *N*-methyl-d-aspartate type of glutamate receptors) controls seizures and improves outcome. Treatment of severely affected patients is generally unsuccessful. High-dose benzoate therapy can aid in seizure control but does not prevent severe mental retardation.

Dinopoulos A et al: Atypical variants of nonketotic hyperglycinemia. Mol Genet Metab 2005;86:61 [PMID: 16157495].

Hennermann JB et al: Prediction of long-term outcome in glycine encephalopathy: A clinical survey. J Inherit Metab Dis 2011 [in press].

Suzuki Y et al: Nonketotic hyperglycinemia: Proposal of a diagnostic and treatment strategy. Pediatr Neurol 2010;43:221 [PMID: 20691948].

Patient and parent support group web site with useful information for families: http://www.nkh-network.org

ORGANIC ACIDEMIAS

ESSENTIALS OF DIAGNOSIS & TYPICAL FEATURES

- Consider in any child presenting with metabolic acidosis and ketosis in early infancy.

Organic acidemias are disorders of amino and fatty acid metabolism in which nonamino organic acids accumulate in serum and urine. These conditions are usually diagnosed by examining organic acids in urine, a complex procedure that requires considerable interpretive expertise and is usually performed only in specialized laboratories. Table 36–4 lists the clinical features of organic acidemias, together with the urine organic acid patterns typical of each. Additional details about some of the more important organic acidemias are provided in the sections that follow.

PROPIONIC & METHYLMALONIC ACIDEMIA (KETOTIC HYPERGLYCINEMIAS)

The oxidation of threonine, valine, methionine, and isoleucine results in propionyl-CoA, which propionyl-CoA carboxylase converts into l-methylmalonyl-CoA, which is metabolized through methylmalonyl-CoA mutase to succinyl-CoA. Gut bacteria and the breakdown of odd-chain-length fatty acids also substantially contribute to propionyl-CoA production. Propionic acidemia is due to a defect in the biotin-containing enzyme propionyl-CoA carboxylase, and methylmalonic aciduria is due to a defect in methylmalonyl-CoA mutase. In most cases the latter is due to a defect in the mutase apoenzyme, but in others it is due to a defect in the biosynthesis of its adenosyl-B_{12} coenzyme. In some of these defects, only the synthesis of adenosyl-B_{12} is blocked; in others, the synthesis of methyl-B_{12} is also blocked, and hence homocysteine is also elevated in blood in addition to methylmalonic acid.

Clinical symptoms in propionic and methylmalonic acidemia vary according to the location and severity of the enzyme block. Children with severe blocks present with acute, life-threatening metabolic acidosis, hyperammonemia, and bone marrow depression in early infancy or with metabolic acidosis, vomiting, and failure to thrive during the first few months of life. Most patients with severe disease have mild or moderate mental retardation. Late complications include pancreatitis, cardiomyopathy, and basal ganglia stroke, and in methylmalonic aciduria, interstitial nephritis.

All forms of propionic and methylmalonic acidemia are autosomal recessive traits and can be diagnosed in utero.

Diagnosis

Laboratory findings consist of increases in urinary organic acids derived from propionyl-CoA or methylmalonic acid (see Table 36–4). Hyperglycinemia can be present. In some forms of abnormal B_{12} metabolism, homocysteine can be elevated. Confirmation is by molecular analysis or by assays in fibroblasts.

Treatment

Patients with enzyme blocks in B_{12} metabolism usually respond to massive doses of vitamin B_{12} given intramuscularly. Vitamin B_{12} nonresponsive methylmalonic acidemia and propionic acidemia require amino acid restriction, strict

Table 36–4. Clinical and laboratory features of organic acidemias.

Disorder	Enzyme Defect	Clinical and Laboratory Features
Isovaleric acidemia	Isovaleryl-CoA dehydrogenase	Acidosis and odor of sweaty feet in infancy, or growth retardation and episodes of vomiting, lethargy, and acidosis. Persistent isovalerylglycine and intermittent 3-hydroxyisovaleric acid in urine.
3-Methylcrotonyl-CoA carboxylase deficiency	3-Methylcrotonyl-CoA carboxylase	Usually asymptomatic. Acidosis and feeding problems in infancy, or Reye-like episodes in older child. 3-Methylcrotonylglycine and 3-hydroxyisovaleric acid in urine.
Combined carboxylase deficiency	Holocarboxylase synthetase	Hypotonia and lactic acidosis in infancy. 3-Hydroxyisovaleric acid in urine, often with small amounts of 3-hydroxypropionic and methylcitric acids. Often biotin-responsive.
Biotinidase deficiency	Biotinidase	Alopecia, seborrheic rash, seizures, and ataxia in infancy or childhood. Urine organic acids as above. Always biotin-responsive.
3-Hydroxy-3-methylglutaric acidemia	3-Hydroxy-3-methylglutaryl-CoA lyase	Hypoglycemia and acidosis in infancy; Reye-like episodes with nonketotic hypoglycemia or leukodystrophy in older children. 3-Hydroxy-3-methylglutaric, 3-methylglutaconic, and 3-hydroxyisovaleric acids in urine.
3-Ketothiolase deficiency	3-Ketothiolase	Episodes of vomiting, severe metabolic acidosis (hyperketosis), and encephalopathy. 2-Methyl-3-hydroxybutyric and 2-methylacetoacetic acids and tiglylglycine in urine, especially after isoleucine load.
Propionic acidemia	Propionyl-CoA carboxylase	Hyperammonemia and metabolic acidosis in infancy; ketotic hyperglycinemia syndrome later. 3-Hydroxypropionic and methylcitric acids in urine, with 3-hydroxy- and 3-ketovaleric acids during ketotic episodes.
Methylmalonic acidemia	Methylmalonyl-CoA mutase	Clinical features same as in propionic acidemia. Methylmalonic acid in urine, often with 3-hydroxypropionic and methylcitric acids.
	Defects in B_{12} biosynthesis	Clinical features same as above when only adenosyl-B_{12} synthesis is decreased; early neurologic features prominent when accompanied by decreased synthesis of methyl-B_{12}. In latter instance, hypomethioninemia and homocystinuria accompany methylmalonic aciduria.
Pyroglutamic acidemia	Glutathione synthetase	Acidosis and hemolytic anemia in infancy; chronic acidosis later. Pyroglutamic acid in urine.
Glutaric acidemia type I	Glutaryl-CoA dehydrogenase	Progressive extrapyramidal movement disorder in childhood, with episodes of acidosis, vomiting, and encephalopathy. Glutaric acid and 3-hydroxyglutaric acid in serum and urine.
Glutaric acidemia type II	Electron transfer flavoprotein (ETF) ETF:ubiquinone oxidoreductase (ETF dehydrogenase)	Hypoglycemia, acidosis, hyperammonemia, and odor of sweaty feet in infancy, often with polycystic and dysplastic kidneys. Later onset may be with episodes of hypoketotic hypoglycemia, liver dysfunction, or slowly progressive skeletal myopathy. Glutaric, ethylmalonic, 3-hydroxyisovaleric, isovalerylglycine, and 2-hydroxyglutaric acids in urine, often with sarcosine in serum.
4-Hydroxybutyric acidemia	Succinic semialdehyde dehydrogenase	Seizures, ataxia, and developmental retardation. 4-Hydroxybutyric acid in urine.

CoA, coenzyme A.

prevention of catabolism, and carnitine supplementation to enhance propionylcarnitine excretion. Intermittent metronidazole can help reduce the propionate load from the gut. In the acute setting, hemodialysis or hemofiltration may be needed. Combined liver-renal transplantation is an option for patients with renal insufficiency, and liver transplantation has shown promise for patients with life-threatening cardiomyopathy.

Carrillo-Carrasco N et al: Combined methylmalonic acidemia and homocystinuria, cblC type. I. Clinical presentations, diagnosis, and management. J Inherit Metab Dis 2011;Jul 12 [Epub ahead of print] [PMID: 21748409].

Carrillo-Carrasco N et al: Combined methylmalonic acidemia and homocystinuria, cblC type. II. Complications, pathophysiology, and outcomes. J Inherit Metab Dis 2011;Jul 12 [Epub ahead of print] [PMID: 21748408].

Chen PW et al: Stabilization of blood methylmalonic acid level in methylmalonic acidemia after liver transplantation. Pediatr Transplant 2010;14:337 [PMID: 19686300].

Dionisi-Vici C et al: "Classical" organic acidurias, propionic aciduria, methylmalonic aciduria and isovaleric aciduria: Long-term outcome and effects of expanded newborn screening using tandem mass spectrometry. J Inherit Metab Dis 2006;29:383 [PMID: 16763906].

Fowler B et al: Causes of and diagnostic approach to methylmalonic acidurias. J Inherit Metab Dis 2008;31:350 [PMID: 18563633].

Hörster F et al: Long-term outcome in methylmalonic acidurias is influenced by the underlying defect (mut0, mut-, cblA, cblB). Pediatr Res 2007;62:225 [PMID: 17597648].

Johnson JA et al: Propionic acidemia: Case report and review of neurologic sequelae. Pediatr Neurol 2009;40:317 [PMID: 19302949].

Knerr I et al: Advances and challenges in the treatment of branched-chain amino/keto acid metabolic defects. J Inherit Metab Dis 2011;Feb 3 [Epub ahead of print] [PMID: 21290185].

Vara R et al: Liver transplantation for propionic acidemia in children. Liver Transpl 2011;17:661 [PMID: 21618686].

Patient and parent support group web site with useful information for families: http://www.oaanews.org and www.pafoundation.com

ISOVALERIC ACIDEMIA

Isovaleric acidemia, caused by deficiency of isovaleryl-CoA dehydrogenase in the leucine oxidative pathway, was the first organic acidemia to be described in humans. Patients with this disorder usually present with poor feeding, metabolic acidosis, seizures, and an odor of sweaty feet during the first few days of life, with coma and death occurring if the condition is not recognized and treated. Other patients have a more chronic course, with episodes of vomiting and lethargy, hair loss, and pancreatitis precipitated by intercurrent infections or increased protein intake. The condition is autosomal recessive and can be diagnosed in utero.

Diagnosis

Isovalerylglycine is consistently detected in the urine by organic acid chromatography.

Treatment

Providing a low-protein diet or a diet low in leucine is effective. Conjugation with either glycine or carnitine helps in maintaining metabolic stability by removing toxic isovaleryl-CoA. Outcome is usually good.

Ensenauer R et al: Newborn screening for isovaleric acidemia using tandem mass spectrometry: Data from 1.6 million newborns. Clin Chem 2011;57:623 [PMID: 21335445].

CARBOXYLASE DEFICIENCY

Isolated pyruvate carboxylase deficiency presents with lactic acidosis and hyperammonemia in early infancy. Even if biochemically stabilized, the neurologic outcome is dismal. Isolated 3-methylcrotonyl-CoA carboxylase deficiency is frequently recognized on newborn screening using acylcarnitine analysis. It is usually a benign condition that only rarely causes symptoms of acidosis and neurologic depression. All carboxylases require biotin as a cofactor. Holocarboxylase synthetase and biotinidase are two enzymes of biotin metabolism. Holocarboxylase synthetase covalently binds biotin to the apocarboxylases for pyruvate, 3-methylcrotonyl-CoA, and propionyl-CoA; and biotinidase releases biotin from these proteins and from proteins in the diet. Recessively inherited deficiency of either enzyme causes deficiency of all three carboxylases (ie, multiple carboxylase deficiency). Patients with holocarboxylase synthetase deficiency usually present as neonates with hypotonia, skin problems, and massive acidosis. Those with biotinidase deficiency present later with a syndrome of ataxia, seizures, seborrhea, and alopecia. Untreated patients can develop mental retardation, hearing loss, and optic nerve atrophy. Newborn screening is justified because the neurologic sequellae of the disorder in many patients are preventable if treated early.

Diagnosis

This diagnosis should be considered in patients with typical symptoms or in those with primary lactic acidosis. Urine organic acids are usually but not always abnormal (see Table 36–4). Diagnosis is made by enzyme assay often carboxylase activity in fibroblasts or leucocytes. Biotinidase can be assayed in serum, and holocarboxylase synthetase in leukocytes or fibroblasts.

Treatment

Oral administration of biotin in large doses often reverses the organic aciduria within days and the clinical symptoms within days to weeks. Hearing loss can occur in patients with biotinidase deficiency despite treatment.

Arnold GL et al: A Delphi-based consensus clinical practice protocol for the diagnosis and management of 3-methylcrotonyl CoA carboxylase deficiency. Mol Genet Metab 2008;93:363 [PMID: 18155630].

Tammachote R et al: Holocarboxylase synthetase deficiency: Novel clinical and molecular findings. Clin Genet 2010;78:88 [PMID: 20095979].

Wolf B: Clinical issues and frequent questions about biotinidase deficiency. Mol Genet Metab 2010;100:6 [PMID: 20129807].

GLUTARIC ACIDEMIA TYPE I

ESSENTIALS OF DIAGNOSIS & TYPICAL FEATURES

- Suspect in children with acute basal ganglia necrosis and macrocrania with subdural bleeds.

- Presymptomatic diagnosis by newborn screening and treatment reduces the incidence of acute encephalopathic crises.

Glutaric acidemia type I is due to deficiency of glutaryl-CoA dehydrogenase. Patients have frontotemporal atrophy with enlarged sylvian fissures and macrocephaly. Sudden or chronic neuronal degeneration in the caudate and putamen causes an extrapyramidal movement disorder in childhood with dystonia and athetosis. Children with glutaric acidemia type I may present with retinal hemorrhages and intracranial bleeding and may thus be falsely considered victims of child abuse. Severely debilitated children often die in the first decade, but several reported patients have had only mild neurologic abnormalities. Most patients develop symptoms in the first 6 years of life. The condition is autosomal recessive and prenatal diagnosis is possible.

Diagnosis

Glutaric acidemia type I should be suspected in patients with acute or progressive dystonia in the first 6 years of life. Magnetic resonance imaging of the brain is highly suggestive. The diagnosis is supported by finding glutaric, 3-hydroxyglutaric acid, and glutarylcarnitine in urine or serum. Demonstration of deficiency of glutaryl-CoA dehydrogenase in fibroblasts, or a mutation in the GCDH gene confirms the diagnosis. Prenatal diagnosis is by enzyme assay, quantitative metabolite analysis in amniotic fluid, or mutation analysis.

Treatment

Strict catabolism prevention during any intercurrent illness is very important and supplementation with large amounts of carnitine may prevent degeneration of the basal ganglia, warranting newborn screening. Early diagnosis via newborn screening does not prevent neurologic disease in all patients, but clearly reduces the risk. Dietary lysine and tryptophan are frequently restricted in young patients. Neurologic symptoms, once present, do not resolve. Symptomatic treatment of severe dystonia is important for affected patients.

Bijarnia S et al: Glutaric aciduria type I: Outcome following detection by newborn screening. J Inherit Metab Dis 2008;31:503 [PMID: 18683078].

Boneh A et al: Newborn screening for glutaric aciduria type I in Victoria: Treatment and outcome. Mol Genet Metab 2008;94:287 [PMID: 18411069].

Kölker S et al: Decline of acute encephalopathic crises in children with glutaryl-CoA dehydrogenase deficiency identified by newborn screening in Germany. Pediatr Res 2007;62:357 [PMID: 17622945].

Kölker S et al: Diagnosis and management of glutaric aciduria type I—revised recommendations. J Inherit Metab Dis 2011;34:677 [PMID: 21431622].

Zinnanti WJ et al: Mechanism of age-dependent susceptibility and novel treatment strategy in glutaric acidemia type I. J Clin Invest 2007;117:3258 [PMID: 17932566].

DISORDERS OF FATTY ACID OXIDATION & CARNITINE

FATTY ACID OXIDATION DISORDERS

ESSENTIALS OF DIAGNOSIS & TYPICAL FEATURES

- Obtain an acylcarnitine profile for any child with hypoglycemia to evaluate for a fatty acid oxidation defect.
- Early diagnosis and treatment can prevent cardiomyopathy in affected children.

Deficiencies of very-long-chain and medium-chain acyl-CoA dehydrogenase (VLCAD, MCAD) and long-chain 3-hydroxyacyl-CoA dehydrogenase (LCHAD), three enzymes of fatty acid β-oxidation, usually cause Reye-like episodes of hypoketotic hypoglycemia, mild hyperammonemia, hepatomegaly, and encephalopathy. Sudden death in infancy is a less common presentation. The long-chain defects, which also include carnitine palmitoyltransferase deficiency I and II and carnitine-acylcarnitine translocase deficiency, often also cause skeletal myopathy with hypotonia and cardiomyopathy, and ventricular arrhythmias. Less severe defects present with recurrent episodes of rhabdomyolysis. LCHAD deficiency may produce progressive liver cirrhosis, peripheral neuropathy, and retinitis pigmentosa. Mothers of affected infants can have acute fatty liver of pregnancy or HELLP syndrome (hemolysis, elevated liver enzymes, and low platelets). Mild carnitine palmitoyltransferase I deficiency may cause renal tubular acidosis and hypertriglyceridemia. MCAD deficiency is common, occurring in perhaps 1:9000 live births. Reye-like episodes may be fatal or cause residual neurologic damage. Episodes tend to become less frequent and severe with time. After the diagnosis is made and treatment instituted, morbidity decreases and mortality is avoided in MCAD deficiency.

Short-chain acyl-CoA dehydrogenase (SCAD) deficiency is characterized by the presence of ethylmalonic acid in the urine, and although some patients have symptoms similar to those in MCAD deficiency, many are asymptomatic. Glutaric acidemia type II results from defects in the transfer of electrons from fatty acid oxidation and some amino acid oxidation into the respiratory chain. Some patients with glutaric acidemia type II have a clinical presentation resembling MCAD deficiency. Patients with a severe neonatal presentation also have renal cystic disease and dysmorphic features. The least affected patients can present with late-onset myopathy and be riboflavin responsive. Some develop cardiomyopathy or leukodystrophy. Deficiency of the ketogenic enzyme 3-hydroxymethylglutaryl-CoA synthase presents with hypoketotic hypoglycemia. These conditions are autosomal recessive.

Diagnosis

The hypoglycemic presentation of Reye-like episodes is associated with a lack of an appropriate ketone response to fasting. Urine organic acid analysis in patients with MCAD deficiency reveals dicarboxylic acids and increased hexanoylglycine, suberylglycine, and phenylpropionylglycine. The finding of normal urine organic acids does not exclude these conditions, because the excretion of these acids is intermittent. Urine and blood findings in glutaric acidemia type II and SCAD deficiency are often diagnostic. The analysis of acylcarnitine esters is a first-line diagnostic test used in neonatal screening because it reveals diagnostic metabolites regardless of clinical status. MCAD deficiency is characterized by elevated octanoylcarnitine. A typical pattern can be recognized in deficiencies of VLCAD, LCHAD, carnitine-acylcarnitine translocase, and severe carnitine palmitoyltransferase. Further confirmation can be obtained from analysis of fatty acid oxidation in fibroblasts. Molecular sequencing is available for each defect with MCAD and LCHAD deficiencies, each having a common mutation. Assays for each enzyme can be done on fibroblasts in specialized laboratories.

Treatment

Management involves prevention of hypoglycemia by avoiding prolonged fasting (> 8–12 hours). This includes providing carbohydrate snacks before bedtime and vigorous treatment of fasting associated with intercurrent infections. Because fatty acid oxidation can be compromised by associated carnitine deficiency, young patients with MCAD deficiency usually receive oral carnitine. Restriction of dietary long-chain fats is not necessary in MCAD deficiency, but is required for severe VLCAD and LCHAD deficiencies. Medium-chain triglycerides are contraindicated in MCAD deficiency but are an essential energy source for patients with severe VLCAD and LCHAD deficiencies or carnitine-acylcarnitine translocase deficiency. Riboflavin may be beneficial in some patients with glutaric acidemia type II. Outcome in MCAD deficiency is excellent, but is more guarded in patients with the other disorders.

Arnold GL et al: A Delphi clinical practice protocol for the management of very long chain acyl-CoA dehydrogenase deficiency. Mol Genet Metab 2009;96:85 [PMID: 19157942].

Arnold GL et al: Lack of genotype-phenotype correlations and outcome in MCAD deficiency diagnosed by newborn screening in New York State. Mol Genet Metab 2010;99:263 [PMID: 20036593].

Bennett MJ: Pathophysiology of fatty acid oxidation disorders. J Inherit Metab Dis 2010;33:533 [PMID: 20824345].

Bonnefont J-P et al: Bezafibrate for an inborn mitochondrial beta-oxidation defect. N Engl J Med 2009;360:838 [PMID: 19228633].

Bonnefont JP et al: Long-term follow-up of bezafibrate treatment in patients with the myopathic form of carnitine palmitoyl-transferase 2 deficiency. Clin Pharmacol Ther 2010;88:101 [PMID: 20505667].

Houten SM, Wanders RJ: A general introduction to the biochemistry of mitochondrial fatty acid beta-oxidation. J Inherit Metab Dis 2010;33:469 [PMID: 20195903].

Lindner M et al: Newborn screening for disorders of fatty-acid oxidation: Experience and recommendations from an expert meeting. J Inherit Metab Dis 2010;33:521 [PMID: 20373143].

Schatz UA, Ensenauer R: The clinical manifestation of MCAD deficiency: Challenges toward adulthood in the screened population. J Inherit Metab Dis 2010;33:513 [PMID: 20532824].

Spiekerkoetter U et al: Current issues regarding treatment of mitochondrial fatty acid oxidation disorders. J Inherit Metab Dis 2010;33:555 [PMID: 20830526].

Spiekerkoetter U et al: Management and outcome in 75 individuals with long-chain fatty acid oxidation defects: Results from a workshop. J Inherit Metab Dis 2009;32:488 [PMID: 19399638].

Spiekerkoetter U: Mitochondrial fatty acid oxidation disorders: Clinical presentation of long-chain fatty acid oxidation defects before and after newborn screening. J Inherit Metab Dis 2010;33:527 [PMID: 20449660].

Spiekerkoetter U et al: Treatment recommendations in long-chain fatty acid oxidation defects: Consensus from a workshop. J Inherit Metab Dis 2009;32:498 [PMID: 19452263].

van Maldegem BT et al: Clinical aspects of short-chain acyl-CoA dehydrogenase deficiency. J Inherit Metab Dis 2010;33:507 [PMID: 20429031].

Wilcken B: Fatty acid oxidation disorders: outcome and long-term prognosis. J Inherit Metab Dis 2010;33:501 [PMID: 20049534].

Yusupov R et al: Sudden death in medium chain acyl-coenzyme a dehydrogenase deficiency (MCADD) despite newborn screening. Mol Genet Metab 2010;101:33 [PMID: 20580581].

Patient and parent support group web site with useful information for families: http://www.fodsupport.org

CARNITINE

Carnitine is an essential nutrient found in highest concentration in red meat. Its primary function is to transport long-chain fatty acids into mitochondria for oxidation. Primary defects of carnitine transport may manifest as Reye syndrome, cardiomyopathy, or skeletal myopathy with hypotonia. These disorders are rare compared with secondary carnitine deficiency, which may be due to diet (especially intravenous alimentation or ketogenic diet), renal losses, drug therapy (especially valproic acid), and other metabolic disorders (especially disorders of fatty acid oxidation and organic acidemias). The prognosis depends on the cause of the carnitine abnormality. Primary carnitine deficiency is one of the most treatable causes of dilated cardiomyopathy in children.

Free and esterified carnitine can be measured in blood. Muscle carnitine may be low despite normal blood levels, particularly in respiratory chain disorders. If carnitine insufficiency is suspected, the patient should be evaluated to rule out disorders that might cause secondary carnitine deficiency.

Oral or intravenous L-carnitine is used in carnitine deficiency or insufficiency in doses of 25–100 mg/kg/d or higher. Treatment is aimed at maintaining normal carnitine levels. Carnitine supplementation in patients with some disorders of fatty acid oxidation and organic acidosis may also augment excretion of accumulated metabolites, although supplementation may not prevent metabolic crises in such patients.

Amat di San Filippo C et al: Cardiomyopathy and carnitine deficiency. Mol Genet Metab 2008;94:162 [PMID: 18337137].

Lee NC et al: Diagnoses of newborns and mothers with carnitine uptake defects through newborn screening. Mol Genet Metab 2010;100:46 [PMID: 20074989].

Li FY et al: Molecular spectrum of SLC22A5 (OCTN2) gene mutations detected in 143 subjects evaluated for systemic carnitine deficiency. Hum Mutat 2010;31:e1632 [PMID: 20574985].

Nasser M et al: Carnitine supplementation for inborn errors of metabolism. Cochrane Database Syst Rev 2009;2:CD006659 [PMID: 19370646].

PURINE METABOLISM DISORDERS

Hypoxanthine-guanine phosphoribosyltransferase is an enzyme that converts the purine bases hypoxanthine and guanine to inosine monophosphate and guanosine monophosphate, respectively. Hypoxanthine-guanine phosphoribosyltransferase deficiency (Lesch-Nyhan syndrome) is an X-linked recessive disorder. The complete deficiency is characterized by central nervous system dysfunction and purine overproduction with hyperuricemia and hyperuricosuria. Depending on the residual activity of the mutant enzyme, male hemizygous individuals may be severely disabled by choreoathetosis, spasticity, and compulsive, mutilating lip and finger biting, or they may have only gouty arthritis and urate ureterolithiasis. Enzyme deficiency can be measured in erythrocytes, fibroblasts, and cultured amniotic cells; this disorder can thus be diagnosed in utero. Adenylosuccinate lyase deficiency involves a defect in the synthesis of purines. Patients present with static mental retardation, hypotonia, and seizures.

Diagnosis

Diagnosis of Lesch-Nyhan syndrome is made by demonstrating an elevated uric acid-creatinine ratio in urine, followed by demonstration of enzyme deficiency in red blood cells or fibroblasts. Screening for adenylosuccinate lyase deficiency is by measurement of succinylpurines using the Bratton-Marshal colorimetric test, with confirmation by further metabolite and molecular assays.

Treatment

Hyperhydration and alkalinization are essential to prevent kidney stones and urate nephropathy. Allopurinol and probenecid may be given to reduce hyperuricemia and prevent gout but do not affect the neurologic status. Physical restraints are often more effective than neurologic medications for automutilation. No effective treatment exists for adenylosuccinate lyase deficiency.

Camici M et al: Pediatric neurological syndromes and inborn errors of purine metabolism. Neurochem Int 2010;56:367 [PMID: 20005278].

Jinnah HA et al: Attenuated variants of Lesch-Nyhan disease. Brain 2010;133(Pt 3):671 [PMID: 20176575].

Micheli V et al: Neurological disorders of purine and pyrimidine metabolism. Curr Top Med Chem 2011;11:923 [PMID: 21401501].

LYSOSOMAL DISEASES

Lysosomes are cellular organelles in which complex macromolecules are degraded by specific acid hydrolases. Deficiency of a lysosomal enzyme causes its substrate to accumulate in the lysosomes, resulting in a characteristic clinical picture. These storage disorders are classified as mucopolysaccharidoses, lipidoses, or mucolipidoses, depending on the nature of the stored material. Two additional disorders, cystinosis and Salla disease, are caused by defects in lysosomal proteins that normally transport material from the lysosome to the cytoplasm. Table 36–5 lists clinical and laboratory features of these conditions. Most are inherited as autosomal recessive traits, and all can be diagnosed in utero.

Diagnosis

The diagnosis of mucopolysaccharidosis is suggested by certain clinical and radiologic findings (dysostosis multiplex, which includes enlarged sella turcia, scaphocephaly, broad ribs, hook shaped vertebrae [L1 and L2 most affected], and prominent pointing of the metacarpals and broad phalanges). Urine screening tests can detect increased mucopolysaccharides and further identify which specific mucopolysaccharides are present. Diagnosis must be confirmed by enzyme assays of leukocytes or cultured fibroblasts. Analysis of urinary oligosaccharides indicates a specific disorder prior to enzymatic testing. Lipidoses present with visceral symptoms or neurodegeneration. The pattern of the leukodystrophy associated with many lipidoses can indicate a specific condition. Diagnosis is made by appropriate enzyme assays of peripheral leukocytes or cultured skin fibroblasts. Molecular analysis is also available for most conditions.

Treatment

Most conditions cannot be treated effectively, but new avenues have given hope in many conditions. Hematopoietic stem cell transplantation can greatly improve the course of some lysosomal diseases and is first-line treatment in some, such as infantile Hurler syndrome. Several disorders are treated with infusions of recombinant modified enzyme. Treatment of Gaucher disease is very effective and long-term data suggest excellent outcome. Similar treatments have been developed for Fabry disease, several mucopolysaccharidoses, and Pompe disease. Substantial improvements in these conditions have been reported but with limitations. New avenues for treatment through substrate inhibition and chaperone therapy are being developed. Treatment of cystinosis

Table 36–5. Clinical and laboratory features of lysosomal storage diseases.

Disorder	Enzyme Defect	Clinical and Laboratory Features	Available Therapies
I. Mucopolysaccharidoses			
Hurler syndrome	α-Iduronidase	Autosomal recessive. Mental retardation, hepatosplenomegaly, umbilical hernia, coarse facies, corneal clouding, dorsolumbar gibbus, severe heart disease. Heparan sulfate and dermatan sulfate in urine.	HSCT ERT
Scheie syndrome	α-Iduronidase (incomplete)	Autosomal recessive. Corneal clouding, stiff joints, normal intellect. Clinical types intermediate between Hurler and Scheie common. Heparan sulfate and dermatan sulfate in urine.	ERT
Hunter syndrome	Sulfoiduronate sulfatase	X-linked recessive. Coarse facies, hepatosplenomegaly, mental retardation variable. Corneal clouding and gibbus not present. Heparan sulfate and dermatan sulfate in urine.	HSCT ERT
Sanfilippo syndrome:		Autosomal recessive. Severe mental retardation and hyperactivity, with comparatively mild skeletal changes, visceromegaly, and facial coarseness. Types cannot be differentiated clinically. Heparan sulfate in urine.	
Type A	Sulfamidase		
Type B	α-*N*-Acetylglucosaminidase		
Type C	Acetyl-CoA: α-glucosaminide-*N*-acetyltransferase		
Type D	α-*N*-acetylglucosamine-6-sulfatase		
Morquio syndrome	*N*-Acetylgalactosamine-6-sulfatase	Autosomal recessive. Severe skeletal changes, platyspondylisis, corneal clouding. Keratan sulfate in urine.	
Maroteaux-Lamy syndrome	*N*-Acetylgalactosamine-4-sulfatase	Autosomal recessive. Coarse facies, growth retardation, dorsolumbar gibbus, corneal clouding, hepatosplenomegaly, normal intellect. Dermatan sulfate in urine.	HSCT ERT
β-Glucuronidase deficiency	β-Glucuronidase	Autosomal recessive. Varies from mental retardation, dorsolumbar gibbus, corneal clouding, and hepatosplenomegaly to mild facial coarseness, retardation, and loose joints. Hearing loss common. Dermatan sulfate or heparan sulfate in urine.	HSCT
II. Oligosaccharidoses			
Mannosidosis	α-Mannosidase	Autosomal recessive. Varies from severe mental retardation, coarse facies, short stature, skeletal changes, and hepatosplenomegaly to mild facial coarseness and loose joints. Hearing loss common. Abnormal oligosaccharides in urine.	HSCT
Fucosidosis	α-Fucosidase	Autosomal recessive. Variable: coarse facies, skeletal changes, hepatosplenomegaly, occasional angiokeratomas. Abnormal oligosaccharides in urine.	HSCT
I-cell disease (mucolipidosis II)	*N*-Acetylglucosaminyl-phosphotransferase	Autosomal recessive; severe and mild forms known. Very short stature, mental retardation, early facial coarsening, clear cornea, and stiffness of joints. Increased lysosomal enzymes in serum. Abnormal sialyl oligosaccharides in urine.	HSCT
Sialidosis	*N*-Acetylineuraminidase (sialidase)	Autosomal recessive. Mental retardation, coarse facies, skeletal dysplasia, myoclonic seizures, macular cherry-red spot. Abnormal sialyl oligosaccharides in urine.	
III. Lipidoses			
Niemann-Pick disease	Sphingomyelinase	Autosomal recessive. Acute and chronic forms known. Acute neuronopathic form common in eastern European Jews. Accumulation of sphingomyelin in lysosomes of RE system and CNS. Hepatosplenomegaly, developmental retardation, macular cherry-red spot. Death by 1–4 y in severe type A; mild type B develops respiratory insufficiency usually in adulthood.	HSCT[a]

(*Continued*)

Table 36–5. Clinical and laboratory features of lysosomal storage diseases. (*Continued*)

Disorder	Enzyme Defect	Clinical and Laboratory Features	Available Therapies
Metachromatic leukodystrophy	Arylsulfatase A	Autosomal recessive. Late infantile form, with onset at 1–4 y, most common. Accumulation of sulfatide in white matter with central leukodystrophy and peripheral neuropathy. Gait disturbances (ataxia), motor incoordination, absent deep tendon reflexes, and dementia. Death usually in first decade.	HSCT[a]
Krabbe disease (globoid cell leukodystrophy)	Galactocerebroside α-galactosidase	Autosomal recessive. Globoid cells in white matter. Onset at 3–6 mo with seizures, irritability, retardation, and leukodystrophy. Death by 1–2 y. Juvenile and adult forms are rare.	HSCT
Fabry disease	α-Galactosidase A	X-linked recessive. Storage of trihexosylceramide in endothelial cells. Pain in extremities, angiokeratoma and (later) poor vision, hypertension, and renal failure.	ERT
Farber disease	Ceramidase	Autosomal recessive. Storage of ceramide in tissues. Subcutaneous nodules, arthropathy with deformed and painful joints, and poor growth and development. Death within first year.	HSCT[a]
Gaucher disease	Glucocerebroside β-glucosidase	Autosomal recessive. Accumulation of glucocerebroside in lysosomes of RE system and CNS. Acute neuronopathic form: retardation, hepatosplenomegaly, macular cherry-red spot, and Gaucher cells in bone marrow. Death by 1–2 y. Chronic form common in eastern European Jews. Hepatosplenomegaly and flask-shaped osteolytic bone lesions. Consistent with normal life expectancy.	ERT SIT
G_{M1} gangliosidosis	G_{M1} ganglioside β-galactosidase	Autosomal recessive. Accumulation of G_{M1} ganglioside in lysosomes of RE system and CNS. Infantile form: abnormalities at birth with dysostosis multiplex, hepatosplenomegaly, macular cherry-red spot, and death by 2 y. Juvenile form: normal development to 1 y of age, then ataxia, weakness, dementia, and death by 4–5 y. Occasional inferior beaking of vertebral bodies of L1 and L2.	HSCT[a]
G_{M2} gangliosidoses Tay-Sachs disease Sandhoff disease	 β-*N*-Acetylhexosaminidase A β-*N*-Acetylhexosaminidase A and B	Autosomal recessive. Tay-Sachs disease common in eastern European Jews; Sandhoff disease is panethnic. Clinical phenotypes are identical, with accumulation of G_{M2} ganglioside in lysosomes of CNS. Onset at age 3–6 mo, with hypotonia, hyperacusis, retardation, and macular cherry-red spot. Death by 2–3 y. Juvenile and adult onset forms of Tay-Sachs disease are rare.	
Wolman disease	Acid lipase	Autosomal recessive. Accumulation of cholesterol esters and triglycerides in lysosomes of reticuloendothelial system. Onset in infancy with gastrointestinal symptoms and hepatosplenomegaly, and death in the first year. Adrenals commonly enlarged and calcified.	HSCT
Niemann-Pick disease type C	*NPC1* gene (95%), *NPC2* gene (5%)	Autosomal recessive. Blocked transport of lipids and cholesterol from late endosomes to lysosomes. Infantile cholestatic liver disease, or later neurodegeneration with vertical supranuclear gaze palsy, ataxia, seizures, spasticity and loss of speech. Some have splenomegaly.	SIT

[a]May be useful in selected patients.
CNS, central nervous system; ERT, enzyme replacement therapy; HSCT, hematopoietic stem cell transplantation; SIT, substrate inhibition therapy; RE, reticuloendothelial.

with cysteamine results in depletion of stored cystine and prevention of complications including renal disease.

Anson DS et al: Therapies for neurological disease in the mucopolysaccharidoses. Curr Gene Ther 2011;11:132 [PMID: 21291356].

Bellettato CM, Scarpa M: Pathophysiology of neuropathic lysosomal storage disorders. J Inherit Metab Dis 2010;33:347 [PMID: 20429032].

Brunetti-Pierri N, Scaglia F: GM1 gangliosidosis: Review of clinical, molecular, and therapeutic aspects. Mol Genet Metab 2008;94:391 [PMID: 18524657].

Caciotti A et al: GM1 gangliosidosis and Morquio B disease: An update on genetic alterations and clinical findings. Biochim Biophys Acta 2011;1812:782 [PMID: 21497194].

Charrow J: Enzyme replacement therapy for Gaucher disease. Expert Opin Biol Ther 2009;9:121 [PMID: 19063698].

Clarke LA et al: Long-term efficacy and safety of laronidase in the treatment of mucopolysaccharidosis I. Pediatrics 2009;123:229 [PMID: 19117887].

Dierks T et al: Molecular basis of multiple sulfatase deficiency, mucolipidosis II/III and Niemann-Pick C1 disease—lysosomal storage disorders caused by defects of non-lysosomal proteins. Biochim Biophys Acta 2009;1793:710 [PMID: 19124046].

Fesslova V et al: The natural course and the impact of therapies of cardiac involvement in the mucopolysaccharidoses. Cardiol Young 2009;19:170 [PMID: 19195419].

Geer JS et al: Mucolipidosis type IV: A subtle pediatric neurodegenerative disorder. Pediatr Neurol 2010;42:223 [PMID: 20159435].

Germain DP: Fabry disease. Orphanet J Rare Dis 2010;5:30 [PMID: 21092187].

Gieselmann V, Krägeloh-Mann I: Metachromatic leukodystrophy—an update. Neuropediatrics 2010;41:1 [PMID: 20571983].

Hopkin RJ et al: Characterization of Fabry disease in 352 pediatric patients in the Fabry Registry. Pediatr Res 2008;64:550 [PMID: 18596579].

Lidove O et al: Effects of enzyme replacement therapy in Fabry disease—a comprehensive review of the medical literature. Genet Med 2010;12:668 [PMID: 20962662].

Martin AM et al: Recommendations on diagnosis, treatment, and monitoring for Gaucher disease. J Pediatr 2009;155(Suppl 4): S10 [PMID: 19765407].

Montano AM et al: International Morquio A Registry: Clinical manifestation and natural course of Morquio A disease. J Inherit Metab Dis 2007;30:165 [PMID: 17347914].

Muenzer J et al: Idursulfase treatment of Hunter syndrome in children younger than 6 years: Results from the Hunter Outcome Survey. Genet Med 2011;13:102 [PMID: 21233716].

Muenzer J et al: Mucopolysaccharidosis I: Management and treatment guidelines. Pediatrics 2009;123:19 [PMID: 19117856].

Muenzer J et al: Multidisciplinary management of Hunter syndrome. Pediatrics 2009;124:e1228 [PMID: 19901005].

Pintos-Morell G, Beck M: Fabry disease in children and the effects of enzyme replacement treatment. Eur J Pediatr 2009;168:1355 [PMID: 19242721].

Prasad VK, Kurtzberg J: Transplant outcome in mucopolysaccharidoses. Semin Hematol 2010;47:59 [PMID: 20109613].

Staretz-Chacham O et al: Lysosomal storage disorders in newborns. Pediatrics 2009;123:1191 [PMID: 19336380].

Valayannopoulos V et al: Mucopolysaccharidosis VI. Orphanet J Rare Dis 2010;5:5 [PMID: 20385007].

Vanier MT: Niemann-Pick disease type C. Orphanet J Rare Dis 2010;5:16 [PMID: 20525256].

Wang RY et al: Lysosomal storage diseases: Diagnostic confirmation and management of presymptomatic individuals. Genet Med 2011;13:457 [PMID: 21502868].

Patient and parent support group web site with useful information for families: http://www.mpssociety.org, www.ulf.org, www.lysosomallearning.com, www.fabry.org, www.gaucherdisease.org, and www.ntsad.org

PEROXISOMAL DISEASES

Peroxisomes are intracellular organelles that contain a large number of enzymes, many of which are oxidases linked to catalase. Among the enzyme systems in peroxisomes one is for β-oxidation of very-long-chain fatty acids, phytanic acid, and bile acids, and one for plasmalogen biosynthesis. In addition, peroxisomes contain oxidases for d- and l-amino acids, pipecolic acid, and phytanic acid, and an enzyme (alanine-glyoxylate aminotransferase) that affects transamination of glyoxylate to glycine.

In some peroxisomal diseases, many enzymes are deficient. Zellweger (cerebrohepatorenal) syndrome, the best known among these, is caused by severe defects in organelle assembly. Patients present in infancy with seizures, hypotonia, characteristic facies with a large forehead, and cholestatic hepatopathy. At autopsy renal cysts and absent peroxisomes are seen. Patients with a similar but milder biochemical and clinical phenotype have neonatal adrenoleukodystrophy or neonatal Refsum disease. They often have detectable peroxisomes.

In other peroxisomal diseases, only a single enzyme is deficient. Primary hyperoxaluria (alanine-glyoxylate aminotransferase deficiency) causes renal stones and nephropathy. Mutations in the X-linked very-long-chain fatty acid transporter gene, *ABCD1,* cause either a rapid leukodystrophy with loss of function (adrenoleukodystrophy), slow progressive spasticity and neuropathy (adrenomyeloneuropathy), or adrenal insufficiency. Defective phytanic acid oxidation in adult Refsum disease causes ataxia, leukodystrophy, cardiomyopathy, neuropathy, and retinal dystrophy. Other isolated enzyme deficiencies can mimic Zellweger syndrome.

Abnormalities of plasmalogen synthesis are clinically associated with rhizomelic chondrodysplasia punctata. Except for adrenoleukodystrophy, all peroxisomal diseases are autosomal recessive and can be diagnosed in utero.

Diagnosis

The best screening test for Zellweger syndrome and other biogenesis disorders is determination of very-long-chain fatty acids in serum or plasma. Urine bile acids are abnormal in other peroxisomal disorders. Phytanic acid and plasmalogens can also be measured. Together, these studies identify most peroxisomal diseases. Fibroblast enzyme assays followed by molecular analysis are needed for confirmation, especially when the parents plan further pregnancies.

Treatment

Bone marrow transplantation may be an effective treatment at the early stages of adrenoleukodystrophy, and close monitoring of affected males is necessary. Adrenal insufficiency requires hydrocortisone substitution. Lorenzo's oil, a mixture of glyceryl-trierucate and glyceryl-trioleate that suppresses endogenous very-long-chain fatty acid synthesis, in combination with a very-low-fat diet and essential fatty acid supplementation, is ineffective in patients with established symptoms, but is under evaluation for prevention of neurologic symptoms in presymptomatic males with adrenoleukodystrophy. Dietary treatment is used and effective for adult Refsum disease. Liver transplantation protects the kidneys in severe primary hyperoxaluria.

Cappa M et al: Adrenoleukodystrophy. Endocr Dev 2011;20:149 [PMID: 21164268].

Ebberink MS et al: Genetic classification and mutational spectrum of more than 600 patients with a Zellweger syndrome spectrum disorder. Hum Mutat 2011;32:59 [PMID: 21031596].

Ferrer I et al: General aspects and neuropathology of X-linked adrenoleukodystrophy. Brain Pathol 2010;20:817 [PMID: 20626743].

Kemp S, Wanders R: Biochemical aspects of X-linked adrenoleukodystrophy. Brain Pathol 2010;20:831 [PMID: 20626744].

Van Veldhoven PP: Biochemistry and genetics of inherited disorders of peroxisomal fatty acid metabolism. J Lipid Res 2010;51:2863 [PMID: 20558530].

CONGENITAL DISORDERS OF GLYCOSYLATION

Many proteins, including many enzymes, require glycosylation for normal function. The carbohydrate-deficient glycoprotein syndromes are an ever-increasing family of disorders that result from defects in the synthesis of glycans or in the attachment of glycans to other compounds. N-linked, O-linked, and combined N- and O-linked glycosylation defects have been described. The most common N-linked defect is phosphomannomutase 2 deficiency or congenital disorders of glycosylation type Ia (CDG-Ia). Children with type Ia disease usually present with prenatal growth disturbance, often with abnormal fat distribution, cerebellar hypoplasia, typical facial dysmorphic features, and mental retardation. The typical course includes chronic liver disease, peripheral neuropathy, endocrinopathies, retinopathy, and in some patients, acute life-threatening events. Patients with type Ib disease have a variable combination of liver fibrosis, protein-losing enteropathy, and hypoglycemia. More than a dozen other forms are characterized by additional key symptoms, including coloboma, cutis laxa, severe epilepsy, ichthyosis, and Dandy-Walker malformation. Biochemical differences and variations in clinical course (eg, the absence of peripheral neuropathy) characterize the other types. Pathophysiology probably relates to defects of those biochemical pathways that require glycosylated proteins. Recently, O-linked glycosylation defects have been found to underlie more classically described genetic syndromes such as multiple exostoses syndrome, Walker-Warburg syndrome, muscle-eye-brain disease, and a number of α-dystroglycanopathies. The syndromes appear to be inherited in an autosomal recessive manner with the exception of multiple exostoses syndrome which is autosomal dominant. The frequency of N-linked glycosylation defects is estimated to be as high as 1:20,000 in northern Europe.

Diagnosis

Diagnosis is supported by finding altered levels of glycosylated enzymes or other proteins such as transferrin, thyroxine-binding globulin, lysosomal enzymes, and clotting factors (IX, XI, antithrombin III, and proteins C and S). However, these levels may be normal in carbohydrate-deficient glycoprotein syndromes or abnormal in other conditions. Diagnosis is confirmed by finding typical patterns of abnormal glycosylation of selected proteins. Most diagnostic laboratories examine serum transferrin to screen for N-linked defects and apoC1 for O-linked defects. Confirmatory diagnosis is by assaying enzyme activity, analysis of lipid-linked oligosaccharides in fibroblasts, and mutation analysis.

Treatment

Treatment is supportive, including monitoring and providing early treatment for expected clinical features. Mannose treatment is curative for patients with type Ib deficiency only.

Foulquier F: COG defect, birth and rise. Biochim Biophys Acta 2009;1792:896 [PMID: 19028570].

Grünewald S: The clinical spectrum of phosphomannomutase 2 deficiency (CDG-Ia). Biochim Biophys Acta 2009;1792:827 [PMID: 19272306].

Haeuptle MA, Hennet T: Congenital disorders of glycosylation: An update on defects affecting the biosynthesis of dolichol-linked oligosaccharides. Hum Mutat 2009;30:1628 [PMID: 19862844].

Jaeken J: Congenital disorders of glycosylation (CDG): It's (nearly) all in it! J Inherit Metab Dis 2011;34:853.

Mercuri E et al: Congenital muscular dystrophies with defective glycosylation of dystroglycan: A population study. Neurology 2009;72:1802 [PMID: 19299310].

Morava E et al: Congenital disorder of glycosylation type Ix: A review of clinical spectrum and diagnostic steps. J Inherit Metab Dis 2008;31:450 [PMID: 18500572].

Patient and parent support group web site with useful information for families: http://www.cdgs.com

SMITH-LEMLI-OPITZ SYNDROME & DISORDERS OF CHOLESTEROL SYNTHESIS

ESSENTIALS OF DIAGNOSIS & TYPICAL FEATURES

- Elevated 7- and 8-dehydrocholesterol in serum and other tissue is diagnostic in SLO syndrome which presents with developmental delay and malformations.
- Chondrodysplasia punctata, skin defects, and neurological symptoms can indicate other cholesterol synthetic defects.

Several defects of cholesterol synthesis are associated with malformations and neurodevelopmental disability. SLO syndrome is an autosomal recessive disorder caused by a deficiency of the enzyme 7-dehydrocholesterol Δ7-reductase. It is characterized by microcephaly, poor growth, mental retardation, typical dysmorphic features of face and extremities (particularly two- to three-toe syndactyly), and often malformations of the heart and genitourinary system. It is further described in Chapter 37. Other cholesterol synthetic defects are seen in Conradi Hünnermann syndrome, which includes chondrodysplasia punctata and atrophic skin. Cholestanolosis (cerebrotendinous xanthomatosis) manifests with progressive ataxia and cataracts.

Diagnosis

In SLO, elevated 7- and 8-dehydrocholesterol in serum or other tissues, including amniotic fluid, is diagnostic. Serum cholesterol levels may be low or in the normal range. Enzymes of cholesterol synthesis may be assayed in cultured fibroblasts or amniocytes, and mutation analysis is possible.

Treatment

Although postnatal treatment does not resolve prenatal injury, supplementation with cholesterol in SLO improves growth and behavior. The role of supplemental bile acids is controversial. Simvastatin reduces 7- and 8-dehydrocholesterol and increases cholesterol levels by induction of its synthetic enzymes, but its effect on clinical symptoms is limited.

Porter FD: Smith-Lemli-Opitz syndrome: Pathogenesis, diagnosis, and management. Eur J Hum Genet 2008;16:535 [PMID: 18285838].

Porter FD, Herman GE: Malformation syndromes caused by disorders of cholesterol synthesis. J Lipid Res 2011;52:6 [PMID: 20929975].

Tierney E et al: Analysis of short-term behavioral effects of dietary cholesterol supplementation in Smith-Lemli-Opitz syndrome. Am J Med Genet A 2010;152A:91 [PMID: 20014133].

Patient and parent support group web site with useful information for families: http://www.smithlemliopitz.org

DISORDERS OF NEUROTRANSMITTER METABOLISM

ESSENTIALS OF DIAGNOSIS & TYPICAL FEATURES

- Movement disorder, especially dystonia and oculogyric crises.
- Severe seizures, abnormal tone, ataxia, and mental retardation occur in severely affected infants.
- Mildly affected patients have dopa-responsive dystonia with diurnal variability.
- Deficient serine synthesis causes microcephaly, seizures, and failure of myelination in neonates.

Abnormalities of neurotransmitter metabolism are increasingly recognized as causes of significant neurodevelopmental disabilities. Affected patients may present with movement disorders (especially dystonia and oculogyric crises), seizures, abnormal tone, or mental retardation, and are often considered to have cerebral palsy. Patients may be mildly affected (eg, dopa-responsive dystonia with diurnal variation) or severely affected (eg, intractable seizures with profound mental retardation). Deficient serine synthesis leads to congenital microcephaly, infantile seizures, and failure of myelination.

Pyridoxine-dependent epilepsy manifests as a severe seizure disorder in the neonatal or early infantile period that responds to high doses of pyridoxine. The disorder is caused by deficient activity of the enzyme α-amino adipic semialdehyde dehydrogenase resulting from mutations in the antiquitin (*ALDH7A1*) gene. Pyridoxal-phosphate–responsive encephalopathy manifests as a severe seizure disorder in infancy that responds to pyridoxal-phosphate. This disorder is caused by mutations in the *PNPO* gene encoding pyridox(am)ine oxidase, which is necessary for activation of pyridoxine.

Diagnosis

Although some disorders can be diagnosed by examining serum amino acids or urine organic acids (eg, 4-hydroxybutyric aciduria), in most cases, diagnosis requires analysis of CSF. Spinal fluid samples for neurotransmitter analysis require special collection and handling, as the neurotransmitter levels are graduated along the axis of the central nervous system and are highly unstable once the sample is collected. A phenylalanine loading test can be diagnostic for mild defects in GTP-cyclohydrolase deficiency, in which neurotransmitter analysis may be insufficiently sensitive. Analysis of CSF shows elevated threonine and decreased pyridoxal-phosphate in pyridoxalphosphate–responsive disease, and decreased serine and glycine in serine biosynthetic defects. Urine α-aminoadipic acid or piperideine-6-carboxylate can be used to identify infants with seizures that may be pyridoxine dependent.

Treatment

For some conditions, such as pyridoxine-responsive seizures, pyridoxal-phosphate–responsive encephalopathy, or dopa-responsive dystonia, response to treatment can be dramatic. For others, response to therapy is less satisfactory in part because of poor penetration of the blood-brain barrier. Supplementation with serine and glycine can substantially improve outcome in serine deficiency.

Hyland K et al: Cerebral folate deficiency. J Inherit Metab Dis 2010;33:563 [PMID: 20668945].

Kurian MA et al: The monoamine neurotransmitter disorders: An expanding range of neurological syndromes. Lancet Neurol 2011;10:721 [PMID: 21777827].

Leen WG et al: Glucose transporter-1deficiency syndrome: The expanding clinical and genetic spectrum of a treatable disorder. Brain 2010;133(Pt 3):655 [PMID: 20129935].

Pearl PL: New treatment paradigms in neonatal metabolic epilepsies. J Inherit Metab Dis 2009;32:204 [PMID: 19234868].

Stockler S et al: Pyridoxine dependent epilepsy and antiquitin deficiency: Clinical and molecular characteristics and recommendations for diagnosis, treatment and follow-up. Mol Genet Metab 2011 May 24 [Epub ahead of print] [PMID: 21704546].

CREATINE SYNTHESIS DISORDERS

Creatine and creatine phosphate are essential for storage and transmission of phosphate-bound energy in muscle and brain. They spontaneously convert to creatinine. Three disorders of creatine synthesis are now known: arginine:glycine amidinotransferase (AGAT) deficiency, guanidinoacetate methyltransferase (GAMT) deficiency, and creatine transporter (CrT1) deficiency. GAMT and AGAT deficiencies are autosomal recessive disorders, whereas CrT1 deficiency is X-linked. All patients demonstrate developmental delay, mental retardation, autistic behavior, seizures, and severe expressive language disturbance. Patients may also show developmental regression and brain atrophy. Patients with GAMT deficiency have more severe seizures and an extrapyramidal movement disorder. The seizure disorder is milder in CrT1-deficient patients. Some female heterozygotes of CrT1 deficiency may also show developmental delay or learning disabilities.

Diagnosis

The common feature of all creatine synthesis defects is a severe depletion of creatine and creatinephosphate in the brain demonstrable by reduction to absence of signal on magnetic resonance spectroscopy. In GAMT deficiency, guanidinoacetate accumulates, whereas in AGAT deficiency, guanidinoacetate is decreased, particularly in urine. Guanidinoacetate seems to be responsible for the severe seizures and movement disorder found in GAMT deficiency. Blood, urine, and CSF creatine levels are decreased in GAMT deficiency but normal in AGAT deficiency. Urine excretion of creatine is elevated in CrT1 deficiency. Enzyme and molecular analyses are available for diagnostic confirmation.

Treatment

Treatment with oral creatine supplementation is in part successful in GAMT and AGAT deficiencies. It is not beneficial in CrT1 deficiency. Treatment by combined arginine restriction and ornithine substitution in GAMT deficiency can decrease guanidinoacetate concentrations and improve the clinical course.

Arias A et al: Creatine transporter deficiency: Prevalence among patients with mental retardation and pitfalls in metabolite screening. Clin Biochem 2007;40:1328 [PMID: 17825809].

Braissant O et al: Creatine deficiency syndromes and the importance of creatine synthesis in the brain. Amino Acids 2011;40: 1315 [PMID: 21390529].

Gordon N: Guanidinoacetate methyltransferase deficiency (GAMT). Brain Dev 2010;32:79 [PMID: 19289269].

Longo N et al: Disorders of creatine transport and metabolism. Am J Med Genet C Semin Med Genet 2011;157:72 [PMID: 21308988].

Nasrallah F et al: Creatine and creatine deficiency syndromes: Biochemical and clinical aspects. Pediatr Neurol 2010;42:163 [PMID: 20159424].

Sun Q, O'Brien WE: Diagnosis of creatine metabolism disorders by determining creatine and guanidinoacetate in plasma and urine. Methods Mol Biol 2010;603:175 [PMID: 20077070].

Valayannopoulos V et al: Treatment by oral creatine, L-arginine and L-glycine in six severely affected patients with creatine transporter defect. J Inherit Metab Dis 2011;Jun 10 [Epub ahead of print] [PMID: 21660517].

QUALITY INITIATIVES IN THE FIELD OF METABOLIC DISEASE

Expanded newborn screening has had a large impact on the field of metabolic disorders. As desired, patients are being diagnosed earlier, and for some patients, this dramatically reduces the disease burden. Expanded newborn screening, however, has also uncovered problems or revealed unexpected consequences that need to be addressed. For example, the clinical spectrum of many disorders is being expanded to include mildly affected or asymptomatic patients. This raises care questions particularly in regard to the need for aggressive management in the more mildly affected patients or if therapy is needed at all for some patients. It is unclear whether some patients diagnosed who are on the more mild end of a disease spectrum would have ever become symptomatic or are those patients representative of a portion of the disease population who may never have presented to care. Consequently, for some disorders, disease incidence appears to be changing. In addition, newborn screening for several conditions has brought to light our ability to detect maternal disease. Disorders such as maternal B12 deficiency and maternal carnitine uptake deficiency pose management as well as risk questions for this largely asymptomatic population. Conditions, felt by most to be benign, are also being diagnosed as a consequence of expanded newborn screening. Further, due to limitations in diagnostic testing, patients who may be carriers for a condition are now being treated, as the carrier status cannot be entirely confirmed nor the condition entirely excluded. This is particularly true for disorders such as glutaric acidemia, type I, and very-long-chain acyl-CoA dehydrogenase deficiency (VLCAD). This not only adds to parental anxiety, but treatment of an unaffected child may entail risk to the child or to family dynamics.

Improvement in diagnostic testing, especially the sensitivity of molecular and enzymatic testing, may help improve the diagnostic conundrum. National initiatives are underway in an attempt to clarify other issues. Initiated under regional programs and now under the guidance of the American College of Medical Genetics and the Newborn Screening Translational Research Network (NBSTRN), uniform clinical data sets for disorders diagnosed via newborn screening have been developed. The hope is also for a national database for data collection integrating clinical care, public health, and state laboratories. The overall goal is to track the long-term outcome of individuals diagnosed with inborn errors of metabolism, to define best practice guidelines, and to determine the benefit of newborn screening. In addition, the NBSTRN seeks to stimulate research in newborn screening, advocate pilot screening programs, and establish a national, virtual dried blood spot repository for research. This national initiative is inclusive of all disorders for which newborn screening occurs, not just inborn errors of metabolism.

Another national focus is the expansion of newborn screening to other genetic disorders. Currently, some states are beginning to implement newborn screening for severe combined immunodeficiency (SCID) and for lysosomal storage disorders such as Pompe disease, Fabry disease, Gaucher disease, and Krabbe disease. A pilot study is also underway for screening for spinal muscular atrophy, and screening for disorders such as Fragile X syndrome and Prader Willi syndrome is being considered. As technology for early detection and treatment strategies advance, more disorders will likely be considered candidates for newborn screening. Additionally, some conditions being considered for screening affect an individual after the newborn period. Second tier, childhood screening for such late onset disorders may be a consideration in the future. Careful consideration will need to be given regarding the risks and benefits to screening for such conditions. The U.S. Secretary for Health and Human Services' Advisory Committee on Heritable Disorders in Newborns and Children has established a rigorous process for disease review before recommending a disorder be considered for screening.

Hinton CF et al: What questions should newborn screening long-term follow-up be able to answer? A statement of the U.S. Secretary for Health and Human Services' Advisory Committee on Heritable Disorders in Newborns and Children. Genet Med 2011;Jun 28 [Epub ahead of print] [PMID: 21716119].

Kemper AR et al: Weighing the evidence for newborn screening for early-infantile Krabbe disease. Genet Med 2010;12:539 [PMID: 20601893].

Levy HL: Newborn screening conditions: what we know, what we do not know, and how will we know it. Genet Med 2010;12 (Suppl 12):S213 [PMID: 21150366].

Lloyd-Puryear MA, Brower A: Long-term follow-up in newborn screening: A systems approach for improving health outcomes. Genet Med 2010;12(Suppl 12):S256 [PMID: 21150372].

Marsden D, Levy H: Newborn screening for lysosomal storage disorders. Clin Chem 2010;56:1071 [PMID: 20489136].

Nakamura K et al: Newborn screening for lysosomal storage disorders. Am J Med Genet C Semin Med Genet 2011;157:63 [PMID: 21312327].

Wilcken B: Expanded newborn screening: Reducing harm, assessing benefit. J Inherit Metab Dis 2010;33(Suppl 2):S205 [PMID: 20440650].

37 Genetics & Dysmorphology

Anne Chun-Hui Tsai, MD, MSc
David K. Manchester, MD
Ellen R. Elias, MD

Genetics is an exciting and rapidly evolving field that has significant relevance to the understanding of human embryology, physiology, and disease processes. Tremendous advances in molecular biology and biochemistry are allowing more comprehensive understanding of mechanisms inherent in genetic disorders, as well as improved diagnostic tests and management options. Many of the newer technologies and terms may be unfamiliar to the clinician in practice. Thus, the topics in the first part of the chapter serve as an introduction and review of the basic principles of genetics, including basic knowledge of cytogenetics and molecular biology. The second part discusses principles of inherited human disorders, encompassing different genetic mechanisms as well as how to obtain a genetic history and pedigree. Topics in the third part of the chapter focus on applied clinical genetics which include dysmorphology, teratology, and perinatology. Common clinical disorders, with descriptions of the diseases, discussion of their pathogenesis, diagnosis, and management are also included.

FOUNDATIONS OF GENETIC DIAGNOSIS

CYTOGENETICS

Cytogenetics is the study of genetics at the chromosome level. Chromosomal anomalies occur in 0.4% of all live births and are a common cause of intellectual disabilities (formerly called mental retardation) and congenital anomalies. The prevalence of chromosomal anomalies is much higher among spontaneous abortions and stillbirths.

Chromosomes

Human chromosomes consist of DNA (the blueprint of genetic material), specific proteins forming the backbone of the chromosome (called histones), and other chromatin structural and interactive proteins. Chromosomes contain most of the genetic information necessary for growth and differentiation. The nuclei of all normal human cells, with the exception of gametes, contain 46 chromosomes, consisting of 23 pairs (Figure 37–1). Of these, 22 pairs are called autosomes. They are numbered according to their size; chromosome 1 is the largest and chromosome 22 the smallest. In addition, there are two sex chromosomes: two X chromosomes in females and one X and one Y chromosome in males. The two members of a chromosome pair are called homologous chromosomes. One homolog of each chromosome pair is maternal in origin (from the egg); the second is paternal (from the sperm). The egg and sperm each contain 23 chromosomes (haploid cells). During formation of the zygote, they fuse into a cell with 46 chromosomes (diploid cell).

Cell Division

Cells undergo cycles of growth and division that are controlled according to their needs and functions.

Mitosis is a kind of cell division, occurring in stages, during which DNA replication takes place and two daughter cells, genetically identical to the original parent cells, are formed. This cell division is typical for all somatic cells (cells other than the sperm or egg, which are called germline cells). There are four phases of mitosis: interphase, prophase, metaphase, and anaphase. In interphase, chromosomes are long, thin, and nonvisible. At this time, the genetic material is replicated. In prophase, the chromosomes are more condensed. During metaphase (the phase following DNA replication but preceding cell division), individual chromosomes can be visualized. Each arm consists of two identical parts, called chromatids. Chromatids of the same chromosome are called sister chromatids. In anaphase, the genetic material is separated into two cells.

Meiosis is a kind of cell division during which eggs and sperm are formed; it is a cell division limited to gametes. During meiosis, three unique processes take place:

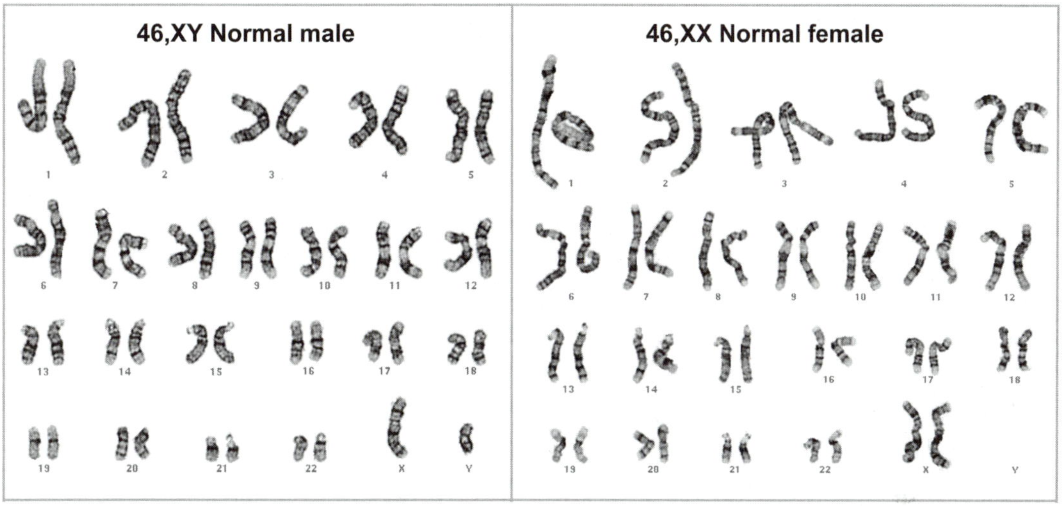

▲ **Figure 37–1.** Normal male and female human karyotype. (Courtesy of the Colorado Genetics Laboratory.)

1. Crossing over of genetic material between two homologous chromosomes (this recombination, or exchange of genetic material increases the viability of human beings).
2. Random assortment of maternally and paternally derived homologous chromosomes into the daughter cells.
3. Two cell divisions, the first of which is a reduction division—that is, separation between the homologous chromosomes. The second meiotic division is like mitosis, separating two sister chromatids into two daughter cells.

Chromosome Preparation & Analysis

Chromosome structure is visible only during mitosis, most often achieved in the laboratory by stimulating a blood lymphocyte culture with a mitogen for 3 days. Other tissues used for this purpose include skin, products of conception, cartilage, and bone marrow. Chorionic villi or amniocytes are used for prenatal diagnosis. Spontaneously dividing cells without a mitogen are present in bone marrow, and historically, bone marrow biopsy was done when immediate identification of a patient's chromosome constitution was necessary for appropriate management (eg, to rule out trisomy 13 in a newborn with a complex congenital heart disease). However, this invasive test has been replaced by the availability of the FISH technique (see following discussion).

Cells processed for routine chromosome analysis are stained on glass slides to yield a light-and-dark band pattern across the arms of the chromosomes (see Figure 37–1). This band pattern is characteristic and reproducible for each chromosome, allowing the chromosomes to be identified. Using different staining techniques, different banding patterns result: G, Q, and R banding. The most commonly used is G banding. The layout of chromosomes on a sheet of paper in a predetermined order is called a **karyotype**. High-resolution chromosome analysis is the study of more elongated chromosomes in prometaphase. Although the bands can be visualized in greater detail, subtle chromosomal rearrangements less than 5 million base pair (5 Mb) can still be missed.

Fluorescence in situ hybridization (FISH) is a powerful technique that labels a known chromosome sequence with DNA probes attached to fluorescent dyes, thus enabling visualization of specific regions of chromosomes by fluorescent microscopy. There are many different kinds of probes, including paint probes (a mixture of sequences throughout one chromosome), sequence-specific probes, centromere probes, and telomere probes. A cocktail of differently colored probes, one color for each chromosome, called multicolor FISH, or M-FISH, can detect complex rearrangements between chromosomes. FISH can detect submicroscopic structural rearrangements undetectable by classic cytogenetic techniques and can identify marker chromosomes. (For pictures of FISH studies, go to http://www.kumc.edu/gec/prof/cytogene.html.)

Interphase FISH allows noncultured cells (lymphocytes, amniocytes) to be rapidly screened for numerical abnormalities such as trisomy 13, 18, or 21, and sex chromosome anomalies. However, because of the possible background or contamination of the signal, the abnormality must be confirmed by conventional chromosome analysis in aneuploidy cases. Six hundred–cell FISH can also be used to ascertain mosaicism.

Chromosomal Microarray Analysis (CMA)

Advances in computer technology and bioinformatics have led to the development of new genetic testing using comparative genomic hybridization with microarray technique. This technique allows detection of very small genetic imbalances anywhere in the genome. Its usefulness has been well documented in cancer research and more recently in assessing small chromosomal rearrangements. In particular, it has been used to detect interstitial and subtelomeric submicroscopic imbalances, to characterize their size at the molecular level, and to define the breakpoints of translocations. Clinically available arrays include (1) 0.5- to 1-Mb bacterial artificial chromosome arrays that can pick up rearrangements greater than 0.5 Mb, (2) oligonucleotide arrays using special probes that can pick up changes as small as 3 Kb, and (3) single nucleotide polymorphism (SNP) arrays, which are used more widely in research settings. Although this powerful new technology can identify extremely subtle DNA rearrangements and changes, many human polymorphisms, including small deletions and duplications, are not totally understood. Therefore, special caution and parental studies are often required in interpreting the results.

Van den Veyver IB et al: Clinical use of array comparative genomic hybridization (aCGH) for prenatal diagnosis in 300 cases. Prenat Diagn 2009 Jan;29(1):29–39.

Stankiewicz P, Beaudet AL: Use of array CGH in the evaluation of dysmorphology, malformations, developmental delay, and idiopathic mental retardation. Curr Opin Genet Dev 2007 Jun;17(3):182–192 [Epub 2007 Apr 30] [Review].

Chromosome Nomenclature

Visible under the microscope is a constriction site on the chromosome called the centromere, which separates the chromosome into two arms: p, for petite, refers to the short arm, and q, the letter following p, refers to the long arm. Each arm is further subdivided into numbered bands visible using different staining techniques. Centromeres are positioned at different sites on different chromosomes and are used to differentiate the chromosome structures seen during mitosis as **metacentric** (p arm and q arm of almost equal size), **submetacentric** (p arm shorter than q arm), and **acrocentric** (almost no p arm). The use of named chromosome arms and bands provides a universal method of chromosome description. Common symbols include *del* (deletion), *dup* (duplication), *inv* (inversion), *ish* (in situ hybridization), *i* (isochromosome), *pat* (paternal origin), *mat* (maternal origin), and *r* (ring chromosome). These terms are further defined under the section on Chromosomal Abnormalities.

Chromosomal Abnormalities

There are two types of chromosomal anomalies: numerical and structural.

A. Abnormalities of Chromosomal Number

When a human cell has 23 chromosomes, such as human ova or sperm, it is in the haploid state (n). After conception, in cells other than the reproductive cells, 46 chromosomes are present in the diploid state (2n). Any number that is an exact multiple of the haploid number—for example, 46(2n), 69(3n), or 92(4n)—is referred to as euploid. Polyploid cells are those that contain any number other than the usual diploid number of chromosomes. Polyploid conceptions are usually not viable except in a "mosaic state," with the presence of more than one cell line in the body (see later text for details).

Cells deviating from the multiple of the haploid number are called aneuploid, meaning not euploid, indicating an abnormal number of chromosomes. Trisomy, an example of aneuploidy, is the presence of three of a particular chromosome rather than two. It results from unequal division, called nondisjunction, of chromosomes into daughter cells. Trisomies are the most common numerical chromosomal anomalies found in humans (eg, trisomy 21 [Down syndrome], trisomy 18, and trisomy 13). Monosomies, the presence of only one member of a chromosome pair, may be complete or partial. Complete monosomies may result from nondisjunction or anaphase lag. All complete autosomal monosomies appear to be lethal early in development and only survive in mosaic forms. Sex chromosome monosomy, however, can be viable.

B. Abnormalities of Chromosomal Structure

Many different types of structural chromosomal anomalies exist. Figure 37–2 displays the formal nomenclature as well as the ideogram demonstrating chromosomal anomalies. In clinical context, the sign (+) or (–) *preceding* the chromosome number indicates increased or decreased number, respectively, of that particular whole chromosome in a cell. For example, 47, XY+21 designates a male with three copies of chromosome 21. The sign (+) or (–) *after* the chromosome number signifies extra material or missing material, respectively, on one of the arms of the chromosome. For example, 46,XX, 8q– denotes a deletion on the long arm of chromosome 8. Detailed nomenclature, such as 8q11, is required to further demonstrate a specific missing region so that genetic counseling can be provided.

1. Deletion (del) (see Figure 37–2A)—This refers to an absence of normal chromosomal material. It may be terminal (at the end of a chromosome) or interstitial (within a chromosome). The missing part is described using the code "del," followed by the number of the chromosome involved in parentheses, and a description of the missing region of that chromosome, also in parentheses, for example, 46,XX,del(1) (p36.3). This chromosome nomenclature describes the loss of genetic material from band 36.3 of the short arm of chromosome 1, which results in 1p36.3 deletion syndrome. Some more common deletions result in clinically

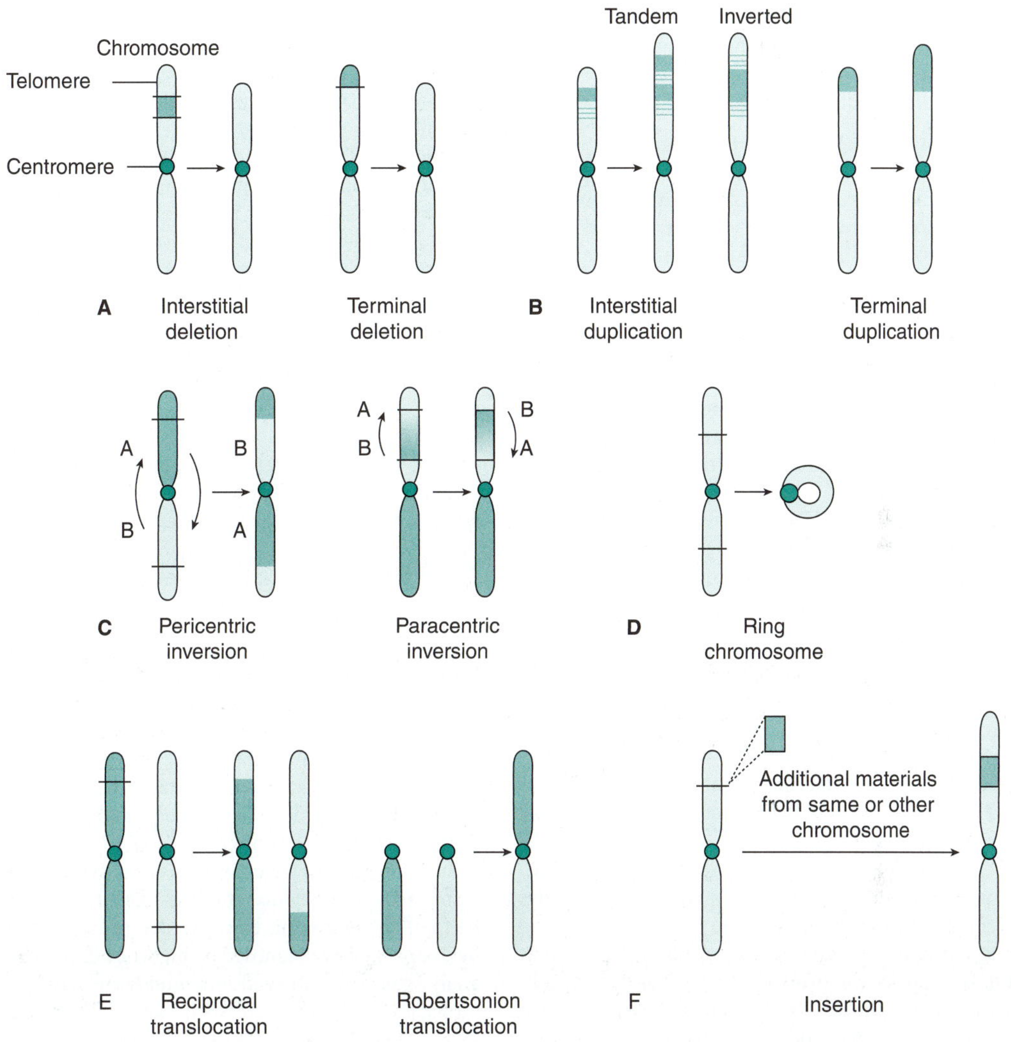

▲ **Figure 37–2.** Examples of structural chromosomal abnormalities: deletion, duplication, inversion, ring chromosome, translocation, and insertion.

recognizable conditions associated with intellectual disabilities and characteristic facial features. (See descriptions of common genetic disorders caused by chromosomal deletions later in the chapter.)

2. Duplication (dup) (see Figure 37–2B)—An extra copy of a chromosomal segment can be tandem (genetic material present in the original direction) or inverted (genetic material present in the opposite direction). A well-described duplication of chromosome 22q11 causes Cat eye syndrome, resulting in iris coloboma and anal or ear anomalies.

3. Inversion (inv) (see Figure 37–2C)—In this aberration, a rearranged section of a chromosome is inverted. It can be paracentric (not involving the centromere) or pericentric (involving the centromere).

4. Ring chromosome (r) (see Figure 37–2D)—Deletion of the normal telomeres (and possibly other subtelomeric sequences) leads to subsequent fusion of both ends to form a circular chromosome. Ring chromosomal anomalies often cause growth retardation and intellectual disability.

5. Translocation (trans) (see Figure 37–2E)—This interchromosomal rearrangement of genetic material may be balanced (the cell has a normal content of genetic material arranged in a structurally abnormal way) or unbalanced (the cell has gained or lost genetic material as a result of chromosomal interchange). Balanced translocations may further be described as reciprocal, the exchange of genetic material between two nonhomologous chromosomes, or robertsonian, the fusion of two acrocentric chromosomes.

6. Insertion (ins) (see Figure 37–2F)—Breakage within a chromosome at two points and incorporation of another piece of chromosomal material is called insertion. This requires three breakpoints and may occur between two chromosomes or within the same chromosome. The clinical presentation or phenotype depends on the origin of the inserted materials.

C. Sex Chromosomal Anomalies

Abnormalities involving sex chromosomes, including aneuploidy and mosaicism, are relatively common in the general population. The most common sex chromosome anomalies include 45,X (Turner syndrome), 47,XXX, 47,XXY (Klinefelter syndrome), 47,XYY, and different mosaic states. (See later text for clinical discussion.)

D. Mosaicism

Mosaicism is the presence of two or more different chromosome constitutions in different cells of the same individual. For example, a patient may have some cells with 47 chromosomes and others with 46 chromosomes (46,XX/47,XX,+21 indicates mosaicism for trisomy 21; similarly, 45,X/46,XX/47,XXX indicates mosaicism for a monosomy and a trisomy X). Mosaicism should be suspected if clinical symptoms are milder than expected in a nonmosaic patient with the same chromosomal abnormality, or if the patient's skin shows unusual pigmentation. The prognosis is frequently better for a patient with mosaicism than for one with a corresponding chromosomal abnormality without mosaicism. In general, the smaller the proportion of the abnormal cell line, the better the prognosis. In the same patient, however, the proportion of normal and abnormal cells in various tissues, such as skin, brain, internal organs, and peripheral blood, may be significantly different. Therefore, the prognosis for a patient with chromosomal mosaicism can seldom be assessed reliably based on the karyotype in peripheral blood alone.

E. Uniparental Disomy

Under normal circumstances, one member of each homologous pair of chromosomes is of maternal origin from the egg and the other is of paternal origin from the sperm (Figure 37–3A). In uniparental disomy (UPD), both copies of a particular chromosome pair originate from the same parent. If UPD is caused by an error in the first meiotic division, both homologous chromosomes of that parent will be present in the gamete—a phenomenon called heterodisomy (see Figure 37–3B). If the disomy is caused by an error in the second meiotic division, two copies of the same chromosome will be present through the mechanism of rescue, duplication, and complementation (see Figure 37–3C through 37–3E)—a phenomenon called isodisomy. Isodisomy may also occur as a postfertilization error (see Figure 37–3F).

A chromosomal analysis would not reveal an abnormality, but DNA analysis would reveal that the child inherited two copies of DNA of a particular chromosome from one parent without the contribution from the other parent. Possible mechanisms for the adverse effects of UPD include homozygosity for deleterious recessive genes and the consequences of imprinting (see discussion in the Imprinting section, later). It is suspected that UPD of some chromosomes is lethal.

UPD has been documented for certain human chromosomes, including chromosomes 7, 11, 15, and X, and has been found in patients with Prader-Willi, Angelman, and Beckwith-Wiedemann syndromes (BWS). In addition, cystic fibrosis with only one carrier parent (caused by maternal isodisomy) has been reported. UPD may cause severe prenatal and postnatal growth retardation.

F. Contiguous Gene Syndromes

Contiguous gene syndromes result when a deletion causes the loss of genes adjacent to each other on a chromosome. Although many genes may be missing, the deletion may still be too small to be detected by routine karyotype. Therefore, contiguous gene syndromes are sometimes called "microdeletion syndromes." The genes involved in these syndromes are related only through their linear placement on the same chromosome segments and may not influence each other's functions directly. Table 37–1 lists examples of some currently known contiguous gene syndromes and their associated chromosomal abnormalities. These deletions may be familial (passed on by a parent), or occur de novo. The deletions may be diagnosed by high-resolution chromosome analysis in some affected individuals, or may be submicroscopic and detectable only with FISH or DNA analysis.

G. Chromosome Fragility

Disorders of DNA repair are associated with chromosomal breakage and death of somatic cells. Most are autosomal recessive. Phenotypes vary considerably (Table 37–2). As a group these disorders typically affect growth and CNS development. They show increased toxicity to mutagen exposures in vitro. Photosensitivity, increased cancer risks, and premature aging are prevalent. Treatment is largely supportive and focuses on surveillance for complications but in at least one disorder, Fanconi anemia, bone marrow transplant can be beneficial. See www.genereviews.org for excellent reviews of these disorders.

H. Chromosomal Abnormalities in Cancer

Numerical and structural chromosomal abnormalities are often identified in hematopoietic and solid-tumor neoplasms in individuals with otherwise normal chromosomes.

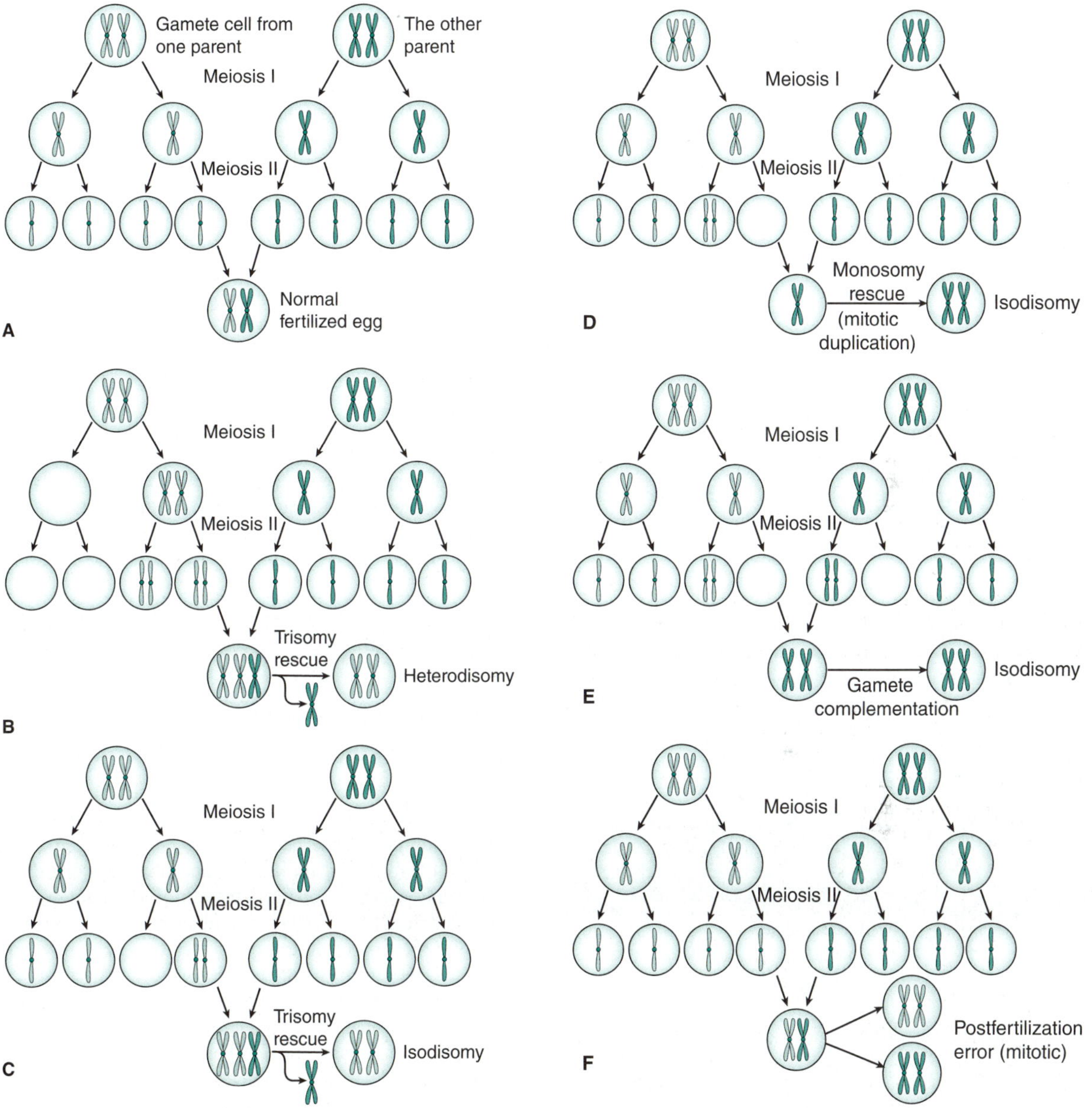

▲ **Figure 37–3.** The assortment of homologous chromosomes during normal gametogenesis and uniparental disomy. **A:** Fertilization of normal gametes. **B:** Heterodisomy by trisomy rescue. **C:** Isodisomy by trisomy rescue. **D:** Isodisomy by monosomy rescue (mitotic duplication). **E:** Gamete complementation. **F:** Postfertilization error.

These cytogenetic abnormalities have been categorized as primary and secondary. In primary abnormalities, their presence is necessary for initiation of the cancer; an example is 13q– in retinoblastoma. Secondary abnormalities appear de novo in somatic cells only after the cancer has developed, for example, Philadelphia chromosome, t(9;22)(q34;q11), in acute and chronic myeloid leukemia. Primary and secondary chromosomal abnormalities are specific for particular neoplasms and can be used for diagnosis or prognosis. For example, the presence of the Philadelphia chromosome is a good prognostic sign in chronic myelogenous leukemia and indicates a poor prognosis in acute lymphoblastic leukemia. The sites of chromosome breaks coincide with the known loci of oncogenes and antioncogenes.

Table 37–1. Examples of common contiguous gene syndromes.

Syndrome	Abnormal Chromosome Segment
Prader-Willi/Angelman syndrome	del 15q11
Shprintzen/DiGeorge spectrum	del 22q11
Williams syndrome	del 7q11
Smith-Magenis syndrome	del 17p11

MOLECULAR GENETICS

Advances in molecular biology have revolutionized human genetics, as they allow for the localization, isolation, and characterization of genes that encode protein sequences. As the Human Genome Project has moved into the postcloning era, the function of gene products and their interaction with one another has become the main theme of molecular genetics. Molecular genetics can help explain the complex underlying biology involved in many human diseases.

Table 37–2. DNA repair disorders.

Disorder	Phenotype
Fanconi anemia	Radial ray limb anomalies, short stature, pigment changes, mild cognitive deficiencies, increased chromosome breakage in vitro, increased cancer risk.
Ataxia-telangiectasia	Ataxia (onset by 1 y), cutaneous/conjunctival telangiectasia, cerebellar hypoplasia, sinusitis, bronchiectasis, diabetes, elevated α-fetoprotein, increased cancer risk.
Bloom syndrome	Short stature, chronic lung disease, sun exposure induced facial telangiectasia, increased sister chromatid exchange, increased cancer risk.
Cockayne syndrome	Severe growth deficiency, microcephaly, photosensitivity, aged facies, cataracts, pigmentary retinopathy, cognitive deficiency, cerebral atrophy, death frequently in early childhood, no increase in cancer risk.
Trichothiodystrophy	Brittle hair with diagnostic microscopic changes in polarized light, microcephaly, short stature, aged appearance, photosensitivity, no increase in cancer risk.
Xeroderma pigmentosum	Severe skin photosensitivity, normal cognitive function, increased risk for skin cancers including melanoma.
Seckel syndrome	Extreme growth deficiency, microcephaly, characteristic facies, pancytopenia, increased sister chromatid exchange.

Molecular diagnosis can be achieved using the following technology: **Southern blot analysis** is the molecular genetic technique used to look for changes in genomic DNA. A similar technique, called **Northern blot analysis**, is used to look for RNA abnormalities. **Western blot analysis** is used to look for protein changes. The **polymerase chain reaction (PCR)** replicates fragments of DNA between predetermined primers so that sufficient DNA is obtained for characterization or sequencing in the space of a few hours. **Quantitative fluorescent PCR** combines PCR amplification with fluorescent DNA probes to provide real-time replication and rapid determination of gene copy number and dosage effects. **DNA sequencing** is the process of determining the nucleotide order of a given DNA fragment. A new generation of sequencing technologies, has provided unprecedented opportunities for high-throughput functional genomic research. To date, these technologies have been applied in a variety of contexts, including whole-genome sequencing which can be performed in 1 week; however, the interpretation of the sequencing requires more bioinformatics information. National Institutes of Health (NIH) predicted the eventual cost for whole genome can be reduced to $1000.

ten Bosch JR, Grody WW: Keeping up with the next generation: Massively parallel sequencing in clinical diagnostics. J Mol Diagn 2008 Nov;10(6):484–492.

Molecular Biology in Clinical Genetics & Genetic Diagnosis

Genetic diagnosis can be performed by direct detection of a mutant gene or by indirect methods. Direct detection is possible only when the gene causing the disease and the nature of the mutation are known. The advantage of a diagnostic study using the direct detection of a mutant gene is that it requires the affected individual only and need not involve the testing of other family members. The methods of direct DNA diagnosis include restriction analysis, direct sequencing with assistance of PCR, heteroduplex assay, and protein truncation assay. The molecular mechanisms causing human diseases include point mutations, deletions, and insertions, and the unstable expansion of trinucleotide repeats, which leads to genetic anticipation. Some disorders that may be diagnosed via direct DNA mutational analysis include Duchenne muscular dystrophy, hemophilia, cystic fibrosis, and fragile X syndrome.

Indirect detection of abnormal genes is used when the gene is known but there is extensive heterogeneity of the molecular defect between families, or when the gene responsible for a disease is unknown but its chromosome location is known. One form of indirect analysis is the linkage method. Linkage traces the inheritance of the abnormal gene between members in a kindred. This method requires that the affected individual be studied, as well as parents and other relatives, both affected and unaffected. Linkage analysis is performed by using markers such as a restriction fragment length polymorphisms. Microsatellite polymorphisms are being used in sibling research studies to identify the multiple genes that contribute to polygenic traits such as diabetes and obesity. They are also used increasingly to identify gene changes in tumors.

Neurofibromatosis is an example of a disorder in which both the direct and indirect assay may be used. An estimated 90%–95% of patients with neurofibromatosis type 1 have a mutation or deletion that can be identified using a direct assay of the neurofibromin gene (*NF1*). The other cases must rely on indirect methods such as linkage analysis for prenatal diagnosis.

Molecular Biology in Prevention & Treatment of Human Diseases

Molecular diagnosis can prevent genetic disease by detection of mutation and permitting prenatal diagnosis. As diseases often present in spectrums and clinical features among disorders can overlap, molecular testing is useful to confirm a diagnosis. Family studies can also clarify the mode of inheritance, thus allowing more accurate determination of recurrence risks and appropriate options. For example, differentiation of gonadal mosaicism from decreased penetrance of a dominant gene has important implications for genetic counseling. In the past, the diagnosis of a genetic disease characterized by late onset of symptoms (eg, Huntington disease) could not be made prior to the appearance of clinical symptoms. In some inborn errors of metabolism, diagnostic tests (eg, measurement of enzyme activities) could be conducted only on inaccessible tissues. Gene identification (mutation analysis) techniques can enormously enhance the ability to diagnose both symptomatic and presymptomatic individuals, heterozygous carriers of gene mutations, and affected fetuses. However, presymptomatic DNA testing is associated with psychological, ethical, and legal implications and therefore should be used only with informed consent. Formal genetic counseling is indicated to best interpret the results of molecular testing.

A normal gene introduced into an individual affected with a serious inherited disorder during embryonic life (germline therapy) in principle has the potential to be transmitted to future generations, whereas its introduction into somatic cells (somatic therapy) affects only the recipient. Experimental gene therapy by bone marrow transplantation is being tried for adenosine deaminase deficiency. Recombinant enzyme replacement has been successfully applied in treating the non-neurologic form of Gaucher disease, Fabry disease, Pompe disease, mucopolysaccharidosis types I and II, and some types of lysosomal storage disease.

Proteomics is the large-scale study of proteins, particularly their structures and functions. The term "proteomics" was first coined in 1997 as an analogy to genomics, the study of the genes. "Proteome" means a blend of "**prote**in" and "genome." Understanding the proteome, the structure and function of each protein and the complexities of protein-protein interactions will be critical for developing effective diagnostic techniques and disease treatments. One of the most promising roles of proteomics has been the identification of potential new drugs for the treatment of disease. This relies on genome and proteome information to identify proteins associated with a disease, which computer software can then use as targets for new drugs. For example, in Alzheimer disease, elevations in beta secretase create amyloid/beta-protein, which causes plaque to build up in the patient's brain, which is thought to play a role in dementia. Targeting this enzyme decreases the amyloid/beta-protein and so slows the progression of the disease.

Pharmacogenomics is a new field offering enormous promise for predicting drug response in patients. For example, by DNA analysis of two specific genes, *CYP2C9* and *VKORC1,* it is now possible to predict response to warfarin anticoagulation therapy and to individualize the dose, saving the patient multiple blood tests and dosage adjustments. It is also possible to predict which patients would be at risk for hearing loss after receiving aminoglycoside treatment, based on mutations in the mitochondrial 12S rRNA gene.

Ma Q et al: Pharmacogenetics, pharmacogenomics, and individualized medicine. Pharmacol Rev 2011 Jun;63(2):437–459 [Epub 2011 Mar 24].

Garcia DA et al: Estimation of the warfarin dose with clinical and pharmacogenetic data. NEJM 2009;360:753–764.

PRINCIPLES OF INHERITED HUMAN DISORDERS

MENDELIAN INHERITANCE

Traditionally, autosomal single-gene disorders follow the principles explained by Mendel's observations. To summarize, the inheritance of genetic traits through generations relies on segregation and independent assortment. **Segregation** is the process through which gene pairs are separated during gamete formation. Each gamete receives only one copy of each gene (allele). **Independent assortment** refers to the idea that the segregation of different alleles occurs independently.

Victor McKusick's catalog, *Mendelian Inheritance in Man,* lists more than 10,000 entries in which the mode of inheritance is presumed to be autosomal dominant, autosomal recessive, X-linked dominant, X-linked recessive, and Y-linked. Single genes at specific loci on one or a pair of chromosomes cause these disorders. An understanding of inheritance terminology is helpful in approaching mendelian disorders. Analysis of the pedigree and the pattern of transmission in the family, identification of a specific condition, and knowledge of that condition's mode of inheritance usually allow for explanation of the inheritance pattern.

Terminology

The following terms are important in understanding heredity patterns.

1. Dominant and recessive—As defined by Mendel, concepts for dominant and recessive refer to the **phenotypic expression** of alleles and are not intrinsic characteristics of gene loci. Therefore, it is inappropriate to discuss "a dominant locus."

2. Genotype—Genotype means the genetic status, that is, the alleles an individual carries.

3. Phenotype—Phenotype is the expression of an individual's genotype including appearance, physical features, organ structure, and biochemical and physiologic nature. It may be modified by environment.

4. Pleiotropy—Pleiotropy refers to the phenomenon whereby a single mutant allele can have widespread effects or expression in different tissues or organ systems. In other words, an allele may produce more than one effect on the phenotype. For example, Marfan syndrome has manifestations in different organ systems (skeletal, cardiac, ophthalmologic, etc) due to a single mutation within the *fibrillin* gene.

5. Penetrance—Penetrance refers to the proportion of individuals with a particular genotype that express the same phenotype. Penetrance is a proportion that ranges between 0 and 1.0 (or 0 and 100%). When 100% of mutant individuals express the phenotype, penetrance is **complete**. If some mutant individuals do not express the phenotype, penetrance is said to be **incomplete**, or **reduced**. Dominant conditions with incomplete penetrance, therefore, are characterized by "skipped" generations with unaffected, obligate gene carriers.

6. Expressivity—Expressivity refers to the variability in degree of phenotypic expression (severity) seen in different individuals with the same mutant genotype. Expressivity may be extremely variable or fairly consistent, both within and between families. Intrafamilial variability of expression may be due to factors such as epistasis, environment, genetic anticipation, presence of phenocopies, mosaicism, and chance (stochastic factors). Interfamilial variability of expression may be due to the previously mentioned factors, but may also be due to allelic or locus genetic heterogeneity.

7. Genetic heterogeneity—Several different genetic mutations may produce phenotypes that are identical or similar enough to have been traditionally considered as one diagnosis. "Anemia" or "mental retardation" are examples of this. There are two types of genetic heterogeneity, locus heterogeneity and allelic heterogeneity.

A. LOCUS HETEROGENEITY—Locus heterogeneity describes a phenotype caused by mutations at more than one genetic locus; that is, mutations at different loci cause the same phenotype or a group of phenotypes that appear similar enough to have been previously classified as a single disease, clinical "entity," or diagnostic spectrum. An example would be Sanfilippo syndrome (mucopolysaccharidosis types IIIA, B, C, and D), in which the same phenotype is produced by four different enzyme deficiencies.

B. ALLELIC HETEROGENEITY—This term is applied to a phenotype causing different mutations at a single-gene locus. As an example, cystic fibrosis may be caused by many different genetic changes, such as homozygosity for the common *ΔF508* mutation, or *ΔF508* and an *R117H* mutation. The latter example represents **compound heterozygosity**.

8. PHENOTYPIC HETEROGENEITY OR "CLINICAL HETEROGENEITY"—This term describes the situation in which more than one phenotype is caused by different allelic mutations at a single locus. For example, different mutations in the *FGFR2* gene can cause different craniosynostosis disorders, including Crouzon syndrome, Jackson-Weiss syndrome, Pfeiffer syndrome, and Apert syndrome. These syndromes are clinically distinguishable and are due to the presence of a variety of genetic mutations within single genes.

9. HOMOZYGOUS—A cell or organism that has identical alleles at a particular locus is said to be homozygous. For example, a cystic fibrosis patient with a *ΔF508* mutation on both alleles would be called homozygous for that mutation.

10. HETEROZYGOUS—A cell or organism that has nonidentical alleles at a genetic locus is said to be heterozygous. In autosomal dominant conditions, a mutation of only one copy of the gene pair is all that is necessary to result in a disease state. However, an individual who is heterozygous for a recessive disorder will not manifest symptoms (see next section).

Online Mendelian Inheritance in Man: http://www.ncbi.nlm.nih.gov/entrez/query.fcgi?db=OMIM

Hereditary Patterns

A. Autosomal Dominant Inheritance

Autosomal dominant inheritance has the following characteristics:

1. If a parent is affected, the risk for each offspring of inheriting the abnormal dominant gene is 50%, or 1:2. This is true whether the gene is penetrant or not in the parent.
2. Affected individuals in the same family may experience variable expressivity.
3. Nonpenetrance is common, and the penetrance rate varies for each dominantly inherited condition.
4. Both males and females can pass on the abnormal gene to children of either sex, although the manifestations may vary according to sex. For example, pattern baldness is a dominant trait but affects only males. In this case, the trait is said to be sex-limited.

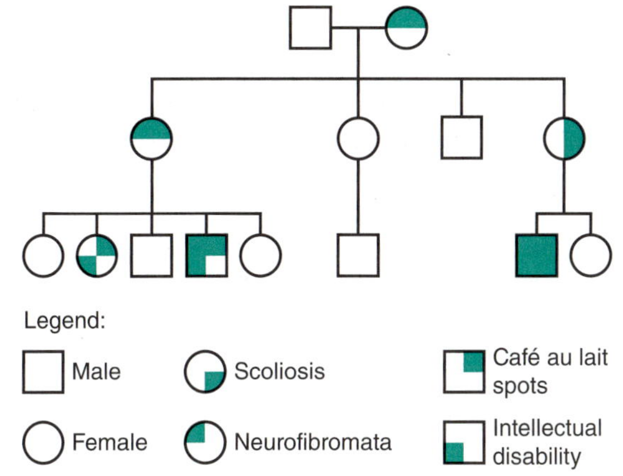

▲ **Figure 37–4.** Autosomal dominant inheritance. Variable expressivity in Neurofibromatosis type 1.

5. Dominant inheritance is typically said to be vertical, that is, the condition passes from one generation to the next in a vertical fashion (Figure 37–4).
6. In some cases, the patient appears to be the first affected individual in the family. This spontaneous appearance is often caused by a new mutation. The mutation rate increases with advancing paternal age (particularly after age 40 years).
7. Explanations for a negative family history include
   a. Nonpaternity.
   b. Decreased penetrance or mild manifestations in one of the parents.
   c. Germline mosaicism (ie, mosaicism in the germ cell line of either parent). Germline mosaicism may mimic autosomal recessive inheritance, because it leads to situations in which two children of completely normal parents are affected with a genetic disorder. The best example of this is osteogenesis imperfecta type II.
   d. The abnormality present in the patient may be a phenocopy, or it may be a similar but genetically different abnormality with a different mode of inheritance.
8. As a general rule, dominant traits are more often related to structural abnormalities of a protein.
9. If an abnormality represents a new mutation of a dominant trait, the parents of the affected individual run a low risk during subsequent pregnancies. The risk for an affected sibling is still slightly increased over the general population, because of the possibility of germline mosaicism.
10. Prevention options available for future pregnancies include prenatal diagnosis, artificial insemination, and egg or sperm donation, depending on which parent has the abnormal gene.

B. Autosomal Recessive Inheritance

Autosomal recessive inheritance also has some distinctive characteristics:

1. The recurrence risk for parents of an affected child is 25%, or 1:4 for each pregnancy. The gene carrier frequency in the general population can be used to assess the risk of having an affected child with a new partner, for unaffected siblings, and for the affected individuals themselves.
2. There is less variability among affected persons. Parents are carriers and are clinically normal. (There are, however, exceptions to this rule. For example, carriers of sickle cell trait may become symptomatic if they become hypoxic.)
3. Males and females are affected equally.
4. Inheritance is horizontal; siblings may be affected (Figure 37–5).
5. The family history is usually negative, with the exception of siblings. However, in common conditions such as cystic fibrosis, a second- or third-degree relative may be affected.
6. Recessive conditions are frequently associated with enzyme defects.
7. In rare instances, a child with a recessive disorder and a normal karyotype may have inherited both copies of the abnormal gene from one parent and none from the

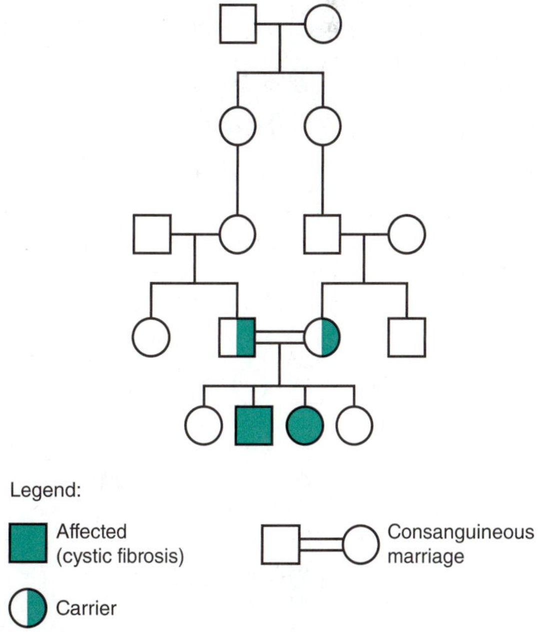

▲ **Figure 37–5.** Autosomal recessive inheritance: cystic fibrosis.

other. This UPD was first described in a girl with cystic fibrosis and growth retardation.

8. Options available for future pregnancies include prenatal diagnosis, adoption, artificial insemination, and egg or sperm donation.

C. X-Linked Inheritance

When a gene for a specific disorder is on the X chromosome, the condition is said to be X-linked, or sex-linked. Females may be either homozygous or heterozygous, because they have two X chromosomes. Males, by contrast, have only one X, and a male is said to be hemizygous for any gene on his X chromosome. The severity of any disorder is greater in males than in females (within a specific family). According to the Lyon hypothesis, because one of the two X chromosomes in each cell is inactivated, and this inactivation is random, the clinical picture in females depends on the percentage of mutant versus normal alleles inactivated. The X chromosome is not inactivated until about 14 days of gestation, and parts of the short arm remain active throughout life.

1. X-linked recessive inheritance—The following features are characteristic of X-linked recessive inheritance:

1. Males are affected, and heterozygous females are either normal or have mild manifestations.
2. Inheritance is diagonal through the maternal side of the family (Figure 37–6A).

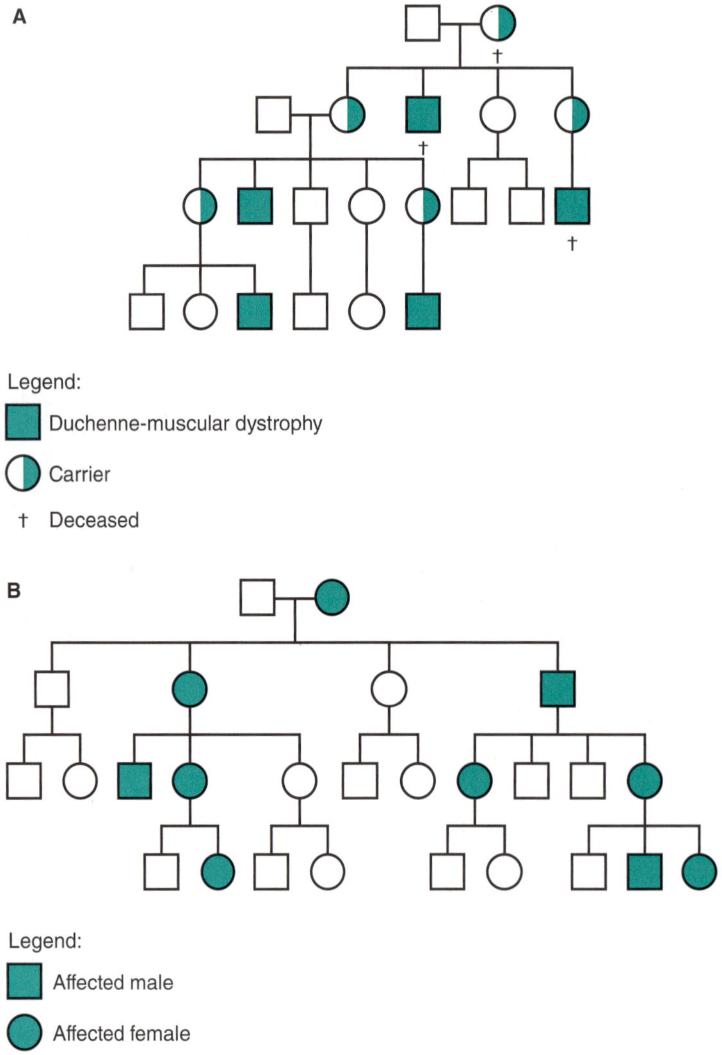

▲ **Figure 37–6. A:** X-linked recessive inheritance. **B:** X-linked dominant inheritance.

3. A female carrier has a 50% chance that each daughter will be a carrier and a 50% chance that each son will be affected.
4. All of the daughters of an affected male are carriers, and none of his sons are affected.
5. The mutation rate is high in some X-linked disorders, particularly when the affected male dies or is so incapacitated by the disorder that reproduction is unlikely. In such instances, the mutation is thought to occur as a new mutation in the affected male, and in the mother, each one-third of the time and to be present in earlier generations one-third of the time. For this reason, genetic counseling may be difficult in families with an isolated case.
6. On rare occasions, a female may be fully affected. Several possible mechanisms may account for a fully affected female: (a) unfavorable lyonization; (b) 45,X karyotype; (c) homozygosity for the abnormal gene; (d) an X-autosome translocation, or other structural abnormality of one X chromosome, in which the X chromosome of normal structure is preferentially inactivated; (e) UPD; and (f) nonrandom inactivation, which may be controlled by an autosomal gene.

2. X-linked dominant inheritance—The X-linked dominant inheritance pattern is much less common than the X-linked recessive type. Examples include incontinentia pigmenti and hypophosphatemic or vitamin D–resistant rickets. The following features are characteristic of X-linked dominant inheritance:

1. The heterozygous female is symptomatic, and the disease is twice as common in females because they have two X chromosomes that can have the mutation.
2. Clinical manifestations are more variable in females than in males.
3. The risk for the offspring of heterozygous females to be affected is 50% regardless of sex.
4. All of the daughters but none of the sons of affected males will have the disorder (see Figure 37–6B).
5. Although a homozygous female is possible (particularly in an inbred population), she would be severely involved. All of her children would also be affected but more mildly.
6. Some disorders (eg, incontinentia pigmenti) are lethal in males (and in homozygous females). Affected women have twice as many daughters as sons and an increased incidence of miscarriages, because affected males will be spontaneously aborted. A 47,XXY karyotype has allowed affected males to survive.

D. Y-Linked Inheritance

In Y-linked inheritance, also known as "holandric" inheritance, a disorder is caused by genes located on the Y chromosome. These conditions are relatively rare with only about 40 entries listed in McKusick's catalog. Male-to-male transmission is seen in this category, with all sons of affected males being affected and no daughters or females being affected.

MULTIFACTORIAL INHERITANCE

Many common attributes, such as height, are familial, and are the result of the actions of multiple rather than single genes. Inheritance of these traits is described as **polygenic** or **multifactorial**. The latter term recognizes that environmental factors such as diet also contribute to these traits. Geneticists are now finding that multiple genes are often expressed in hierarchies, in which the action of a small number of genes, two or three, explains much of the variation observed within affected populations.

Studies of twins have proven useful in determining the relative importance of genetic versus environmental factors in the expression of polygenic traits. If genetic factors are of little or no importance, then the concordance between monozygotic and dizygotic twins should be the same. (Dizygotic twins are no more genetically similar to each other than to other siblings.) If an abnormality is completely genetic, the concordance between identical twins should be 100%. In polygenic conditions, the concordance rate for identical twins is usually higher than that seen in dizygotic twins but is still not 100%, indicating that both genetic and environmental factors are playing a role.

Many disorders and congenital abnormalities that are clearly familial but do not segregate as mendelian traits (eg, autosomal dominant, recessive) show polygenic inheritance. For the most part, these conditions become manifest when thresholds of additive gene actions or contributing environmental factors are exceeded. Many common disorders ranging from hypertension, stroke, and thrombophlebitis to behavioral traits such as alcoholism demonstrate multifactorial (polygenic) inheritance. Some common birth defects, including isolated congenital heart disease, cleft lip and palate, and neural tube defects, also demonstrate polygenic inheritance. Neural tube defects provide a good model illustrating how identification of both environmental and genetic contributions to multifactorial traits can lead to preventive measures.

Polygenic or multifactorial inheritance has several distinctive characteristics:

1. The risk for relatives of affected persons is increased. The risk is higher for first-degree relatives (those who have 50% of their genes in common) and lower for more distant relations, although the risk for the latter is higher than for the general population (Table 37–3).
2. The recurrence risk varies with the number of affected family members. For example, after one child is born with a neural tube defect, the recurrence risk is 2%–3%. If a second affected child is born, the risk for any future child increases to 10%–12%. This is in contrast to

Table 37–3. Empiric risks for some congenital disorders.

Anencephaly and spina bifida: incidence (average) 1:1000	
One affected child: 2%–3%	
Two affected children: 10%–12%	
One affected parent: 4%–5%	
Hydrocephalus: incidence 1:2000 newborns	
Occasional X-linked recessive	
Often associated with neural tube defect	
Some environmental etiologies (eg, toxoplasmosis)	
Recurrence risk, one affected child	
Hydrocephalus: 1%	
Some central nervous system abnormality: 3%	
Nonsyndromic cleft lip and/or palate: incidence (average) 1:1000	
One affected child: 2%–4%	
One affected parent: 2%–4%	
Two affected children: 10%	
One affected parent, one affected child: 10%–20%	
Nonsyndromic cleft palate: incidence 1:2000	
One affected child: 2%	
Two affected children: 6%–8%	
One affected parent: 4%–6%	
One affected parent, one affected child: 15%–20%	
Congenital heart disease: incidence 8:1000	
One affected child: 2%–3%	
One affected parent, one affected child: 10%	
Clubfoot: incidence 1:1000 (male: female = 2:1)	
One affected child: 2%–3%	
Congenital dislocated hip: incidence 1:1000	
(female > male) with marked regional variation	
One child affected: 2%–14%	
Pyloric stenosis: Incidence, males: 1:200; females: 1:1000	
Male index patient	
Brothers	3.2%
Sons	6.8%
Sisters	3.0%
Daughters	1.2%
Female index patient	
Brothers	13.2%
Sons	20.5%
Sisters	2.5%
Daughters	11.1%

single-gene disorders, in which the risk is the same no matter how many family members are affected.

3. The risk is higher if the defect is more severe. In Hirschsprung disease, another polygenic condition, the longer the aganglionic segment, the higher is the recurrence risk.
4. Sex ratios may not be equal. If a marked discrepancy exists, the recurrence risk is higher if a child of the less commonly affected sex has the disorder. This assumes that more genetic factors are required to raise the more resistant sex above the threshold. For example, pyloric stenosis is more common in males. If the first affected child is a female, the recurrence risk is higher than if the child is a male.
5. The risk for the offspring of an affected person is approximately the same as the risk for siblings, assuming that the spouse of the affected person has a negative family history. For many conditions, however, assortative mating, "like marrying like," adds to risks in offspring.

NONMENDELIAN INHERITANCE

Epigenetic Regulation

Although development is regulated by genes, it is initiated and sustained by nongenetic processes. Epigenetic events are points of interaction between developmental programs and the physicochemical environments in differentiating cells. Genetic imprinting and DNA methylation are examples of epigenetic processes that affect development. Certain genes important in regulation of growth and differentiation are themselves regulated by chemical modification that occurs in specific patterns in gametes. For example, genes that are methylated are "turned off" and not transcribed. The pattern of which genes are methylated may be determined or affected by the sex of the parent of origin (see next section). Expression of imprinted genes may sometimes be limited to specific organs (eg, the brain), and imprinting may be relaxed and methyl groups lost as development progresses. Disruption of imprinting is now recognized as contributing to birth defect syndromes (described later in this chapter). Certain techniques developed to assist infertile couples (advanced reproductive technology) may affect epigenetic processes and lead to genetic disorders in the offspring conceived via these methods.

Niemitz EL, Feinberg AP: Epigenetics and assisted reproductive technology: A call for investigation. Am J Hum Genet 2004;74:599 [PMID: 14991528].

Imprinting

Although the homologs of chromosome pairs may appear identical on routine karyotype analysis, it is now known that the parental origin of each homolog can affect which genes are actually transcribed and which are inactivated. The term *imprinting* refers to the process by which preferential transcription of certain genes takes place, depending on the parental origin, that is, which homolog (maternal or paternal) the gene is located on. Certain chromosomes, particularly chromosome X, and the autosomes 15, 11, and 7, have imprinted regions where some genes are only read from one homolog (ie, either the maternal or paternal allele) under normal circumstances, and the gene on the other homolog is normally inactivated. Errors in imprinting may arise because of UPD (in which a copy from one parent is missing), by a chromosomal deletion causing loss of the gene normally transcribed, or by mutations in the imprinting genes that normally code for transcription or inactivation of other genes downstream. A good example of how imprinting may affect human disease is Beckwith-Wiedemann Syndrome, the gene for which is located on chromosome 11p15.

Cohen MM et al: *Overgrowth Syndromes*. Oxford University Press, 2002.

Genetic Anticipation

Geneticists coined the term "anticipation" to describe an unusual pattern of inheritance in which symptoms became manifest at earlier ages and with increasing severity as traits are passed to subsequent generations. Mapping of the genes responsible for these disorders led to the discovery that certain repeat sequences of DNA at disease loci were not stable when passed through meiosis. Repeated DNA sequences, in particular triplets (eg, CGG and CAG), tended to increase their copy number. As these runs of triplets expanded, they eventually affected the expression of genes and produced symptoms. Curiously, all the disorders undergoing triplet repeat expansion detected thus far produce neurologic symptoms. Most are progressive. In general, the size of the triplet expansion is roughly correlated with the timing and severity of symptoms. The reasons for the meiotic instability of these sequences are not yet understood. The mechanisms appear to involve interactions between DNA structure (eg, formation of hairpin loops) and replication enzymes (DNA polymerase complexes) during meiosis.

Triplet repeat instability can modify the inheritance of autosomal dominant, autosomal recessive, and X-linked traits. Autosomal dominant disorders include several spinal cerebellar atrophies, Huntington disease, and myotonic dystrophy. Unstable triplet repeat expansion contributes to at least one autosomal recessive disorder, Friedreich ataxia. The most common X-linked disorder demonstrating triplet repeat instability and expansion is Fragile X syndrome.

Mitochondrial Inheritance

Mitochondrial disorders can be caused by both nuclear and mitochondrial genes. The former would follow Mendelian inheritance, either AR, AD, or X-Linked while the latter demonstrates mitochondrial inheritance. Mitochondrial DNA is double-stranded, circular, and smaller than nuclear DNA, and is found in the cytoplasm. It codes for enzymes involved in oxidative phosphorylation, which generates adenosine triphosphate. Since the 1990s, enormous advances in technology and improved clinical documentation have led to a better understanding of the interesting disorders caused by mutations in mitochondrial DNA (mtDNA).

Mitochondrial disorders can be associated with point mutations, deletions, or duplications in mtDNA. However, there is a threshold effect depending on the heteroplasmy (see next). Because of the difficulty in predicting mitochondrial DNA disorders and the variability of the clinical course, it is often difficult to calculate specific recurrence risks.

Mitochondrial disorders related to mtDNA have the following characteristics:

1. They show remarkable phenotypic variability.
2. They are maternally inherited, because only the egg has any cytoplasmic material, and during early embryogenesis any sperm-born mitochondrial material will be eliminated.
3. In most mitochondrial disorders, cells are heteroplasmic (Figure 37–7). That is, all cells contain both normal and mutated or abnormal mtDNA. The proportion of normal to abnormal mtDNA in the mother's egg seems to determine the severity of the offspring's disease and the age at onset in most cases.
4. Those tissues with the highest adenosine triphosphate requirements—specifically, central nervous system (CNS) and skeletal muscle—seem to be most susceptible to mutations in mtDNA.
5. Somatic cells show an increase in mtDNA mutations and a decline in oxidative phosphorylation function with age. This explains the later onset of some of these disorders and may indeed be a clue to the whole aging process.

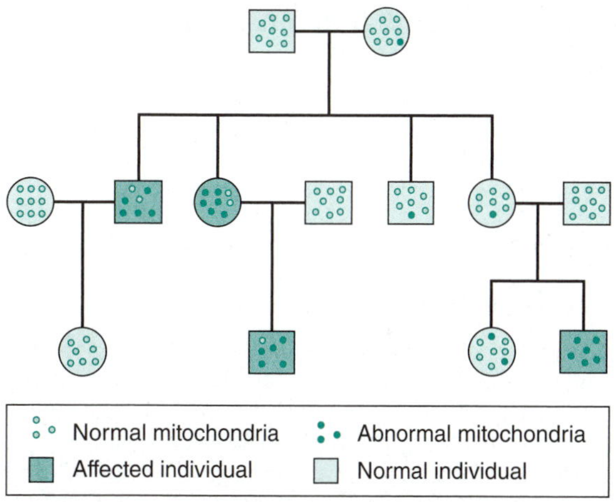

▲ Figure 37–7. Mitochondrial inheritance. Mutations are transmitted through the maternal line.

Rahman S, Hanna MG: Diagnosis and therapy in neuromuscular disorders: Diagnosis and new treatments in mitochondrial diseases. J Neurol Neurosurg Psychiatry 2009 Sep;80(9):943–953.

Wong LJ et al: Current molecular diagnostic algorithm for mitochondrial disorders. Mol Genet Metab 2010 Jun;100(2):111–117.

FAMILY HISTORY & PEDIGREE

The first step in the collection of information regarding the genetics of a syndromic diagnosis is the construction of a family tree or pedigree. Underused by most medical personnel, the pedigree is a valuable record of genetic and medical information, which is much more useful in visual form than in list form. Tips for pedigree preparation include the following:

- Start with the proband—the patient's siblings and parents, and obtain a three-generational history if possible.
- Always ask about consanguinity.
- Obtain data from both sides of the family.
- Ask about spontaneous abortions, stillbirths, infertility, children relinquished for adoption, and deceased individuals.

In the course of taking the family history, one may find information that is not relevant in elucidating the cause of the patients' problem but may indicate a risk for other important health concerns. Such information should be appropriately followed and addressed. Such conditions that may arise are an overwhelming family history of early-onset breast and ovarian cancer, or multiple pregnancy losses necessitating chromosome analyses.

Bennett RL et al: Standardized human pedigree nomenclature: Update and assessment of the recommendations of the National Society of genetic counselors. J Genet Couns 2008;17:424–433.

DYSMORPHOLOGY & HUMAN EMBRYOLOGY

Birth defects are the leading cause of death in the first year of life. They are evident in 2%–3% of newborn infants and in up to 7% of adults. Many are now detected by ultrasound prior to birth. Clinical investigation of the causes and consequences of birth defects is called dysmorphology.

MECHANISMS

Developmental Biology

Cell proliferation and programmed cell death (apoptosis) both contribute to embryonic structural formation. The genes that control these processes are being identified. Products of other genes establish regulatory pathways in which positive and negative signaling loops initiate and maintain cell differentiation with precise timing. Cell biology now provides techniques that allow experimental access to developmental pathways. Embryology has become more experimental than descriptive and practitioners can expect systems biology to soon begin to inform them about the origins of specific birth defects. This level of understanding will open the door to interventions that may well prevent birth defects or treat them prenatally.

Cellular Interactions

The picture emerging from experimental studies of morphogenesis is one of a hierarchy of gene expression during development. Morphogenesis begins with expression of genes encoding transcription factors. These proteins bind to DNA in undifferentiated embryonic cells and recruit them into developmental fields, groups of cells primed to respond to specific signals later in development. This recruitment also establishes spatial relationships and orients cells with respect to their neighbors. As fields differentiate into identifiable tissues (eg, ectoderm, mesoderm, and endoderm), cellular proliferation, migration, and further differentiation are mediated through genes encoding cell signaling proteins.

Signaling proteins include growth factors and their receptors, cellular adhesion molecules, and extracellular matrix proteins that both provide structure and position signals to developing tissues. The emerging field of systems biology is beginning to describe and quantitate these interactions over time.

Environmental Factors

The effects of exogenous agents during development are also mediated through genetically regulated pathways. At the cellular level, xenobiotics (compounds foreign to nature) cause birth defects either because they disrupt cell signaling and thereby misdirect morphogenesis, or because they are cytotoxic and lead to cell death in excess of the usual developmental program.

In general, drug receptors expressed in embryos and fetuses are the same molecules that mediate pharmacologic effects in adults. However, effector systems may be different, reflecting incomplete morphogenesis and differences between fetal and postnatal physiology. These circumstances allow prediction of dose-response relationships during development on the one hand, but call for caution about predicting effects on the other.

Xenobiotics must traverse the placenta to affect embryonic and fetal tissues. The human placenta is a relatively good barrier against microorganisms, but it is ineffective at excluding drugs and many chemicals. The physicochemical properties (eg, molecular size, solubility, and charge) that allow foreign chemicals to be absorbed into the maternal circulation also allow them to cross the placenta. The placenta can metabolize some xenobiotics but it is most active against steroid hormones and low-level environmental contaminants than drugs.

The timing of xenobiotic exposures is an important determinant of their effects. Morphogenic processes express so-called critical periods, during which developing organs they produce are particularly susceptible to maldevelopment. Critical periods of susceptibility are not all confined to early gestation. In particular, the developing brain is susceptible to toxicity throughout pregnancy.

As discussed, over-the-counter, prescribed, and abused drugs that are pharmacologically active in mothers will be active across the placenta. Exposure to agents achieving cytotoxic levels in adults are likely to be teratogenic (ie, cause birth defects). Abused substances such as alcohol that are toxic to adults are predictably toxic to embryos and fetuses. Drugs generally safe in adults will be generally safe for fetuses. However, keeping in mind that embryonic and fetal physiology may differ from that of an adult with respect to drug action, some risk for abnormal development must always be considered. Risk assessment requires continuous monitoring of populations exposed to drugs during pregnancy.

Effects of toxic environmental contaminants on the embryo and fetus are also dose-dependent. Thus, the level of exposure to a toxin frequently becomes the primary determinant of its risk. Exposures producing symptoms in mothers can be assumed to be potentially toxic to the fetus.

Environmental mutagens present a special problem. Animal experiments indicate that high levels of exposure to mutagenic agents are also teratogenic. Most effects are mediated through increased apoptosis responding to DNA damage. This is especially true for the developing brain. At lower doses attempts to repair DNA damage in embryonic or fetal cells may lead to somatic mutations that can contribute to carcinogenesis or be expressed as mosaic organ dysgenesis.

Transplacental pharmacologic effects can also be therapeutic. The potential for embryonic and fetal drug therapies during pregnancy is increasing. For example, folic acid supplementation can lower risks for birth defects such as spina bifida, and maternally administered corticosteroids can induce fetal synthesis and secretion of pulmonary surfactants prior to delivery.

Mechanical Factors

Much of embryonic development and all of fetal growth occurs normally within the low pressure and space provided by amniotic fluid. Loss or inadequate production of amniotic fluid can have disastrous effects, as can disruption of placental membranes. Disruption of placental membranes in early gestation leads to major structural distortion and most often lethal. Later, deformation or even amputation of fetal extremities (amniotic band sequence) can occur.

Movement is also important for morphogenesis. Fetal movement is necessary for normal development of joints and is the principal determinant of folds and creases present at birth in the face, hands, feet, and other areas of the body. Clubfoot is an etiologically heterogeneous condition in which the foot is malpositioned at birth. It more often results from mechanical constraint secondary to intrauterine crowding, weak fetal muscles, or abnormal neurologic function than from primary skeletal maldevelopment.

Lung and kidney development are particularly sensitive to mechanical forces. Constriction of the chest through maldevelopment of the ribs, lack of surrounding amniotic fluid, or lack of movement (fetal breathing) leads to varying degrees of pulmonary hypoplasia in which lungs are smaller than normal and develop fewer alveoli. Mechanically induced pulmonary hypoplasia is a common cause of respiratory distress at birth and may be lethal.

Cystic renal dysplasia is frequently associated with obstruction ureters or bladder outflow. As pressure within obstructed renal collecting systems increases, it distorts cell interactions and alters histogenesis. Developing kidneys exposed to increased internal pressures for long periods eventually become nonfunctional.

CLINICAL DYSMORPHOLOGY

The most important task for the clinician presented with an infant with a birth defect is to determine whether the problem is isolated or part of a larger embryopathy (syndromic).

Terminology

Classification of dysmorphic features strives to reflect mechanisms of maldevelopment. However, much of the terminology that describes abnormal development in humans remains historical and documents recognition of patterns prior to understanding of their biology. For example, birth defects are referred to as **malformations** when they result from altered genetic or developmental processes. When physical forces interrupt or distort morphogenesis, their effects are termed **disruptions** and **deformations**, respectively. The term **dysplasia** is used to denote abnormal histogenesis. Malformations occurring together more frequently than would be expected by chance alone may be classified as belonging to **associations**. Those in which the order of maldevelopment is understood may be referred to as **sequences**. For example, Robin sequence (or Pierre Robin anomalad) is used to describe cleft palate that has occurred because poor growth of the jaw (retrognathia) has displaced the tongue and prevented posterior closure of the palate. **Syndromes** are simply recurrent patterns of maldevelopment, which have in many cases a known genetic cause.

Evaluation of the Dysmorphic Infant

Caring for infants with birth defects can be very stressful. The extent of an infant's abnormalities may not be immediately apparent, and parents who feel grief and guilt are often desperate for information. However, as with any medical problem the history and physical examination provide most of the clues to diagnosis. Special aspects of these procedures are outlined in the following sections.

A. History

Pregnancy histories nearly always contain important clues to the diagnosis. Parental recall after delivery of an abnormal infant is better than recall after a normal birth. An obstetric wheel can help document gestational age and events of the first trimester: the last menstrual period, the onset of symptoms of pregnancy, the date of diagnosis of the pregnancy, the date of the first prenatal visit, and the physician's impressions of fetal growth at that time. Family histories should always be reviewed. Environmental histories should include descriptions of parental habits and work settings in addition to medications and use of drugs, tobacco, and alcohol.

B. Physical Examination

Meticulous physical examination is crucial for accurate diagnosis in dysmorphic infants and children. In addition to the routine procedures described in Chapter 2, special attention should be paid to the neonate's physical measurements (Figure 37–8). Photographs are helpful and should include a ruler for reference.

C. Imaging and Laboratory Studies

Radiologic and ultrasonographic examinations can be extremely helpful in the evaluation of dysmorphic infants. Films of infants with apparent limb or skeletal anomalies should include views of the skull and all of the long bones in addition to frontal and lateral views of the axial skeleton. Chest and abdominal films should be obtained when indicated. The pediatrician should consult a radiologist for further workup. Computed tomography (CT), magnetic resonance imaging (MRI), and ultrasonography are all useful diagnostic tools, but their interpretation in the face of birth defects may require considerable experience.

Traditional cytogenetic analysis provides specific diagnoses in approximately 5% of dysmorphic infants who survive the neonatal period. Chromosomal abnormalities are recognized in 10%–15% of infants who die. With the availability of chromosomal microarray at least 10%–15% additional subtle chromosomal anomalies has been identified. Of note, many copy number variations (CNV) exist in different individuals; therefore, interpretation is sometimes difficult and may require parental samples for clarification. Common disorders such as trisomies 21 and 18 can be determined rapidly through use of FISH, but this technique should always be accompanied by a complete karyotype. A normal karyotype does not rule out the presence of significant genetic disease. Any case requiring rapid diagnosis should be discussed with an experienced clinical geneticist.

D. Perinatal Autopsy

When a dysmorphic infant dies, postmortem examination can provide important diagnostic information. The pediatrician should discuss the case thoroughly with the pathologist, and photographs should always be taken. Radiologic imaging should be included whenever limb anomalies or disproportionate growth is present. Tissue, most often skin, should be submitted for cytogenetic analysis. Fibroblasts from these studies should routinely be frozen and preserved for future studies. The pediatrician and the pathologist should also consider whether samples of blood, urine, or other tissue should be obtained for biochemical analyses. Placental as well as fetal tissue can be used for viral culture.

Hudgins L, Cassidy SB: Congenital anomalies: In Martin RJ et al (editors): *Fanaroff and Martin's Neonatal-Perinatal Medicine—Diseases of the Fetus and Infant,* 8th ed. Elsevier Mosby, Philadelphia, 2006:561–582.

CHROMOSOMAL DISORDERS: ABNORMAL NUMBER

TRISOMIES

1. Trisomy 21 (Down Syndrome)

ESSENTIALS OF DIAGNOSIS & TYPICAL FEATURES

- Characteristic features include upslanting palpebral fissures, epicanthal folds, midface hypoplasia, and small, dysplastic pinnae.
- Generalized hypotonia.
- Cognitive disabilities (usually mild to moderate).
- Associated with congenital heart disease and gastrointestinal anomalies.

Down syndrome occurs in about 1:760 newborns. Cognitive disabilities are characteristic of Down syndrome, as is generalized hypotonia. The affected newborn may have prolonged physiologic jaundice, polycythemia, and a transient leukemoid reaction. Feeding problems are common during infancy. Problems which may be seen during childhood include thyroid dysfunction, visual issues, hearing loss, obstructive sleep apnea, celiac disease, and atlanto-occipital instability. Leukemia is 12–20 times more common in Down syndrome patients.

Clinical Findings

The principal physical findings include a flattened occiput, characteristic facies (upslanting palpebral fissures, epicanthal folds, midface hypoplasia, and small, dysplastic pinnae), and minor limb abnormalities. About one-third to one-half of children with Down syndrome have congenital heart disease, most often endocardial cushion defects or other septal defects. Anomalies of the gastrointestinal tract, including

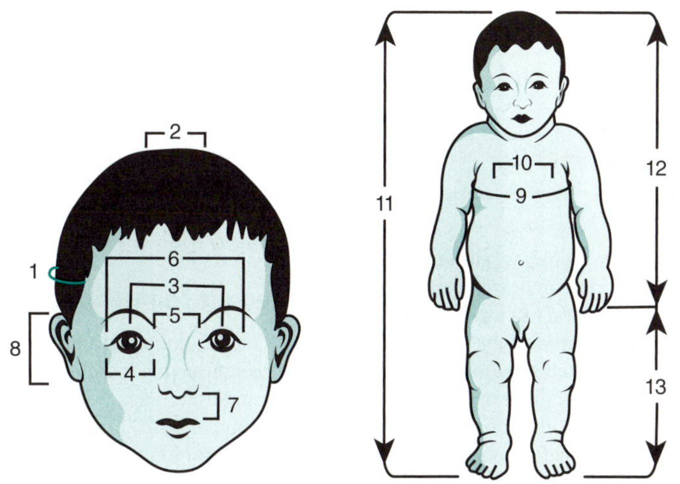

Measurement	Range (cm)	
	Term (38–40 wk)	Preterm (32–37 wk)
1 Head circumference	32–37	27–32
2 Anterior fontanelle $\left(\frac{L-W}{2}\right)$	0.7–3.7	. . .
3 Interpupillary distance	3.3–4.5	3.1–3.9
4 Palpebral fissure	1.5–2.1	1.3–1.6
5 Inner canthal distance	1.5–2.5	1.4–2.1
6 Outer canthal distance	5.3–7.3	3.9–5.1
7 Philtrum	0.6–1.2	0.5–0.9
8 Ear length	3–4.3	2.4–3.5
9 Chest circumference	28–38	23–29
10 Internipple distance*	6.5–10	5–6.5
11 Height	47–55	39–47
12/13 Ratio $\frac{\text{Upper body segment}}{\text{Lower body segment}}$	1.7	. . .
14 Hand (palm to middle finger)	5.3–7.8	4.1–5.5
15 Ratio of middle finger to hand	0.38–0.48	0.38–0.5
16 Penis (pubic bone to tip of glans)	2.7–4.3	1.8–3.2

*Internipple distance should not exceed 25% of chest circumference.

▲ **Figure 37–8.** Neonatal measurements.

esophageal and duodenal atresias, are seen in about 15% of cases.

Information regarding health care guidelines for patients with Down syndrome. Available at: http://www.downsyn.com/guidelines/healthcare.html

2. Trisomy 18 Syndrome

The incidence of trisomy 18 syndrome is about 1:4000 live births, and the ratio of affected males to females is approximately 1:3. Trisomy 18 is characterized by prenatal and postnatal growth retardation that is often severe, and hypertonicity. Complications are related to associated birth defects. Death is often caused by heart failure or pneumonia and usually occurs in infancy or early childhood, although a small percentage of patients reach adulthood. Surviving children show significant cognitive disabilities.

Clinical Findings

Infants with trisomy 18 are often small for gestational age and have dysmorphic features including a characteristic facies and extremities (overlapping fingers and rockerbottom feet), and congenital heart disease (often ventricular septal defect or patent ductus arteriosus). To see clinical pictures of patients with trisomy 18, visit the following web site: http://medgen.genetics.utah.edu/photographs/pages/trisomy_18.htm.

3. Trisomy 13 Syndrome

The incidence of trisomy 13 is about 1:12,000 live births, and 60% of affected individuals are female. Most infants with trisomy 13 have congenital anomalies that are incompatible with survival. Surviving children demonstrate failure to thrive, cognitive disabilities, apneic spells, seizures, and deafness. Death usually occurs in early infancy or by the second year of life, commonly as a result of heart failure or infection.

Clinical Findings

The symptoms and signs include characteristic features, often a normal birth weight, CNS malformations, eye malformations, cleft lip and palate, polydactyly or syndactyly, and congenital heart disease. The facies of an infant with trisomy 13 can be viewed at the following web site: www.trisomy.org.

Treatment of Trisomies

A. Medical Therapy

Interventions for specific issues such as surgery or medications for heart problems, antibiotics for infections, serial thyroid function tests, infant stimulation programs, special education, and physical, occupational, and speech therapies are all indicated. The goal of treatment is to help affected children develop to their full potential. Parents' participation in support groups such as the local chapter of the National Down Syndrome Congress should be encouraged. See the following web site: http://www.ndss.org/.

There is no treatment, other than general supportive care, for trisomy 13 or 18. Rapid confirmation of suspected Trisomy 13 or 18 can be made by FISH. A support group for families of children with trisomies 13 and 18 who survive beyond infancy is called SOFT. See the following web site: http://www.trisomy.org/.

B. Genetic Counseling

Most parents of trisomic infants have normal karyotypes. The risk of having a child affected with a trisomy increases with maternal age. For example, age-specific risks are approximately 1:2000 for mothers younger than 25 years; and 1:100 for mothers at age 40. The recurrence risk for trisomy in future pregnancies is equal to 1:100 plus the age-specific maternal risk.

If the child has a trisomy resulting from a translocation, and the parent has an abnormal karyotype, the risks are increased. When the mother is the carrier of a balanced robertsonian translocation, there is a 10%–15% chance that the child will be affected and a 33% chance that the child will be a balanced translocation carrier. When the father is the carrier, there is a smaller than 0.5% chance of having another affected child. If the child has a 21/21 translocation and one parent has the translocation, the recurrence risk is 100%.

The mother's age at the time of conception and the nature of the chromosomal abnormality are important in genetic counseling, which is indicated for parents of all children with chromosomal abnormalities. Prenatal diagnosis is available.

SEX CHROMOSOME ABNORMALITIES

1. Turner Syndrome (Monosomy X, Gonadal Dysgenesis)

ESSENTIALS OF DIAGNOSIS & TYPICAL FEATURES

- Webbed neck, triangular facies, short stature, wide-set nipples, amenorrhea, and absence of secondary sex characteristics.
- Associated with coarctation of the aorta and genitourinary malformations.
- IQ is usually normal but learning disabilities are common.
- Mosaic individuals may manifest only short stature and amenorrhea.

The incidence of Turner syndrome is 1:10,000 females. However, it is estimated that 95% of conceptuses with monosomy X are miscarried and only 5% are liveborn.

Clinical Findings

Newborns with Turner syndrome may have webbed neck, edema of the hands and feet, coarctation of the aorta, and a characteristic triangular facies. Later symptoms include short stature, a shield chest with wide-set nipples, streak ovaries, amenorrhea, absence of secondary sex characteristics, and infertility. Some affected girls, particularly those with mosaicism, have only short stature and amenorrhea, without dysmorphic features.

Complications relate primarily to coarctation of the aorta, when present. Malformations of the urinary tract may be seen. Learning disabilities are common, secondary to difficulties in perceptual motor integration.

Treatment

In Turner syndrome the identification and treatment of perceptual difficulties before they become problematic is very important. Estrogen replacement therapy permits development of secondary sex characteristics and normal menstruation, and prevents osteoporosis. Growth hormone therapy has been used to increase the height of affected girls. Females with 45,X or 45,X mosaicism have a low fertility rate, and those who become pregnant have a high risk of fetal wastage (spontaneous miscarriage, ~30%; stillbirth, 6%–10%). Furthermore, their liveborn offspring have an increased frequency of chromosomal abnormalities involving either sex chromosomes or autosomes, and congenital malformations. Thus, prenatal ultrasonography and chromosome analysis are indicated for the offspring of females with sex chromosome abnormalities.

2. Klinefelter Syndrome (XXY)

ESSENTIALS OF DIAGNOSIS & TYPICAL FEATURES

- Diagnosis is rarely made before puberty.
- Key findings include microorchidism; lack of libido; minimal facial hair; and tall, eunuchoid build.
- IQ can vary (normal to borderline with a small percentage showing cognitive disabilities).

The incidence of Klinefelter syndrome in the newborn population is roughly 1:1000, but it is about 1% among intellectual disabilities males and about 3% among males seen at infertility clinics. The maternal age at birth is often advanced. Unlike Turner syndrome, Klinefelter syndrome is rarely the cause of spontaneous abortions. The diagnosis is seldom made before puberty except as a result of prenatal diagnosis, because prepubertal boys have a normal phenotype.

Clinical Findings

The characteristic findings after puberty include microorchidism associated with otherwise normal external genitalia, azoospermia, sterility, gynecomastia, normal to borderline IQ, diminished facial hair, lack of libido and potency, and a tall, eunuchoid build. In chromosome variants with three or four X chromosomes (XXXY and XXXXY), intellectual disabilities may be severe, and radioulnar synostosis may be present as well as anomalies of the external genitalia and cryptorchidism. In general, the physical and mental abnormalities associated with Klinefelter syndrome increase as the number of sex chromosomes increases.

Treatment

Males with Klinefelter syndrome require testosterone replacement therapy. The presence of the extra X chromosome may allow expression of what might normally be a lethal X-linked disorder to occur.

3. XYY Syndrome

Newborns with XYY syndrome in general are normal. Affected individuals may on occasion exhibit an abnormal behavior pattern from early childhood and may have mild intellectual disabilities. Fertility may be normal. Many males with an XYY karyotype are normal. There is no treatment.

4. XXX Syndrome

The incidence of females with an XXX karyotype is approximately 1:1000. Females with XXX are phenotypically normal. However, they tend to be taller than usual and to have lower IQs than their normal siblings. Learning and behavioral issues are relatively common. This is in contrast to individuals with XXXX, a much rarer condition causing more severe developmental issues, and a dysmorphic phenotype reminiscent of Down syndrome.

Jones KL: *Smith's Recognizable Patterns of Human Malformation*, 6th ed. Elsevier, 2006.

CHROMOSOMAL ABNORMALITIES: ABNORMAL STRUCTURE

Chromosomal abnormalities most often present in newborns as multiple congenital anomalies in association with intrauterine growth retardation. In addition to trisomies as just described, other more subtle chromosomal abnormalities are also common. In some cases, a chromosomal rearrangement is too subtle to be detected by karyotype, but can be detected by FISH. The newest technology, comparative genomic hybridization array (microarray), enables screening for multiple submicroscopic chromosomal abnormalities simultaneously, and is a very helpful tool in evaluating the child with a suspected chromosomal abnormality.

Although most cases of severe chromosomal abnormality such as trisomy are lethal, some individuals may survive if the abnormality exists in mosaic form. Two examples of this include trisomy 8 and Cat eye syndrome, caused by extra genetic material, which is derived from a portion of chromosome 22.

Miller DT, Adam MP, Aradhya S, et al. Consensus statement: Chromosomal microarray is a first-tier clinical diagnostic test for individuals with developmental disabilities or congenital anomalies. Am J Hum Genet 2010;86:749–764.

CHROMOSOME DELETION DISORDERS

Three common chromosomal deletion disorders that were previously detected on routine karyotype analysis, and confirmed via FISH assay, but are now detected with microarray, are 1p36– syndrome, Wolf-Hirschhorn syndrome (4p–), and cri du chat syndrome (5p–). Microdeletion or contiguous gene syndrome are referring to those small deletion not readily picked up by karyotype but detected by microarray or FISH.

1. Deletion 1p36 Syndrome

Microcephaly and a large anterior fontanelle are characteristic features of 1p36– syndrome. Cardiac defects are common, and dilated cardiomyopathy may present in infancy. Intellectual disability, hypotonia, hearing loss, and seizures are usually seen.

2. Wolf-Hirschhorn Syndrome

Also known as 4p– (deletion of 4p16), this syndrome is characterized by microcephaly and unusual development of the nose and orbits that produces an appearance suggesting an ancient Greek warrior's helmet. Other anomalies commonly seen include cleft lip and palate, and cardiac and renal defects. Seizure disorders are common, and the majority of patients have severe intellectual disability.

3. Cri du Chat Syndrome

Also known as 5p–(deletion of terminal chromosome 5p), this disorder is characterized by unique facial features, growth retardation, and microcephaly. Patients have an unusual catlike cry. Most patients have major organ anomalies and significant intellectual disability.

4. Contiguous Gene Disorders

Three common contiguous gene disorders which are usually suspected on the basis of an abnormal phenotype and then confirmed by FISH or microarray assay, are Williams syndrome, Smith-Magenis syndrome, and Velocardiofacial syndrome. The meiotic mechanisms responsible for interstitial chromosomal deletions causing these disorders also result in duplications. We now understand that interstitial chromosomal duplications in the following regions also produce abnormal phenotypes:

i. Williams Syndrome

Williams syndrome is a contiguous gene disorder that deletes the gene for elastin and other neighboring genes at 7q11.2. It is characterized by short stature; congenital heart disease (supravalvular aortic stenosis); coarse, elfin-like facies with prominent lips; hypercalcemia or hypercalciuria in infancy; developmental delay; and neonatal irritability evolving into an overly friendly personality. Calcium restriction may be necessary in early childhood to prevent nephrocalcinosis. The hypercalcemia often resolves during the first year of life. The natural history includes progression of cardiac disease and predisposition to hypertension and spinal osteoarthritis in adults. Most patients have mild to moderate intellectual deficits.

Duplication of chromosome 7q11.2 results in a syndrome that includes speech delay, and features of autistic spectrum disorders. Physical features are less consistent than in Williams syndrome.

Van der Aa et al: Fourteen new cases contribute to the characterization of the 7q11.23 microdupliction syndrome. Europ J Med Genet 2009;52:94 [PMID: 19249392].

ii. Smith-Magenis Syndrome

This syndrome is associated with microdeletion of 17p11 and is characterized by prominent forehead, deep-set eyes, cupid-shaped upper lip, self-mutilating behavior, sleep disturbance, and intellectual disabilities. Some patients also have seizure disorders, hearing loss, thyroid disease, and immunological and lipid abnormalities.

Duplication of 17p11 produces Potocki-Lupski syndrome that is characterized by growth failure, variable levels of cognitive deficiencies, autistic features, and, occasionally, structural abnormalities of the heart.

Potocki L et al: Characterization of Potocki-Lupksi syndrome ([Dup(17)(p11.2p11.2]) and delineation of a dosage sensitive critical interval that can convey an autism phenotype. Am J Hum Genet 2007;80:633 [PMID: 17357070].

iii. Velocardiofacial Syndrome (Deletion 22q11 Syndrome)

Also known as DiGeorge syndrome, this condition was originally described in newborns presenting with cyanotic congenital heart disease, usually involving great vessel abnormalities; thymic hypoplasia leading to immunodeficiency; and hypocalcemia due to absent parathyroid glands. This chromosomal abnormality is associated with a highly variable phenotype. Characteristics include mild microcephaly, palatal clefting or incompetence, speech and language delays, and congenital heart disease (Great vessel abnormalities, tetralogy of Fallot, and a variety of other abnormalities). Some affected individuals are predisposed to psychosis.

Duplication of the 22q11 region produces a mild and highly variable phenotype that ranges from developmental delays and learning disabilities to functionally normal.

Ou Z et al: Microduplications of 22q11.2 are frequently inherited and are associated with variable phenotypes. Genet Med 2008;10:267 [PMID: 18414210].

MENDELIAN DISORDERS

AUTOSOMAL DOMINANT DISORDERS

Neurofibromatosis, Marfan syndrome, achondroplasia, osteogenesis imperfecta, and the craniosynostoses are among the most well-known autosomal dominant disorders. There are many other common autosomal dominant disorders, including Treacher Collins syndrome, associated with a distinct craniofacial phenotype including malar and mandibular hypoplasia, and Noonan syndrome, which has a phenotype similar to Turner syndrome and is characterized by short stature and a webbed neck. Two other common genetic disorders whose causative genes were recently identified and found to be dominant mutations are CHARGE syndrome and Cornelia de Lange syndrome.

1. Neurofibromatosis Type 1

Neurofibromatosis type 1 (NF-1) is one of the most common autosomal dominant disorders, occurring in 1:3000 births and seen in all races and ethnic groups. In general, the disorder is progressive, with new manifestations appearing over time. Neurofibromatosis type 2 (NF-2), characterized by bilateral acoustic neuromas, with minimal or no skin manifestations, is a different disease caused by a different gene.

The gene for NF-1 is on the long arm of chromosome 17 and seems to code for a protein similar to a tumor suppresser factor. NF results from many different mutations of this gene. Approximately half of all NF cases are caused by new mutations. Careful evaluation of the parents is necessary to provide accurate genetic counseling. Recent evidence suggests that penetrance is close to 100% in those who carry the gene if individuals are examined carefully.

Café au lait macules may be present at birth, and about 80% of individuals with NF-1 will have more than six by age 1 year. Neurofibromas are benign tumors consisting of Schwann cells, nerve fibers, and fibroblasts; they may be discrete or plexiform. The incidence of Lisch nodules, which can be seen with a slit lamp, also increases with age. Affected individuals commonly have a large head, bony abnormalities on radiographic studies, scoliosis, and a wide spectrum of developmental problems. Although the average IQ is within the normal range, it is lower than in unaffected family members. (For more details of medical evaluation and treatment, see Chapter 25 of this book.) Useful information is provided on the following web site: http://www.nfinc.org.

Hyperpigmented macules can occur in other conditions such as Albright, Noonan, Leopard, and Banayan-Riley-Ruvalcaba (BRR) syndromes. The genes for NF-1, Noonan, and Leopard syndromes are molecules which control cell cycling through the RAS-MAPK signal transduction pathways; therefore, it is not surprising that some features can be shared.

2. Marfan Syndrome

ESSENTIALS OF DIAGNOSIS & TYPICAL FEATURES

- Skeletal abnormalities (Ghent criteria).
- Lens dislocation.
- Dilation of the aortic root.
- Dural ectasia.
- Positive family history.

Clinical Findings

Genetic testing is available for mutations causing Marfan syndrome, but the diagnosis remains largely clinical and is based on the Ghent criteria (available at: http://www.genetests.org). Children most often present with a positive family history, suspicious skeletal findings, or ophthalmologic complications. Motor milestones are frequently delayed due to joint laxity and mild myopathy. Adolescents are prone to spontaneous pneumothorax. Dysrhythmias may be present. Aortic and valvular complications are not common in children but are more likely in sporadic cases. The characteristic facies is long and thin, with down-slanting palpebral fissures. The palate is high arched, and dentition is often crowded. The uvula may be bifid.

Marfan syndrome is genetically heterogeneous. Mutations in the gene for fibrillin-1 proteins (*FBN1*) are most common but mutations in (*FBN2*) and in transforming growth factor b receptors (*TGFBR1* and *2*) can also produce phenotypes that fit criteria for a clinical diagnosis of Marfan syndrome.

Differential Diagnosis

Homocystinuria should be excluded through metabolic testing in all individuals with marfanoid skeletal features. An X-linked recessive disorder, **Lujan syndrome**, combines marfanoid habitus with cognitive disability. Other connective tissue disorders, **Ehlers-Danlos syndrome**, and **Stickler syndrome** should also be considered.

Genes mutated in Marfan syndrome can also be mutated in related disorders: **Beal syndrome** (*FBN2*), **Shprintzen-Goldberg**

syndrome (*FBN1*), and the recently described **Loeys-Dietz syndrome** (*TGFBR1* and *TGFBR2*). The reader is referred to reviews available at http://www.genetests.org for descriptions of these disorders.

Complications

The skeletal problems including scoliosis are progressive. Astigmatism and myopia are very common and surveillance for lens dislocation is necessary.

The most serious associated medical problems involve the heart. Although many patients with Marfan syndrome have mitral valve prolapse, the most serious concern is progressive aortic root dilation, which may lead to aneurysmal rupture and death, and progressive or acute valvular (aortic more frequently than mitral) incompetency.

Families and practitioners seeking additional information about Marfan syndrome can be referred to the National Marfan Foundation (http://www.marfan.org).

Treatment

A. Medical Therapy

Medical treatment for patients with Marfan syndrome includes surveillance for and appropriate management of the ophthalmologic, orthopedic, and cardiac issues. Serial echocardiograms are indicated to diagnose and follow the degree of aortic root enlargement, which can be managed medically or surgically, in more severe cases. Prophylactic β-adrenergic blockade can slow the rate of aortic dilation and reduce the development of aortic complications.

Interest in the effects of deficient extracellular fibrillin-1 has led to the discovery that the mild myopathy in Marfan syndrome reflects excessive signaling by transforming growth factor β (TGFβ), an inhibitor of myoblast differentiation. Animal studies suggest that aortic aneurysm can be prevented by TGFβ antagonists, including blockers of angiotensin II type 1 receptors. Research studies are currently underway using this approach in human patients.

B. Genetic Counseling

Genetic testing for mutations in *FBN1* and *FBN2* and in *TGFBR1* and *TGFBR2* should be considered in all individuals with Marfan syndrome as penetrance is variable and apparently unaffected family members can carry and pass on mutations.

3. Achondroplasia

Achondroplasia, the most common form of skeletal dysplasia, is caused by a mutation in *FGFR3*.

Clinical Findings

The classic phenotype includes relative macrocephaly, midface hypoplasia, short-limbed dwarfism, and trident-shaped hands. The phenotype is apparent at birth. Individuals with achondroplasia are cognitively normal.

Treatment

A. Medical Therapy

Orthopedic intervention is necessary for spinal problems including severe lumbar lordosis and gibbus deformity. Long bone lengthening surgery may help to improve upper extremity function.

Head circumference during infancy must be closely monitored and plotted on a diagnosis-specific head circumference chart. Bony overgrowth at the level of the foramen magnum may lead to progressive hydrocephalus and brainstem compression, and may warrant neurosurgical intervention.

Many patients find support through organizations such as the Little People of America, at the following web site: http://www.lpaonline.org.

B. Genetic Counseling

The vast majority of cases (approximately 90%) represent a new mutation. Two hemizygous parents with achondroplasia have a 25% risk of having a child homozygous for *FGFR3* mutations, which is a lethal disorder.

4. Osteogenesis Imperfecta

Osteogenesis imperfecta (OI), or brittle bone disease, is a relatively common disorder. The more common forms are caused by mutations in type I collagen.

Clinical Findings

A number of types of OI have now been described, but the four most common types of OI are

- Type I, a mild form, with increased incidence of fracturing and blue sclerae.
- Type II, usually lethal in the newborn period with multiple congenital fractures and severe lung disease.
- Type III, a severe form causing significant bony deformity secondary to multiple fractures (many of which are congenital), blue sclerae, short stature, and mild restrictive lung disease.
- Type IV, another mild form with increased incidence of fracturing after birth; dentinogenesis imperfecta is common.

Treatment

A. Medical Therapy

A major advancement in the treatment of OI patients has been the use of pamidronate, a bisphosphonate compound, which has been reported to lead to a reduced incidence of fracture and improvement in bone density. Patients should be followed by an experienced orthopedist, as rodding of long bones and surgery to correct scoliosis are often required. Hearing assessments are indicated, because of the association between OI and deafness. Close dental follow-up is also necessary.

B. Genetic Counseling

The four main types of OI are associated with mutations in the genes coding for type I collagen. Collagen analysis performed in skin fibroblasts can confirm the diagnosis. DNA analysis in blood is also possible. The milder forms may be seen as the result of dominant inheritance, while the more severe forms of OI generally result from new mutations.

5. Craniosynostoses Syndromes

The craniosynostoses disorders are common dominant disorders associated with premature fusion of cranial sutures. This class of disorders is now known to be caused by various mutations in *FGFR* genes.

Crouzon syndrome is the most common of these disorders and is associated with multiple suture fusions, but with normal limbs. Other craniosynostosis disorders have limb as well as craniofacial anomalies, and include Pfeiffer, Apert, Jackson-Weiss, and Saethre-Chotzen syndromes.

Patients with craniosynostosis often have shallow orbits, midface narrowing that may result in upper airway obstruction, and hydrocephalus that may require shunting. Children with craniosynostosis may require multiple-staged craniofacial and neurosurgical procedures to address these issues, but usually have normal intelligence.

6. CHARGE Syndrome

CHARGE syndrome affects structures derived from rostral neural crest cells but also includes abnormal development of the eyes and midbrain. The acronym CHARGE serves as a mnemonic for associated abnormalities that include **c**olobomas, congenital **h**eart disease, choanal **a**tresia, growth **r**etardation, **g**enital abnormalities (hypogenitalism), and **e**ar abnormalities, with deafness. Facial asymmetry is a common finding. CHARGE is now known to be caused by mutations in the *CHD7* gene on chromosome 8q. A web site with information on CHARGE syndrome is available at http://www.chargesyndrome.org/.

Bergman JE et al: CHD7 mutations and CHARGE syndrome: The clinical implications of an expanding phenotype. J Med Genet 2011 May;48(5):334–342 [Epub 2011 Mar 4].

7. Cornelia de Lange Syndrome

Cornelia de Lange syndrome is characterized by severe growth retardation; limb, especially hand, reduction defects (50%); congenital heart disease (25%); and stereotypical facies with hirsutism, medial fusion of eyebrows (synophrys), and thin, down-turned lips. The course and severity are variable, but the prognosis for survival and normal development is poor.

Heterozygous mutations in the cohesin regulator, NIPBL, or the cohesin structural components SMC1A and SMC3, have been identified in approximately 65% of individuals with CdLS. Cohesin regulates sister chromatid cohesion during mitotis and meiosis. In addition, cohesin has been demonstrated to play a critical role in the regulation of gene expression. Furthermore, multiple proteins in the cohesin pathway are also involved in additional fundamental biological events such as double strand DNA break repair, chromatin remodeling and maintaining genomic stability.

Liu J et al: Cornelia de Lange syndrome. Adv Exp Med Biol 2010;685:111–123.

Jones KL: *Recognizable Patterns of Human Malformation*, 6th ed. Elsevier, 2006.

8. Noonan Syndrome

Noonan syndrome is an autosomal dominant disorder characterized by short stature, congenital heart disease, abnormalities of cardiac conduction and rhythm, webbed neck, down-slanting palpebral fissures, hearing loss, and low-set ears. The phenotype evolves with age and may be difficult to recognize in older patients. Mild developmental delays are often present. Recent advances in molecular genetic research have led to the definition of the RAS-mitogen-activated protein kinase (MAPK) pathway disorders or "RASopathies." They comprise Noonan syndrome and related disorders (cardio-facio-cutaneous and Costello syndromes), as well as neurofibromatosis type 1.

Products of proto-oncogenes help control cell cycling through RAS-MAPK signal transduction pathways. Cell cycling controls are also affected by mutations in other genes that produce more complicated Noonan-like disorders (ie, Costello and cardiofaciocutaneous syndromes) in which cardiomyopathies are prominent. Because mutations causing NF-1 also affect RAS proto-oncogene signaling, it is not surprising that there is an NF-1 subtype with a so-called Noonan phenotype.

Constitutional overactivation at various levels of the RAS-MAPK pathway causes overlapping syndromes, comprising characteristic facial features, cardiac defects, cutaneous abnormalities, growth deficit, neurocognitive delay, and predisposition to malignancies. Each syndrome also exhibits unique features that probably reflect genotype-related specific biological effects.

Zenker M: Clinical manifestations of mutations in RAS and related intracellular signal transduction factors. Curr Opin Pediatr 2011 Aug;23(4):443–451.

AUTOSOMAL RECESSIVE DISORDERS

1. Cystic Fibrosis

The gene for cystic fibrosis, *CFTR,* is found on the long arm of chromosome 7. Approximately 1 in 22 persons are carriers. Many different mutations have been identified; the most common mutation in the Caucasian population is known as Δ *F508.*

Cloning of the gene for cystic fibrosis and identification of the mutation in the majority of cases have completely changed genetic counseling and prenatal diagnosis for this disorder, although the sweat chloride assay is still important in confirming the diagnosis.

The identification of the mutation in the cystic fibrosis gene has also raised the issue of mass newborn screening, because of the high frequency of this gene in the Caucasian population. Some states, such as Colorado, have offered newborn screening by trypsinogen assay, which can detect 70% of patients with cystic fibrosis. Although early detection can ensure good nutritional status starting at birth, newborn screening is controversial as there is no cure for cystic fibrosis. (For more details of medical management, see Chapters 19 and 22.)

2. Smith-Lemli-Opitz Syndrome

Smith-Lemli-Opitz syndrome is caused by a metabolic error in the final step of cholesterol production, resulting in low cholesterol levels and accumulation of the precursor 7-dehydrocholesterol (7-DHC). Because cholesterol is a necessary precursor for sterol hormones, bile acids and CNS myelin, and cholesterol content is crucial for the integrity of all cell membranes, the medical consequences of both cholesterol deficiency and 7-DHC accumulation are complex and severe. A number of other genetic disorders involving cholesterol biosynthesis more proximally in the pathway have been recently described (ie, Desmosterolosis) but are quite rare with a very severe and often lethal phenotype.

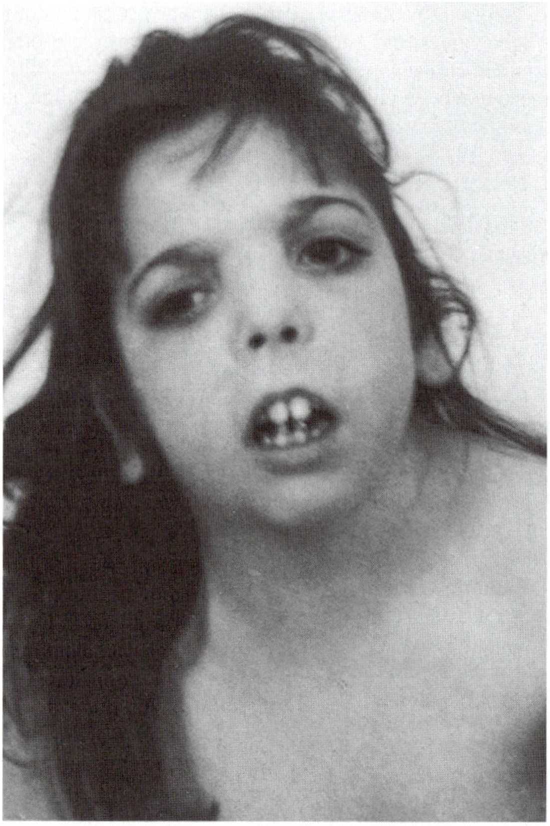

▲ **Figure 37–9.** Child with Smith-Lemli-Opitz syndrome, featuring bitemporal narrowing, upturned nares, ptosis, and small chin.

Clinical Findings

Patients with Smith-Lemli-Opitz syndrome present with a characteristic phenotype, including dysmorphic facial features (Figure 37–9), multiple congenital anomalies, hypotonia, growth failure, and intellectual disability. The diagnosis can be confirmed via a simple blood test looking for the presence of the precursor, 7-DHC. This blood test can only be done in special laboratories. Prenatal testing is available.

Treatment

Treatment with cholesterol can ameliorate the growth failure and lead to improvement in medical issues, although treatment does not cure this complex disorder.

3. Sensorineural Hearing Loss

Although there is marked genetic heterogeneity in causes of sensorineural hearing loss, including dominant, recessive, and X-linked patterns, nonsyndromic, recessively inherited deafness is the predominant form of severe inherited childhood deafness. Several hundred genes are known to cause hereditary hearing loss and deafness. The hearing loss may be conductive, sensorineural, or a combination of both; syndromic or nonsyndromic; and prelingual (before language develops) or postlingual (after language develops). The genetic forms of hearing loss are diagnosed by otologic, audiologic, and physical examination; family history; ancillary testing (such as CT examination of the temporal bone); and molecular genetic testing. Molecular genetic tests are available for many types of syndromic and nonsyndromic deafness, but often only on a research basis. In the clinical setting, molecular genetic testing is available for some recessive conditions including Usher syndrome types 2A (*USH2A* gene) and 3 (one mutation in *USH3A*), and at least six other rare forms of genetically caused deafness.

Testing for deafness-causing mutations in two more common genes, *GJB2* (which encodes the protein connexin 26) and *GJB6* (which encodes the protein connexin 30), plays a prominent role in diagnosis and genetic counseling. Mutations in connexin 26 are present in 49% of cases of prelingual deafness.

Nance WE: The genetics of deafness. Ment Retard Dev Disabil Res Rev 2003;9:109 [PMID: 12784229].

4. Spinal Muscular Atrophy

Spinal muscular atrophy (SMA) is an autosomal recessive neuromuscular disorder in which anterior horn cells in the spinal cord degenerate. The mechanism for the loss of cells appears to involve apoptosis of neurons in the absence of the product of the SMN1 (survival motor neuron) gene located on chromosome 5q. Loss of anterior horn cells leads to progressive atrophy of skeletal muscle. The disorder has an incidence of approximately 1 in 12,000, with the majority of the cases presenting in infancy. Carrier frequencies approach 1 in 50 in populations with European ancestry.

Clinical Findings

Three clinical subtypes are recognized based on age of onset and rate of progression. SMA I is the most devastating. Mild weakness may be present at birth but is clearly evident by 3 months and is accompanied by loss of reflexes and fasciculations in affected muscles. Progression of the disorder leads to eventual respiratory failure, usually by age 1 year. Symptoms of SMA II begin later, with weakness and decreased reflexes generally apparent by age 2 years. Children affected with SMA III begin to become weak as they approach adolescence.

Homozygous deletion of exon 7 of *SMN1* is detectable in approximately 95%–98% of cases of all types of SMA and confirms the diagnosis. The *SMN1* region on chromosome 5q is complex and variability in presentation of the disorder involves expression of up to three copies of the neighboring *SMN2* gene. More severe phenotypes have fewer *SMN2* copies. Approximately 2%–5% of patients affected with SMA will be compound heterozygotes in whom there is one copy of *SMN1* with exon 7 deleted and a second copy with a point mutation.

Prenatal diagnosis is available through genetic testing, but careful molecular analysis of the proband and demonstration of carrier status in parents is advised since, in addition to the problem of potential compound heterozygosity, 2% of cases occur as a result of a de novo mutation in one *SMN1* allele. In this case, one of the parents is not a carrier and recurrence risks are low. Carrier testing is further complicated by a duplication of *SMN1* in 4% of the population that results in there being two *SMN1* genes on one of their chromosomes. Hence, reproductive risk assessment, carrier testing, and prenatal diagnosis of SMA are best undertaken in the context of careful genetic counseling.

5. Metabolic Disorders

Most inborn errors of metabolism are inherited in an autosomal recessive pattern. (See Chapter 36 for detailed explanations of these disorders.)

X-LINKED DISORDERS

1. Duchenne & Becker Muscular Dystrophies

Duchenne muscular dystrophy (DMD) results from failure of synthesis of the muscle cytoskeletal protein dystrophin, the gene for which is located on the X chromosome, Xp12. Approximately 1 in 4000 male children is affected. Mutations in the same gene that result in partial expression of the dystrophin protein produce a less severe phenotype, Becker muscular dystrophy (BMD). In both DMD and BMD, progressive degeneration of skeletal and cardiac muscle occurs. Boys with DMD exhibit proximal muscle weakness and pseudo-hypertrophy of calf muscles by age 5–6 years. Patients become nonambulatory by age 13. Serum creatine kinase levels are markedly elevated. Boys with DMD frequently die in their 20s of respiratory failure and cardiac dysfunction. The prognosis for BMD is more variable. Although corticosteroids are useful in maintaining strength, they do not slow progression of the disorder.

The gene for dystrophin is very large and a common target for mutation. Large deletions or duplications can be detected in the gene for dystrophin in 65% of cases. Methods for detecting small and even point mutations have now been developed. Mutation testing and careful clinical assessment are replacing muscle biopsies in making the diagnosis of DMD.

One-third of DMD cases presenting with a negative family history are likely to be new mutations. Genetic counseling is complicated by the fact that germline mosaicism for mutations in the dystrophin gene occur in approximately 15%–20% of families. Therefore, if a mutation has been detected in a proband, prenatal diagnosis is routinely offered to his mother regardless of her apparent carrier status. It is also necessary to look for mutations in all sisters of affected boys. Since mutations are now detected in the great majority of DMD cases, there is considerably less need for estimating carrier risks based on creatine kinase levels or using genetic linkage for prenatal diagnosis. Nonetheless, counseling and prenatal diagnosis remain difficult in some families. (Additional information about muscular dystrophies is included in Chapter 25.)

2. Hemophilia

Hemophilia A is an X-linked, recessive, bleeding disorder caused by a deficiency in the activity of coagulation factor VIII. Affected individuals develop a variable phenotype of hemorrhage into joints and muscles, easy bruising, and prolonged bleeding from wounds. The disorder is caused by heterogeneous mutations in the factor VIII gene, which maps to Xq28. Carrier detection and prenatal diagnosis are possible. Replacement of factor VIII is done using a variety of preparations derived from human plasma or recombinant techniques. Although replacement therapy is effective in most cases, 10%–15% of treated individuals develop neutralizing antibodies that decrease its effectiveness. (See Chapter 30 for additional discussion.)

3. Metabolic Disorders

Some important inborn errors are inherited as X-linked disorders, such as adrenoleukodystrophy. (See Chapter 36 for more detailed descriptions.)

NONMENDELIAN DISORDERS

DISORDERS OF IMPRINTING

1. Beckwith-Wiedemann Syndrome

The association of macrosomia (enlarged body size), macroglossia (enlarged tongue), and omphalocele constitutes the Beckwith-Wiedemann syndrome (BWS), now known to be related to abnormal expression of genes located on chromosome 11p15. Other associated findings include hypertelorism, unusual ear creases, infantile hypoglycemia due to transient hyperinsulinemia, multiple congenital anomalies (cleft palate and genitourinary anomalies common), and increased risk for certain malignancies, especially Wilms tumor (7%–10%).

A growth factor gene, *IGF2,* is imprinted such that the maternal allele is ordinarily not expressed during intrauterine development. Chromosomal abnormalities such as duplication of the paternal 11p15 region, or paternal UPD, are associated with BWS. Paternal UPD may also lead to loss of expression of a tumor suppressor gene (*H19*), normally read from the maternal homolog, contributing to the increased predisposition to cancer seen in this disorder. Children affected with BWS should undergo tumor surveillance protocols, including an abdominal ultrasound every 3 months until they reach age 7 years, as diagnosing malignancy at early stages leads to a significant improvement in outcome.

2. Prader-Willi Syndrome

Prader-Willi syndrome results from lack of expression of several imprinted genes, including *SNRPn,* located on chromosome 15q11. Clinical characteristics include severe hypotonia in infancy, often necessitating placement of a feeding gastrostomy tube. In older children, characteristic facies evolve over time, including almond-shaped eyes, along with frequent strabismus. Short stature, obesity, hypogenitalism, and small hands and feet with tapering fingers are felt to be associated with growth hormone deficiency and GH treatment is now offered to PWS patients. Obsessive hyperphagia (usual onset 3–4 years) is the hallmark of this disorder.

Deletion of the paternally inherited allele of chromosome 15q11 (detected by FISH or microarray) is the most common chromosomal abnormality causing Prader-Willi syndrome, followed by maternal UPD, diagnosed by DNA methylation studies.

3. Angelman Syndrome

Angelman syndrome also involves imprinting and results from a variety of mutations that inactivate a ubiquitin-protein ligase gene, *UBE3A,* located in the same region of chromosome 15 as *SNRPn,* the maternally imprinted gene involved in Prader-Willi syndrome (see preceding section). *UBE3A* is paternally imprinted, and during normal development the maternal allele is expressed only in the brain. The classic phenotype includes severe intellectual disability with prognathism, seizures, and marked delay in motor milestones, abnormal gait and posturing, poor language development, and paroxysmal laughter and tongue thrusting.

Angelman syndrome is most commonly caused when sequences detectable by microarray or FISH on 15q11 are deleted from the maternal homolog. Uniparental paternal disomy 15 is the least common cause. Mutations in *UBE3A* cause the disorder in about one-fourth of cases. Imprinting errors, which may be associated with advanced reproductive techniques, may also result in Angelman syndrome.

Niemitz EL, Feinberg AP: Epigenetics and assisted reproductive technology: A call for investigation. Am J Hum Genet 2004;74:599 [PMID: 14991528].

Iliadou AN, Janson PC, Cnattingius S: Epigenetics and assisted reproductive technology. J Intern Med 2011;270(5):414–420 [PMID: 21848664].

DISORDERS ASSOCIATED WITH ANTICIPATION

1. (Autosomal Dominant) Myotonic Dystrophy

Most myotonic dystrophy, an autosomal dominant condition characterized by muscle weakness and tonic muscle spasms (myotonia) along with hypogonadism, frontal balding, cardiac conduction abnormalities, and cataracts, presents in adults. This disorder occurs when a CTG repeat in the *DMPK* gene on chromosome 19 expands to 50 or more copies. Normal individuals have from 5 to 35 CTG repeat copies. Individuals carrying 35–49 repeats are generally asymptomatic, but repeat copies greater than 35 are meiotically unstable and tend to further expand when passed to subsequent generations. Individuals with 50–100 copies may be only mildly affected (eg, cataracts). Most individuals with repeat copies greater than 100 will have symptoms or electrical myotonia as adults.

As unstable alleles continue to expand and copy numbers approach 400, symptoms become evident in children. Expansion from greater than 1000 copies produces fetal and neonatal disease that can be lethal. Expansion from approximately 200 to 400 repeat copies produces mild, often clinically undetected symptoms, while very large copy numbers (800–2000) are associated with fetal manifestations (polyhydramnios and arthrogryposis). This occurs most frequently when the unstable repeats are passed through an affected mother. Therefore, an important component in the workup of the floppy or weak infant is a careful neurologic assessment of both parents for evidence of weakness or myotonia. Molecular testing that measures the number of CTG repeats is diagnostic clinically and prenatally. (See Chapter 25 for additional discussion.)

2. (Autosomal Recessive) Friedreich Ataxia

Symptoms of Friedreich ataxia include loss of coordination (cerebellar dysfunction) with both motor and sensory findings beginning in preadolescence and typically progressing through the teenage years. The gene involved, *FDRA*, is located on chromosome 9. Normal individuals carry 7–33 GAA repeats at this locus. Close to 96% of affected patients are homozygous for repeat expansions that exceed 66 copies. However, point mutations in the gene also occur. Meiotic instability for GAA repeats is more variable than for others and contractions occur more frequently than do expansions. Relationships between genotype and phenotype are also more complex. Molecular diagnostic testing requires careful interpretation with respect to prognosis and reproductive risks. (See Chapter 25 for additional discussion.)

3. (X-Linked) Fragile X Syndrome

Fragile X syndrome, present in approximately 1 in 1000 males, is the most common cause of cognitive disabilities in males. The responsible gene is *FMR1*, which has unstable CGG repeats at the 5′ end. Normal individuals have up to 50 CGG repeats. Individuals with 51–200 CGG repeats have a premutation and may manifest symptoms including developmental, behavioral, and physical traits, premature ovarian failure in a subset of females; and a progressive, neurologic deterioration in older males called FXTAS (fragile X–associated tremor-ataxia syndrome). Affected individuals with fragile X syndrome (full mutation) have more than 200 CGG repeats and also have hypermethylation of both the CGG expansion and an adjacent CpG island. This methylation turns off the FMR1 gene. DNA analysis, rather than cytogenetic testing, is the method of choice for confirming the diagnosis of fragile X syndrome.

Clinical Features

Most males with fragile X syndrome present with intellectual disabilities, oblong facies with large ears, and large testicles after puberty. Other physical signs include symptoms suggestive of a connective tissue disorder (eg, hyperextensible joints or mitral valve prolapse). Many affected individuals are hyperactive and exhibit infantile autism or autistic-like behavior.

Unlike other X-linked disorders where female heterozygotes are asymptomatic, females with a full mutation may exhibit a phenotype ranging from normal IQ to intellectual disability, and autism, and may manifest other behavioral problems.

Clinical expression of fragile X differs in male and female offspring depending on which parent is transmitting the gene. The premutation can change into the full mutation only when passed through a female. Identification of the abnormal DNA amplification by direct DNA analysis can confirm the diagnosis of fragile X in an affected individual and can detect asymptomatic gene carriers of both sexes. Therefore, DNA analysis is a reliable test for prenatal and postnatal diagnosis of fragile X syndrome and facilitates genetic counseling. (Management considerations for patients with fragile X syndrome are described in Chapter 3.)

Hagerman PJ, Hagerman RJ: The fragile-X premutation: A maturing perspective. Am J Hum Genet 2004;74:805 [PMID: 15052536].

MITOCHONDRIAL DISORDERS

More than 100 point mutations and rearrangements of mtDNA have been identified, which are associated with a large number of human diseases. Symptoms of mitochondrial disorders are secondary to deficiency in the respiratory chain enzymes of oxidative phosphorylation, which supply energy to all cells. Mitochondrial diseases are usually progressive disorders with neurologic dysfunction including hypotonia, developmental delay, and seizures. Ophthalmologic issues, hearing loss, gastrointestinal tract dysfunction with growth failure, renal, endocrine, cardiac, and autonomic dysfunction are some of the many issues which can affect patients with mitochondrial diseases. The following disorders are three of the more common ones.

1. MELAS

MELAS is an acronym for mitochondrial encephalopathy, lactic acidosis, and strokelike episodes. Symptoms occur in the pediatric age group and include recurrent episodes resembling stroke (blindness, paralysis), headache, vomiting, weakness of proximal muscles, and elevated blood lactate. (***Note:*** Lactate may be falsely elevated secondary to technical difficulties in obtaining a free-flowing blood specimen or delay in laboratory measurement.) The most common mutation causing MELAS is in the $tRNA^{Leu}$ gene (*A3243G*).

2. MERRF

MERRF is an acronym for **m**yoclonus **e**pilepsy with **r**agged **r**ed **f**ibers. Children with MERRF present with a variety of neurologic symptoms, including myoclonus, deafness, weakness of muscles, and seizures. Eighty percent of cases are due to a missense mutation in the mitochondrial $tRNA^{Lys}$ gene (*A8344G*).

3. Leigh Subacute Necrotizing Encephalomyelopathy

Multiple different abnormalities in respiratory chain function lead to Leigh disease, a very severe disorder associated with progressive loss of developmental milestones, along with extrapyramidal symptoms and brainstem dysfunction. Episodes of deterioration are frequently associated with an intercurrent febrile illness. Symptoms include hypotonia, unusual choreoathetoid hand movements, feeding dysfunction with failure to thrive, and seizures. Focal necrotic lesions of the brainstem and thalamus are hallmarks on MRI scan. Mitochondrial mutations affecting the respiratory chain, especially complexes I, II, and IV, and nuclear DNA mutations affecting complex II have been identified as causing Leigh disease.

Wong LJ, Scaglia F, Graham BH, Craigen WJ: Current molecular diagnostic algorithm for mitochondrial disorders. Mol Genet Metab 2010 Jun;100(2):111–117 [PMID: 20359921].

DISORDERS OF MULTIFACTORIAL INHERITANCE

CLEFT LIP & CLEFT PALATE

ESSENTIALS OF DIAGNOSIS & TYPICAL FEATURES

- Cleft lip is more common in males, cleft palate in females.
- Cleft lip and palate may be isolated defects (nonsyndromic) or associated with other anomalies as part of a genetic disorder (syndromic).
- Pierre Robin sequence, the association of cleft palate, micrognathia, and glossoptosis may lead to severe airway complications in young infants, necessitating tracheostomy.

General Considerations

From a genetic standpoint, cleft lip with or without cleft palate is distinct from isolated cleft palate. Although both can occur in a single family, particularly in association with certain syndromes, this pattern is unusual. Racial background is a factor in the incidence of facial clefting. Among Asians, Caucasians, and blacks, the incidence is 1.61, 0.9, and 0.31, respectively, per 1000 live births.

Clinical Findings

A cleft lip may be unilateral or bilateral and complete or incomplete. It may occur with a cleft of the entire palate or just the primary (anterior and gingival ridge) or secondary (posterior) palate. An isolated cleft palate can involve only the soft palate or both the soft and hard palates. It can be a V-shaped or a wide horseshoe, U-shaped cleft. When the cleft palate is associated with micrognathia and glossoptosis (a tongue that falls back and causes respiratory or feeding problems), it is called the **Pierre Robin sequence**. Among individuals with facial clefts—more commonly those with isolated cleft palate—the incidence of other congenital abnormalities is increased, with up to a 60% association with other anomalies or syndromes. The incidence of congenital heart disease, for example, is 1%–2% in liveborn infants, but among those with Pierre Robin sequence it can be as high as 15%. Associated abnormalities should be looked for in the period immediately after birth and before surgery.

Differential Diagnosis

A facial cleft may occur in many different circumstances. It may be an isolated abnormality or part of a more generalized syndrome. Prognosis, management, and accurate determination of recurrence risks all depend on accurate diagnosis. In evaluating a child with a facial cleft, the physician must determine if the cleft is nonsyndromic or syndromic.

A. Nonsyndromic

In the past, nonsyndromic cleft lip or cleft palate was considered a classic example of polygenic or multifactorial inheritance. Several recent studies have suggested that one or more major autosomal loci, both recessive and dominant may be involved. Empirically, however, the recurrence risk is still in the range of 2%–3% because of nonpenetrance or the presence of other contributing genes.

B. Syndromic

Cleft lip, with or without cleft palate, and isolated cleft palate may occur in a variety of syndromes that may be environmental, chromosomal, single gene, or of unknown origin (Table 37–4). Prognosis and accurate recurrence risks depend on the correct diagnosis.

Complications

Problems associated with facial clefts include early feeding difficulties, which may be severe; airway obstruction necessitating tracheostomy; recurrent serous otitis media associated with fluctuating hearing and language delays; speech problems, including language delay, hypernasality, and articulation errors; and dental and orthodontic complications.

Treatment

A. Medical Therapy

Long-term management ideally should be provided through a multidisciplinary cleft palate clinic.

Table 37–4. Syndromic isolated cleft palate (CP) and cleft lip with or without cleft palate (CL/CP).

Environmental
Maternal seizures, anticonvulsant usage (CL/CP or CP)
Fetal alcohol syndrome (CP)
Amniotic band syndrome (CL/CP)
Chromosomal
Trisomies 13 and 18 (CL/CP)
Wolf-Hirschhorn or 4p- syndrome (CL/CP)
Shprintzen or 22q11.2 deletion syndrome (CP)
Single-gene disorders
Treacher Collins syndrome, AD (CP)
Stickler syndrome, AD (CP—particularly Pierre-Robin)
Smith-Lemli-Opitz, AR (CP)
Unknown cause
Moebius syndrome (CP)

AD, autosomal dominant; AR, autosomal recessive.

B. Genetic Counseling

Accurate counseling depends on accurate diagnosis and the differentiation of syndromic from nonsyndromic clefts. A complete family history must be taken, and the patient and both parents must be examined. The choice of laboratory studies is guided by the presence of other abnormalities and clinical suspicions, and may include microarray analysis and metabolic and DNA studies. Clefts of both the lip and the palate can be detected on detailed prenatal ultrasound.

NEURAL TUBE DEFECTS

ESSENTIALS OF DIAGNOSIS & TYPICAL FEATURES

- Various defects, ranging from anencephaly to open or skin-covered lesions of the spinal cord, may occur in isolation or as part of a syndrome.
- Myelomeningocele is usually associated with hydrocephalus, Arnold-Chiari II malformation, neurogenic bladder and bowel, and congenital paralysis in the lower extremities.
- Anomalies of the CNS, heart, and kidneys may also be seen.
- MRI helps determine the extent of the anatomic defect in skin covered lesions.

General Considerations

Neural tube defects comprise a variety of malformations, including anencephaly, encephalocele, spina bifida (myelomeningocele), sacral agenesis, and other spinal dysraphisms. Evidence suggests that the neural tube develops via closure at multiple closure sites and that each closure site is mediated by different genes and affected by different teratogens. Hydrocephalus associated with the Arnold-Chiari type II malformation commonly occurs with myelomeningocele. Sacral agenesis, also called the caudal regression syndrome, occurs more frequently in infants of diabetic mothers.

Clinical Findings

At birth, neural tube defects can present as an obvious rachischisis (open lesion), or as a more subtle skin-covered lesion. In the latter case, MRI should be conducted to better define the anatomic defect. The extent of neurologic deficit depends on the level of the lesion and may include clubfeet, dislocated hips, or total flaccid paralysis below the level of the lesion. Hydrocephalus may be apparent at birth or may develop after the back has been surgically repaired. Neurogenic bladder and bowel are commonly seen. Other anomalies of the CNS may be present, as well as anomalies of the heart or kidneys.

Differential Diagnosis

Neural tube defects may occur in isolation (nonsyndromic) or as part of a genetic syndrome. They may result from teratogenic exposure to alcohol or the anticonvulsant valproate. Any infant with dysmorphic features or other major anomalies in addition to a neural tube defect should be evaluated by a geneticist, and a microarray analysis should be performed.

Treatment

A. Neurosurgical Measures

Infants with an open neural tube defect should be placed in prone position, and the lesion kept moist with sterile dressing. Neurosurgical closure should occur within 24–48 hours after birth to reduce risk of infection. The infant should be monitored closely for signs of hydrocephalus. Shunts are required in about 85% of cases of myelomeningocele and are associated with complications including malfunction and infection. Symptoms of the Arnold-Chiari II malformation include feeding dysfunction, abducens nerve palsy, vocal cord paralysis with stridor, and apnea. Shunt malfunction may cause an acute worsening of Arnold-Chiari symptoms that may be life-threatening.

B. Orthopedic Measures

The child's ability to walk varies according to the level of the lesion. Children with low lumbar and sacral lesions walk with minimal support, while those with high lumbar and thoracic lesions are rarely functional walkers. Orthopedic input is necessary to address foot deformities and scoliosis. Physical therapy services are indicated.

C. Urologic Measures

Neurogenic bladders have variable presentations. Urodynamic studies are recommended early on to define bladder function, and management is guided by the results of these studies. Continence can often be achieved by the use of anticholinergic or sympathomimetic agents, clean intermittent catheterization, and a variety of urologic procedures. Renal function should be monitored regularly, and an ultrasound examination should be periodically repeated. Symptomatic infections should be treated.

Symptoms of neurogenic bowel include incontinence and chronic constipation and are managed with a combination of dietary modifications, laxatives, stool softeners, and rectal stimulation. A surgical procedure called ACE (antegrade continence enema) may be recommended for patients with severe constipation that is unresponsive to conservative management.

D. Genetic Counseling

Most isolated neural tube defects are polygenic, with a recurrence risk of 2%–3% in future pregnancies. The recurrence risk for siblings of the parents and siblings of the patients is 1%–2%. A patient with spina bifida has a 5% chance of having an affected child. Prenatal diagnosis is possible. In fetuses with open neural tube defects, maternal serum α-fetoprotein levels measured at 16–18 weeks' gestation are elevated. α-Fetoprotein and acetylcholine esterase levels in amniotic fluid are also elevated. Ultrasound studies alone can detect up to 90% of neural tube defects.

Prophylactic folic acid can significantly lower the incidence and recurrence rate of neural tube defects, if the intake of the folic acid starts at least 3 months prior to conception and continues for the first month of pregnancy, at a dose of 4 mg/d for women at increased risk. For women of childbearing age without a family history of neural tube defects, the dose is 0.4 mg of folic acid daily. Folic acid supplementation prior to conception may also lower the incidence of other congenital malformations such as conotruncal heart defects.

Special Issues & Prognosis

All children requiring multiple surgical procedures (ie, patients with spina bifida or urinary tract anomalies) have a significant risk for developing hypersensitivity type I (IgE-mediated) allergic reactions to latex. For this reason, nonlatex medical products are now routinely used when caring for patients with neural tube defects.

Most individuals with spina bifida are cognitively normal, but learning disabilities are common. Individuals with encephalocele or other CNS malformations generally have a much poorer intellectual prognosis. Individuals with closed spinal cord abnormalities (eg, sacral lipomas) have more mild issues in general, and intelligence is usually normal. Spinal cord tethering may present later with symptoms of back pain, progressive scoliosis, and changes in bowel or bladder function. This often requires neurosurgical intervention.

Individuals with neural tube defects have lifelong medical issues, requiring the input of a multidisciplinary medical team. A good support for families is the national Spina Bifida Association, at the following web site: http://www.sbaa.org.

COMMON RECOGNIZABLE DISORDERS WITH VARIABLE OR UNKNOWN CAUSE

The text that follows describes several important and common human malformation syndromes. The best illustrations of these syndromes are found in *Smith's Recognizable Patterns of Human Malformation*. An excellent Internet site at the University of Kansas Medical Center can be consulted for further information: http://www.kumc.edu/gec/support.

1. Arthrogryposis Multiplex

The term *arthrogryposis* is often used as shorthand to describe multiple congenital contractures that affect two or more different areas of the body. Arthrogryposis is not a specific diagnosis, but rather a clinical finding, and it is a characteristic of more than 300 different disorders. Causes most often involve constraint, CNS maldevelopment or injury, and neuromuscular disorders. Polyhydramnios is often present as a result of lack of fetal swallowing. Pulmonary hypoplasia may also be present, reflecting lack of fetal breathing. The workup includes brain imaging, careful consideration of metabolic disease, neurologic consultation, and, in some cases, electrophysiologic studies and muscle biopsy. The parents should be examined, and a family history reviewed carefully for findings such as muscle weakness or cramping, cataracts, and early-onset heart disease, suggesting myotonic dystrophy. Mutations in at least five genes (*TNNI2*, *TNNT3*, *TPM2*, *MYH3*, and *MYH8*) that encode components of the contractile apparatus of fast-twitch myofibers can cause distal arthrogryposis.

Bamshad M et al: Arthrogryposis: A Review and Update. J Bone Joint Surg Am 2009 July 1;91(Suppl 4):40–46.

2. Goldenhar Syndrome

Goldenhar syndrome, also known as vertebro-auriculofacial syndrome, is an association of multiple anomalies involving the head and neck. The classic phenotype includes hemifacial microsomia (one side of the face smaller than the other), and abnormalities of the pinna on the same side with associated deafness. Ear anomalies may be quite severe and include anotia. A characteristic benign fatty tumor in the outer eye, called an epibulbar dermoid, is frequently present, as are preauricular ear tags. Vertebral anomalies, particularly of the cervical vertebrae, are common. The Arnold-Chiari type I malformation (herniation of the cerebellum into the cervical spinal canal) is a common associated anomaly. Cardiac anomalies and hydrocephalus are seen in more severe cases. Most patients with Goldenhar syndrome have normal intelligence. The cause is unknown; however, there is significant overlap with the Townes-Brocks syndrome, caused by mutations in the *SALL1* gene. (See Craniofacial Microsomia Overview, Gene Reviews, www.genereviews.org for an excellent discussion and differential diagnosis.)

3. Oligohydramnios Sequence (Potter Sequence)

This condition presents in newborns as severe respiratory distress due to pulmonary hypoplasia in association with positional deformities of the extremities, usually bilateral clubfeet, and typical facies consisting of suborbital creases, depressed nasal tip and low-set ears, and retrognathia. The sequence may be due to prolonged lack of amniotic fluid. Most often it is due to leakage, renal agenesis, or severe obstructive uropathy.

4. Overgrowth Syndromes

Overgrowth syndromes are becoming increasingly recognized as important childhood conditions. They may present at birth and are characterized by macrocephaly, motor delays (cerebral hypotonia), and occasional asymmetry of extremities. Bone age may be advanced. The most common overgrowth syndrome is **Sotos syndrome**. Patients with Sotos syndrome have a characteristic facies with a prominent forehead and down-slanting palpebral features. Mutations in NSD1 cause Sotos syndrome. Patients have a small but increased risk of cancer.

Other overgrowth syndromes include BWS, described earlier, and two single-gene disorders, Simpson-Golabi-Behmel syndrome and Bannayan-Riley-Ruvalcaba syndrome. Patients with **Simpson-Golabi-Behmel syndrome** exhibit a BWS-like phenotype, but with additional anomalies, including polydactyly and more severe facial dysmorphism. Unlike patients with BWS, who have normal intelligence, patients with Simpson-Golabi-Behmel syndrome often have developmental delay. It is inherited as an X-linked disorder. Patients with **Bannayan-Riley-Ruvalcaba syndrome** have macrosomia, macrocephaly, and unusual freckling of the penis. They may present with autism. They may develop hemangiomatous or lymphangiomatous growths and have a predisposition to certain malignancies (thyroid, breast, colon cancer). The cause of Bannayan-Riley-Ruvalcaba syndrome is a mutation of the *PTEN* gene implicated in Cowden syndrome, the association of intestinal polyposis with malignant potential. Proteus syndrome was recently found to caused by mosaic AKT-1 mutation.

Lindhurst MJ et al: A mosaic activating mutation in AKT1 associated with the Proteus syndrome. N Engl J Med 2011 Aug 18;365(7):611–619 [Epub 2011 Jul 27].

5. Syndromic Short Stature

Short stature is an important component of numerous syndromes, or it may be an isolated finding. In the absence of nutritional deficiencies, endocrine abnormalities, evidence of skeletal dysplasia (disproportionate growth with abnormal skeletal films), or a positive family history, intrinsic short stature can be due to UPD. The phenotype of Russell-Silver syndrome—short stature with normal head growth (pseudo-hydrocephalus), normal development, and minor dysmorphic features (especially fifth finger clinodactyly)—has been associated in some cases with maternal UPD7.

6. VACTERL Association

ESSENTIALS OF DIAGNOSIS & TYPICAL FEATURES

VACTERL association is described by an acronym denoting the association of the following:

- Vertebral defects (segmentation anomalies).
- Imperforate anus.
- Cardiac malformation (most often ventricular septal defect).
- Tracheoesophageal fistula.
- Renal anomalies.
- Limb (most often radial ray) anomalies.

The disorder is sporadic, and some of the defects may be life-threatening. The prognosis for normal development is good. The cause is unknown, but a high association with monozygotic twinning suggests a mechanism dating back to events perhaps as early as blastogenesis.

Careful examination and follow-up are important, because numerous other syndromes have overlapping features. Microarray studies and genetic consultation are warranted.

7. Kabuki syndrome

Kabuki syndrome (KS) is characterized by typical facial features (elongated palpebral fissures with eversion of the lateral third of the lower eyelid; arched and broad eyebrows; short columella with depressed nasal tip; large, prominent, or cupped ears), minor skeletal anomalies, persistence of fetal fingertip pads, mild to moderate intellectual disability, and postnatal growth deficiency. Other findings may include: congenital heart defects, genitourinary anomalies, cleft lip and/or palate, gastrointestinal anomalies including anal atresia, ptosis and strabismus, and widely spaced teeth and hypodontia. Functional differences can include: increased susceptibility to infections and autoimmune disorders, seizures, endocrinologic abnormalities including isolated premature thelarche in females, feeding problems, and hearing loss. Molecular genetic testing for *MLL2*, the only gene in which mutations are known to cause KS, is available on a clinical basis. The cause is heterogeneous, not all individuals with Kabuki syndrome was found to have a MLL2 mutation.

Adam MP et al: Kabuki syndrome. Gene review.

GENETIC EVALUATION OF THE CHILD WITH DEVELOPMENTAL DISABILITIES

Cognitive disabilities or developmental delays affect 8% of the population. Disorders associated with symptoms of delayed development are heterogeneous but frequently include heritable components. Evaluation should be multidisciplinary; Table 37–5 lists the main features of developmental delay, emphasizing the major clinical and genetic considerations. (See Chapter 3 for additional information about developmental delay and intellectual disability.)

Obtaining a detailed history, including pertinent prenatal and perinatal events, is critical. Feeding issues and slow growth velocity are seen in many genetic disorders causing developmental delay. Rate of developmental progress and particularly a history of loss of skills are important clues, as the latter might suggest a metabolic disorder with a neurodegenerative component. Family history can provide clues to suggest possible genetic etiologies, particularly if there is a history of consanguinity or a family pattern of other affected individuals.

Physical examination provides helpful clues. Referral to a clinical geneticist is indicated whenever unusual features are encountered. Neurologic, ophthalmologic, and audiologic consultation should be sought when indicated. Brain imaging should be requested in cases involving unexplained deviations from normal head growth. Neuroimaging and skeletal studies may also be indicated when dysmorphic features are present.

Metabolic and genetic testing procedures other than those listed in the Table 37–5 may also be indicated.

Table 37–5. Evaluation of the child with developmental delay.

History
Pregnancy history
Growth parameters at birth
Neonatal complications
Feeding history
History of somatic growth
Motor, language, and psychosocial milestones
Seizures
Loss of skills
Abnormal movements
Results of previous tests and examinations
Family history
Developmental and educational histories
Psychiatric disorders
Pregnancy outcomes
Medical history
Consanguinity
Physical examination
General pediatric examination, including growth parameters
Focused dysmorphologic evaluation including measurement of facial features and limbs
Complete neurologic examination
Parental growth parameters (especially head circumferences) and dysmorphic features should also be assessed
Imaging studies
See text
Laboratory assessment[a]
Microarray analysis (this has replaced chromosome analysis and FISH testing in most cases)
Fragile X testing (analysis of *FMR1* gene for triplet repeats)
Other blood analyses: comprehensive metabolic panel, acylcarnitine profile creatinine kinase (CK), lactate, pyruvate (this testing is helpful in the case of hypotonia)
Other metabolic tests may be helpful as second tier tests, including:
Serum amino acid analysis
Urine amino and organic acid analyses
Urine analysis for mucopolysaccharides (if coarse features and organomegaly)

Interpretation & Follow-Up

Clinical experience indicates that specific diagnoses can be made in approximately half of patients evaluated according to the protocol presented here. With specific diagnosis comes prognosis, ideas for management, and insight into recurrence risks. Prenatal diagnosis may also become possible.

Follow-up is important both for patients in whom diagnoses have been made and for those patients initially lacking a diagnosis. Genetic information is accumulating rapidly and can be translated into new diagnoses and better understanding with periodic review of clinical cases.

Autism

Autism is a developmental disorder comprising abnormal function in three domains: language development, social development, and behavior. The majority of patients with autism also have cognitive disabilities and might be appropriately evaluated according to the recommendations above. However, given the enormous increase in prevalence of autism in the past decade, it is worth discussing the genetic evaluation of autism separately.

There are multiple known genetic causes of autism. Advances in molecular diagnosis, understanding of metabolic derangements, and technologies such as microarray are allowing more patients with autism to be identified with specific genetic disorders. This allows more accurate genetic counseling for recurrence risk, as well as diagnosis-specific interventions which may improve prognosis.

With this in mind, recommendations for the genetic evaluation of a child with autism include the following:

1. Genetic referral if dysmorphic features or cutaneous abnormalities are present (ie, hypopigmented spots such as those seen in patients with **tuberous sclerosis**).
2. Laboratory testing to include the following:
   a. Microarray.
   b. Molecular testing for **fragile X syndrome**.
   c. Methylation testing for UPD15 if phenotype is suggestive of **Angelman syndrome**.
   d. Measurement of cholesterol and 7-DHC if syndactyly is present between the second and third toes, to rule out mild form of **Smith-Lemli-Opitz syndrome**.
   e. MECP2 testing if clinical course is suggestive of **Rett syndrome** (ie, neurodegenerative course, progressive microcephaly, and seizures in a female patient).
   f. PTEN molecular testing if the head circumference is greater than 2 standard deviations above the mean, plus evidence of penile freckling, lipomatous lesions, or a strong family history of certain malignancies.

Autism spectrum disorders are discussed in more detail in Chapter 3.

PERINATAL GENETICS

TERATOGENS

1. Drug Abuse & Fetal Alcohol Syndrome

Fetal alcohol syndrome results from excessive exposure to alcohol during gestation and affects 30%–40% of offspring of mothers whose daily intake of alcohol exceeds 3 ounces. Features of the syndrome include short stature, poor head growth (may be postnatal in onset), developmental delay, and midface hypoplasia characterized by a poorly developed long philtrum, narrow palpebral fissures, and short nose with anteverted nares. Facial findings may be subtle, but careful measurements and comparisons with standards (see Figure 37–8) are helpful. Structural abnormalities occur in half of affected children. Cardiac anomalies and neural tube defects are commonly seen. Genitourinary tract anomalies are frequent. Neurobehavioral effects also occur and may be stereotypic with poor judgment and inappropriate social interactions such as lack of stranger anxiety in toddlers commonly found. Cognitive deficiencies and behavioral problems may occur without other classic features of fetal alcohol syndrome and constitute an alcohol related neurological disorder (ARND).

Maternal abuse of drugs and other psychoactive substances is also associated with increased risks for adverse perinatal outcomes including miscarriage, preterm delivery, growth retardation, and increased risk for injury to the developing CNS. Methamphetamine and crack cocaine appear to be particularly dangerous. Maternal abuse of inhalants such as glue appears to be associated with findings similar to those of fetal alcohol syndrome. For most abused substances, the link between exposures and specific adverse outcomes is less well demonstrated than with alcohol. Multiple factors are probably involved, and it should be recognized that substance abuse often involves more than one drug.

Careful evaluation for other syndromes and chromosomal disorders should be included in the workup of exposed infants. Behavioral abnormalities in older children may be the result of maternally abused substances but they may also reflect evolving psychiatric disorders. Psychiatric disorders, many recognized as heritable, affect large numbers of men and women with substance abuse problems. Fetal alcohol spectrum disorders are discussed in more detail in Chapter 3.

2. Maternal Anticonvulsant Effects

Anticonvulsant exposure during pregnancy is associated with adverse outcomes in approximately 10% of children born to women treated with these agents. A syndrome characterized by small head circumference, anteverted nares, cleft lip and palate (occasionally), and distal digital hypoplasia was first described in association with maternal use of phenytoin but also occurs with other anticonvulsants. Risks for spina bifida are increased, especially in pregnancies exposed to valproic acid.

3. Retinoic Acid Embryopathy

Vitamin A and its analogs are potent morphogens that have considerable teratogenic potential. Developmental toxicity occurs in approximately one-third of pregnancies exposed in the first trimester to the synthetic retinoid isotretinoin, commonly prescribed to treat acne. Exposure disrupts migration of rostral neural crest cells and produces CNS maldevelopment, especially of the posterior fossa; ear anomalies (often absence of pinnae); congenital heart disease (great vessel anomalies); and tracheoesophageal fistula. These findings constitute a partial phenocopy of DiGeorge syndrome and demonstrate the continuum of contributing genetic and environmental factors in morphogenesis. It is now recognized that vitamin A itself, when taken as active retinoic acid in doses exceeding 25,000 IU/d during pregnancy, can produce similar fetal anomalies. For safety, vitamin A intake is therefore limited to 10,000 IU/d of retinoic acid. Maternal ingestion of large amounts of vitamin A taken as retinol during pregnancy, however, does not increase risks, because conversion of this precursor to active retinoic acid is internally regulated.

ASSISTED REPRODUCTION

Assisted reproductive technologies including in vitro fertilization are now utilized in a significant number of pregnancies. Although healthy live births are accepted as the usual outcomes resulting from successful application of these procedures, the actual number of viable embryos is limited and questions about the risks of adverse effects continue to be raised. Increased rates of twinning, both monozygotic and dizygotic, are well recognized while the possibility of increased rates of birth defects remains controversial. Abnormal genetic imprinting appears to be associated with in vitro fertilization. Evidence supports increased prevalence of Beckwith-Wiedemann and Angelman syndromes among offspring of in vitro pregnancies.

PRENATAL DIAGNOSIS

Prenatal screening for birth defects is now routinely offered to pregnant women of all ages. Prenatal diagnosis for specific genetic disorders is indicated in 7%–8% of pregnancies. Prenatal diagnosis introduces options for management including termination of abnormal pregnancies, preparation for specialized perinatal care, and, in some cases, fetal therapies.

Prenatal assessment of the fetus includes techniques that screen maternal blood, image the conceptus, and sample fetal and placental tissues.

Maternal Blood Analysis

Elevated levels of maternal serum α-fetoprotein correlate with open neural tube defects but low levels are associated with Down syndrome and other chromosomal abnormalities. First trimester measurements of PAPA (pregnancy-associated plasma protein A) and the free β-subunit of human chorionic gonadotropin screen for trisomies 21 and 18. In the second trimester maternal α-fetoprotein, human chorionic gonadotropin, unconjugated estradiol, and inhibin ("quad screen") combine to estimate risks for trisomies 21 and 18. Low estradiol levels can also predict cases of Smith-Lemli-Opitz syndrome, a devastating autosomal recessive disorder discussed earlier.

Fetal cells, including lymphocytes, trophoblasts, and nucleated red blood cells, circulate at low frequency in maternal blood and may eventually provide access to direct information about the conceptus.

Analysis of Fetal Samples

A. Amniocentesis

Whereas maternal blood levels are screened for fetal abnormalities, genetic amniocentesis is applied to make specific diagnoses. This procedure samples fluid surrounding the fetus; the cells obtained are cultured for cytogenetic, molecular, or metabolic analyses. α-Fetoprotein and other chemical markers can also be measured. This is a safe procedure with a complication rate (primarily for miscarriage) of less than 0.01% in experienced hands.

B. Chorionic Villus Sampling (Placental)

Chorionic villus sampling is generally performed at 11–12 weeks' gestation. Tissue obtained by chorionic villus sampling provides DNA for molecular analysis and contains dividing cells (cytotrophoblasts) that can be rapidly evaluated by FISH. However, direct cytogenetic preparations may be of poor quality and placental fibroblasts must be routinely grown and analyzed. In addition, chromosomal abnormalities detected by this technique may be confined to the placenta (**confined placental mosaicism**) and be less informative than amniocentesis.

C. Fetal Blood and Tissue

Fetal blood can be sampled directly in late gestation through ultrasound-guided percutaneous umbilical blood sampling (PUBS). A wide range of diagnostic tests ranging from biochemical to comparative genomic hybridization can be applied. Fetal urine sampled from the bladder or dilated proximal structures can provide important information about fetal renal function.

It is occasionally necessary to obtain biopsy specimens of fetal tissues such as liver or muscle for accurate prenatal diagnosis. These procedures are available in only a few perinatal centers.

D. Preimplantation Genetic Diagnosis (PGD)

With the advent of single-cell PCR techniques as well as interphase FISH it is now possible to make genetic diagnoses in preimplantation human embryos by removing and analyzing blastocyst cells. Using this procedure parents can now consider selecting pregnancies for positive attributes such as becoming donors for transplantation of tissues to siblings affected by genetic disorders.

Fetal Imaging

Fetal ultrasonography has become routine and MRI imaging is becoming increasingly common during pregnancy while fetal x-rays are seldom employed. Ultrasonography has joined maternal blood sampling as a screening technique for common chromosomal aneuploidies, neural tube defects, and other structural anomalies. Pregnancies at increased risk for CNS anomalies, skeletal dysplasias, and structural defects of the heart and kidneys should be monitored by careful ultrasound examinations. Fetal MRI has become routine in the workup of suspected fetal CNS abnormalities as well as in an increasing number of other fetal anomalies.

Allergic Disorders

38

Ronina A. Covar, MD
David M. Fleischer, MD
Mark Boguniewicz, MD

Allergic disorders are among the most common problems seen by pediatricians and primary care physicians, affecting over 25% of the population in developed countries. In the most recent National Health and Nutrition Examination Survey, 46% of the population had positive test responses to one or more allergens. In children, the increased prevalence of asthma, allergic rhinitis, and atopic dermatitis has been accompanied by significant morbidity and school absenteeism, with adverse consequences for school performance and quality of life, as well as economic burden measured in billions of dollars. In this chapter, atopy refers to a genetically determined predisposition to develop IgE antibodies found in patients with asthma, allergic rhinitis, and atopic dermatitis.

ASTHMA

ESSENTIALS OF DIAGNOSIS & TYPICAL FEATURES

- Episodic symptoms of airflow obstruction including wheezing, cough, and chest tightness.
- Airflow obstruction at least partially reversible.
- Exclusion of alternative diagnoses.

General Considerations

Asthma is the most common chronic disease of childhood, affecting over 7.1 million children in the United States. While current prevalence rates for asthma have increased in the past decade, the rate of asthma attack in the past year has been stable. One of 10 children has current asthma, and nearly two out of every three children affected have had at least one attack due to asthma in the past year. There is still a disproportionately higher health care utilization for asthma among children compared to adults affected by this disease. The burden of hospitalizations and emergency department or ambulatory and office visits, all indicators of severe asthma and risk factors for fatal asthma, impose significant costs to the health care system and to families, caretakers, schools, and parents' employers. Indirect costs primarily from loss of productivity due to school/work absences are harder to measure, yet considerable. Asthma remains a potentially life-threatening disease for children; the rate of asthma deaths was 0.3 per 10,000 children with current asthma. The prevalence and morbidity and mortality rates for asthma are higher among minority and inner city populations. The reasons for this are unclear but may be related to a combination of more severe disease, poor access to health care, lack of asthma education, delay in use of appropriate controller therapy, and environmental factors (eg, irritants including smoke and air pollutants, and perennial allergen exposure).

Up to 80% of children with asthma develop symptoms before their fifth birthday. Atopy (personal or familial) is the strongest identifiable predisposing factor. Sensitization to inhalant allergens increases over time and is found in the majority of children with asthma. The principal allergens associated with asthma are perennial aeroallergens such as dust mite, animal dander, cockroach, and *Alternaria* (a soil mold). Rarely, foods may provoke isolated asthma symptoms.

About 40% of infants and young children who have wheezing with viral infections in the first few years of life will have continuing asthma through childhood. Viral infections (eg, respiratory syncytial virus [RSV], rhinovirus, parainfluenza and influenza viruses, metapneumovirus) are associated with wheezing episodes in young children. RSV may be the predominant pathogen of wheezing infants in the emergency room setting, but rhinovirus can be detected in the majority of older wheezing children. Furthermore, RSV and parainfluenza have been associated with more severe respiratory illnesses, but in general, rhinovirus is the most commonly identified respiratory virus with wheezing episodes. It is uncertain if these viruses contribute to the development of chronic asthma, independent of atopy. Severe RSV bronchiolitis in infancy has been linked to asthma and allergy in later in childhood. Although speculative, individuals with lower airways vulnerability to common respiratory viral pathogens may be at risk for persistent asthma.

Exposure to tobacco smoke, especially from the mother, is also a risk factor for asthma. Other triggers include exercise, cold air, cigarette smoke, pollutants, strong chemical odors, and rapid changes in barometric pressure. Aspirin sensitivity is uncommon in children. Recent evidence suggests that acetaminophen exposure increases the risk of wheezing and asthma. Psychological factors may precipitate asthma exacerbations and place the patient at high risk from the disease.

Pathologic features of asthma include shedding of airway epithelium, edema, mucus plug formation, mast cell activation, and collagen deposition beneath the basement membrane. The inflammatory cell infiltrate includes eosinophils, lymphocytes, and neutrophils, especially in fatal asthma exacerbations. Airway inflammation contributes to airway hyperresponsiveness, airflow limitation, and disease chronicity. Persistent airway inflammation can lead to airway wall remodeling and irreversible changes.

Clinical Findings

A. Symptoms and Signs

The diagnosis of asthma in children is based largely on clinical judgment and an assessment of symptoms, activity limitation, and quality of life. For example, if a child with asthma refrains from participating in physical activities so as not to trigger asthma symptoms, their asthma would be inadequately controlled but not detected by the standard questions. In the National Asthma Education and Prevention Program (NAEPP) clinical guidelines, asthma control is introduced as an approach to assess the adequacy of current treatment, and to improve care and outcomes for children with asthma. For children with asthma, numerous validated instruments and questionnaires for assessing health-related quality of life and asthma control have been developed. The Asthma Control Test (ACT, www.asthmacontrol.com), the Asthma Control Questionnaire (ACQ, www.qoltech.co.uk/Asthma1.htm), and the Asthma Therapy Assessment Questionnaire (ATAQ, www.ataqinstrument.com) for children 12 years of age and older, and the Childhood ACT for children 4–11 years of age are examples of self-administered questionnaires that have been developed with the objective of addressing multiple domains of asthma control such as frequency of daytime and nocturnal symptoms, use of reliever medications, functional status, missed school or work, and so on. A five-item caregiver-administered instrument, the Test for Respiratory and Asthma Control in Kids (TRACK), has been validated as a tool to assess both impairment and risk presented in the NAEPP EPR3 guidelines in young children with recurrent wheezing or respiratory symptoms consistent with asthma.

Wheezing is the most characteristic sign of asthma, although some children may have recurrent cough and shortness of breath. Complaints may include "chest congestion," prolonged cough, exercise intolerance, dyspnea, and recurrent bronchitis or pneumonia. If symptoms are absent or mild, chest auscultation during forced expiration may reveal prolongation of the expiratory phase and wheezing. As the obstruction becomes more severe, wheezes become more high-pitched and breath sounds diminished. With severe obstruction, wheezes may not be heard because of poor air movement. Flaring of nostrils, intercostal and suprasternal retractions, and use of accessory muscles of respiration are signs of severe obstruction. Cyanosis of the lips and nail beds may be seen with underlying hypoxia. Tachycardia and pulsus paradoxus also occur. Agitation and lethargy may be signs of impending respiratory failure.

B. Laboratory Findings

Bronchial hyperresponsiveness, reversible airflow limitation, and airway inflammation are key features of asthma. Documentation of all these components is not always necessary, unless the presentation is rather atypical.

Bronchial hyperresponsiveness to nonspecific stimuli is a hallmark of asthma. These include inhaled pharmacologic agents such as histamine and methacholine as well as physical stimuli such as exercise and cold air. Airways may exhibit hyperresponsiveness or twitchiness even when baseline pulmonary function tests are normal. Giving increasing amounts of a bronchoconstrictive agent to induce a decrease in lung function (usually a 20% drop in forced expiratory volume in 1 second [FEV_1]) is the most common method of testing airway responsiveness. Hyperresponsiveness in normal children younger than age 5 years is greater than in older children. The level of airway hyperresponsiveness usually correlates with the severity of asthma. Bronchoprovocation challenges may help to establish a diagnosis of asthma when the history, examination, and pulmonary function tests are not definitive.

Recent asthma clinical guidelines reinforce the use of spirometry over peak expiratory flow rate (PEFR) measurements, in the evaluation of airflow limitation in asthma. This can be measured by reduction in FEV_1 and FEV_1/FVC values compared to reference or predicted values. By itself, it is not adequate in establishing a diagnosis, but it can be an important parameter to monitor asthma activity and treatment response. In children, FEV_1 may be normal, despite frequent symptoms. Spirometric measures of airflow limitation can be associated with symptom severity, likelihood of exacerbation, hospitalization, or respiratory compromise. Regular monitoring of pre- and/or postbronchodilator FEV_1 can be used to track lung growth patterns over time. During acute asthma exacerbations, FEV_1 is diminished and the flow-volume curve shows a "scooping out" of the distal portion of the expiratory portion of the loop (Figure 38–1).

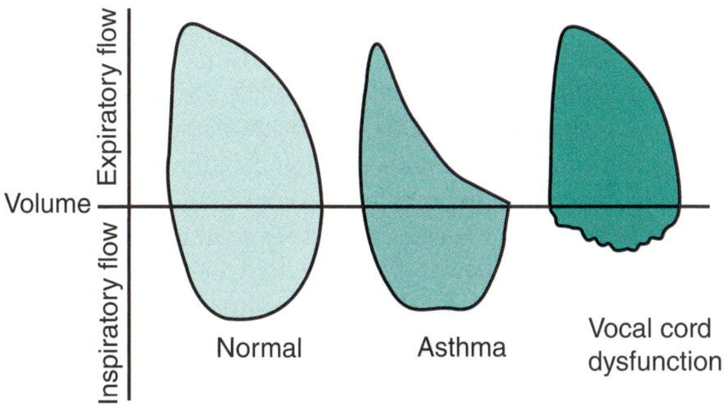

▲ **Figure 38–1.** Representative flow-volume loops in persons with normal lung function, asthma, and vocal cord dysfunction.

Lung function assessment using body box plethysmography to determine lung volume measurements can also be informative. The residual volume, functional residual capacity, and total lung capacity are usually increased, while the vital capacity is decreased. Reversal or significant improvement of these abnormalities in response to inhaled bronchodilator therapy or with anti-inflammatory therapy can be observed.

PEFR monitoring can be a simple and reproducible tool to assess asthma activity in children with moderate or severe asthma, a history of severe exacerbations, or poor perception of airflow limitation or worsening condition. Significant changes in PEFR may occur before symptoms become evident. In more severe cases, PEFR monitoring enables earlier recognition of suboptimal asthma control. Infant pulmonary function can be measured in sedated children with compression techniques. The forced oscillation technique can be used to measure airway resistance even in younger children.

Hypoxemia is present early with a normal or low Pco_2 level and respiratory alkalosis. Hypoxemia may be aggravated during treatment with a β_2-agonist due to ventilation-perfusion mismatch. Oxygen saturation less than 91% is indicative of significant obstruction. Respiratory acidosis and increasing CO_2 tension may ensue with further airflow obstruction and signal impending respiratory failure. Hypercapnia is usually not seen until the FEV_1 falls below 20% of predicted value. Metabolic acidosis has also been noted in combination with respiratory acidosis in children with severe asthma and indicates imminent respiratory failure. Pao_2 less than 60 mm Hg despite oxygen therapy and $Paco_2$ over 60 mm Hg and rising more than 5 mm Hg/h are relative indications for mechanical ventilation in a child in status asthmaticus.

Pulsus paradoxus may be present with moderate or severe asthma exacerbation. In moderate asthma exacerbation in a child, this may be between 10 and 25 mm Hg, and in severe asthma exacerbation between 20 and 40 mm Hg. Absence of pulsus paradoxus in a child with severe asthma exacerbation may signal respiratory muscle fatigue.

Clumps of eosinophils on sputum smear and blood eosinophilia are frequent findings. Their presence tends to reflect disease activity and does not necessarily mean that allergic factors are involved. Leukocytosis is common in acute severe asthma without evidence of bacterial infection and may be more pronounced after epinephrine administration. Hematocrit can be elevated with dehydration during prolonged exacerbations or in severe chronic disease. Noninvasive measures of airway inflammation include exhaled nitric oxide concentrations, serum eosinophil cationic protein levels, and induced sputum. Each test has its strengths and weaknesses.

C. Imaging

Evaluation of asthma usually does not need chest radiographs (posteroanterior and lateral views) since they often appear normal, although subtle and nonspecific findings of hyperinflation (flattening of the diaphragms), peribronchial thickening, prominence of the pulmonary arteries, and areas of patchy atelectasis may be present. Atelectasis may be misinterpreted as the infiltrates of pneumonia. Some lung abnormalities, such as bronchiectasis, which may point to a different diagnosis implicating an asthma masquerader, such as cystic fibrosis, allergic bronchopulmonary mycoses (aspergillosis), ciliary dyskinesias, or immune deficiencies, can be better appreciated with high-resolution, thin-section chest computed tomography (HRCT) scans. HRCT has been used to quantify hyperinflation and bronchial wall thickening as a marker of airway remodeling in children with severe asthma and define peripheral airways disease. It is useful in ruling out certain diagnoses in patients with difficult to manage asthma but radiation exposure should be considered when ordering HRCT.

Allergy testing is discussed in the section on General Measures under Treatment, Chronic Asthma.

▶ Differential Diagnosis

Diseases that may be mistaken for asthma are often related to the patient's age (Table 38–1). Congenital abnormalities must be excluded in infants and young children. Asthma can be confused with croup, acute bronchiolitis, pneumonia, and pertussis. Immunodeficiency may be associated with cough and wheezing. Foreign bodies in the airway may cause dyspnea or wheezing of sudden onset, and on auscultation wheezing may be unilateral. Asymmetry of the lungs secondary to air trapping may be seen on a chest radiograph, especially with forced expiration. Cystic fibrosis can be associated with or mistaken for asthma.

Vocal cord dysfunction is an important masquerader of asthma, although the two can coexist. It is characterized by the paradoxic closure of the vocal cords that can result in dyspnea and wheezing. Diagnosis is made by direct visualization of the vocal cords. In normal individuals, the vocal cords abduct during inspiration and may adduct slightly during expiration. Asthmatic patients may have narrowing of the glottis during expiration as a physiologic adaptation to

Table 38–1. Differential diagnosis of asthma in infants and children.

Viral bronchiolitis
Aspiration
Laryngotracheomalacia
Vascular rings
Airway stenosis or web
Enlarged lymph nodes
Mediastinal mass
Foreign body
Bronchopulmonary dysplasia
Obliterative bronchiolitis
Cystic fibrosis
Vocal cord dysfunction
Cardiovascular disease

airway obstruction. In contrast, patients with isolated vocal cord dysfunction typically show adduction of the anterior two-thirds of their vocal cords during inspiration, with a small diamond-shaped aperture posteriorly. Because this abnormal vocal cord pattern may be intermittently present, a normal examination does not exclude the diagnosis. Exercise or methacholine challenges can precipitate symptoms of vocal cord dysfunction. The flow-volume loop may provide additional clues to the diagnosis of vocal cord dysfunction. Truncation of the inspiratory portion can be demonstrated in most patients during an acute episode, and some patients continue to show this pattern even when they are asymptomatic (see Figure 38–1). Children with vocal cord dysfunction, especially adolescents, tend to be overly competitive, primarily in athletics and scholastics. A psychiatric consultation may help define underlying psychological issues and provide appropriate therapy. Treatment of isolated vocal cord dysfunction includes education regarding the condition and appropriate breathing exercises. Hypnosis, biofeedback, and psychotherapy have been effective for some patients.

Conditions That May Increase Asthma Severity

Chronic hyperplastic sinusitis is frequently found in association with asthma. Upper airway inflammation has been shown to contribute to the pathogenesis of asthma, and asthma may improve after treatment of sinusitis. However, sinus surgery is usually not indicated for initial treatment of chronic mucosal disease associated with allergy.

A significant correlation has been observed between nocturnal asthma and gastroesophageal reflux. Patients may not complain of burning epigastric pain or have other reflux symptoms—cough may be the only sign. For patients with poorly controlled asthma, particularly with a nocturnal component, investigation for gastroesophageal reflux may be warranted even in the absence of suggestive symptoms.

Population studies have demonstrated associations between obesity and asthma. Obesity has been linked not only to the development of asthma but also with asthma control and severity. What contributes to these associations or to what extent inflammation or physiologic impairment relates to both obesity and asthma is less established. It becomes difficult to determine if a child's trouble breathing is a result of obesity itself, its comorbidities (eg, gastroesophageal reflux or obstructive sleep apnea), and/or asthma. A management approach targeting weight reduction in obese children is encouraged to improve asthma control or its assessment.

The risk factors for death from asthma include psychological and sociological factors. They are probably related to the consequences of illness denial as well as to nonadherence with prescribed therapy. Recent studies have shown that less than 50% of inhaled asthma medications are taken as prescribed and that compliance does not improve with increasing severity of illness. Moreover, children requiring hospitalization for asthma, or their caregivers, have often failed to institute appropriate home treatment.

Complications

With acute asthma, complications are primarily related to hypoxemia and acidosis and can include generalized seizures. Pneumomediastinum or pneumothorax can be a complication in status asthmaticus. With chronic asthma, recent studies point to airway wall remodeling and loss of pulmonary function with persistent airway inflammation. Childhood asthma independent of any corticosteroid therapy has been shown to be associated with delayed maturation and slowing of prepubertal growth velocity. However, attainment of final predicted adult height does not appear to be compromised.

Treatment

A. Chronic Asthma

1. General measures—Optimal asthma management includes an assessment and regular monitoring of disease activity, education and partnership to improve the child's and his/her family's knowledge and skills for self-management, identification and management of triggers and conditions that may worsen asthma, and appropriate medications selected to address the patient's needs. The objective of asthma management is the attainment of the best possible asthma control.

An assessment of asthma severity (ie, the intrinsic intensity of disease) is generally most accurate in patients not receiving controller therapy. Hence, assessing asthma severity directs the level of initial therapy. For those already on treatment, asthma severity can be classified according to the level or intensity of medication requirement to maintain adequate asthma control. The two general categories are intermittent and persistent asthma, the latter further subdivided into mild, moderate, and severe (Table 38–2). In contrast, asthma

Table 38–2. Assessing severity and initiating treatment for patients who are not currently taking long-term control medications.

Components of Severity		Classification of Asthma Severity			
			Persistent		
		Intermittent	Mild	Moderate	Severe
Impairment	Daytime symptoms	≤ 2 d/wk	> 2 d/wk but not daily	Daily	Throughout the day
	Nighttime awakenings				
	Age 0–4 y	0	1–2 ×/mo	3–4 ×/mo	> 1 ×/wk
	Age ≥ 5 y	≤ 2 ×/mo	3–4 ×/mo	> 1 ×/wk but not nightly	Often 7 ×/wk
	SABA use for symptoms (not prevention of EIB)	≤ 2 d/wk	> 2 d/wk but not daily, and not more than 1 × on any day	Daily	Several times per d
	Interference with normal activity	None	Minor limitation	Some limitation	Extremely limited
	Lung function				
	FEV_1% predicted	Normal FEV_1 between exacerbations			
	Age ≥ 5 y	> 80% predicted	≥ 80% predicted	60%–80% predicted	< 60% predicted
	FEV_1/FVC ratio				
Normal FEV_1/FVC: 8–19 y, 85% 20–39 y, 80%	Age 5–11 y	> 85%	> 80%	75%–80%	< 75%
	Age ≥ 12 y	Normal	Normal	Reduced 5%	Reduced > 5%
Risk	Exacerbations requiring systemic corticosteroids				
	Age 0–4 y	0–1/y (see note)	≥ 2 exacerbations in 6 mo requiring systemic corticosteroids OR ≥ 4 wheezing episodes/year lasting > 1 d and risk factors for persistent asthma		
	Age ≥ 5 y	0–1/y (see note)	≥ 2/y (see note)		
		Consider severity and interval since last exacerbation. Frequency and severity may fluctuate over time for patients in any severity category. Relative annual risk of exacerbations may be related to FEV_1.			
Recommended step for initiating therapy		Step 1	Step 2	Age 0–4 y	
				Step 3	Step 3
				Age 5–11 y	
				Step 3, medium-dose ICS option	Step 3, medium-dose ICS option, OR step 4
				Age ≥12 y	
				Step 3	Step 4 or 5
				Consider a short course of systemic corticosteroids	
		In 2–6 wk, evaluate level of asthma control that is achieved and adjust therapy accordingly. If no clear benefit is observed within 4–6 wk, consider adjusting therapy or alternative diagnoses.			

Notes:

- The stepwise approach is meant to assist, not replace, the clinical decision making required to meet individual patient needs.
- Level of severity is determined by both impairment and risk. Assess impairment domain by patient's/caregiver's recall of previous 2–4 weeks. Symptom assessment for longer periods should reflect a global assessment such as inquiring whether a patient's asthma is better or worse since the last visit. Assign severity to the most severe category in which any feature occurs.

Table 38–2. Assessing severity and initiating treatment for patients who are not currently taking long-term control medications. (*Continued*)

- At present, there are inadequate data to correspond frequencies of exacerbations with different levels of asthma severity. For treatment purposes, patients who had ≥ 2 exacerbations requiring oral systemic corticosteroids in the past 6 months, or ≥ 4 wheezing episodes in the past year, and who have risk factors for persistent asthma may be considered the same as patients who have persistent asthma, even in the absence of impairment levels consistent with persistent asthma.
- EIB, exercise-induced bronchospasm; FEV_1, forced expiratory volume in 1 second; FVC, forced vital capacity; ICS, inhaled corticosteroids; SABA, short-acting β_2-agonist.

Adapted from the National Asthma Education and Prevention Program: Expert Panel Report 3 (EPR 3): Guidelines for the Diagnosis and Management of Asthma—Summary Report 2007. Available at: http://www.nhlbi.nih.gov/guidelines/asthma/asthgdln.htm

control refers to the degree to which symptoms, ongoing functional impairments, and risk of adverse events are minimized and goals of therapy are met. Assessment of asthma control should be done at every visit as this is important in adjusting therapy. It is categorized as "well controlled", "not well controlled", and "very poorly controlled" (Table 38–3). Responsiveness to therapy is the ease with which asthma control is attained by treatment. It can also encompass monitoring for adverse effects related to medication use.

Classification of either asthma severity or control is based on the domains of current impairment and risk, recognizing that these domains may respond differently to treatment. The level of asthma severity or control is established upon the most severe component of impairment or risk. Generally, the assessment is symptom based, except for the use of lung function for school-aged children and youths. Impairment includes an assessment of the patient's recent symptom frequency and intensity and functional limitations (ie, nighttime awakenings, need for short-acting β_2-agonists for quick relief, work or school days missed, ability to engage in normal or desired activities, and quality-of-life assessments) and airflow compromise using preferably spirometry. On the other hand, risk refers to an evaluation of the patient's likelihood of developing asthma exacerbations, reduced lung growth in children (or progressive decline in lung function in adults), or risk of untoward effects from medications.

Education is important and partnership with the child's family involving shared treatment decision making is a key component in the management to improve adherence and outcomes. The patient and family must understand the role of asthma triggers, the importance of disease activity even without obvious symptoms, how to use objective measures to gauge disease activity, and the importance of airway inflammation—and they must learn to recognize the warning signs of worsening asthma, allowing for early intervention. A stepwise care plan should be developed for all patients with asthma. Providing asthma action plans is currently a requirement that is tracked by many hospitals and others to document that educational instruction for chronic disease management has been given. Asthma action plans should be provided to school personnel and all those who care for children with asthma.

Because the degree of airflow limitation is poorly perceived by many patients, peak flow meters can aid in the assessment of airflow obstruction and day-to-day disease activity. Peak flow rates may provide early warning of worsening asthma. They are also helpful in monitoring the effects of medication changes. Spacer devices optimize delivery of medication from metered-dose inhalers (MDIs) to the lungs and, with inhaled steroids, minimize side effects. Large-volume spacers are preferred. Poor understanding by patients and families of proper device use can lead to inadequate delivery and treatment with inhaled medications, especially inhaled controllers. Short instructive videos for device use can be provided to educate families and other caregivers (URL: http://www.thechildrenshospital.org/conditions/lung/asthmavideos.aspx).

Patients should avoid exposure to tobacco smoke and allergens to which they are sensitized, exertion outdoors when levels of air pollution are high, β-blockers, and sulfite-containing foods. Patients with persistent asthma should be given the inactivated influenza vaccine yearly unless they have a contraindication.

For patients with persistent asthma, the clinician should use the patient's history to assess sensitivity to seasonal allergens and *Alternaria* mold; use skin testing or in vitro testing to assess sensitivity to perennial indoor allergens; assess the significance of positive tests in the context of the patient's history; and identify relevant allergen exposures. For dust mite–allergic children, important environmental control measures include encasing the pillow and mattress in an allergen-impermeable cover and washing the sheets and blankets on the patient's bed weekly in hot water. Other measures include keeping indoor humidity below 50%, minimizing the number of stuffed toys, and washing such toys weekly in hot water. Children allergic to furred animals or feathers should avoid indoor exposure to pets, especially for prolonged periods of time. If removal of the pet is not possible, the animal should be kept out of the bedroom with the door closed. Carpeting and upholstered furniture should be removed. While a high-efficiency particle-arresting filter unit in the bedroom may reduce allergen levels, symptoms may persist if the pet remains indoors. For cockroach-allergic children, control measures need to be instituted

Table 38–3. Assessing asthma control and adjusting therapy in children.

Components of Control		Classification of Asthma Control		
		Well Controlled	**Not Well Controlled**	**Very Poorly Controlled**
Impairment	Symptoms	≤ 2 d/wk but not more than once on each day	> 2 d/wk or multiple times on ≤ 2 d/wk	Throughout the day
	Nighttime awakenings			
	Age 0–4 y	≤ 1 × /mo	> 1 × /mo	> 1 × /wk
	Age 5–11 y	≤ 1 × /mo	≥ 2 × /mo	≥ 2 × /wk
	Age ≥ 12 y	≤ 2 × /mo	1–3 × /wk	≥ 4 × /wk
	SABA use for symptoms (not EIB pretreatment)	≤ 2 d/wk	> 2 d/wk	Several times per d
	Interference with normal activity	None	Some limitation	Extremely limited
	Lung function			
	Age 5–11 y			
	FEV_1% predicted or peak flow	> 80% predicted or personal best	60%–80% predicted or personal best	< 60% predicted or personal best
	FEV_1/FVC	> 80%	75–80%	< 75%
	Age ≥ 12 y			
	FEV_1% predicted or peak flow	> 80% predicted or personal best	60%–80% predicted or personal best	< 60% predicted or personal best
	Validated questionnaires			
	Age ≥ 12 y			
	ATAQ	0	1–2	3–4
	ACQ	≤ 0.75[a]	≤ 1.5	N/A
	ACT	≥ 20	16–19	≤ 15
Risk	Exacerbations requiring systemic corticosteroids			
	Age 0–4 y	0–1 y	2–3/y	> 3/y
	Age ≥ 5 y	0–1 y	≥ 2/y (see note)	
	Consider severity and interval since last exacerbation.			
	Treatment-related adverse effects	Medication side effects can vary in intensity from none to very troublesome and worrisome. The level of intensity does not correlate to specific levels of control but should be considered in the overall assessment of risk.		
	Reduction in lung growth or progressive loss of lung function	Evaluation requires long-term follow-up care.		
Recommended action for treatment		• Maintain current step. • Regular follow-up every 1–6 mo to maintain control. • Consider step-down if well controlled for at least 3 mo.	• Step up (1 step) and • Reevaluate in 2–6 wk. • If no clear benefit in 4–6 wk consider alternative diagnoses or adjusting therapy. • For side effects, consider alternative options.	• Consider short course of oral corticosteroids. • Step up (1–2 steps), and • Reevaluate in 2 wk. • If no clear benefit in 4–6 wk, consider alternative diagnoses or adjusting therapy. • For side effects, consider alternative options.

Notes:

- The stepwise approach is meant to assist, not replace, the clinical decision making required to meet individual patient needs.
- The level of control is based on the most severe impairment or risk category. Assess impairment domain by caregiver's recall of previous 2–4 weeks. Symptom assessment for longer periods should reflect a global assessment such as inquiring whether the patient's asthma is better or worse since the last visit.
- At present, there are inadequate data to correspond frequencies of exacerbations with different levels of asthma control. In general, more frequent and intense exacerbations (eg, requiring urgent, unscheduled care, hospitalization, or ICU admission) indicate poorer disease control. For treatment purposes, patients who had ≥ 2 exacerbations requiring oral systemic corticosteroids in the past year may be considered the same as patients who have not-well-controlled asthma, even in the absence of impairment levels consistent with not-well-controlled asthma.

Table 38–3. Assessing asthma control and adjusting therapy in children. (*Continued*)

- Validated questionnaires for the impairment domain (the questionnaires do not assess lung function or the risk domain):
  a. ATAQ = Asthma Therapy Assessment Questionnaire
  b. ACQ = Asthma Control Questionnaire
  c. ACT = Asthma Control Test
  d. Minimal Important Difference: 1.0 for ATAQ; 0.5 for the ACQ; not determined for ACT; [a]ACQ values of 0.76–1.40 are indeterminate regarding well-controlled asthma.
- Before step-up therapy:
  a. Review adherence to medications, inhaler technique, and environmental control.
  b. If alternative treatment option was used in a step, discontinue it and use preferred treatment for that step. EIB, exercise-induced bronchospasm; FEV_1, forced expiratory volume in 1 second; FVC, forced vital capacity.

Adapted from the National Asthma Education and Prevention Program: Expert Panel Report 3 (EPR 3): Guidelines for the Diagnosis and Management of Asthma—Summary Report 2007. Available at: http://www.nhlbi.nih.gov/guidelines/asthma/asthgdln.htm

when infestation is present in the home. Poison baits, boric acid, and traps are preferred to chemical agents, which can be irritating if inhaled by asthmatic individuals. Indoor molds are especially prominent in humid or damp environments. Measures to control dampness or fungal growth in the home may be of benefit. Patients can reduce exposure to outdoor allergens by staying in an air-conditioned environment. Allergen immunotherapy may be useful for implicated aeroallergens that cannot be avoided. However, it should be administered only in facilities staffed and equipped to treat life-threatening reactions.

Patients should be treated for rhinitis, sinusitis, or gastroesophageal reflux, if present. Treatment of upper respiratory tract symptoms is an integral part of asthma management. Intranasal corticosteroids are recommended to treat chronic rhinosinusitis in patients with persistent asthma because they reduce lower airway hyperresponsiveness and asthma symptoms. Intranasal cromolyn reduces asthma symptoms during the ragweed season but less so than intranasal corticosteroids. Treatment of rhinosinusitis includes medical measures to promote drainage and the use of antibiotics for acute bacterial infections (see Chapter 18). Medical management of gastroesophageal reflux includes avoiding eating or drinking 2 hours before bedtime, elevating the head of the bed with 6- to 8-in blocks, and using appropriate pharmacologic therapy.

2. Pharmacologic therapy—A revised stepwise approach to pharmacologic therapy, broken down by age categories, is recommended in the NAEPP *Expert Panel Report 3* (http://www.nhlbi.nih.gov) (Table 38–4). This approach is based on the concepts of asthma severity and asthma control. A separate set of recommendations for younger children is provided given the lack of tools which can be used to assess lung function and quality of life otherwise available for older children. Treatment recommendations for older children and adults are better supported by stronger evidence from available clinical trials, whereas those for younger children have been extrapolated from studies in older children and adults.

The choice of initial therapy is based on assessment of asthma severity, and for patients who are already on controller therapy, treatment can be adjusted based on assessment of asthma control and responsiveness to therapy. The goals of therapy are to reduce the components of both impairment (eg, preventing chronic and troublesome symptoms, allowing infrequent need of quick-relief medications, maintaining "normal" lung function, maintaining normal activity levels including physical activity and school attendance, meeting families' expectations and satisfaction with asthma care) and risk (eg, preventing recurrent exacerbations, reduced lung growth, and medication adverse effects).

1. The stepwise approach is meant to assist, not replace, the clinical decision making required to meet individual patient needs.
2. In the absence of persistent symptoms, the new clinical guidelines recommend considering initiation of long-term controller therapy for infants and younger children who have risk factors for asthma (ie, modified asthma predictive index: parental history of asthma, physician-diagnosed atopic dermatitis, or sensitization to aeroallergens or two of the following: wheezing apart from colds, sensitization to foods, or peripheral eosinophilia) *and* four or more episodes of wheezing over the past year that lasted longer than 1 day and affected sleep or two or more exacerbations in 6 months requiring systemic corticosteroids.
3. Inhaled corticosteroids, either as monotherapy or in combination with adjunctive therapy, are preferred treatment for all levels of persistent asthma.
4. Along with medium-dose inhaled corticosteroids, combination therapy with inhaled corticosteroids plus any of the following adjunctive therapies—long-acting inhaled β_2-agonists (LABAs), leukotriene modifying agents, cromones, and theophylline—is recommended as step 3 treatment for moderate persistent asthma, or as step-up therapy for uncontrolled persistent asthma

Table 38–4. Stepwise approach for managing asthma in children.

	Intermittent	Persistent Asthma: Daily Medication					
	Step 1	Step 2	Step 3	Step 4	Step 5	Step 6	Step down if possible (and asthma is well controlled at least 3 mo) **Assess Control** Step up if needed (first check inhaler technique, adherence, environmental control, and comorbid condition)
Age 0–4 y	*Preferred* SABA PRN	*Preferred* Low-dose ICS *Alternative* Cromolyn or montelukast	*Preferred* Medium-dose ICS	*Preferred* Medium-dose ICS + either LABA or LTRA	*Preferred* High-dose ICS + either LABA or LTRA	*Preferred* High-dose ICS + either LABA or LTRA AND oral corticosteroid	
Age 5–11 y	*Preferred* SABA PRN	*Preferred* Low-dose ICS *Alternative* Cromolyn, LTRA, nedocromil, or theophylline	*Preferred* EITHER Low-dose ICS + either LABA, LTRA, or theophylline OR medium-dose ICS	*Preferred* Medium-dose ICS + LABA *Alternative* Medium-dose ICS + either LTRA or theophylline	*Preferred* High-dose ICS + LABA *Alternative* High-dose ICS + either LTRA or theophylline	*Preferred* High-dose ICS + LABA AND oral corticosteroid *Alternative* High-dose ICS + either LTRA or theophylline AND oral corticosteroid	
Age ≥ 12 y	*Preferred* SABA PRN	*Preferred* Low-dose ICS *Alternative* Cromolyn, LTRA, nedocromil, or theophylline	*Preferred* Low-dose ICS + LABA OR medium-dose ICS *Alternative* Low-dose ICS + either LTRA, theophylline, or zileuton	*Preferred* Medium-dose ICS + LABA *Alternative* Medium-dose ICS + either LTRA or theophylline or zileuton	*Preferred* High-dose ICS + LABA AND consider omalizumab for patients with allergies	*Preferred* High-dose ICS + LABA + oral corticosteroid AND consider omalizumab for patients with allergies	

Each step: Patient education, environmental control, and management of comorbidities.

Age ≥ 5 y: Steps 2–4: Consider subcutaneous allergen immunotherapy for patients who have allergic asthma.

Quick-Relief Medication for All Patients

- SABA as needed for symptoms. Intensity of treatment depends on severity of symptoms: up to three treatments at 20-minute intervals as needed. Short course of oral systemic corticosteroids may be needed.
- Caution: Use of SABA > 2 d/wk for symptom relief (not prevention of EIB) generally indicates inadequate control and the need to step up treatment.
- For ages 0–4 years: With viral respiratory infection: SABA q4-6h up to 24 hours (longer with physician consult). Consider short course of systemic corticosteroids if exacerbation is severe or patient has history of previous severe exacerbations.

Alphabetical order is used when more than one treatment option is listed within either preferred or alternative therapy.

Notes:

- The stepwise approach is meant to assist, not replace, the clinical decision making required to meet individual patient needs.
- If alternative treatment is used and response is inadequate, discontinue it and use the preferred treatment before stepping up.
- If clear benefit is not observed within 4–6 weeks and patient/family medication technique and adherence are satisfactory, consider adjusting therapy or alternative diagnosis.
- Studies on children aged 0–4 years are limited. Step 2 therapy is based on Evidence A. All other recommendations are based on expert opinion and extrapolation from studies in older children.
- For age 5–11 years, steps 1 and 2 medications are based on Evidence A. Step 3 ICS + adjunctive therapy and ICS are based on Evidence B for efficacy of each treatment and extrapolation from comparator trials in older children and adults—comparator trials are not available for this age group; steps 4–6 are based on expert opinion and extrapolation from studies in older children and adults.

Table 38–4. Stepwise approach for managing asthma in children. (*Continued*)

- For ages ≥ 12 years, steps 1, 2 and 3 preferred therapies are based on Evidence A; step 3 alternative therapy is based on Evidence A for LTRA, Evidence B for theophylline, and Evidence D for zileuton. Step 4 preferred therapy is based on Evidence B, and alternative therapy is based on Evidence B for LTRA and theophylline and Evidence D for zileuton. Step 5 preferred therapy is based on Evidence B. Step 6 preferred therapy is based on (EPR-1 1997) and Evidence B for omalizumab. In step 6, before oral systemic corticosteroids are introduced, a trial of high-dose ICS + LABA + either LTRA, theophylline, or zileuton may be considered, although this approach has not been studied in clinical trials.
- Clinicians who administer immunotherapy or omalizumab should be prepared and equipped to identify and treat anaphylaxis that may occur.
- Theophylline is a less desirable alternative due to the need to monitor serum concentration levels.
- Zileuton is less desirable alternative due to limited studies as adjunctive therapy and the need to monitor liver function.
- Immunotherapy for steps 2–4 is based on Evidence B for house dust mites, animal danders, and pollens; evidence is weak or lacking for molds and cockroaches. Evidence is strongest for immunotherapy with single allergens. The role of allergy in asthma is greater in children than in adults.
- ICS, inhaled corticosteroid; LABA, inhaled long-acting β_2-agonist; LTRA, leukotriene receptor antagonist; prn, as needed; SABA, inhaled short-acting β_2-agonist.

Adapted from the National Asthma Education and Prevention Program: Expert Panel Report 3 (EPR 3): Guidelines for the Diagnosis and Management of Asthma—Summary Report 2007. Available at: http://www.nhlbi.nih.gov/guidelines/asthma/asthgdln.htm.

for school-aged children and youths. In children aged 0–4 years, medium-dose inhaled corticosteroids as monotherapy remain the step 3 therapy, and combination therapy to be initiated only as a step 4 treatment. A rescue course of systemic corticosteroids may be necessary at any step.

Asthma medications are classified as long-term controller medications and quick-relief medications. The former includes anti-inflammatory agents, leukotriene modifiers, and long-acting bronchodilators. Although LABAs (salmeterol, formoterol) are β-agonists, they are considered to be daily controller medications, but unlike the other asthma controller medications with primarily anti-inflammatory properties, LABAs cannot be administered as monotherapy.

Inhaled corticosteroids are the most potent inhaled anti-inflammatory agents currently available. Different inhaled corticosteroids are not equivalent on a per puff or microgram basis (Table 38–5). Early intervention with inhaled corticosteroids can improve asthma control and prevent exacerbations during treatment, but they do not prevent the development of persistent asthma nor do they alter its natural history. Long-term inhaled corticosteroids may be associated with early slowing of growth velocity in children. Possible risks from inhaled corticosteroids need to be weighed against the risks from undertreated asthma. The adverse effects from inhaled corticosteroids are generally dose and duration dependent, so that greater risks for systemic adverse effects are expected with high doses. The various inhaled corticosteroids are delivered in different devices such as MDI (beclomethasone, ciclesonide, fluticasone, flunisolide, and triamcinolone), dry powder inhaler (DPI) (fluticasone Diskus™, budesonide Flexhaler™, and mometasone Twisthaler™), and nebulized aerosol suspensions (budesonide respules). Inhaled medications delivered in MDI now use the more ozone-friendly hydrofluoroalkane (HFA) propellant, which has replaced chlorofluorocarbons (CFC). See instructions for different device use at the following URL: http://www.thechildrenshospital.org/conditions/lung/asthmavideos.aspx.

Only inhaled corticosteroids have been shown to be effective in long-term clinical studies with infants. Nebulized budesonide is approved for children as young as 12 months. The suspension (available in quantities of 0.25 mg/2 mL, 0.5 mg/2 mL, and 1.0 mg/2 mL) is usually administered either once or twice daily in divided doses. For effective drug delivery, it is critical that the child have a mask secured on the face for the entire treatment, as blowing it in the face is not effective and yet a common practice by parents. Notably, this drug should not be given by ultrasonic nebulizer. Limited data suggest that inhaled corticosteroids may be effective even in very young children when delivered by MDI with a spacer and mask.

Fewer data are available with nedocromil, although data from the Childhood Asthma Management Program study showed that an inhaled corticosteroid was superior to nedocromil with respect to several efficacy parameters, including rate of hospitalization, symptom-free days, need for albuterol rescue, and longer time to treatment with prednisone, when each was compared to a placebo.

Theophylline is rarely used. Sustained-release theophylline, an alternative long-term control medication for older children, may have particular risks of adverse effects in infants, who frequently have febrile illnesses that increase theophylline concentrations. Hence, if theophylline is used, it requires monitoring of serum concentration to prevent numerous dose-related acute toxicities.

Table 38–5. Estimated comparative inhaled corticosteroid doses.

Drug	Low Daily Dose			Medium Daily Dose			High Daily Dose		
	0–4 y	5–11 y	≥ 12 y	0–4 y	5–11 y	≥ 12 y	0–4 y	5–11 y	≥ 12 y
Beclomethasone HFA, 40 or 80 mcg/puff	NA	80–160 mcg	80–240 mcg	NA	> 160–320 mcg	> 240–480 mcg	NA	> 320 mcg	> 480 mcg
Budesonide DPI 90, 80, or 200 mcg/inhalation	NA	180–400 mcg	180–600 mcg	NA	> 400–800 mcg	> 600–1200 mcg	NA	> 800 mcg	> 1200 mcg
Budesonide inhaled suspension for nebulization, 0.25-, 0.5-, and 1.0-mg dose	0.25–0.5 mg	0.5 mg	NA	> 0.5–1.0 mg	1.0 mg	NA	> 1.0 mg	2.0 mg	NA
Flunisolide, 250 mcg/puff	NA	500–750 mcg	500–1000 mcg	NA	1000–1250 mcg	> 1000–2000 mcg	NA	> 1250 mcg	> 2000 mcg
Flunisolide HFA, 80 mcg/puff	NA	160 mcg	320 mcg	NA	320 mcg	> 320–640 mcg	NA	≥ 640 mcg	> 640 mcg
Fluticasone HFA/MDI, 44, 110, or 220 mcg/puff	176 mcg	88–176 mcg	88–264 mcg	> 176–352 mcg	> 176–352 mcg	> 264–440 mcg	> 352 mcg	> 352 mcg	> 440 mcg
Fluticasone DPI, 50, 100, or 250 mcg/inhalation	NA	100–200 mcg	100–300 mcg	NA	> 200–400 mcg	> 300–500 mcg	NA	> 400 mcg	> 500 mcg
Mometasone DPI, 220 mcg/inhalation	NA	NA	220 mcg	NA	NA	440 mcg	NA	NA	> 440 mcg
Triamcinolone acetonide, 75 mcg/puff	NA	300–600 mcg	300–750 mcg	NA	> 600–900 mcg	> 750–1500 mcg	NA	> 900 mcg	> 1500 mcg

DPI, dry powder inhaler; HFA, hydrofluoroalkane; MDI, metered-dose inhaler; NA, not approved and no data available for this age group. Adapted from the National Asthma Education and Prevention Program: Expert Panel Report 3 (EPR 3): Guidelines for the Diagnosis and Management of Asthma—Summary Report 2007. Available at: http://www.nhlbi.nih.gov/guidelines/asthma/asthgdln.htm.

For school aged children whose asthma is uncontrolled on low dose inhaled corticosteroid (ie, requiring Step 3 guidelines therapy), majority are likely to respond to a step up combination therapy with a long-acting β2-agonist bronchodilator (eg, salmeterol and formoterol), although some respond best either to an increased dose of inhaled corticosteroid or to an addition of a leukotriene receptor antagonist. *LABAs should not be used for treatment of acute symptoms, nor should they be used without any inhaled corticosteroid therapy, even if the patient feels better.* Salmeterol is available as an inhalation powder (one inhalation twice daily for patients aged 4 years and older). It is also available combined with fluticasone (50 mcg salmeterol with 100, 250, or 500 mcg fluticasone in a DPI or 21 mcg salmeterol with 45, 115, or 230 mcg fluticasone in an MDI). For children 12 years and older, one inhalation DPI or two inhalations MDI can be taken twice daily. (***Note:*** The 100/50 fluticasone/salmeterol combination is approved in children aged 4 and older.) It can also be used 30 minutes before exercise (but not in addition to regularly used LABAs). Formoterol has a more rapid onset of action and is available singly as a DPI (Aerolizer, 12 mcg) or combined with an inhaled corticosteroid (formoterol fumarate, either 4.5 mcg with budesonide [80 or 160 mcg] or 5 mcg with mometasone [100 or 200 mcg], in an MDI). Formoterol DPI is approved for use in children 5 years and older, one inhalation (12 mcg) twice daily, while the combination product is approved for children 12 years and older, two inhalations twice daily. For long-term control, formoterol should be used in combination with an anti-inflammatory agent. It can be used for exercise-induced bronchospasm in patients 5 years and older, one inhalation at least 15 minutes before exercise (but not in addition to regularly used LABAs). Of note, the U.S. Food and Drug Administration (FDA) has requested the manufacturers of Advair Diskus and HFA (salmeterol and fluticasone), Serevent Diskus (salmeterol xinafoate), Foradil Aerolizer (formoterol fumarate), Symbicort HFA, and Brovana (arformoterol tartrate inhalation solution, a LABA approved for chronic obstructive pulmonary disease) to update their product information warning sections regarding an increase in severe asthma episodes associated with these agents. This action is in response to data showing an increased number of asthma-related deaths in patients receiving LABA therapy in addition to their usual asthma care as compared with patients not receiving LABAs. This notice is also intended to reinforce the appropriate use of LABAs in the management of asthma. Specifically, LABA products should not be initiated as first-line asthma therapy, used with worsening wheezing, or used for acute control of bronchospasm. No data are available regarding safety concerns in patients using these products for exercise-induced bronchoconstriction. Additional information, including copies of the Patient and Healthcare Professional information sheets, can be found at: http://www.fda.gov/cder/drug/infopage/LABA/default.htm.

Montelukast and zafirlukast are leukotriene-receptor antagonists available in oral formulations. Montelukast is given once daily and has been approved for treatment of chronic asthma in children aged 1 year and older, as an alternative step 2 monotherapy and add-on therapy for steps 3–6. It is also indicated for seasonal allergic rhinitis in patients 2 years and older, and for perennial allergic rhinitis in patients 6 months and older. To date, no drug interactions have been noted. The dosage is 4 mg for children 1–5 years (oral granules are available for children aged 12–23 months), 5 mg for children aged 6–14 years, and 10 mg for those aged 15 years and older. The drug is given without regard to mealtimes, preferably in the evening. Zafirlukast is approved for patients aged 5 years and older. The dose is 10 mg twice daily for those 5–11 years and 20 mg twice daily for those 12 years and older. It should be taken 1 hour before or 2 hours after meals. Zileuton is a 5-lipoxygenase inhibitor indicated for chronic treatment in children 12 years of age and older, available in regular 600 mg dose tablet four times a day or extended release 600 mg dose tablet, 2 tablets twice a day. Patients need to have hepatic transaminase levels evaluated at initiation of therapy, then once a month for the first 3 months, every 2–3 months for the remainder of the first year, and periodically thereafter if receiving long-term zileuton therapy. Rare cases of Churg-Strauss syndrome have been reported in adult patients with severe asthma whose steroid dosage was being tapered during concomitant treatment with leukotriene-receptor antagonists (as well as inhaled corticosteroids), but no causal link has been established. Both zafirlukast and zileuton are microsomal P-450 enzyme inhibitors that can inhibit the metabolism of drugs such as warfarin and theophylline. The FDA has requested that manufacturers include a precaution in the drug prescribing information (drug labeling) regarding neuropsychiatric events (agitation, aggression, anxiousness, dream abnormalities and hallucinations, depression, insomnia, irritability, restlessness, suicidal thinking and behavior, and tremor) based on postmarket reports of patients taking leukotriene modifying agents. Of note, in a study of children with mild to moderate persistent asthma that looked at whether responses to an inhaled corticosteroid and a leukotriene-receptor antagonist are concordant for individuals or whether asthmatic patients who do not respond to one medication respond to the other, response to fluticasone and montelukast were found to vary considerably. Children with low pulmonary function or high levels of markers associated with allergic inflammation responded better to the inhaled corticosteroid.

Quick-relief medications include short-acting inhaled β_2-agonists (SABAs) such as albuterol, levalbuterol, pirbuterol, or terbutaline. Albuterol can be given by nebulizer, 0.05 mg/kg (with a minimal dose of 0.63 mg and a maximum of 5 mg) in 2–3 mL saline (although it is also available in a 0.63 mg/3 mL and 1.25 mg/3 mL dosing) or by MDI. It is better to use SABAs as needed rather than on a regular basis. Increasing use, including more than one canister per month, may signify inadequate asthma control and the need to intensify anti-inflammatory therapy. Levalbuterol, the (*R*)-enantiomer of racemic albuterol, is available in solution for nebulization in patients aged 6–11 years, 0.31 mg every 8 hours, and in patients 12 years and older, 0.63–1.25 mg every 8 hours. It has recently become available in an HFA formulation for children 4 years and older, two inhalations (90 mcg) every 4–6 hours as needed. Anticholinergic agents such as ipratropium, 1–3 puffs or 0.25–0.5 mg by nebulizer every 6 hours, may provide additive benefit when used together with an inhaled SABA. Systemic corticosteroids such as prednisone, prednisolone, and methylprednisolone can be given in a dosage of 1–2 mg/kg, usually up to 60 mg/d in single or divided doses for 3–10 days. There is no evidence that tapering the dose following a "burst" prevents relapse.

Anti-IgE (omalizumab) is a recombinant DNA-derived humanized IgG_1 monoclonal antibody that selectively binds to human IgE. It inhibits the binding of IgE to the high-affinity IgE receptor (FcεRI) on the surface of mast cells and basophils. Reduction in surface-bound IgE on FcεRI-bearing cells limits the degree of release of mediators of the allergic response. Treatment with omalizumab also reduces the number of FcεRI receptors on basophils in atopic patients. Omalizumab is indicated for patients 12 years of age and older with moderate to severe persistent asthma who have a positive skin test or in vitro reactivity to a perennial aeroallergen with total serum IgE of 30–700 IU/mL, and whose symptoms are inadequately controlled with medium to high dose inhaled corticosteroids and a LABA. Omalizumab has been shown to decrease the incidence of asthma exacerbations and improve asthma control in these patients. Dosing is based on the patient's weight and serum IgE level and is given subcutaneously every 2–4 weeks. The FDA has ordered a black box warning to the label because of new reports of serious and life-threatening anaphylactic reactions (bronchospasm, hypotension, syncope, urticaria, and angioedema of the throat or tongue) in patients after treatment with Xolair (omalizumab). Based on reports from approximately 39,500 patients, anaphylaxis following Xolair treatment occurred in at least 0.1% of treated people. Although these reactions occurred within 2 hours of receiving a Xolair subcutaneous injection, they also included reports of serious delayed reactions 2–24 hours or even longer after receiving the injections. Anaphylaxis occurred after any dose of Xolair (including the first dose), even in patients with no allergic reaction to previous doses. Omalizumab-treated patients should be observed in the facility for an extended period after the drug is given, and medical providers who administer the injection should be prepared to manage life-threatening anaphylactic reactions. Patients who receive omalizumab should be fully informed about the signs and symptoms of anaphylaxis, their chance of developing delayed anaphylaxis following each injection, and how to treat it, including the use of autoinjectable epinephrine.

Immunotherapy (discussed in more detail in a subsequent section) can be considered for children 5 years and older with allergic asthma who require steps 2, 3, and 4 therapy.

Continual monitoring is necessary to ensure that control of asthma is achieved and sustained. Once control is established, gradual reduction in therapy is appropriate and may help determine the minimum amount of medication necessary to maintain control. Regular follow-up visits with the clinician are important to assess the degree of control and consider appropriate adjustments in therapy. At each step, patients should be instructed to avoid or control exposure to allergens, irritants, or other factors that contribute to asthma severity.

Referral to an asthma specialist for consultation or comanagement is recommended if there are difficulties in achieving or maintaining control. For children younger than age 5 years, referral is recommended for moderate persistent asthma or if the patient requires step 3 or 4 care and should be considered if the patient requires step 2 care. For children 5 years and older, consultation with a specialist is recommended if the patient requires step 4 care or higher and should be considered at step 3. Referral is also recommended if allergen immunotherapy or anti-IgE therapy is being considered.

3. Exercise-induced bronchospasm—Exercise-induced bronchospasm should be anticipated in all asthma patients. It typically occurs during or minutes after vigorous activity, reaches its peak 5–10 minutes after stopping the activity, and usually resolves over the next 20–30 minutes. Participation in physical activity should be encouraged in children with asthma, although the choice of activity may need to be modified based on the severity of illness, presence of other triggers such as cold air, and, rarely, confounding factors such as osteoporosis. Poor endurance or exercise-induced bronchospasm can be an indication of poorly controlled persistent asthma. If symptoms occur during usual play activities, either initiation of or a step-up in long-term therapy is warranted. However, for those with exercise-induced bronchospasm as the only manifestation of asthma despite otherwise being "well-controlled," treatment immediately prior to vigorous activity or exercise is usually effective. SABAs, leukotriene receptor antagonists, cromolyn, or nedocromil can be used before exercise. The combination of a SABA with either cromolyn or nedocromil is more effective than either drug alone. Salmeterol and formoterol may block exercise-induced bronchospasm for up to 12 hours (as discussed earlier). However, decreased duration of protection against exercise-induced bronchospasm can be expected with regular use. Montelukast may be effective up to 24 hours. An extended warm-up period may induce a refractory state, allowing patients to exercise without a need for repeat medications.

B. Acute Asthma

1. General measures—The most effective strategy in managing asthma exacerbations involves early recognition of warning signs and early treatment. For patients with moderate or severe persistent asthma or a history of severe exacerbations, this should include a written action plan. The latter usually defines the patient's green, yellow, and red zones based on symptoms (and PEFR for patients with poor symptom perception) with corresponding measures to take according to the state the patient is in. PEFR cut-off values are conventionally set as > 80% (green), 50%–80% (yellow), and < 50% (red) of the child's personal best. Prompt communication with the clinician is indicated with severe symptoms or a drop in peak flow or with decreased response to SABAs. At such times, intensification of therapy may include a short course of oral corticosteroids. The child should be removed from exposure to any irritants or allergens that could be contributing to the exacerbation.

2. Management at home—Early treatment of asthma exacerbations may prevent hospitalization and a life-threatening event. Initial treatment should be with a SABA such as albuterol or levalbuterol; 2–6 puffs from an MDI can be given every 20 minutes up to three times, or a single treatment can be given by nebulizer (0.05 mg/kg [minimum dose, 1.25 mg; maximum, 2.5 mg] of 0.5% solution of albuterol in 2–3 mL saline; or 0.075 mg/kg [minimum dose, 1.25 mg; maximum, 5 mg] of levalbuterol). If the response is good as assessed by sustained symptom relief or improvement in PEFR to over 80% of the patient's best, the SABA can be continued every 3–4 hours for 24–48 hours. Patients should be advised to seek medical care once excessive doses of bronchodilator therapy are used or for prolonged periods (eg, > 12 puffs/d for > 24 hours). Doubling the dose of inhaled corticosteroids is not proven sufficient to prevent worsening of exacerbations; however, recent evidence indicates that quadrupling the inhaled corticosteroid dose at the early sign of deterioration might be effective. If the patient does not completely improve from the initial therapy or PEFR falls between 50% and 80% predicted or personal best, the SABA should be continued, an oral corticosteroid should be added, and the patient should contact the physician urgently. If the child experiences marked distress or if PEFR persists at 50% or less, the patient should repeat the SABA immediately and go to the emergency department or call 911 or another emergency number for assistance.

3. Management in the office or emergency department— Functional assessment of the patient includes obtaining objective measures of airflow limitation with PEFR or FEV_1 and monitoring the patient's response to treatment; however, very severe exacerbations and respiratory distress may prevent the execution of lung function measurements using maximal expiratory maneuver. Flow-volume loops should be obtained to differentiate upper and lower airway obstruction, especially in patients with atypical presentation. Other tests may include oxygen saturation and blood gases. Chest radiographs are not recommended routinely but should be considered to rule out pneumothorax, pneumomediastinum, pneumonia, or lobar atelectasis. If the initial FEV_1 or PEFR is over 40%, initial treatment can be with a SABA by inhaler (albuterol, 4–8 puffs) or nebulizer (0.15 mg/kg of albuterol 0.5% solution; minimum dose, 2.5 mg), up to three doses in the first hour. Oxygen should be given to maintain oxygen saturation at greater than 90%. Oral corticosteroids (1–2 mg/kg/d in divided doses; maximum of 60 mg/d for children aged ≤ 12 years and 80 mg/d for those > 12 years) should be instituted if the patient responds poorly to therapy or if the patient has recently been on oral corticosteroids. Sensitivity to adrenergic drugs may improve after initiation of corticosteroids. If the initial FEV_1 or PEFR is under 40%, initial treatment should be with a high-dose SABA plus ipratropium bromide (0.25–0.5 mg every 20 minutes) by nebulizer or continuously for the first hour (0.5 mg/kg/h). Oxygen should be given to maintain oxygen saturation at greater than 90%, and systemic corticosteroids should be administered. For patients with severe exacerbation having no response to initial aerosolized therapy, or for those who cannot cooperate with or who resist inhalation therapy, adjunctive therapies such as intravenous magnesium sulfate (25–75 mg/kg up to 2 g in children) and heliox-driven albuterol nebulization should be considered. Epinephrine 1:1000 or terbutaline 1 mg/mL (both 0.01 mg/kg up to 0.3–0.5 mg) may be administered subcutaneously every 20 minutes for three doses; although the use of intravenous β_2-agonists is still unproven. For impending or ongoing respiratory arrest, patients should be intubated and ventilated with 100% oxygen, given intravenous corticosteroids, and admitted to an intensive care unit (ICU). Potential indications for ICU admission also include any FEV_1 or PEFR less than 25% of predicted that improves less than 10% after treatment or values that fluctuate widely. (See Asthma [life-threatening] in Chapter 14.) Further treatment is based on clinical response and objective laboratory findings. Hospitalization should be considered strongly for any patient with a history of respiratory failure.

4. Hospital management—For patients who do not respond to outpatient and emergency department treatment, admission to the hospital becomes necessary for more aggressive care and support. The decision to hospitalize should also be based on presence of risk factors for mortality from asthma, duration and severity of symptoms, severity of airflow limitation, course and severity of previous exacerbations, medication use at the time of the exacerbation, access to medical care, and home and psychosocial conditions. Fluids should be given at maintenance requirements unless the patient has poor oral intake secondary to respiratory distress or vomiting, because overhydration may contribute to pulmonary edema associated with high intrapleural pressures generated in severe asthma. Potassium requirements should be kept in mind because both corticosteroids and β_2-agonists can cause potassium loss. Moisturized oxygen should be titrated by oximetry to maintain oxygen saturation above 90%. Inhaled β_2-agonist should be continued by nebulization in single doses as needed or by continuous therapy, along with systemic corticosteroids (as discussed earlier). Ipratropium is no longer recommended during hospitalization. In addition, the role of methylxanthines in hospitalized children remains controversial. Antibiotics may be necessary to treat coexisting bacterial infection. Sedatives and anxiolytic agents are contraindicated in severely ill patients owing to their depressant effects on respiration. Chest physiotherapy is usually not recommended for acute exacerbations.

5. Patient discharge—Criteria for discharging patients home from the office or emergency department should include a sustained response of at least 1 hour to bronchodilator therapy with FEV_1 or PEFR greater than 70% of predicted or personal best and oxygen saturation greater than 90% in room air. Prior to discharge, the patient's or caregiver's ability to continue therapy and assess symptoms appropriately needs to be considered. Patients should be given an action plan for management of recurrent symptoms or exacerbations, and instructions about medications should be reviewed. The inhaled SABA and oral corticosteroids should be continued, the latter for 3–10 days. Finally, the patient or caregiver should be instructed about the follow-up visit, typically within 1 week. Hospitalized patients should receive more intensive education prior to discharge. Referral to an asthma specialist should be considered for all children with severe exacerbations or multiple emergency department visits or hospitalizations.

Prognosis

Since the 1970s, morbidity rates for asthma have increased, but mortality rates may have stabilized. Mortality statistics indicate that a high percentage of deaths have resulted from underrecognition of asthma severity and undertreatment, particularly in labile asthmatic patients and in asthmatic patients whose perception of pulmonary obstruction is poor. Long-term outcome studies suggest that children with mild symptoms generally outgrow their asthma, while patients with more severe symptoms, marked airway hyperresponsiveness, and a greater degree of atopy tend to have persistent disease. Data from an unselected birth cohort from New Zealand showed more than one in four children had wheezing that persisted from childhood to adulthood or that relapsed after remission. Recent evidence suggests that early intervention with anti-inflammatory therapy does not alter the development of persistent asthma, and it is also unclear if such intervention or environmental control measures influence the natural history of childhood asthma. Nonetheless, the pediatrician or primary care provider together with the asthma specialist has the responsibility to optimize control and, it is hoped, reduce the severity of asthma in children. Interventions that can have long-term effects such as halting progression or inducing remission are necessary to decrease the public health burden of this common condition.

Resources for health care providers, patients, and families include:

Asthma and Allergy Foundation of America
1233 20th St NW, Suite 402
Washington, DC 20036; (800) 7-ASTHMA
http://www.aafa.org/

Asthma and Allergy Network/Mothers of Asthmatics
2751 Prosperity Avenue, Suite 150
Fairfax, VA 22031; (800) 878-4403
http://www.aanma.org/

Lung Line (800) 222-LUNG
Asthma Device Training:
http://www.thechildrenshospital.org/conditions/lung/asthmavideos.aspx

Agency for Healthcare Research and Quality. 2006 Hospital Discharges by age groups.
http://hcupnet.ahrq.gov/. Accessed May 15, 2009.

Akinbami LJ, Moorman JE, Liu X: Asthma prevalence, health care use, and mortality: United States, 2005–2009. Natl Health Stat Report 2011 Jan 12;(32):1–14 [PMID: 21355352].

Center for Disease Control and Prevention. National Center for Health Statistics. Health Data Interactive. Available at: http://www.cdc.gov/nchs/fastats/asthma.htm. Accessed Aug 1, 2011.

Covar RA et al: Childhood Asthma Management Program Research Group. Predictors of remitting, periodic, and persistent childhood asthma. J Allergy Clin Immunol 2010 Feb;125(2):359–366 e3 [PMID: 20159245].

Guilbert T et al: Long-term inhaled corticosteroids in preschool children at high risk for asthma. N Engl J Med 2006;354:1985 [PMID: 16687711].

Lemanske RF Jr et al: Childhood Asthma Research and Education (CARE) Network of the National Heart, Lung, and Blood Institute. Step-up therapy for children with uncontrolled asthma receiving inhaled corticosteroids. N Engl J Med 2010 Mar 18;362(11):975–985 [PMID: 20197425].

National Asthma Education and Prevention Program: Expert Panel Report 3 (EPR 3): Guidelines for the Diagnosis and Management of Asthma—Summary Report 2007. J Allergy Clin Immunol 2007;120(Suppl):S94 [PMID: 17983880]. Available at: http://www.nhlbi.nih.gov/guidelines/asthma/asthgdln.htm.

ALLERGIC RHINOCONJUNCTIVITIS

ESSENTIALS OF DIAGNOSIS & TYPICAL FEATURES

After exposure to allergen:

- Sneezing.
- Itching of nose and eyes.
- Clear rhinorrhea or nasal congestion.

General Considerations

Allergic rhinoconjunctivitis is the most common allergic disease and significantly affects quality of life as well as school performance and attendance. It frequently coexists with asthma, can impact asthma control, and is a risk factor for subsequent development of asthma. Over 80% of patients with asthma have rhinitis and 10%–14% of patients with rhinitis have asthma. About 80% of individuals with allergic rhinitis develop their symptoms before age 20 years. It is estimated that 13% of children had a physician diagnosis of allergic rhinitis. Prevalence of this disease increases during childhood, peaking at 15% in the postadolescent years. Although allergic rhinoconjunctivitis is more common in boys during early childhood, there is little difference in incidence between the sexes after adolescence. Race and socioeconomic status are not considered to be important factors.

The pathologic changes in allergic rhinoconjunctivitis are chiefly hyperemia, edema, and increased serous and mucoid secretions caused by mediator release, all of which lead to variable degrees of nasal obstruction and conjunctival injection, nasal and ocular pruritus, or nasal and ocular discharge. Ocular allergies can occur in isolation, but more commonly they are in conjunction with nasal symptoms. This process may involve other structures, including the sinuses and possibly the middle ear. Inhalant allergens are primarily responsible for symptoms, but food allergens can cause symptoms as well. Children with allergic rhinitis seem to be more susceptible to—or at least may experience more symptoms from—upper respiratory infections, which, in turn, may aggravate the allergic rhinitis.

Allergic rhinoconjunctivitis has been classified as perennial, seasonal (hay fever), or episodic; however, there are areas where pollens and soil molds may be present year round while exposure to typical perennial allergens such as indoor furred animals may be intermittent. For this reason, the preferred terms are *intermittent* (ie, symptoms present < 4 days a week or for < 4 weeks) and *persistent* (ie, symptoms present > 4 days a week and for > 4 weeks). In addition, severity should be noted as *mild* (ie, without impairment or disturbance of sleep, daily activities, leisure, sport, school, or work, or without troublesome symptoms) or *moderate-severe* (ie, presence of one or more of the aforementioned). The major pollen groups in the temperate zones include trees (late winter to early spring), grasses (late spring to early summer), and weeds (late summer to early fall), but seasons can vary significantly in different parts of the country. Mold spores also cause seasonal allergic rhinitis, principally in the summer and fall. Seasonal allergy symptoms may be aggravated by coincident exposure to perennial allergens.

Clinical Findings

A. Symptoms and Signs

Patients may complain of itching of the nose, eyes, palate, or pharynx and loss of smell or taste. Nasal itching can cause paroxysmal sneezing and epistaxis. Repeated rubbing of the nose (so-called allergic salute) may lead to a horizontal crease across the lower third of the nose. Nasal obstruction is associated with mouth breathing, nasal speech, allergic salute, and snoring. Nasal turbinates may appear pale blue and swollen with dimpling or injected with minimal edema. Typically, clear and thin nasal secretions are increased, with anterior rhinorrhea, sniffling, postnasal drip, and congested cough. Nasal secretions often cause poor appetite, fatigue, and pharyngeal irritation. Conjunctival injection, tearing, periorbital edema, and infraorbital cyanosis (so-called allergic shiners) are frequently observed. Increased pharyngeal lymphoid tissue ("cobblestoning") from chronic drainage and enlarged tonsillar and adenoidal tissue may be present.

B. Laboratory Findings

Eosinophilia often can be demonstrated on smears of nasal secretions or blood. This is a frequent but nonspecific finding and may occur in nonallergic conditions. Although serum IgE may be elevated, measurement of total IgE is a poor screening tool owing to the wide overlap between atopic and nonatopic subjects. Skin testing to identify allergen-specific IgE is the most sensitive and specific test for inhalant allergies; alternatively, the Phadia ImmunoCAP assay, radioallergosorbent test (RAST), or other in vitro tests can be done for suspected allergens.

Differential Diagnosis

Disorders that need to be differentiated from allergic rhinitis include infectious rhinosinusitis. Foreign bodies and structural abnormalities such as choanal atresia, marked septal deviation, nasal polyps, and adenoidal hypertrophy may cause chronic symptoms. Overuse of topical nasal decongestants may result in rhinitis medicamentosa (rebound congestion). Use of medications such as propranolol, clonidine, and some psychoactive drugs may cause nasal congestion. Illicit drugs such as cocaine can cause rhinorrhea. Spicy or hot foods may cause gustatory rhinitis. Nonallergic rhinitis with eosinophilia syndrome is usually not seen in young children. Vasomotor rhinitis is associated with persistent symptoms but without allergen exposure. Less common causes of symptoms that may be confused with allergic rhinitis include pregnancy, congenital syphilis, hypothyroidism, tumors, and cerebrospinal fluid rhinorrhea.

As in the differential diagnoses for allergic rhinitis, infectious conjunctivitis (secondary to viral, bacterial, or chlamydial etiology) can mimic allergic eye disorders. In this case, it typically develops in one eye first, and symptoms include stinging or burning sensation (rather than pruritus) with a foreign body sensation and eye discharge (watery, mucoid, or purulent). Nasolacrimal duct obstruction, foreign body, blepharoconjunctivitis, dry eye, uveitis, and trauma are other masqueraders of ocular allergy.

The other conditions which comprise allergic eye diseases, presenting with bilateral conjunctivitis, include atopic keratoconjunctivitis, vernal conjunctivitis, and giant papillary conjunctivitis. Except for giant papillary conjunctivitis, the three (allergic conjunctivitis, atopic keratoconjunctivitis, and vernal conjunctivitis) are associated with allergic sensitization. Atopic keratoconjunctivitis and vernal conjunctivitis are both vision-threatening. Atopic keratoconjunctivitis is rarely seen before late adolescence and it most commonly involves the lower tarsal conjunctiva. Ocular symptoms (itching, burning, and tearing) are more severe than in allergic conjunctivitis and persist all year round, with accompanying eyelid eczema with erythema and thick, dry scaling skin, which can extend to the periorbital skin and cheeks. Vernal conjunctivitis is characterized by giant papillae, described as cobblestoning, seen in the upper tarsal conjunctiva. It affects boys more often than girls and patients of Asian and African descent are more predisposed. It affects individuals in temperate areas, with exacerbations in the spring and summer months. In addition to severe pruritus which can be exacerbated by exposure to irritants, light, or perspiration, other accompanying signs and symptoms include photophobia, foreign body sensation, lacrimation, and presence of stringy or thick, ropey discharge, transient yellow-white points in the limbus (Trantas dots) and conjunctiva (Horner points), corneal "shield" ulcers, Dennie lines (prominent skin folds that extend in an arc form from the inner canthus beneath and parallel to the lower lid margin), and prominently long eyelashes. Giant papillary conjunctivitis is associated with exposure to foreign bodies such as contact lenses, ocular prostheses, and sutures. It is characterized by mild ocular itching, tearing, and mucoid discharge especially on awakening. Trantas dots, limbal infiltration, bulbar injection, and edema may also be found. One eye condition, contact allergy, which can also involve the conjunctivae especially when associated with use of topical medications, contact lens solutions, and preservatives, typically affects the eyelids.

Complications

Sinusitis may accompany allergic rhinitis. Allergic mucosal swelling of the sinus ostia can obstruct sinus drainage, interfering with normal sinus function and predisposing to chronic mucosal disease. Nasal polyps due to allergy are unusual in children, and cystic fibrosis should be considered if they are present. Unlike vision-threatening complications associated with atopic keratoconjunctivitis and vernal conjunctivitis, allergic conjunctivitis manifests primarily with significant pruritus and discomfort affecting the patients' quality of life.

Treatment

A. General Measures

The value of identification and avoidance of causative allergens cannot be overstated. Reducing indoor allergens through environmental control measures as discussed in the section on asthma can be very effective. Nasal saline irrigation may be useful. For ocular allergies, cold compresses and lubrication are also important.

B. Pharmacologic Therapy

Pharmacologic management of mild intermittent rhinitis includes oral or intranasal H_1 antihistamines and intranasal decongestants (for < 10 days and not to be repeated more than twice a month). Oral decongestants are not usually recommended in children. Options for moderate-severe intermittent rhinitis are oral or intranasal antihistamines, oral H_1 antihistamines and decongestants, intranasal corticosteroids, and cromones. The same medication options are available for persistent rhinitis, but a stepwise approach is proposed both for treatment of mild and moderate-severe persistent rhinitis. For mild persistent rhinitis, reassessment after 2–4 weeks is recommended and treatment should be continued, with a possible reduction in intranasal corticosteroids, even if the symptoms have abated. If, however, the patient has persistent mild symptoms while on H_1 antihistamines or cromones, an intranasal corticosteroid is appropriate. For moderate-severe persistent disease, use of intranasal corticosteroids as first-line therapy is recommended. For severe nasal congestion, either a short 1- to 2-week course of an oral corticosteroid or an intranasal decongestant for less than 10 days may be added. If the patient improves, the treatment should last for at least 3 months or until the pollen season is over. If the patient does not improve within 2–4 weeks despite adequate compliance and use of medications, comorbidities such as nasal polyps, sinusitis, and significant allergen exposure should be considered, as well as the possibility of misdiagnosis. Once these are ruled out, options include increasing the dose of the intranasal corticosteroid, combination therapy with an H_1 antihistamine (particularly if major symptoms are sneezing, itching, or rhinorrhea), ipratropium bromide (if major symptom is rhinorrhea), or an oral H_1 antihistamine and decongestant. Referral to a specialist may be considered if the treatment is not sufficient.

For allergic rhinoconjunctivitis, topical nasal corticosteroids also reduce ocular symptoms, presumably through a naso-ocular reflex. For ocular allergies which persist or occur independent of rhinitis, pharmacologic treatment includes use of oral or topical antihistamines, topical decongestants, mast cell stabilizers, and anti-inflammatory agents. In general, topical ophthalmic drops should not be used with contact lenses. Topical decongestants relieve erythema, congestion, and edema but do not affect the allergic response. Combined therapy with an antihistamine and a vasoconstrictive agent is more effective than either agent alone. Topical medications with both antihistamine and mast cell blocking properties provide the most benefits which incorporate fast-acting symptom relief and anti-inflammatory action. Refrigerating ophthalmic drops before use can provide soothing relief as well. However, children can get wary of eye drops and prefer oral preparations. Avoiding contamination by preventing the applicator tip from touching the eye or eyelid is important. Severe ocular allergy can be treated with topical, or rarely, oral corticosteroids. In such a case, a referral to an ophthalmologist is warranted, as these treatments can be associated with elevation of the intraocular pressure, viral infections, and cataract formation.

Allergen immunotherapy can be very effective in allergic rhinoconjunctivitis and may decrease the requirement for medications to control the symptoms in the long term.

1. Antihistamines—Antihistamines help control itching, sneezing, and rhinorrhea. Sedating antihistamines include diphenhydramine, chlorpheniramine, hydroxyzine, and clemastine. Sedating antihistamines may cause daytime somnolence and negatively affect school performance and other activities, especially driving. Second-generation antihistamines include loratadine, desloratadine, cetirizine, and fexofenadine. Cetirizine is approved for use in children aged 6–23 months (2.5 mg daily), 2–5 years (2.5–5.0 mg/d or 2.5 mg twice a day), and 6 years or older (5–10 mg/d). It is now available without a prescription. Loratadine is approved for use in children aged 2–5 years (5 mg/d) and 6 years or older (10 mg/d), and is available without prescription in tablet, rapidly disintegrating tablet, and liquid formulations. Desloratadine is approved for use in children aged 6–11 months (1 mg/d), 1–5 years (1.25 mg/d), and for 12 years and older (5 mg/d). Fexofenadine is approved for children aged 6–23 months (15 mg twice a day), 2–11 years (30 mg twice a day), and 12 years or older (60 mg twice a day or 180 mg once daily), and is also now available without a prescription. Levocetirizine (5 mg/d) is approved for children aged 6 years and older. Loratadine, fexofenadine, and cetirizine are available in combination with pseudoephedrine for patients aged 12 years or older, although regular use of these combination products is not recommended. Azelastine is available in nasal and ophthalmic formulations. Levocabastine and emedastine are available as ophthalmic preparations. They should not be used for treatment of contact lens–related irritation and caution should be implemented with concomitant use of soft contact lenses.

2. Mast cell stabilizers—Intranasal ipratropium can be used as adjunctive therapy for rhinorrhea. Intranasal cromolyn may be used alone or in conjunction with oral antihistamines and decongestants. It is most effective when used prophylactically, one to two sprays/nostril, four times a day. This dose may be tapered if symptom control is achieved. Rarely, patients complain of nasal irritation or burning. Most patients find complying with four-times-daily dosing difficult. Cromolyn is also available in an ophthalmic solution. (See also Chapter 16.) It can be used to treat giant papillary and vernal conjunctivitis. Other ophthalmic mast cell stabilizers include lodoxamide 0.1% solution (can be used for vernal keratoconjunctivitis as well), one to two drops four times a day; nedocromil sodium 2%, one to two drops two times a day; and pemirolast potassium 0.1%, one to two drops four times a day.

3. Decongestants and vasoconstrictor agents—Nasal α-adrenergic agents help to relieve nasal congestion and ophthalmic vasoconstrictors relieve ocular erythema, edema, and congestion. Topical nasal decongestants such as phenylephrine and oxymetazoline should not be used for more than 4 days for severe episodes because prolonged use may be associated with rhinitis medicamentosa. As with nasal decongestants, a rebound phenomenon (ie, conjunctivitis medicamentosa with hyperemia and stinging/burning) can occur with chronic use of ophthalmic vasoconstrictive agents such as naphazoline and tetrahydrozoline. Oral decongestants, including pseudoephedrine, phenylephrine, and phenylpropanolamine, are often combined with antihistamines or expectorants and cough suppressants in over-the-counter (OTC) cold medications, but there are no convincing data to support the use of oral decongestants for upper respiratory illnesses in children nor for regular use in patients with allergic rhinitis. They may cause insomnia, agitation, tachycardia, and, rarely, cardiac arrhythmias. Of note, the FDA has recommended the removal of phenylpropanolamine from all drug products due to a public health advisory concerning the risk of hemorrhagic stroke associated with its use.

4. Corticosteroids—Intranasal corticosteroid sprays are effective in controlling allergic rhinitis if used chronically. They are minimally absorbed in usual doses and are available in pressurized nasal inhalers and aqueous sprays. Mometasone and fluticasone furoate nasal sprays have been approved for use in children as young as age 2 years (one spray in each nostril once daily) and in children 12 years or older (two sprays/nostril once daily). Fluticasone propionate nasal spray is approved for children 4 years or older, and budesonide and triamcinolone nasal sprays are approved for those 6 years or older (one to two sprays/nostril once daily). Flunisolide is approved for ages 6–14 years (one spray/nostril three times a day or two sprays/nostril twice a day). Ciclesonide is approved for seasonal allergic rhinitis in children 6 years and older and those with perennial allergic rhinitis for children 12 years and older, two sprays in each nostril once daily. Side effects include nasal irritation, soreness, and bleeding, although epistaxis occurs commonly in patients with allergic rhinitis if corticosteroids are used chronically. Rarely, these drugs can cause septal perforation. Excessive doses may produce systemic effects, especially if used together with orally inhaled steroids for asthma. Onset of action is within hours, although clinical benefit is usually not observed for a week or more. They may be effective alone or together with antihistamines.

Use of oral or topical (eg, loteprednol etabonate) corticosteroids for the treatment of ocular allergy should be worked out in conjunction with an ophthalmologist due to potential complications mentioned in the preceding section.

5. Other pharmacologic agents—Montelukast is approved for perennial allergic rhinitis in children aged 6 months and older (4 mg/d for ages 6–23 months) and seasonal allergic rhinitis in children 2 years and older in doses as discussed in the preceding section on Pharmacologic Therapy under Treatment, Chronic Asthma. Oral antihistamines are also available in combination with a decongestant. Ketorolac, a nonsteroidal anti-inflammatory drug (NSAID), is available as an ophthalmic solution but should be avoided in patients with aspirin or NSAID sensitivity and should be used with caution in those with complicated eye surgeries, corneal denervation or epithelial defects, ocular surface diseases, diabetes mellitus, or rheumatoid arthritis. Combination ophthalmic preparations are available. Both antazoline and pheniramine are antihistamine/vasoconstrictor formulations. Olopatadine 0.1%, epinastine 0.05%, and ketotifen 0.025% ophthalmic solutions have antihistamine and mast cell–stabilizing actions and can be given to children older than age 3 years as one drop twice a day (8 hours apart) for olopatadine and every 8–12 hours for ketotifen, respectively. Ketotifen fumarate 0.025% is now available as an OTC ophthalmic medication. Olopatadine 0.2% is the first once-daily ophthalmic medication available for the treatment of ocular pruritus associated with allergic conjunctivitis.

C. Surgical Therapy

Surgical procedures, including turbinectomy, polypectomy, and functional endoscopic sinus surgery, are rarely indicated in allergic rhinitis or chronic hyperplastic sinusitis.

D. Immunotherapy

Allergen immunotherapy should be considered when symptoms are severe and due to unavoidable exposure to inhalant allergens, especially if symptomatic measures have failed. Immunotherapy is the only form of therapy that may alter the course of the disease. It should not be prescribed by sending the patient's serum to a laboratory where extracts based on in vitro tests are prepared for the patient (ie, the remote practice of allergy). Subcutaneous immunotherapy should be done in a facility where a physician prepared to treat anaphylaxis is present. Patients with concomitant asthma should not receive an injection if their asthma is not under good control (ie, peak flows preinjection are below 80% of personal best), and the patient should wait for 25–30 minutes after an injection before leaving the facility. Outcomes with single allergen immunotherapy show success rates of approximately 80%. The optimal duration of therapy is unknown, but data suggest that immunotherapy for 3–5 years may have lasting benefit. Sublingual immunotherapy has been developed and recommended in Europe, Argentina, Brazil, the Gulf States, and South Africa, for treatment of allergic rhinitis caused by pollens in both adults and children, and for allergic rhinitis caused by dust mites only in adults. Although local adverse effects are common (in about 35%), this form of immunotherapy allows for a less stringent administration as this can be given at home. This is still considered experimental in the United States, as extracts have not been FDA-approved.

Prognosis

Allergic rhinoconjunctivitis associated with sensitization to indoor allergens tends to be protracted unless specific allergens can be identified and eliminated from the environment. In seasonal allergic rhinoconjunctivitis, symptoms are usually most severe from adolescence through mid-adult life. After moving to a region devoid of problem allergens, patients may be symptom-free for several years, but they can develop new sensitivities to local aeroallergens.

Bousquet J, Khaltaev N, Cruz AA: Allergic Rhinitis and its Impact on Asthma (ARIA) 2008 update (in collaboration with the World Health Organization, GA(2)LEN and AllerGen). Allergy 2008 Apr;63(Suppl 86):8–160 [PMID: 18331513].

Brozek JL et al: Global Allergy and Asthma European Network; Grading of Recommendations Assessment, Development, and Evaluation Working Group. Allergic Rhinitis and its Impact on Asthma (ARIA) guidelines: 2010 revision. J Allergy Clin Immunol 2010 Sep;126(3):466–476 [PMID: 20816182].

Meltzer EO et al: Burden of allergic rhinitis: Results from the pediatric allergies in America survey. J Allergy Clin Immunol 2009;124:S43–S70 [PMID: 19592081].

Simons FER: Advances in H1-antihistamines. N Engl J Med 2004;351:2203 [PMID: 15548781].

ATOPIC DERMATITIS

ESSENTIALS OF DIAGNOSIS & TYPICAL FEATURES

- Pruritus.
- Facial and extensor involvement in infants and young children.
- Flexural lichenification in older children and adolescents.
- Chronic or relapsing dermatitis.
- Personal or family history of atopic disease.

General Considerations

Atopic dermatitis is a chronically relapsing inflammatory skin disease typically associated with respiratory allergy. Over half of patients with atopic dermatitis will develop asthma and allergic rhinitis. A subset of patients with atopic dermatitis has been shown to have mutations in the gene encoding filaggrin, a protein essential for normal epidermal barrier function. These patients have early-onset, more severe, and persistent disease. Mutations in filaggrin have also been associated with increased risk for asthma, but only in patients with atopic dermatitis. Atopic dermatitis may result in significant morbidity, leading to school absenteeism, occupational disability, and emotional stress. The disease presents in early childhood, with onset prior to age 5 years in approximately 90% of patients.

Clinical Findings

A. Symptoms and Signs

Atopic dermatitis has no pathognomonic skin lesions or laboratory parameters. Diagnosis is based on the clinical features, including severe pruritus, a chronically relapsing course, and typical morphology and distribution of the skin lesions. Acute atopic dermatitis is characterized by intensely pruritic, erythematous papules associated with excoriations, vesiculations, and serous exudate; subacute atopic dermatitis by erythematous, excoriated, scaling papules; and chronic atopic dermatitis by thickened skin with accentuated markings (lichenification) and fibrotic papules. Patients with chronic atopic dermatitis may have all three types of lesions present concurrently. Patients usually have dry, "lackluster" skin. During infancy, atopic dermatitis involves primarily the face, scalp, and extensor surfaces of the extremities. The diaper area is usually spared. When involved, it may be secondarily infected with *Candida*. In older patients with long-standing disease, the flexural folds of the extremities are the predominant location of lesions.

B. Laboratory Findings

Identification of allergens involves taking a careful history and performing selective immediate hypersensitivity skin tests or in vitro tests when appropriate. Negative skin tests with proper controls have a high predictive value for ruling out a suspected allergen. Positive skin tests have a lower correlation with clinical symptoms in suspected food allergen–induced atopic dermatitis and should be confirmed with double-blind, placebo-controlled food challenges unless there is a coincidental history of anaphylaxis to the suspected food. Alternatively, specific IgE levels to milk, egg, peanut, and fish proteins have been established with the Phadia ImmunoCAP assay correlating with a greater than 95% chance of a clinical reaction.

Elevated serum IgE levels can be demonstrated in 80%–85% of patients with atopic dermatitis, and a similar number have positive immediate skin tests or in vitro tests with food and inhalant allergens. Several well-controlled studies suggest that specific allergens can influence the course of this disease. However, triggers for clinical disease cannot be predicted simply by performing allergy testing. Double-blind, placebo-controlled food challenges show that food allergens can cause exacerbations in a subset of patients with atopic dermatitis. Although lesions induced by single positive challenges are usually transient, repeated challenges, more typical of real-life exposure, can result in eczematous lesions. Furthermore, elimination of food allergens results in amelioration of skin disease and a decrease in spontaneous basophil histamine release. Exacerbation of atopic dermatitis can occur with exposure to aeroallergens such as house dust mites, and environmental control measures have been shown to result in clinical improvement. Patients can make specific IgE directed at *Staphylococcus aureus* toxins secreted on the skin, and this correlates with clinical severity better than total serum IgE levels. Eosinophilia may occur. Routine skin biopsy does not differentiate atopic dermatitis from other eczematous processes but may be helpful in atypical cases. Tests for the most common filaggrin gene mutations using DNA from buccal swabs or blood are available. Testing may identify patients who would be at increased risk for more severe, persistent atopic dermatitis and be more likely to develop allergic sensitizations and asthma.

Differential Diagnosis

Scabies can present as a pruritic skin disease. However, distribution in the genital and axillary areas and the presence of linear lesions as well as skin scrapings may help to distinguish it from atopic dermatitis. Seborrheic dermatitis may be distinguished by a lack of significant pruritus; its predilection for the scalp (so-called cradle cap); and its coarse, yellowish scales. Allergic contact dermatitis may be suggested by the distribution of lesions with a greater demarcation of dermatitis than in atopic dermatitis. Occasionally, allergic contact dermatitis superimposed on atopic dermatitis may appear as an acute flare of the underlying disease. Nummular eczema is characterized by coin-shaped plaques. Although unusual in children, mycosis fungoides or cutaneous T-cell lymphoma has been described and is diagnosed by skin biopsy. Eczematous rash has been reported in patients with human immunodeficiency virus (HIV) infection. Other disorders that may resemble atopic dermatitis include Wiskott-Aldrich syndrome, severe combined immunodeficiency disease, hyper-IgE syndrome, IPEX (immune dysregulation, polyendocrinopathy, enteropathy, X-linked) syndrome, zinc deficiency, phenylketonuria, and Letterer-Siwe disease.

Complications

Ocular complications associated with atopic dermatitis can lead to significant morbidity. Atopic keratoconjunctivitis is always bilateral, and symptoms include itching, burning, tearing, and copious mucoid discharge. It is frequently associated with eyelid dermatitis and chronic blepharitis, and may result in visual impairment from corneal scarring. (See Chapter 16.) Keratoconus in atopic dermatitis is believed to result from persistent rubbing of the eyes in patients with atopic dermatitis and allergic rhinitis. Anterior subcapsular cataracts may develop during adolescence or early adult life.

Patients with atopic dermatitis have increased susceptibility to infection or colonization with a variety of organisms. These include viral infections with herpes simplex, molluscum contagiosum, and human papillomavirus. Of note, even a past history of atopic dermatitis is considered a contraindication for receiving the current smallpox (vaccinia) vaccine. Superimposed dermatophytosis may cause atopic dermatitis to flare. *S aureus* can be cultured from the skin of more than 90% of patients with atopic dermatitis, compared with only 5% of normal subjects. Patients with atopic dermatitis often have toxin-secreting *S aureus* cultured from their skin and can make specific IgE antibodies against the toxins found on their skin. *S aureus* toxins can act as superantigens, contributing to persistent inflammation or exacerbations of atopic dermatitis. Patients without obvious superinfection may show a better response to combined antistaphylococcal and topical corticosteroid therapy than to corticosteroids alone. Although recurrent staphylococcal pustulosis can be a significant problem in atopic dermatitis, invasive *S aureus* infections occur rarely and should raise the possibility of an immunodeficiency such as hyper-IgE syndrome. Patients with atopic dermatitis may be predisposed to colonization and infections by microbial organisms due to decreased synthesis of antimicrobial peptides in the skin, which may be mediated by increased levels of TH2-type cytokines.

Patients with atopic dermatitis often have a nonspecific hand dermatitis. This is frequently irritant in nature and aggravated by repeated wetting.

Nutritional disturbances may result from unwarranted and unnecessarily vigorous dietary restrictions imposed by physicians and parents.

Poor academic performance and behavioral disturbances may be a result of uncontrolled intense or frequent itching, sleep loss, and poor self-image. Severe disease may lead to problems with social interactions and self-esteem.

Treatment

A. General Measures

Patients with atopic dermatitis have a lowered threshold of irritant responsiveness. Avoidance of irritants such as detergents, chemicals, and abrasive materials as well as extremes of temperature and humidity is important in managing this disease. New clothing should be washed to reduce the content of formaldehyde and other chemicals. Because residual laundry detergent in clothing may be irritating, using a liquid rather than a powder detergent and adding an extra rinse cycle is beneficial. Occlusive clothing should be avoided in favor of cotton or cotton blends. Temperature in the home and work environments should be controlled to minimize sweating. Swimming is usually well tolerated; however, because swimming pools are treated with chlorine or bromine, patients should shower and use a mild cleanser to remove these chemicals, then apply a moisturizer or occlusive agent. Sunlight may be beneficial to some patients with atopic dermatitis, but nonsensitizing sunscreens should be used to avoid sunburn. Prolonged sun exposure can cause evaporative losses, overheating, and sweating, all of which can be irritating.

In children who have undergone controlled food challenges, eggs, milk, peanuts, soy, wheat, and fish account for approximately 90% of the food allergens that exacerbate atopic dermatitis. Avoidance of foods implicated in controlled challenges can lead to clinical improvement. Extensive elimination diets, which can be nutritionally unsound and burdensome, are almost never warranted because even patients with multiple positive skin tests rarely react to more than three foods on blinded challenges.

In patients who demonstrate specific IgE to dust mite allergen, environmental control measures aimed at reducing the dust mite load improve atopic dermatitis. These include use of dust mite–proof covers on pillows and mattresses, washing linens weekly in hot water, decreasing indoor humidity levels, and in some cases removing bedroom carpeting.

Counseling may be of benefit when dealing with the frustrations associated with atopic dermatitis. Relaxation, behavioral modification, or biofeedback training may help patients with habitual scratching. Patients with severe or disfiguring disease may require psychotherapy.

Clinicians should provide the patient and family with both general information and specific written skin care recommendations. The patient or parent should demonstrate an appropriate level of understanding to help ensure a good outcome. Educational pamphlets and a video about atopic dermatitis can be obtained from the National Eczema Association, a national nonprofit, patient-oriented organization, at: (800) 818-7546; http://www.nationaleczema.org.

B. Hydration

Patients with atopic dermatitis have evaporative losses due to a defective skin barrier, so soaking the affected area or bathing for 10–15 minutes in warm water, then applying an occlusive agent to retain the absorbed water, is an essential component of therapy. Oatmeal or baking soda added to the bath may feel soothing to certain patients but does not improve water absorption. Atopic dermatitis of the face or neck can be treated by applying a wet facecloth or towel to the involved area. The washcloth may be more readily accepted by a child if it is turned into a mask and also allows the older patient to remain functional. Lesions limited to the hands or feet can be treated by soaking in a basin. Daily baths may be needed and increased to several times daily during flares of atopic dermatitis, while showers may be adequate for patients with mild disease. It is important to use an occlusive preparation within a few minutes after soaking the skin to prevent evaporation, which is both drying and irritating.

C. Moisturizers and Occlusives

An effective emollient combined with hydration therapy will help skin healing and can reduce the need for topical corticosteroids. Moisturizers are available as lotions, creams, and ointments. Because lotions contain more water than creams, they are more drying because of their evaporative effect. Preservatives and fragrances in lotions and creams may cause skin irritation. Moisturizers often need to be applied several times daily on a long-term basis and should be obtained in the largest size available. Crisco shortening can be substituted as an inexpensive alternative. Petroleum jelly (Vaseline) is an effective occlusive agent when used to seal in water after bathing. Topical nonsteroidal creams approved as medical devices (thus, currently requiring prescriptions) for relief and management of signs and symptoms of dermatoses include Atopiclair, MimyX, EpiCeram, and Eletone.

D. Corticosteroids

Corticosteroids reduce the inflammation and pruritus in atopic dermatitis. Topical corticosteroids can decrease *S aureus* colonization. Systemic corticosteroids, including oral prednisone, should be avoided in the management of this chronic relapsing disease. The dramatic improvement observed with systemic corticosteroids may be associated with an equally dramatic flaring of atopic dermatitis following their discontinuation. Topical corticosteroids are available in a wide variety of formulations, ranging from extremely high-potency to low-potency preparations (see Table 15–3). Choice of a particular product depends on the severity and distribution of skin lesions. Patients need to be counseled regarding the potency of their corticosteroid preparation and its potential side effects. In general, the least potent agent that is effective should be used. However, choosing a preparation that is too weak may result in persistence or worsening of the atopic dermatitis. Side effects include thinning of the skin, telangiectasias, bruising, hypopigmentation, acne, and striae, although these occur infrequently when low- to medium-potency topical corticosteroids are used appropriately. In contrast, use of potent topical corticosteroids for prolonged periods—especially under occlusion—may result in significant atrophic changes as well as systemic side effects. The face (especially the eyelids) and intertriginous areas are especially sensitive to corticosteroid side effects, and only low-potency preparations should be used routinely on these areas. Because topical corticosteroids are commercially available in a variety of bases, including ointments, creams, lotions, solutions, gels, and sprays, there is no need to compound them. Ointments are most occlusive and in general provide better delivery of the medication while preventing evaporative losses. However, in a humid environment, creams may be better tolerated than ointments because the increased occlusion may cause itching or even folliculitis. Creams and lotions, while easier to spread, can contribute to skin dryness and irritation. Solutions can be used on the scalp and hirsute areas, although they can be irritating, especially to open lesions. With clinical improvement, a less potent corticosteroid should be prescribed and the frequency of use decreased. Topical corticosteroids can be discontinued when inflammation resolves, but hydration and moisturizers need to be continued. Several topical steroids including fluticasone 0.05% cream and desonide 0.05% hydrogel have been approved in infants as young as 3 months of age for up to 28 days.

E. Topical Calcineurin Inhibitors

Tacrolimus and pimecrolimus are immunomodulatory agents that inhibit the transcription of proinflammatory cytokines as well as other allergic mediators and target key cells in allergic inflammation. They are available in topical formulations, and long-term studies have confirmed both efficacy and safety. Local burning at the site of application, which occurs more frequently with tacrolimus ointment, has been the most common side effect, although this is usually a transient problem. Tacrolimus ointment—0.03% for children 2–15 years of age and 0.1% for older patients—is approved for twice-daily short-term and intermittent long-term use in moderate to severe atopic dermatitis. Pimecrolimus 1% cream is approved for patients 2 years of age or older who have mild to moderate atopic dermatitis. As a precaution, patients should wear sunscreen with both drugs. In Europe, tacrolimus ointment is approved as twice weekly maintenance therapy for patients 2 years and older whose eczema lesions have cleared with re-evaluation of need for continued therapy after 12 months.

Although there is no evidence of a causal link between cancer and the use of topical calcineurin inhibitors, the FDA has issued a boxed warning for pimecrolimus cream and tacrolimus ointment because of a lack of long-term safety data (see U.S. package inserts for Elidel [Novartis] and Protopic [Astellas]). The new labeling states that these drugs are recommended as second-line treatment for short-term and noncontinuous chronic treatment and that their use in children younger than the age of 2 years is currently not recommended.

F. Tar Preparations

Tar preparations are used primarily in shampoos and rarely as bath additives. Side effects associated with tar products include skin dryness or irritation, especially if applied to inflamed skin, and, less commonly, photosensitivity reactions and folliculitis.

G. Wet Dressings

Wet dressings are used together with hydration and topical corticosteroids for the treatment of severe atopic dermatitis. They can serve as an effective barrier against the persistent scratching that often undermines therapy. Total body dressings can be applied by using wet pajamas or long underwear with dry pajamas or a sweat suit on top. Hands and feet can be covered by wet tube socks with dry tube socks on top. Alternatively, wet gauze with a layer of dry gauze over it can be used and secured in place with an elastic bandage. Dressings can be removed when they dry out, usually after several hours, and are often best tolerated at bedtime. Incorrect use of wet dressings can result in chilling, maceration of the skin, or secondary infection.

H. Anti-Infective Therapy

Systemic antibiotic therapy may be important when treating atopic dermatitis secondarily infected with *S aureus*. For limited areas of involvement, a topical antibiotic such as mupirocin or retapamulin ointment may be effective. A first- or second-generation cephalosporin or semisynthetic penicillin is usually the first choice for oral therapy, as erythromycin-resistant organisms are fairly common. Overuse may result in colonization by methicillin-resistant *S aureus*. Some pediatric dermatologists have recommended bleach baths (6% sodium hypochlorite, ½ cup in a full tub of water) two times per week in combination with nasal mupirocin (twice daily for 5 consecutive days per month) for patients with recurrent methicillin-resistant *S aureus*.

Disseminated eczema herpeticum usually requires treatment with systemic acyclovir. Patients with recurrent cutaneous herpetic lesions can be given prophylactic oral acyclovir. Superficial dermatophytosis and *Malassezia sympodialis* infection can be treated with topical or (rarely) systemic antifungal agents.

I. Antipruritic Agents

Pruritus is usually the least well-tolerated symptom of atopic dermatitis. Oral antihistamines and anxiolytics may be effective owing to their tranquilizing and sedating effects and can be taken mostly in the evening to avoid daytime somnolence. Nonsedating antihistamines may be less effective in treating pruritus, although beneficial effects have been reported in blinded studies. Use of topical antihistamines and local anesthetics should be avoided because of potential sensitization.

J. Recalcitrant Disease

Patients who are erythrodermic or who appear toxic may need to be hospitalized. Hospitalization may also be appropriate for those with severe disease who fail outpatient management. Marked clinical improvement often occurs when the patient is removed from environmental allergens or stressors. In the hospital, compliance with therapy can be monitored, the patient and family can receive intense education, and controlled provocative challenges can be conducted to help identify triggering factors.

Limited published data are available on use of cyclosporine in children treated with both continuous and intermittent therapy (5 mg/kg daily) for up to 1 year. Patients treated with this agent should have their dose titrated to the lowest effective dose after the disease is brought under control with appropriate monitoring, under the care of a specialist familiar with the drug. Mycophenolate mofetil has also been shown to be safe and effective in children with severe atopic dermatitis although this was a retrospective case series.

Ultraviolet light therapy can be useful for chronic recalcitrant atopic dermatitis in a subset of patients under the supervision of a dermatologist. Photochemotherapy with oral methoxypsoralen therapy followed by UVA (ultraviolet A) has been used in a limited number of children with severe atopic dermatitis unresponsive to other therapy, and significant improvement has been noted. However, the increased long-term risk of cutaneous malignancies from this therapy prevents its widespread use.

K. Experimental and Unproved Therapies

Subcutaneous desensitization to dust mite allergen has been shown to improve atopic dermatitis in adult patients and one blinded, placebo-controlled study of sublingual desensitization in dust mite allergic children showed benefit in mild-moderate atopic dermatitis; however, further controlled trials are needed before this form of therapy can be recommended for atopic dermatitis. Treatment of atopic dermatitis with high-dose intravenous immunoglobulin and omalizumab is currently investigational. Although disturbances in the metabolism of essential fatty acids have been reported in patients with atopic dermatitis, controlled trials with fish oil and evening primrose have shown no clinical benefit.

Prognosis

While many children, especially those with mild disease will outgrow their atopic dermatitis, patients with Filaggrin gene mutations are more likely to have more persistent and severe disease. In addition, these patients appear to be the ones at greater risk for developing asthma and allergic sensitizations.

Akdis CA et al: Diagnosis and treatment of atopic dermatitis in children and adults: European Academy of Allergology and Clinical Immunology/American Academy of Allergy, Asthma and Immunology/PRACTALL Consensus Report. J Allergy Clin Immunol 2006;118:152 [PMID: 16815151].

Boguniewicz M et al: A multidisciplinary approach to evaluation and treatment of atopic dermatitis. Semin Cutan Med Surg 2008;27:115 [PMID: 18620133].

Boguniewicz M et al: Recent insights into atopic dermatitis and implications for management of infectious complications. J Allergy Clin Immunol 2010;125:4 [PMID: 20109729].

Huang JT et al: Treatment of *Staphylococcus aureus* colonization in atopic dermatitis decreases disease severity. Pediatrics 2009;123:e808 [PMID: 19403473].

URTICARIA & ANGIOEDEMA

ESSENTIALS OF DIAGNOSIS & TYPICAL FEATURES

- Urticaria: erythematous, blanchable, circumscribed, pruritic, edematous papules ranging from 1 to 2 mm to several centimeters in diameter and involving the superficial dermis. Individual lesions can coalesce.
- Angioedema: edema extending into the deep dermis or subcutaneous tissues.
- Both resolve without sequelae—urticaria usually within hours (individual lesions rarely lasting up to 24 hours), angioedema within 72 hours.

General Considerations

Urticaria and angioedema are common dermatologic conditions, occurring at some time in up to 25% of the population. About half of patients will have concomitant urticaria and angioedema, whereas 40% will have only urticaria and 10% only angioedema. Urticarial lesions are arbitrarily designated as acute, lasting less than 6 weeks, or chronic, lasting more than 6 weeks. Acute versus chronic urticaria can also be distinguished by differences in histologic features. A history of atopy is common with acute urticaria or angioedema. In contrast, atopy does not appear to be a factor in chronic urticaria.

Mast cell degranulation, dilated venules, and dermal edema are present in most forms of urticaria or angioedema. The dermal inflammatory cells may be sparse or dense depending on the chronicity of the lesions. Mast cells are thought to play a critical role in the pathogenesis of urticaria or angioedema through release of a variety of vasoactive mediators. Mast cell activation and degranulation can be triggered by different stimuli, including cross-linking of Fc receptor–bound IgE by allergens or anti-FcεRI antibodies. Non–IgE-mediated mechanisms have also been identified, including complement anaphylatoxins (C3a, C5a), radiocontrast dyes, and physical stimuli. Chronic urticarial lesions have greater numbers of perivascular mononuclear cells, consisting primarily of T cells. There is also a marked increase in cutaneous mast cells. The cause of acute disease can be identified in about half of patients and includes allergens such as foods, aeroallergens, latex, drugs, and insect venoms. Infectious agents, including streptococci, mycoplasmas, hepatitis B virus, and Epstein-Barr virus, can cause acute urticaria. Urticaria or angioedema can occur after the administration of blood products or immunoglobulin. This results from immune complex formation with complement activation, vascular alterations, and triggering of mast cells by anaphylatoxins. Opiate analgesics, polymyxin B, tubocurarine, and radiocontrast media can induce acute urticaria by direct mast cell activation. These disorders can also occur following ingestion of aspirin or nonsteroidal anti-inflammatory agents (see later section on Adverse Reactions to Drugs & Biologicals).

Physical urticarias represent a heterogeneous group of disorders in which urticaria or angioedema is triggered by physical stimuli, including pressure, cold, heat, water, or vibrations. Dermographism is the most common form of physical urticaria, affecting up to 4% of the population and occurring at skin sites subjected to mechanical stimuli. Many physical urticarias are considered to be acute because the lesions are usually rapid in onset, with resolution within hours. However, symptoms can recur for months to years. The cause of chronic urticaria is usually not due to allergies and typically cannot be determined. It can be associated with an underlying systemic disease such as thyroid disease. Some studies have demonstrated IgG autoantibodies directed at the high-affinity receptor for IgE or at IgE, suggesting that chronic urticaria may be an autoimmune disease.

Clinical Findings

A. Symptoms and Signs

Cold-induced urticaria or angioedema can occur within minutes of exposure to a decreased ambient temperature or as the skin is warmed following direct cold contact. Systemic features include headache, wheezing, and syncope. If the entire body is cooled, as may occur during swimming, hypotension and collapse can occur. Two forms of dominantly inherited cold urticaria have been described. The immediate form is known as familial cold urticaria, in which erythematous macules appear rather than wheals, along with fever, arthralgias, and leukocytosis. The delayed form consists of erythematous, deep swellings that develop 9–18 hours after local cold challenge without immediate lesions.

In solar urticaria, which occurs within minutes after exposure to light of appropriate wavelength, pruritus is followed by morbilliform erythema and urticaria.

Cholinergic urticaria occurs after increases in core body and skin temperatures and typically develops after a warm bath or shower, exercise, or episodes of fever. Occasional episodes are triggered by stress or the ingestion of certain foods. The eruption appears as small punctate wheals surrounded by extensive areas of erythema. Rarely, the urticarial lesions become confluent and angioedema develops. Associated features can include one or more of the following: headache, syncope, bronchospasm, abdominal pain, vomiting, and diarrhea. In severe cases, systemic anaphylaxis may develop. In pressure urticaria or angioedema, red, deep, painful swelling occurs immediately or 4–6 hours after the skin has been exposed to pressure. The immediate form is often associated with dermographism. The delayed form, which may be associated with fever, chills, and arthralgias, may be accompanied by elevated erythrocyte sedimentation rate and leukocytosis. Lesions are frequently diffuse, tender, and painful rather than pruritic. They typically resolve within 48 hours.

B. Laboratory Findings

Laboratory tests are selected on the basis of the history and physical findings. Testing for specific IgE antibody to food or inhalant allergens may be helpful in implicating a potential cause. Specific tests for physical urticarias, such as an ice cube test or a pressure test, may be indicated. Intradermal injection of methacholine reproduces clinical symptoms locally in about one-third of patients with cholinergic urticaria. A throat culture for streptococcal infection may be warranted with acute urticaria. In chronic urticaria, selected screening studies to look for an underlying disease may be indicated, including a complete blood count, erythrocyte sedimentation rate, biochemistry panel, and urinalysis. Antithyroid antibodies may be considered. Intradermal testing with the patient's serum has been suggested as a method of detecting histamine-releasing activity, including autoantibodies (autologous serum skin test). Basophil and mast cell activation markers including CD63 and CD203c have been shown to be upregulated in patients with well-characterized autoimmune urticaria. Other tests should be done based on suspicion of a specific underlying disease. If the history or appearance of the urticarial lesions suggests vasculitis, a skin biopsy for immunofluorescence is indicated. Patient diaries occasionally may be helpful to determine the cause of recurrent hives. A trial of food or drug elimination may be considered.

Differential Diagnosis

Urticarial lesions are usually easily recognized—the major dilemma is the etiologic diagnosis. Lesions of urticarial vasculitis typically last for more than 24 hours. "Papular urticaria" is a term used to characterize multiple papules from insect bites, found especially on the extremities, and is not true urticaria. Angioedema can be distinguished from other forms of edema because it is transient, asymmetrical, and nonpitting and does not occur predominantly in dependent areas. Hereditary angioedema is a rare autosomal dominant disorder caused by a quantitative or functional deficiency of C1-esterase inhibitor and characterized by episodic, frequently severe, nonpruritic angioedema of the skin, gastrointestinal tract, or upper respiratory tract. Life-threatening laryngeal angioedema may occur.

Complications

In severe cases of cholinergic urticaria, systemic anaphylaxis may develop. In cold-induced disease, sudden cooling of the entire body as can occur with swimming can result in hypotension and collapse.

Treatment

A. General Measures

The most effective treatment is identification and avoidance of the triggering agent. Underlying infection should be treated appropriately. Patients with physical urticarias should avoid the relevant physical stimulus. Patients with cold urticaria should be counseled not to swim alone and prescribed autoinjectable epinephrine in case of generalized mast cell degranulation with immersion in cold water or other widespread cold exposures.

B. Antihistamines

For the majority of patients, H_1 antihistamines given orally or systemically are the mainstay of therapy. Antihistamines are more effective when given on an ongoing basis rather than after lesions appear. For breakthrough symptoms, the dose may need to be increased. In the case of cold urticaria, the best treatment appears to be cyproheptadine. Cholinergic urticaria can be treated with hydroxyzine and dermographism with hydroxyzine or diphenhydramine. The addition of H_2 antihistamines may benefit some patients who fail to respond to H_1-receptor antagonists alone. Second-generation antihistamines (discussed previously under Allergic Rhinoconjunctivitis) are long acting, show good tissue levels, are non- or minimally sedating at usual dosing levels, and lack anticholinergic effects. In adolescents who are of driving age or operate machinery, nonsedating antihistamines should be used during the day and sedating antihistamines at bedtime, if needed. Patients with urticaria may require treatment with higher than usual doses of antihistamines.

C. Corticosteroids

Although corticosteroids are usually not indicated in the treatment of acute or chronic urticaria, severe recalcitrant cases may require alternate-day therapy in an attempt to diminish disease activity and facilitate control with antihistamines. Systemic corticosteroids may also be needed in the treatment of urticaria or angioedema secondary to necrotizing vasculitis, an uncommon occurrence in patients with serum sickness or collagen-vascular disease.

D. Other Pharmacologic Agents

Limited studies suggest that some patients may benefit from treatment with a leukotriene-receptor antagonist. The tricyclic antidepressant doxepin blocks both H_1 and H_2 histamine receptors and may be particularly useful in chronic urticaria, although its use may be limited by the sedating side effect. A limited number of patients—including euthyroid patients—with chronic urticaria and antithyroid antibodies have improved when given thyroid hormone, although this treatment remains controversial. Treatment of chronic urticaria with hydroxychloroquine, sulfasalazine, cyclosporine, intravenous immune globulin, or omalizumab should be considered investigational.

Prognosis

Spontaneous remission of urticaria and angioedema is frequent, but some patients have a prolonged course, especially those with physical urticaria. In one natural history study, approximately 58% of children with chronic urticaria became symptom free after 6 months. Reassurance is important, because this disorder can cause significant frustration. Periodic follow-up is indicated, particularly for patients with laryngeal edema, to monitor for possible underlying cause.

Zuberbier T et al: EAACI/GA2LEN/EDF/WAO guideline: Definition, classification and diagnosis of urticaria. Allergy 2009:64:1417 [PMID: 19772512].

Zuberbier T et al: EAACI/GA2LEN/EDF/WAO guideline: Management of urticaria. Allergy 2009;64:1427 [PMID: 19772513].

ANAPHYLAXIS

ESSENTIALS OF DIAGNOSIS & TYPICAL FEATURES

- Serious allergic reaction that is rapid in onset and may cause death after exposure to allergen in a previously sensitized person.
- Generalized pruritus, anxiety, urticaria, angioedema, throat fullness, wheezing, dyspnea, hypotension, and collapse.

General Considerations

Anaphylaxis is an acute life-threatening clinical syndrome that occurs when large quantities of inflammatory mediators are rapidly released from mast cells and basophils after exposure to an allergen in a previously sensitized patient. Anaphylactoid reactions mimic anaphylaxis but are not mediated by IgE antibodies. They may be mediated by anaphylatoxins such as C3a or C5a or through nonimmune mast cell degranulating agents. Some of the common causes of anaphylaxis or anaphylactoid reactions are listed in Table 38–6. Idiopathic anaphylaxis by definition has no recognized external cause. The clinical history is the most important tool in making the diagnosis of anaphylaxis.

Clinical Findings

A. Symptoms and Signs

The history is the most important tool to determine whether a patient has had anaphylaxis. The symptoms and signs of anaphylaxis depend on the organs affected. Onset typically occurs within minutes after exposure to the offending agent and can be short-lived, protracted, or biphasic, with recurrence after several hours despite treatment.

Anaphylaxis is highly likely when any one of the following three criteria is fulfilled:

1. Acute onset of an illness (minutes to several hours) with involvement of the skin, mucosal tissue, or both

Table 38–6. Common causes of systemic allergic and pseudoallergic reactions.

Causes of anaphylaxis
Drugs
Antibiotics
Anesthetic agents
Foods
Peanuts, tree nuts, shellfish, and others
Biologicals
Latex
Insulin
Allergen extracts
Antisera
Blood products
Enzymes
Monoclonal antibodies (eg, omalizumab)
Insect venoms
Radiocontrast media
Aspirin and other nonsteroidal anti-inflammatory drugs
Anesthetic agents
Idiopathic

(eg, generalized hives, pruritus or flushing, swollen lips-tongue-uvula) *and at least one of the following*:

a. Respiratory compromise (eg, dyspnea, wheeze-bronchospasm, stridor, reduced peak expiratory flow, hypoxemia)
b. Reduced blood pressure or associated symptoms of end-organ dysfunction (eg, hypotonia [collapse], syncope, incontinence)

2. Two or more of the following that occur rapidly after exposure to a *likely* allergen for that patient (minutes to several hours):
   a. Involvement of the skin-mucosal tissue (eg, generalized urticaria, itch-flush, swollen lips-tongue-uvula)
   b. Respiratory compromise (eg, dyspnea, wheeze-bronchospasm, stridor, reduced PEFR, hypoxemia)
   c. Reduced blood pressure or associated symptoms (eg, hypotonia [collapse], syncope, incontinence)
   d. Persistent gastrointestinal symptoms (eg, crampy abdominal pain, vomiting)
3. Reduced blood pressure after exposure to a *known* allergen for that patient (minutes to several hours)
   a. Infants and children: low systolic blood pressure (age specific) or greater than 30% decrease in systolic pressure
   b. Low systolic blood pressure in children, defined as less than 70 mm Hg in those aged from 1 month to 1 year, less than (70 mm Hg + [2 × age]) in those 1–10 years of age, and less than 90 mm Hg in those 11–17 years

B. Laboratory Findings

An absence of laboratory findings does not rule out anaphylaxis. Tryptase released by mast cells can be measured in the serum and may be helpful when the diagnosis of anaphylaxis is in question. The blood sample should be obtained within 3 hours of onset of the reaction, although tryptase levels are often normal, particularly in individuals with food-induced anaphylaxis. The complete blood count may show an elevated hematocrit due to hemoconcentration. Elevation of serum creatine kinase, aspartate aminotransferase, and lactic dehydrogenase may be seen with myocardial involvement. Electrocardiographic abnormalities may include ST-wave depression, bundle branch block, and various arrhythmias. Arterial blood gases may show hypoxemia, hypercapnia, and acidosis. The chest radiograph may show hyperinflation.

Differential Diagnosis

Although shock may be the only sign of anaphylaxis, other diagnoses should be considered, especially in the setting of sudden collapse without typical allergic findings. Other causes of shock along with cardiac arrhythmias must be ruled out. (See Chapters 12 and 14.) Respiratory failure associated with asthma may be confused with anaphylaxis. Mastocytosis, hereditary angioedema, scombroid poisoning, vasovagal reactions, vocal cord dysfunction, and anxiety attacks may cause symptoms mistaken for anaphylaxis.

Complications

Depending on the organs involved and the severity of the reaction, complications may vary from none to aspiration pneumonitis, acute tubular necrosis, bleeding diathesis, or sloughing of the intestinal mucosa. With irreversible shock, heart and brain damage can be terminal. Risk factors for fatal or near-fatal anaphylaxis include age (adolescents and young adults), reactions to peanut or tree nuts, associated asthma, strenuous exercise, and ingestion of medications such as β-blockers.

Prevention

Strict avoidance of the causative agent is extremely important. An effort to determine its cause should be made, beginning with a thorough history. Typically there is a strong temporal relationship between exposure and onset of symptoms. Testing for specific IgE to allergens with either in vitro or skin testing may be indicated. With exercise-induced anaphylaxis, patients should be instructed to exercise with another person and to stop exercising at the first sign of symptoms. If prior ingestion of food has been implicated, eating within 4 hours—perhaps up to 12 hours—before exercise should be avoided. Patients with a history of anaphylaxis should carry epinephrine for self-administration, preferably in the form of an autoinjector (eg, EpiPen, Twinject, or Adrenaclick in 0.15- and 0.3-mg doses), and they and all caregivers should be instructed on its use. When epinephrine autoinjectors are unavailable or unaffordable, patients in some communities have been provided with unsealed syringes containing premeasured epinephrine doses, but this is not the recommended form since it needs to be replaced every few months on a regular basis due to lack of stability and the use of a syringe is more unwieldy in an emergent situation. They should also carry an oral antihistamine such as diphenhydramine, preferably in liquid or fast-melt preparation to hasten absorption, and consider wearing a medical alert bracelet. Patients with idiopathic anaphylaxis may require prolonged treatment with oral corticosteroids. Specific measures for dealing with food, drug, latex, and insect venom allergies as well as radiocontrast media reactions are discussed in the next sections.

Treatment

A. General Measures

Anaphylaxis is a medical emergency that requires rapid assessment and treatment. Exposure to the triggering agent should be discontinued. Airway patency should be maintained and blood pressure and pulse monitored. Simultaneously and promptly, emergency medical services or a call for help to a resuscitation team should be made. The patient should be placed in a supine position with the legs elevated unless precluded by shortness of breath or emesis. Oxygen should be delivered by mask or nasal cannula with pulse oximetry monitoring. If the reaction is secondary to a sting or injection into an extremity, a tourniquet may be applied proximal to the site, briefly releasing it every 10–15 minutes.

B. Epinephrine

Epinephrine is the treatment of choice for anaphylaxis. Epinephrine 1:1000, 0.01 mg/kg to a maximum of 0.5 mg in adults and 0.3 mg in children, should be injected intramuscularly in the midanterolateral thigh, without delay. This dose may be repeated at intervals of 5–15 minutes as necessary for controlling symptoms and maintaining blood pressure. If the precipitating allergen has been injected intradermally or subcutaneously, absorption may be delayed by giving 0.1 mL of epinephrine subcutaneously at the injection site unless the site is a digit. There is no precisely established dosing regimen for intravenous epinephrine in anaphylaxis, but a 5–10 mcg intravenous bolus for hypotension and 0.1–0.5 mg intravenously for cardiovascular collapse has been suggested.

C. Antihistamines

Diphenhydramine, an H_1-blocker, 1–2 mg/kg up to 50 mg, can be given intramuscularly or intravenously. Intravenous antihistamines should be infused over a period of 5–10 minutes to avoid inducing hypotension. Addition of ranitidine, an H_2-blocker, 1 mg/kg up to 50 mg intravenously, may be more effective than an H_1-blocker alone, especially for hypotension, but histamine blockers should be considered second-line treatment for anaphylaxis.

D. Fluids

Treatment of persistent hypotension despite epinephrine requires restoration of intravascular volume by fluid replacement, initially with a crystalloid solution, 20–30 mL/kg in the first hour.

E. Bronchodilators

Nebulized β_2-agonists such as albuterol 0.5% solution, 2.5 mg (0.5 mL) diluted in 2–3 mL saline, or levalbuterol, 0.63 mg or 1.25 mg, may be useful for reversing bronchospasm. Intravenous methylxanthines are generally not recommended because they provide little benefit over inhaled β_2-agonists and may contribute to toxicity.

F. Corticosteroids

Although corticosteroids do not provide immediate benefit, when given early they may prevent protracted or biphasic anaphylaxis. Intravenous methylprednisolone, 50–100 mg (adult) or 1 mg/kg, maximum 50 mg (child), can be given every 4–6 hours. Oral prednisone, 1 mg/kg up to 50 mg, might be sufficient for less severe episodes.

G. Vasopressors

Hypotension refractory to epinephrine and fluids should be treated with intravenous vasopressors such as noradrenaline, vasopressin, or dopamine. (See Chapter 14.)

H. Observation

The patient should be monitored after the initial symptoms have subsided, because biphasic or protracted anaphylaxis can occur despite ongoing therapy. Biphasic reactions occur in 1%–20% of anaphylactic reactions, but no reliable clinical predictors have been identified. Observation periods should be individualized based on the severity of the initial reaction, but a reasonable time for observation is 4–6 hours in most patients, with prolonged observation or admission for severe or refractory symptoms.

Prognosis

Anaphylaxis can be fatal. In two reports describing children, adolescents, and adults who died from food-induced anaphylaxis (eg, from peanuts, tree nuts, fish, shellfish, and milk) over the past 12 years, treatment with epinephrine was delayed for more than 1 hour after onset as it was not readily accessible in the majority of subjects. The prognosis, however, is good when signs and symptoms are recognized promptly and treated aggressively, and the offending agent is subsequently avoided. Exercise-induced and idiopathic anaphylaxis may be recurrent. Because accidental exposure to the causative agent may occur, patients, parents, and caregivers must be prepared to recognize and treat anaphylaxis (emergency action plan).

Allergy Clin Immunol 2010;126(3):477–480; e1–42 [PMID: 20692689].
Simons FE et al: World Allergy Organization. World Allergy Organization anaphylaxis guidelines: Summary. J Allergy Clin Immunol 2011;127(3):587–593 e1–22 [PMID: 21377030].

ADVERSE REACTIONS TO DRUGS & BIOLOGICALS

ESSENTIALS OF DIAGNOSIS & TYPICAL FEATURES

- Most adverse drug reactions are not allergic although patients or caregivers often report them as a drug allergy.
- Antibiotics constitute the most frequent cause of allergic drug reactions.
- Reliable testing for most drugs other than penicillins and a few large protein molecules is not available.

The majority of adverse drug reactions are not immunologically mediated and may be due to idiosyncratic reactions, overdosage, pharmacologic side effects, nonspecific release of pharmacologic effector molecules, or drug interactions.

Patients or caregivers often describe an adverse drug reaction as being allergic in nature, and clinicians may document a drug allergy in the patient's medical record based solely on this history. Adverse drug reactions are any undesirable and unintended response elicited by a drug. Allergic or hypersensitivity drug reactions are adverse reactions involving immune mechanisms. Although hypersensitivity reactions account for only 5%–10% of all adverse drug reactions, they are the most serious, with 1:10,000 resulting in death. Clinicians can report adverse drug reactions and get updated information on drugs, vaccines, and biologics at the FDA's MedWatch web site.

1. Antibiotics

Antibiotics constitute the most frequent cause of allergic drug reactions. Amoxicillin, trimethoprim–sulfamethoxazole, and ampicillin are the most common causes of cutaneous drug reactions.

Most antibiotics and their metabolites are low-molecular-weight compounds that do not stimulate immunity until they have become covalently bound to a carrier protein. The penicillins and other β-lactam antibiotics, including cephalosporins, carbacephems, carbapenems, and monobactams, share a common β-lactam ring structure and a marked propensity to couple to carrier proteins. Penicilloyl is the predominant metabolite of penicillin and is called the major determinant. The other penicillin metabolites are present in low concentrations and are referred to as minor determinants. Sulfonamide reactions are mediated presumably by a reactive metabolite (hydroxylamine) produced by cytochrome P-450 oxidative metabolism. Slow acetylators appear to be at increased risk. Other risk factors for drug reactions include previous exposure, previous reaction, age (20–49 years), route (parenteral), and dose of administration (high, intermittent). Atopy does not predispose to development of a reaction, but atopic individuals have more severe reactions.

Immunopathologic reactions to antibiotics include type I (IgE-mediated) reactions resulting from a drug or metabolite interaction with preformed specific IgE bound to the surfaces of tissue mast cells or circulating basophils. Release of mediators such as histamine and leukotrienes contributes to the clinical development of angioedema, urticaria, bronchospasm, or anaphylaxis. Type II (cytotoxic) reactions involve IgG or IgM antibodies that recognize drug bound to cell membranes. In the presence of serum complement, the antibody-coated cell is either cleared or destroyed, causing drug-induced hemolytic anemia or thrombocytopenia. Type III (immune complex) reactions are caused by soluble complexes of drug or metabolite with IgG or IgM antibody. If the immune complex is deposited on blood vessel walls and activates the complement cascade, serum sickness may result. Type IV (T-cell–mediated) reactions require activated T lymphocytes that recognize a drug or its metabolite as seen in allergic contact dermatitis. Sensitization usually occurs via the topical route of administration. Immunopathologic reactions not fitting into the types I–IV classification include Stevens-Johnson syndrome, exfoliative dermatitis, and the maculopapular rash associated with penicillin or ampicillin. The prevalence of morbilliform rashes in patients given ampicillin is between 5.2% and 9.5% of treatment courses. However, patients given ampicillin during Epstein-Barr virus and cytomegalovirus infections or with acute lymphoblastic anemia have a 69%–100% incidence of non–IgE-mediated rash. Serum sickness–like reactions resemble type III reactions, although immune complexes are not documented; β-lactams, especially cefaclor, and sulfonamides have been implicated most often. They may result from an inherited propensity for hepatic biotransformation of drug into toxic or immunogenic metabolites. The incidence of "allergic" cutaneous reactions to trimethoprim–sulfamethoxazole in patients with AIDS has been reported to be as high as 70%. The mechanism is thought to relate to the severe immune dysregulation, although it may be due to glutathione deficiency resulting in toxic metabolites.

Clinical Findings

A. Symptoms and Signs

Allergic reactions can result in pruritus, urticaria, angioedema, or anaphylaxis. Serum sickness is characterized by fever, rash, lymphadenopathy, myalgias, and arthralgias. Cytotoxic drug reactions can result in symptoms and signs associated with the underlying anemia or thrombocytopenia. Delayed-type hypersensitivity may cause contact dermatitis.

B. Laboratory Findings

Skin testing is the most rapid, useful, and sensitive method of demonstrating the presence of IgE antibody to a specific allergen. Skin testing to nonpenicillin antibiotics may be difficult, however, because many immunologic reactions are due to metabolites rather than to the parent drug and because the relevant metabolites for most drugs other than penicillin have not been identified. Because metabolites are usually low-molecular-weight haptens, they must combine with carrier proteins to be useful for diagnosis. In the case of contact sensitivity reactions to topical antibiotics, a 48-hour patch test can be useful.

Solid-phase in vitro immunoassays for IgE to penicillins are available for identification of IgE to penicilloyl but are considerably less sensitive and give less information than skin testing. Assays for specific IgG and IgM have been shown to correlate with a drug reaction in immune cytopenias, but in most other instances such assays are not clinically useful. Skin testing for immediate hypersensitivity is helpful only in predicting reactions caused by IgE antibodies. Most nonpruritic maculopapular rashes will not be predicted by skin testing.

Approximately 80% of patients with a history of penicillin allergy will have negative skin tests. Penicillin therapy in patients with a history of an immediate hypersensitivity reaction to penicillin, but with negative skin tests to both penicilloyl and the minor determinant mixture, is accompanied by a 1%–3% chance of urticaria or other mild allergic reactions at some time during therapy, with anaphylaxis occurring in less than 0.1% of patients. In contrast, the predictive value of a positive skin test is approximately 60%. Testing with penicilloyl linked to polylysine (PPL) alone has a sensitivity of about 76%; use of both PPL and penicillin G (used as a minor determinant) increases sensitivity to about 95%. Not using the minor determinant mixture in skin testing can result in failure to predict potential anaphylactic reactions. Unfortunately, the minor determinant mixture is still not commercially available, although most academic allergy centers make their own. Approximately 4% of subjects tested who have no history of penicillin allergy have positive skin tests, and most fatalities occur in patients with no prior history of reaction. Rarely, patients may have skin test reactivity only to a specific semisynthetic penicillin. Resensitization in skin test–negative children occurs infrequently (< 1%) after a course of oral antibiotic. Of note, the manufacturing of the major determinant of penicillin testing reagent Pre-Pen (penicilloyl-polylysine) in the United States was discontinued for several years. AllerQuest received approval from the FDA in January 2008 to manufacture Pre-Pen and the product is once again available (distributed by ALK-Abello, Inc).

The degree of cross-reactivity of determinants formed from cephalosporins with IgE to other β-lactam drugs remains unresolved, especially because haptens that may be unique to cephalosporin metabolism remain unknown. The degree of clinical cross-reactivity is much lower than the invitro cross-reactivity. A clinical adverse reaction rate of 3%–7% for cephalosporins may be expected in patients with positive histories of penicillin allergy. Antibodies to the second- and third-generation cephalosporins appear to be directed at the unique side chains rather than at the common ring structure. The present literature suggests that a positive skin test to a cephalosporin used at a concentration of 1 mg/mL would place the patient at increased risk for an allergic reaction to that antibiotic. However, a negative skin test would not exclude sensitivity to a potentially relevant metabolite. One review concluded that there is no increased incidence of allergy to second- and third-generation cephalosporins in patients with penicillin allergy and that penicillin skin testing does not identify patients who develop cephalosporin allergy. However, another study suggested that although only 2% of penicillin-allergic patients would react to a cephalosporin, they would be at risk for anaphylaxis.

Carbacephems (loracarbef) are similar to cephalosporins, although the degree of cross-reactivity is undetermined. Carbapenems (imipenem) represent another class of β-lactam antibiotics with a bicyclic nucleus and a high degree of cross-reactivity with penicillin although recent prospective studies suggest an incidence of cross-reactivity on skin testing of approximately 1%. Monobactams (aztreonam) contain a monocyclic rather than bicyclic ring structure, and limited data suggest that aztreonam can be safely administered to most penicillin-allergic subjects. In contrast, administration of aztreonam to a patient with ceftazidime allergy may be associated with increased risk of allergic reaction due to similarity of side chains.

Skin testing for non–β-lactam antibiotics is less reliable, because the relevant degradation products are for the most part unknown or multivalent reagents are unavailable.

Treatment

A. General Measures

Withdrawal of the implicated drug is usually a central component of management. Acute IgE-mediated reactions such as anaphylaxis, urticaria, and angioedema are treated according to established therapeutic guidelines that include the use of epinephrine, H_1- and H_2-receptor blocking agents, volume replacement, and systemic corticosteroids (see previous sections). Antibiotic-induced immune cytopenias can be managed by withdrawal of the offending agent or reduction in dose. Drug-induced serum sickness can be suppressed by drug withdrawal, antihistamines, and corticosteroids. Contact allergy can be managed by avoidance and treatment with antihistamines and topical corticosteroids. Reactions such as toxic epidermal necrolysis and Stevens-Johnson syndrome require immediate drug withdrawal and supportive care.

B. Alternative Therapy

If possible, subsequent therapy should be with an alternative drug that has therapeutic actions similar to the drug in question but with no immunologic cross-reactivity.

C. Desensitization

Administering gradually increasing doses of an antibiotic either orally or parentally over a period of hours to days may be considered if alternative therapy is not acceptable. This should be done only by a physician familiar with desensitization, typically in an intensive care setting. Of note, desensitization is only effective for the course of therapy for which the patient was desensitized, unless maintained on a chronic prophylactic dose of the medication as patients revert from a desensitized to allergic state after the drug is discontinued. In addition, desensitization does not reduce or prevent non–IgE-mediated reactions. Patients with Stevens-Johnson syndrome should not be desensitized because of the high mortality rate.

Prognosis

The prognosis is good when drug allergens are identified early and avoided. Stevens-Johnson syndrome and toxic epidermal necrolysis may be associated with a high mortality rate.

2. Latex Allergy

General Considerations

Allergic reactions to latex and rubber products have become increasingly common since the institution of universal precautions for exposure to bodily fluids. Children with spina bifida appear to have a unique sensitivity to latex, perhaps because of early and frequent latex exposure as well as altered neuroimmune interactions. Atopy—especially symptomatic latex allergy—appears to be significantly increased in patients with spina bifida experiencing anaphylaxis during general anesthesia. Other conditions requiring chronic or recurrent exposure to latex such as urogenital anomalies and ventriculoperitoneal shunt have also been associated with latex hypersensitivity. The combination of atopy and frequent exposure seems to synergistically increase the risk of latex hypersensitivity.

Latex is the milky fluid obtained by tapping the cultivated rubber tree, *Hevea brasiliensis*. During manufacture of latex products, various antioxidants and accelerators such as thiurams, carbamates, and mercaptobenzothiazoles are added. IgE from latex-sensitized individuals reacts with different protein components, supporting the notion that more than one clinically important latex antigen exists. New allergenic epitopes are generated during the manufacturing process. Thus, polypeptides from latex glove extracts vary both quantitatively and qualitatively with different brands and lots of gloves. Identification of the causative antigens is important because it may be possible to alter the manufacturing process to reduce the final allergen content.

Latex is ubiquitous in medical settings, and many sources may be inconspicuous. Synthetic alternatives to some latex products—including gloves, dressings, and tape—are available. Avoidance of contact with latex-containing items, however, may be insufficient to prevent allergic reactions, because lubricating powders may serve as vehicles for aerosolized latex antigens. The use of powder-free latex gloves is an important control measure for airborne latex allergen.

Nonmedical sources of latex are also common and include balloons, toys, rubber bands, erasers, condoms, and shoe soles. Pacifiers and bottle nipples have also been implicated as sources of latex allergen, although these products are molded rather than dipped, and allergic reactions to molded products are less common. Latex-allergic patients and their caregivers must be continuously vigilant for hidden sources of exposure.

Clinical Findings

A. Symptoms and Signs

The clinical manifestations of IgE-mediated reactions to latex can involve the full spectrum of symptoms associated with mast cell degranulation. Localized pruritus and urticaria occur after cutaneous contact; conjunctivitis and rhinitis can result from aerosol exposure or direct facial contact. Systemic reactions, including bronchospasm, laryngospasm, and hypotension, may occur with more substantial exposure or in extremely sensitive individuals. Finally, vascular collapse and shock leading to fatal cardiovascular events may occur. Intraoperative anaphylaxis represents a common and serious manifestation of latex allergy.

Allergic contact dermatitis to rubber products typically appears 24–48 hours after contact. The primary allergens include accelerators and antioxidants used in the manufacturing process. The diagnosis is established by patch testing. Shoe soles are an important source of exposure. The skin lesions appear primarily as a patchy eczema on exposed surfaces, although reactions can become generalized.

B. Laboratory Findings

Epicutaneous prick testing is a rapid, inexpensive, and sensitive test that detects the presence of latex-specific IgE on skin mast cells although a standardized antigen is not yet commercially available. Reports of life-threatening anaphylactic events have been associated with skin testing to latex, and intradermal testing may be especially dangerous.

Immunoassay testing involves the in vitro measurement of specific IgE, which binds latex antigens. Antigen sources used for testing have included native plant extracts, raw latex, and finished products. When compared with a history of latex-induced symptoms or positive skin tests, the sensitivity of immunoassays testing for latex antigens ranges from 50% to 100% with specificity between 63% and 100%. These broad ranges may reflect the patient population studied and the source of latex antigen as well as the assay employed. A positive immunoassay test to latex in the presence of a highly suggestive latex allergy history is useful and may circumvent the potential concerns associated with prick skin testing in certain patients. Patch testing with standardized T.R.U.E. Test or other sources of antigens can identify antigens used in the manufacturing of latex products that can cause allergic contact dermatitis.

Cross-reactivity has been demonstrated between latex and a number of other antigens such as foods. Banana, avocado, and chestnut have been found to be antigenically similar to latex both immunologically and clinically.

Complications

Complications may be similar to those caused by other allergens. Prolonged exposure to aerosolized latex may lead to persistent asthma. Chronic allergic contact dermatitis, especially on the hands, can lead to functional disability.

Treatment

Avoidance remains the cornerstone of treatment for latex allergy. Prevention and supportive therapy are the most common methods for managing this problem. Patients identified as being allergic to latex may need to have a personal supply of vinyl or latex-free gloves for use when visiting a physician or dentist. "Hypoallergenic gloves" are poorly classified with respect to their ability to induce IgE-mediated reactions; the FDA currently uses this term to designate products that have a reduced capacity to induce contact dermatitis. Nonlatex gloves include nitrile and vinyl ones. A glove made from guayule latex has been approved by the FDA. Autoinjectable epinephrine and medical identification bracelets may be prescribed for latex-allergic patients along with avoidance counseling.

Prophylactic premedication of latex-allergic individuals has been used in some surgical patients at high risk for latex allergy. The rationale for this therapy is derived from the pretreatment protocols developed for iodinated radiocontrast media and anesthetic reactions. Although there has been some success using this regimen, anaphylaxis has occurred despite pretreatment. This approach should not substitute for careful avoidance measures.

Prognosis

Owing to the ubiquitous nature of natural rubber, the prognosis is guarded for patients with severe latex allergy. Chronic exposure to airborne latex particles may lead to chronic asthma. Chronic dermatitis can lead to functional disability.

3. Vaccines

Mumps-measles-rubella (MMR) vaccine has been shown to be safe in egg-allergic patients (although rare reactions to gelatin or neomycin can occur). Although the amount of ovalbumin in influenza vaccine is variable, content does not appear to predict risk of reaction and several studies suggest that egg allergic children can safely receive influenza vaccine injection as a single full dose. While skin prick testing is no longer recommended, administration in a 2-step protocol (1/10 dose, 30 minute observation, 9/10 dose, 30 minute observation) is an option. In addition, the live intranasal influenza vaccine is contraindicated in egg-allergic children.

4. Radiocontrast Media

Non–IgE-mediated anaphylactoid reactions may occur with radiocontrast media with up to a 30% reaction rate on reexposure. Management involves using a low-molarity agent and premedication with prednisone, diphenhydramine, and possibly an H_2-blocker.

5. Insulin

Approximately 50% of patients receiving insulin have positive skin tests, but IgE-mediated reactions occur rarely. Insulin resistance is mediated by IgG. If less than 24 hours has elapsed after an allergic reaction to insulin, do not discontinue insulin but rather reduce the dose by one-third, then increase by 2–5 units per injection. Skin testing and desensitization are necessary if the interval between the allergic reaction and subsequent dose is greater than 24 hours.

6. Local Anesthetics

Less than 1% of reactions to local anesthetics are IgE-mediated. Management involves selecting a local anesthetic from another class. Esters of benzoic acid include benzocaine and procaine; amides include lidocaine and mepivacaine. Alternatively, the patient can be skin tested with the suspected agent, followed by a provocative challenge. To rule out paraben sensitivity, skin testing can be done with 1% lidocaine from a multidose vial.

7. Aspirin & Other Nonsteroidal Anti-Inflammatory Drugs

Adverse reactions to aspirin and nonsteroidal anti-inflammatory drugs (NSAIDs) include urticaria and angioedema; rhinosinusitis, nasal polyps, and asthma; anaphylactoid reactions; and NSAID-related hypersensitivity pneumonitis. After a systemic reaction, a refractory period of 2–7 days occurs. Most aspirin-sensitive patients tolerate sodium salicylate. All NSAIDs inhibiting cyclooxygenase (COX) cross-react with aspirin. Cross-reactivity between aspirin and tartrazine (yellow dye No. 5) has not been substantiated in controlled trials. No skin test or in vitro test is available to diagnose aspirin sensitivity. Oral challenge can induce severe bronchospasm. Desensitization and cross-desensitization to NSAIDs can be achieved in most patients and maintained for a long term. Leukotriene-receptor antagonists or 5-lipoxygenase inhibitors attenuate the reaction to aspirin challenge and may be beneficial adjunct treatment in aspirin-sensitive asthmatic patients. Studies suggest that COX-2 inhibitors may be tolerated by patients with ASA-induced asthma.

8. Biological Agents

In recent years, a growing number of biological agents have become available for the treatment of autoimmune, neoplastic, cardiovascular, infectious, and allergic diseases, among others. Their use may be associated with a variety of adverse reactions, including hypersensitivity reactions. The FDA issued a boxed warning regarding risk of anaphylaxis and need for patient monitoring with use of omalizumab (see section on Pharmacologic Therapy under Treatment, Chronic Asthma, earlier). Updated information can be found at the FDA's MedWatch web site under Vaccines, Blood, and Biologics.

9. Hypersensitivity to Retroviral Agents

Adverse drug reactions are being reported with increasing frequency to antiretroviral agents, including reverse transcriptase inhibitors, protease inhibitors, and fusion inhibitors. Hypersensitivity to abacavir is a well-described, multiorgan, potentially life-threatening reaction that occurs in HIV-infected children. The reaction is independent of dose with onset generally within 9–11 days of initiation of drug therapy. Rechallenge can be accompanied by significant hypotension and given a mortality rate of 0.03%; hypersensitivity to abacavir is an absolute contraindication for subsequent use. Prophylaxis with prednisolone does not appear to prevent hypersensitivity reactions to abacavir. Importantly, genetic susceptibility appears to be conferred by the HLA-B*5701 allele with a positive predictive value of > 70% and negative predictive value of 95%–98%. Genetic screening would be cost-effective in Caucasians, but not in African or Asian populations as their HLA-B*5701 allele frequency is < 1%.

10. Adverse Reactions to Chemotherapeutic Agents

A number of chemotherapeutic agents, including monoclonal antibodies, have been implicated in hypersensitivity reactions. Rapid desensitization to unrelated agents, including carboplatin, paclitaxel, and rituximab, has been reported. This 12-step protocol appeared to be successful in both IgE- and non–IgE-mediated reactions.

Centers for Disease Control and Prevention, National Immunization Program. Available at: http://www.cdc.gov/nip

Cernadas JR et al: General considerations on rapid desensitization for drug hypersensitivity—a consensus statement. Allergy 2010:65:1357 [PMID: 20716314].

Davis CM et al: Diagnosis and management of HIV drug hypersensitivity. J Allergy Clin Immunol 2008;121:826 [PMID: 18190954].

FDA MedWatch. Available at: http://www.fda.gov/medwatch/index.html

Greenhawt MJ et al: Administering influenza vaccine to egg allergic recipients: A focused practice parameter update. 2011;106:11 [PMID: 21195939].

Joint Task Force on Practice Parameters et al: Drug allergy: An updated practice parameter. Ann Allergy Asthma Immunol 2010;105:259 [PMID: 20934625].

Kelso JM et al: Adverse reactions to vaccines. Ann Allergy Asthma Immunol 2009;103:S1 [PMID: 19886402].

Pichichero ME: A review of evidence supporting the American Academy of Pediatrics recommendation for prescribing cephalosporin antibiotics for penicillin-allergic patients. Pediatrics 2005;115:1048 [PMID: 15805383].

Romano A et al: Diagnosis and management of drug hypersensitivity reactions. J Allergy Clin Immunol 2011;127:S67 [PMID: 21354502].

Segal AR et al: Cutaneous reactions to drugs in children. Pediatrics 2007;120:e1082 [PMID: 17908729].

Vultaggio A et al: Immediate adverse reactions to biologicals: From pathogenic mechanisms to prophylactic management. Curr Opin Allergy Clin Immunol 2011;11:262 [PMID: 21460715].

FOOD ALLERGY

ESSENTIALS OF DIAGNOSIS & TYPICAL FEATURES

- Temporal relationship between ingestion of a suspected food and onset of allergic symptoms.
- For IgE-mediated reactions, positive prick skin test or invitro test to a suspected food allergen confirmed by a double-blind, placebo-controlled food challenge (except in cases of anaphylaxis).

General Considerations

The recently released Guidelines for the Diagnosis and Management of Food Allergy in the United States: Report of the NIAID-Sponsored Expert Panel (henceforth referred to as the Food Allergy Guidelines) defines a food allergy as an adverse health effect arising from a specific immune response that occurs reproducibly on exposure to a given food. Food allergy affects approximately 8% of young children and 3%–4% of adults. The most common IgE-associated food allergens in children are milk egg, peanut, soy, wheat, tree nuts, fish, and shellfish. In older patients, fish, shellfish, peanut, and tree nuts are most often involved in allergic reactions, and may be lifelong allergies. The highest prevalence of food allergy is found in children with moderate to severe atopic dermatitis, with approximately 35% affected, whereas chronic conditions such as urticaria and asthma are much less likely due solely to food allergy. Of note, food allergy can be caused by non–IgE-mediated mechanisms, in conditions such as food protein–induced enterocolitis or proctocolitis. It can also be caused by mixed IgE- and non–IgE-mediated mechanisms, as in eosinophilic esophagitis and gastroenteritis (Table 38–7).

Table 38–7. Food allergy disorders.

IgE-mediated
Gastrointestinal: pollen-food allergy syndrome, immediate GI anaphylaxis
Cutaneous: urticaria, angioedema, morbilliform rashes, and flushing
Respiratory: acute rhinoconjunctivitis, acute wheezing
Generalized: anaphylactic shock
Mixed IgE- and non-IgE-mediated
Gastrointestinal: eosinophilic esophagitis/gastroenteritis/colitis
Cutaneous: atopic dermatitis
Respiratory: asthma
Non-IgE-mediated
Gastrointestinal: food protein-induced enterocolitis, proctocolitis, and enteropathy syndromes; celiac disease
Cutaneous: contact dermatitis, dermatitis herpetiformis
Respiratory: food-induced pulmonary hemosiderosis (Heiner syndrome)

Some adverse reactions diagnosed by patients or physicians as food allergy involve non–immune-mediated mechanisms such as pharmacologic and metabolic mechanisms, reactions to food toxins, or intolerances (eg, lactose intolerance). These will not be covered in this chapter.

Clinical Findings

A. Symptoms and Signs

A thorough medical history is crucial in identify symptoms associated with potential food allergy; a history of a temporal relationship between the ingestion of a suspected food and onset of a reaction—as well as the nature and duration of symptoms observed—is important in establishing the diagnosis. For all IgE-mediated reactions, reactions to foods occur within minutes and up to 2 hours after ingestion. For the non–IgE-mediated and mixed disorders, reactions can be delayed in onset for more than several hours, such as in food protein–induced enterocolitis, to possibly days later with onset of vomiting or an eczema flare after food exposure due to eosinophilic esophagitis or atopic dermatitis, respectively. At times, acute symptoms may occur, but the cause may not be obvious because of hidden food allergens. A symptom diary kept for 7–14 days may be helpful in establishing an association between ingestion of foods and symptoms and also provides a baseline observation for the pattern of symptom expression. It is important to record both the form in which the food was ingested and the foods ingested concurrently.

Hives, flushing, facial angioedema, and mouth or throat itching are common. In severe cases, angioedema of the tongue, uvula, pharynx, or upper airway can occur. Contact urticaria can occur without systemic symptoms in some children. Gastrointestinal symptoms include abdominal discomfort or pain, nausea, vomiting, and diarrhea. Children with food allergy may occasionally have isolated rhinoconjunctivitis or wheezing. Rarely, anaphylaxis to food may involve only cardiovascular collapse (see section on Anaphylaxis, earlier).

B. Laboratory Findings

Typically, fewer than 50% of histories of food allergy will be confirmed by blinded food challenge (although this percentage is much higher in food-induced anaphylaxis). Prick skin testing is useful to rule out a suspected food allergen, because the predictive value is high for a properly performed negative test with an extract of good quality (negative predictive accuracy of > 95%). In contrast, the predictive value for a positive test is approximately 50%. Serum food-specific IgE tests have lower specificity and positive predictive values. In contrast, food-specific IgE levels to milk, egg, peanut, and fish proteins have been established with the Phadia ImmunoCAP assay correlating with a greater than 95% chance of a clinical reaction, but values have not been established for other foods. A list of nonstandardized and unproven procedures for the diagnosis of food allergy, including the measurement of allergen-specific-IgG to foods, is provided in the Food Allergy Guidelines.

The double-blind, placebo-controlled food challenge is considered the gold standard for diagnosing food allergy, except in severe reactions. If there is high suspicion of possible allergic reactivity to a food with a negative skin test or an undetectable serum IgE level (or both), a food challenge may be necessary to confirm the presence or absence of allergy. Even when multiple food allergies are suspected, most patients will test positive to three or fewer foods on blinded challenge. Therefore, extensive elimination diets are almost never indicated, and an evaluation by an allergist is preferred before multiple foods are eliminated from the diet unnecessarily. Elimination without controlled challenge is a less desirable but at times more practical approach for suspected food allergy. Elimination diets and food challenges may also be the only tools for evaluation of suspected non–IgE-mediated food reactions.

Differential Diagnosis

Repeated vomiting in infancy may be due to pyloric stenosis or gastroesophageal reflux. With chronic gastrointestinal symptoms, enzyme deficiency (eg, lactase), cystic fibrosis, celiac disease, chronic intestinal infections, gastrointestinal malformations, and irritable bowel syndrome should be considered.

Treatment

Treatment consists of eliminating and avoiding foods that have been documented to cause allergic reactions. This involves educating the patient, parent, and caregivers regarding hidden food allergens, the necessity for reading labels, and the signs and symptoms of food allergy and its appropriate management (emergency action plan; a copy of this plan is provided in the Food Allergy Guidelines). New food labeling laws went into effect in January 2006 requiring simple terms to indicate the presence of the major food allergens listed previously (eg, milk instead of casein).

Consultation with a dietitian familiar with food allergy may be helpful, especially when common foods such as milk, egg, peanut, soy, or wheat are involved. All patients with a history of IgE-mediated food allergy should carry self-injectable epinephrine (see section on Anaphylaxis) and a fast-acting antihistamine, and consider wearing medical identification jewelry. Clinical trials of oral and sublingual immunotherapy have been used as potential future treatments of food allergy. However, diets containing extensively heated (baked) milk and egg are potential alternative approaches to food oral immunotherapy and are changing the previous standard of strict avoidance diets for patients with food allergy.

Prognosis

The prognosis is good if the offending food can be identified and avoided. Unfortunately, accidental exposure to food allergens in severely allergic patients can result in death. Most children outgrow their food allergies to milk, egg, wheat, and soy but not to peanut or tree nuts (only 20% and 10% of children may outgrow peanut and tree nut allergy, respectively). The natural history of food allergy can be followed by measuring food-specific IgE levels and performing food challenges when indicated. Approximately 3%–4% of children will have food allergy as adults. Resources for food-allergic patients include the Food Allergy and Anaphylaxis Network, at: (800) 929-4040; http://www.foodallergy.org, and the Food Allergy Initiative, at (212) 207-1974; http://www.faiusa.org.

Boyce JA et al: Guidelines for the Diagnosis and Management of Food Allergy in the United States: Report of the NIAID-Sponsored Expert Panel. J Allergy Clin Immunol 2010; 126(Suppl 1):1–58 [PMID: 21134576].

Kim EH et al: Sublingual immunotherapy for peanut allergy: Clinical and immunologic evidence of desensitization. J Allergy Clin Immunol 2011;127(3):640–646 [PMID: 21281959].

Kim JS, Nowak-Wêgrzyn A, Sicherer SH, Noone S, Moshier EL, Sampson HA: Dietary baked milk accelerates the resolution of cow's milk allergy in children. J Allergy Clin Immunol 2011;128(1):125–131 [PMID: 21601913].

INSECT ALLERGY

ESSENTIALS OF DIAGNOSIS & TYPICAL FEATURES

- Local or systemic allergic signs and symptoms after insect sting.

Allergic reactions to insects include symptoms of respiratory allergy as a result of inhalation of particulate matter of insect origin, local cutaneous reactions to insect bites, and anaphylactic reactions to stings. The latter are almost exclusively caused by Hymenoptera and result in approximately 40 deaths each year in the United States. The order Hymenoptera includes honeybees, yellow jackets, yellow hornets, white-faced hornets, wasps, and fire ants. Africanized honeybees, also known as killer bees, are a concern because of their aggressive behavior and excessive swarming, not because their venom is more toxic. Rarely, patients sensitized to reduviid bugs (also known as kissing bugs) may have episodes of nocturnal anaphylaxis. Lepidopterism refers to adverse effects secondary to contact with larval or adult butterflies and moths. Salivary gland antigens are responsible for immediate and delayed skin reactions in mosquito-sensitive patients.

Clinical Findings

A. Symptoms and Signs

Insect bites or stings can cause local or systemic reactions ranging from mild to fatal responses in susceptible persons. The frequency increases in the summer months and with outdoor exposure. Local cutaneous reactions include urticaria as well as papulovesicular eruptions and lesions that resemble delayed hypersensitivity reactions. Papular urticaria is almost always the result of insect bites, especially of mosquitoes, fleas, and bedbugs. Toxic systemic reactions consisting of gastrointestinal symptoms, headache, vertigo, syncope, convulsions, or fever can occur following multiple stings. These reactions result from histamine-like substances in the venom. In children with hypersensitivity to fire ant venom, sterile pustules occur at sting sites on a nonimmunologic basis due to the inherent toxicity of piperidine alkaloids in the venom. Mild systemic reactions include itching, flushing, and urticaria. Severe systemic reactions may include dyspnea, wheezing, chest tightness, hoarseness, fullness in the throat, hypotension, loss of consciousness, incontinence, nausea, vomiting, and abdominal pain. Delayed systemic reactions occur from 2 hours to 3 weeks following the sting and include serum sickness, peripheral neuritis, allergic vasculitis, and coagulation defects.

B. Laboratory Findings

Skin testing is indicated for children with systemic reactions. Venoms of honeybee, yellow jacket, yellow hornet, white-faced hornet, and wasp are available for skin testing and treatment. Fire ant venom is not yet commercially available, but an extract made from fire ant bodies appears adequate to establish the presence of IgE antibodies to fire ant venom. Of note, venom skin test results can be negative in patients with systemic allergic reactions, especially in the first few weeks after a sting, and the tests may need to be repeated. The presence of a positive skin test denotes prior sensitization but does not predict whether a reaction will occur with the patient's next sting, nor does it differentiate between local and systemic reactions. It is common for children who have had an allergic reaction to have positive skin tests to more than one venom. This might reflect sensitization from prior stings that did not result in an allergic reaction or cross-reactivity between closely related venoms. In vitro testing (compared with skin testing) has not substantially improved the ability to predict anaphylaxis. With venom RAST, there is a 15%–20% incidence of both false-positive and false-negative results. Tests for mosquito saliva antigens or other insect allergy are not commercially available.

Complications

Secondary infection can complicate allergic reactions to insect bites or stings. Serum sickness, nephrotic syndrome, vasculitis, neuritis, and encephalopathy may be seen as late sequelae of reactions to stinging insects.

Treatment

For cutaneous reactions caused by biting insects, symptomatic therapy includes cold compresses, antipruritics (including antihistamines), and occasionally potent topical corticosteroids. Treatment of stings includes careful removal of the stinger, if present, by flicking it away from the wound and not by grasping in order to prevent further envenomation. Topical application of monosodium glutamate, baking soda, or vinegar compresses is of questionable efficacy. Local reactions can be treated with ice, elevation of the affected extremity, oral antihistamines, and NSAIDs as well as potent topical corticosteroids. Large local reactions, in which swelling extends beyond two joints or an extremity, may require a short course of oral corticosteroids. Anaphylactic reactions following Hymenoptera stings should be managed essentially the same as anaphylaxis (see section on Anaphylaxis). Children who have had severe or anaphylactic reactions to Hymenoptera stings—or their parents and caregivers—should be instructed in the use of epinephrine. Patients at risk for anaphylaxis from an insect sting should also wear a medical alert bracelet indicating their allergy. Children at risk from insect stings should avoid wearing bright-colored clothing and perfumes when outdoors and should wear long pants and shoes when walking in the grass. Patients who experience severe systemic reactions and have a positive skin test should receive venom immunotherapy. Immunotherapy is not indicated for children with only urticarial or local reactions.

Prognosis

Children generally have milder reactions than adults after insect stings, and fatal reactions are extremely rare. Patients aged 3–16 years with reactions limited to the skin, such as urticaria and angioedema, appear to be at low risk for more severe reactions with subsequent stings.

Golden D: Outcomes of allergy to insect stings in children, with and without venom immunotherapy. N Engl J Med 2004;351:668 [PMID: 15306668].

39 Antimicrobial Therapy

John W. Ogle, MD

PRINCIPLES OF ANTIMICROBIAL THERAPY

Antimicrobial therapy of infections is arguably the most important scientific development of 20th-century medicine. It contributes significantly to the quality of life of many people and reduces the morbidity and mortality due to infectious disease. The remarkable success of antimicrobial therapy has been achieved with comparatively little toxicity and expense. The relative ease of administration and the widespread availability of these drugs have led many to adopt a philosophy of broad-spectrum empiric antimicrobial therapy for many common infections.

Unfortunately this era of cheap, safe, and reliable therapy is being limited by the increasing frequency of antimicrobial resistance in previously susceptible microorganisms. The problem of antimicrobial resistance is not new—resistance was recognized for sulfonamides and penicillins shortly after their introduction. What is new is the worldwide dissemination of resistant clones of microorganisms, such as *Streptococcus pneumoniae* and *Staphylococcus aureus*, which are more virulent and commonly cause serious infections, not only among hospitalized patients, but also among outpatients.

Until recently the recognition of new resistant clones was balanced by the promise of newer and more potent antimicrobial agents. Today, because fewer new agents are under development, clinicians are beginning to encounter limitations in their ability to treat some serious bacterial infections. Many factors contribute to the selection of resistant clones. Our success in treating chronic diseases and immune-compromising conditions, which has resulted in additional years of life for patients, has increased opportunities for selection of resistant strains in inpatient units and chronic care facilities. Overuse of antimicrobial agents also contributes to the selection of resistant strains. Examples include antimicrobial treatment of mildly ill patients with self-limited conditions, such as viral infections, and administration of broad-spectrum antimicrobials to patients whose conditions could be treated with narrow-spectrum agents. Similarly, failure to document infection with cultures obtained prior to starting therapy limits our willingness to stop or narrow the spectrum of antimicrobials. Insufficient research has been conducted to determine the optimal duration of therapy for many infections, with the result that we probably often treat longer than is necessary. Prophylactic strategies, as used for prevention of recurrent otitis media or urinary tract infection, create a selection pressure for antibiotic resistance.

The decision-making process for choosing an appropriate antimicrobial agent is summarized in Table 39–1. Accurate clinical diagnosis is based on the history, physical examination, and initial laboratory tests. The clinical diagnosis then leads to a consideration of the organisms most commonly associated with the clinical condition, the usual pattern of antimicrobial susceptibility of these organisms, and past experience with successful treatment regimens.

Cultures should be obtained in potentially serious infections. Empiric antimicrobial therapy may be initiated and then modified according to the patient's response and the culture results. Often several equally safe and efficacious antimicrobials are available. In this circumstance, the relative cost and ease of administration of these choices should be considered.

Other important considerations include the patient's age, immune status, and exposure history. Neonates and young infants may present with nonspecific signs of infection, making the differentiation of serious disease from mild illness difficult. In older children, clinical diagnosis is more precise, which may permit therapy to be avoided or allow use of a narrower-spectrum antibiotic. Immune deficiency may increase the number and types of potential infecting organisms that need to be considered, including organisms that are usually avirulent, but in the altered host may cause serious infections that are difficult to treat. An abnormal immune response may also diminish the severity of the clinical signs and symptoms of infection, leading to underestimation of the severity of illness. The exposure history may suggest the greater likelihood of certain types of infecting organisms.

Table 39–1. Steps in decision making for use of antimicrobial agents.

Step	Action	Example
1	Determine diagnosis	Septic arthritis
2	Consider age and preexisting condition	Previously healthy 2-year-old child
3	Consider common organisms	*Staphylococcus aureus, Kingella kingae*
4	Consider organism susceptibility	Penicillin- or ampicillin-resistant; frequency MRSA[a] in community
5	Obtain proper cultures[b]	Blood, joint fluid
6	Initiate empiric therapy based on above considerations and past experience (eg, personal, literature)	Nafcillin and cefotaxime, substitute vancomycin for nafcillin if obviously ill or MRSA prevalent.
7	Modify therapy based on culture results and patient response	*S aureus* isolated. Discontinue cefotaxime. Substitute nafcillin for vancomycin if susceptible.
8	Follow clinical response	Interval physical examination
9	Stop therapy	Clinically improved or well, minimum 3–4 wk

[a]Methicillin-resistant *S aureus*.
[b]Indicated for serious or unusual infections or those with unpredictable clinical response to empiric therapy.

This history includes exposures from family members, classmates, and day care environments, and exposure to unusual organisms by virtue of travel, diet, or contact with animals.

Final important considerations are the pace and seriousness of the illness. A rapidly progressive and severe illness should be treated initially with broad-spectrum antimicrobials until a specific etiologic diagnosis is made. A mildly ill outpatient should receive treatment preferentially with narrow-spectrum antimicrobials.

Antimicrobial susceptibility, antimicrobial families, and dosing recommendations are listed in Tables 39–2 to 39–6.

ANTIMICROBIAL SUSCEPTIBILITY TESTING

Cultures and other diagnostic material must be obtained prior to initiating antimicrobial therapy—especially when the patient has a serious infection, initial attempts at therapy have failed, a patient has an unusual exposure, or multiagent therapy is anticipated. Whenever cultures identify the causative organism, therapy can be narrowed or optimized according to susceptibility results. Antimicrobial susceptibility testing should be done in a laboratory using carefully defined procedures (as defined by the Clinical and Laboratory Standards Institute).

There are several ways to test antimicrobial susceptibility. Identification of an antibiotic-destroying enzyme (eg, β-lactamase) implies resistance to β-lactam–containing antimicrobial agents. Tube or microtiter broth dilution techniques can be used to determine the minimum inhibitory concentration (MIC) of an antibiotic, which is the amount of antibiotic (in mcg/mL) necessary to inhibit the organism under specific laboratory conditions. Disk susceptibility testing (also performed under carefully controlled conditions) yields similar results. The E-test is a standardized test for some organisms that correlates well with MICs. Clinical laboratories usually define antimicrobial susceptibility (susceptible, intermediate, and resistant) in relation to levels of the test antibiotic achievable in the blood or another body fluid (cerebrospinal fluid [CSF] or urine).

Organisms are usually considered susceptible to an antibiotic if the MIC of the antibiotic for the organism is significantly lower than levels of that agent achieved in the blood using appropriate parenteral dosages. This assumption of susceptibility should be reconsidered whenever the patient has a focus of infection (eg, meningitis, osteomyelitis, or abscess) in which poor antibiotic penetration might occur, because the levels of antibiotic in such areas might be lower than the MIC. Conversely, although certain organisms may be reported to be resistant to an antibiotic because sufficiently high blood concentrations cannot be achieved, urine concentrations may be much higher. If so, a urinary tract infection might respond to an antibiotic that would not be adequate for treatment of septicemia.

Thus, antimicrobial susceptibility testing, although a very important part of therapeutic decision making, reflects assumptions that the clinician must understand, especially for serious infections. Ultimately the true test of the efficacy of therapy is patient response. Patients who do not respond to seemingly appropriate therapy may require reassessment, including reconsidering the diagnosis, reculturing, and repeat susceptibility testing, to determine whether resistant strains have evolved or superinfection with a resistant organism is present. Antimicrobial therapy cannot be expected to cure some infections unless additional supportive treatment (usually surgical) is undertaken.

ALTERATION OF DOSE & MEASUREMENT OF BLOOD LEVELS

Certain antimicrobial agents have not been approved (and often not tested) for use in newborns. For those that have been approved, it is important to recognize that both dose and frequency of administration may need to be altered (see Tables 39–4 and 39–5), especially in young (7 days or younger) or low-birth-weight neonates (≤ 2000 g).

Antimicrobial agents are excreted or metabolized through various physiologic mechanisms (eg, renal, hepatic). It is important to consider these routes of excretion and alter the antimicrobial dosage appropriately in any patient with some

Table 39–2. Susceptibility of some common pathogenic microorganisms to various antimicrobial drugs.

Organism	Potentially Useful Antibiotics[a]
Bacteria	
Anaerobic bacteria[b]	Cefotetan,[c] cefoxitin,[c] clindamycin, doripenem,[c] ertapenem, imipenem, meropenem, metronidazole, penicillins with or without β-lactamase inhibitor, tigecycline[c]
Bacillus anthracis	Amoxicillin, ciprofloxacin, clindamycin, doxycycline, levofloxacin, rifampin, vancomycin
Bartonella henselae	Azithromycin, ciprofloxacin, clarithromycin, doxycycline, erythromycin, rifampin
Bordetella pertussis	Amoxicillin, azithromycin, clarithromycin, erythromycin, trimethoprim-sulfamethoxazole
Borrelia burgdorferi	Amoxicillin, cefuroxime, cephalosporins (III),[d] clarithromycin, doxycycline
Campylobacter spp	Azithromycin, carbapenems, erythromycin, fluoroquinolones,[c,e] tetracyclines
Clostridium spp	Clindamycin, metronidazole, penicillins, tetracyclines
Clostridium difficile	Bacitracin (PO), metronidazole, vancomycin (PO)
Corynebacterium diphtheriae	Clindamycin, erythromycin, penicillins
Enterobacteriaceae[f]	Aminoglycosides,[g] ampicillin, aztreonam, carbapenems, cefepime, cephalosporins, fluoroquinolones,[c,e] tigecycline, trimethoprim-sulfamethoxazole
Enterococcus	Ampicillin (with aminoglycoside), carbapenems (not E faecium), linezolid, quinupristin-dalfopristin[c] (E faecium only), tigecycline, vancomycin
Haemophilus influenzae	Amoxicillin-clavulanate, ampicillin (if β-lactamase-negative),[h] cephalosporins (II and III),[d] chloramphenicol, fluoroquinolones,[c,e] rifampin, trimethoprim-sulfamethoxazole
Listeria monocytogenes	Ampicillin with aminoglycoside, trimethoprim-sulfamethoxazole, vancomycin
Moraxella catarrhalis	Amoxicillin-clavulanate, ampicillin (if β-lactamase-negative),[h] cephalosporins (II and III),[d] erythromycin, fluoroquinolones, trimethoprim-sulfamethoxazole
Neisseria gonorrhoeae	Ampicillin (if β-lactamase-negative),[h] cephalosporins (II and III),[d] penicillins, selected fluoroquinolones (only if known susceptible),[c,e] spectinomycin
Neisseria meningitidis	Ampicillin, cephalosporins (II and III),[d] fluoroquinolones,[c,e] penicillins, rifampin
Nocardia asteroides	Tetracycline, trimethoprim-sulfamethoxazole (+ amikacin for severe infections), Meropenem or cephalosporins (II and III)[d] for brain abscess
Pasteurella multocida	Amoxicillin-clavulanate, ampicillins, penicillins, tetracyclines
Pseudomonas aeruginosa	Aminoglycosides,[g] anti-*Pseudomonas* penicillins,[c] aztreonam, cefepime, ceftazidime, ciprofloxacin,[c] doripenem, imipenem, meropenem
Salmonella spp	Ampicillin, azithromycin, cephalosporins (III),[d] fluoroquinolones,[c,e] trimethoprim-sulfamethoxazole
Shigella spp	Ampicillin, azithromycin, cephalosporins (III),[d] fluoroquinolones,[c,e] tetracyclines, trimethoprim-sulfamethoxazole
Staphylococcus aureus	Antistaphylococcal penicillins,[i] cefepime, cephalosporins (I and II), ciprofloxacin, clindamycin, erythromycin, rifampin, trimethoprim-sulfamethoxazole, vancomycin
S aureus (methicillin-resistant)	Clindamycin, daptomycin,[c] linezolid, quinupristin-dalfopristin,[c] tigecycline,[c] trimethoprim-sulfamethoxazole, vancomycin
Staphylococci (coagulase-negative)	Cephalosporins (I and II),[j] clindamycin, rifampin, vancomycin
Streptococci (most species)	Ampicillin, cephalosporins, clindamycin, enhanced fluoroquinolones,[c,k] erythromycin, meropenem, penicillins, vancomycin
Streptococcus pneumoniae[l]	Ampicillin, cephalosporins, enhanced fluoroquinolones,[c,k] erythromycin, meropenem, penicillin, vancomycin

(*Continued*)

Table 39–2. Susceptibility of some common pathogenic microorganisms to various antimicrobial drugs. (*Continued*)

Organism	Potentially Useful Antibiotics[a]
Intermediate organisms	
Chlamydia spp	Clarithromycin, erythromycin, levofloxacin,[c] ofloxacin,[c] tetracyclines
Mycoplasma spp	Azithromycin, clarithromycin, erythromycin, fluoroquinolones,[c,e] tetracyclines
Rickettsia spp	Fluoroquinolones,[c,e] tetracyclines
Fungi	
Candida spp	Amphotericin B, anidulafungin, caspofungin, fluconazole, flucytosine, itraconazole, ketoconazole, micafungin, nystatin, posaconazole, voriconazole
Fungi, systemic[b]	Amphotericin B, anidulafungin, caspofungin, fluconazole, 5-fluorocytosine,[b] itraconazole, ketoconazole, micafungin, posaconazole, voriconazole
Dermatophytes	Butenafine, ciclopirox olamine, clotrimazole, econazole, fluconazole, griseofulvin, itraconazole, ketoconazole, miconazole, naftifine, oxiconazole, terbinafine
Pneumocystis jiroveci	Atovaquone, clindamycin-primaquine, dapsone, pentamidine, trimethoprim-sulfamethoxazole
Viruses	
Herpes simplex	Acyclovir, cidofovir, penciclovir,[c] famciclovir, foscarnet,[o] trifluridine, valacyclovir
Human immunodeficiency virus	Six classes: (1) nucleoside reverse transcriptase inhibitors, (2) non-nucleoside reverse transcriptase inhibitors, (3) protease inhibitors, (4) fusion inhibitors, (5) integrase inhibitors, (6) CCR-5 co-receptor antagonists; optimally combinations of ≥ 3 drugs from 2 different classes should be used (see Chapter 41)
Influenza virus	Amantadine,[m] oseltamivir, rimantidine,[m] zanamivir
Respiratory syncytial virus	Ribavirin[n]
Varicella-zoster virus	Acyclovir, famciclovir, foscarnet,[o] valacyclovir
Cytomegalovirus	Cidofovir, fomivirsen (topical or intravitreal), foscarnet, ganciclovir, valganciclovir
Hepatitis B[c]	Adefovir, entecavir, interferon-α, lamivudine, telbivudine, tenofovir
Hepatitis C[c]	Interferon-α, ribavirin

[a]In alphabetical order. Selection depends on patient's age, diagnosis, site of infection, severity of illness, antimicrobial susceptibility of suspected organism, and drug risk.
[b]Species-dependent, 5-fluorocytosine is used in combinations with other agents.
[c]Not FDA-approved for use in children.
[d]Refer to second- (II) or third- (III) generation cephalosporins.
[e]Includes ciprofloxacin, levofloxacin, lomefloxacin, norfloxacin, ofloxacin, moxifloxacin, gatifloxacin, gemifloxacin.
[f]Includes *E coli*, *Klebsiella* spp, *Enterobacter* spp, and others; antimicrobial susceptibilities should always be measured.
[g]Amikacin, gentamicin, kanamycin, tobramycin.
[h]Also applies to amoxicillin and related compounds.
[i]Cloxacillin, dicloxacillin, methicillin, nafcillin, oxacillin.
[j]Only if the coagulase-negative *Staphylococcus* is also methicillin- or oxacillin-sensitive.
[k]Includes levofloxacin, lomefloxacin, moxifloxacin, gatifloxacin, gemifloxacin.
[l]Because of increasing frequency of *S pneumoniae* strains resistant to penicillin and cephalosporins, presumptive therapy for severe infections (eg, meningitis) should include vancomycin until susceptibility studies are available.
[m]Influenza A only. Resistance is common, currently recommended in the United States only for seasonal H1N1 strains.
[n]FDA-approved for therapy of respiratory syncytial virus by aerosol, but clinical studies show variable efficacy.
[o]Used to treat infections with acyclovir-resistant virus.

Table 39–3. Groups of common antibacterial agents.

Group	Examples	Some Common Susceptible Organisms[a]	Common Resistant Organisms	Common or Unique Adverse Reactions
Penicillin group				
Penicillins	Penicillin G, V	*Streptococcus, Neisseria*	*Staphylococcus, Haemophilus,* Enterobacteriaceae	Rash, anaphylaxis, drug fever, bone marrow suppression
Ampicillins	Ampicillin, amoxicillin	(Same as penicillins), plus *Haemophilus* (β-lactamase negative), *Escherichia coli, Enterococcus*	*Staphylococcus*, many Enterobacteriaceae	Diarrhea
Antistaphylococcal penicillins	Cloxacillin, dicloxacillin, methicillin, nafcillin, oxacillin	*Streptococcus, Staphylococcus aureus*	Gram-negative, *Staphylococcus* (coagulase-negative), *Enterococcus*	Renal (interstitial nephritis)
Anti-*Pseudomonas* penicillins	Azlocillin, piperacillin, ticarcillin	(Same as ampicillins), plus *Pseudomonas*	(Same as ampicillins)	Decreased platelet adhesiveness, hypokalemia, hypernatremia, high sodium load
Penicillins with β-lactamase inhibitor combination	Amoxicillin–clavulanate, ampicillin–sulbactam, ticarcillin–clavulanate	Broad-spectrum	Some Enterobacteriaceae, *Pseudomonas*	Diarrhea
Carbapenems	Imipenem–cilastatin meropenem, ertapenem, doripenem	Broad-spectrum, gram-negative rods, anaerobes, *Pseudomonas*	MRSA,[b] many enterococci	Central nervous system (CNS), seizures
Cephalosporin group				
First-generation (I)	Cefazolin, cephalexin, cephalothin, cephapirin, cephradine	Gram-positive	Gram-negative, *Enterococcus*, some *Staphylococcus* (coagulase-negative)	Rash; anaphylaxis, drug fever
Second-generation (II)	Cefaclor, cefamandole, cefprozil, cefonicid, cefuroxime, loracarbef	Gram-positive, some *Haemophilus*, some Enterobacteriaceae	*Enterococcus, Pseudomonas*, some *Staphylococcus* (coagulase-negative)	Serum sickness (cefaclor)
	Cefoxitin, cefotetan	Same as second-generation plus anaerobes		
Third-generation (III)	Cefotaxime, ceftizoxime, ceftriaxone, cefpodoxime, ceftibuten, cefdinir	*Streptococcus, Haemophilus,* Enterobacteriaceae, *Neisseria*	*Pseudomonas, Staphylococcus*	Biliary sludging (ceftriaxone) rash
	Ceftazidime, cefepime	(Same as other third-generation cephalosporins), plus *Pseudomonas*, some *Staphylococcus*		
Other drugs				
Clindamycin	Clindamycin	Gram-positive, anaerobes, some MRSA	Gram-negative, *Enterococcus*	Nausea, vomiting, hepatotoxicity
Vancomycin	Vancomycin	Gram-positive	Gram-negative	"Red man" syndrome, shock, ototoxicity, renal

(*Continued*)

Table 39–3. Groups of common antibacterial agents. (*Continued*)

Group	Examples	Some Common Susceptible Organisms[a]	Common Resistant Organisms	Common or Unique Adverse Reactions
Macrolides and azalides	Erythromycin, clarithromycin, azithromycin	Gram-positive *Bordetella, Haemophilus, Mycoplasma, Chlamydia, Legionella, Salmonella, Shigella*	Some gram-negative	Nausea and vomiting
Monobactams	Aztreonam	Gram-negative aerobes, *Pseudomonas*	Gram-positive cocci	Rash, diarrhea
Oxazolidinones	Linezolid	Gram-positive aerobes	Gram-negative aerobes	Diarrhea, thrombocytopenia
Streptogramins	Quinupristin–dalfopristin	Gram-positive aerobes	Gram-negative aerobes	Arthralgia, myalgia
Fluoroquinolones[c]	Ciprofloxacin, ofloxacin	Gram-negative, *Chlamydia, Mycoplasma, Pseudomonas* (ciprofloxacin)	*Enterococcus, Streptococcus, S pneumoniae*, anaerobes, *Staphylococcus*	Gastrointestinal (GI), rash, CNS
	Gatifloxacin, levofloxacin, moxifloxacin	Gram-negative, streptococci, *Streptococcus pneumoniae*, staphylococci	Some *Enterococcus*	GI, rash, CNS
Tetracyclines	Chlortetracycline, tetracycline, doxycycline, minocycline	Anaerobes, *Mycoplasma, Chlamydia, Rickettsia, Ehrlichia*	Many Enterobacteriaceae, *Staphylococcus*	Teeth stained,[d] rash, flora overgrowth, hepatotoxicity, pseudotumor cerebri
Sulfonamides	Many	Gram-negative (urine)	Gram-positive	Rash, renal, bone marrow suppression, Stevens-Johnson syndrome
Trimethoprim–sulfamethoxazole	Trimethoprim–sulfamethoxazole	*S aureus*, gram-negative, *S pneumoniae, Haemophilus influenzae*	*Streptococcus, Pseudomonas*, anaerobes	Rash, renal, bone marrow suppression, Stevens-Johnson syndrome
Rifampin	Rifampin	*Neisseria, Haemophilus, Staphylococcus, Streptococcus*	Resistance develops rapidly if used as sole agent	Rash, GI, hepatotoxicity, CNS, bone marrow suppression, alters metabolism of other drugs
Aminoglycosides	Amikacin, gentamicin, kanamycin, streptomycin, tobramycin	Gram-negative, including *Pseudomonas aeruginosa*	Gram-positive, anaerobes, some pseudomonads	Nephrotoxicity, ototoxicity, potentiates neuromuscular blocking agents

[a]Not all strains susceptible; always obtain antimicrobial susceptibility tests on significant isolates.
[b]MRSA = methicillin-resistant *S aureus*.
[c]Fluoroquinolones are used with caution in children.
[d]Dose-dependent in children younger than age 9 years.

degree of organ dysfunction. (See Chapter 24.) As indicated in Table 39–4, an assessment of renal or hepatic function may routinely be necessary for patients receiving certain drugs (eg, renal function for aminoglycosides, hepatic function for erythromycin or clindamycin); otherwise, harmful drug levels may accumulate. In some circumstances a patient may be receiving multiple drugs where the drug interactions are unknown. If significant organ dysfunction is present, drug clearance may be delayed and dosage modification may be necessary (see detailed descriptions in individual drug information packets), and measurement of drug levels may be indicated.

Serum levels of drugs posing a high risk of toxicity (eg, aminoglycosides) are ordinarily measured. Measurement of other drugs (eg, vancomycin) may be useful in selected circumstances (see following discussion). For certain serious bacterial infections (eg, bacterial endocarditis), measurement of the serum concentration of an antimicrobial may be important to determine optimal therapy.

Certain drug interactions may require modification of drug dosage or other therapeutic alterations. For example, rifampin stimulates the metabolism of warfarin, progesterone, prednisone, and anticonvulsants by stimulating the cytochrome P-450 (CYP-450) metabolic pathway. Dosage adjustments or alternative medications may be necessary to avoid significant adverse events. Another common example is erythromycin, which may inhibit the metabolism of

Table 39–4. Guidelines for use of common parenteral antibacterial agents[a] in children age 1 month or older.

Agent	Route	Dose[b] (mg/kg/d)	Maximum Daily Dose	Interval (h)	Adjustment[c]	Blood Levels[d] (mcg/mL)	
						Peak	Trough
Amikacin	IM, IV	15–22.5	1.5 g	8	R	15–25	< 10
Ampicillin	IM, IV	100–400	12 g	4–6	R		
Aztreonam	IM, IV	90–120	6 g	6–8	R		
Cefazolin	IM, IV	50–100	6 g	8	R		
Cefepime	IM, IV	100–150	4–6 g	8–12	R		
Cefotaxime	IM, IV	100–200	12 g	6–8	R		
Cefoxitin	IM, IV	80–160	12 g	4–6	R		
Ceftazidime	IM, IV	100–150	6 g	8	R		
Ceftizoxime	IM, IV	150–200	12 g	6–8	R		
Ceftriaxone	IM, IV	50–100	4 g	12–24	R		
Cefuroxime	IM, IV	100–150	6 g	6–8	R		
Cephalothin	IM, IV	75–125	12 g	4–6	R		
Cephradine	IM, IV	50–100	8 g	6	R		
Clindamycin	IM, IV	25–40	4 g	6–8	R, H		
Gentamicin	IM, IV	3–7.5	300 mg	8	R	5–10	< 2
Linezolid	IV, PO	20	1.2 g	12	R		
Meropenem	IV	60–120	2 g	8	R		
Metronidazole	IV	30	4 g	6	H		
Nafcillin	IM, IV	150	12 g	6	H		
Penicillin G	IM, IV	100,000–250,000 U/kg	20 million units	4–6	H, R		
Penicillin G (benzathine)	IM	50,000 U/kg	2.4 million units	Single dose	None		
Penicillin G (procaine)	IM	25,000–50,000 U/kg	4.8 million units	12–24	R		
Tetracycline[e]	IV[e]	20–30	2 g	12	R		
Ticarcillin	IV	200–300	24 g	4–6	R		
Tobramycin	IM, IV	3–6	300 mg	8	R	5–10	< 2
Vancomycin	IV	40–60	2 g	6	R	20–40[f]	5–10[f]

[a]Not including some newly released drugs, ones not recommended for use in children, or ones not widely used.
[b]Always consult package insert for complete prescribing information. Dosage may differ for alternative routes, newborns (see Table 39–6), or patients with liver or renal failure (see Adjustment column) and may not be recommended for use in pregnant women or newborns. Maximum dosage may be indicated only in severe infections or by parenteral routes.
[c]Mode of excretion (R = renal, H = hepatic) of antimicrobial agent should be assessed at the onset of therapy and dosage modified or levels determined as indicated in package insert.
[d]Suggested levels to reduce toxicity.
[e]Use with caution in children younger than age 9 years because of tooth staining with repeated doses.
[f]Target peak and trough vancomycin levels are not well correlated with either toxicity or outcome. Measure selectively in meningitis, impaired or changing renal function, or altered volume of distribution.

Table 39–5. Guidelines for use of common oral antibacterial agents in children age 1 month or older.

Agent[a]	Dose[b] (mg/kg/d)	Interval (h)	Other Considerations
Amoxicillin	40	8-12	Gastrointestinal (GI) side effects
Amoxicillin[c] (high dose)	80-90	12	GI side effects
Amoxicillin-clavulanate[d]	45	8-12	GI side effects
Ampicillin	50	6	GI side effects
Azithromycin	10 (first dose) then 5; 12 for pharyngitis	24	GI side effects
Cefaclor	40	8	Serum sickness-like illness
Cefadroxil	30	12	
Cefdinir	14	12-24	GI side effects
Cefpodoxime	10	12	Taste (suspension)
Cefprozil	30	12	GI side effects
Ceftibuten	9	24	GI side effects
Cefuroxime	30-40	12	GI side effects
Cephalexin	25-50	6	
Ciprofloxacin	20-30	12	
Clarithromycin	15	12	GI side effects
Clindamycin	20-30	6	GI side effects
Dicloxacillin	12-25	6	GI side effects
Doxycycline[d]	2-4	12-24	Teeth stained < 9 y
Erythromycin[f]	20-50	6-12	GI side effects
Erythromycin-sulfisoxazole	40 (erythromycin)	6-8	
Levofloxacin			
< 5 y	20	12	
> 5 y	10	24	
Linezolid	20	12	GI side effects
Loracarbef	15; 30 for otitis	12	
Metronidazole	15-35	8	
Nitrofurantoin	5-7	6	
Oxacillin	50-100	6	
Penicillin V	25-50	6	Taste (suspension)
Rifampin	10-20	12-24	
Sulfisoxazole	120-150	6	
Tetracycline[e]	25-50[c]	6	Teeth stained < 9 y
Trimethoprim-sulfamethoxazole	8-12 (TMP)	12	Stevens-Johnson syndrome

[a]Not including some newly released drugs, ones not recommended for use in children, or ones not widely used.
[b]Always consult package insert for complete prescribing information. Dosage may differ for alternative routes, newborns (see Table 39–6), or patients with liver or renal failure (see Table 39–4, Adjustment column) and may not be recommended for use in pregnant women or newborns. Maximum dosage may be indicated only in severe infections or by parenteral routes.
[c]Higher dose amoxicillin indicated for therapy of otitis media in regions where rates of penicillin-resistant *S pneumoniae* are high.
[d]Several formulations with differing clavulanate concentrations available.
[e]Use with caution in children younger than age 9 years because of tooth staining with repeated doses.
[f]Preparation-dependent.

Table 39–6. Guidelines for use of selected antimicrobial agents in newborns.

			Maximum Dosage (mg/kg/d) [Frequency]				Blood Levels (mcg/mL)	
	Route	Body Wt (g)	< 7 Days	Interval (h)	8–30 Days	Interval (h)	Peak	Trough
Amikacin[a]	IV, IM	< 2000	15	12	22.5	8	15–25	5–10
		> 2000	20	12	30	8		
Ampicillin	IV, IM	< 2000	100	12	150	8		
		> 2000	150	8	200	6		
Cefotaxime	IV, IM		100	12	150	8		
Ceftazidime	IV, IM	< 2000	100	12	150	8		
		> 2000	100	8	150	8		
Clindamycin	IV, IM, PO	< 2000	10	12	15	8		
		> 2000	15	8	20	6		
Erythromycin	PO	< 2000	20	12	30	8		
		> 2000	20	12	40	8		
Gentamicin[a]	IV, IM		5	12–18	7.5	8	5–10	< 2
Nafcillin	IV	< 2000	50	12	75	8		
		> 2000	75	8	150	6		
Oxacillin	IV, IM	< 2000	100	12	150	8		
		> 2000	50	8	8200	6		
Penicillin G[b]	IV	< 2000	100,000	12	150,000	8		
		> 2000	150,000	8	200,000	6		
Ticarcillin-clavulanate	IV, IM	< 2000	150	12	225	8		
		> 2000	225	8	300	6		
Tobramycin[a]	IV, IM		5	12–18	7.5	8	5–10	< 2
Vancomycin[c]	IV		20	12	30	8	20–40	5–10

[a]Neonates weighting < 1200 g may require even smaller doses. Antibiotic levels should be closely monitored.
[b]Penicillin dosages are in U/kg/d. Other preparations (eg, benzathine penicillin) may be given IM. See specific diseases for dosage.
[c]Target peak and trough vancomycin levels are not well correlated with either toxicity or outcome. For some resistant organisms trough levels of 10-15 mcg/ml may be indicated.

theophylline, resulting in toxic theophylline levels. Although many drug interactions are known and well documented, it may be difficult to predict interactions that result from a combination of four, five, or more different medications. A high level of suspicion regarding adverse clinical events should be maintained.

THE USE OF NEW ANTIMICROBIAL AGENTS

New antibiotics are introduced frequently, often with claims about unique features that distinguish these usually more expensive products from existing compounds. Often these drugs share many properties with existing drugs. The role that any new antimicrobial will play can only be determined over time, during which new or previously unrecognized side effects might be described and the clinical efficacy established. Clinical trials may not be confirmed in the larger number of patients subsequently treated in practice. Because this may take many years, a conservative approach to using new antibiotics seems fitting, especially because their costs are often higher, and appropriate antimicrobial choices for most common infections already exist. It is appropriate to ask if a new antimicrobial has been proved to be as effective as (or more effective than) the current drug of choice, and whether its side effects are comparable (or less common) and its cost reasonable. The withdrawal of moxalactam and trovafloxacin due to unexpected serious side effects, which were not anticipated despite extensive premarket testing, highlight the caution necessary before using new antimicrobials. The heavy marketing of new cephalosporins and fluoroquinolones, which are very similar to existing drugs, is typical of the difficulty in evaluating antimicrobials.

The development of new antibiotics is important as a response to the emergence of resistant organisms and for treatment of infections that are clinically difficult to treat (eg, viruses, fungi, and some resistant bacteria). Fortunately, these infections are either rare or (usually) self-limited in immunocompetent hosts.

PROPHYLACTIC ANTIMICROBIAL AGENTS

Antimicrobials can be used to decrease the incidence of postoperative infections (Table 39–7). A dose of an antimicrobial given 30 minutes to 2 hours prior to surgery can reduce postoperative wound infection. The goal is to achieve high levels in the serum at the time of incision and by this means—along with good surgical technique—to minimize viable bacterial contamination of the wound. During a lengthy procedure, a second dose may be given. No evidence exists that multiple subsequent doses of antimicrobials confer additional benefit. The antimicrobial(s) used for

Table 39–7. Antimicrobial prophylaxis and preferred prophylactic agents: selected conditions and pathogens.[a]

Pathogen (Indication)	Prophylactic Agent
Bacillus anthracis[b]	Amoxicillin (if proved susceptible), ciprofloxacin, doxycycline
Bacterial endocarditis[c]	Ampicillin, ampicillin and gentamicin, amoxicillin, or other approved regimens
Bordetella pertussis (exposure to respiratory secretions)	Azithromycin, clarithromycin, erythromycin
Chlamydia trachomatis (genital contact)	Azithromycin, doxycycline
Haemophilus influenzae type b[d] (household exposure)	Rifampin
Mycobacterium tuberculosis (household exposure)	Isoniazid or rifampin
Neisseria meningitidis (household exposure)	Rifampin, ciprofloxacin
Neisseria gonorrhoeae (ophthalmia neonatorum)	Erythromycin, silver nitrate ophthalmic, povidone-iodine
N gonorrhoeae (sexual contact)	Ceftriaxone, cefixime, cefpodoxime
Treponema pallidum (sexual contact)	Penicillin
Streptococcus pneumoniae (sickle cell disease, asplenia)	Penicillin
Postoperative wound infection[e]	Cefazolin, Vancomycin other regimens[e]
Group A streptococci (rheumatic fever)[f]	Benzathine penicillin G, penicillin, sulfadiazine
Group B streptococcal sepsis	Ampicillin to mother prior to delivery
Pneumonic *Yersinia pestis*[g] (exposure)	Tetracycline[h]
Francisella tularensis[g] (aerosolized exposure)	Tetracycline[h]
Vibrio cholera	Tetracycline,[h] trimethoprim-sulfamethoxazole
Recurrent urinary tract infection	Nitrofurantoin, trimethoprim-sulfamethoxazole
Pneumocystis jiroveci—(HIV, some immunocompromised patients)	Atovaquone, clindamycin-primaquine, dapsone, trimethoprim-sulfamethoxazole, pentamidine

[a]Decisions for prophylaxis must take a number of factors into account, including the evidence for efficacy of therapy, the degree of the exposure to an infecting agent, the risk and consequences of infection, the susceptibility of the infecting agent to antimicrobials, and the patient's ability to tolerate and comply with the antimicrobial agent. See individual chapters for discussion.
[b]Decisions for prophylaxis should be made in accordance with the responsible public health department recommendations.
[c]See discussion in Chapter 20.
[d]Prophylaxis provided to family if contacts include children younger than age 4 years. Some experts provide prophylaxis in day care settings after one case and some after two cases of Hib infection.
[e]Alternative regimens may be used, depending on the site of surgery and the degree of contamination. Vancomycin may be used when the patient is known to be colonized with MRSA or if MRSA is a common postoperative infection.
[f]Oral prophylaxis may be indicated in some patients. Alternative regimens indicated for penicillin-allergic patients. See discussion in chapter.
[g]Prophylaxis not well established. Carefully assess risk on a case-by-case basis.
[h]Usually not indicated for children younger than age 9 years because of tooth staining with repeated doses.

prophylaxis are directed toward the flora that most commonly cause postoperative infection at a given anatomic site. Gram-positive cocci, such as *S aureus*, are usually targeted, and a first-generation cephalosporin (eg, cefazolin) is a cost-effective choice. Third-generation cephalosporins and other broad-spectrum agents are more expensive and offer less benefit because they are less active than cefazolin against *S aureus*. Cefoxitin or cefotetan is useful for procedures, such as colorectal surgery, although cefazolin is appropriate for most gynecologic patients. In colorectal surgery, orally administered antimicrobials such as neomycin and erythromycin may be as effective as parenteral antimicrobials.

In hospitals where the predominant *S aureus* strains are methicillin-resistant or in cases where the patient is allergic to penicillin and cephalosporins, vancomycin can be considered. However, prophylactic vancomycin has caused hypotension at the time of induction of general anesthesia. Frequent use of vancomycin as a prophylactic antimicrobial will contribute to the development of vancomycin-resistant strains such as *Enterococcus faecalis*. For these reasons, vancomycin should generally not be used for prophylaxis, although it might prove useful for individual patients at extremely high risk.

Prophylactic antimicrobials are given in several other circumstances. Endocarditis prophylaxis is indicated during dental, colorectal, or genitourinary procedures in patients with high-risk heart lesions, such as prosthetic cardiac valves, surgically corrected systemic pulmonary shunts, and mitral valve prolapse with regurgitation. Patients with indwelling vascular catheters, such as Broviac catheters, should receive prophylaxis during similar procedures, which are likely to induce a transient bacteremia. Prophylaxis against infection with group A streptococci reduces the recurrence rate for acute rheumatic fever. Postexposure prophylaxis is given after exposure to pertussis, *Haemophilus influenzae* type b (Hib) infection (depending on age), meningococcus, gonococcus, tuberculosis (household exposure), plague, aerosolized tularemia or anthrax, and other high-risk infections. Family or close contacts of patients with severe invasive streptococcal disease may benefit from prophylaxis. Silver nitrate, erythromycin, povidone–iodine, and tetracycline are used in ophthalmic preparations for prevention of gonococcal ophthalmia neonatorum. Children with asplenia or sickle cell disease receive prophylactic penicillin to protect against overwhelming *S pneumoniae* sepsis, usually started immediately with the onset of fever.

Prophylactic antimicrobials are sometimes used for some children at high risk for recurrent urinary tract infection, but the rate of infection has not been proven to decrease.

INITIAL EMPIRIC ANTIMICROBIAL CHOICES FOR SELECTED CONDITIONS

General recommendations for specific conditions are as follows. A specific selection depends on the patient's age, diagnosis, site of infection, severity of illness, antimicrobial susceptibility of bacterial isolates, and history of drug allergy. Always consult the package insert for detailed prescribing information. Tables 39–2 to 39–6 include further information.

Neonatal Sepsis & Meningitis

The newborn with sepsis may have signs of focal infection, such as pneumonia or respiratory distress syndrome, or may have subtle nonfocal signs. Group B streptococci, *Escherichia coli*, and other gram-negative rods are commonly encountered. *Listeria monocytogenes* is now uncommon in many nurseries, but a recent nationwide outbreak demonstrates the pathogenic potential of this organism. Ampicillin and gentamicin (or another aminoglycoside) are preferred. If meningitis is present, many clinicians substitute a third-generation cephalosporin for the aminoglycoside. *S pneumoniae* is an uncommon cause of meningitis in neonates. However, if the Gram stain shows gram-positive cocci suggesting *S pneumoniae*, substitution of vancomycin for ampicillin should be considered. In the newborn with cellulitis, *S aureus* including methicillin-resistant *S aureus* (MRSA) and group A streptococci are additional considerations. Nafcillin, oxacillin, or a first-generation cephalosporin is usually added. Vancomycin is added if MRSA is common in the geographic area. Omphalitis is often polymicrobial, and *Enterococcus* species, gram-negative aerobes, and anaerobes may be causative. Clindamycin, ampicillin, and an aminoglycoside or cefotaxime cover the most likely organisms; early surgical intervention is indicated.

Sepsis in an Infant

S pneumoniae and *Neisseria meningitidis* are most commonly encountered in infants. Hib infection may occur in unimmunized children. A third-generation cephalosporin is appropriate. Intermediate-level penicillin and cephalosporin resistance in *S pneumoniae* usually do not cause therapy to fail unless meningitis or another difficult-to-treat infection, such as endocarditis or osteomyelitis, is present.

Occult bacteremia may be encountered in young infants with high fever. Prior to immunization with vaccines effective against Hib, persistent bacteremia and complications including meningitis were seen in approximately 50% of children infected with occult Hib bacteremia. With widespread use of Hib vaccine, Hib is a very uncommon cause of occult bacteremia in young children with fever. Similarly, prior to the introduction of the conjugate pneumococcal vaccines vaccine, *S pneumonia* bacteremia was demonstrated in 3%–5% of infants aged 3–36 months with fever of 39°C or greater, no identified source for fever on examination, and white blood cell count (WBC) of 15,000/mm^3. The risk of bacteremia was 6%–10% in younger children with progressively high fever and high WBCs. The risk of developing meningitis due to persistent *S pneumoniae* is estimated at 3% of those who are known to be bacteremic. The risk of *S pneumoniae* bacteremia and its complications is significantly reduced in children immunized with the conjugate pneumococcal vaccines. In clinical trials and subsequent national surveillance for the incidence of disease, the 7 valent pneumococcal vaccine reduced the incidence of invasive pneumococcal diseases by approximately 90%. Studies are underway with the newer 13 valent pneumococcal vaccines. Observation without antimicrobials, but with appropriate plans for follow-up examinations, is appropriate for most febrile young children who are fully immunized.

Nosocomial Sepsis

Many bacterial pathogens can cause infection in hospitalized patients. Recent local experience is usually the best guide to etiologic diagnosis. For example, some intensive care units experience frequent infections due to *Enterobacter cloacae*, whereas in other units *Klebsiella pneumoniae* is the most common nosocomial isolate. Initial therapy should include antibiotics effective for MRSA and resistant *Pseudomonas aeruginosa* if these are frequent isolates. *E faecalis* is a common cause of nosocomial bacteremia in patients with central catheters, particularly in units where cephalosporins are heavily used. Coagulase-negative staphylococci are commonly isolated from patients with indwelling central catheters. In seriously ill patients, when the local experience suggests that *Enterococcus* species or coagulase-negative staphylococci are common, the initial regimen should include vancomycin. Because *Enterococcus* species and coagulase-negative staphylococci commonly cause fever without significant morbidity or mortality, initial regimens without vancomycin are appropriate, with adjustment of treatment after susceptibility is known. If *P aeruginosa* or other resistant gram-negative rods are common, ceftazidime or cefepime should be included in initial therapy. *Candida* is a common isolate from blood cultures from immunocompromised or seriously ill patients in the intensive care unit. Empiric antifungal therapy is initiated in some high-risk patients.

Meningitis

Bacterial meningitis in neonates is usually caused by infection with group B streptococci, *E coli*, other gram-negative rods, or *L monocytogenes*. A combination of ampicillin and a third-generation cephalosporin is started initially. In an infant or older child, *S pneumoniae* or *N meningitidis* are the most common isolates. Hib is uncommon now because of widespread immunization. Increasingly, *S pneumoniae* with resistance to a third-generation cephalosporin (MIC > 2 mcg/mL) may occur in 3%–5% of isolates.

In bacterial meningitis, peak CSF antimicrobial concentrations 10 or more times greater than the MIC of the organism are desirable, but this may be difficult to achieve if organisms are resistant. The therapeutic problem is complicated if dexamethasone, which reduces the entry of some antimicrobials into the CSF, is also given. Thus, initial therapy of bacterial meningitis in an older child should include vancomycin and a third-generation cephalosporin. Alternatively, meropenem has also been successful. A lumbar puncture should be considered 24–48 hours after the start of therapy to assess the sterility of the CSF. Rifampin should be added if the Gram stain or cultures of CSF are positive on repeated lumbar puncture, if the child fails to improve, or if an organism with a very high MIC to ceftriaxone is isolated. The optimal therapy of highly resistant *S pneumoniae* meningitis is not well established.

Meningitis in a child with a ventriculoperitoneal shunt is most commonly caused by coagulase-negative staphylococci, many of which are methicillin-resistant, or *Corynebacterium* species, which are resistant to many antimicrobials. In many of these patients who are not seriously ill, therapy should be postponed while awaiting the appropriate shunt fluid for Gram stain and culture. Seriously ill patients should initially be given vancomycin and a third-generation cephalosporin, because *S aureus* and gram-negative rods are also possible and can cause serious infection.

Urinary Tract Infection

E coli is the most common isolate from the urinary tract. Outpatients with symptoms of lower urinary tract disease or with mild illness can be given ampicillin, cephalexin, or trimethoprim–sulfamethoxazole (TMP–SMX). Local experience and resistance rates should guide initial therapy. In selected patients with pyelonephritis, outpatient therapy is effective using parenteral aminoglycosides or ceftriaxone once per day. Oral cefixime and amoxicillin–clavulanate can be used in place of ceftriaxone for outpatient therapy. Ciprofloxacin has been approved by the U.S. Food and Drug Administration for therapy of urinary tract infection in children older than 1 year, but it should be reserved for complicated cases. For hospitalized patients with urinary tract infection and suspected bacteremia, ampicillin and gentamicin or a third-generation cephalosporin is appropriate. Gram stain should be used to guide the initial choice. For patients with known or suspected resistant organisms, such as *P aeruginosa*, or for patients with urosepsis, an aminoglycoside and ceftazidime, cefepime, or ticarcillin may be started. Unit-specific data on typical bacterial species and their patterns of susceptibility should guide the antimicrobial choice for nosocomial urinary tract infections.

Bacterial Pneumonia

Bacterial pneumonia in newborns generally should be treated with the same antimicrobial choices as sepsis. Infants and older children are frequently infected with *S pneumoniae*. Ampicillin and amoxicillin are effective in most patients eligible for outpatient therapy. Children who require hospitalization may benefit from a second- or third-generation cephalosporin. The broader initial coverage is indicated because of the greater severity of disease. A rapidly progressive pneumonia, with pneumatoceles or large pleural effusions, may be due to MRSA or group A streptococci, Hib, or another gram-negative rod. Vancomycin should be used in addition to a third-generation cephalosporin in these instances.

Children aged 6 years and older frequently have infection with *Mycoplasma pneumoniae*, *Chlamydia pneumoniae*, or *S pneumoniae*. Erythromycin, clarithromycin, or azithromycin is usually indicated for initial empiric therapy.

Skin & Soft Tissue Infections

S aureus and *Streptococcus pyogenes* are the most common causes of skin and soft tissue infections (SSTIs) in children. Community-acquired MRSA infections are common in many communities and complicate clinical decision making. Culture and susceptibility testing of abscesses, cellulitis, and more serious SSTIs is very important for optimal clinical management. Children with cellulitis more commonly have infection with group A streptococci, and empiric outpatient therapy with cephalexin or dicloxacillin is preferred. Children with small (< 5 cm) abscesses usually are effectively treated with incision and drainage without an antimicrobial. Outpatient therapy of large (> 5 cm) abscesses includes incision and drainage and empiric clindamycin or TMP–SMX, depending on local susceptibility patterns. However, in many communities, 50% or more of MRSA isolates are also resistant to clindamycin, fluoroquinolones, and erythromycin. Knowledge of the local resistance pattern of community-acquired MRSA is helpful in choosing initial antimicrobial therapy. Adequate cultures, the thoroughness of drainage procedures, and careful outpatient follow-up are needed to ensure optimal outcomes. Group A streptococcal infections are not adequately treated with TMP–SMX.

SPECIFIC ANTIMICROBIAL AGENTS

PENICILLINS

Aminopenicillins

Penicillin remains the drug of choice for streptococcal infections, acute rheumatic fever prophylaxis, syphilis, oral anaerobic infections, dental infections, *N meningitidis* infection, leptospirosis, rat-bite fever, actinomycosis, and infections due to *Clostridium* and *Bacillus* species. For oral therapy of minor infections, amoxicillin or ampicillin is usually equivalent. For systemic therapy, aqueous penicillin G is preferable. For treatment of streptococcal pharyngitis, some experts recommend a first-generation cephalosporin. Amoxicillin is preferred therapy for pneumonia and otitis media due to *S pneumoniae*. Amoxicillin is preferred for oral therapy of Lyme disease in children. For dog or cat bites, where *Pasteurella multocida* is commonly encountered, amoxicillin–clavulanate provides good coverage of *Pasteurella* as well as *Staphylococcus*. An alternative is separate prescriptions for penicillin and an antistaphylococcal drug such as cephalexin, or clindamycin and TMP–SMX in penicillin-allergic patients. For human bites, amoxicillin–clavulanate provides adequate therapy for *Eikenella corrodens* and other mixed oral aerobes and anaerobes. The β-lactamase inhibitor sulbactam combined with ampicillin is given parenterally for human and animal bites, and some other infections due to organisms from the oral flora, in which mixed aerobic and anaerobic bacteria may be resistant to ampicillin due to β-lactamase production.

Penicillinase-Resistant Penicillins

S aureus is usually resistant to penicillin and amoxicillin owing to penicillinase production. Nafcillin, oxacillin, methicillin, and first- and second-generation cephalosporins are stable to penicillinase and are usually equivalent for intravenous therapy. Methicillin is associated with more frequent interstitial nephritis. Oxacillin and methicillin are renally excreted, whereas nafcillin is excreted through the biliary tract. These properties are occasionally considered in children with renal or liver failure. Cost should usually be the deciding factor for choosing an agent. Often both *S aureus* and *S pyogenes* are suspected initially (eg, in cellulitis or postoperative wound infections). The penicillinase-resistant penicillins (PRPs) and first- and second-generation cephalosporins are efficacious for most streptococcal infections, although penicillin remains the drug of choice.

MRSA is an increasingly common and serious community-acquired infection in children and may cause nosocomial infection. MRSA infections are also resistant to other PRPs and to other cephalosporins. Vancomycin is effective against MRSA and coagulase-negative staphylococci. *S aureus* infections range in severity from minor infections treated on an outpatient basis to life-threatening infections. Severe infections due to MRSA are a serious concern in many communities. It is important to culture and determine antimicrobial susceptibility of suspected *S aureus* infections. In communities with frequent MRSA infections in children, initial therapy of seriously ill children should include vancomycin. MRSA may also be resistant to macrolides and clindamycin by alteration in the bacterial 23s-ribosomal RNA. Many strains reported as clindamycin-susceptible and erythromycin-resistant are truly resistant to clindamycin. This inducible resistance to clindamycin may be detected in erythromycin-resistant MRSA that demonstrates a D-zone in disk susceptibility testing to clindamycin. Community-acquired MRSA is more likely to be susceptible to TMP–SMX, clindamycin, and tetracyclines than hospital-acquired infections.

For outpatient therapy, cloxacillin, dicloxacillin, and first- or second-generation cephalosporins are usually equally effective for infections due to susceptible *S aureus*. Cost may determine the choice between drugs.

Anti-*Pseudomonas* Penicillins

Ticarcillin, mezlocillin, and piperacillin are active intravenously against streptococci, ampicillin-susceptible enterococci,

H influenzae, gram-negative rods (including more resistant gram-negative rods such as *Enterobacter*, *Proteus*, and *P aeruginosa*), and gram-negative anaerobes such as *Bacteroides fragilis. P aeruginosa* is inherently resistant to most antimicrobials, and high levels of these drugs are usually required. The combination of ticarcillin or piperacillin and an aminoglycoside is synergistic against *P aeruginosa* and many other enteric gram-negative rods. Ticarcillin in a fixed combination with clavulanic acid has activity against β-lactamase–producing strains of *Klebsiella*, *S aureus*, and *Bacteroides*. Piperacillin is more active in vitro against many gram-negative enteric infections and may be advantageous in some circumstances, but it is not approved in children. Piperacillin–tazobactam is another combination antimicrobial and β-lactamase inhibitor that has enhanced activity against many β-lactamase producers.

Antipseudomonal penicillins cause the same toxicities as penicillin and therefore are usually very safe. Carbenicillin, ticarcillin, and piperacillin contain large amounts of sodium, which may cause problems for some patients with cardiac or renal disease.

GLYCOPEPTIDE AGENTS

Vancomycin and teicoplanin are glycopeptide antimicrobial agents active against the cell wall of gram-positive organisms. Only vancomycin is licensed in the United States. Vancomycin is useful for parenteral therapy of resistant gram-positive cocci such as penicillin- and cephalosporin-resistant *S pneumoniae*, MRSA, methicillin-resistant coagulase-negative staphylococci, and ampicillin-resistant enterococci. Vancomycin is also used orally for therapy of colitis due to *Clostridium difficile*, although it should not be used as the drug of first choice.

The empiric use of vancomycin has increased tremendously over the last decade. As a result, vancomycin-resistant enterococci (VRE) and coagulase-negative staphylococci have become problems, particularly in inpatient units, intensive care units, and oncology wards. *S aureus* with increased MICs to vancomycin has been reported in the United States and Japan. This resistance is of concern because of the inherent virulence of many *S aureus* strains. Vancomycin use should be monitored carefully in hospitals and their intensive care units. It should not be used empirically when an infection is mild or when other antimicrobial agents are likely to be effective. Vancomycin should be stopped promptly if infection is found to be due to organisms susceptible to other antimicrobials.

Rapid infusion of vancomycin is associated with the "red man syndrome," characterized by diffuse red flushing, at times pruritus, and occasionally tachycardia and hypotension. As a result, vancomycin is infused slowly over 1 hour or longer in some cases. Diphenhydramine or hydrocortisone (or both) may also be used as premedication.

Measurement of peak-and-trough serum vancomycin concentrations is not necessary in most clinical situations, because the levels achieved with standard dosing are usually predictable and nontoxic. Measurement of serum concentrations is helpful in patients with abnormal or unpredictable renal function; in those with altered volume of distribution, as occurs in nephrotic syndrome or shock; and in those receiving higher-dose therapy (eg, for meningitis or other difficult-to-treat infections). For patients receiving antimicrobials for weeks to months, weekly monitoring of clinical signs and symptoms and of urinalysis, creatinine, and complete blood count will allow detection of toxicity.

OXAZOLIDINONES

Linezolid is the first drug in this new class of antimicrobials which have a distinct new mechanism of action; they bind to the 50s-ribosomal RNA subunit and prevent initiation of protein synthesis. Because of this unique mechanism, there is no cross-resistance with other classes of antimicrobials. The in vitro development of resistance has also been uncommon.

Linezolid is active against aerobic gram-positive organisms, including streptococci, staphylococci, enterococci, and pneumococci. Because linezolid is active against gram-positive organisms resistant to other antimicrobials (eg, MRSA, methicillin-resistant coagulase-negative staphylococci, VRE, and penicillin-resistant *S pneumoniae*), it is useful for these difficult-to-treat infections.

Linezolid is safe and well tolerated in children. Gastrointestinal symptoms are the most commonly encountered side effect. Neutropenia and thrombocytopenia have been reported, and linezolid should therefore be used with monitoring in patients at increased risk for these problems or in patients receiving therapy for 2 weeks or longer. Linezolid is an inhibitor of monoamine oxidase (MAO) and should not be used in patients taking MAO inhibitors, or in patients taking phenylpropanolamine or pseudoephedrine.

Linezolid should be used only for infections due to a proven gram-positive pathogen that is known or strongly suspected to be resistant to other available agents.

QUINUPRISTIN–DALFOPRISTIN

Quinupristin and dalfopristin are two antimicrobials of the streptogramin class, which individually are bacteriostatic, but in combination are synergistic and bacteriocidal. These drugs are combined in a fixed ratio of 70:30, known as Synercid. Streptogramins inhibit protein synthesis by binding to the 50s-ribosomal subunit. The streptogramins were discovered many years ago, but interest has increased only recently due to the activity of these agents against some very difficult-to-treat gram-positive infections.

The quinupristin–dalfopristin combination has activity against staphylococci, streptococci, pneumococci, and some enterococci. Quinupristin–dalfopristin is primarily indicated for serious infections due to vancomycin-resistant *Enterococcus faecium* and MRSA. Quinupristin–dalfopristin is not active against *E faecalis* and, therefore, differentiation of these strains from *E faecium* is important prior to initiating therapy.

Quinupristin–dalfopristin is not approved for therapy in children. Nonetheless, therapy has been initiated under a compassionate release program in some pediatric patients seriously ill with difficult-to-treat infections due to resistant organisms.

Arthralgias and myalgias have at times been severe in adult patients. Other significant side effects include elevated bilirubin and inflammation at intravenous sites.

Quinupristin–dalfopristin is a significant inhibitor of CYP-450 3A4 and, therefore, must be used with caution in patients receiving drugs metabolized by this mechanism (eg, clarithromycin, itraconazole, erythromycin, and many others).

CEPHALOSPORINS

Cephalosporin agents make up a large and often confusing group of antimicrobials. Many of these drugs are similar in antibacterial spectrum and side effects and may have similar names. Clinicians should learn well the properties of one or two drugs in each class. Cephalosporins are often grouped as "generations" to signify their similar antimicrobial activity. First-generation cephalosporins such as cefazolin intravenously and cephalexin orally are useful mainly for susceptible *S aureus* infection and urinary tract infection due to susceptible *E coli*. Second-generation cephalosporins, such as cefuroxime intravenously and cefprozil and cefuroxime orally, have somewhat reduced, but acceptable, activity against gram-positive cocci, and greater activity against some gram-negative rods compared with first-generation cephalosporins. They are active against *H influenzae* and *Moraxella catarrhalis*, including strains that produce β-lactamase capable of inactivating ampicillin. Third-generation cephalosporins have substantially less activity against gram-positive cocci, such as *S aureus*, but greatly augmented activity against aerobic gram-negative rods. Cefotaxime and ceftriaxone are examples of intravenous drugs, whereas cefpodoxime and ceftibuten are representative oral drugs. Cefepime is a new antimicrobial often described as fourth-generation because of its broad activity against gram-positive and gram-negative organisms, including *P aeruginosa*. Cefepime is stable to β-lactamase degradation and is a poor inducer of β-lactamase. Cefepime will be most useful for organisms resistant to other drugs.

No cephalosporin agent has substantial activity against *L monocytogenes*, enterococci, or MRSA. The only cephalosporins useful for treating anaerobic infections are cefoxitin and cefotetan, which are second-generation cephalosporins with excellent activity against *B fragilis*. Ceftazidime and cefepime are cephalosporins with activity against *P aeruginosa*.

Allergy to β-lactam antimicrobials is reported commonly by parents. Immediate hypersensitivity reactions, including anaphylaxis or hives, most commonly predict IgE-mediated allergy. In contrast, most delayed reactions and nonspecific rashes are likely due to the underlying infection or nonallergic reactions. (See Chapter 38.) Cephalosporins should be used with caution in children with immediate hypersensitivity reactions to penicillins or cephalosporins.

Resistance to cephalosporins is common among aerobic gram-negative rods. The presence of inducible cephalosporinases in some gram-negative rod organisms, such as *P aeruginosa*, *Serratia marcescens*, *Citrobacter*, and *Enterobacter*, has led to clinical failures because of the emergence of resistance during therapy. Extended-spectrum β-lactamases mediate broad resistance to all penicillins, aminopenicillins, cephalosporins, and monobactams. Carbapenems, fluoroquinolones, or combinations including these drugs are used for serious infections due to gram-negative organisms with these enzymes. Active laboratory-based surveillance is necessary to detect resistance in these gram-negative organisms.

AZTREONAM

Aztreonam is the only monobactam antimicrobial agent approved in the United States. Although it is not approved for use in children younger than age 9 months, there is considerable pediatric experience with its use, including in neonates and premature infants. Aztreonam is active against aerobic gram-negative rods, including *P aeruginosa*. Aztreonam has activity against *H influenzae* and *M catarrhalis*, including those that are β-lactamase producers. Most patients with allergy to penicillin or cephalosporins are not sensitized to aztreonam, except that children with prior reactions to ceftazidime may have reactions to aztreonam because aztreonam and ceftazidime have a common side chain.

CARBAPENEMS

Meropenem, ertapenem, doripenem, and imipenem are broad-spectrum β-lactam antimicrobials. Imipenem–cilastatin is a combination of an active antibiotic and cilastatin, which inhibits the metabolism of imipenem in the kidneys and thereby results in high serum and urine levels of imipenem. These carbapenems are also active against *S pneumoniae*, including many penicillin- and cephalosporin-resistant strains. Carbapenems have been used successfully to treat meningitis and may be considered if vancomycin is not tolerated. An increased frequency of seizures is encountered when central nervous system infections are treated with carbapenems. These agents are broadly active against streptococci, methicillin-susceptible *S aureus*, some enterococci, and gram-negative rods such as *P aeruginosa*, β-lactamase–producing *H influenzae*, and gram-negative anaerobes. Ertapenem has less activity against *P aeruginosa*, *Acinetobacter* species, and *Enterococcus* species than meropenem and imipenem. Because carbapenems are active against so many species of bacteria, there is a strong temptation to use them as single-drug empiric therapy. Units that have used carbapenems heavily have encountered resistance in many different species of gram-negative rods.

MACROLIDES & AZALIDES

Erythromycin was once the most commonly used macrolide antimicrobial agent, but now azithromycin and clarithromycin are preferred because of decreased side effects. It is active against many bacteria that are resistant to cell wall–active antimicrobials, and is the drug of choice for *Bordetella pertussis*, *Legionella pneumophila*, *C pneumoniae*, *M pneumoniae*, and *Chlamydia trachomatis* infections (in children in whom tetracycline is not an option). Erythromycin is used for outpatient therapy of streptococcal and staphylococcal infections in patients with penicillin allergy. More serious infections due to streptococci and staphylococci are usually treated with penicillins, clindamycin, PRPs, or cephalosporins because of a significant incidence of erythromycin resistance in both species. *S pneumoniae* resistant to erythromycin and the related macrolides are now frequent in many communities. This limits the ability of macrolide antimicrobials for therapy of otitis media and sinusitis. Gastrointestinal side effects are common. Interactions with theophylline, carbamazepine, terfenadine, cycloserine, and other drugs may require dosage modifications of erythromycin and clarithromycin. Significant interactions with azithromycin are less common. Erythromycin exposure is associated with pyloric stenosis in newborns, so azithromycin is preferred in most neonates.

Erythromycin is available in many formulations, including the base, estolate, ethyl succinate, and stearate. Transient hepatic toxicity occurs in adults, but is much less common in children. Erythromycin base and stearate should be taken with meals for best absorption.

Clarithromycin and azithromycin, macrolide and azalide antimicrobials, respectively, are much less likely than erythromycin to cause nausea, vomiting, and diarrhea. These agents are useful in children who cannot tolerate erythromycin. Clarithromycin is more active than erythromycin against *H influenzae*, *M catarrhalis*, and *Neisseria gonorrhoeae* and is the drug of choice, usually in combination, for some nontuberculous mycobacterial infections. Azithromycin has a prolonged tissue half-life that achieves a prolonged antimicrobial effect. Azithromycin is dosed once daily for 5 days, but must be taken 1 hour before or 2 hours after meals because food interferes with absorption. Although azithromycin is active against *H influenzae*, some authors report poor eradication of *H influenzae* from the middle ear. Azithromycin can be used for single-dose therapy of *C trachomatis* infections. It is beneficial in adolescents when compliance with erythromycin or tetracycline is a concern. Azithromycin is useful for therapy of *Shigella* and *Salmonella* infections, including typhoid fever resistant to ampicillin and TMP–SMX. Alternatives include third-generation cephalosporins and fluoroquinolones. Clarithromycin is effective against Lyme disease, but amoxicillin is the drug of choice in young children. Clarithromycin and azithromycin are alternative drugs for toxoplasmosis in sulfonamide-allergic patients and as alternatives to erythromycin in legionellosis. In vitro and limited clinical experience in providing treatment to contacts of pertussis patients suggests efficacy equal to that of erythromycin. Clarithromycin and azithromycin are considerably more expensive than most erythromycin formulations, and for that reason are usually preferred, but they are advantageous by virtue of their twice-daily and once-daily dosing, respectively. Some failures of the newer macrolides have occurred in *S pneumoniae* sepsis and meningitis, perhaps because of low serum levels despite the high tissue levels achieved. High rates of resistance to macrolides and azalides have been encountered in some communities. The frequent use of azithromycin for respiratory infections and acute otitis media has contributed to selection of resistant strains.

CLINDAMYCIN

Clindamycin is active against *S aureus*, some MRSA, *S pyogenes*, other streptococcal species except enterococci, and both gram-positive and gram-negative anaerobes. Clindamycin or metronidazole is frequently combined with other antimicrobials for empiric therapy of suspected anaerobic or mixed anaerobic and aerobic infections. Empiric use of clindamycin is justified in suspected anaerobic infections because cultures frequently cannot be obtained and, if obtained, may be slow in confirming anaerobic infection. Examples are pelvic inflammatory disease, necrotizing enterocolitis, other infections in which the integrity of the gastrointestinal or genitourinary tracts is compromised, and sinusitis. Clindamycin does not achieve high levels in CSF, but brain abscesses, toxoplasmosis, and other central nervous system infections, where disruption of the blood-brain barrier occurs, can be successfully treated with clindamycin. Clindamycin should be added to regimens for treatment of serious streptococcal and staphylococcal infections, such as necrotizing fasciitis and toxic shock syndrome. Both in vitro and clinical data suggest increased bactericidal killing, and improved outcomes occur with clindamycin. For most oral anaerobes (eg, in a dental abscess), penicillin is more active than clindamycin. Clindamycin has been associated with the occurrence of *C difficile*–related pseudomembranous colitis. Although diarrhea is a frequent side effect, pseudomembranous colitis is uncommonly due to clindamycin in children.

SULFONAMIDES

Sulfonamides—the oldest class of antimicrobials—remain useful for treatment of urinary tract infections, and for other infections due to *E coli* and for *Nocardia*. Although useful for rheumatic fever prophylaxis in penicillin-allergic patients, sulfonamides fail to eradicate group A streptococci and cannot be used for treatment of acute infections.

TMP–SMX is a fixed combination that is more active than either drug alone. Gram-positive cocci, including some *S pneumoniae*, many staphylococci, *Haemophilus*, and many gram-negative rods, are susceptible. Unfortunately, resistance to TMP–SMX has become more common. *S pneumoniae* resistant to penicillin and cephalosporins is often also resistant to TMP–SMX and erythromycin. In communities, where *Shigella* and *Salmonella enteritidis* strains remain susceptible, as do most *E coli* strains, TMP–SMX is very useful for treatment of both urinary tract infections and bacterial dysentery. TMP–SMX is also the drug of choice for treatment or prophylaxis against *Pneumocystis jiroveci* infection. Myelosuppressive side effects especially anemia limit the use of TMP–SMX in some children infected with HIV.

Sulfonamide is associated with several cutaneous reactions, including urticaria, photosensitivity, Stevens-Johnson syndrome, purpura, and maculopapular rashes. Hematologic side effects such as leukopenia, thrombocytopenia, and hemolytic anemia are uncommon. Common gastrointestinal side effects are nausea and vomiting. The dermatologic and hematologic side effects are thought to be more common and more severe with TMP–SMX than with sulfonamide alone.

TETRACYCLINES

Tetracyclines, which are effective against a broad range of bacteria, are not commonly used in children because alternative effective drugs are available. Many different tetracycline formulations are available. Tetracyclines are effective against *B pertussis* and *E coli* and many species of *Rickettsia*, *Chlamydia*, and *Mycoplasma*. Doxycycline or minocycline is the drug of choice for eradication of *C trachomatis* in pelvic inflammatory disease and nongonococcal urethritis.

Staining of permanent teeth was noted in young children given repeated courses of tetracyclines. As a result, tetracyclines are generally not given to children younger than age 9 years unless alternative drugs are unavailable. A single course of tetracycline does not pose a significant risk of tooth staining. Mucous membrane candidiasis, photosensitivity, nausea, and vomiting are other common side effects. Tetracycline should be taken on an empty stomach, either 1 hour before or 2 hours after a meal. Doxycycline is well absorbed even in the presence of food; administration with food may minimize gastrointestinal side effects. Doxycycline is often preferred because it is better tolerated than tetracycline, and twice-daily administration is convenient.

Tetracycline is used for therapy of rickettsial infections such as Rocky Mountain spotted fever, ehrlichiosis, rickettsialpox, murine typhus, and Q fever; as an alternative to erythromycin for *M pneumoniae* and *C pneumoniae* infections; and for treatment of psittacosis, brucellosis, *P multocida* infection, and relapsing fever.

Tigecycline is a new polyketide antimicrobial that is an analogue of tetracycline and a bacteriostatic inhibitor of protein synthesis. Tigecycline is active against gram-negative aerobes, anaerobes, and many gram-positive cocci including MRSA. It is approved for intravenous therapy of adults with complicated SSTIs and complicated intra-abdominal infections.

AMINOGLYCOSIDES

The aminoglycosides bind to ribosomal subunits and inhibit protein synthesis. They are active against aerobic gram-negative rods, including *P aeruginosa*. Streptomycin was the first drug in this class, but today it is used only to treat tuberculosis and the occasional cases of plague and tularemia.

Aminoglycosides are used to treat serious gram-negative infections and are given intravenously or intramuscularly. They are also used to treat pyelonephritis, suspected gram-negative sepsis, and in other settings where *P aeruginosa* infections are common, such as cystic fibrosis and burns. Aminoglycosides have activity against gram-positive organisms and, combined with penicillin or ampicillin, may achieve synergistic killing of *L monocytogenes* and group B streptococci. Penicillin, ampicillin, or vancomycin combined with gentamicin is indicated for therapy of serious enterococcal infections, such as sepsis or endocarditis because of more rapid clinical improvement with combined therapy. Aminoglycosides have activity against *S aureus*, but are always used in combination with other antistaphylococcal antibiotics.

Aminoglycosides are not active in an acidic environment and may not be effective against abscesses. Aminoglycosides diffuse poorly into the CSF and achieve only about 10% of serum concentrations. As a result, a third-generation cephalosporin is preferred for treatment of meningitis.

Aminoglycosides kill bacteria in a concentration-dependent manner. They also have a prolonged suppressive effect on the regrowth of susceptible organisms (postantibiotic effect). These principles have led some investigators to establish guidelines for once-daily dosing of aminoglycosides, using larger initial doses given every 24 hours. Although aminoglycosides are associated with both renal and eighth nerve toxicity, the entry of the drug into renal and cochlear cells is saturable. It therefore was predicted that once-daily dosing would result in less toxicity than traditional twice-daily or three-times-daily dosing. Studies in adult patients confirm that once-daily dosing is as efficacious as traditional dosing and is associated with less toxicity. Although there is extensive experience with dosing intervals of 18–36 hours in premature infants, small total daily doses are customarily used (2.0–2.5 mg/kg per dose of gentamicin or tobramycin). A convenient and cost-effective approach in children is based on the experience with adult patients and uses larger daily doses (4–7 mg/kg per dose every 24 hours). Nevertheless, traditional twice-daily or three-times-daily dosing regimens of aminoglycosides, with monitoring of serum levels, are still widely used. Careful monitoring is necessary, particularly in children with abnormal or changing renal function, premature infants, and infants with rapidly changing volumes of distribution. Aminoglycosides are usually infused over 30–45 minutes, and the peak serum concentration is measured 30–45 minutes after the end of the infusion. A trough serum concentration is measured prior to the next dose. The efficacious and nontoxic serum concentrations for gentamicin and tobramycin are trough less than 2 mcg/mL and peak 5–10 mcg/mL; for amikacin, trough less than 10 mcg/mL and peak 15–25 mcg/mL (see Table 39–4). Aminoglycoside levels and creatinine levels should be measured in children expected to receive more than 3 days of therapy, and repeated weekly in children on long-term therapy, even when renal function is normal and stable.

FLUOROQUINOLONES

Modification of the quinolone structure of nalidixic acid has led to many new compounds called fluoroquinolones, which are well absorbed after oral administration and possess excellent antibacterial activity against resistant gram-negative pathogens. The currently available fluoroquinolones vary in their activity against specific organisms. Fluoroquinolones are active against most of the Enterobacteriaceae, including *E coli*, *Enterobacter*, *Klebsiella*, in some cases *P aeruginosa*, and many other gram-negative bacteria such as *H influenzae*, *M catarrhalis*, *N gonorrhoeae*, and *N meningitidis*. Some fluoroquinolones (ofloxacin and levofloxacin) are active against *C trachomatis* and *Mycoplasma*. The fluoroquinolones are active against some enterococci, *S aureus*, MRSA, and coagulase-negative staphylococci. The newer quinolones have good activity against penicillin and cephalosporin-resistant *S pneumonia*.

Ciprofloxacin and its otic and ophthalmic preparations are the only fluoroquinolone antimicrobials currently approved for use in children older than 1 year, although fluoroquinolones offer very attractive alternatives to approved agents. The objection to quinolones is based on the recognition that nalidixic acid and other quinolones cause arthropathy when tested experimentally in newborn animals of many species. The fear that children would also be more susceptible than adults to cartilage injury has not been realized in clinical experience. Both retrospective long-term follow-up studies of children given nalidixic acid and prospective studies of children receiving treatment under protocols with fluoroquinolones have shown similar rates of toxicity compared with adult patients. Arthropathy occurs uncommonly, although tendon rupture is a reported rare, serious complication. For these reasons, quinolones should be considered for use in children when the benefit clearly outweighs the risk, when no alternative drug is available, and after discussion with the parents.

Ciprofloxacin is useful for oral therapy of resistant gram-negative urinary tract infections, such as those caused by *P aeruginosa*. Fluoroquinolones are no longer recommended for single-dose therapy of gonorrhea due to frequent resistance, but ofloxacin and levofloxacin are an alternative therapy for treating Chlamydia infections and pelvic inflammatory disease. Ciprofloxacin and ofloxacin are used as therapy of resistant cases of shigellosis. Levofloxacin and ciprofloxacin are usually the drugs of choice for treatment of traveler's diarrhea. Ciprofloxacin is useful for treatment of *P aeruginosa* infection in patients with cystic fibrosis, and as therapy for chronic suppurative otitis media. Several quinolones are used as therapy for pneumonia due to *Legionella*, *Mycoplasma*, or *C pneumoniae*, although a macrolide is often preferred, and as prophylactic therapy of meningococcal infection. Ofloxacin and levofloxacin are used for treatment of some cases of *Mycobacterium tuberculosis* and some atypical mycobacterial infections.

METRONIDAZOLE

Metronidazole has excellent activity against most anaerobes, particularly gram-negative anaerobes, such as *Bacteroides* and *Fusobacterium*, and against gram-positive anaerobes such as *Clostridium*, *Prevotella*, and *Porphyromonas*. Gram-positive anaerobic cocci such as *Peptococcus* and *Peptostreptococcus* are often more susceptible to penicillin or to clindamycin. Because metronidazole lacks activity against aerobic organisms, it is usually given with one or more other antibiotics. Metronidazole is well absorbed after oral administration and has excellent penetration into the central nervous system. Metronidazole is the drug of choice for bacterial vaginosis and for *C difficile* enterocolitis. It is active against many parasites, including *Giardia lamblia* and *Entamoeba histolytica*.

DAPTOMYCIN

Daptomycin has broad bactericidal activity against gram-positive cocci. Daptomycin is a lipopeptide that binds to bacterial cell membranes, resulting in membrane depolarization and cell death. Daptomycin is active against methicillin-sensitive and -resistant *S aureus*, *S pyogenes*, and *Streptococcus agalactiae*, as well as *E faecium* (including vancomycin-resistant strains) and *E faecalis* (vancomycin-sensitive strains). Daptomycin is given as a once-daily intravenous infusion of 4 mg/kg and is approved for therapy of complicated SSTIs in adults, but has not been sufficiently studied in children younger than 18 years to make recommendations for dosing and use. Daptomycin therapy of pneumonia was unsuccessful in a large percentage of cases, and should not be used. Daptomycin is excreted renally, so a modification of dosing is needed in patients with impaired renal function. Nausea, constipation, and headache are the most common side effects of therapy. In patients with muscle pain, monitoring creatinine phosphokinase levels should be done.

REFERENCES

Bradley JS et al: The management of community-acquired **pneumonia** in infants and children older than 3 months of age: clinical practice guidelines by the Pediatric Infectious Diseases Society and the Infectious Diseases Society of America. Clin Infect Dis 2011;53(7):e25–e76 [PMID: 21880587].

Bradley JS, Nelson JB: Nelson's Pocketbook of Pediatric Antimicrobial Therapy, 18th ed. American Academy of Pediatrics, 2010–2011.

Chen AE et al: Randomized controlled trial of cephalexin versus clindamycinin for uncomplicated pediatric skin infections. Pediatrics 2011;127:e573 [PMID: 21339275].

Elliot DJ et al: Empiric antimicrobial therapy for pediatric skin and soft-tissue infections in the era of methicillin-resistant *Staphylococcus aureus*. Pediatrics 2009;123(6):e959 [PMID: 19470525].

Gilbert DN et al: The Sanford Guide to Antimicrobial Therapy, 41st ed. Antimicrobial Therapy, Inc., 2011.

Web Resources

Alliance for the Prudent Use of Antibiotics: http://www.tufts.edu/med/apua

CDC Antibiotic and Antimicrobial Resistance page: http://www.cdc.gov/drugresistance

Infectious Diseases Society of America: http://www.idsociety.org/

Infections: Viral & Rickettsial

40

Myron J. Levin, MD
Adriana Weinberg, MD

VIRAL INFECTIONS

Viruses cause most pediatric infections. Mixed viral or viral-bacterial infections of the respiratory and intestinal tracts are rather common, as is prolonged asymptomatic shedding of some viruses in childhood. Thus, the detection of a virus is not always proof that it is the cause of a given illness. Viruses are often a predisposing factor for bacterial respiratory infections (eg, otitis, sinusitis, and pneumonia).

Many respiratory and herpesviruses can now be detected within 24–48 hours by combining culture and monoclonal antibody techniques ("rapid culture technique"). Diagnosis of many viral illnesses is also possible through antigen or nucleic acid detection techniques. These techniques are more rapid than isolation of viruses in tissue culture and in most cases are equally sensitive or more so. Polymerase chain reaction (PCR) amplification of viral genes has led to recognition of previously undetected infections. New diagnostic tests have changed some basic concepts about viral diseases and made diagnosis of viral infections both more certain and more complex. Only laboratories with excellent quality-control procedures should be used, and the results of new tests must be interpreted cautiously. The availability of specific antiviral agents increases the value of early diagnosis for some serious viral infections. Table 40–1 lists viral agents associated with common clinical signs, and Table 40–2 lists diagnostic tests. The viral diagnostic laboratory should be contacted for details regarding specimen collection, handling, and shipping. Table 40–3 lists common causes of red rashes in children that should be considered in the differential diagnosis of certain viral illnesses.

RESPIRATORY INFECTIONS

Many viral infections cause both upper or lower respiratory tract signs and symptoms. Those that produce a predominance of these signs and symptoms are described in the text that follows. Many so-called respiratory viruses can also produce distinct nonrespiratory disease (eg, enteritis or cystitis caused by adenoviruses; parotitis caused by parainfluenza viruses). Respiratory viruses can cause disease in any area of the respiratory tree. Thus, they can cause coryza, pharyngitis, sinusitis, tracheitis, bronchitis, bronchiolitis, and pneumonia—although certain viruses tend to be closely associated with one anatomic area (eg, parainfluenza with croup, respiratory syncytial virus [RSV] with bronchiolitis) or discrete epidemics (eg, influenza, RSV, parainfluenza). Nevertheless it is impossible on clinical grounds to be certain of the viral cause of an infection in a given child. This information is provided by the virology laboratory and is often important for epidemiologic, therapeutic, and preventive reasons. In immunocompromised patients these annoying, but otherwise benign, viruses can cause severe pneumonia.

VIRUSES CAUSING THE COMMON COLD

The common cold syndrome (also called upper respiratory infection) is characterized by combinations of runny nose, nasal congestion, sore throat, tearing, cough, and sneezing. Low-grade fever may be present. The causal agent is usually not sought or determined. Epidemiologic studies indicate that rhinoviruses, which are the most common cause (30%–40%; much more in some series), are present throughout the year, but are more prevalent in the colder months in temperate climates. Adenoviruses also cause colds in all seasons and epidemics are common. Respiratory syncytial virus, parainfluenza viruses, human metapneuomovirus, and influenza viruses cause the cold syndrome during epidemics from late fall through winter. Multiple strains of coronaviruses account for 5%–10% of colds in winter. Equally prevalent in aggregate are other newly identified respiratory viruses such as the human bocavirus (a parvovirus) and several polyomaviruses. The precise role of these newly discovered viruses in childhood disease is under study. Enteroviruses cause the "summer cold." One outcome of these infections is morbidity continuing for 5–7 days. It is also likely that changes in respiratory epithelium, local mucosal swelling,

Table 40–1. Some viral causes of clinical syndromes.

Rash
- Enterovirus
- Adenovirus
- Measles
- Rubella
- Human herpesvirus type 6[a] or 7[a]
- Varicella
- Parvovirus B19[b]
- Epstein-Barr virus
- Dengue and other arboviral diseases
- Human immunodeficiency virus (HIV), acute syndrome

Fever
- Enterovirus
- Epstein-Barr virus
- Human herpesvirus type 6[a] or 7[a]
- Cytomegalovirus
- Influenza
- Rhinovirus
- Arboviruses
- Most others

Conjunctivitis
- Adenovirus
- Enterovirus 70
- Measles
- Herpes simplex virus[c]

Parotitis
- Mumps
- Parainfluenza
- Enterovirus
- Cytomegalovirus
- Epstein-Barr virus
- HIV

Pharyngitis
- Adenovirus
- Enterovirus
- Epstein-Barr virus
- Herpes simplex virus[d]
- Influenza
- Other respiratory viruses

Adenopathy
- Epstein-Barr virus
- Cytomegalovirus
- Rubella[e]
- HIV

Croup
- Parainfluenza
- Influenza
- Adenovirus
- Other respiratory viruses

Bronchiolitis
- Respiratory syncytial virus[f]
- Adenovirus
- Parainfluenza
- Influenza
- Human metapneumovirus

Pneumonia
- Respiratory syncytial virus
- Adenovirus
- Parainfluenza
- Hantavirus
- Measles
- Varicella[g]
- Cytomegalovirus[h,i]
- Influenza

Enteritis
- Rotavirus
- Enteric adenovirus
- Enterovirus
- Astrovirus
- Calicivirus
- Norovirus
- Cytomegalovirus[i]

Hepatitis
- Hepatitis A,[j] B, C, D, E
- Epstein-Barr virus
- Adenovirus
- Cytomegalovirus
- Varicella[k]
- Parvovirus B19

Arthritis (Arthralgia)
- Parvovirus B19
- Rubella
- Hepatitis B
- Dengue and chikungunya fever

Congenital or perinatal infection
- Adenovirus
- Cytomegalovirus
- Hepatitis B
- Hepatitis C[l]
- Rubella
- HIV
- Parvovirus B19
- Enterovirus
- Varicella
- Herpes simplex virus

Meningoencephalitis
- Enterovirus
- Mumps
- Arboviruses (includes West Nile virus)
- Herpes simplex virus
- Cytomegalovirus[i]
- Lymphocytic choriomeningitis virus
- Measles
- Varicella
- Adenovirus
- HIV
- Epstein-Barr virus
- Influenza
- Rabies

[a]Roseola agents.
[b]Erythema infectiosum agent.
[c]Conjunctivitis rare, only in primary infections; keratitis in older patients.
[d]May cause isolated pharyngeal vesicles at any age.
[e]May cause adenopathy without rash; especially postauricular.
[f]Over 70% of cases.
[g]Immunosuppressed, pregnant, rarely other adults.
[h]Usually only in young infants.
[i]Severely immunosuppressed at risk.
[j]Anicteric cases more common in children; these may resemble viral gastroenteritis.
[k]Common, but only mild laboratory abnormalities; severe in immunosuppressed.
[l]Especially when the mother is HIV-positive.

Table 40–2. Diagnostic tests for viral infections.

Agent	Rapid Antigen Detection (Specimen)	Tissue Culture Mean Days to Positive (Range)	Serology		PCR	Comments
			Acute	Paired		
Adenovirus	+ (respiratory and enteric)	10 (1–21)	–	+	+	"Enteric" strains detected by culture on special cell line, antigen detection, or PCR
Arboviruses	–	–	+	+	+	Acute serum may diagnose many forms
Astrovirus	–	–	–	–	+	Diagnosis by electron microscopy
Calicivirus	– RL	–	–	–	+	Diagnosis by electron microscopy; PCR generally available for norovirus; present in RL for others
Colorado tick virus	On RBC	–	–	RL, CDC	+	
Coronavirus	–	RL	–	+	+	
Cytomegalovirus	+ (tissue biopsy, urine, blood, respiratory secretions)	2 (2–28)	+	+	+	Diagnosis by presence of IgM antibody; rapid culture method generally available; low avidity antibody indicates recent infection.
Dengue	–	5 days (RL)	+	+	+	Testing at CDC; 90% seropositive at 6 days
Enterovirus	–	3 (2–8) Coxsackie A difficult to culture	–	+	+	
Epstein-Barr virus	–	–	+	+	+	Single serologic panel defines infection status; heterophil antibodies less sensitive
Hantavirus	–	–	+	ND	RL	Diagnosis by presence of IgM antibody
Hepatitis A virus	–	–	+	ND	RL	Diagnosis by presence of IgM antibody
Hepatitis B virus	+ (blood)	–	+	ND	+	Diagnosis by presence of surface antigen or anticore IgM antibody
Hepatitis C virus	–	–	+	ND	+	Positive serology suggests that hepatitis C could be the causative agent; PCR is confirmatory. PCR may be positive before serology
Herpes simplex virus	+ (mucosa, tissue biopsy, respiratory secretions, skin)	1 (1–7)	+	+	+	Serology rarely used for herpes simplex; IgM antibody used in selected cases
Human herpesvirus 6 and 7	–	2 (RL)	+	+	+	Roseola agent
Human immunodeficiency virus	+ (blood) (acid dissociation of immune complexes); not done in the United States	15 (5–28)	+	ND	+	Antibody proves infection unless passively acquired (maternal antibody gone by age 15 mo); culture not widely available; PCR definitive for early diagnosis in infant (detect RNA or DNA)
Human metapneumovirus	+	2	–	+	+	
Influenza virus	+ (respiratory secretions)	2 (2–14)	–	+	+	Antigen detection 40%–90% sensitive (varies with virus strain)
Lymphocytic choriomeningitis virus	–	–	–	+	RL	Can be isolated in suckling mice
Measles virus	+ (respiratory secretions)	–	+	+	+	Difficult to grow; IgM serology diagnostic
Mumps virus	–	> 5	+	+	+	IgM ELISA antibody may allow single-specimen diagnosis

(*Continued*)

Table 40–2. Diagnostic tests for viral infections. (*Continued*)

Agent	Rapid Antigen Detection (Specimen)	Tissue Culture Mean Days to Positive (Range)	Serology		PCR	Comments
			Acute	Paired		
Parvovirus B19	–	–	+	ND	+	Erythema infectiosum agent; IgM serology is often diagnostic, but may be positive for a prolonged period
Parainfluenza virus	+ (respiratory secretions)	2 (2–14)	–	+	+	
Rabies virus	+ (skin, conjunctiva, suspected animal source tissue biopsy)	–	+	+	CDC	Usually diagnosed by antigen detection
Respiratory syncytial virus	+ (respiratory secretions)	2 (2–21)	–	+	+	Rapid antigen detection; 90% sensitive; PCR has excellent sensitivity
Rhinovirus	–	4 (2–7)	–	–	+	Too many strains to type serologically
Rotavirus	+ (feces)	–	–	–	+	Rapid assay methods are usually reliable
Rubella virus	–	> 10	+	+	+	Recommended that paired sera be tested simultaneously
Varicella-zoster virus	+ (skin scraping)	3 (3–21) RL	+	+	+	
West Nile virus	–	RL	+	+	+	IgM antibody usually detected by 1 wk; PCR is useful only on CSF

Plus signs signify commercially or widely available; **minus signs** signify not commercially available. ***Note:*** Results from some commercial laboratories are unreliable. **RL** indicates research laboratory only; **CDC:** Specific antibody titers or PCR available by arrangement with individual research laboratories or the Centers for Disease Control and Prevention. **ND:** Not done.
CSF, cerebrospinal fluid; ELISA, enzyme-linked immunosorbent assay; PCR, polymerase chain reaction; RBC, red blood cell.

and altered local immunity are sometimes the precursors of more severe illnesses such as otitis media, pneumonia, and sinusitis. During and following a cold, the bacterial flora changes and bacteria are found in normally sterile areas of the upper airway. Asthma attacks are frequently provoked by any of the viruses that cause the common cold. These "cold viruses" are a common cause of lower respiratory tract infection in young children. There is no evidence that antibiotics will prevent complications of the common cold, and the unjustified widespread use of antibiotics for cold symptoms has contributed to the emergence of antibiotic-resistant respiratory flora.

In 5%–10% of children, symptoms from these virus infections persist for more than 10 days. This overlap with the symptoms of bacterial sinusitis presents a difficult problem for clinicians, especially because colds can produce an abnormal computed tomography (CT) scan of the sinuses. Viruses that cause a minor illness in immunocompetent children, such as rhinoviruses, influenza, RSV, and metapneumovirus, can cause severe lower respiratory disease in immunologically or anatomically compromised children.

There is no evidence that symptomatic relief for children can be achieved with oral antihistamines, decongestants, or cough suppressants. The FDA has recommended that such over-the-counter medications not be used in children less than 2 years old. Topical decongestants provide temporary improvement in nasal symptoms. Vitamin C has not been shown to have a significant preventative or therapeutic role. Zinc therapy of the common cold and prevention with zinc is effective, but there is great uncertainty about dosing and some adverse effects.

Bonzel L, Tenenbaum T, Schroten H et al: Frequent detection of viral coinfection in children hospitalized with acute respiratory tract infection using a real-time polymerase chain reaction. Ped Infect Dis J 2008;27:589.

Olenec JP, Kim WK, Lee WM et al: Weekly monitoring of children with asthma for infections and illness during common cold seasons. J Allergy & Clin Immunol 2010;125(5):1001 [PMID: 20392488].

Singh M, Das RR: Zinc for the common cold. Cochrane Database of Systematic Rev 2011;2:CD001 364 [PMID: 21328251].

Techasaensiri B, Techasaensiri C et al: Viral coinfections in children with invasive pneumococcal disease. Ped Infect Dis J 2010;29:2010.

Winther B: Rhinovirus infections in the upper airway. Proc Am Thoracic Soc 2011;8(1):79 [PMID: 21364225].

Table 40–3. Some red rashes in children.

Condition	Incubation Period (d)	Prodrome	Rash	Laboratory Tests	Comments, Other Diagnostic Features
Adenovirus	4–5	URI; cough; fever	Morbilliform (may be petechial)	Normal; may see leukopenia or lymphocytosis	Upper or lower respiratory symptoms are prominent. No Koplik spots. No desquamation.
Drug allergy	—	None, or fever alone, or with myalgia, pruritus	Macular, maculopapular, urticarial, or erythroderma	Leukopenia, eosinophilia	Rash variable. Severe reactions may resemble measles, scarlet fever; Kawasaki disease; marked toxicity possible.
Enterovirus	2–7	Variable fever, chills, myalgia, sore throat	Usually macular, maculopapular on trunk or palms, soles; vesicles or petechiae also seen	Variable; PCR	Varied rashes may resemble those of many other infections. Pharyngeal or hand-foot-mouth vesicles may occur.
Ehrlichiosis (monocytic)	5–21	Fever; headache; flulike; myalgia; GI symptoms	Variable; maculopapular, petechial, scarlatiniform, vasculitic	Leukopenia, thrombocytopenia, abnormal liver function. Serology for diagnosis; morulae in monocytes	Geographic distribution is a clue; seasonal; tick exposure; rash present in only 45%.
Erythema multiforme	—	Usually none or related to underlying cause	Discrete, red maculopapular lesions; symmetrical, distal, palms and soles; target lesions classic	Normal or eosinophilia	Reaction to drugs (especially sulfonamides), or infectious agents (*Mycoplasma*; herpes simplex virus). Urticaria, arthralgia also seen.
Infectious mononucleosis (EBV infection)	30–60	Fever, malaise	Macular, scarlatiniform, or urticarial in 5% to almost 100% who are on penicillins and related drugs (not a penicillin allergy)	Atypical lymphocytosis; heterophil antibodies; EBV-specific antibodies in an acute pattern EBV; abnormal liver function tests	Pharyngitis, lymphadenopathy, hepatosplenomegaly.
Juvenile rheumatoid arthritis (systemic; Still diseases)	—	High fever, malaise	Evanescent salmon-pink macules, especially in pressure areas (prominent when fever is present)	Increased inflammatory markers; leukocytosis; thrombocytosis	Oligo- or polyarticular arthritis; asymptomatic anterior uveitis.
Kawasaki disease	Unknown	Fever, cervical adenopathy, irritability	Polymorphous (may be erythroderma) on trunk and extremities; red palms and soles, conjunctiva, lips, tongue, pharynx. Late desquamation is common. Some of these findings may be absent with atypical disease	Leukocytosis, thrombocytosis, elevated ESR or CRP; pyuria; decreased albumin; negative cultures and streptococcal serology; resting tachycardia	Swollen hands, feet; prolonged illness; uveitis; aseptic meningitis; no response to antibiotics. Vasculitis and aneurysms of coronary and other arteries occur (cardiac ultrasound).
Leptospirosis	4–19	Fever (biphasic), myalgia, chills	Variable erythroderma	Leukocytosis; hematuria, proteinuria; hyperbilirubinemia	Conjunctivitis; hepatitis, aseptic meningitis may be seen. Rodent, dog contact.
Measles	9–14	Cough, rhinitis, conjunctivitis	Maculopapular; face to trunk; lasts 7–10 d; Koplik spots in mouth	Leukopenia; antimeasles IgM	Toxic. Bright red rash becomes confluent, may desquamate. Fever falls after rash appears. Inadequate measles vaccination.

(*Continued*)

Table 40–3. Some red rashes in children. (*Continued*)

Condition	Incubation Period (d)	Prodrome	Rash	Laboratory Tests	Comments, Other Diagnostic Features
Parvovirus (erythema infectiosum)	10–17 (rash)	Mild (flulike)	Maculopapular on cheeks ("slapped cheek"), forehead, chin; then down limbs, trunk, buttocks; may fade and reappear for several weeks	IgM-EIA; PCR	Purpuric stocking-glove rash is rare, but distinctive; aplastic crisis in patients with chronic hemolytic anemia. May cause arthritis or arthralgia.
Rocky Mountain spotted fever	3–12	Headache (retro-orbital); toxic; GI symptoms; high fever; flulike	Onset 2–6 d after fever; palpable maculopapular on palms, soles, extremities, with spread centrally; petechial	Leukopenia; thrombocytopenia; abnormal liver function; CSF pleocytosis; serology positive at 7–10 d of rash; biopsy will give earlier diagnosis	Eastern seaboard and southeastern United States; April–September; tick exposure.
Roseola (exanthem subitum) (HHV-6)	10–14	Fever (3–4 d)	Pink, macular rash occurs at the end of febrile period; transient	Normal	Fever often high; disappears when rash develops; child appears well. Usually occurs in children 6 mo–3 y of age. Seizures may complicate.
Rubella	14–21	Usually none	Mild maculopapular; rapid spread face to extremities; gone by day 4	Normal or leukopenia	Postauricular, occipital adenopathy common. Polyarthralgia in some older girls. Mild clinical illness. Inadequate rubella vaccination.
Staphylococcal scalded skin	Variable	Irritability, absent to low fever	Painful erythroderma, followed in 1–2 d by cracking around eyes, mouth; bullae form with friction (Nikolsky sign)	Normal if only colonized by staphylococci; leukocytosis and sometimes bacteremia if infected	Normal pharynx. Look for focal staphylococcal infection. Usually occurs in infants.
Staphylococcal scarlet fever	1–7	Variable fever	Diffuse erythroderma; resembles streptococcal scarlet fever except eyes may be hyperemic and no "strawberry" tongue; pharynx spared	Leukocytosis is common because of infected focus	Focal infection usually present.
Stevens-Johnson syndrome	—	Pharyngitis, conjunctivitis, fever, malaise	Bullous erythema multiforme; may slough in large areas; hemorrhagic lips; purulent conjunctivitis	Leukocytosis	Classic precipitants are drugs (especially sulfonamides); *Mycoplasma pneumoniae* and herpes simplex infections. Pneumonitis and urethritis also seen.
Streptococcal scarlet fever	1–7	Fever, abdominal pain, headache, sore throat	Diffuse erythema, "sandpaper" texture; neck, axillae, inguinal areas; spreads to rest of body; desquamates 7–14 d; eyes not red	Leukocytosis; positive group A *Streptococcus* culture of throat or wound; positive streptococcal antigen test in pharynx	Strawberry tongue, red pharynx with or without exudate. Eyes, perioral and periorbital area, palms, and soles spared. Pastia lines. Cervical adenopathy. Usually occurs in children 2–10 y of age.
Toxic shock syndrome	Variable	Fever, myalgia, headache, diarrhea, vomiting	Nontender erythroderma; red eyes, palms, soles, pharynx, lips	Leukocytosis; abnormal liver enzymes and coagulation tests; proteinuria	*Staphylococcus aureus* infection; toxin-mediated multiorgan involvement. Swollen hands, feet. Hypotension or shock.

CSF, cerebrospinal fluid; CRP, C-reactive protein, EIA, enzyme immunoassay; ESR, erythrocyte sedimentation rate; GI, gastrointestinal; HHV-6, human herpesvirus 6; IFA, immunofluorescent assay; PCR, polymerase chain reaction; URI, upper respiratory infection.

INFECTIONS DUE TO ADENOVIRUSES

ESSENTIALS OF DIAGNOSIS & TYPICAL FEATURES

- Multiple syndromes, depending on the type of adenovirus.
- Upper respiratory infections; most notable is severe pharyngitis with tonsillitis and cervical adenopathy.
- Conjunctivitis.
- Pneumonia.
- Enteric adenoviruses cause mild diarrheal illnesses.
- Definitive diagnosis by antigen detection, PCR, or culture.

There are over 50 types of adenoviruses, which account for 5%–10% of all respiratory illnesses in childhood, usually pharyngitis or tracheitis, but occasionally pneumonia. Adenoviral infections, which are common early in life, occur 3–10 days after exposure to respiratory droplets or fomites. Enteric adenoviruses are an important cause of childhood diarrhea. Epidemic respiratory disease occurs in winter and spring, especially in closed environments such as day care centers and institutions. Because of latent infection in lymphoid tissue, asymptomatic shedding from the respiratory or intestinal tract is common.

Specific Adenoviral Syndromes

A. Pharyngitis

Pharyngitis is the most common adenoviral disease, and the most common viral cause of severe pharyngitis in children. Fever and adenopathy are common. Tonsillitis may be exudative. Rhinitis and an influenza-like systemic illness may be present. Laryngotracheitis or bronchitis may accompany pharyngitis.

B. Pharyngoconjunctival Fever

Conjunctivitis may occur alone and be prolonged, but most often is associated with preauricular adenopathy, fever, pharyngitis, and cervical adenopathy. Foreign body sensation and other symptoms last less than a week. Lower respiratory symptoms are uncommon.

C. Epidemic Keratoconjunctivitis

Symptoms are severe conjunctivitis with punctate keratitis and occasionally visual impairment. A foreign body sensation, photophobia, and swelling of conjunctiva and eyelids are characteristic. Preauricular adenopathy and subconjunctival hemorrhage are common.

D. Pneumonia

Severe pneumonia may occur at all ages. It is especially common in young children (< age 3 years). Chest radiographs show bilateral peribronchial and patchy ground-glass interstitial infiltrates in the lower lobes. Symptoms persist for 2–4 weeks. Adenoviral pneumonia can be necrotizing and cause permanent lung damage, especially bronchiectasis. A pertussis-like syndrome with typical cough and lymphocytosis can occur with lower respiratory tract infection. A new variant of adenovirus serotype 14 can cause unusually severe, sometimes fatal pneumonia in children and adults.

E. Rash

A diffuse morbilliform (rarely petechial) rash resembling measles, rubella, or roseola may be present. Koplik spots are absent.

F. Diarrhea

Enteric adenoviruses (types 40 and 41) cause 3%–5% of cases of short-lived diarrhea in afebrile children, especially in those less than 4 years old.

G. Mesenteric Lymphadenitis

Fever and abdominal pain may mimic appendicitis. Pharyngitis is often associated. Adenovirus-induced adenopathy may be a factor in appendicitis and intussusception.

H. Other Syndromes

Immunosuppressed patients, including neonates, may develop severe or fatal pulmonary or gastrointestinal infections or multisystem disease. Other rare complications include encephalitis, hepatitis, and myocarditis. Adenoviruses have been implicated in the syndrome of idiopathic myocardiopathy. Hemorrhagic cystitis can be a serious problem in immunocompromised children.

Laboratory & Diagnostic Studies

Diagnosis can be made by conventional culture of conjunctival, respiratory, or stool specimens, but several days to weeks are required. Viral culture using the rapid culture technique with immunodiagnostic reagents detects adenovirus in 48 hours. Adenovirus infection can also be diagnosed using these reagents directly on respiratory secretions. This is quicker, but less sensitive, than the culture methods. PCR is an important, relatively rapid and sensitive diagnostic method for adenovirus infections. Special cells are needed to isolate enteric adenoviruses. ELISA tests rapidly detect enteric adenoviruses in diarrheal specimens. Respiratory adenovirus infections can be detected retrospectively by comparing acute and convalescent sera, but this is not helpful during an acute illness.

Treatment

There is no specific treatment for adenovirus infections. Intravenous immune globulin (IVIG) may be tried in immunocompromised patients with severe pneumonia. There are anecdotal reports of successful treatment of immunocompromised patients with cidofovir, which inhibits adenovirus in vitro.

Marcos MA et al: Viral pneumonia. Curr Opin Infect Dis 2009;22:143 [PMID: 19276881].

Pavia AT: Viral infections of the lower respiratory tract: Old viruses, new viruses, and the role of diagnosis. Clin Infect Dis 2011;52(Suppl 4):S284 [PMID: 21460286].

INFLUENZA

ESSENTIALS OF DIAGNOSIS & TYPICAL FEATURES

- Fever, cough, pharyngitis, malaise, congestion.
- Pneumonia.
- Encephalitis.
- Seasonal: late fall through mid-spring.
- Detection of virus, viral antigens, or nucleic acid in respiratory secretions.

Symptomatic infections are common in children because they lack immunologic experience with influenza viruses. Infection rates in children are greater than in adults and are instrumental in initiating community outbreaks. Epidemics occur in fall and winter. Three main types of influenza viruses (A/H1N1, A/H3N2, B) cause most human epidemics, with antigenic drift ensuring a supply of susceptible hosts of all ages. In recent years, avian influenza A/H5N1 has caused isolated human outbreaks in Asia that are associated with high rates of hospitalization and death. A swine-origin influenza A/H1N1 initiated a human pandemic in the spring of 2009. Almost 50 million Americans were infected with this virus in 2009. Illnesses caused by this virus tend to be more severe in older children and young adults. In addition, the rates of hospitalization and death are higher than typically observed with seasonal influenza.

Clinical Findings

Spread of influenza occurs by way of airborne respiratory secretions. The incubation period is 2–7 days.

A. Symptoms and Signs

Influenza infection in older children and adults produces a characteristic syndrome of sudden onset of high fever, severe myalgia, headache, and chills. These symptoms overshadow the associated coryza, pharyngitis, and cough. Usually absent are rash, marked conjunctivitis, adenopathy, exudative pharyngitis, and dehydrating enteritis. Fever, diarrhea, vomiting, and abdominal pain are common in young children. Infants may develop a sepsis-like illness and apnea. Chest examination is usually unremarkable. Unusual clinical findings include croup (most severe with type A influenza), exacerbation of asthma, myositis (especially calf muscles), myocarditis, parotitis, encephalopathy (distinct from Reye syndrome), nephritis, and a transient maculopapular rash. Acute illness lasts 2–5 days. Cough and fatigue may last several weeks. Viral shedding may persist for several weeks in young children.

B. Laboratory Findings

The leukocyte count is normal to low, with variable shift. Influenza infections may be more difficult to recognize in children than in adults even during epidemics, and therefore a specific laboratory test is highly recommended. The virus can be found in respiratory secretions by direct fluorescent antibody staining of nasopharyngeal epithelial cells, ELISA, optic immunoassay (OIA), and PCR. It can also be cultured within 3–7 days from pharyngeal swabs or throat washings. Many laboratories use the rapid culture technique by centrifuging specimens onto cultured cell layers and detecting viral antigen after 48 hours. Other body fluids or tissues (except lung) rarely yield the virus in culture and are more appropriately tested by PCR, which, due to its high sensitivity, can increase influenza detection in respiratory specimens. A late diagnosis may be made with paired serology, using hemagglutination inhibition assays.

C. Imaging

The chest radiograph is nonspecific; it may show hyperaeration, peribronchial thickening, diffuse interstitial infiltrates, or bronchopneumonia in severe cases. Hilar nodes are not enlarged. Pleural effusion is rare in uncomplicated influenza.

Differential Diagnosis

The following may be considered: all other respiratory viruses, *Mycoplasma pneumoniae* or *Chlamydia pneumoniae* (longer incubation period, prolonged illness), streptococcal pharyngitis (pharyngeal exudate or petechiae, adenitis, no cough), bacterial sepsis (petechial or purpuric rash may occur), toxic shock syndrome (rash, hypotension), and rickettsial infections (rash, different season, insect exposure). High fever, the nature of preceding or concurrent illness in family members, and the presence of influenza in the community are distinguishing features from parainfluenza or RSV infections.

Complications & Sequelae

Lower respiratory tract symptoms are most common in children younger than age 5 years. Hospitalization rates are highest in children younger than 2 years. Influenza can cause croup in these children. Secondary bacterial infections (classically staphylococcal) of the middle ear, sinuses, or lungs (pneumococcal was common in the swine-origin H1N1 pandemic of 2009) are most common. Of the viral infections that precede Reye syndrome, varicella and influenza (usually type B) are most notable. During an influenza outbreak, ill children who develop protracted vomiting or irrational behavior should be evaluated for Reye syndrome. Influenza can also cause viral or postviral encephalitis, with cerebral symptoms much more prominent than those of the accompanying respiratory infection. Although the myositis is usually mild and resolves promptly, severe rhabdomyolysis and renal failure have been reported.

Children with underlying cardiopulmonary, metabolic, neuromuscular, or immunosuppressive disease may develop severe viral pneumonia. During the H1N1 pandemic, new high risk conditions were described: obesity and the first 2 weeks of postpartum.

Prevention

The inactivated influenza vaccine is moderately protective in older children (see Chapter 10). A live attenuated influenza vaccine (FluMist) is significantly more efficacious in children and is currently recommended for immunocompetent children 2 years of age or older. It is currently recommended that all children and adults 6 months and older should be immunized and that two doses be administered during the first year of immunization. Widespread resistance to adamantanes of seasonal influenza A H3N2 and pandemic influenza A H1N1/2009 and resistance to oseltamivir of seasonal influenza A H1N1 complicate chemoprophylaxis. Zanamivir (10 mg daily inhalations) can be used in children older than age 5 years and covers both pandemic and seasonal influenza viruses. Alternatively, rimantadine or amantadine (1–9 years 6.6 mg/kg in two doses or a single daily dose; > 10 years 200 mg in two doses or single daily dose) can be used in combination with oseltamivir (children < 15 kg, 30 mg daily; those 15–23 kg, 45 mg daily; those 23–40 kg, 60 mg daily; and those > 40 kg, 75 mg daily). For outbreak prophylaxis, therapy should be maintained for 2 weeks or more and for 1 week after the last case of influenza is diagnosed. Chemoprophylaxis should be considered during an epidemic for high-risk children who cannot be immunized or who have not yet developed immunity (about 6 weeks after primary vaccination or 2 weeks after a booster dose).

Treatment & Prognosis

Treatment consists of general support and management of pulmonary complications, especially bacterial superinfections. Antivirals are of some benefit against seasonal influenza in immunocompetent hosts if begun within 48 hours after symptom onset. Treatment duration is 5 days and the doses are twice as much as those used for prophylaxis (see earlier). Antivirals are recommended for all children with pandemic influenza A H1N1/2009. Studies in lung transplant patients indicate that oseltamivir might be useful for treatment of influenza in this immunocompromised population.

Recovery is usually complete unless severe cardiopulmonary or neurologic damage has occurred. Fatal cases occur in immunodeficient and anatomically compromised children.

Effective treatment or prophylaxis of influenza in children markedly reduces the incidence of acute otitis media and antibiotic usage during the flu season.

Prevention and control of influenza. Recommendations of the Advisory Committee on Immunization Practices (ACIP). MMWR Recomm Rep 2011;60(33):1128–1132.

Jain S et al: Hospitalized patients with 2009 H1N1 influenza in the United States, April–June 2009. N Engl J Med 2009;361:1935 [PMID: 19815859].

PARAINFLUENZA (CROUP)

ESSENTIALS OF DIAGNOSIS & TYPICAL FEATURES

- Fever, nasal congestion, sore throat, cough.
- Croup.
- Detection of live virus, antigens, or nucleic acid in respiratory secretions.

Parainfluenza viruses (types 1–4) are the most important cause of croup. Most infants are infected with type 3 within the first 3 years of life, often in the first year. Type 3 appears annually, with a peak in the spring or summer. Infection with types 1 and 2 is experienced gradually over the first 5 years of life, usually during outbreaks in the fall; most primary infections are symptomatic and frequently involve the lower respiratory tract. The concept that parainfluenza 4 has reduced pathogenicity is currently being reevaluated. Its epidemiology seems to overlap with that of parainfluenza 3.

Clinical Findings

A. Symptoms and Signs

Clinical diseases include febrile upper respiratory infection (especially in older children with reexposure), laryngitis, tracheobronchitis, croup, and bronchiolitis (second most common cause after RSV). The relative incidence of these manifestations is type-specific. Parainfluenza viruses (especially type 1) cause 65% of cases of croup in young children, 25% of tracheobronchitis, and 50% of laryngitis. Croup is characterized by a barking cough, inspiratory stridor (especially when agitated), and hoarseness. Type 2 parainfluenza is more likely to cause bronchiolitis. Parainfluenza virus can cause pneumonia in infants and immunodeficient children, and causes particularly high mortality among stem cell recipients. Onset is acute. Most children are febrile. Symptoms of upper respiratory tract infection often accompany croup.

B. Laboratory Findings

Diagnosis is often based on clinical findings. These viruses can be identified by conventional or rapid culture techniques (48 hours), by direct immunofluorescence on nasopharyngeal epithelial cells in respiratory secretions (< 3 hours), or by PCR (< 24 hours).

Differential Diagnosis

Parainfluenza-induced respiratory syndromes are difficult to distinguish from those caused by other respiratory viruses. Viral croup must be distinguished from epiglottitis caused by *Haemophilus influenzae* (abrupt onset, toxicity and high fever, drooling, dyspnea, little cough, left shift of blood smear, and a history of inadequate immunization).

Treatment

No specific therapy or vaccine is available. Croup management is discussed in Chapter 19. Ribavirin is active in vitro and has been used in immunocompromised children, but its efficacy is unproved.

Ren L et al: Human parainfluenza virus type 4 infection in Chinese children with lower respiratory tract infections: A comparison study. Journal of Clinical Virology 2011 Jul;51(3):209–212.

Fry AM et al: Seasonal trends of human parainfluenza viral infections: United States, 1990–2004. Clin Infect Dis 2006;43:1016 [PMID: 16983614].

RESPIRATORY SYNCYTIAL VIRUS DISEASE

ESSENTIALS OF DIAGNOSIS & TYPICAL FEATURES

- Diffuse wheezing and tachypnea following upper respiratory symptoms in an infant (bronchiolitis).
- Epidemics in late fall to early spring (January–February peak).
- Hyperinflation on chest radiograph.
- Detection of RSV antigen or nucleic acid in nasal secretions.

General Considerations

RSV is a ubiquitous infection of early childhood. Almost all children develop upper respiratory symptoms; of these 20%–30% will develop evidence of lower respiratory infection. RSV is the most important cause of lower respiratory tract illness in young children, accounting for more than 70% of cases of bronchiolitis and 40% of cases of pneumonia. Outbreaks occur annually, and attack rates are high; 60% of children are infected in the first year of life, and 90% by age 2 years. During peak season (cold weather in temperate climates), the clinical diagnosis of RSV infection in infants with bronchiolitis is as accurate as most laboratory tests. Despite the presence of serum antibody, reinfection is common. Two distinct genotypes can co-circulate or one may predominate in a community. Yearly shift in prevalence of these genotypes is a partial explanation for reinfection. However, reinfection generally causes only upper respiratory symptoms in anatomically normal children. No vaccine is available. Immunosuppressed patients may develop progressive severe pneumonia. Children with congenital heart disease with increased pulmonary blood flow, children with chronic lung disease (eg, cystic fibrosis), and premature infants younger than age 6 months (especially when they have chronic lung disease of prematurity) are also at higher risk for severe illness.

Clinical Findings

A. Symptoms and Signs

Initial symptoms are those of upper respiratory infection. Low-grade fever may be present. The classic disease is bronchiolitis, characterized by diffuse wheezing, variable fever, cough, tachypnea, difficulty feeding, and, in severe cases, cyanosis. Hyperinflation, crackles, prolonged expiration, wheezing, and retractions are present. The liver and spleen may be palpable because of lung hyperinflation, but are not enlarged. The disease usually lasts 3–7 days in previously healthy children. Fever is present for 2–4 days; it does not correlate with pulmonary symptoms and may be absent during the height of lung involvement.

Apnea, poor feeding, and lethargy may be presenting manifestations, especially in premature infants, in the first few months of life. Apnea usually resolves after a few days, often being replaced by obvious signs of bronchiolitis.

RSV infection in subsequent years is more likely to cause tracheobronchitis or upper respiratory tract infection. Exceptions are immunocompromised children and those with severe chronic lung or heart disease, who may have especially severe or prolonged primary infections and are subject to additional attacks of severe pneumonitis.

B. Laboratory Findings

Rapid detection of RSV antigen in nasal or pulmonary secretions by fluorescent antibody staining or ELISA requires only several hours and is more than 90% sensitive and specific. Rapid tissue culture methods take 48 hours and have comparable sensitivity.

C. Imaging

Diffuse hyperinflation and peribronchiolar thickening are most common; atelectasis and patchy infiltrates also occur in uncomplicated infection, but pleural effusions are rare. Consolidation (usually subsegmental) occurs in 25% of children with lower respiratory tract disease.

Differential Diagnosis

Although almost all cases of bronchiolitis are due to RSV during an epidemic, other viruses, including parainfluenza, rhinovirus, and especially human metapneumovirus, cannot be excluded. Mixed infections with other viruses, chlamydiae, or bacteria can occur. Wheezing may be due to asthma, a foreign body, or other airway obstruction. RSV infection may closely resemble chlamydial pneumonitis when fine crackles are present and fever and wheezing are not prominent. The two may also coexist. Cystic fibrosis may resemble RSV infection; a positive family history or failure to thrive associated with hyponatremia or hypoalbuminemia should prompt a sweat chloride test. Pertussis should also be considered in this age group, especially if cough is prominent and the infant is younger than age 6 months. A markedly elevated leukocyte count should suggest bacterial superinfection (neutrophilia) or pertussis (lymphocytosis).

Complications

RSV commonly infects the middle ear. Symptomatic otitis media is more likely when secondary bacterial infection is present (usually due to pneumococci or *H influenzae*). This is the most common complication (10%–20%). Bacterial pneumonia complicates only 0.5%–1% of hospitalized patients. Sudden exacerbations of fever and leukocytosis should suggest bacterial infection. Respiratory failure or apnea may require mechanical ventilation, but occurs in less than 2% of hospitalized previously healthy full-term infants. Cardiac failure may occur as a complication of pulmonary disease or myocarditis. RSV commonly causes exacerbations of asthma. Nosocomial RSV infection is so common during outbreaks that elective hospitalization or surgery, especially for those with underlying illness, should be postponed. Well-designed hospital programs to prevent nosocomial spread are imperative (see next section).

Prevention & Treatment

Children who are very hypoxic or cannot feed because of respiratory distress must be hospitalized and given humidified oxygen as directed by oxygen saturation and tube or intravenous feedings. Antibiotics, decongestants, and expectorants are of no value in routine infections. RSV-infected children should be kept in respiratory isolation. Cohorting ill infants in respiratory isolation during peak season (with or without rapid diagnostic attempts) and emphasizing good hand washing may greatly decrease nosocomial transmission.

The utility of bronchodilator therapy alone has not been consistently demonstrated. Often a trial of bronchodilator therapy is given to determine response and is subsequently discontinued if there is no improvement. Racemic epinephrine occasionally works when albuterol fails. This therapeutic trial should only be undertaken in a hospital setting and care taken to observe children for an extended period after a positive response. The use of corticosteroids is also controversial. A meta-analysis of numerous studies of corticosteroid therapy indicated a significant effect on hospital stay, especially in those most ill at the time of treatment, but use of a single dose of corticosteroids had no lasting effect on respiratory status and did not prevent hospitalization. The combined use of racemic epinephrine and 5 days of oral dexamethasone significantly reduced hospitalization in one trial.

Ribavirin is the only licensed antiviral therapy used for RSV infection. It is given by continuous aerosolization. It is rarely used in infants without significant anatomic or immunologic defects. At best, there is a very modest effect on disease severity in immunocompetent infants with no underlying anatomic abnormality. Even in high-risk infants, clinical response to ribavirin therapy was not demonstrated in several studies. Nevertheless, ribavirin is sometimes used in severely ill children who are immunologically or anatomically compromised and in those with severe cardiac disease.

Monthly intramuscular administration of humanized RSV monoclonal antibody is now recommended to prevent severe disease in selected high-risk patients during epidemic periods. Monthly administration should be considered during the RSV season for high-risk children, as described in Chapter 10. Use of passive immunization for immunocompromised children is logical but not established. RSV antibody is not effective for treatment of established infection.

Prognosis

Although mild bronchiolitis does not produce long-term problems, 30%–40% of patients hospitalized with this infection will wheeze later in childhood, and RSV infection in infancy may be one important precursor to asthma. Chronic restrictive lung disease and bronchiolitis obliterans are rare sequelae.

Krilov LR: Respiratory syncytial virus disease: Update on treatment and prevention. Exert Rev Antiinfective Therapy 2011;9(1):27–32 [PMID: 21171875].

Plint AC et al: Epinephrine and dexamethasone in children with bronchiolitis. N Engl J Med 2009;360:2079 [PMID: 19439742].

Simoes EA et al: Palivizumab prophylaxis, respiratory syncytial virus, and subsequent recurrent wheezing. J Pediatr 2007;151:34 [PMID: 17586188].

Wright M, Piedmonte G: Respiratory syncytial virus prevention and therapy: Past, present, and future. Ped Pulmonology 2011;46(4):324 [PMID: 21438168].

HUMAN METAPNEUMOVIRUS INFECTION

ESSENTIALS OF DIAGNOSIS & TYPICAL FEATURES

- Cough, coryza, sore throat.
- Bronchiolitis.
- Detection of viral antigens or nucleic acid in respiratory secretions.

General Considerations

Human metapneumovirus (hMPV) is a common agent of respiratory tract infections that is very similar to RSV in epidemiologic and clinical characteristics. Like RSV, parainfluenza, mumps, and measles, hMPV belongs to the paramyxovirus family. Humans are its only known reservoir. Seroepidemiologic surveys indicate that the virus has worldwide distribution. More than 90% of children contract hMPV infection by age 5 years, typically during late autumn through early spring outbreaks. hMPV accounts for 15%–25% of the cases of bronchiolitis and pneumonia in children younger than 2 years. Older children and adults can also develop symptomatic infection.

Clinical Findings

A. Symptoms and Signs

The most common symptoms are fever, cough, rhinorrhea, and sore throat. Bronchiolitis and pneumonia occur in 40%–70% of the children who acquire hMPV before the age of 2 years. Asymptomatic infection is uncommon. Other manifestations include otitis, conjunctivitis, diarrhea, and myalgia. Acute wheezing has been associated with hMPV in children of all ages, raising the possibility that this virus, like RSV, might trigger reactive airway disease. Dual infection with hMPV and RSV or other respiratory viruses seems to be a common occurrence and may increase morbidity and mortality.

B. Laboratory Findings

The virus has very selective tissue culture tropism, which accounts for its late discovery in spite of its presence in archived specimens from the mid-1950s. The preferred method of diagnosis is PCR performed on respiratory specimens. Rapid shell vial culture is an acceptable, albeit less sensitive, alternative. Antibody tests are available, but are most appropriately used for epidemiologic studies.

C. Imaging

Lower respiratory tract infection frequently shows hyperinflation and patchy pneumonitis on chest radiographs.

Treatment & Prognosis

No antiviral therapies are available to treat hMPV. Ribavirin has in vitro activity against human metapneumovirus, but there are no data to support its therapeutic value. Children with lower respiratory tract disease may require hospitalization and ventilatory support, but less frequently than with RSV-associated bronchiolitis. Duration of hospitalization in hMPV is typically shorter than in RSV.

Barenfanger J et al: Prevalence of human metapneumovirus in central Illinois in patients thought to have respiratory viral infections. J Clin Microbiol 2008;46:1489.

Mammas IN et al: Detection of human metapneumovirus in infants with acute respiratory tract infection. Mol Medicine Rep 2011;4(2):267 [PMID: 21468562].

INFECTIONS DUE TO ENTEROVIRUSES

ESSENTIALS OF DIAGNOSIS & TYPICAL FEATURES

- Acute febrile illness with headache and sore throat.
- Summer–fall epidemics.
- Other common features: rash, nonexudative pharyngitis.
- Common cause of aseptic meningitis.
- Complications: myocarditis, neurologic damage, life-threatening illness in newborns.

Enteroviruses are a major cause of illness in young children. The multiple types have similar nucleic acid and protein components, and may produce identical syndromes. The multiplicity of types makes vaccine development impractical and has hindered development of antigen detection and serologic tests. However, common RNA sequences and group antigens have led to diagnostic tests for viral nucleic acid and proteins. A PCR assay is available in many medical centers, but tissue culture is still used in some centers as a diagnostic method for echoviruses, polioviruses, and coxsackie B viruses. Although cultures may turn positive in 2–4 days, the relatively rapid answer obtained with PCR facilitates clinical decisions, particularly in cases of meningoencephalitis and severe unexplained illness in neonates.

Parechoviruses are a genus of the family picornaviruses which were formerly considered to be enteroviruses (echoviruses 22 and 23). It is now realized that these are responsible for a significant number of pediatric infections. Some of the 15 types of parechovirures infect almost every child before the age of 2 years; others before age 5 years.

Transmission of enteroviruses is fecal-oral or from upper respiratory secretions. Multiple enteroviruses circulate in the community at any one time; summer–fall outbreaks are common in temperate climates, but infections are seen year-round. After poliovirus, coxsackie B virus is most virulent, followed by echovirus. Neurologic, cardiac, and overwhelming neonatal infections are the most severe forms of illness.

ACUTE FEBRILE ILLNESS

Accompanied by nonspecific upper respiratory or enteric symptoms, the sudden onset of fever and irritability in infants or young children is often enteroviral in origin, especially in late summer and fall. More than 90% of enteroviral infections are not distinctive. Occasionally a petechial rash is seen; more often a diffuse maculopapular or morbilliform eruption (often prominent on palms and soles) occurs on the second to fourth day of fever. Rapid recovery is the rule. More than one febrile enteroviral illness can occur in the same patient in one season. The leukocyte count is usually normal. Infants, because of fever and irritability, may undergo an evaluation for bacteremia or meningitis and be hospitalized to rule out sepsis. Approximately half of these infants have aseptic meningitis. In the summer months enterovirus infection is more likely than human herpesvirus 6 (HHV-6) to cause an acute medical visit for fever. Duration of illness is 4–5 days.

Sawyer MH: Enterovirus infections: Diagnosis and treatment. Semin Pediatr Infect Dis 2002;13:40 [PMID: 12118843].

Harvala H, Simmonds P: Human parechoviruses: Biology, epidemiology and clinical significance. J Clin Virol 2009;45(1):1 [PMID: 19372062].

RESPIRATORY TRACT ILLNESSES

1. Febrile Illness with Pharyngitis

This syndrome is most common in older children, who complain of headache, sore throat, myalgia, and abdominal discomfort. The usual duration is 3–4 days. Vesicles or papules may be seen in the pharynx. There is no exudate. Occasionally, enteroviruses are the cause of croup, bronchitis, or pneumonia. They may also exacerbate asthma.

2. Herpangina

Herpangina is characterized by an acute onset of fever and posterior pharyngeal grayish white vesicles that quickly form ulcers (< 20 in number), often linearly arranged on the posterior palate, uvula, and tonsillar pillars. Bilateral faucial ulcers may also be seen. Dysphagia, vomiting, abdominal pain, and anorexia also occur and, rarely, parotitis or vaginal ulcers. Symptoms disappear in 4–5 days. The epidemic form is due to several coxsackie A viruses; coxsackie B viruses and echoviruses cause sporadic cases.

The differential diagnosis includes primary herpes simplex gingivostomatitis (ulcers are more prominent anteriorly, and gingivitis is present), aphthous stomatitis (fever absent, recurrent episodes, anterior lesions), trauma, hand-foot-and-mouth disease (see later discussion), and Vincent angina (painful gingivitis spreading from the gum line, underlying dental disease). If the enanthema is missed, tonsillitis might be incorrectly diagnosed.

3. Acute Lymphonodular Pharyngitis

Coxsackievirus A10 has been associated with a febrile pharyngitis characterized by nonulcerative yellow-white posterior pharyngeal papules in the same distribution as herpangina. The duration is 1–2 weeks; therapy is supportive.

4. Pleurodynia (Bornholm Disease, Epidemic Myalgia)

Caused by coxsackie B virus (epidemic form) or many nonpolio enteroviruses (sporadic form), pleurodynia is associated with an abrupt onset of unilateral or bilateral spasmodic pain of variable intensity over the lower ribs or upper abdomen. Associated symptoms include headache, fever, vomiting, myalgias, and abdominal and neck pain. Physical findings include fever, chest muscle tenderness, decreased thoracic excursion, and occasionally a friction rub. The chest radiograph is normal. Hematologic tests are nondiagnostic. The illness generally lasts less than 1 week.

This is a disease of muscle, but the differential diagnosis includes bacterial pneumonia, bacterial and tuberculous effusion, and endemic fungal infections (all excluded radiographically and by auscultation), costochondritis (no fever or other symptoms), and a variety of abdominal problems, especially those causing diaphragmatic irritation.

There is no specific therapy. Potent analgesic agents and chest splinting alleviate the pain.

RASHES (INCLUDING HAND-FOOT-AND-MOUTH DISEASE)

The rash may be macular, maculopapular, urticarial, scarlatiniform, petechial, or vesicular. One of the most characteristic is that of hand-foot-and-mouth disease (caused by coxsackieviruses, especially types A5, A10, and A16), in which vesicles or red papules are found on the tongue, oral mucosa, hands, and feet. Often they appear near the nails and on the heels. Associated fever, sore throat, and malaise are mild. The rash may appear when fever abates, simulating roseola.

Cardiac Involvement

Myocarditis and pericarditis may be caused by a number of nonpolio enteroviruses, particularly type B coxsackieviruses. Most commonly, upper respiratory symptoms are followed by substernal pain, dyspnea, and exercise intolerance. A friction rub or gallop may be detected. Ultrasound will define ventricular dysfunction or pericardial effusion, and electrocardiography may show pericarditis or ventricular irritability. Creatine phosphokinase may be elevated. The disease may be mild or fatal; most children recover completely. In infants, other organs may be involved at the same time; in older patients, cardiac disease is usually the sole manifestation (see Chapter 20 for therapy). Enteroviral RNA is present in cardiac tissue in some cases of dilated cardiomyopathy or myocarditis; the significance of this finding is unknown. Epidemics of enterovirus 71, which occur in Asia, as well as sporadic cases in the United States, are associated with severe left ventricular dysfunction and pulmonary edema following typical mucocutaneous manifestations of enterovirus infection. Enterovirus 71 also can cause isolated severe neurologic disease or neurologic disease in combination with myocardial disease.

Chang LY: Enterovirus 71 in Taiwan. Pediatr Neonatol 2008;49:103 [PMID: 19054914].

Chapman NM, Kim KS: Persistent coxsackievirus infection: Enterovirus persistence in chronic myocarditis and dilated cardiomyopathy. Curr Topics Microbiol Immunol 2008;323:275 [PMID: 18357775].

Severe Neonatal Infection

Sporadic and nosocomial nursery cases of severe systemic enteroviral disease occur. Clinical manifestations include combinations of fever, rash, pneumonitis, encephalitis, hepatitis, gastroenteritis, myocarditis, pancreatitis, and myositis. The infants, usually younger than 1 week, may appear septic, with cyanosis, dyspnea, and seizures. The differential diagnosis includes bacterial and herpes simplex infections, necrotizing enterocolitis, other causes of heart or liver failure, and metabolic diseases. Diagnosis is suggested by the finding of cerebrospinal fluid (CSF) mononuclear pleocytosis and confirmed by the isolation of virus or detection of enteroviral RNA in urine, stool, CSF, or pharynx. Therapy is supportive. IVIG is often administered, but its value is uncertain. Passively acquired maternal antibody may protect newborns from severe disease. For this reason, labor should not be induced in pregnant women near term who have suspected enteroviral disease. Some of these infections are now known to be caused by parechoviruses.

Tebruegge M, Curtis N: Enterovirus infections in neonates. Semin Fetal Noenatal Med 2009;14:222 [PMID: 19303380].

CENTRAL NERVOUS SYSTEM ILLNESSES

1. Poliomyelitis

ESSENTIALS OF DIAGNOSIS & TYPICAL FEATURES

- Inadequate immunization or underlying immune deficiency.
- Headache, fever, muscle weakness.
- Aseptic meningitis.
- Asymmetrical, flaccid paralysis; muscle tenderness and hyperesthesia; intact sensation; late atrophy.

General Considerations

Poliovirus infection is subclinical in 90%–95% of cases; it causes nonspecific febrile illness in about 5% of cases and aseptic meningitis, with or without paralytic disease, in 1%–3%. In endemic areas, most older children and adults are immune because of prior inapparent infections. Occasional cases in the United States occur in patients who travel to foreign countries or come in contact with visitors from areas that have poliovirus outbreaks. Severe poliovirus infection was a rare complication of OPV (oral poliovirus vaccine) vaccination as a result of reversion of the vaccine virus. The incidence of vaccine-associated paralytic poliomyelitis (VAPP) in the United States was 1:750,000 and 1:2.4 million doses for the first and second dose of OPV, respectively. Although rare, VAPP became more common than wild-type poliomyelitis in the United States in the 1980s. This led to a change in the recommended immunization regimen, substituting inactivated poliovirus vaccine (IPV) for OPV (see Chapter 10).

Clinical Findings

A. Symptoms and Signs

The initial symptoms are fever, myalgia, sore throat, and headache for 2–6 days. In less than 10% of infected children, several symptom-free days are followed by recurrent fever and signs of aseptic meningitis: headache, stiff neck, spinal rigidity, and nausea. Mild cases resolve completely. In only 1%–2% of these children do high fever, severe myalgia, and anxiety portend progression to loss of reflexes and subsequent flaccid paralysis. Sensation remains intact, although hyperesthesia of skin overlying paralyzed muscles is common and pathognomonic.

Paralysis is usually asymmetrical. Proximal limb muscles are more often involved than distal, and lower limb involvement is more common than upper. Bulbar involvement affects swallowing, speech, and cardiorespiratory function and accounts for most deaths. Bladder distention and marked constipation characteristically accompany lower limb paralysis. Paralysis is usually complete by the time the temperature normalizes. Weakness often resolves completely. Atrophy is usually apparent by 4–8 weeks. Most improvement of muscle paralysis occurs within 6 months.

B. Laboratory Findings

In patients with meningeal symptoms, the CSF contains up to several hundred leukocytes (mostly lymphocytes) per microliter; the glucose level is normal, and protein concentration is mildly elevated. Poliovirus is easy to grow in cell culture and can be readily differentiated from other enteroviruses. It is rarely isolated from spinal fluid but is often present in the throat and stool for several weeks following infection. Paired serology is also diagnostic. Laboratory methods are available to differentiate wild from attenuated vaccine isolates.

Differential Diagnosis

Aseptic meningitis due to poliovirus is indistinguishable from that due to other viruses. Paralytic disease in the United States is usually due to nonpolio enteroviruses. Polio may resemble Guillain-Barré syndrome (minimal sensory loss, ascending symmetrical loss of function; minimal pleocytosis, high protein concentration in spinal fluid), polyneuritis (sensory loss), pseudoparalysis due to bone or joint problems (eg, trauma, infection), botulism, or tick paralysis.

Complications & Sequelae

Complications are the result of the acute and permanent effects of paralysis. Respiratory, pharyngeal, bladder, and bowel malfunction are most critical. Deaths are usually due to complications arising from respiratory dysfunction. Limbs injured near the time of infection, such as by intramuscular injections, excessive prior use, or trauma, tend to be most severely involved and have the worst prognosis for recovery (provocation paralysis).

Treatment & Prognosis

Therapy is supportive. Bed rest, fever and pain control (heat therapy is helpful), and careful attention to progression of weakness (particularly of respiratory muscles) are important. No intramuscular injections should be given during the acute phase. Intubation or tracheostomy for secretion control and catheter drainage of the bladder may be needed. Assisted ventilation and enteral feeding may also be needed. Disease is worse in adults and pregnant women than in children. Postpolio muscular atrophy occurs in 30%–40% of paralyzed limbs 20–30 years later, characterized by increasing weakness and fasciculations in previously affected, partially recovered limbs.

2. Nonpolio Viral Meningitis

Nonpolio enteroviruses cause over 80% of cases of aseptic meningitis at all ages. In the summer and fall, multiple cases may be seen associated with circulation of neurotropic strains. Nosocomial outbreaks also occur.

Clinical Findings

The usual enteroviral incubation period is 4–6 days. Because many enteroviral infections are subclinical or not associated with central nervous system (CNS) symptoms, a history of contact with a patient with meningitis is unusual. Neonates may acquire infection from maternal blood, vaginal secretions, or feces at birth; occasionally the mother has had a febrile illness just prior to delivery.

A. Symptoms and Signs

Incidence is much greater in children younger than age 1 year. Onset is usually acute with variable fever, marked irritability, and lethargy in infants. Older children also describe frontal headache, photophobia, and myalgia. Abdominal pain, diarrhea, and vomiting may occur. The incidence of rash varies with the infecting strain. If rash occurs, it is usually seen after several days of illness and is diffuse, macular or maculopapular, occasionally petechial, but not purpuric. Oropharyngeal vesicles and rash on the palms and soles suggest an enterovirus. The anterior fontanelle may be full. Meningismus may be present. The illness may be biphasic, with nonspecific symptoms and signs preceding those related to the CNS. In older children, it is easier to demonstrate meningeal signs. Seizures are unusual, and focal neurologic findings, which are rare, should lead to a search for an alternative cause. Frank encephalitis, which is uncommon at any age, occurs most often in neonates. Because of the overall frequency of enteroviral disease in children, 5%–10% of all cases of encephalitis of proved viral origin are caused by enteroviruses. Enteroviruses tend to cause less severe encephalitis than other viral agents. However, parechoviruses, which have recently been demonstrated to be a significant cause of aseptic meningitis, sometimes cause white matter defects.

Enterovirus 71 infections that begin with typical mucocutaneous manifestations of enteroviruses can be complicated by severe brainstem encephalitis and polio-like flaccid paralysis. Enterovirus 70 outbreaks have resulted in hemorrhagic conjunctivitis together with paralytic poliomyelitis. Other nonpolio enteroviruses cause sporadic cases of acute motor weakness similar to that seen with poliovirus infection. Children with congenital immune deficiency, especially agammaglobulinemia, are subject to chronic enteroviral meningoencephalitis that is often fatal or associated with severe sequelae.

B. Laboratory Findings

Blood leukocyte counts are often normal. The spinal fluid leukocyte count is 100–1000/μL. Early in the illness, polymorphonuclear cells predominate; a shift to mononuclear cells occurs within 8–36 hours. In about 95% of cases, spinal fluid parameters include a total leukocyte count less than 3000/μL, protein less than 80 mg/dL, and glucose more than 60% of serum values. Marked deviation from any of these findings should prompt consideration of another diagnosis (see following section). The syndrome of inappropriate secretion of antidiuretic hormone may occur, but is rarely clinically significant.

Culture of CSF may yield an enterovirus within a few days (< 70%). However, PCR for enteroviruses is the most useful diagnostic method in many centers (sensitivity > 90%) and can give an answer within 24–48 hours. Parechoviruses will be detected by most PCR methods, but will be identified as "enterovirus." Virus may be detected in acellular

CSF. Detection of an enterovirus from throat or stool suggests, but does not prove, enteroviral meningitis. Vaccine-strain poliovirus present in feces in infants being evaluated for aseptic meningitis (outside of the United States) may confuse the diagnosis, but can usually be distinguished by growth characteristics.

C. Imaging

Cerebral imaging is not often indicated; if done, it is usually normal. Subdural effusions, infarcts, edema, or focal abnormalities seen in bacterial meningitis are absent except for the rare case of focal encephalitis.

Differential Diagnosis

The leading cause of aseptic meningitis is enteroviruses, especially in the summer and fall. Other causative viruses are mosquito-borne viruses (flavivirus, bunyavirus). These are usually considered during an investigation of encephalitis, but many of them are more likely to cause isolated meningitis and should be considered when seasonal clusters of viral meningitis occur. Primary herpes simplex infection can cause aseptic meningitis in adolescents who have a genital herpes infection. In neonates, early herpes simplex meningoencephalitis may mimic enteroviral disease (see section on Infections Due to Herpesviruses, later). This is an important alternative diagnosis to exclude because of the need for urgent antiviral therapy. Lymphocytic choriomeningitis virus causes meningitis in children in contact with rodents (pet or environmental exposure). Meningitis occurs in some patients at the time of infection with human immunodeficiency virus (HIV).

Other causes of aseptic meningitis that may resemble enteroviral infection include partially treated bacterial meningitis (recent antibiotic treatment, CSF parameters resembling those seen in bacterial disease and bacterial antigen sometimes present); parameningeal foci of bacterial infection such as brain abscess, subdural empyema, mastoiditis (predisposing factors, glucose level in CSF may be lower, focal neurologic signs, and characteristic imaging); tumors or cysts (malignant cells detected by cytologic examination, a history of neurologic symptoms, higher protein concentration or lower glucose level in CSF); trauma (presence, without exception, of red blood cells, which may be erroneously assumed to be due to traumatic lumbar puncture, but are crenated and fail to clear); vasculitis (other systemic or neurologic signs, found in older children); tuberculous or fungal meningitis (see Chapters 42 and 43); cysticercosis; parainfectious encephalopathies (*M pneumoniae*, cat-scratch disease, respiratory viruses [especially influenza]); Lyme disease; leptospirosis; and rickettsial diseases.

Prevention & Treatment

No specific therapy exists. Infants are usually hospitalized, isolated, and treated with fluids and antipyretics. Moderately to severely ill infants are given appropriate antibiotics for bacterial pathogens until cultures are negative for 48–72 hours. This practice is changing somewhat, and hospital stay shortened, in areas where the PCR assay for enteroviruses is available. If patients, especially older children, are mildly ill, antibiotics may be withheld and the child observed. The illness usually lasts less than 1 week. Codeine compounds or other strong analgesics may be needed. C-reactive protein and lactate levels are usually low in the CSF of children with viral meningitis; both may be elevated with bacterial infection. With clinical deterioration, repeat lumbar puncture, cerebral imaging, neurologic consultation, and more aggressive diagnostic tests should be considered. Herpesvirus encephalitis is an important consideration in such cases, particularly in infants younger than age 1 month, and often warrants empiric acyclovir therapy until an etiologic diagnosis is made.

Prognosis

In general, enteroviral meningitis has no significant short-term neurologic or developmental sequelae. Developmental delay may follow severe neonatal infections. Unlike mumps, enterovirus infections rarely cause hearing loss.

Centers for Disease Control and Prevention: Progress toward interruption of wild poliovirus transmission—worldwide, January 2010–March 2011. MMWR – Morbidity and Mortality Weekly Report 2011;60(18):582 [PMID: 21566559].

Ooi MH, Wong SC et al: Clinical features, diagnosis, and management of enterovirus 71. Lancet Neurology 2010;9(11):1097 [PMID: 20965438].

Poh CL, Tan EL: Detection of enteroviruses from clinical specimens. Meth Molecular Biol 2011;665:65 [PMID: 21116796].

Rhoades RE et al: Enterovirus infections of the central nervous system. Virology 2011;411(2):288 [PMID: 21251690].

Salvarangan R et al: Human parechovirus 3 causing sepsis-like illness in children from Midwestern United States. Oed Infect Dis J 2011;30(3):238.

INFECTIONS DUE TO HERPESVIRUSES

HERPES SIMPLEX INFECTIONS

ESSENTIALS OF DIAGNOSIS & TYPICAL FEATURES

- Grouped vesicles on an erythematous base, typically in or around the mouth or genitals.
- Tender regional adenopathy, especially with primary infection.
- Fever and malaise with primary infection.
- Recurrent episodes in many patients.

General Considerations

There are two types of herpes simplex viruses (HSVs). Type 1 (HSV-1) causes most cases of oral, skin, and cerebral disease in older children. Type 2 (HSV-2) causes most (> 50%, especially in adolescents and young adults) genital and many congenital infections. Latent infection is routinely established in sensory ganglia during primary infection. Recurrences may be spontaneous or induced by external events (eg, fever, menstruation, or sunlight) or immunosuppression. Transmission is by direct contact with infected secretions. HSVs are very susceptible to antiviral drugs.

Primary infection with HSV-1 often occurs early in childhood, although many adults (20%–50%) never get infected. Primary infection with HSV-1 is subclinical in 80% of cases and causes gingivostomatitis in the remainder. HSV-2, which is transmitted sexually, is also usually (65%) subclinical or produces mild, nonspecific symptoms. Infection with one type of HSV may prevent or attenuate clinically apparent infection with the other type, but individuals can be infected at different times with both HSV-1 and HSV-2. Recurrent episodes are due to reactivation of latent HSV.

The source of primary infection is usually an asymptomatic excreter. Most previously infected individuals shed HSV at irregular intervals. At any one time (point prevalence), more than 5% of normal seropositive adults excrete HSV-1 in the saliva; the percentage is higher in recently infected children, and detection of viral DNA exceeds 12%. HSV-2 shedding in genital secretions occurs with a similar or higher point prevalence exceeding 15%, depending on the method of detection (viral isolation vs PCR) and the interval since the initial infection. A history of contact with an active HSV infection is unusual.

Clinical Findings

A. Symptoms and Signs

1. Gingivostomatitis—High fever, irritability, and drooling occur in infants. Multiple oral ulcers are seen on the tongue and on the buccal and gingival mucosa, occasionally extending to the pharynx. Pharyngeal ulcers may predominate in older children and adolescents. Diffusely swollen red gums that are friable and bleed easily are typical. Cervical nodes are swollen and tender. Duration is 7–14 days. Herpangina, aphthous stomatitis, thrush, and Vincent angina should be excluded.

2. Vulvovaginitis or urethritis (See Chapter 44)—Genital herpes (especially HSV-2) in a prepubertal child should suggest sexual abuse. Vesicles or painful ulcers on the vulva, vagina, or penis, and tender adenopathy are seen. Systemic symptoms (fever, flulike illness, myalgia) are common with the initial episode. Painful urination is frequent, especially in females. Primary infections last 10–14 days before healing. Lesions may resemble trauma, syphilis (ulcers are painless), or chancroid (ulcers are painful and nodes are erythematous and fluctuant) in the adolescent, and bullous impetigo or severe chemical irritation in younger children.

3. Cutaneous infections—Direct inoculation onto cuts or abrasions may produce localized vesicles or ulcers. A deep HSV infection on the finger (called herpetic whitlow) may be mistaken for a bacterial felon or paronychia; surgical drainage is of no value and is contraindicated. HSV infection of eczematous skin may result in extensive areas of vesicles and shallow ulcers (eczema herpeticum), which may be mistaken for impetigo or varicella.

4. Recurrent mucocutaneous infection—Recurrent oral shedding is asymptomatic. Perioral recurrences often begin with a prodrome of tingling or burning limited to the vermilion border, followed by vesiculation, scabbing, and crusting around the lips over 3–5 days. Recurrent intraoral lesions are rare. Fever, adenopathy, and other symptoms are absent. Recurrent cutaneous herpes most closely resembles impetigo, but the latter is often outside the perinasal and perioral region, recurs infrequently in the same area of skin, responds to antibiotics, yields a positive result on Gram stain, and *Streptococcus pyogenes* or *Staphylococcus aureus* can be isolated. Recurrent genital disease is common after the initial infection with HSV-2. It is shorter (5–7 days) and milder (mean, four lesions) than primary infection and is not associated with systemic symptoms. Recurrent genital disease, which may also recur on the thighs and buttocks, is also preceded by a cutaneous sensory prodrome.

5. Keratoconjunctivitis—Keratoconjunctivitis may be part of a primary infection due to spread from infected saliva. Most cases are caused by reactivation of virus latent in the ciliary ganglion. Keratoconjunctivitis produces photophobia, pain, and conjunctival irritation. With recurrences, dendritic corneal ulcers may be demonstrable with fluorescein staining. Stromal invasion may occur. Corticosteroids should never be used for unilateral keratitis without ophthalmologic consultation. Other causes of these symptoms include trauma, bacterial infections, and other viral infections (especially adenovirus if pharyngitis is present; bilateral involvement makes HSV unlikely) (see Chapter 16).

6. Encephalitis—Although unusual in infants outside the neonatal period, encephalitis may occur at any age, usually without cutaneous herpes lesions. In older children, HSV encephalitis can follow a primary infection, but often represents reactivation of latent virus. HSV is the most common cause of sporadic severe encephalitis. Diagnosing this cause of encephalitis is very important because it can be treated with specific antiviral therapy. Acute onset is associated with fever, headache, behavioral changes, and focal neurologic deficits and/or focal seizures. Mild mononuclear pleocytosis is typically present along with an elevated protein concentration, which continues to rise on repeat lumbar punctures. In older children, hypodense areas with a medial and inferior temporal lobe predilection are seen on CT scan, especially after 3–5 days, but the findings in infants may be more diffuse. Magnetic resonance imaging (MRI) is more sensitive and is positive sooner. Periodic focal epileptiform discharges are seen on electroencephalograms, but are not diagnostic of HSV infection. Viral cultures of CSF are rarely positive. The PCR assay to detect HSV DNA in CSF is a sensitive and specific rapid test. Without early antiviral therapy, the prognosis is poor. The differential diagnosis includes mumps, mosquito-borne and other viral encephalitides, parainfectious and postinfectious encephalopathy, brain abscess, acute demyelinating syndromes, and bacterial meningoencephalitis.

7. Neonatal infections—Infection is acquired by ascending spread prior to delivery (< 5% of cases) or most often at the time of vaginal delivery from a mother with genital infection. Eight to fifteen percent of HSV-2–seropositive pregnant women at delivery have HSV-2 detected by PCR in the genital tract, although neonatal infection is rarely acquired from mothers with infection in the distant past. This is because transplacentally acquired antibody is usually protective. Occasionally, the infection is acquired in the postpartum period from oral secretions of family members or hospital personnel. A history of genital herpes in the mother is usually absent. Within a few days and up to 6 weeks (most often within 4 weeks), skin vesicles appear (especially at sites of trauma, such as where scalp monitors were placed). Some infants (45%) have infection limited to the skin, eye, or mouth. Other infants are acutely ill, presenting with jaundice, shock, bleeding, or respiratory distress (20%). Some infants appear well initially, but dissemination of the infection to the brain or other organs becomes evident during the ensuing week if it is untreated. HSV infection (and empiric therapy) should be strongly considered in newborns with the sepsis syndrome that is unresponsive to antibiotic therapy and has negative bacterial cultures. Some infected infants exhibit only neurologic symptoms at 2–3 weeks after delivery: apnea, lethargy, fever, poor feeding, or persistent overt seizures. The brain infection in these children is often diffuse and is best diagnosed by MRI. The skin lesions may resemble impetigo, bacterial scalp abscesses, or miliaria. Skin lesions may be absent at the time of presentation or may never develop. Skin lesions may recur over weeks or months after recovery from the acute illness. Progressive culture–negative pneumonitis is another manifestation of neonatal HSV. Most cases of neonatal herpes infection are acquired from mothers with undiagnosed genital herpes, most of whom acquired the infection during the pregnancy—especially near term.

B. Laboratory Findings

With multisystem disease, abnormalities in platelets, clotting factors, and liver function tests are often present. A finding of lymphocytic pleocytosis and elevated CSF protein indicates viral meningitis or encephalitis. Virus may be cultured from infected epithelial sites (vesicles, ulcers, or conjunctival scrapings) and from infected tissue (skin, brain) obtained by biopsy. Cultures of CSF yield positive results in about 50% of neonatal cases, but are uncommon in older children. HSV will be detected within 2 days by rapid tissue culture methods, but PCR is the preferred diagnostic method for all specimens. A positive test from skin, throat, eye, or stool of a newborn is diagnostic. Vaginal culture of the mother may offer circumstantial evidence for the diagnosis, but may be negative.

Rapid diagnostic tests include immunofluorescent stains or ELISA to detect viral antigen in skin or mucosal scrapings. The PCR assay for HSV DNA is positive (> 95%) in the CSF when there is brain involvement. Serum is often positive in the presence of multisystem disease. Typing of genital HSV isolates from adolescents has prognostic value, since HSV-1 genital infection rarely recurs, whereas recurrence of genital HSV-2 is frequent.

Complications, Sequelae, & Prognosis

Gingivostomatitis may result in dehydration due to dysphagia; severe chronic oral disease and esophageal involvement may occur in immunosuppressed patients. Primary vulvovaginitis may be associated with aseptic meningitis, paresthesias, autonomic dysfunction due to neuritis (urinary retention, constipation), and secondary candidal infection. HIV transmission from individuals who are seropositive for HSV infection is increased, and HIV acquisition is enhanced in HSV infected contacts. Extensive cutaneous disease (as in eczema) may be associated with dissemination and bacterial superinfection. Keratitis may result in corneal opacification or perforation. Untreated encephalitis is fatal in 70% of patients and causes severe damage in most of the remainder. When acyclovir treatment is instituted early, 20% of patients die and 40% are neurologically impaired.

Disseminated neonatal infection (25% of cases) is fatal for 30% of neonates in spite of therapy, and 20% of survivors are often impaired. Infants with CNS infection (30% of cases) have a 5% mortality with therapy and 70% of survivors are impaired; treated neonates with infection limited to skin, eye, and mouth survive, very often without sequelae.

Treatment

A. Specific Measures

HSV is sensitive to antiviral therapy.

1. Topical antivirals—Antiviral agents are effective for corneal disease and include 1% trifluridine and 3% acyclovir (1–2 drops five times daily). These agents should be used with the guidance of an ophthalmologist and used concurrently with oral antiviral therapy.

2. Mucocutaneous HSV infections—These infections respond to administration of oral nucleoside analogues (acyclovir, valacyclovir, or famciclovir). The main indications are severe genital HSV infection in adolescents (see Chapter 44; acyclovir, 400 mg three times daily for 7–10 days) and severe gingivostomatitis in young children. Antiviral therapy is beneficial for primary disease when begun early. Recurrent disease rarely requires therapy. Frequent genital recurrences may be suppressed by oral administration of nucleoside analogues (acyclovir, 400 mg twice daily), but this approach should be used sparingly. Other forms of severe cutaneous disease, such as eczema herpeticum, respond to these antivirals. Intravenous acyclovir may be required when disease is extensive in immunocompromised children (10–20 mg/kg or 500 mg/m^2 every 8 hours for 14–21 days). Oral acyclovir, which is available in suspension, is also used within 72–96 hours for severe primary gingivostomatitis in immunocompetent young children (20 mg/kg per dose [maximum of 400 mg per dose] four times a day for 7 days). Antiviral therapy does not alter the incidence or severity of subsequent recurrences of oral or genital infection. Development of resistance to antivirals, which is very rare after treating immunocompetent patients, occurs in immunocompromised patients who receive frequent and prolonged therapy.

3. Encephalitis—Treatment consists of intravenous acyclovir, 10–20 mg/kg (500 mg/m^2) every 8 hours for 21 days.

4. Neonatal infection—Newborns receive intravenous acyclovir, 20 mg/kg every 8 hours for 21 days (14 days if infection is limited to skin, eye, or mouth). Therapy should not be discontinued in neonates with CNS disease unless a repeat CSF HSV PCR assay is negative near the end of treatment. The value of subsequent prolonged oral prophylactic antiviral therapy in survivors is being studied.

B. General Measures

1. Gingivostomatitis—Gingivostomatitis is treated with pain relief and temperature control measures. Maintaining hydration is important because of the long duration of illness (7–14 days). Nonacidic, cool fluids are best. Topical anesthetic agents (eg, viscous lidocaine or an equal mixture of kaolin–attapulgite [Kaopectate], diphenhydramine, and viscous lidocaine) may be used as a mouthwash for older children who will not swallow it; ingested lidocaine may be toxic to infants or may lead to aspiration. Antiviral therapy is indicated in normal hosts with severe disease. Antibiotics are not helpful.

2. Genital infections—Genital infections may require pain relief, assistance with voiding (warm baths, topical anesthetics, rarely catheterization), and psychological support. Lesions should be kept clean; drying may shorten the duration of symptoms. Sexual contact should be avoided during the interval from prodrome to crusting stages. Because of the frequency of asymptomatic shedding, the only effective way to prevent spread is the use of condoms.

3. Cutaneous lesions—Skin lesions should be kept clean, dry, and covered if possible to prevent spread. Systemic analgesics may be helpful. Secondary bacterial infection is uncommon in patients with lesions on the mucosa or involving small areas. Secondary infection should be considered and treated if necessary (usually with an antistaphylococcal agent) in patients with more extensive lesions. Candidal superinfection occurs in 10% of women with primary genital infections.

4. Recurrent cutaneous disease—Recurrent disease is usually milder than primary infection. Sun block lip balm helps prevent labial recurrences that follow intense sun exposure. There is no evidence that the many popular topical or vitamin therapies are efficacious.

5. Keratoconjunctivitis—An ophthalmologist should be consulted regarding the use of cycloplegics, anti-inflammatory agents, local debridement, and other therapies.

6. Encephalitis—Extensive support will be required for obtunded or comatose patients. Rehabilitation and psychological support are often needed for survivors.

7. Neonatal infection—The affected infant should be isolated and given acyclovir. Cesarean delivery is indicated if the mother has obvious cervical or vaginal lesions, especially if these represent primary infection (35%–50% transmission rate). With infants born vaginally to mothers who have active lesions of recurrent genital herpes, appropriate cultures should be obtained at 24–48 hours after birth, and the infants should be observed closely. Treatment is given to infants whose culture results are positive or who have suggestive signs or symptoms. Infants born to mothers with obvious primary genital herpes should receive therapy before the culture results are known. For women with a history of genital herpes infection, but no genital lesions, vaginal delivery with peripartum cultures of maternal cervix is the standard. Clinical follow-up of the newborn is recommended when maternal culture results are positive. Repeated cervical cultures during pregnancy are not useful.

A challenging problem is the newborn, especially in the first 3 weeks of life, that presents with fever (or hypothermia) and a sepsis-like picture. This is further confounded in the late summer by the existence of circulating enteroviruses. These infants should be considered for empiric acyclovir therapy, pending results of PCR studies, given the poor outcome of disseminated herpes in the newborn. The index of suspicion is increased when there is a CSF pleocytosis, elevated hepatic transaminase levels, a very ill-appearing infant, rash, or respiratory distress.

Corey L, Wald A: Maternal and neonatal herpes simplex virus infections. N Engl J Med 2009;361:1376 [PMID: 19797284].

De Tiege X, Rozenberg F, Heron B: The spectrum of herpes encephalitis in children. J Europ Paed Neuroogy Soc 2008;12:72.

Long SS, Pool TE, Vodzak J et al: Herpes simplex virus infection in young infants during 2 decades of empiric acyclovir therapy. Ped Infect Dis J 2011;30(7):556.

Thompson C, Whitley R: Neonatal herpes simplex virus infections: Where are we now? Adv Experimental Med & Biology 2011;697:221 [PMID: 21120729].

VARICELLA & HERPES ZOSTER

ESSENTIALS OF DIAGNOSIS & TYPICAL FEATURES

- Varicella (chickenpox):
  - Exposure to varicella or herpes zoster 10–21 days previously; no prior history of varicella.
  - Widely scattered red macules and papules concentrated on the face and trunk, rapidly progressing to clear vesicles on an erythematous base, pustules, and then crusts, over 5–6 days.
  - Variable fever and nonspecific systemic symptoms.
- Herpes zoster (shingles):
  - History of varicella.
  - Dermatomal paresthesias and pain prior to eruption (more common in older children).
  - Dermatomal distribution of grouped vesicles on an erythematous base.

General Considerations

Primary infection with varicella-zoster virus results in varicella, which generally confers lifelong immunity; the virus remains latent in sensory ganglia. Herpes zoster, which represents reactivation of this latent virus, occurs in 30% of individuals at some time in their life. The incidence of herpes zoster is highest in elderly individuals and in immunosuppressed patients, but herpes zoster occurs in immune competent children. Spread of varicella from a close contact is by respiratory secretions or fomites from vesicles or pustules, with an 85% infection rate in susceptible persons. Exposure to herpes zoster is about one-third as likely to cause varicella in a susceptible host. Over 95% of young adults with a history of varicella are immune, as are 90% of native-born Americans who are unaware of having had varicella. Many individuals from tropical or subtropical regions fail to develop varicella in their childhood and remain susceptible through early adulthood. Humans are the only reservoir.

Clinical Findings

Exposure to varicella or herpes zoster has usually occurred 14–16 days previously (range, 10–21 days). Contact may not have been recognized, since the index case of varicella is infectious 1–2 days before rash appears. Although varicella is the most distinctive childhood exanthem, inexperienced observers may mistake other diseases for varicella. A 1- to 3-day prodrome of fever, malaise, respiratory symptoms, and headache may occur, especially in older children. The unilateral, dermatomal vesicular rash and pain of herpes zoster is very distinctive for that disease. The preeruptive pain of herpes zoster may last several days and be mistaken for other illnesses.

A. Symptoms and Signs

1. Varicella—The usual case consists of mild systemic symptoms followed by crops of red macules that rapidly become small vesicles with surrounding erythema (described as a "dew drop on a rose petal"), form pustules, become crusted, and then scab over and leave no scar. The rash appears predominantly on the trunk and face. Lesions occur in the scalp, and sometimes in the nose, mouth (where they are nonspecific ulcers), conjunctiva, and vagina. The magnitude of systemic symptoms usually parallels skin involvement. Up to five crops of lesions may be seen. New crops usually stop forming after 5–7 days. Pruritus is often intense. If varicella occurs in the first few months of life, it is often mild as a result of persisting maternal antibody. Once crusting begins, the patient is no longer contagious. A modified form of varicella occurs in about 15% of vaccinated children exposed to varicella, in spite of receiving a single dose of varicella vaccine. This is usually much milder than typical varicella, with fewer lesions that heal rapidly. Cases of modified varicella are contagious, especially if the modified case has 50 or more skin lesions.

2. Herpes zoster—The eruption of shingles involves a single dermatome (thus unilateral), usually truncal or cranial. Especially in older children this is preceded by neuropathic pain or itching in the same area (designated the "prodrome"). The rash does not cross the midline. Ophthalmic zoster may be associated with corneal involvement. The closely grouped vesicles, which resemble a localized version of varicella or herpes simplex, often coalesce. Crusting occurs in 7–10 days. Postherpetic neuralgia is rare in children. A few vesicles are occasionally seen outside the involved dermatome. Herpes zoster is a common problem in HIV-infected or other immunocompromised children, and is also common in children who had varicella in early infancy or whose mothers had varicella during pregnancy.

B. Laboratory Findings

Leukocyte counts are normal or low. Leukocytosis suggests secondary bacterial infection. The virus can be identified by fluorescent antibody staining of a lesion smear. Rapid culture methods take 48 hours. When the etiology is critical, as in immune compromised children with atypical disease, PCR is definitive. Diagnosis made with paired serology is not clinically useful. Serum aminotransferase levels may be modestly elevated during normal varicella.

C. Imaging

Varicella pneumonia classically produces numerous bilateral nodular densities and hyperinflation. This is very rare in immunocompetent children. Abnormal chest radiographs are seen more frequently in adults and immunocompromised children.

Differential Diagnosis

Varicella is usually distinctive. Similar rashes include those of coxsackievirus infection (fewer lesions, lack of crusting), impetigo (fewer lesions, smaller area, no classic vesicles, positive Gram stain, perioral or peripheral lesions), papular urticaria (insect bite history, nonvesicular rash), scabies (burrows, no typical vesicles; failure to resolve), parapsoriasis (rare in children < 10 years, chronic or recurrent, often a history of prior varicella), rickettsialpox (eschar where the mite bites, smaller lesions, no crusting), dermatitis herpetiformis (chronic, urticaria, residual pigmentation), and folliculitis. Herpes zoster is sometimes confused with a linear eruption of herpes simplex or a contact dermatitis (eg, *Rhus* dermatitis).

Complications & Sequelae

A. Varicella

Secondary bacterial infection with staphylococci or group A streptococci is most common, presenting as impetigo, cellulitis or fasciitis, abscesses, scarlet fever, or sepsis. Bacterial superinfection occurs in 2%–3% of children. Before a vaccine became available, hospitalization rates associated with varicella were 1:750–1:1000 cases in children and 10-fold higher in adults.

Protracted vomiting or a change in sensorium suggests Reye syndrome or encephalitis. Because Reye syndrome usually occurs in patients who are also receiving salicylates, these should be avoided in patients with varicella. Encephalitis occurs in less than 0.1% of cases, usually in the first week of illness, and is usually limited to cerebellitis with ataxia, which resolves completely. Diffuse encephalitis can be severe.

Varicella pneumonia usually afflicts immunocompromised children (especially those with leukemia or lymphoma or those receiving high doses of corticosteroids or chemotherapy) and adults; pregnant women may be at special risk. Cough, dyspnea, tachypnea, rales, and cyanosis occur several days after onset of rash. Varicella may be life-threatening in immunosuppressed patients. In addition to pneumonitis, their disease may be complicated by hepatitis and encephalitis. The acute illness in these children often begins with unexplained severe abdominal pain. Varicella exposure in severely varicella-naïve immunocompromised children must be evaluated immediately for postexposure prophylaxis (see Chapter 10).

Hemorrhagic varicella lesions may be seen without other complications. This is most often caused by autoimmune thrombocytopenia, but hemorrhagic lesions can occasionally represent idiopathic disseminated intravascular coagulation (purpura fulminans).

Neonates born to mothers who develop varicella from 5 days before to 2 days after delivery are at high risk for severe or fatal (5%) disease and must be given varicella-zoster immune globulin (VariZIG) and followed closely (see Chapter 10).

Varicella occurring during the first 20 weeks of pregnancy may cause (2% incidence) congenital infection associated with cicatricial skin lesions, associated limb anomalies, and cortical atrophy.

Unusual complications of varicella include optic neuritis, myocarditis, transverse myelitis, orchitis, and arthritis.

B. Herpes Zoster

Complications of herpes zoster include secondary bacterial infection, motor or cranial nerve paralysis, meningitis, encephalitis, keratitis, and dissemination in immunosuppressed patients. These complications are rare in immune competent children, and they do not develop prolonged pain. Postherpetic neuralgia does occur in immunocompromised children.

Prevention

Varicella-specific hyperimmune globulin is available for postexposure prevention of varicella of high-risk susceptible persons (see Chapter 10). Postexposure prophylaxis with acyclovir is effective when it is started at 7–9 days after exposure and is continued for 7 days. Varicella vaccine is also useful for postexposure prophylaxis when given within 3–5 days of the exposure. Two doses of the live attenuated varicella vaccine are now part of routine childhood immunization, and "catch-up" immunization is recommended for all other susceptible children and adults.

Treatment

A. General Measures

Supportive measures include maintenance of hydration, administration of acetaminophen for discomfort, cool soaks or antipruritics for itching (diphenhydramine, 1.25 mg/kg every 6 hours, or hydroxyzine, 0.5 mg/kg every 6 hours), and observance of general hygiene measures (keep nails trimmed and skin clean). Care must be taken to avoid overdosage with antihistaminic agents. Topical or systemic antibiotics may be needed for bacterial superinfection.

B. Specific Measures

Acyclovir is the preferred drug for varicella and herpes zoster infections. Recommended parenteral acyclovir dosage for severe disease is 10 mg/kg (500 mg/m^2) intravenously every 8 hours, each dose infused over 1 hour, for 7–10 days. Parenteral therapy should be started early in immunocompromised patients or high-risk infected neonates. Hyperimmune globulin is of no value for established disease. The effect of oral acyclovir (80 mg/kg/d, divided in four doses) on varicella in immunocompetent children was modestly beneficial and nontoxic, but only when administered within 24 hour after the onset of varicella. Oral acyclovir should be used selectively in immunocompetent children (eg, when intercurrent illness is present; possibly when the index case is a sibling or when the patient is an adolescent—both of which are associated with more severe disease) and in children with underlying chronic illnesses. Valacyclovir and famciclovir are superior antiviral agents because of better absorption; only acyclovir is available as a pediatric suspension. Herpes zoster in an immunocompromised child should be treated with intravenous acyclovir when it is severe, but oral valacyclovir or famciclovir can be used in immunocompromised children when the nature of the illness and the immune status support this decision.

Prognosis

Except for secondary bacterial infections, serious complications are rare and recovery complete in immune competent hosts.

Shah SS, Wood SM, Luan X, Ratner AJ: Decline in varicella-related ambulatory visits and hospitalizations in the United States since routine immunization against varicella. Ped Infect Dis J 2010;29(3):199.

Shapiro ED et al: Effectiveness of 2 doses of varicella vaccine in children. J Infect Dis 2011;203(3):312 [PMID: 21208922].

ROSEOLA INFANTUM (EXANTHEM SUBITUM)

ESSENTIALS OF DIAGNOSIS & TYPICAL FEATURES

- High fever in a child aged 6–36 months.
- Minimal toxicity.
- Rose-pink maculopapular rash appears when fever subsides.

General Considerations

Roseola infantum is a benign illness caused by HHV-6 or HHV-7. HHV-6 is a major cause of acute febrile illness in young children. Its significance is that it may be confused with more serious causes of high fever and its role in inciting febrile seizures.

Clinical Findings

The most prominent historical feature is the abrupt onset of fever, often reaching 40.6°C, which lasts up to 8 days (mean, 4 days) in an otherwise mildly ill child. The fever then ceases abruptly, and a characteristic rash may appear. Roseola occurs predominantly in children aged 6 months to 3 years, with 90% of cases occurring before the second year. HHV-7 infection tends to occur somewhat later in childhood. These viruses are the most common recognized cause of exanthematous fever in this age group and are responsible for 20% of emergency department visits by children aged 6–12 months.

A. Symptoms and Signs

Mild lethargy and irritability may be present, but generally there is a dissociation between systemic symptoms and the febrile course. The pharynx, tonsils, and tympanic membranes may be injected. Conjunctivitis and pharyngeal exudate are notably absent. Diarrhea and vomiting occur in one-third of patients. Adenopathy of the head and neck often occurs. The anterior fontanelle is bulging in one-quarter of HHV-6–infected infants. If rash appears (20%–30% incidence), it coincides with lysis of fever and begins on the trunk and spreads to the face, neck, and extremities. Rose-pink macules or maculopapules, 2–3 mm in diameter, are nonpruritic, tend to coalesce, and disappear in 1–2 days without pigmentation or desquamation. Rash may occur without fever.

B. Laboratory Findings

Leukopenia and lymphocytopenia are present early. Laboratory evidence of hepatitis occurs in some patients, especially adults.

Differential Diagnosis

The initial high fever may require exclusion of serious bacterial infection. The relative well-being of most children and the typical course and rash soon clarify the diagnosis. The erythrocyte sedimentation rate is normal. If the child has a febrile seizure, it is important to exclude bacterial meningitis. The CSF is normal in children with roseola. In children who receive antibiotics or other medication at the beginning of the fever, the rash may be attributed incorrectly to drug allergy.

Complications & Sequelae

Febrile seizures occur in up to 10% of patients (even higher percentages in those with HHV-7 infections). There is evidence that HHV-6 can directly infect the CNS, causing meningoencephalitis or aseptic meningitis. Multiorgan disease (pneumonia, hepatitis, bone marrow suppression, encephalitis) may occur in immunocompromised patients.

Treatment & Prognosis

Fever is managed readily with acetaminophen and sponge baths. Fever control should be a major consideration in children with a history of febrile seizures. Roseola infantum is otherwise entirely benign.

Kainth MK, Caserta MT: Molecular diagnostic tests for human herpesvirus 6. Ped Infect Dis J 2011;30(7):604.

Laina I, Syriopoulou VP, Daikos GL et al: Febrile seizures and primary human herpesvirus 6 infection. Ped Neurology 2010;42(1):28 [PMID: 20004859].

Prober CG: Human herpesvirus 6. Adv Exper Med & Biol 2011;697:87 [PMID: 21120721].

CYTOMEGALOVIRUS INFECTIONS

ESSENTIALS OF DIAGNOSIS & TYPICAL FEATURES

- Primary infection:
  - Asymptomatic or minor illness in young children.
  - Mononucleosis-like syndrome without pharyngitis in postpubertal individuals.
- Congenital infection:
  - Intrauterine growth retardation.
  - Microcephaly with intracerebral calcifications and seizures.
  - Retinitis and encephalitis.
  - Hepatosplenomegaly with thrombocytopenia.
  - "Blueberry muffin" rash.
  - Sensorineural deafness.
- Immunocompromised hosts:
  - Retinitis and encephalitis.
  - Pneumonitis.
  - Enteritis and hepatitis.
  - Bone marrow suppression.

General Considerations

Cytomegalovirus (CMV) is a ubiquitous herpesvirus transmitted by many routes. It can be acquired in utero following maternal viremia or postpartum from birth canal secretions or maternal milk. Young children are infected by the saliva of playmates; older individuals are infected by sexual partners (eg, from saliva, vaginal secretions, or semen). Transfused blood products and transplanted organs can be a source of CMV infection. Clinical illness is determined largely by the patient's immune competence. Immunocompetent individuals usually develop a mild self-limited illness, whereas immunocompromised children can develop severe, progressive, often multiorgan disease. In utero infection can be teratogenic.

1. In Utero Cytomegalovirus Infection

Approximately 0.5%–1.5% of children are born with CMV infections acquired during maternal viremia. CMV infection is asymptomatic in over 90% of these children, who are usually born to mothers who had experienced reactivation of latent CMV infection during the pregnancy. Symptomatic infection occurs predominantly in infants born to mothers with primary CMV infection, but can also result from recurrent, most likely, reinfection during pregnancy. Even when exposed to a primary maternal infection, less than 50% of fetuses are infected, and in only 10% of those infants is the infection symptomatic at birth. Primary infection in the first half of pregnancy poses the greatest risk for severe fetal damage.

Clinical Findings

A. Symptoms and Signs

Severely affected infants are born ill; they are often small for gestational age, floppy, and lethargic. They feed poorly and have poor temperature control. Hepatosplenomegaly, jaundice, petechiae, seizures, and microcephaly are common. Characteristic signs are a distinctive chorioretinitis and periventricular calcification. A purpuric (so-called blueberry muffin) rash similar to that seen with congenital rubella may be present. The mortality rate is 10%–20%. Survivors usually have significant sequelae, especially mental retardation, neurologic deficits, retinopathy, and hearing loss. Isolated hepatosplenomegaly or thrombocytopenia may occur. Even mildly affected children may subsequently manifest mental retardation and psychomotor delay. However, most infected infants (90%) are born to mothers with preexisting immunity that had a reactivation of latent CMV during pregnancy. These children have no clinical manifestations at birth. Of these, 10%–15% develop sensorineural hearing loss, which is often bilateral and may appear several years after birth.

B. Laboratory Findings

In severely ill infants, anemia, thrombocytopenia, hyperbilirubinemia, and elevated aminotransferase levels are common. Lymphocytosis occurs occasionally. Pleocytosis and an elevated protein concentration are found in CSF. The diagnosis is readily confirmed by isolation of CMV from urine or saliva within 48 hours, using rapid culture methods combined with immunoassay. The presence in the infant of IgM-specific CMV antibodies suggests the diagnosis. Some commercial ELISA kits are 90% sensitive and specific for these antibodies. Universal screening of asymptomatic children using blood or saliva CMV PCR during the first weeks of life is being evaluated for early detection of children at high risk of developing hearing loss.

C. Imaging

Head radiologic examinations may show microcephaly, periventricular calcifications, and ventricular dilation. These findings strongly correlate with neurologic sequelae and retardation. Long bone radiographs may show the "celery stalk" pattern characteristic of congenital viral infections. Interstitial pneumonia may be present.

Differential Diagnosis

CMV infection should be considered in any newborn that is seriously ill shortly after birth, especially once bacterial sepsis, metabolic disease, intracranial bleeding, and cardiac disease have been excluded. Other congenital infections to be considered in the differential diagnosis include toxoplasmosis (serology, more diffuse calcification of the CNS, specific type of retinitis, macrocephaly), rubella (serology, specific type of retinitis, cardiac lesions, eye abnormalities), enteroviral infections (time of year, maternal illness, severe hepatitis, PCR), herpes simplex (skin lesions, cultures, severe hepatitis, PCR), and syphilis (serology for both infant and mother, skin lesions, bone involvement).

Prevention & Treatment

Support is rarely required for anemia and thrombocytopenia. Most children with symptoms at birth have significant neurologic, intellectual, visual, or auditory impairment. Ganciclovir, 5 mg/kg every 12 hours, is recommended for children with severe, life- or sight-threatening disease, or if end-organ disease recurs or progresses. Duration is up to 6 weeks or until symptoms resolve. This approach decreases viral shedding and limits progression of symptoms, including hearing loss, during treatment. However, some of the therapeutic advantage is progressively lost over time after treatment is discontinued. Studies are currently ongoing to determine if early and more prolonged treatment (6 months) with valganciclovir decreases the risk or magnitude of hearing loss, which affects 6%–23% of children with asymptomatic CMV at birth in addition to the symptomatic ones.

Recent developments in the diagnosis of primary CMV infection during pregnancy using anti-CMV IgM and low-avidity IgG assays followed by quantitative CMV PCR testing of the amniotic fluid at 20–24 weeks' gestation have made possible the diagnosis of congenital CMV infection before birth. Many pregnant women elect to terminate gestation under these circumstances, but a recent study has also shown that passive immunoprophylaxis with hyperimmune CMV IgG may prevent development of congenital disease. A subunit CMV vaccine administered to CMV-seronegative pregnant women had a 50% efficacy for prevention of congenital CMV infection.

2. Perinatal Cytomegalovirus Infection

CMV infection can be acquired from birth canal secretions or shortly after birth from maternal milk. In some socioeconomic groups, 10%–20% of infants are infected at birth and excrete CMV for many months. Infection can also be acquired in the postnatal period from unscreened transfused blood products.

Clinical Findings

A. Symptoms and Signs

Ninety percent of immunocompetent infants infected by their mothers at birth develop subclinical illness (ie, virus excretion only) or a minor illness within 1–3 months. The remainder develop an illness lasting several weeks characterized by hepatosplenomegaly, lymphadenopathy, and interstitial pneumonitis in various combinations. The severity of the pneumonitis may be increased by the simultaneous presence of *Chlamydia trachomatis*. Infants who receive blood products are often premature and immunologically impaired. If they are born to CMV-negative mothers and subsequently receive CMV-containing blood, they frequently develop severe infection and pneumonia after a 2- to 6-week incubation period.

B. Laboratory Findings

Lymphocytosis, atypical lymphocytes, anemia, and thrombocytopenia may be present, especially in premature infants. Liver function is abnormal. CMV can be isolated from urine and saliva. Secretions obtained at bronchoscopy contain CMV and epithelial cells bearing CMV antigens. Serum levels of CMV antibody rise significantly.

C. Imaging

Chest radiographs show a diffuse interstitial pneumonitis in severely affected infants.

Differential Diagnosis

CMV infection should be considered as a cause of any prolonged illness in early infancy, especially if hepatosplenomegaly, lymphadenopathy, or atypical lymphocytosis is present. This must be distinguished from granulomatous or malignant diseases and from congenital infections (syphilis, toxoplasmosis, hepatitis B) not previously diagnosed. Other viruses (Epstein-Barr virus [EBV], HIV, adenovirus) can cause this syndrome. CMV is a recognized cause of viral pneumonia in this age group. Because asymptomatic CMV excretion is common in early infancy, care must be taken to establish the diagnosis and to rule out concomitant pathogens such as *Chlamydia* and RSV. Severe CMV infection in early infancy may indicate that the child has a congenital or acquired immune deficiency.

Prevention & Treatment

The self-limited disease of normal infants requires no therapy. Severe pneumonitis in premature infants requires oxygen administration and often intubation. Very ill infants should receive ganciclovir (6 mg/kg every 12 hours). CMV infection acquired by transfusion can be prevented by excluding CMV-seropositive blood donors. Milk donors should also be screened for prior CMV infection. It is likely that high-risk infants receiving large doses of IVIG for other reasons will be protected against severe CMV disease.

3. Cytomegalovirus Infection Acquired in Childhood & Adolescence

Young children are readily infected by playmates, especially because CMV continues to be excreted in saliva and urine for many months after infection. The cumulative annual incidence of CMV excretion by children in day care centers exceeds 75%. In fact, young children in a family are often the source of primary CMV infection of their mothers during subsequent pregnancies. An additional peak of CMV infection takes place when adolescents become sexually active. Sporadic acquisition of CMV occurs after blood transfusion and transplantation.

Clinical Findings

A. Symptoms and Signs

Most young children who acquire CMV are asymptomatic or have a minor febrile illness, occasionally with adenopathy. They provide an important reservoir of virus shedders that facilitates spread of CMV. Occasionally a child may have prolonged fever with hepatosplenomegaly and adenopathy. Older children and adults, many of whom are infected during sexual activity, are more likely to be symptomatic in this fashion and can present with a syndrome that mimics the infectious mononucleosis syndrome that follows EBV infection (1–2 weeks of fever, malaise, anorexia, splenomegaly, mild hepatitis, and some adenopathy; see next section). This syndrome can also occur 2–4 weeks after transfusion of CMV-infected blood.

B. Laboratory Findings

In the CMV mononucleosis syndrome, lymphocytosis and atypical lymphocytes are common, as is a mild rise in aminotransferase levels. CMV is present in saliva and urine; CMV DNA can be uniformly detected in plasma or blood.

Differential Diagnosis

In older children, CMV infection should be included as a possible cause of fever of unknown origin, especially when lymphocytosis and atypical lymphocytes are present. CMV infection is distinguished from EBV infection by the absence of pharyngitis, the relatively minor adenopathy, and the absence of serologic evidence of acute EBV infection. Mononucleosis syndromes also are caused by *Toxoplasma gondii*, rubella virus, adenovirus, hepatitis A virus, and HIV.

Prevention

Screening of transfused blood or filtering blood (thus removing CMV-containing white blood cells) prevents cases related to this source.

4. Cytomegalovirus Infection in Immunocompromised Children

In addition to symptoms experienced during primary infection, immunocompromised hosts develop symptoms with reinfection or reactivation of latent CMV. This is clearly seen in children with acquired immunodeficiency syndrome (AIDS), after transplantation, or with congenital immunodeficiencies. However, in most immunocompromised patients, primary infection is more likely to cause severe symptoms than is reactivation or reinfection. The severity of the resulting disease is generally proportionate to the degree of immunosuppression.

Clinical Findings

A. Symptoms and Signs

A mild febrile illness with myalgia, malaise, and arthralgia may occur, especially with reactivation disease. Severe disease often includes subacute onset of dyspnea and cyanosis as manifestations of interstitial pneumonitis. Auscultation reveals only coarse breath sounds and scattered rales. A rapid respiratory rate may precede clinical or radiographic evidence of pneumonia. Hepatitis without jaundice or hepatomegaly is common. Diarrhea, which can be severe, occurs with CMV colitis, and CMV can cause esophagitis with symptoms of odynophagia or dysphagia. These enteropathies are most common in AIDS, as is the presence of a retinitis that often progresses to blindness. Encephalitis and polyradiculitis also occur in AIDS.

B. Laboratory Findings

Neutropenia and thrombocytopenia are common. Atypical lymphocytosis is infrequent. Serum aminotransferase levels are often elevated. The stools may contain occult blood if enteropathy is present. CMV is readily isolated from saliva, urine, buffy coat, and bronchial secretions. Results are available in 48 hours. Interpretation of positive cultures is made difficult by asymptomatic shedding of CMV in saliva and urine in many immunocompromised patients. CMV disease correlates more closely with the presence of CMV in the blood or lung lavage fluid. Monitoring for the appearance of CMV DNA in plasma or CMV antigen in blood mononuclear cells is used as a guide to early antiviral ("preemptive") therapy.

C. Imaging

Bilateral interstitial pneumonitis is present on chest radiographs.

Differential Diagnosis

The initial febrile illness must be distinguished from treatable bacterial or fungal infection. Similarly, the pulmonary disease must be distinguished from intrapulmonary hemorrhage; drug-induced or radiation pneumonitis; pulmonary edema; and bacterial, fungal, parasitic, and other virus infections.

CMV infection causes bilateral and interstitial abnormalities seen on chest radiographs, cough is nonproductive, chest pain is absent, and the patient is not usually toxic. *Pneumocystis jiroveci* infection may have a similar presentation. These patients may have polymicrobial disease. It is suspected that bacterial and fungal infections are enhanced by the neutropenia that can accompany CMV infection. Infection of the gastrointestinal tract is diagnosed by endoscopy. This will exclude candidal, adenoviral, and herpes simplex infections and allows tissue confirmation of CMV-induced mucosal ulcerations.

Prevention & Treatment

Blood donors should be screened to exclude those with prior CMV infection, or blood should be filtered. Ideally, seronegative transplant recipients should receive organs from seronegative donors. Severe symptoms, most commonly pneumonitis, often respond to early therapy with intravenous ganciclovir (5 mg/kg every 12 hours for 14–21 days). Neutropenia is a frequent side effect of this therapy. Foscarnet and cidofovir are alternative therapeutic agents recommended for patients with ganciclovir-resistant virus. Prophylactic use of oral or intravenous ganciclovir or foscarnet may prevent CMV infections in organ transplant recipients. A new drug with an excellent safety profile, maribavir, has shown efficacy in hematopoietic stem cell recipients. Additional studies are being conducted in solid organ transplant recipients. Preemptive therapy can be used in transplant recipients by monitoring CMV in blood by PCR and instituting therapy when the results reach a certain threshold regardless of clinical signs or symptoms. CMV-seropositive children with AIDS and low CD4 counts (< 50/μL) should have funduscopic examinations and plasma CMV DNA measurements every 3 months.

Boppana SB et al: Dried blood spot real-time polymerase chain reaction assays to screen newborns for congenital cytomegalovirus infection. JAMA 2010;303:1375.

Mussi-Pinhata MM et al: Birth prevalence and natural history of congenital cytomegalovirus infection in a highly seroimmune population. Clin Infect Dis 2009;49:522.

Pass RF et al: Vaccine prevention of maternal cytomegalovirus infection. N Engl J Med 2009;360:1191.

Rosenthal LS et al: Cytomegalovirus shedding and delayed sensorineural hearing loss. Pediatr Infect Dis J 2009;28:515.

INFECTIOUS MONONUCLEOSIS (EPSTEIN-BARR VIRUS)

ESSENTIALS OF DIAGNOSIS & TYPICAL FEATURES

- Prolonged fever.
- Exudative pharyngitis.
- Generalized adenopathy.
- Hepatosplenomegaly.
- Atypical lymphocytes.
- Heterophil antibodies.

General Considerations

Mononucleosis is the most characteristic syndrome produced by EBV infection. Young children infected with EBV have either no symptoms or a mild nonspecific febrile illness. As the age of the host increases, EBV infection is more likely to produce the typical features of the mononucleosis syndrome, including 20%–25% of infected adolescents. EBV is acquired readily from asymptomatic carriers (15%–20% of whom excrete the virus in saliva on any given day) and from recently ill patients, who excrete virus for many months. Young children are infected from the saliva of playmates and family members. Adolescents may be infected through sexual activity. EBV can also be transmitted by blood transfusion and organ transplantation.

Clinical Findings

A. Symptoms and Signs

After an incubation period of 1–2 months, a 2- to 3-day prodrome of malaise and anorexia yields, abruptly or insidiously, to a febrile illness with temperatures exceeding 39°C. The major complaint is pharyngitis, which is often (50%) exudative. Lymph nodes are enlarged, firm, and mildly tender. Any area may be affected, but posterior and anterior cervical nodes are almost always enlarged. Splenomegaly is present in 50%–75% of patients. Hepatomegaly is common (30%), and the liver is frequently tender. Five percent of patients have a rash, which can be macular, scarlatiniform, or urticarial. Rash is almost universal in patients taking penicillin or ampicillin. Soft palate petechiae and eyelid edema are also observed.

B. Laboratory Findings

1. Peripheral blood—Leukopenia may occur early, but an atypical lymphocytosis (comprising over 10% of the total leukocytes at some time in the illness) is most notable. Hematologic changes may not be seen until the third week of illness and may be entirely absent in some EBV syndromes (eg, neurologic ones).

2. Heterophil antibodies—These nonspecific antibodies appear in over 90% of older patients with mononucleosis, but in fewer than 50% of children younger than age 5 years. They may not be detectable until the second week of illness and may persist for up to 12 months after recovery. Rapid screening tests (slide agglutination) are usually positive if the titer is significant; a positive result strongly suggests but does not prove EBV infection.

3. Anti-EBV antibodies—It may be necessary to measure specific antibody titers and/or PCR when heterophil antibodies fail to appear, as in young children. Acute EBV infection is established by detecting IgM antibody to the viral capsid antigen (VCA) or by detecting a greater than or equal to fourfold change of IgG anti-VCA titers (in normal hosts, IgG antibody peaks by the time symptoms appear; in immunocompromised hosts, the tempo of antibody production may be delayed). The absence of anti–Epstein-Barr nuclear antigen (EBNA) antibodies, which are typically first detected longer than or equal to 4 weeks after the initiation of symptoms, may also be used to diagnose acute infection in immunocompetent hosts. However, immunocompromised hosts may fail to develop anti-EBNA antibodies.

4. EBV PCR—Detection of EBV DNA is the method of choice for the diagnosis of CNS and ocular infections. Quantitative EBV PCR in peripheral blood mononuclear cells has been used to diagnose EBV-related lymphoproliferative disorders in transplant patients.

Differential Diagnosis

Severe pharyngitis may suggest group A streptococcal infection. Enlargement of only the anterior cervical lymph nodes, a neutrophilic leukocytosis, and the absence of splenomegaly suggest bacterial infection. Although a child with a positive throat culture result for *Streptococcus* usually requires therapy, up to 10% of children with mononucleosis are asymptomatic streptococcal carriers. In this group, penicillin therapy is unnecessary and often causes a rash. Severe primary herpes simplex pharyngitis, occurring in adolescence, may also mimic infectious mononucleosis. In this type of pharyngitis, some anterior mouth ulcerations should suggest the correct diagnosis. Adenoviruses are another cause of severe, often exudative pharyngitis. EBV infection should be considered in the differential diagnosis of any perplexing prolonged febrile illness. Similar illnesses that produce atypical lymphocytosis include rubella (pharyngitis not prominent, shorter illness, less adenopathy and splenomegaly), adenovirus (upper respiratory symptoms and cough, conjunctivitis, less adenopathy, fewer atypical lymphocytes), hepatitis A or B (more severe liver function abnormalities, no pharyngitis, no lymphadenopathy), and toxoplasmosis (negative heterophil test, less pharyngitis). Serum sickness–like drug reactions and leukemia (smear morphology is important) may be confused with infectious mononucleosis. CMV mononucleosis is a close mimic except for minimal pharyngitis and less adenopathy; it is much less common. Serologic tests for EBV and CMV should clarify the correct diagnosis. The acute initial manifestation of HIV infection can be a mononucleosis-like syndrome.

Complications

Splenic rupture is a rare complication, which usually follows significant trauma. Hematologic complications, including hemolytic anemia, thrombocytopenia, and neutropenia, are more common. Neurologic involvement can include aseptic meningitis, encephalitis, isolated neuropathy such as Bell palsy, and Guillain-Barré syndrome. Any of these may appear prior to or in the absence of the more typical signs and symptoms of infectious mononucleosis. Rare complications include myocarditis, pericarditis, and atypical pneumonia. Recurrence or persistence of EBV-associated symptoms for 6 months or longer characterizes chronic active EBV. This disease is due to continuous viral replication and warrants specific antiviral therapy. Rarely EBV infection becomes a progressive lymphoproliferative disorder characterized by persistent fever, multiple organ involvement, neutropenia or pancytopenia, and agammaglobulinemia. Hemocytophagia is often present in the bone marrow. An X-linked genetic defect in immune response has been inferred for some patients (Duncan syndrome, X-linked lymphoproliferative disorder). Children with other congenital immunodeficiencies or chemotherapy-induced immunosuppression can also develop progressive EBV infection, EBV-associated lymphoproliferative disorder or lymphoma, and other malignancies.

Treatment & Prognosis

Bed rest may be necessary in severe cases. Acetaminophen controls high fever. Potential airway obstruction due to swollen pharyngeal lymphoid tissue responds rapidly to systemic corticosteroids. Corticosteroids may also be given for hematologic and neurologic complications, although no controlled trials have proved their efficacy in these conditions. Fever and pharyngitis disappear by 10–14 days. Adenopathy and splenomegaly can persist several weeks longer. Some patients complain of fatigue, malaise, or lack of well-being for several months. Although corticosteroids may shorten the duration of fatigue and malaise, their long-term effects on this potentially oncogenic viral infection are unknown, and indiscriminate use is discouraged. Patients with splenic enlargement should avoid contact sports for 6–8 weeks. Acyclovir, valacyclovir, penciclovir, ganciclovir, and foscarnet are active against EBV and are indicated in the treatment of chronic active EBV.

Management of EBV-related lymphoproliferative disorders relies primarily on decreasing the immunosuppression whenever possible. Adjunctive therapy with acyclovir, ganciclovir, or another antiviral active against EBV as well as γ globulin has been used without scientific evidence of efficacy.

Hakim H et al: Comparison of various blood compartments and reporting units for the detection and quantification of Epstein Barr virus in peripheral blood. J Clin Microbiol 2007;45:2151.

Higgins CD et al: A study of risk factors for acquisition of Epstein Barr virus and its subtypes. J Infect Dis 2007;195:474 [PMID: 17230406].

VIRAL INFECTIONS SPREAD BY INSECT VECTORS

In the United States, mosquitoes are the most common insect vectors that spread viral infections (Table 40–4). As a consequence, these infections—and others that are spread by ticks—tend to occur as summer–fall epidemics that coincide with the seasonal breeding and feeding habits of the vector, and the etiologic agent varies by region. Other insect-borne viral infections are seen in international travelers. Thus, a careful travel and exposure history is critical for correct diagnostic workup.

ENCEPHALITIS

ESSENTIALS OF DIAGNOSIS & TYPICAL FEATURES

- Fever and headache.
- Change in mental status or behavior (or both), with or without focal neurologic deficits.
- CSF shows a mononuclear cell pleocytosis, elevated protein level, and normal glucose level.

Encephalitis is a common severe manifestation of many infections spread by insects (see Table 40–4). With many viral pathogens, the infection is most often subclinical, or a mild CNS disease such as meningitis is present. These infections have some distinguishing features in terms of subclinical infection rate, unique neurologic syndromes, associated systemic symptoms, and prognosis. The diagnosis is generally made clinically during recognized outbreaks and is confirmed by virus-specific serology. Prevention consists of control of mosquito vectors and precautions with proper clothing and insect repellents to minimize mosquito and tick bites. It is essential before making the diagnosis of arboviral encephalitis, which is not treatable, to exclude herpes encephalitis, which warrants specific antiviral therapy. Delay in administering this therapy may have dire consequences.

West Nile Virus Encephalitis

This flavivirus was the most important arbovirus infection in the United States, in 2003, when it caused more than 10,000 clinically apparent infections, more than 2900 nervous system infections, and 265 deaths, in 47 states. Prevalence has declined to less than 150 cases reported in recent 2 years, but West Nile virus remains the major cause of endemic arboviral encephalitis in the United States. The reservoir of West Nile virus includes more than 160 species of birds whose migration explains the extent of endemic disease. Epidemics occur in summer–fall; most infected individuals are asymptomatic. Approximately 20% develop West Nile fever, which is characterized by fever, headache, retro-orbital pain, nausea and vomiting, lymphadenopathy, and a maculopapular rash (20%–50%). Less than 1% of infected patients develop meningitis or encephalitis, but 10% of these cases are fatal (0.1% of all infections). Children are most likely to have neuroinvasive disease limited to meningitis. The major risk factor for severe disease is age older than 50 years and immune compromise. Children, especially adolescents, develop West Nile fever; and less than one-third of children with clinically apparent infection have neuroinvasive disease. The neurologic manifestations are most often those found with other meningoencephalitides. However, distinguishing atypical features include polio-like flaccid paralysis, movement disorders (parkinsonism, tremor, myoclonus), brainstem symptoms, polyneuropathy, and optic neuritis. Muscle weakness, facial palsy, and hyporeflexia are common (20% of each finding). Recovery is slow and serious sequelae occur in some severely affected patients. Diagnosis is best made by detecting IgM antibody (enzyme immunoassay [EIA]) to the virus in CSF. This will be present by 5–6 days (95%) after onset. PCR is a specific diagnostic tool, but is less sensitive than antibody detection. Antibody rise in serum can also be used for diagnosis.

Treatment is supportive, although various antivirals and specific immune globulin are being studied. The infection is not spread between contacts, but can be spread by donated organs and blood and breast milk, and transplacentally.

Rossi SL, Ross TM, Evans JD: West Nile virus. Clin Lab Med 2010;30(1):47 [PMID: 20513541].

Rizzo C, Esposito S et al: West Nile virus infections in children: A disease pediatricians should think about. Ped Infect Dis J 2011;30(1):65 [PMID: 21173677].

DENGUE

ESSENTIALS OF DIAGNOSIS & TYPICAL FEATURES

- Travel or residence in an endemic area.
- First infection (first episode) results in nonspecific rash and fever; retro-orbital pain, severe myalgia, and arthralgia may occur.
- Subsequent infection with a different (heterotypic) serotype of dengue may result in dengue hemorrhagic fever (thrombocytopenia, bleeding, plasma leak syndrome); this may progress to shock (dengue shock syndrome).

In endemic areas, 50–100 million cases of dengue occur each year, often in severe forms. In the United States, > 400 cases

Table 40–4. Some insect-borne viral diseases occurring in the United States or in returning U.S. travelers.

Disease	Natural Reservoir (Vector)	Geographic Distribution	Incubation Period	Clinical Presentations	Laboratory Findings	Complications, Sequelae	Diagnosis, Therapy, Comments
Flaviviruses							
St. Louis encephalitis (SLE)	Birds (*Culex* mosquitoes)	Southern Canada, central and southern United States, Texas, Caribbean, South America	2–5 d (up to 3 wk)	Second most common cause of arbovirus encephalitis. Abrupt onset of fever, chills, headache, nausea, vomiting; may develop generalized weakness, seizures, coma, ataxia, cranial nerve palsies. Aseptic meningitis is common in children.	Modest leukocytosis, neutrophilia, elevated liver enzymes. CSF: 100–200 WBCs/μL; PMNs predominate early.	Mortality rate 2%–5% at age < 5 or > 50 y. Neurologic sequelae in 1%–20%.	~15 cases/y, < 2% symptomatic. (Worse in elderly.) Therapy: supportive. Diagnosis: serology. Specific antibody often present within 5 d.
Dengue	Humans (*Aedes* mosquitoes)	Asia, Africa, Central and South America, Caribbean; observed in Texas/Mexico border area and Key West, Florida	4–7 d (range, 3–14 d)	Fever, headache, myalgia, joint and bone pain, retroocular pain, nausea and vomiting; maculopapular or petechial rash in 50%, sparing palms and soles; adenopathy. Biphasic course may occur Meningoencephalitis in 5%–10% of children.	Leukopenia, thrombocytopenia. CSF: 100–500 mononuclear cells/μL if neurologic signs are present.	Hemorrhagic fever, shock syndrome, prolonged weakness, encephalitis.	High infection rate. 100–150 cases occur in the U.S. travelers to endemic areas. Therapy: supportive. Diagnosis: serology; IgM-EIA antibody by day 6.
West Nile	Birds (*Culex* mosquitoes); small mammals	North Africa, Middle East, parts of Asia, Europe, continental United States	2–14 d	Abrupt onset of fever, headache, sore throat, myalgia, retroocular pain, conjunctivitis; 20%–50% with rash; adenopathy. Meningitis alone is most common in children. Encephalitis may be accompanied by muscle weakness, flaccid paralysis, or movement disorders.	Mild leukocytosis; 10%–15% lymphopenic or thrombocytopenic; CSF pleocytosis with < 500 cells; may be neutrophils early.	Mortality rate 10%, of those with CNS symptoms, but rare in children; weakness and myalgia may persist for an extended period.	Most important mosquito-borne encephalitis in the United States. (~150 cases reposted each year.) Diagnosis: IgM-EIA serology; cross-reacts with St. Louis encephalitis; positive by 5–6 d after onset of CNS symptoms. Diagnosis by PCR is less sensitive. Therapy: supportive.
Japanese encephalitis	Birds, large mammals; reptiles (*Culex* mosquitos)	SE Asia; Australasia	5–14 d	Onset with fever, cough, coryza, headache. Aseptic meningitis is common in children.	CSF: 10–100 lymphocytes/μL; atypical lymphocytes may be present; protein may reach 200 mg/dL.	Seizures are common in children; when encephalitis occurs, it can result in lasting motor, learning, and behavioral abnormalities.	Vaccination is an important consideration for children visiting or residing in endemic areas.
Alpha toga viruses							
Eastern equine encephalitis	Birds (*Culiseta* mosquitoes)	Eastern seaboard United States, Caribbean, South America	2–5 d	Similar to that of St. Louis encephalitis, but more severe. Progresses rapidly in one-third to coma and death.	Leukocytosis with neutrophilia. CSF: 500–2000 WBCs/μL; PMNs predominate early.	Mortality rate 20%–50%; neurologic 50% of children.	< 10 cases/y. Only 3%–10% of cases are symptomatic, but sequelae are common in young children who develop symptoms. Therapy: supportive. Diagnosis: serology. Titers often positive in the first week. Equine deaths may signal an outbreak.

(*Continued*)

Table 40–4. Some insect-borne viral diseases occurring in the United States or in returning U.S. travelers. (*Continued*)

Disease	Natural Reservoir (Vector)	Geographic Distribution	Incubation Period	Clinical Presentations	Laboratory Findings	Complications, Sequelae	Diagnosis, Therapy, Comments
Western equine encephalitis	Birds (*Culiseta* mosquitoes)	Canada, Mexico, and United States west of Mississippi River	2–5 d	Similar to that of St. Louis encephalitis. Most infections are subclinical.	Variable white counts. CSF: 10–300 WBCs/μL.	Permanent brain damage, 10% overall; most severe in older adults.	No reported cases in the United States in recent years. Case/infection is 1:1000 for older adults and 1:1 for infants. Equine illness precedes human outbreaks. Diagnosis: IgM antibody in the first week. Therapy: supportive.
Venezuelan equine encephalitis	Horses (10 species of mosquitoes)	South and Central America, Texas	1–6 d	Similar to that of St. Louis encephalitis.	Lymphopenia, mild thrombocytopenia, abnormal liver function tests. CSF: 50–200 mononuclear cells/μL	Severe disease more common in infants; 20% fatality rate for encephalitis.	Most infections do not cause encephalitis. No cases in the United States in recent years. Vaccination of horses will stop epidemic. Therapy: supportive. Diagnosis: IgM antibody (EIA).
Bunyavirus							
California encephalitis serogroup (LaCrosse, Jamestown Canyon, California)	Chipmunks and other small mammals (*Aedes* mosquitoes)	Northern and mid-central United States, southern Canada	3–7 d	Second most common arbovirus etiology, especially LaCrosse. Symptoms are similar to those of St. Louis encephalitis; sore throat and respiratory symptoms are common; focal neurologic signs in up to 25%. Seizures prominent. Prepubertal children are most likely to have severe disease. Can mimic herpes simplex encephalitis.	Variable white counts. CSF: 30–200 up to 600 WBCs/μL; variable PMNs; protein often normal.	Mortality rate < 2%. Seizures may occur during acute illness.	~75 cases/y in the United States, 5% symptomatic. > 10% with sequelae. Therapy: supportive. Diagnosis: serology. Up to 90% have specific IgM antibody in the first week; 25% of population in certain regions has IgG antibody.
Coltivirus							
Colorado tick fever	Small mammals (*Dermacentor andersoni*, or wood tick)	Rocky Mountain region of United States and Canada	3–4 d (range, 2–14 d)	Fever, chills, myalgia, conjunctivitis, headache, retro-orbital pain; rash in < 10%. No respiratory symptoms. Biphasic fever in 50%.	Leukopenia (maximum at 4–6 d), mild thrombocytopenia.	Rare encephalitis, coagulopathy.	Patient may have no known tick bite. Acute illness lasts 7–10 d; prolonged fatigue in adults. Therapy: supportive. Diagnosis: serology, direct FA staining of red cells for viral antigen, PCR.

CNS, central nervous system; CSF, cerebrospinal fluid; EIA, enzyme immunoassay; FA, fluorescent antibody; PCR, polymerase chain reaction; PMN, polymorphonuclear neutrophil; WBC, white blood cell.

are diagnosed, most often in travelers from the Caribbean or Asia and less often in those visiting Central and South America, making it the most common arboviral disease in travelers. Dengue is the second most common cause of fever (after malaria) in returning travelers. Dengue occurs in Mexico, and Texas has sporadic indigenous outbreaks. The spread of dengue requires the requisite species (which is present in the United States) of mosquito, which transmits virus from a reservoir of viremic humans in endemic areas. Most patients have mild disease, especially young children, who may have a nonspecific fever and rash. Severity is a function of age, and prior infection with other serotypes of dengue virus is a prerequisite for severe hemorrhagic complications.

Clinical Findings

A. Symptoms and Signs

Dengue fever begins abruptly 4–7 days after transmission (range, 3–14 days) with fever, chills, severe retro-orbital pain, severe muscle and joint pain, nausea, and vomiting. Erythema of the face and torso may occur early. After 3–4 days, a centrifugal maculopapular rash appears in half of the patients. The rash can become petechial, and mild hemorrhagic signs (epistaxis, gingival bleeding, microscopic blood in stool or urine) may be noted. The illness lasts 5–7 days, although rarely fever may reappear for several additional days. Fever may become relatively lower on the third day, only to become higher until defervescence.

B. Laboratory Findings

Leukopenia and a mild drop in platelets are common. Liver function tests are usually normal. Diagnosis is made by viral culture of plasma (50% sensitive up to the fifth day), by detecting IgM-specific ELISA antibodies (90% sensitive at the sixth day), or by detecting a rise in type-specific antibody. PCR testing is available for diagnosis in some areas.

Differential Diagnosis

This diagnosis should be considered for any traveler to an endemic area who has symptoms suggestive of a systemic viral illness, although less than 1 in 1000 travelers to these areas develops dengue. Often the areas visited have other unique pathogens circulating (eg, malaria, typhoid fever, leptospirosis, other endemic alphaviruses and flaviviruses, and measles). Especially relevant in travelers from India and the Indian ocean islands is chikungunya fever, which also presents with fever, and rash. This illness is associated with arthralgia/arthritis, rather than myalgia as is seen with dengue. EBV, influenza, enteroviruses, and acute HIV infection may produce a similar illness. Dengue is not associated with sore throat or cough. An illness that starts 2 weeks after the trip ends or that lasts longer than 2 weeks is not dengue or chikungunya fever.

Complications

Rarely dengue fever is associated with meningoencephalitis (5%–10%) or hepatic damage. More common in endemic areas is the appearance of dengue hemorrhagic fever, which is defined by significant thrombocytopenia (< 100,000 platelets/μL, bleeding, and a plasma leak syndrome [hemoconcentration = hematocrit > 20% higher than baseline], hypoalbuminemia, and pleural or peritoneal effusions). This is the consequence of circulating antibody and other immune responses acquired from a prior dengue virus infection; thus, it is rarely seen in typical travelers. Failure to recognize and treat this complication may lead to dengue shock syndrome, which is defined by signs of circulatory failure and hypotension or shock, and has a high fatality rate (10%). Dengue can be transmitted in utero from a pregnant woman infected within 2 weeks prior to delivery.

Prevention

Prevention of dengue fever involves avoiding high-risk areas and using conventional mosquito avoidance measures. The main vector is a daytime feeder. A vaccine to prevent dengue is being tested.

Treatment

Dengue fever is treated by oral replacement of fluid lost from gastrointestinal symptoms. Analgesic therapy, which is often necessary, should not include drugs that affect platelet function. Recovery is complete without sequelae. The hemorrhagic syndrome requires prompt fluid therapy with plasma expanders and isotonic saline.

Centers for Disease Control and Prevention: Key West, Florida, 2009–2010. MMWR-Morbidity and Mortality Weekly Report 2010;59(19):577 [PMID: 20489680].

Chen LH, Wilson ME: Dengue and chikungunya infections in travelers. Curr Opinion in Infect Dis 2010;23:438.

Morens D: Dengue fever and dengue hemorrhagic fever. Ped Infect Dis J 2009;28:635.

COLORADO TICK FEVER

ESSENTIALS OF DIAGNOSIS & TYPICAL FEATURES

- Travel in endemic area; tick bite.
- Fever, chills, headache, retro-orbital pain, myalgia.
- Biphasic fever curve.
- Leukopenia early in the illness.

Colorado tick fever is endemic in the high plains and mountains of the central and northern Rocky Mountains and northern Pacific coast of the United States. The reservoir of the virus consists of squirrels and chipmunks. Many hundreds of cases of Colorado tick fever occur each year in visitors or laborers entering this region, primarily from May through July.

Clinical Findings

A. Symptoms and Signs

After a 3- to 4-day incubation period (maximum, 14 days), fever begins suddenly together with chills, lethargy, headache, ocular pain, myalgia, abdominal pain, and nausea and vomiting. Conjunctivitis may be present. A nondistinctive maculopapular rash occurs in 5%–10% of patients. The illness lasts 7–10 days, and half of patients have a biphasic fever curve with several afebrile days in the midst of the illness.

B. Laboratory Findings

Leukopenia is characteristic early in the illness. Platelets are modestly decreased. Specific ELISA testing is available, but 3–4 weeks may elapse before seroconversion. Fluorescent antibody staining will detect virus-infected erythrocytes during the illness and for weeks after recovery.

Differential Diagnosis

Early findings, especially if rash is present, may suggest enterovirus, measles, or rubella infection. Enteric fever may be an early consideration because of the presence of leukopenia and thrombocytopenia. A history of tick bite, which is often obtained; information about local risk; and the biphasic fever pattern will help with the diagnosis. Because of the wilderness exposure, diseases such as leptospirosis, borreliosis, tularemia, ehrlichiosis, and Rocky Mountain spotted fever will be considerations.

Complications

Meningoencephalitis occurs in 3%–7% of patients. Cardiac and pulmonary complications are rare.

Prevention & Treatment

Prevention involves avoiding endemic areas and using conventional means to avoid tick bite. Therapy is supportive. Do not use analgesics that modify platelet function.

Romero JR, Simonsen KA: Powassan encephalitis and Colorado tick fever. Infect Dis Clin North Am 2008;22:545 [PMID: 18755390].

OTHER MAJOR VIRAL CHILDHOOD EXANTHEMS

See the earlier section on Infections Due to Herpesviruses for a discussion of varicella and roseola, the two other major childhood exanthems.

ERYTHEMA INFECTIOSUM

ESSENTIALS OF DIAGNOSIS & TYPICAL FEATURES

- Fever and rash with "slapped-cheek" appearance, followed by a symmetrical, full-body maculopapular rash.
- Arthritis in older children.
- Profound anemia in patients with impaired erythrocyte production.
- Nonimmune hydrops fetalis following infection of pregnant women.

General Considerations

This benign exanthematous illness of school-aged children is caused by the human parvovirus designated B19. Spread is respiratory, occurring in winter–spring epidemics. A nonspecific mild flulike illness may occur during the viremia at 7–10 days; the characteristic rash occurring at 10–17 days represents an immune response. The patient is viremic and contagious prior to—but not after—the onset of rash.

Approximately half of infected individuals have a subclinical illness. Most cases (60%) occur in children between ages 5 and 15 years, with an additional 40% occurring later in life. Forty percent of adults are seronegative. The disease is mildly contagious; the secondary attack rate in a school or household setting is 50% among susceptible children and 20%–30% among susceptible adults.

Clinical Findings

Owing to the nonspecific nature of the exanthem and the many subclinical cases, a history of contact with an infected individual is often absent or unreliable. Recognition of the illness is easier during outbreaks.

A. Symptoms and Signs

Typically, the first sign of illness is the rash, which begins as raised, fiery red maculopapular lesions on the cheeks that coalesce to give a "slapped-cheek" appearance. The lesions are warm, nontender, and sometimes pruritic. They may be scattered on the forehead, chin, and postauricular areas, but the circumoral region is spared. Within 1–2 days, similar lesions appear on the proximal extensor surfaces of the extremities and spread distally in a symmetrical fashion. Palms and soles are usually spared. The trunk, neck, and buttocks are also commonly involved. Central clearing of confluent lesions produces a characteristic lacelike pattern. The rash fades in several days to several weeks but frequently reappears in response to local irritation, heat (bathing), sunlight, and stress. Nearly 50% of infected children have some rash remaining (or recurring) for 10 days. Fine desquamation may be present. Mild systemic symptoms occur in up to 50% of children. These symptoms include low-grade fever, mild malaise, sore throat, and coryza. They appear for 2–3 days and are followed by a week-long asymptomatic phase before the rash appears.

Purpuric stocking-glove rashes, neurologic disease, and severe disorders resembling hemolytic-uremic syndrome have also been described in association with parvovirus B19.

B. Laboratory Findings

A mild leukopenia occurs early in some patients, followed by leukocytosis and lymphocytosis. Specific IgM and IgG serum antibody tests are available, but care must be used in choosing a reliable laboratory for this test. IgM antibody is present in 90% of patients at the time of the rash. Nucleic acid detection tests are often definitive, but parvovirus DNA may be detectable in blood for as long as 9 months after infection. The disease is not diagnosed by routine viral culture.

Differential Diagnosis

In children immunized against measles and rubella, parvovirus B19 is the most frequent agent of morbilliform and rubelliform rashes. The characteristic rash and the mild nature of the illness distinguish erythema infectiosum from other childhood exanthems. It lacks the prodromal symptoms of measles and the lymphadenopathy of rubella. Systemic symptoms and pharyngitis are more prominent with enteroviral infections and scarlet fever.

Complications & Sequelae

A. Arthritis

Arthritis is more common in older patients, beginning with late adolescence. Approximately 10% of children have severe joint symptoms. Girls are affected more commonly than boys. Pain and stiffness occur symmetrically in the peripheral joints. Arthritis usually follows the rash and may persist for 2–6 weeks but resolves without permanent damage.

B. Aplastic Crisis and Other Hematologic Abnormalities

Parvovirus B19 replicates primarily in erythroid progenitor cells. Consequently, reticulocytopenia occurs for approximately 1 week during the illness. This goes unnoticed in individuals with a normal erythrocyte half-life, but results in severe anemia in patients with chronic hemolytic anemia. The rash of erythema infectiosum follows the hemolysis in these patients.

Pure red cell aplasia, leukopenia, pancytopenia, idiopathic thrombocytopenic purpura, and a hemophagocytic syndrome have also been described. Patients with HIV infection and other immunosuppressive illnesses may develop prolonged anemia or pancytopenia. Patients with hemolytic anemia and aplastic crisis, or with immunosuppression, may be contagious and should be isolated while in the hospital.

C. Other End-Organ Infections

Parvovirus is under study as a potential cause of a variety of collagen-vascular diseases. Parvovirus has been associated with neurologic syndromes, hepatitis, and suppression of bone marrow lineages. It is an accepted cause of myocarditis.

D. In Utero Infections

Infection of susceptible pregnant women may produce fetal infection with hydrops fetalis. Fetal death occurs in about 6% of cases; most fatalities occur in the first 20 weeks. This is higher than the rate of fetal loss expected in typical pregnancies. Congenital anomalies have not been associated with parvovirus B19 infection during pregnancy.

Treatment & Prognosis

Erythema infectiosum is a benign illness for immunocompetent individuals. Patients with aplastic crisis may require blood transfusions. It is unlikely that this complication can be prevented by quarantine measures, because acute parvovirus infection in contacts is often unrecognized and is most contagious prior to the rash. Pregnant women who are exposed to erythema infectiosum or who work in a setting in which an epidemic occurs should be tested for evidence of prior infection. Susceptible pregnant women should then be followed up for evidence of parvovirus infection. Approximately 1.5% of women of childbearing age are infected during pregnancy. If maternal infection occurs, the fetus should be followed by ultrasonography for evidence of hydrops and distress. In utero transfusion or early delivery may salvage some fetuses. Pregnancies should not be terminated because of parvovirus infection. The risk of fetal death among exposed pregnant women of unknown serologic status is less than 2.5% for homemakers and less than 1.5% for school-teachers.

Intramuscular immune globulin is not protective. High-dose IVIG has stopped viremia and led to marrow recovery in some cases of prolonged aplasia. Its role in immunocompetent patients and pregnant women is unknown.

Enders M, Klingel K, Weidner A et al: Risk of fetal hydrops and non-hydropic late intrauterine fetal death after gestational parvovirus B19 infection. J Clin Virol 2010;49(3):163 [PMID: 20729141].

Gutermuth J, Nadas K, Seifert F et al: Papular-purpuric gloves and sicks syndrome. Lancet 2011;378(9786):198 [PMID: 21742170].

Lackner H, Sovinz P, Benesch M et al: The spectrum of parvovirus B19 infection in a pediatric hemato-ocologic ward. Ped Infect Dis J 2011;30(5):440 [PMID: 21502929].

MEASLES (RUBEOLA)

ESSENTIALS OF DIAGNOSIS & TYPICAL FEATURES

- Exposure to measles 9–14 days previously.
- Prodrome of fever, cough, conjunctivitis, and coryza.
- Koplik spots (few to many small white papules on a diffusely red base on the buccal mucosa) 1–2 days prior to and after onset of rash.
- Maculopapular rash spreading down from the face and hairline to the trunk over 3 days and later becoming confluent.
- Leukopenia.

General Considerations

This childhood exanthem is rarely seen in the United States because of universal vaccination (< 100 cases in 2010, all of which were imported or related to imported cases). Sporadic clusters of cases are the result of improper immunization rather than of vaccine failures. It is recommended that all children be revaccinated prior to entry into primary or secondary school (see Chapter 10). The attack rate in susceptible individuals is extremely high; spread is via respiratory droplets. Morbidity and mortality rates in the developing world are substantial because of underlying malnutrition and secondary infections. Because humans are the sole reservoir of measles, there is the potential to eliminate this disease worldwide.

Clinical Findings

A history of contact with a suspected case may be absent because airborne spread is efficient and patients are contagious during the prodrome. Contact with an imported case may not be recognized. In temperate climates, epidemic measles is a winter–spring disease. Many suspected cases are misdiagnoses of other viral infections.

A. Symptoms and Signs

High fever and lethargy are prominent. Sneezing, eyelid edema, tearing, copious coryza, photophobia, and harsh cough ensue and worsen. Koplik spots are white macular lesions on the buccal mucosa, typically opposite the lower molars. These are almost pathognomonic for rubeola, although they may be absent. A discrete maculopapular rash begins when the respiratory symptoms are maximal and spreads quickly over the face and trunk, coalescing to a bright red. As it involves the extremities, it fades from the face and is completely gone within 6 days; fine desquamation may occur. Fever peaks when the rash appears and usually falls 2–3 days thereafter.

B. Laboratory Findings

Lymphopenia is characteristic. Total leukocyte counts may fall to 1500/μL. The diagnosis is usually made by detection of measles IgM antibody in serum drawn at least 3 days after the onset of rash or later by detection of a significant rise in antibody. Direct detection of measles antigen by fluorescent antibody staining of nasopharyngeal cells is a useful rapid method. PCR testing of oropharyngeal secretions or urine is extremely sensitive, specific, and can detect infection up to 5 days before symptoms.

C. Imaging

Chest radiographs often show hyperinflation, perihilar infiltrates, or parenchymal patchy, fluffy densities. Secondary consolidation or effusion may be visible.

Differential Diagnosis

Table 40–3 lists other illnesses that may resemble measles.

Complications & Sequelae

A. Respiratory Complications

These complications occur in up to 15% of patients. Bacterial superinfection of the lungs, middle ear, sinus, and cervical nodes are most common. Fever that persists after the third or fourth day of rash suggests such a complication, as does leukocytosis. Bronchospasm, severe croup, and progressive viral pneumonia or bronchiolitis (in infants) also occur. Immunosuppressed patients are at much greater risk for fatal pneumonia than are immunocompetent patients.

B. Cerebral Complications

Encephalitis occurs in 1 in 2000 cases. Onset is usually within a week after appearance of rash. Symptoms include combativeness, ataxia, vomiting, seizures, and coma. Lymphocytic pleocytosis and a mildly elevated protein concentration are usual CSF findings, but the fluid may be normal. Forty percent of patients so affected die or have severe neurologic sequelae.

Subacute sclerosing panencephalitis (SSPE) is a slow measles virus infection of the brain that becomes symptomatic years later in about 1 in 100,000 previously infected children. This progressive cerebral deterioration is associated with myoclonic jerks and a typical electroencephalographic pattern. It is fatal in 6–12 months. High titers of measles antibody are present in serum and CSF.

C. Other Complications

These include hemorrhagic measles (severe disease with multiorgan bleeding, fever, cerebral symptoms), thrombocytopenia, appendicitis, keratitis, myocarditis, and premature delivery or stillbirth. Mild liver function test elevation is detected in up to 50% of cases in young adults; frank jaundice may also occur. Measles causes transient immunosuppression; thus, reactivation or progression of tuberculosis (including transient cutaneous anergy) can occur in children with untreated tuberculosis.

Prevention

The current two-dose active vaccination strategy is successful. Vaccine should not be withheld for concurrent mild acute illness, tuberculosis or positive tuberculin skin test, breast feeding, or exposure to an immunodeficient contact. The vaccine is recommended for HIV-infected children without severe HIV complications and adequate CD4 cells (≥ 15%).

Treatment & Prognosis

Vaccination prevents the disease in susceptible exposed individuals if given within 72 hours (see Chapter 10). Immune globulin (0.25 mL/kg intramuscularly; 0.5 mL/kg if immunocompromised) will prevent or modify measles if given within 6 days. Suspected cases should be diagnosed promptly and reported to the local health department.

Recovery generally occurs 7–10 days after onset of symptoms. Therapy is supportive: eye care, cough relief (avoid opioid suppressants in infants), and fever reduction (acetaminophen, lukewarm baths; avoid salicylates). Secondary bacterial infections should be treated promptly; antimicrobial prophylaxis is not indicated. Ribavirin is active in vitro and may be useful in infected immunocompromised children. In malnourished children, vitamin A supplementation should be given to attenuate the illness.

Garg RK: Subacute sclerosing panencephalitis. J Neurol 2008;255:1861.

Orenstein W et al: Measles elimination in United States. J Infect Dis 2004;189(Suppl):S1 [PMID: 15106120].

RUBELLA

ESSENTIALS OF DIAGNOSIS & TYPICAL FEATURES

- History of rubella vaccination usually absent.
- Prodromal nonspecific respiratory symptoms and adenopathy (postauricular and occipital).
- Maculopapular rash beginning on face, rapidly spreading to the entire body, and disappearing by fourth day.
- Few systemic symptoms.
- Congenital infection.
  - Retarded growth, development.
  - Cataracts, retinopathy.
  - Purpuric "blueberry muffin" rash at birth.
  - Jaundice, thrombocytopenia.
  - Deafness.
  - Congenital heart defect.

General Considerations

If it were not teratogenic, rubella would be of little clinical importance. Clinical diagnosis is difficult in some cases because of its variable expression. In one study, over 80% of infections were subclinical. Rubella is transmitted by aerosolized respiratory secretions. Patients are infectious 5 days before until 5 days after the rash. Endemic rubella is absent in the United States and congenital rubella, in infants born to unimmunized women and the occasional woman who is reinfected in pregnancy, is now very rare. Sporadic cases occur in migrants to the United States.

Clinical Findings

The incubation period is 14–21 days. The nondistinctive signs may make exposure history unreliable. A history of immunization makes rubella unlikely but still possible. Congenital rubella usually follows maternal infection in the first trimester.

A. Symptoms and Signs

1. Infection in children—Young children may only have rash. Older patients often have a nonspecific prodrome of low-grade fever, ocular pain, sore throat, and myalgia. Postauricular and suboccipital adenopathy (sometimes generalized) is characteristic. This often precedes the rash or may occur without rash. The rash consists of erythematous discrete maculopapules beginning on the face. A "slapped-cheek" appearance or pruritus may occur. Scarlatiniform or morbilliform rash variants may occur. The rash spreads quickly to the trunk and extremities after fading from the face; it is gone by the fourth day. Enanthema is usually absent.

2. Congenital infection—More than 80% of women infected in the first 4 months of pregnancy (25% near the end of the second trimester) deliver an affected infant; congenital disease occurs in less than 5% of women infected later in pregnancy. Later infections can result in isolated defects, such as deafness. The main manifestations are as follows:

A. GROWTH RETARDATION—Between 50% and 85% of infants are small at birth and remain so.

B. CARDIAC ANOMALIES—Pulmonary artery stenosis, patent ductus arteriosus, ventricular septal defect.

C. OCULAR ANOMALIES—Cataracts, microphthalmia, glaucoma, retinitis.

D. DEAFNESS—Sensorineural (> 50% of cases).

E. CEREBRAL DISORDERS—Chronic encephalitis; retardation.

F. HEMATOLOGIC DISORDERS—Thrombocytopenia, dermal nests of extramedullary hematopoiesis or purpura ("blueberry muffin" rash), lymphopenia.

G. OTHERS—Hepatitis, osteomyelitis, immune disorders, malabsorption, diabetes.

B. Laboratory Findings

Leukopenia is common, and platelet counts may be low. Congenital infection is associated with low platelet counts, abnormal liver function tests, hemolytic anemia, and CSF pleocytosis. Total serum IgM is elevated, and IgA and IgG levels may be depressed.

Virus may be isolated from throat or urine from 1 week before to 2 weeks after onset of rash. Children with congenital infection are infectious for months. For optimal virus isolation, the virus laboratory must be notified that rubella is suspected. Serologic immunoassay diagnosis is best made by demonstrating a fourfold rise in antibody titer between specimens drawn 1–2 weeks apart. The first should be drawn promptly, because titers increase rapidly after onset of rash, and both specimens must be tested simultaneously by a single laboratory. Very high rubella IgM antibody titers are also present. Because the decision to terminate a pregnancy is usually based on serologic results, testing must be done carefully.

C. Imaging

Pneumonitis and bone metaphyseal longitudinal lucencies may be present in radiographs of children with congenital infection.

Differential Diagnosis

Rubella may resemble infections due to enterovirus, adenovirus, measles, EBV, roseola, parvovirus, and *T gondii*. Drug reactions may also mimic rubella. Because public health implications are great, sporadic suspected cases should be confirmed serologically or virologically.

Congenital rubella must be differentiated from congenital CMV infection, toxoplasmosis, and syphilis.

Complications & Sequelae

A. Arthralgia and Arthritis

Both occur more often in adult women. Polyarticular involvement (fingers, knees, wrists), lasting a few days to weeks, is typical. Frank arthritis occurs in a small percentage of patients. It may resemble acute rheumatoid arthritis.

B. Encephalitis

With an incidence of about 1:6000, this is a nonspecific parainfectious encephalitis associated with a low mortality rate. A syndrome resembling SSPE (see section on Measles, earlier) has also been described in congenital rubella.

C. Rubella in Pregnancy

Infection in the mother is self-limited and not severe.

Prevention

Rubella is one of the infections that could be eradicated (see Chapter 10 for the indication and efficacy of rubella vaccine). Standard prenatal care should include rubella antibody testing. Seropositive mothers are at no risk; seronegative mothers are vaccinated after delivery.

A pregnant woman possibly exposed to rubella should be tested immediately; if seropositive, she is immune and need not worry. If she is seronegative, a second specimen should be drawn in 4 weeks, and both specimens should be tested simultaneously. Seroconversion in the first trimester suggests high fetal risk; such women require counseling regarding therapeutic abortion.

When pregnancy termination is not an option, some experts recommend intramuscular administration of 20 mL of immune globulin within 72 hours after exposure in an attempt to prevent infection. (This negates the value of subsequent antibody testing.) The efficacy of this practice is unknown.

Treatment & Prognosis

Symptomatic therapy is sufficient. Arthritis may improve with administration of anti-inflammatory agents. The prognosis is poor in congenitally infected infants, in whom most defects are irreversible or progressive. The severe cognitive defects in these infants seem to correlate closely with the degree of growth failure.

Berger BE, Omer SB: Could the United States experience rubella outbreaks as a result of vaccine refusal and disease importation? Human Vaccines 2010;6(12):1016 [PMID: 21150305].

Meints L, Chescheir N: Screening for infectious disease in pregnant, foreign-born women from multiple global areas. J Reproduct Med 2010;55(9–10):382 [PMID: 21043363].

INFECTIONS DUE TO OTHER VIRUSES

HANTAVIRUS CARDIOPULMONARY SYNDROME

ESSENTIALS OF DIAGNOSIS & TYPICAL FEATURES

- Influenza-like prodrome (fever, myalgia, headache, cough).
- Rapid onset of unexplained pulmonary edema and myocardiopathy.
- Residence or travel in endemic area; exposure to aerosols from deer mouse droppings or secretions.

General Considerations

Hantavirus cardiopulmonary syndrome is the first native bunyavirus infection endemic in the United States. This syndrome is distinctly different in mode of spread (no arthropod vector) and clinical picture from other bunyavirus diseases.

Clinical Findings

The initial cases of hantavirus cardiopulmonary syndrome involved travel to or residence in a limited area in the southwestern United States where there was a potential for exposure to the reservoir, the deer mouse. Since this and many other related rodents live in many other locales, the disease has been confirmed in more than 30 states and Canada. Epidemics occur when environmental conditions favor large increases in the rodent population and increased prevalence of virus in this reservoir.

A. Symptoms and Signs

After an incubation period of 1–3 weeks, onset is sudden, with a nonspecific virus-like prodrome: fever; back, hip, and leg pain; chills; headache; and nausea and vomiting. Abdominal pain may be present. Sore throat, conjunctivitis, rash, and adenopathy are absent, and respiratory symptoms are absent or limited to a dry cough. After 1–10 days (usually 3–7), dyspnea, tachypnea, and evidence of a pulmonary capillary leak syndrome appear. This often progresses rapidly over a period of hours. Hypotension is common, not only from hypoxemia but also from myocardial dysfunction. Copious, amber-colored, nonpurulent secretions are common. Decreased cardiac output due to myocardiopathy and elevated systemic vascular resistance distinguish this disease from early bacterial sepsis.

B. Laboratory Findings

The hemogram shows leukocytosis with a prominent left shift and immunoblasts, thrombocytopenia, and hemoconcentration. Lactate dehydrogenase (LDH) is elevated, as are liver function tests; serum albumin is low. Creatinine is elevated in some patients, and proteinuria is common. Lactic acidosis and low venous bicarbonate are poor prognostic signs. A serum IgM ELISA test is positive early in the illness. Otherwise, the diagnosis is made by specific staining of tissue or PCR, usually at autopsy.

C. Imaging

Initial chest radiographs are normal. Subsequent radiographs show bilateral interstitial infiltrates with the typical butterfly pattern of acute pulmonary edema, bibasilar airspace disease, or both. Significant pleural effusions are often present. These findings contrast with those of other causes of acute respiratory distress syndrome.

Differential Diagnosis

In some geographic areas, plague and tularemia may be possibilities. Infections with viral respiratory pathogens and *Mycoplasma* have a slower tempo, do not elevate the LDH level, and do not cause the hematologic changes seen in this syndrome. Q fever, psittacosis, toxin exposure, legionellosis, and fungal infections are possibilities, but the history, tempo of the illness, and blood findings, as well as the exposure history, should be distinguishing features. Hantavirus cardiopulmonary syndrome is a consideration in previously healthy persons with a febrile illness associated with unexplained pulmonary edema.

Treatment & Prognosis

Ribavirin, to which hantaviruses and other bunyaviruses are susceptible, has not been demonstrated to alter the course of the illness. Management should concentrate on oxygen therapy and mechanical ventilation as required. Because of capillary leakage, Swan-Ganz catheterization to monitor cardiac output and inotropic support—rather than fluid therapy—should be used to maintain perfusion. Venoarterial extracorporeal membrane oxygenation can provide short-term support for selected patients. The strains of virus present in North America are not spread by person-to-person contact. No isolation is required. The case fatality rate is 30%–40%. Guidelines are available for reduction of exposure to the infectious agent.

Centers for Disease Control and Prevention. Hantavirus pulmonary syndrome in five pediatric patients—four states, 2009. MMWR - Morbidity & Mortality Weekly Reports 2009;58(50):1409 [PMID: 20032925].

MacNeil A, Ksiazek TG, Rollin PE: Hantavirus pulmonary syndrome, United States, 1993–2009. Emerg Infect Dis 2011;17:1195.

Simpson SQ, Spikes L et al: Hantavirus pulmonary syndrome. Infect Dis Clin NAmer 2010;24(1):159 [PMID: 20171551].

MUMPS

ESSENTIALS OF DIAGNOSIS & TYPICAL FEATURES

- No prior mumps immunization.
- Parotid gland swelling.
- Aseptic meningitis with or without parotitis.

General Considerations

Mumps was one of the classic childhood infections; virus spread by the respiratory route attacked almost all unimmunized children (asymptomatically in 30%–40% of cases), and produced lifelong immunity. The vaccine is so efficacious that clinical disease is rare in immunized children. As a result of subclinical infections or childhood immunization, 95% of adults are immune, although immunity can wane in late adolescence. When susceptibles accumulate occasional epidemics (> 2300 cases in 2010) can occur, which are aborted by reimmunization of the at-risk population. Infected patients can spread the infection from 1 to 2 days prior to the onset of symptoms and for 5 additional days. The incubation period is 14–21 days.

A history of exposure to a child with parotitis is not proof of mumps exposure. In an adequately immunized individual, parotitis is usually due to another cause. Currently in the United States, less than one case is reported per 100,000 population.

Clinical Findings

A. Symptoms and Signs

1. Salivary gland disease—Tender swelling of one or more glands, variable fever, and facial lymphedema are typical. Parotid involvement is most common; this is bilateral in 70% of patients. The ear is displaced upward and outward; the mandibular angle is obliterated. Systemic toxicity is usually absent. Parotid stimulation with sour foods may be quite painful. The orifice of the Stensen duct may be red and swollen; yellow secretions may be expressed, but pus is absent. Parotid swelling dissipates after 1 week.

2. Meningoencephalitis—Prior to widespread immunization, mumps was the most common cause of aseptic meningitis, which is usually manifested by mild headache or asymptomatic mononuclear pleocytosis. Fewer than 10% of patients have clinical meningitis or encephalitis. Cerebral symptoms do not correlate with parotid symptoms, which are absent in many patients with meningoencephalitis. Although neck stiffness, nausea, and vomiting can occur, encephalitic symptoms are rare (1:4000 cases of mumps); recovery in 3–10 days is the rule.

3. Pancreatitis—Abdominal pain may represent transient pancreatitis. Because salivary gland disease may elevate serum amylase, specific markers of pancreatic function (lipase, amylase isoenzymes) are required for assessing pancreatic involvement.

4. Orchitis, oophoritis—Involvement of the gonads is associated with fever, local tenderness, and swelling. Epididymitis is usually present. Orchitis is unusual in young children, but occurs in up to one-third of affected postpubertal males. Usually, it is unilateral and resolves in 1–2 weeks. Although one-third of infected testes atrophy, bilateral involvement and sterility are rare.

5. Other—Thyroiditis, mastitis (especially in adolescent females), arthritis, and presternal edema (occasionally with dysphagia or hoarseness) may be seen.

B. Laboratory Findings

Peripheral blood leukocyte count is usually normal. Up to 1000 cells/μL (predominantly lymphocytes) may be present in the CSF, with mildly elevated protein and normal to slightly decreased glucose. Viral culture or PCR tests of saliva, throat, urine, or spinal fluid may be positive for at least 1 week after onset. Paired sera assayed by ELISA or a single positive IgM antibody test are currently used for diagnosis.

Differential Diagnosis

Mumps parotitis may resemble the following conditions: cervical adenitis (the jaw angle may be obliterated, but the ear does not usually protrude; the Stensen duct orifice is normal; leukocytosis and neutrophilia are observed), bacterial parotitis (pus in the Stensen duct, toxicity, exquisite tenderness), recurrent parotitis (idiopathic or associated with calculi), tumors or leukemia, and tooth infections. Many viruses, including parainfluenza, enteroviruses, EBV, CMV, and influenza virus, can cause parotitis. Parotid swelling in HIV infection is less painful and tends to be bilateral and chronic, but bacterial parotitis occurs in some children with HIV infection.

Unless parotitis is present, mumps meningitis resembles that caused by enteroviruses or early bacterial infection. An elevated amylase level is a useful clue in this situation. Isolated pancreatitis is not distinguishable from many other causes of epigastric pain and vomiting. Mumps is a classic cause of orchitis, but torsion, bacterial or chlamydial epididymitis, *Mycoplasma* infection, other viral infections, hematomas, hernias, and tumors must also be considered.

Complications

The major neurologic complication is nerve deafness (usually unilateral) which can result in inability to hear high tones. It may occur without meningitis. Permanent damage is rare, occurring in less than 0.1% of cases of mumps. Aqueductal stenosis and hydrocephalus (especially following congenital infection), myocarditis, transverse myelitis, and facial paralysis are other rare complications.

Treatment & Prognosis

Treatment is supportive and includes provision of fluids, analgesics, and scrotal support for orchitis. Systemic corticosteroids have been used for orchitis, but their value is anecdotal.

Deeks SL, Lim GH, Gubbay GL et al: An assessment of mumps vaccine effectiveness by dose during an outbreak in Canada. Canad Med Assoc J 2011;183(9):1014 [PMID: 21576295].

Barskey AE, Glasser JW, LeBaron CW: Mumps resurgences in the United States: A historical perspective on unexpected elements. Vaccine 2009;27(44):6186 [PMID: 19815120].

Ternavasio-de la Vega HG et al: Mumps orchitis in the post-vaccine era (1967-2009): A single-center series of 67 patients and review of clinical outcome and trenes. Medicine 2010;89(2):96 [PMID: 20517181].

RABIES

ESSENTIALS OF DIAGNOSIS & TYPICAL FEATURES

- History of animal bite 10 days to 1 year (usually < 90 days) previously.
- Paresthesias or hyperesthesia in bite area.
- Progressive limb and facial weakness in some patients (dumb rabies; 30%).
- Irritability followed by fever, confusion, combativeness, muscle spasms (especially pharyngeal with swallowing) in all patients (furious rabies).
- Rabies antigen detected in corneal scrapings or tissue obtained by brain or skin biopsy; Negri bodies seen in brain tissue.

General Considerations

Rabies remains a potentially serious public health problem wherever animal immunization is not widely practiced or when humans play or work in areas with sylvan rabies. Although infection does not always follow a bite by a rabid animal (about 40% infection rate), infection is almost invariably fatal. Any warm-blooded animal may be infected, but susceptibility and transmissibility vary with different species. Bats often carry and excrete the virus in saliva or feces for prolonged periods; they are the major cause of rabies in the United States. Dogs and cats are usually clinically ill within 10 days after becoming contagious (the standard quarantine period for suspect animals). Valid quarantine periods or signs of illness are not fully known for many species. Rodents rarely transmit infection. Animal vaccines are very effective when properly administered, but a single inoculation may fail to produce immunity in up to 20% of dogs.

The risk is assessed according to the type of animal (bats are always considered to have a high likelihood of being rabid; raccoons, skunks, foxes in many areas), wound extent and location (infection more common after head or hand bites, or if wounds have extensive salivary contamination or are not quickly and thoroughly cleaned), geographic area (urban rabies is rare to nonexistent in the U.S. cities; rural rabies is possible, especially outside the United States), and animal vaccination history (risk low if documented). Most rabies in the United States is caused by genotypes found in bats, yet a history of bat bite is rarely obtained. Aerosolized virus in caves inhabited by bats has caused infection.

Clinical Findings

A. Symptoms and Signs

Paresthesias at the bite site are usually the first symptoms. Nonspecific anxiety, excitability, or depression follows, then muscle spasms, drooling, hydrophobia, delirium, and lethargy. Swallowing or even the sensation of air blown on the face may cause pharyngeal spasms. Seizures, fever, cranial nerve palsies, coma, and death follow within 7–14 days after onset. In a minority of patients, the spastic components are initially absent and the symptoms are primarily flaccid paralysis and cranial nerve defects. The furious components appear subsequently.

B. Laboratory Findings

Leukocytosis is common. CSF is usually normal or may show elevation of protein and mononuclear cell pleocytosis. Cerebral imaging and electroencephalography are not diagnostic.

Infection in an animal may be determined by use of the fluorescent antibody test to examine brain tissue for antigen. Rabies virus is excreted in the saliva of infected humans, but the diagnosis is usually made by antigen detection in scrapings or tissue samples of richly innervated epithelium, such as the cornea or the hairline of the neck. Classic Negri cytoplasmic inclusion bodies in brain tissue are not always present. Seroconversion occurs after 7–10 days.

Differential Diagnosis

Failure to elicit the bite history in areas where rabies is rare may delay diagnosis. Other disorders to be considered include parainfectious encephalopathy; encephalitis due to herpes simplex, mosquito-borne viruses, other viruses; and Guillain-Barré syndrome.

Prevention

See Chapter 10 for information regarding vaccination and postexposure prophylaxis. Rabies immune globulin and diploid cell vaccine have made prophylaxis more effective and minimally toxic. Because rabies is almost always fatal, presumed exposures must be managed carefully.

Treatment & Prognosis

Survival is rare, but has been reported in patients receiving meticulous intensive care and a variety of antiviral therapies of unproven benefit. Early diagnosis is important for the protection and prophylaxis of individuals exposed to the patient.

Wilde H et al: Management of human rabies. Trans R Soc Trop Med Hyg 2008;102:979.

RICKETTSIAL INFECTIONS

Rickettsiae are pleomorphic, gram-negative coccobacilli that are obligate intracellular parasites. Rickettsial diseases are often included in the differential diagnosis of febrile rashes. Q fever, which was formerly classified as a Rickettsial organism, is not characterized by rash. Severe headache, myalgia, and pulmonary symptoms are prominent manifestations of rickettsial disease. The endothelium is the primary target tissue, and the ensuing vasculitis is responsible for severe illness.

All rickettsioses except Q fever are transmitted by cutaneous arthropod contact (ticks, fleas, mice, lice—depending on the disease), either by bite or by contamination of skin breaks with vector feces. In all except Rocky Mountain spotted fever and murine typhus, there is a characteristic eschar at the bite site, called the *tache noire*. Evidence of such contact by history or physical examination may be completely lacking, especially in young children. The geographic distribution of the vector is often the primary determinant for suspicion of these infections. Therapy often must be empiric. Many new broad-spectrum antimicrobials are inactive against these cell wall–deficient organisms; tetracycline is usually effective.

HUMAN EHRLICHIOSIS

ESSENTIALS OF DIAGNOSIS & TYPICAL FEATURES

- Residing or travel in endemic area when ticks are active.
- Tick bite noted (~75%).
- Fever, headache, rash (~67%), gastrointestinal symptoms.
- Leukopenia, thrombocytopenia, elevated serum transaminases, hypoalbuminemia.
- Definitive diagnosis by specific serology.

In humans, *Ehrlichia sennetsu* is responsible for a mononucleosis-like syndrome seen in Japan and Malaysia. One agent of North American human ehrlichiosis is *Ehrlichia chaffeensis*. The reservoir hosts are probably wild rodents, deer, and sheep; ticks are the vectors. Most cases caused by this agent are reported in the south-central, southeastern, and middle Atlantic states. Arkansas, Missouri, Kentucky, Tennessee, and North Carolina are high-prevalence areas. Almost all cases occur between March and October, when ticks are active.

A second ehrlichiosis syndrome, seen in the upper Midwest and Northeast (Connecticut, Wisconsin, Minnesota, and New York are high-prevalence areas), is caused by *Anaplasma phagocytophilum* and *Ehrlichia ewingii*. Anaplasmosis also occurs in the western United States. New pathogenic Ehrlichia species have been discovered in the past two years.

E chaffeensis has a predilection for mononuclear cells, whereas *A phagocytophilum* and *E ewingii* infect and produce intracytoplasmic inclusions in granulocytes. Hence, diseases caused by these agents are referred to as human monocytic ehrlichiosis or human granulocytic ehrlichiosis, respectively. Ehrlichiosis, Lyme disease, and babesiosis share some tick vectors; thus, dual infections are common and should be considered in patients who fail to respond to therapy.

Clinical Findings

In approximately 75% of patients, a history of tick bite can be elicited. The majority of the remaining patients report having been in a tick-infested area. The usual incubation period is 5–21 days.

A. Symptoms and Signs

Fever is universally present and headache is common (less so in children). Gastrointestinal symptoms (abdominal pain, anorexia, nausea and vomiting) are reported in most pediatric patients. Distal limb edema may occur. Chills, photophobia, conjunctivitis, and myalgia occur in more than half of patients. Rash occurs in two-thirds of children with monocytic ehrlichiosis, but is less common (~50%) in granulocytic ehrlichiosis. Rash may be erythematous, macular, papular, petechial, scarlatiniform, or vasculitic. Meningitis occurs. Interstitial pneumonitis, acute respiratory distress syndrome, and renal failure occur in severe cases. Physical examination reveals rash (not usually palms and soles), mild adenopathy, and hepatomegaly. In children without a rash, infection may present as a fever of unknown origin.

B. Laboratory Findings

Laboratory abnormalities include leukopenia with left shift, lymphopenia, thrombocytopenia, and elevated aminotransferase levels. Hypoalbuminemia and hyponatremia are common. Disseminated intravascular coagulation can occur in severe cases. Anemia occurs in one-third of patients. CSF pleocytosis (mononuclear cells; increased protein) is common. The definitive diagnosis is made serologically, either by a single high titer or a fourfold rise in titer. The Centers for Disease Control and Prevention uses appropriate antigens in an immunofluorescent antibody test in order to distinguish between the etiologic agents. Intracytoplasmic inclusions (morulae) may occasionally be observed in mononuclear cells in monocytic ehrlichiosis, and are usually observed in polymorphonuclear cells from the peripheral blood or bone marrow in granulocytic ehrlichiosis. Specific PCR testing is available for diagnosis.

Differential Diagnosis

In regions where these infections exist, ehrlichiosis should be included in the differential diagnosis of children who present during tick season with fever, leukopenia or thrombocytopenia (or both), and increased serum transaminase levels. The differential diagnosis includes septic or toxic shock, other rickettsial infections (especially Rocky Mountain spotted fever), Colorado tick fever, leptospirosis, Lyme borreliosis, relapsing fever, EBV, CMV, viral hepatitis and other viral infections, Kawasaki disease, systemic lupus erythematosus, and leukemia.

Treatment & Prognosis

Asymptomatic or clinically mild and undiagnosed infections are common in some endemic areas. The disease may last several weeks if untreated. One-quarter of hospitalized children require intensive care. Meningoencephalitis and persisting neurologic deficits occur in 5%–10% of patients. Doxycycline, 2 mg/kg every 12 hours (IV or PO; maximum 100 mg per dose) for 7–10 days, is the treatment of choice. Patients with suspected disease must be treated concurrently with attempts to establish the diagnosis. Response to therapy should be evident in 24–48 hours. Deaths are uncommon in children but do occur. Immune compromise is a risk factor for severe disease.

Ismail N, Bloch KC, McBride JW: Human ehrlichiosis and anaplasmosis. Clin Lab Medicine 2010;30(1):261 [PMID: 20513551].

Thomas RJ, Dumier JS, Carylon JA: Current management of human granulocytic anaplasmosis, human monocytic ehrlichiosis and Ehrlichia ewingii ehrlichiosis. Expert Rev Antiinfective Therapy 2009;7(6):709 [PMID: 19681699].

ROCKY MOUNTAIN SPOTTED FEVER

ESSENTIALS OF DIAGNOSIS & TYPICAL FEATURES

- Residing or travel in endemic area when ticks are active.
- Fever, rash (palms and soles), gastrointestinal symptoms, headache.
- Tick bite (50%).
- Thrombocytopenia, hyponatremia.
- Definitive diagnosis by specific serology.

Rickettsia rickettsii causes one of many similar tick-borne illnesses characterized by fever and rash that occur worldwide. Most are named after their geographic area. Dogs and rodents, as well as large mammals, are reservoirs of *R rickettsii*.

Rocky Mountain spotted fever is the most severe rickettsial infection and the most important (~1000 cases per year) in the United States. It occurs predominantly along the eastern seaboard; in the southeastern states; and in Arkansas, Texas, Missouri, Kansas, and Oklahoma. It is much less common in the west. Most cases occur in children exposed in rural areas from April to September. Because tick attachment lasting 6 hours or longer is needed, frequent tick removal is a preventive measure.

Clinical Findings

A. Symptoms and Signs

After the incubation period of 3–12 days (mean, 7 days), there is high fever (> 40°C, often hectic), usually of abrupt onset, myalgia, severe and persistent headache (retro-orbital), toxicity, photophobia, vomiting, abdominal pain and diarrhea. A rash occurs in more than 95% of patients and appears 2–6 days after fever onset as macules and papules; most characteristic (65%) is involvement of the palms, soles, and extremities. The rash becomes petechial and spreads centrally from the extremities. Conjunctivitis, splenomegaly, edema, meningismus, irritability, and confusion may occur.

B. Laboratory Findings

Laboratory findings are nonspecific and reflect diffuse vasculitis: thrombocytopenia, hyponatremia, early mild leukopenia, proteinuria, mildly abnormal liver function tests, hypoalbuminemia, and hematuria. CSF pleocytosis is common. Serologic diagnosis is achieved with indirect fluorescent or latex agglutination antibody methods, but generally is informative only 7–10 days after onset of the illness. Skin biopsy with specific fluorescent staining may give the diagnosis within the first week of the illness.

Differential Diagnosis

The differential diagnosis includes meningococcemia, measles, meningococcal meningitis, staphylococcal sepsis, enteroviral infection, leptospirosis, Colorado tick fever, scarlet fever, murine typhus, Kawasaki disease, and ehrlichiosis.

Treatment & Prognosis

To be effective, therapy for Rocky Mountain spotted fever must be started early, often on the basis of a presumptive diagnosis prior to rash onset in endemic areas. It is important to remember that atypical presentations, such as the absence of pathognomonic rash, often lead to delay in appropriate therapy. Doxycycline is the treatment of choice for children, regardless of age. Dosing is 2 mg/kg every 12 hours (IV or PO; maximum 100 mg per dose) for 2 or 3 days after the temperature has returned to normal for a full day. A minimum of 10 days of therapy is recommended.

Complications and death result from severe vasculitis, especially in the brain, heart, and lungs. The mortality rate is 5%–7%. Persistent neurologic deficits occur. Delay in therapy is an important determinant of mortality.

Buckingham SC et al: Clinical and laboratory features, hospital course, and outcome of Rocky Mountain spotted fever. J Pediatr 2007;150:180 [PMID: 17236897].

Minniear TD, Buckingham SC: Managing rocky mountain spotted fever. Expert Rev Antiinfective Therapy 2009;7(9):1131 [PMID: 19883333].

ENDEMIC TYPHUS (MURINE TYPHUS)

ESSENTIALS OF DIAGNOSIS & TYPICAL FEATURES

- Residing in endemic area.
- Fever for 10–14 days.
- Headache, chills, myalgia.
- Maculopapular rash spreading from trunk to extremities (not on palms and soles) 3–7 days after fever onset.
- Definitive diagnosis by serology.

Endemic typhus is present in the southern United States, mainly in southern Texas, and in Southern California, and in Hawaii. The disease is transmitted by fleas from infected rodents or by inhalation. Domestic cats, dogs, and opossums may play a role in the transmission of suburban cases. No eschar appears at the inoculation site, which may go unnoticed. The incubation period is 6–14 days. Headache, myalgia and arthralgia, and chills slowly worsen. Fever may last 10–14 days. After 3–7 days, a rash appears. Truncal macules and papules spread to the extremities; the rash is rarely petechial. The rash resolves in less than 5 days. The location of the rash in typhus, with sparing of the palms and soles, helps distinguish the disease from Rocky Mountain spotted fever. Rash may be absent in 20%–40% of patients. Hepatomegaly may be present. Intestinal and respiratory symptoms may occur. Mild thrombocytopenia and elevated liver enzymes may be present. The illness is usually self-limited and milder than epidemic typhus. More prolonged neurologic symptoms have been described. Doxycycline is the drug of choice, which should be continued for 3 days after evidence of clinical improvement. Fluorescent antibody and ELISA tests are available.

Gikas A et al: Murine typhus in children: clinical and laboratory features from 41 cases in Crete, Greece. Clin Microbiol & Infection 2009;15(Suppl 2):211 [PMID: 19374652].

Green JS et al: A cluster of pediatric endemic typhus cases in Orange County, California. Ped Infect Dis J 2011;30(2):163 [PMID: 21298850].

Q FEVER

ESSENTIALS OF DIAGNOSIS & TYPICAL FEATURES

- Exposure to farm animals (sheep, goats, cattle) and pets.
- Flulike illness (fever, severe headache, myalgia).
- Cough; atypical pneumonia.
- Hepatomegaly and hepatitis.
- Diagnosis by serology.

Coxiella burnetii is transmitted by inhalation rather than by an arthropod bite. Q fever is also distinguished from rickettsial diseases by the infrequent occurrence of cutaneous manifestations and by the prominence of pulmonary disease. The birth tissues and excreta of domestic animals and of some rodents are major infectious sources. The organisms may be carried long distances in fine particle aerosols. Unpasteurized milk from infected animals may also transmit disease.

Clinical Findings

A. Symptoms and Signs

Most patients have a self-limited flulike syndrome of chills, fever, severe headache, and myalgia of abrupt onset occurring 10–25 days after exposure. Abdominal pain, vomiting, chest pain, and dry cough are prominent in children. Examination of the chest may produce few findings, as in other atypical pneumonias. Hepatosplenomegaly is common. The illness lasts 1–4 weeks and frequently is associated with weight loss.

B. Laboratory Findings

Leukopenia with left shift is characteristic. Thrombocytopenia is unusual and another distinction from rickettsial diseases. Aminotransferase and γ-glutamyl transferase levels are elevated. Diagnosis is made by finding an antibody response (fourfold rise or single high titer in ELISA; IFA, or CF antibody assay) to the phase II organism. Chronic infection is indicated by antibody against the phase I organism. IgM ELISA and specific PCR tests are also available.

C. Imaging

Pneumonitis occurs in 50% of patients. Multiple segmental infiltrates are common, but the radiographic appearance is not pathognomonic. Consolidation and pleural effusion are rare.

Differential Diagnosis

In the appropriate epidemiologic setting, Q fever should be considered in evaluating causes of atypical pneumonias, such as *M pneumoniae*, viruses, *Legionella*, and *C pneumoniae*. It should also be included among the causes of mild to moderate hepatitis without rash or adenopathy in children with exposure to farm animals.

Treatment & Prognosis

Typically the illness lasts 1–2 weeks without therapy. The course of the uncomplicated illness is shortened with doxycycline. Therapy is continued for several days after the patient becomes afebrile (usually 10–14 days). Quinolones are also effective.

One complication is chronic disease, which often implies myocarditis or granulomatous hepatitis. Meningoencephalitis is a rare complication. *C burnetii* is also one of the causes of so-called culture-negative endocarditis. Coxiella endocarditis often occurs in the setting of valve abnormalities and is difficult to treat; mortality approaches 50%.

Gikas A et al: Q fever: Clinical manifestations and treatment. Expert Rev of Antiinfective Therapy 2010;8(5):529 [PMID: 20455682].

Marrie TJ: Q fever pneumonia. Infect Dis Clin NA 2010;24(1):27 [PMID: 20171543].

41 Human Immunodeficiency Virus Infection

Elizabeth J. McFarland, MD

General Considerations

Human immunodeficiency virus (HIV) is a retrovirus that primarily infects cells of the immune system. Within 48 hours of infection, replicating virus is found throughout the lymphoid tissue. The function and number of CD4 T lymphocytes (helper cells) and other affected cells are diminished by HIV infection, with profound effects on both humoral and cell-mediated immunity. In the absence of treatment, HIV infection causes generalized immune incompetence, leading to conditions that meet the definition of acquired immunodeficiency syndrome (AIDS) (Centers for Disease Control and Prevention [CDC] category C diagnoses; Table 41–1) and eventually death. Treatment with highly active antiretroviral therapy (HAART) can transform this disease from uniformly fatal within years of diagnosis to a chronic illness. Optimal treatment outcomes rely on early diagnosis. Unfortunately an estimated 25% of HIV-infected people in the United States are undiagnosed. In an effort to increase the number of HIV-infected people in care, the CDC recommends HIV testing at least once as part of routine medical care for all patients over age 16 years and annually for patients with exposure risks. Primary care physicians are encouraged to participate in the care of HIV-infected children in collaboration with centers staffed by personnel with expertise in pediatric HIV issues.

Worldwide there are over 34 million people living with HIV, with children accounting for 3.4 million. The great majority live in resource limited settings, primarily sub-Saharan Africa (http://www.who.int/hiv/data/en/). HIV is transmitted by sexual contact, percutaneous exposure to contaminated blood (eg, injecting drug use or transfusion with contaminated blood products), and mother-to-child transmission (MTCT). New approaches to prevention hold promise for slowing the rates of transmission if they can be successfully implemented.

PREVENTION

Prevention of Mother-to-Child-Transmission (PMTCT)

Mother-to-child transmission of HIV may occur in utero, at the time of labor and delivery, and via breastmilk. Without intervention and with breastfeeding, transmission rates are 20%–40%. However, the rate of MTCT can be reduced to less than 1%–2% by providing antenatal, peripartum, postnatal antiretroviral medications and avoidance of breastfeeding. In the United States, as a result of these interventions, the number of vertically acquired HIV cases is very low (< 200 cases annually). Most transmissions involve women who do not receive antiretroviral (ARV) therapy during pregnancy, either because the infection is undiagnosed or because of lack of prenatal care. Modified interventions that are feasible in resource-limited settings have demonstrated efficacy, resulting in 2%–5% transmission rates. Unfortunately due to barriers to the scale-up of these interventions, the World Health Organization (WHO) estimated in 2010 that only 59% of HIV infected pregnant women received treatment for PMTCT and that there were 390,000 new pediatric infections worldwide.

Key to PMTCT is identification of pregnant women with HIV infection. The CDC and the American College of Obstetrics and Gynecology recommend routine HIV testing, with an option to refuse, early in gestation for all pregnant women. Women with ongoing risk factors for HIV acquisition (multiple partners, STDs, substance use) should be retested later in gestation. A woman presenting in labor without previously documented HIV testing should have rapid HIV testing (results within 60 minutes). Antiretroviral medications, even if implemented within 48 hours postpartum, may reduce transmission by as much as 50%.

In the United States, all HIV-infected pregnant women are prescribed HAART during pregnancy, infant zidovudine

Table 41–1. Centers for Disease Control and Prevention Clinical Categories of Children with Human immunodeficiency Virus Infection.

Category N: Not symptomatic
No signs or symptoms or only one of the conditions listed in category A
Category A: Mildly symptomatic
Having two or more of the following conditions:
Lymphadenopathy
Hepatomegaly
Splenomegaly
Dermatitis
Parotitis
Recurrent or persistent upper respiratory infection, sinusitis, or otitis media
Category B: Moderately symptomatic
Having symptoms attributed to HIV infection other than those in category A or C
Examples:
Anemia, neutropenia, thrombocytopenia
Bacterial meningitis, pneumonia, sepsis (single episode)
Candidiasis, oropharyngeal, persisting > 2 mo
Cardiomyopathy
Cytomegalovirus infection with onset < age 1 mo
Diarrhea, recurrent or chronic
Hepatitis
Herpes simplex virus recurrent stomatitis, bronchitis, pneumonitis, esophagitis at < 1 mo of age
Herpes zoster, two or more episodes or more than one dermatome
Leiomyosarcoma
Lymphoid interstitial pneumonia
Nephropathy
Nocardiosis
Persistent fever
Toxoplasmosis with onset < age 1 mo
Varicella, complicated
Category C: Severely symptomatic
Serious bacterial infections, multiple or recurrent
Candidiasis, esophageal or pulmonary
Coccidioidomycosis, disseminated
Cryptosporidiosis or isosporiasis with diarrhea > age 1 mo
Cytomegalovirus infection with onset > age 1 mo
Encephalopathy
Herpes simplex virus: persistent oral lesions, or bronchitis, pneumonitis, esophagitis at > age 1 mo
Histoplasmosis
Kaposi sarcoma
Lymphoma
Mycobacterium tuberculosis, extrapulmonary
Mycobacterium infection, other species, disseminated
Pneumocystis jiroveci pneumonia
Progressive multifocal leukoencephalopathy
Salmonella septicemia, recurrent
Toxoplasmosis of the brain with onset > age 1 mo
Wasting syndrome

Adapted from MMWR Recomm Rep 1994;43(RR-12):6, 8.

for six weeks, and avoidance of breastfeeding. For women who are identified late or who fail to have viral suppression on treatment (plasma virus ≥ 1000 copies/mL), an elective C-section prior to labor will reduce transmission risk by 50%.

WHO recommends HAART for women who require treatment for their own health. For women who do not meet in-country guidelines for treatment, WHO provides two options—(A) maternal zidovudine (AZT) from 14 weeks gestation with infant peripartum prophylaxis and daily infant nevirapine for the duration of breasfeeding or (B) maternal HAART during pregnancy and for the duration of breastfeeding with infant peripartum prophylaxis.

In the United States, HIV-infected women should not breastfeed as there is access to formula and a safe water supply. In many resource-limited countries, breastfeeding has a survival benefit despite the risk of HIV transmission. Therefore, breastfeeding is recommended in those settings. Transmission via breast milk can be substantially reduced by either infant ARV prophylaxis or maternal ARV treatment continued throughout the breastfeeding period. Unfortunately, many women are not able to access these medications.

Chasela CS, Hudgens MG, Jamieson DJ et al: Maternal or infant antiretroviral drugs to reduce HIV-1 transmission. N Engl J Med 2010 Jun 17;362(24):2271–2281.

Mahy M et al: What will it take to achieve virtual elimination of mother-to-child transmission of HIV? An assessment of current progress and future needs. Sex Transm Infect 2010 Dec;86(Suppl 2):ii48–55.

Panel on Treatment of HIV-Infected Pregnant Women and Prevention of Perinatal Transmission: Recommendations for Use of Antiretroviral Drugs in Pregnant HIV-1-Infected Women for Maternal Health and Interventions to Reduce Perinatal HIV Transmission in the United States. 2011 Sep 14;1–207. Available at: http://aidsinfo.nih.gov/contentfiles/PerinatalGL.pdf. Accessed November 6, 2011.

World Health Organization: Antiretroviral Drugs for Treating Pregnant women and preventing HIV infection in infants—Recommendations for a public health approach, 2010 version. Available at: http://whqlibdoc.who.int/publications/2010/9789241599818_eng.pdf. Accessed December 6, 2011.

Prevention of Sexual Transmission

Sexual activity, both heterosexual and men-having-sex-with-men (MSM), is the main mode of infection after puberty, with a smaller number of cases resulting from the sharing of contaminated needles. As a result of careful donor screening and testing of donated blood, HIV transmission resulting from blood products is now extremely rare in the United States (1:2,000,000 transfusions). Latex condoms used consistently and correctly are highly effective in preventing sexual transmission. Behavioral interventions to increase use of condoms and other safer sex practices are a cornerstone of prevention efforts. The success rate with behavioral interventions varies in different populations. Recently, several biomedical prevention interventions have demonstrated efficacy in randomized clinical trials (summaries at http://www.cdc.gov/hiv/prep/). These include (1) male circumcision—approximately 50% reduction in female-to-male transmission; (2) preexposure prophylaxis (PrEP) for HIV-uninfected partners using selected daily antiretroviral drugs—44%–70% reduction for MSM and 60%–70% reduction for discordant heterosexual couples; (3) ARV treatment of HIV-infected individuals—96% reduction in the risk of transmission to their partners. Finally, postexposure prophylaxis (PEP) using combination antiretroviral drugs initiated within 72 hours after a known HIV exposure was associated with reduced transmission in case-cohort studies. The CDC funds a hotline for questions regarding postexposure prophylaxis (PEPline, 888-488-4911).

Centers for Disease Control and Prevention: Antiretroviral postexposure prophylaxis after sexual, injection-drug use, or other nonoccupational exposure to HIV in the United States: Recommendations from the U.S. Department of Health and Human Services. MMWR 2005;54(RR-2):1–16.

Centers for Disease Control and Prevention: Interim Guidance: Preexposure Prophylaxis for the Prevention of HIV Infection in Men Who Have Sex with Men. MMWR 2011;60:65–68.

Centers for Disease Control and Prevention Guidelines: Revised Recommendations for HIV Testing of Adults, Adolescents, and Pregnant Women in Health-Care Setting. MMWR 2006 Sep 22;55(RR-14):1–17.

Grant RM et al for the iPrEx Study Team: Preexposure Chemoprophylaxis for HIV Prevention in Men Who Have Sex with Men. N Engl J Med 2010;363:2587–2599.

PERINATALLY HIV-EXPOSED INFANT

ESSENTIALS OF DIAGNOSIS

Children < age 18 months and born to an HIV-infected mother:

- Definitively infected:
  - Positive results on two separate determinations on blood or tissue (excluding cord blood) for one or more of the following HIV detection tests: HIV nucleic acid detection (DNA or RNA), HIV antigen (p24), HIV culture.
- Definitively uninfected:
  - Two negative HIV nucleic acid (DNA or RNA) detection tests from separate specimens, one obtained at age > 1 month and another at age ≥ 4 months.

  Or

  - Two negative HIV antibody tests from separate specimens obtained at age ≥ 6 months.

  And

  - No other laboratory (prior positive nucleic acid tests) or clinical evidence of HIV infection/AIDS (see Table 41–1).
- Presumptively uninfected:
  - Two negative HIV nucleic acid detection (DNA or RNA) tests from separate specimens, one obtained at age ≥ 14 days and another at age ≥ 1 month.

  Or

  - One negative HIV nucleic acid detection test obtained at age ≥ 8 weeks.

  And

  - No other laboratory (prior positive nucleic acid tests) or clinical evidence of HIV infection/AIDS (see Table 41–1).

Clinical Findings

Newborns with perinatal HIV infection are rarely symptomatic at birth and there is no recognized primary infection syndrome in these infants. Birth size and physical features are not different from uninfected neonates. However, approximately 30%–80% of infected infants have disease progression within the first year of life. Hepatomegaly, splenomegaly, lymphadenopathy, parotitis, and recurrent respiratory tract infections are signs associated with mild disease. Severe bacterial infections, progressive neurologic disease, anemia, and fever are associated with shorter survival. Early antiretroviral therapy can slow or prevent disease progression. Hence, early diagnosis is critical and can be accomplished using laboratory testing during the first months of life.

Laboratory Diagnosis

Infants born to HIV-infected mothers will have HIV antibody until 6–18 months—regardless of infection status—owing to transplacental passage of maternal antibody. Therefore, diagnosis must be made by direct detection of virus. The preferred test for infant diagnosis is detection of HIV DNA or RNA in blood, collectively referred to as nucleic acid amplication testing (NAT). HIV NAT is positive in blood at birth for the fraction of infants infected in utero. The majority of infected infants, with in utero or peripartum acquisition, will have detectable HIV by 2 weeks of life and over 95% will have detectable virus by 4 weeks. Thus, infection can be presumptively excluded, in the absence of breastfeeding, by 1 month of age. Definitive absence of infection is defined by negative HIV NAT at greater than 1 and 4 months. Breast-fed infants may acquire HIV at any time until they are fully weaned and virus may first be detectable as much as 6 weeks after the exposure. Thus, these infants should be retested at 6 weeks after their last exposure to identify or presumptively exclude infection. Positive HIV NAT at any age requires repeat testing for confirmation since false positives may occur.

After 12–18 months of age, many clinicians will obtain HIV antibody testing to demonstrate reversion to seronegative status, thereby confirming the absence of infection.

Complications

HIV-infected infants have a high risk of suffering from *Pneumocystis jiroveci* pneumonia (PCP) with the peak incidence at age 2–6 months. Thus, prophylaxis for *P jiroveci* pneumonia is given to infants born to HIV-infected mothers beginning at age 4–6 weeks until they are found to be presumptively uninfected. Infants with ongoing HIV exposure via breastfeeding are recommended to continue PCP prophylaxis until HIV infection has been excluded after cessation of breastfeeding. Infants who meet the criteria for being presumptively uninfected prior to age 6 weeks do not need to start prophylaxis.

With successful implementation of PMTC, the majority of HIV-exposed infants are uninfected. During the period of ARV prophylaxis, some infants have a reversible anemia or neutropenia that is usually not clinically significant. Subsequently, children who have been exposed to HIV and to antiretroviral drug prophylaxis are generally healthy with no persistent serious adverse outcomes yet proven to be related to HIV or ARV exposure. However, studies are ongoing to examine exposed children for rare, subtle and/or late effects that might alter growth, neurocognitive development, immune and organ function. Some studies of children born to HIV-infected mothers have found symptoms consistent with mitochondrial toxicity. There is biological plausibility for this toxicity because the nucleoside analogue drugs used during pregnancy and postnatally to prevent transmission can cause mitochondrial toxicity in some cases with prolonged use. However, other studies have failed to confirm the findings. The issue remains controversial, but at present it is clear that the benefit of prenatal and postnatal treatment to prevent HIV transmission outweighs the potential risk.

Centers for Disease Control and Prevention: Revised surveillance case definitions for HIV infection among adults, adolescents, and children aged < 18 months and for HIV infection and AIDS among children aged 18 months to < 13 years—United States, 2008. MMWR Recomm Rep 2008;57(RR-10):1–9.

Havens PL, Mofenson LM: Committee on Pediatric AIDS: Evaluation and management of the infant exposed to HIV-1 in the United States. Pediatrics 2009;123:175–187.

HIV INFECTION ACQUIRED AFTER INFANCY

ESSENTIALS OF DIAGNOSIS

Any of the following tests demonstrated on at least two separate occasions:

- Positive HIV EIA antibody test with a positive confirmatory test (Western blot, immune fluorescent antibody, antibody test) test for children age > 18 months.
- Positive HIV rapid antibody test with confirmation by a second antibody test from a different manufacture using a different antigen or test principle.
- Positive HIV nucleic acid amplification test (HIV DNA or RNA).

Clinical Findings

A. Symptoms and Signs

1. Primary acute infection—Among adolescents and adults with acute infection, nonspecific symptoms (eg, flu- or mild mononucleosis-like illness) beginning 2–4 weeks after exposure occur in 30%–90% of new infections but are frequently not severe enough to be brought to medical attention. *Acute retroviral syndrome* with symptoms of fever, malaise, and pharyngitis is often indistinguishable from other similar viral illnesses. Less common but more distinguishing features are generalized lymphadenopathy, rash, oral and genital ulcerations, aseptic meningitis, and thrush. Additional information on behaviorally acquired HIV is found in Chapter 44.

2. Established infection—After acute infection, levels of HIV peak in the bloodstream at 1–2 months. In adults, the level of viremia declines without therapy coincident with the appearance of an HIV-specific host immune response, and plasma viremia usually reaches a steady-state level about 6 months after primary infection. The amount of virus present in the plasma at that point and thereafter is predictive of the rate of disease progression for the individual. Perinatally-infected infants typically have a more gradual decline in circulating virus, reaching a set point after several years of infection.

Despite ongoing virus replication, for most adults/adolescents and for some children, a period of clinical latency occurs, lasting from 1 year to more than 12 years during which the infected person is asymptomatic. The virus and anti-HIV immune responses are in a steady state, with high levels of virus production and destruction balanced against production and destruction of CD4 lymphocytes. Eventually, the balance favors the virus, and the viral burden increases as the CD4 lymphocyte count declines associated with progression to clinical disease.

3. Disease staging—The CDC has developed disease staging criteria for HIV-infected children (see Tables 41–1 and 41–2). The criteria incorporate clinical symptoms ranging from no symptoms to mild, moderate, and severe symptoms (categories N, A, B, and C, respectively) and age-adjusted CD4 lymphocyte counts (immunologic categories 1, 2, or 3, corresponding to no, moderate, or severe immune suppression, respectively). Each child is classified both by

Table 41–2. Immunologic categories based on age-specific CD4 lymphocyte counts and percentages of total lymphocytes.

	Age of Child					
	< 12 mo		1–5 y		6–12 y	
Immunologic Category	Cells/µL	%	Cells/µL	%	Cells/µL	%
1. No evidence of suppression	≥ 1500	≥ 25	≥ 1000	≥ 25	≥ 500	≥ 25
2. Evidence of moderate suppression	750–1499	15–24	500–999	15–24	200–499	15–24
3. Evidence of severe suppression	< 750	< 15	< 500	< 15	< 200	< 15

Adapted from MMWR Recomm Rep 1994;43(RR-12):4.

CD4 lymphocyte count and by clinical category. The WHO has established a similar clinical staging system that is used widely outside the United States (Table 41–3). Both staging criteria assess the degree of disease progression and have been shown to be predictive of mortality risk for children over age two who not receiving antiretroviral therapy. Disease stage is used in determining when to initiate antiretroviral therapy.

The clinical diagnosis of AIDS is made when an HIV-infected child develops any of the opportunistic infections, malignancies, or conditions listed in category C of the CDC disease staging criteria (see Table 41–1). In adults and adolescents, the criteria for a diagnosis of AIDS also include absolute CD4 lymphocyte counts of 200/µL or less.

Table 41–3. World Health Organization clinical staging of HIV for infants and children with established HIV infection.

Clinical stage 1: Asymptomatic
- Asymptomatic
- Persistent generalized lymphadenopathy

Clinical stage 2: Mild symptoms
- Unexplained persistent hepatosplenomegaly
- Papular pruritic eruptions
- Fungal nail infection
- Angular cheilitis
- Lineal gingival erythema
- Extensive wart virus infection
- Extensive molluscum contagiosum
- Recurrent oral ulcerations
- Unexplained persistent parotid enlargement
- Herpes zoster
- Recurrent or chronic upper respiratory tract infections (otitis media, otorrhea, sinusitis or tonsillitis)

Clinical stage 3: Advanced symptoms
- Unexplained moderate malnutrition or wasting not adequately responding to standard therapy
- Unexplained persistent diarrhea
- Unexplained persistent fever
- Persistent oral candidiasis (after first 6–8 wks of life)
- Oral hairy leukoplakia
- Acute necrotizing ulcerative gingivitis or periodontitis
- Lymph node tuberculosis
- Pulmonary tuberculosis
- Severe recurrent bacterial pneumonia
- Symptomatic lymphoid interstitial pneumonitis
- Chronic HIV-associated lung disease including brochiectasis
- Unexplained anemia, neutropenia, thrombocytopenia

Clinical stage 4: Severe symptoms
- Unexplained severe wasting, stunting or severe malnutrition not responding to standard therapy
- Pneumocystis pneumonia
- Recurrent severe bacterial infections (such as empyema, pyomyositis, bone or joint infection, or meningitis but excluding pneumonia)
- Chronic herpes simplex infection
- Esophageal candidiasis (or candidiasis of trachea, bronchi or lungs)
- Extrapulmonary tuberculosis
- Kaposi sarcoma
- Cytomegalovirus infection: retinitis or cytomegalovirus infection affecting another organ, with onset at age older than one month
- Central nervous system toxoplasmosis (after one month of life)
- Extrapulmonary cryptococcosis
- HIV encephalopathy
- Disseminated endemic mycosis (coccidiomycosis or histoplasmosis)
- Disseminated non-tuberculous mycobacterial infection
- Chronic cryptosporidiosis (with diarrhea)
- Chronic isosporiasis
- Cerebral or B-cell non-Hodgkin lymphoma
- Progressive multifocal leukoencephalopathy
- Symptomatic HIV-associated nephropathy or HIV-associated cardiomyopathy

Adapted from http://www.who.int/hiv/pub/guidelines/HIVstaging150307.pdf

4. Infections related to immunodeficiency—Progressive immune dysfunction in both humoral and cell-mediated responses results in susceptibility to infection. Bouts of bacteremia, especially due to *Streptococcus pneumoniae*, occur at rates of 3 per 100 child-years without HAART and decrease to 0.36 per 100 child-years with HAART, but this remains at least three times higher than in HIV-uninfected children. Infections with *Mycobacterium tuberculosis* are a major cause of morbidity in countries with high rates of endemic tuberculosis (TB). Given the frequency of coinfection, diagnosis of *M tuberculosis* in a child is an indication for HIV testing. Likewise, children with HIV infection and their family members should have regular evaluation for *M tuberculosis* exposure and testing if appropriate. Herpes zoster (shingles) occurs 10 times more frequently among untreated HIV-infected children compared with age-matched healthy children. Late-stage immunodeficiency is accompanied by susceptibility to a variety of opportunistic pathogens. Pneumonia caused by *P jiroveci* is a common AIDS-defining diagnosis in children with unrecognized HIV infection and therefore not receiving PCP prophylaxis. The incidence is highest between ages 2 and 6 months and is often fatal during this period. Symptoms are difficult to distinguish from those of viral or atypical pneumonia. (See Chapter 43.) Persistent candidal mucocutaneous infections (oral, cutaneous, and vaginal) are common. Candidal esophagitis occurs with more advanced disease. In children with severe immunosuppression, cytomegalovirus (CMV) infections may result in disseminated disease, hepatitis, gastroenteritis, retinitis, and encephalitis.

Disseminated infection with *Mycobacterium avium* complex (MAC), presenting with fever, night sweats, weight loss, diarrhea, fatigue, lymphadenopathy, hepatomegaly, anemia, and granulocytopenia, occurs in infected children who have CD4 lymphocyte counts below 50–100/μL. A variety of diarrheal pathogens that cause mild, self-limited symptoms in healthy persons may result in severe, chronic diarrhea in HIV-infected persons. These include *Cryptosporidium parvum*, *Microsporidia*, *Cyclospora*, *Isospora belli*, *Giardia lamblia*, and bacterial pathogens. Chronic parvovirus infection manifested by anemia can occur.

5. Organ system disease—HIV infection may directly affect a variety of organ systems and produce disease manifestations that include encephalopathy, pneumonitis, hepatitis, diarrhea, hematologic suppression, nephropathy, and cardiomyopathy. On average, HIV-infected children have lower than normal neuropsychological functioning. In many children, neuropsychological deficits do not normalize when antiretroviral therapy is started, despite suppression of viremia. Symptoms include acquired microcephaly, progressive motor deficit, ataxia, pseudobulbar palsy, and failure to attain (or loss of) developmental milestones.

Lymphoid interstitial pneumonitis, which is common in untreated children with HIV infection, is characterized by a diffuse peribronchial and interstitial infiltrate composed of lymphocytes and plasma cells. It may be asymptomatic or associated with dry cough, hypoxemia, dyspnea or wheezing on exertion, and clubbing of the digits. Children with this disorder frequently have enlargement of the parotid glands and generalized lymphadenopathy.

6. Malignancy—Children with HIV are at increased risk of malignancy. The most commonly occurring tumors are non-Hodgkin lymphomas which may occur at unusual extranodal sites (central nervous system, bone, gastrointestinal tract, liver, or lungs). Cervical infection with human papillomavirus is more likely to progress to neoplasia in adolescent females with HIV infection and the rate of progression is not altered by HAART. Carcinoma due to anal human papillomavirus is also a concern. Kaposi's sarcoma, a skin/mucus membrane malignancy, common in HIV infected gay males with advanced disease, is also observed among HIV-infected African children but is rare in children in the United States.

B. Laboratory Findings

Established HIV infection in children > 18 months may be diagnosed by detecting HIV antibody by enzyme-linked immunosorbent assay (ELISA) or by rapid antibody tests. A confirmatory test, usually a Western blot, immune fluorescent antibody, or a second rapid test from a different manufacture using a different antigen or test principle, must be performed because rare individuals have cross-reacting antibodies which result in a false-positive ELISA or rapid test. In the early weeks after acute HIV infection acquired by high-risk behaviors, HIV antibody may be absent. Most patients will seroconvert by 6 weeks, but occasionally seroconversion does not occur for 3–6 months. When acute HIV infection is suspected, nucleic acid amplification tests will detect circulating HIV (see Laboratory Diagnosis above).

The hallmark of HIV disease progression is decline in the absolute number and percentage of CD4 T lymphocytes and an increasing percentage of CD8 T lymphocytes. The CD4 T-lymphocyte values are predictive of the child's risk of opportunistic infections. Healthy infants and children have CD4 T-lymphocyte numbers that are much higher than in adults; these gradually decline to adult levels by age 5–6 years. Hence, age-adjusted values must be used when assessing a child's absolute CD4 T-lymphocyte count (see Table 41–2).

Hypergammaglobulinemia of IgG, IgA, and IgM is characteristic. Late in the disease, some individuals may become hypogammaglobulinemic. Hematologic abnormalities (anemia, neutropenia, and thrombocytopenia) may occur due to effects of HIV disease. With brain involvement, the cerebrospinal fluid may either be normal or may be associated with elevated protein and a mononuclear pleocytosis.

Differential Diagnosis

HIV infection should be in the differential diagnosis for children being evaluated for immunodeficiency. Depending on the degree of immunosuppression, the presentation in HIV infection may be similar to that of B-cell, T-cell, or combined immunodeficiencies, such as hypogammaglobinemia and severe combined immunodeficiency (see Chapter 33). HIV infection should also be considered in the evaluation of children with failure to thrive, developmental delay, and *M tuberculosis* infection. Children or adolescents with chronic HIV infection may present with generalized lymphadenopathy or hepatosplenomegaly resembling infections with viruses such as EBV or CMV. Because blood tests are definitive for the diagnosis of HIV infection, the diagnosis can be readily established or excluded. In rare cases, HIV-infected children with hypogammaglobulinemia have falsely negative antibody tests but may be diagnosed with a nucleic acid–based test. Absence of maternal risk factors or history of negative test results during pregnancy, particularly if documentation of the results is lacking, should not dissuade from testing for HIV if the patient has signs consistent with the HIV-associated disease.

Centers for Disease Control and Prevention: Guidelines for the Prevention and Treatment of Opportunistic Infections Among HIV-Exposed and HIV-Infected Children. MMWR 2009;58(RR-11):2–61.

Centers for Disease Control and Prevention: 1994 Revised classification system for human immunodeficiency virus infection in children less than 13 years of age. MMWR Recomm Rep 1994;43(RR-12):1 [PMID: 7908403].

Gona P et al: Incidence of opportunistic and other infections in HIV-infected children in the HAART era. JAMA 2006;296:292 [PMID: 16849662].

Hecht FM, Busch MP, Rawal B et al: Use of laboratory tests and clinical symptoms for identification of primary HIV infection. AIDS 2002;16(8):1119–1129.

Steenhoff AP et al: Invasive pneumococcal disease among human immunodeficiency virus-infected children, 1989–2006. Pediatr Infect Dis J 2008;27:886–891.

Treatment

HIV infection calls for specific antiretroviral treatment to prevent progressive deterioration of the immune system, as well as prophylactic measures at late stages of HIV infection to prevent opportunistic infections. Guidelines for the treatment of HIV developed by a national working group of pediatric HIV specialists are published by the U.S. Public Health System at: http://www.aidsinfo.nih.gov. The treatment paradigm changes frequently; therefore, prior to initiating treatment, expert consultation should be obtained.

A. Specific Measures

1. Antiretroviral medications—The U.S. Food and Drug Administration (FDA) has approved 24 drugs categorized into five different drug classes for the treatment of HIV. All but one drug are in oral form; one must be injected subcutaneously (Enfuvirtide). Only one of the drugs is available for intravenous administration (Zidovudine). Many of the drugs have pediatric indications; several others have sufficient pharmacokinetic data for pediatric dosing recommendations in the absence of formal FDA approval for children. The mechanism of action of the each class is described briefly below. Specific drugs in each class are listed in Table 41-4.

A. NUCLEOSIDE AND NUCLEOTIDE REVERSE TRANSCRIPTASE INHIBITORS (NRTIs)—The NRTIs act as nucleotide analogues, which are incorporated into HIV DNA during transcription by the HIV reverse transcriptase. The result is chain termination and failure to complete provirus, preventing integration of HIV genome into cellular DNA.

B. NON-NUCLEOSIDE REVERSE TRANSCRIPTASE INHIBITORS (NNRTIs)—NNRTIs also inhibit HIV DNA synthesis

Table 41–4. U.S. Food and Drug Administration approved antiretroviral drug class (*mechanism of action*) and specific drugs in class.

Nucleoside/ Nucleotide Reverse Transcriptase Inhibitors (NRTIs)	Non-nucleoside Reverse Transcriptase Inhibitors (NNRTIs)	Protease Inhibitors (PIs)
(Chain termination of HIV DNA)	*(Synthesis of HIV DNA inhibited)*	*(Production of noninfectious virions)*
Abacavir (ABC; Ziagen)[a]	Delavirdine (DLV, Rescriptor)	Atazanavir (ATV, Reyataz)[a]
Didanosine (ddI; Videx)[a]	Efavirenz (EFV, Sustiva)[a]	Darunavir (DRV, Prezista)[a]
Emtricitabine (FTC; Emtriva)[a]	Etravirine (ERV, Intelence)	Fosamprenavir (FPV, Lexiva)[a]
Lamivudine (3TC; Epivir)[a]	Nevirapine (NVP, Viramune)[a]	Indinavir (IDV, Crixivan)
Stavudine (d4T; Zerit)[a]	Rilpivirine (RPV, Edurant)	Lopinavir/ritonavir (LPV/r, Kaletra)[a]
Tenofovir (TDF; Viread)		Nelfinavir (NFV, Viracept)[a]
Zidovudine (ZDV, AZT; Retrovir)[a]		Ritonavir (RTV, Norvir)[a]
		Saquinavir (SQV, Invirase)
		Tipranavir (TPV, Aptivus)[a]
Integrase Inhibitor	**Entry Inhibitors**	
(Integration of viral nucleic acid in host genome prevented)	*(Viral-cell membrane fusion inhibited)*	
Raltegravir (RAL, Isentress)	Enfuvirtide (T-20, Fuzeon)[a] *(CCR5 co-receptor antagonist)*	
	Maraviroc (MVC, Selzentry)	

[a]FDA-approved drug for use in pediatric populations.

but act at a different site on the viral reverse transcriptase enzyme so that cross-resistance with NRTIs does not occur.

c. Protease inhibitors (PIs)—PIs bind the HIV protease and interfere with assembly of infectious virions. Most are given in combination ("boosted") with a low dose of ritonavir, a second protease inhibitor, which inhibits their metabolism and thereby increases plasma levels.

d. Integrase inhibitor—This drug inhibits the viral integrase enzyme and prevents integration of HIV-1 nucleic acid into the host genome.

e. Entry inhibitors—There are two approved entry inhibitors. Enfuvirtide binds to the viral envelope protein and interferes with HIV fusion with the host cell plasma membrane, thereby preventing entry of the virus into the cell. Enfuvirtide must be administered parenterally which limits tolerability. Maraviroc is a chemokine receptor antagonist that binds one of the HIV co-receptor proteins (CCR5) on the host CD4 T cell. This blocks viral binding and prevents cell entry for virus that uses that receptor.

2. Principles of HIV treatment—Treatment of HIV is aimed at suppressing viral replication and thereby increasing/maintaining immune function. Antiretroviral treatment that reduces HIV replication is associated with an increase in CD4 T-lymphocyte count, reconstitution of immune function, and arrest of disease progression. Avoiding emergence of drug resistant HIV during therapy is key to long-term treatment success. HIV has a high spontaneous mutation rate that leads to emergence of drug resistance if viral suppression is incomplete. Prevention of resistance mutations requires that virus is not replicating and has no opportunity to generate new mutations.

The current standard regimen to achieve complete viral suppression is a combination of three drugs, including at least two drugs with different mechanisms of action. Optimally, children on ARV treatment will have laboratory monitoring every 3–4 months to confirm viral suppression and maintenance of CD4 T cells. If plasma virus becomes consistently detectable (viral rebound), the underlying cause must be determined and, if necessary, a change in the medication combination is made. Unfortunately, regular viral load and CD4 T cell testing is cost-prohibitive in many resource-limited settings. Monitoring with only clinical assessment increases the risk of continuing a regimen that is not fully suppressive. However, given the survival benefit, treatment should not be withheld on the basis of limited access to laboratory monitoring. Strict adherence to the prescribed treatment is critical. A wide range of issues will impact adherence including convenience and tolerability as well as psychosocial factors such as developmental stages, mental health of child and caregiver, HIV knowledge, and beliefs about treatment. Programs and services that enhance adherence are essential adjuncts of any HIV treatment regimen.

Within 3–6 months of successful ARV treatment, circulating HIV declines to below the limit of detection and CD4 T cell counts improve and may normalize. However, HIV persists in long-lived resting cells and cessation of antiretroviral treatment results in resumption of viremia and decline in CD4 lymphocytes. Therefore, treatment for HIV with currently available modalities must be a lifelong endeavor.

3. Criteria for initiation of antiretroviral medications—The paradigm for when to initiate treatment has shifted in past years as new evidence is available to determine the risk/benefit ratio for treatment. Early treatment has the potential advantage of more complete immune reconstitution and reduced risk of HIV disease complications but also presents risks related to medication toxicity and development of viral resistance. Children with clinical progression (CDC category B or C and WHO Stages 3 and 4) are at high risk of further progression and should start treatment promptly. Up to 30%–50% of infants (age <12–24 months) are at high risk of rapid progression and there are no tests that reliably identify rapid progressors. Consequently, early treatment, after expedited adherence counseling, is strongly recommended for all infants younger than 12 months per U.S. guidelines and 24 months per WHO guidelines, irrespective of clinical or immunologic progression. A randomized trial of early versus deferred treatment for infants has demonstrated a survival benefit for early treatment. For children and adolescents, clinical status, CD4 percent and count, and viral load are considered in the decision to initiate treatment. Recommendations for children living in the United States are summarized in Table 41–5. WHO recommendations

Table 41–5. United States guidelines for indications to start antiretroviral therapy HIV-infected.

Age	Criteria	Recommendation
Age < 12 mo	Regardless of clinical symptoms, immune status, or viral load	Treat
Age 1 to < 5y	• Clinical category B or C	Treat
	• CD4 < 25%	Treat
	• Clinical category A or N and CD4 ≥ 25% with:	
	• HIV RNA ≥ 100,000 copies/mL	Treat
	• HIV RNA < 100,000 copies/mL	Consider treatment
≥ 5 y	• Clinical category B or C	Treat
	• CD4 ≤ 500 cells/m³	Treat
	• Clinical category A or N and CD4 > 500 cells/m³ with:	
	• HIV RNA ≥ 100,000 copies/mL	Treat
	• HIV RNA < 100,000 copies/mL	Consider treatment

Adapted from Panel on Antiretroviral Therapy and Medical Management of HIV-Infected Children. Guidelines for the Use of Antiretroviral Agents in Pediatric HIV Infection. August 11, 2011. Available at: http://www.aidsinfo.nih.gov.

are found at http://www.who.int/hiv/topics/paediatric/en/index.html.

4. Complications of antiretroviral medications—After initiation of ARV treatment, patients must be monitored for complications. Each medication has specific toxicities which are described in detail at http://www.aidsinfo.nih.gov/guidelines/html/2/pediatric-treatment-guidelines/0/. Common adverse events are gastrointestinal distress, hematologic toxicity (anemia, neutropenia), elevated liver enzymes, dyslipidemia (elevated LDL-cholesterol and triglycerides), glucose intolerance, and abnormal fat distribution (lipodystrophy). Reduced bone mineral content and renal dysfunction may result from drug effects as well as from direct effects of HIV. Several drugs (eg, nevirapine, abacavir) have been associated with severe hepatitis sometimes associated with a systemic hypersensitivity reaction which may be life threatening if not identified early or upon challenge with the same medication. The human mitochondrial DNA polymerase has limited affinity for the nucleotide analogues. Incorporation of the analogue into mitochondrial DNA is one mechanism thought to lead to many of the adverse effects observed with these drugs. Mitochondrial toxicity can lead to lactic acidosis which is a rare, but potentially fatal, complication. During the initial weeks of treatment, children may have a worsening or unmasking of symptoms due to underlying infection with other organisms such as *M tuberculosis* as a result of immune restoration, an event termed immune reconstitution inflammatory syndrome (IRIS).

Bartlett JA, Shao JF: Successes, challenges, and limitations of current antiretroviral therapy in low-income and middle-income countries. Lancet Infect Dis 2009;9:637–649.

Boulware DR, Callens S, Pahwa S: Pediatric HIV immune reconstitution inflammatory syndrome. Curr Opin HIV AIDS 2008;3(4):461–467.

Chadwick EG, Yogev R, Alvero CG et al: Long-term outcomes for HIV-infected infants less than 6 months of age at initiation of lopinavir/ritonavir combination antiretroviral therapy. AIDS 2011;25(5):643–649.

Jacobson DL, Lindsey JC, Gordon CM, Moye J, Hardin DS, Mulligan K, Aldrovandi GM: Pediatric AIDS Clinical Trials Group P1045 team. Total body and spinal bone mineral density across Tanner stage in perinatally HIV-infected and uninfected children and youth in PACTG 1045. AIDS 2010 Mar 13;24(5):687–696.

Panel on Antiretroviral Therapy and Medical Management of HIV-Infected Children: Guidelines for the Use of Antiretroviral Agents in Pediatric HIV Infection. August 11, 2011;1–268. Available at: http://aidsinfo.nih.gov/ContentFiles/PediatricGuidelines.pdf. Accessed November 6, 2011.

Puthanakit T, Oberdorfer P, Akarathum N et al: Immune reconstitution syndrome after highly active antiretroviral therapy in human immunodeficiency virus-infected Thai children. Pediatr Infect Dis J 2006;25:53–58.

Rhoads MP, Lanigan J, Smith CJ et al: Effect of specific antiretroviral therapy (ART) drugs on lipid changes and the need for lipid management in children with HIV. J Acquir Immune Defic Syndr 2011 Apr 14 [Epub ahead of print].

Van Dyke RB, Patel K, Siberry GK et al: Antiretroviral Treatment of U.S. Children with Perinatally-Acquired HIV Infection: Temporal Changes in Therapy between 1991 and 2009 and Predictors of Immunologic and Virologic Outcomes. J Acquir Immune Defic Syndr 2011;57(2):165–173.

World Health Organization: Antiretroviral therapy for HIV infection in infants and children: Towards universal access. Recommendations for a public health approach: 2010 revision 1–206. http://www.who.int/hiv/pub/paediatric/infants2010/en/index.html.

B. General Measures

1. Immunizations—All inactivated vaccines that are recommended for healthy children in the United States are also indicated for HIV-infected children. In general, vaccine responses will be more robust when administered to children with suppressed plasma virus and restored CD4 T-cell counts.

Varicella and mumps-measles-rubella (MMR) vaccines are recommended for HIV-infected children, provided they are asymptomatic or only mildly symptomatic and have CD4 T-cell parameters consistent with category 1 or 2 (see Table 41–2). Rotavirus vaccine has not been extensively studied in immunocompromised infants. However, the majority of HIV-exposed infants will be eligible for rotavirus vaccine prior to definitive exclusion of HIV. Since the majority of infants born in the United States will be uninfected, the benefit of initiating the vaccine series outweighs the undocumented risk and is therefore recommended. Annual influenza vaccination after age 6 months, preferably with the inactivated vaccine, is recommended for HIV-infected children and their close contacts. Close contacts may receive the live attenuated influenza vaccine. For other live vaccines (eg, Bacille Calmette-Guérin [BCG], yellow fever) the risk-benefit ratio must be considered

Vaccines against encapsulated bacteria may reduce the risk of these infections in HIV-infected children. Most experts recommend two doses of meningococcal conjugate vaccine (MCV) given soon after age 2 years, rather than deferring to age 11 years. Children who have not received pneumococcal conjugate vaccine (PCV13) and *Haemophilus influenzae* type b (Hib) vaccine series as infants (eg, immigrants) may benefit from two doses of Hib vaccine and two doses of PCV13 (separated by 8 weeks) even when given after the usual cutoff age of 60 months. The 23-valent pneumococcal polysaccharide vaccine (PPSV) should also be given after age 2 years with a second dose 3–5 years later. The response to hepatitis B vaccine is particularly unreliable in people with HIV. Therefore, a test for hepatitis B surface antibody should be obtained after the three-dose series. If the titer is less than 10 mIU/mL, a second series of three vaccinations is recommended.

2. Prophylaxis for infections—Children with suppressed CD4 lymphocyte numbers benefit from prophylactic treatment to prevent opportunistic infections. Children who have

Table 41–6. Drug regimens for *Pneumocystis jiroveci* prophylaxis for children older than 4 weeks.

Recommended regimen
Trimethoprim-sulfamethoxazole, 150 mg TMP/m^2/d plus 750 mg SMX/m^2/d, administered orally, divided into two doses per d/3 d a wk on consecutive days
Alternative (same total daily dosages):
Single daily dose 3 d a wk on consecutive days
Divided twice-daily doses 7 d a wk
Divided twice-daily doses 3 d a wk on alternate days
Alternative if trimethoprim-sulfamethoxazole is not tolerated
Dapsone, 2 mg/kg/d (not to exceed 100 mg) orally once daily or 4 mg/kg (not to exceed 200 mg) orally once wkly
Atovaquone, age 1–3 mo and > 24 mo, 30 mg/kg orally once daily; age 4–24 mo, 45 mg/kg orally once daily
Aerosolized pentamidine (children > age 5 y), 300 mg via Respirgard II inhaler monthly

Adapted from Centers for Disease Control and Prevention: Guidelines for the Prevention and Treatment of Opportunistic Infections Among HIV-Exposed and HIV-Infected Children. MMWR Recomm Rep 2009;58(RR-11):127. Available at: http://www.aidsinfo.nih.gov/guidelines.

had their CD4 counts restored with antiretroviral therapy to category 1 or 2 for over 3 months can be taken off prophylactic treatments.

Antibiotic prophylaxis for *P jiroveci* pneumonia has been extremely effective. HIV-infected infants should receive Pneumocystis prophylaxis until age 12 months, after which prophylaxis is based on assessment of symptoms and age-adjusted CD4 lymphocyte counts every 3 months. Children with CDC Immune Category 3 CD4 T cell parameters (Table 41–2) should begin PCP prophylaxis. Published guidelines from the CDC for *P jiroveci* pneumonia prophylaxis are summarized in Table 41–6.

4. Psychosocial support and mental health—Evaluation and support for psychosocial needs of HIV-affected families is imperative. As with other chronic illnesses, HIV infection affects all family members, and it also carries additional social stigma. Emotional concerns and financial needs, which are more prominent than medical needs at many stages of the disease process, influence the family's ability to comply with a medical treatment regimen. HIV-infected children often have comorbid mental health conditions. Rates of attention-deficit/hyperactivity disorder range from 20% to 50% in various studies. Hospital admissions for mental health disorders are more frequent among HIV-infected children. In one study, dual diagnosis of HIV and a mental health disorder occurred in 85% of adolescents who acquired HIV infection through high-risk behaviors. Ideally, care should be coordinated by a team of caregivers that is familiar with HIV disease and its comorbidities, newest therapies, and community resources.

5. Universal precautions—The infant or child who is well enough to attend day care or school should not be treated differently from other children. The exception may be a toddler with uncontrollable biting behavior or bleeding lesions that cannot be covered adequately; in these situations, the child may be withheld from group day care. Families may choose to make the school health care provider and teacher aware of the diagnosis, but there is no legal requirement that any individual at the school or day care center be informed. The parents and child may prefer to keep the diagnosis confidential, because the stigma associated with HIV infection remains difficult to overcome. Because undiagnosed HIV-infected infants and children might be enrolled, all schools and day care centers should have policies with simple guidelines for using universal precautions to prevent transmission of HIV infection in these settings.

Horizontal transmission (in the absence of sexual contact or injecting drug use) of HIV is exceedingly rare and is associated with exposure of broken skin or mucous membranes to HIV-infected blood or bloody secretions. Several cases have resulted from HIV-infected caregivers feeding children premasticated food; hence, families should be advised against this practice. Saliva, tears, urine, and stool are not contagious if they do not contain gross blood. A barrier protection (eg, latex or rubber gloves or thick pads of fabric or paper) should be used when possible contact with blood or bloody body fluids occurs. Objects that might be contaminated with blood, such as razors or toothbrushes, should not be shared. No special care is required for dishes, towels, toys, or bedclothes. Blood-soiled clothing may be washed routinely with hot water and detergent. Contaminated surfaces may be disinfected easily with a variety of agents, including household bleach (1:10 dilution), some commercial disinfectants (eg, Lysol), or 70% isopropyl alcohol.

Crane HM, Dhanireddy S, Kim HN, Ramers C, Dellit TH, Kitahata MM, Harrington RD: Optimal timing of routine vaccination in HIV-infected persons. Current HIV/AIDS Reports 2009;6(2):93–99.

Chernoff M et al: IMPAACT P1055 Study Team: Mental health treatment patterns in perinatally HIV-infected youth and controls. Pediatrics 2009;124:627–636.

42

Infections: Bacterial & Spirochetal

John W. Ogle, MD
Marsha S. Anderson, MD

BACTERIAL INFECTIONS

GROUP A STREPTOCOCCAL INFECTIONS

ESSENTIALS OF DIAGNOSIS & TYPICAL FEATURES

- Streptococcal pharyngitis:
  - Clinical diagnosis based entirely on symptoms; signs and physical examination unreliable.
  - Throat culture or rapid antigen detection test positive for group A streptococci.
- Impetigo:
  - Rapidly spreading, highly infectious skin rash.
  - Erythematous denuded areas and honey-colored crusts.
  - Group A streptococci are grown in culture from most (not all) cases.

General Considerations

Group A streptococci (GAS) are common gram-positive bacteria producing a wide variety of clinical illnesses, including acute pharyngitis, impetigo, cellulitis, and scarlet fever, the generalized illness caused by strains that elaborate erythrogenic toxin. GAS can also cause pneumonia, septic arthritis, osteomyelitis, meningitis, and other less common infections. GAS infections may also produce nonsuppurative sequelae (rheumatic fever and acute glomerulonephritis).

The cell walls of streptococci contain both carbohydrate and protein antigens. The C-carbohydrate antigen determines the group, and the M- or T-protein antigens determine the specific type. In most strains, the M protein appears to confer virulence, and antibodies developed against the M protein are protective against reinfection with that type.

Almost all GAS are β-hemolytic. These organisms may be carried without symptoms on the skin and in the pharynx, rectum, and vagina. Between 10% and 15% of school-aged children in some studies are asymptomatic pharyngeal carriers of GAS. Streptococcal carriers are individuals who do not mount an immune response to the organism and are therefore believed to be at low risk for nonsuppurative sequelae. All GAS are sensitive to penicillin. Resistance to erythromycin is common in some countries and has increased in the United States.

Prevention

GAS pharyngitis usually occurs after contact with respiratory secretions of a person infected with GAS. Crowding facilitates spread of GAS and outbreaks of pharyngitis and impetigo can be seen. Prompt recognition and institution of antibiotics may decrease spread. Treatment with antibiotics prevents acute rheumatic fever.

Clinical Findings

A. Symptoms and Signs

1. Respiratory infections

A. Infancy and early childhood (age < 3 years)—The onset is insidious, with mild symptoms (low-grade fever, serous nasal discharge, and pallor). Otitis media is common. Exudative pharyngitis and cervical adenitis are uncommon in this age group.

B. Childhood type—Onset is sudden, with fever and marked malaise and often with repeated vomiting. The pharynx is sore and edematous, and generally there is tonsillar exudate. Anterior cervical lymph nodes are tender and enlarged. Small petechiae are frequently seen on the soft palate. In **scarlet fever**, the skin is diffusely erythematous and appears sunburned and roughened (sandpaper rash). The rash is most intense in the axillae, groin, and on the abdomen and trunk. It blanches except in the skin folds, which do not blanch and are pigmented (Pastia sign). The rash usually appears 24 hours after the onset of fever and rapidly spreads over the next 1–2 days. Desquamation begins on the face at the end of the first week and becomes generalized by the third week. Early in the course of infection, there is circumoral pallor and the surface of the tongue is coated white, with the papillae enlarged and bright red (white strawberry tongue). Subsequently desquamation occurs, and the tongue appears beefy red (strawberry tongue). Petechiae may be seen on all mucosal surfaces.

c. Adult type—The adult type of GAS is characterized by exudative or nonexudative tonsillitis with fewer systemic symptoms, lower fever, and no vomiting. Scarlet fever is uncommon in adults.

2. Impetigo—Streptococcal impetigo begins as a papule that vesiculates and then breaks, leaving a denuded area covered by a honey-colored crust. Both *Staphylococcus aureus* and GAS are isolated in some cases. The lesions spread readily and diffusely. Local lymph nodes may become swollen and inflamed. Although the child often lacks systemic symptoms, a high fever and toxicity may be present. If flaccid bullae are noted, the disease is called bullous impetigo and is caused by an epidermolytic toxin-producing strain of *S aureus*.

3. Cellulitis—The portal of entry is often an insect bite or superficial abrasion. A diffuse, rapidly spreading cellulitis occurs that involves the subcutaneous tissues and extends along the lymphatic pathways with only minimal local suppuration. Local acute lymphadenitis occurs. The child is usually acutely ill, with fever and malaise. In classic erysipelas, the involved area is bright red, swollen, warm, and very tender. The infection may extend rapidly from the lymphatics to the bloodstream.

Streptococcal perianal cellulitis is an entity peculiar to young children. Pain with defecation often leads to constipation, which may be the presenting complaint. The child is afebrile and otherwise well. Perianal erythema, tenderness, and painful rectal examination are the only abnormal physical findings. Scant rectal bleeding with defecation may occur. A perianal swab culture usually yields heavy growth of GAS. A variant of this syndrome is streptococcal vaginitis in prepubertal girls. Symptoms are dysuria and pain; marked erythema and tenderness of the introitus and blood-tinged discharge are seen.

4. Necrotizing fasciitis—This dangerous disease is reported sporadically and may occur as a complication of varicella infection. About 20%–40% of cases are due to GAS; 30%–40% are due to *S aureus*; and the rest are a result of mixed bacterial infections. The disease is characterized by extensive necrosis of superficial fasciae, undermining of surrounding tissue, and usually systemic toxicity. Initially the skin overlying the infection is tender and pale red without distinct borders, resembling cellulitis. Blisters or bullae may appear. The color deepens to a distinct purple or in some cases becomes pale. Tenderness out of proportion to the clinical appearance, skin anesthesia (due to infarction of superficial nerves), or "woody" induration suggest necrotizing fasciitis. Involved areas may develop mild to massive edema. Early recognition and aggressive debridement of necrotic tissue are essential.

5. Group A streptococcal infections in newborn nurseries—GAS epidemics occur occasionally in nurseries. The organism may be introduced into the nursery from the vaginal tract of a mother or from the throat or nose of a mother or a staff member. The organism then spreads from infant to infant. The umbilical stump is colonized while the infant is in the nursery. Like staphylococcal infections, there may be no or few clinical manifestations while the infant is still in the nursery. Most often, a colonized infant develops a chronic oozing omphalitis days later. The organism may spread from the infant to other family members. Serious and even fatal infections may develop, including sepsis, meningitis, empyema, septic arthritis, and peritonitis.

6. Streptococcal sepsis—Serious illness from GAS sepsis is now more common both in children and in adults. Rash and scarlet fever may be present. Prostration and shock result in high mortality rates. Pharyngitis is uncommon as an antecedent illness. Underlying disease is a predisposing factor.

7. Streptococcal toxic shock syndrome (STSS)—Toxic shock syndrome caused by GAS has been defined. Like *S aureus*–associated toxic shock, multiorgan system involvement is a prominent part of the illness. The diagnostic criteria include (1) isolation of GAS from a normally sterile site, (2) hypotension or shock, and (3) at least two of the following: renal impairment (creatinine > two times the upper limit of normal for age), thrombocytopenia (< 100,000/mm^3), or coagulopathy, liver involvement (transaminases > two times normal), acute respiratory distress syndrome, generalized erythematous macular rash or soft tissue necrosis (myositis, necrotizing fasciitis, gangrene). In cases that otherwise meet clinical criteria, isolation of GAS from a nonsterile site (throat, wound, or vagina) is indicative of a probable cause.

B. Laboratory Findings

Leukocytosis with a marked shift to the left is seen early. Eosinophilia regularly appears during convalescence. β-Hemolytic streptococci are cultured from the throat or site of infection. The organism may be cultured from the skin and by needle aspiration from subcutaneous tissues and other involved sites such as infected nodes. Occasionally blood cultures are positive. Newer rapid antigen detection tests such as optical immunoassays and DNA chemiluminescence probes are very specific, and in some cases are almost as sensitive as traditional throat culture. However, sensitivity varies with the type of test used and the experience level of the laboratory or office. Many experts recommend backup throat culture in patients with negative rapid strep antigen tests. Patients with positive rapid strep antigen tests do not need a confirmation by throat culture, since the specificity of antigen tests are high.

Antistreptolysin O (ASO) titers rise about 150 units within 2 weeks after acute infection. Elevated ASO and anti-DNase B titers are useful in documenting prior throat infections in cases of acute rheumatic fever. The streptozyme test detects antibodies to streptolysin O, hyaluronidase, streptokinase, DNase B, and NADase. It is somewhat more sensitive than the measurement of ASO titers.

Proteinuria, cylindruria, and minimal hematuria may be seen early in children with streptococcal infection. True poststreptococcal glomerulonephritis is seen 1–4 weeks after the respiratory or skin infection.

Differential Diagnosis

Streptococcal infection in early childhood must be differentiated from adenovirus and other respiratory virus infections. The pharyngitis in herpangina (coxsackievirus A) is vesicular or ulcerative. Herpes simplex also causes ulcerative lesions, which most commonly involve the anterior pharynx, tongue, and gums. In infectious mononucleosis, the pharyngitis is also exudative, but splenomegaly and generalized adenopathy are typical, and laboratory findings are often diagnostic (atypical lymphocytes, elevated liver enzymes, and a positive heterophil or other serologic test for mononucleosis). Uncomplicated streptococcal pharyngitis improves within 24–48 hours if penicillin is given and by 72–96 hours without antimicrobials.

Group G and group C streptococci are uncommon causes of pharyngitis but have been implicated in epidemics of sore throat in college students. Acute rheumatic fever does not occur following group G or group C infection, although acute glomerulonephritis (AGN) is a complication. *Arcanobacterium hemolyticum* may cause pharyngitis with scarlatina-like or maculopapular truncal rash. In diphtheria, systemic symptoms, vomiting, and fever are less marked; pharyngeal pseudomembrane is confluent and adherent; the throat is less red; and cervical adenopathy is prominent. Pharyngeal tularemia causes white rather than yellow exudate. There is little erythema, and cultures for β-hemolytic streptococci are negative. A history of exposure to rabbits and a failure to respond to antimicrobials may suggest the diagnosis. Leukemia and agranulocytosis may present with pharyngitis and are diagnosed by bone marrow examination.

Scarlet fever must be differentiated from other exanthematous diseases (principally rubella), erythema due to sunburn, drug reactions, Kawasaki disease, toxic shock syndrome (TSS), and staphylococcal scalded skin syndrome (see also Table 40–3).

Complications

Suppurative complications of GAS infections include sinusitis, otitis, mastoiditis, cervical lymphadenitis, pneumonia, empyema, septic arthritis, and meningitis. Spread of streptococcal infection from the throat to other sites—principally the skin (impetigo) and vagina—is common and should be considered in every instance of chronic vaginal discharge or chronic skin infection, such as that complicating childhood eczema. Both acute rheumatic fever and AGN are nonsuppurative complications of GAS infections.

A. Acute Rheumatic Fever (See Chapter 20)

B. Acute Glomerulonephritis

AGN can follow streptococcal infections of either the pharynx or the skin—in contrast to rheumatic fever, which follows pharyngeal infection only. AGN may occur at any age, even infancy. In most reports of AGN, males predominate by a ratio of 2:1. Rheumatic fever occurs with equal frequency in both sexes. Certain M types are associated strongly with poststreptococcal glomerulonephritis (nephritogenic types). The serotypes producing disease on the skin often differ from those found in the pharynx.

The incidence of AGN after streptococcal infection is variable and has ranged from 0% to 28%. Several outbreaks of AGN in families have involved 50%–75% of siblings of affected patients in 1- to 7-week periods. Second attacks of glomerulonephritis are rare. The median period between infection and the development of glomerulonephritis is 10 days. In contrast, acute rheumatic fever occurs after a median of 18 days.

C. Poststreptococcal Reactive Arthritis

Following an episode of group A streptococcal pharyngitis, a reactive arthritis develops in some patients. This reactive arthritis is believed to be due to immune complex deposition and is seen about 1–2 weeks following the acute infection. Patients with poststreptococcal reactive arthritis do not have the full constellation of clinical and laboratory criteria needed to fulfill the Jones criteria for a diagnosis of acute rheumatic fever.

Treatment

A. Specific Measures

Treatment is directed toward both eradication of acute infection and prevention of rheumatic fever. In patients with pharyngitis, antibiotics should be started early to relieve symptoms and should be continued for 10 days to prevent rheumatic fever. Although early therapy has not been shown to prevent AGN, it seems advisable to treat impetigo promptly in sibling contacts of patients with poststreptococcal nephritis. Neither sulfonamides nor trimethoprim–sulfamethoxazole is effective in the treatment of streptococcal infections. Although topical therapy for impetigo with antimicrobial ointments (especially mupirocin) is as effective as systemic therapy, it does not eradicate pharyngeal carriage and is less practical for extensive disease.

1. Penicillin—Except for penicillin-allergic patients, penicillin V (phenoxymethyl penicillin) is the drug of choice. Penicillin resistance has never been documented. For children weighing less than 27 kg, the regimen is 250 mg, given orally two or three times a day for 10 days. For heavier children, adolescents, or adults 500 mg two or three times a day is recommended. Giving penicillin V (250 mg) twice daily is as effective as more frequent oral administration or intramuscular therapy. Once-daily oral amoxicillin (50 mg/kg, maximum 1000 mg) has been shown to be as effective as penicillin V given three times a day. Another alternative for treatment of pharyngitis and impetigo is a single dose of benzathine penicillin G, given intramuscularly (600,000 units for children weighing < 60 lb [27.2 kg] and 1.2 million units for children weighing > 60 lb [27.2 kg]). Intramuscular delivery ensures compliance, but is painful. Parenteral therapy is indicated if vomiting or sepsis is present. Mild cellulitis due to GAS may be treated orally or intramuscularly.

Cellulitis requiring hospitalization can be treated with aqueous penicillin G (150,000 U/kg/d, given intravenously in four to six divided doses) or cefazolin (100 mg/kg/d, given intravenously in three divided doses) until there is marked improvement. Penicillin V (50 mg/kg/d in four divided doses) or cephalexin (50–75 mg/kg/d in four divided doses) may then be given orally to complete a 10-day course. Acute cervical lymphadenitis may require incision and drainage. Treatment of necrotizing fasciitis requires emergency surgical debridement followed by high-dose parenteral antibiotics appropriate to the organisms cultured.

2. Other antibiotics—Cephalexin, ceftibuten, cefdinir, and cefadroxil are other effective oral antimicrobials. For penicillin-allergic patients with pharyngitis or impetigo the following alternative regimens have been used: azithromycin (12 mg/kg/d) once daily for 5 days, or clindamycin (20 mg/kg/day in 3 divided doses; maximum 1.8 g/d) for 10 days. Patients with immediate, anaphylactic hypersensitivity to penicillin should not receive cephalosporins, because up to 15% will also be allergic to cephalosporins. Erythromycin resistance, although not currently widespread in the United States, was reported in 48% of strains tested in Pittsburgh in 2001. In most studies, bacteriologic failures after cephalosporin therapy are less frequent than failures following penicillin. However, cephalosporins are generally more expensive than penicillin. Additionally, there are few conclusive data on the ability of these agents to prevent rheumatic fever. Therefore, penicillin remains the agent of choice for nonallergic patients. Many strains are resistant to tetracycline.

For infections requiring intravenous therapy, aqueous penicillin G (250,000 U/kg in six divided doses) given intravenously is usually the drug of choice. Cefazolin (100 mg/kg/d intravenously or intramuscularly in three divided doses); clindamycin (25–40 mg/kg/d intravenously in four divided doses); and vancomycin (40 mg/kg/d intravenously in four divided doses) are alternatives in penicillin-allergic patients. Clindamycin is preferred by many experts and may be superior to penicillin for necrotizing fasciitis if the organism is susceptible to it. Clindamycin should not be used alone empirically for severe, suspected GAS infections because a small percentage of isolates in the United States are resistant to it. Some physicians use both penicillin and clindamycin in patients with necrotizing fasciitis or STSS.

3. Serious GAS disease—Serious GAS infections, such as pneumonia, osteomyelitis, septic arthritis, sepsis, endocarditis, meningitis, and STSS, require parenteral antimicrobial therapy. Penicillin G is the drug of choice for these invasive infections. Clindamycin, in addition to penicillin G, is advocated by many experts for STSS or necrotizing fasciitis. Necrotizing fasciitis requires prompt surgical debridement. In STSS, volume status and blood pressure should be monitored and patients evaluated for a focus of infection, if not readily apparent. Intravenous immune globulin (in addition to antibiotics) has been used in severe cases.

4. Treatment failure—Even when compliance is perfect, organisms will be found in cultures in 5%–15% of children after cessation of therapy. Reculture is indicated only in patients with relapse or recrudescence of pharyngitis or those with a personal or family history of rheumatic fever. Repeat treatment at least once with an oral cephalosporin or clindamycin is indicated in patients with recurrent culture-positive pharyngitis.

5. Prevention of recurrences in rheumatic individuals—The preferred prophylaxis for rheumatic individuals is benzathine penicillin G, 1.2 million units (600,000 units for patients weighing less than 27 kg) intramuscularly every 4 weeks. If the risk of streptococcal exposure is high, every-3-week dosing is preferred. One of the following alternative oral prophylactic regimens may be used: sulfadiazine, 0.5 g once a day (if < 27 kg) or 1 g once a day (if > 27 kg); penicillin V, 250 mg twice daily; or erythromycin, 250 mg twice daily. Continued prophylaxis is recommended for at least 5 years or until age 21 years (whichever is longer) if carditis is absent. Prophylaxis should be continued if the risk of contact with persons with GAS is high (eg, parents of school-aged children, pediatric nurses, and teachers). In the presence of carditis without residual heart or valvular disease, a minimum of 10 years (or well into adulthood, whichever is longer) is the minimum duration. If the patient has residual valvular heart disease, many recommend lifelong prophylaxis. These patients should be at least 10 years from their last episode of rheumatic disease and at least 40 years of age before considering discontinuation of prophylaxis. A similar approach to the prevention of recurrences of glomerulonephritis may be used during childhood when there is a suspicion that repeated streptococcal infections coincide with flareups of glomerulonephritis.

6. Poststreptococcal reactive arthritis—In contrast to rheumatic fever, nonsteroidal agents may not dramatically improve joint symptoms. However, like patients with rheumatic fever, some patients with poststreptococcal reactive arthritis have developed carditis several weeks to months after their arthritis symptoms began. Therefore, some experts recommend antibiotic prophylaxis of these patients for 1 year and monitoring for signs of carditis (see recommendations for prevention of recurrences of rheumatic fever, above). If carditis does not develop, prophylaxis could then be discontinued.

If carditis develops, the patient should be considered to have acute rheumatic fever and prophylaxis continued as described above.

B. General Measures

Acetaminophen is useful for pain or fever. Local treatment of impetigo may promote earlier healing. Crusts should first be soaked off. Areas beneath the crusts should then be washed with soap daily.

C. Treatment of Complications

Rheumatic fever is best prevented by early and adequate penicillin treatment of the streptococcal infection.

D. Treatment of Carriers

Identification and treatment of GAS carriers is difficult. There are no established clinical or serologic criteria for differentiating carriers from the truly infected. Some children receive multiple courses of antimicrobials, with persistence of GAS in the throat, leading to a "streptococcal neurosis" on the part of families.

In certain circumstances, eradication of carriage may be desirable: (1) when a family member has a history of rheumatic fever; (2) when an episode of STSS or necrotizing fasciitis has occurred in a household contact; (3) multiple, recurring, documented episodes of GAS in family members despite adequate therapy; and (4) during an outbreak of rheumatic fever or GAS-associated glomerulonephritis. Clindamycin (20 mg/kg/d, given orally in three divided doses, to a maximum of 1.8 g/d) or a combination of rifampin (20 mg/kg/d, given orally for 4 days) and penicillin in standard dosage given orally has been used to attempt eradication of carriage.

Prognosis

Death is rare except in infants or young children with sepsis or pneumonia. The febrile course is shortened and complications eliminated by early and adequate treatment with penicillin.

Tanz RR, Shulman ST: Chronic pharyngeal carriage of group A streptococci. Pediatr Infect Dis J 2007;26:175 [PMID: 17259882].

Wessels MR: Clinical practice: Streptococcal pharyngitis. N Engl J Med 2011;364:648–655 [PMID: 21323542].

GROUP B STREPTOCOCCAL INFECTIONS

ESSENTIALS OF DIAGNOSIS & TYPICAL FEATURES

- Early-onset neonatal infection:
  - Newborn younger than age 7 days, with rapidly progressing overwhelming sepsis, with or without meningitis.
  - Pneumonia with respiratory failure is frequent; chest radiograph resembles that seen in hyaline membrane disease.
  - Leukopenia with a shift to the left.
  - Blood or cerebrospinal fluid (CSF) cultures growing group B streptococci (GBS).
- Late-onset Infection:
  - Meningitis, sepsis, or other focal infection in a child aged 1–16 weeks with blood or CSF cultures growing GBS.

Prevention

Many women of childbearing age possess type-specific circulating antibody to the polysaccharide antigens for GBS. These antibodies are transferred to the newborn via the placental circulation. GBS carriers delivering healthy infants have significant serum levels of IgG antibody to this antigen. In contrast, women delivering infants who develop either early- or late-onset GBS disease rarely have detectable antibody in their sera.

Monovalent and bivalent vaccines with type II or III polysaccharide antigens have been studied in pregnant women, with 80%–90% of vaccine recipients developing fourfold or greater increases in GBS capsular polysaccharide type-specific IgG. These reports suggest that a multivalent vaccine could be developed and given to pregnant women to prevent many cases of early-onset GBS disease.

The Centers for Disease Control and Prevention (CDC) has issued culture-based maternal guidelines for the prevention of early-onset GBS disease.

CDC Recommendations for Prevention of Perinatal GBS Disease

1. All pregnant women should be screened at 35–37 weeks' gestation with a vaginal and rectal culture for GBS. *Exceptions:* Women with known GBS bacteriuria during the current pregnancy or women who have delivered a previous infant with GBS disease do not need screening—all these women need intrapartum prophylaxis.
2. If GBS status is unknown at onset of labor or rupture of membranes, intrapartum chemoprophylaxis should be administered to women with any of the following:

   a. Gestation less than 37 weeks

   b. Rupture of membranes >18 hours

c. Intrapartum temperature of greater than 38°C (100.4°F). If chorioamnionitis is suspected, broad spectrum antibiotics that include coverage for Group B Streptococcus should replace GBS intrapartum prophylaxis.

3. Intrapartum antibiotic prophylaxis (IAP) to prevent GBS disease is not routinely recommended for cesarean deliveries performed prior to the onset of labor and prior to rupture of amniotic membranes, regardless of the woman's GBS colonization status or the gestational age of the pregnancy.
4. IAP recommendations (Table 42–1).
5. Empiric treatment of a neonate whose mother received IAP for prevention of GBS (Figure 42–1).

Clinical Findings

The incidence of perinatal GBS disease has declined dramatically since screening of pregnant mothers and provision of intrapartum chemoprophylaxis began. Although most patients with GBS disease are infants younger than age 3 months, cases are seen in infants aged 4–5 months. Serious infection also occurs in women with puerperal sepsis, immunocompromised patients, patients with cirrhosis and spontaneous peritonitis, and diabetic patients with cellulitis. Two distinct clinical syndromes distinguished by differing perinatal events, age at onset, and serotype of the infecting strain occur in infants.

Risk factors for early-onset group GBS disease include maternal GBS colonization, gestational age less than 37 weeks, rupture of membranes > 18 hours prior to presentation, young maternal age, history of a previous infant with invasive GBS disease, African-American or Hispanic ethnic origin, and low or absent maternal GBS anticapsular antibodies.

A. Early-Onset Infection

"Early-onset" illness is observed in newborns younger than 7 days old. The onset of symptoms in the majority of these infants occurs in the first 48 hours of life, and most are ill within 6 hours. Apnea is often the first sign. Sepsis, shock, meningitis, apnea, and pneumonia are the most common clinical presentations. There is a high incidence of associated maternal obstetric complications, especially premature labor and prolonged rupture of the membranes. Newborns with early-onset disease are severely ill at the time of diagnosis, and more than 50% die. Although most infants with early-onset infections are full-term, premature infants are at increased risk for the disease. Newborns with early-onset infection acquire GBS in utero as an ascending infection or during passage through the birth canal. When early-onset infection is complicated by meningitis, more than 80% of the bacterial isolates belong to serotype III. Postmortem examination of infants with early-onset disease usually reveals pulmonary inflammatory infiltrates and hyaline membranes containing large numbers of GBS.

Table 42–1. Centers for Disease Control and Prevention recommended regimens for intrapartum antimicrobial prophylaxis for perinatal group B streptococcal (GBS) disease.[a]

Recommended	Penicillin G, 5 million units IV initial dose, then 2.5–3 million units IV q4h until delivery
Alternative	Ampicillin, 2 g IV initial dose, then 1 g IV q4h until delivery
If penicillin allergic[b]	
Patients not at high risk for anaphylaxis	Cefazolin, 2 g IV initial dose, then 1 g IV q8h until delivery
Patients at high risk for anaphylaxis[c]	
GBS susceptible to clindamycin and erythromycin[d]	Clindamycin, 900 mg IV q8h until delivery
GBS resistant to clindamycin or erythromycin or susceptibility unknown	Vancomycin,[e] 1 g IV q12h until delivery

[a]Broader-spectrum agents, including an agent active against GBS, may be necessary for treatment of chorioamnionitis.
[b]History of penicillin allergy should be assessed to determine whether a high risk for anaphylaxis is present. Penicillin-allergic patients with a history of anaphylaxis, angioedema, respiratory distress, or urticaria after receiving penicillin or a cephalosporin are at high risk for anaphylaxis and should not receive penicillin, ampicillin, or cefazolin for GBS intrapartum prophylaxis.
[c]If laboratory facilities are adequate, clindamycin and erythromycin susceptibility testing should be performed on prenatal GBS isolates from penicillin-allergic women at high risk for anaphylaxis.
[d]Resistance to erythromycin is often, but not always, associated with clindamycin resistance. If a strain is resistant to erythromycin, but appears susceptible to clindamycin, it may have inducible resistance to clindamycin.
[e]Cefazolin is preferred over vancomycin for women with a history of penicillin allergy other than immediate hypersensitivity reactions, and pharmacologic data suggest it achieves effective intra-amniotic concentrations. Vancomycin should be reserved for penicillin-allergic women at high risk for anaphylaxis.
Reprinted, with permission, from Schrag S et al: Prevention of perinatal Group B streptococcal disease. Revised guidelines from CDC. MMWR Recomm Rep 2002;51(RR-11):1.

B. Late-Onset Infection

"Late-onset" infection occurs in infants between ages 7 days and 4 months (median age at onset, about 4 weeks). Maternal obstetric complications are not usually associated with late-onset infection. These infants are usually not as ill at the time of diagnosis as those with early-onset disease, and the mortality rate is lower. In recent series, about 37% of patients have meningitis and 46% have sepsis. Septic arthritis and osteomyelitis, meningitis, occult bacteremia, otitis media,

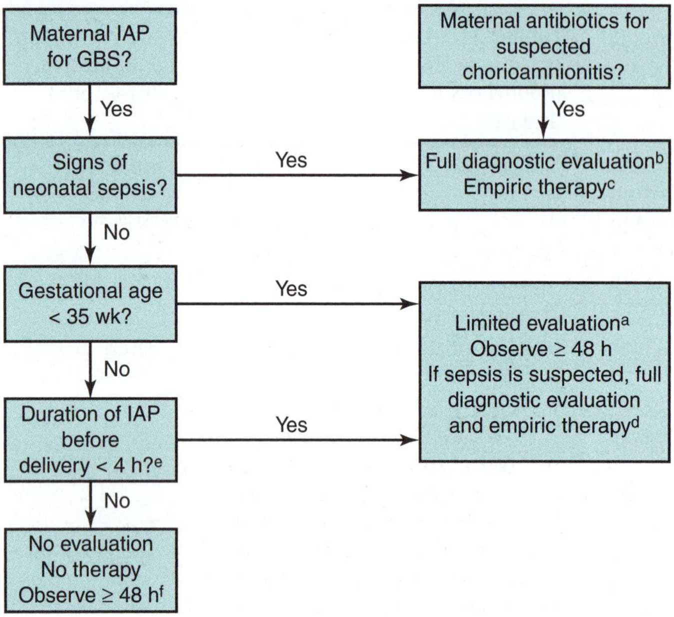

[a] If no maternal intrapartum prophylaxis for GBS was administered despite an indication being present, data are insufficient on which to recommend a single management strategy.

[b] Includes complete blood cell count and differential, blood culture, and chest radiograph if respiratory abnormalities are present. When signs of sepsis are present, a lumbar puncture, if feasible, should be performed.

[c] Duration of therapy varies depending on results of blood culture, cerebrospinal fluid findings, if obtained, and the clinical course of the infant. If laboratory results and clinical course do not indicate bacterial infection, duration may be as short as 48 h.

[d] CBC with differential and blood culture.

[e] Applies only to penicillin, ampicillin, or celazoin and assumes recommended dosing regimens.

[f] A healthy-appearing infant who was 38 weeks' gestation at delivery and whose mother received 4 h of intrapartum prophylaxis before delivery may be discharged home after 24 h if other discharge criteria have been met and a person able to comply fully with instructions for home observation will be present. If any one of these conditions is not met, the infant should be observed in the hospital for at least 48 h and until criteria for discharge are achieved.

▲ **Figure 42–1.** Algorithm for treatment of a newborn whose mother received intrapartum antimicrobial prophylaxis (IAP) for prevention of group B streptococci (GBS) or suspected chorioamnionitis. This algorithm is not an exclusive course of management. Variations that incorporate individual circumstance or institutional preferences may be appropriate. (Reproduced, with permission, from Schrag S et al: Prevention of perinatal group B streptococcal disease, revised guidelines from CDC. MMWR Recomm Rep 2002;51[RR-11]:1.)

ethmoiditis, conjunctivitis, cellulitis (particularly of the face or submandibular area), lymphadenitis, breast abscess, empyema, and impetigo have been described. Strains of GBS possessing the capsular type III polysaccharide antigen are isolated from more than 95% of infants with late-onset disease, regardless of clinical manifestations. The exact mode of transmission of the organisms is not well defined.

C. Laboratory Findings

Culture of GBS from a normally sterile site such as blood, pleural fluid, or CSF provides proof of diagnosis. Frequent false-positive results limit the usefulness of testing for GBS antigen in urine and CSF.

Treatment

Intravenous ampicillin and an aminoglycoside is the initial regimen of choice for newborns with presumptive invasive GBS disease. For neonates younger than 7 days of age with meningitis, the recommended ampicillin dosage is 200–300 mg/kg/d, given intravenously in three divided doses. For infants older than 7 days of age, the recommended ampicillin dosage is 300 mg/kg/d, given intravenously in four divided doses.

Penicillin G can be used alone once GBS is identified and clinical and microbiologic responses have occurred. GBS are less susceptible than other streptococci to penicillin, and high doses are recommended, especially for meningitis. In infants with meningitis, the recommended dosage of penicillin G varies with age: for infants age 7 days or younger, 250,000–450,000 U/kg/d, given intravenously in three divided doses; for infants older than age 7 days, 450,000–500,000 U/kg/d, given intravenously in four to six divided doses.

A second lumbar puncture after 24–48 hours of therapy is recommended by some experts to assess efficacy. Duration of therapy is 2–3 weeks for meningitis; at least 4 weeks for osteomyelitis, cerebritis, ventriculitis, or endocarditis; and 10–14 days for bacteremia and most other infections. Therapy does not eradicate carriage of the organism.

Although streptococci have been universally susceptible to penicillins, increasing minimum inhibitory concentrations (MICs) have been observed in some isolates. In one U.S. study, 10 of 574 rectovaginal isolates obtained from pregnant women in South Carolina were not fully penicillin-susceptible. However, all isolates were vancomycin-susceptible. Resistance of isolates to clindamycin and erythromycin has increased significantly worldwide in the past few years.

Centers for Disease Control and Prevention (CDC): Prevention of Perinatal Group B Streptococcal Disease Revised Guidelines from CDC, 2010. MMWR 2010:59(RR10);1–32.

http://www.cdc.gov/mmwr/preview/mmwrhtml/rr5910a1.htm?s_cid=rr5910a1_w

Centers for Disease Control and Prevention (CDC): Group B Streptococcus Algorithms and Tables. Available at: http://www.cdc.gov/groupbstrep/guidelines/algorithms-tables.html.

STREPTOCOCCAL INFECTIONS WITH ORGANISMS OTHER THAN GROUP A OR B

Streptococci of groups other than A and B are part of the normal flora of humans and can occasionally cause disease. Group C or group G organisms occasionally produce pharyngitis (with an ASO rise), but without risk of subsequent rheumatic fever. AGN may occasionally occur. Group D streptococci and *Enterococcus* species are normal inhabitants of the gastrointestinal tract and may produce urinary tract infections, meningitis, and sepsis in the newborn, as well as endocarditis. Nosocomial infections caused by *Enterococcus* are frequent in neonatal and oncology units and in patients with central venous catheters. Nonhemolytic aerobic streptococci and β-hemolytic streptococci are normal flora of the mouth. They are involved in the production of dental plaque and probably dental caries and are the most common cause of subacute infective endocarditis. Finally, there are numerous anaerobic and microaerophilic streptococci, normal flora of the mouth, skin, and gastrointestinal tract, which alone or in combination with other bacteria may cause sinusitis, dental abscesses, brain abscesses, and intra-abdominal or lung abscesses.

Treatment

A. Enterococcal Infections

Enterococcus faecalis and *Enterococcus faecium* are the two most common and most important strains causing human infections. In general, *E faecalis* is more susceptible to antibiotics than *E faecium*, but antibiotic resistance is commonly seen with both species.

1. Infections with ampicillin-susceptible enterococci— Lower tract urinary infections can be treated with oral amoxicillin. Pyelonephritis should be treated intravenously with ampicillin and gentamicin (gentamicin dosing may need to be adjusted for altered renal function). Sepsis or meningitis in the newborn should be treated intravenously with a combination of ampicillin (100–200 mg/kg/d in three divided doses) and gentamicin (3 mg/kg/d in three divided doses). Peak serum gentamicin levels of 3–5 mcg/mL are adequate as gentamicin is used as a synergistic agent. Endocarditis requires 6 weeks of intravenous treatment. Ampicillin or penicillin in combination with Gentamicin is used in susceptible strains. Consult the American Heart Association guidelines for infective endocarditis for treatment recommendations for endocarditis.

2. Infections with ampicillin-resistant or vancomycin-resistant enterococci—Ampicillin-resistant enterococci are often susceptible to vancomycin (40–60 mg/kg/d in four divided doses). Vancomycin-resistant enterococci are usually also resistant to ampicillin. Two agents are effective against vancomycin-resistant enterococci and approved for use in adults. Quinupristin–dalfopristin (Synercid) is approved for infections with vancomycin-resistant *E faecium* (not effective against *E faecalis*). Linezolid (Zyvox) is approved for vancomycin-resistant *E faecalis* and *E faecium* infections. Both agents are bacteriostatic against enterococci. Isolates resistant to these newer agents have been reported. Infectious disease consultation is recommended when use of these drugs is entertained or when vancomycin-resistant enterococcal infections are identified.

B. Viridans Streptococci Infections (Subacute Infective Endocarditis)

It is important to determine the penicillin sensitivity of the infecting strain as early as possible in the treatment of viridans streptococcal endocarditis. Resistant organisms are most commonly seen in patients receiving penicillin prophylaxis for rheumatic heart disease. Treatment of endocarditis varies depending on whether the patient has native valves or prosthetic valves/material and whether the organism is penicillin susceptible. Refer to the American Heart Guidelines on Infective Endocarditis for a complete discussion and recommendations.

C. Other Viridans Streptococci–Related Infections

Viridans streptococci are normal flora of the gastrointestinal tract, respiratory tract, and the mouth. In many cases, isolation of viridans streptococci from a blood culture is considered to be a "contaminant" in the absence of signs or symptoms of endocarditis or other invasive disease. However, in children who are immunocompromised, have congenital or acquired valvular heart disease, or those who have indwelling lines, these viridans streptococci may be a cause of serious morbidity. About one-third of bacteremias in patients with malignancies may be due to bacteria from the *Streptococcus* viridans group. Mucositis and gastrointestinal toxicity from chemotherapy are among the risk factors for developing disease. Even in children with normal immune systems, viridans streptococci sometimes cause serious infections. For example, viridans streptococci isolated from an abdominal abscess after sustained rupture of the appendix represents a true pathogen. *Streptococcus anginosus,* a member of the *Streptococcus* viridans group, is seen as a cause of intracranial abscess (often as a complication of sinusitis) and abdominal abscesses. In patients with risk factors or signs/symptoms for subacute endocarditis, isolation of one of the members of the *Streptococcus* viridans group should prompt consideration and evaluation for possible endocarditis (see previous section).

Increasing prevalence of antibiotic resistance has been seen over the last 10 years in isolates of the streptococci viridans group. Penicillin resistance varies with geographic region, institution, and the populations tested, but has ranged from 30% to 70% in oncology patients. Cephalosporin resistance is also relatively common. Therefore, it is important to obtain antibiotic susceptibilities to the organism to select effective therapy. Vancomycin, linezolid, and quinupristin-dalfopristin are still effective against most isolates.

Baddour M: Infective endocarditis: Diagnosis and management. Circulation 2005;111:3167 [PMID: 15956145].

Butler KM: Enterococcal infection in children. Semin Pediatr Infect Dis 2006;17:128 [PMID: 16934707].

PNEUMOCOCCAL INFECTIONS

ESSENTIALS OF DIAGNOSIS & TYPICAL FEATURES

- Bacteremia:
  - High fever (> 39.4°C).
  - Leukocytosis (> 15,000/μL).
  - Age 6–24 months.
- Pneumonia:
  - Fever, leukocytosis, and tachypnea.
  - Localized chest pain.
  - Localized or diffuse rales. Chest radiograph may show lobar infiltrate (with effusion).
- Meningitis:
  - Fever, leukocytosis.
  - Bulging fontanelle, neck stiffness.
  - Irritability and lethargy.
- All types:
  - Diagnosis confirmed by cultures of blood, CSF, pleural fluid, or other body fluid.

General Considerations

Sepsis, sinusitis, otitis media, pneumonitis, meningitis, osteomyelitis, cellulitis, arthritis, vaginitis, and peritonitis are all part of a spectrum of pneumococcal infection. Clinical findings that correlate with occult bacteremia in ambulatory patients include age (6–24 months), degree of temperature elevation (> 39.4°C), and leukocytosis (> 15,000/μL). Although each of these findings is in itself nonspecific, a combination of them should arouse suspicion. This constellation of findings in a child who has no focus of infection may be an indication for blood cultures and antibiotic therapy. The cause of most of such bacteremic episodes is pneumococci.

Streptococcus pneumoniae is a common cause of acute purulent otitis media and is the organism responsible for most cases of acute bacterial pneumonia in children. The disease is indistinguishable on clinical grounds from other bacterial pneumonias. Effusions are common, although frank empyema is less common. Abscesses also occasionally occur.

The incidence rate of pneumococcal meningitis has decreased since incorporation of the pneumococcal conjugate vaccine into the infant vaccine schedule. However, pneumococcal meningitis is still more common than *Haemophilus influenzae* type b meningitis. Pneumococcal meningitis, sometimes recurrent, may complicate serious head trauma, particularly if there is persistent leakage of CSF. This has led some physicians to recommend the prophylactic administration of penicillin or other antimicrobials in such cases.

Children with sickle cell disease, other hemoglobinopathies, congenital or acquired asplenia, and some immunoglobulin and complement deficiencies are unusually susceptible to pneumococcal sepsis and meningitis. They often have a catastrophic illness with shock and disseminated intravascular coagulation (DIC). Even with excellent supportive care, the mortality rate is 20%–50%. The spleen is important in the control of pneumococcal infection by clearing organisms from the blood and producing an opsonin that enhances phagocytosis. Autosplenectomy may explain why children with sickle cell disease are at increased risk of developing serious pneumococcal infections. Children with cochlear implants are at higher risk for pneumococcal meningitis.

Children who have, or who are planning to receive, a cochlear implant should receive age-appropriate pneumococcal vaccination (> 2 weeks prior to surgery if possible).

S pneumoniae rarely causes serious disease in the neonate. Although *S pneumoniae* does not normally colonize the vagina, transient colonization does occur. Serious neonatal disease—including pneumonia, sepsis, and meningitis—may occur and clinically is similar to GBS infection.

Historically, penicillin was the agent of choice for pneumococcal infections, and some strains are still highly susceptible to penicillin. However, pneumococci with moderately increased resistance to penicillin are found in most communities. The prevalence of these relatively penicillin-resistant strains in North America varies geographically. Pneumococci with high-level resistance to penicillin and multiple other drugs are increasingly encountered throughout the United States. Pneumococci from normally sterile body fluids should be routinely tested for susceptibility to penicillin as well as other drugs.

Pneumococci have been classified into more than 90 serotypes based on capsular polysaccharide antigens. The frequency distribution of serotypes varies at different times, in different geographic areas, and with different sites of infection. Prior to institution of pneumococcal conjugate vaccine (PCV), serotypes 4, 6B, 9V, 14, 18C, 19F, and 23F caused about 80%–85% of invasive pneumococcal infections in young children. Since routine immunization with PCV-7, serotype 19A is the most common cause of invasive pneumococcal infections in PCV-7 immunized children.

Prevention

The first pneumococcal conjugate vaccine was licensed in the United States in 2000 and was a 7-valent vaccine recommended for immunization of young children. The serotypes in the vaccine caused the bulk of pediatric invasive pneumococcal disease. A 13-valent pneumococcal conjugate vaccine was licensed in 2010. This vaccine confers expanded protection to an additional 6 serotypes, and is the vaccine currently recommended for routine use in the infant and childhood immunization schedule. Use of the protein conjugate vaccine is important in the prevention of pneumococcal disease because young children (age < 2 years), who are most at risk for the disease, are unable to immunologically mount a predictable response to the 23-valent polysaccharide vaccine. The 13-valent vaccine is currently recommended for (1) infant primary series and booster dosing (replaces the 7 valent vaccine), (2) routine vaccination of children aged 2–59 months, and (3) use in children aged 60–71 months who have underlying medical conditions that increase risk for pneumococcal disease or complications. This vaccine is discussed in detail in Chapter 10. For certain children >2 years of age who are at high risk for pneumococcal disease (sickle cell anemia, anatomic or functional asplenia, HIV infected children, and persons with certain chronic illnesses), the 23-valent pneumococcal vaccine is recommended following completion of the pneumococcal conjugate vaccine series (see Chapter 10).

Clinical Findings

A. Symptoms and Signs

In pneumococcal sepsis, fever usually appears abruptly, often accompanied by chills. There may be no respiratory symptoms. In pneumococcal sinusitis, mucopurulent nasal discharge may occur. In infants and young children with pneumonia, fever and tachypnea without auscultatory changes are the usual presenting signs. Respiratory distress is manifested by nasal flaring, chest retractions, and tachypnea. Abdominal pain is common. In older children, the adult form of pneumococcal pneumonia with signs of lobar consolidation may occur, but sputum is rarely bloody. Thoracic pain (from pleural involvement) is sometimes present, but is less common in children. With involvement of the right hemidiaphragm, pain may be referred to the right lower quadrant, suggesting appendicitis. Vomiting is common at onset but seldom persists. Convulsions are relatively common at onset in infants.

Meningitis is characterized by fever, irritability, convulsions, and neck stiffness. The most important sign in very young infants is a tense, bulging anterior fontanelle. In older children, fever, chills, headache, and vomiting are common symptoms. Classic signs are nuchal rigidity associated with positive Brudzinski and Kernig signs. With progression of untreated disease, the child may develop opisthotonos, stupor, and coma.

B. Laboratory Findings

Leukocytosis is often pronounced (20,000–45,000/μL), with 80%–90% polymorphonuclear neutrophils. Neutropenia may be seen early in very serious infections. The presence of pneumococci in the nasopharynx is not a helpful finding, because up to 40% of normal children carry pneumococci in the upper respiratory tract. Large numbers of organisms are seen on Gram-stained smears of endotracheal aspirates from patients with pneumonia. In meningitis, CSF usually shows an elevated white blood cell (WBC) count of several thousand, chiefly polymorphonuclear neutrophils, with decreased glucose and elevated protein levels. Gram-positive diplococci may be seen on some (but not all) stained smears of CSF sediment. Antigen detection tests are not useful.

Differential Diagnosis

There are many causes of high fever and leukocytosis in young infants; 90% of children presenting with these features have a disease other than pneumococcal bacteremia, such as human herpesvirus 6, enterovirus, or other viral infection; urinary tract infection; unrecognized focal infection elsewhere in the body; or early acute shigellosis.

Infants with upper respiratory tract infection who subsequently develop signs of lower respiratory disease are most likely to be infected with a respiratory virus. Hoarseness or wheezing is often present. A radiograph of the chest typically shows perihilar infiltrates and increased bronchovascular markings. Viral respiratory infection often precedes pneumococcal pneumonia; therefore, the clinical picture may be mixed.

Staphylococcal pneumonia may be indistinguishable early in its course from pneumococcal pneumonia. Later, pulmonary cavitation and empyema occur. Staphylococcal pneumonia is most common in infants.

In primary pulmonary tuberculosis, children do not have a toxic appearance, and radiographs show a primary focus associated with hilar adenopathy and often with pleural involvement. Miliary tuberculosis presents a classic radiographic appearance.

Pneumonia caused by *Mycoplasma pneumoniae* is most common in children aged 5 years and older. Onset is insidious, with infrequent chills, low-grade fever, prominent headache and malaise, cough, and, often, striking radiographic changes. Marked leukocytosis (> 18,000/μL) is unusual.

Pneumococcal meningitis is diagnosed by lumbar puncture. Without a Gram-stained smear and culture of CSF, it is not distinguishable from other types of acute bacterial meningitis.

Table 42–2. Penicillin breakpoints (minimum inhibitory concentrations [MIC]) for *Streptococcus pneumoniae* by susceptibility category—Clinical and Laboratory Standards Institute, 2008.

Drug	Clinical Syndrome and Drug Route	Susceptibility Category MIC (mcg/mL)		
		Susceptible	Intermediate	Resistant
Penicillin	Meningitis, intravenous penicillin	≤ 0.06	None*	≥ 0.12
	Nonmeningitis, intravenous penicillin	≤ 2	4	≥ 8
	Nonmeningitis, oral penicillin	≤ 0.06	0.12–1	≥ 2
Cefotaxime or Ceftriaxone	Meningitis, intravenous cefotaxime or ceftriaxone	≤ 0.5	1	≥ 2
	Nonmeningitis, intravenous cefotaxime or ceftriaxone	≤ 1	2	≥ 4

*There is no intermediate category for meningitis.

Complications

Complications of sepsis include meningitis and osteomyelitis; complications of pneumonia include empyema, parapneumonic effusion, and, rarely, lung abscess. Mastoiditis, subdural empyema, and brain abscess may follow untreated pneumococcal otitis media. Both pneumococcal meningitis and peritonitis are more likely to occur independently without coexisting pneumonia. Shock, DIC, and Waterhouse-Friderichsen syndrome resembling meningococcemia are occasionally seen in pneumococcal sepsis, particularly in asplenic patients. Hemolytic-uremic syndrome may occur as a complication of pneumococcal pneumonia or sepsis.

Treatment

A. Specific Measures

All *S pneumoniae* isolated from normally sterile sites should be tested for antimicrobial susceptibility. The term "nonsusceptible" is used to describe both intermediate and resistant isolates. Strains that are nonsusceptible to penicillin, ceftriaxone (or cefotaxime), and other antimicrobials are increasingly common globally. Antimicrobial susceptibility breakpoints for *S pneumoniae* to penicillin and ceftriaxone/cefotaxime are based on whether the patient has meningitis and the drug route (oral vs intravenous), see Table 42–2. Therapy of meningitis, empyema, osteomyelitis, and endocarditis due to nonsusceptible *S pneumoniae* is challenging, because penetration of antimicrobials to these sites is limited. Infectious disease consultation is recommended for advice regarding these problems. For empiric therapy of serious or life-threatening infections pending susceptibility test results, vancomycin and ceftriaxone (or cefotaxime) are recommended.

1. Bacteremia—In studies done prior to immunization of young children with conjugated pneumococcal vaccine, 3%–5% of blood cultures in patients younger than 2 years of age yielded *S pneumoniae*. These percentages decreased with the addition of conjugated pneumococcal vaccine to the vaccine schedule. The current 13-valent pneumococcal vaccine contains antigens to the pneumococcal serotypes that cause about 65% of invasive pneumococcal disease. Many experts treat suspected bacteremia with ceftriaxone (50 mg/kg, given intramuscularly or intravenously). Compared with oral amoxicillin (80–90 mg/kg/d), ceftriaxone may reduce fever and the need for hospitalization. However, meningitis occurs with the same frequency despite presumptive therapy. All children with blood cultures that grow pneumococci should be reexamined as soon as possible. The child who has a focal infection, such as meningitis, or who appears septic should be admitted to the hospital to receive parenteral antimicrobials. If the child is afebrile and appears well or mildly ill, outpatient management is appropriate. Severely ill or immunocompromised children, in whom infection with *S pneumoniae* is suspected, should be treated with vancomycin (if meningitis is also suspected use ceftriaxone or cefotaxime in addition to vancomycin) until the susceptibilities of the organism are known.

2. Pneumonia—For infants (1 month of age or older) with susceptible organisms appropriate regimens include aqueous penicillin G (250,000–400,000 U/kg/d, given intravenously in four to six divided doses), cefotaxime (50 mg/kg every 8 hours), or ceftriaxone (50 mg/kg every 12–24 hours). If susceptibilities are not known and the patient is severely ill or immunocompromised, vancomycin (10 mg/kg every 6 hours) should be used as part of the regimen to provide coverage for penicillin- or cephalosporin-resistant pneumococcus. Once results of susceptibility testing are available, the regimen can be tailored. Mild pneumonia may be treated with amoxicillin (80–90 mg/kg/d) for 7–10 days. Alternative regimens include oral macrolides and cephalosporins.

3. Otitis media—Most experts recommend oral amoxicillin (80–90 mg/kg/d, divided in two doses) as first-line therapy. The standard course of therapy is 10 days; however, many physicians treat uncomplicated, mild cases in children 6 years of age or older for 5–7 days. Treatment failures may be treated with amoxicillin–clavulanate (80–90 mg/kg/d of the amoxicillin component in the 14:1 formulation), intramuscular ceftriaxone, cefuroxime axetil, or cefdinir. Azithromycin can also be used.

4. Meningitis—Until bacteriologic confirmation and susceptibility testing are completed, patients should receive vancomycin (60 mg/kg/d, given intravenously in four divided doses) and cefotaxime (225–300 mg/kg/d intravenously in four divided doses), or vancomycin (see previous dosage) and ceftriaxone (100 mg/kg/d, given intravenously in two divided doses). Patients with beta-lactam antibiotic allergy (penicillins, cephalosporins) can be treated with a combination of vancomycin (see previous dosage) and rifampin (20 mg/kg/day in 2 divided doses). Use of vancomycin alone or use of rifampin alone is not recommended. Corticosteroids (dexamethasone, 0.6 mg/kg/d, in four divided doses for 4 days) are controversial but are recommended by many experts as adjunctive therapy for pneumococcal meningitis. A repeat lumbar puncture at 24–48 hours should be considered to ensure sterility of the CSF if dexamethasone is given, if resistant pneumococci are isolated, or if the patient is not demonstrating expected improvement after 24–48 hours on therapy.

If the isolate is determined to be penicillin-susceptible, aqueous penicillin G can be administered (300,000–400,000 U/kg/d, given intravenously in four to six divided doses for 10–14 days). Alternatively, use of ceftriaxone or cefotaxime is acceptable alternative therapy in penicillin- and cephalosporin-susceptible isolates. Consult an infectious disease specialist or the *Red Book* (American Academy of Pediatrics, 2009) for a complete discussion of pneumococcal meningitis and for therapeutic options for isolates that are nonsusceptible to penicillin or cephalosporins.

Prognosis

In children, case fatality rates of less than 1% should be achieved except for meningitis, where rates of 5%–20% still prevail. The presence of large numbers of organisms without a prominent CSF inflammatory response or meningitis due to a penicillin-resistant strain indicates a poor prognosis. Serious neurologic sequelae, particularly hearing loss, are frequent following pneumococcal meningitis.

Advisory Committee on Immunization Practices: Pneumococcal vaccination for cochlear implant candidates and recipients: Updated recommendations of the Advisory Committee on Immunization Practices. MMWR Morb Mortal Wkly Rep 2003;52:739 [PMID: 12908457].

CDC: ACIP provisional recommendations for use of 13-valent pneumococcal conjugate vaccine (PCV13) among infants and children. Available at: http://www.cdc.gov/vaccines/recs/provisional/downloads/pcv13-mar-2010-508.pdf

CDC: Preventing pneumococcal disease among infants and young children: Recommendations of the Advisory Committee on Immunization Practices (ACIP). MMWR 2000;49(RR-9). http://www.cdc.gov/mmwr/preview/mmwrhtml/rr4909a1.htm#tab8

Pickering LK, Baker CJ, Kimberlin DW, Long SS (editors): *Red Book 2009 Report of the Committee on Infectious Diseases.* 28th ed. Elk Grove Village, IL: American Academy of Pediatrics; 2009.

STAPHYLOCOCCAL INFECTIONS

Staphylococcal infections are common in childhood and range from local mild infections to overwhelming systemic infections. Examples of disease caused by Staphylococci include, but are not limited to, furuncles, carbuncles, scalded skin syndrome, osteomyelitis, pyomyositis, septic arthritis, pneumonia, bacteremia, endocarditis, meningitis, and toxic shock syndrome. Staphylococci are the major cause of osteomyelitis and of septic arthritis and are an uncommon but important cause of bacterial pneumonia. A toxin produced by certain strains causes staphylococcal food poisoning. Staphylococci are responsible for many infections of artificial heart valves. Finally, they are found in infections at all ages and in multiple sites, particularly when infection is introduced from the skin or upper respiratory tract or when closed compartments become infected (pericarditis, sinusitis, cervical adenitis, surgical wounds, abscesses in the liver or brain, and abscesses elsewhere in the body).

Staphylococci that do not produce the enzyme coagulase are termed *coagulase-negative* and are seldom speciated in the clinical microbiology laboratory. Most *S aureus* strains produce coagulase. *S aureus* and coagulase-negative staphylococci are normal flora of the skin and respiratory tract. The latter rarely cause disease except in compromised hosts, the newborn, or patients with plastic indwelling lines.

Most strains of *S aureus* elaborate β-lactamase that confers penicillin resistance. This can be overcome in clinical practice by the use of a cephalosporin or a penicillinase-resistant penicillin, such as methicillin, oxacillin, nafcillin, cloxacillin, or dicloxacillin. Methicillin-resistant *S aureus* (MRSA) are resistant in vivo to all of these penicillinase-resistant penicillins and cephalosporins. MRSA has dramatically increased in prevalence globally as both a health care–associated and a community-associated pathogen. Health care–associated infections are likely to be multidrug resistant. Community-associated MRSA may be susceptible to clindamycin and/or trimethoprim/sulfamethoxazole, but resistance rates to these agents vary widely geographically. MRSA strains with intermediate susceptibility to vancomycin are occurring more frequently and occasionally vancomycin-resistant strains are isolated. The existence of such strains is of concern because of the inherent virulence of most strains of *S aureus* and because of the limited choices for therapy.

S aureus produces a variety of exotoxins, most of which are of uncertain importance. Two toxins are recognized as playing a central role in specific diseases: exfoliatin and staphylococcal enterotoxin. The former is largely responsible for the various clinical presentations of scalded skin syndrome. Enterotoxin causes staphylococcal food poisoning. The exoprotein toxin most commonly associated with TSS has been termed TSST-1. Panton-Valentine leukocidin (PVL) is an exotoxin produced by some clinical isolates of methicillin-susceptible *S aureus* (MSSA) and MRSA strains. PVL is a virulence factor that causes leukocyte destruction and tissue necrosis. PVL-producing *S aureus* strains are often community-acquired, and have most commonly produced boils and abscesses. However, they also have been associated with severe cellulitis, osteomyelitis, and deaths from necrotizing pneumonia in otherwise healthy children and young adults.

Prevention

No licensed vaccines are available. Patients with recurrent skin infections with *S aureus* should practice good skin hygiene to try to prevent recurrences. Keeping fingernails short, good skin hygiene, not sharing towels or other personal items, and use of a clean towel daily may help prevent recurrences.

Clinical Findings

A. Symptoms and Signs

1. Staphylococcal skin diseases—Dermal infection with *S aureus* causes pustules, furuncles, carbuncles, or cellulitis. Community-associated MRSA and MSSA frequently cause skin and soft tissue infections. Currently MRSA furuncles and abscesses are extraordinarily common in clinical practice. Parents initially may think the child has a spider bite. Skin lesions can be seen anywhere on the body but are commonly seen on the buttocks in infants and young children. Factors that facilitate transmission of MRSA or MSSA include crowding, compromised skin (eg, eczema), participation on contact sports teams, day care attendance, bare skin contact with surfaces used by others (exercise mats, sauna benches), and sharing towels or other personal items.

S aureus are often found along with streptococci in impetigo. If the strains produce exfoliatin, localized lesions become bullous (bullous impetigo).

Scalded skin syndrome is a toxin-mediated illness caused by exfoliative toxins A and B produced by certain strains of *S aureus*. The initial infection may begin at any site but is in the respiratory tract in most cases. There is a prodromal phase of erythema, often beginning around the mouth, accompanied by fever and irritability. The involved skin becomes tender, and a sick infant will cry when picked up or touched. A day or so later, exfoliation begins, usually around the mouth. The inside of the mouth is red, and a peeling rash is present around the lips, often in a radial pattern. Generalized, painful peeling may follow, involving the limbs and trunk but often sparing the feet. More commonly, peeling is confined to areas around body orifices. If erythematous but unpeeled skin is rubbed sideways, superficial epidermal layers separate from deeper ones and slough (Nikolsky sign). Generally, if secondary infection does not occur, there is healing without scarring. In the newborn, the disease is termed *Ritter disease* and may be fulminant.

2. Osteomyelitis and septic arthritis—(See Chapter 26.) MRSA invasive disease, including osteomyelitis and septic arthritis is being seen increasingly.

3. Staphylococcal pneumonia—Staphylococcal pneumonia in infancy is characterized by abdominal distention, high fever, respiratory distress, and toxemia. It may occur without predisposing factors or after minor skin infections. The organism is necrotizing, producing bronchoalveolar destruction. Pneumatoceles, pyopneumothorax, and empyema are frequently encountered. Rapid progression of disease is characteristic. Frequent chest radiographs to monitor the progress of disease are indicated. Presenting symptoms may be typical of paralytic ileus, suggestive of an abdominal catastrophe.

Invasive MRSA infections are on the rise and increasing numbers of MRSA pneumonias have been reported in all age groups. Many of these reports are in patients who develop MRSA pneumonia as a complication of influenza. MRSA or MSSA pneumonias are rapidly progressive, severe, and often devastating. Complicated pneumonias are frequent including necrotizing pneumonia, pneumatoceles, and/or empyemas. Purulent pericarditis occurs by direct extension in about 10% of cases, with or without empyema.

4. Staphylococcal food poisoning—Staphylococcal food poisoning is a result of ingestion of enterotoxin produced by staphylococci growing in uncooked and poorly refrigerated food. The disease is characterized by vomiting, prostration, and diarrhea occurring 2–6 hours after ingestion of contaminated foods.

5. Staphylococcal endocarditis—*S aureus* may produce infection of normal heart valves, of valves or endocardium in children with congenital or rheumatic heart disease, or of artificial valves. About 25% of all cases of endocarditis are due to *S aureus*. The great majority of artificial heart valve infections involve either *S aureus* or coagulase-negative staphylococci. Infection usually begins in an extracardiac focus, often the skin. Involvement of the endocardium should be considered when blood cultures grow *S aureus*, particularly when cultures are persistently positive. Suspicion must be highest in the presence of congenital heart disease, particularly ventricular septal defects with aortic insufficiency but also simple ventricular septal defect, patent ductus arteriosus, and tetralogy of Fallot.

The presenting symptoms in staphylococcal endocarditis are fever, weight loss, weakness, muscle pain or diffuse skeletal pain, poor feeding, pallor, and cardiac decompensation. Signs include splenomegaly, cardiomegaly, petechiae, hematuria, and a new or changing murmur. The course of *S aureus* endocarditis is rapid, although subacute disease occurs occasionally. Peripheral septic embolization and uncontrollable cardiac failure are common, even when optimal antibiotic therapy is administered, and may be indications for surgical intervention (see later discussion).

6. Toxic shock syndrome—TSS is characterized by fever, blanching erythroderma, diarrhea, vomiting, myalgia, prostration, hypotension, and multiorgan dysfunction. It is due to *S aureus* focal infection, usually without bacteremia. Large numbers of cases have been described in menstruating adolescents and young women using vaginal tampons. TSS has also been reported in boys and girls with focal staphylococcal infections and in individuals with wound infections due to *S aureus*. Additional clinical features include sudden onset; conjunctival suffusion; mucosal hyperemia; desquamation of skin on the palms, soles, fingers, and toes during convalescence; DIC in severe cases; renal and hepatic functional abnormalities; and myolysis. The mortality rate with early treatment is now about 2%. Recurrences are seen during subsequent menstrual periods in as many as 60% of untreated women who continue to use tampons. Recurrences occur in up to 15% of women given antistaphylococcal antibiotics who stop using tampons. The disease is caused by strains of *S aureus* that produce TSST-1 or one of the related enterotoxins.

7. Coagulase-negative staphylococcal infections—Localized and systemic coagulase-negative staphylococcal infections occur primarily in immunocompromised patients, high-risk newborns, and patients with plastic prostheses or catheters. Coagulase-negative staphylococci are the most common nosocomial pathogen in hospitalized low-birth-weight neonates in the United States. Intravenous administration of lipid emulsions and indwelling central venous catheters are risk factors contributing to coagulase-negative staphylococcal bacteremia in newborn infants. In patients with an artificial heart valve, a Dacron patch, a ventriculoperitoneal shunt, or a central venous catheter, coagulase-negative staphylococci are a common cause of sepsis or catheter infection, often necessitating removal of the foreign material and protracted antibiotic therapy. Because blood cultures are frequently contaminated by this organism, diagnosis of genuine localized or systemic infection is often difficult.

B. Laboratory Findings

Moderate leukocytosis (15,000–20,000/μL) with a shift to the left is occasionally found, although normal counts are common, particularly in infants. The sedimentation rate is elevated. Blood cultures are frequently positive in systemic staphylococcal disease and should always be obtained when it is suspected. Similarly, pus from sites of infection should always be aspirated or obtained surgically, examined with Gram stain, and cultured both aerobically and anaerobically. There are no useful serologic tests for staphylococcal disease.

Differential Diagnosis

Staphylococcal skin disease takes many forms; therefore, the differential list is long. Staphylococcal skin abscesses, furuncles, and carbuncles are often confused initially with a spider bite. Bullous impetigo must be differentiated from chemical or thermal burns, from drug reactions, and, in the very young, from the various congenital epidermolytic syndromes or even herpes simplex infections. Staphylococcal scalded skin syndrome may resemble scarlet fever, Kawasaki disease, Stevens-Johnson syndrome, erythema multiforme, and other drug reactions. A skin biopsy may be critical in establishing the diagnosis. Varicella lesions may become superinfected with exfoliatin-producing staphylococci and produce a combination of the two diseases (bullous varicella).

Severe, rapidly progressing pneumonia with formation of abscesses, pneumatoceles, and empyemas is typical of *S aureus* infection and GAS but may occasionally be produced by pneumococci, *H influenzae*, and GAS.

Staphylococcal food poisoning is often epidemic. It is differentiated from other common-source gastroenteritis syndromes (*Salmonella*, *Clostridium perfringens*, and *Vibrio parahaemolyticus*) by the short incubation period (2–6 hours), the prominence of vomiting (as opposed to diarrhea), and the absence of fever.

Endocarditis is suspected with *S aureus* bacteremia, particularly when a significant heart murmur or preexisting cardiac disease is present. (See Chapter 20.)

Newborn infections with *S aureus* can resemble infections with streptococci and a variety of gram-negative organisms. Umbilical and respiratory tract colonization occurs with many pathogenic organisms (GBS, *Escherichia coli*, and *Klebsiella*), and both skin and systemic infections occur with virtually all of these organisms.

TSS must be differentiated from Rocky Mountain spotted fever, leptospirosis, Kawasaki disease, drug reactions, adenovirus, and measles (see also Table 40–3).

Treatment

A. Specific Measures

Community-acquired MRSA infections are on the rise. The incidence of community-acquired MRSA isolates varies greatly geographically, but in many communities in the United States MRSA is the most common pathogen isolated from patients with skin and soft tissue infections. For empiric coverage of potentially life threatening infections with suspected *Staphylococcus aureus* (in which susceptibilities are not known) initial therapy should include vancomycin in combination with either nafcillin or oxacillin. Antibiotic therapy can then be adjusted based on identification of the organism and susceptibility results.

Currently, most community-acquired MRSA strains are susceptible to trimethoprim–sulfamethoxazole (TMP–SMX) and some are susceptible to clindamycin. Less serious infections in nontoxic patients may be initially treated using one of these agents while awaiting cultures and susceptibility data. Knowledge of the community MRSA susceptibility patterns is useful in guiding empiric therapy while awaiting susceptibility test results.

For MSSA strains, a β-lactamase–resistant penicillin is the drug of choice (oxacillin, nafcillin, or methicillin). In serious systemic disease, in osteomyelitis, and in the treatment of large abscesses, intravenous therapy is indicated initially (oxacillin or nafcillin, 100–150 mg/kg/d in four divided doses, or methicillin, 200–300 mg/kg/d in four divided doses). When high doses over a long period are required, it is preferable to avoid use of methicillin, because of the frequency with which interstitial nephritis occurs. In serious or life-threatening illness, an aminoglycoside antibiotic (gentamicin or tobramycin) or rifampin may be used in addition for its possible synergistic action. Consultation with an infectious disease physician is recommended in these situations.

Cephalosporins may be considered for MSSA infections in patients with a history of penicillin sensitivity unless there is a history of type 1 hypersensitivity reaction (ie, anaphylaxis, wheezing, edema, and hives). Cefazolin, 100–150 mg/kg/d, given intravenously in three divided doses, or cephalexin, 50–100 mg/kg/d, given orally in four divided doses, can be used once a child is able to take oral antibiotics. The third-generation cephalosporins should not generally be used for staphylococcal infections.

For nonmeningeal, suspected nosocomially acquired MRSA infections, vancomycin (40 mg/kg/d intravenously in three or four divided doses) should be used until results of susceptibility testing are available (frequently clindamycin and TMP–SMX–resistant). Infections due to MRSA do not respond to cephalosporins despite in vitro testing that suggests susceptibility. For treatment of meningitis, vancomycin must be given in higher doses (60 mg/kg/d divided into four doses). The addition of rifampin is advocated by some (rifampin should not be used alone to treat this condition).

1. Skin infections—Treatment of skin and soft tissue infections depends, in part, on the extent of the lesion, immunocompetence of the host, and the toxicity of the patient. Afebrile, well-appearing patients with small abscesses may do well with incision and drainage (with or without the addition of oral antimicrobials). More serious infections or infections in immunocompromised patients should be treated more aggressively. Hospitalization and intravenous antibiotics may be required. Culture and susceptibility testing help guide therapy regardless of whether the patient initially is started on antibiotics. Results of these tests facilitate therapeutic decisions in cases in which patients do not respond to initial management or empiric intravenous antibiotic therapy was initiated.

For patients who are not sick enough to require hospitalization or intravenous therapy, selection of the best empiric antimicrobial depends on local rates of MRSA and local susceptibilities. β-Lactam antibiotics, such as penicillins and cephalosporins, can no longer be depended on as single agents for the majority of cases in communities with high MRSA rates. TMP–SMX and clindamycin (depending on local susceptibility patterns) may be used for empiric staphylococcal coverage. However, GAS are generally resistant to TMP–SMX and in a small number of cases may also be resistant to clindamycin. Many clinicians empirically use a combination of TMP–SMX and cefazolin for initial treatment until susceptibilities are known. Linezolid is another option, although the cost of this drug is high.

2. Osteomyelitis and septic arthritis—Treatment should be begun intravenously, with antibiotics selected to cover the most likely organisms (staphylococci in hematogenous osteomyelitis; meningococci, pneumococci, staphylococci in children younger than age 3 years with septic arthritis; staphylococci and gonococci in older children with septic arthritis). Knowledge of local MRSA rates will help guide empiric therapy. Antibiotic levels should be kept high at all times.

In osteomyelitis, clinical studies support the use of intravenous treatment until fever and local symptoms and signs have subsided—usually after at least 3–5 days—followed by oral therapy (for susceptible strains, dicloxacillin, 100–150 mg/kg/d in four divided doses; or cephalexin, 100–150 mg/kg/d in four divided doses) for at least 3 additional weeks. Longer treatment may be required, particularly when radiographs show extensive involvement. Treatment of community-acquired MRSA osteomyelitis should be based on susceptibility results; however, isolates are frequently susceptible to TMP–SMX or clindamycin. Vancomycin can be used as part of an empiric regimen while awaiting susceptibilities in seriously ill patients or in areas where MRSA rates are high. In arthritis, where drug diffusion into synovial fluid is good, intravenous therapy need be given only for a few days, followed by adequate oral therapy for at least 3 weeks. In all instances, oral therapy should be administered with careful attention to compliance, either in the hospital or at home.

The erythrocyte sedimentation rate (ESR) is a good indicator of response to therapy. Surgical drainage of osteomyelitis or septic arthritis is often required. (See Chapter 26.)

3. Staphylococcal pneumonia—In the few areas of the country where MRSA is not prevalent, or if the isolate is known to be MSSA, nafcillin and oxacillin are the usual drugs of choice. Vancomycin can be used empirically until results of cultures and susceptibility tests are obtained. Linezolid has recently been reported to be as efficacious as vancomycin for the treatment of resistant gram-positive pneumonia and soft tissue infections (cure rates: 95% linezolid vs 94% vancomycin).

Empyema and pyopneumothorax require drainage. The choice of chest tube versus thoracoscopic drainage depends on the practitioner's experience and skill. If staphylococcal pneumonia is treated promptly and empyema drained, resolution in children often is complete.

4. Staphylococcal food poisoning—Therapy is supportive and usually not required except in severe cases or for small infants with marked dehydration.

5. Staphylococcal endocarditis—The treatment of Staphylococcal endocarditis depends on whether the patient has a prosthetic valve or material in the heart and on the susceptibilities of the organism. High-dose, prolonged parenteral treatment is indicated. Methicillin-susceptible isolates, in the absence of prosthetic material, are often treated with oxacillin or nafcillin. Some experts also recommend addition of gentamicin for the first 3–5 days. In penicillin-allergic patients (type 1 hypersensitivity or anaphylaxis) or patients with MRSA isolates, vancomycin should be used.

For patients (without penicillin allergy) with prosthetic material in the heart and who have methicillin susceptible isolates, nafcillin (or oxacillin) plus rifampin is used; gentamicin is added during the first 2 weeks. For patients with MRSA endocarditis with prosthetic material present, vancomycin plus rifampin is recommended; gentamicin is added for the first 2 weeks. Therapy lasts in all instances for at least 6 weeks. Please see the American Heart Association's Guidelines on Infective Endocarditis: Diagnosis and Management and consult an infectious disease physician for this serious and sometimes complicated problem.

Occasionally, medical treatment fails. Signs of treatment failure are (1) recurrent fever without apparent treatable other cause (eg, thrombophlebitis, respiratory or urinary tract infection, drug fever), (2) persistently positive blood cultures, (3) intractable and progressive congestive heart failure, and (4) recurrent (septic) embolization. In such circumstances—particularly (2), (3), and (4)—evaluation for valve replacement becomes necessary. Antibiotics are continued for at least another 4 weeks. Persistent or recurrent infection may require a second surgical procedure.

6. Toxic shock syndrome—Treatment is aimed at expanding blood volume, maintaining perfusion pressure with inotropic agents, ensuring prompt drainage of a focus of infection (or removal of tampons or foreign bodies), and giving intravenous antibiotics.

Vancomycin, in addition to a β-lactam antibiotic (oxacillin or nafcillin), can be used for empiric therapy. Some experts also add clindamycin, since clindamycin is a protein synthesis inhibitor and may turn off toxin production. Clindamycin should not be used empirically as a single agent until susceptibilities (when an isolate grows) are known; some strains of *S aureus* are clindamycin-resistant.

Intravenous immune globulin has been used as adjunctive therapy. Some experts believe that corticosteroid therapy may be effective if given to patients with severe illness early in the course of their disease. Successful antibiotic treatment reduces risk of recurrence.

7. Vancomycin-resistant *S aureus* infections (VRSA)—Reports of VRSA isolates are rare but are likely to increase in frequency in the future. Such isolates are sometimes susceptible to clindamycin or TMP–SMX. If not, therapeutic options are limited and include use of quinupristin–dalfopristin, linezolid, and daptomycin. Experience is very limited with daptomycin in pediatric patients. Consultation with an infectious disease specialist is recommended.

8. Coagulase-negative staphylococcal infections—Bacteremia and other serious coagulase-negative staphylococcal infections are treated initially with vancomycin. Coagulase-negative staphylococci are uncommonly resistant to vancomycin. (See Chapter 39 for dosing.) Strains susceptible to methicillin are treated with methicillin, oxacillin, or cefazolin.

Baddour M: Infective Endocarditis: Diagnosis and Management. Circulation 2005;111:3167 [PMID: 15956145]. Available at: http://circ.ahajournals.org/content/111/23/e394.full.pdf

Daum RS: Clinical practice. Skin and soft-tissue infections caused by methicillin-resistant *Staphylococcus aureus*. N Engl J Med 2007;357:380 [PMID: 17652653].

Liu et al: Clinical Practice Guidelines by the Infectious Diseases Society of America for the Treatment of Methicillin-Resistant Staphylococcus Aureus Infections in Adults and Children. Clin Infect Dis 2011;52:285–322 [PMID: 21217178]. Available at: http://cid.oxfordjournals.org/content/52/3/e18.long

MENINGOCOCCAL INFECTIONS

ESSENTIALS OF DIAGNOSIS & TYPICAL FEATURES

- Fever, headache, vomiting, convulsions, shock (meningitis).
- Fever, shock, petechial or purpuric skin rash (meningococcemia).
- Diagnosis confirmed by culture of normally sterile body fluids.

General Considerations

Meningococci (*Neisseria meningitidis*) may be carried asymptomatically for many months in the upper respiratory tract. Less than 1% of carriers develop disease. Meningitis and sepsis are the two most common forms of illness, but septic arthritis, pericarditis, pneumonia, chronic meningococcemia, otitis media, conjunctivitis, and vaginitis also occur. The incidence of invasive diseases in the United States is about 1.2 cases per 100,000 people. An estimated 2400–3000 cases occur in the United States annually. The highest attack rate for meningococcal meningitis is in the first year of life. There also is an elevated attack rate during the teen years. The development of irreversible shock with multiorgan failure is a significant factor in the fatal outcome of acute meningococcal infections.

Meningococci are gram-negative organisms containing endotoxin in their cell walls. Endotoxins cause capillary vascular injury and leak as well as DIC. Meningococci are classified serologically into groups: A, B, C, Y, and W-135 are the groups most commonly implicated in systemic disease. The serologic groups serve as markers for studying outbreaks and transmission of disease. Currently in the United States, serogroups B, C, and Y each account for about 30% of cases. Serogroup A causes periodic epidemics in developing countries, but only occasionally is associated with cases of meningococcal disease in the United States. Sulfonamide resistance is common in non–serotype-A strains. *N meningitidis* with increased MICs to penicillin G are reported from South Africa and Spain. A small number of these isolates are reported in the United States. The resistance in these strains is low-level and not due to β-lactamase. Resistant isolates are susceptible to third-generation cephalosporins. Few isolates are resistant to rifampin.

Children develop immunity from asymptomatic carriage of meningococci (usually nontypeable, nonpathogenic strains) or other cross-reacting bacteria. Patients deficient in one of the late components of complement (C6, C7, C8, or C9) are uniquely susceptible to meningococcal infection, particularly group A meningococci. Deficiencies of early and alternate pathway complement components also are associated with increased susceptibility.

Clinical Findings

A. Symptoms and Signs

Many children with clinical meningococcemia also have meningitis, and some have other foci of infection. All children with suspected meningococcemia should have a lumbar puncture.

1. Meningococcemia—A prodrome of upper respiratory infection is followed by high fever, headache, nausea, marked toxicity, and hypotension. Purpura, petechiae, and occasionally bright pink, tender macules or papules over the extremities and trunk are seen. The rash usually progresses rapidly. Occasional cases lack rash. Fulminant meningococcemia (Waterhouse-Friderichsen syndrome) progresses rapidly and is characterized by DIC, massive skin and mucosal hemorrhages, and shock. This syndrome also may be caused by *H influenzae, S pneumoniae,* or other bacteria. Chronic meningococcemia is characterized by periodic bouts of fever, arthralgia or arthritis, and recurrent petechiae. Splenomegaly often is present. Patients may be free of symptoms between bouts. Chronic meningococcemia occurs primarily in adults and mimics Henoch-Schönlein purpura.

2. Meningitis—In many children, meningococcemia is followed within a few hours to several days by symptoms and signs of acute purulent meningitis, with severe headache, stiff neck, nausea, vomiting, and stupor. Children with meningitis generally fare better than children with meningococcemia alone, probably because they have survived long enough to develop clinical signs of meningitis.

B. Laboratory Findings

The peripheral WBC count may be either low or elevated. Thrombocytopenia may be present with or without DIC. (See Chapter 30.) If petechial or hemorrhagic lesions are present, meningococci can sometimes be seen microscopically in tissue fluid expressed from a punctured lesion. CSF is generally cloudy and contains more than 1000 WBCs/μL, with many polymorphonuclear neutrophils and gram-negative intracellular diplococci. A total hemolytic complement assay may reveal absence of late components as an underlying cause.

Differential Diagnosis

The skin lesions of *H influenzae* or pneumococci, enterovirus infection, endocarditis, leptospirosis, Rocky Mountain spotted fever, other rickettsial diseases, Henoch-Schönlein purpura, and blood dyscrasias may be similar to meningococcemia. Severe *S aureus* sepsis has been reported in some patients to present with purpura. Other causes of sepsis and meningitis are distinguished by appropriate Gram stain and cultures.

Complications

Meningitis may lead to permanent central nervous system (CNS) damage, with deafness, convulsions, paralysis, or impaired intellectual function. Hydrocephalus may develop and requires ventriculoperitoneal shunt. Subdural collections of fluid are common but usually resolve spontaneously. Extensive skin necrosis, loss of digits or extremities, intestinal hemorrhage, and late adrenal insufficiency may complicate fulminant meningococcemia.

Prevention

A. Chemoprophylaxis

Household contacts, day care center contacts, and hospital personnel directly exposed to the respiratory secretions of patients are at increased risk for developing meningococcal infection and should be given chemoprophylaxis with rifampin. The secondary attack rate among household members is 1%–5% during epidemics and less than 1% in nonepidemic situations. Children between the ages of 3 months and 2 years are at greatest risk, presumably because they lack protective antibodies. Secondary cases may occur in day care centers and in classrooms. Hospital personnel are not at increased risk unless they have had contact with a patient's oral secretions, for example, during mouth-to-mouth resuscitation, intubation, or suctioning procedures. Approximately 50% of secondary cases in households have their onset within 24 hours of identification of the index case. Exposed contacts should be notified promptly. If they are febrile, they should be fully evaluated and given high doses of penicillin or another effective antimicrobial pending the results of blood cultures.

All high-risk contacts should receive chemoprophylaxis for meningococcal disease as soon as an index case is identified. High risk contacts are defined as:

- All household contacts (especially children < 2 yrs of age)
- Persons with child care or preschool contact with the index patient at any time in the 7 days prior to illness onset
- Persons with direct exposure to index patients secretions (sharing of drinks, straws, cigarettes, toothbrushes, eating utensils, kissing, etc) at any time in the 7 days prior to illness onset
- Persons who have performed mouth-to-mouth resuscitation or performed unprotected endotracheal intubation of the index patient at any time in the 7 days prior to illness onset
- Persons who have slept in the same dwelling as the index patient within 7 days of illness onset
- Passengers who were seated directly next to the index patient on a flight of more than 8 hours duration.

The most commonly used agent for meningococcal chemoprophylaxis is rifampin, given orally in the following dosages twice daily for 2 days: 600 mg for adults; 10 mg/kg for children *older* than 1 month (maximum dosage 600 mg); and 5 mg/kg for infants *younger* than 1 month. Rifampin may stain a patient's tears (and contact lenses), sweat, and urine orange; it may also affect the reliability of oral contraceptives, and alternative contraceptive measures should therefore be employed when rifampin is administered. Rifampin should not be given to pregnant women. Instead, intramuscular ceftriaxone is the preferred agent: 125 mg given as a single dose if the patient is younger than 15 years; 250 mg given as a single dose if older than 15 years. Penicillin and most other antibiotics (even with parenteral administration) are not effective chemoprophylactic agents, because they do not eradicate upper respiratory tract carriage of meningococci. Ciprofloxacin (20 mg/kg as a single dose, maximum dose 500 mg) effectively eradicates nasopharyngeal carriage in adults and children but is not approved for use in children or in pregnant women. Throat cultures to identify carriers are not useful.

B. Vaccine

Two types of vaccines are currently licensed in the United States. A quadrivalent polysaccharide vaccine (MSPV-4) prepared from purified meningococcal polysaccharides (A, C, Y, and W-135) is available in the United States for children older than 2 years of age. Quadrivalent meningococcal conjugate vaccines (see Chapter 10) are licensed for use in children and adults between the ages of 9 months and 55 years, and meningococcal conjugate vaccine is preferred over the polysaccharide vaccine. In general, conjugate vaccines provide longer-lasting immunity and a more robust immune response than polysaccharide vaccines. See Chapter 10 for a discussion on meningococcal vaccines.

Treatment

Blood cultures should be obtained for all children with fever and purpura or other signs of meningococcemia, and antibiotics should be administered immediately as an emergency procedure. There is a good correlation between survival rates and prompt initiation of antibiotic therapy. Purpura and fever should be considered a medical emergency.

Children with meningococcemia or meningococcal meningitis should be treated as though shock were imminent even if their vital signs are stable when they are first seen. If hypotension already is present, supportive measures should be aggressive, because the prognosis is grave in such situations. Treatment should be started emergently and in an intensive care setting but should not be delayed for the sake of transporting the patient. Shock may worsen following antimicrobial therapy due to endotoxin release. To minimize the risk of nosocomial transmission, patients should be placed in respiratory isolation for the first 24 hours of antibiotic treatment.

A. Specific Measures

Antibiotics should be initiated promptly. Because other bacteria, such as *S pneumoniae, S aureus,* or other gram-negative organisms, can cause identical syndromes, initial therapy should be broad. Vancomycin and cefotaxime (or ceftriaxone) are preferred initial coverage. Once *N meningitidis* has been isolated, penicillin G, cefotaxime, or ceftriaxone intravenously for 7 days are the drugs of choice. Relative penicillin resistance is uncommon but has been reported in the United States.

B. General Measures

Most cases of invasive meningococcal disease are treated with intravenous antibiotics for 7 days.

1. Cardiovascular—(See Chapter 14 for management of septic shock.) Corticosteroids are not beneficial. Sympathetic blockade and topically applied nitroglycerin have been used locally to improve perfusion.

2. Hematologic—Adjunctive therapy with heparin is controversial. Because hypercoagulability is frequently present in patients with meningococcemia, some experts believe heparin should be considered for those with DIC. A loading dose of 50 U/kg is followed by 15 U/kg/h as a continuous infusion. The patient is monitored by following the partial thromboplastin time and heparin assay. Recombinant tissue plasminogen activator, concentrated antithrombin III, and recombinant protein-C infusions have been tried experimentally to reverse coagulopathy. (See Chapter 30 for the management of DIC.)

Prognosis

Unfavorable prognostic features include shock, DIC, and extensive skin lesions. The case fatality rate in fulminant meningococcemia is over 30%. In uncomplicated meningococcal meningitis, the fatality rate is much lower (10%–20%).

Bilukha OO, Rosenstein N; National Center for Infectious Diseases, Centers for Disease Control and Prevention (CDC): Prevention and control of meningococcal disease. Recommendations of the Advisory Committee on Immunization Practices (ACIP). MMWR Recomm Rep 2005;54(RR-7):1 [PMID: 15917737]. Available at: http://www.cdc.gov/mmwr/preview/mmwrhtml/rr5407a1.htm

Brayer AF, Humiston SF: Invasive meningococcal disease in childhood. Pediatrics in Review 2011;32:152–161.

GONOCOCCAL INFECTIONS

ESSENTIALS OF DIAGNOSIS & TYPICAL FEATURES

- Purulent urethral discharge with intracellular gram negative diplococci on smear in male patients (usually adolescents).
- Purulent, edematous, sometimes hemorrhagic conjunctivitis with intracellular gram-negative diplococci in 2- to 4-day-old infants.
- Fever, arthritis (often polyarticular) or tenosynovitis, and maculopapular peripheral rash that may be vesiculopustular or hemorrhagic.
- Positive culture of blood, pharyngeal, or genital secretions.

General Considerations

Neisseria gonorrhoeae is a gram-negative diplococcus. Although morphologically similar to other neisseriae, it differs in its ability to grow on selective media and to ferment carbohydrates. The cell wall of *N gonorrhoeae* contains endotoxin, which is liberated when the organism dies and is responsible for the production of a cellular exudate. The incubation period is short, usually 2–5 days.

Nearly 301,000 cases of gonorrhea were reported in the United States in 2009. Gonococcal disease in children may be transmitted sexually or nonsexually. Prepubertal gonococcal infection outside the neonatal period should be considered presumptive evidence of sexual contact or child abuse. Prepubertal girls usually manifest gonococcal vulvovaginitis because of the neutral to alkaline pH of the vagina and thin vaginal mucosa.

In the adolescent or adult, the workup of every case of gonorrhea should include a careful and accurate inquiry into the patient's sexual practices, because pharyngeal infection resulting from oral sex must be detected if present and may be difficult to eradicate. Efforts should be made to identify and provide treatment to all sexual contacts. When prepubertal children are infected, epidemiologic investigation should be thorough.

Antimicrobial-resistant gonococci are a serious problem. *N gonorrhoeae* infections resistant to tetracyclines, penicillins, and fluoroquinolones are common. Fluoroquinolone antimicrobials are no longer recommended for therapy in the United States. In some cases, clinicians will have very limited choices for therapy. Many clinical laboratories do not routinely perform antimicrobial susceptibility tests on *N gonorrhoeae*, and many infections are documented by nonculture methods.

Clinical Findings

A. Symptoms and Signs

1. Asymptomatic gonorrhea—The ratio of asymptomatic to symptomatic gonorrheal infections in adolescents and adults is probably 3–4:1 in women and 0.5–1:1 in men. Asymptomatic infections are as infectious as symptomatic ones.

2. Uncomplicated genital gonorrhea

A. MALE WITH URETHRITIS—Urethral discharge is sometimes painful and bloody and may be white, yellow, or green. There may be associated dysuria. The patient usually is afebrile.

B. PREPUBERTAL FEMALE WITH VAGINITIS—The only clinical findings initially may be dysuria and polymorphonuclear neutrophils in the urine. Vulvitis characterized by erythema, edema, and excoriation accompanied by a purulent discharge may follow.

C. POSTPUBERTAL FEMALE WITH CERVICITIS—Symptomatic disease is characterized by a purulent, foul-smelling vaginal discharge, dysuria, and occasionally dyspareunia. Fever and abdominal pain are absent. The cervix is frequently hyperemic and tender when touched. This tenderness is not worsened by moving the cervix, nor are the adnexa tender to palpation.

d. Rectal gonorrhea—Rectal gonorrhea often is asymptomatic. There may be purulent discharge, edema, and pain during evacuation.

3. Pharyngeal gonorrhea—Pharyngeal infection usually is asymptomatic. There may be some sore throat and, rarely, acute exudative tonsillitis with bilateral cervical lymphadenopathy and fever.

4. Conjunctivitis and iridocyclitis—Copious, usually purulent exudate is characteristic of gonococcal conjunctivitis. Newborns are symptomatic on days 2–4 of life. In the adolescent or adult, infection probably is spread from infected genital secretions by the fingers.

5. Pelvic inflammatory disease (salpingitis)—The interval between initiation of genital infection and its ascent to the uterine tubes is variable and may range from days to months. Menses frequently are the initiating factor. With the onset of a menstrual period, gonococci invade the endometrium, causing transient endometritis. Subsequently salpingitis may occur, resulting in pyosalpinx or hydrosalpinx. Rarely infection progresses to peritonitis or perihepatitis. Gonococcal salpingitis occurs in an acute, a subacute, or a chronic form. All three forms have in common tenderness on gentle movement of the cervix and bilateral tubal tenderness during pelvic examination.

Gonococci or *Chlamydia trachomatis* are the cause of about 50% of cases of pelvic inflammatory disease. A mixed infection caused by enteric bacilli, *Bacteroides fragilis,* or other anaerobes occur in the other 50%.

6. Gonococcal perihepatitis (Fitz-Hugh and Curtis syndrome)—In the typical clinical pattern, the patient presents with right upper quadrant tenderness in association with signs of acute or subacute salpingitis. Pain may be pleuritic and referred to the shoulder. Hepatic friction rub is a valuable but inconstant sign.

7. Disseminated gonorrhea—Dissemination follows asymptomatic more often than symptomatic genital infection and often results from gonococcal pharyngitis or anorectal gonorrhea. The most common form of disseminated gonorrhea is polyarthritis or polytenosynovitis, with or without dermatitis. Monarticular arthritis is less common, and gonococcal endocarditis and meningitis are fortunately rare.

a. Polyarthritis—Disease usually begins with the simultaneous onset of low-grade fever, polyarthralgia, and malaise. After a day or so, joint symptoms become acute. Swelling, redness, and tenderness occur, frequently over the wrists, ankles, and knees but also in the fingers, feet, and other peripheral joints. Skin lesions may be noted at the same time. Discrete, tender, maculopapular lesions 5–8 mm in diameter appear that may become vesicular, pustular, and then hemorrhagic. They are few in number and noted on the fingers, palms, feet, and other distal surfaces and may be single or multiple. In patients with this form of the disease, blood cultures are often positive, but joint fluid rarely yields organisms. Skin lesions often are positive by Gram stain but rarely by culture. Genital, rectal, and pharyngeal cultures must be performed.

b. Monarticular arthritis—In this somewhat less common form of disseminated gonorrhea, fever is often absent. Arthritis evolves in a single joint. Dermatitis usually does not occur. Systemic symptoms are minimal. Blood cultures are negative, but joint aspirates may yield gonococci on smear and culture. Genital, rectal, and pharyngeal cultures must be performed.

B. Laboratory Findings

Demonstration of gram-negative, kidney-shaped diplococci in smears of urethral exudate in males is presumptive evidence of gonorrhea. Positive culture confirms the diagnosis. Negative smears do not rule out gonorrhea. Gram-stained smears of cervical or vaginal discharge in girls are more difficult to interpret because of normal gram-negative flora, but they may be useful when technical personnel are experienced. In girls with suspected gonorrhea, both the cervical os and the anus should be cultured. Gonococcal pharyngitis requires culture for diagnosis.

Cultures for *N gonorrhoeae* are plated on a selective chocolate agar containing antibiotics (eg, Thayer-Martin agar) to suppress normal flora. If bacteriologic diagnosis is critical, suspected material should be cultured on chocolate agar as well. Because gonococci are labile, agar plates should be inoculated immediately and placed without delay in an atmosphere containing CO_2 (candle jar). When transport of specimens is necessary, material should be inoculated directly into Transgrow medium prior to shipment to an appropriate laboratory. In cases of possible sexual molestation, notify the laboratory that definite speciation is needed, because nongonococcal *Neisseria* species can grow on the selective media.

Nucleic acid amplification tests on urine or genital specimens now enable detection of *N gonorrhoeae* and *C trachomatis*. These tests have excellent sensitivity and are replacing culture in many laboratories. All children or adolescents with a suspected or established diagnosis of gonorrhea should have serologic tests for syphilis and HIV.

Differential Diagnosis

Urethritis in the male may be gonococcal or nongonococcal (NGU). NGU is a syndrome characterized by discharge (rarely painful), mild dysuria, and a subacute course. The discharge is usually scant or moderate in amount but may be profuse. *C trachomatis* is the only proven cause of NGU.

Doxycycline (100 mg orally twice a day for 7 days) is efficacious. Single-dose azithromycin, 1 g orally, may achieve better compliance. *C trachomatis* has been shown to cause epididymitis in males and salpingitis in females.

Vulvovaginitis in a prepubertal female may be due to infection caused by miscellaneous bacteria, including *Shigella* and GAS, *Candida,* and herpes simplex. Discharges may be caused by trichomonads, *Enterobius vermicularis* (pin-worm), or foreign bodies. Symptom-free discharge (leukorrhea) normally accompanies rising estrogen levels.

Cervicitis in a postpubertal female, alone or in association with urethritis and involvement of Skene and Bartholin glands, may be due to infection caused by *Candida,* herpes simplex, *Trichomonas,* or discharge resulting from inflammation caused by foreign bodies (usually some form of contraceptive device). Leukorrhea may be associated with birth control pills.

Salpingitis may be due to infection with other organisms. The symptoms must be differentiated from those of appendicitis, urinary tract infection, ectopic pregnancy, endometriosis, or ovarian cysts or torsion.

Disseminated gonorrhea presents a differential diagnosis that includes meningococcemia, acute rheumatic fever, Henoch-Schönlein purpura, juvenile rheumatoid arthritis, lupus erythematosus, leptospirosis, secondary syphilis, certain viral infections (particularly rubella, but also enteroviruses and parvovirus), serum sickness, type B hepatitis (in the prodromal phase), infective endocarditis, and even acute leukemia and other types of cancer. The fully evolved skin lesions of disseminated gonorrhea are remarkably specific, and genital, rectal, or pharyngeal cultures, plus cultures of blood and joint fluid, usually yield gonococci from at least one source.

Prevention

Prevention of gonorrhea is principally a matter of sex education, condom use, and identification and treatment of contacts.

Treatment

A. Uncomplicated Urethral, Endocervical, or Rectal Gonococcal Infections in Adolescents

Ceftriaxone (250 mg intramuscularly in a single dose) or cefixime (400 mg orally in a single dose), and doxycycline (100 mg orally twice a day for 7 days), or azithromycin (1 g orally in a single dose) is recommended unless *C trachomatis* is ruled out. Ceftizoxime, cefotaxime, and cefotetan parenterally are alternative single-dose therapies. Fluoroquinolones are no longer recommended for therapy due to increasing rates of resistance.

Tetracyclines should be avoided in pregnancy, and repeated doses may stain the teeth of young children. Erythromycin or amoxicillin is recommended for therapy of *C trachomatis* in pregnant women; azithromycin is an alternative regimen. Repeat testing 3 weeks after completion of therapy is recommended in pregnant women.

Spectinomycin (2 g intramuscularly in a single dose) is used for penicillin- and cephalosporin-allergic patients, but is not currently available in the United States. A repeat culture after completion of therapy is not necessary in asymptomatic adolescents after the ceftriaxone–doxycycline regimen. A repeat culture after completion of therapy should be obtained from infants and children.

B. Pharyngeal Gonococcal Infection

Ceftriaxone (250 mg intramuscularly in a single dose) and Azithromycin 1 gram is a single dose or Doxycycline 100 mg twice daily for 7 days should be used; neither spectinomycin nor amoxicillin is recommended.

C. Disseminated Gonorrhea

Recommended regimens include ceftriaxone (1 g intramuscularly or intravenously once daily) or cefotaxime (1 g intravenously every 8 hours or ceftixozime (1 g intravenously every 8 hours). Oral therapy may follow parenteral therapy 24–48 hours after improvement. Recommended regimens include cefixime (400 mg) twice daily to complete 7 days of therapy. Fluoroquinolones are not recommended. If concurrent infection with *Chlamydia* is present or has not been excluded, a course of doxycycline, azithromycin, or erythromycin should also be prescribed.

D. Pelvic Inflammatory Disease

Doxycycline (100 mg twice a day orally) and either cefoxitin (2 g intramuscularly or intravenously every 6 hours) or cefotetan (2 g intramuscularly or intravenously every 12 hours) are given until the patient is clinically improved, then doxycycline is administered by mouth to complete 14 days of therapy. Clindamycin and gentamicin given intravenously until the patient improves clinically may be used rather than cefoxitin. Many other regimens have been used for therapy of pelvic inflammatory disease, although comparative efficacy data are limited.

E. Prepubertal Gonococcal Infections

1. Uncomplicated genitourinary, rectal, or pharyngeal infections—These infections may be treated with ceftriaxone (50 mg/kg/d to a maximum of 125 mg intramuscularly in a single dose). Children older than age 8 years should also receive doxycycline (100 mg orally twice daily for 7 days). The physician should evaluate all children for evidence of sexual abuse and coinfection with syphilis, *Chlamydia,* and HIV.

2. Disseminated gonorrhea—This should be treated with ceftriaxone (50 mg/kg once daily parenterally for 7 days).

Centers for Disease Control and Prevention (CDC) et al: Sexually transmitted diseases treatment guidelines, 2010. MMWR 2010;59(RR12):1 [PMID: 21160459].

BOTULISM

ESSENTIALS OF DIAGNOSIS & TYPICAL FEATURES

- Dry mucous membranes.
- Nausea and vomiting.
- Diplopia; dilated, unreactive pupils.
- Descending paralysis.
- Difficulty in swallowing and speech occurring within 12–36 hours after ingestion of toxin-contaminated food.
- Multiple cases in a family or group.
- Hypotonia and constipation in infants.
- Diagnosis by clinical findings and identification of toxin in blood, stool, or implicated food.

Prevention

Infant botulism is acquired by ingestion of botulism spores which then sporulate into *C botulinum* organisms that can form botulinum toxin. Honey can contain botulism spores so it is recommended that honey not be consumed by infants less than 12 months of age. Corn syrups that have not been pasteurized may pose a theoretical risk and some organizations (American Academy of Pediatrics) recommend that infants less than 12 months should not consume unpasteurized corn syrup.

Food-borne botulism is acquired by ingesting preformed botulism toxin in food. In the United States, food-borne botulism is most commonly seen with ingestion of home canned foods of low acidity (ie, corn, asparagus, green beans). However, baked potatoes wrapped in aluminum foil that have not been kept hot and home-fermented fish have also been associated with cases of botulism. Persons who eat home-canned foods should consider boiling foods for at least 10 minutes (can destroy potential toxin). Safe food handling practices include keeping foods either refrigerated (< 45°F) or hot (> 185°F), and disposing of any cracked jars or bulging/dented cans.

General Considerations

Botulism is a paralytic disease caused by *Clostridium botulinum,* an anaerobic, gram-positive, spore-forming bacillus normally found in soil. The organism produces an extremely potent neurotoxin. Of the seven types of toxin (A–G), types A, B, and E cause most human diseases. The toxin, a polypeptide, is so potent that 0.1 mg is lethal for humans.

Food-borne botulism usually results from ingestion of toxin-containing food. Preformed toxin is absorbed from the gut and produces paralysis by preventing acetylcholine release from cholinergic fibers at myoneural junctions. In the United States, home-canned vegetables are usually the cause. Commercially canned foods rarely are responsible. Virtually any food will support the growth of *C botulinum* spores into vegetative toxin-producing bacilli if an anaerobic, nonacid environment is provided. The food may not appear or taste spoiled. The toxin is heat-labile, but the spores are heat-resistant. Inadequate heating during processing (temperature < 115°C) allows the spores to survive and later resume toxin production. Boiling of foods for 10 minutes or heating at 80°C for 30 minutes before eating will destroy the toxin.

Infant botulism is seen in infants younger than age 6 months (median, 10 weeks). The initial symptoms are usually constipation and progressive, often severe hypotonia. Infants younger than age 2 weeks rarely develop botulism. The toxin appears to be produced by *C botulinum* organisms residing in the gastrointestinal tract. In some instances, honey has been the source of spores. Clinical findings include constipation, weak suck and cry, pooled oral secretions, cranial nerve deficits, generalized weakness, and, on occasion, apnea. The characteristic electromyographic pattern of brief, small, abundant motor-unit action potentials (BSAPs) may help confirm the diagnosis.

Annually, 10–15 cases of wound botulism are reported. Most cases occur in drug abusers with infection in intravenous or intramuscular injection sites.

Botulism, as a result of aerosolization of botulinum toxin, also could occur as the result of a bioterrorism event. Only three such cases of botulism have been reported; the incubation period was not well-defined, but was about 72 hours in the reported cases.

Clinical Findings

A. Symptoms and Signs

The incubation period for food-borne botulism is 8–36 hours. The initial symptoms are lethargy and headache. These are followed by double vision, dilated pupils, ptosis, and, within a few hours, difficulty with swallowing and speech. Pharyngeal paralysis occurs in some cases, and food may be regurgitated. The mucous membranes often are very dry. Descending skeletal muscle paralysis may be seen. Death usually results from respiratory failure.

Botulism patients present with a "classic triad": (1) afebrile; (2) symmetrical, flaccid, descending paralysis with prominent bulbar palsies; and (3) clear sensorium. Recognition of this triad is important in making the clinical diagnosis. Botulism is caused by a toxin, thus there is no fever unless secondary infection (eg, aspiration pneumonia) occurs. Common bulbar palsies seen include dysphonia, dysphagia, dysarthria, and diplopia (four "Ds").

B. Laboratory Findings

The diagnosis is made by demonstration of *C botulinum* toxin in stool, gastric aspirate or vomitus, or serum. Serum and stool samples can be sent for toxin confirmation (done by toxin neutralization mouse bioassay at CDC or state health departments). Foods that are suspected to be contaminated should be kept refrigerated and given to public health personnel for testing. Laboratory findings, including CSF examination, are usually normal. Electromyography suggests the diagnosis if the characteristic BSAP abnormalities are seen. A nondiagnostic electromyogram does not exclude the diagnosis.

Differential Diagnosis

Guillain-Barré syndrome is characterized by ascending paralysis, sensory deficits, and elevated CSF protein without pleocytosis.

Other illnesses that should be considered include poliomyelitis, post diphtheritic polyneuritis, certain chemical intoxications, tick paralysis, and myasthenia gravis. The history and elevated CSF protein characterize postdiphtheritic polyneuritis. Tick paralysis presents with a flaccid ascending motor paralysis. An attached tick should be sought. Myasthenia gravis usually occurs in adolescent girls. It is characterized by ocular and bulbar symptoms, normal pupils, fluctuating weakness, absence of other neurologic signs, and clinical response to cholinesterase inhibitors.

Complications

Difficulty in swallowing leads to aspiration pneumonia. Serious respiratory paralysis may be fatal despite assisted ventilation and intensive supportive measures.

Treatment

A. Specific Measures

Early treatment of botulism with antitoxin (food-borne or wound botulism) or passive human botulism immune globulin (infant botulism) is beneficial. Treatment should begin as soon as the clinical diagnosis is made (prior to microbiologic or toxin confirmation).

For suspected wound or food-borne botulism (non-infant botulism), patients should be treated with the heptavalent botulinum antitoxin (HBAT), which is only available from the CDC under an investigational new drug protocol. HBAT is an equine derived antitoxin and contains antibodies to all 7 known botulinum toxin types (A through G). The treatment protocol (available from the CDC) includes detailed instructions for intravenous administration of antitoxin. The CDC ([770] 488-7100) can be contacted for help in obtaining the product and for consultation. In addition, epidemic assistance, and laboratory testing services are available from the CDC through state health departments.

For treatment of infant botulism, intravenous human botulism immune globulin (Baby-BIG) is approved by the U.S. Food and Drug Administration (FDA) for use. Baby-BIG is a product containing high titers of neutralizing antibodies against type A and B toxin and is made from pooled plasma of adults who were immunized with a botulism toxoid vaccine. Results of a placebo-controlled clinical trial of use in infant botulism showed reduction in the mean hospital stay (2.5 weeks in treated patients vs 5.5 weeks in the placebo group) and decrease in mechanical ventilation time in the Baby-BIG–treated group. Although the cost of the preparation is very high, it still is cost-saving since there is a substantial reduction in hospital days, intensive care unit stay, and ventilator time in treated infants. Baby-BIG is not indicated for use in any form of botulism (wound, food-borne) other than infant botulism. To obtain Baby-BIG (in any state), contact the California Department of Public Health at: (510) 231-7600.

B. General Measures

General and supportive therapy consists of bed rest, ventilatory support (if necessary), fluid therapy, and enteral or parenteral nutrition. Aminoglycoside antimicrobials and clindamycin may exacerbate neuromuscular blockage and should be avoided.

Prognosis

The mortality rate has declined substantially in recent years and currently is at 6%. In nonfatal cases, symptoms subside over 2–3 months and recovery is usually complete.

Centers for Disease Control and Prevention (CDC): Botulism Technical Information. Available at: http://www.cdc.gov/nczved/divisions/dfbmd/diseases/botulism/technical.html

Centers for Disease Control and Prevention (CDC): Investigational Heptavalent Botulinum Antitoxin (HBAT) to Replace Licensed Botulinum Antitoxin AB and Investigational Botulinum Antitoxin E. MMWR 2010;59(10);299 [PMID: 20300057].

Lawrence DT et al: Food poisoning. Emerg Med Clin North Am 2007;25(2):357 [PMID: 17482025].

Long SS: Infant botulism and treatment with BIG-IV (BabyBIG). Pediatr Infect Dis J 2007;26:261 [PMID: 17484226].

Underwood K et al: Infant botulism: A 30-year experience spanning the introduction of botulism immune globulin intravenous in the intensive care unit at Childrens Hospital Los Angeles. Pediatrics 2007;120:e1380–e1385 [PMID: 18055655].

TETANUS

ESSENTIALS OF DIAGNOSIS & TYPICAL FEATURES

- Nonimmunized or partially immunized patient.
- History of skin wound.
- Spasms of jaw muscles (trismus).
- Stiffness of neck, back, and abdominal muscles, with hyperirritability and hyperreflexia.

- Episodic, generalized muscle contractions.
- Diagnosis is based on clinical findings and the immunization history.

General Considerations

Tetanus is caused by *Clostridium tetani,* an anaerobic, gram-positive bacillus that produces a potent neurotoxin. In unimmunized or incompletely immunized individuals, infection follows contamination of a wound by soil containing clostridial spores from animal manure. The toxin reaches the CNS by retrograde axon transport, is bound to cerebral gangliosides, and appears to increase reflex excitability in neurons of the spinal cord by blocking function of inhibitory synapses. Intense muscle spasms result. Two-thirds of cases in the United States follow minor puncture wounds of the hands or feet. In many cases, no history of a wound can be obtained. Injecting substances and drug abuse may be risk factors (in individuals who are not tetanus-immune). In the newborn, usually in underdeveloped countries, infection generally results from contamination of the umbilical cord. The incubation period typically is 4–14 days but may be longer. In the United States, cases in young children are due to failure to immunize. Eighty-five percent of cases occur in adults older than 25 years.

Prevention

A. Tetanus Toxoid

Active immunization with tetanus toxoid prevents tetanus. Immunity is almost always achieved after the third dose of vaccine. Tetanus immune globulin (TIG) is an additional agent used to prevent tetanus in persons who have received less than 3 doses of tetanus toxoid or in immunocompromised patients who do not make sufficient antibody (ie, HIV infection; see Chapter 10). A tetanus toxoid booster at the time of injury is needed if none has been given in the past 10 years—or within 5 years for heavily contaminated wounds. Nearly all cases of tetanus (99%) in the United States are in nonimmunized or incompletely immunized individuals. Many adolescents and adults lack protective antibody.

B. Wound Care and Prophylaxis for Tetanus-Prone Wounds

Wounds that are contaminated with soil, debris, feces, or saliva are at increased risk for tetanus. Puncture wounds or wounds that contain devitalized tissue are at increased risk of infection with *C tetani.* This includes wounds that result from crush injury, frostbite, burns, or avulsion. All wounds should be adequately cleaned, foreign material removed, and debrided if necrotic or devitalized tissue is present or if residual foreign matter is present. The decision to use tetanus toxoid–containing vaccine or human TIG depends on the type of injury and the tetanus immunization status of the patient. (See Chapter 10; Table 10–5.) TIG should be used in children with fewer than three previous tetanus toxoid immunizations (DPT, DPaT, DT, Td, Tdap) who have tetanus-prone wounds, and should be administered to HIV-infected children with tetanus-prone wounds, regardless of their immunization history. When TIG is indicated for wound, prophylaxis 250 units are given intramuscularly regardless of age. If tetanus immunization is incomplete, a dose of age-appropriate vaccine should be given. When both are indicated, tetanus toxoid and TIG should be administered concurrently at different sites using different syringes. (See Chapter 10.)

Prophylactic antimicrobials are useful if the child is unimmunized and TIG is not available.

Clinical Findings

A. Symptoms and Signs

The first symptom often is mild pain at the site of the wound, followed by hypertonicity and spasm of the regional muscles. Characteristically, difficulty in opening the mouth (trismus) is evident within 48 hours. In newborns, the first signs are irritability and inability to nurse. The infant may then develop stiffness of the jaw and neck, increasing dysphagia, and generalized hyperreflexia with rigidity and spasms of all muscles of the abdomen and back (opisthotonos). The facial distortion resembles a grimace (risus sardonicus). Difficulty in swallowing and convulsions triggered by minimal stimuli such as sound, light, or movement may occur. Individual spasms may last seconds or minutes. Recurrent spasms are seen several times each hour, or they may be almost continuous. In most cases, the temperature is normal or only mildly elevated. A high or subnormal temperature is a bad prognostic sign. Patients are fully conscious and lucid. A profound circulatory disturbance associated with sympathetic overactivity may occur on the second to fourth day, which may contribute to the mortality rate. This is characterized by elevated blood pressure, increased cardiac output, tachycardia (> 20 beats/min), and arrhythmia.

B. Laboratory Findings

The diagnosis is made on clinical grounds. There may be a mild polymorphonuclear leukocytosis. The CSF is normal with the exception of mild elevation of opening pressure. Serum muscle enzymes may be elevated. Transient electrocardiographic and electroencephalographic abnormalities may occur. Anaerobic culture and microscopic examination of pus from the wound can be helpful, but *C tetani* is difficult to grow, and the drumstick-shaped gram-positive bacilli often cannot be found.

Differential Diagnosis

Poliomyelitis is characterized by asymmetrical paralysis in an incompletely immunized child. The history of an animal bite and the absence of trismus may suggest rabies. Local infections of the throat and jaw should be easily recognized. Bacterial meningitis, phenothiazine reactions, decerebrate posturing, narcotic withdrawal, spondylitis, and hypocalcemic tetany may be confused with tetanus.

Complications

Complications include sepsis, malnutrition, pneumonia, atelectasis, asphyxial spasms, decubitus ulcers, and fractures of the spine due to intense contractions. They can be prevented in part by skilled supportive care.

Treatment

A. Specific Measures

Human TIG in a single dose of 3000–6000 units, intramuscularly, is given to children and adults. Doses of 500 units have been used in infants. Infiltration of part of the TIG dose around the wound is recommended. If TIG is indicated, but not available, intravenous immune globulin in a dose of 200–400 mg/kg intravenously can be used (although it is not licensed for this indication). In countries where TIG or immune globulin are not available, equine tetanus antitoxin may be available. Surgical debridement of wounds is indicated, but more extensive surgery or amputation to eliminate the site of infection is not necessary. Antibiotics are given to attempt to decrease the number of vegetative forms of the bacteria to decrease toxin production: oral or intravenous metronidazole (30 mg/kg/d in four divided doses; maximum 4 g/d) for 10–14 days is the preferred agent.

B. General Measures

The patient is kept in a quiet room with minimal stimulation. Control of spasms and prevention of hypoxic episodes are crucial. Benzodiazepines can be used to help control spasms and provide some sedation. Mechanical ventilation and muscle paralysis are necessary in severe cases. Nasogastric or intravenous feedings should be used to limit stimulation of feedings and prevent aspiration.

Prognosis

The fatality rate in newborns and heroin-addicted individuals is high. The overall mortality rate in the United States is 11%. The fatality rate depends on the quality of supportive care, the patient's age, and the patient's vaccination history. Many deaths are due to pneumonia or respiratory failure. If the patient survives 1 week, recovery is likely.

Brook I: Current concepts in the management of *Clostridium tetani* infection. Expert Rev Anti Infect Ther 2008;6(3):327–336 [PMID: 18588497].

Gibson K, Bonaventure UJ, Kiviri W: Tetanus in developing countries: A case series and review. Can J Anaesth 2009;56(4): 307–315 [PMID: 19296192].

Centers for Disease Control and Prevention (CDC): Tetanus. Available at: http://www.cdc.gov/vaccines/pubs/pinkbook/downloads/tetanus.pdf

GAS GANGRENE

ESSENTIALS OF DIAGNOSIS & TYPICAL FEATURES

- Contamination of a wound with soil or feces.
- Massive edema, skin discoloration, bleb formation, and pain in an area of trauma.
- Serosanguineous exudate from wound.
- Crepitation of subcutaneous tissue.
- Rapid progression of signs and symptoms.
- Clostridia cultured or seen on stained smears.

General Considerations

Gas gangrene (clostridial myonecrosis) is a necrotizing infection that follows trauma or surgery and is caused by several anaerobic, gram-positive, spore-forming bacilli of the genus *Clostridium*. Occasionally the source is the gastrointestinal tract and muscles are hematogenously seeded. The spores are found in soil, feces, and vaginal secretions. In devitalized tissue, the spores germinate into vegetative bacilli that proliferate and produce toxins, causing thrombosis, hemolysis, and tissue necrosis. *C perfringens*, the species causing approximately 80% of cases of gas gangrene, produces at least eight such toxins. The areas involved most often are the extremities, abdomen, and uterus. *Clostridium septicum* may also cause myonecrosis and causes septicemia in patients with neutropenia. Nonclostridial infections with gas formation can mimic clostridial infections and are more common. Neutropenia is a risk factor for this severe infection.

Prevention

Gas gangrene can be prevented by the adequate cleansing and debridement of all wounds. It is essential that foreign bodies and dead tissue be removed. A clean wound does not provide a suitable anaerobic environment for the growth of clostridial species.

Clinical Findings

A. Symptoms and Signs

The onset of gas gangrene usually is sudden, often 1 day after trauma or surgery (mean, 3–4 days), but can be delayed up to 20 days. The skin around the wound becomes discolored, with hemorrhagic bullae, serosanguineous exudate, and crepitus may be observed the subcutaneous tissues. The absence of crepitus does not rule out the diagnosis. Pain and swelling usually are intense. Systemic illness appears early and progresses rapidly to intravascular hemolysis, jaundice, shock, toxic delirium, and renal failure.

B. Laboratory Findings

Isolation of the organism requires anaerobic culture. Gram-stained smears may demonstrate many gram-positive rods and few inflammatory cells.

C. Imaging

Radiographs may demonstrate gas in tissues, but this is a late finding and is also seen in infections with other gas-forming organisms or may be due to air introduced into tissues during trauma or surgery.

D. Operative Findings

Direct visualization of the muscle at surgery may be necessary to diagnose gas gangrene. Early, the muscle is pale and edematous and does not contract normally; later, the muscle may be frankly gangrenous.

Differential Diagnosis

Gangrene and cellulitis caused by other organisms and clostridial cellulitis (not myonecrosis) must be distinguished. Necrotizing fasciitis may resemble gas gangrene.

Treatment

A. Specific Measures

Penicillin G (300,000–400,000 U/kg/d intravenously in six divided doses) should be given, usually combined with clindamycin or metronidazole. Clindamycin, metronidazole, meropenem, and imipenem–cilastatin are alternatives for penicillin-allergic patients. Some experts recommend a combination of penicillin and clindamycin. Clindamycin is a protein synthesis inhibitor and may inhibit toxin production.

B. Surgical Measures

Surgery should be prompt and extensive, with removal of all necrotic tissue. Compartment syndromes can occur even if there are few cutaneous findings. Checking compartment pressures in patients with severe pain and any signs of compartment syndrome is prudent.

C. Hyperbaric Oxygen

Hyperbaric oxygen therapy has been shown to be effective, but is not a substitute for surgery. A patient may be exposed to 2–3 atm in pure oxygen for 1- to 2-hour periods for as many sessions as necessary until clinical remission occurs.

Prognosis

Clostridial myonecrosis is fatal if untreated. With early diagnosis, antibiotics, and surgery, the mortality rate is 20%–60%. Involvement of the abdominal wall, leukopenia, intravascular hemolysis, renal failure, and shock are ominous prognostic signs.

Langham M, Arnold L: Clostridial myonecrosis in an adolescent male. Pediatrics 2005;116:e737 [PMID: 16199671]. Available at: http://pediatrics.aappublications.org/content/116/5/e735.full.pdf

Smith-Slatas CL et al: Clostridium septicum infections in children: A case report and review of the literature. Pediatrics 2006;117:e796 [PMID: 16567392].

DIPHTHERIA

ESSENTIALS OF DIAGNOSIS & TYPICAL FEATURES

- Gray, adherent pseudomembrane, most often in the pharynx but also in the nasopharynx or trachea.
- Sore throat, serosanguinous nasal discharge, hoarseness, and fever in a nonimmunized child.
- Peripheral neuritis or myocarditis.
- Positive culture.
- Treatment should not be withheld pending culture results.

General Considerations

Diphtheria is an acute infection of the upper respiratory tract or skin caused by toxin-producing *Corynebacterium diphtheriae*. Diphtheria in the United States is rare; five cases have been reported since 2000; none since 2003. However, significant numbers of elderly adults and unimmunized children are susceptible to infection. Diphtheria still occurs in epidemics in countries where immunization is not universal. Travelers to these areas may acquire the disease.

Corynebacteria are gram-positive, club-shaped rods with a beaded appearance on Gram stain. The capacity to produce exotoxin is conferred by a lysogenic bacteriophage and is not present in all strains of *C diphtheriae*. In immunized communities, infection probably occurs through spread of the phage among carriers of susceptible bacteria rather than through spread of phage-containing bacteria themselves. Diphtheria toxin kills susceptible cells by irreversible inhibition of protein synthesis.

The toxin is absorbed into the mucous membranes and causes destruction of epithelium and a superficial inflammatory response. The necrotic epithelium becomes embedded in exuding fibrin and WBCs and RBCs (red blood cells), forming a grayish pseudomembrane over the tonsils, pharynx, or larynx. Any attempt to remove the membrane exposes and tears the capillaries, resulting in bleeding. The diphtheria bacilli within the membrane continue to produce toxin, which is absorbed and may result in toxic injury to heart muscle, liver, kidneys, and adrenals, and is sometimes accompanied by hemorrhage. The toxin also produces neuritis, resulting in paralysis of the soft palate, eye muscles, or extremities. Death may occur as a result of respiratory obstruction or toxemia and circulatory collapse. The patient may succumb after a somewhat longer time as a result of cardiac damage. The incubation period is 2–7 days.

Clinical Findings

A. Symptoms and Signs

1. Pharyngeal diphtheria—Early manifestations of diphtheritic pharyngitis are mild sore throat, moderate fever, and malaise, followed fairly rapidly by prostration and circulatory collapse. The pulse is more rapid than the fever would seem to justify. A pharyngeal membrane forms and may spread into the nasopharynx or the trachea, producing respiratory obstruction. The membrane is tenacious and gray and is surrounded by a narrow zone of erythema and a broader zone of edema. The cervical lymph nodes become swollen, and swelling is associated with brawny edema of the neck (so-called bull neck). Laryngeal diphtheria presents with stridor, which can progress to obstruction of the airway.

2. Other forms—Cutaneous, vaginal, and wound diphtheria account for up to one-third of cases and are characterized by ulcerative lesions with membrane formation.

B. Laboratory Findings

Diagnosis is clinical. Direct smears are unreliable. Material is obtained from the nose, throat, or skin lesions, if present, for culture, but specialized culture media are required. Between 16 and 48 hours is required before identification of the organism. A toxigenicity test is then performed. Cultures may be negative in individuals who have received antibiotics. The WBC count usually is normal, but hemolytic anemia and thrombocytopenia are frequent.

Differential Diagnosis

Pharyngeal diphtheria resembles pharyngitis secondary to β-hemolytic streptococcus, Epstein-Barr virus, or other viral respiratory pathogens. A nasal foreign body or purulent sinusitis may mimic nasal diphtheria. Other causes of laryngeal obstruction include epiglottitis and viral croup. Guillain-Barré syndrome, poliomyelitis, or acute poisoning may mimic the neuropathy of diphtheria.

Complications

A. Myocarditis

Diphtheritic myocarditis is characterized by a rapid, thready pulse; indistinct heart sounds, ST-T wave changes, conduction abnormalities, dysrhythmias, or cardiac failure; hepatomegaly; and fluid retention. Myocardial dysfunction may occur from 2 to 40 days after the onset of pharyngitis.

B. Polyneuritis

Neuritis of the palatal and pharyngeal nerves occurs during the first or second week. Nasal speech and regurgitation of food through the nose are seen. Diplopia and strabismus occur during the third week or later. Neuritis may also involve peripheral nerves supplying the intercostal muscles, diaphragm, and other muscle groups. Generalized paresis usually occurs after the fourth week.

C. Bronchopneumonia

Secondary pneumonia is common in fatal cases.

Prevention

A. Immunization

Immunization with diphtheria toxoid combined with pertussis and tetanus toxoids (DTaP) should be used routinely for infants and children. (See Chapter 10.)

B. Care of Exposed Susceptibles

Children exposed to diphtheria should be examined, and nose and throat cultures obtained. If signs and symptoms of early diphtheria are found, antibiotic treatment should be instituted. Immunized asymptomatic individuals should receive diphtheria toxoid if a booster has not been received within 5 years. Unimmunized close contacts should receive either erythromycin orally (40 mg/kg/d in four divided doses) for 7 days or benzathine penicillin G intramuscularly (25,000 U/kg), active immunization with diphtheria toxoid, and observation daily.

Treatment

A. Specific Measures

1. Antitoxin—To be effective, diphtheria antitoxin should be administered within 48 hours. (See Chapter 9.)

2. Antibiotics—Penicillin G (150,000 U/kg/d intravenously or intramuscularly) should be given for 14 days. For penicillin-allergic patients, erythromycin (40 mg/kg/d) is given orally for 14 days.

B. General Measures

Bed rest in the hospital for 10–14 days is usually required. All patients must be strictly isolated for 1–7 days until respiratory secretions are noncontagious. Isolation may be discontinued when two successive nose and throat cultures at 24-hour intervals are negative. These cultures should not be taken until at least 24 hours have elapsed since the cessation of antibiotic treatment.

C. Treatment of Carriers

All carriers should receive treatment. Erythromycin (40 mg/kg/d orally in three or four divided doses), penicillin V potassium (50 mg/kg/d) for 10 days, or benzathine penicillin G (600,000–1,200,000 units intramuscularly) should be given. All carriers must be quarantined. Before they can be released, carriers must have two negative cultures of both the nose and the throat taken 24 hours apart and obtained at least 24 hours after the cessation of antibiotic therapy.

Prognosis

Mortality varies from 3% to 25% and is particularly high in the presence of early myocarditis. Neuritis is reversible; it is fatal only if an intact airway and adequate respiration cannot be maintained. Permanent heart damage from myocarditis occurs rarely.

Centers for Disease Control and Prevention (CDC): Diphtheria. Available at: http://www.cdc.gov/ncidod/dbmd/diseaseinfo/diphtheria_t.htm

Halasa NB et al: Poor immune responses to a birth dose of diphtheria, tetanus, and acellular pertussis vaccine. J Pediatr 2008;153(3):327 [PMID: 18534242].

INFECTIONS DUE TO ENTEROBACTERIACEAE

ESSENTIALS OF DIAGNOSIS & TYPICAL FEATURES

- Diarrhea by several different mechanisms due to *E coli*.
- Hemorrhagic colitis and hemolyticuremic syndrome.
- Neonatal sepsis or meningitis.
- Urinary tract infection.
- Opportunistic infections.
- Diagnosis confirmed by culture.

General Considerations

Enterobacteriaceae are a family of gram-negative bacilli that are normal flora in the gastrointestinal tract and are also found in water and soil. They cause gastroenteritis, urinary tract infections, neonatal sepsis and meningitis, and opportunistic infections. *E coli* is the organism in this family that most commonly causes infection in children, but *Klebsiella, Morganella, Enterobacter, Serratia, Proteus,* and other genera are also important, particularly in the compromised host. Shigella and Salmonella are discussed in separate sections.

E coli strains capable of causing diarrhea were originally termed enteropathogenic *E coli* (EPEC) and were recognized by serotype. It is now known that *E coli* may cause diarrhea by several distinct mechanisms. Classic EPEC strains cause a characteristic histologic injury in the small bowel termed adherence and effacement. Enterotoxigenic *E coli* (ETEC) causes a secretory, watery diarrhea. ETEC adheres to enterocytes and secretes one or more plasmid-encoded enterotoxins. One of these, heat-labile toxin, resembles cholera toxin in structure, function, and mechanism of action. Enteroinvasive *E coli* (EIEC) are very similar to *Shigella* in their pathogenetic mechanisms. Enterohemorrhagic *E coli* (EHEC) cause hemorrhagic colitis and the hemolytic-uremic syndrome. The most common EHEC serotype is O157:H7, although several other serotypes cause the same syndrome. These strains elaborate one of several cytotoxins, closely related to Shiga toxin produced by *Shigella dysenteriae*. Outbreaks of hemolytic-uremic syndrome associated with EHEC have followed consumption of inadequately cooked ground beef. Thorough heating to 68–71°C is necessary. Unpasteurized fruit juice, various uncooked vegetables, and contaminated water also have caused infections and epidemics. The common source for EHEC in all of these foods and water is the feces of cattle. Person-to-person spread including spread in day care centers by the fecal-oral route has been reported.

E coli that aggregate on the surface of hep cells in tissue culture are termed enteroaggregative *E coli* (EAggEC). EAggEC cause diarrhea by a distinct but unknown mechanism.

Eighty percent of *E coli* strains causing neonatal meningitis possess specific capsular polysaccharide (K1 antigen), which, alone or in association with specific somatic antigens, confers virulence. Approximately 90% of urinary tract infections in children are caused by *E coli*. *E coli* binds to the uroepithelium by P-fimbriae, which are present in more than 90% of *E coli* that cause pyelonephritis. Other bacterial cell surface structures, such as O and K antigens, and host factors are also important in the pathogenesis of urinary tract infections.

Klebsiella, Enterobacter, Serratia, and *Morganella* are normally found in the gastrointestinal tract and in soil and water. *Klebsiella* may cause a bronchopneumonia with cavity formation. *Klebsiella, Enterobacter,* and *Serratia* are often hospital-acquired opportunists associated with antibiotic usage, debilitated states, and chronic respiratory conditions. They frequently cause urinary tract infection or sepsis. In many newborn nurseries, nosocomial outbreaks caused by antimicrobial-resistant *Klebsiella* or *Enterobacter* species are a major problem.

Many of these infections are difficult to treat because of antibiotic resistance. Antibiotic susceptibility tests are necessary. Parenteral third-generation cephalosporins are usually more active than ampicillin, but resistance due to high-level production of chromosomal cephalosporinase may occur. *Enterobacter* and *Serratia* strains broadly resistant to cephalosporins also cause infections in hospitalized newborns and children. Aminoglycoside antibiotics are usually effective but require monitoring of serum levels to ensure therapeutic and nontoxic levels.

Clinical Findings

A. Symptoms and Signs

1. *E coli* gastroenteritis—*E coli* may cause diarrhea of varying types and severity. ETEC usually produce mild, self-limiting illness without significant fever or systemic toxicity, often known as traveler's diarrhea. However, diarrhea may be severe in newborns and infants, and occasionally an older child or adult will have a cholera-like syndrome. EIEC strains cause a shigellosis-like illness, characterized by fever, systemic symptoms, blood and mucus in the stool, and leukocytosis, but currently are uncommon in the United States. EHEC strains cause hemorrhagic colitis. Diarrhea initially is watery and fever usually is absent. Abdominal pain and cramping occur; diarrhea progresses to blood streaking or grossly bloody stools. Hemolytic-uremic syndrome occurs within a few days of diarrhea in 2%–5% of children and is characterized by microangiopathic hemolytic anemia, thrombocytopenia, and renal failure. (See Chapter 24.)

2. Neonatal sepsis—Findings include jaundice, hepatosplenomegaly, fever, temperature lability, apneic spells, irritability, and poor feeding. Respiratory distress develops when pneumonia occurs; it may appear indistinguishable from respiratory distress syndrome in preterm infants. Meningitis is associated with sepsis in 25%–40% of cases. Other metastatic foci of infection may be present, including pneumonia and pyelonephritis. Sepsis may lead to severe metabolic acidosis, shock, DIC, and death.

3. Neonatal meningitis—Findings include high fever, full fontanelles, vomiting, coma, convulsions, pareses or paralyses, poor or absent Moro reflex, opisthotonos, and occasionally hypertonia or hypotonia. Sepsis coexists or precedes meningitis in most cases. Thus, signs of sepsis often accompany those of meningitis. CSF usually shows a cell count of over 1000/μL, mostly polymorphonuclear neutrophils, and bacteria on Gram stain. CSF glucose concentration is low (usually less than half that of blood), and the protein is elevated above the levels normally seen in newborns and premature infants (> 150 mg/dL).

4. Acute urinary tract infection—Symptoms include dysuria, increased urinary frequency, and fever in the older child. Nonspecific symptoms such as anorexia, vomiting, irritability, failure to thrive, and unexplained fever are seen in children younger than age 2 years. Young infants may present with jaundice. As many as 1% of school-aged girls and 0.05% of boys have asymptomatic bacteriuria. Screening for and treatment of asymptomatic bacteriuria is not recommended.

B. Laboratory Findings

Because *E coli* are normal flora in the stool, a positive stool culture alone does not prove that the *E coli* in the stool are causing disease. Serotyping, tests for enterotoxin production or invasiveness, and tests for P-fimbriae are performed in research laboratories. MacConkey agar with sorbitol substituted for lactose (SMAC agar) is useful to screen stool for EHEC. Serotyping and testing for enterotoxin are available at many state health departments and increasingly from commercial and hospital laboratories. Blood cultures are positive in neonatal sepsis. Cultures of CSF and urine should also be obtained. The diagnosis of urinary tract infections is discussed in Chapter 24.

Differential Diagnosis

The clinical picture of EPEC infection may resemble that of salmonellosis, shigellosis, or viral gastroenteritis. Neonatal sepsis and meningitis caused by *E coli* can be differentiated from other causes of neonatal infection only by blood and CSF culture.

Treatment

A. Specific Measures

1. *E coli* gastroenteritis—Gastroenteritis due to EPEC seldom requires antimicrobial treatment. Fluid and electrolyte therapy, preferably given orally, may be required to avoid dehydration. Bismuth subsalicylate reduces stool volume by about one-third in infants with watery diarrhea, probably including ETEC. In nursery outbreaks, *E coli* gastroenteritis has been treated with neomycin (100 mg/kg/d orally in three divided doses for 5 days). Clinical efficacy is not established. Traveler's diarrhea may be treated with TMP–SMX in children and with fluoroquinolones in adults, although resistance to these drugs is increasing. Azithromycin is an alternative. The risk of hemolytic-uremic syndrome is not proven to be increased by antimicrobial therapy of EHEC cases, but most experts recommend no treatment of suspected cases.

2. *E coli* sepsis and pneumonia—The drugs of choice are ampicillin (150–200 mg/kg/d, given intravenously or intramuscularly in divided doses every 4–6 hours), cefotaxime (150–200 mg/kg/d, given intravenously or intramuscularly in divided doses every 6–8 hours), ceftriaxone (50–100 mg/kg/d, given intramuscularly as single dose or in two divided doses), and gentamicin (5.0–7.5 mg/kg/d, given intramuscularly or intravenously in divided doses every 8 hours). Initial therapy often includes at least two drugs until microbial etiology is established and susceptibility testing is completed. Treatment is continued for 10–14 days. Amikacin or tobramycin may be used instead of gentamicin if the strain is susceptible. Third-generation cephalosporins are often an attractive alternative as single-drug therapy and do not require monitoring for toxicity.

3. *E coli* meningitis—Third-generation cephalosporins such as cefotaxime (200 mg/kg/d intravenously in four divided doses) are given for a minimum of 3 weeks. Ampicillin (200–300 mg/kg/d intravenously in four to six divided doses) and gentamicin (5.0–7.5 mg/kg/d intramuscularly or intravenously in three divided doses) also are effective for susceptible strains. Treatment with intrathecal and intraventricular aminoglycosides does not improve outcome. Serum levels need to be monitored.

4. Acute urinary tract infection—(See Chapter 24.)

Prognosis

Death due to gastroenteritis leading to dehydration can be prevented by early fluid and electrolyte therapy. Neonatal sepsis with meningitis is still associated with a mortality rate of over 50%. Most children with recurrent urinary tract infections do well if they have no underlying anatomic defects. The mortality rate in opportunistic infections usually depends on the severity of infection and the underlying condition.

Anjay MA et al: Leukocytosis as a predictor for progression to haemolytic uraemic syndrome in *Escherichia coli* O157:H7 infection. Arch Dis Child 2007;92:820 [PMID: 17715449].

Centers for Disease Control and Prevention (CDC): Diarrheagenic *Escherichia coli*. Available at: http://www.cdc.gov/nczved/divisions/afbmd/diseases/diarrheagenic_ecoli/technical.html

DuPont HL: Therapy for and prevention of traveler's diarrhea. Clin Infect Dis 2007;45(Suppl 1):S78 [PMID: 17582576].

Qazi SA, Stsoll BJ: Neonatal sepsis: A major global public health challenge. Pediatr Infect Dis J 2009;28(Suppl 1):S1–S2 [PMID: 19106756].

Raffaelli RM et al: Child care-associated outbreak of *Escherichia coli* O157: H7 and hemolytic uremic syndrome. Pediatr Infect Dis 2007;26(10):951 [PMID: 17901803].

Wendel AM et al: Multistate outbreak of *Escherichia coli* O157:H7 infection associated with consumption of packaged spinach, August-September 2006: The Wisconsin Investigation. Clinical Infect Dis 2009;48(8):1079 [PMID: 19265476].

Zaidi AK et al: Pathogens associated with sepsis in newborns and young infants in developing countries. Pediatr Infect Dis J 2009;28(Suppl 1):S10 [PMID: 19106757].

PSEUDOMONAS INFECTIONS

ESSENTIALS OF DIAGNOSIS & TYPICAL FEATURES

- Opportunistic infection.
- Confirmed by cultures.

General Considerations

Pseudomonas aeruginosa is an aerobic gram-negative rod with versatile metabolic requirements. The organism may grow in distilled water and in commonly used disinfectants, complicating infection control in medical facilities. *P aeruginosa* is both invasive and destructive to tissue as well as toxigenic due to secreted exotoxins, all factors that contribute to virulence. Other genera previously classified as Pseudomonas frequently cause nosocomial infections and infections in immunocompromised children. *Stenotrophomonas maltophilia* (previously *Pseudomonas maltophilia*) and *Burkholderia cepacia* (previously *Pseudomonas cepacia*) are the most frequent.

P aeruginosa is an important cause of infection in children with cystic fibrosis, neoplastic disease, neutropenia, or extensive burns and in those receiving antibiotic therapy. Infections of the urinary and respiratory tracts, ears, mastoids, paranasal sinuses, eyes, skin, meninges, and bones are seen. *Pseudomonas* pneumonia is a common nosocomial infection in patients receiving assisted ventilation.

P aeruginosa sepsis may be accompanied by characteristic peripheral lesions called ecthyma gangrenosum. Ecthyma gangrenosum also may occur by direct invasion through intact skin in the groin, axilla, or other skinfolds. *P aeruginosa* is an infrequent cause of sepsis in previously healthy infants and may be the initial sign of underlying medical problems. *P aeruginosa* osteomyelitis often complicates puncture wounds of the feet. *P aeruginosa* is a frequent cause of malignant external otitis media and of chronic suppurative otitis media. Outbreaks of vesiculopustular skin rash have been associated with exposure to contaminated water in whirlpool baths and hot tubs.

P aeruginosa infects the tracheobronchial tree of nearly all patients with cystic fibrosis. Mucoid exopolysaccharide, an exuberant capsule, is characteristically overproduced by isolates from patients with cystic fibrosis. Although bacteremia seldom occurs, patients with cystic fibrosis ultimately succumb to chronic lung infection with *P aeruginosa*. Infection due to *B cepacia* has caused a rapidly progressive pulmonary disease in some colonized patients and may be spread by close contact.

Osteomyelitis of the calcaneus or other foot bones occurs after punctures such as stepping on a nail and is commonly due to *P aeruginosa*.

Clinical Findings

The clinical findings depend on the site of infection and the patient's underlying disease. Sepsis with these organisms resembles gram-negative sepsis with other organisms, although the presence of ecthyma gangrenosum suggests the diagnosis. The diagnosis is made by culture. Pseudomonas infection should be suspected in neonates and neutropenic patients with clinical sepsis. A severe necrotizing pneumonia occurs in patients on ventilators.

Patients with cystic fibrosis have a persistent bronchitis that progresses to bronchiectasis and ultimately to respiratory failure. During exacerbations of illness, cough and sputum production increase with low-grade fever, malaise, and diminished energy.

The purulent aural drainage without fever in patients with chronic suppurative otitis media is not distinguishable from that due to other causes.

Prevention

A. Infections in Debilitated Patients

Colonization of extensive second- and third-degree burns by *P aeruginosa* can lead to fatal septicemia. Aggressive debridement and topical treatment with 0.5% silver nitrate solution, 10% mafenide cream, or silver sulfadiazine will greatly inhibit *P aeruginosa* contamination of burns. (See Chapter 12 for a discussion of burn wound infections and prevention.)

B. Nosocomial Infections

Faucet aerators, communal soap dispensers, disinfectants, improperly cleaned inhalation therapy equipment, infant incubators, and many other sources that usually are associated with wet or humid conditions all have been associated with Pseudomonas epidemics. Infant-to-infant transmission by nursery personnel carrying Pseudomonas on the hands is frequent in neonatal units. Careful maintenance of equipment and enforcement of infection control procedures are essential to minimize nosocomial transmission.

C. Patients with Cystic Fibrosis

Chronic infection of the lower respiratory tract occurs in nearly all patients with cystic fibrosis. The infecting organism is seldom cleared from the respiratory tract, even with intensive antimicrobial therapy, and the resultant injury to the lung eventually leads to pulmonary insufficiency. Treatment is aimed at controlling signs and symptoms of the infection.

Treatment

P aeruginosa is inherently resistant to many antimicrobials and may develop resistance during therapy. Mortality rates in hospitalized patients exceed 50%, owing both to the severity of underlying illnesses in patients predisposed to Pseudomonas infection and to the limitations of therapy. Antibiotics effective against Pseudomonas include the amino-glycosides, ureidopenicillins (ticarcillin and piperacillin), β-lactamase inhibitor with a ureidopenicillin (ticarcillin–clavulanate and piperacillin–tazobactam), expanded-spectrum cephalosporins (ceftazidime and cefepime), imipenem, meropenem, and ciprofloxacin. Colistin has been used in some children with multi-drug resistance. Antimicrobial susceptibility patterns vary from area to area, and resistance tends to appear as new drugs become popular. Treatment of infections is best guided by clinical response and susceptibility tests.

Gentamicin or tobramycin (5.0–7.5 mg/kg/d, given intramuscularly or intravenously in three divided doses) or amikacin (15–22 mg/kg/d, given in two or three divided doses) in combination with ticarcillin (200–300 mg/kg/d, given intravenously in four to six divided doses) or with another antipseudomonal β-lactam antibiotic is recommended for treatment of serious Pseudomonas infections. Ceftazidime (150–200 mg/kg/d, given in four divided doses) or cefepime (150 mg/kg/d, given in three divided doses) has excellent activity against *P aeruginosa*. Treatment should be continued for 10–14 days. Treatment with two active drugs is recommended for all serious infections.

Pseudomonas osteomyelitis due to punctures requires thorough surgical debridement and antimicrobial therapy for 2 weeks. *Pseudomonas* folliculitis does not require antibiotic therapy.

Oral or intravenous ciprofloxacin is also effective against susceptible *P aeruginosa,* but is not approved by the FDA for use in children except in the case of urinary tract infection. Nonetheless, in some circumstances of antimicrobial resistance, or when the benefits clearly outweigh the small risks, ciprofloxacin may be used.

Chronic suppurative otitis media responds to intravenous ceftazidime (150–200 mg/kg/d in three or four divided doses) given until the drainage has ceased for 3 days. Twice-daily ceftazidime with aural debridement and cleaning given on an outpatient basis has also been successful. Swimmer's ear may be caused by *P aeruginosa* and responds well to topical drying agents (alcohol–vinegar mix) and cleansing.

Prognosis

Because debilitated patients are most frequently affected, the mortality rate is high. These infections may have a protracted course, and eradication of the organisms may be difficult.

Falagas ME et al: Intravenous colistimethate (colistin) use in critically ill children without cystic fibrosis. Pediatr Infect Dis J 2009;28(2):123 [PMID: 19115501].

Hengge UR, Bardeli V: Images in clinical medicine: Green nails. N Eng J Med 2009;360(11):1125 [PMID: 19279344].

Lahiri T: Approaches to the treatment of initial *Pseudomonas aeruginosa* infection in children who have cystic fibrosis. Clin Chest Med 2007;28:307 [PMID: 17467550].

Vitaliti SM et al: Neonatal sepsis caused by *Ralstonia pickettii*. Pediatr Infect Dis J 2008;27(3):283 [PMID: 18277913].

Yu Y et al: Hot tub folliculitis or hot hand-foot syndrome caused by *Pseudomonas aeruginosa*. J Am Acad Dermatol 2007;57:596 [PMID: 17658195].

SALMONELLA GASTROENTERITIS

ESSENTIALS OF DIAGNOSIS & TYPICAL FEATURES

- Nausea, vomiting, headache, meningismus.
- Fever, diarrhea, abdominal pain.
- Culture or organism from stool, blood, or other specimens.

General Considerations

Salmonellae are gram-negative rods that frequently cause food-borne gastroenteritis and occasionally bacteremic infection of bone, meninges, and other foci. Approximately 2400 serotypes of *Salmonella enterica* are recognized. *Salmonella typhimurium* is the most frequently isolated serotype in most parts of the world. Although 49,000 cases were reported in 2009, it is estimated that 100 or more occur for each one reported. This yields an estimate or more than 4 million cases yearly in the United States.

Salmonellae are able to penetrate the mucin layer of the small bowel and attach to epithelial cells. Organisms penetrate the epithelial cells and multiply in the submucosa. Infection results in fever, vomiting, and watery diarrhea; the diarrhea occasionally includes mucus and polymorphonuclear neutrophils in the stool. Although the small intestine is generally regarded as the principal site of infection, colitis also occurs. *S typhimurium* frequently involves the large bowel.

Salmonella infections in childhood occur in two major forms: (1) gastroenteritis (including food poisoning), which may be complicated by sepsis and focal suppurative complications; and (2) enteric fever (typhoid fever and paratyphoid fever) (see section on Typhoid Fever and Parathyroid Fever). Although the incidence of typhoid fever has decreased in the United States, the incidence of *Salmonella* gastroenteritis has greatly increased in the past 15–20 years. The highest attack rates occur in children younger than age 6 years, with a peak in the age group from 6 months to 2 years.

Salmonellae are widespread in nature, infecting domestic and wild animals. Fowl and reptiles have a particularly high carriage rate. Transmission results primarily from ingestion of contaminated food. Transmission from human to human occurs by the fecal-oral route via contaminated food, water, and fomites. Numerous foods, including meats, milk, cheese, ice cream, chocolate, contaminated egg powder, and frozen whole egg preparations used to make ice cream, custards, and mayonnaise are associated with outbreaks. Eggs with contaminated shells that are consumed raw or undercooked have been incriminated in outbreaks and sporadic cases. Animal contact also can be a source for salmonella.

Because salmonellae are susceptible to gastric acidity, the elderly, infants, and patients taking antacids or H_2-blocking drugs are at increased risk for infection. Most cases of *Salmonella* meningitis (80%) and bacteremia occur in infancy. Newborns may acquire the infection from their mothers during delivery and may precipitate outbreaks in nurseries. Newborns are at special risk for developing meningitis.

Epidemiologic studies suggest that 100 mild cases of *Salmonella* infection occur for each case detected by a positive culture.

Clinical Findings

A. Symptoms and Signs

There is a very wide range of severity of infection. Infants usually develop fever, vomiting, and diarrhea. The older child also may complain of headache, nausea, and abdominal pain. Stools are often watery or may contain mucus and, in some instances, blood, suggesting shigellosis. Drowsiness and disorientation may be associated with meningismus. Convulsions occur less frequently than with shigellosis. Splenomegaly occasionally occurs. In the usual case, diarrhea is moderate and subsides after 4–5 days, but it may be protracted.

B. Laboratory Findings

Diagnosis is made by isolation of the organism from stool, blood, or, in some cases, from urine, CSF, or pus from a suppurative lesion. The WBC count usually shows a polymorphonuclear leukocytosis but may show leukopenia. Salmonella isolates should be reported to public health authorities for epidemiologic purposes.

Differential Diagnosis

In staphylococcal food poisoning, the incubation period is shorter (2–4 hours) than in Salmonella food poisoning (12–24 hours). Fever is absent, and vomiting rather than diarrhea is the main symptom. In shigellosis, many polymorphonuclear leukocytes usually are seen on a stained smear of stool, and the peripheral WBC count is more likely to slow a marked left shift, although some cases of salmonellosis are indistinguishable from shigellosis. *Campylobacter* gastroenteritis commonly resembles salmonellosis clinically. Culture of the stools is necessary to distinguish the causes of bacterial gastroenteritis.

Complications

Unlike most types of infectious diarrhea, salmonellosis is frequently accompanied by bacteremia, especially in newborns and infants. Septicemia with extraintestinal infection is seen, most commonly with *Salmonella choleraesuis* but also with *Salmonella enteritidis, S typhimurium,* and *Salmonella paratyphi* B and C. The organism may spread to any tissue and may cause arthritis, osteomyelitis, cholecystitis, endocarditis, meningitis, pericarditis, pneumonia, or pyelonephritis. Patients with sickle cell anemia or other hemoglobinopathies have a predilection for the development of osteomyelitis. Severe dehydration and shock are more likely to occur with shigellosis but may occur with *Salmonella* gastroenteritis.

Prevention

Measures for the prevention of *Salmonella* infections include thorough cooking of foodstuffs derived from contaminated sources, adequate refrigeration, control of infection among domestic animals, and meticulous meat and poultry inspections. Raw and undercooked fresh eggs should be avoided. Food handlers and child care workers with salmonellosis should have three negative stool cultures before resuming work. Asymptomatic children, who have recovered from *Salmonella* infection, do not need exclusion.

Treatment

A. Specific Measures

In uncomplicated *Salmonella* gastroenteritis, antibiotic treatment does not shorten the course of the clinical illness and may prolong convalescent carriage of the organism. Colitis or secretory diarrhea due to Salmonella may improve with antibiotic therapy.

Because of the higher risk of sepsis and focal disease, antibiotic treatment is recommended in infants younger than age 3 months, in severely ill children, and in children with sickle cell disease, liver disease, recent gastrointestinal surgery, cancer, depressed immunity, or chronic renal or cardiac disease. Infants younger than age 3 months with positive stool cultures or suspected salmonellosis sepsis should be admitted to the hospital, evaluated for focal infection including cultures of blood and CSF, and given treatment intravenously. A third-generation cephalosporin is usually recommended due to frequent resistance to ampicillin and TMP–SMX. Older patients developing bacteremia during the course of gastroenteritis should receive parenteral treatment initially, and a careful search should be made for additional foci of infection. After signs and symptoms subside, these patients should receive oral medication. Parenteral and oral treatment should last a total of 7–10 days. Longer treatment is indicated for specific complications. If susceptibility tests indicate resistance to ampicillin, third-generation cephalosporins or TMP–SMX should be given. Fluoroquinolones also are efficacious but are not approved for administration to children. Fluoroquinolones or azithromycin are used for strains resistant to multiple other drugs.

Empiric therapy of gram-negative meningitis is with meropenem (120 mg/kg/d) intravenously in three divided doses or cefepime (150 mg/kg/d) in three divided doses with adjustment based on culture and susceptibility testing.

Often ampicillin (200–300 mg/kg/d intravenously in four to six divided doses) or a third-generation cephalosporin (cefotaxime, ceftriaxone) is used for 4–6 weeks to complete therapy.

Outbreaks on pediatric wards are difficult to control. Strict hand washing, cohorting of patients and personnel, and ultimately closure of the unit may be necessary.

B. Treatment of the Carrier State

About half of patients may have positive stool cultures after 4 weeks. Infants tend to remain convalescent carriers for up to a year. Antibiotic treatment of carriers is not effective.

C. General Measures

Careful attention must be given to maintaining fluid and electrolyte balance, especially in infants.

Prognosis

In gastroenteritis, the prognosis is good. In sepsis with focal suppurative complications, the prognosis is more guarded. The case fatality rate of *Salmonella* meningitis is high in infants. There is a strong tendency to relapse if treatment is not continued for at least 4 weeks.

Centers for Disease Control and Prevention (CDC): FoodNet. Available at: http://www.cdc.gov/foodnet

Centers for Disease Control and Prevention (CDC): *Salmonella* infection (salmonellosis). Available at: http://www.cdc.gov/salmonella/

Hendriksen RS et al: Emergence of multidrug-resistant salmonella concord infections in Europe and the United States in children adopted from Ethiopia, 2003–2007. Pediatr Infect Dis J 2009;28(9):814 [PMID: 19710587].

Jain S et al: Multistate outbreak of *Salmonella typhimurium* and saintpaul infections associated with unpasteurized orange juice—United States, 2005. Clin Infect Dis 2009;48(8):1065 [PMID: 19281328].

Maki DG: Coming to grips with foodborne infection—peanut butter, peppers, and nationwide salmonella outbreaks. N Engl J Med 2009;360(10):949 [PMID: 19213675].

Sotir MJ et al: Salmonella Wandsworth Outbreak Investigation Team: Outbreak of *Salmonella* Wandsworth and Typhimurium infections in infants and toddlers traced to a commercial vegetable-coated snack food. Pediatr Infect Dis J 2009;28(12):1 [PMID: 19779390].

TYPHOID FEVER & PARATYPHOID FEVER

ESSENTIALS OF DIAGNOSIS & TYPICAL FEATURES

- Insidious or acute onset of headache, anorexia, vomiting, constipation or diarrhea, ileus, and high fever.
- Meningismus, splenomegaly, and rose spots.
- Leukopenia; positive blood, stool, bone marrow, and urine cultures.

General Considerations

Typhoid fever is caused by the gram-negative bacillus *Salmonella typhi*. Paratyphoid fevers, which are usually milder but may be clinically indistinguishable, are caused by *S paratyphi* A, *Salmonella schottmülleri*, or *Salmonella hirschfeldii* (formerly *S paratyphi* A, B, and C). Children have a shorter incubation period than do adults (usually 5–8 days instead of 8–14 days). The organism enters the body through the walls of the intestinal tract and, following a transient bacteremia, multiplies in the reticuloendothelial cells of the liver and spleen. Persistent bacteremia and symptoms then follow. Reinfection of the intestine occurs as organisms are excreted in the bile. Bacterial emboli produce the characteristic skin lesions (rose spots). Typhoid fever is transmitted by the fecal-oral route and by contamination of food or water. Unlike other *Salmonella* species, there are no animal reservoirs of *S typhi*; each case is the result of direct or indirect contact with the organism or with an individual who is actively infected or a chronic carrier.

About 400 cases per year were reported in the United States in 2009, 80% of which are acquired during foreign travel.

Clinical Findings

A. Symptoms and Signs

In children, the onset of typhoid fever usually is sudden rather than insidious, with malaise, headache, crampy abdominal pains and distention, and sometimes constipation followed within 48 hours by diarrhea, high fever, and toxemia. An encephalopathy may be seen with irritability, confusion, delirium, and stupor. Vomiting and meningismus may be prominent in infants and young children. The classic lengthy three-stage disease seen in adult patients often is shortened in children. The prodrome may last only 2–4 days, the toxic stage only 2–3 days, and the defervescence stage 1–2 weeks.

During the prodromal stage, physical findings may be absent, but abdominal distention and tenderness, meningismus, mild hepatomegaly, and minimal splenomegaly may be present. The typical typhoidal rash (rose spots) is present in 10%–15% of children. It appears during the second week of the disease and may erupt in crops for the succeeding 10–14 days. Rose spots are erythematous maculopapular lesions 2–3 mm in diameter that blanch on pressure. They are found principally on the trunk and chest and they generally disappear within 3–4 days. The lesions usually number fewer than 20.

B. Laboratory Findings

Typhoid bacilli can be isolated from many sites, including blood, stool, urine, and bone marrow. Blood cultures are positive in 50%–80% of cases during the first week and less often later in the illness. Stool cultures are positive in about 50% of cases after the first week. Urine and bone marrow cultures also are valuable. Most patients will have negative cultures (including stool) by the end of a 6-week period. Serologic tests (Widal reaction) are not as useful as cultures because both false-positive and false-negative results occur. Leukopenia is common in the second week of the disease, but in the first week, leukocytosis may be seen. Proteinuria, mild elevation of liver enzymes, thrombocytopenia, and DIC are common.

Differential Diagnosis

Typhoid and paratyphoid fevers must be distinguished from other serious prolonged fevers. These include typhus, brucellosis, malaria, tularemia, tuberculosis, psittacosis, vasculitis, lymphoma, mononucleosis, and Kawasaki disease. The diagnosis of typhoid fever often is made clinically in developing countries, but the accuracy of clinical diagnosis is variable. In developed countries, where typhoid fever is uncommon and physicians are unfamiliar with the clinical picture, the diagnosis often is not suspected until late in the course. Positive cultures confirm the diagnosis.

Complications

The most serious complications of typhoid fever are gastrointestinal hemorrhage (2%–10%) and perforation (1%–3%). They occur toward the end of the second week or during the third week of the disease.

Intestinal perforation is one of the principal causes of death. The site of perforation generally is the terminal ileum or cecum. The clinical manifestations are indistinguishable from those of acute appendicitis, with pain, tenderness, and rigidity in the right lower quadrant.

Bacterial pneumonia, meningitis, septic arthritis, abscesses, and osteomyelitis are uncommon complications, particularly if specific treatment is given promptly. Shock and electrolyte disturbances may lead to death.

About 1%–3% of patients become chronic carriers of *S typhi*. Chronic carriage is defined as excretion of typhoid bacilli for more than a year, but carriage is often lifelong. Adults with underlying biliary or urinary tract disease are much more likely than children to become chronic carriers.

Prevention

Routine typhoid vaccine is not recommended in the United States but should be considered for foreign travel to endemic areas. An attenuated oral typhoid vaccine produced from strain Ty21a has better efficacy and causes minimal side effects but is not approved for children younger than age 6 years. The vaccine is repeated after 5 years. A capsular polysaccharide vaccine (ViCPS) requires one intramuscular injection and may be given to children age 2 years and older. (See Chapter 10.)

Treatment

A. Specific Measures

Third-generation cephalosporins such as cefotaxime (150 mg/kg divided in three doses), azithromycin (10 mg/kg on day 1, followed by 5 mg/kg for 7 days), or a fluoroquinolone are used for presumptive therapy. Antimicrobial susceptibility testing and local experience are used to direct subsequent therapy. Equally effective regimens for susceptible strains include the following: TMP–SMX

(10 mg/kg trimethoprim and 50 mg/kg sulfamethoxazole per day orally in two or three divided doses), amoxicillin (100 mg/kg/d orally in four divided doses), and ampicillin (100–200 mg/kg/d intravenously in four divided doses). Aminoglycosides and first- and second-generation cephalosporins are clinically ineffective regardless of in vitro susceptibility results. Ciprofloxacin or other fluoroquinolones are efficacious but not approved in children, but may be used for multiply resistant strains. Treatment duration is 14–21 days. Patients may remain febrile for 3–5 days even with appropriate therapy.

B. General Measures

General support of the patient is exceedingly important and includes rest, good nutrition and hydration, and careful observation, with particular regard to evidence of intestinal bleeding or perforation. Blood transfusions may be needed even in the absence of frank hemorrhage.

Prognosis

A prolonged convalescent carrier stage may occur in children. Three negative cultures after all antibiotics have been stopped are required before contact precautions are stopped. With early antibiotic therapy, the prognosis is excellent, and the mortality rate is less than 1%. Relapse occurs 1–3 weeks later in 10%–20% of patients despite appropriate antibiotic treatment.

Bhutta ZA, Threlfall J: Addressing the global disease burden of typhoid fever. JAMA 2009;302(8):898 [PMID: 19706867].

Levine MM: Typhoid vaccines ready for implementation. N Engl J Med 2008;361(4):403 [PMID: 19625721].

Martinez-Roig A et al: Pancreatitis in typhoid fever relapse. Pediatr Infect Dis J 2009;28(1):74 [PMID: 19034060].

Parry CM et al: Randomized controlled comparison of ofloxacin, azithromycin, and an ofloxacin-azithromycin combination for treatment of multidrug-resistant and nalidixic acid-resistant typhoid fever. Antimicrob Agents Chemother 2007;51:819 [PMID: 17145784].

SHIGELLOSIS (BACILLARY DYSENTERY)

ESSENTIALS OF DIAGNOSIS & TYPICAL FEATURES

- Cramps and bloody diarrhea.
- High fever, malaise, convulsions.
- Pus and blood in diarrheal stools examined microscopically.
- Diagnosis confirmed by stool culture.

General Considerations

Shigellae are nonmotile gram-negative rods of the family Enterobacteriaceae and are closely related to *E coli*. The genus *Shigella* is divided into four species: *S dysenteriae, Shigella flexneri, Shigella boydii,* and *Shigella sonnei*. Approximately 15,000 to 20,000 cases of shigellosis are reported each year in the United States. *S sonnei* followed by *S flexneri* are the most common isolates.

S dysenteriae, which causes the most severe diarrhea of all species and the greatest number of extraintestinal complications, accounts for less than 1% of all *Shigella* infections in the United States.

Shigellosis may be a serious disease, particularly in young children, and without supportive treatment an appreciable mortality rate results. In older children and adults, the disease tends to be self-limited and milder. *Shigella* is usually transmitted by the fecal-oral route. Food- and water-borne outbreaks are increasing in occurrence, but are less important overall than person-to-person transmission. The disease is very communicable—as few as 200 bacteria can produce illness in an adult. The secondary attack rate in families is high, and shigellosis is a serious problem in day care centers and custodial institutions. *Shigella* organisms produce disease by invading the colonic mucosa, causing mucosal ulcerations and microabscesses. A plasmid-encoded gene is required for enterotoxin production, chromosomal genes are required for invasiveness, and smooth lipopolysaccharides are required for virulence. An experimental vaccine is under development and is safe and immunogenic in young children.

Clinical Findings

A. Symptoms and Signs

The incubation period of shigellosis is usually 2–4 days. Onset is abrupt, with abdominal cramps, urgency, tenesmus, chills, fever, malaise, and diarrhea. Hallucinations and seizures sometimes accompany high fever. In severe forms, blood and mucus are seen in small stools (dysentery), and meningismus and convulsions may occur. In older children, the disease may be mild and may be characterized by watery diarrhea without blood. In young children, a fever of 39.4–40°C is common. Rarely there is rectal prolapse. Symptoms generally last 3–7 days.

B. Laboratory Findings

The total WBC count varies, but often there is a marked shift to the left. The stool may contain gross blood and mucus, and many neutrophils are seen if mucus from the stool is examined microscopically. Stool cultures are usually positive; however, they may be negative because the organism is somewhat fragile and present in small numbers late in the disease, and because laboratory techniques are suboptimal for the recovery of shigellae.

Differential Diagnosis

Diarrhea due to rotavirus infection is a winter rather than a summer disease. Usually children with viral gastroenteritis are not as febrile or toxic as those with shigellosis, and the stool does not contain gross blood or neutrophils. Intestinal infections caused by Salmonella or Campylobacter are differentiated by culture. Grossly bloody stools in a patient without fever or stool leukocytes suggest *E coli* O157:H7 infection. Amebic dysentery is diagnosed by microscopic examination of fresh stools or sigmoidoscopy specimens. Intussusception is characterized by an abdominal mass (so-called currant jelly stools) without leukocytes, and by absence of initial fever. Mild shigellosis is not distinguishable clinically from other forms of infectious diarrhea.

Complications

Dehydration, acidosis, shock, and renal failure are the major complications. In some cases, a chronic form of dysentery occurs, characterized by mucoid stools and poor nutrition. Bacteremia and metastatic infections are rare but serious complications. Febrile seizures are common. Fulminating fatal dysentery and hemolytic-uremic syndrome occur rarely. Reiter syndrome may follow *S flexneri* infection.

Treatment

A. Specific Measures

Resistance to TMP–SMX (10 mg/kg/d trimethoprim and 50 mg/kg/d sulfamethoxazole, given in two divided doses orally for 5 days) and ampicillin (100 mg/kg/d divided in four doses) is common and limits the use of these drugs to cases where results of susceptibility testing are known. Amoxicillin is not effective. Parenteral ceftriaxone and oral cefixime are both effective. Azithromycin (12 mg/kg/d on day 1, then 6 mg/kg/d for 4 days) was superior to cefixime in one study. Ciprofloxacin (500 mg, given twice daily for 5 days) is efficacious in adults but is not approved for use in children. However, it may be used in children who remain symptomatic and in need of therapy, and when multiply resistant strains limit other preferred choices. Successful treatment reduces the duration of fever, cramping, and diarrhea and terminates fecal excretion of *Shigella*. Tetracycline and chloramphenicol are also effective, but resistance is common. Presumptive therapy should be limited to children with classic shigellosis or known outbreaks. Afebrile children with bloody diarrhea are more commonly infected with EHEC. Antimicrobial therapy of EHEC may increase the likelihood of hemolytic-uremic syndrome, and is not recommended.

B. General Measures

In severe cases, immediate rehydration is critical. A mild form of chronic malabsorption syndrome may supervene and require prolonged dietary control.

Prognosis

The prognosis is excellent if vascular collapse is treated promptly by adequate fluid therapy. The mortality rate is high in very young, malnourished infants who do not receive fluid and electrolyte therapy. Convalescent fecal excretion of *Shigella* lasts 1–4 weeks in patients not receiving antimicrobial therapy. Long-term carriers are rare.

Arvelo W et al: Transmission risk factors and treatment of pediatric shigellosis during a large daycare center-associated outbreak of multidrug resistant *Shigella sonnei*. Pediatr Infect Dis J 2009;28(11):1 [PMID: 19738503].

Niyogi SK: Increasing antimicrobial resistance—an emerging problem in the treatment of shigellosis. Clin Microbiol Infect 2007;13:1141 [PMID: 17953700].

Centers for Disease Control and Prevention (CDC): Shigellosis. Available at: www.cdc.gov/nczved/divisions/dfbmd/shigellosis/

CHOLERA

ESSENTIALS OF DIAGNOSIS & TYPICAL FEATURES

- Sudden onset of severe watery diarrhea.
- Persistent vomiting without nausea or fever.
- Extreme and rapid dehydration and electrolyte loss, with rapid development of vascular collapse.
- Contact with a case of cholera or with shellfish, or the presence of cholera in the community.
- Diagnosis confirmed by stool culture.

General Considerations

Cholera is an acute diarrheal disease caused by the gram-negative organism *Vibrio cholerae*. It is transmitted by contaminated water or food, especially contaminated shellfish. Epidemics are common in impoverished areas where hygiene and safe water supply are limited. Typical disease is generally so dramatic that in endemic areas the diagnosis is obvious. Individuals with mild illness and young children may play an important role in transmission of the infection.

Asymptomatic infection is far more common than clinical disease. In endemic areas, rising titers of vibriocidal antibody are seen with increasing age. Infection occurs in individuals with low titers. The age-specific attack rate is highest in children younger than age 5 years and declines with age. Cholera is unusual in infancy.

Cholera toxin is a protein enterotoxin that is primarily responsible for symptoms. Cholera toxin binds to a regulatory subunit of adenylyl cyclase in enterocytes, causing increased cyclic adenosine monophosphate and an outpouring of NaCl and water into the lumen of the small bowel.

Nutritional status is an important factor determining the severity of the diarrhea. Duration of diarrhea is prolonged in adults and children with severe malnutrition.

Cholera is endemic in India and southern and Southeast Asia and in parts of Africa. The most recent pandemic, caused by the El Tor biotype of *V cholerae* 01, began in 1961 in Indonesia. Epidemic cholera spread in Central and South America, with a total of 1 million cases and 9500 deaths reported through 1994. A severe cholera outbreak is ongoing in Haiti since October 2010. More than 500,000 cases and 6000 deaths are estimated. Cases in the United States occurred in the course of foreign travel or as a result of consumption of contaminated imported food. Cholera is increasingly associated with consumption of shellfish. Interstate shipment of oysters has resulted in cholera in several inland states. Cholera is now rare in the United States with fewer than 10 cases per year reported.

V cholerae is a natural inhabitant of shellfish and copepods in estuarine environments. Seasonal multiplication of *V cholerae* may provide a source of outbreaks in endemic areas. Chronic cholera carriers are rare. The incubation period is short, usually 1–3 days.

Clinical Findings

A. Symptoms and Signs

Many patients infected with *V cholerae* have mild disease, with 1%–2% developing severe diarrhea. During severe cholera, there is a sudden onset of massive, frequent, watery stools, generally light gray in color (so-called rice-water stools) and containing some mucus but no pus. Vomiting may be projectile and is not accompanied by nausea. Within 2–3 hours, the tremendous loss of fluids results in life-threatening dehydration, hypochloremia, and hypokalemia, with marked weakness and collapse. Renal failure with uremia and irreversible peripheral vascular collapse will occur if fluid therapy is not administered. The illness lasts 1–7 days and is shortened by appropriate antibiotic therapy.

B. Laboratory Findings

Markedly elevated hemoglobin (20 g/dL) and marked acidosis, hypochloremia, and hyponatremia are seen. Stool sodium concentration may range from 80 to 120 mEq/L. Cultural confirmation requires specific media and takes 16–18 hours for a presumptive diagnosis and 36–48 hours for a definitive bacteriologic diagnosis.

Prevention

Cholera vaccine is available outside of the United States and provides 50%–75% efficacy. Protection lasts 3–6 months. Cholera vaccine is not generally recommended for travelers. Tourists visiting endemic areas are at little risk if they exercise caution in what they eat and drink and maintain good personal hygiene. In endemic areas, all water and milk must be boiled, food protected from flies, and sanitary precautions observed. Simple filtration of water is highly effective in reducing cases. Thorough cooking of shellfish prevents transmission. All patients with cholera should be isolated.

Chemoprophylaxis is indicated for household and other close contacts of cholera patients. It should be initiated as soon as possible after the onset of the disease in the index patient. Tetracycline (500 mg/d for 5 days) is effective in preventing infection. TMP–SMX may be substituted in children.

Treatment

Physiologic saline or lactated Ringer solution should be administered intravenously in large amounts to restore blood volume and urine output and prevent irreversible shock. Potassium supplements are required. Sodium bicarbonate, given intravenously, also may be needed initially to overcome profound metabolic acidosis from bicarbonate loss in the stool. Moderate dehydration and acidosis can be corrected in 3–6 hours by oral therapy alone, because the active glucose transport system of the small bowel is normally functional. The optimal composition of the oral solution (in milliequivalents per liter [mEq/L]) is as follows: Na^+, 90; Cl^-, 80; and K^+, 20 (with glucose, 110 mmol/L).

Treatment with tetracycline (50 mg/kg/d orally in four divided doses for 2–5 days) or azithromycin (10 mg/kg/d in one dose for 1–5 days) shortens the duration of the disease in children and prevents clinical relapse but is not as important as fluid and electrolyte therapy. Tetracycline resistance occurs in some regions, and ciprofloxacin may be used depending on local resistance patterns. TMP–SMX or azithromycin should be used in children younger than age 9 years.

Prognosis

With early and rapid replacement of fluids and electrolytes, the case fatality rate is 1%–2% in children. If significant symptoms appear and no treatment is given, the mortality rate is over 50%.

Chin CS et al: The origin of the Haitian cholera outbreak strain. N Engl J Med 2011;364:33–42 [PMID: 21142692].

Nelson EJ et al: Antibiotics for both moderate and severe cholera. N Engl J Med 2011;364:5–7 [PMID: 21142691].

Roy SK et al: Zinc supplementation in children with cholera in Bangladesh: Randomized controlled trial. BMJ 2008;336(7638):227 [PMID: 18184631].

Walton DA, Ivers CL: Responding to cholera in post-earthquake Haiti. N Engl J Med 2011;364:3–5 [PMID: 21142690].

CAMPYLOBACTER INFECTION

ESSENTIALS OF DIAGNOSIS & TYPICAL FEATURES

- Fever, vomiting, abdominal pain, diarrhea.
- Presumptive diagnosis by darkfield or phase contrast microscopy of stool wet mount or modified Gram stain.
- Definitive diagnosis by stool culture.

General Considerations

Campylobacter species are small gram-negative, curved or spiral bacilli that are commensals or pathogens in many animals. *Campylobacter jejuni* frequently causes acute enteritis in humans. In the 1990s, *C jejuni* was responsible for 3%–11% of cases of acute gastroenteritis in North America and Europe. In many areas, enteritis due to *C jejuni* is more common than that due to *Salmonella* or *Shigella*. *Campylobacter fetus* causes bacteremia and meningitis in immunocompromised patients. *C fetus* may cause maternal fever, abortion, stillbirth, and severe neonatal infection. *Helicobacter pylori* (previously called *Campylobacter pylori*) causes gastritis and peptic ulcer disease in both adults and children. (See Chapter 21.)

Campylobacter colonizes domestic and wild animals, especially poultry. Numerous cases have been associated with sick puppies or other animal contacts. Contaminated food and water, improperly cooked poultry, and person-to-person spread by the fecal-oral route are common routes of transmission. Outbreaks associated with day care centers, contaminated water supplies, and raw milk have been reported. Newborns may acquire the organism from their mothers at delivery.

Clinical Findings

A. Symptoms and Signs

C jejuni enteritis can be mild or severe. In tropical countries, asymptomatic stool carriage is common. The incubation period is usually 1–7 days. The disease usually begins with sudden onset of high fever, malaise, headache, abdominal cramps, nausea, and vomiting. Diarrhea follows and may be watery or bile-stained, mucoid, and bloody. The illness is self-limiting, lasting 2–7 days, but relapses may occur. Without antimicrobial treatment, the organism remains in the stool for 1–6 weeks.

B. Laboratory Findings

The peripheral WBC count generally is elevated, with many band forms. Microscopic examination of stool reveals erythrocytes and pus cells.

Isolation of *C jejuni* from stool is not difficult but requires selective agar, incubation at 42°C rather than 35°C, and incubation in an atmosphere of about 5% oxygen and 5% CO_2 (candle jar is satisfactory).

Differential Diagnosis

Campylobacter enteritis may resemble viral gastroenteritis, salmonellosis, shigellosis, amebiasis, or other infectious diarrheas. Because it also mimics ulcerative colitis, Crohn disease, intussusception, and appendicitis, mistaken diagnosis can lead to unnecessary diagnostic testing or surgery.

Complications

The most common complication is dehydration. Other uncommon complications include erythema nodosum, convulsions, reactive arthritis, bacteremia, urinary tract infection, and cholecystitis. Guillain-Barré syndrome may follow *C jejuni* infection by 1–3 weeks.

Prevention

No vaccine is available. Hand washing and adherence to basic food sanitation practices help prevent disease. Hand washing and cleaning of kitchen utensils after contact with raw poultry are important.

Treatment

Treatment of fluid and electrolyte disturbances is important. Antimicrobial treatment with erythromycin in children (30–50 mg/kg/d orally in four divided doses for 5 days), azithromycin for 5 days, or ciprofloxacin terminates fecal excretion. Fluoroquinolone-resistant *C jejuni* are now common worldwide. Therapy given early in the course of the illness will shorten the duration of symptoms but is unnecessary if given later. Antimicrobials used for shigellosis, such as TMP–SMX and ampicillin, are inactive against Campylobacter. Supportive therapy is sufficient in most cases.

Prognosis

The outlook is excellent if dehydration is corrected and misdiagnosis does not lead to inappropriate diagnostic or surgical procedures.

Jones TF: Changing challenges of bacterial enteric infection in the United States. J Infect Dis 2009;199(4):465 [PMID: 19281301].

Kalra V et al: Association of *Campylobacter jejuni* infection with childhood Guillain-Barre syndrome: A case-control study. J Child Neuro 2009;24(6):664 [PMID: 19491112].

Ternhag A et al: A meta-analysis on the effects of antibiotic treatment on duration of symptoms caused by infection with *Campylobacter* species. Clin Infect Dis 2007;44:696 [PMID: 17278062].

Centers for Disease Control and Prevention (CDC): *Campylobacter* infections. Available at: http://www.cdc.gov/nczved/divisions/dfbmd/diseases/campylobacter

TULAREMIA

ESSENTIALS OF DIAGNOSIS & TYPICAL FEATURES

- A cutaneous or mucous membrane lesion at the site of inoculation and regional lymph node enlargement.
- Sudden onset of fever, chills, and prostration.
- History of contact with infected animals, principally wild rabbits, or history of tick exposure.
- Positive culture or immunofluorescence from mucocutaneous ulcer or regional lymph nodes.
- High serum antibody titer.

General Considerations

Tularemia is caused by *Francisella tularensis*, a gram-negative organism usually acquired directly from infected animals (principally wild rabbits) or by the bite of an infected tick. Occasionally infection is acquired from infected domestic dogs or cats; by contamination of the skin or mucous membranes with infected blood or tissues; by inhalation of infected material; by bites of fleas or deer flies that have been in contact with infected animals; or by ingestion of contaminated meat or water. The incubation period is short, usually 3–7 days, but may vary from 2 to 25 days.

Ticks are the most important vector of tularemia and rabbits are the classic vector. It is important to seek a history of rabbit hunting, skinning, or food preparation in any patient who has a febrile illness with tender lymphadenopathy, often in the region of a draining skin ulcer.

Prevention

Children should be protected from insect bites, especially those of ticks, fleas, and deer flies, by the use of proper clothing and repellents. Because rabbits are the source of most human infections, the dressing and handling of such game should be performed with great care. Rubber gloves should be worn by hunters or food handlers when handling carcasses of wild rabbits. If contact occurs, thorough washing with soap and water is indicated. For postexposure prophylaxis from an intentional release of *F tularensis* (bioterrorism), a 14-day course of doxycycline or ciprofloxacin is recommended (children less than 8 years should not receive doxycycline unless benefits outweigh risks; in children less than 18 years ciprofloxacin is not approved for this indication—weigh benefits and risk).

Clinical Findings

A. Symptoms and Signs

Several clinical types of tularemia occur in children. Sixty percent of infections are of the ulceroglandular form and start as a reddened papule that may be pruritic, quickly ulcerates, and is not very painful. Soon, the regional lymph nodes become large and tender. Fluctuance quickly follows. There may be marked systemic symptoms, including high fever, chills, weakness, and vomiting. Pneumonitis occasionally accompanies the ulceroglandular form or may be seen as the sole manifestation of infection (pneumonic form). A detectable skin lesion may be absent, and localized lymphoid enlargement may exist alone (glandular form). Oculoglandular and oropharyngeal forms also occur. The latter is characterized by tonsillitis, often with membrane formation, cervical adenopathy, and high fever. In the absence of a primary ulcer or localized lymphadenitis, a prolonged febrile disease reminiscent of typhoid fever can occur (typhoidal form). Splenomegaly is common in all forms.

B. Laboratory Findings

F tularensis can be recovered from ulcers, regional lymph nodes, and sputum of patients with the pneumonic form. However, the organism grows only on an enriched medium (blood-cystine-glucose agar), and laboratory handling is dangerous owing to the risk of airborne transmission to laboratory personnel. Immunofluorescent staining of biopsy material or aspirates of involved lymph nodes is diagnostic, although it is not widely available.

The WBC count is not remarkable. Agglutinins are present after the second week of illness, and in the absence of a positive culture their development confirms the diagnosis. A tube agglutination titer of 1:160 or greater or a microagglutination titer of 1:128 or higher is considered positive. PCR of blood, lymph node aspirate, or tissue may be available through State Health Departments.

Differential Diagnosis

The typhoidal form of tularemia may mimic typhoid, brucellosis, miliary tuberculosis, Rocky Mountain spotted fever, and mononucleosis. Pneumonic tularemia resembles atypical or mycotic pneumonitis. The ulceroglandular type of tularemia resembles pyoderma caused by staphylococci or streptococci, plague, anthrax, and cat-scratch fever. The oropharyngeal type must be distinguished from streptococcal or diphtheritic pharyngitis, mononucleosis, herpangina, or other viral pharyngitides.

Treatment

A. Specific Measures

Historically, streptomycin was the drug of choice. Gentamicin and amikacin also are efficacious, more available, and familiar to clinicians. A 10-day course is usually sufficient, although more severe infections may need longer therapy. Doxycycline is effective, but relapse rates are higher. Doxycycline is not usually recommended for children younger than 8 years of age unless benefits of use outweigh the risk of dental staining. Doxycycline is a static (as opposed to cidal) agent and should be given for at least 14 days. Ciprofloxacin also can be used in patients with less severe disease. Ciprofloxacin is not approved for children younger than 18 years, and is not usually recommended in children unless benefits outweigh risks.

B. General Measures

Antipyretics and analgesics may be given as necessary. Skin lesions are best left open. Glandular lesions occasionally require incision and drainage.

Prognosis

The prognosis is excellent in cases of tularemia that are recognized early and treated appropriately.

Ellis J, Oyston PCF, Green M, Titball RW: Tularemia. Clin Micro Rev;15(4):61–646 [PMID: 12364373]. Available at: http://cmr.asm.org/cgi/content/full/15/4/631?view=long&pmid=12364373

Lieberman JM: North American zoonoses. Pediatr Ann 2009;38(4):193–198 [PMID: 19455948].

Center for Disease Control (CDC) and Prevention. Available at: http://www.cdc.gov/tularemia/

PLAGUE

ESSENTIALS OF DIAGNOSIS & TYPICAL FEATURES

- Sudden onset of fever, chills, and prostration.
- Regional lymphadenitis with suppuration of nodes (bubonic form).
- Hemorrhage into skin and mucous membranes and shock (septicemia).
- Cough, dyspnea, cyanosis, and hemoptysis (pneumonia).
- History of exposure to infected animals.

General Considerations

Plague is an extremely serious acute infection caused by a gram-negative bacillus, *Yersinia pestis*. It is a disease of rodents that is transmitted to humans by flea bites. Plague bacilli have been isolated from ground squirrels, prairie dogs, and other wild rodents in many of the western and southwestern states in the United States. Most cases have come from New Mexico, Arizona, Colorado, and California. Direct contact with rodents, rabbits, or domestic cats may transmit fleas infected with plague bacilli. Most cases occur from June through September. Human plague in the United States appears to occur in cycles that reflect cycles in wild animal reservoirs.

Prevention

Proper disposal of household and commercial wastes and chemical control of rats are basic elements of plague prevention. Flea control is instituted and maintained with liberal use of insecticides. Children vacationing in remote camping areas should be warned not to handle dead or dying animals. Domestic cats that roam freely in suburban areas may contact infected wild animals and acquire infected fleas. There is no commercially available vaccine for plague.

All persons who have been exposed to plague in the previous 6 days (via personal contact with an infected person, contact with plague infected fleas, or exposure to infected tissues) should be given antimicrobial prophylaxis or be instructed to closely monitor themselves for fever or other symptoms and report any illness or any fever to their physician. Persons who have close personal contact (< 2 m) with a person with pneumonic plague should receive antimicrobial prophylaxis for 7 days from the last exposure. Doxycycline or ciprofloxacin are the recommended agents for prophylaxis. For children younger than 8 years, TMP–SMX is an alternative agent but the efficacy is unknown. Chloramphenicol is also an alternative agent. For persons who have had a known or suspected exposure to plague-infected fleas in the previous week, the same antimicrobial regimen can be used for prophylaxis. Patients on prophylaxis should still seek prompt medical care for onset of fever or other illness.

Clinical Findings

A. Symptoms and Signs

Plague assumes several clinical forms; the two most common are bubonic and septicemic. Pneumonic plague, the form that occurs when organisms enter the body through the respiratory tract, is uncommon.

1. Bubonic plague—Bubonic plague begins after an incubation period of 2–8 days with a sudden onset of high fever, chills, headache, vomiting, and marked delirium or clouding of consciousness. A less severe form also exists, with a less precipitous onset, but with progression over several days to severe symptoms. Although the flea bite is rarely seen, the regional lymph node, usually inguinal and unilateral, is/are painful and tender, 1–5 cm in diameter. The node usually suppurates and drains spontaneously after 1 week. The plague bacillus produces endotoxin that causes vascular necrosis. Bacilli may overwhelm regional lymph nodes and enter the circulation to produce septicemia. Severe vascular necrosis results in widely disseminated hemorrhage in skin, mucous membranes, liver, and spleen. Myocarditis and circulatory collapse may result from damage by the endotoxin. Plague meningitis or pneumonia may occur following bacteremic spread from an infected lymph node.

2. Septicemic plague—Plague may initially present as septicemia without evidence of lymphadenopathy. In some series, 25% of cases are initially septicemic. Septicemic plague carries a worse prognosis than bubonic plague, largely because it is not recognized and treated early. Patients may present initially with a nonspecific febrile illness characterized by fever, myalgia, chills, and anorexia. Plague is frequently complicated by secondary seeding of the lung causing plague pneumonia.

3. Primary pneumonic plague—Inhalation of *Y pestis* bacilli causes primary plague pneumonia. This form of plague has been transmitted to humans from cats with pneumonic plague and would be the form of plague most likely seen after aerosolized release of *Y pestis* in a bioterrorist incident. After an incubation of 1–6 days, the patient develops fever, cough, shortness of breath, and the production of bloody, watery, or purulent sputum. Gastrointestinal symptoms are sometimes prominent. Because the initial focus of infection is the lung, buboes are usually absent; occasionally cervical buboes may be seen.

B. Laboratory Findings

Aspirate from a bubo contains bipolar-staining gram-negative bacilli. Pus, sputum, and blood all yield the organism. Rapid diagnosis can be made with fluorescent antibody detection or polymerase chain reaction (PCR) on clinical specimens. Confirmation is made by culture or serologic testing. Laboratory infections are common enough to make bacterial isolation dangerous. Cultures are usually positive within 48 hours. Paired acute and convalescent sera may be tested for an antibody rise in those cases with negative cultures.

Differential Diagnosis

The septic phase of the disease may be confused with illnesses such as meningococcemia, sepsis caused by other bacteria, and rickettsioses. The bubonic form resembles tularemia, anthrax, cat-scratch fever, streptococcal adenitis, and cellulitis. Primary gastroenteritis and appendicitis may have to be distinguished.

Treatment

A. Specific Measures

Streptomycin (30 mg/kg/d intramuscularly in two to three divided doses) or gentamicin (7.5 mg/kg/d intravenously in three divided doses) for 7–10 days after defervescence is effective. For patients not requiring parenteral therapy, doxycycline, ciprofloxacin or chloramphenicol may be given. Doxycycline is not usually recommended for children younger than 8 years of age and ciprofloxacin is not usually recommended for children less than 18 years of age unless benefits of use outweigh the risk. However, plague is a potentially life-threatening condition and benefits of use of these agents outweigh potential risks. Plague bacilli that are multiply resistant to antimicrobials are uncommon but of serious concern.

Mortality is extremely high in septicemic and pneumonic plague if specific antibiotic treatment is not started in the first 24 hours of the disease.

Every effort should be made to effect resolution of buboes without surgery. Pus from draining lymph nodes should be handled with gloves.

B. General Measures

Pneumonic plague is highly infectious, and droplet isolation is required until the patient has been on effective antimicrobial therapy for 48 hours. All contacts should receive prophylaxis with oral doxycycline 2.2 mg/kg per dose (maximum dose 100 mg) given twice a day for 7 days. State health officials should be notified immediately about suspected cases of plague.

Prognosis

The mortality rate in untreated bubonic plague is about 50%. The mortality rate for treated pneumonic plague is 50%–60%. Recent mortality rates in New Mexico were 3% for bubonic plague and 71% for the septicemic form.

Lieberman JM: North American zoonoses. Pediatr Ann 2009;38(4):193–198 [PMID: 19455948].

Prentice MB, Rahalison L: Plague. Lancet 2007;369:1196 [PMID: 17416264].

Centers for Disease Control and Prevention (CDC): Plague. Available at: http://www.cdc.gov/ncidod/dvbid/plague

HAEMOPHILUS INFLUENZAE TYPE B INFECTIONS

ESSENTIALS OF DIAGNOSIS & TYPICAL FEATURES

- Purulent meningitis in children younger than age 4 years with direct smears of CSF showing gram-negative pleomorphic rods.
- Acute epiglottitis: high fever, drooling, dysphagia, aphonia, and stridor.
- Septic arthritis: fever, local redness, swelling, heat, and pain with active or passive motion of the involved joint in a child 4 months to 4 years of age.
- Cellulitis: sudden onset of fever and distinctive cellulitis in an infant, often involving the cheek or periorbital area.
- In all cases, a positive culture from the blood, CSF, or aspirated pus confirms the diagnosis.

General Considerations

H influenzae type b (Hib) has become uncommon because of widespread immunization in early infancy. The 99% reduction in incidence seen in many parts of the United States is due to high rates of vaccine coverage and reduced nasopharyngeal carriage after vaccination. Forty percent of cases occur in children younger than 6 months who are too young to have completed a primary immunization series. Hib may cause meningitis, bacteremia, epiglottitis (supraglottic croup), septic arthritis, periorbital and facial cellulitis, pneumonia, and pericarditis.

Disease due to *H influenzae* types a, c, d, e, f, or unencapsulated strains is rare, but it now accounts for a larger proportion of positive culture results. Third-generation cephalosporins are preferred for initial therapy of Hib infections. Ampicillin is adequate for culture-proved Hib susceptible strains.

Unencapsulated, nontypeable *H influenzae* frequently colonize the mucous membranes and cause otitis media, sinusitis, bronchitis, and pneumonia in children and adults. Bacteremia is uncommon. Neonatal sepsis similar to early-onset GBS is recognized. Obstetric complications of chorioamnionitis and bacteremia are usually the source of neonatal cases.

Ampicillin resistance occurs in 25%–40% of nontypeable *H influenzae.*

Prevention

Several carbohydrate protein conjugate Hib vaccines are currently available (see Chapter 10).

The risk of invasive Hib disease is highest in unimmunized, or partially immunized, household contacts who are younger than 4 years of age. The following situations require rifampin chemoprophylaxis of all household contacts (except pregnant women) to eradicate potential nasopharyngeal colonization with Hib and limit risk of invasive disease: (1) families where at least one household contact is younger than age 4 years and either unimmunized or incompletely immunized against Hib; (2) an immunocompromised child (of any age or immunization status) resides in the household; or (3) a child younger than age 12 months resides in the home and has not received the primary series of the Hib vaccine. Preschool and day care center contacts may need prophylaxis if more than one case has occurred in the center in the previous 60 days (discuss with state health officials). The index case also needs chemoprophylaxis in these situations to eradicate nasopharyngeal colonization unless treated with ceftriaxone or cefotaxime (both are effective in eradication of Hib from the nasopharynx). Household contacts and index cases older than 1 month of age who need chemoprophylaxis should be given rifampin, 20 mg/kg per dose (maximum adult dose, 600 mg) orally, once daily for 4 successive days. Infants who are younger than 1 month should be given oral rifampin (10 mg/kg per dose once daily for 4 days). Rifampin should not be used in pregnant females.

Clinical Findings

A. Symptoms and Signs

1. Meningitis—Infants usually present with fever, irritability, lethargy, poor feeding with or without vomiting, and a high-pitched cry.

2. Acute epiglottitis—The most useful clinical finding in the early diagnosis of Hib epiglottitis is evidence of dysphagia, characterized by a refusal to eat or swallow saliva and by drooling. This finding, plus the presence of a high fever in a toxic child—even in the absence of a cherry-red epiglottis on direct examination—should strongly suggest the diagnosis and lead to prompt intubation. Stridor is a late sign. (See Chapter 19.)

3. Septic arthritis—Hib is a common cause of septic arthritis in unimmunized children younger than age 4 years in the United States. The child is febrile and refuses to move the involved joint and limb because of pain. Examination reveals swelling, warmth, redness, tenderness on palpation, and severe pain on attempted movement of the joint.

4. Cellulitis—Cellulitis due to Hib occurs almost exclusively in children between the ages of 3 months and 4 years but is now uncommon as a result of immunization. Fever is usually noted at the same time as the cellulitis, and many infants appear toxic. The cheek or periorbital (preseptal) area is usually involved.

B. Laboratory Findings

The WBC count in Hib infections may be high or normal with a shift to the left. Blood culture is frequently positive. Positive culture of aspirated pus or fluid from the involved site proves the diagnosis. In untreated meningitis, CSF smear may show the characteristic pleomorphic gram-negative rods.

C. Imaging

A lateral view of the neck may suggest the diagnosis in suspected acute epiglottitis, but misinterpretation is common. Intubation should not be delayed to obtain radiographs. Haziness of maxillary and ethmoid sinuses occurs with orbital cellulitis.

Differential Diagnosis

A. Meningitis

Meningitis must be differentiated from head injury, brain abscess, tumor, lead encephalopathy, and other forms of meningoencephalitis, including mycobacterial, viral, fungal, and bacterial agents.

B. Acute Epiglottitis

In croup caused by viral agents (parainfluenza 1, 2, and 3, respiratory syncytial virus, influenza A, adenovirus), the child has more definite upper respiratory symptoms, cough, hoarseness, slower progression of obstructive signs, and lower fever. Spasmodic croup usually occurs at night in a child with a history of previous attacks. Sudden onset of choking and paroxysmal coughing suggests foreign body aspiration. Retropharyngeal abscess may have to be differentiated from epiglottitis.

C. Septic Arthritis

Differential diagnosis includes acute osteomyelitis, prepatellar bursitis, cellulitis, rheumatic fever, and fractures and sprains.

D. Cellulitis

Erysipelas, streptococcal cellulitis, insect bites, and trauma (including Popsicle panniculitis or other types of freezing injury) may mimic Hib cellulitis. Periorbital cellulitis must be differentiated from paranasal sinus disease without cellulitis, allergic inflammatory disease of the lids, conjunctivitis, and herpes zoster infection.

Complications

A. Meningitis (See Chapter 25)

B. Acute Epiglottitis

The disease may rapidly progress to complete airway obstruction with complications owing to hypoxia. Mediastinal emphysema and pneumothorax may occur.

C. Septic Arthritis

Septic arthritis may result in rapid destruction of cartilage and ankylosis if diagnosis and treatment are delayed. Even with early treatment, the incidence of residual damage and disability after septic arthritis in weight-bearing joints may be as high as 25%.

D. Cellulitis

Bacteremia may lead to meningitis or pyarthrosis.

Treatment

All patients with bacteremic or potentially bacteremic Hib diseases require hospitalization for treatment. The drugs of choice in hospitalized patients are a third-generation cephalosporin (cefotaxime or ceftriaxone) until the sensitivity of the organism is known. Meropenem is an alternative choice.

Persons with invasive Hib disease should be in droplet isolation for 24 hours after initiation of parenteral antibiotic therapy.

A. Meningitis

Therapy is begun as soon as bacterial meningitis has been identified and CSF, blood, and other appropriate cultures have been obtained. Empiric intravenous therapy recommended for meningitis (until organism identified) is Vancomycin in combination with either cefotaxime or ceftriaxone. Once the organism has been identified as *Haemophilus influenza* and the susceptibilities are known, the antibitiotic regimen can be tailored accordingly. Most isolates will be susceptible to ceftriaxone or cefotaxime. Meropenem is an alternative agent. Therapy should preferably be given intravenously for the entire course. Ceftriaxone may be given intramuscularly if venous access becomes difficult.

Duration of therapy is 10 days for uncomplicated meningitis. Longer treatment is reserved for children who respond slowly or in whom complications have occurred.

Dexamethasone given immediately after diagnosis and continued for 4 days may reduce the incidence of hearing loss in children with Hib meningitis. The use of dexamethasone is controversial, but when it is used the dosage is 0.6 mg/kg/d in four divided doses for 4 days. Starting dexamethasone more than 6 hours after antibiotics have been initiated is unlikely to provide benefits.

Repeated lumbar punctures are usually not necessary in Hib meningitis. They should be obtained in the following circumstances: unsatisfactory or questionable clinical response, seizure occurring after several days of therapy, and prolonged (7 days) or recurrent fever if the neurologic examination is abnormal or difficult to evaluate.

B. Acute Epiglottitis (See Chapter 19)

C. Septic Arthritis

Initial therapy should include an effective antistaphylococcal antibiotic and cefotaxime or ceftriaxone (dosage as for meningitis) until identification of the organism is made. Cefotaxime or ceftriaxone are the usual agents used once the isolate is known to be Haemophilus and susceptibilities are known. Ampicillin resistance is now common in the United States. Occasionally isolates are resistant to third generation cephalosporins. Meropenem, if the isolate is susceptible, can be used as an alternative. If a child is improved following initial intravenous therapy, transition to oral therapy based on susceptibilities can occur. Possible oral agents include amoxicillin/clavulanate (75–100 mg/kg/d of amoxicillin component in four divided doses every 6 hours) may be administered under careful supervision to complete a 4-week course. Alternative agents include second- or third-generation cephalosporins. Drainage of infected joint fluid is an essential part of treatment. In joints other than the hip, this can often be accomplished by one or more needle aspirations. In hip infections—and in arthritis of other joints when treatment is delayed or clinical response is slow—surgical drainage is advised. The joint should be immobilized.

D. Cellulitis, Including Orbital Cellulitis

Initial therapy for orbital cellulitis should be broad spectrum antibiotic therapy. The most likely pathogens may include

Streptococcus pneumonia, Streptococcus angionosus, Group A *Streptococcus, Staphylococcus aureus, Haemophilus influenzae,* and anaerobes. Once the organism is known to be *H influenzae* orbital and susceptibilities are known, cefotaxime, ceftriaxone, or Meropenem can be used depending on susceptibilities. Therapy is given parenterally for at least 3–7 days (some clinicians treat up to 2 weeks intravenously) followed by oral treatment. There is usually marked improvement after 72 hours of treatment. Antibiotics should be given for at approximately 21 days based on the severity of infection and response to therapy.

Prognosis

The case fatality rate for Hib meningitis is less than 5%. Young infants have the highest mortality rate. One of the most common neurologic sequelae, developing in 5%–10% of patients with Hib meningitis, is sensorineural hearing loss. Patients with Hib meningitis should have their hearing checked during the course of the illness or shortly after recovery. Children in whom invasive Hib infection develops despite appropriate immunization should have tests to investigate immune function and to rule out HIV. The case fatality rate in acute epiglottitis is 2%–5%. Deaths are associated with bacteremia and the rapid development of airway obstruction. The prognosis for the other diseases requiring hospitalization is good with the institution of early and adequate antibiotic therapy.

Centers for Disease Control and Prevention. Available at: http://www.cdc.gov/vaccines/pubs/pinkbook/downloads/hib.pdf

Tristram S, Jacobs MR, Appelbaum AP: Antimicrobial resistance in *Haemophilus influenzae.* Clin Microbiol Rev 2007;20:368 [PMID: 17428889].

PERTUSSIS (WHOOPING COUGH)

ESSENTIALS OF DIAGNOSIS & TYPICAL FEATURES

- Prodromal catarrhal stage (1–3 weeks) characterized by mild cough and coryza, but without fever.
- Persistent staccato, paroxysmal cough ending with a highpitched inspiratory "whoop."
- Leukocytosis with absolute lymphocytosis.
- Diagnosis confirmed by PCR or culture of nasopharyngeal secretions.

General Considerations

Pertussis is an acute, highly communicable infection of the respiratory tract caused by *Bordetella pertussis* and characterized by severe bronchitis. Children usually acquire the disease from symptomatic family contacts. Adults and adolescents who have mild respiratory illness, not recognized as pertussis, frequently are the source of infection. Asymptomatic carriage of *B pertussis* is not recognized. Infectivity is greatest during the catarrhal and early paroxysmal cough stage (for about 4 weeks after onset).

Pertussis cases have increased in the United States since 1980. In 2007, about 10,000 cases were reported; increased to more than 15,000 cases in 2009. The morbidity and mortality of pertussis is greatest in young children. Fifty percent of children younger than age 1 year with a diagnosis of pertussis are hospitalized. Deaths occur primarily in children less than one year and are increasing in frequency.

The duration of active immunity following natural pertussis is not known. Reinfections are usually milder. Immunity following vaccination wanes in 5–10 years. The majority of young adults in the United States are susceptible to pertussis infection, and disease is probably common but unrecognized. Decreased efficacy of acellular vaccines compared to whole cell vaccines and low rates of immunization in some communities has led to increasing numbers of cases.

Bordetella parapertussis causes a similar but milder syndrome.

B pertussis organisms attach to the ciliated respiratory epithelium and multiply there; deeper invasion does not occur. Disease is due to several bacterial toxins, the most potent of which is pertussis toxin, which is responsible for the typical lymphocytosis.

Clinical Findings

A. Symptoms and Signs

The onset of pertussis is insidious, with catarrhal upper respiratory tract symptoms (rhinitis, sneezing, and an irritating cough). Slight fever may be present; temperature greater than 38.3°C suggests bacterial superinfection or another cause of respiratory tract infection. After about 2 weeks, cough becomes paroxysmal, characterized by 10–30 forceful coughs ending with a loud inspiration (the whoop). Infants and adults with otherwise typical severe pertussis often lack characteristic whooping. Vomiting commonly follows a paroxysm. Coughing is accompanied by cyanosis, sweating, prostration, and exhaustion. This stage lasts for 2–4 weeks, with gradual improvement. Cough suggestive of chronic bronchitis lasts for another 2–3 weeks. Paroxysmal coughing may continue for some months and may worsen with intercurrent viral respiratory infection. In adults, older children, and partially immunized individuals, symptoms may consist only of irritating cough lasting 1–2 weeks. Clinical pertussis is milder in immunized children.

B. Laboratory Findings

WBC counts of 20,000–30,000/μL with 70%–80% lymphocytes typically appear near the end of the catarrhal stage; and the degree of lymphocytosis correlates with the severity of disease. Severe pulmonary hypertension and hyperleukocytosis (greater than 70,000/μL) are associated with severe disease and death in young children with pertussis. Many older children and adults with mild infections never demonstrate lymphocytosis. The blood picture may resemble lymphocytic leukemia or leukemoid reactions. Identification of *B pertussis* by culture or PCR from nasopharyngeal swabs or nasal wash specimens proves the diagnosis. The organism may be found in the respiratory tract in diminishing numbers beginning in the catarrhal stage and ending about 2 weeks after the beginning of the paroxysmal stage. After 4–5 weeks of symptoms, cultures are almost always negative. Culture requires specialized media and careful attention to specimen collection and transport. PCR detection has replaced culture in most pediatric centers because of improved sensitivity, decreased time to diagnosis, and cost. Enzyme-linked immunosorbent assays (ELISAs) for detectionof antibody to pertussis toxin or filamentous hemagglutinin may be useful for diagnosis but interpretation of antibody titers may be difficult in previously immunized patients. The chest radiograph reveals thickened bronchi and sometimes shows a "shaggy" heart border.

Differential Diagnosis

The differential diagnosis of pertussis includes bacterial, tuberculous, chlamydial, and viral pneumonia. The absence of fever in pertussis differentiates this disease from most bacterial infections. Cystic fibrosis and foreign body aspiration may be considerations. Adenoviruses and respiratory syncytial virus may cause paroxysmal coughing with an associated elevation of lymphocytes in the peripheral blood, mimicking pertussis.

Complications

Bronchopneumonia due to superinfection is the most common serious complication. It is characterized by abrupt clinical deterioration during the paroxysmal stage, accompanied by high fever and sometimes a striking leukemoid reaction with a shift to predominantly polymorphonuclear neutrophils. Atelectasis is a second common pulmonary complication. Atelectasis may be patchy or extensive and may shift rapidly to involve different areas of lung. Intercurrent viral respiratory infection is also a common complication and may provoke worsening or recurrence of paroxysmal coughing. Otitis media is common. Residual chronic bronchiectasis is infrequent despite the severity of the illness. Apnea and sudden death may occur during a particularly severe paroxysm. Seizures complicate 1.5% of cases, and encephalopathy occurs in 0.1%. The encephalopathy frequently is fatal. Anoxic brain damage, cerebral hemorrhage, or pertussis neurotoxins are hypothesized, but anoxia is most likely the cause. Epistaxis and subconjunctival hemorrhages are common.

Prevention

Active immunization (see Chapter 10) with DTaP vaccine should be given in early infancy. The occurrence and increased recognition of disease in adolescents and adults contributes to the increasing number of cases. A booster dose of vaccine in adolescents between the ages of 11 and 18 years is recommended. Subsequent booster doses of Tdap are recommended for adults aged 18–60 years to replace Td boosters. Immunization of pregnant women, new mothers, care givers of infants less than 6 months, and health care workers of young children is also recommended.

Chemoprophylaxis with azithromycin or clarithromycin should be given to exposed family, household and hospital contacts, particularly those younger than age 2 years, although data to support the efficacy of such preventive therapy are not strong. Hospitalized children with pertussis should be isolated because of the great risk of transmission to patients and staff. Several large hospital outbreaks have been reported.

Treatment

A. Specific Measures

Antibiotics may ameliorate early infections but have no effect on clinical symptoms in the paroxysmal stage. Azithromycin is the drug of choice because it promptly terminates respiratory tract carriage of *B pertussis*. Resistance to macrolides has been rarely reported. Clarithromycin may also be used. Erythromycin given 4 times daily for 14 days is acceptable but not preferred. Ampicillin (100 mg/kg/d in four divided doses) may also be used for erythromycin-intolerant patients. Azithromycin is often preferred due to ease of compliance and decreased gastrointestinal side effects. Erythromycin has been associated with pyloric stenosis in infants less than 1 month of age. Azithromycin is recommended for therapy or prophylaxis in infants less than 1 month.

Corticosteroids reduce the severity of disease but may mask signs of bacterial superinfection. Albuterol (0.3–0.5 mg/kg/d in four doses) has reduced the severity of illness, but tachycardia is common when the drug is given orally, and aerosol administration may precipitate paroxysms.

B. General Measures

Nutritional support during the paroxysmal phase is important. Frequent small feedings, tube feeding, or parenteral fluid supplementation may be needed. Minimizing stimuli that trigger paroxysms is probably the best way of controlling cough. In general, cough suppressants are of little benefit.

C. Treatment of Complications

Respiratory insufficiency due to pneumonia or other pulmonary complications should be treated with oxygen and assisted ventilation if necessary. Convulsions are treated with oxygen and anticonvulsants. Bacterial pneumonia or otitis media requires additional antibiotics.

Prognosis

The prognosis for patients with pertussis has improved in recent years because of excellent nursing care, treatment of complications, attention to nutrition, and modern intensive care. However, the disease is still very serious in infants younger than age 1 year; most deaths occur in this age group. Children with encephalopathy have a poor prognosis.

Committee on Infectious Diseases: Additional recommendations for use of tetanus toxoid, reduced-content diphtheria toxoid, and acellular pertussis vaccine (tdap). Pediatrics 2011;128(4):809–812 [PMID: 21949151].

Haberling DL et al: Infant and maternal risk factors for pertussis-related infant mortality in the United States, 1999 to 2004. Pediatr Infect Dis J 2009;28(3):194 [PMID: 19209089].

Halasa NB et al: Fatal pulmonary hypertension associated with pertussis in infants: Does extracorporeal membrane oxygenation have a role? Pediatrics 2003;112:1274 [PMID: 14654596].

Munoz F, Englund J: Infant pertussis: Is cocooning the answer? Clin Infet Dis 2011;53(9):893–896 [PMID: 21946188].

Nicholson CE: Early exchange and pheresis therapies in critical pertussis. Pediatr Crit Care Med 2011;12(2):240–241 [PMID: 21646959].

Robbins JB et al: Pertussis vaccine: A critique. Pediatr Infect Dis J 2009;28(3):237 [PMID: 19165133].

Rowlands HE et al: Impact of rapid leukodepletion on the outcome of severe clinical pertussis in young infants. Pediatrics 2010;126(4):e816–e827 [PMID: 20819895].

Sin MA et al: Pertussis outbreak in primary and secondary schools in Ludwigslut, Germany, demonstrating the role of waning immunity. Pediatr Infect Dis J 2009;28(3):242 [PMID: 19209094].

LISTERIOSIS

ESSENTIALS OF DIAGNOSIS & TYPICAL FEATURES

- Early-onset neonatal disease:
  - Signs of sepsis a few hours after birth in an infant born with fetal distress and hepatosplenomegaly; maternal fever.
- Late-onset neonatal disease:
  - Meningitis, sometimes with monocytosis in the CSF and peripheral blood.
  - Onset at age 9–30 days.

General Considerations

Listeria monocytogenes is a gram-positive, non–spore-forming aerobic rod distributed widely in the animal kingdom and in food, dust, and soil. It causes systemic infections in newborn infants and immunosuppressed older children. In pregnant women, infection is relatively mild, with fever, aches, and chills, but is accompanied by bacteremia and sometimes results in intrauterine or perinatal infection with grave consequences for the fetus or newborn. One-fourth of cases occur in pregnant women, and 20% of their pregnancies end in stillbirth or neonatal death. Listeria is present in the stool of approximately 10% of the healthy population. Persons in contact with animals are at greater risk. Outbreaks of listeriosis have been traced to contaminated cabbage in coleslaw, soft cheese, hot dogs, luncheon meats, and milk. Listeria infections have decreased since the adoption of strict regulations for ready-to-eat foods; 850 cases were reported in 2009. A large multistate outbreak due to contaminated cantaloupe has caused more than 20 deaths in elderly and immunocompromised patients in 2011, and demonstrates the potential of this organism to cause serious illness.

Like GBS infections, Listeria infections in the newborn can be divided into early and late forms. Early infections are more common, leading to a severe congenital form of infection. Later infections are often characterized by meningitis.

Clinical Findings

A. Symptoms and Signs

In the early neonatal form, symptoms of listeriosis usually appear on the first day of life and always by the third day. Fetal distress is common, and infants frequently have signs of severe disease at birth. Respiratory distress, diarrhea, and fever occur. On examination, hepatosplenomegaly and a papular rash are found. A history of maternal fever is common. Meningitis may accompany the septic course. The late neonatal form usually occurs after age 9 days and can occur as late as 5 weeks. Meningitis is common, characterized by irritability, fever, and poor feeding.

Listeria infections are rare in older children and usually are associated with immunodeficiency. Several recent cases were associated with tumor necrosis factor-α neutralizing agents. Signs and symptoms are those of meningitis, usually with insidious onset.

B. Laboratory Findings

In all patients except those receiving white cell depressant drugs, the WBC count is elevated, with 10%–20% monocytes. When meningitis is found, the characteristic CSF cell count is high (> 500/μL) with a predominance of polymorphonuclear neutrophils in 70% of cases. Monocytes may predominate in up to 30% of cases. Gram-stained smears of CSF are usually negative, but short gram-positive rods may be seen. The chief pathologic feature in severe neonatal sepsis is miliary granulomatosis with microabscesses in liver, spleen, CNS, lung, and bowel.

Culture results are frequently positive from multiple sites, including blood from the infant and the mother.

Differential Diagnosis

Early-onset neonatal disease resembles hemolytic disease of the newborn, GBS sepsis or severe cytomegalovirus infection, rubella, or toxoplasmosis. Late-onset disease must be differentiated from meningitis due to echovirus and coxsackievirus, GBS, and gram-negative enteric bacteria.

Prevention

Immunosuppressed, pregnant, and elderly patients can decrease the risk of Listeria infection by avoiding soft cheeses, by thoroughly reheating or avoiding delicatessen and ready-to-eat foods, by avoiding raw meat and milk, and by thoroughly washing fresh vegetables.

Treatment

Ampicillin (150–300 mg/kg/d every 6 hours intravenously) is the drug of choice in most cases of listeriosis. Gentamicin (2.5 mg/kg every 8 hours intravenously) has a synergistic effect with ampicillin and should be given in serious infections and to patients with immune deficits. Vancomycin may be substituted for ampicillin when empirically treating meningitis. If ampicillin cannot be used, TMP–SMX also is effective. Cephalosporins are not effective. Treatment of severe disease should continue for at least 2 weeks; meningitis is treated 2–3 weeks.

Prognosis

In a recent outbreak of early-onset neonatal disease, the mortality rate was 27% despite aggressive and appropriate management. Meningitis in older infants has a good prognosis. In immunosuppressed children, prognosis depends to a great extent on that of the underlying illness.

Gillespie IA et al: Disease presentation in relation to infection foci for non-pregnancy-associated human listeriosis in England and Wales, 2001 to 2007. J Clin Microbiol 2009;47(10):3301 [PMID: 19675217].

Guevara RE, Mascola L, Sorvillo F: Risk factors for mortality among patients with nonperinatal listeriosis in Los Angeles County, 1992–2004. Clin Infect Dis 2009;48(11):1507 [PMID: 19400687].

Mitja O et al: Predictors of mortality and impact of aminoglycosides on outcome in listeriosis in a retrospective cohort study. J Antimicrob Chemother 2009;64(2):416 [PMID: 19468027].

Centers for Disease Control and Prevention (CDC): Listeriosis. Available at: http://www.cdc.gov/nczved/dfbmd/disease_listing/listeriosis_gi.html

Center for Disease Control and Prevention (CDC): Multistate Outbreak of Listeriosis Associated with Jensen Farms Cantaloupe—United States, Aug–Sep 2011. MMWR 2011;60: 1357–1358 [PMID: 21976119].

TUBERCULOSIS

ESSENTIALS OF DIAGNOSIS & TYPICAL FEATURES

- All types: positive tuberculin test in patient or members of household, suggestive chest radiograph, history of contact, and demonstration of organism by stain and culture.
- Pulmonary: fatigue, irritability, and undernutrition, with or without fever and cough.
- Glandular: chronic cervical adenitis.
- Miliary: classic snowstorm appearance of chest radiograph.
- Meningitis: fever and manifestations of meningeal irritation and increased intracranial pressure. Characteristic CSF.

General Considerations

Tuberculosis is a granulomatous disease caused by *Mycobacterium tuberculosis*. It is a leading cause of death throughout the world. Children younger than age 3 years are most susceptible. Lymphohematogenous dissemination through the lungs to extrapulmonary sites, including the brain and meninges, eyes, bones and joints, lymph nodes, kidneys, intestines, larynx, and skin, is more likely to occur in infants. Increased susceptibility occurs again in adolescence, particularly in girls within 2 years of menarche. Following substantial increases in disease during the 1980s, tuberculosis incidence has decreased since 1992 due to increased control measures. More than 11,500 new cases were reported in 2009; only 646 of these were in children less than 14 years old. High-risk groups include ethnic minorities, foreign-born persons, prisoners, residents of nursing homes, indigents, migrant workers, and health care providers. However, 50% of cases occurred in U.S.–born persons. HIV infection is an important risk factor for both development and spread of disease. Pediatric tuberculosis incidence mirrors the trends seen in adults.

Exposure to an infected adult is the most common risk factor in children. The primary complex in infancy and childhood consists of a small parenchymal lesion in any area of the lung with caseation of regional nodes and calcification. Postprimary tuberculosis in adolescents and adults commonly occurs in the apices of the lungs and is likely to cause chronic progressive cavitary pulmonary disease with less tendency for hematogenous dissemination. *Mycobacterium bovis* infection is clinically identical to *M tuberculosis*. *M bovis* may be acquired from unpasteurized dairy products obtained outside the United States.

Clinical Findings

A. Symptoms and Signs

1. Pulmonary—(See Chapter 19.)

2. Miliary—Diagnosis is usually based on the classic "snowstorm" or "millet seed" appearance of lung fields on radiograph, although early in the course of disseminated tuberculosis the chest radiograph may show no or only subtle abnormalities. Choroidal tubercles are sometimes seen on funduscopic examination. Other lesions may be present and produce osteomyelitis, arthritis, meningitis, tuberculomas of the brain, enteritis, or infection of the kidneys and liver.

3. Meningitis—Symptoms include fever, vomiting, headache, lethargy, and irritability, with signs of meningeal irritation and increased intracranial pressure, cranial nerve palsies, convulsions, and coma.

4. Lymphatic—The primary complex may be associated with a skin lesion drained by regional nodes or chronic cervical node enlargement or infection of the tonsils. Involved nodes may become fixed to the overlying skin, suppurate, and drain.

B. Laboratory Findings

The tuberculin skin test (TST; 0.1 mL of intermediate-strength purified protein derivative inoculated intradermally) is positive at 48–72 hours if there is significant induration (Table 42–3). Parental reporting of skin test results is often inaccurate. All tests should be read by professionals trained to interpret TST. False-negative results occur in malnourished patients, in those with overwhelming disease, and in 10% of children with isolated pulmonary disease. Temporary suppression of tuberculin reactivity may be seen with viral infections (eg, measles, influenza, varicella, and mumps), after live virus immunization, and during corticosteroid or other immunosuppressive drug therapy. For these reasons, a negative TST test does not exclude the diagnosis of tuberculosis. When tuberculosis is suspected in a child, household members and adult contacts (eg, teachers and caregivers) also should be tested immediately. Multiple puncture tests (tine tests) should not be used because they are associated with false-negative and false-positive reactions, and because standards for interpretation of positive results do not exist. γ-Interferon release assays (IGRAs) are approved to replace TST tests in adults and older children. These assays have much higher specificity due to less common false-positive results from nontuberculosis mycobacteria and BCG. They are done on blood obtained by venipuncture and are further advantageous in requiring only a single visit; however, on children older than 5 years these tests may be used rather than TST.

IGRA are reported as positive, negative or indeterminate. They are most useful in BCG immunized children where false positive TSTs are common.

Table 42–3. Interpretation of tuberculin skin test reactions.[a]

Degree of Risk	Risk Factors	Positive Reaction
High	Recent close contact with a case of active tuberculosis Chest radiograph compatible with tuberculosis Immunocompromise HIV infection	≥ 5 mm induration
Medium	Current or previous residence in high-prevalence area (Asia, Africa, Latin America) Skin test converters within past 2 y Intravenous drug use Homelessness or residence in a correctional institution Recent weight loss or malnutrition Leukemia, Hodgkin disease, or diabetes mellitus Age < 4 y	≥ 10 mm induration
Low	Children ≥ 4 y without any risk factor	≥ 15 mm induration

[a]Standard intradermal Mantoux test, 5 test units. Measure perpendicular to the long axis of the arm. Induration only, not erythema, is measured.

The ESR is usually elevated. Cultures of pooled early morning gastric aspirates from three successive days will yield *M tuberculosis* in about 40% of cases. Biopsy may be necessary to establish the diagnosis. Therapy should not be delayed in suspected cases. The CSF in tuberculous meningitis shows slight to moderate pleocytosis (50–300 WBCs/μL, predominantly lymphocytes), decreased glucose, and increased protein.

The direct detection of mycobacteria in body fluids or discharges is best done by staining specimens with auramin-erhodamine and examining them with fluorescence microscopy; this method is superior to the Ziehl-Neelsen method.

C. Imaging

Chest radiograph should be obtained in all children with suspicion of tuberculosis at any site or with a positive skin test. Segmental consolidation with some volume loss and hilar adenopathy are common findings in children. Paratracheal adenopathy is a classic presentation. Pleural effusion also occurs with primary infection. Cavities and apical disease are unusual in children but are common in adolescents and adults.

Differential Diagnosis

Pulmonary tuberculosis must be differentiated from fungal, parasitic, mycoplasmal, and bacterial pneumonias; lung abscess; foreign body aspiration; lipoid pneumonia; sarcoidosis; and mediastinal cancer. Cervical lymphadenitis is most likely due to streptococcal or staphylococcal infections. Cat-scratch fever and infection with atypical mycobacteria may need to be distinguished from tuberculous lymphadenitis. Viral meningoencephalitis, head trauma (child abuse), lead poisoning, brain abscess, acute bacterial meningitis, brain tumor, and disseminated fungal infections must be excluded in tuberculous meningitis. A positive TST or IGRA in the patient or family contacts is frequently valuable in suggesting the diagnosis of tuberculosis. A negative TST or IGRA does not exclude tuberculosis.

Prevention

A. BCG Vaccine

Bacille Calmette–Guérin (BCG) vaccines are live-attenuated strains of *M bovis*. Although neonatal and childhood administration of BCG is carried out in countries with a high prevalence of tuberculosis, protective efficacy varies greatly with vaccine potency and method of delivery. BCG given to infants decreases disseminated tuberculosis but does not protect against pulmonary tuberculosis later in childhood or adolescence. Because the great majority of children who have received BCG still have negative TST tests, the past history of BCG vaccination should be ignored in interpreting the skin test. In the United States, BCG vaccination is not recommended. IGRAs give negative results in patients with false-positive PPDs due to BCG.

B. Isoniazid Chemoprophylaxis

Daily administration of isoniazid (10 mg/kg/d orally; maximum 300 mg) is advised for children who are exposed by prolonged close or household contact with adolescents or adults with active disease. Isoniazid is given until 2 months after last contact. At the end of this time, a Mantoux test should be done, and therapy should be continued for an additional 7 months if the test is positive.

C. Other Measures

Tuberculosis in infants and young children is evidence of recent exposure to active infection in an adult, usually a family member or household contact. The source contact (index case) should be identified, isolated, and given treatment to prevent other secondary cases. Reporting cases to local health departments is essential for contact tracing. Exposed tuberculin-negative children should usually receive isoniazid chemoprophylaxis. If a repeated skin test is negative 2–3 months following the last exposure, isoniazid may be stopped. Routine tuberculin skin testing is not recommended for children without risk factors who reside in communities with a low incidence of tuberculosis. Children with no personal risk for tuberculosis but who reside in communities with a high incidence of tuberculosis should be given a skin test at school entry and then again at age 11–16 years. Children with a risk factor for acquiring tuberculosis should be tested every 2–3 years. Incarcerated adolescents and children living in a household with HIV-infected persons should have annual skin tests.

Children who immigrate into the United States from a country with a high incidence of infection should receive a skin test on entry to the United States or upon presentation to health care providers. A past history of BCG vaccine should not delay skin testing. IGRAs may be used in chidren ≥ 5 years.

Treatment

A. Specific Measures

Most children with active tuberculosis in the United States are hospitalized initially. If the infecting organism has not been isolated from the presumed contact for susceptibility testing, reasonable attempts should be made to obtain it from the child using morning gastric aspirates, sputum, bronchoscopy, thoracentesis, or biopsy when appropriate. Unfortunately, cultures are frequently negative in children, and the risk of these procedures must be weighed against the yield. Therapy is given daily for 14 days and then reduced to two to three times per week for the duration of the course. Directly observed administration of all doses of antituberculosis therapy by a trained health care professional is essential to ensure compliance with therapy.

Children with positive skin tests (see Table 42–3) without symptoms and a normal chest radiograph have latent tuberculosis and should receive 9 months of isoniazid (10 mg/kg/d orally; maximum 300 mg) therapy. Rifampin (10–15 mg/kg ld orally; maximum 600 mg) for 4 months is efficacious and compliance is easier with the shorter duration of therapy. In children with active pulmonary disease, therapy for 6 months using isoniazid (10 mg/kg/d), rifampin (15 mg/kg/d), and pyrazinamide (25–30 mg/kg/d) in a single daily oral dose for 2 months, followed by isoniazid plus rifampin (either in a daily or twice-weekly regimen) for 4 months appears effective for eliminating isoniazid-susceptible organisms. For more severe disease, such as miliary or CNS infection, duration is increased to 12 months or more, and a fourth drug (streptomycin or ethambutol) is added for the first 2 months. In communities with resistance rates greater than 4%, initial therapy should usually include four drugs.

1. Isoniazid—The hepatotoxicity from isoniazid seen in adults and some adolescents is rare in children. Transient elevation of aminotransferases (up to three times normal) may be seen at 6–12 weeks, but therapy is continued unless clinical illness occurs. Routine monitoring of liver function tests is unnecessary unless prior hepatic disease is known or the child is severely ill. Peripheral neuropathy associated with pyridoxine deficiency is rare in children, and it is not necessary to add pyridoxine unless significant malnutrition coexists or if the child is strictly breastfed.

2. Rifampin—Although it is an excellent bactericidal agent, rifampin is never used alone owing to rapid development of resistance. Hepatotoxicity may occur but rarely with recommended doses. The orange discoloration of secretions is benign but may stain contact lenses or clothes.

3. Pyrazinamide—This excellent sterilizing agent is most effective during the first 2 months of therapy. With the recommended duration and dosing, it is well tolerated. Although pyrazinamide elevates the uric acid level, it rarely causes symptoms of hyperuricemia in children. Use of this drug is now common for tuberculous disease in children, and resistance is uncommon. Oral acceptance and CNS penetration are good.

4. Ethambutol—Because optic neuritis is the major side effect in adults, ethambutol has usually been given only to children whose vision can be reliably tested for loss of color differentiation. Optic neuritis is rare and usually occurs in those receiving more than the recommended dosage of 25 mg/kg/d. Documentation of optic toxicity in children is lacking despite considerable worldwide experience. Therefore, many four-drug regimens for children now include ethambutol.

5. Streptomycin—Streptomycin (20–30 mg/kg/d, given intramuscularly in one or two doses) should be given for 1 or 2 months in severe disease. The child's hearing should be tested periodically during use as ototoxicity is common.

B. Chemotherapy for Drug-Resistant Tuberculosis

The incidence of drug resistance is increasing and reaches 10%–20% in some areas of the United States. Transmission of multiple drug-resistant and extensively drug-resistant strains to contacts has occurred in some epidemics. Consultation with local experts in treating tuberculosis is important in these difficult cases. Therapy should continue for 18 months or longer. Often, four to six first- and second-line medications are needed.

C. General Measures

Corticosteroids may be used for suppressing inflammatory reactions in meningeal, pleural, and pericardial tuberculosis and for the relief of bronchial obstruction due to hilar adenopathy. Prednisone is given orally, 1 mg/kg/d for 2 weeks, with gradual withdrawal over the next 4–6 weeks. The use of corticosteroids may mask progression of disease. Accordingly, the clinician needs to be sure that an effective regimen is being used.

Prognosis

If bacteria are sensitive and treatment is completed, most children are cured with minimal sequelae. Repeat treatment is more difficult and less successful. With antituberculosis chemotherapy (especially isoniazid), there should now be nearly 100% recovery in miliary tuberculosis. Without treatment, the mortality rate in both miliary tuberculosis and tuberculous meningitis is almost 100%. In the latter form, about two-thirds of patients receiving treatment survive. There may be a high incidence of neurologic abnormalities among survivors if treatment is started late.

American Thoracic Society, CDC, Infectious Diseases Society of America: Treatment of tuberculosis. MMWR Recomm Rep 2003;52(RR-11):1 [PMID: 12836625].

Cattamanchi A et al: Clinical characteristics and treatment outcomes of patients with isoniazid-monoresistant tuberculosis. Clin Infect Dis 2009;48(2):179 [PMID: 19086909].

Centers for Disease Control and Prevention (CDC): Trends in tuberculosis—United States, 2010. MMWR Morb Mortal Wkly Rep 2011;60(11):333–337 [PMID: 21430636].

Ho CC et al: Safety of fluoroquinolone use in patients with hepa totoxicity induced by anti-tuberculosis regimens. Clin Infect Dis 2009;48(11):1526 [PMID: 19400686].

Lighter J: Latent tuberculosis diagnosis in children by using the QuantiFERON-TB Gold In-Tube test. Pediatrics 2009;123(1): 30–37 [PMID: 19117857].

Long R et al: Empirical treatment of community-acquired pneumonia and the development of fluoroquinolone-resistant tuberculosis. Clin Infect Dis 2009;48(10):1354 [PMID: 19348594].

Mazurek GH et al: Centers for Disease Control and Prevention (CDC): Updated guidelines for using Interferon Gamma Release Assays to detect Mycobacterium tuberculosis infection—United States, 2010. MMWR Recomm Rep 2010;59(RR-5):1–25 [PMID: 20577159].

INFECTIONS WITH NONTUBERCULOUS MYCOBACTERIA

ESSENTIALS OF DIAGNOSIS & TYPICAL FEATURES

- Chronic unilateral cervical lymphadenitis.
- Granulomas of the skin.
- Chronic bone lesion with draining sinus (chronic osteomyelitis).
- Reaction to PPD-S (standard) of 5–8 mm, negative chest radiograph, and negative history of contact with tuberculosis.
- Diagnosis by positive acid-fast stain or culture.
- Disseminated infection in patients with AIDS.

General Considerations

Many species of acid-fast mycobacteria other than *M tuberculosis* may cause subclinical infections and occasionally clinical disease resembling tuberculosis. Strains of nontuberculous mycobacteria are common in soil, food, and water. Organisms enter the host by small abrasions in skin, oral mucosa, or gastrointestinal mucosa. Strain cross-reactivity with *M tuberculosis* can be demonstrated by simultaneous skin testing (Mantoux) with PPD-S (standard) and PPD prepared from one of the atypical antigens. Unfortunately, reagents prepared for routine nontuberculosis skin testing are not available to clinicians.

Mycobacterium avium complex (MAC), *Mycobacterium kansasii, Mycobacterium fortuitum, Mycobacterium abscessus, Mycobacterium marinum,* and *Mycobacterium chelonae* are most commonly encountered. *M fortuitum, M abscessus,* and *M chelonae* are "rapid growers" requiring 3–7 days for recovery, whereas other mycobacteria require several weeks. After inoculation they form colonies closely resembling *M tuberculosis* morphologically.

Clinical Findings

A. Symptoms and Signs

1. Lymphadenitis—In children, the most common form of infection due to mycobacteria other than *M tuberculosis* is cervical lymphadenitis. MAC is the most common organism. A submandibular or cervical node swells slowly and is firm and initially somewhat tender. Low-grade fever may occur. Over time, the node suppurates and may drain chronically. Nodes in other areas of the head and neck and elsewhere are sometimes involved.

2. Pulmonary disease—In the western United States, pulmonary disease is usually due to *M kansasii.* In the eastern United States, it may be due to MAC. In other countries, disease is usually caused by MAC. In adults, there is usually underlying chronic pulmonary disease. Immunologic deficiency may be present. Presentation is clinically indistinguishable from that of tuberculosis. Adolescents with cystic fibrosis may be infected with nontuberculous mycobacteria.

3. Swimming pool granuloma—This is due to *M marinum.* A solitary chronic granulomatous lesion with satellite lesions develops after minor trauma in infected swimming pools or other aquatic sources. Minor trauma in home aquariums or other aquatic environments may also lead to infection.

4. Chronic osteomyelitis—Osteomyelitis is caused by *M kansasii, M fortuitum,* or other rapid growers. Findings include swelling and pain over a distal extremity, radiolucent defects in bone, fever, and clinical and radiographic evidence of bronchopneumonia. Such cases are rare.

5. Meningitis—Disease is due to *M kansasii* and may be indistinguishable from tuberculous meningitis.

6. Disseminated infection—Rarely, apparently immunologically normal children develop disseminated infection due to nontuberculous mycobacteria. Children are ill, with fever and hepatosplenomegaly, and organisms are demonstrated in bone lesions, lymph nodes, or liver. Chest radiographs are usually normal. Between 60% and 80% of patients with AIDS will acquire MAC infection, characterized by fever, night sweats, weight loss, and diarrhea. Infection usually indicates severe immune dysfunction and is associated with CD4 lymphocyte counts less than 50/μL.

B. Laboratory Findings

In most cases, there is a small reaction (< 10 mm) when Mantoux testing is done. Larger reactions may be seen particularly with *M marinum* infection. The chest radiograph is negative, and there is no history of contact with a case of tuberculosis. Needle aspiration of the node excludes bacterial infection and may yield acid-fast bacilli on stain or culture. Fistulization should not be a problem because total excision is usually recommended for infection due to atypical mycobacteria. Cultures of any normally sterile body site may yield MAC in immunocompromised patients with disseminated disease. Blood cultures are positive, with a large density of bacteria.

Differential Diagnosis

See section on differential diagnosis in the previous discussion of tuberculosis and in Chapter 19.

Treatment

A. Specific Measures

The usual treatment of lymphadenitis is complete surgical excision. Occasionally excision is impossible because of proximity to branches of the facial or other nerves of the salivary glands. Chemotherapy may then be necessary. Response of extensive adenopathy or other forms of infection varies according to the infecting species and susceptibility. Usually, combinations of two to four medications administered for months are required. Isoniazid, rifampin, and ethambutol (depending on sensitivity to isoniazid) will result in a favorable response in almost all patients with *M kansasii* infection. Chemotherapeutic treatment of MAC is much less satisfactory because resistance to isoniazid, rifampin, and pyrazinamide is common. Susceptibility testing is necessary to optimize therapy. Most clinicians favor surgical excision of involved tissue if possible and treatment with at least three drugs to which the organism has been shown to be sensitive. Disseminated disease in patients with AIDS calls for a combination of three or more active drugs. Clarithromycin or azithromycin and ethambutol is started, in addition to one or more of the following drugs: ethionamide, capreomycin, amikacin, rifabutin, or ciprofloxacin. *M fortuitum* and *M chelonei* are usually susceptible to amikacin plus cefoxitin or meropenem followed by clarithromycin, azithromycin, or doxycycline, and may be successfully treated with such combinations. Swimming pool granuloma due to *M marinum* is usually treated with doxycycline (in children older than 9 years) or rifampin, plus ethambutol, clarithromycin, or TMP–SMX for a minimum of 3 months. Surgery may also be beneficial.

B. General Measures

Isolation of the patient is usually not necessary. General supportive care is indicated for the child with disseminated disease.

Prognosis

The prognosis is good for patients with localized disease, although fatalities occur in immunocompromised patients with disseminated disease.

Blyth CC et al: Nontuberculosis mycobacterial infection in children. Pediatr Infect Dise J 2009;28(9):801 [PMID: 19636280].

Centers for Disease Control and Prevention (CDC): *Mycobacterium avium* complex. Available at: www.cdc.gov/ncidod/dbmd/diseaseinfo/mycobacteriumavium_t.htm

Cruz AT et al: Mycobacterial infections in Texas children: A 5-year case series. Pediatr Infect Dis J 2010;29(8):772–774 [PMID: 20661106].

Timmerman MK et al: Treatment of non-tuberculous mycobacterial cervicofacial lymphadenitis in children: Critical appraisal of the literature. Clin Otolaryngol 2008;33(6):546–552 [PMID: 19126128].

LEGIONELLA INFECTION

ESSENTIALS OF DIAGNOSIS & TYPICAL FEATURES

- Severe progressive pneumonia in a child with compromised immunity.
- Diarrhea and neurologic signs are common.
- Positive culture requires buffered charcoal yeast extract media and proves infection.
- Direct fluorescent antibody staining of respiratory secretions proves infection.

General Considerations

Legionella pneumophila is a ubiquitous gram-negative bacillus that causes two distinct clinical syndromes: Legionnaire disease and Pontiac fever. Usually Legionnaire disease is an acute, severe pneumonia that is frequently fatal in immunocompromised patients. Pontiac fever is a mild, flulike illness that spares the lungs and is characterized by fever, headache, myalgia, and arthralgia. The disease is self-limited and is described in outbreaks in otherwise healthy adults.

Over 40 species of Legionella have been discovered, but not all cause disease in humans. *L pneumophila* causes most infections. Legionella is present in many natural water sources as well as domestic water supplies (faucets and showers). Contaminated cooling towers and heat exchangers have been implicated in several large institutional outbreaks. Person-to-person transmission has not been documented.

Few cases of Legionnaire disease have been reported in children. Most were in children with compromised cellular immunity. In adults, risk factors include smoking, underlying cardiopulmonary or renal disease, alcoholism, and diabetes.

L pneumophila is thought to be acquired by inhalation of a contaminated aerosol. The bacteria are phagocytosed but proliferate within macrophages. Cell-mediated immunity is necessary to activate macrophages to kill intracellular bacteria.

Prevention

No vaccine is available. Hyperchlorination and periodic superheating of water supplies in hospitals have been shown to reduce the number of organisms and the risk of infection.

Clinical Findings

A. Symptoms and Signs

Onset of fever, chills, anorexia, and headache is abrupt. Pulmonary symptoms appear within 2–3 days and progress rapidly. The cough is nonproductive early. Purulent sputum occurs late. Hemoptysis, diarrhea, and neurologic signs (including lethargy, irritability, tremors, and delirium) are seen.

B. Laboratory Findings

The WBC count is usually elevated. Chest radiographs show rapidly progressive patchy consolidation. Cavitation and large pleural effusions are uncommon. Cultures from sputum, tracheal aspirates, or bronchoscopic specimens, when grown on specialized media are positive in 70%–80% of patients at 3–7 days. Direct fluorescent antibody staining of sputum or other respiratory specimens is only 50–70% sensitive but 95% specific. A false-positive test can be seen in patients with tularemia. A negative result on culture or direct fluorescent antibody staining of sputum or tracheal secretions does not rule out disease due to Legionella. PCR detection of respiratory secretions for Legionella is available at some centers. A urine immunoassay for Legionella antigen is about 70% sensitive and is highly specific. Serologic tests are available, but a maximum rise in titer may require 6–8 weeks.

Differential Diagnosis

Legionnaire disease is usually a rapidly progressive pneumonia in a patient who appears very ill with unremitting fevers. Other bacterial pneumonias, viral pneumonias, *Mycoplasma* pneumonia, and fungal disease are all possibilities and may be difficult to differentiate clinically in an immunocompromised patient.

Complications

In sporadic untreated cases, mortality rates are 5%–25%. In immunocompromised patients with untreated disease, mortality approaches 80%. Hematogenous dissemination may result in extrapulmonary foci of infection, including pericardium, myocardium, and kidneys. Legionella may be the cause of culture-negative endocarditis.

Treatment

Intravenous azithromycin, 10 mg/kg/d given as a once-daily dose (maximum dose 500 mg), is the drug of choice. Rifampin (20 mg/kg/d divided in two doses) may be added to the regimen in gravely ill or immunocompromised patients. Ciprofloxacin and levofloxacin are effective in adults but are not approved for use in children. Duration of therapy is 5–10 days if azithromycin is used; for other antibiotics a 14- to 21-day course is recommended. Oral therapy may be substituted for intravenous therapy as the patient's condition improves.

Prognosis

Mortality rate is high if treatment is delayed. Malaise, problems with memory, and fatigue are common after recovery.

Centers for Disease Control and Prevention. Available at: http://www.cdc.gov/legionella/

Diederen BM: Legionella spp. and Legionnaires' disease. J Infect 2008;56(1):1–12 [PMID: 17980914].

PSITTACOSIS (ORNITHOSIS) & *CHLAMYDOPHILA PNEUMONIAE* INFECTION

ESSENTIALS OF DIAGNOSIS & TYPICAL FEATURES

- Fever, cough, malaise, chills, headache.
- Diffuse rales; no consolidation.
- Long-lasting radiographic findings of bronchopneumonia.
- Isolation of the organism or rising titer of complement fixing antibodies.
- Exposure to infected birds (ornithosis).

General Considerations

Psittacosis is caused by *Chlamydia psittaci*. When the agent is transmitted to humans from psittacine birds (parrots, parakeets, cockatoos, and budgerigars), the disease is called psittacosis or parrot fever. However, other avian genera (eg, pigeons and turkeys) are common sources of infection in the United States, and the general term ornithosis often is used. The agent is an obligate intracellular parasite. Human-to-human spread rarely occurs. The incubation period is 5–14 days. The bird from which the disease was transmitted may not be clinically ill.

Chlamydophila pneumoniae (formerly *Chlamydia pneumoniae*) may cause atypical pneumonia similar to that due to *M pneumoniae*. Transmission is by respiratory spread. Infection appears to be most prevalent during the second decade; half of surveyed adults are seropositive. Only a small percentage of infections result in clinical pneumonia. The disease may be more common than atypical pneumonia due to *M pneumoniae*. Lower respiratory tract infection due to *C pneumoniae* is uncommon in infants and young children.

Prevention

Persons cleaning bird cages should use caution when cleaning cages or disposing of bird droppings to avoid aerosolization of *C psittaci*. *C psittaci* is susceptible to 1% Lysol or a 1:100 dilution of household bleach and one of these can be used to disinfect cages. Sick birds should be evaluated by a veterinarian and can be treated with antimicrobials. *C pneumoniae* is transmitted person to person by infected respiratory tract secretions. Prevention involves avoidance of known infected persons, using good hand hygiene (both infected persons and noninfected persons), and encouraging good respiratory hygiene (covering mouth with coughing, disposing of tissues contaminated with respiratory secretions).

Clinical Findings

A. Symptoms and Signs

1. *C psittaci*—The disease is extremely variable but tends to be mild in children. The onset is rapid or insidious, with fever, chills, headache, backache, malaise, myalgia, and dry cough. Signs include pneumonitis, altered percussion notes and breath sounds, and rales. Pulmonary findings may be absent early. Dyspnea and cyanosis may occur later. Splenomegaly, epistaxis, prostration, and meningismus are occasionally seen. Delirium, constipation or diarrhea, and abdominal distress may occur.

2. *C pneumoniae*—Clinically, *C pneumoniae* infection is similar to *M pneumoniae* infection. Most patients have mild upper respiratory infections. Lower respiratory tract infection is characterized by fever, sore throat (perhaps more severe with *C pneumoniae*), cough, and bilateral pulmonary findings and infiltrates.

B. Laboratory Findings

1. *C psittaci*—In psittacosis, the WBC count is normal or decreased, often with a shift to the left. Proteinuria is common. *C psittaci* is present in the blood and sputum during the first 2 weeks of illness but culture is avoided since it can represent a hazard to laboratory workers. A diagnosis can be made if *C psittaci* IgM is greater than or equal to 1:16 (microimmunofluorescent assay), a culture is positive for the organism, there is a fourfold rise in complement fixation titers in specimens obtained at least 2 weeks apart, or there is a single titer above 1:32 (microimmunofluorescent or complement fixation assay). The titer rise may be blunted or delayed by therapy. Infection with *C pneumoniae* may lead to diagnostic confusion because cross-reactive antibody may cause false-positive *C psittaci* titers. Microimmunofluorescence and PCR assays are specific but usually not available for *C psittaci*.

2. *C pneumoniae*—A fourfold rise in IgG titer (microimmunofluorescence antibody test) or an IgM titer above 1:16 is evidence of infection. IgG antibody peaks 6–8 weeks after infection. *C pneumoniae* can be isolated from nasal wash or throat swab specimens after inoculation into cell culture. A PCR assay also is available.

C. Imaging

The radiographic findings in psittacosis are those of central pneumonia that later becomes widespread or migratory. Psittacosis is indistinguishable from viral pneumonias by radiograph. Signs of pneumonitis may appear on radiograph in the absence of clinical suspicion of pulmonary involvement.

Differential Diagnosis

Psittacosis can be differentiated from viral or mycoplasmal pneumonias only by the history of contact with potentially infected birds. In severe or prolonged cases with extrapulmonary involvement the differential diagnosis is broad, including typhoid fever, brucellosis, and rheumatic fever.

Complications

Complications of psittacosis include myocarditis, endocarditis, hepatitis, pancreatitis, and secondary bacterial pneumonia. *C pneumoniae* infection may be prolonged or may recur.

Treatment

Psittacosis—Doxycycline should be given for 14 days after defervescence to patients older than 8 years with psittacosis. Alternatively, erythromycin or azithromycin, may be used in younger children. Supportive oxygen may be needed. A 14–21 day course is recommended.

Chlamydophila pneumonia—*C pneumoniae* responds to macrolides (azithromycin, erythromycin) or doxycycline: a 10–14 day course is recommended for erythromycin or docycycline; when using azithromycin the treatment length is 5 days.

Centers for Disease Control and Prevention. Available at: http://www.cdc.gov/ncidod/dbmd/diseaseinfo/chlamydiapneumonia_t.htm

Cunha BA: The atypical pneumonias: Clinical diagnosis and importance. Clin Microbiol Infect 2006;12(Suppl 3):12–24 [PMID: 16669925].

CAT-SCRATCH DISEASE

ESSENTIALS OF DIAGNOSIS & TYPICAL FEATURES

- History of a cat scratch or cat contact.
- Primary lesion (papule, pustule, or conjunctivitis) at site of inoculation.
- Acute or subacute regional lymphadenopathy.
- Aspiration of sterile pus from a node.
- Laboratory studies excluding other causes.
- Biopsy of node or papule showing histopathologic findings consistent with cat-scratch disease and occasionally characteristic bacilli on Warthin-Starry stain.
- Positive cat-scratch serology (antibody to *Bartonella henselae*).

General Considerations

The causative agent of cat-scratch disease is *B henselae,* a gram-negative bacillus that also causes bacillary angiomatosis. Cat-scratch disease is usually a benign, self-limited form of lymphadenitis. Patients often report a cat scratch (67%) or contact with a cat or kitten (90%). The cat almost invariably is healthy. The clinical picture is that of a regional lymphadenitis associated with an erythematous papular skin lesion without intervening lymphangitis. The disease occurs worldwide and is more common in the fall and winter. It is estimated that more than 20,000 cases per year occur in the United States. The most common systemic complication is encephalitis.

Clinical Findings

A. Symptoms and Signs

About 50% of patients with cat-scratch disease develop a primary lesion at the site of the wound. The lesion usually is a papule or pustule that appears 7–10 days after injury and is located most often on the arm or hand (50%), head or leg (30%), or trunk or neck (10%). The lesion may be conjunctival (10%). Regional lymphadenopathy appears 10–50 days later and may be accompanied by mild malaise, lassitude, headache, and fever. Multiple sites are seen in about 10% of cases. Involved nodes may be hard or soft and 1–6 cm in diameter. They are usually tender, warm, and erythematous and 10–20% of them suppurate. Lymphadenopathy usually resolves in about 2 months but may persist for up to 8 months.

Unusual manifestations include erythema nodosum, thrombocytopenic purpura, conjunctivitis (Parinaud oculoglandular fever), parotid swelling, pneumonia, osteolytic lesions, mesenteric and mediastinal adenitis, neuroretinitis, peripheral neuritis, hepatitis, granulomata of the liver and spleen, and encephalopathy.

Immunocompetent patients may develop an atypical systemic form of cat-scratch disease. These patients have prolonged fever, fatigue, and malaise. Lymphadenopathy may be present. Hepatosplenomegaly or low-density hepatic or splenic lesions visualized by ultrasound or computed tomography scan are seen in some patients.

Infection in immunocompromised individuals may take the form of bacillary angiomatosis, presenting as vascular tumors of the skin and subcutaneous tissues. Immunocompromised patients may also have bacteremia or infection of the liver (peliosis hepatis).

B. Laboratory Findings

Serologic evidence of Bartonella infection by indirect immunofluorescent antibody or ELISA with a titer above 1:64 is supportive of the diagnosis. PCR assays are available. Cat-scratch skin test antigens are not recommended.

Histopathologic examination of involved tissue may show pyogenic granulomas or bacillary forms demonstrated by Warthin-Starry silver stain (but bacillary forms on stain are not specific for cat scratch disease). Later in the course necrotizing granulomas may be seen. There usually is some elevation in the ESR. In patients with CNS involvement, the CSF is usually normal but may show a slight pleocytosis and modest elevation of protein.

Differential Diagnosis

Cat-scratch disease must be distinguished from pyogenic adenitis, tuberculosis (typical and atypical), tularemia, plague, brucellosis, lymphoma, primary toxoplasmosis, infectious mononucleosis, lymphogranuloma venereum, and fungal infections.

Treatment

Treatment of cat-scratch disease adenopathy is controversial because the disease usually resolves without therapy and the patient is typically not exceedingly ill. Treatment of typical cat-scratch disease with a 5-day course of azithromycin has been shown to speed resolution of lymphadenopathy in some patients. The best therapy is reassurance that the adenopathy is benign and will subside spontaneously with time (mean duration of illness is 14 weeks). In cases of nodal suppuration, needle aspiration under local anesthesia relieves the pain. Excision of the involved node is indicated in cases of chronic adenitis. In some reports, azithromycin, ciprofloxacin, rifampin, or TMP–SMX have been useful. Azithromycin is used by many experts if treatment of adenopathy is desired because it is given once a day, is reasonably priced, and was studied in one randomized placebo-controlled trial. In that trial, lymph node volume decreased faster than placebo by 1 month; there was no difference in long-term resolution in the azithromycin and placebo groups.

Immunocompromised patients with evidence of infection should be treated with antibiotics: long-term therapy (months) in these patients with azithromycin, erythromycin, or doxycycline often is needed to prevent relapses. Immunocompetent patients with more severe disease or evidence of systemic infection (eg, hepatic or splenic lesions) should also be treated with antibiotics.

Prognosis

The prognosis is good if complications do not occur.

Centers for Disease Control and Prevention. Available at: http://wwwnc.cdc.gov/travel/yellowbook/2012/chapter-3-infectious-diseases-related-to-travel/bartonella-associated-infections.htm

English R: Cat-scratch disease. Pediatr Rev 2006;27:123 [PMID: 16581952].

SPIROCHETAL INFECTIONS

SYPHILIS

ESSENTIALS OF DIAGNOSIS & TYPICAL FEATURES

- Congenital:
  - All types: history of untreated maternal syphilis, a positive serologic test, and a positive darkfield examination.
  - Newborn: hepatosplenomegaly, characteristic radiographic bone changes, anemia, increased nucleated red cells, thrombocytopenia, abnormal spinal fluid, jaundice, edema.
  - Young infant (3–12 weeks): snuffles, maculopapular skin rash, mucocutaneous lesions, pseudoparalysis (in addition to radiographic bone changes).
  - Children: stigmata of early congenital syphilis, interstitial keratitis, saber shins, gummas of nose and palate.
- Acquired:
  - Chancre of genitals, lip, or anus in child or adolescent.
  - History of sexual contact.

General Considerations

Syphilis is a chronic, generalized infectious disease caused by a spirochete, *Treponema pallidum*. In the acquired form, the disease is transmitted by sexual contact. Primary syphilis is characterized by the presence of an indurated painless chancre, which heals in 7–10 days. A secondary eruption involving the skin and mucous membranes appears in 4–6 weeks. After a long latency period, late lesions of tertiary syphilis involve the eyes, skin, bones, viscera, CNS, and cardiovascular system.

Congenital syphilis results from transplacental infection. Infection may result in stillbirth or produce illness in the newborn, in early infancy, or later in childhood. Syphilis occurring in the newborn and young infant is comparable to secondary disease in the adult but is more severe and life-threatening. Late congenital syphilis (developing in childhood) is comparable to tertiary disease.

The incidence of primary and secondary syphilis is increasing in the United States particularly among men. Nearly, 14,000 new cases of primary and secondary syphilis, 400 cases of congenital syphilis and nearly 45,000 total cases were reported in 2009.

Prevention

A serologic test for syphilis should be performed at the initiation of prenatal care and repeated at delivery in women at increased risk for syphilis. Serologic tests may be negative on both the mother and infant at the time of birth if the mother acquires syphilis near term. Adequate treatment of mothers with secondary syphilis before the last month of pregnancy reduces the incidence of congenital syphilis from 90% to less than 2%. Examination and serologic testing of sexual partners and siblings should also be done.

Clinical Findings

A. Symptoms and Signs

1. Congenital Syphilis

A. NEWBORNS—Most newborns with congenital syphilis are asymptomatic. If infection is not detected and treated, symptoms develop within weeks to months. When clinical signs are present, they usually consist of jaundice, anemia with or without thrombocytopenia, increase in nucleated red blood cells, hepatosplenomegaly, and edema. Overt signs of meningitis (bulging fontanelle or opisthotonos) may be present, but subclinical infection with CSF abnormalities is more common.

B. YOUNG INFANTS (3–12 WEEKS)—The infant may appear normal for the first few weeks of life only to develop mucocutaneous lesions and pseudoparalysis of the arms or legs. Shotty lymphadenopathy may be felt. Hepatomegaly is universal, with splenomegaly in 50% of patients. Other signs of disease similar to those seen in the newborn may be present. Anemia has been reported as the only presenting manifestation of congenital syphilis in this age group. "Snuffles" (syphilitic rhinitis), characterized by a profuse mucopurulent discharge, are present in 25% of patients. A syphilitic rash is common on the palms and soles but may occur anywhere on the body. The rash consists of bright red, raised maculopapular lesions that gradually fade. Moist lesions occur at the mucocutaneous junctions (nose, mouth, anus, and genitals) and lead to fissuring and bleeding.

Syphilis in the young infant may lead to stigmata recognizable in later childhood, such as rhagades (scars) around the mouth or nose, a depressed bridge of the nose (saddle nose), and a high forehead (secondary to mild hydrocephalus associated with low-grade meningitis and frontal periostitis). The permanent upper central incisors may be peg-shaped with a central notch (Hutchinson teeth), and the cusps of the sixth-year molars may have a lobulated mulberry appearance.

C. CHILDREN—Bilateral interstitial keratitis (at age 6–12 years) is characterized by photophobia, increased lacrimation, and vascularization of the cornea associated with exudation. Chorioretinitis and optic atrophy may also be seen. Meningovascular syphilis (at age 2–10 years) is usually slowly progressive, with mental retardation, spasticity, abnormal pupillary response, speech defects, and abnormal CSF. Deafness sometimes occurs. Thickening of the periosteum of the anterior tibias produces saber shins. A bilateral effusion in the knee joints may occur but is not associated with sequelae. Soft inflammatory growths called gummas may develop in the nasal septum, palate, long bones, and subcutaneous tissues.

2. Acquired syphilis—The primary chancre of the genitals, mouth, or anus may occur from genital, anal, or oral sexual contact. If the chancre is missed, signs of secondary syphilis, such as rash, fever, headache, and malaise, may be the first manifestations.

B. Laboratory Findings

1. Darkfield microscopy—Treponemes can be seen in scrapings from a chancre and from moist lesions.

2. Serologic tests for syphilis—There are two general types of serologic tests for syphilis: treponemal and nontreponemal. There are two types of nontreponemal tests: Venereal Disease Research Laboratory (VDRL) and the rapid plasma reagin (RPR). The VDRL and RPR are inexpensive, rapid tests that are useful for screening and following disease activity or adequacy of therapy. These tests provide quantitative results if the test is positive. False-positive nontreponemal tests can occur in patient with measles, hepatitis, mononucleosis, lymphoma, tuberculosis, endocarditis, pregnancy, and intravenous drug abuse. When evaluating a newborn infant for potential syphilis, umbilical cord blood specimens should not be used for nontreponemal tests: a false-positive test may result from Wharton jelly contamination of the sample. Conversely, a false-negative test may be seen in the setting where maternal infection occurred late in pregnancy.

Positive nontreponemal tests should be confirmed with a more specific treponemal test such as the fluorescent treponemal antibody absorbed (FTA-ABS) test or the *T pallidum* particle agglutination (TP-PA) test. False-positive FTA-ABS tests are uncommon except with other spirochetal diseases such as leptospirosis, rat bite fever, and Lyme disease.

One or two weeks after the onset of primary syphilis (chancre), the FTA-ABS test becomes positive. The VDRL or a similar nontreponemal test usually turns positive a few days later. By the time the secondary stage has been reached, virtually all patients show both positive FTA-ABS and positive nontreponemal tests. During latent and tertiary syphilis, the VDRL may become negative, but the FTA-ABS test usually remains positive. The quantitative VDRL or a similar nontreponemal test should be used to follow-up treated cases (see following discussion).

EIA tests specific for *T pallidun* are available in many laboratories and are replacing FTA-ABS, TP-PA tests. As these are rapid, inexpensive tests with greater specificity, a different screening strategy is now often used. The initial screen is done with EIA test followed by the RPR or VDRL, if positive.

In infants, positive serologic tests in cord sera may represent passively transferred antibody rather than congenital infection and therefore must be supplemented by a combination of clinical and laboratory data. Elevated total cord IgM is a helpful but nonspecific finding. A specific IgM–FTA-ABS is available, but negative results are not conclusive and should not be relied on. Demonstration of characteristic treponemes by darkfield examination of material from a moist lesion (skin; nasal or other mucous membranes) is definitive. Mouth lesions would be best examined by direct fluorescent antibody to distinguish *T pallidum* from nonpathogenic treponemes commonly found in the mouth. Serial measurement of quantitative RPR or VDRL is also very useful, because passively transferred antibody in the absence of active infection should decay with a normal half-life of about 18 days (see discussion of evaluation of infants for congenital syphilis section on Initial Evaluation and Treatment under Congenital Syphilis).

For evaluation of possible neurosyphilis, the CSF should be examined for cell count, glucose, protein, and a CSF VDRL. A negative CSF VDRL does not rule out neurosyphilis.

C. Imaging

Radiographic abnormalities are present in 90% of infants with symptoms of congenital syphilis and in 20% of asymptomatic infants. Metaphyseal lucent bands, periostitis, and a widened zone of provisional calcification may be present. Bilateral symmetrical osteomyelitis with pathologic fractures of the medial tibial metaphyses (Wimberger sign) is almost pathognomonic.

Differential Diagnosis

A. Congenital Syphilis

1. Newborns—Sepsis, congestive heart failure, congenital rubella, toxoplasmosis, disseminated herpes simplex, cytomegalovirus infection, and hemolytic disease of the newborn have to be differentiated. A positive Coombs test and blood group incompatibility distinguish hemolytic disease.

2. Young infants—Injury to the brachial plexus, poliomyelitis, acute osteomyelitis, and septic arthritis must be differentiated from pseudoparalysis. Coryza due to viral infection often responds to symptomatic treatment. Rash (ammoniacal diaper rash) and scabies may be confused with a syphilitic eruption.

3. Children—Interstitial keratitis and bone lesions of tuberculosis are distinguished by positive tuberculin reaction and chest radiograph. Arthritis associated with syphilis is unaccompanied by systemic signs, and joints are nontender. Mental retardation, spasticity, and hyperactivity are shown to be of syphilitic origin by strongly positive serologic tests.

B. Acquired Syphilis

Herpes genitalis, traumatic lesions, and other venereal diseases must be differentiated from primary chancers.

Treatment

A. Specific Measures

Penicillin is the drug of choice for *T pallidum* infection. If the patient is allergic to penicillin, azithromycin, ceftriaxone or one of the tetracyclines may be used, but are of unknown efficacy.

1. Congenital syphilis

A. INITIAL EVALUATION AND TREATMENT—Newborns should not be discharged from the hospital until the mother's serologic status for syphilis has been determined. Infants born to seropositive mothers require careful examination and quantitative nontreponemal (VDRL, RPR) syphilis testing. The same quantitative antitreponemal test used in evaluating the mother should be used in the infant so the titers can be compared. Maternal records regarding any prior diagnosis of syphilis, treatment, and follow-up titers should be reviewed. Infants should be further evaluated for congenital syphilis in any of the following circumstances:

- The maternal titer has increased fourfold.
- The infant's titer is at least fourfold greater than the maternal titer.
- Signs of syphilis are found on examination.
- Maternal syphilis was not treated or was inadequately treated during pregnancy.
- Maternal syphilis was treated with a nonpenicillin regimen, or the regimen or dose of medication is undocumented.
- Maternal syphilis was treated during pregnancy, but therapy was completed less than 4 weeks prior to delivery.
- Maternal syphilis was treated appropriately during pregnancy, but without the appropriate decrease in maternal nontreponemal titers after treatment.

The complete evaluation of an infant for possible congenital syphilis includes complete blood count, liver function tests, long bone radiographs, CSF examination (cell counts, glucose, and protein), CSF VDRL, and quantitative serologic tests. In addition, the placenta and umbilical cord should be examined pathologically using fluorescent antitreponemal antibody, if available. An ophthalmologic examination may also be done.

Treatment for congenital syphilis is indicated for infants with physical signs; umbilical cord or placenta positive for DFA-TP staining or darkfield examination; abnormal radiographs; elevated CSF protein or cell counts; reactive CSF VDRL; or serum quantitative nontreponemal titer that is more than fourfold higher than the maternal titer (using same test). Infants with proved or suspected congenital syphilis should receive either (1) aqueous crystalline penicillin G, 50,000 U/kg per dose intravenously every 12 hours (if < 1 week old) or (2) every 8 hours (if 1–4 weeks old) for 10 days. Procaine penicillin G, 50,000 U/kg in a single daily dose for 10 days is an alternative if compliance is assured. All infants diagnosed after age 4 weeks should receive 50,000 U/kg per dose aqueous crystalline penicillin intravenously every 4–6 hours for 10 days.

Additionally, treatment should be given to infants whose mothers have inadequately treated syphilis, to those whose mothers received treatment less than 1 month before delivery, to those whose mothers have undocumented or inadequate serologic response to therapy, and to those whose mothers were given nonpenicillin drugs to treat syphilis. In these instances, if the infant is asymptomatic, has a normal physical examination, normal CSF parameters, nonreactive CSF VDRL, normal bone films, quantitative nontreponemal titer less than fourfold of the mother's titer, and good follow-up is certain, some experts would give a single dose of penicillin G benzathine, 50,000 U/kg intramuscularly. If there is any abnormality in the preceding evaluation or if the CSF testing is not interpretable, the full 10 days of intravenous penicillin should be given. Close clinical and serologic monthly follow-up is necessary.

Asymptomatic, seropositive infants with normal physical examinations born to mothers who received adequate syphilis treatment (completed > 4 weeks prior to delivery) and whose mothers have an appropriate serologic response (fourfold or greater decrease in titer) to treatment may be at lower risk for congenital syphilis. Some experts believe complete laboratory and radiographic evaluation in these infants (CSF and long bone films) is not necessary. Infants who meet the preceding criteria, who have nontreponemal titers less than fourfold higher than maternal titers, and for whom follow-ups are certain can be given benzathine penicillin G, 50,000 U/kg, administered intramuscularly in a single dose. Infants should be followed with quantitative serologic tests and physical examinations until the nontreponemal serologic test is negative (see discussion of follow-up, next). Rising titers or clinical signs usually occur within 4 months in infected infants, requiring a full evaluation (including CSF studies and long bone radiographs) and institution of intravenous penicillin therapy.

B. Follow-up for congenital syphilis—Children treated for congenital syphilis need physical examinations every 2–3 months after completion of therapy, and both physical examinations and quantitative VDRL or RPR tests should be performed until the tests become nonreactive. Repeat CSF examination, including a CSF VDRL test, every 6 months until normal is indicated for infants with a positive CSF VDRL reaction or with abnormal cell counts or protein in the CSF. A reactive CSF VDRL test at the 6-month interval is an indication for retreatment. Titers decline with treatment and are usually negative by 6 months. Repeat treatment is indicated for children with rising titers or stable titers that do not decline.

2. Acquired syphilis of less than 1 year's duration— Benzathine penicillin G (50,000 U/kg, given intramuscularly, to a maximum of 2.4 million units) is given to adolescents with primary, secondary, or latent disease of less than 1 year's duration. All children should have a CSF examination (with CSF VDRL) prior to commencing therapy, to exclude neurosyphilis. Adolescents and adults need a CSF examination if clinical signs or symptoms suggest neurologic involvement or if they are HIV-infected.

3. Syphilis of more than 1 year's duration (late latent disease)—Syphilis of more than 1 year's duration (without evidence of neurosyphilis) requires weekly intramuscular benzathine penicillin G therapy for 3 weeks. CSF examination and VDRL test should be done on all children and patients with coexisting HIV infection or neurologic symptoms. In addition, patients who have failed treatment or who were previously treated with an agent other than penicillin need a CSF examination and CSF VDRL.

4. Neurosyphilis—Aqueous crystalline penicillin G is recommended, 200,000–300,000 U/kg/d in four to six divided doses, given intravenously for 10–14 days. The maximum adult dose is 4 million units per dose. Some experts recommend following this regimen with an intramuscular course of benzathine G penicillin, 50,000 U/kg given once a week for 3 consecutive weeks, to a maximum dose of 2.4 million units.

B. General Measures

Penicillin treatment of early congenital or secondary syphilis may result in a dramatic systemic febrile illness termed the Jarisch-Herxheimer reaction. Treatment is symptomatic, with careful follow-up. Transfusion may be necessary in infants with severe hemolytic anemia.

Prognosis

Severe disease, if undiagnosed, may be fatal in the newborn. Complete cure can be expected if the young infant is given penicillin. Serologic reversal usually occurs within 1 year.

Treatment of primary syphilis with penicillin is curative. Permanent neurologic sequelae may occur in meningovascular syphilis.

Chakraborty R, Luck S: Managing congenital syphilis again? The more things change. Curr Opin Infect Dis 2007;20:247 [PMID: 17471033].

Centers for Disease Control and Prevention (CDC) et al: Sexually transmitted diseases treatment guidelines, 2010. MMWR Recomm Rep 2010;59(RR-12) [PMID: 21160459].

Woods CR: Congenital syphilis-persisting pestilence. Pediatr Infect Dis J 2009;28(6):536–537 [PMID: 19483520].

RELAPSING FEVER

ESSENTIALS OF DIAGNOSIS & TYPICAL FEATURES

- Episodes of fever, chills, malaise.
- Occasional rash, arthritis, cough, hepatosplenomegaly, conjunctivitis.
- Diagnosis suggested by direct microscopic identification of spirochetes in smears of peripheral blood. Diagnosis confirmed with serologic testing.

General Considerations

Relapsing fever is a vector-borne disease caused by spirochetes of the genus Borrelia. Epidemic relapsing fever is transmitted to humans by body lice (*Pediculus humanus*) and endemic relapsing fever by soft-bodied ticks (genus *Ornithodoros*). Tick-borne relapsing fever is endemic in the western United States. Although several hundred cases are reported per year, substantial underdiagnosis occurs. Transmission usually takes place during the warm months, when ticks are active and recreation or work brings people into contact with *Ornithodoros* ticks. *B hermsii* causes most tick-borne infection in the United States. Infection is often acquired in mountain camping areas and cabins. The ticks are nocturnal feeders and remain attached for only 5–20 minutes. Consequently, the patient seldom remembers a tick bite. Rarely, neonatal relapsing fever results from transplacental transmission of Borrelia. Both louse-borne and tick-borne relapsing fever may be acquired during foreign travel.

Clinical Findings

A. Symptoms and Signs

The incubation period is 2–18 days. The attack is sudden, with high fever, chills, tachycardia, nausea and vomiting, headache, myalgia, and arthralgia. After 3–10 days, the fever falls. The disease is characterized by relapses at intervals of 1–2 weeks and lasting 3–5 days. The relapses duplicate the initial attack but become progressively less severe. In louse-borne relapsing fever, there is usually a single relapse. In tick-borne infection, two to six relapses occur.

Hepatomegaly, splenomegaly, pneumonitis, meningitis, and mycocarditis may appear later in the course of the disease. An erythematous rash may be seen over the trunk and extremities, and petechiae may be present. Jaundice, iritis, conjunctivitis, cranial nerve palsies, and hemorrhage occur more commonly during relapses.

B. Laboratory Findings

During febrile episodes, the patient's urine contains protein, casts, and occasionally erythrocytes; a marked polymorphonuclear leukocytosis is present; and about 25% of patients have a false-positive serologic test for syphilis. Spirochetes can be found in the peripheral blood by direct microscopy in approximately 70% of cases by darkfield examination or by Wright, Giemsa, or acridine orange staining of thick and thin smears. Spirochetes are not found during afebrile periods. Immunofluorescent antibody (or ELISA confirmed by Western blot) can help establish the diagnosis serologically. However, high titers of *Borrelia hermsii* can cross-react with *Borrelia burgdorferi* (the agent in Lyme disease) or Leptospira in immunofluorescent antibody assay, ELISA, and Western blots. Serologic specimens can be sent to the Division of Vector-Borne Infectious Diseases, Centers for Disease Control and Prevention, Fort Collins, CO 80522.

Differential Diagnosis

Relapsing fever may be confused with malaria, leptospirosis, dengue, typhus, rat-bite fever, Colorado tick fever, Rocky Mountain spotted fever, collagen-vascular disease, or any fever of unknown origin.

Complications

Complications include facial paralysis, iridocyclitis, optic atrophy, hypochromic anemia, pneumonia, nephritis, myocarditis, endocarditis, and seizures. CNS involvement occurs in 10%–30% of patients.

Treatment

For children younger than age 8 years who have tick-borne relapsing fever, standard dosages of penicillin or erythromycin should be given for 10 days. Older children may be given doxycycline. Chloramphenicol is also efficacious and was often used in the past.

Severely ill patients should be hospitalized. Patients may experience a Jarisch-Herxheimer reaction (usually noted in the first few hours after commencing antibiotics). Isolation precautions are not necessary for relapsing fever. Contact precautions are recommended for patients with louse infestations.

Prognosis

The mortality rate in treated cases of relapsing fever is very low, except in debilitated or very young children. With treatment, the initial attack is shortened and relapses prevented. The response to antimicrobial therapy is dramatic.

Centers for Disease Control. Available at: http://www.cdc.gov/ncidod/dvbid/relapsingfever/

Dworkin MS et al: Tick-borne relapsing fever. Infect Dis Clin North Am 2008;22(3):449–468 [PMID: 18755384].

LEPTOSPIROSIS

ESSENTIALS OF DIAGNOSIS & TYPICAL FEATURES

- Biphasic course lasting 2–3 weeks.
- Initial phase: high fever, headache, myalgia, and conjunctivitis.
- Apparent recovery for 2–3 days.
- Return of fever associated with meningitis.
- Jaundice, hemorrhages, and renal insufficiency (severe cases).
- Culture of organism from blood and CSF (early) and from urine (later), or direct microscopy of urine or CSF.
- Positive leptospiral agglutination test.

General Considerations

Leptospirosis is a zoonosis caused by many antigenically distinct but morphologically similar spirochetes. The organism enters through the skin or respiratory tract. Classically the severe form (Weil disease), with jaundice and a high mortality rate, was associated with infection with *Leptospira icterohaemorrhagiae* after immersion in water contaminated with rat urine. It is now known that a variety of animals (eg, dogs, rats, and cattle) may serve as reservoirs for pathogenic *Leptospira,* that a given serogroup may have multiple animal species as hosts, and that severe disease may be caused by many different serogroups.

In the United States, leptospirosis usually occurs after contact with dogs. Cattle, swine, or rodents may transmit the organism. Sewer workers, farmers, slaughterhouse workers, animal handlers, and soldiers are at risk for occupational exposure. Outbreaks have resulted from swimming in contaminated streams and harvesting field crops. In the United States, about 100 cases are reported yearly, about one-third of them in children.

Clinical Findings

A. Symptoms and Signs

1. Initial phase—The incubation period is 4–19 days (mean, 10 days). Chills, fever, headache, myalgia (especially lumbar area and calves), conjunctivitis without exudate-photophobia, cervical lymphadenopathy, and pharyngitis commonly occur. The initial leptospiremic phase lasts for 3–7 days.

2. Phase of apparent recovery—Symptoms typically (but not always) subside for 2–3 days.

3. Systemic phase—Fever reappears and is associated with headache, muscular pain, and tenderness in the abdomen and back, and nausea and vomiting. Conjunctivitis and uveitis are common. Lung, heart, and joint involvement occasionally occur. These manifestations are due to extensive vasculitis.

A. CNS INVOLVEMENT—The CNS is involved in 50%–90% of cases. Severe headache and mild nuchal rigidity are usual, but delirium, coma, and focal neurologic signs may be seen.

B. RENAL AND HEPATIC INVOLVEMENT—In about 50% of cases, the kidney or liver is affected. Gross hematuria and oliguria or anuria is sometimes seen. Jaundice may be associated with an enlarged and tender liver.

C. GALLBLADDER INVOLVEMENT—Leptospirosis may cause acalculous cholecystitis in children, demonstrable by abdominal ultrasound as a dilated, nonfunctioning gallbladder. Pancreatitis is unusual.

D. HEMORRHAGE—Petechiae, ecchymoses, and gastrointestinal bleeding may be severe.

E. RASH—A rash is seen in 10%–30% of cases. It may be maculopapular and generalized or may be petechial or purpuric. Occasionally erythema nodosum is seen. Peripheral desquamation of the rash may occur. Gangrenous areas are sometimes noted over the distal extremities. In such cases, skin biopsy demonstrates the presence of severe vasculitis involving both the arterial and the venous circulations.

B. Laboratory Findings

Leptospires are present in the blood and CSF only during the first 10 days of illness. They appear in the urine during the second week, where they may persist for 30 days or longer. Culture is difficult and requires specialized media and conditions. The WBC count often is elevated, especially when there is liver involvement. Serum bilirubin levels usually remain below 20 mg/dL. Other liver function tests may be abnormal, although the aspartate transaminase usually is elevated only slightly. An elevated serum creatine kinase is frequently found. CSF shows moderate pleocytosis (< 500/μL)—predominantly mononuclear cells—increased protein (50–100 mg/dL), and normal glucose. Urine often shows microscopic pyuria, hematuria, and, less often, moderate proteinuria (++ or greater). The ESR is elevated markedly. Chest radiograph may show pneumonitis.

Serologic antibodies measured by enzyme immunoassay may be demonstrated during or after the second week of illness. The confirmatory test of choice is a microscopic agglutination test, performed at some reference laboratories. Leptospiral agglutinins generally reach peak levels by the third to fourth week. A 1:100 titer is considered suspicious; a fourfold or greater rise is diagnostic. A PCR assay may be available at specialized research centers or through the CDC.

Differential Diagnosis

Fever and myalgia associated with the characteristic conjunctival injection should suggest leptospirosis. During the prodrome, malaria, typhoid fever, typhus, rheumatoid arthritis, brucellosis, and influenza may be suspected. Later, depending on the organ systems involved, a variety of other diseases need to be distinguished, including encephalitis, viral or tuberculous meningitis, viral hepatitis, glomerulonephritis, viral or bacterial pneumonia, rheumatic fever, subacute infective endocarditis, acute surgical abdomen, and Kawasaki disease (see Table 40–3).

Prevention

Preventive measures include avoidance of contaminated water and soil, rodent control, immunization of dogs and other domestic animals, and good sanitation. Immunization or antimicrobial prophylaxis with doxycycline may be of value to certain high-risk occupational groups.

Treatment

A. Specific Measures

Aqueous penicillin G (150,000 U/kg/d, given in four to six divided doses intravenously for 7–10 days) should be given when the diagnosis is suspected. Alternative agents include parenteral cefotaxime, ceftriaxone, or doxycycline. Studies in severely ill patients indicate a benefit even if treatment is started 4 days after onset. A Jarisch-Herxheimer reaction may occur. Oral doxycycline may be used for mildly ill patients. Doxycycline should not be used in children < 8 years or pregnant women.

B. General Measures

Symptomatic and supportive care is indicated, particularly for renal and hepatic failure and hemorrhage. Contact isolation is recommended, due to potential transmission from contact with urine.

Prognosis

Leptospirosis is usually self-limiting and not characterized by jaundice. The disease usually lasts 1–3 weeks but may be more prolonged. Relapse may occur. There are usually no permanent sequelae associated with CNS infection, although headache may persist. The mortality rate in the United States is 5%, usually from renal failure. The mortality rate may reach 20% or more in elderly patients who have severe kidney and hepatic involvement.

Levett P: Leptospirosis. Clin Microbiol Rev 2001;14(2):296–326 [PMID: 11292640]. Available at: http://cmr.asm.org/cgi/reprint/14/2/296

Palaniappan RU et al: Leptospirosis: Pathogenesis, immunity, and diagnosis. Curr Opin Infect Dis 2007;20:284 [PMID: 17471039].

Pavli A, Maltezou HC: Travel-acquired leptospirosis. J Travel Med 2008;15(6):447–453 [PMID: 19090801].

LYME DISEASE

ESSENTIALS OF DIAGNOSIS & TYPICAL FEATURES

- Characteristic skin lesion (erythema migrans) 3–30 days after tick bite.
- Arthritis, usually pauciarticular, occurring about 4 weeks after appearance of skin lesion. Headache, chills, and fever.
- Residence or travel in an endemic area during the late spring to early fall.

General Considerations

Lyme disease is a subacute or chronic spirochetal infection caused by *B burgdorferi* and transmitted by the bite of an infected deer tick (*Ixodes* species). The disease was known in Europe for many years as tick-borne encephalomyelitis, often associated with a characteristic rash (erythema migrans). Discovery of the agent and vector followed investigation of an outbreak of pauciarticular arthritis in Lyme, Connecticut, in 1977.

Although cases are reported from many countries, the most prominent endemic areas in the United States include the Northeast, upper Midwest, and West Coast. The northern European countries also have high rates of infection. Nearly 40,000 confirmed or probable cases were reported in the United States in 2009. Knowledge of the local epidemiology is important as Lyme disease is common in some areas of northeastern United States, but rare in the mountain states. The disease is spreading as a result of increased infection in and distribution of the tick vector. Most cases with rash are recognized in spring and summer, when most tick bites occur; however, because the incubation period for joint and neurologic disease may be months, cases may present at any time. *Ixodes* ticks are very small, and their bite is often unrecognized.

Clinical Findings

A. Symptoms and Signs

Erythema chronicum migrans, the most characteristic feature of Lyme disease, is recognized in 60%–80% of patients. Between 3 and 30 days after the bite, a ring of erythema develops at the site and spreads over days. It may attain a diameter of 20 cm. The center of the lesion may clear (resembling tinea corporis), remain red, or become raised (suggesting a chemical or infectious cellulitis). Mild tenderness may occur. Many patients are otherwise asymptomatic. Some have fever (usually low-grade), headache, and myalgias. Multiple satellite skin lesions, urticaria, or diffuse erythema may occur. Untreated, the rash lasts days to 3 weeks.

In up to 50% of patients, arthritis develops several weeks to months after the bite. Recurrent attacks of migratory, monarticular, or pauciarticular arthritis involving the knees and other large joints occur. Each attack lasts for days to a few weeks. Fever is common and may be high. Complete resolution between attacks is typical. Chronic arthritis develops in less than 10% of patients, more often in those with the DR4 haplotype.

Neurologic manifestations develop in up to 20% of patients and usually consist of Bell palsy, aseptic meningitis (which may be indistinguishable from viral meningitis), or polyradiculitis. Peripheral neuritis, Guillain-Barré syndrome, encephalitis, ataxia, chorea, and other cranial neuropathies are less common. Seizures suggest another diagnosis. Untreated, the neurologic symptoms are usually self-limited but may be chronic or permanent. Although fatigue and nonspecific neurologic symptoms may be prolonged in a few patients, Lyme disease is not a cause of chronic fatigue syndrome. Self-limited heart block or myocardial dysfunction occurs in about 5% of patients.

B. Laboratory Findings

Most patients with only rash have normal laboratory tests. Children with arthritis may have moderately elevated ESRs and WBC counts; the antinuclear antibodies and rheumatoid factor tests are negative or nonspecific; streptococcal antibodies are not elevated. Circulating IgM cryoglobulins may be present. Joint fluid may show up to 100,000 cells with a polymorphonuclear predominance, normal glucose, and elevated protein and immune complexes; Gram stain and culture are negative. In patients with CNS involvement, the CSF may show lymphocytic pleocytosis and elevated protein; the glucose and all cultures and stains are normal or negative. Abnormal nerve conduction may be present with peripheral neuropathy.

C. Diagnosis

Lyme disease is a clinical diagnosis. Local epidemiology, history of travel to endemic areas, physical examination, and laboratory features are important to consider. The causative organism is difficult to culture. Serologic testing may support the clinical diagnosis. Antibody testing should be performed in experienced laboratories. Serologic diagnosis of Lyme disease is based on a two-test approach: an ELISA and an immunoblot to confirm a positive or indeterminate ELISA. Antibodies may not be detectable until several weeks after infection has occurred; therefore, serologic testing in children with a typical rash is not recommended. Therapy early in disease may blunt antibody titers. Recent studies have shown considerable intralaboratory and interlaboratory variability in titers reported. Serologic testing of patients with nonspecific complaints from low prevalence areas results in falsely positive tests. Overdiagnosis of Lyme disease based on atypical symptoms and positive serology appears to be common. Sera from patients with syphilis, HIV, and leptospirosis may give false-positive results. Patients who receive appropriate treatment for Lyme disease may remain seropositive for years. Diagnosis of CNS disease requires objective abnormalities of the neurologic examination, laboratory or radiographic studies, and consistent positive serology.

Differential Diagnosis

Aside from the disorders already mentioned, the rash may resemble pityriasis, erythema multiforme, a drug eruption, or erythema nodosum. Erythema chronicum migrans is nonscaly, minimally tender or nontender, and persists longer in the same place than many of the more common childhood erythematous rashes. The arthritis may resemble juvenile rheumatoid arthritis, reactive arthritis, septic arthritis, reactive effusion from a contiguous osteomyelitis, rheumatic fever, leukemic arthritis, systemic lupus erythematosus, and Henoch-Schönlein purpura. Spontaneous resolution in a few days to weeks helps differentiate Lyme disease from juvenile rheumatoid arthritis, in which arthritis lasting a minimum of 6 weeks is required for diagnosis. The neurologic signs may suggest idiopathic Bell palsy, viral or parainfectious meningitis or meningoencephalitis, lead poisoning, psychosomatic illness, and many other conditions.

Prevention

Prevention consists of avoidance of endemic areas, wearing long sleeves and pants, frequent checks for ticks, and application of tick repellents. Ticks usually are attached for 24–48 hours before transmission of Lyme disease occurs. Ticks should be removed with a tweezer by pulling gently without twisting or excessive squeezing of the tick. Permethrin sprayed on clothing decreases tick attachment. Repellents containing high concentrations of *N*, *N*-Diethyl-meta-toluamide (DEET) may be neurotoxic and should be used cautiously in young children and infants and washed off when tick exposure ends. The CDC does not recommend prophylactic antibiotics for tick bites in asymptomatic individuals.

Treatment

Antimicrobial therapy is beneficial in most cases of Lyme disease. It is most effective if started early. Prolonged treatment is important for all forms. Relapses occur in some patients on all regimens.

A. Rash, Early Infections

Amoxicillin, 50 mg/kg/d orally in two divided doses (to a maximum of 2 g/d) for 14–21 days can be used for children of all ages. Doxycycline (100 mg orally twice a day) for 14–21 days may be used for children older than age 8 years. Erythromycin (30 mg/kg/d) or cefuroxime is used in penicillin-allergic children, although erythromycin may be less effective than amoxicillin.

B. Arthritis

The amoxicillin or doxycycline regimen (same dosage as for the rash) should be used, but treatment should continue for 4 weeks. Parenteral ceftriaxone (75–100 mg/kg/d) or penicillin G (300,000 U/kg/d, given intravenously in four divided doses for 2–4 weeks) is used for persistent arthritis.

C. Bell Palsy

The same oral drug regimens may be used for 3–4 weeks.

D. Other Neurologic Disease or Cardiac Disease

Parenteral therapy for 2–3 weeks is recommended with either ceftriaxone (75–100 kg/d in one daily dose) or penicillin G (300,000 U/kg/d intravenously in four divided doses).

Halperin JJ et al: Practice parameter: Treatment of nervous system Lyme disease (an evidence-based review): Report of the Quality Standards Subcommittee of the American Academy of Neurology. Neurology 2007;69:91 [PMID: 17522387].

Lantos PM et al: Final report of the Lyme disease review panel of the Infectious Diseases Society of America. Clin Infect Dis 2010;51(1):1–5 [PMID: 20504239].

Skogman BH et al: Lyme neuroborreliosis in children: A prospective study of clinical features, prognosis and outcome. Pediatr Infect Dis J 2008;27(12):1089 [PMID: 19008771].

Tuerlinckx D et al: Prediction of lyme meningitis based on a logistic regression model using clinical and cerebrospinal fluid analysis: A European study. Pediatr Infect Dis J 2009;28(5):394 [PMID: 19295463].

Wormser GP et al: The clinical assessment, treatment and prevention of lyme disease by the Infectious Diseases Society of America. Clin Infect Dis 2006;43(11):1089 [PMID: 17029130].

Centers for Disease Control and Prevention (CDC): Lyme disease. Available at: http://www.cdc.gov/ncidod/dvbid/lyme/index.htm

Infections: Parasitic & Mycotic

43

Samuel R. Dominguez, MD, PhD
Myron J. Levin, MD

PARASITIC INFECTIONS

Parasitic diseases are common and may present clinically in a variety of ways (Table 43–1). Although travel to endemic areas suggests particular infections, many are transmitted through fomites or acquired from contact with human carriers and can occur anywhere. Some of the less common parasitic infections and those seen primarily in the developing world are presented in abbreviated form in Table 43–2.

Selection of Patients for Evaluation

The incidence of parasitic infections varies greatly with geographic area. Children who have traveled or lived in areas where parasitic infections are endemic are at risk for infection with a variety of intestinal and tissue parasites. Children who have resided only in developed countries are usually free of tissue parasites (except *Toxoplasma*). Searching for intestinal parasites is expensive for the patient and time-consuming for the laboratory. More than 90% of ova and parasite examinations performed in most hospital laboratories in the United States are negative; many have been ordered inappropriately. An approach to determining which children with diarrhea need such examinations is presented in Figure 43–1. It can be more cost-effective to treat symptomatic U.S. immigrants with albendazole or nitazoxanide, broad-spectrum antiparasitic drugs, and to investigate only those whose symptoms persist.

Immunodeficient children are very susceptible to protozoal intestinal infections. Multiple opportunists are frequently identified, and the threshold for ordering tests should be low for these children.

Specimen Processing

For tissue parasites, contact the laboratory for proper collection procedures. Diarrheal stools may contain trophozoites that die rapidly during transport. The specimen should be either examined immediately or placed in a stool fixative such as polyvinyl alcohol. Fixative vials for home collection of stool are commercially available. They may contain toxic compounds, so they should be stored safely. Fixed specimens are stable at room temperature. Formed stools usually contain cysts that are more stable. It is also best to fix these after collection, although they may be reliably examined after transport at room temperature.

Eosinophilia & Parasitic Infections

Although certain parasites commonly cause eosinophilia, in developed countries other causes are much more common and include allergies, drugs, and other infections. Heavy intestinal nematode infections cause eosinophilia; they are easily detected on a single ova and parasite examination. Light nematode infections and common protozoal infections—giardiasis, cryptosporidiosis, and amebiasis—rarely cause eosinophilia. Eosinophilia is also unusual or minimal in more serious infections such as amebic liver abscess and malaria.

The most common parasitic infection in the United States that causes significant eosinophilia with negative stool examination is toxocariasis. In a young child with unexplained eosinophilia and a negative stool examination, a serologic test for *Toxocara* may be the next appropriate test. Trichinosis, which is a rare parasitic infection, causes marked eosinophilia; strongyloidiasis is a cause of eosinophilia that may be difficult to diagnose with stool examinations. The differential

Table 43–1. Signs and symptoms of parasitic infection.

Sign/Symptom	Agent	Comments[a]
Abdominal pain	*Anisakis*	Shortly after raw fish ingestion.
	Ascaris	Heavy infection may obstruct bowel, biliary tract.
	Clonorchis	Heavy, early infection. Hepatomegaly later.
	Entamoeba histolytica	Hematochezia, variable fever, diarrhea.
	Fasciola hepatica	Diarrhea, vomiting.
	Hookworm	Iron deficiency anemia with heavy infection.
	Strongyloides	Eosinophilia, pruritus. May resemble peptic disease.
	Trichinella	Myalgia, periorbital edema, eosinophilia.
	Trichuris	Diarrhea, dysentery with heavy infection.
Cough	*Ascaris*	Wheezing, eosinophilia during migration phase.
	Paragonimus westermani	Hemoptysis; chronic. May mimic tuberculosis.
	Strongyloides	Wheezing, pruritus, eosinophilia during migration or dissemination.
	Toxocara	Affects ages 1–5 y; hepatosplenomegaly; eosinophilia.
	Tropical eosinophilia	Pulmonary infiltrates, eosinophilia.
Diarrhea	*Blastocystis*	Possibly with heavy infection in immunosuppressed or immunocompetent individuals.
	Cyclospora	Watery; severe in immunosuppressed individuals.
	Cryptosporidium	Watery; chronic in immunosuppressed individuals.
	Dientamoeba fragilis	Only with heavy infection.
	E histolytica	Hematochezia, variable fever; no eosinophilia.
	Giardia	Afebrile, chronic; anorexia.
	Schistosoma	Chronic; hepatosplenomegaly (some types).
	Strongyloides	Abdominal pain; eosinophilia.
	Trichinella	Myalgia, periorbital edema, eosinophilia.
	Trichuris	With heavy infection.
Dysentery	*Balantidium coli*	Swine contact.
	E histolytica	Few to no leukocytes in stool; fever; hematochezia.
	Schistosoma	During acute infection.
	Trichuris	With heavy infection.
Dysuria	*Enterobius*	Usually girls with worms in urethra, bladder; nocturnal, perianal pruritus.
	Schistosoma (*S haematobium*)	Hematuria. Exclude bacteriuria, stones (some types).
Headache (and other cerebral symptoms)	*Angiostrongylus*	Eosinophilic meningitis.
	Baylisascaris procyonis	Eosinophilic meningitis
	Gnathostoma	Eosinophilic meningitis
	Naegleria	Freshwater swimming; rapidly progressive meningoencephalitis.
	Plasmodium	Fever, chills, jaundice, splenomegaly. Cerebral ischemia (with *P falciparum*).
	Taenia solium	Cysticercosis. Focal seizures, deficits; hydrocephalus, aseptic meningitis.
	Toxoplasma	Meningoencephalitis (especially in infants and the immunosuppressed); focal lesions in immunosuppressed; hydrocephalus in infants.
	Trypanosoma	African forms. Chronic lethargy (sleeping sickness).
Pruritus	*Ancylostoma braziliense*	Creeping eruption; dermal serpiginous burrow.
	Enterobius	Perianal, nocturnal.
	Filaria	Variable; seen in many filarial diseases; eosinophilia.
	Hookworm	Local at penetration site in heavy exposure.
	Strongyloides	Diffuse with migration; may be recurrent.
	Trypanosoma	African forms; one of many nonspecific symptoms.

(*Continued*)

Table 43–1. Signs and symptoms of parasitic infection. (*Continued*)

Sign/Symptom	Agent	Comments[a]
Rash	Hookworm	Pruritic, papulovesicular rash at site of penetration.
	Schistosoma	Maculopapular rash at site of penetration.
	Strongyloides	Pruritic rash at site of penetration.
	Toxoplasma	Maculopapular rash seen with congential and sometimes acquired infection.
Fever	*E histolytica*	With acute dysentery or liver abscess.
	Leishmania donovani	Hepatosplenomegaly, anemia, leukopenia.
	Plasmodium	Chills, headache, jaundice; periodic.
	Toxocara	Cough, hepatosplenomegaly, eosinophilia.
	Toxoplasma	Generalized adenopathy; splenomegaly.
	Trichinella	Myalgia, periorbital edema, eosinophilia.
	Trypanosoma	Early stage, African forms; lymphadenopathy.
Anemia	*Diphyllobothrium*	Megaloblastic due to vitamin B_{12} deficiency; rare.
	Hookworm	Iron deficiency.
	L donovani	Fever, hepatosplenomegaly, leukopenia (kala-azar).
	Plasmodium	Hemolysis.
	Trichuris	Heavy infection; due to iron loss.
Eosinophilia	*Angiostrongylus*	Eosinophilic meningitis.
	Baylisascaris procyonis	Eosinophilic meningitis
	Fasciola	Abdominal pain.
	Gnathostoma	Eosinophilic meningitis
	Filaria	Microfilariae in blood; lymphadenopathy.
	Onchocerca	Skin nodules, keratitis.
	Schistosoma	Chronic; intestinal or genitourinary symptoms.
	Strongyloides	Abdominal pain, diarrhea.
	Toxocara	Hepatosplenomegaly, cough; affects ages 1–5 y.
	Trichinella	Myalgia, periorbital edema.
	Tropical pulmonary eosinophilia	Cough; pulmonary infiltrates.
	T solium (cysticercosis)	Eosinophils in CSF.
Hematuria	*Schistosoma*	*S haematobium*. Bladder, urethral granulomas. Exclude stones.
Hemoptysis	*P westermani*	Lung fluke. Variable chest pain; chronic.
Hepatomegaly	*Clonorchis*	Heavy infection. Tenderness early; cirrhosis late.
	Echinococcus	Chronic; cysts.
	E histolytica	Toxic hepatitis or abscess. No eosinophilia.
	L donovani	Splenomegaly, fever, pancytopenia.
	Schistosoma (not *haematobium*)	Chronic; hepatic fibrosis, splenomegaly (some types).
	Toxocara	Splenomegaly, eosinophilia, cough; no adenopathy.
Splenomegaly	*L donovani*	Hepatomegaly, fever, anemia.
	Plasmodium	Fever, chills, jaundice, headache.
	Schistosoma (not *haematobium*)	Hepatomegaly.
	Toxocara	Eosinophilia, hepatomegaly.
	Toxoplasma	Lymphadenopathy, other symptoms.
Lymphadenopathy	Filaria	Inguinal typical; chronic.
	L donovani	Hepatosplenomegaly, pancytopenia, fever.
	Schistosoma	Acute infection; fever, rash, arthralgia, hepatosplenomegaly.
	Toxoplasma	Cervical common; may involve single group of nodes; splenomegaly.
	Trypanosoma	Localized near bite or generalized; hepatosplenomegaly (Chagas disease); generalized (especially posterior cervical) in African forms.

[a]Symptoms usually related to degree of infestation. Infestation with small numbers of organisms is often asymptomatic.

Table 43–2. Some parasitic infections rarely seen in developed regions.

Agent (Disease)	Geographic Region	Vector	Symptoms and Signs	Laboratory Findings	Diagnosis	Therapy and Comments
Angiostrongylus cantonensis (eosinophilic meningitis)	Hawaii, Asia, Pacific Islands	Snails, slugs	Ingestion (usually inadvertent) followed in 1–4 wk by meningitis of variable severity. Paresthesias.	Eosinophils in CSF and blood	Positive serology. Larvae may be present in CSF.	Fever absent or low. No focal lesions on CNS imaging. No specific therapy. Steroids may be beneficial. Mebendazole may help.
Clonorchis sinensis (liver fluke infection)	Asia	Raw fish	Adult flukes obstruct biliary tree. Acute: hepatomegaly, fever, jaundice, urticaria. Late: cirrhosis, carcinoma.	Variable liver function abnormalities	Ova in feces.	Praziquantel. Advanced disease not treatable. Liver transplant.
Gnathostoma spinigerum (eosinophilic meningitis)	Southeast Asia, Mexico, Central and South America	Raw or undercooked fish, frogs, pigs, snakes, fowl, eels	Painful, recurrent, pruritic, erythematous rashes. Can invade eye causing pain, uveitis, and blindness. Recurrent meningitis with radicular pain and paresthesias.	Peripheral and CNS eosinophilia	Identification of organism in host tissue. ELISA and Western blot.	Albendazole, ivermectin. Symptoms can recur for 10–12 y.
Leishmania braziliensis, L mexicana (chiclero ulcer)	South America	Sandfly	Painful mucocutaneous ulcers or granulomas. Nasolabial lesions common.	—	Skin biopsy. Positive skin test, serology.	Sodium stibogluconate, meglumine antimonate, pentamidine, amphotericin; ketoconazole.
Leishmania donovani (kala-azar)	Mideast, India, Mediterranean, South and Central America	Sandfly	Fever, generalized adenopathy, hepatosplenomegaly weeks to months after infection.	Pancytopenia, hypergammaglobulinemia	Organisms in skin biopsy. Positive skin test, serology.	Sodium stibogluconate, meglumine antimonate, pentamidine, amphotericin B.
Leishmania tropica (Oriental sore)	Asia, India, North Africa	Sandfly	Papule at bite site (usually on face, limbs) develops after weeks to months, then ulcerates and scars.	—	Organisms in skin biopsy. Positive skin test, serology.	Sodium stibogluconate, meglumine antimonate, pentamidine, amphotericin.
Paragonimus westermani (lung fluke infection)	Asia, South America, Africa	Raw crabs, crustaceans	Cough, hemoptysis. Rarely seizures, other CNS signs if migration to brain occurs.	—	Large ova in concentrated fecal specimens. Cystic nodular lesions on chest radiograph or CNS imaging.	Resembles pulmonary tuberculosis. Praziquantel very effective.
Trypanosoma brucei (sleeping sickness)	Africa	Tsetse fly	Hepatosplenomegaly, adenopathy. Nodule at bite site (resolves). Recurrent fever, headache, myalgia, progressive encephalitis.	Elevated ESR, anemia, CSF pleocytosis	Organisms in marrow, nodes. Positive serology.	Suramin, eflornithine, pentamidine, melarsoprol.
Trypanosoma cruzi (Chagas disease)	South and Central America, Mexico	Reduviid bug	Acute: painful red nodule at bite site, conjunctivitis, periorbital edema (Romaña sign), fever, local ± generalized adenitis. Late: myocarditis, megaesophagus, megacolon.	Mononuclear leukocytosis	Organisms in peripheral blood. Positive serology.	Nifurtimox or benznidazole may help early. No therapy for late disease. May be transmitted by blood transfusion or congenitally.
Wuchereria, Brugia (filariasis)	Tropics, subtropics	Mosquito	Chronic adenopathy, often inguinal. Obstructive lymphedema.	Eosinophilia	Concentrated blood smears for larvae. Positive serology.	Diethylcarbamazine kills larvae. Surgery for lymphatic obstruction.

CNS, central nervous system; CSF, cerebrospinal fluid; ESR, erythrocyte sedimentation rate.

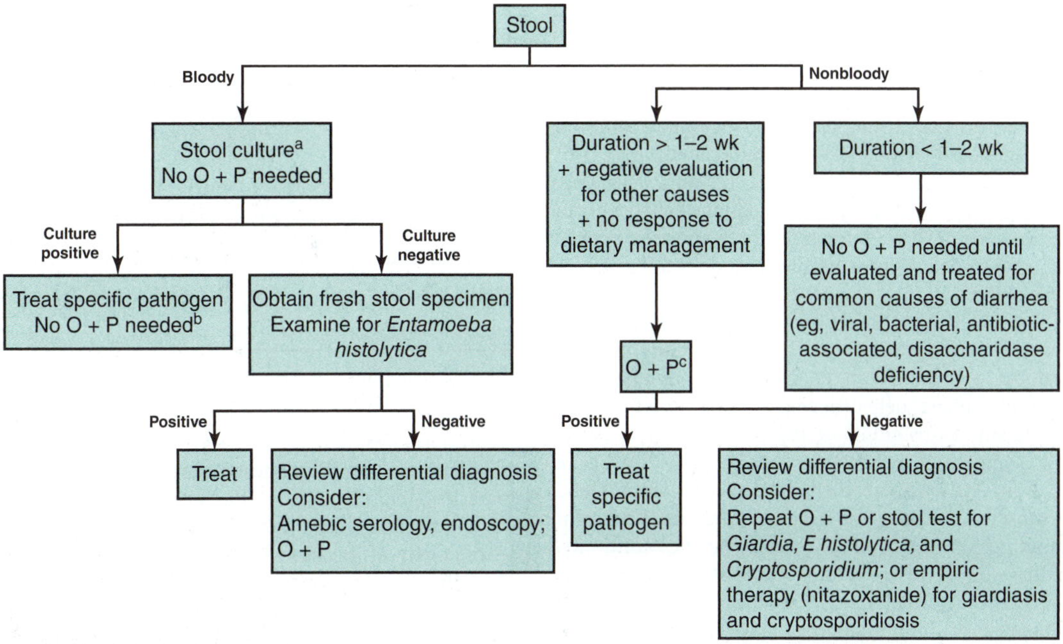

O + P = Ova and parasite examination.
[a]*Shigella, Salmonella, Campylobacter, Escherichia coli* O 157, *Yersinia*: assay for *Clostridium difficile* toxin if recent antimicrobial use.
[b]Unless critically ill, from endemic area for amebiasis, or unresponsive to standard therapy.
[c]Include examination for *Cryptosporidium* and *Cyclospora*; immediate stool fixation needed if stool is diarrheal.

▲ **Figure 43–1.** Parasitologic evaluation of acute diarrhea.

diagnosis of eosinophilia is broad for patients who have been in developing countries (see Table 43–1).

PROTOZOAL INFECTIONS

SYSTEMIC INFECTIONS

1. Malaria

ESSENTIALS OF DIAGNOSIS & TYPICAL FEATURES

- Residence in or travel to an endemic area (fever in the returning traveler)
- Cyclic paroxysms of chills, fever, and intense sweating.
- Headache, backache, cough, abdominal pain, nausea, vomiting, diarrhea.
- Coma, seizures.
- Splenomegaly, anemia.
- Malaria parasites in peripheral blood smear.

General Considerations

Malaria kills a million children worldwide each year and is undergoing a resurgence in areas where it was previously controlled. Approximately 1000 imported cases are diagnosed in the United States each year; local transmission may occasionally take place from imported cases. Human malaria was known to be caused by four Plasmodium species—*Plasmodium vivax* (most common), *Plasmodium falciparum* (most virulent), *Plasmodium ovale* (similar to *P vivax*), and *Plasmodium malariae*. Recently a fifth species, *Plasmodium knowlesi*, which causes malaria in macaques, has been recognized as a cause of malaria in humans. The majority of cases of malaria due to *P knowlesi* have been from people or travelers to Malaysia or neighboring countries in Southeast Asia.

The female anopheline mosquito transmits the parasites. The gametocytes ingested from infected humans form sporozoites in the mosquito; when these are inoculated into a susceptible host and they subsequently infect hepatocytes. The initial hepatic (preerythrocytic) phase is about 1–2 weeks for all but *P malariae* infection (3–5 weeks), but the initial symptoms may be delayed for up to a year in *P falciparum*, 4 years in *P vivax*, and decades in *P malariae* infections. Merozoites released into the circulation from hepatocytes infect red cells (young cells by *P vivax* and *P ovale*, old cells by *P malariae*, and all cells by *P falciparum* and *P knowlesi*) and begin the synchronous erythrocytic cycles, rupturing the infected cells at regular 48- or 72-hour intervals. Asynchronous cycles causing daily fevers are most common in early stages of infection. Survival is associated with a progressive decrease in intensity of cycles; relapses years later may occur from persistent hepatic infection, which occurs in *P vivax* and *P ovale* infections. Infection acquired congenitally or from transfusions or needlesticks does not result in a hepatic phase.

Susceptibility varies genetically; certain red cell phenotypes are partially resistant to *P falciparum* infection (hemoglobin S, hemoglobin F, thalassemia, and possibly glucose-6-phosphate dehydrogenase [G6PD] deficiency). The worldwide distribution of the four species is determined to some extent by host genetic factors. The absence of *P vivax* from Africa reflects the lack of specific Duffy blood group substances among most native Africans. Recurrent infections result in acquired species-specific immunity, which does not prevent infection, but decreases parasitemia and symptoms. Normal splenic function is an important factor because of the immunologic and filter functions of the spleen. Asplenic persons develop rapidly progressive malaria with many circulating infected erythrocytes (including mature forms of *P falciparum*). Maternal immunity protects the neonate.

Table 43–3. Differentiation of malaria parasites on blood smears.

	Plasmodium falciparum	*P vivax, P ovale*
Multiple infected erythrocytes	Common	Rare
Mature trophozoites or schizonts	Absent[a]	Common
Schüffner dots	Absent	Common
Enlarged erythrocytes	Absent	Common
Banana-shaped gametocytes	Common	Absent

[a]Usually sequestered in the microcirculation. Rare cases with circulating forms have extremely high parasitemia and a poor prognosis.

Clinical Findings

A. Symptoms and Signs

Clinical manifestations vary according to species, strain, and host immunity. The infant presents with recurrent bouts of fever, irritability, poor feeding, vomiting, jaundice, and splenomegaly. Rash is usually absent, which helps distinguish malaria from viral infections in patients presenting with similar symptoms. In older children, the pathognomonic constellation of headache, backache, chills, myalgia, and fatigue is more easily elicited. Fever may be cyclic (every 48 hours for all but *P malariae* infection, in which it occurs every 72 hours) or irregular (most commonly observed with *P falciparum*). Between attacks, patients may look quite well. If the disease is untreated, relapses cease within a year in *P falciparum* and within several years in *P vivax* infections, but may recur decades later with *P malariae* infection. Infection during pregnancy often causes intrauterine growth restriction or premature delivery but rarely true fetal infection.

Physical examination in patients with uncomplicated cases may show only mild splenomegaly and anemia.

B. Laboratory Findings

The diagnosis of malaria relies on detection of one or more of the four human plasmodia in blood smears. Most acute infections are caused by *P vivax*, *P ovale*, or *P falciparum*, although 5%–7% are due to multiple species. Giemsa-stained thick smears offer the highest diagnostic accuracy for malaria parasites. Identification of the *Plasmodium* species relies on morphologic criteria (Table 43–3) and requires an experienced observer. Because the early trophozoites of *P knowlesi* resemble the ring form of *P falciparum* and its later stages mimic those of *P malariae*, *P knowlesi* is often misdiagnosed. Accordingly, as *P knowlesi* infection is potentially life threatening, it should always be suspected in cases in which microscopic examination suggests *P malariae*, but in which the patient has severe malaria, considerable parasitemia, and/or a recent history of travel to Southeast Asia.

Alternative techniques of similar or higher diagnostic accuracy for *P falciparum* include enzyme-linked immunosorbent assay (ELISA), DNA hybridization, and polymerase chain reaction (PCR). Rapid antigen detection tests (RDTs) have recently been developed and are starting to be used in malaria-endemic areas in Africa. A unique feature of the microscopic examination is the semiquantitative estimate of the parasitemia, which is best done on thin smears. This information is particularly useful in the management of infections caused by *P falciparum*, in which high parasitemia ($>$ 10% infected erythrocytes or $>$ 500,000 infected erythrocytes/μL) is associated with high morbidity and mortality and requires hospitalization. Treatment response of *P falciparum* and chloroquine-resistant *P vivax* infections is best monitored by daily parasitemia assays. Constant or increased number of infected erythrocytes after 48 hours of treatment or after the second hemolytic crisis suggests an inadequate therapeutic response. Other laboratory findings that reflect the severity of hemolysis include decreased hematocrit, hemoglobin, and haptoglobin levels; increased reticulocyte count; hyperbilirubinemia; and increased lactate dehydrogenase. Thrombocytopenia is common, but the incidence of leukocytosis is variable.

Differential Diagnosis

Relapsing fever may be associated with borreliosis, brucellosis, sequential common infections, Hodgkin disease, juvenile rheumatoid arthritis, or rat-bite fever. Other common causes of high fever and headache include influenza, *Mycoplasma pneumoniae* or enteroviral infection, sinusitis, meningitis, enteric fever, tuberculosis, occult pneumonia, or bacteremia. Fever, headache, and jaundice in a patient returning from tropical areas indicate that leptospirosis and yellow fever should be included in the differential diagnosis. Malaria may also coexist with other diseases.

Complications & Sequelae

Severe complications are limited to *P falciparum* and *P knowlesi* infection and result from microvascular obstruction and tissue ischemia. Impaired consciousness and seizures are the most common complications of malaria in children. In addition, respiratory failure, renal impairment, severe bleeding, and shock are associated with a poor prognosis. Among the laboratory abnormalities, hypoglycemia, acidosis, elevated aminotransferases, and parasitemia greater than 10% characterize severe malaria.

Prevention

Malaria chemoprophylaxis should be instituted 2 weeks (weekly regimens) to 2 days (daily regimens) before traveling to an area of endemic infection to permit alternatives if the drug is not tolerated. Because the antimalarial drugs recommended for prophylaxis do not kill sporozoites, therapy should be continued for 1 week (atovaquone–proguanil) or 4 weeks (all other regimens) after returning from an endemic area to cover infection acquired at departure.

No drug regimen guarantees protection against malaria. If fever develops within 1 year (particularly within 2 months) after travel to an endemic area, patients should be advised to seek medical attention. Insect repellents, insecticide-impregnated bed nets, and proper clothing are important adjuncts for malaria prophylaxis.

For a full discussion regarding currently recommended medications for malaria prophylaxis, please see the corresponding section in Chapter 45.

Treatment

Treatment for malaria includes a variety of supportive strategies in addition to the antimalarial drugs. It is advisable to hospitalize nonimmune patients infected with *P falciparum* until a decrease in parasitemia is demonstrated, indicating that treatment is effective and severe complications are unlikely to occur. Malaria due to *P knowlesi* should be treated like *P falciparum* malaria as it might progress rapidly into severe disease.

Partially immune patients with uncomplicated *P falciparum* infection and nonimmune persons infected with *P vivax*, *P ovale*, or *P malariae* can receive treatment as outpatients if follow-up is reliable. For children, hydration and treatment of hypoglycemia are of utmost importance. Anemia, seizures, pulmonary edema, and renal failure require conventional management. Corticosteroids are contraindicated for cerebral malaria because of increased mortality. In severe malaria, exchange transfusion can be lifesaving, particularly in nonimmune persons with parasitemia greater than 15%.

Choice of antimalarial treatment depends on the immune status of the person, plasmodium species, degree of parasitemia, and geographical region of acquisition. An algorithm for the treatment of malaria is shown in Figure 43–2 and a description of the recommended antimalarial drugs available in the United States is provided in Table 43–4. Updated treatment guidelines are available at the Centers for Disease Control and Prevention (CDC) (http://www.cdc.gov/malaria/diagnosis_treatment/treatment.html). Artemisinin derivatives, which clear parasites very rapidly and are widely used as key components and often as first line therapy in malaria treatment worldwide, are available in the United States only for the treatment of severe malaria through the CDC (www.cdc.gov/malaria/features/artesunate_now_available.htm).

Chen LH et al: Controversies and misconceptions in malaria chemoprophylaxis for travelers. JAMA 2007;297:2251 [PMID: 17519415].

Griffith KS et al: Treatment of malaria in the United States. JAMA 2007;297:2264 [PMID: 17519416].

Kantele A et al: Review of cases with the emerging fifth human malaria parasite, Plasmodium knowlesi. CID 2011;52:1356–1362 [PMID: 21596677].

Rosenthal PJ: Artesunate for the treatment of severe falciparum malaria. N Engl J Med 2008;358:1829–1836 [PMID: 18434652].

Sinclair D et al: Artesunate versus quinine for treating severe malaria. Cochrane Database of Systematic Reviews 2011;issue 3:Art No CD005967 [PMID: 214128920].

Taylor SM et al: Does this patient have malaria? JAMA 2010;304:2048–2056 [PMID: 21057136].

2. Babesiosis

Babesia microti is a malaria-like protozoan that infects and lyses erythrocytes of wild and domestic animals in North America and Europe. In the United States, human babesiosis occurs in the coastal areas of New England, northern California and Washington State, and in the lakes region of the upper Midwest. Humans accidentally enter the cycle when bitten by *Ixodes scapularis* (deer tick), one of the intermediate hosts and vectors of *B microti*. After inoculation, the protozoan penetrates erythrocytes and starts an asynchronous cycle that causes hemolysis. Babesia infection is also a transfusion-transmissible disease.

Clinical Findings

A. Symptoms and Signs

The incubation period is 1–3 weeks, but may extend up to 6 weeks. Many times the tick bite is unnoticed. Symptoms are nonspecific and include sustained or cyclic fever up to 40°C,

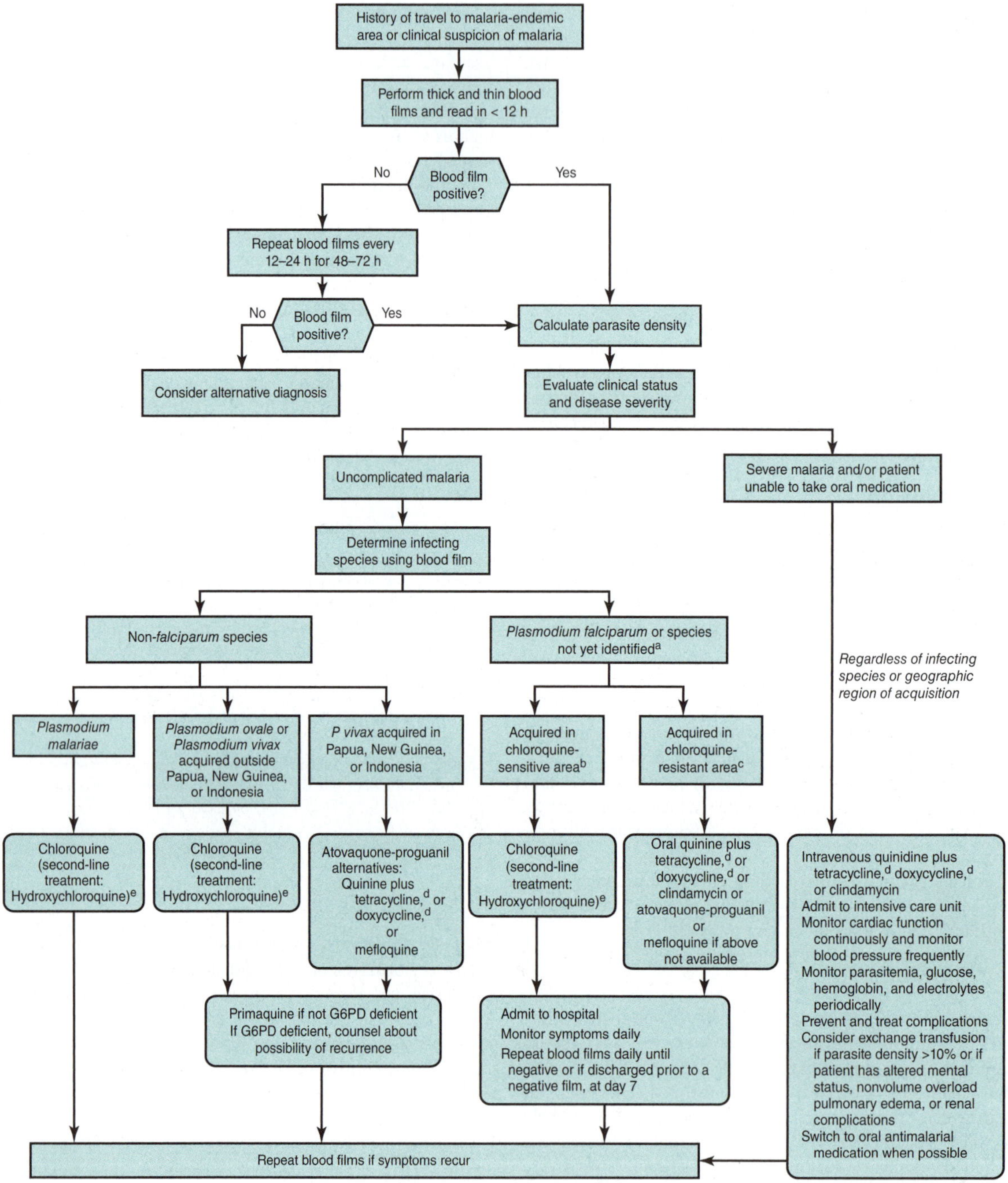

[a]If species not yet identified is subsequently diagnosed as a non-*falciparum* infection, then complete treatment as per the identified species recommendations. G6PD indicates glucose-6-phosphate dehydrogenase.
[b]Central America west of the Panama Canal, Mexico, Hispaniola, parts of China, and the Middle East.
[c]All malaria-endemic countries except those listed in second footnote.
[d]Contraindicated in pregnant women and children younger than 8 years of age.
[e]Drug options for chloroquine-resistant *P falciparum* may also be used if chloroquine or hydroxychloroquine cannot be used.

▲ **Figure 43–2.** Malaria treatment algorithm. (Adapted from Centers for Disease Control and Prevention. Malaria. http://www.cdc.gov/malaria/resources/pdf/algorithm.pdf. Accessed May 4, 2012.)

Table 43–4. Antimalarial drugs available in the United States recommended for use in the treatment of malaria.

Drug	Indication	Adult Dosage	Pediatric Dosage[a]	Potential Adverse Effects	Comments
Atovaquone–proguanil (oral)	*Plasmodium falciparum* from chloroquine-resistant areas	Adult tablet = 250 mg atovaquone/100 mg proguanil 4 adult tablets orally per day × 3 d	Pediatric tablet = 62.5 mg atovaquone/25 mg proguanil 5–8 kg: 2 pediatric tablets orally per day × 3 d > 8–10 kg: 3 pediatric tablets orally per day × 3 d > 10–20 kg: 1 adult tablet orally per day × 3 d > 20–30 kg: 2 adult tablets orally per day × 3 d > 30–40 kg: 3 adult tablets orally per day × 3 d > 40 kg: 4 adult tablets orally per day × 3 d	Abdominal pain, nausea, vomiting, diarrhea, headache, rash, mild reversible elevations in liver amino-transferase levels	Not indicated for use in pregnant women due to limited data Contraindicated if hypersensitivity to atovaquone or proguanil; severe renal impairment (creatine clearance < 30 mL/min) Should be taken with food to increase absorption of atovaquone
Chloroquine phosphate	*P falciparum* from chloroquine-sensitive areas *P vivax* from chloroquine-sensitive areas All *P ovale*; all *P malariae*	600-mg base (= 1000 mg salt) orally immediately, followed by 300-mg base (= 500 mg salt) orally at 5, 24, and 48 h Total dose: 1500-mg base (= 2500 mg salt)	10-mg base/kg orally immediately, followed by 6-mg base/kg orally at 6, 24, and 48 h Total dose: 25-mg base/kg	Nausea, vomiting, rash, headache, dizziness, urticaria, abdominal pain, pruritus	Safe in children and pregnant women Give for chemoprophylaxis (500 mg salt orally every week) in pregnant women with chloroquine-sensitive *P vivax* Contraindicated if retinal or visual field change; hypersensitivity to 4-aminoquinolines Use with caution in those with impaired liver function since the drug is concentrated in the liver
Clindamycin (oral or IV)	*P falciparum* from chloroquine-resistant areas *P vivax* from chloroquine-resistant areas (in combination with quinine or quinidine)	Oral: 20-mg base/kg/d orally divided 3 times daily × 7 d IV: 10-mg base/kg loading dose IV followed by 5-mg base/kg IV every 8 h; switch to oral clindamycin (oral dose as above) as soon as patient can take oral medication; treatment course = 7 d	Oral: 20-mg base/kg/d orally divided 3 times daily × 7 d IV: 10-mg base/kg loading dose IV followed by 5-mg base/kg IV every 8 h; switch to oral clindamycin (oral dose as above) as soon as patient can take oral medication; treatment course = 7 d	Diarrhea, nausea, rash	Always use in combination with quinine or quinidine Safe in children and pregnant women

(*Continued*)

Table 43–4. Antimalarial drugs available in the United States recommended for use in the treatment of malaria. (*Continued*)

Drug	Indication	Adult Dosage	Pediatric Dosage[a]	Potential Adverse Effects	Comments
Doxycycline (oral or IV)	*P falciparum* from chloroquine-resistant areas	Oral: 100 mg orally twice daily × 7 d	Oral: 2.2 mg/kg orally every 12 h × 7 d	Nausea, vomiting, diarrhea, abdominal pain, dizziness, photosensitivity, headache, esophagitis, odynophagia	Always use in combination with quinine or quinidine
	P vivax from chloroquine-resistant areas (in combination with quinine or quinidine)	IV: 100 mg IV every 12 h and then switch to oral doxycycline (as above) as soon as patient can take oral medication; treatment course = 7 d	IV: IV only if patient is not able to take oral medication; for children < 45 kg, give 2.2 mg/kg IV every 12 h and then switch to oral doxycycline (dose as above) as soon as patient can take oral medication; for children ≥ 45 kg, use same dosing as for adults; treatment course = 7 d	Rarely, hepatotoxicity, pancreatitis, and benign intracranial hypertension seen with tetracycline class of drugs	Contraindicated in children ≤ 8 y, pregnant women, and persons with hypersensitivity to tetracyclines While food, milk, and divalent and trivalent cations decrease the absorption of tetracycline, doxycycline can be taken with food, including milk products, which helps to decrease gastrointestinal disturbances To prevent esophagitis, the tetracyclines should be taken with large amounts of fluids, and patients should not lie down for 1 h after taking the drugs Concurrent treatment with barbiturates, carbamazepine, or phenytoin may cause a reduction in serum concentrations of doxycycline
Hydroxychloroquine (oral)	Second-line alternative for treatment of:	620-mg base (= 800 mg salt) orally immediately, followed by 310-mg base (= 400 mg salt) orally at 6, 24, and 48 h	10-mg base/kg orally immediately, followed by 5-mg base/kg orally at 6, 24, and 48 h	Nausea, vomiting, rash, headache, dizziness, urticaria, abdominal pain, pruritus[b]	Safe in children and pregnant women Give for chemoprophylaxis (310-mg base orally every week) in pregnant women with chloroquine-sensitive *P vivax* Contraindicated if retinal or visual field change; hypersensitivity to 4-aminoquinolines Use with caution in those with impaired liver function
	P falciparum from chloroquine-sensitive areas *P vivax* from chloroquine-sensitive areas All *P ovale*; all *P malariae*	Total dose: 1550-mg base (= 2000 mg salt)	Total dose: 25-mg base/kg		
Mefloquine[c]	*P falciparum* from chloroquine-resistant areas, except Thailand-Burmese and Thailand-Cambodian border regions	684-mg base (= 750 mg salt) orally as initial dose, followed by 456-mg base (= 500 mg salt) orally given 6-12 h after initial dose	13.7-mg base/kg (= 15 mg salt/kg) orally as initial dose, followed by 9.1-mg base/kg (= 10 mg salt/kg) orally given 6–12 h after initial dose	Gastrointestinal complaints (nausea, vomiting, diarrhea, abdominal pain), mild neuropsychiatric complaints (dizziness, headache, somnolence, sleep disorders), myalgia, mild skin rash, and fatigue; moderate to severe	Contraindicated if hypersensitive to the drug or to related compounds; cardiac conduction abnormalities; psychiatric disorders; seizure disorders

				neuropsychiatric reactions, electrocardiographic changes, including sinus arrhythmia, sinus bradycardia, first degree atrioventricular block, prolongation of QTc interval, and abnormal T waves	
	P vivax from chloroquine-resistant areas	Total dose = 1250 mg salt	Total dose = 25 mg salt/kg		Do not administer if patient has received related drugs (chloroquine, quinine, quinidine) < 12 h earlier May be used for chemoprophylaxis (250 mg salt orally every week) in pregnant women with chloroquine-resistant *P vivax*
Primaquine phosphate	Radical cure of *P vivax* and P ovale (to eliminate hypnozoites)	30-mg base orally per day × 14 d	0.5-mg base/kg orally per day × 14 d	Gastrointestinal disturbances, methemoglobinemia (self-limited), hemolysis in persons with G6PD deficiency	Must screen for G6PD deficiency prior to use Contraindicated in persons with G6PD deficiency; pregnant women Should take with food to minimize gastrointestinal adverse effects
Quinine sulfate (oral)	*P falciparum* from chloroquine-resistant areas	542-mg base (= 650 mg salt)[d] orally 3 times daily × 3 d (infections acquired outside Southeast Asia) to 7 d (infections acquired in Southeast Asia)	8.3-mg base/kg (= 10 mg salt/kg) orally 3 times daily × 3 d (infections acquired outside Southeast Asia) to 7 d (infections acquired in Southeast Asia)	Cinchonism,[e] sinus arrhythmia, junctional rhythms, atrioventricular block, prolonged QT interval ventricular tachycardia, ventricular fibrillation (these are rare and more commonly seen with quinidine), hypoglycemia	Combine with tetracycline, doxycycline, or clindamycin, except for *P vivax* infections in children ≤ 8 y or pregnant women
	P vivax from chloroquine-resistant areas				Contraindicated in hypersensitivity including history of blackwater fever, thrombocytopenic purpura, or thrombocytopenia associated with quinine or quinidine use; many cardiac conduction defects and arrhythmias[f]; myasthenia gravis; optic neuritis

(*Continued*)

Table 43–4. Antimalarial drugs available in the United States recommended for use in the treatment of malaria. (*Continued*)

Drug	Indication	Adult Dosage	Pediatric Dosage[a]	Potential Adverse Effects	Comments
Quinidine gluconate (IV)	Severe malaria (all species, independently of chloroquine resistance)	6.25-mg base/kg (= 10 mg salt/kg) loading dose IV over 1-2 h, then 0.0125-mg base/kg/min (= 0.02 mg salt/kg/min) continuous infusion for at least 24 h	Same as adult	Cinchonism, tachycardia, prolongation QRS and QTc intervals, flattening of T wave (effects are often transient)	Combine with tetracycline, doxycycline, or clindamycin
	Patient unable to take oral medication	Alternative regimen: 15-mg base/kg (= 24 mg salt/kg) loading dose IV infused over 4 h), followed by 7.5 mg base/kg (= 12 mg salt/kg) infused over 4 h every 8 h, starting 8 h after the loading dose (see package insert); once parasite density < 1% and patient can take oral medication, complete treatment with oral quinine, dose as above		Ventricular arrhythmias, hypotension, hypoglycemia	Contraindicated in hypersensitivity; thrombocytopenic purpura or thrombocytopenia associated with quinine or quinidine use; many cardiac conduction defects and arrhythmias[g]; myasthenia gravis; optic neuritis
	Parasitemia > 10%	Quinidine or quinine course = 7 d in Southeast Asia (3 d in Africa or South America)			
Tetracycline (oral or IV)	*P falciparum* from chloroquine-resistant areas	Oral: 250 mg orally 4 times daily × 7 d	25 mg/kg/d orally divided 4 times daily × 7 d	See doxycycline	See doxycycline
	P vivax from chloroquine-resistant areas (in combination with quinine-quinidine)	IV: dosage same as for oral	IV: dosage same as for oral		

[a]Pediatric dosage should never exceed adult dosage.
[b]Extrapolated from chloroquine literature.
[c]Mefloquine should not be used to treat *P falciparum* infections acquired in the following areas: borders of Thailand with Burma (Myanmar) and Cambodia, western provinces of Cambodia, eastern states of Burma (Myanmar), border between Burma and China, Laos along borders of Laos and Burma (and adjacent parts of Thailand-Cambodia border), and southern Vietnam due to resistant strains.
[d]Quinine sulfate capsule manufactured in the United States is in a 324-mg dose; therefore, two capsules should be sufficient for adult dosing.
[e]Nausea, vomiting, headache, tinnitus, deafness, dizziness, and visual disturbances.
[f]Refer to quinine sulfate, package insert (Mutual Pharmaceutical Inc, Philadelphia, PA, August 2005).
[g]Refer to quinidine gluconate, package insert (Eli Lily Co, Indianapolis, Ind, February 2002).
G6PD, glucose-6-phosphate dehydrogenase; IV, intravenous.
Data from Centers for Disease Control and Prevention. Malaria. http://www.cdc.gov/malaria/resources/pdf/treatmenttable.pdf. Accessed May 4, 2012.

shaking chills, malaise, myalgias, headache, and dark urine. Hepatosplenomegaly is an uncommon finding. The disease is usually self-limited, but severe cases have been described in asplenic patients and immunocompromised hosts. Because they share a common vector, physicians should consider the possibility of coinfection with *Borrelia burgdorferi* or *Anaplasma phagocytophilum* in any patient diagnosed with *Babesia* infection.

B. Laboratory Findings

The diagnosis is made in a patient with viral infection–like symptoms by identifying babesial parasites in blood by microscopic evaluation of thin or thick blood smears or by PCR amplification of babesial DNA. *Babesia* parasites are intraerythrocytic organisms that resemble *P falciparum* ring forms. Specific serologic tests are also available through the CDC.

Treatment

Clindamycin (7–10 mg/kg, up to 600 mg, every 8 hours) in combination with quinine (8 mg/kg, up to 650 mg, every 8 hours) or azithromycin (10 mg/kg up to 500 mg on the first day, followed by 5 mg/kg up to 250 mg/d) in combination with atovaquone (20 mg/kg, up to 750 mg, twice a day) for 7–10 days are the treatments of choice. For mild to moderate disease, azithromycin plus atovaquone is preferred because it is efficacious and causes fewer adverse side effects. Partial or complete RBC exchange transfusion is indicated for persons with severe babesiosis, as indicated by high-grade parasitemia (≥ 10%), significant hemolysis, or renal, hepatic, or pulmonary compromise.

Gubernot DM et al: Babesia infection through blood transfusion: Reports received by the US Food and Drug Administration, 1997–2007. Clin Infect Dis 2009;48:25–30 [PMID: 19035776].

Vannier E, Gewurz BE, Krause PJ: Human babesiosis. Infect Dis Clin North Am 2008;22:469–488 [PMID: 18755385].

Vannier E, Krause PJ: Update on babesiosis. Interdiscip Perspect Infect Dis 2009;2009:984568 [Epub 2009 Aug 27] [PMID: 19727410].

3. Toxoplasmosis

ESSENTIALS OF DIAGNOSIS & TYPICAL FEATURES

- Congenital toxoplasmosis: chorioretinitis, microphthalmia, strabismus, microcephaly, hydrocephaly, convulsions, psychomotor retardation, intracranial calcifications, jaundice, hepatosplenomegaly, abnormal blood cell counts.
- Acquired toxoplasmosis in an immunocompetent host: lymphadenopathy, hepatosplenomegaly, rash.
- Acquired or reactivated toxoplasmosis in an immunocompromised host: encephalitis, chorioretinitis, myocarditis, and pneumonitis.
- Ocular toxoplasmosis: chorioretinitis.
- Serologic evidence of infection with *Toxoplasma gondii* or demonstration of the agent in tissue or body fluids.

General Considerations

T gondii is a worldwide parasite of animals and birds. Felines, the definitive hosts, excrete oocysts in their feces. Ingested mature oocysts or tissue cysts lead to tachyzoite invasion of the intestinal cells. Intracellular replication of the tachyzoites causes cell lysis and spread of the infection to adjacent cells or to other tissues via the bloodstream. In chronic infection, *T gondii* appears in bradyzoite-containing tissue cysts that do not trigger an inflammatory reaction. In immunocompromised hosts, tachyzoites are released from the cysts and begin a new cycle of infection.

The two major routes of *Toxoplasma* transmission to humans are oral and congenital. Oocysts survive for up to 18 months in moist soil. Oral infection occurs after ingestion of cysts on contaminated surfaces (including pica) and in undercooked meat or other food products. Oocyst survival is limited in dry, very cold, or very hot conditions, and at high altitude, which probably accounts for the lower incidence of toxoplasmosis in these climatic regions. In the United States, less than 1% of cattle and 25% of sheep and pigs are infected with toxoplasmosis. In humans, depending on geographic area, seropositivity increases with age from 0%–10% in children younger than age 10 years, to 3%–70% in adults.

Congenital transmission occurs during acute infection of pregnant women. Rarely, fetal infection has been documented in immunocompromised mothers who have chronic toxoplasmosis. Treatment during pregnancy decreases transmission by 60%.

Clinical Findings

Clinical toxoplasmosis can be divided into four groups: (1) congenital infection, (2) acquired in the immunocompetent host, (3) acquired or reactivated in the immunocompromised host, and (4) ocular disease.

A. Congenital Toxoplasmosis

Congenital toxoplasmosis is the result of acute infection during pregnancy and occurs in 1 in 3000 to 1 in 10,000 live births in the United States. The rate of transmission and disease severity in the baby vary according to when in pregnancy the infection is acquired. First-trimester infections lead to congenital infections about 10%–20% of the time, but the clinical disease is severe with microcephaly or hydrocephaly, severe chorioretinitis, hearing loss, convulsions, abnormal cerebrospinal fluid (CSF) (xanthochromia and mononuclear pleocytosis), cerebral calcifications, and mental retardation.

Other findings include strabismus, eye palsy, maculopapular rash, pneumonitis, myocarditis, hepatosplenomegaly, jaundice, thrombocytopenia, lymphocytosis and monocytosis, and an erythroblastosis-like syndrome. Infection of a mother in the third trimester results in 70%–90% rate of congenital infection, but the majority of these children are asymptomatic at birth. Many of these children, however, will go on to develop ocular disease later and some will have subtle neurologic deficits.

B. Acquired *Toxoplasma* Infection in the Immunocompetent Host

Typically, acquired infection in the immunocompetent host is asymptomatic. About 10%–20% of patients, however, may develop lymphadenopathy and/or a flulike illness. The nodes are discrete, variably tender, and do not suppurate. Cervical lymph nodes are most frequently involved, but any nodes may be enlarged. Less common findings include fever, malaise, myalgias, fatigue, hepatosplenomegaly, low lymphocyte counts (usually < 10%), and liver enzyme elevations. Unilateral chorioretinitis may occur. The disease is self-limited, although lymph node enlargement may persist or may wax and wane for a few months to 1 or more years.

Toxoplasmic lymphadenitis must be distinguished from other causes of infectious mononucleosis-like syndromes (<1% are caused by *Toxoplasma*). Recovery typically occurs without any specific antiparasitic treatment.

C. Acute Toxoplasmosis in the Immunodeficient Host

Patients infected with human immunodeficiency virus (HIV), and those with lymphoma, leukemia, or transplantation, are at high risk for developing severe disease (most commonly central nervous system [CNS] disease, but also chorioretinitis, myocarditis, or pneumonitis) following acute infection or reactivation. Toxoplasmic encephalitis is one of the most common causes of mass lesions in the brains of persons with HIV/AIDS.

D. Ocular Toxoplasmosis

Ocular toxoplasmosis is an important cause of chorioretinitis in the United States. It may result from congenital infection, but it is believed that acquired infection is the cause of the majority of ocular toxoplasmosis. Congenitally infected individuals are usually asymptomatic until the second or third decade of life when symptomatic eye disease occurs due to the rupture of tissue cysts and the release of bradyzoites and tachyzoites into the retina. Typically, ocular toxoplasmosis presents as a focal necrotizing retinochoroiditis often associated with a preexistent chorioretinal scar, and variable involvement of the vitreous, retinal blood vessels, optic nerve, and anterior segment of the eye. The appearance of the ocular lesion is not specific and mimics other granulomatous ocular diseases.

E. Diagnostic Findings

Serologic tests are the primary means of diagnosis, but results must be interpreted carefully. Reference laboratories with special expertise in toxoplasma serologic assays and their interpretation are essential for establishing a diagnosis and should be preferred. Active infection can also be diagnosed by PCR of blood or body fluids; by visualization of tachyzoites in histologic sections or cytology preparations, or cysts in placenta or fetal tissues; or by characteristic lymph node histology. IgG antibodies, become detectable 1–2 weeks after infection, peak at 1–2 months, and thereafter persist for life. IgM antibodies, measured by ELISA or particle agglutination, appear earlier and decline faster than IgG antibodies, but can last for 12–18 months after acute infection. Absence of both serum IgG and IgM virtually rules out the diagnosis of toxoplasmosis. Acute toxoplasmosis in an immunocompetent host is best documented by analyzing IgG and IgM in paired blood samples drawn 3 weeks apart. Because high antibody titers (IgM or IgG) can persist for several months after acute infection, a single high-titer determination is nondiagnostic; seroconversion or a fourfold increase in titer confirms the diagnosis. In the immunocompromised host, serologic tests are not sensitive, and active infection is documented by PCR or finding tachyzoites by histologic examination.

The diagnosis of toxoplasmosis in the older child with visual complaints is usually made by finding *T gondii* IgG or IgM antibodies in the serum combined with the presence of a typical eye lesion. The diagnosis can be confirmed by demonstrating high antibody titers or by detecting *T gondii* DNA by PCR in the aqueous humor.

Diagnosis of congenital infection, which can be difficult, is made by a combination of serologic testing, parasite isolation, and clinical findings. Evaluation of the baby should include *Toxoplasma*-specific IgG, IgM, IgA, and IgE of the newborn and mother. IgM antibodies indicate an immune response by the infant. Persistence of the other antibodies also indicate infection of the infant. Blood, CSF, and amniotic fluid specimens should be assayed by PCR in a reference laboratory for the presence of *T gondii*. In addition, the child should have thorough ophthalmologic, auditory, and neurologic evaluation; a lumbar puncture; and computed tomographic (CT) scan of the head (to detect CNS calcifications). A congenital infection is confirmed serologically by detecting persistent or increasing IgG antibody levels compared to the mother, persistently positive IgG antibodies beyond the first year of life, and/or a positive *T gondii*–specific IgM or IgA antibody test.

Differential Diagnosis

Congenital toxoplasmosis must be differentiated from infection with cytomegalovirus, rubella, herpes simplex, syphilis, Lyme disease, listeriosis, erythroblastosis, and the encephalopathies that accompany degenerative diseases. Acquired infection mimics viral, bacterial, or lymphoproliferative disorders.

Prevention

Primary prevention of toxoplasmosis in pregnant women (and immunocompromised patients) is an essential public health goal and guidelines have been published by the Centers for Disease Control and Prevention. These include (1) cook meat to safe temperature (beef, lamb, and veal to at least 145°F; pork, ground meat, and wild game to 160°F; poultry to 180°F), (2) peel and/or wash fruits and vegetables thoroughly before eating, (3) wash hands and cutting boards, dishes, and the like after contact with raw meat, (4) wear gloves when gardening or coming in contact with soil or sand, as cat feces may contaminate them, and (5) if possible, pregnant women should avoid changing cat litter. If they cannot avoid changing cat litter, they should change it daily as oocysts require 48–72 hours to sporulate and become infectious. Serologic screening of pregnant women remains a controversial tool in the prevention of congenital toxoplasmosis, but is probably cost-effective and warranted in areas of high prevalence.

Treatment

Treatment of acute toxoplasmosis in the immunocompetent host does not require specific therapy, unless the infection occurs during pregnancy. Toxoplasmic chorioretinitis presenting beyond infancy is treated the same way regardless of whether it is due to reactivation or primary infection. Treatment consists of oral pyrimethamine (2 mg/kg maximum 200 mg loading dose followed by 1 mg/kg daily, maximum 75 mg) plus sulfadiazine (100 mg/kg daily, maximum 1500 mg), given with leucovorin (10–20 mg three times a week). In addition, corticosteroids (prednisone 1 mg/kg daily) are given when lesions threaten vision. Treatment is given for 1–2 weeks after the resolution of symptoms. The duration of additional therapy should be guided by frequent ophthalmologic examinations. Pyrimethamine can cause gastrointestinal upset, leukopenia, thrombocytopenia, and rarely, agranulocytosis; weekly complete blood counts should be checked while on therapy.

A year of treatment is recommended for all congenitally infected infants. Children treated with pyrimethamine (loading dose 2 mg/kg daily for 2 days followed by 1 mg/kg daily for 6 months followed by 1 mg/kg every Monday, Wednesday, and Friday for 6 months) plus sulfadiazine (100 mg/kg divided in doses for 12 months) plus leucovorin (10 mg 3 times a week) have better neurodevelopmental and visual outcomes than historical controls. While on therapy, infants should be monitored for bone marrow toxicity.

In primary infection during pregnancy, spiramycin is started immediately. Pyrimethamine plus sulfadiazine, alternating every 3 weeks with spiramycin, are used when fetal infection has been documented.

Dubey JP, Jones JL: *Toxoplasma gondii* infection in humans and animals in the United States. Int J Parasitol 2008;38:1257–1278 [PMID: 18508057].

McAuley JB: Toxoplasmosis in children. Pediatr Infect Dis J 2008;27:161–162 [PMID: 18227714].

Petersen E: Toxoplasmosis. Semin Fetal Neonatal Med 2007;12:214 [PMID: 17321812].

Vasconcelos-Santos DV et al: Review for disease of the year: Differential diagnosis of ocular toxoplasmosis. Ocular Immunology & Inflammation 2011;19:171–179 [PMID: 21595533].

GASTROINTESTINAL INFECTIONS

1. Amebiasis

ESSENTIALS OF DIAGNOSIS & TYPICAL FEATURES

- Acute dysentery: diarrhea with blood and mucus, abdominal pain, tenesmus.

  Or
- Chronic nondysenteric diarrhea.

  Or
- Hepatic abscess.
- Amebas or cysts in stool or abscesses; amebic antigen in stool.
- Serologic evidence of amebic infection.

General Considerations

Amebiasis is defined as an infection with *Entamoeba histolytica* regardless of symptoms. This parasite is found worldwide, but has a particularly high prevalence in areas with poor socioeconomic and sanitary conditions. In the United States, infections are seen in travelers to and emigrants from endemic areas. The majority of infections are asymptomatic (> 90%), but tissue invasion can result in amebic colitis, hepatic abscess, and hematogenous spread to other organs. Transmission is usually fecal-oral. Infections with two other *Entamoeba* species, *E dispar* and *E moshkovskii*, which are morphologically indistinguishable from *E histolytica* are recognized in humans. Infections with these species are thought to be about 10 times more common than infection with *E histolytica*, but are not thought to cause human disease.

Clinical Findings

A. Symptoms and Signs

Patients with intestinal amebiasis can have asymptomatic cyst passage, or be symptomatic with acute amebic proctocolitis, chronic nondysenteric colitis, or ameboma. Because all *E dispar* and *E moshkovskii* infections and up to 90% of *E histolytica* infections are asymptomatic, carriage is the most common manifestation of amebiasis. Patients with acute amebic colitis typically have a 1- to 2-week history of watery stools containing blood and mucus, abdominal pain, and tenesmus. A minority of patients are febrile or dehydrated. Abdominal examination may reveal pain over the lower abdomen. Fulminant colitis is an unusual complication of amebic dysentery that is associated with a grave prognosis (> 50% mortality), and is characterized by severe bloody diarrhea, fever, and diffuse abdominal pain. Children younger than age 2 years are at increased risk for this condition. Chronic amebic colitis is clinically indistinguishable from idiopathic inflammatory bowel disease; patients present with recurrent episodes of bloody diarrhea over a period of years. Ameboma is a localized amebic infection, usually in the cecum or ascending colon, which presents as a painful abdominal mass.

The most common complications of intestinal amebiasis are intestinal perforation, toxic megacolon, and peritonitis. Perianal ulcers, a less common complication, are painful, punched-out lesions that usually respond to medical therapy. Infrequently, colonic strictures may develop following colitis.

Extraintestinal amebiasis can result in liver, lung, and cerebral abscesses, and rarely genitourinary disease. Patients with amebic liver abscess, the most common form of extraintestinal amebiasis, present with recent-onset fever and right upper quadrant tenderness. The pain may be dull or pleuritic or referred to the right shoulder. Physical examination reveals liver enlargement in less than 50% of affected patients. Some patients have a subacute presentation lasting 2 weeks to 6 months. In these patients, hepatomegaly, anemia, and weight loss are common findings, and fever is less common. Jaundice and diarrhea are rarely associated with an amebic liver abscess. In children with fever of unknown origin who live in, or travel to, endemic areas, amebic liver abscess should be considered in the differential diagnosis.

The most common complication of amebic liver abscess is pleuropulmonary amebiasis due to rupture of a right liver lobe abscess. Lung abscesses may occur from hematogenous spread. Cough, dyspnea, and pleuritic pain can also be caused by the serous pleural effusions and atelectasis that frequently accompany amebic liver abscesses. Rupture of hepatic abscesses can lead to peritonitis and more rarely to pericarditis. Cerebral amebiasis is an infrequent manifestation. Genitourinary amebiasis, which is also uncommon, results from rupture of a liver abscess, hematogenous dissemination, or lymphatic spread.

B. Diagnostic Findings

The differential diagnosis of acute amebic colitis includes bacterial (eg, *Salmonella* spp, *Shigella* spp, *E coli* spp, *Mycobacterium tuberculosis*), parastitic (eg, *Schistosoma mansoni*, *Balantidium coli*), and noninfectious (eg, inflammatory bowel disease, diverticulitis, ischemic colitis) causes of dysentery. Chronic amebic colitis has to be distinguished from inflammatory bowel disease and *Cyclospora*. Occult blood is present in virtually all cases of amebic colitis and can be used as an inexpensive screening test. Fecal leukocytes are uncommon. The presence of hematophagous trophozoites in feces indicates pathogenic *E histolytica* infection.

Intestinal amebiasis is diagnosed by detecting the parasite on stool examination or mucosal biopsy. Ideally, a wet mount preparation of the stool should be examined within 20 minutes after collection to detect motile trophozoites. Otherwise, specimens should be fixed with polyvinyl alcohol or refrigerated to avoid disintegration of the trophozoites. Examination of three separate stool specimens on three different days has 90% sensitivity for the diagnosis of amebic dysentery. However, infection of the ascending colon, amebomas, and extraintestinal infections frequently yield negative stool examinations. The antigen detection test for stool is very sensitive and more specific, because it detects *E histolytica*–specific antigens that do not cross-react with *E dispar*. Colonoscopy and biopsy are most helpful in diagnosing amebic colitis when stool samples lack ova or parasites. Barium studies are contraindicated for patients with suspected acute amebic colitis because of the risk of perforation.

The presence of antibodies against *E histolytica* can differentiate *E histolytica* from *E dispar* infections. Specific antibody is induced by both intestinal and extraintestinal invasive amebiasis. ELISA and indirect hemagglutination assays are positive in 85%–95% of invasive *E histolytica* colitis or amebic abscess. However, these antibodies persist for years, and a positive result does not distinguish between acute and past infection, but are useful in a traveler from a nonendemic area who is returning from a trip to an endemic area. Noninvasive imaging studies have greatly improved the diagnosis of hepatic abscesses. Ultrasonographic examination and CT are sensitive techniques that can guide fine-needle aspiration to obtain specimens for definitive diagnosis. Because an amebic abscess may take up to 2 years to completely resolve on CT scans, imaging techniques are not recommended for therapeutic evaluation. PCR-based testing has the highest sensitivity and specificity for the diagnosis of *E histolytica*, but is only available in certain research and reference laboratories.

Prevention & Treatment

Travelers to endemic areas need to follow the precautions for preventing enteric infections—drink bottled or boiled water and eat cooked or peeled vegetables and fruits.

Treatment of amebic infection is complex because different agents are required for eradicating the parasite from the bowel or tissue (Table 43–5). Whether treatment of asymptomatic cyst passers is indicated is a controversial issue. The prevalent opinion is that asymptomatic infection with *E histolytica*, as evidenced by amebic cysts in the stool and a positive serologic test, should be treated in nonendemic areas. If serologic tests are negative, the cysts are more likely to represent infection with the nonpathogenic *E dispar*,

Table 43–5. Treatment of amebiasis.

Type of Infection	Drug of Choice	Dosage
Asymptomatic	Paromomycin	25–35 mg/kg/d in three doses for 7 d
	or	
	Iodoquinol	30–40 mg/kg/d (maximum, 2 g) in three doses for 20 d
	or	
	Diloxanide furoate[a]	20 mg/kg/d up to 1.5 g/d in three doses for 10 d
Intestinal disease and hepatic abscess[b]	Metronidazole	35–50 mg/kg/d up to 2.25 g/d in three doses for 10 d
	or	
	Tinidazole[c]	50 or 60 mg/kg up to 2 g/d for 3 d

[a]Diloxanide furoate is available from the CDC Drug Service: (404) 639–3670.
[b]Treatment should be followed by iodoquinol or paromomycin.
[c]Not marketed in the United States; higher dosage.

which does not require treatment. Noninvasive infections may be treated with paromomycin, a nonabsorbable aminoglycoside that can be used safely during pregnancy and causes only mild intestinal side effects, including flatulence and increased number of stools. Diloxanide furoate is relatively nontoxic and used widely outside the United States. The treatment of invasive amebiasis requires metronidazole. Metronidazole has a disulfiram-like effect and should be avoided in patients receiving ethanol-containing medications. Tinidazole, a more potent nitroimidazole against amebic infection, can be used for shorter treatment courses and is well tolerated in children.

Treatment of invasive amebiasis should always be followed with an intraluminal cysticidal agent, even if the stool examination is negative. Metronidazole and paromomycin should not be given concurrently, because the diarrhea that is a common side effect of paromomycin may make it difficult to assess response to therapy. Patients with large, thin-walled hepatic abscesses may need therapeutic aspiration to avoid abscess rupture. Patients with amebiasis should be placed under enteric precautions.

Fotedar R et al: Laboratory diagnostic techniques for *Entamoeba* species. Clin Micro Rev 2007;20:511–532 [PMID: 17630338].

Mortimer L et al: The immunopathogenesis of Entamoeba histolytica. Exp Parasitol 2010 Nov;126(3):366–380 [PMID: 20303955].

Pritt BS, Clark CG: Amebiasis. Mayo Clin Proc 2008;83:1154–1160 [PMID: 18828976].

Ximénez C et al: Novelties on amoebiasis: A neglected tropical disease. J Global Infect Dis 2011 Apr;3(2):166–174 [PMID: 21731305].

2. Giardiasis

ESSENTIALS OF DIAGNOSIS & TYPICAL FEATURES

- Chronic relapsing diarrhea, flatulence, bloating, anorexia, poor weight gain.
- No fever or hematochezia.
- Detection of trophozoites, cysts, or *Giardia* antigens in stool.

General Considerations

Giardiasis, caused by *Giardia lamblia*, is the most common intestinal protozoal infection in children in the United States and in most of the world. Endemic worldwide, the infection is classically associated with drinking contaminated water, either in rural areas or in areas with faulty purification systems. Even ostensibly clean urban water supplies can be contaminated intermittently, and infection has been acquired in swimming pools. Fecal-oral contamination allows person-to-person spread. Day care centers are a major source of infection, with an incidence of up to 50% reported in some centers. No symptoms occur in 25% of infected persons, facilitating spread to household contacts. Food-borne outbreaks also occur. Although infection is rare in neonates, giardiasis may occur at any age.

Clinical Findings

A. Symptoms and Signs

Giardia infection is followed by asymptomatic cyst passage, acute self-limited diarrhea, or a chronic syndrome of diarrhea, malabsorption, and weight loss. Acute diarrhea occurs 1–2 weeks after infection and is characterized by abrupt onset of diarrhea with greasy, malodorous stools; malaise; flatulence; bloating; and nausea. Fever and vomiting occur in a few patients. Urticaria, reactive arthritis, biliary tract disease, gastric infection, and constipation have occasionally been reported. The disease has a protracted course (> 1 week) and frequently leads to weight loss. Patients who develop chronic diarrhea complain of profound malaise, lassitude, headache, and diffuse abdominal pain in association with bouts of diarrhea—most typically foul-smelling, greasy stools—intercalated with periods of constipation or normal bowel habits. This syndrome can persist for months until specific therapy is administered or until it subsides spontaneously. Chronic diarrhea frequently leads to malabsorption, steatorrhea, vitamins A and B_{12} deficiencies, and disaccharidase depletion. Lactose intolerance, which develops in 20%–40% of patients and can persist for several weeks after treatment, needs to be differentiated from relapsing giardiasis or reinfection.

B. Laboratory Findings

The diagnosis of giardiasis relies on finding the parasite in stool or detecting *Giardia* antigen in feces. For ova and parasite examination, a fresh stool provides the best results. Liquid stools have the highest yield of trophozoites, which are more readily found on wet mounts. With semiformed stools, the examiner should look for cysts in fresh or fixed specimens, preferably using a concentration technique. When these techniques are applied carefully, one examination has a sensitivity of 50%–70%; three examinations increase the sensitivity to 90%. *Giardia* antigen detection by means of ELISAs, nonenzymatic immunoassays, and direct fluorescence antibody tests are the standard diagnostic tests in the United States. They are comparable in cost to a stool ova and parasite examination, have a more rapid return of results, and are 85%–90% sensitive and 95%–100% specific. With a careful stool ova and parasite examination or with the use of a new antigen test, direct sampling of duodenal aspirates or biopsy, which was utilized in the past, is now restricted to particularly difficult cases.

Prevention

The prevention of giardiasis requires proper treatment of water supplies and interruption of person-to-person transmission. Where water might be contaminated, travelers, campers, and hikers should use methods to make water safe for drinking. Boiling is the most reliable method; the time of boiling (1 minute at sea level) will depend on the altitude. Chemical disinfection with iodine or chlorine and filtration are alternative methods of water treatment.

Sexual transmission is prevented by avoiding oral-anal and oral-genital sex. Interrupting fecal-oral transmission requires strict hand washing. However, outbreaks of diarrhea in day care centers might be particularly difficult to eradicate. Reinforcing hand washing and treating the disease in both symptomatic and asymptomatic carriers may be necessary.

Treatment

Metronidazole, tinidazole, and nitazoxanide are the drugs of choice for treatment of giardiasis. When given at 5 mg/kg (up to 250 mg) three times a day for 5 days, metronidazole has 80%–95% efficacy. The drug is well tolerated in children. It has a disulfiram-like effect and should be avoided in patients receiving ethanol-containing medication. Metronidazole can be administered safely during pregnancy. Tinidazole has an efficacy approaching 90% when given as a single dose of 50 mg/kg (up to 2 g). Nitazoxanide is available in liquid formulation and requires only 3 days of treatment. Recommended doses are 100 mg (5 mL) every 12 hours for children 12–47 months of age and 200 mg (10 mL) for 4- to 11-year-olds. Furazolidone is sometimes used in children because it is available in suspension. Administered at 1.5 mg/kg (up to 100 mg) four times daily for 7–10 days, it has only 80% efficacy. Furazolidone may cause gastrointestinal side effects, turn urine red, and cause mild hemolysis in patients with G6PD deficiency. For patients who do not respond to therapy, or who suffer relapse, a second course with the same drug or switching to another drug is equally effective. In cases of repeated treatment failure, albendazole (400 mg/d for 5–10 days), although not specifically recommended in the United States for the treatment of giardiasis, is an effective option.

Escobedo AA et al: Giardiasis: The ever-present threat of a neglected disease. Infect Disord Drug Targets 2010;10(5):329–348 [PMID: 20701575].

Huang DB et al: An updated review on *Cryptosporidium* and *Giardia*. Gastroenterol Clin North Am 2006;35:291 [PMID: 16880067].

3. Cryptosporidiosis

Cryptosporidia are intracellular protozoa that have gained importance because they cause severe and devastating diarrhea in patients with acquired immunodeficiency syndrome (AIDS) and in other immunodeficient persons. This ubiquitous parasite infects and reproduces in the epithelial cell lining of the digestive and respiratory tracts of humans and most other vertebrate animals. Humans acquire the infection from contaminated water supplies, including swimming pools and lake water, or from close contact with infected humans or animals. Most human infections are caused by *C parvum* or *C hominis*, although other species have been reported to cause human disease.

Clinical Findings

A. Symptoms and Signs

Immunocompetent persons infected with *Cryptosporidium* spp usually develop self-limited diarrhea (2–26 days) with or without abdominal cramps. Diarrhea can be mild and intermittent or continuous, watery, and voluminous. Low-grade fever, nausea, vomiting, loss of appetite, and malaise may accompany the diarrhea. Children younger than age 2 years are more susceptible to infection than older children. Immunocompromised patients (either cellular or humoral deficiency) tend to develop a severe, prolonged, chronic diarrhea which can often result in severe malnutrition, and subsides only after the immunodeficiency is corrected. Other clinical manifestations associated with cryptosporidiosis in immunocompromised hosts include cholecystitis, pancreatitis, hepatitis, biliary tree involvement, and respiratory symptoms.

B. Laboratory Findings

Cryptosporidiosis has no characteristic laboratory features other than identification of the microorganism in feces or on biopsy. ELISA and PCR tests are more sensitive than staining of stool specimens or concentrates.

Prevention & Treatment

Prevention of *Cryptosporidium* infection is limited by oocyst resistance to some of the standard water purification procedures and to common disinfectants. Enteric precautions are recommended for infected persons. Boiled or bottled drinking water may be considered for those at high risk for developing chronic infection (eg, inadequately treated patients with AIDS).

Immunocompetent patients and those with temporary immunodeficiencies respond to treatment with nitazoxanide, antidiarrheal agents, and hydration. Immunocompromised patients usually require more intense supportive care with parenteral nutrition in addition to hydration and nonspecific antidiarrheal agents. Octreotide acetate, a synthetic analogue of somatostatin that inhibits secretory diarrhea, has been associated with symptomatic improvement but not with parasitologic cure. Among the antiparasitic agents, nitazoxanide is the treatment of choice. Regimens using paromomycin, azithromycin, and/or rifabutin have met with limited success. For patients with AIDS, institution of effective anti-retroviral therapy results in elimination of symptomatic cryptosporidiosis.

Cabada MM et al: Treatment of cryptosporidiosis: Do we know what we think we know? Curr Opin Infect Dis 2010;23:494–499 [PMID: 20689422].

Davies AP et al: Cryptosporidiosis. BMJ 2009;399:963–967 [PMID: 19841008].

Huang DB et al: An updated review on *Cryptosporidium* and *Giardia*. Gastroenterol Clin North Am 2006;35:291 [PMID: 16880067].

4. Cyclosporiasis

Cyclospora spp are ubiquitous coccidian parasites that infect both humans and a variety of animals worldwide. *Cyclospora cayetanensis* is the only species known to infect humans. Cyclosporiasis is seen in three main epidemiologic settings: sporadic cases in endemic areas (particularly Haiti, Guatemala, Peru, and Nepal), travelers to endemic areas, and in food- or water-borne outbreaks in nonendemic areas, particularly in relation to importation of fresh produce. The incubation period is 1–14 days (average, 7 days). Infection may be asymptomatic, cause mild to moderate self-limiting diarrhea, or cause protracted or severe diarrhea. In the immunocompetent host, diarrhea usually lasts 10–25 days but may be followed by a relapsing pattern that can last several months. Diarrhea (5–15 movements per day) is usually watery, sometimes explosive, and often accompanied by nausea, vomiting, abdominal cramping, and bloating. Profound fatigue, anorexia, and myalgias have also been reported. The infection can be unusually severe in immunocompromised patients. Although the illness is self-limited, it may last for several weeks. Diagnosis is based on finding oocysts 8–10 mm in diameter on examination of stool specimens stained with acid-fast stain. The treatment of choice is trimethoprim–sulfamethoxazole for 7 days.

Hall et al: Surveillance for laboratory-confirmed sporadic cases of cyclosporiasis—United States, 1997–2008. MMWR 2011;60(2):1–11 [PMID: 21471951].

Ortega et al: Update on Cyclospora cayetanensis, a food-borne and waterborne parasite. Clin Micro Rev 2011;23:218–234 [PMID: 20065331].

5. Free-Living Amebas

ESSENTIALS OF DIAGNOSIS & TYPICAL FEATURES

- Acute meningoencephalitis: fever, headache, meningismus, acute mental deterioration.
- Swimming in warm, freshwater in an endemic area.
- Chronic granulomatous encephalitis: insidious onset of focal neurologic deficits.
- Keratitis: pain, photophobia, conjunctivitis, blurred vision.

General Considerations

Infections with free-living amebas are uncommon. *Naegleria* species, *Acanthamoeba* species, and *Balamuthia* amebas have been associated with human disease, primarily infections of the central nervous system.

Acute meningoencephalitis, caused by *Naegleria fowleri*, occurs mostly in children and young adults. Patients present with abrupt fever, headache, nausea and vomiting, meningismus, and decreased mental status a few days to 2 weeks after swimming in warm freshwater lakes. Swimming history may be absent. CNS invasion occurs after nasal inoculation of *N fowleri*. The disease is rapidly progressive, and death ensues within 1 week of onset.

Chronic granulomatous encephalitis, caused by *Acanthamoeba* or *Balamuthia*, can occur in immunocompetent patients, but occurs more commonly in patients who are immunocompromised from corticosteroid use, chemotherapy, or HIV. There is no association with freshwater swimming. This disease has an insidious onset of focal neurologic deficits, and approximately 50% of patients present with headache. Skin, sinus, or lung infections with *Acanthamoeba* precede many of the CNS infections and may still be present at the onset of neurologic disease. The granulomatous encephalitis progresses to fatal outcome over a period of weeks to months (average 6 weeks).

Acanthamoeba keratitis is a corneal infection associated with minor trauma or use of soft contact lenses in otherwise healthy persons. Clinical findings of *Acanthamoeba* keratitis include radial keratoconjunctivitis and stromal ring infiltrate. Amebic keratitis usually follows an indolent course and initially may resemble herpes simplex or bacterial keratitis; delay in diagnosis is associated with worse outcomes.

Clinical Findings & Differential Diagnosis

Amebic encephalitis should be included in the differential diagnosis of acute meningoencephalitis in children with a history of recent freshwater swimming. The CSF is usually hemorrhagic, with leukocyte counts that may be normal early in the disease but later range from 400 to 2600/mL with neutrophil predominance, low to normal glucose, and elevated protein. The etiologic diagnosis relies on finding trophozoites on a wet mount of the CSF.

Granulomatous encephalitis is diagnosed by brain biopsy of CT-identified nonenhancing lucent areas. The CSF of these patients is usually nondiagnostic with a lymphocytic pleocytosis, mild to severe elevation of protein (> 1000 mg/dL), and normal or low glucose. *Acanthamoeba* and *Balamuthia* amebas have only rarely been found in the CSF; however, they can be visualized in brain biopsies or grown from brain or other infected tissues. Immunofluorescent and PCR-based diagnostic assays are available through the Centers for Disease Control and Prevention.

Acanthamoeba keratitis is diagnosed by finding the trophozoites in corneal scrapings or by isolating the parasite from corneal specimens or contact lens cultures.

Prevention

Because primary amebic meningitis occurs infrequently, active surveillance of lakes for *N fowleri* is not warranted. However, in the presence of a documented case, it is advisable to close the implicated lake to swimming. *Acanthamoeba* keratitis can be prevented by heat disinfection of contact lenses, by storage of lenses in sterile solutions, and by not wearing lenses when swimming in freshwater.

Treatment

Treatment of acute amebic meningoencephalitis caused by *N fowleri* should be attempted with high-dose intravenous amphotericin B with the possible addition of miconazole and rifampin. Successful treatment of *Balamuthia* encephalitis has been reported using a combination of flucytosine, pentamidine, fluconazole, sulfadiazine, and a macrolide. *Acanthamoeba* encephalitis should be treated with a combination of pentamidine, an azole compound, flucytosine, and sulfadiazine.

Acanthamoeba keratitis responds well to surgical debridement followed by 3–4 weeks of topical 1% miconazole; 0.1% propamidine isethionate; and polymyxin B sulfate, neomycin, and bacitracin (Neosporin).

Centers for Disease Control and Prevention: *Balamuthia* amebic encephalitis. Morb Mort Weekly Report 2008;57:768.

Visvesvara GS: Amebic meningoencephalitides and keratitis: Challenges in diagnosis and treatment. Curr Opin Infect Dis 2010;23:590–594 [PMID: 2082332].

Visvesvara GS et al: Pathogenic and opportunistic free-living amoebae: *Acanthamoeba* spp., *Balamuthia mandrillaris*, *Naegleria fowleri*, and *Sappinia diploidea*. FEMS Immunol Med Microbiol 2007;50:1–26 [PMID: 17428307].

TRICHOMONIASIS

Trichomonas vaginalis infection is discussed in Chapter 44.

METAZOAL INFECTIONS

NEMATODE INFECTIONS

1. Enterobiasis (Pinworms)

ESSENTIALS OF DIAGNOSIS & TYPICAL FEATURES

- Anal pruritus.
- Worms in the stool or eggs on perianal *skin*.

General Considerations

This worldwide infection is caused by *Enterobius vermicularis*. The adult worms are about 5–10 mm long and lives in the colon; females deposit eggs on the perianal area, primarily at night, which cause intense pruritus. Scratching contaminates the fingers and allows transmission back to the host (autoinfection) or to contacts.

Clinical Findings

A. Symptoms and Signs

Although blamed for many types of symptoms, pinworms are definitely associated only with localized pruritus. Adult worms may migrate within the colon or up the urethra or vagina in girls. They can be found within the bowel wall, in the lumen of the appendix (usually an incidental finding by the pathologist), in the bladder, and even in the peritoneal cavity of girls. The granulomatous reaction that may be present around these ectopic worms is usually asymptomatic. Worm eradication may correspond with the cure of recurrent urinary tract infections in some young girls.

B. Laboratory Findings

The usual diagnostic test consists of pressing a piece of transparent tape on the child's anus in the morning prior to bathing, then placing it on a drop of xylene on a slide. Microscopic examination under low power usually demonstrates the ova. Occasionally, eggs or adult worms are seen in fecal specimens. Parents may also notice adult worms.

Differential Diagnosis

Nonspecific irritation or vaginitis, streptococcal perianal cellulitis (usually painful with marked erythema), and vaginal or urinary bacterial infections may at times resemble pinworm infection, although the symptoms of pinworms are often so suggestive that a therapeutic trial is justified without a confirmed diagnosis.

Treatment

A. Specific Measures

Treat all household members at the same time to prevent reinfections. Because the drugs are not active against the eggs, therapy should be repeated after 2 weeks to kill the recently hatched adults.

Pyrantel pamoate is given as a single dose (11 mg/kg; maximum 1 g); it is safe and very effective. Mebendazole (100 mg) and albendazole (400 mg) in a single dose are highly effective for this infection at all ages.

B. General Measures

Personal hygiene must be emphasized. Nails should be kept short and clean. Children should wear undergarments to bed to diminish contamination of fingers; bedclothes should be laundered frequently; infected persons should bathe in the morning, thereby removing a large proportion of eggs. Although eggs may be widely dispersed in the house and multiple family members infected, the disease is mild and treatable.

Brown MD: *Enterobius vermicularis.* N Engl J Med 2006;354:e12 [PMID: 16571876].

2. Ascariasis

ESSENTIALS OF DIAGNOSIS & TYPICAL FEATURES

- Abdominal cramps and discomfort.
- Large, white or reddish, round worms, or ova in the feces.

General Considerations

Together with the whipworm and hookworms (see below), *Ascaris* comprises the group of "soil-transmitted helminths." These parasites cause human infection through contact with eggs or larvae that thrive in the moist soil of the tropics and subtropics. Worldwide, more than a billion people are infected with at least one of these parasites, and, especially in less developed countries, it is not uncommon for children to be chronically infected with all three worms. These parasites are strongly associated with acute poverty and epidemiologic evidence suggests that exposure to infectious eggs shared by household members are important determinants of individual infections and household clustering. Children infected with these worms are at increased risk for malnutrition, stunted growth, intellectual retardation, and cognitive and education deficits. Together, the soil-transmitted helminths are one of the world's most important causes of physical and intellectual growth retardation.

Ascaris lumbricoides is a worldwide human parasite. Ova passed by carriers may remain viable for months under the proper soil conditions. The ova contaminate food or fingers and are subsequently ingested by a new host. The larvae hatch, penetrate the intestinal wall, enter the venous system, reach the alveoli, are coughed up, and return to the small intestine, where they mature. The female lays thousands of eggs daily.

Clinical Findings

A. Symptoms and Signs

The majority of infections with *A lumbricoides* are asymptomatic, although moderate to heavy infections are associated with abdominal pain, weight loss, anorexia, diarrhea, and vomiting, and may lead to malnutrition. During the larval migratory phase, an acute transient eosinophilic pneumonitis (Löffler syndrome) may occur. Acute intestinal obstruction has been associated with heavy infections, which is more common in children due to their smaller intestinal diameter and their higher worm burden. Rarely, worm migration can cause peritonitis or appendicitis, secondary to intestinal wall perforation, and common bile duct obstruction, resulting in biliary colic, cholangitis, or pancreatitis.

B. Laboratory Findings

The diagnosis is made by observing the large roundworms (1.5–4 cm) in the stool or by microscopic detection of the ova.

Treatment

Because the adult worms live less than a year, asymptomatic infection need not be treated. Mebendazole (100 mg twice a day for 3 days or 500 mg once), pyrantel pamoate (a single dose of 11 mg/kg; maximum 1 g), and albendazole (400 mg in a single dose, or 200 mg in children 1–2 years of age) are highly and equally effective. In cases of intestinal or biliary obstruction, piperazine (150 mg/kg initially, followed by six doses of 65 mg/kg every 12 hours by nasogastric tube) is recommended because it narcotizes the worms and helps relieve obstruction. However, surgical removal is occasionally required.

Bethony J et al: Soil-transmitted helminth infections: Ascariasis, trichuriasis, and hookworm. Lancet 2006;367:1521 [PMID: 16679166].

Keiser J et al: Efficacy of current drugs against soil-transmitted helminth infections. JAMA 2008;299:1937–1948 [PMID: 18430913].

Walker et al: Individual predisposition, household clustering, and risk factors for human infection with *Ascaris lumbricoides*: New epidemiological insights. PLoS NTD 2011;5:e1047 [PMID: 21541362].

3. Trichuriasis (Whipworm)

Trichuris trichiura is a widespread human and animal parasite common in children living in warm, humid areas conducive to survival of the ova. Ingested infective eggs hatch in the upper small intestine. The adult worms live in the cecum and colon; the ova are passed and become infectious after several weeks in the soil. Unlike *Ascaris*, *Trichuris* does not have a migratory tissue phase. Symptoms are not present unless the infection is severe, in which case pain, diarrhea, iron deficient anemia, and mild abdominal distention are present. Massive infections may also cause rectal prolapse and dysentery. Detection of the characteristic barrel-shaped ova in the feces confirms the diagnosis. Adult worms may be seen in the prolapsed rectum or at proctoscopy; their thin heads are buried in the mucosa, and the thicker posterior portions protrude. Mild to moderate eosinophilia may be present.

Treatment of trichuriasis with currently available anthelminthic agents is unsatisfactory. Nevertheless, mebendazole (100 mg orally twice a day for 3 days or 500 mg once) or albendazole (400 mg in a single dose for 3 days, or 200 mg in children 1–2 years of age) tends to improve gastrointestinal symptoms.

Bethony J et al: Soil-transmitted helminth infections: Ascariasis, trichuriasis, and hookworm. Lancet 2006;367:1521 [PMID: 16679166].

Keiser J et al. Efficacy of current drugs against soil-transmitted helminth infections. JAMA 2008;299:1937–1948 [PMID: 18430913].

4. Hookworm

ESSENTIALS OF DIAGNOSIS & TYPICAL FEATURES

- Iron-deficiency anemia.
- Abdominal discomfort, weight loss.
- Ova in the feces.

General Considerations

The common human hookworms are *Ancylostoma duodenale* and *Necator americanus*. Both are widespread in the tropics and subtropics, with an estimated 600–700 million people infected worldwide. Most infections occur in the Asian countries of Indonesia, Bangladesh, and India, followed by Nigeria, the Democratic Republic of the Congo, and Brazil. The larger *A duodenale* is more pathogenic because it consumes more blood, up to 0.5 mL per worm per day.

The adults live in the jejunum. Eggs are passed in the feces and develop and hatch into infective larvae in warm, damp soil within 2 weeks. The larvae penetrate human skin on contact, enter the blood, reach the alveoli, are coughed up and swallowed, and develop into adults in the intestine. The adult worms attach with their mouth parts to the mucosa, from which they suck blood. Blood loss is the major sequel of infection. Infection rates reach 90% in areas without sanitation.

Separate species, *Ancylostoma braziliense* and *Ancylostoma caninum* (the dog and cat hookworm), cause creeping eruption (cutaneous larva migrans). Larvae produce pruritic, reddish papules at the site of skin entry and an intensely pruritic, serpiginous tracks or bullae are formed as they migrate through the skin. Larval can move up to a few centimeters a day and activity can continue for several weeks, but eventually the rash is self-limiting. An advancing, intensely pruritic, serpiginous tunnel in the skin is pathognomonic. Cutaneous larva migrans is a disease of children and others who come in contact with soil contaminated with cat and dog feces. In the United States, the disease is most prevalent in the Southeast. Most cases in the United States are imported by travelers returning from tropical and subtropical areas.

Clinical Findings

A. Symptoms and Signs

Patients with hookworm infection usually are asymptomatic or have complaints of diarrhea; chronic hookworm infection, however, is a common cause of moderate and severe hypochromic microcytic anemia, and heavy infection can cause hypoproteinemia with edema. Chronic hookworm infection in children may lead to growth delay, deficits in cognition, and developmental delay. The larvae usually penetrate the skin of the feet and cause a stinging or burning sensation, followed by an intense local itching (ground itch) and a papulovesicular rash that may persist for 1–2 weeks. Pneumonitis associated with migrating larvae is uncommon and usually mild, except during heavy infections. Colicky abdominal pain, nausea, and/or diarrhea and marked eosinophilia may be observed.

B. Laboratory Findings

The large ova of both species of hookworm are found in feces and are indistinguishable. Microcytic anemia, hypoalbuminemia, eosinophilia, and hematochezia occur in severe cases.

Prevention

Fecal contamination of soil and skin contact with potentially contaminated soil should be avoided. Vaccines that target the nutritional and metabolic requirements of the adult hookworm are currently under development.

Treatment

A. Specific Measures

In a recent meta-analysis, albendazole (400 mg orally in a single dose, or 200 mg in children 1–2 years of age) was significantly more efficacious than mebendazole or pyrantel pamoate, and is considered the drug of choice for treatment of hookworm infections. Mebendazole (100 mg orally twice a day for 3 days) and pyrantel pamoate (11 mg/kg, to a maximum of 1 g, daily for 3 days) are second-line options.

B. General Measures

Iron therapy may be as important as worm eradication.

Prognosis

The outcome after therapy is usually excellent.

Becker SL et al: Diagnosis, clinical features, and self-reported morbidity of *Strongyloides stercoralis* and hookworm infection in a co-endemic setting. PLoS NTD 2011;5(8):e1292 [PMID: 21886853].

Hortez PJ et al: Developing vaccines to combat hookworm infection and intestinal schistosomiasis. Nature Reviews Micro 2010;8:814–826 [PMID: 20948553].

Keiser J et al: Efficacy of current drugs against soil-transmitted helminth infections. JAMA 2008;299:1937–1948 [PMID: 18430913].

5. Strongyloidiasis

ESSENTIALS OF DIAGNOSIS & TYPICAL FEATURES

- Abdominal pain, diarrhea.
- Eosinophilia.
- Larvae in stools and duodenal aspirates.
- Serum antibodies.

General Considerations

Strongyloides stercoralis is unique in having both parasitic and free-living forms; the latter can survive in the soil for several generations. The parasite is found in most tropical and sub-tropical regions of the world. The adults live in the submucosal tissue of the duodenum and occasionally elsewhere in the intestines. Eggs deposited in the mucosa hatch rapidly; the first-stage (rhabditiform) larvae, therefore, are the predominant form found in duodenal aspirates and feces. The larvae mature rapidly to the tissue-penetrating filariform stage and initiate internal autoinfection. The filariform larvae also inhabit the soil and can penetrate the skin of another host, subsequently migrating into veins and pulmonary alveoli, reaching the intestine when coughed up and swallowed.

Older children and adults are infected more often than are young children. Even low worm burden can result in significant clinical symptoms. Immunosuppressed patients may develop fatal disseminated strongyloidiasis, known as the *hyperinfection syndrome*. Autoinfection can result in persistent infection for decades.

Clinical Findings

A. Symptoms and Signs

Chronic *S stercorali* infections can be asymptomatic or cause cutaneous, gastrointestinal, and/or pulmonary symptoms. At the site of skin penetration, a pruritic rash may occur. Large numbers of migrating larvae can cause wheezing, cough, shortness of breath, and hemoptysis. Although one-third of intestinal infections are asymptomatic, the most prominent features of strongyloidiasis include abdominal pain, distention, diarrhea, vomiting, and occasionally malabsorption.

Patients with cellular immunodeficiencies and those on corticosteroid therapy may develop disseminated infection, involving the intestine, the lungs, and the meninges. Gram-negative sepsis may complicate disseminated strongyloidiasis.

B. Laboratory Findings

There is no gold standard for diagnosis, which can be difficult because of low parasite load and irregular larval output. Finding larvae in the feces, duodenal aspirates, or sputum is diagnostic. IgG antibodies measured by ELISA or immunoblot are relatively sensitive (83%–93%). The presence of specific antibody, however, does not distinguish between past and present infection and *Strongyloides* antibody assays can cross-react with other helminth infections. Marked eosinophilia is common. Because the rate of detection of *Strongyloides* larvae in a single fecal sample is low (~25%), all patients who have visited an endemic area and present with GI symptoms should be evaluated with three serial stool samples (for ova and parasites), and serology (ELISA) for *S stercoralis* should be performed. Patients with pulmonary symptoms with suspected strongyloides infection should have sputum samples evaluated for the detection of *S stercoralis*.

Differential Diagnosis

Strongyloidiasis should be differentiated from peptic disease, celiac disease, regional or tuberculous enteritis, and hookworm infections. The pulmonary phase may mimic asthma or bronchopneumonia. Patients with severe infection can present with an acute abdomen.

Prevention & Treatment

Ivermectin (two doses of 0.2 mg/kg given 1 to 14 days apart) is the drug of choice. Tiabendazole at a dose of 25 mg/kg orally twice orally twice a day for three days is an alternative therapy. Albendazole has a much lower efficacy. Relapses are common. In the hyperinfection syndrome, 1–3 weeks of therapy with ivermectin may be necessary and multiple follow-up stool studies for 2 weeks after therapy are indicated to assure clearance of larvae. Patients from endemic areas should be tested for specific antibodies and receive treatment before undergoing immunosuppression.

Becker SL et al: Diagnosis, clinical features, and self-reported morbidity of *Strongyloides stercoralis* and hookworm infection in a co-endemic setting. PLoS NTD 2011;5(8):e1292 [PMID: 21886853].

Montes M et al: Strongyloides stercoralis: There but not seen. Curr Opin Infect Dis 2010;23:500–502 [PMID: 20733481].

Segarra-Newnham M: Manifestations, diagnosis, and treatment of *Strongyloides stercoralis* infection. Ann Pharmacother 2007;41:1992–2001 [PMID: 17940124].

6. Visceral Larva Migrans (Toxocariasis)

ESSENTIALS OF DIAGNOSIS & TYPICAL FEATURES

- Visceral involvement, including hepatomegaly, marked eosinophilia, and anemia.
- Posterior or peripheral ocular inflammatory mass.
- Elevated antibody titers in serum or aqueous fluid; demonstration of *Toxocara* larvae in biopsy specimen.

General Considerations

Visceral larva migrans is a worldwide disease. The agent is the cosmopolitan intestinal ascarid of dogs and cats, *Toxocara canis* or *Toxocara cati*. The eggs passed by infected animals contaminate parks and other areas that young children frequent. Children with pica are at increased risk. In the United States, seropositivity ranges from 2.8% in unselected populations to 23% in southern states to 54% in rural areas. Ingested eggs hatch and penetrate the intestinal wall, then migrate to the liver. Most of the larvae are retained in the liver, but some may pass through the organ reaching the lungs, eyes, muscles and/or the CNS, where they die and incite a granulomatous inflammatory reaction.

Clinical Findings

A. Visceral Larva Migrans

Toxocariasis is usually asymptomatic, but young children (aged 1–5 years) sometimes present with anorexia, fever, fatigue, pallor, abdominal pain and distention, nausea, vomiting, and cough. Hepatomegaly is common, splenomegaly is unusual, and adenopathy is absent. Lung involvement, usually asymptomatic, can be demonstrated readily by radiologic examination. Seizures are common, but more severe neurologic abnormalities are infrequent. Eosinophilia with leukocytosis, anemia, and elevated liver function tests are typical. ELISA is sensitive, specific, and useful in confirming the clinical diagnosis. Most patients recover spontaneously, but disease may last up to 6 months.

B. Ocular Larva Migrans

This condition occurs in older children and adults who present with a unilateral posterior or peripheral inflammatory eye mass. History of visceral larva migrans and eosinophilia are typically absent. Anti-*Toxocara* antibody titers are low in the serum and high in vitreous and aqueous fluids.

C. Diagnostic Findings

Hypergammaglobulinemia and elevated isohemagglutinins sometimes result from cross-reactivity between *Toxocara* antigens and human group A and B blood antigens. The diagnosis is confirmed by finding larvae in granulomatous lesions. High ELISA serology and the exclusion of other causes of hypereosinophilia provide a presumptive diagnosis to be made in typical cases.

Differential Diagnosis

Diseases associated with hypereosinophilia must be considered. These include trichinosis (enlarged liver not common; muscle tenderness common), eosinophilic leukemia (rare in children; eosinophils are abnormal in appearance), collagen-vascular disease (those associated with eosinophilia are rare in young children), strongyloidiasis (no organomegaly; enteric symptoms are common), early ascariasis, tropical eosinophilia (occurring mainly in India), allergies, and hypersensitivity syndromes.

Prevention & Treatment

A. Specific Measures

The clinical benefit of specific anthelmintic therapy is not defined. Treatment with albendazole (400 mg twice a day for 5 days) or mebendazole (100–200 mg twice a day for 5 days) is indicated for severe complications involving the brain, lung, or heart.

B. General Measures

Treating any cause of pica, such as iron deficiency, is important. Corticosteroids are used to treat marked inflammation of lungs, eyes, or other organs. Pets should be dewormed routinely. Other children in the household may be infected. Mild eosinophilia and positive serologic tests may be the only clue to their infection. Therapy is not necessary for these individuals.

Rubingsy-Elefant G et al: Human toxocariasis: Diagnosis, worldwide seroprevalences, and clinical expression of the systemic and ocular forms. Annals of Tropical Medicine and Parsitology 2010;104:3–23 [PMID: 20149289].

7. Trichinosis

ESSENTIALS OF DIAGNOSIS & TYPICAL FEATURES

- Vomiting, diarrhea, and pain within 1 week of eating infected meat.
- Fever, periorbital edema, myalgia, and marked eosinophilia.

GENERAL CONSIDERATIONS

Trichinella are small roundworms that inhabit hogs and several other meat-eating animals. Currently, there are eight recognized *Trichinella* species, with *Trichinella spiralis* being the most commonly recognized and most adapted to domestic and wild swine. The most important source of human infection worldwide is the domestic pig, but in Europe meat from wild boars and horses caused several prominent outbreaks. The human cycle begins with ingestion of viable larvae in undercooked meat. In the intestine, the larvae develop into adult worms that mate and produce hundreds of larvae. The larvae enter the bloodstream and migrate to the striated muscle where they continue to grow and eventually encyst. Symptoms are caused by the inflammatory response in the intestines or muscle.

Clinical Findings

A. Symptoms and Signs

Most infections are asymptomatic. The severity of clinical disease is strongly correlated with the number of ingested larvae. Infection can be divided into two phases: an intestinal phase and a muscular (or systemic) phase. The initial bowel penetration may cause fever, headache, chills, and gastrointestinal complaints within 1 week after ingestion of contaminated meat. This may progress to the classic myopathic form, which consists of fever, eyelid or facial edema, myalgia, and weakness. Complications, including myocarditis, thromboembolic disease, and encephalitis, occasionally occur. The leading pathologic process of trichinellosis is vasculitis, which can be manifest as a maculopapular exanthem, subungual bleeding, conjunctivitis and subconjunctival hemorrhages, headaches, dry cough, and painful movement of the eye muscles. Severe cerebral involvement or myocarditis can be fatal. Symptoms usually peak after 2–3 weeks but may last for months. Children typically have milder clinical and laboratory findings than adults.

B. Diagnosis

The diagnosis of trichinosis should be based on three main criteria: (1) clinical findings (fever; myalgias; eyelid and/or facial edema; gastrointestinal symptoms; and subconjunctival, subungual, and retinal hemorrhages); (2) laboratory findings (nonspecific eosinophilia and increased levels of muscle enzymes, antibody detection, and/or detection of larvae in a muscle biopsy); and (3) epidemiologic investigation.

Differential Diagnosis

The classic symptoms are pathognomonic if one is aware of this disease. It has to be distinguished from gastrointestinal pathogens, serum sickness, dermatomyositis, typhoid fever, sinusitis (facial swelling is unilateral), influenza with myopathy, toxocariasis, and invasive schistosomiasis.

Prevention

Because a microscopic examination must be performed, meat in the United States is not inspected for trichinosis. Although all states require the cooking of hog swill, hog-to-hog or hog-to-rat cycles may continue. All pork and sylvatic meat (eg, bear or walrus) should be cooked at least 65°C. Freezing meat to at least −15°C for 3 weeks may also prevent transmission. Animals used for food should not be fed or allowed access to raw meat.

Treatment

Albendazole is the drug of choice for treatment of trichinosis as plasma levels are more reliably attained than with mebendazole. The recommended dose of albendazole is 400 mg twice daily for 8–14 days. Mebendazole is an acceptable alternative and can be given at a dose of 200–400 mg three times a day for 3 days followed by 400–500 mg three times a day for 10 days. Concurrent corticosteroids (prednisone 30–60 mg/d for 10–15 days) are used for treatment of severe symptoms. Administration of analgesics is sometimes required.

Prognosis

Prognosis for severe cases with cardiac and cerebral complications is poor, with a mortality rate around 5%. In milder cases, prognosis is good, and most patients' symptoms disappear within 2–6 months.

Gottstein B et al: Epidemiology, diagnosis, treatment, and control of trichinellosis. Clin Micro Rev 2009;22:127–145 [PMID: 19136437].

Ozdemir D et al: Acute trichinellosis in children compared with adults. Pediatr Infect Dis J 2005:24:897 [PMID: 16220088].

8. Raccoon Roundworm Infections

ESSENTIALS OF DIAGNOSIS & TYPICAL FEATURES

- Eosinophilic meningoencephalitis or encephalopathy.
- Ocular larva migrans.
- Contact with raccoons or raccoon feces.

General Considerations

Human infections with *Baylisascaris procyonis*, the raccoon roundworm, are increasingly recognized, particularly in children. The definitive host of this ascarid is the raccoon. Humans who ingest the eggs excreted in raccoon feces become intermediate hosts when the larvae penetrate the gut and disseminate via the bloodstream to the brain, eyes, viscera, and muscles. Young age, pica, and exposure to raccoon feces (eg, while camping) represent the main risk factors for this infection. Most of the infections are asymptomatic, but cases of severe encephalitis (neural larva migrans) and endophthalmitis (ocular larva migrans) occur. Symptoms typically begin 2–4 weeks after inoculation. CNS infections characteristically present as acute, rapidly progressive encephalitis with eosinophilic pleocytosis of the CSF (varies from 4% to 68% eosinophils in mild pleocytosis between 1 and 125 cells/mm^3). Both CNS and ocular infections resemble other larva migrans infections such as toxocariasis; therefore, *B procyonis* should be considered in the differential diagnosis of these infections when *Toxocara* serology is negative. The diagnosis of *B procyonis* is established by observing the larvae on examination of tissue biopsies or by serology (of serum or CSF), and should be considered in the differential diagnosis in anyone with CSF eosinophilia. Antihelmintic drugs have not been shown to have any beneficial effect for the treatment of baylisascariasis, since they lack larvicidal effects in human tissues. Nevertheless, albendazole (20–40 mg/kg/d for 1–4 weeks) has been used to treat most cases, together with anti-inflammatory drugs. Complete resolution of symptoms has not been achieved thus far. Immediate prophylactic treatment with albendazole should be considered for those with significant exposures to raccoon latrines or cages.

Gavin PJ et al: Baylisascariasis. Clin Microbiol Rev 2005;18:703 [PMID: 16223954].

Graeff-Teixeira C et al: Update on eosinophilic meningoencephalitis and its clinical relevance. Clin Microbiol Rev 2009;22: 322–348 [PMID: 19366917].

CESTODE INFECTIONS (FLUKES)

1. Taeniasis & Cysticercosis

ESSENTIALS OF DIAGNOSIS & TYPICAL FEATURES

- Mild abdominal pain; passage of worm segments (taeniasis).
- Focal seizures, headaches (neurocysticercosis).
- Cysticerci present in biopsy specimens, on plain films (as calcified masses), or on CT scan or magnetic resonance imaging (MRI).
- Proglottids and eggs in feces; specific antibodies in serum or CSF.

General Considerations

Pigs are the usual intermediate host of the tapeworm *Taenia solium*. Human cysticercosis occurs when the eggs, which are excreted in the feces of a person infected with the parasite, are ingested. Importantly, cysticercosis cannot be acquired by eating pork. Ingestion of infected pork results in adult tapeworm infection (taeniasis) because infected pork contains the larval cysts that develop into the adult tapeworm but does not contain the eggs which cause cysticercosis.

Larvae released from ingested eggs enter the circulation to encyst in a variety of tissues, especially muscle and brain. Full larval maturation occurs in 2 months, but the cysts cause little inflammation until the larvae die months to years later. Inflammatory edema ensues with calcification or disappearance of the cyst. A slowly expanding mass of sterile cysts at the base of the brain may cause obstructive hydrocephalus (racemose cysticercosis).

T solium and the beef tapeworm (*Taenia saginata*), which can causes taeniasis but not cysticercosis, are distributed worldwide. Contamination of foods by eggs in human feces allows person-to-person spread without exposure to meat or travel to endemic areas. Asymptomatic cases are common, but *T solium* is the most common helminth infection of the CNS and a leading cause of acquired epilepsy in the world.

Clinical Findings

A. Symptoms and Signs

1. Taeniasis—In most tapeworm infections, the only clinical manifestation is the passage of fecal proglottids, which are white, motile bodies 1–2 cm in size. They occasionally crawl out onto the skin and down the leg, especially the larger *T saginata*. Children may harbor the adult worm for years and complain of abdominal pain, anorexia, and diarrhea.

2. Cysticercosis—In the parenchymatous form, the parasite lodges in the brain as a single or multiple cysts. Pericystic inflammation results in granuloma formation, which is the cause of seizures in most patients. There are four stages of development of a parenchymal larval cyst: vesicular, colloidal, nodular, and calcified. The vesicular cyst is viable, where the scolex exists within the cyst and there is minimal or no enhancement due to a limited host immune response. As the scolex dies, due to either the host immune response or cysticidal treatment, fluid migrates from the degenerating cysts into the surrounding parenchyma and incites a strong immune response, characterized by strong enhancement on CT or MRI. This cyst, which lacks a well-defined scolex, is the colloidal cyst. As the cyst further degenerates, it develops into a nodular cyst and then calcifies, which is recognized as punctuate calcification on CT scan. Brain cysts may remain silent or cause seizures, headache, hydrocephalus, and basilar meningitis. Rarely, the spinal cord is involved. Neurocysticercosis manifests an average of 5 years after exposure, but may cause symptoms in the first year of life. In the eyes, cysts cause bleeding, retinal detachment, and uveitis. Definitive diagnosis requires histologic demonstration of larvae or cyst membrane. Presumptive diagnosis is often made by the characteristics of the cysts seen on CT scan or MRI. The presence of *T solium* eggs in feces, which is uncommon with cysticercosis, supports the diagnosis.

B. Laboratory Findings

Neuroimaging is the mainstay of diagnosis of neurocysticercosis. The diagnosis should be suspected in any patient who has lived in an endemic area and presents with a compatible clinical picture and suggestive lesions on CT scans.

Eggs or proglottids may be found in feces or on the perianal skin (using the tape method employed for pinworms). Eggs of both *Taenia* species are identical. The species are identified by examination of proglottids.

Peripheral eosinophilia is minimal or absent. CSF eosinophilia is seen in 10%–75% of cases of neurocysticercosis; its presence supports an otherwise presumptive diagnosis.

ELISA antibody titers are eventually positive in up to 98% of serum specimens and over 75% of CSF specimens from patients with neurocysticercosis. Solitary cysts are associated with seropositivity less often than are multiple cysts. High titers tend to correlate with more severe disease. CSF titers are higher if cysts are near the meninges.

The differential diagnosis of neurocysticercosis includes tuberculous granuloma, microabscesses, focal meningoencephalitis, arachnoid cyst, neoplasms, and vascular lesions.

Treatment

A. Taeniasis

Praziquantel (5–10 mg/kg once) and albendazole are equally effective. Feces free of segments or ova for 3 months suggest cure.

B. Cysticercosis

The treatment modalities available for neurocysticercosis include cysticidal agents (to kill larvae), corticosteroids (to decrease or prevent the inflammatory reaction), antiepileptic drugs (if seizures are present), and surgery (to remove cysts or for placement of a shunt for hydrocephalus). The use of cysticidal therapy is somewhat controversial, but most experts would recommend treatment with a cysticidal agent in most cases of neurocysticercosis, except in patients with inactive, calcified lesions. In patients with viable parenchymal cysts, cysticidal therapy decreases the burden of parasites and the number of seizures. Similarly, cysticidal therapy is associated with more complete and faster resolution on imaging and fewer seizures in patients with a single small enhancing lesion.

Albendazole, 15 mg/kg/d (maximum, 800 mg) divided in two doses daily for 8–15 days, is the treatment of choice. Larval death may result in clinical worsening because of inflammatory edema. A short course of dexamethasone may decrease these symptoms. Corticosteroids are mandatory treatment for large intraventricular cysts and encephalitis (dexamethasone 0.1 mg/kg/day d or prednisolone 1 mg/kg/d for as long as needed). Giant subarachnoidal cysts may require more than one cycle of therapy or surgery (or both). Minimally invasive neurosurgery (neuroendoscopic extraction) is the currently recommended management of intraventricular cysts. Follow-up scans every several months help assess the response to therapy.

Prevention

Prevention requires proper cooking of meat, careful washing of raw vegetables and fruits, treating intestinal carriers, avoiding the use of human excrement for fertilizer, and providing proper sanitary facilities.

Prognosis

The prognosis is good in intestinal taeniasis. Symptoms associated with a few cerebral cysts may disappear in a few months; heavy brain infections may cause death or chronic neurologic impairment.

Garcia HH et al: Cysticercosis of the central nervous system: How should it be managed? Curr Opin Infect Dis 2011;24:423–427 [PMID: 21788891].

Graeff-Teixeira C et al: Update on eosinophilic meningoencephalitis and its clinical relevance. Clin Microbiol Rev 2009;22:322–348 [PMID: 19366917].

Sinha S, Sharma BS: Neurocysticercosis: A review of current status and management. J Clin Neurosci 2009;16:867–876 [PMID: 19394828].

2. Hymenolepiasis

Hymenolepis nana, the cosmopolitan human tapeworm, is a common parasite of children; *Hymenolepis diminuta*, the rat tapeworm, is rare. The former is capable of causing autoinfection. Larvae hatched from ingested eggs penetrate the intestinal wall and then reenter the lumen to mature into adults. Their eggs are immediately infectious for the same or a new host. The adult is only a few centimeters long. Finding the characteristic eggs in feces is diagnostic.

H diminuta has an intermediate stage in rat fleas and other insects; children are infected when they ingest these insects.

Light infections with either tapeworm are usually asymptomatic; heavy infection can cause diarrhea and abdominal pain. Therapy is with praziquantel (25 mg/kg once).

3. Echinococcosis

ESSENTIALS OF DIAGNOSIS & TYPICAL FEATURES

- Cystic tumors of liver, lungs, kidneys, bones, brain, and other organs.
- Eosinophilia.
- Urticaria and pruritus if cysts rupture.
- Protoscoleces or daughter cysts in the primary cyst.
- Positive serology.
- Epidemiologic evidence of exposure.

General Considerations

Dogs, cats, and other carnivores are the hosts for *Echinococcus granulosus*. Cystic and alveolar echinococcosis (hydatid disease) cause significant morbidity and mortality worldwide. Endemic areas include Australia, New Zealand, and the southwestern United States, including Native American reservations where shepherding is practiced. The adult tapeworm lives in sheep intestines, and eggs are passed in the feces. When ingested by humans, the eggs hatch, and the larvae penetrate the intestinal mucosa and disseminate via the bloodstream to produce cysts; the primary sites of involvement are the liver (60%–70%) and the lungs (20%–25%). A unilocular cyst is most common. Over time, the cyst may reach 25 cm in diameter, although most are much smaller. The cysts of *Echinococcus multilocularis* are multilocular and demonstrate more rapid growth.

Clinical Findings

A. Symptoms and Signs

The clinical manifestations of echinococcosis are variable and depend primarily on the site, size, and condition of the cysts. The rates of growth of cysts are variable, and range between 1 and 5 cm in diameter per year. A slowly growing cyst is tolerated fairly well until it causes dysfunction due to its size. Liver cysts can cause hepatomegaly, right upper quadrant pain, nausea, and vomiting. If a cyst ruptures, the sudden release of its contents can result in a severe allergic reaction. Cysts may cause biliary obstruction. Most hepatic cysts are in the right lobe.

Rupture of a pulmonary cyst causes coughing, dyspnea, wheezing, urticaria, chest pain, and hemoptysis; cyst and worm remnants are found in sputum. Brain cysts may cause focal neurologic signs and convulsions; renal cysts cause pain and hematuria; bone cysts cause pain.

B. Laboratory Findings

The presence of a cyst-like mass in a person with appropriate epidemiologic exposure supports the diagnosis. CT, MRI, and ultrasonography are useful for the diagnosis of deep-seated lesions. Abdominal ultrasonography is the most widely used diagnostic tool. Antibody assays are useful to confirm a presumptive diagnosis, but some patients with echinococcosis do not have a detectable immune response (related to the integrity of the cyst and sequestration of echinococcal antigens inside the cyst). ELISA is the method most widely used for antibody testing.

Confirmation may be obtained by ultrasonography-guided fine-needle aspiration coupled with parasitologic examination for protoscoleces, rostellar hooks, antigens, or DNA. Eosinophilia is present in only about 25% of patients. Serologic tests are useful for diagnosis and follow-up of therapy.

C. Imaging

Pulmonary or bone cysts may be visible on plain films. Other imaging techniques are preferred for cysts in other organs. Visualization of daughter cysts is highly suggestive of echinococcosis.

Differential Diagnosis

Tumors, bacterial or amebic abscess, cavitary tuberculosis (pulmonary), mycoses, and benign cysts must be considered.

Complications

Sudden cyst rupture with anaphylaxis and death is the worst complication. If the patient survives, secondary infections from seeding of daughter cysts may occur. Segmental lung collapse, secondary bacterial infections, effects of increased intracranial pressure, and severe renal damage due to renal cysts are other potential complications.

Treatment

There is no "best" treatment option for cystic echinococcus and no clinical trial has compared all the different treatment modalities. Treatment indications are complex and based on cyst characteristics, available medical/surgical expertise and equipment, and adherence of patients to long-term monitoring. Because treatment involves a variety of options and expertise, patients should be referred to recognized reference and national/regional treatment centers, whenever available. Definitive therapy of *E multilocularis* requires meticulous surgical removal of the cysts. A surgeon familiar with this disease should be consulted. Medical therapy may be of additional benefit, particularly in disseminated disease, and chemotherapy alone has been shown to cure about one-third of patients. Albendazole (10–15 mg/kg/d for 3 months), sometimes with the addition of praziquantel, is the regimen of choice. A third treatment option is a four-step procedure (PAIR; puncture, aspiration, injection, and reaspiration). This procedure consists of (1) percutaneous puncture using ultrasound guidance, (2) aspiration of liquid contents, (3) injection of a protoscolicidal agents (95% ethanol or hypertonic saline for at least 15 minutes), and (4) reaspiration. PAIR is indicated for those who cannot undergo surgery. If the cyst leaks or ruptures, the allergic symptoms must be managed immediately. For alveolar echinococcus, radical surgery for complete resection of the cyst is the goal. In some patients (particularly in those in whom complete resection is not possible), lifetime chemotherapy may be required.

Prognosis

Patients with large liver cysts may be asymptomatic for years. Surgery is often curative for lung and liver cysts, but not always for cysts in other locations.

Brunetti E et al: Expert consensus for the diagnosis and treatment of cystic and alveolar echinococcosis in humans. Acta Trop 2010;114:1–16 [PMID: 19931502].

Kern P: Clinical features and treatment of alveolar echinococcosis. Curr Opin Infect Dis 2010;23:505–512 [PMID: 20683265].

Moro P, Schantz PM: Echinococcosis: A review. Int J Infect Dis 2009;13:125–133.

TREMATODE INFECTIONS

Schistosomiasis

ESSENTIALS OF DIAGNOSIS & TYPICAL FEATURES

- Transient pruritic rash after exposure to freshwater.
- Fever, urticaria, arthralgias, cough, lymphadenitis, and eosinophilia.
- Weight loss, anorexia, hepatosplenomegaly or hematuria, dysuria.
- Eggs in stool, urine, or rectal biopsy specimens.

General Considerations

One of the most common serious parasitic diseases, schistosomiasis, is caused by several species of *Schistosoma* flukes. *Schistosoma japonicum*, *Schistosoma mekongi*, and *S mansoni* involve the intestines and *Schistosoma haematobium*, the urinary tract. The first two species are found in eastern and southeastern Asia; *S mansoni* in tropical Africa, the Caribbean, and parts of South America; and *S haematobium* in northern Africa. Important transmission sites include Lake Malawi and Lake Victoria in Africa, Poyang and Dongting Lakes in China, and along the Mekong River in Laos.

Infection is caused by free-swimming larvae (cercariae), which emerge from the intermediate hosts, certain species of freshwater snails. The cercariae penetrate human skin, migrate to the liver, and mature into adults, which then migrate through the portal vein to lodge in the bladder veins (*S haematobium*), superior mesenteric veins (*S mekongi* and *S japonicum*), or inferior mesenteric veins (*S mansoni*). Clinical disease results primarily from inflammation caused by the many eggs that are laid in the perivascular tissues or that embolize to the liver. Escape of ova into bowel or bladder lumen allows microscopic visualization and diagnosis from stool or urine specimens, as well as contamination of freshwater and infection of the snail hosts that ingest them.

Clinical Findings

Much of the population in endemic areas is infected but asymptomatic. Only heavy infections produce symptoms.

A. Symptoms and Signs

Schistosomiasis progresses in three distinct phases: acute, chronic, and advanced disease. The cercarial penetration may cause a maculopapular, pruritic rash, comprising discrete, erythematous, raised lesions that vary in size from 1 to 3 cm. The symptoms of acute schistosomiasis (Katayama syndrome) can last from days to weeks, and can include fever, malaise, cough, diarrhea, hematuria, and right upper quadrant pain. The differential diagnosis of acute schistosomiasis includes gastroenteritis, hepatitis A, B, and C, HIV, salmonellosis and urinary tract infection. The chronic stages of disease caused by the parasite in mesenteric veins are characterized by hepatic fibrosis, portal hypertension, splenomegaly, ascites, and bleeding from esophageal varices. The chronic inflammation in the urinary tract associated with *S haematobium* infections may result in obstructive uropathy, stones, infection, bladder cancer, fistulas, and anemia due to chronic hematuria. Spinal cord granulomas and paraplegia due to egg embolization into the Batson plexus have been reported.

B. Laboratory Findings

The diagnosis is made by finding the species-specific eggs in feces (*S japonicum*, *S mekongi*, *S mansoni*, and occasionally

S haematobium) or urine (*S haematobium* and occasionally *S mansoni*). If no eggs are found, concentration methods should be used. Because the shedding of eggs can vary, three specimens should be obtained. Urine specimens should be collected between 10 AM and 2 PM to coincide with the timing of maximal egg secretion. Testing should wait until 2 months after the last known freshwater contact as this is the time required for worms to start producing eggs following infection. A rectal biopsy may reveal *S mansoni* and should be done if other specimens are negative. Serological tests are also available and may be helpful in making the diagnosis in patients who are not excreting eggs. Peripheral eosinophilia is common, and eosinophils may be seen in urine.

Prevention

The best prevention is to avoid contact with contaminated freshwater in endemic areas. Efforts to destroy the snail hosts have been successful in areas of accelerated economic development.

Treatment

A. Specific Measures

Praziquantel is the treatment of choice for schistosomiasis. A dosage of 40 mg/kg/d in two or three divided doses (*S mansoni* or *S haematobium*) over one day or 20 mg/kg three times a day (*S japonicum* or *S mekongi*) over one day is very effective and nontoxic. Praziquantel has no effect on eggs and immature worms and therefore a repeat dose 4–6 weeks later is sometimes needed.

B. General Measures

Therapy of nutritional deficiency or secondary bacterial infections may be needed. The patient's urinary tract should be evaluated carefully in *S haematobium* infection; reconstructive surgery may be needed. Hepatic fibrosis requires careful evaluation of the portal venous system and surgical management of portal hypertension when appropriate.

Prognosis

Therapy decreases the worm burden and liver size, despite continued exposure in endemic areas. Early disease responds well to therapy, but once significant scarring or severe inflammation has occurred, eradication of the parasites is of little benefit.

Gary DJ et al: Diagnosis and management of schistosomiasis. BMJ 2011;342:d2651 [PMID: 21586478].

Gryseels B et al: Human schistosomiasis. Lancet 2006;368:1106 [PMID: 16997665].

Hortez PJ et al: Developing vaccines to combat hookworm infection and intestinal schistosomiasis. Nature Reviews Micro 2010;8:814–826 [PMID: 20948553].

MYCOTIC INFECTIONS

Fungi can be classified as yeasts, which are unicellular and reproduce by budding; as molds, which are multicellular and consist of tubular structures (hyphae) and grow by elongation and branching; or as dimorphic fungi, which can exist either as yeasts or molds depending on environmental conditions. Categorization according to anatomic and epidemiologic features is shown in Table 43–6.

In the United States, systemic disease in normal hosts is commonly caused by three organisms—*Coccidioides*, *Histoplasma*, and *Blastomyces*—which are restricted to certain geographic areas. Prior residence in or travel to these areas, even for a brief time, is a prerequisite for inclusion in a differential diagnosis. Of these three, *Histoplasma* most often relapses years later in patients who are immunosuppressed.

Immunosuppression (especially of T-cell–mediated immunity), foreign bodies (eg, central catheters), ulceration of gastrointestinal and respiratory mucosa, severe burns, broad-spectrum antimicrobial therapy, malnutrition, HIV infection, and neutropenia or neutrophil defects are major risk factors for opportunistic fungal disease.

Laboratory diagnosis may be difficult because of the small number of fungi present in some lesions, slow growth of some organisms, and difficulty in distinguishing normal colonization of mucosal surfaces from infection. A tissue biopsy with fungal stains and culture is the best method for diagnosing systemic disease with some fungi. Repeat blood cultures may be negative even in the presence of intravascular infections. Serologic tests are useful for diagnosing coccidioidomycosis and histoplasmosis, and antigen detection is useful for diagnosing histoplasmosis, cryptococcosis, and aspergillosis in limited circumstances.

The common superficial fungal infections of the hair and skin are discussed in Chapter 15.

Montenegro BL, Arnold JC: North American dimorphic fungal infections in children. Pediatrics in Review 2010;31(6):e40 [PMID: 20516233].

Kuyucu N: Amphotericin B use in children: Conventional and lipid-based formulations. Exp Rev of Antiinfective Therapy 2011;9(3):357 [PMID: 21417875].

Chen SC, Playford EG, Sorrell TC: Antifungal therapy in invasive fungal infections. Cur Opinion in Pharmacology 2010;10(5):522 [PMID: 20598943].

Oz Y, Kiraz N: Diagnostic methods for fungal infections in pediatric patients: Microbiological, serological, and molecular methods. Exp Rev of Antiinfective Therapy 2011;9(3):289 [PMID: 21417868].

Somer A, Torun SH, Salman N: Caspofungin therapy in immunocompromised children and neonates. Exp Rev of Antiinfective Therapy 2011;9(3):347 [PMID: 21417874].

Table 43–6. Pediatric fungal infections.

Type	Agents	Incidence	Diagnosis	Diagnostic Tests	Therapy	Prognosis
Superficial	*Candida*[a] Dermatophytes *Malassezia*	Very common	Simple	KOH prep	Topical	Good
Subcutaneous	*Sporothrix*[a]	Uncommon	Simple[b]	Culture	Oral	Good
Systemic: normal host (endemic)	*Coccidioides* *Histoplasma* *Blastomyces*	Common: regional	Often presumptive	Chest radiograph; serology, antigen detection (histoplasmosis; blastomycosis); histology; culture of body fluids or tissue	None[c] or systemic	Good
Systemic: opportunistic infection	*Candida*[a] *Pneumocystis*[d] *Aspergillus* Mucorales *Malassezia* *Pseudallescheria* *Cryptococcus*	Uncommon	Difficult[e]	Tissue biopsy, culture, antigen detection (cryptococcosis)	Systemic, prolonged	Poor if therapy is delayed and in severely immune compromised hosts

[a]*Candida* and *Sporothrix* in immunocompromised patients may cause severe, rapidly progressive disease and require systemic therapy.
[b]Sporotrichosis may require biopsy for diagnosis.
[c]Often self-limited in normal host.
[d]Asymptomatically infects many normal hosts.
[e]Except *Cryptococcus,* which is often diagnosed by antigen detection.
KOH, potassium hydroxide.

BLASTOMYCOSIS

ESSENTIALS OF DIAGNOSIS & TYPICAL FEATURES

- Residence in, or travel to, an endemic area.
- In immunocompetent patients, most often a self-limited flu-like illness; acute pneumonia occurs in a minority of cases.
- Complications include progressive pneumonia and disseminated disease (CNS, skin, bone and joints, genitourinary tract).
- Diagnosis by culture of specimens from bronchoscopy, skin, or other tissue.

General Considerations

The causative fungus, *Blastomyces dermatitidis*, is found in soil primarily in the Mississippi and Ohio River valleys, additional southeastern and south central states, and the states bordering the Great Lakes. Transmission is by inhalation of spores. Subclinical disease is common. Severe disease is much more common in adults and males. In children, infection rates are similar in both sexes.

Clinical Findings

A. Symptoms and Signs

Primary infection is often unrecognized or produces pneumonia. Acute symptoms include cough, chest pain, headache, weight loss, and fever. These occur several weeks to months after inoculation. Infection is most often self-limited in immunocompetent patients. In some patients an indolent progressive pulmonary disease occurs after an incubation period of 30–45 days. Cutaneous lesions usually represent disseminated disease; local primary inoculation is rare. Skin lesions are slowly progressive and ulcerative with a sharp, heaped-up border or verrucous appearance. Bone disease resembles other forms of chronic osteomyelitis. Lytic skull lesions in children are typical, but long bones, vertebrae, and the pelvis may be involved. Extrapulmonary disease occurs in 25%–40% of patients with progressive disease. A total body radiographic examination is advisable when blastomycosis is diagnosed in the skin or another nonpulmonary site. Lymph nodes, and brain may be involved, but the genitourinary tract involvement characteristic of dissemination in adults is rare in prepubertal children.

B. Laboratory Findings

An initial suppurative response is followed by an increase in the number of mononuclear cells, and then formation of noncaseating granulomas. Diagnosis requires isolation or visualization of the fungus. Pulmonary specimens (sputum, tracheal aspirates, or lung biopsy) may be positive using conventional stains or fungal cell wall stains. The budding yeasts are thick-walled, have refractile walls, and are very large and distinctive (figure-of-eight appearance). The fungus can be grown readily in most laboratories, but 1–2 weeks are required. Sputum specimens are positive in more than 80% of cases and in almost all bronchial washings, and skin lesions are positive in 80%–100%. Serologic tests are generally not helpful for diagnosis. An ELISA antigen detection method, similar to that used for histoplasmosis, can detect *Blastomyces* antigen in urine and other body fluids, but there is cross-reactivity with histoplamosis.

C. Imaging

Radiographic consolidation and fibronodular interstitial and alveolar infiltrates are typical; effusions, hilar nodes, and cavities are less common. The paucity of cavitation distinguishes acute blastomycosis from histoplasmosis and tuberculosis. Miliary patterns also occur with acute infection. Chronic disease can develop in the upper lobes, with cavities and fibronodular infiltrations similar to those seen in tuberculosis, but unlike in tuberculosis or histoplasmosis, these lesions rarely caseate or calcify.

Differential Diagnosis

Primary pulmonary infection resembles acute viral, bacterial, or mycoplasmal infections. Blastomycosis should be considered when a significant pulmonary infection in an endemic area fails to respond to antibiotic therapy. Subacute infection mimics tuberculosis, histoplasmosis, and coccidioidomycosis. Chronic pulmonary or disseminated disease must be differentiated from cancer, tuberculosis, or other fungal infections.

Treatment

Recommended therapy for moderately severe or life-threatening (especially in the immunocompromised patient) or CNS infections is amphotericin B (0.7–1.0 mg/kg intravenously) for 1–2 weeks or until improved or a lipid formulation (3–5 mg/kg/d intravenously). This is followed by oral itraconazole (6–8 mg/kg/d) for 6 months. Itraconazole drug levels are valuable for monitoring therapy in severely ill patients. Mild pulmonary blastomycosis does not require treatment. However, mild to moderate blastomycosis is often treated with oral itraconazole alone for 6–12 months. Bone disease may require a full year of itraconazole therapy. Surgical debridement is required for devitalized bone, drainage of large abscesses, and pulmonary lesions not responding to medical therapy.

Smuth JA, Kauffman CA: Blastomycosis. Proc Am Thoracic Soc 2010;7(3):173 [PMID: 20463245].

Hage CA, Knox KS, Davis TE, Wheat LJ: Antigen detection in bronchoalveolar lavage fluid for diagnosis of fungal pneumonia. Curr Opinion in Pulmonary Med 2011;17(3):167 [PMID: 21311331].

Saccente M, Woods GL: Clinical and laboratory update on blastomycosis. Clin Microbiol Rev 2010;23(2):367 [PMID: 20375357].

CANDIDIASIS

ESSENTIALS OF DIAGNOSIS & TYPICAL FEATURES

- In normal or immunosuppressed individuals: superficial infections (oral thrush or ulcerations, vulvovaginitis, erythematous intertriginous rash with satellite lesions); fungemia related to intravascular devices.
- In immunosuppressed individuals: systemic infections (candidemia with renal, hepatic, splenic, pulmonary, or cerebral abscesses); chorioretinitis; cutaneous nodules.
- In either patient population: budding yeast and pseudohyphae are seen in biopsy specimens, body fluids, or scrapings of lesions; positive culture.

General Considerations

Disease due to *Candida* is caused by *Candida albicans* in 60%–80% of cases; similar systemic infection may be due to *Candida tropicalis*, *Candida parapsilosis*, *Candida glabrata*, and a few other *Candida* species. Speciation is important because of differences in pathogenicity and response to azole therapy. In tissue, pseudohyphae or budding yeast (or both) are seen. *Candida* grows on routine media more slowly than many bacteria; growth is usually evident on agar after 2–3 days and in blood culture media in 2–7 days.

C albicans is ubiquitous, usually in small numbers, on skin, mucous membranes, or in the intestinal tract. Normal bacterial flora, intact epithelial barriers, neutrophils and macrophages in conjunction with antibody and complement, and normal lymphocyte function are factors in preventing invasion. Disseminated infection is almost always preceded by prolonged broad-spectrum antibiotic therapy, instrumentation (including intravascular catheters), and/or immunosuppression. Patients with diabetes mellitus are especially prone to superficial *Candida* infection; thrush and vaginitis are most common. *Candida* is the fourth most common blood isolate in hospitals in the United States and is a common cause of catheter-related urinary tract infection.

Clinical Findings

A. Symptoms and Signs

1. Oral candidiasis (thrush)—Adherent creamy white plaques on the buccal, gingival, or lingual mucosa are seen.

These may be painful. Lesions may be few and asymptomatic, or they may be extensive, extending into the esophagus. Thrush is very common in otherwise normal infants in the first weeks of life; it may last weeks despite topical therapy. Spontaneous thrush in older children is unusual unless they have recently received antimicrobials. Corticosteroid inhalation for asthma predisposes patients to thrush. HIV infection should be considered if there is no other reason for oral thrush, or if it is persistent or recurrent. Angular cheilitis is the name given to painful erythematous fissures caused by *Candida* at the corners of the mouth, often in association with a vitamin or iron deficiency.

2. Vaginal infection—Vulvovaginitis occurs in sexually active girls, in diabetic patients, and in girls receiving antibiotics. Thick, odorless, cheesy discharge with intense pruritus is typical. The vagina and labia are usually erythematous and swollen. Outbreaks are more frequent before menses.

3. Skin infection

A. Diaper dermatitis—Diaper dermatitis is often due entirely or partly to *Candida*. Pronounced erythema with a sharply defined margin and satellite lesions is typical. Pustules, vesicles, papules, or scales may be seen. Weeping, eroded lesions with a scalloped border are common. Any moist area, such as axillae, and inguinal or neck folds, may be involved.

B. Congenital skin lesions—These lesions may be seen in infants born to women with *Candida* amnionitis. A red maculopapular or pustular rash is seen. Dissemination may occur in premature infants or in term infants after prolonged rupture of membranes.

C. Scattered red papules or nodules—Such findings in immunocompromised patients may represent cutaneous dissemination.

D. Paronychia and onychomycosis—These conditions occur in immunocompetent children, but are often associated with immunosuppression, hypoparathyroidism, or adrenal insufficiency (*Candida* endocrinopathy syndrome). The selective absence of specific innate and T-cell responses to *Candida* can lead to marked, chronic skin and nail infections called *chronic mucocutaneous candidiasis*.

E. Chronic draining otitis media—This problem may occur in patients who have received multiple courses of antibiotics and are superinfected with *Candida*.

4. Enteric infection—Esophageal involvement in immunocompromised patients is the most common enteric manifestation. It is manifested by substernal pain, dysphagia, painful swallowing, and anorexia. Nausea and vomiting are common in young children. Most patients do not have thrush. Stomach or intestinal ulcers also occur.

5. Pulmonary infection—Because the organism frequently colonizes the respiratory tract, it is commonly isolated from respiratory secretions. Thus, demonstration of tissue invasion is needed to diagnose *Candida* pneumonia or tracheitis. It is rare, seen mainly in immunosuppressed patients and patients intubated for long periods, usually while taking antibiotics. The infection may cause fever, cough, abscesses, nodular infiltrates, and effusion.

6. Renal infection—Candiduria may be the only manifestation of disseminated disease. More often, candiduria is associated with instrumentation, an indwelling catheter, or anatomic abnormality of the urinary tract. Symptoms of cystitis may be present. Masses of *Candida* may obstruct ureters and cause obstructive nephropathy. *Candida* casts in the urine suggest renal tissue infection.

7. Other infections—Myocarditis, meningitis, and osteomyelitis usually occur only in immunocompromised patients or neonates. Endocarditis may occur on an artificial or abnormal heart valve, especially when an intravascular line is present.

8. Disseminated candidiasis—Skin and mucosal colonization precedes, but does not predict dissemination. Too often, dissemination is confused with bacterial sepsis. This occurs in neonates—especially premature infants—in an intensive care unit setting, and is recognized when the infant fails to respond to antibiotics or when candidemia is documented. Invasive disease can occur in >50% of very low birth weight infants. These infants often have unexplained feeding intolerance, cardiovascular instability, apnea, new or worsening respiratory failure, glucose intolerance, thrombocytopenia, or hyperbilirubinemia. A careful search should be carried out for lesions suggestive of disseminated *Candida* (retinal cotton-wool spots or chorioretinitis; nodular dermal abscesses). If these findings are absent, diagnosis is often based presumptively on the presence of a compatible illness in an immunocompromised patient, a burn patient, or a patient with prolonged postsurgical or intensive care unit course who has no other cause for the symptoms, who fails to respond to antimicrobials, and who usually has *Candida* colonization of mucosal surfaces. Treatment for presumptive infection is often undertaken because candidemia is not identified antemortem in many such patients.

Hepatosplenic and renal candidiasis occurs in immunosuppressed patients. The typical case consists of a severely neutropenic patient who develops chronic fever, variable abdominal pain, and abnormal liver function tests. No bacteria are isolated, and there is no response to antimicrobials. Symptoms persist even when neutrophils return. Ultrasound or CT scan of the liver, spleen and kidney demonstrates multiple round lesions. Biopsy is needed to confirm the diagnosis.

B. Laboratory Findings

Budding yeast cells are easily seen in scrapings or other samples. A wet mount preparation of vaginal secretions is 40%–50% sensitive; this is increased to 50%–70% with the addition of 10% potassium hydroxide to the sample. The use of a Gram-stained smear is 70%–100% sensitive. The presence of pseudohyphae suggests tissue invasion. Culture is definitive. Ninety-five percent of positive blood cultures will be detected within 3 days, but cultures may remain negative (10%–40%) even with disseminated disease or endocarditis. *Candida* should never be considered a contaminant in cultures from normally sterile sites. *Candida* in any number in appropriately collected urine suggests true infection. Antigen tests are not sensitive or specific enough for clinical use. The ability of yeast to form germ tubes when incubated in human serum gives a presumptive speciation for *C albicans*.

Differential Diagnosis

Thrush may resemble formula (which can be easily wiped away with a tongue blade or swab, revealing normal mucosa without underlying erythema or erosion), other types of ulcers (including herpes), burns, or oral changes induced by chemotherapy. Skin lesions may resemble contact, allergic, chemical, or bacterial dermatitis; miliaria; folliculitis; or eczema. Candidemia and systemic infection should be considered in any seriously ill patient with the risk factors previously mentioned.

Complications

Failure to recognize disseminated disease early is the greatest complication. Arthritis and meningitis occur more often in neonates than in older children. Blindness from retinitis, massive emboli from large vegetations of endocarditis, and abscesses in any organ are other complications. The greater the length or extent of immunosuppression and the longer the delay before therapy, the more likely that complications will occur.

Treatment

A. Oral Candidiasis

In infants, oral nystatin suspension (100,000 units four to six times a day in the buccal fold after feeding until resolution) usually suffices. Nystatin must come in contact with the lesions because it is not absorbed systemically. Older children may use it as a mouthwash (200,000–500,000 units five times a day), although it is poorly tolerated because of its taste. Clotrimazole troches (10 mg) four times a day are an alternative in older children. Prolonged therapy with either agent or more frequent dosing may be needed. Painting the lesions with a cotton swab dipped in gentian violet (0.5%–1%) is visually dramatic and messy, but may help refractory cases. Eradication of *Candida* from pacifiers, bottle nipples, toys, or the mother's breasts (if the infant is breast-feeding and there is candidal infection of the nipples) may be helpful.

Oral azoles, such as fluconazole (6 mg/kg/d), are effective in older children with candidal infection refractory to nystatin. Discontinuation of antibiotics or corticosteroids is advised when possible.

B. Skin Infection

Cutaneous infection usually responds to a cream or lotion containing nystatin, amphotericin B, or an imidazole (miconazole, clotrimazole, others). Associated inflammation, such as severe diaper dermatitis, is helped by concurrent use of a topical mild corticosteroid cream, such as 1% hydrocortisone. One approach is to keep the involved area dry; a heat lamp and nystatin powder may be used. Suppression of intestinal *Candida* with nystatin and eradicating thrush may speed recovery and prevent recurrence of the diaper dermatitis.

C. Vaginal Infections

Vulvovaginal candidiasis (see Chapter 44) is treated with clotrimazole, miconazole, triazoles, or nystatin (cheapest if generic is used) suppositories or creams, usually applied once nightly for 3–7 days. A high-dose clotrimazole formulation need be given for only a single night. *Candida* balanitis in sexual partners should be treated. Oral azole therapy is equally effective. A single 150-mg oral dose of fluconazole is effective for vaginitis. It is more expensive, but very convenient. No controlled study has shown that treating colonization of male sexual partners prevents recurrence in females. Frequent recurrent infections may require elimination of risk factors, the use of oral therapy, or some prophylactic antifungal therapy, such as a single dose of fluconazole weekly for 6 months.

D. Renal Infection

Candiduria in an immune competent host with a urinary catheter may respond to its removal. Candiduria is treated in all high-risk patients, usually with a 7- to 14-day course of fluconazole (3–6 mg/kg/d), which is concentrated in the urine. Amphotericin B may be required in patients with fluconazole-resistant organisms. Renal abscesses or ureteral fungus balls require intravenous antifungal therapy. Surgical debridement may be required. Removal of an indwelling catheter is imperative.

E. Systemic Infection

1. Disseminated Candida infection—Systemic infection is dangerous and resistant to therapy. Surgical drainage of abscesses and removal of all infected tissue (eg, a heart valve) are required for cure. Hepatosplenic candidiasis should be treated until all lesions have disappeared or are calcified on imaging studies. Treatment of systemic infection has traditionally utilized amphotericin B. Lipid forms of amphotericin B retain the antifungal potency of the free drug but are much better tolerated. Although they are much more expensive than amphotericin B, they are indicated for patients who are intolerant of conventional therapy and for those whose infection is refractory to treatment or who have a high likelihood of developing renal toxicity from such therapy.

Flucytosine (50–75 mg/kg/d orally in four doses; keep serum levels < 75 mcg/mL) may be additive or synergistic to amphotericin B. Unlike amphotericin B, flucytosine penetrates tissues well. It should not be used as a single agent in serious infections because resistance develops rapidly.

Fluconazole and itraconazole (best absorbed from the liquid solution) and newer azole drugs, such as voriconazole and posiconazole, and a new class of drugs, echinocandins, are used interchangeably or in conjunction with amphotericin. They are often preferred because in general they are less toxic. They are acceptable alternatives for serious *C albicans* infections in nonneutropenic patients and are often effective as first-line therapy in immunocompromised patients. Fluconazole is well absorbed (oral and intravenous therapy are equivalent), reasonably nontoxic, and effective for a variety of *Candida* infections. Fluconazole dosage is 8–12 mg/kg/d in a single daily dose for initial therapy of severely ill children. Selected patients with prolonged immunosuppression (eg, after bone marrow transplantation) should receive prophylactic azole, echinocandin, or intermittent amphotericin B prophylaxis. The decision to use systemic azole therapy should include consideration of the local experience with azole-resistant *Candida* and if the patient had recent prophylaxis or treatment with azoles. Susceptibility testing for *Candida* species is now available to guide this decision. *C glabrata* and *C krusei* are common isolates that may be resistant to fluconazole; these are often susceptible to the newer azoles and echinocandins. *C lusitaniae* is usually resistant to amphotericin.

Correction of predisposing factors is important (eg, discontinuing antibiotics and immunosuppressives, improving control of diabetes, and removing infected devices and lines).

2. Candidemia—Infected central venous lines must be removed immediately; this alone often is curative. If the infection is considered limited to the line and environs, a 14-day course (after the last positive culture) of a systemic antifungal agent following line removal is recommended for nonneutropenic patients. This is because of the late occurrence of focal *Candida* infection, especially retinal infection, in some cases. Persistent fever and candidemia suggest infected thrombus, endocarditis, or tissue infection.

Prognosis

Superficial disease in normal hosts has a good prognosis; in abnormal hosts, it may be refractory to therapy. Early therapy of systemic disease is often curative if the underlying immune response is adequate. The outcome is poor when therapy is delayed or when host response is inadequate.

Katragkou A, Roilides E: Best practice in treating infants and children with proven, probable or suspected invasive fungal infections. Curr Opinion in Infect Dis 2011;24(3):225 [PMID: 21455060].

Moudgal V, Sobel J: Antifungals to treat Candida albicans. Expert Opinion on Pharmacotherapy 2010;11(12):2037 [PMID: 20536294].

Pappas PG et al: Clinical practice guidelines for the management of candidiasis: 2009 update by the Infectious Diseases Society of America. Clin Infect Dis 2009;48:503 [PMID: 19191635].

Zaoutis T: Candidemia in children. Curr Med Research & Opinion 2010;26(7):1761 [PMID: 20513207].

COCCIDIOIDOMYCOSIS

ESSENTIALS OF DIAGNOSIS & TYPICAL FEATURES

- Residence in, or travel to, an endemic area.
- Primary pulmonary form: fever, chest pain, cough, anorexia, weight loss, and often a macular rash, erythema nodosum, or erythema multiforme.
- Primary cutaneous form: skin trauma followed in 1–3 weeks by an ulcer and regional adenopathy.
- Spherules seen in pus, sputum, CSF, joint fluid; positive culture.
- Appearance of precipitating (early) and complement-fixing antibodies (late).

General Considerations

Coccidioidomycosis is caused by the dimorphic fungus *Coccidioides* (*immitis* or *posadasii*), which are endemic in the Sonoran Desert areas of western parts of Texas, southern New Mexico and Arizona, southern California, northern Mexico, and South America. Infection results from inhalation or inoculation of arthrospores (highly contagious and readily airborne in the dry climate). Even brief travel in or through an endemic area, especially during windy seasons, may result in infection. Human-to-human transmission does not occur. More than half of all infections are asymptomatic, and less than 5%–10% are associated with significant pulmonary disease. Chronic pulmonary disease or dissemination occurs in less than 1% of cases.

Clinical Findings

A. Symptoms and Signs

1. Primary disease—The incubation period is 10–16 days (range, 7–28 days). Symptoms vary from those of a mild fever and arthralgia to severe influenza-like illness with high fever, nonproductive cough, pleurisy, myalgias, arthralgias, headache, night sweats, and anorexia. Upper respiratory tract signs are uncommon. Severe pleuritic chest pain suggests this diagnosis. Signs vary from none to rash, rales, pleural rubs, and signs of pulmonary consolidation. Weight loss may occur.

2. Skin disease—Up to 10% of children develop erythema nodosum or erythema multiforme. These manifestations imply a favorable host response to the organism. Less specific maculopapular eruptions occur in a larger number of children. Skin lesions can occur following fungemia. Primary skin inoculation sites develop indurated ulcers with local adenopathy. Contiguous involvement of skin from deep infection in nodes or bone also occurs. The presence of chronic skin lesions with this fungus should lead to a search for other areas of infection (eg, lungs).

3. Chronic pulmonary disease—This is uncommon in children. Chronic disease is manifested by chronic cough (occasionally with hemoptysis), weight loss, pulmonary consolidation, effusion, cavitation, or pneumothorax.

4. Disseminated disease—This is less common in children than adults. It is more common in infants, neonates, pregnant women (especially during the third trimester), blacks, Filipinos, American Indians, and patients with HIV or other types of immunosuppression. More than one organ may be involved. The most common sites involved are bone or joint (usually a single bone or joint; subacute or chronic swelling, pain, redness), nodes, meninges (slowly progressive meningeal signs, ataxia, vomiting, headache, and cranial neuropathies), and kidneys (dysuria and urinary frequency). As with most fungal diseases, the evolution of the illness is usually slow.

B. Laboratory Findings

Direct examination of respiratory secretions, pus, CSF, or tissue may reveal large spherules (30–60 μm) containing endospores. These are the product of coccidioidal spores germinating in tissue. Phase-contrast microscopy is useful for demonstrating these refractile bodies. The organism is detected by using periodic acid–Schiff reagent, methenamine silver, and calcofluor stains. Fluffy, gray-white colonies grow within 2–5 days on routine fungal and many other media. CSF cultures are often negative.

Routine laboratory tests are nonspecific. The sedimentation rate is usually elevated. Eosinophilia may occur, particularly prior to dissemination, and is more common in coccidioidomycosis than in many other conditions with similar symptoms. Meningitis causes a mononuclear pleocytosis (70% contain eosinophils) with elevated protein and mild hypoglycorrhachia.

Within 2–21 days, most patients develop a delayed hypersensitivity reaction to coccidioidin skin test antigen (Spherulin, 0.1 mL intradermally, should produce 5-mm induration at 48 hours) but test antigen is often unavailable in the United States. Erythema nodosum predicts strong reactivity; when this reaction is present, the antigen should be diluted 10–100 times before use. The skin test may be negative in immunocompromised patients or in those with disseminated disease. Positive reactions may remain for years and do not prove active infection.

Antibodies consist of precipitins (usually measurable by 2–3 weeks in 90% of cases and gone by 12 weeks) and complement-fixing antibodies (delayed for several weeks; appear as the precipitins are falling and disappear by 8 months, unless dissemination or chronic infection occurs). Thus, serum precipitins usually indicate acute infection. The extent of the complement-fixing antibody response reflects the severity of infection. Persistent high levels suggest dissemination. Excellent ELISA assays, which are now available to detect IgM and IgG antibodies against coccidioidal antigens, become positive in some patients as early as 1–3 weeks after onset of symptoms. The presence of antibody in CSF indicates CNS infection; CSF and serum antibody titers correlate with disease progression and response to therapy. Tests to detect coccidioidal antigen in urine are being validated.

C. Imaging

Approximately half of symptomatic infections are associated with abnormal chest radiographs—usually infiltrates with hilar adenopathy. Pulmonary consolidation, effusion, and thin-walled cavities may be seen. About 5% of infected patients have asymptomatic nodules or cysts after recovery. Unlike tuberculosis reactivation, apical disease is not prominent. Bone infection causes osteolysis that enhances with technetium. Cerebral imaging may show hydrocephalus and meningitis; intracranial abscesses and calcifications are unusual. Radiographic evolution of all lesions is slow.

Differential Diagnosis

Primary pulmonary infection resembles acute viral, bacterial, or mycoplasmal infections; subacute presentation mimics tuberculosis, histoplasmosis, and blastomycosis. Chronic pulmonary or disseminated disease must be differentiated from cancer, tuberculosis, or other fungal infections.

Complications

Dissemination of primary pulmonary disease is associated with permissive ethnic background, prolonged fever (> 1 month), a negative skin test, high complement-fixation antibody titer, and marked hilar adenopathy. Local pulmonary complications include effusion, empyema, and pneumothorax. Cerebral infection can cause noncommunicating hydrocephalus due to basilar meningitis.

Treatment

A. Specific Measures

Mild pulmonary infections in most normal patients require no therapy. These patients should be assessed for 1–2 years to document resolution and to identify any complications. Antifungal therapy is used for prolonged fever, weight loss (> 10%), prolonged duration of night sweats, severe pneumonitis (especially if persisting for 4–6 weeks), or any form of disseminated disease. Neonates, pregnant women, and patients with high antibody titer also receive treatment. Therapy is often utilized for pregnant women and patients that are at high-risk because of their race.

Amphotericin B is used to treat severe disease (1 mg/kg/d until improvement, then reduce dose; total duration, 2–3 months). Lipid formulations are used at 2–5 mg/kg/d. In general, the more rapidly progressive the infection, the more compelling the case for amphotericin B therapy. However, posaconazole and voriconazole are effective and their role as first-line therapy is being determined. For less severe disease and for meningeal disease, fluconazole or itraconazole are preferred (duration of therapy is > 6 months, and is indefinite for meningeal disease). Measurement of serum levels is suggested to monitor therapy. Chronic fibrocavitary pneumonia is treated for at least 12 months. Lifelong suppressive therapy is recommended after treating coccidioidal meningitis. Itraconazole may be superior to fluconazole. Refractory meningitis may require prolonged intrathecal or intraventricular amphotericin B therapy. Pregnant patients should not receive azoles.

B. General Measures

Most pulmonary infections require only symptomatic therapy, self-limited activity, and good nutrition. Patients are not contagious.

C. Surgical Measures

Excision of chronic pulmonary cavities or abscesses may be needed. Infected nodes, sinus tracts, and bone are other operable lesions. Azole therapy should be given prior to surgery to prevent dissemination and should be continued for 4 weeks arbitrarily or until other criteria for cure are met.

Prognosis

Most patients recover. Even with amphotericin B, however, disseminated disease may be fatal, especially in those racially predisposed to severe disease. Reversion of the skin test to negative or a rising complement-fixing antibody titer is an ominous sign. Individuals who later in life undergo immunosuppressive therapy or develop HIV may experience reactivation of dormant disease. Thus, some transplant and oncology programs determine prior infection by serology and either provide prophylaxis or observe patients closely during periods of intense immune suppression.

Homans JD, Spencer L: Itraconazole treatment of nonmeningeal coccidioidomycosis in children: Two case reports and review of the literature. Ped Infect Dis J 2010;29(1):65 [PMID: 19884875].

Mathisen G, Shelub A, Truong J, Wigen C: Coccidiodal meningitis: Clinical presentation and management in the fluconazole era. Medicine 2010;89(5):251 [PMID: 20827104].

Montenegro BL, Arnold JC: North American dimorphic fungal infections in children. Pediatrics in Review 2010;31(6):e40 [PMID: 20516233].

Shehab ZM: Coccidioidomycosis. Adv Pediatrics 2010;57(1):269 [PMID: 21056742].

CRYPTOCOCCOSIS

ESSENTIALS OF DIAGNOSIS & TYPICAL FEATURES

- Acute pneumonitis in immunocompetent individuals.
- Immunosuppressed patients especially vulnerable to CNS infection (headache, vomiting, cranial nerve palsies, meningeal signs; mononuclear cell pleocytosis).
- Cryptococcal antigen detected in CSF; also in serum and urine in some patients.
- Readily isolated on routine media.

General Considerations

Cryptococcus neoformans (sometimes *C gattii*) is a ubiquitous soil yeast. It appears to survive better in soil contaminated with bird excrement, especially that of pigeons. However, most infections in humans are not associated with a history of significant contact with birds. Inhalation is the presumed route of inoculation. Infections in children are rare, even in heavily immunocompromised patients such as those with HIV infection. Immunocompetent individuals can also be infected. Asymptomatic carriage does not occur.

Clinical Findings

A. Symptoms and Signs

1. Pulmonary disease—Pulmonary infection precedes dissemination to other organs. It is frequently asymptomatic (ie, many older children and adults have serologic evidence of prior infection) and less often clinically apparent than cryptococcal meningitis. Pneumonia is the primary manifestation in one-third of patients; CNS disease is the primary manifestation in 50%. Cryptococcal pneumonia may coexist with cerebral involvement. Symptoms are nonspecific and subacute—cough, weight loss, and fatigue.

2. Meningitis—The most common clinical disease is meningitis, which follows hematogenous spread from a pulmonary focus. This is much more likely to occur in an immunosuppressed patient (especially HIV) than in one that is immune competent. Symptoms of headache, vomiting, and fever occur over days to months. Meningeal signs and papilledema are common. Cranial nerve dysfunction and seizures may occur.

3. Other forms—Cutaneous forms are usually secondary to dissemination. Papules, pustules, and ulcerating nodules are typical. Bones (rarely joints) may be infected; osteolytic areas are seen, and the process may resemble osteosarcoma. Many other organs, especially the eyes, can be involved with dissemination.

B. Laboratory Findings

The CSF usually has a lymphocytic pleocytosis; it may be completely normal in immunosuppressed patients with meningeal infection. Direct microscopy may reveal organisms in sputum, CSF, or other specimens. The capsular antigen can be detected by latex agglutination or ELISA, which are both sensitive (> 90%) and specific. Serum, CSF, and urine may be tested. The serum may be negative if the only organ infected is the lung. False-negative CSF tests have been reported. The organism grows well after several days on many routine media; for optimal culture, collecting and concentrating a large amount of CSF (10 mL) is recommended, because the number of organisms may be low.

C. Imaging

Radiographic findings are usually lower lobe infiltrates or nodular densities; less often effusions; and rarely cavitation, hilar adenopathy, or calcification. Single or multiple focal mass lesions (cryptococcoma) may be detected in the CNS on CT or MRI scan.

Differential Diagnosis

Cryptococcal meningitis may mimic tuberculosis, viral meningoencephalitis, meningitis due to other fungi, or a space-occupying CNS lesion. Lung infection is difficult to differentiate from many causes of pneumonia.

Complications

Hydrocephalus may be caused by chronic basilar meningitis. Symptomatic intracranial hypertension is common. Significant pulmonary or osseous disease may accompany the primary infection or dissemination.

Treatment

Patients with symptomatic pulmonary disease should receive fluconazole for 3–6 months. All immunocompromised patients with cryptococcal pulmonary disease should have a lumbar puncture to rule out CNS infection; this should also be done for immunocompetent patients with cryptococcal antigen in the serum. Severely ill patients should receive amphotericin B (0.7 mg/kg/d). Meningitis is treated with amphotericin B (increase dose to 1 mg/kg/d) and flucytosine (100 mg/kg/d). This combination is synergistic and allows lower doses of amphotericin B to be used. Therapy is usually 6 weeks for CNS infections (or for 1 month after sterilization) and 8 weeks for osteomyelitis. An alternative is to substitute fluconazole (10 mg/kg/d) after 2 weeks of the combination therapy and continue fluconazole alone for 8–10 weeks. Fluconazole is the preferred maintenance therapy to prevent relapses in high-risk (eg, HIV) patients. CSF antigen levels should be checked after 2 weeks of therapy. Intracranial hypertension is treated by frequent spinal taps or a lumbar drain.

Prognosis

Treatment failure, including death, is common in immunosuppressed patients, especially those with AIDS. Lifelong maintenance therapy may be required in these patients. Poor prognostic signs are the presence of extrameningeal disease, fewer than 20 cells/μL of initial CSF, and initial CSF antigen titer greater than 1:32.

Joshi NS et al: Epidemiology of cryptococcal infection in hospitalized children. Ped Infect Dis J 2010;29(12):e91 [PMID: 20935590].

Perfect JR et al: Clinical guidelines for the management of cryptococcal disease: 2010 update by the Infectious Diseases Society of America. Clin Infect Dis 2010;50(3):291 [PMID: 20047480].

HISTOPLASMOSIS

ESSENTIALS OF DIAGNOSIS & TYPICAL FEATURES

- Residence in or travel to an endemic area.
- Pneumonia with flulike illness.
- Hepatosplenomegaly, anemia, leukopenia if disseminated.
- Histoplasmal antigen in urine, blood, bronchoalveolar lavage fluid or CSF.
- Detection by staining the organism in smears or tissue, or by culture.

General Considerations

The dimorphic fungus *Histoplasma capsulatum* is found in the central and eastern United States (Ohio and Mississippi River valleys), Mexico, and most of South America. Soil contamination is enhanced by the presence of bat or bird feces. The small yeast form is seen in infected tissues, especially within macrophages. Infection is acquired by inhaling spores that transform into the pathogenic yeast phase. Infections in endemic areas are very common at all ages and are usually asymptomatic. Over two-thirds of children are infected in these areas. Reactivation is rare in children, but occurs after treatment with immune suppressive agents, such as biological response modifiers and chemotherapy. Reactivation may occur years after primary infection. Reinfection also occurs.

The extent of symptoms with primary or reinfection is influenced by the size of the infecting inoculum.

Clinical Findings

Because human-to-human transmission does not occur, infection requires exposure in the endemic area—usually within prior weeks or months. Congenital infection does not occur.

A. Symptoms and Signs

1. Asymptomatic infection (90% of infections)—Asymptomatic histoplasmosis is usually diagnosed by the presence of scattered calcifications in lungs or spleen and a positive skin test or serology. The calcification may resemble that caused by tuberculosis, but may be more extensive than the usual Ghon complex.

2. Pneumonia—Approximately 5% of patients have mild to moderate disease. The cause of this illness is usually not recognized as being due to histoplasma. Acute pulmonary disease may resemble influenza, with fever, myalgia, arthralgia, and cough occurring 1–3 weeks after exposure. The subacute form resembles infections such as tuberculosis, with cough, weight loss, night sweats, and pleurisy. Chronic disease is unusual in children. Physical examination may be normal, or rales may be heard. A small number of patients may have immune-mediated signs such as arthritis, pericarditis, and erythema nodosum. The usual duration of the disease is less than 2 weeks, followed by complete resolution. Symptoms may last several months before resolving without antifungal therapy.

3. Disseminated infection (5% of infections)—Fungemia during primary infection probably occurs in the first 2 weeks of all infections, including those with minimal symptoms. Transient hepatosplenomegaly may occur, but resolution is the rule in immunocompetent individuals. Heavy exposure, severe underlying pulmonary disease, and immunocompromise are risk factors for progressive reticuloendothelial cell infection, with anemia, fever, weight loss, organomegaly, bone marrow involvement, and death. Dissemination may occur in otherwise immunocompetent children; usually they are younger than age 2 years.

4. Other forms—Ocular involvement consists of multifocal choroiditis. This usually occurs in immune competent adults who exhibit other evidence of disseminated disease. Brain, pericardium, intestine, and skin (oral ulcers and nodules) are other sites that can be involved. Adrenal gland involvement is common with systemic disease.

B. Laboratory Findings

Routine tests are normal or nonspecific in the benign forms. Pancytopenia is present in many patients with disseminated disease. The diagnosis can be made by demonstrating the organism by histology or culture. Tissue yeast forms are small and may be mistaken for artifact. They are usually found in macrophages, occasionally in peripheral blood leukocytes in severe disease, but rarely in sputum, urine, or CSF. Cultures of infected fluids or tissues may yield the organism after 1–6 weeks of incubation on fungal media, but even cultures of bronchoalveolar lavage or transbronchial biopsy specimens in immunocompromised patients are often negative (15%). Thus, bone marrow and tissue specimens are needed. Detection of histoplasmal antigen in blood, urine, CSF, and bronchoalveolar lavage fluid is the most sensitive diagnostic test (90% positive in the urine with disseminated disease, 75% positive with acute pneumonia) but false negative results may occur. The level of antigen correlates with the extent of the infection, and antigen levels can be used to follow the response to therapy and to indicate low-grade infection persisting after completion of therapy (eg, in a child with HIV infection).

Antibodies may be detected by immunodiffusion and complement fixation; the latter rises in the first 2–6 weeks of illness and falls thereafter unless dissemination occurs. Cross-reactions occur with some other endemic fungi. A single high titer or rising titer indicates a high likelihood of disease. Antigen detection has replaced serology as a rapid diagnostic test.

C. Imaging

Scattered pulmonary calcifications in a well child are typical of past infection. Bronchopneumonia (focal midlung infiltrates) occurs with acute disease, often with hilar and mediastinal adenopathy, occasionally with nodules, but seldom with effusion. Apical cavitation occurs with chronic infection, often on the background of preexisting pulmonary infection.

Differential Diagnosis

Pulmonary disease resembles viral infection, tuberculosis, coccidioidomycosis, and blastomycosis. Systemic disease resembles disseminated fungal or mycobacterial infection, leukemia, histiocytosis, or cancer.

Treatment

Mild infections do not require therapy. Treatment is indicated for severe pulmonary disease (diffuse radiographic involvement); disseminated disease; or when endovascular, CNS, or chronic pulmonary disease is present; and for children younger than age 1 year. Treatment should also be considered for patients who do not improve after 1 month. Disseminated disease in infants may respond to as few as 10 days of amphotericin B, although 4–6 weeks (or 30 mg/kg total dosage) is usually recommended. Amphotericin B is the preferred therapy for moderately severe forms of the disease. Patients with severe disease (especially pulmonary) may benefit from a short course of corticosteroid therapy. Surgical excision of chronic pulmonary lesions is rarely required.

Itraconazole (3–5 mg/kg/d for 6–12 weeks; achieve peak serum level of > 1.0 mcg/mL) appears to be equivalent to amphotericin B therapy for mild disease and can be substituted in severe disease after a favorable initial (2 weeks) response to amphotericin B. With chronic pulmonary, CNS, or disseminated disease, prolonged therapy may be required.

Quantitation of fungal antigen is useful for directing therapy, and should be monitored for one year after successful treatment of severe disease. Histoplasmosis can reactivate in previously infected individuals who subsequently become immunosuppressed. Chronically immunosuppressed patients (eg, those with HIV) may require lifelong maintenance therapy with itraconazole.

Prognosis

Patients with mild and moderately severe infections have a good prognosis. With early diagnosis and treatment, infants with disseminated disease usually recover; the prognosis worsens if the immune response is poor.

Hage CA, Knox CS, Davis TE, Wheat LJ: Antigen detection in bronchoalveolar fluid for diagnosis of fungal pneumonia. Curr Opinion in Pulmonary Med 2011;17(3):167 [PMID: 21311331].

Knox KS, Hage CA: Histoplasmosis. Proc Am Thoracic Soc 2010;7(3):169 [PMID: 20463244].

Wheat LJ: Approach to the diagnosis of endemic mycoses. Clin Chest Med 2009;30:379 [PMID: 19375642].

SPOROTRICHOSIS

ESSENTIALS OF DIAGNOSIS & TYPICAL FEATURES

- Subacute cutaneous ulcers.
- New lesions appearing proximal to existing lesions along a draining lymphatic.
- Absence of systemic symptoms.
- Isolation of *Sporothrix schenckii* from wound drainage or biopsy.

General Considerations

Sporotrichosis is caused by *Sporothrix schenckii*, a dimorphic fungus present as a mold in soil, plants, and plant products from most areas of North and South America. Spores of the fungus can cause infection when they breach the skin at areas of minor trauma. Sporotrichosis has been transmitted from cutaneous lesions of pets.

Clinical Findings

Cutaneous disease is by far the most common manifestation. Typically at the site of inapparent skin injury, an initial papular lesion will slowly become nodular and ulcerate. Subsequent new lesions develop in a similar fashion proximally along lymphatics draining the primary lesion. This sequence of developing painless, chronic ulcers in a linear pattern is strongly suggestive of the diagnosis. Solitary lesions may exist and some lesions may develop a verrucous character. Systemic symptoms are absent and laboratory evaluations are normal, except for acute phase reactants. The fungus rarely disseminates in immunocompetent hosts, but bone and joint infections have been described. Cavitary pneumonia is an uncommon manifestation when patients inhale the spores. Immunocompromised patients, especially those with HIV infection, may develop disseminated skin lesions and multiorgan disease with extensive pneumonia.

Differential Diagnosis

The differential diagnosis of nodular lymphangitis (sporotrichoid infection) includes other endemic fungi and some bacteria, especially atypical mycobacteria, pyoderma gangrenosum, nocardiosis, and syphilis. Diagnosis is made by culture. Biopsy of skin lesions will demonstrate a suppurative response with granulomas and provides the best source for laboratory isolation. Occasionally, the characteristic yeast will be seen in the biopsy.

Treatment & Prognosis

Treatment is with itraconazole (200 mg/d or 5 mg/kg/d) for 2–4 weeks after lesions heal; usually 3–6 months. Prognosis is excellent with lymphocutaneous disease in immunocompetent children. Pulmonary or osteoarticular disease, especially in immunocompromised individuals, requires longer therapy. Amphotericin B may be required for disseminated disease, CNS disease, and severe pulmonary disease. Surgical debridement may be required.

Barros MD et al: Endemic of zoonotic sporotrichosis: Profile of cases in children. Ped Infect Dis J 2008;27(3):246.

Montenegro BL, Arnold JC: North American dimorphic fungal infections in children. Pediatrics in Review 2010;31(6):e40 [PMID: 20516233].

PNEUMOCYSTIS AND OTHER OPPORTUNISTIC FUNGAL INFECTIONS

The name of this category indicates that fungi that are normally not pathogenic, or do not cause severe disease, may do so when given the *opportunity* by changes in host defenses. They occur most commonly when patients are treated with corticosteroids, antineoplastic drugs, or radiation, thereby reducing the number or function of neutrophils and T-cells. Inborn errors in immune function (combined immune deficiency or chronic granulomatous disease) may also be complicated by these fungal infections. Opportunistic infections are facilitated by altering the normal flora with antibiotics and by disruption of mucous membranes or skin with antineoplastic therapy or indwelling lines and tubes.

Table 43–7 indicates that filamentous fungi are prominent causes of severe systemic fungal disease in immunocompromised patients. *Aspergillus* species (usually *fumigatus*) and Zygomycetes (usually Mucorales) cause subacute pneumonia and sinusitis and should be considered when these conditions do not respond to antibiotics in immunocompromised patients. *Aspergillus* species also commonly cause invasive disease in patients with chronic granulomatous disease. Mucormycosis is especially likely to produce severe sinusitis in patients with chronic acidosis, usually when the diabetes is poorly controlled. This fungus may invade the orbit and cause brain infection. Mucormycosis also occurs in patients receiving iron chelation therapy. These fungal infections may disseminate widely. Imaging procedures may suggest the etiology, but they are best diagnosed by aspiration or biopsy of infected tissues. A characteristic CT finding is the "halo sign," which is a ground-glass opacity surrounding a pulmonary nodule or mass. The "reversed halo sign" is a focal rounded ground-glass opacity surrounded by a crescent or complete ring of consolidation. Detection of mannose in blood and alveolar fluid is sometimes useful for the diagnosis of aspergillosis and detection of β-D-glucan in blood and alveolar fluid should soon be available for the diagnosis of other opportunistic pathogens.

Although *Cryptococcus* can cause disease in the immune competent hosts, it is more likely to be clinically apparent and severe in immunocompromised patients. This yeast causes

Table 43–7. Unusual fungal infections in children.

Organism	Predisposing Factors	Route of Infection	Clinical Disease	Diagnostic Tests	Therapy and Comments
Aspergillus species	None	Inhalation of spores	Allergic bronchopulmonary aspergillosis; wheezing, cough, migratory infiltrates, eosinophilia.	Organisms in sputum; positive skin test; specific IgE antibody; elevated IgE levels.	Hypersensitivity to fungal antigens. Use steroids. Antifungals may not be needed.
	Immunosuppression	Inhalation of spores	Progressive pulmonary disease: consolidation, nodules, abscesses. Sinusitis Disseminated disease: usually lung, brain; occasionally intestine, kidney, heart, bone. Invades blood vessels.	Demonstrate fungus in tissues by stain or culture; septate hyphae branching at 45-degree angle; antigen detection may be useful.	Amphotericin B, voriconazole, and oral caspofungin are equally effective; these can be used in combination.
Malassezia furfur, M pachydermatis	Central venous catheter, usually lipid infusion (can occur in the absence of lipid)	Line infection from skin colonization	Sepsis; pneumonitis, thrombocytopenia.	Culture of catheter or blood on lipid-enriched media (for *M furfur; M pachydermatis* does not need lipid). Fungus may be seen in buffy coat.	Discontinuation of lipid may be sufficient. Remove catheter. Short-term amphotericin B may be added. Organism ubiquitous on normal skin; requires long-chain fatty acids for growth.
Mucorales (*Mucor, Rhizopus, Absidia*)	Immunosuppression, diabetic acidosis, iron overload	Inhalation, mucosal colonization	Rhinocerebral: sinus, nose, necrotizing vasculitis; central nervous system spread. Pulmonary. Disseminated: any organ.	Demonstrate broad aseptate hyphae branching at 90-degree angles in tissues by stain Culture: rapidly growing, fluffy fungus.	Amphotericin B, surgical debridement; voriconazole and posaconazole may also be effective or can be used as a second agent for combined therapy. Poor prognosis.
Scedosporium spp	Immunosuppression	Inhalation	Disseminated abscesses (lung, brain, liver, spleen, other).	Culture of pus or tissue.	Surgical drainage; voriconazole or caspofungin.
	Minor trauma	Cutaneous	Mycetoma (most common).	Yellow-white granules in pus. Culture.	Aggressive surgery. Amputation may be needed.

pneumonia and is a prominent cause of fungal meningitis. *Candida* species in these patients cause fungemia and multiorgan disease, with lungs, esophagus, liver, and spleen frequently affected (see the section on disseminated Candida, earlier).

Opportunistic fungal infections should always be included in the differential diagnosis of unexplained fever or pulmonary infiltrates in immunocompromised patients. These pathogens should be aggressively pursued with imaging studies and with tissue sampling when clues are available. *Cryptococcus* and *Aspergillus* may be demonstrated with specific antigen tests. Opportunistic infections are difficult to treat because of the deficiencies in host immune response. Treatment should be undertaken with consultants who are expert in managing these infections. Voriconazole is the drug of choice for many mold infections, but both echinocandins and amphotericin B are good alternatives. Combinations of current antifungal drugs are being tested to improve the outcome. Many children who will have depressed phagocytic and T-cell–mediated immune function for long periods (eg, after hematopoietic stem cell transplants) should receive antifungal prophylaxis during the period of severe immune suppression, most often fluconazole or itraconazole. Very-low birth weight infants, who are at high risk for systemic Candida infection, often receive similar prophylaxis for prolonged periods.

Malassezia furfur is a yeast that normally causes the superficial skin infection known as tinea versicolor (see Chapter 15). This organism is considered an opportunist when it is associated with prolonged intravenous therapy, especially when central lines used for hyperalimentation. The yeast, which requires skin lipids for its growth, can infect lines when lipids are present in the infusate. Some species will grow in the absence of lipids. Unexplained fever and thrombocytopenia are common. Pulmonary infiltrates may be present. The diagnosis is facilitated by alerting the bacteriology laboratory to add olive oil to culture media. The infection will respond to removal of the line or the lipid supplement. Amphotericin B may hasten resolution.

Georgiadou SP et al: The diagnostic value of halo and reversed halo signs for invasive mold infections in compromised hosts. Clin Infect Dis 2011; 52(9):1144 [PMID: 21467021].

Karageorgopoulos DE et al: β-D-Glucan assay for the diagnosis of invasive fungal infections: A meta-analysis. Clin Infect Dis 2011;52(6):750.

Katragkou A, Roilides E: Best practice in treating infants and children with proven, probable, or suspected invasive fungal infections. Curr Opinion in Infectious Dis 2011;24(3):225 [PMID: 21455060].

Maertens J et al: European guidelines for antifungal management in leukemia and hematopoietic stem cell transplant recipients: Summary of the ECIL 3—2009 update. Bone Marrow Transplantation 2011;46(5):709 [PMID: 20661235].

Spellberg B et al: Recent advances in the management of mucormycosis: From bench to bedside. Clin Infect Dis 2009;48:1743.

Oz Y, Kiraz N: Diagnostic methods for fungal infections in pediatric patients: microbiological, serological and molecular methods. Exp Rev of Antiinfective Therapy 2011;9(3):289 [PMID: 21417868].

PNEUMOCYSTIS JIROVECI INFECTION

ESSENTIALS OF DIAGNOSIS & TYPICAL FEATURES

- Significant immunosuppression.
- Fever, tachypnea, cough, dyspnea.
- Hypoxemia; diffuse interstitial infiltrates.
- Detection of the organism in specimens of pulmonary origin.

General Considerations

Although classified as a fungus on the basis of structural and nucleic acid characteristics, Pneumocystis responds readily to antiprotozoal drugs and antifols. It is a ubiquitous pathogen. Initial infection is presumed to occur asymptomatically via inhalation, usually in early childhood, and to become a clinical problem upon reactivation during immune suppression. There is evidence that person-to-person transmission may contribute to symptomatic disease in immune compromised individuals. In the normal host clinical disease rarely occurs. A syndrome of afebrile pneumonia similar to that caused by *Chlamydia trachomatis* in normal infants has been described, but its etiology is rarely appreciated. Whether by reactivation or new exposure, severe signs and symptoms occur chiefly in patients with abnormal T-cell function, such as hematologic malignancies and organ transplantation. Pneumocystis also causes severe pneumonia in patients with γ-globulin deficiency and is an AIDS-defining illness for children with advanced HIV infection. Prophylaxis usually prevents this infection (see Chapter 41).

Prolonged, high-dose corticosteroid therapy for any condition is a risk factor; onset of illness as steroids are tapered is a typical presentation. Severely malnourished infants with no underlying illness may also develop this infection, as can those with congenital immunodeficiency. The incubation period is usually at least 1 month after onset of immunosuppressive therapy.

Infection is generally limited to the lower respiratory tract. In advanced disease, spread to other organs occurs.

Clinical Findings

A. Symptoms and Signs

In most patients, a gradual onset of fever, tachypnea, dyspnea, and mild, nonproductive cough occurs over 1–4 weeks.

Initially the chest is clear, although retractions and nasal flaring are present. At this stage the illness is nonspecific. Hypoxemia out of proportion to the clinical and radiographic signs is an early finding; however, even minimally decreased arterial oxygen pressure values should suggest this diagnosis in immunosuppressed children. Tachypnea, nonproductive cough, and dyspnea progress. Respiratory failure and death occur without treatment. In some children with AIDS or severe immunosuppression from chemotherapy or organ transplantation, the onset may be abrupt and progression more rapid. Acute dyspnea with pleuritic pain may indicate the related complication of pneumothorax.

The general examination is unremarkable except for tachypnea and tachycardia; rales may be absent. There are no upper respiratory signs, conjunctivitis, organomegaly, enanthem, or rash.

B. Laboratory Findings

Laboratory findings reflect the individual child's underlying illness and are not specific. Serum lactate dehydrogenase levels may be elevated markedly as a result of pulmonary damage. In moderately severe cases, the arterial oxygen pressure is less than 70 mm Hg or the alveolar-arterial gradient is less than 35 mm Hg.

C. Imaging

Early chest radiographs are normal. The classic pattern in later films is that of bilateral, interstitial, lower lobe alveolar disease starting in the perihilar regions, without effusion, consolidation, or hilar adenopathy. High-resolution CT scanning may reveal extensive ground-glass attenuation or cystic lesions. Older HIV-infected patients present with other patterns, including nodular infiltrates, lobar pneumonia, cavities, and upper lobe infiltrates.

D. Diagnostic Findings

Diagnosis requires finding characteristic round (6–8 mm) cysts in a lung biopsy specimen, bronchial brushings, alveolar washings, induced sputum, or tracheal aspirates. Tracheal aspirates are less sensitive, but are more rapidly and easily obtained. They are more often negative in children with leukemia compared with those with HIV infection; presumably, greater immunosuppression permits replication of a larger numbers of organisms. Because pneumonia in immunosuppressed patients may have many causes, negative results from tracheal secretions should prompt more aggressive diagnostic attempts. Bronchial washing using fiberoptic bronchoscopy is usually well tolerated and rapidly performed.

Several rapid stains—as well as the standard methenamine silver stain—are useful. The indirect fluorescent antibody method is most sensitive. These methods require competent laboratory evaluation, because few organisms may be present and many artifacts may be found.

Differential Diagnosis

In immunocompetent infants, *C trachomatis* pneumonia is the most common cause of the afebrile pneumonia syndrome described for Pneumocystis. In older immunocompromised children, the differential diagnosis includes influenza, respiratory syncytial virus, cytomegalovirus, adenovirus, and other viral infections; bacterial and fungal pneumonia; pulmonary emboli or hemorrhage; congestive heart failure; and *Chlamydia pneumoniae* and *M pneumoniae* infections. Lymphoid interstitial pneumonitis, which occurs in older infants with untreated HIV infection, is more indolent and the patient's lactate dehydrogenase level is normal (see Chapter 41). *Pneumocystis* pneumonia is rare in children who are complying with prophylactic regimens.

Prevention

Children at high risk for developing Pneumocystis infection should receive prophylactic therapy. Children at risk include those with hematologic malignancies, children who for other reasons are receiving intensive chemotherapy or high-dose corticosteroids, and children with organ transplants or advanced HIV infection. All children born to HIV-infected mothers should receive prophylaxis against Pneumocystis starting at age 6 weeks until HIV infection has been ruled out or, if the infant is infected for the first year of life, when the patient's immunologic status will determine additional prophylaxis (see Chapter 41). The prophylaxis of choice is trimethoprim–sulfamethoxazole (150 mg/m^2/d of trimethoprim and 750 mg/m^2/d of sulfamethoxazole) for 3 consecutive days of each week. Alternatives to this prophylaxis regimen are described in Chapter 41.

Treatment

A. General Measures

Supplemental oxygen and nutritional support may be needed. The patient should be in respiratory isolation.

B. Specific Measures

Trimethoprim–sulfamethoxazole (20 mg/kg/d of trimethoprim and 100 mg/kg/d of sulfamethoxazole in four divided doses intravenously or orally if well tolerated) is the treatment of choice. Improvement may not be seen for 3–5 days. Duration of treatment is 3 weeks in HIV-infected children. Methylprednisolone (2–4 mg/kg/d in four divided doses intravenously) should also be given to HIV-infected patients with moderate to severe infection (partial oxygen pressure < 70 mm Hg or alveolar-arterial gradient > 35) for the first 5 days of treatment. The dosage is reduced by 50% for the next 5 days and further by 50% until antibiotic treatment is completed. If trimethoprim–sulfamethoxazole is not tolerated or there is no clinical response in 5 days, pentamidine isethionate (4 mg/kg once daily by slow intravenous infusion) should be given. Clinical efficacy is similar with pentamidine, but adverse reactions are more common.

These reactions include dysglycemia, pancreatitis, nephrotoxicity, and leukopenia. Other effective alternatives utilized in adults include atovaquone, trimethoprim plus dapsone, and primaquine plus clindamycin.

Prognosis

The mortality rate is high in immunosuppressed patients who receive treatment late in the illness.

Calderon EJ et al: Pneumocystis infection in humans: Diagnosis and treatment. Exp Rev of Antiinfective Therapy 2010;8(6):683 [PMID: 20521896].

Carmona EM, Limper AH: Update on the diagnosis and treatment of Pneumocystis pneumonia. Therap Adv in Respir Dis 2011;5(1):41 [PMID: 20736243].

Catherinot E et al: Pneumocystis jirovecii pneumonia. Infect Dis Clinics N Amer 2010;24(1):107 [PMID: 20171548].

Sexually Transmitted Infections

44

Daniel H. Reirden, MD
Ann-Christine Nyquist, MD, MSPH

The rate of sexually transmitted infections (STIs) acquired during adolescence remains high despite widespread educational programs and increased access to health care. By senior year in high school, nearly half of youth will have had sexual intercourse. The highest age-specific rates for gonorrhea, chlamydia, and human papillomavirus (HPV) infection occur in adolescents and young adults (15–24 years of age). While this population accounts for only 25% of the sexually active population, these youth account for almost half of the incident STI infections. Adolescents contract STIs at a higher rate than adults because of sexual risk taking, age-related biologic factors, and barriers to health care access. In every state and the District of Columbia, adolescents can provide consent for the diagnosis and treatment of STIs without parental consent. Only one state requires the notification of a parent in the event of a positive test; 17 others allow for the disclosure to a parent. In many states, adolescents can also provide consent for human immunodeficiency virus (HIV) counseling and testing. Since individual state laws vary, practitioners should be knowledgeable about the legal definitions regarding age of consent and confidentiality requirements in their respective state.

Providers should screen sexually experienced adolescents for STIs and use this opportunity to discuss risk reduction. Since not all adolescents receive regular preventive care, providers should consider using acute care visits to offer screening and education. Health education counseling should be nonjudgmental and appropriate for the developmental level, yet sufficiently thorough to identify risk behaviors because many adolescents may not readily acknowledge engaging in these behaviors.

ADOLESCENT SEXUALITY

The spectrum of sexual behavior includes holding hands and kissing, touching, mutual masturbation, oral-genital contact, and vaginal and anal intercourse. Each has its associated risks. A small, but statistically significant, trend has occurred in the epidemiology of sexual risk taking toward less sexual involvement and later onset of vaginal intercourse. The most recent Youth Risk Behavior Survey (2009) reports that 46% of high school students have had vaginal intercourse; 7% percent of teenagers initiated sex by age 13. Racial and gender differences exist; non-Hispanic Black adolescents report a higher prevalence of sexual activity and an earlier age of initiation. Thirty-four percent of students had sex in the 3 months prior to the survey—49% of twelfth-graders and 21% of ninth-graders. Nearly 14% of students reported having had four or more lifetime sexual intercourse partners. Nationally 61% of youth reported that either they or their partner had used a condom during their last sexual intercourse. Paradoxically, condom use decreases with age—64% of ninth-graders report condom use at their last intercourse compared with 55% of twelfth-graders. Substance use contributes to an increase in risky sexual activity and 22% of sexually active youth report that they used alcohol or drugs prior to their last intercourse.

Oral sex has not been as well studied. One study reports that 38% of boys and 42% of girls in the tenth grade engaged in oral sex, with only 17% of those engaged in oral sex using any protection. Anal intercourse occurs in both hetero- and homosexual populations. Nonconsensual sexual activity may occur in both male and female adolescents.

Adolescent development is a time of exploration, including one's sexual orientation. Frequently, teenagers may not identify themselves as gay, lesbian, or bisexual; thus, sensitive, nonjudgmental history taking is necessary to elicit a history of same-sex partners. Adolescents struggling with their emerging sexual orientation and associated stigma may engage in sexual activity with partners of both sexes or use substances to cope thereby impairing their decision-making abilities.

Centers for Disease Control and Prevention: Youth risk behavior surveillance—United States 2009. MMWR Surveill Summ 2010;59(SS-5) [PMID: 20520591].

Shafii T, Burstein G: The adolescent sexual health visit. Obstet Gynecol Clin N Am 2009;36:99 [PMID: 19344850].

State Policies in Brief: Minor's Access to STI Services as of July1, 2011. Guttmacher Organization web site. Available at: http://www.guttmacher.org/media/nr/2011/06/27/index.html. Accessed July 19, 2011.

RISK FACTORS

Certain behaviors and experiences put the adolescent at higher risk for developing STIs. These include early age at sexual debut, lack of condom use, multiple partners, prior STI, history of STI in a partner, and sex with a partner who is 3 or more years older. The type of sex affects risk as well, with intercourse being riskier than oral sex. Other risk-taking behaviors associated with STIs in adolescents are smoking, alcohol use, drug use, dropping out of school, pregnancy, and depression.

The adolescent female is especially predisposed to chlamydia, gonorrhea, and HPV infection because the cervix during adolescence has an exposed squamocolumnar junction. The rapidly dividing cells in this area are especially susceptible to microorganism attachment and infection. During early to midpuberty, this junction slowly invaginates as the uterus and cervix mature, and by the late teens to early 20s the squamocolumnar junction is inside the cervix.

Centers for Disease Control and Prevention: Youth risk behavior surveillance—United States 2009. MMWR Surveill Summ 2010;59(SS-5) [PMID: 20520591].

Gavin L et al: Sexual and reproductive health of persons aged 10–24 years—United States, 2002–2007. MMWR Surveill Summ 2009;58:1 [PMID: 19609250].

Halpern-Flesher BL et al: Oral versus vaginal sex among adolescents: Perceptions, attitudes, and behavior. Pediatrics 2005; 115:845 [PMID: 15805354].

Khan MR et al: Depression, sexually transmitted infection, and sexual risk behavior among young adults in the United States. Arch Pediatr Adolesc Med 2009;163:644 [PMID: 19581548].

PREVENTION OF SEXUALLY TRANSMITTED INFECTIONS

Efforts to reduce STI risk behavior should begin before the onset of sexual experimentation: first by helping youth personalize their risk for STIs and encouraging positive behaviors that minimize these risks, and then by enhancing communication skills with sexual partners about STI prevention, abstinence, and condom use.

Primary prevention focuses largely on education and risk-reduction techniques. It is essential to recognize that a key task of adolescence is developing sexual identity. Teenagers are sexual beings that will decide if, when, and how they are going to initiate sexual involvement. Health care providers should routinely address sexuality as part of well-adolescent checkups. Being open and frank about the risks and benefits of each specific type of sexual activity will help youth think about their decision and the consequences. Although more than 90% of students have been taught about HIV infection and other STIs in school, adolescents still have a difficult time personalizing risk. Discussing prevalence, symptoms, and sequelae of STIs can raise awareness and help teenagers make informed decisions about initiating sexual activity and the use of safer sex techniques. Abstinence is theoretically an effective method of preventing sexually transmitted infections. However, many studies have failed to show sustainable protection. Making condoms available reiterates the message that safer sex is vital to health. Discussing condoms, dental dams, and the proper use of lubrication also facilitates safer sex practices. Condoms may prevent infections with HIV, HPV, gonorrhea, *Chlamydia*, and herpes simplex virus (HSV). They are probably effective in preventing other STIs as well.

Secondary prevention requires identifying and treating STIs (see the next section on Screening for Sexually Transmitted Infections) before infected individuals transmit infection to others. Access to medical care is critical to this objective. Identifying and treating STIs in partners is essential in limiting the spread of these infections. Cooperation with the state or county health department is valuable, because these agencies assume the responsibility for locating the contacts of infected persons and ensuring appropriate treatment.

Tertiary prevention is directed toward complications of a specific illness. Examples of tertiary prevention would be treating pelvic inflammatory disease (PID) before infertility develops, following the serologic response to syphilis to prevent late-stage syphilis, treating cervicitis to prevent PID, or treating a chlamydial infection before epididymitis ensues.

Finally, preexposure vaccination against hepatitis B, hepatitis A, and HPV reduces the risk for these preventable STIs. All adolescents should have prior or current immunization against hepatitis B. (See Chapter 10.) However, because hepatitis B infection is frequently sexually transmitted, this vaccine is especially critical for all unvaccinated patients being evaluated for an STI. Hepatitis A vaccination is recommended for all individuals. Preexposure vaccination for HPV will decrease the risk for cervical dysplasia and cervical cancer in females, and decreases the risk for genital warts in males and females. (See Chapter 10.)

Delisi K, Gold MA: The initial adolescent preventive care visit. Clin Obstet Gyn 2008;51:190 [PMID: 18463451].

Rietmeijer CA: Risk reduction counseling for prevention of sexually transmitted infections: How it works and how to make it work. Sex Transm Infect 2007;83:2 [PMID: 17283359].

Shafii T, Burstein GR: The adolescent sexual health visit. Obstet Gynecol Clin North Am 2009;36:99 [PMID: 19344850].

SCREENING FOR SEXUALLY TRANSMITTED INFECTIONS

The ability of the health care provider to obtain an accurate sexual history is crucial in prevention and control efforts.

Teenagers should be asked open-ended questions about their sexual experiences to assess their risk for STIs. Questions must be explicit and understandable to the youth. If the adolescent has ever engaged in sexual activity, the provider needs to determine what kind of sexual activity (mutual masturbation or oral, anal, or vaginal sex); whether it has been opposite-sex, same-sex, or both; whether birth control and condoms were used; and whether it has been consensual or forced. During the interview the clinician should take the opportunity to discuss risk-reduction techniques regardless of the history obtained from the youth.

A routine laboratory screening process is warranted if the patient has engaged in intercourse, presents with STI symptoms, or reports a partner with an STI. The availability of nucleic acid amplification tests (NAATs), primarily for *Chlamydia* and *Neisseria gonorrhoeae*, has changed the nature of STI screening and intervention. These amplification tests are more than 95% sensitive and more than 99% specific, using either urine or cervical/urethral swabs. Annual screening of all sexually active females aged 25 years or younger is recommended for *Chlamydia trachomatis*. Routine chlamydial testing should be considered for all adolescent males, especially for males who have sex with men, have new or multiple sex partners, or are in correctional facilities. For men who have sex with men, consideration should be given to testing oropharyngeal and rectal sites, as asymptomatic infections are common. Use of NAAT is recommended for samples from these sites, but such tests are not currently FDA-approved and providers must locate a laboratory that has performed the necessary validation studies.

Initial screening for urethritis in males begins with a physical examination. A first-catch urine sample (the first 10–40 mL of voided urine collected after not voiding for 2 hours) should be sent for *Chlamydia* and *N gonorrhoeae* testing if there are no signs (urethral discharge or lesions) or symptoms. With signs or symptoms of urethritis, a urethral swab should be sent to test for both *N gonorrhoeae* and *Chlamydia*. A wet mount preparation should then be done on a spun urine sample or from urethral discharge, evaluating for the presence of *Trichomonas vaginalis*.

Screening asymptomatic females is more complicated because a variety of approaches are available. Generally, either a first-void urine specimen or a cervical swab is used to screen for *Chlamydia* and *N gonorrhoeae* by NAAT. Any vaginal discharge symptoms should include evaluation of wet mount of vaginal secretions to check for bacterial vaginosis and trichomoniasis, and a potassium hydroxide (KOH) preparation to screen for yeast infections. The Papanicolaou (Pap) smear serves to evaluate the cervix for the presence of dysplasia. The first Pap smear should be performed at age 21 years and then annually. HPV typing is not recommended.

In urban areas with a relatively high rate of syphilis or in males who have sex with men, an RPR/VDRL (rapid plasma reagin/Venereal Disease Research Laboratory) test should be drawn yearly. RPR and HIV antibody tests should be done in all individuals in whom a concomitant STI is present.

Centers for Disease Control and Prevention: Sexually Transmitted Diseases Guidelines, 2010. MMWR 2010;59(RR-12):10–11 [PMID: 21160459].

Henry-Reid LM et al: Current pediatrician practices in identifying high-risk behaviors of adolescents. Pediatrics 2010;125:e741 [PMID: 20308220].

Kent CK et al: Prevalence of rectal, urethral, and pharyngeal *Chlamydia* and gonorrhea detected in 2 clinical settings among men who have sex with men: San Francisco, California, 2003. Clin Infect Dis 2005;41:67 [PMID: 15937765].

SIGNS & SYMPTOMS

The most common symptoms in males are dysuria and penile discharge resulting from urethral inflammation. However, providers should be aware that many urethral infections are asymptomatic. Less common symptoms are scrotal pain, hematuria, proctitis, and pruritus in the pubic region. Signs include epididymitis, orchitis, and urethral discharge. Rarely do males develop systemic symptoms. For females, the most common symptoms are vaginal discharge and dysuria. Again, infection may be asymptomatic. Vaginal itching and irregular menses or spotting are also common. Abdominal pain, fever, and vomiting, although less common and specific, are signs of PID. Pain in the genital region and dyspareunia may be present.

Signs that can be found in both males and females with an STI include genital ulcerations, adenopathy, and genital warts.

THE MOST COMMON ANTIBIOTIC-RESPONSIVE SEXUALLY TRANSMITTED INFECTIONS

C trachomatis and *N gonorrhoeae* are STIs that are epidemic in the United States and are readily treated when appropriate antibiotics are administered in a timely fashion.

CHLAMYDIA TRACHOMATIS INFECTION

General Considerations

C trachomatis is the most common bacterial cause of STIs in the United States. In 2009, over 1 million cases in adolescents and young adults were reported to the CDC. *C trachomatis* is an obligate intracellular bacterium that replicates within the cytoplasm of host cells. Destruction of *Chlamydia*-infected cells is mediated by host immune responses.

Clinical Findings

A. Symptoms and Signs

Clinical infection in females manifests as dysuria, urethritis, vaginal discharge, cervicitis, irregular vaginal bleeding, or PID. The presence of mucopus at the cervical os (mucopurulent cervicitis) is a sign of chlamydial infection or gonorrhea. Chlamydial infection is asymptomatic in 75% of females.

Chlamydial infection may be asymptomatic in 70% of males or manifest as dysuria, urethritis, or epididymitis. Some patients complain of urethral discharge. On clinical examination, a clear white discharge may be found after milking the penis. Proctitis or proctocolitis from *Chlamydia* may occur in adolescents practicing receptive anal intercourse.

B. Laboratory Findings

NAAT is the most sensitive (92%–99%) way to detect *Chlamydia*. Enzyme-linked immunosorbent assay (ELISA) or direct fluorescent antibody (DFA) tests are less sensitive, but may be the only testing option in some centers.

A cervical swab, using the manufacturer's swab provided with the specific test, or first-void urine specimen should be obtained. For urine screening, yields of testing are maximized when collecting between 10 and 20 mL of urine and ensuring that patient has not voided for 2 hours. Often a single swab can be used to collect both the *Chlamydia* and *N gonorrhoeae* specimen. To optimize detection of *Chlamydia* from the cervix, columnar cells need to be collected by inserting the swab in the os and rotating it 360 degrees. NAAT is not licensed for rectal samples but some laboratories have validated testing on rectal specimens for *C trachomatis*. Thus, when a rectal specimen is obtained, this must often be evaluated by less sensitive culture methods unless there is access to a laboratory that has performed validation testing of NAAT for nongenital sites.

The first-void urine test for leukocyte esterase was previously used for screening asymptomatic, sexually active males. Because of the high false-positive rate, this screening technique is now less commonly used. In symptomatic males, examination of the urine sediment for white blood cells (WBCs) provides a screen for urethritis, although it is often impractical to perform in a clinical setting. In general, a first-void urine sample, or urethral swab for NAAT, should be obtained at least annually. Some studies suggest that more frequent screenings—every 6 months—in higher-prevalence populations can decrease the rate of chlamydial infection. Evaluation of the symptomatic male patient or an asymptomatic contact for *Chlamydia* is the same.

For both males and females, testing urine allows for more frequent screening and simplifies screening in large group settings, such as schools and correctional facilities.

Complications

Epididymitis is a complication in males. Reiter syndrome occurs in association with chlamydial urethritis. This should be suspected in male patients who are sexually active and present with low back pain (sacroiliitis), arthritis (polyarticular), characteristic mucocutaneous lesions, and conjunctivitis. PID is an important complication in females.

Treatment

Infected patients and their contacts, regardless of the extent of signs or symptoms, need to receive treatment (Table 44–1). Because adolescents have a high risk of acquiring a repeat chlamydial infection within several months of the first infection, all infected females and males should be retested approximately 3 months after treatment.

Baraitser P, Alexander S, Sheringham J: Chlamydia trachomatis screening in young women. Curr Opin Obstet Gynecol 2011;23:315 [PMID: 21897235].

Bebear C, de Barbeyrac B: Genital *Chlamydia trachomatis* infections. Clin Micro Infect 2009;15:4 [PMID: 19220334].

Centers for Disease Control and Prevention: Sexually Transmitted Diseases Guidelines, 2010. MMWR 2010;59(RR-12):44–47 [PMID: 21160459].

NEISSERIA GONORRHOEAE INFECTION

General Considerations

Gonorrhea is the second most prevalent bacterial STI in the United States, where an estimated 700,000 new *N gonorrhoeae* infections occur each year. While the overall rates have decreased, gonorrhea rates continue to be highest among adolescents and young adults. Among females in 2009, 15- to 19-year-olds and 20- to 24-year-olds had the highest rates of gonorrhea; among males, 20- to 24-year-olds had the highest rate.

Sites of infection include the cervix, urethra, rectum, and pharynx. In addition, gonorrhea is a cause of PID. Humans are the natural reservoir. Gonococci are present in the exudate and secretions of infected mucous membranes.

Clinical Findings

A. Symptoms and Signs

In uncomplicated gonococcal cervicitis, females are symptomatic 23%–57% of the time, presenting with vaginal discharge and dysuria. Urethritis and pyuria may also be present. Mucopurulent cervicitis with a yellowish discharge may be found, and the cervix may be edematous and friable. Other symptoms include abnormal menstrual periods and dyspareunia. Approximately 15% of females with endocervical gonorrhea have signs of involvement of the upper genital tract. Compared with chlamydial infection, pelvic inflammation with gonorrhea has a shorter duration, but an increased intensity of symptoms, and is more often associated with fever. Symptomatic males usually have a yellowish-green urethral discharge and burning on urination, but most males (55%–67%) with *N gonorrhoeae* are asymptomatic. Both males and females can develop gonococcal proctitis and pharyngitis after appropriate exposure.

Table 44–1. Treatment regimens for sexually transmitted infections.

	Recommended Regimens	Pregnancy[a] [Category]
Pelvic inflammatory disease (PID)		
Parenteral therapy regimen A ***Note***: Therapy should be continued for 24–48 h after patient has improved; therapy can then be switched to either oral regimen to complete a 14-d course.	Cefotetan, 2 g IV every 12 h or Cefoxitin, 2 g IV every 6 h plus Doxycycline, 100 mg IV or orally every 12 h	Safe [B] Safe [B] Contraindicated [D]
Parenteral therapy regimen B ***Note***: Once clinically improved for 48 h, patients can continue doxycycline, 100 mg PO bid for 14 d total.[b]	Clindamycin, 900 mg IV every 8 h plus Gentamicin, 2 mg/kg IV loading dose, then 1.5 mg/kg IV every 8 h	Safe [B] Safe [B]
Alternative parenteral regimens	Ampicillin/sulbactam, 3 g IV every 6 h plus Doxycycline, 100 mg IV or orally every 12 h	Safe [A] Contraindicated [D]
Recommended outpatient regimen ***Note***: Pregnant patients with PID and women with tubo-ovarian abscesses should be hospitalized and given parenteral antibiotics.[b]	Ceftriaxone, 250 mg IM once plus Doxycycline, 100 mg orally twice a day for 14 d with or without Metronidazole, 500 mg orally twice a day for 14 d or Cefoxitin, 2 g IM once plus probenecid, 1 g orally as a single dose plus Doxycycline, 100 mg orally twice a day for 14 d with or without Metronidazole, 500 mg orally twice a day for 14 d or Other parenteral third-generation cephalosporin (eg, ceftizoxime or cefotaxime) plus Doxycycline, 100 mg orally twice a day for 14 d with or without Metronidazole, 500 mg orally twice a day for 14 d	Safe [B] Contraindicated [D] Safe [B] Safe [B] Contraindicated [D] Safe [B] Safe [B] Contraindicated [D] Safe [B]
Cervicitis		
Chlamydia	Azithromycin, 1 g orally as single dose or Doxycycline, 100 mg orally twice a day for 7 d	Safe [B] Contraindicated [D]
Gonorrhea, uncomplicated		
Cervicitis, urethritis, rectal, pharyngitis ***Note***: Empiric treatment for *Chlamydia trachomatis* with azithromycin or doxycycline is recommended due to coexisting infection in 20%–40% of patients with gonorrhea infection.	Ceftriaxone, 250 mg IM as single dose or, if not an option Cefixime, 400 mg orally as single dose or Cephalosporins single-dose regimens[c] plus Azithromycin, 1 g orally as single dose or Doxycycline, 100 mg orally twice a day for 7 d	Safe [B] Safe [B] Safe [B] Safe [B] Contraindicated [D]
Gonorrhea, disseminated		
Note: Treat IV until clinically improved (usually 48 h; then switch to PO); complete at least a 7-d course.	Ceftriaxone, 1 g IV or IM every 24 h	Safe [B]
Alternative regimens	Cefotaxime, 1 g IV every 8 h or Ceftizoxime, 1 g IV every 8 h	Safe [B] Safe [B]

(*Continued*)

Table 44–1. Treatment regimens for sexually transmitted infections. (*Continued*)

	Recommended Regimens	Pregnancy[a] [Category]
Oral regimen[d]	Cefixime, 400 mg orally twice a day	Safe [B]
	or	
	Cefixime suspension, 400 mg by suspension (200 mg/5 mL) orally twice a day	Safe [B]
Nongonococcal, nonchlamydial urethritis		
	Azithromycin, 1 g orally as single dose	Safe [B]
	or	
	Doxycycline, 100 mg orally twice a day for 7 d	Contraindicated [D]
Alternative regimens	Erythromycin base, 500 mg orally four times a day for 7 d	Safe [B]
	or	
	Erythromycin ethylsuccinate, 800 mg orally four times a day for 7 d	Safe [B]
	or	
	Ofloxacin, 300 mg orally twice a day for 7 d	Contraindicated [C]
	or	
	Levofloxacin, 500 mg orally once daily for 7 d	Contraindicated [C]
Recurrent or persistent urethritis	Metronidazole, 2 g orally as single dose	Safe [B]
	or	
	Tinidazole, 2 g orally as single dose	Contraindicated [C]
	plus	
	Azithromycin, 1 g orally as single dose (if not used for initial episode)	Safe [B]
Proctitis, proctocolitis, and enteritis		
	Ceftriaxone, 250 mg IM	Safe [B]
	plus	
	Doxycycline, 100 mg orally twice a day for 7 d	Contraindicated [D]
Trichomonas vaginalis vaginitis or urethritis		
	Metronidazole, 2 g orally as single dose	Safe [B]
	or	
	Tinidazole, 2 g orally as single dose	Contraindicated [C]
Alternative regimen	Metronidazole, 500 mg orally twice a day for 7 d	Safe [B]
Bacterial vaginosis		
	Metronidazole, 500 mg orally twice a day for 7 d	Safe [B]
	or	
	Metronidazole, 0.75% gel, 5 g intravaginally once daily for 5 d	Safe [B]
	or	
	Clindamycin cream, 2%, one applicator intravaginally at bedtime for 7 d	Safe [B]
Alternative regimen	Clindamycin, 300 mg orally twice a day for 7 d	Safe [B]
	or	
	Clindamycin ovule, 100 mg intravaginally once at bedtime for 3 d	Safe [B]
	or	
	Tinidazole, 2 g orally once daily for 2 d	Contraindicated [C]
	or	
	Tinidazole, 1 g orally once daily for 5 d	Contraindicated [C]
Vulvovaginal candidiasis		
	Butoconazole, clotrimazole, miconazole, terconazole or tioconazole, intravaginally for 1, 3, or 7 d	Safe [B]
	or	
	Butoconazole sustained-release, 5 g once intravaginally	Safe [B]
	or	
	Fluconazole, 150 mg oral tablet, in single dose	Contraindicated [C]

(*Continued*)

Table 44–1. Treatment regimens for sexually transmitted infections. (*Continued*)

	Recommended Regimens	Pregnancy[a] [Category]
Syphilis		
Early (primary, secondary, or latent < 1 y)	Benzathine penicillin G, 2.4 million units IM (for patients > 40 kg)	Safe [B]
	or	
	Benzathine penicillin G, 50,000 U/kg IM (for patients < 40 kg); up to 2.4 million units in one dose	Safe [B]
Late (> 1-y duration or of unknown duration)	Benzathine penicillin G, 7.2 million units total, administered as three doses of 2.4 million units IM each at 1-wk intervals	Safe [B]
	or	
	Benzathine penicillin G, 50,000 U/kg IM (for patients < 40 kg) once a week for 3 consecutive wk; up to 2.4 million units in one dose	Safe [B]
Neurosyphilis		
	Aqueous crystalline penicillin G, 18–24 million U/d, administered as 3–4 million units IV every 4 h or continuous infusion for 10–14 d	Safe [B]
	or	
Alternative regimen (if compliance can be assured)	Procaine penicillin, 2.4 million units IM once daily plus	Safe [B]
	Probenicid 500 mg orally four times a day for 10–14 d	Safe [B]
Epididymitis		
Most likely caused by gonococcal or chlamydial infection	Ceftriaxone, 250 mg IM as single dose	
	plus	
	Doxycycline, 100 mg orally twice a day for 10 d	
Most likely caused by enteric organisms; patient > 35 y or allergies to cephalosporins or tetracyclines (or both)	Ofloxacin, 300 mg orally twice a day for 10 d	
	or	
	Levofloxacin, 500 mg orally once daily for 10 d	
***C trachomatis* infection**		
Cervicitis or urethritis	Azithromycin, 1 g orally as single dose	Safe [B]
	or	
	Doxycycline, 100 mg orally twice a day for 7 d	Contraindicated [D]
Alternative regimen[b]	Erythromycin, 500 mg orally four times a day for 7 d	Safe [B]
	or	
	Erythromycin ethylsuccinate, 800 mg orally four times a day for 7 d	Safe [B]
	or	
	Ofloxacin, 300 mg orally twice a day for 7 d	Contraindicated [C]
	or	
	Levofloxacin 500 mg orally once daily for 7 d	Contraindicated [C]
Granuloma inguinale		
	Doxycycline, 100 mg orally twice a day for 3 wk or longer	Contraindicated [D]
Alternative regimen	Ciprofloxacin, 750 mg orally twice a day for at least 3 wk	Contraindicated [C]
	or	
	Erythromycin base, 500 mg orally four times a day for at least 3 wk	Safe [B]
	or	
	Azithromycin, 1 g orally once a week for at least 3 wk	Safe [B]
	or	
	Trimethoprim–sulfamethoxazole, one double-strength tablet orally twice a day for at least 21 d	Contraindicated [C]
Lymphogranuloma venereum		
	Doxycycline, 100 mg orally twice a day for 21 d	Contraindicated [C]
Alternative regimen	Erythromycin, 500 mg orally four times a day for 21 d	Safe [B]

(*Continued*)

Table 44–1. Treatment regimens for sexually transmitted infections. (*Continued*)

	Recommended Regimens	Pregnancy[a] [Category]
Herpes simplex infection		
First episode, genital	Acyclovir, 400 mg orally three times a day for 7–10 d	Safe [B]
	or	
	Acyclovir, 200 mg orally five times a day for 7–10 d	Safe [B]
	or	
	Famciclovir, 250 mg orally three times a day for 7–10 d	Safe [B]
	or	
	Valacyclovir, 1 g orally twice a day for 7–10 d	Safe [B]
Episodic therapy for recurrent genital herpes	Acyclovir, 400 mg orally three times a day for 5 d	Safe [B]
	or	
	Acyclovir, 800 mg orally twice a day for 5 d	Safe [B]
	or	
	Acyclovir, 800 mg orally three times a day for 2 d	Safe [B]
	or	
	Famciclovir, 125 mg orally twice a day for 5 d	Safe [B]
	or	
	Famciclovir, 1000 mg orally twice a day for 1 d	Safe [B]
	or	
	Famciclovir, 500 mg once orally, followed by 250 mg orally twice a day for 2 d	Safe [B]
	or	
	Valacyclovir, 500 mg orally twice a day for 3 d	Safe [B]
	or	
	Valacyclovir, 1 g orally once daily for 5 d	Safe [B]
Suppressive therapy for recurrent genital herpes	Acyclovir, 400 mg orally twice a day	Safe [B]
	or	
	Famciclovir, 250 mg orally twice a day	Safe [B]
	or	
	Valacyclovir, 500 mg orally daily (if < 10 recurrences per year; if ≥ 10 recurrences, use 1 g daily)	Safe [B]
Chancroid		
	Azithromycin, 1 g orally as single dose	Safe [B]
	or	
	Ceftriaxone, 250 mg IM once	Safe [B]
	or	
	Ciprofloxacin, 500 mg orally twice a day for 3 d	Contraindicated [D]
	or	
	Erythromycin base, 500 mg orally three times a day for 7 d	Safe [B]
Human papillomavirus infection		
External lesions ***Note***: Topical therapies usually require weekly treatments for 4 consecutive wks	Podophyllin, 25% in benzoin tincture applied directly to warts; wash off in 1–4 h; weekly [contraindicated for urethral or intravaginal lesions]	Contraindicated [X]
	or	
	Trichloroacetic acid (85%) or Bicholoracetic acid; apply directly to warts; wash off in 6–8 h; weekly	Safe
	or	
	Podofilox, 0.5% solution; apply twice a day for 3 d; used by patient at home; practitioner needs to demonstrate how compound is applied (to be used only on external lesions)	Contraindicated [C]
	or	
	Imiquimod 5% cream, applied 3 times a week overnight (maximum of 16 wk)	Contraindicated [C]
	or	
	Sinecatechins 15% ointment, applied 3 times daily (maximum of 16 wk)	Unknown safety
	or	
	Cryotherapy: liquid nitrogen, cryoprobe safe laser surgery	Safe

(*Continued*)

Table 44–1. Treatment regimens for sexually transmitted infections. (*Continued*)

	Recommended Regimens	Pregnancy[a] [Category]
Ectoparasitic infections		
Pubic lice[d]	Permethrin 1% creme rinse: wash off after 10 min or Pyrethrins with piperonyl butoxide: apply, wash off after 10 min	Safe [B] Safe [B]
Alternative regimen	Malathion 0.5% lotion: wash off after 8–12 h or Ivermectin, 250 mcg/kg repeated in 2 wk	Safe [B] Contraindicated [C]
Scabies[d]	Permethrin cream 5%: apply to entire body from the neck down, wash off after 8–14 h or Ivermectin, 200 mcg/kg orally, repeat in 2 wk	Safe [B] Contraindicated [C]
Alternative regimen	Lindane (1%): apply to entire body from neck down, wash off after 8 h	Contraindicated [C]

[a]FDA use in pregnancy ratings: [A] *Controlled studies show no risk*. Adequate, well-controlled studies in pregnant women have failed to demonstrate a risk to the fetus in any trimester of pregnancy. [B] *No evidence of risk in humans*. Adequate, well-controlled studies in pregnant women have not shown increased risk of fetal abnormalities despite adverse findings in animals, in the absence of adequate human studies, animal studies show no fetal risk. The chance of fetal harm is remote but remains a possibility. [C] *Risk cannot be ruled out*. Adequate, well-controlled human studies are lacking, and animal studies have shown a risk to the fetus or are lacking as well. There is a chance of fetal harm if the drug is administered during pregnancy; but the potential benefits outweigh the potential risk. [D] *Positive evidence of risk*. Studies in humans, or investigational or postmarketing data, have demonstrated fetal risk. Nevertheless, potential benefits from the use of the drug may outweigh the potential risk. For example, the drug may be acceptable if needed in a life-threatening situation or serious disease for which safer drugs cannot be used or are ineffective. [X] *Contraindicated in pregnancy*. Studies in animals or humans, or despite adverse findings in animals, or investigational or postmarketing reports have demonstrated positive evidence of fetal abnormalities or risk that clearly outweighs any possible benefit to the patient.
[b]Doxycycline is contraindicated in pregnancy. Alternative therapies during pregnancy which include erythromycin, azithromycin, and amoxicillin are not as effective, but are clinically useful if the recommended regimens cannot be used due to allergy or pregnancy.
[c]Single-dose cephalosporin regimens include ceftizoxime (500 mg IM) or cefoxitin (2 g IM) administered with probenecid (1 g PO) or cefotaxime (500 mg IM). Some evidence indicates that cefpodoxime (400 mg) and cefuroxime axetil (1 g) might be oral alternatives.
[d]Bedding and clothing need to be decontaminated by washing in hot water or by dry cleaning. Regimen may be repeated in 1 week if complete response is not achieved.
IM, intramuscular; IV, intravenous; NAAT, nucleic acid amplification test.

B. Laboratory Findings

A first void urine sample or cervical swab from females should be sent for NAAT. Culture or NAAT for *N gonorrhoeae* in males can be achieved with a swab of the urethra or first-void urine. Urethral culture is less sensitive (85%) compared with the 95%–99% sensitivity using NAAT methods on either urethral or urine specimens. Gram stain of urethral discharge showing gram-negative intracellular diplococci indicates gonorrhea in a male.

If proctitis is present, appropriate cultures should be obtained and treatment for both gonorrhea and chlamydial infection given. If oral exposure to gonorrhea is suspected, cultures should be taken and the patient given empiric treatment. If there is access to a laboratory that has performed validation studies of NAAT for oropharyngeal or rectal specimens, this will substantially increase detection over culture methods.

Differential Diagnosis

Gonococcal pharyngitis needs to be differentiated from pharyngitis caused by streptococcal infection, herpes simplex, adenovirus, and infectious mononucleosis. Chlamydial infection needs to be differentiated from gonococcal infection.

Complications

Disseminated gonococcal infection occurs in a minority (0.5%–3%) of patients with untreated gonorrhea. Hematogenous spread most commonly causes arthritis and dermatitis. The joints most frequently involved are the wrist, metacarpophalangeal joints, knee, and ankle. Skin lesions are typically tender, with hemorrhagic or necrotic pustules or bullae on an erythematous base occurring on the distal extremities. Disseminated disease occurs more frequently in females than in males. Risk factors include pregnancy and gonococcal pharyngitis. Gonorrhea is complicated occasionally by perihepatitis.

Treatment (see Table 44–1)

In 2010, the CDC made two significant changes to gonorrhea treatment recommendations: dual treatment and treatment with ceftriaxone 250 mg IM regardless of anatomic site involved. These changes reflect increasing resistance to cephalosporins; the frequency of coinfection with Chlamydia; and the need to increase consistency of treatment regimens.

Their guidelines also state that *N gonorrhoeae* and *C trachomatis* do not require tests of cure when they are treated with first-line medications, unless the patient remains symptomatic. If retesting is indicated, it should be delayed for 1 month after completion of therapy if NAATs are used. Retesting might also be considered for sexually active adolescents likely to be reinfected. Patients should be advised to abstain from sexual intercourse until both they and their partners have completed a course of treatment. Treatment for disseminated disease may require hospitalization. Quinolones should no longer be used to treat gonorrhea due to high levels of quinolone resistance in all populations in the United States. Failure of initial treatment should prompt reevaluation of the patient and consideration of retreatment with ceftriaxone.

Centers for Disease Control and Prevention: Sexually Transmitted Diseases Guidelines, 2010. MMWR 2010;59(RR-12):49–55 [PMID: 21160459].

THE SPECTRUM OF SIGNS & SYMPTOMS OF SEXUALLY TRANSMITTED INFECTIONS

The patient presenting with an STI usually has one or more of the signs or symptoms described in this section. Management considerations for STIs include assessing the patient's adherence to therapy and ensuring follow-up, treating STIs in partners, and determining pregnancy risk. Treatment of each STI is detailed in Table 44–1.

CERVICITIS

General Considerations

In most cases of cervicitis no organism is isolated. The most common causes include *C trachomatis* or *N gonorrhoeae*. HSV, *T vaginalis*, and *Mycoplasma genitalium* are less common causes. Bacterial vaginosis is now recognized as a cause of cervicitis. Cervicitis can also be present without an STI.

Clinical Findings

A. Symptoms and Signs

Two major diagnostic signs characterize cervicitis: (1) purulent or mucopurulent endocervical exudate visible in the endocervical canal or on an endocervical swab and (2) easily induced bleeding with the passage of a cotton swab through the cervical os. Cervicitis is often asymptomatic, but many patients with cervicitis have an abnormal vaginal discharge or postcoital bleeding.

B. Laboratory Findings

Although endocervical Gram stain may show an increased number of polymorphonuclear leukocytes, this finding has a low positive predictive value and is not recommended for diagnosis. Patients with cervicitis should be tested for *C trachomatis*, *N gonorrhoeae*, and trichomoniasis by using the most sensitive and specific tests available at the site.

Complications

Persistent cervicitis is difficult to manage and requires reassessment of the initial diagnosis and reevaluation for possible re-exposure to an STI. Cervicitis can persist despite repeated courses of antimicrobial therapy. Presence of a large ectropion can contribute to persistent cervicitis.

Treatment

Empiric treatment for both gonorrhea and chlamydial infection is recommended because coinfection is common. If the patient is asymptomatic except for cervicitis, then treatment may wait until diagnostic test results are available (see Table 44–1). Follow-up is recommended if symptoms persist. Patients should be instructed to abstain from sexual intercourse until they and their sex partners are cured and treatment is completed.

Lusk MJ, Konecny P: Cervicitis: A review. Curr Opin Infect Dis 2008;21:49 [PMID: 18192786].

PELVIC INFLAMMATORY DISEASE

General Considerations

Pelvic inflammatory disease (PID) is defined as inflammation of the upper female genital tract and may include endometritis, salpingitis, tubo-ovarian abscess, and pelvic peritonitis. It is the most common gynecologic disorder necessitating hospitalization for female patients of reproductive age in the United States. Over 1 million females develop PID annually, 60,000 are hospitalized, and over 150,000 are evaluated in outpatient settings. The incidence is highest in the teen population. Teenage girls who are sexually active have a high risk (1 in 8) of developing PID, whereas women in their 20s have one-tenth the risk. Predisposing risk factors include multiple sexual partners, younger age of initiating sexual intercourse, prior history of PID, and lack of condom use. Lack of protective antibody from previous exposure to sexually transmitted organisms and cervical ectopy contribute to the development of PID. Many adolescents with subacute or asymptomatic disease are never identified.

PID is a polymicrobial infection. Causative agents include *N gonorrhoeae*, *Chlamydia*, anaerobic bacteria that reside in the vagina, and genital mycoplasmas. Vaginal douching and other mechanical factors such as an intrauterine device or prior gynecologic surgery increase the risk of PID by providing access of lower genital tract organisms to pelvic organs. Recent menses and bacterial vaginosis have been associated with the development of PID.

Clinical Findings

A. Symptoms and Signs

Acute PID is difficult to diagnose because of the wide variation in the symptoms and signs. No single historical, clinical, or laboratory finding has both high sensitivity and specificity for the diagnosis. Diagnosis of PID is usually made clinically (Table 44–2). Typical patients have lower abdominal pain, nausea, vomiting, and fever. However, the patient may be afebrile. Vaginal discharge is variable. Cervical motion tenderness, uterine or adnexal tenderness, or signs of peritonitis are often present. Mucopurulent cervicitis is present in 50% of patients. Tubo-ovarian abscesses can often be detected by careful physical examination (feeling a mass or fullness in the adnexa).

B. Laboratory Findings

Laboratory findings include elevated WBCs with a left shift and elevated acute phase reactants (erythrocyte sedimentation rate or C-reactive protein). A positive test for *N gonorrhoeae* or *C trachomatis* is supportive, although 25% of the time neither of these bacteria is detected. Pregnancy needs to be ruled out, because patients with an ectopic pregnancy can present with abdominal pain.

C. Diagnostic Studies

Laparoscopy is the gold standard for detecting salpingitis. It is used if the diagnosis is in question or to help differentiate PID from an ectopic pregnancy, ovarian cysts, or adnexal torsion. Endometrial biopsy should be performed in women undergoing laparoscopy who do not have visual evidence of salpingitis as some women may only have endometritis. The clinical diagnosis of PID has a positive predictive value for salpingitis of 65%–90% in comparison with laparoscopy. Pelvic ultrasonography also is helpful in detecting tubo-ovarian abscesses, which are found in almost 20% of teens with PID. Transvaginal ultrasound is more sensitive than abdominal ultrasound. All women who have acute PID should be tested for *N gonorrhoeae* and *C trachomatis* and should be screened for HIV infection.

Table 44–2. Diagnostic criteria for pelvic inflammatory disease.

Minimum criteria
Empiric treatment of PID should be initiated in sexually active young women and others at risk for sexually transmitted infections if one or more of the following minimum criteria are present:
• They are experiencing pelvic or lower abdominal pain and no other cause(s) for the illness can be identified
• Cervical motion tenderness or uterine tenderness or adnexal tenderness
Additional supportive criteria
Oral temperature > 38.3°C (101°F)
Abnormal cervical or vaginal mucopurulent discharge
Presence of white blood cells on microscopic evaluation of vaginal secretions diluted in saline
Elevated erythrocyte sedimentation rate or elevated C-reactive protein
Laboratory documentation of infection with *Neisseria gonorrhoeae* or *Chlamydia trachomatis*
Definitive criteria (selected cases)
Histopathologic evidence of endometritis on endometrial biopsy
Tubo-ovarian abscess on sonography or other radiologic tests
Laparoscopic abnormalities consistent with PID

Adapted, with permission, from Centers for Disease Control and Prevention: Sexually transmitted diseases treatment guidelines 2010. MMWR Recomm Rep 2010;59(RR-12).

Differential Diagnosis

Differential diagnosis includes other gynecologic illnesses (ectopic pregnancy, threatened or septic abortion, adnexal torsion, ruptured and hemorrhagic ovarian cysts, dysmenorrhea, endometriosis, or mittelschmerz), gastrointestinal illnesses (appendicitis, cholecystitis, hepatitis, gastroenteritis, or inflammatory bowel disease), and genitourinary illnesses (cystitis, pyelonephritis, or urinary calculi).

Complications

Scarring of the fallopian tubes is one of the major sequelae of PID. After one episode of PID, 17% of patients become infertile, 17% develop chronic pelvic pain, and 10% will have an ectopic pregnancy. Infertility rates increase with each episode of PID; three episodes of PID result in a 73% infertility rate. Duration of symptoms appears to be the largest determinant of infertility. Hematogenous or lymphatic spread of organisms from the fallopian tubes rarely causes Fitz-Hugh-Curtis syndrome. Inflammation of the liver capsule (perihepatitis) results in symptoms of right upper quadrant pain and elevation of liver function tests.

Treatment

The objectives of treatment are both to achieve a clinical cure and to prevent long-term sequelae. There are no differences in short- and long-term clinical and microbiologic response rates between parenteral and oral therapy. PID is frequently managed at the outpatient level, although some clinicians argue that all adolescents with PID should be hospitalized because of the rate of complications. Severe systemic symptoms and toxicity, signs of peritonitis, inability to take fluids, pregnancy, nonresponse or intolerance of oral antimicrobial therapy, and tubo-ovarian abscess favor hospitalization. In addition, if the health care provider believes that the patient will not adhere to treatment, hospitalization is warranted. Surgical drainage may be required for adequate treatment of tubo-ovarian abscesses.

The antibiotic regimens described in Table 44–1 are broad spectrum to cover the numerous microorganisms associated with PID. All treatment regimens should be effective against *N gonorrhoeae* and *C trachomatis* because negative endocervical screening tests do not rule out upper reproductive tract infection with these organisms. Outpatient treatment should be reserved for compliant patients who have classic signs of PID without systemic symptoms. Patients with PID who receive outpatient treatment should be reexamined within 24–48 hours, with phone contact in the interim, to detect persistent disease or treatment failure. Patients should have substantial improvement within 48–72 hours. An adolescent should be reexamined 7–10 days after the completion of therapy to ensure the resolution of symptoms.

Haggerty CL, Ness RB: Newest approaches to treatment of pelvic inflammatory disease: A review of recent randomized clinical trials. Clin Infect Dis 2007;44:953 [PMID: 17342647].

Sweet RL: Treatment strategies for pelvic inflammatory disease. Exp Opin Pharmacother 2009;10:823 [PMID: 19351231].

Trig BG, Kerndt PR, Aynalem G: Sexually transmitted infections and pelvic inflammatory disease in women. Med Clin North Am 2008;92:1083 [PMID: 18721654].

Walker CK, Wiesenfeld HC: Antibiotic therapy for acute pelvic inflammatory disease: The 2006 Centers for Disease Control and Prevention sexually transmitted diseases treatment guidelines. Clin Infect Dis 2007;44:S111 [PMID: 17342664].

URETHRITIS

General Considerations

The most common bacterial causes of urethritis in males are *N gonorrhoeae* and *C trachomatis*. Additionally, *T vaginalis*, HSV, *Ureaplasma urealyticum*, and *M genitalium* cause urethritis. Approximately 15%–25% of nongonococcal, nonchlamydial urethritis can be attributed both to *M genitalium* and *U urealyticum*. Coliforms may cause urethritis in males practicing insertive anal intercourse. Mechanical manipulation or contact with irritants can also cause transient urethritis. It is important to recognize that urethritis in both males and females is frequently asymptomatic.

Females often present with symptoms of a urinary tract infection and "sterile pyuria" (no enteric bacterial pathogens isolated), which reflects urethritis caused by the organisms described above.

Clinical Findings

A. Symptoms and Signs

If symptomatic, males present most commonly with a clear or purulent discharge from the urethra, dysuria, or urethral pruritus. Hematuria and inguinal adenopathy can occur. Most infections caused by *C trachomatis* and *T vaginalis* are asymptomatic, while 70% of males with *M genitalium* and 23%–90% with gonococcal urethritis are symptomatic.

B. Laboratory Findings

In a symptomatic male a positive leukocyte esterase test on first-void urine, or microscopic examination of first-void urine demonstrating more than 10 WBCs per high-power field, is suggestive of urethritis. Gram stain of urethral secretions demonstrating more than 5 WBCs per high-power field is also suggestive. Gonococcal urethritis is established by documenting the presence of WBCs containing intracellular gram-negative diplococci. Urethral swab or first-void urine for NAAT should be sent to the laboratory to detect *N gonorrhoeae* and *C trachomatis*. Evaluation for *T vaginalis* should be considered when the other test results are negative. Microscopic examination of urethral discharge is not a sensitive test. Specific PCR testing of urine is available for *Mycoplasma* and *Ureaplasma*, though it is not often clinically utilized.

Complications

Complications include recurrent or persistent urethritis, epididymitis, prostatitis, or Reiter syndrome.

Treatment (See Table 44–1)

Patients with objective evidence of urethritis should receive empiric treatment for gonorrhea and chlamydial infection, ideally directly observed in the office. Some data suggests better outcomes for treatment of *Mycoplasma genitalium* with azithromycin. If the infection is unresponsive to initial treatment and the infection is NAAT-negative, trichomoniasis should be ruled out and nongonococcal, nonchlamydial urethritis should be suspected and treated appropriately. Patients should be instructed to return for evaluation if symptoms persist or recur after completion of initial empiric therapy. Symptoms alone, without documentation of signs or laboratory evidence of urethral inflammation, are not a sufficient basis for retreatment. Sexual partners should either be evaluated or treated for gonorrhea and chlamydial infection.

Centers for Disease Control and Prevention. Sexually Transmitted Diseases Guidelines, 2010. MMWR 2010;59(RR-12):40–42 [PMID: 21160459].

Gaydos C et al: *Mycoplasma genitalium* compared to *Chlamydia*, gonorrhoea and *Trichomonas* as an aetiological agent of urethritis in men attending STD clinics. Sex Transm Infect 2009;85:438 [PMID: 19383597].

Mena LA et al: A randomized comparison of azithromycin and doxycycline for the treatment of *Mycoplasma genitalium*-positive urethritis in men. Clin Infect Dis 2009;48:1649 [PMID: 19438399].

EPIDIDYMITIS

General Considerations

Epididymitis in a male who is sexually active is most often caused by *C trachomatis* or *N gonorrhoeae*. Epididymitis caused by *Escherichia coli* occurs among males who are the insertive partners during anal intercourse and in males who have urinary tract abnormalities.

Clinical Findings

A. Symptoms and Signs

Epididymitis presents as a constellation of pain, swelling, and inflammation of the epididymis. In many cases, the testis is also involved.

B. Laboratory and Diagnostic Studies

Diagnosis is generally made clinically. Color Doppler ultrasound can help make the diagnosis. Although often not available, radionuclide scanning of the scrotum is the most accurate method of diagnosis. Laboratory evaluation is identical to evaluation for suspected urethritis.

Differential Diagnosis

Acute epididymitis must be distinguished from orchitis due to infarct, testicular torsion, viral infection, testicular cancer, tuberculosis, or fungal infection.

Complications

Infertility is rare, and chronic local pain is uncommon.

Treatment

Empiric therapy (see Table 44–1) is indicated before culture results are available. As an adjunct to therapy, bed rest, scrotal elevation, and analgesics are recommended until fever and local inflammation subside. Lack of improvement of swelling and tenderness within 3 days requires reevaluation of both the diagnosis and therapy. Sex partners should be evaluated and treated for gonorrhea and chlamydial infections.

Bohm MK, Gift TL, Tao G: Patterns of single and multiple claims of epididymitis among young privately-insured males in the United States, 2001 to 2004. Sex Transm Dis 2009;36:490 [PMID: 19455076].

Centers for Disease Control and Prevention: Sexually Transmitted Diseases Guidelines, 2010. MMWR 2010;59(RR-12):67–69 [PMID: 21160459].

PROCTITIS, PROCTOCOLITIS, & ENTERITIS

General Considerations

Proctitis occurs predominantly among persons who participate in anal intercourse. Enteritis occurs among those whose sexual practices include oral-fecal contact. Proctocolitis can be acquired by either route depending on the pathogen. Common sexually transmitted pathogens causing proctitis or proctocolitis include *C trachomatis* (including lymphogranuloma venereum [LGV] serovars), *Treponema pallidum*, HSV, *N gonorrhoeae*, *Giardia lamblia*, and enteric organisms. As many as 85% of rectal infections with *N gonorrhoeae* and *C trachomatis* are asymptomatic. The presence of symptomatic or asymptomatic proctitis may facilitate the transmission of HIV infection.

Clinical Findings

A. Symptoms and Signs

Proctitis, defined as inflammation limited to the distal 10–12 cm of the rectum, is associated with anorectal pain, tenesmus, and rectal discharge. Acute proctitis among persons who have recently practiced receptive anal intercourse is most often sexually transmitted. The symptoms of proctocolitis combine those of proctitis, plus diarrhea or abdominal cramps (or both), because of inflamed colonic mucosa more than 12 cm from the anus. Enteritis usually results in diarrhea and abdominal cramping without signs of proctitis or proctocolitis.

B. Laboratory and Diagnostic Studies

Evaluation may include anoscopy or sigmoidoscopy, stool examination, culture or NAAT for appropriate organisms, and serology for syphilis.

Treatment

Management will be determined by the etiologic agent. (See Table 44–1 and Chapter 42.) Reinfection may be difficult to distinguish from treatment failure.

Centers for Disease Control and Prevention: Sexually Transmitted Diseases Guidelines, 2010. MMWR 2010;59(RR-12):87–88 [PMID: 21160459].

Felt-Bersma RJ, Bartelsman JF: Haemorrhoids, rectal prolapse, anal fissure, peri-anal fistulae and sexually transmitted diseases. Best Pract Res Clin Gastroenterol 2009;23:575 [PMID: 19647691].

VAGINAL DISCHARGE

Adolescent girls may have a normal physiologic leukorrhea, secondary to turnover of vaginal epithelium. Infectious causes of discharge include *T vaginalis*, *C trachomatis*, *N gonorrhoeae*, and bacterial vaginosis pathogens. Candidiasis is a yeast infection that produces vaginal discharge, but is not usually sexually transmitted. Vaginitis is characterized by vaginal discharge, vulvar itching, and irritation, and sometimes with vaginal odor. Discharge may be white, gray, or yellow. Physiologic leukorrhea is usually white, homogeneous, and not associated with itching, irritation, or foul odor. Mechanical, chemical, allergic, or other noninfectious irritants of the vagina may cause vaginal discharge.

1. Bacterial Vaginosis

General Considerations

Bacterial vaginosis is a polymicrobial infection of the vagina caused by an imbalance of the normal bacterial vaginal flora. The altered flora has a paucity of hydrogen peroxide–producing lactobacilli and increased concentrations of anaerobic bacteria (*Mobiluncus* sp), and *Gardnerella vaginalis, Ureaplasma,* and *Mycoplasma.* It is unclear whether bacterial vaginosis is sexually transmitted, but it is associated with having multiple sex partners and women with bacterial vaginosis are at increased risk for other STIs.

Clinical Findings

A. Symptoms and Signs

The most common symptom is a copious, malodorous, homogeneous thin gray-white vaginal discharge. Patients may report vaginal itching or dysuria. The fishy odor may be more noticeable after intercourse or during menses, when the high pH of blood or semen volatilizes the amines.

B. Laboratory Findings

Bacterial vaginosis is most often diagnosed by the use of clinical criteria, which include (1) presence of thin, white discharge that smoothly coats the vaginal walls, (2) fishy (amine) odor before or after the addition of 10% KOH (whiff test), (3) pH of vaginal fluid greater than 4.5 determined with narrow-range pH paper, and (4) presence of "clue cells" on microscopic examination. Clue cells are squamous epithelial cells that have multiple bacteria adhering to them, making their borders irregular and giving them a speckled appearance. Diagnosis requires three out of four criteria, although many female patients who fulfill these criteria have no discharge or other symptoms.

Complications

Bacterial vaginosis during pregnancy is associated with adverse outcomes such as premature labor, preterm delivery, intraamniotic infection, and postpartum endometritis. In the nonpregnant individual, it may be associated with PID and urinary tract infections.

Treatment

All female patients who have symptomatic disease should receive treatment to relieve vaginal symptoms and signs of infection (see Table 44–1). Pregnant patients should receive treatment to prevent adverse outcomes of pregnancy. Treatment for patients who do not complain of vaginal discharge or itching, but who demonstrate bacterial vaginosis on routine pelvic examination, is unclear. Because some studies associate bacterial vaginosis and PID, the recommendation is to have a low threshold for treating asymptomatic bacterial vaginosis. Follow-up visits are unnecessary if symptoms resolve. Recurrence of bacterial vaginosis is not unusual. Follow-up examination 1 month after treatment for high-risk pregnant patients is recommended.

Males do not develop infection equivalent to bacterial vaginosis and are often asymptomatic. Treatment of male partners has no effect on the course of infection in females although treatment is recommended for female partners.

Brotman RM et al: Findings associated with recurrence of bacterial vaginosis among adolescents attending sexually transmitted diseases clinics. J Pediatr Adolesc Gynecol 2007;20:225 [PMID: 17673134].

Fethers KA et al: Sexual risk factors and bacterial vaginosis: A systematic review and meta-analysis. Clin Infect Dis 2008;47:1426 [PMID: 18947329].

2. Trichomoniasis

General Considerations

Trichomoniasis is caused by *T vaginalis*, a flagellated protozoan that infects 5–7 million people annually in the United States.

Clinical Findings

A. Symptoms and Signs

Fifty percent of females with trichomoniasis develop a symptomatic vaginitis with vaginal itching, a green-gray malodorous frothy discharge, and dysuria. Occasionally postcoital bleeding and dyspareunia may be present. The vulva may be erythematous and the cervix friable.

B. Laboratory Findings

Mixing the discharge with normal saline facilitates detection of the flagellated protozoan on microscopic examination (wet preparation). This has a sensitivity of only 60%–70% even with immediate evaluation of the slide to achieve optimal results. Culture and PCR testing are available when the diagnosis is unclear. PCR tests are sensitive, but expensive, and not readily available. Two FDA-approved, point-of-care antigen-based detection assays for *T vaginalis* are available, but false positive results are problematic in low disease prevalence populations. Both antigen assays are performed on vaginal secretions and have a sensitivity greater than 83.3% and a specificity greater than 97%. Trichomonal urethritis frequently causes a positive urine leukocyte esterase test and WBCs on urethral smear.

Complications

Male partners of females diagnosed with trichomoniasis have a 22% chance of having trichomoniasis. Half of males with trichomoniasis will have urethritis. *Trichomonas* infection in females has been associated with adverse pregnancy outcomes. Rescreening for *T vaginalis* at 3 months following initial infection is recommended for women due to the high rate of reinfection.

Treatment

See Table 44–1 for treatment recommendations.

Nanda N et al: Trichomoniasis and its treatment. Expert Rev Anti Infect Ther 2006;4:125 [PMID: 16441214].

Pattullo L et al: Stepwise diagnosis of Trichomonas vaginalis infection in adolescent women. J Clin Microbiol 2009;47:59 [PMID: 18987174].

Wendel KA, Workowski KA: Trichomoniasis: Challenges to appropriate management. Clin Infect Dis 2007;44:S123 [PMID: 17342665].

3. Vulvovaginal Candidiasis

General Considerations

Vulvovaginal candidiasis is caused by *Candida albicans* in 85%–90% of cases. Most females will have at least one episode of vulvovaginal candidiasis in their lifetime, and almost half will have two or more episodes. The highest incidence is between ages 16 and 30 years. Predisposing factors include recent use of antibiotics, diabetes, pregnancy, and HIV. Risk factors include vaginal intercourse, especially with a new sexual partner, use of oral contraceptives, and use of spermicide. This disease is usually caused by unrestrained growth of *Candida* that normally colonizes the vagina asymptomatically or is infected secondarily from *Candida* present in the GI tract. Recurrences reflect reactivation of colonization.

Clinical Findings

A. Symptoms and Signs

Typical symptoms include pruritus and a white, cottage cheese-like vaginal discharge without odor. The itching is more common midcycle and shortly after menses. Other symptoms include vaginal soreness, vulvar burning, vulvar edema and redness, dyspareunia, and dysuria (especially after intercourse).

B. Laboratory Findings

The diagnosis is usually made by visualizing yeast or pseudohyphae with 10% KOH (90% sensitive) or Gram stain (77% sensitive) in the vaginal discharge. Fungal culture can be used if symptoms and microscopy are not definitive or if disease is unresponsive or recurrent. However, culture is not very specific as colonization is common in asymptomatic females. Vaginal pH is normal with yeast infections.

Complications

The only complication of vulvovaginal candidiasis is recurrent infections. Most females with recurrent infection have no apparent predisposing or underlying conditions.

Treatment

Short-course topical formulations effectively treat uncomplicated vaginal yeast infections (see Table 44–1). The topically applied azole drugs are more effective than nystatin. Treatment with azoles results in relief of symptoms and negative cultures in 80%–90% of patients who complete therapy. Oral fluconazole as a one-time dose is an effective oral treatment. Patients should be instructed to return for follow-up visits only if symptoms persist or recur. Six-month prophylaxis regimens have been effective in many female patients with persistent or recurrent yeast infection. Recurrent disease is usually due to *C albicans* that remains susceptible to azoles, and should be treated for 14 days with oral azoles. Some non-albicans *Candida* will respond to itraconazole or boric acid gelatin capsules (600 mg daily for 14 days) intravaginally. Treatment of sex partners is not recommended, but may be considered for females who have recurrent infection.

GENITAL ULCERATIONS

In the United States, young, sexually active patients who have genital ulcers have genital herpes or syphilis. The relative frequency of each disease differs by geographic area and patient population; however, in most areas, genital herpes is the most prevalent of these diseases. More than one of these diseases could be present in a patient with genital ulcers. All ulcerative diseases are associated with an increased risk for HIV infection. Oral and genital lesions may be presenting symptoms during primary HIV infection (acute retroviral syndrome). Less common causes of genital ulceration include chancroid and donovanosis.

Location of the ulcers is dependent on the specific type of sexual behavior. Ulcers may be vaginal, vulvar, cervical, penile, or rectal. Oral lesions may occur concomitantly with genital ulcerations or as stand-alone lesions in HSV infection and syphilis. Each etiologic agent has specific characteristics that are described in the following sections. Lesion pain, inguinal lymphadenopathy, and urethritis may be found in association with the ulcers.

1. Herpes Simplex Virus Infection

General Considerations

HSV is the most common cause of visible genital ulcers. HSV-1 and HSV-2 are viruses that infect primarily humans. HSV-1 is commonly associated with infections of the face, including the eyes, pharynx, and mouth. HSV-2 is most commonly associated with anogenital infections. However, each serotype is capable of infecting either region. HSV-1 infections are frequently established in children by age 5; lower socioeconomic groups have higher infection rates. Both HSV-1 and HSV-2 are STIs. The prevalence of both infections in the United States increases during teen years. Rates of HSV-2 seroprevalence reach 20%–40% in 40-year-olds. HSV infections are chronic as a result of latent infection of sensory ganglia. Latent infection is life long, although many individuals infected with HSV-2 infections have not been diagnosed or have had mild or unrecognized symptoms. Nevertheless, these individuals can still asymptomatically shed virus and thereby unknowingly transmit the infection, and they can reactivate the virus to cause clinical infection in themselves.

Clinical Findings

A. Symptoms and Signs

Symptomatic initial genital HSV infection causes vesicles of the vulva, vagina, cervix, penis, rectum, or urethra, which are quickly followed by shallow, painful ulcerations. Atypical presentation of HSV infection includes vulvar erythema and fissures. Urethritis may occur. Initial infection can be severe, lasting up to 3 weeks, and be associated with fever and malaise, as well as localized tender adenopathy. The pain and dysuria can be extremely uncomfortable, requiring sitz baths, topical anesthetics, and occasionally catheterization for urinary retention.

Symptoms tend to be more severe in females. Recurrence in the genital area with HSV-2 is likely (65%–90%). Approximately 40% of individuals infected with HSV-2 will experience more than or equal to six recurrences per year in the early years after initial infection. Prodromal pain in the genital, buttock, or pelvic region is common prior to recurrences. Recurrent genital herpes is of shorter duration (5–7 days), with fewer lesions and usually no systemic symptoms. Commonly, there is decreased frequency and severity of recurrences over time, although approximately one-third of individuals fail to demonstrate this time-dependent improvement. First-episode genital herpes infection caused by HSV-1 is usually the consequence of oral-genital sex. Primary HSV-1 infection is as severe as HSV-2 infection, and treatment is the same. Recurrence of HSV-1 happens in less than 50% of patients, and the frequency of recurrences is much less than in those patients with prior HSV-2 infection.

B. Laboratory Findings

Diagnosis of genital HSV infection is often made presumptively, but in one large series this diagnosis was incorrect for 20% of cases. Several laboratory tests can aid in confirmation of the diagnosis. Viral culture has been the gold standard and can provide results in as few as 48 hours. Culture must be obtained by unroofing an active vesicle and swabbing the base of the lesion. DFA testing can provide results within hours. DFA can also determine serotype, which is important for prognosis. NAAT of viral DNA is becoming a more common diagnostic method.

Differential Diagnosis

Genital HSV infections must be distinguished from other ulcerative STI lesions, including syphilis, chancroid, and lymphogranuloma venereum. Non-STIs might include herpes zoster, Behçet syndrome, or lichen sclerosis. (See next sections on Syphilis and Chancroid.)

Complications

Complications, almost always with the first episode of genital HSV infection, include viral meningitis, urinary retention, transmission to newborns at birth, and pharyngitis. Infection with genital HSV, whether active or not, greatly increases the likelihood of transmitting or acquiring HIV infection within couples discordant for HIV.

Prevention

All patients with active lesions should be counseled to abstain from sexual contact. Almost all patients have very frequent periodic asymptomatic shedding of HSV, and most cases of genital HSV infection are transmitted by persons who are unaware that they have the infection or are asymptomatic when transmission occurs. Reactivation with asymptomatic shedding occurs even in individuals who were asymptomatically infected. Individuals with prior HSV infection should be encouraged to use condoms to protect susceptible partners. Antiviral prophylaxis of infected individuals reduces shedding and significantly reduces the chance of transmission to their sexual partners.

Treatment

Antiviral drugs administered within the first 5 days of primary infection decrease the duration and severity of HSV infection (see Table 44–1). The effect of antivirals on the severity or duration of recurrent disease is limited. For best results, therapy should be started with the prodrome or during the first day of the attack. Patients should have a prescription at home to initiate treatment. If recurrences are frequent and cause significant physical or emotional discomfort, patients may elect to take antiviral prophylaxis on a daily basis to reduce the frequency (70%–80% decrease) and duration of recurrences. Treatment of first or subsequent attacks will not prevent future attacks, but recurrence frequency and severity decrease in many individuals over time.

Centers for Disease Control and Prevention: Sexually Transmitted Diseases Guidelines, 2010. MMWR 2010;59(RR-12):20–25 [PMID: 21160459].

Cernik C, Gallina K, Brodell RT: The treatment of herpes simplex infections: An evidence-based review. Arch Intern Med 2008;168:1137 [PMID: 18541820].

Chayavichitsilp P et al: Herpes simplex. Pediatr Rev 2009;119 [PMID: 19339385].

2. Syphilis

General Considerations

Syphilis is an acute and chronic STI caused by infection with *T pallidum*. The national rate of syphilis has increased annually since reaching an all time low in 2000. Increases have been observed in both genders, but predominantly in males who have sex with men, who now account for 62% of primary and secondary cases reported to the CDC. In 2009, the number of syphilis cases reached almost 14,000, nearly a 4% increase from the previous year. Men between the ages of 15–24 years have the highest rates of syphilis.

Clinical Findings

A. Symptoms and Signs

Skin and mucous membrane lesions characterize the acute phase of primary and secondary syphilis. Lesions of the bone, viscera, aorta, and central nervous system predominate in the chronic phase (tertiary syphilis) (see Chapter 42). Prevention of syphilis is also important because syphilitic mucosal lesions facilitate transmission of HIV.

Primary syphilis usually presents as a solitary chancre at the point of inoculum. Characteristically, the chancre presents as a painless, indurated, nonpurulent ulcer with a clean base and associated nontender, firm adenopathy. The chancre appears on average 21 days (range: 3–90 days) after exposure and resolves spontaneously 4–8 weeks later. Because it is painless, it may go undetected, especially if the lesion is within the vagina, oropharynx, urethra, or rectum. Chancres may occur on the genitalia, anus, or oropharynx. Secondary syphilis occurs 4–10 weeks after the chancre appears, with generalized malaise, adenopathy, and a nonpruritic maculopapular rash that often includes the palms and soles. Secondary syphilis resolves in 1–3 months, but can recur. Verrucous lesions known as condylomata lata may develop on the genitalia. These must be distinguished from genital warts.

B. Laboratory Findings

If the patient has a suspect primary lesion, is at high risk, is a contact, or may have secondary syphilis, a nontreponemal serum screen—either RPR or VDRL—should be performed. If the nontreponemal test is positive, then a specific treponemal test—a fluorescent treponemal antibody-absorbed (FTAABS) or microhemagglutination-*T pallidum* (MHA-TP) test—is done to confirm the diagnosis. An additional diagnostic tool is darkfield microscopy, which can be used to detect spirochetes in scrapings of the chancre base. Darkfield examinations and DFA tests of lesion exudate or tissue are the definitive methods for diagnosing early syphilis.

If a patient is engaging in high-risk sexual behavior or is living in an area in which syphilis is endemic, RPRs should be drawn yearly to screen for asymptomatic infection. Annual RPR testing among high-risk groups is essential to distinguish between early latent syphilis (1 year or less post-infection), late latent syphilis (> 1 year postinfection), or syphilis of unknown duration, as treatment recommendations vary. Syphilis is reportable to state health departments, and all sexual contacts need to be evaluated. Patients also need to be evaluated for other STIs, especially HIV, because HIV-infected patients have increased rates of failure with some treatment regimens.

Complications

Untreated syphilis can lead to tertiary complications with serious multiorgan involvement, including aortitis and neurosyphilis. Transmission to the fetus can occur from an untreated pregnant individual (see Chapters 2 and 42).

Treatment

See Table 44–1 for treatment recommendations. Patients should be reexamined clinically and serologically with nontreponemal tests at 6 and 12 months after treatment. If signs or symptoms persist or recur, or patients do not have a fourfold decrease in their nontreponemal test titer, they should be considered to have failed treatment or be reinfected and need retreatment.

Centers for Disease Control and Prevention: *2009 Sexually Transmitted Diseases Surveillance*. Atlanta, GA: U.S. Department of Health and Human Services, Centers for Disease Control and Prevention. Available at: http://www.cdc.gov/std/stats09/Syphilis.htm. Accessed September 10, 2011.

Kent ME, Romanelli F: Reexamining syphilis: An update on epidemiology, clinical manifestations, and management. Ann Pharmacother 2008;42:226 [PMID: 18212261].

3. Chancroid

General Considerations

Chancroid is caused by *Haemophilus ducreyi*. It is relatively rare outside of the tropics and subtropics, but is endemic in some urban areas in the United States, and has been associated with HIV infection, drug use, and prostitution. A detailed history, including travel, may prove to be important in identifying this infection.

Clinical Findings

A. Symptoms and Signs

The typical lesion begins as a papule that erodes after 24–48 hours into an ulcer. The ulcer is painful and has ragged, sharply demarcated edges and a purulent base (unlike syphilis). The ulcer is typically solitary and somewhat deeper than HSV infection. The lesions may occur anywhere on the genitals and are more common in men than in women. Tender, fluctuant (unlike syphilis and HSV) inguinal adenopathy is present in 50% of patients. A painful ulcer in combination with suppurative inguinal adenopathy is very often chancroid.

B. Laboratory Findings

Gram stain shows gram-positive cocci arranged in a boxcar formation. Culture, which has a sensitivity of less than 80%, can be performed on a special medium that is available in academic centers. PCR testing may improve laboratory diagnosis in areas where such testing is available.

Differential Diagnosis

Chancroid is distinguished from syphilis by the painful nature of the ulcer and the associated tender suppurative adenopathy. HSV vesicles often produce painful ulcers, but these are multiple, smaller, and shallower than chancroid ulcers. Adenopathy associated with initial HSV infection does not suppurate. A presumptive diagnosis of chancroid should be considered in a patient with typical painful genital ulcers and regional adenopathy when the test results for syphilis and HSV are negative.

Treatment

Symptoms improve within 3 days after therapy (see Table 44–1). Most ulcers resolve in 7 days, although large ulcers may take 2 weeks to heal. All sexual contacts need to be examined and given treatment, even if asymptomatic. Individuals with HIV coinfection may have slower rates of healing or treatment failures.

Centers for Disease Control and Prevention: Sexually Transmitted Diseases Guidelines, 2010. MMWR 2010;59(RR-12):19–20 [PMID: 21160459].

Kaliaperumal K: Recent advances in management of genital ulcer disease and anogenital warts. Dermatol Ther 2008;21:196 [PMID: 18564250].

4. Lymphogranuloma Venereum

General Considerations

Lymphogranuloma venereum (LGV), caused by *C trachomatis* serovars L1, L2, or L3, is generally rare in the United States. The disease is endemic in Southeast Asia, the Caribbean, Latin America, and areas of Africa. Since 2003, an increased number of cases in the United States, Western Europe, and Canada have occurred primarily among men who have sex with men and have been associated with HIV coinfection.

Clinical Findings

A. Symptoms and Signs

Patients with LGV present with a painless vesicle or ulcer that heals spontaneously, followed by development of tender adenopathy, either unilateral or bilateral. A classic finding is the groove sign—an inguinal crease created by concomitant involvement of inguinal and femoral nodes. These nodes become matted and fluctuant and may rupture. LGV can cause proctocolitis with rectal ulceration, purulent anal discharge, fever, tenesmus, and lower abdominal pain, primarily in men who have sex with men.

B. Laboratory Findings

Diagnosis of LGV can be difficult. It generally requires a clinical suspicion based on physical examination findings. Lesion swabs and lymph node aspirates can be tested for *Chlamydia* by culture, DFA, or nucleic acid amplification. NAAT is not FDA cleared for rectal specimens. Additional genotyping is necessary to differentiate LGV from non-LGV serovars of *Chlamydia*. In the absence of laboratory testing to confirm the diagnosis, one should treat for LGV if clinical suspicion is high.

Differential Diagnosis

Differential diagnosis during the adenopathy phase includes bacterial adenitis, lymphoma, and cat-scratch disease. Differential diagnosis during the ulcerative phase encompasses all causes of genital ulcers.

Treatment

See Table 44–1 for treatment recommendations. Despite effectiveness of azithromycin for non-LGV chlamydial infections, there have been no controlled treatment trials to recommend its use in LGV. HIV-infected individuals are treated the same as non-HIV infected individuals, but should be monitored closely to assess response to treatment.

McLean CA, Stoner BP, Workowski KA: Treatment of lymphogranuloma venereum. Clin Infect Dis 2007;44(Suppl 3):S147 [PMID: 17342667].

Richardson D, Goldmeier D: Lymphogranuloma venereum: An emerging cause of proctitis in men who have sex with men. Int J STD AIDS 2007;18:11 [PMID: 17326855].

White JA: Manifestations and management of lymphogranuloma venereum. Curr Opin Infect Dis 2009;22:57 [PMID: 19532081].

5. Other Ulcerations

Granuloma inguinale, or donovanosis, is caused by *Klebsiella granulomatis*, a gram-negative bacillus that is rare in the United States, but is endemic in India, the Caribbean, and southern Africa. An indurated subcutaneous nodule erodes to form a painless, friable ulcer with granulation tissue. Diagnosis is based on clinical suspicion and supported by a Wright or Giemsa stain of the granulation tissue that reveals intracytoplasmic rods (Donovan bodies) in mononuclear cells. See Table 44–1 for treatment recommendations. Relapse may occur 6–18 months even following effective treatment with a 3-week course of doxycycline.

Kaliaperumal K: Recent advances in management of genital ulcer disease and anogenital warts. Dermatol Ther 2008;21:196 [PMID: 18564250].

GENITAL WARTS & HUMAN PAPILLOMAVIRUS

General Considerations

Condylomata acuminata, or genital warts, are caused by HPV, which can also cause cervical dysplasia and cervical cancer. HPV is transmitted sexually. An estimated 20 million people are infected annually with HPV, including approximately more than 9 million sexually active adolescents and young adults 15–24 years of age. The majority (74%) of new HPV infections occurs among those 15–24 years of age;

in females younger than age 25 years, the prevalence ranges between 28% and 46%. It is estimated that 32%–50% of adolescent females having sexual intercourse in the United States have HPV infections, though only 1% may have visible lesions. Thirty to 60% of males whose partners have HPV have evidence of condylomata on examination. An estimated 1 million new cases of genital warts occur every year in the United States.

Although there are almost 100 serotypes of HPV, types 6 and 11 cause approximately 90% of genital warts, and HPV types 16 and 18 cause more than 70% of cervical dysplasia and cervical cancer. The infection is more common in persons with multiple partners and in those who initiate sexual intercourse at an early age.

Pap smears should be obtained by age 21. Thereafter, annual cervical screening should be performed using conventional Pap smears. Sexually active HIV-infected should have Pap smears as soon as they become sexually active if that is before age 21.

Clinical Findings

A. Symptoms and Signs

For males, verrucous lesions are found on the shaft or corona of the penis. Lesions also may develop in the urethra or rectum. Lesions do not produce discomfort. They may be single or found in clusters. Females develop verrucous lesions on any genital mucosal surface, either internally or externally, and often develop perianal lesions.

B. Laboratory Findings

External, visible lesions have unique characteristics that make the diagnosis straightforward. Condylomata acuminata can be distinguished from condylomata lata (syphilis), skin tags, and molluscum contagiosum by application of 5% acetic acid solution. Acetowhitening is used to indicate the extent of cervical infection.

Pap smears detect cervical abnormalities. HPV infection is the most frequent cause of an abnormal smear. Pap smear findings are graded by the atypical nature of the cervical cells. These changes range from atypical squamous cells of undetermined significance (ASCUS) to low-grade squamous intraepithelial lesions (LSIL) and high-grade squamous intraepithelial lesions (HSIL). LSIL encompasses cellular changes associated with HPV and mild dysplasia. HSIL includes moderate dysplasia, severe dysplasia, and carcinoma in situ.

Follow-up for ASCUS is controversial, as only 25% progress to dysplasia, and the remainder are unchanged or regress. New recommendations suggest repeat cytology in 12 months and no HPV testing. If the HPV test is performed, then the result should not be used for deciding upon colposcopy, and patients should be observed with annual cytology for up to a period of 2 years. If the grade of the atypical squamous cells remains uncertain or if there is HSIL, colposcopy is recommended. If LSIL is detected, colposcopy is not needed, but a repeat Pap smear should be done in 1 year, and if LSIL or HSIL are subsequently detected, the patient should be referred for colposcopy for direct visualization or biopsy of the cervix (or both). If a Pap smear shows signs of inflammation only, and concomitant infection such as vaginitis or cervicitis is present, the smear should be repeated after the inflammation has cleared.

Differential Diagnosis

The differential diagnosis includes normal anatomic structures (pearly penile papules, vestibular papillae, and sebaceous glands), molluscum contagiosum, seborrheic keratosis, and syphilis.

Complications

Because genital warts can proliferate and become friable during pregnancy, many experts advocate their removal during pregnancy. HPV types 6 and 11 can cause laryngeal papillomatosis in infants and children. Complications of appropriate treatment include scarring with changes in skin pigmentation or pain at the treatment site. Pap smears with persistent or high-grade dysplasia require biopsy and/or resection, which may result in cervical abnormalities that complicate pregnancy. Cervical cancer is the most common and important sequelae of HPV.

Prevention

The use of condoms significantly reduces, but does not eliminate, the risk for transmission to uninfected partners. The quadrivalent HPV vaccine is 96%–100% effective in preventing HPV-6 and 11–related genital warts and HPV-16 and 18–related cervical dysplasia. It is recommended for girls and women aged 9–26 years and approved for males aged 9–26 years. Males are protected against genital warts, and anal cancer, which has a significantly increased incidence in males who practice anal sex. The bivalent HPV vaccine is greater than 93% effective in preventing HPV-16 and 18–related cervical dysplasia. It is recommended only for girls aged 10–25 years. (See Chapter 10.)

Treatment

Penile and external vaginal or vulvar lesions can be treated topically. Treatment may need to occur weekly for 4–6 weeks. An experienced practitioner should treat internal and cervical lesions (see Table 44–1). Treatment may clear the visible lesions, but not reduce the presence of virus, nor is it clear whether transmission of HPV is reduced by treatment.

Warts may resolve or remain unchanged if left untreated or they may increase in size or number. Treatment can induce wart-free periods in most patients. Most recurrences occur within the 3 months following completion of a treatment regimen. Appropriate follow-up of abnormal Pap smears is essential to detect any progression to malignancy.

Centers for Disease Control and Prevention: Quadrivalent human papillomavirus vaccine: Recommendations of the Advisory Committee on Immunization Practices (ACIP). MMWR Morb Mortal Wkly Rep 2007;56:1 [PMID: 17380109].

Hager WD: Human papilloma virus infection and prevention in the adolescent population. J Pediatr Adoles Gynecol 2009;22:197 [PMID: 19481480].

Moscicki AB: Management of adolescents who have abnormal cytology and histology. Obstet Gynecol Clin North Am 2008;35:633 [PMID: 19061822].

ASCCP Consensus Guidelines for Management of Abnormal Cervical Cytology: http://www.asccp.org/ConsensusGuidelines/AbnormalCervicalScreeningTests/tabid/5958/Default.aspx. Accessed September 15, 2011.

OTHER VIRAL INFECTIONS

1. Hepatitis (See also Chapter 22)

General Considerations

In the United States, viral hepatitis is linked primarily to three viruses: Hepatitis A (HAV); Hepatitis B (HBV); and Hepatitis C (HCV). Each virus has the potential to be spread through sexual activity. HAV is spread via fecal-oral transmission and oral-anal contact. Both HBV and HCV are spread through contact with blood or body fluids. Sexual transmission of HBV is believed to be much more efficient than that of HCV.

Universal immunization recommendations for HAV and HBV have contributed to the decline in prevalence of these diseases. However, individuals born before implementation of routine vaccination, especially those in high-risk groups (multiple sexual partners or men who have sex with men), should receive vaccination.

Daniels D, Grytdal S, Wasley A: Surveillance for acute viral hepatitis—United States, 2007. MMWR Surveill Summ 2009 May 22;58(3):1–27 [PMID: 19478727].

2. Human Immunodeficiency Virus (See also Chapter 41)

General Considerations

Approximately, 35% of the 42,800 newly diagnosed HIV-infections occurring in 2009 in the United States are in youth and young adults aged 13–29 years. Because of the long latency period between infection with HIV and progression to AIDS, it is felt that many HIV-positive young adults contracted HIV during adolescence. CDC prevalence data indicate that young men who have sex with men continue to be the highest-risk group, particularly young men of color. Young women account for approximately one-third of the infections in this age group with Black and Hispanic women bearing a disproportionate burden of the disease. Risk factors for contracting HIV include a prior STI, infrequent condom use, practicing insertive or receptive anal sex (both males and females), prior genital HSV infection, practicing survival sex (ie, trading sex for money or drugs), intravenous drug or crack cocaine use, crystal methamphetamine use, homelessness, and being the victim of sexual abuse (males).

HIV infection should be considered in all sexually active youth, whether they have sex with males, females, or both. The CDC recommends that all sexually active individuals older than 13 be offered HIV testing at least once. Individual risk factors should then be used to determine the frequency of repeat testing. Opportunities for HIV screening in adolescents should include STI screening or treatment, pregnancy testing, or routine health evaluations. Most states allow adolescents to consent to HIV testing and treatment, but providers should be aware of their particular State's laws.

Clinical Findings

A. Symptoms and Signs

Adolescents may be asymptomatic with recent HIV infection or may present with the acute retroviral syndrome, which is evident 2–6 weeks after exposure. The acute clinical syndrome, present in about 50% of patients, is generally indistinguishable from other viral illnesses with respect to fever, malaise, and upper respiratory symptoms. Distinguishing features include generalized lymphadenopathy, rash, oral and genital ulcerations, aseptic meningitis, and thrush.

After the acute illness, signs and symptoms may be absent for many years.

B. Laboratory Findings

If acute HIV infection is suspected, HIV testing should be done by HIV RNA PCR testing or HIV DNA PCR testing. Routine serological testing may not be positive for 6 weeks or longer. Viral load values of less than 10,000 copies/mL by RNA PCR may indicate a false positive in this setting and repeat testing would be indicated.

Routine HIV screening may be conducted either by blood or by oral fluids. The testing relies on ELISA screening and a positive ELISA test must be confirmed by Western Blot testing. These methods have high degrees of sensitivity and specificity, but positive predictive values rely on underlying prevalence in individual communities.

Treatment

The most important aspect of identifying adolescents and young adults with HIV infection is linking them to care. Data support the treatment of youth with HIV infection in care settings that provide comprehensive, multidisciplinary care.

These settings will be best equipped to provide emotional support, preventative care, access to research, and guidance on the appropriate timing of antiretroviral therapies.

Centers for Disease Control and Prevention: Sexually Transmitted Diseases Guidelines, 2010. MMWR 2010;59(RR-12):14–18 [PMID: 21160459].

Simpkins EP, Siberry GK, Hutton N: Thinking about HIV infection. Pediatr Rev 2009;30:337 [PMID: 19726700].

3. HIV Post-Sexual Exposure Prophylaxis

Adolescents may present to health care providers seeking post-exposure prophylaxis (nPEP) following an assault or a high-risk sexual encounter. The risk of acquiring HIV infection through sexual assault or abuse is low but present. The risk for HIV transmission from a positive contact per episode of receptive penile-anal sexual exposure is estimated at 0.5%–3%; the risk per episode of receptive vaginal exposure is estimated at less than 0.1%–0.2%. HIV transmission also occurs from receptive oral exposure, but the risk is unknown. The risk of HIV transmission may be increased in certain conditions: trauma, including bleeding, with vaginal, anal, or oral penetration; site of exposure to ejaculate; HIV viral load in ejaculate; duration of HIV infection in the assailant or partner; and presence of an STI, prior genital HSV infection, or genital lesions in either partner.

Health care providers that consider offering PEP should take into account the likelihood that exposure to HIV occurred, the potential benefits and risks of such therapy, and the interval between the exposure and initiation of therapy. It will be helpful to know the HIV status of the sexual contact. The CDC provides an algorithm for consideration of PEP. In general, PEP is not recommended when more than 72 hours have passed since exposure. If the patient decides to take PEP, clinical management should be implemented according to published CDC guidelines. Providers should be aware that structural barriers exist to obtaining PEP, and that adolescent assault victims have a high discontinuation rate due to adverse effects from the medication.

Bryant J, Baxter L, Hird S: Non-occupational postexposure prophylaxis for HIV: A systematic review. Health Technol Assess 2009;13:1 [PMID: 19236820].

Centers for Disease Control and Prevention: Antiretroviral postexposure prophylaxis after sexual, injection-drug use, or other nonoccupational exposure to HIV in the United States: Recommendations from the U.S. Department of Health and Human Services. MMWR Recomm Rep 2005;54(RR-2) [PMID: 15660015].

Neu N et al: Postexposure prophylaxis for HIV in children and adolescents after sexual assault: A prospective observational study in an urban medical center. Sex Transm Dis 2007;34:65 [PMID: 16794560].

ECTOPARASITIC INFECTIONS

1. Pubic Lice

Pthirus pubis, the pubic louse, lives in pubic hair. The louse or the nits can be transmitted by close contact from person to person. Patients complain of itching and they may report having seen the insect. Examination of the pubic hair may reveal the louse crawling around or attached to the hair. Closer inspection may reveal the nit or sac of eggs, which is a gelatinous material (1–2 mm) stuck to the hair shaft. See Table 44–1 for treatment recommendations.

2. Scabies

Sarcoptes scabiei, the causative organism in scabies, is smaller than the louse. It can be identified by the classic burrow, which is created by the organism laying eggs and traveling just below the skin surface. Scabies can be sexually transmitted by close skin-to-skin contact and can be found in the pubic region, groin, lower abdomen, or upper thighs. The rash is intensely pruritic, especially at night, erythematous, and scaly.

See Table 44–1 for treatment options. Ivermectin is an oral therapeutic option for scabies that may hold particular promise in the treatment of severe infestations or in epidemic situations. When treating with lotion or shampoo, the entire area needs to be covered for the time specified by the manufacturer. One treatment usually clears the infestation, although a second treatment may be necessary. Bed sheets and clothes must be washed in hot water. Both sexual and close personal or household contacts within the preceding month should be examined and treated.

Hicks MI, Elston DM: Scabies. Dermatol Ther 2009;22:279 [PMID: 19580575].

Leone PA: Scabies and pediculosis pubis: An update of treatment regimens and general review. Clin Infect Dis 2007;44:S153 [PMID: 17342668].

REFERENCES

Centers for Disease Control and Prevention: Sexually transmitted diseases treatment guidelines 2010. MMWR Recomm Rep 2010;59(RR-12):1 [PMID: 21160459]. Available at: http://www.cdc.gov/std/treatment

Erb T, Beigi RH: Update on infectious diseases in adolescent gynecology. J Pediatr Adolesc Gyn 2008;21:135 [PMID: 18549965].

Sanfilippo JS, Lara-Torre E: Adolescent gynecology. Obstet Gyn 2009;113:935 [PMID: 19305342].

Trigg BG, Kerndt PR, Aynalem G: Sexually transmitted infections and pelvic inflammatory disease in women. Med Clin North Am 2008;92:1083 [PMID: 18721654].

Workowski KA, Berman SA: Centers for Disease Control and Prevention sexually transmitted diseases treatment guidelines. Clin Infect Dis 2007;44:S73 [PMID: 17342670].

45 Travel Medicine

Suchitra Rao, MBBS
Sarah K. Parker, MD

INTRODUCTION

Twenty-seven million people from the United States travel internationally per year; one-third of them travel to developing nations. Fifty to seventy percent of travelers become ill during their travel overseas. The number of children traveling with families continues to increase. Children are usually more susceptible to infectious diseases, trauma, and other health problems, which vary with the destination. Preparation for travel with children and infants includes consideration of the destination-specific risks, underlying medical problems, and administration of both routine and travel-related vaccines. The physician involved in pretravel counseling should focus on the issues listed in Table 45–1.

PREPARING CHILDREN AND INFANTS FOR TRAVEL

Travel Plans

Parents and care providers should be advised that travel with children and infants is much more enjoyable when the number of journeys in a single trip is limited; travel time is kept relatively short; and travel delays are anticipated. Planning for delays and other problems should include bringing new or favorite toys or games for distraction, and carrying extra food and drink, changes of clothing, and fever medications.

Medical Care During Travel

It is useful to obtain the names and addresses of local health care providers at the family's destination. This is available from travel medicine practitioners or from the membership directory of the International Society of Travel Medicine. The International Association for Medical Assistance to Travelers web site (www.iamat.org) is another useful resource with a worldwide directory of providers proficient in English. Travel insurance is highly encouraged. Insurance providers not only cover medical care at the destination, but provide 24-hour help lines with information regarding English-speaking physicians and hospitals, and can arrange and pay for evacuation to a medical facility that provides necessary treatment if not available locally. In emergencies, parents and caretakers should take their children to the largest medical facility in the area, which is more likely to have a pediatric unit and trauma services.

Trauma

Trauma is the most common cause of morbidity and mortality in traveling children. Parents should rent larger, safer vehicles, and should use car seats whenever possible. However, in many developing countries, car seats are not available, so caretakers may need to travel with their own. Taxis often do not have seatbelts, so it may be necessary to request taxis with seatbelts by calling in advance.

Air Travel

Healthy term infants can travel by commercial pressurized airplane. Children at higher risk during air travel may include premature infants and those with chronic cardiac or pulmonary disease, so appropriate counseling with their specialist is indicated. Many parents request advice regarding sedation of their child during travel, and while not recommended, the most widely used agent is diphenhydramine. It is advisable to try a test dose prior to travel as idiosyncratic reactions and overdosing leading to an anticholinergic syndrome or a paradoxical stimulating effect can occur.

Ear Pain

Children and infants often have pain during ascent and descent of commercial airplanes due to changes in middle ear pressure causing retraction or protrusion of the tympanic membrane. Methods said to alleviate or minimize ear pain during these times include chewing, swallowing, nursing, and bottle feeding.

Table 45–1. Preparing for travel—issues specific to travel as indicated.

Vaccinations (indications, safety, and tolerability)
Insect precautions (use of protective clothing, repellants, bed nets, insecticides)
Malaria chemoprophylaxis (benefits of a particular regimen vs potential adverse reactions)
Food and water precautions and environmental risks from water-borne disease
Traveler's diarrhea and self-treatment
Health insurance/Evacuation insurance
Trauma prevention and car seats
Access to medical care during travel
Altitude sickness
Disease outbreaks in destination
Climate
Jetlag
Animal exposure, trauma from animals
General health and routine illness
Clothing and footwear
Copies of prescriptions, vaccination documentation, physician's letter, list of medications
Travel-specific medications
Safe sex counseling
First aid kits
Crime and safety

Motion Sickness

Almost 60% of children will experience motion sickness during travel. While older children have symptoms similar to those in adults (such as nausea, epigastric discomfort, headache, general discomfort), children less than 5 years of age may have gait abnormalities as the predominant symptom. Nonpharmacologic strategies include eating a light meal at least 3 hours before travel; avoiding dairy products and foods high in calories, protein, and sodium before travel; sitting in the middle of the back seat or in the front seat if age-appropriate; focusing on a stable object or the horizon; avoiding reading or other visual stimuli; eye closure; fresh air; and limiting excessive head movement. Pharmacologic intervention has not been well studied in children, but if necessary, antihistamines such as diphenhydramine is recommended in children less than 12 years of age, and scopolamine is acceptable for children older than 12 years of age. These measures, however, are not evidence-based.

High Altitude

Acute mountain sickness is as common in children as in adults, but may go unrecognized due to its subtle presentation, such as unexplained fussiness or change in appetite and sleep patterns. High-altitude pulmonary edema (HAPE) is seen in children traveling to high altitudes; it also occurs in children who live at high altitude, descend for a period of time, and return to altitude. Mild symptoms of altitude sickness can be treated with rest and hydration, or analgesics such as ibuprofen or acetaminophen. Acetazolamide has not been studied in children for acute mountain sickness, but is safe in this age group, and is used for both prophylaxis and treatment. The recommended dose is 5 mg/kg/day (125 mg maximum) divided twice daily, starting 1 day before ascent, and continued for 2 days at high altitude.

Medications/First Aid Kit

A small medical kit is useful to take when traveling. Included in this kit should be medications for illnesses that the child experiences at home, trip-specific items, and the usual first aid kit items (Table 45–2). Medications should be purchased prior to travel, as those obtained at some destinations may be of poor quality or contain toxic substances.

Stauffer W, Christenson JC, Fischer PR: Preparing children for international travel. Travel Med Infect Dis 2008 May;6(3):101–113 [PMID: 18486064].

Christenson JC: Preparing children for travel to tropical and developing regions. Pediatr Ann 2004 Oct;33(10):676–684 [PMID: 15515354].

Table 45–2. First aid kit for international travel.

Medications
Malaria prophylaxis
Acetaminophen and ibuprofen
Antibiotics
Antihistamines
Topical formulations
Hydrocortisone ointment
Antibiotic and antifungal ointment
Insect repellants
Sunscreen
Antibacterial soap/alcohol-based hand sanitizer
Antiseptic wipes
Other
Bed nets
Thermometer
Medicine spoon and cup
Oral rehydration salts in powder form
Sterile cotton balls, cotton tip applicators
Tweezers
Water purification tablets
Gauze bandages
Tape—hypoallergenic, waterproof
Triangular bandage/sling/splint
Tongue depressor
Adhesive bandages
Flashlight
First aid book
Copies of prescriptions

VACCINATIONS—ROUTINE CHILDHOOD VACCINES MODIFIED FOR TRAVEL

Many vaccine-preventable diseases remain prevalent in developing countries, and outbreaks still occur in areas where these diseases are considered rare. The schedule for some vaccines may be accelerated for travel and some vaccines can be given earlier than the recommended age. The rationale for recommended intervals is to balance the high-risk age for disease with the infant immunologic response. Barriers to some early immunizations are: antibody from the mother interfering with an infant's ability to mount an antibody response, particularly to live vaccines, and the lack of a T-cell dependent immune response in those under 2 years. For children traveling to highly endemic areas, however, it is preferable to vaccinate prior to the recommended age despite the possible need for repeat vaccination at a later date.

Vaccination pertaining to children traveling follows the routine vaccination schedule as outlined in Chapter 10 (Immunization). It may be necessary to accelerate routine pediatric vaccinations due to travel. The recommended minimum interval between doses is listed in Table 45–3. However, longer intervals are preferable. Minor febrile illnesses are not a contraindication to routine or travel vaccines, and should not lead to their postponement. Live vaccines should be given together or separated by 30 days or more.

Table 45–3. Accelerated vaccinations.

Vaccine	Minimum Age for First Dose	Minimum Time to Second Dose (wk)	Minimum Time to Third Dose (wk)	Minimum Time for Fourth Dose (wk)
MMR	12 mo[a]	4	–	–
Hepatitis B	Birth	4	8[b]	–
DTP/DTaP	6 wk	4	4	6 mo
Hib	6 wk	4	4	8[c]
IPV	6 wk	4	4	4[d]
MCV	2 y			
MPS4	3 mo	5 y		
PCV	4 wk	4	4	8
Varicella	12 mo	4	–	–
Rotavirus	4 wk[e]	4	4	–
Hepatitis A	1 y	6 mo	–	–

[a]Children traveling abroad may be vaccinated as early as 6 months of age. Before departure, children aged 6–11 months should receive the first dose of MMR vaccine. This will not count towards their series and they will still require 2 doses after 12 months of age.
[b]The third dose should be given at least 4 months after the first dose and at a minimum of 6 months of age.
[c]If third dose is given after 4 years, the fourth dose is not required.
[d]Recommended at 6–18 months of age.
[e]This differs from the package insert but is validated by data held by the manufacturer.
DTaP, diphtheria-tetanus-acellular pertussis; DTP, diphtheria-tetanuspertussis; Hib, *Haemophilus influenzae* type b; IPV, inactivated polio vaccine; MCV, meningococcal conjugate vaccine; MMR, measles, mumps, rubella; MPS4, meningococcal polysaccharide.

Diptheria-Tetanus-Acellular Pertussis (DTaP) Vaccine

Immunization is recommended prior to travel to developing countries because of the greater risk of disease from diphtheria, tetanus, and pertussis. Tetanus risk is high in several areas of the developing world where fecal contamination of soil is extensive. Infants should receive their first DTaP at 6 weeks of age for an adequate immune response, with a 4-week interval between the subsequent two doses. The fourth dose may be given 6–12 months after the third dose provided that the child is 12 months of age or older. Appropriate protection is achieved after the third dose. Tdap is licensed for children at least 11 years of age. Adolescents and adult caretakers, who are prominent vectors in the spread of pertussis to young children, should receive a single Tdap booster. If more than 5 years has elapsed since the last dose, a booster should be considered for children and adolescents to minimize tetanus risk. Tdap is preferred to Td in children older than 11 years of age if they have not received Tdap previously.

Haemophilus influenzae Type b (Hib) Vaccine

The indications for vaccination of Hib in children traveling are the same as for United States residents. If previously unvaccinated, infants less than 15 months of age should receive at least 2 doses prior to travel. An accelerated schedule can start at a minimum of 6 weeks of age, with a 4-week interval between the first, second, and third doses, and at least 8 weeks between third and fourth doses.

Hepatitis A Vaccine

Hepatitis A is one of the most common vaccine-preventable illnesses globally, and vaccination should be provided prior to travel to developing countries. In many developing countries, more than 90% of local children have hepatitis A antibodies by 6 years of age. The disease is much less common in children from the developed world, so they are likely to be susceptible when traveling to high-risk areas. Although two doses of the vaccine are recommended 6–12 months apart, a single dose will provide protection during the trip if given at least 2 weeks prior to departure. The earliest age of administration is 1 year in the United States. Immune serum globulin (0.02 mL/kg IM) can be given for protection of children younger than 1 year of age, or if travel will occur within 2 weeks after vaccination. This interferes with MMR and varicella vaccination, so these vaccines should be given 2 weeks prior to immunoglobulin.

Hepatitis B Vaccine

Areas of high endemicity for hepatitis B include most of Asia, the Middle East, Africa, and the Amazon Basin. Unimmunized children are at risk if they receive blood transfusions that have not been screened for HBV surface antigen (HBsAg), are exposed to unsterilized medical or dental equipment. Children traveling to developing countries should be vaccinated before departure. An accelerated schedule is possible, with the second dose given with a minimum 4-week interval, and the third dose given at least 8 weeks after the second dose. The third dose should not be given before 24 weeks of age.

Influenza Vaccine

Children are at high risk of respiratory infection during travel. The influenza vaccine is recommended for travel during the influenza season, which is between September and March in the Northern Hemisphere, and between April and August in the Southern Hemisphere, and year round in the tropics. The vaccine may not protect against new strains circulating in the Southern Hemisphere. Influenza vaccine is recommended for children at least 6 months of age; those younger than 9 years of age will need two doses of vaccine 4 weeks apart. It is preferable to be vaccinated at least 2 weeks prior to departure. The annual seasonal influenza vaccine may not be routinely available in the United States from the late spring to early fall, when it may be needed for travelers, but may be available at some travel clinics. Revaccination is not recommended for those who will be traveling during April through September and were vaccinated the preceding fall.

Measles, Mumps, Rubella (MMR) Vaccine

While measles is no longer endemic in the United States, measles is still prevalent in many parts of the world, including Europe. Children as young as 6 months of age traveling outside the United States are recommended to receive the vaccine, but any doses given prior to 12 months do not count toward an adequate two-dose series, as maternal antibodies may interfere with the immune response. These infants will still require one dose of MMR at 12–15 months of age and a second dose at 4–6 years of age. The second dose is to protect those individuals (~5%) who did not respond the first time. If an accelerated schedule is required, two doses must be separated by minimum of 4 weeks.

Meningococcal Vaccine

There are two meningococcal vaccines available. The conjugated quadrivalent (MCV4) vaccine is approved for use in persons aged 2–55 years. This vaccine is recommended for those visiting the meningitis belt of Africa (sub-Saharan region) or who live in areas with high rates of meningitis. It must be given at least 10 days before international travel. The quadrivalent meningococcal polysaccharide vaccine (MPSV4) is licensed for persons aged 2–55 years. Both vaccines protect against serotypes A, C, Y, and W-135. The duration of protection is 3 years in children and 5 years in adults. MPSV4 should be used for persons older than 55 years of age and is safe to give to children aged 3 months to 2 years who require vaccination. Meningococcal vaccination is required by the Saudi Arabian government for pilgrims undertaking the Hajj or Umra pilgrimage to Mecca and Medina, because of the international outbreak of *Neisseria meningitidis* W-135 in 2000 and 2001. Further information concerning geographic areas recommended for meningococcal vaccination can be obtained from http://www.cdc.gov/travel.

Pneumococcal Vaccine

Streptococcus pneumoniae infection is prevalent worldwide, and children less than 2 years of age have the highest rates of disease. The 13-valent pneumococcal conjugate vaccine (PCV 13) is recommended for routine use in children 5 years of age or less. In addition, the pneumococcal polysaccharide (PPSV23) is recommended for children and adults 2 years of age or older who have certain underlying medical conditions, and for all adults 65 years of age or older. For children aged 5 years or less who have completed the PCV 7 series, a single additional dose of PCV 13 is recommended. The minimal interval is 4 weeks between the first three doses, and 8 weeks between the third and fourth dose.

Polio Vaccine

Transmission of polio still occurs in regions of Asia and Africa. Adequate immunization with inactivated polio vaccine (IPV) should be administered prior to travel to developing countries. The minimum age of administration is 6 weeks of age for IPV. The recommended interval between the first and second dose is 4 weeks as well as between the second and third dose, and 4 weeks between subsequent doses. One additional lifetime dose (a fifth dose) of the IPV should be given to caretakers who are traveling to areas with recent circulating polio.

Rotavirus Vaccine

Rotavirus is the most common cause of severe gastroenteritis in infants and young children worldwide, and vaccination with the complete series is recommended prior to travel if age-appropriate. The minimum and maximum age for the first dose is 4 weeks and 14 weeks, 6 days respectively. There is insufficient data on the safety in older infants. The minimum interval between doses is 4 weeks.

Greenwood CS, Greenwood NP, Fischer PR: Immunization issues in pediatric travelers. Expert Rev Vaccines 2008 Jul;7(5): 651–661 [PMID: 18564019].

Hill DR et al: The practice of travel medicine: Guidelines by the Infectious Diseases Society of America. Clin Infect Dis 2006 Dec 15;43(12):1499–1539 [PMID: 17109284].

VACCINATIONS—TRAVEL-SPECIFIC

Japanese Encephalitis Vaccine

Japanese encephalitis (JE) is caused by a flavivirus transmitted by the night-biting Culex mosquito. The risk of contracting severe JE is low, especially for travelers that will have a brief stay in an endemic area, as the infection rate in Culex mosquitoes is 3% or lower, and only 1 in 200 infections with JE lead to neuroinvasive disease. The symptoms of JE include seizures, paralysis, coma, and mental status changes; residual neurological damage occurs in 50% of those with clinical disease. The case fatality rate is 30% in those with severe disease. Most symptomatic cases occur in children less than 10 years of age, and in the elderly. The areas at risk include most of Asia, Eastern Russia, some areas of the Western Pacific, and the Torres Strait Islands of Australia. The peak season is between April and October, during and just after the rainy season. The JE vaccine reduces the risk for disease among those who will be in a high risk setting, as determined by the destination, duration, and season of travel. However, the immunization options for children are now limited since the inactivated whole virus vaccine based on the Nakayama strain (approved for children aged 1 to 18 years of age) is no longer available in the United States. It has been replaced by a new JE vaccine (Ixiaro), which is an inactivated cell culture–derived vaccine approved for adult travelers (≥ 17 years of age). It is given as two doses, at least 28 days apart, and is associated with fewer adverse effects than the inactivated Nakayama strain vaccine. Pediatric safety and immunogenicity studies of this vaccine is underway, but it will likely be several years before Ixiaro is licensed in the United States for use in children. The manufacturer is studying a 6 ug per 0.5 mL dose for children ages 3 years and older and a 3 ug per 0.25 mL for children aged 2 months to 2 years of age. For health care providers interested in obtaining the JE vaccine for children traveling for extended periods of time, options include: enrolling children in the clinical trial; administering Ixiaro off-label; or referring children to an international traveler's health clinic in Asia.

Rabies Vaccine

Rabies is found worldwide and contracted through the bite or saliva-contaminated scratch of infected animals. In parts of Africa, Asia, and Central and South America, canine rabies is highly endemic (Rabnet—www.who.int/rabies/rabnet/en/—provides country-specific animal and human data), where 40% of rabies occurs in children less than 14 years of age. This increased risk is due to the fact that children are attracted to animals; are more likely to be bitten; and may not report minor encounters with animals. Most cases of rabies in travelers occur through the bite of an infected dog, cat, or monkey (particularly those that live near temples in parts of Asia). Bats, mongooses, and foxes are other animals that can transmit disease.

The rabies vaccine is recommended for travelers to areas in which rabies is endemic and for those who will have occupational or recreational exposure (such as cavers), especially if access to medical care will be limited when traveling. The risk of a bite from a potentially rabid animal is up to 2% for travelers to the developing world. There are three types of inactivated virus vaccine available, which are administered prior to exposure in three doses at days 0, 7, and 21 or 28. Vaccination prior to exposure may not be completely protective; further doses are required if a high-risk bite occurs. The minimum age of administration is 1 year, and duration of protection is 2 years. Malaria chemoprophylaxis with mefloquine or chloroquine should begin 1 month after completing the rabies vaccine series to avoid interference with the immune response.

It is important to counsel travelers about: animal avoidance; thorough cleansing of a bite wound with irrigation for at least 5 minutes; and the need to seek additional vaccination on days 0 and 3 if an exposure occurs.

In the event of a bite in a nonvaccinated individual, rabies immunoglobulin and four doses of vaccine at days 0, 3, 7, and 14 are required.

Yellow Fever Vaccine

Yellow fever is a flavivirus transmitted by mosquitoes, found in urban and rural areas in sub-Saharan Africa and equatorial South America. Of those infected with the virus, 15% have moderate to severe infection. The licensed 17D strain live attenuated vaccine is highly effective. It must be administered 10 days before travel to an endemic region for the development of protective antibodies. It is required by many countries for reentry after travel to an endemic area, and receipt of the vaccine should be documented in the International Certificate of Vaccination that became available in December 2007 (wwwnc.cdc.gov/travel/yellowbook provides an updated list of countries in which Yellow Fever vaccination is recommended). For this reason, it is only administered at certified clinics. The vaccine is given subcutaneously, and a booster is required every 10 years (but immunity may be lifelong after a single dose). The recommended minimum age of administration is 9 months of age, and vaccine should not be administered to at-risk infants less than 6 months of age, due to the increased risk of encephalitis (0.5–4 per 1000 vaccinees). The risk of severe vaccine-related disease is also higher in adult caretakers over 60 years of age. The decision to immunize infants who are 6–8 months of age must balance the infant's risk for exposure with the risk for vaccine-associated encephalitis. In addition to age limitations, the vaccine should not be administered to those who are pregnant, have egg allergy or immunosuppression (including a history of thymus disorder or thymectomy). A letter of medical exemption may be required for these travelers. Adverse effects include encephalitis (15 per million doses for those over 60 years of age) and multisystem disease (5 per million doses).

Cholera Vaccine

The cholera vaccine is no longer produced in the United States and is no longer recommended for international travel, as the disease is rare in travelers. There are live and killed vaccines available in other countries, but these confer only slight protection.

Typhoid Vaccine

The risk of typhoid fever in travelers is 1–10:100,000, depending on the destination. Areas at risk include South Asia, West and North Africa, South America, and Latin America.

Travelers to the Indian subcontinent are at greatest risk. The vaccine is recommended for long-term travelers traveling to an endemic area, those traveling off standard tourist routes, immunocompromised travelers, those of south Indian ancestry, and patients with cholelithiasis. There are currently two vaccines available, a capsular polysaccharide (ViCPS) and a live attenuated (Ty21a) vaccine. The ViCPS is given intramuscularly 2 weeks prior to travel. The minimum age of administration for this vaccine is 2 years; efficacy is 75% over 2 years. The Ty21a is an oral vaccine given as four doses every second day, which needs to be completed more than 1 week prior to travel to be effective. It is licensed for children over the age of 6 years; efficacy is 80% over 5 years. It is contraindicated in immunodeficient populations. Antibiotics interfere with growth of the vaccine strain bacteria. Mefloquine, chloroquine, and prophylactic doses of atovaquone-proguanil can be given concurrently with the typhoid vaccine. Fever, headache, and severe local pain and swelling are reported with the ViCPS more frequently than with other vaccines.

Tuberculosis

Tuberculosis risk is increased for travelers, especially for those visiting Africa, Asia, Latin America, and the former Soviet Union. The risk is higher in long-term travelers to countries with a high incidence of tuberculosis, and is highest among health care workers. Bacillus Calmette-Guérin (BCG) vaccination is given soon after birth in many countries, but not in the United States. It protects against miliary and meningeal tuberculosis (it does not protect against pulmonary disease), with efficacy only established in children less than 1 year. It may be considered in children less than 5 years of age who will be in a high-risk area for a prolonged period. BCG is not widely available in the United States, and may be administered in the destination country. A preferred alternative is that travelers to high prevalence areas have a PPD skin test prior to travel and 3 months after return. It should be noted that live virus vaccines can create an anergic state, in which PPD skin tests can be falsely negative. Therefore, PPD testing should be performed on the same day as any live vaccine administration, or 28 or more days later.

The World Health Organization (WHO) has published recommendations related to tuberculosis and guidelines for tuberculosis prevention and management during air travel (www.who.int/docstore/gtb/publications/aircraft/PDF/98_256.pdf).

Giovanetti F: Immunisation of the travelling child. Travel Med Infect Dis Nov 2007;5(6):349–364 [PMID: 17983974].

Greenwood CS, Greenwood NP, Fischer PR: Immunization issues in pediatric travelers. Expert Rev Vaccines 2008 Jul;7(5):651–661 [PMID: 18564019].

Hill DR et al: The practice of travel medicine: Guidelines by the Infectious Diseases Society of America. Clin Infect Dis 2006 Dec 15;43(12):1499–1539 [PMID: 17109284].

Ritz N, Connell TG, Curtis N: To BCG or not to BCG? Preventing travel-associated tuberculosis in children. Vaccine 2008 Nov 5; 26(47):5905–5910 [PMID: 18804139].

Wilder-Smith A: Meningococcal vaccines: A neglected topic in travel medicine? Expert Rev Vaccines 2009 Oct;8(10):1343–1350 [PMID: 19803757].

CDC Traveler's Health Yellow Book. Available at: http://www.nc.cdc.gov/travel/yellowbook/2012/chapter-7-international-travel-infants-children/vaccine-recommendations-for-infants-and-children.htm

TRAVELER'S DIARRHEA

Diarrhea is one of the most common illnesses in travelers to the developing world. Children are at highest risk, usually having more severe and prolonged illness than adults. Traveler's diarrhea is defined in adults as three or more loose stools in a 24-hour period, plus either fever, nausea, vomiting, or abdominal cramping. There is no strict definition in child travelers, as the pattern, consistency, and frequency of stools vary during the course of childhood. A useful definition to use for traveling children is: a recent change in normal stool patterns, with an increase in frequency (at least three stools per 24 hours) and a decrease in consistency to an unformed state. Most illness usually resolves over a 3- to 5-day period and occurs in the first 2 weeks of travel. Enterotoxigenic *Escherichia coli* (ETEC) is the most common cause, accounting for up to one-third of cases. Other pathogens implicated are listed in Table 45–4. Counseling prior to travel includes education and caution with food handling and food and water consumption, and provision for self-treatment in the event of illness.

Prevention

Travelers should be advised to seek restaurants with a good safety reputation; to eat hot thoroughly cooked food; to

Table 45–4. Pathogens causing traveler's diarrhea.

Bacterial
Enterotoxigenic *Escherichia coli* (ETEC)
Enteroaggregative *E coli*
Salmonella spp
Shigella spp
Campylobacter jejuni
Aeromonas spp
Plesiomonas spp
Vibrio cholera
Non-cholerae *Vibrio* spp
Enterotoxigenic *Bacteroides fragilis*
Viral
Rotavirus
Noroviruses
Sapoviruses
Parasistic
Giardia lamblia
Cyclospora cayetanensis
Cryptosporidium hominis
Entamoeba histolytica

eat fruits and vegetables that can be peeled by the traveler; and to avoid tap water. They should also avoid ice cubes, fruit juices, fresh salads, unpasteurized dairy products, cold sauces and toppings, open buffets, undercooked foods, and food or beverages from street vendors. They should check the integrity of caps before buying bottled water to avoid bottles filled with tap water. It is also useful to remind the travelers about hand-washing after using the toilet and before eating. Families can consider using alcohol-containing hand sanitizers as an alternative to soap and water when access is limited during travel. Milk that is pasteurized or boiled is considered safe provided that it is stored at the appropriate temperature. It may be necessary to bring powdered milk to mix it with safe drinking water if the quality of milk is questionable. While these measures seem logical and should be recommended, there is little evidence that they prevent traveler's diarrhea, both in adults and in children.

Chemoprophylaxis and Treatment

The principles of treatment include adequate hydration and a short course of antibiotics when warranted; medical attention should be sought for severe or prolonged disease.

For mild disease, hydration may be all that is necessary, without any diet restriction. This can be achieved with oral rehydration therapy to supplement a regular diet. Packets of dry rehydration powder to be mixed with water are available from pharmacies, either prior to travel or at the destination. If this is not available, parents can be instructed on how to make oral rehydration solution (Table 45–5) or to use a sports drink such as Gatorade as a suitable alternative in older children and toddlers. The breast-fed infant should continue to breast feed, in addition to receiving oral rehydration therapy.

Table 45–5. Recipe for oral rehydration solution.

- ¼ teaspoon (1.25 cc) salt
- ¼ teaspoon (1.25 cc) bicarbonate of soda[a]
- 2 tablespoons (30 cc) sugar
- 1 L of water

[a]If bicarbonate of soda is not available, substitute an additional ¼ teaspoon (1.25 cc) of salt.

The vomiting child is at greater risk of dehydration, so aggressive rehydration is crucial. Parents should be reassured that some fluid will be absorbed even if vomiting is ongoing. This is best achieved with small amounts of fluid given often to prevent further vomiting.

The antimotility agent loperamide, which is often used in adults to minimize symptom duration, is not advised for children due to the risk of adverse events such as toxic megacolon, ileus, coma, and lethargy. Bismuth subsalicylate decreases the number of unformed stools in adults. Its routine use is not recommended in pediatrics, as aspirin is contraindicated in children less than 18 years of age due to the risk of Reye syndrome, and dosing of bismuth has not been established for children.

For children with signs and symptoms of bacterial gastroenteritis, such as fever or blood in the stool, empiric antibiotic therapy should be considered. The drug of choice in children is azithromycin (10 mg/kg orally once a day for 3 days). It is available in a powdered form that can be reconstituted and stored without refrigeration. It is a good choice because of the growing resistance of many gastroenteritis-causing bacteria to ciprofloxacin. There are no pediatric trials of empiric azithromycin, so the dosing recommendations are based on pharmacokinetic data and studies involving the treatment of diarrhea in Africa and Thailand. Ciprofloxacin is not recommended in children less than 1 year of age due to the occurrence of arthropathy in animal studies. There are no definitive data in children to support an increased risk of arthropathy, but this is generally reserved for treatment in adults (the pediatric dose is 20 mg/kg/d orally in two divided doses for 3 days).

Trimethoprim–sulfamethoxazole (TMP–SMX) has been used to treat traveler's diarrhea in children, but is no longer recommended because of increasing antibiotic resistance. Rifaximin, a nonabsorbable derivative of rifamycin, is effective in treating ETEC and other noninvasive enteropathogens. Since it is not absorbed, high concentrations are achieved in the intestinal lumen. It is licensed for patients 12 years of age and older at a treatment dose of 200 mg three times a day for 3 days.

The use of prophylactic antibiotics is not recommended due to the risk of adverse events to prevent a disease of limited morbidity, as well as the effect of prophylaxis in contributing to the emergence of antibiotic resistance. Rifaximin, however, is showing promise in adult studies as a chemoprophylactic agent, but it is expensive, and requires further study in pediatrics. Probiotics are of unproven benefit for the prevention of traveler's diarrhea, with contradictory reports of efficacy in adult studies.

Ang JY, Mathur A: Traveler's diarrhea: Updates for pediatricians. Pediatr Ann 2008 Dec;37(12):814–820 [PMID: 19143332].

de la Cabada Bauche J, Dupont HL: New developments in traveler's diarrhea. Gastroenterol Hepatol (NY) 2011 Feb;7(2):88–95 [PMID: 21475415].

DuPont HL: Azithromycin for the self-treatment of traveler's diarrhea. Clin Infect Dis 2007 Feb 1;44(3):347–349 [PMID: 17205439].

DuPont HL et al: Expert review of the evidence base for prevention of travelers' diarrhea. J Travel Med 2009 May–Jun;16(3):149–160 [PMID: 19538575].

Hill DR, Ryan ET: Management of travellers' diarrhoea. BMJ 2008;337:a1746 [PMID: 18838421].

MALARIA PROPHYLAXIS AND PREVENTION (SEE ALSO CHAPTER 43)

Malaria is the most common preventable infectious cause of death among travelers, and a common cause of fever in the returned traveler. Children comprise 20% of imported cases of malaria. It is largely a preventable disease in travelers through personal protective measures and chemoprophylaxis. However, no method is 100% protective. The risk of acquiring malaria varies with the season, climate, altitude, number of mosquito bites, and destination, with the highest risk in Oceania, Africa, the Indian subcontinent, and the Amazon.

Prevention of Mosquito Bites

Malaria is transmitted via the night-biting *Anopheles* mosquitoes. Mosquito bites are avoided by staying in well-screened and air-conditioned rooms from dusk until dawn, wearing clothing covering arms and legs, and avoiding scented soaps, shampoos, and perfumes. Mosquito nets are highly effective, and can be used over beds, cribs, playpens, car seats, and strollers. Repellants containing 25%–50% DEET are also recommended, as this concentration confers 5–8 hours of protection. When used appropriately, DEET is safe for infants and children over the age of 2 months. It should not be applied to children's hands, mouth, or near the eyes, and is best washed off upon returning indoors. There have been case reports of seizures and toxic encephalopathy with use of DEET, but these cases occurred with misapplication. Picaridin is an alternative to DEET available in many countries. A concentration of 20% Picaridin is as effective as DEET-containing products. It lacks the corrosiveness and greasy texture of DEET, and has been advised as safe for use in children by the American Academy of Pediatrics. However, because it is relatively new, it lacks the safety profile of DEET, especially for children. Clothing and bed nets may be sprayed with insecticides such as permethrin, which confers protection for 2–6 weeks, even with regular washing. The combination of DEET every 8–12 hours and permethrin on clothing is over 99% effective in prevention of mosquito bites.

Chemoprophylaxis

Prophylactic medications suppress malaria by killing asexual blood stages of the parasite before they cause disease, so protective levels of medication must be present in the blood before developing parasites are released from the liver. Therefore, it is necessary to start prophylaxis before the first possible exposure, and to continue it for a sufficient period after return to a safe area.

The choice of antimalarial depends on the age of the child, resistance patterns, restrictions on the agent of choice, the child's ability to swallow tablets, the frequency of dosing, cost, availability of medication, and access to a compounding pharmacy for adequate dispensing of medication. For most children, once weekly mefloquine is preferable, and is approved for use in children of any age. Atovaquone/proguanil is available in pediatric dosing, although only in tablet formulation. It is currently approved in most countries for children weighing greater than 5 kg. Doxycycline is another alternative, but should be used only in children 8 years or older due to the risk of teeth staining. Chloroquine is the drug of choice in areas of chloroquine sensitivity (Mexico, Hispaniola, Central America, west and north of the Panama Canal, and parts of North Africa, the Middle East, and China). Pediatric and adult dosing, side effects, and other information about malaria chemoprophylaxis are in Table 45–6.

Antimalarial medications (with the exception of atovaquone/proguanil) are bitter, so it may be necessary to grind the medication in a very sweet food, such as chocolate syrup or sweetened condensed milk. Infants may need to have their medication prepared by a compounding pharmacy, where the appropriate dose can be placed in a gelatin capsule, which can then be opened by the caregiver and mixed into food or liquid.

Shetty AK, Woods CR: Prevention of malaria in children. Pediatr Infect Dis J 2006 Dec;25(12):1173–1176 [PMID: 17133165].

Greenwood B: Anti-malarial drugs and the prevention of malaria in the population of malaria endemic areas. Malar J 2010 Dec 13; 9(Suppl 3):S2 [PMID: 21144082].

Chen LH, Wilson ME, Schlagenhauf P: Prevention of malaria in long-term travelers. JAMA 2006 Nov 8;296(18):2234–2244 [PMID: 17090770].

VISITS TO FRIENDS AND RELATIVES (VFR) IN HIGH-RISK AREAS

Individuals who return to their home country are at the highest risk of travel-related infectious diseases. Sixty percent of malaria cases and over 75% of typhoid cases occur in these

Table 45–6. Malaria prophylaxis.

Drug	Usage	Adult Dose	Pediatric Dose	Directions	Comments
Atovaquone/proguanil	Prophylaxis in areas with chloroquine-resistant or mefloquine-resistant *Plasmodium falciparum*.	Adult tabs contain 250 mg atovaquone and 100 mg proguanil hydrochloride. 1 adult tab orally, daily.	Pediatric tabs contain 62.5 mg atovaquone and 25 mg proguanil hydrochloride. 11–20 kg: 1 tab 21–30 kg: 2 tabs 31–40 kg: 3 tabs 41 kg or more: 1 adult tab daily.	Begin 1–2 d before travel to malarious areas. Take daily at the same time each day while in the area and for 7 d after leaving such areas.	Contraindicated in persons with severe renal impairment (creatinine clearance < 30 mL/min). Atovaquone/proguanil should be taken with food or a milky drink. Not recommended for prophylaxis for children < 11 kg, pregnant women, and women breast-feeding infants weighing < 11 kg, but consider if drug resistant area (call CDC). Do not take with tetracycline, metoclopramide, rifampin, or rifabutin (all reduce atovaquone concentration).
Chloroquine phosphate	Prophylaxis only in areas with chloroquine-sensitive *P falciparum*.	150 and 300 mg base tabs (300 and 500 mg salt) orally, once per week (any age or size).	5 mg/kg base (8.3 mg/kg salt) orally, once per week, up to max adult dose. Tabs not scored.	Begin 1–2 wk before travel to malarious areas. Take weekly on the same day of the week while in the area and for 4 wk after leaving such areas.	Contraindicated in persons with prior retinal or visual field changes. May exacerbate psoriasis. Bitter taste. Interferes with rabies vaccine response. Not contraindicated in pregnancy.
Doxycycline	Prophylaxis in areas with chloroquine-resistant or mefloquine-resistant *P falciparum*.	100 mg orally, daily.	8 y of age: 2 mg/kg up to adult dose of 100 mg/d. Syrup available.	Begin 1–2 d before travel to malarious areas. Take daily at the same time each day while in the area and for 4 wk after leaving such areas.	Contraindicated in children < 8 y of age and pregnant women. May decrease oral contraceptive efficacy. Photosensitivity.
Hydroxychloroquine sulfate	An alternative to chloroquine in areas with chloroquine-sensitive *P falciparum*.	310 mg base (400 mg salt) orally, once per week.	5 mg/kg base (6.5 mg/kg salt) orally, once per week, up to max adult dose. Tabs not scored.	Begin 1–2 wk before travel to malarious areas. Take weekly on the same day of the week while in the area and for 4 wk after leaving such areas.	

Mefloquine	Prophylaxis in areas with chloroquine-resistant *P falciparum*.	228 mg base (250 mg salt) orally, once per week.	5–9 kg: 4.6 mg/kg base (5 mg/kg salt) orally, once per week. Tabs scored. 10–19 kg: ¼ tab once per week 20–30 kg: ½ tab once per week 31–45 kg: ¾ tab once per week: 46 kg 1 tab once per week	Begin 1–2 wk before travel to malarious areas. Take weekly on the same day of the week while in the area and for 4 wk after leaving such areas (start 2 wk prior if want to evaluate for side effects that may necessitate change).	Contraindicated in persons allergic to mefloquine or related compounds (eg, quinine and quinidine) and in persons with active depression, a recent history of depression, generalized anxiety disorder, psychosis, schizophrenia, other major psychiatric disorders, or seizures. Use with caution in persons with psychiatric disturbances. Not recommended for persons with cardiac conduction abnormalities. Not contraindicated in pregnancy. Bitter taste. May be able to use in < 5–9 kg; consult with CDC.
Primaquine (posttravel prophylaxis for long-term *Plasmodium vivax and Plasmodium ovale* exposure)	Used for presumptive antirelapse therapy (terminal prophylaxis) to decrease the risk of relapses of *P vivax* and *P ovale*.	30 mg base (52.6 mg salt) orally, once per day for 14 d after departure from the malarious area.	0.6 mg/kg base (1.0 mg/kg salt) up to adult dose orally, once per day for 14 d after departure from the malarious area.	Primaquine presumptive antirelapse therapy is administered for 14 d after the traveler has left a malarious area. When chloroquine, doxycycline, or mefloquine is used for prophylaxis, primaquine is usually taken during the last 2 wk of postexposure prophylaxis, but may be taken immediately after those medications are completed. When atovaquone/proguanil is used for prophylaxis, primaquine may be taken either during the final 7 d of atovaquone/proguanil and then for an additional 7 d, or for 14 d after atovaquone/proguanil is completed.	Indicated for persons who have had prolonged exposure to P vivax and P ovale or both (eg, missionaries or peace corps volunteers). All persons who take primaquine should have a documented normal G6PD (glucose-6-phosphate dehydrogenase) level prior to starting this medication. Contraindicated in persons with G6PD1 deficiency. Also contraindicated during pregnancy and lactation unless the breastfed infant has a documented normal G6PD level. Also an option for prophylaxis in special circumstances.

travelers; and VFR children are at highest risk of hepatitis A. The reasons for this include the following:

- Longer stays and increased likelihood of pregnancy or young age in the traveler
- Travel to remote rural areas
- Intimate contact with the local population
- Decreased likelihood of seeking (or following) pretravel advice because of familiarity with their home country
- Assumed immunity to infections
- Socio-cultural barriers—for example, language barriers, prohibitive cost of vaccines, and medications if lower socioeconomic status, belief systems of illness
- Eating and sleeping in local households, where hygiene may be suboptimal
- Use of high-risk forms of transportation

Thus, certain issues need to be emphasized when discussing travel for VFRs. Given the risk of water-borne infections, they should boil water and milk if other safe drinking water is expensive; consume only piping hot foods and beverages; and follow proper hand-washing techniques at all times. Vaccination recommendations and malaria prophylaxis are of greater importance in VFRs. Similarly, VFRs provide greater opportunity for contracting vaccine-preventable diseases, such as typhoid, rabies, yellow fever, and meningococcal infection. They are associated with a higher risk of exposure to people with tuberculosis, so for this reason PPD testing is recommended after return from travel.

Bacaner N et al: Travel medicine considerations for North American immigrants visiting friends and relatives. JAMA 2004 Jun 16;291(23):2856–2864 [PMID: 15199037].

Leder K et al: Illness in travelers visiting friends and relatives: A review of the GeoSentinel Surveillance Network. Clin Infect Dis 2006;43(9):1185–1193 [PMID: 17029140].

HIV AND SEXUALLY TRANSMITTED DISEASES (SEE ALSO CHAPTER 41)

Adolescent travelers may partake in high-risk activities while traveling, putting them at risk of human immunodeficiency virus (HIV) and other sexually transmitted diseases. The adolescent traveler should be counseled about the risks of sexually transmitted diseases and abstinence or safe sexual practices. Bringing a supply of latex condoms may be appropriate along with instruction on their proper use. They should be advised that HIV and other sexually transmitted diseases can also be contracted via oral sex and in nonsexual activities such as intravenous drug use. They should avoid needles, tattoos, pedicures, and dental care while traveling. There may be a risk of HIV and other virus transmission through blood transfusion, as many developing countries do not have adequate blood banking and transfusion protocols. In fact, 10%–20% of countries have inadequate screening.

Antiretroviral therapy is recommended if there is exposure was from a known HIV-positive contact, and may be considered if the source is unknown. The usual recommended regimens are outlined in Chapter 41.

Further information on HIV can be found in Chapter 41.

Breuner CC: The adolescent traveler. Prim Care 2002 Dec;29(4): 983–1006 [PMID: 12687903].

MMWR: Available at: http://aidsinfo.nih.gov/contentfiles/NonOccupational ExposureGL.pdf

FEVER IN THE RETURNED TRAVELER

More than half of travelers to the developing world experience a health-related travel problem during their trip; 8% require medical attention on return. The majority will develop common medical problems, such as upper respiratory tract infections, pneumonia, urinary tract infections, and otitis media, with the remainder developing travel-related infections. The most common of these diseases are malaria (21%), acute traveler's diarrhea (15%), dengue fever (6%), and typhoid/enteric fever (2%). Children who travel with caretakers visiting friends and relatives are at greatest risk. New pathogens and the changing epidemiology of some infectious diseases pose new risks to travelers—such as avian influenza, multidrug-resistant TB, chikungunya virus, and leishmaniasis.

Symptomatic returning travelers should be urgently and thoroughly evaluated for travel-related illness to prevent serious life-threatening disease and transmission to close contacts. The initial evaluation should include questions directed toward the travel itinerary, with dates of arrival and departure, specific activities, rural versus urban location, and accommodations. Specific information should be obtained regarding fresh water contact (for schistosomiasis in some areas), sexual contacts, animal exposures, activities or hobbies, ill person contacts, and sources of food and water. A complete medication and vaccination history should be sought. It should be noted that despite malaria chemoprophylaxis and protection against mosquitoes, no regimen is 100% protective. A thorough physical examination should include dermatologic examination, eye examination for scleral icterus, conjunctival injection or petechiae, and evaluation for hepatosplenomegaly or lymphadenopathy. Routine laboratory evaluation includes a complete blood count, ESR, CRP, serum chemistry, liver enzyme profile, and urinalysis. The laboratory evaluation should also focus on diseases that are life-threatening, with thick and thin smears for malaria (ideally three that are 12 hours apart), and blood cultures for typhoid fever. Specific testing should be done as directed by findings on history, physical examination, and preliminary laboratory test findings (Table 45–7). It may be necessary to seek the opinion of individuals with experience in international travel medicine, if available.

Table 45–7. Laboratory evaluations to consider for fever in the returned traveler.

Routine
Hematologic
Complete blood count and differential
Thick and thin blood smear (ideally collect 3 at 12 hour intervals)
Sedimentation rate
C-Reactive protein
Electrolytes
Liver function tests
Blood culture
Urine
Urinalysis
Culture
Specific to presentation
Hematologic
Serologies for specific pathogens
Stool
Bacterial culture
Fecal leucocytes
Giardia and *Cryptosporidium* antigen test
Clostridium difficile toxin (if antibiotic exposure)
Ova and parasite examination
Special studies (eg, stool for *Entamoeba histolytica* antigen, special stains)
Cerebrospinal fluid
Cell count with differential, protein, glucose, culture, freeze extra sample
Antibody and polymerase chain reaction tests as appropriate
Imaging studies
Chest radiography and abdominal ultrasound imaging as appropriate
Other specialized tests
Placement of PPD (purified protein derivative)
Morning gastric aspirates or sputum for AFB (acid-fast bacilli) stain
Bronchoscopy
Sigmoidoscopy, colonoscopy
Skin biopsy
Bone marrow aspirate
Skin snips (eg, for *Onchocerciasis*)

Fever is the most common complaint in a child who becomes ill after international travel. The most common travel-related infectious causes of fever are outlined below.

Malaria

Malaria is a medical emergency, as a child infected with *Plasmodium falciparum* may progress from relatively minor symptoms to death in less than 24 hours. A child with malaria presents with paroxysmal high fevers, sweats, rigors, headaches, and malaise. The presence of nausea, vomiting, and abdominal pain in pediatric malaria may mimic acute gastroenteritis. Patients infected with *P falciparum* usually present within 2 months of exposure, whereas patients with *Plasmodium vivax* and *Plasmodium ovale* can present months to years after infection.

A more detailed description of the symptoms of malaria, diagnosis, and treatment are presented in Chapter 43.

Dengue fever

Dengue fever is an important tropical disease frequently encountered in travelers. The incubation period is 3–14 days; therefore, dengue should be considered for a febrile illness within the first 2 weeks after return from travel. It is acquired more commonly during urban travel in the daylight hours because of the biting preference of the vector *Aedes aegypti* mosquito. The classic presentation is high fever, retro-orbital headache, myalgias, arthralgias, diffuse blanching maculopapular, or petechial rash. It is possible for children to present with fever and irritability alone. Further information about dengue fever is presented in Chapter 40.

Typhoid fever

Typhoid fever, which is a relatively common cause of fever in children after travel, is caused by *Salmonella typhi*. A common presentation of typhoid fever is with fever, headache, abdominal pain, and initial diarrhea followed by constipation. Enteric fever has a similar presentation and is caused by other serovars of *Salmonella*. A person with typhoid fever usually appears toxic, and on examination may have hepatosplenomegaly and rarely rose spots. Typhoid fever is discussed in Chapter 42.

Information about other diseases sometimes occurring in the returned traveler is provided in Table 45–8 and Chapter 43.

Centers for Disease Control (CDC) Yellow Book: Available at: http://wwwnc.cdc.gov/travel/content/yellowbook/home-2010.aspx House HR, Ehlers JP: Travel-related infections. Emerg Med Clin North Am 2008 May;26(2):499–516 [PMID: 18406985].

Nield LS, Stauffer W, Kamat D: Evaluation and management of illness in a child after international travel. Pediatr Emerg Care 2005 Mar;21(3):184–195 [PMID: 15744199].

Wilson ME et al: Fever in returned travelers: Results from the GeoSentinel Surveillance Network. Clin Infect Dis 2007 Jun 15;44(12):1560–1568 [PMID: 17516399].

REFERENCES

Web Resources

CDC traveler's health: http://www.cdc.gov/travel/destinat.htm

CDC Yellow Book: http://wwwnc.cdc.gov/travel/content/yellowbook/home-2010.aspx

Table 45–8. Illnesses in the returning traveler.

Disease	Etiology	Common Presenting Symptoms and Signs	Usual Incubation Period	Geographic Location	Mode of Transmission
Malaria	*Plasmodium falciparum*	Fever Headache Myalgias Chills Rigors	7–30 d	More prevalent in sub-Saharan Africa than in other regions of the world, also South East (SE) Asia, South America, Mexico	Bite from *Anopheles* mosquito
Malaria	*Plasmodium vivax*	As for *P falciparum*	10–17 d and up to a year	SE Asia, sub-Saharan Africa, South America, Central America	As for *P falciparum*
Malaria	*Plasmodium ovale*	As for *P falciparum*	16–18 d	West Africa, the Philippines, eastern Indonesia, and Papua New Guinea. It has been reported from Cambodia, India, Thailand, and Vietnam	As for *P falciparum*
Malaria	*Plasmodium malariae*	As for *P falciparum*	16–59 d	Sub-Saharan Africa, much of southeast Asia, Indonesia, on many of the islands of the western Pacific and in areas of the Amazon Basin of South America	As for *P falciparum*
Malaria	*Plasmodium knowlesi*	As for *P falciparum*	10–12 d	SE Asia	
Dengue	Dengue virus	Fever Myalgias Maculopapular or petechial rash Arthralgias	2–7 d	Northern Australia, SE Asia, Mexico, Central America, South America, Puerto Rico, Florida Keys	Bite from *Aedes aegypti* mosquito
Typhoid fever	*Salmonella enterica* serovar *typhi*	Fever Malaise Anorexia Abdominal pain	10–14 d	South Asia, West and North Africa, South America, and Latin America	Ingestion of contaminated food/water
Paratyphoid fever	*S enterica* serovar *paratyphi*	Same as for typhoid fever	Same as for typhoid fever	Same as for typhoid fever	Same as for typhoid fever
Schistosomiasis	*Schistosoma mansoni, Schistosoma hematobium, Schistosoma japonicum*	Urticarial rash Fever Headache Myalgia Respiratory symptoms	23–70 d (average 1 mo)	*S mansoni*—South America, Caribbean *S hematobium*—Africa, Middle East *S japonicum*—Far East	Contaminated water containing freshwater snails

African tick typhus	*Rickettsia conorii*	Fever Headache Myalgia Maculopapular rash Malaise	5–7 d	Africa, Middle East, India, and Mediterranean Basin	Bite from hard ticks
Scrub typhus	*Orientia tsutsugamushi*	Fever Headache Myalgia Possibly a maculopapular rash	10–12 d	"Tsutsugamushi triangle"—from northern Japan and Eastern Russia in the North, to Northern Australia in the South, to Pakistan and Afghanistan in the west	From chigger bites (the larval stage of the biculid mites)
Leptospirosis	*Leptospira* spp	Fever Headache Chills Myalgia Nausea Diarrhea Abdominal pain Uveitis Adenopathy Conjunctival suffusion	5–14 d (average 10 d)	Worldwide	Contact with urine from domestic and wild animals contaminating water and soil
Babesiosis	*Babesia microti, Babesia divergens, Babesia duncani*	Fevers Chills Symptoms similar to malaria	1–4 wk	Europe, United States, sporadic cases in Asia, Mexico, Africa	Bite of *Ixodes* ticks
Yellow fever	Yellow fever virus	Fever Chills Headache Jaundice Backache Myalgias Prostration Nausea Vomiting	3–6 d	Tropical and sub-Tropical Africa and South America, Caribbean (countries that lie within a band 15 degrees north to 10 degrees south of the Equator)	Bite of mosquitoes (*Aedes aegypti* and others)
Chikungunya	CHIK virus	Fever Joint pain Maculopapular rash Headache Nausea Vomiting Myalgias	2–12 d (usually 2–4 d)	Tropical Africa & Asia (SE Asia & India)	Bite from *Aedes* mosquitoes
Amebiasis	*Entamoeba histolytica*	Fever Diarrhea Right upper quadrant pain	7–28 d	Worldwide, but higher incidence in developing countries	Contaminated food and water

Centers for Disease Control (CDC): http://www.cdc.gov/travel/index.htm

GIDEON: http://www.cyinfo.com

International Association for Medical Assistance to Travellers: http://www.iamat.org

International Society of Travel Medicine: http://www.istm.org

International SOS: http://www.internationalsos.com

London School of Hygiene and Tropical Medicine: http://www.lshtm.ac.uk

Malaria information specific to country: www.cdc.gov/malaria/risk_map

ProMED: http://www.promedmail.org

Rabies information specific to country: http://www.who.int/rabies/rabnet/en

Royal Society of Tropical Medicine and Hygiene: http://www.rstmh.org

The Malaria Foundation: http://www.malaria.org

Travax Encompass: http://www.travax.com

United States Department of State: http://www.travel.state.gov

WHO for maps of vaccine preventable diseases: http://www.who.int.ith

General References

Chen LH, Wilson ME: The role of the traveler in emerging infections and magnitude of travel. Med Clin North Am 2008 Nov;92(6):1409–1432 [PMID: 19061759].

Chen LH, Wilson ME, Schlagenhauf P: Prevention of malaria in long-term travelers. JAMA 2006 Nov 8;296(18):2234–2244 [PMID: 17090770].

Giovanetti F: Immunisation of the travelling child. Travel Med Infect Dis 2007 Nov;5(6):349–364 [PMID: 17983974].

Greenwood CS, Greenwood NP, Fischer PR: Immunization issues in pediatric travelers. Expert Rev Vaccines 2008 Jul;7(5):651–661 [PMID: 18564019].

Hill DR et al: The practice of travel medicine: Guidelines by the Infectious Diseases Society of America. Clin Infect Dis 2006 Dec 15;43(12):1499–1539 [PMID: 17109284].

House HR, Ehlers JP: Travel-related infections. Emerg Med Clin North Am 2008 May;26(2):499–516 [PMID: 18406985].

Lee PJ: Vaccines for travel and international adoption. Pediatr Infect Dis J 2008 Apr;27(4):351–354 [PMID: 18379374].

Stauffer W, Christenson JC, Fischer PR: Preparing children for international travel. Travel Med Infect Dis 2008 May;6(3):101–113 [PMID: 18486064].

Chemistry & Hematology Reference Intervals

46

Georgette Siparsky, PhD
Frank J. Accurso, MD

Laboratory tests provide valuable information necessary to evaluate a patient's condition and to monitor recommended treatment. Chemistry and hematology test results are compared with those of healthy individuals or those undergoing similar therapeutic treatment to determine clinical status and progress. In the past, the term *normal ranges* relayed some ambiguity because statistically, the term *normal* also implied a specific (gaussian or normal) distribution and epidemiologically it implied the state of the majority, which is not necessarily the desirable or targeted population. This is most apparent in cholesterol levels, where values greater than 200 mg/dL are common, but not desirable. Use of the term *reference range* or *reference interval* is therefore recommended by the International Federation of Clinical Chemistry (IFCC) and the Clinical and Laboratory Standards Institute (CLSI, formerly the National Committee for Clinical Laboratory Standards [NCCLS]) to indicate that the values relate to a reference population and clinical condition.

Reference ranges are established for a specific age (eg, α-fetoprotein), sex, and sexual maturity (eg, luteinizing hormone and testosterone); they are also defined for a specific pharmacologic status (eg, taking cyclosporine), dietary restrictions (eg, phenylalanine), and stimulation protocol (eg, growth hormone). Similarly, diurnal variation is a factor (eg, cortisol), as is degree of obesity (eg, insulin). Some reference ranges are particularly meaningful when combined with other results (eg, parathyroid hormone and calcium), or when an entire set of analytes is evaluated (eg, lipid profile: triglyceride, cholesterol, high-density lipoprotein, and low-density lipoprotein).

Laboratory tests are becoming more specific and measure much lower concentrations than ever before. Therefore, reference ranges should reflect the analytical procedure as well as reagents and instrumentation used for a specific analysis. As test methodology continues to evolve, reference ranges are modified and updated.

CHALLENGES IN DETERMINING & INTERPRETING PEDIATRIC REFERENCE INTERVALS

The pediatric environment is particularly challenging for the determination of reference intervals since growth and developmental stages do not have a distinct and finite boundary by which test results can be tabulated. Reference ranges may overlap and, in many cases, complicate diagnosis and treatment. Collection and allocation of test results by age for the purpose of establishing a reference range is a convenient and manageable way to report them, but caution is needed in their interpretation and clinical correlation.

A particular difficulty lies in establishing reference ranges for analytes whose levels are changed under scheduled stimulation conditions. The common glucose tolerance test is such an example, but more complex endocrinology tests (eg, stimulation by clonidine and cosyntropin) require skill and extensive experience to interpret. Reference ranges for these serial tests are established over a long period of time and are not easily transferable between test methodologies. Changing analytical technologies adds a new dimension to the challenges of establishing pediatric reference ranges.

Adeli K: Special Issue on Laboratory Reference Intervals. eJIFCC. September 2008. Available at: http://www.ifcc.org/PDF/190201200801.pdf

C28A3: Defining, Establishing, and Verifying Reference Intervals in the Clinical Laboratory; Approved Guideline—Third Edition. Available at: http://www.clsi.org/source/orders

GUIDELINES FOR USE OF DATA IN A REFERENCE RANGE STUDY

The College of American Pathologists provides guidelines for the adoption of reference ranges used in hospitals and commercial clinical laboratories. It recognizes the enormous task of establishing a laboratory's own reference ranges, and recommends alternatives to the process. A laboratory may acquire reference ranges by:

1. Conducting its own study to evaluate a statistically significant number of "healthy" volunteers. It is a monumental task for a laboratory to develop its own pediatric reference ranges, because parental consent and procedural approval by review boards need to be addressed. The numerous age categories to be evaluated also add to the complexity and size of the study.
2. Adopting ranges established by the manufacturer of a particular analytical instrument. The laboratory must validate the data by analyzing a sample of 20 "reference" subjects (patients representing that specific population) to confirm that the adopted range is truly representative of that group.
3. Using reference data in the general medical literature and conferring with physicians to make sure the data agree with their clinical experience. A validation study is also recommended.
4. Analyzing hospital patient data. Laboratory test results from hospital patients have been used to compute reference ranges provided they fulfill stated clinical criteria. Patient records need to indicate that the patient's specific medical condition does not influence the analyte whose reference range is being determined. For example, a child undergoing surgery for bone fracture repair is expected to have normal electrolytes and thyroid function, whereas a child examined for precocious puberty should not be included in a reference range study for luteinizing hormone. In the REALAB Project, Grossi et al chose the "inclusion criterion," whereby tests that have a single laboratory measurement were used; justification was based on the fact that persons with repeated testing had a higher probability of being diseased and their results should be excluded from the study.

Statistically, the sample size of a hospital patient study should be considerably larger than that of a healthy group. A study from a healthy population may require 20 subjects to be statistically significant, whereas a hospital population should evaluate a minimum of 120 patients. At Children's Hospital Colorado, the free thyroxine reference range was recently established using 1480 clinic and hospital patient results in this manner.

Biological Variation Database Reference List: http://www.westgard.com/biological-variation-database-reference-list.htm

College of American Pathologists publication: http://www.cap.org/apps/docs/laboratory_accreditation/sample_checklist.pdf

Grossi E et al: The REALAB Project: A new method for the formulation of reference intervals based on current data. Clin Chem 2005;51:1232 [PMID: 15919879].

Schnabl K, Chan MK, Gong Y, Adeli K: Closing the Gap on Paediatric Reference Intervals: The CALIPER Initiative. Clin Biochem Rev 2008 Aug;29(3):89–96 [PMID: 19107221].

STATISTICAL COMPUTATION OF REFERENCE INTERVALS

The establishment of reference intervals is based on a statistical distribution of test results obtained from a representative population. The CLSI recommendation for data collection and statistical analysis provides guidelines for managing the data. For clinicians, it is not important that they can reproduce the calculation. It is far more critical to understand the benefits and restrictions provided by the described statistical approaches, and to evaluate patient results with these limitations in mind.

In reviewing the statistics, 95% of all results will be inherently included in the reference range. Note that 5% of that population will have "abnormal" results, when in fact they are "healthy" and an integral part of the reference group study. Similarly, an equivalent 5% of the "ill" population will have laboratory results within the reference range. These are inherent features of the statistical computation. Taking that analysis one step further, the probability of a healthy patient having a test result within a calculated reference range is

$$P = 0.95$$

When multiple tests or panels of tests are used, the combined probability of all the test results falling in their respective reference ranges drops dramatically. For example, the probability of all results from 10 tests in the complete metabolic panel being in the reference range is

$$P = (0.95)^{10} = 0.60$$

Therefore, about one-third of healthy patients will have one test result in the panel that is outside the reference range.

A. Parametric Method of Computation

The parametric method of establishing reference intervals is simple, though not always representative, since it is based on the assumption that the data have a gaussian distribution. A mean (x) and standard deviation (s) are calculated; test results of 95% of that specific population will fall within the mean $\pm 1.96s$, as shown in Figure 46–1.

Where the distribution is not gaussian, a mathematical manipulation of the values (eg, plotting the log of the value, instead of the value itself) may give a gaussian distribution. The mean and standard deviation are then converted back to give a usable reference range.

B. Nonparametric Method of Computation

The nonparametric method of establishing reference ranges is currently recommended by CLSI since it defines outliers as those in the extreme 2.5 percentile of the upper

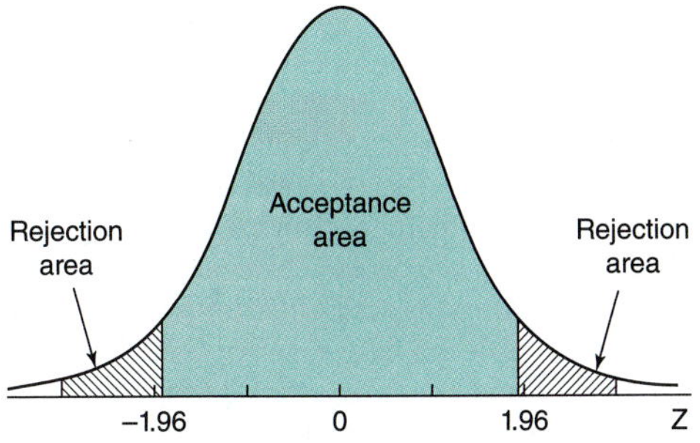

▲ **Figure 46–1.** Gaussian distribution and parametric calculation using $x \pm 1.96s$ to define the range.

and lower limits of data respectively. The number of data points excluded at the limits depends on the skew of the curve, and so the computation accommodates a nongaussian distribution. A histogram depicting the nongaussian distribution of data from a free thyroxine reference range study conducted at Children's Hospital Colorado is shown in Figure 46–2.

Ichihara K, Boyd JC: IFCC Committee on Reference Intervals and Decision Limits (C-RIDL). An appraisal of statistical procedures used in derivation of reference intervals. Clin Chem Lab Med 2010 Nov;48(11):1537–1551 [PMID: 21062226].

WHY REFERENCE INTERVALS VARY

Recent modifications to reference ranges are due to the introduction of new and improved analytical procedures, advanced automated instrumentation, and standardization of reagents and reference materials. Reference ranges are also affected by preanalytical variations that can occur during sample collection, processing, and storage.

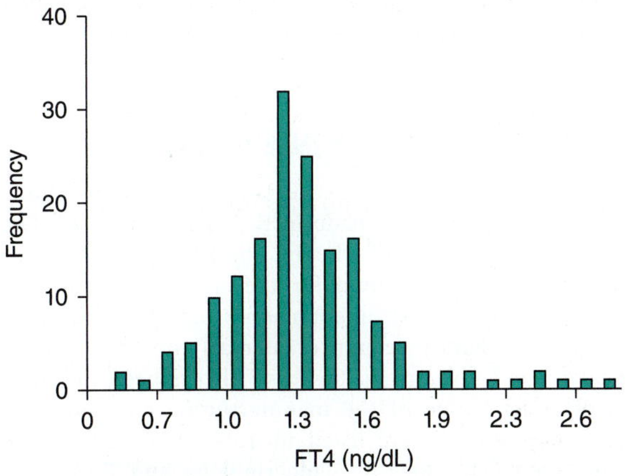

▲ **Figure 46–2.** Histogram of free thyroxine (FT4) using clinic and hospital patients at Children's Hospital Colorado.

Preanalytical variations of biological origin can occur when specimens are drawn in the morning versus in the evening, or from hospitalized recumbent patients versus ambulatory outpatients. Variations also may be caused by metabolic and hemodynamic factors. Preanalytical factors may be a product of the socioeconomic environment or ethnic background (eg, genetic or dietary).

Analytical variations are caused by differences in analytical measurements and depend on the analytical tools as well as an inherent variability in obtaining a quantitative value. Furthermore, scientific progress is constantly introducing new reagents, instruments, and improved testing procedures to the clinical laboratory, and each tool adds an element of variability between tests.

1. **Antigen-antibody reactions** have revolutionized clinical chemistry, but have also added a degree of variability because biologically derived reagents have different specificity and sensitivity. In addition to the targeted analyte, some of its metabolites are also measured, and these may or may not be biologically active.
2. **Reference materials** continue to be reviewed and evaluated by organizations such as the World Health Organization and the National Institute for Standards and Technology. A new standard was recently established for troponin I, and reference ranges were modified to reflect the new standard.
3. **Analytical instrumentation** with advanced electronics and robotics has improved accuracy of results and increased throughput. However, they have added an element of variability between instruments from different manufacturers.
4. **Analytical detection methods** have also made big strides as they have expanded from simple ultraviolet–visible spectrophotometry to fluorescence, nephelometry, radioimmunoassay, and chemiluminescence. For example, the third-generation thyroid-stimulating hormone assays can now measure concentrations as low as 0.001 μIU/mL; the reference range was recently modified to reflect the improved sensitivity of the assay.

Jung B, Adeli K: Clinical laboratory reference intervals in pediatrics: The CALIPER initiative. Clin Biochem 2009 Nov;42 (16–17):1589–1595 [Epub 2009 Jul 7] [PMID: 19591815].

Nakamoto J, Fuqua JS: Laboratory assays in pediatric endocrinology: Common aspects. Pediatr Endocrinol Rev 2007 Oct;5(Suppl 1):539–554 [PMID: 18167465].

Yüksel B et al: J Clin Res Pediatr Endocrinol 2011 Jun;3(2):84–8 [Epub 2011 Jun 8] [PMID: 21750637]. Free PMC Article at: http://www.ncbi.nlm.nih.gov/pmc/articles/PMC3119446/?tool=pubmed

SENSITIVITY & SPECIFICITY

Despite its statistical derivation, a reference interval does not necessarily provide a finite and clear-cut guideline as to whether a patient has a disease. There will always be a segment of the population with test values that fall within the reference interval, but clinical manifestations that indicate disease is present. Similarly, a segment of the population will have test values outside the reference interval, but no clinical signs of disease. The ability of a test and corresponding reference interval to detect individuals with disease is defined by the diagnostic sensitivity of the test. Similarly, the ability of a test to detect individuals without disease is described by the diagnostic specificity. These characteristics are governed by the analytical quality of the test as well as the numerical parameters (reference interval) that define the presence of disease. The tolerance level for the desired sensitivity and specificity of a test requires significant input from clinicians.

Generally, specificity increases as sensitivity decreases. A typical reference range frequency distribution, shown in Figure 46–3 (solid line), provides information on the test results of a number of healthy subjects, or individuals without the disease. A second curve (dashed line) shows test results for individuals with the disease. As with most tests, there is an overlap area. A patient with a test result of 1 is likely healthy, and the result indicates a true negative (TN) for the presence of disease. A patient with a test result of 9 is likely to have the disease and the test result is a true positive (TP). There is a small, but significant, population with a test result of 2–5 in whom the test is not 100% conclusive. A statistical analysis may determine the most likely cutoff for healthy individuals, but the clinically acceptable cutoff depends on the test as well as clinical correlation. Where the treatment is aggressive and has serious side effects, a clinician may choose to err on the side of caution and hold treatment for anyone with a test value of less than 6.

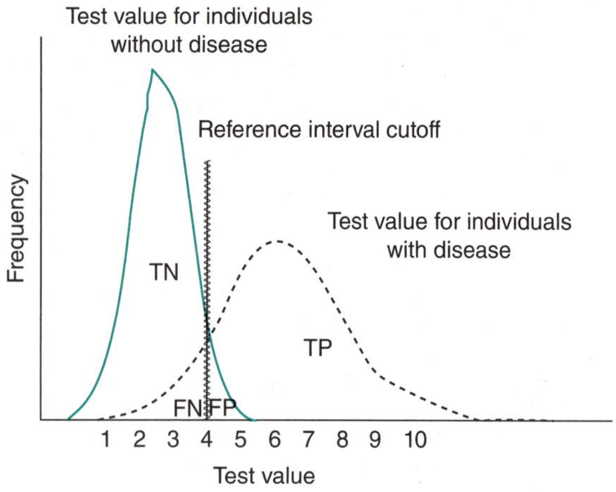

▲ **Figure 46–3.** Frequency distribution of test results for patients with and without disease. FN, false negative; FP, false positive; TN, true negative; TP, true positive.

If cutoff values for the reference interval are such that a test result indicates that a healthy patient has the disease, the result is a false positive (FP). Conversely if a test result indicates that a patient is well when in fact he or she has the disease, the result is a false negative (FN). To define the ability of the test and reference interval to identify a disease state, the diagnostic sensitivity and specificity are measured.

$$\text{Diagnostic sensitivity} = \text{TP}/(\text{TP} + \text{FN})$$

$$\text{Diagnostic specificity} = \text{TN}/(\text{TN} + \text{FP})$$

In the example shown in Figure 46–3, a reference interval of 0.5–3 will provide more TN results and minimize FP results. Alternatively, a reference interval of 0.5–4 will increase the rate of FN. Thus, an increase in sensitivity leads to a decrease in specificity. A medical condition that requires aggressive treatment may necessitate a test and corresponding reference interval with a high sensitivity, which is a measure of the TP rate. This is accomplished at the expense of lowering specificity.

A reference interval is a statistical representation of test results from a finite population, but it is by no means inclusive of every member of the group. It is merely one component in the measure of a patient's status to be viewed in relation to the sensitivity and specificity of the test.

Clinical laboratory data are frequently interpreted using a dynamic approach in which each value is compared with another. In this case, time series analysis of relative values may provide more important information than comparison against a strict reference range. Examples include the evaluation of enzyme activity over time and various stimulation studies for endocrine assessment. Drug monitoring also is a dynamic process.

PEDIATRIC REFERENCE INTERVALS

The establishment of reference ranges is a complex process. Assumptions are made in the management of data processes, regardless of whether "healthy" individuals or hospital patients are used for the accumulation of test results. Analytical instrument manufacturers conduct large studies to identify reference intervals for each specific analyte, and pediatric values have always been the most challenging. Some of the manufacturers' recommended reference intervals are listed in Table 46–1 for general chemistry, Table 46–2 for endocrinology, and Table 46–3 for hematology. The interpretation of chemistry and hematology laboratory results is equally complex and forms a continuous challenge for physicians and the medical community at large.

Table 46–1. General chemistry.

Analyte, Units Specimen Type, Source of Ranges	Age	Methodology	Male Range	Female Range
Albumin (g/dL) S, P	0-7 d	Vitros 5600	2.3-3.8	1.8-3.9
	8-30 d		2.0-4.5	1.8-4.4
	1-2 m		2.0-4.8	1.9-4.2
	3-5 m		2.1-4.9	2.2-4.4
	6-12 m		2.1-4.7	2.2-4.7
	1-3 y		3.4-4.2	3.4-4.2
	4-6 y		3.5-5.2	3.5-5.2
	7-18 y		3.7-5.6	3.7-5.6
	19y-Adult		3.5-5.0	3.5-5.0
ALP (U/L) S, P	0-7 d	Vitros 5600	77-265	65-270
	8-30 d		91-375	65-365
	1-3 m		60-360	80-425
	4-6 m		55-325	80-345
	7-12 m		60-300	60-330
	1-3 y		129-291	129-291
	4-6 y		134-346	134-346
	7-9 y		156-386	156-386
	10-11 y		120-488	116-515
	12-13 y		178-455	93-386
	14-15 y		116-483	62-209
	16-18 y		58-237	45-116
	19y-Adult		38-126	38-126
ALT (U/L) S, P	1-7 d	Vitros 5600	6-40	7-40
	8-30 d		10-40	8-32
	1-3 m		13-39	12-47
	4-6 m		12-42	12-37
	7-12 m		13-45	12-41
	1-3 y		5-45	5-45
	4-6 y		10-25	10-25
	7-9 y		10-35	10-35
	10-11 y		10-35	10-30
	12-13 y		10-55	10-30
	14-15 y		10-45	5-30
	16-18 y		10-40	5-35
	19 y-Adult		21-72	9-52
Ammonia (umol/L) P	0-1 d	Vitros 5600	64-107	64-107
	1-13 y		56-92	56-92
	14 d-17 y		21-50	21-50
	18-Adult		9-33	9-33
Amylase (U/L) S, P	0-2 m	Vitros 5600	0-30	0-30
	3-5 m		0-50	0-50
	6-11 m		0-80	0-80
	1-18 y		30-100	30-100
	19y-Adult		30-110	30-110
AST (U/L) S, P	0-7 d	Vitros 5600	30-100	24-95
	8-30 d		20-70	24-72
	1-3 m		22-63	20-64
	4-6 m		13-65	20-63
	7-12 m		25-55	22-63
	1-3 y		20-60	20-60
	4-6 y		15-50	15-50
	7-9 y		15-40	15-40
	10-11 y		10-60	10-40
	12-15 y		15-40	10-30
	16-18 y		15-45	5-30
	19y-Adult		17-59	14-36

(*Continued*)

Table 46–1. General chemistry. (*Continued*)

Analyte, Units Specimen Type, Source of Ranges	Age	Methodology	Male Range	Female Range
BNP, (ng/L) S, P	0–adult	Vitros 5600	0–99	0–99
BUN (mg/dL) S, P (15)	0–7 d 8–30 d 1–3 m 4–6 m 7–12 m 1–3 y 4–13 y 14–18 y 19–Adult	Vitros 5600	2–13 2–15 2–14 1–13 1–13 5–17 7–17 8–21 7–17	2–13 2–16 2–12 1–14 2–14 5–17 7–17 8–21 9–20
C3 (mg/dL) S, P	0–1 m 1–2 m 2–3 m 3–4 m 4–5 m 5–6 m 6–9 m 9–11 m 11–12 m 1–2 y 2–3 y 3–5 y 5–8 y 8–10y 10–19y > 19 y	Vitros 5600	55–129 61–155 67–136 64–182 67–174 77–178 78–173 76–187 87–181 84–177 80–178 89–173 92–161 93–203 86–184 88–165	55–129 61–155 67–136 64–182 67–174 77–178 78–173 76–187 87–181 84–177 80–178 89–173 92–161 93–203 86–184 88–165
C4 (mg/dL) S, P	0–1 m 1–2 m 2–3 m 3–4 m 4–5 m 5–6 m 6–9 m 9–11 m 11–12 m 1–2 y 2–3 y 3–5 y 5–8 y 8–10 y 10–19 y > 19 yrs	Vitros 5600	9.2–33 9.7–37 11–35 11–50 9.3–47 11–55 12–48 16–51 16–52 12–45 13–47 17–42 16–42 13–52 10–40 14–44	9.2–33 9.7–37 11–35 11–50 9.3–47 11–55 12–48 16–51 16–52 12–45 13–47 17–42 16–42 13–52 10–40 14–44
Ca (mg/dL) S, P	0–8 d 8–30 d 1–3 m 3–6 m 6–12 m 1–4 y 4–10 y 10–12 y 12–14 y 14–16 y 16–19 y > 19 y	Vitros 5600	7.3–11.4 8.6–11.7 8.5–11.3 8.3–11.4 7.7–11.0 8.7–9.8 8.8–10.1 8.9–10.1 8.8–10.6 9.2–10.7 8.9–10.7 8.4–10.2	7.5–11.3 8.4–11.9 8.0–11.1 7.7–11.5 7.8–11.1 8.7–9.8 8.8–10.1 8.9–10.1 8.8–10.6 9.2–10.7 8.9–10.7 8.4–10.2

(*Continued*)

Table 46–1. General chemistry. (*Continued*)

Analyte, Units Specimen Type, Source of Ranges	Age	Methodology	Male Range	Female Range
Chloride (mmol/L) S, P	0-8 d 8 d-6 m 6-12 m 1-19 y > 19 y	Vitros 5600	96-111 96-110 96-108 96-109 98-107	96-111 96-110 96-108 96-109 98-107
Cholesterol (mg/dL) S, P	0 d-2 m 2-7 m 7-12 m > 1 y	Vitros 5600	45-177 60-197 89-208 44-181	63-198 66-218 74-218 44-181
Creatine Kinase (U/L) S, P	0-3 m 3-12 m 1-2 y 2-11 y 11-15 y 15-19 > 19 y	Vitros 5600	28-300 24-170 27-160 30-150 30-150 33-145 55-170	48-470 26-240 24-175 24-175 30-170 27-140 30-135
Creatinine (mg/dL) S, P	0-3 d 3-10 d 10-17 d 17 d-1 y 1-11 y 11-18 y > 18 y	Vitros 5600	0.33-1.08 0.14-0.90 0.14-0.61 0.14-0.52 0.23-0.61 0.42-0.90 0.71-1.18	0.33-1.08 0.14-0.90 0.14-0.61 0.14-0.52 0.23-0.61 0.42-0.90 0.52-0.99
GGT (U/L) S, P	0-8 d 8-30 d 1-4 m 4-7 m 7-12 m 1-4 y 4-7 y 7-10 y 10-12 y 12-14 y 14-16 y 16-19 y > 19 y	Vitros 5600	25-148 23-153 17-130 8-83 10-35 5-16 8-18 11-21 14-25 14-37 10-28 9-29 15-73	19-131 17-124 17-124 15-109 10-54 5-16 8-18 11-21 14-23 12-21 12-22 9-23 12-43
Glucose (mg/dL) S, P	0-30 d > 1 mo	Vitros 5600	40-80 60-105	40-80 60-105
Glucose - CSF (mg/dL), CSF	0 d-Adult	Vitros 5600	40-75	40-75
HDL (mg/dL) S, P	0-2 Y > 2y	Vitros 5600	8-61 > 45	8-61 > 45
IgA (mg/dL) S,P	0-30 d 1-6 m 6-12 m 1-4 y 4-7 y 7-10 y 10-13 y 13-16 y 16-19 y > 19 y	Vitros 5600	0-11 0-40 1-82 9-137 44-187 58-204 46-218 29-251 68-259 70-400	0-10 0-42 6-68 15-111 33-146 28-180 55-193 62-241 69-262 70-400

(*Continued*)

Table 46–1. General chemistry. (*Continued*)

Analyte, Units Specimen Type, Source of Ranges	Age	Methodology	Male Range	Female Range
IgG (mg/dL) S,P	0-30 d 1-6 m 6-12 m 1-4 y 4-7 y 7-10 y 10-13 y 13-16 y 16-19 y > 19 y	Vitros 5600	197–833 140–533 130–823 413–1112 468–1328 582–1441 685–1620 590–1600 522–1703 700–1600	136–872 311–664 325–647 421–1202 560–1319 485–1473 586–1609 749–1640 804–1817 700–1600
IgM (mg/dL) S,P	0-30 d 1-6 m 6-12 m 1-4 y 4-7 y 7-10 y 10-13 y 13-16 y 16-19 y > 19 y	Vitros 5600	0–65 0–84 15–117 30–146 31–151 21–140 27–151 26–184 28–179 40–230	0–57 0–127 0–130 35–184 42–184 30–165 42–211 34–225 42–224 40–230
Iron (µg/dl) S, P	0-7 d 7 d-1 y 1-10 y > 10 y	Vitros 5600	100–250 40–100 50–120 49–181	100–250 40–100 50–120 37–170
LDH (U/L) S,P	0-1 m 1-4 m 4-7 m 7-12 m 1-4 y 4-7 y 7-10 y 10–12 y 12–14 y 14–16 y 16–18 y > 18 y	Vitros 5600	550–2100 480–1220 400–1230 380–1200 500–920 470–900 420–750 432–700 470–750 360–730 340–670 313–618	580–2000 460–1150 460–1150 460–1060 500–920 470–900 420–750 380–700 380–640 390–580 340–670 313–618
Magnesium (mg/dL) S,P	0-7 d 7-30 d 1 m–2 y 2–6 y 6–10 y 10–14 y > 14 y	Vitros 5600	1.2–1.6 1.6–2.4 1.6–2.6 1.5–2.4 1.6–2.3 1.6–2.2 1.5–2.3	1.2–1.6 1.6–2.4 1.6–2.6 1.5–2.4 1.6–2.3 1.6–2.2 1.5–2.3
NT Pro-BNP (pg/mL) S,P	0–Adult	Vitros 5600	0–125	0–125
Potassium (mmol/L) S,P	0-7 d 7 d-3 m 3 m–18 y > 18 y	Vitros 5600	3.7–5.9 4.1–5.3 3.4–4.7 3.5–5.0	3.7–5.9 4.1–5.3 3.4–4.7 3.5–5.0
Prealbumin (mg/dL) S,P	0-1 m 1-6 m 6 m–4 y 4-6 y 6–14 y 14–19 y > 19 y	Vitros 5600	7–22 8–34 7–32 12–30 12–42 22–45 17–42	7–22 8–34 7–32 12–30 12–42 22–45 17–42

(*Continued*)

Table 46–1. General chemistry. (*Continued*)

Analyte, Units Specimen Type, Source of Ranges	Age	Methodology	Male Range	Female Range
Phosphorus (mg/dL) S,P	0–1 m 1-3 m 3-12 m 1-2 y 2-13 y 13-16 y 16-18 y > 18 y	Vitros 5600	2.7-7.2 3.0-6.8 3.0-6.9 2.5-6.4 3.0-6.0 3.0-5.4 3.0-5.2 2.5-4.5	3.0-8.0 3.0-7.5 2.5-7.0 3.0-6.5 2.5-6.0 3.0-5.6 3.0-4.8 2.5-4.5
Sodium (mmol/L) S,P	0-8 d 8-30 d 1-6 m 6-12 m 1-19 y > 19 y	Vitros 5600	133–146 134–144 134–142 133–142 134–143 137–145	133–146 134–144 134–142 133–142 134–143 137–145
Total bilirubin (mg/dL) S,P	0-1 d 1-3 d 3-30 d > 1 m	Vitros 5600	0.1-5.8 0.1-8.5 0.1-11.5 0.2-1.2	0.1-5.8 0.1-8.5 0.1-11.5 0.2-1.2
Troponin I (ng/mL) P	0 d–Adult	Vitros 5600	< 0.12	< 0.12
T4 (μg/dL) S,P	0-3 d 3-30 d 30 d-1 y 1-6 y 6-19 y > 19 y	Vitros 5600	8–20 5–15 6–14 4.5–11 4.5–10 4.5–10	8–20 5–15 6–14 4.5–11 4.5–10 5.5–11
Total protein (g/dL) S,P	0-2 m 2-6 m 6-12 m 1-4 y 4-7 y 7-10 y 10-20 y > 20 y	Vitros 5600	3.9-7.6 4.1-7.9 3.9-7.9 5.9-7.0 5.9-7.8 6.2-8.1 6.3-8.6 6.2-8.2	3.4-7.0 3.9-7.6 4.5-7.8 5.9-7.0 5.9-7.8 6.2-8.1 6.3-8.6 6.2-8.2
Triglycerides (mg/dL) S,P	0–Adult	Vitros 5600	< 75	< 75
TCO2-Bicarb (mmol/L) S,P	0-7 d 7-30 d 1-6 m 6-12 m 1-19 y > 19	Vitros 5600	17–26 17–27 17–29 18–29 20–31 22–30	17–26 17–27 17–29 18–29 20–31 22–30
Uric Acid (mg/dL) S,P	0-30 d 1-12 m 1-10 y 10-12 y 12-14 y 14-16 y 16-18 y > 18 y	Vitros 5600	2.0-5.2 2.5-9.0 1.8-5.0 2.3-5.4 2.7-6.7 2.4-7.8 4.0-8.6 3.5-8.5	2.0-5.2 2.5-9.0 1.8-5.0 3.0-4.7 3.0-5.9 3.0-5.9 3.0-5.9 2.5-7.5

B, whole blood; CSF, spinal fluid; P, plasma; RBC, red blood cells; S, serum; U, urine.
Data source: Children's Hospital, Colorado, Chemistry Laboratory Procedures Manual

Table 46–2. Endocrine chemistry

Analyte, Units, Specimen Type, Source	Age	Methodology	Male Range	Female Range
Cortisol (μg/dL)	0-Adult	Vitros 5600		
S, P	(AM values)		4.5-22.7	4.5-22.7
	(PM values)		1.7-14.1	1.7-14.1
Estradiol (ng/mL)	Prepuberty	Esoterix	< 1.5	< 1.5
S	Tanner 1		0.5-1.1	0.5-2.0
	Tanner 2		0.5-1.6	1.0-2.4
	Tanner 3		0.5-2.5	0.7-6.0
	Tanner 4		1.0-3.6	2.1-8.5
	Tanner 5		1.0-3.6	3.4-17
FSH (mIU/mL)	1-11 m	DPC Immulite	0.16-4.1	0.24-14.2
S, P	1-8 y		0.26-3.0	1.0-4.2
	Tanner Stage1		0.26-3.0	1.0-4.2
	Tanner Stage2		1.8-3.2	1.0-10.8
	Tanner Stage3		1.2-5.8	1.5-12.8
	Tanner Stage4		2.0-9.2	1.5-11.7
	Tanner Stage5		2.6-11.0	1.0-9.2
	Adult		2.0-9.2	
	Follicular			1.8-11.2
	Midcycle			6-35
	Luteal Phase			1.8-11.2
Growth Hormone (ng/mL)	1-8 d	DPC Immulite	1.18-27	2.4-24
S	8d -1y		0.69-17.3	1.07-17.6
	1-3 y		0.43-2.4	0.5-3.5
	4-6 y		0.09-2.5	0.10-2.2
	7-8 y		0.15-3.2	0.16-5.4
	9-10 y		0.09-1.95	0.08-3.1
	11 y		0.08-4.7	0.12-6.9
	12 y		0.12-8.9	0.14-11.2
	13 y		0.10-7.9	0.21-17.8
	14 y		0.09-7.1	0.14-9.9
	15 y		0.10-7.8	0.24-10.0
	16 y		0.08-11.4	0.26-11.7
	17 y		0.22-12.2	0.30-10.8
	18 y		0.97-4.7	0.24-4.3
IGF-1 (ng/mL)	0-7 d	DPC Immulite	1-26	1-26
S, P	8-15 d		11-41	11-41
	16 d-1 y		55-327	55-327
	1 y		55-327	55-327
	2 y		51-303	51-303
	3 y		49-289	49-289
	4 y		49-283	49-283
	5 y		50-286	50-286
	6 y		52-297	52-297
	7 y		57-316	57-316
	8 y		64-345	64-345
	9 y		74-388	74-388
	10 y		88-452	88-452
	11 y		111-551	111-551
	12 y		143-693	143-693
	13 y		183-850	183-850
	14 y		220-972	220-972
	15 y		237-996	237-996
	16 y		226-903	226-903
	17 y		193-731	193-731
	18 y		163-584	163-584
	19 y		141-483	141-483
	20 y		127-424	127-424

(*Continued*)

Table 46–2. Endocrine chemistry (*Continued*)

Analyte, Units, Specimen Type, Source	Age	Methodology	Male Range	Female Range
IGF-BP3 (μg/mL) S, P	0–7 d	DPC Immulite	0.1–0.7	0.1–0.7
	8–15 d		0.5–1.4	0.5–1.4
	16 d–1 y		0.7–3.6	0.7–3.6
	2 y		0.8–3.9	0.8–3.9
	3 y		0.9–4.3	0.9–4.3
	4 y		1.0–4.7	1.0–4.7
	5 y		1.1–5.2	1.1–5.2
	6 y		1.3–5.6	1.3–5.6
	7 y		1.4–6.1	1.4–6.1
	8 y		1.6–6.5	1.6–6.5
	9 y		1.8–7.1	1.8–7.1
	10 y		2.1–7.7	2.1–7.7
	11 y		2.4–8.4	2.4–8.4
	12 y		2.7–8.9	2.7–8.9
	13 y		3.1–9.5	3.1–9.5
	14 y		3.3–10.0	3.3–10.0
	15 y		3.5–10.0	3.5–10.0
	16 y		3.4–9.5	3.4–9.5
	17 y		3.2–8.7	3.2–8.7
	18 y		3.1–7.9	3.1–7.9
	19 y		2.9–7.3	2.9–7.3
	20 y		2.9–7.2	2.9–7.2
LH (mIU/mL) S, P	14 d–11 m	DPC Immulite	0.02–7.0	0.02–7.0
	1–8 y		0.02–0.3	0.02–0.3
	Tanner Stage1		0.02–0.3	0.02–0.18
	Tanner Stage2		0.2–4.9	0.02–4.7
	Tanner Stage3		0.2–5.0	0.10–12.0
	Tanner Stage4		0.4–7.0	0.4–11.7
	Tanner Stage5		0.4–7.0	0.4–11.7
	Adult		1.5–9.0	
	Follicular			2.0–9.0
	Midcycle			18.0–49.0
	Leuteal			2.0–11.0
T4 Free (ng/dL) S, P	0–2 d	Vitros 5600	2.0–5.0	2.0–5.0
	3–30 d		0.9–2.2	0.9–2.2
	1 m–19 y		0.9–2.0	0.9–2.0
	>19 y		0.78–2.19	0.78–2.19
TSH (μIU/mL) S, P	0–3 d	Vitros 5600	1.0–20.0	1.0–20.0
	3–30 d		0.5–8.0	0.5–8.0
	1–6 m		0.5–6.0	0.5–6.0
	6 m–5 y		0.5–6.0	0.5–6.0
	5–13 y		0.5–5.5	0.5–5.5
	>13 y		0.5–5.0	0.5–5.0
Testosterone, Total (ng/dL) S, P	Premature	Vitros 5600	37–198	5–22
	Newborn		75–400	20–64
	Prepubertal		1–10	1–10
	Tanner 1		1–10	1–10
	Tanner 2		18–150	7–28
	Tanner 3		100–320	15–35
	Tanner 4		200–620	13–32
	Tanner 5		350–970	20–38
	Adult (20–49)		132–813	5–77

Data source: Children's Hospital, Colorado, Chemistry Laboratory Procedures Manual.

Table 46–3. Hematology

Analyte, Units, Specimen Type, Source	Age	Methodology	Male Range	Female Range
WBC (x10^9/L) EDTA Whole Blood	0–1 m 1–24 m 2–10 y 10–17 y Adult	Beckman LH750	9.0–32.0 5–13.0 4–12.0 4–10.5 4–10.5	9.0–32.0 5–13.0 4–12.0 4–10.5 4–10.5
RBC (x10^{12}/L) EDTA Whole Blood	0–1 m 1–24 m 2–10 y 10–17 y Adult	Beckman LH750	4.6–6.7 3.8–5.4 4.0–5.3 4.2–5.6 4.7–6.0	4.6–6.7 3.8–5.4 4.0–5.3 4.2–5.6 4.2–5.4
Hemoglobin (g/dL) EDTA Whole Blood	0–1 m 1–24 m 2–10 y 10–17 y Adult	Beckman LH750	13.0–22.0 9.5–14.0 11.5–14.5 11.5–14.5 13.5–18.0	13.0–22.0 9.5–14.0 11.5–14.5 11.5–14.5 13.5–18.0
HCT (%) EDTA Whole Blood	0–1 m 1–24 m 2–10 y 10–17 y Adult	Beckman LH750	42–70 30–41 33–43 36–47 42–52	42–70 30–41 33–43 35–45 37–47
MCV (fL) EDTA Whole Blood	0–1 m 1–24 m 2–10 y 10–17 y Adult	Beckman LH750	90–115 70–90 76–90 78–95 78–100	90–115 70–90 76–90 78–95 78–100
Polys (absolute) EDTA Whole Blood	0–1 m 1–24 m 2–10 y 10–17 y Adult	Beckman LH750	6–23.5 1.1–6.6 1.4–6.6 1.5–6.6 1.5–6.1	6–23.5 1.1–6.6 1.4–6.6 1.5–6.6 1.5–6.6
Bands# (absolute) EDTA Whole Blood	0–1 m 1–24 m 2–10 y 10-Adult	Beckman LH750	< 3.5 < 1.0 < 1.0 < 1.0	< 3.5 < 1.0 < 1.0 < 1.0
Lymphs# (absolute) EDTA Whole Blood	0–1 m 1–24 m 2–10 y 10–17 y Adult	Beckman LH750	2.5–10.5 1.8–9.0 1.0–5.5 1.0–3.5 1.5–3.5	2.5–10.5 1.8–9.0 1.0–5.5 1.0–3.5 1.5–3.5
Monos# (absolute) EDTA Whole Blood	0–1 m 1 m-Adult	Beckman LH750	< 2.0 < 1.0	< 2.0 < 1.0
EOS # (absolute) EDTA Whole Blood	0–1 m 1 m-Adult	Beckman LH750	< 2.0 < 0.7	< 2.0 < 0.7
Basos# (absolute) EDTA Whole Blood	0–1 m 1 m-Adult	Beckman LH750	< 0.4 < 0.1	< 0.4 < 1.0
Platelet (x10^3/uL) EDTA Whole Blood	0 d-Adult	Beckman LH750	150–500	150–500

Data source: Children's Hospital, Colorado, Hematology Laboratory Procedures Manual.

Index

Page references followed by *f* indicate figures; page references followed by *t* indicate tables.